SKELETAL TRAUMA

BASIC SCIENCE, MANAGEMENT, AND RECONSTRUCTION

SKELETAL TRAUMA

BASIC SCIENCE, MANAGEMENT, AND RECONSTRUCTION

FIFTH EDITION

Volume 1

Bruce D. Browner, MD, MHCM, FACS
Adjunct Professor
Department of Orthopaedic Surgery
Duke University School of Medicine
Overseas Coordinator
Tanzania Trauma System Project
Durham, North Carolina

Jesse B. Jupiter, MD
Director, Orthopaedic Hand Service
Massachusetts General Hospital
Hansjörg Wyss/AO Professor
Harvard Medical School
Boston, Massachusetts

Christian Krettek, MD, FRACS, FRCSEd
Professor and Director
Hannover Medical School (MHH)–Trauma Department
Hannover, Germany

Paul A. Anderson, MD
Professor
Department of Orthopedics and Rehabilitation
University of Wisconsin
Madison, Wisconsin

ELSEVIER
SAUNDERS

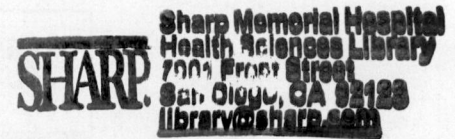

ELSEVIER
SAUNDERS

1600 John F. Kennedy Blvd.
Ste 1800
Philadelphia, PA 19103-2899

Part number: 9996098001 (vol 1)
9996098060 (vol 2)
ISBN: 978-1-4557-7628-3 (set)

SKELETAL TRAUMA: BASIC SCIENCE, MANAGEMENT AND RECONSTRUCTION, FIFTH EDITION

Notices

Knowledge and best practice in this field are constantly changing. As new research and experience broaden our understanding, changes in research methods, professional practices, or medical treatment may become necessary.

Practitioners and researchers must always rely on their own experience and knowledge in evaluating and using any information, methods, compounds, or experiments described herein. In using such information or methods they should be mindful of their own safety and the safety of others, including parties for whom they have a professional responsibility.

With respect to any drug or pharmaceutical products identified, readers are advised to check the most current information provided (i) on procedures featured or (ii) by the manufacturer of each product to be administered, to verify the recommended dose or formula, the method and duration of administration, and contraindications. It is the responsibility of practitioners, relying on their own experience and knowledge of their patients, to make diagnoses, to determine dosages and the best treatment for each individual patient, and to take all appropriate safety precautions.

To the fullest extent of the law, neither the Publisher nor the authors, contributors, or editors, assume any liability for any injury and/or damage to persons or property as a matter of products liability, negligence or otherwise, or from any use or operation of any methods, products, instructions, or ideas contained in the material herein.

Previous editions copyrighted: 2003, 1998, 1992

Library of Congress Cataloging-in-Publication Data

Skeletal trauma : basic science, management, and reconstruction / [edited by] Bruce D. Browner, Jesse B. Jupiter, Christian Krettek, Paul A. Anderson.—Fifth edition.
p. ; cm.
Preceded by Skeletal trauma / [edited by] Bruce D. Browner … [et al.]. 4th ed. 2009.
Includes bibliographical references and index.
ISBN 978-1-4557-7628-3 (set : hardcover : alk. paper)
I. Browner, Bruce D., editor. II. Jupiter, Jesse B., editor. III. Krettek, Christian, 1953-, editor. IV. Anderson, Paul, 1952- , editor.
[DNLM: 1. Fractures, Bone. 2. Bone and Bones—injuries. 3. Dislocations. 4. Ligaments—injuries. WE 175]
RD101
617.4′71044—dc23

2014022019

Executive Content Strategist: Dolores Meloni
Senior Content Development Manager: Maureen Iannuzzi
Publishing Services Manager: Catherine Jackson
Senior Project Manager: Carol O'Connell
Design Direction: Renee Duenow

Printed in Canada

Last digit is the print number: 9 8 7 6 5 4 3 2 1

The Editors Dedicate the Fifth Edition to Their Families and to Fallen and Wounded Warriors

To my wife, Barbara Thea Browner
to my children: Jeremy Todd Browner, Esq., Nina Mikhellasvili Browner, MD,
Nicole Browner Samuel, and Marc Aaron Samuel, Esq.
and to my grandchildren: Benjamin Noah Browner, Zachary Myer Samuel, Dylan Jethro Samuel, Sophia Alexandra Browner, and Emily Jordyn Samuel
In memory of my mother, Mona Alexander Browner
In appreciation for the support and encouragement from
my father, Irwin Eric Browner, and his wife, Adele Doris Browner,
and my mother-in-law, Betty Appleman Jacowsky
Bruce D. Browner

To my wife, Beryl Stephanie Abrams Jupiter
to my daughter, Stacy Deborah Jupiter
In memory of my son, Benjamin Scott Jupiter
In memory of my parents, Miriam and Samuel Jupiter
Jesse B. Jupiter

To my wife, Ulrike Krettek, MD
to my children: Felicitas Krettek and Florian Krettek
In memory of my mother, Felizitas Krettek
In appreciation of her and my father's support and encouragement
Christian Krettek

To my wife, Veronica Anderson,
without whose love and support I could not do all that I do
to my son, Christopher Anderson
to my daughter Meredith Rasco and her husband Kenneth Rasco
and to my grandchildren, Henry and Julian Rasco
In memory of my mother, Shirley G. McCarthy
Paul A. Anderson

We dedicate this text also to the brave men and women in the military who have sacrificed their lives or sustained serious injuries while fighting to preserve the freedom and security of our nations.

Contributors

YVES PASCAL ACKLIN, MD, DMEDSC
Trauma and General Surgery Unit
Department of Surgery
Kantonsspital Graubünden
Chur, Switzerland
47: Fracture of the Humeral Shaft

JULIE E. ADAMS, MD
Department of Orthopaedic Surgery
University of Minnesota
Minneapolis, Minnesota
46: Trauma to the Adult Elbow and Fractures of the Distal Humerus. A: Trauma to the Adult Elbow

LOUIS F. AMOROSA, MD
Clinical Instructor
Department of Orthopaedic Surgery
New York Medical College/Westchester Medical Center
Valhalla, New York
34: Subaxial Cervical Spine Trauma

JONAS ANDERMAHR, MD
Professor of University Clinic of Cologne
Director of Center of Orthopaedic and Trauma Surgery
Kreiskrankenhaus Mechernich GmbH
Mechernich, Germany
49: Fractures and Dislocations of the Clavicle

ROMNEY C. ANDERSEN, MD
COL, MC, U.S. Army
Chairman, Department of Orthopaedics
Walter Reed National Military Medical Center
Professor of Surgery
Uniformed Services University of the Health Sciences
Bethesda, Maryland
72: Amputations in Trauma

CAESAR A. ANDERSON, MD, MPH
Medical Director, Wound and Hyperbaric Medicine
Emergency Medicine and Hyperbaric Medicine
University of California, San Diego
Encinitas, California
14: Medical Management of the Orthopaedic Trauma Patient. D: Substance Abuse Syndromes: Recognition, Prevention, and Treatment

PAUL A. ANDERSON, MD
Professor
Department of Orthopedics and Rehabilitation
University of Wisconsin
Madison, Wisconsin
35: Thoracolumbar Fractures. E: New Concepts in the Management of Thoracolumbar Fractures
37: Osteoporotic Spinal Fractures

BASEM I. AWAD, MD
Assistant Lecturer
Department of Neurological Surgery
Mansoura University School of Medicine
Mansoura, Egypt
31: Pathophysiology and Emergent Treatment of Spinal Cord Injury

CHRISTOPHER S. BAILEY, BPE, MD, FRCSC, MSC
Associate Professor
Department of Surgery, Division of Orthopaedics
Schulich School of Medicine, Western University;
Orthopaedic Spine Consultant
London Health Sciences Centre
London, Ontario, Canada
39: Principles of Orthotic Management

TESSA BALACH, MD
Assistant Professor
Orthopaedic Surgery
University of Connecticut Health Center
Farmington, Connecticut
20: Pathologic Fractures

PAUL C. BALDWIN III, MD
Orthopaedic Surgery Resident
University of Connecticut Health Center
Orthopaedic Surgery Resident
University of Connecticut Health Center
Farmington, Connecticut
21: Osteoporotic Fragility Fractures

CRAIG S. BARTLETT III, MD
Medical Director of Orthopaedic Trauma
Department of Orthopaedics and Rehabilitation
The University of Vermont
Burlington, Vermont
65: Fractures of the Tibial Pilon

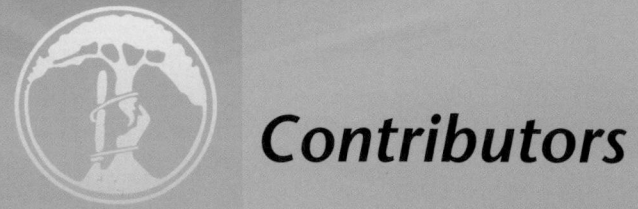

MICHAEL R. BAUMGAERTNER, MD
Professor
Chief of Orthopaedic Trauma
Orthopaedic Trauma and Reconstruction
Department of Orthopaedics and Rehabilitation
Yale University School of Medicine
New Haven, Connecticut
53: Medical Management of the Patient with Hip Fracture
55: Intertrochanteric Hip Fractures

JOAN ELIZABETH BECHTOLD, PHD
Gustilo Professor of Orthopaedic Biomechanics Research
Department of Orthopaedic Surgery
University of Minnesota
Graduate Professor
Mechanical and Biomedical Engineering
University of Minnesota
Director of Research
Minneapolis Medical Research Foundation
Excelen: Center for Bone and Joint Research and Education
Minneapolis, Minnesota
5: Biomechanics of Fractures

ERIC J. BELIN, MD
Assistant Professor
Department of Medicine
College of Medicine
Medical University of South Carolina
Charleston, South Carolina
35: Thoracolumbar Fractures. E: New Concepts in the Management of Thoracolumbar Fractures

CARLO BELLABARBA, MD
Professor, Departments of Orthopaedic and Neurological Surgery
Director, Orthopaedic Spine Service
University of Washington
Acting Chief of Orthopaedics
Harborview Medical Center
Seattle, Washington
33: Craniocervical Injuries. A: Occipital-Cervical Spine Injuries
40: Pelvic Ring Injuries: Parts I and III

EMANUEL D.L. BENNINGER, MD
Department of Orthopaedics and Traumatology
Kantonsspital St. Gallen
Switzerland
48: Proximal Humerus Fractures and Glenohumeral Dislocations. C: Glenohumeral Dislocations and D: Treatment of Fracture Sequelae of the Proximal Humerus

KAVI BHALLA, PHD
Department of International Health
Johns Hopkins Bloomberg School of Public Health
Baltimore, Maryland
2: Global Burden of Musculoskeletal Injuries

RANDY R. BINDRA, MD, FRCS
Professor of Orthopaedic Surgery
Griffith University and Gold Coast University Hospital
Gold Coast, Australia
42: Fractures and Dislocations of the Hand

ROBERT BLEASE, MD
Lieutenant Colonel (LTC)
Medical Department, Army Trauma Training Center
United States Army
Orthopaedic Trauma Surgeon
Orthopaedics Department
Jackson Memorial Hospital
Miami, Florida
19: Gunshot Wounds and Blast Injuries

CHRISTOPHER T. BORN, MD, FAAOS, FACS
Intrepid Heroes Professor of Orthopaedic Surgery
Brown University
Warren Alpert Medical School
Director of Orthopaedic Trauma
Rhode Island Hospital
Providence, Rhode Island
12: Disaster Management

MICHAEL J. BOSSE, MD
Director of Orthopaedic Trauma Surgery
Carolinas Medical Center
Charlotte, North Carolina
29: Psychological, Social, and Functional Manifestations of Orthopaedic Trauma and Traumatic Brain Injury

RICHARD JACKSON BRANSFORD, MD
Associate Professor
Departments of Orthopaedic and Neurological Surgery
University of Washington
Harborview Medical Center
Seattle, Washington
33: Craniocervical Injuries. A: Occipital-Cervical Spine Injuries
40: Pelvic Ring Injuries: Parts I and III

MARK R. BRINKER, MD
Director of Acute and Reconstructive Trauma
Co-Director, The Center for Problem Fractures and Limb Restoration
Texas Orthopedic Hospital
Fondren Orthopedic Group LLP;
Clinical Professor of Orthopaedic Surgery
The University of Texas Medical School at Houston
Houston, Texas;
Clinical Professor of Orthopaedic Surgery
Tulane University School of Medicine
New Orleans, Louisiana
25: Nonunions: Evaluation and Treatment

BRUCE D. BROWNER, MHCM, FACS
Adjunct Professor
Department of Orthopaedic Surgery
Duke University School of Medicine
Overseas Coordinator
Tanzania Trauma System Project
Durham, North Carolina
24: Chronic Osteomyelitis

RYAN CALFEE, MD, MSC
Assistant Professor
Department of Orthopaedic Surgery
Washington University School of Medicine
St. Louis, Missouri
12: Disaster Management

CHARLES CASSIDY, MD
Henry H. Banks Associate Professor and Chairman
Orthopaedics
Tufts Medical Center
Boston, Massachusetts
43: Fractures and Dislocations of the Carpus

RENAN C. CASTILLO, PHD
Department of Health Policy and Management
Johns Hopkins Bloomberg School of Public Health
Baltimore, Maryland
2: Global Burden of Musculoskeletal Injuries

PAUL C. CELESTRE, MD
Clinical Instructor
Department of Orthopaedic Surgery
University of Louisville;
Spine Fellow, Norton Leatherman Spine Center
Louisville, Kentucky
35: Thoracolumbar Fractures. C: Identification, Classification, Mechanism, and Treatment of Thoracolumbar Fracture-Dislocations

RAJIV CHANDAWARKAR, MD
Associate Professor, Plastic Surgery
Adjunct Associate Professor, Orthopedics
Director, Plastic Surgery OSU-East Hospital
The Ohio State University Wexner Medical Center
Columbus, Ohio
18: Soft Tissue Reconstruction

MARK COHEN, MD
Professor
Director, Orthopaedic Education
Director, Hand and Elbow Section
Department of Orthopaedic Surgery
Rush University Medical Center
Chicago, Illinois
44: Fractures of the Distal Radius

PETER A. COLE, MD
Chief
Department of Orthopaedic Surgery
Regions Hospital
St. Paul, Minnesota;
Professor
Orthopaedic Surgery
University of Minnesota
Minneapolis, Minnesota
50: Scapular and Rib Fractures
62: Tibial Plateau Fractures

CHRISTOPHER L. COLTON, MD, FRCS, FRCSED
Senior Consultant in Orthopaedic Trauma (Retired)
Nottingham University Hospital
Nottingham, England
1: The History of Fracture Treatment

LEO M. COONEY, JR., MD
Humana Foundation Professor of Geriatric Medicine
Yale University School of Medicine
Yale-New Haven Hospital
New Haven, Connecticut
53: Medical Management of the Patient with Hip Fracture

BRIAN W. COOPER, MD, FACP
Formerly, Director, Division of Infectious Disease, Allergy, and Immunology
Hartford Hospital
Professor of Clinical Medicine
University of Connecticut School of Medicine
Farmington, Connecticut
13: Occupational Hazards in the Treatment of Orthopaedic Trauma. B: Prevention of Occupationally Acquired Bloodborne Pathogens

R. RICHARD COUGHLIN, MD, MSC
Clinical Professor
Department of Orthopaedic Surgery
University of California, San Francisco;
Director Institute for Global Orthopaedics and Traumatology
Orthopaedic Trauma Institute, San Francisco General Hospital
San Francisco, California
3: The Challenges of Orthopaedic Trauma Care in the Developing World

KRISTIAN DALZELL, MBCHB, FRACS
Orthopaedic Surgery
Christchurch Public Hospital and Burwood Spinal Unit
Christchurch, New Zealand
32: The Timing of Management of Spinal Cord Injuries

NANDITA DAS, PHD
Clinical Research Assistant
Norton Healthcare
Louisville, Kentucky
35: Thoracolumbar Fractures. C: Identification, Classification, Mechanism, and Treatment of Thoracolumbar Fracture-Dislocations

SEBASTIAN DECKER, MD
Resident
Hannover Medical School (MHH)–Trauma Department
Hannover, Germany
33: Craniocervical Injuries. C: C2 Fractures
40: Pelvic Ring Injuries: Parts I-III

CHRISTOPHER W. DIGIOVANNI, MD
Visiting Professor, Harvard Medical School
Chief, Foot and Ankle Service and Fellowship Program
Director, MGH Comprehensive Foot and Ankle Center
Department of Orthopaedic Surgery
Massachusetts General Hospital
Boston, Massachusetts
67: Foot Injuries

JOHN R. DIMAR II, MD
Clinical Professor of Orthopedic Surgery
University of Louisville Department of Orthopedic Surgery
Leatherman Spine Center, Norton Hospital;
Co-director of the Leatherman Spine Center
Chief of Pediatric Orthopedic Surgery
Kosairs Childrens Hospital
Louisville, Kentucky
35: Thoracolumbar Fractures. C: Identification, Classification, Mechanism, and Treatment of Thoracolumbar Fracture-Dislocations

DOUGLAS R. DIRSCHL, MD
Professor and Chairman
Department of Orthopaedic Surgery and Rehabilitation Medicine
University of Chicago Medicine and the Biological Sciences
Chicago, Illinois
28: Professionalism and the Economics of Orthopaedic Trauma Care

RYAN DUFFY, MD
Orthopaedic Trauma Fellow
University of California San Francisco/San Francisco General Hospital
Orthopaedic Trauma Institute
San Francisco, California
65: Fractures of the Tibial Pilon

MICHAEL G. FEHLINGS, MD, PHD, FRCSC, FACS
Professor of Neurosurgery
Krembil Chair in Neural Repair and Regeneration
McLaughlin Scholar in Molecular Medicine
Head Spinal Program
University of Toronto
University Health Network;
Medical Director, Krembil Neuroscience Center
Toronto Western Hospital
Toronto, Ontario, Canada
32: The Timing of Management of Spinal Cord Injuries

DEBORAH FELDMAN, MD
Associate Professor
Obstetrics and Gynecology
University of Connecticut;
Attending Perinatologist
Obstetrics and Gynecology
Hartford Hospital
Hartford, Connecticut
14: Medical Management of the Orthopaedic Trauma Patient. C: Management of the Pregnant Woman

DAVID V. FELICIANO, MD
Battersby Professor and Chief
Division of General Surgery
Indiana University Medical Center
Chief of Surgery
Indiana University Hospital
Indianapolis, Indiana
15: Evaluation and Treatment of Vascular Injuries

MICHAEL FINN, MD
Assistant Professor of Neurological Surgery
Department of Neurosurgery
University of Colorado
Aurora, Colorado
36: Fractures in the Ankylosed Spine

JOHN C. FRANCE, MD
Professor, Vice Chairman, Chief of Spine Surgery
Orthopaedic Surgery
West Virginia University
Morgantown, West Virginia
33: Craniocervical Injuries. B: Atlas Fractures and Atlantoaxial Injuries, C: C2 Fractures

BRETT A. FREEDMAN, MD
LTC, MC, U.S. Army
Chief, Department of Orthopaedics and Rehabilitation
Landstuhl Regional Medical Center
U.S. Army Base—Landstuhl, Germany
16: Compartment Syndromes

RICHARD GANNON, PHARM D
Pharmacy Clinical Specialist–Pain Management
Department of Pharmacy
Hartford Hospital
Hartford, Connecticut;
Assistant Clinical Professor
School of Pharmacy
University of Connecticut
Storrs, Connecticut
14: Medical Management of the Orthopaedic Trauma Patient. A: Acute Pain Management, Regional Anesthesia Techniques, and Management of Complex Regional Pain Syndrome

JOSHUA L. GARY, MD
Assistant Professor
Department of Orthopaedic Surgery
University of Texas Health Science Center—Houston
Houston, Texas
41: Surgical Treatment of Acetabular Fractures

RALPH GAULKE, PRIV-DOZ DR MED
Trauma Department
Hannover Medical School (MHH)–Trauma Department
Hannover, Germany
45: Diaphyseal Fractures of the Forearm

FLORIAN GEBHARD, MD, PHD
Director and Chair
Department of Orthopaedic Trauma
Ulm University
Ulm, Germany
66: Malleolar Fractures and Soft Tissue Injuries of the Ankle

TAD GERLINGER, MD COL, MC, USA (RET)
Associate Professor of Surgery (Orthopaedics), USUHS
Assistant Professor
Rush University
Chicago, Illinois
12: Disaster Management

GEORGE M. GHOBRIAL, MD
Resident Physician
Neurological Surgery
Thomas Jefferson University Hospital
Philadelphia, Pennsylvania
38: Avoiding Complications in Spine Trauma Patients

PETER V. GIANNOUDIS, MBBS, MD, FRCS
Professor of Trauma and Orthopaedic Surgery
School of Medicine,
University of Leeds
Leeds, United Kingdom
58: Femoral Shaft Fractures
69: Periprosthetic Fractures of the Lower Extremity

DANIEL J. GIANOLI, MD
Clinical Instructor
University of Connecticut School of Medicine
Assistant Staff
Hartford Hospital
Hartford, Connecticut
14: Medical Management of the Orthopaedic Trauma Patient. A: Acute Pain Management, Regional Anesthesia Techniques, and Management of Complex Regional Pain Syndrome

PETER GINAITT, BS, RN EMT-C
Director Office of Emergency Preparedness
Rhode Island Hospital
Providence, Rhode Island
12: Disaster Management

RYAN T. GOCKE, MD
CDR, MC, U.S. Navy
Division Head, Spine Surgery
Naval Hospital Camp Lejeune
Camp Lejeune, North Carolina
33: Craniocervical Injuries. C: C2 Fractures

CURTIS GOREHAM-VOSS, PHD
Biomechanics Postdoctoral Fellow
University of Minnesota
Minneapolis, Minnesota
5: Biomechanics of Fractures

THOMAS GÖSLING, MD
Professor
Trauma and Orthopaedic Surgery
General Hospital Braunschweig
Braunschweig, Germany
58: Femoral Shaft Fractures

RICHARD A. GOSSELIN, MD, MPH, MSC, FRCS(C)
Associate Clinical Professor, Department of Orthopedic Surgery
Co-Director, Institute for Global Orthopedics and Traumatology
University of California, San Francisco
San Francisco, California
3: The Challenges of Orthopaedic Trauma Care in the Developing World

JAMES A. GOULET, MD
Professor
Department of Orthopaedic Surgery
University of Michigan Hospitals
Ann Arbor, Michigan
52: Hip Dislocations

MATT L. GRAVES, MD
Hansjörg Wyss AO Medical Foundation Chair of Orthopaedic Trauma
Associate Professor and Residency Program Director
Department of Orthopaedic Surgery, Division of Trauma
University of Mississippi Medical Center
Jackson, Mississippi
8: Principles of Internal Fixation

STUART A. GREEN, MD
Clinical Professor, Orthopaedic Surgery
Orthopaedic Surgery
University of California, Irvine
Irvine, California
1: The History of Fracture Treatment: Gavriil A. Ilizarov and the Discovery of Distraction Osteogenesis
7: Principles and Complications of External Skeletal Fixation

JOHN GREENE, MD
Vice President of Medical Affairs
Hartford Region of Hartford Healthcare
Hartford, Connecticut;
Clinical Professor
Obstetrics and Gynecology
University of Connecticut
Farmington, Connecticut
14: Medical Management of the Orthopaedic Trauma Patient. C: Management of the Pregnant Woman

DAVINA V. GUTIERREZ, PHD
Postdoc Researcher
Department of Neuroscience
MetroHealth Medical Center
Case Western Reserve University
Cleveland, Ohio
31: Pathophysiology and Emergent Treatment of Spinal Cord Injury

JESSE C. HAHN, MD
Orthopaedic Trauma Institute
San Francisco, California
65: Fractures of the Tibial Pilon

GEORGE J. HAIDUKEWYCH, MD
Professor of Orthopaedic Surgery
University of Central Florida
Academic Chairman and Chief of Orthopaedic Trauma and Adult Reconstruction
Orlando Health Orthopaedic Institute
Orlando, Florida
56: Posttraumatic Reconstruction of the Hip Joint

JONATHAN S. HALL, MD
Orthopaedic Surgeon
ProOrtho, a division of Proliance Surgeons
Kirkland, Washington
65: Fractures of the Tibial Pilon

SHANNON HAN, MD
Resident Physician
Jefferson Medical College
Philadelphia, Pennsylvania
38: Avoiding Complications in Spine Trauma Patients

SIGVARD T. HANSEN, JR., MD
Professor and Chairman Emeritus
Department of Orthopaedic Surgery
University of Washington School of Medicine
Former Director
Foot and Ankle Institute
Harborview Medical Center
Seattle, Washington
68: Posttraumatic Reconstruction of the Foot and Ankle

MITCHEL B. HARRIS, MD
Chief, Orthopaedic Trauma Service;
Professor, Harvard Medical School
Department of Orthopaedic Surgery
Brigham and Women's Hospital
Boston, Massachusetts
10: Initial Evaluation of the Spine in Trauma Patients

JAMES S. HARROP, MD
Associate Professor
Neurological Surgery
Jefferson Medical College
Philadelphia, Pennsylvania
38: Avoiding Complications in Spine Trauma Patients

BRANDI HARTLEY, MD
Department of Orthopaedic Surgery
University of Louisville School of Medicine
Louisville, Kentucky
23: Diagnosis and Treatment of Complications

NAEL HAWI, MD
Department of Trauma and Orthopaedics
Hannover Medical School (MHH)–Trauma Department
Hannover, Germany
59: Fractures of the Distal Femur

ROMAN HAYDA, MD, COL (RET)
Associate Professor of Orthopaedic Surgery
Brown University
Warren Alpert Medical School
Co-Director of Orthopaedic Trauma
Rhode Island Hospital
Providence, Rhode Island
12: Disaster Management

JOSEPH R. HSU, MD
Orthopaedic Surgeon, Carolinas Medical Center
Orthopaedic trauma
Charlotte, North Carolina
71: Limb Salvage and Reconstruction

AARON R. JACOBSON, DC
Clinical Research Coordinator
Department of Orthopaedic Surgery
University of Minnesota
Minneapolis, Minnesota;
Department of Orthopaedic Surgery
Regions Hospital
St. Paul, Minnesota
50: Scapular and Rib Fractures

MICHAEL JAGODZINSKI, MD
Professor
Trauma Department
AGAPLESION ev. Krankenhaus Bethel
Bückeburg, Germany
60: Patella Fractures and Extensor Mechanism Injuries
61: Knee Dislocations and Soft Tissue Injuries

SAMEER JAIN, MBCHB MRCS
Specialty Registrar in Trauma and Orthopaedic Surgery
Academic Department of Trauma and Orthopaedic Surgery
Leeds General Infirmary
Leeds, United Kingdom
69: Periprosthetic Fractures of the Lower Extremity

ANDREI F. JOAQUIM, MD, PHD
Assistant Neurosurgeon
Department of Neurology
State University of Campinas (UNICAMP)
Campinas, São Paulo, Brazil
35: Thoracolumbar Fractures. A: Classification

CLIFFORD B. JONES, MD, FACS
Orthopaedic Associates of Michigan
Clinical Professor, Michigan State University College of Human Medicine
Adjunct Professor, Van Andel Research Institute
Grand Rapids, Michigan
17: Open Fractures

MANJUL JOSHIPURA, MBBS, MS (ORTHOPAEDICS)
Director
Academy of Traumatology
Ahmedabad, India
3: The Challenges of Orthopaedic Trauma Care in the Developing World

BERNHARD JOST, MD
Prof. Dr. med.
Department of Orthopaedics and Traumatology
Kantonsspital St. Gallen
Switzerland
48: Proximal Humerus Fractures and Glenohumeral Dislocations

KEVIN L. JU, MD
Harvard Combined Orthopaedics
Department of Orthopaedic Surgery
Brigham and Women's Hospital
Boston, Massachusetts
10: Initial Evaluation of the Spine in Trauma Patients

JESSE B. JUPITER, MD
Director, Orthopaedic Hand Service
Massachusetts General Hospital
Hansjörg Wyss/AO Professor
Harvard Medical School
Boston, Massachusetts
49: Fractures and Dislocations of the Clavicle
51: Replantation

WARREN KADRMAS, MD LTCOL, MC, USAF, FS
San Antonio Military Medical Center
San Antonio, Texas
12: Disaster Management

STEVEN P. KALANDIAK, MD
Assistant Professor
Orthopaedics Department
University of Miami
Miami, Florida
19: Gunshot Wounds and Blast Injuries

STEPHEN L. KATES, MD
Hansjörg Wyss Professor of Orthopaedic Surgery
University of Rochester
Rochester, New York
21: Osteoporotic Fragility Fractures

MELISSA A. KLAUSMEYER, MD
Assistant Professor
Division of Plastic and Reconstructive Surgery
Department of General Surgery
Department of Orthopedic Surgery
University of Colorado, School of Medicine
Aurora, Colorado
51: Replantation

KENNETH J. KOVAL, MD
Director of Orthopaedic Research
Adult Orthopaedics
Orlando Regional Medical Center
Orlando, Florida
21: Osteoporotic Fragility Fractures

CHRISTIAN KRETTEK, MD, FRACS, FRCSED
Professor and Director
Hannover Medical School (MHH)–Trauma Department
Hannover, Germany
33: Craniocervical Injuries. C: C2 Fractures
40: Pelvic Ring Injuries: Part III
59: Fractures of the Distal Femur

ASHESH KUMAR, MD, MSC, FRCSC
Clinical Fellow
Division of Orthopaedic Surgery
St. Michael's Hospital
Toronto, Ontario
6: Closed Fracture Management. E: Humeral Shaft Fractures, F: Proximal Humerus Fractures

RAMESH KUMAR, MD
Neurosurgical House Officer
Department of Neurosurgery
University of Colorado
Aurora, Colorado
36: Fractures in the Ankylosed Spine

JOHN Y. KWON, MD
Department of Orthopaedic Surgery
Massachusetts General Hospital
Boston, Massachusetts
67: Foot Injuries

RICHARD F. KYLE, MD
Professor, University of Minnesota
Chairman, Department of Orthopaedic Surgery
Medical Director, Biomechanics Laboratory
Hennepin County Medical Center
Minneapolis, Minnesota
5: Biomechanics of Fractures

PAUL M. LAFFERTY, MD
Assistant Professor
Department of Orthopaedic Surgery
University of Minnesota;
Orthopaedic Surgeon
Department of Orthopaedic Surgery
Regions Hospital
St. Paul, Minnesota
62: Tibial Plateau Fractures

LOREN L. LATTA, PE, PHD
Professor and Director of Biomechanics Research
Department of Orthopaedics
University of Miami
Miami, Florida;
Director, Max Biedermann Institute for Biomechanics
Mount Sinai Medical Center
Miami Beach, Florida
6: Closed Fracture Management. H: Tibial Fractures

ALEXANDER LERNER, MD, PHD
Head of Department
Orthopaedic Surgery
Ziv Medical Center;
Professor
Faculty of Medicine in Galilee
Bar-Ilan University
Zefat, Israel
71: Limb Salvage and Reconstruction

MICHAEL P. LESLIE, DO
Assistant Professor
Orthopaedic Trauma and Reconstruction
Department of Orthopaedics and Rehabilitation
Yale University School of Medicine
New Haven, Connecticut
55: Intertrochanteric Hip Fractures

PAUL E. LEVIN, MD
Vice-Chairman, Department of Orthopaedic Surgery
Montefiore Medical Center/The Albert Einstein College of Medicine
Bronx, New York
29: Psychological, Social, and Functional Manifestations of Orthopaedic Trauma and Traumatic Brain Injury

BRUCE A. LEVY, MD
Professor of Orthopaedics
Department of Orthopaedic Surgery
Mayo Clinic
Rochester, Minnesota
62: Tibial Plateau Fractures

GEOFFREY S. F. LING, MD, PHD, COL. (RET.) U.S. ARMY
Departments of Anesthesiology and Neurology
Uniformed Services University of the Health Sciences
Bethesda, Maryland
29: Psychological, Social, and Functional Manifestations of Orthopaedic Trauma and Traumatic Brain Injury

STEVEN C. LUDWIG, MD
Associate Professor of Orthopaedics, Chief of Spine Surgery
Department of Orthopaedics
University of Maryland
Baltimore, Maryland
35: Thoracolumbar Fractures. E: New Concepts in the Management of Thoracolumbar Fractures

THUAN V. LY, MD
Assistant Professor
Orthopaedic Surgery
University of Minnesota Regions Hospital
St. Paul, Minnesota
54: Intracapsular Hip Fractures

SUSAN G. MACARTHUR, RN, CIC, CPHQ, MPH
Director, Infection Prevention and Regulatory Readiness
Connecticut Children's Medical Center
Hartford, Connecticut
13: Occupational Hazards in the Treatment of Orthopaedic Trauma. B: Prevention of Occupationally Acquired Bloodborne Pathogens

ELLEN J. MACKENZIE, PHD
Fred and Julie Soper Professor in Health Policy and Management and Chair
Department of Health Policy and Management
Johns Hopkins Bloomberg School of Public Health
Baltimore, Maryland
29: Psychological, Social, and Functional Manifestations of Orthopaedic Trauma and Traumatic Brain Injury

CHRISTIAAN N. MAMCZAK, DO
Staff Orthopaedic Traumatologist
Beacon Orthopaedic Trauma Surgery
Memorial Hospital of South Bend;
Assistant Clinical Instructor
Indiana University School of Medicine
South Bend, Indiana
11: Damage Control Orthopaedic Surgery: A Strategy for the Orthopaedic Care of the Critically Injured Patient

MARK W. MANOSO, MD
Orthopedic Service of the Department Surgery
Madigan Army Medical Center
Tacoma, Washington
33: Craniocervical Injuries. A: Occipital-Cervical Spine Injuries

MEIR T. MARMOR, MD
Assistant Clinical Professor
Orthopaedic Trauma Institute
University of California, San Francisco
San Francisco, California
64: Tibial Shaft Fractures

DEAN MARIANO, DO
Clinical Director
Midstate Medical Center/Spine and Pain Institute
Meriden, Connecticut
14: Medical Management of the Orthopaedic Trauma Patient. A: Acute Pain Management, Regional Anesthesia Techniques, and Management of Complex Regional Pain Syndrome

PETER J. MAS, MS, DABMP
Medical Health Physicist, RSO
Medical Physics
Hartford Hospital
Hartford, Connecticut
13: Occupational Hazards in the Treatment of Orthopaedic Trauma. A: Optimal and Safe Use of C-Arm X-Ray Fluoroscopy Units

AMIR M. MATITYAHU, MD
Associate Clinical Professor
Orthopaedic Trauma Institute
University of California, San Francisco
San Francisco, California
64: Tibial Shaft Fractures

JOEL M. MATTA, MD
The Hip and Pelvis Institute
St. John's Health Center
Santa Monica, California
1: The History of Fracture Treatment: Emile Letournel and the Surgery of Pelvic and Acetabular Fractures

MICHAEL D. MCKEE, MD
Professor of Surgery
St. Michael's Hospital
Toronto, Ontario, Canada
46: Trauma to the Adult Elbow and Fractures of the Distal Humerus. B: Fractures of the Distal Humerus

CHARLES N. MOCK, MD, PHD, FACS
Professor of Surgery
University of Washington
Seattle, Washington
3: The Challenges of Orthopaedic Trauma Care in the Developing World

TIMOTHY MOORE, MD
Associate Professor
Orthopaedic Surgery and Neurosciences
MetroHealth Medical Center
Cleveland, Ohio
35: Thoracolumbar Fractures. D. Fractures of the Low Lumbar Spine

ADRIENNE MORAFF, MD
Resident Physician
Department of Neurosurgery
Stanford University Hospitals
Stanford, California
35: Thoracolumbar Fractures. D. Fractures of the Low Lumbar Spine

VICTOR A. MORRIS, MD
Assistant Professor of Medicine, General Medicine
Director, Hospitalist Service
Director, Medicine Consult Service
Yale University School of Medicine
Yale-New Haven Hospital
New Haven, Connecticut
53: Medical Management of the Patient with Hip Fracture

CALIN S. MOUCHA, MD
Associate Chief, Joint Replacement Surgery
The Mount Sinai Hospital
Assistant Professor
Leni & Peter W. May Department of Orthopaedic Surgery
Icahn School of Medicine at Mount Sinai
New York, New York
22: Surgical Site Infection Prevention

CHRISTIAN W. MÜLLER, MD
Trauma and Orthopaedic Surgeon
Hannover Medical School (MHH)–Trauma Department
Hannover, Germany
33: Craniocervical Injuries. C: C2 Fractures

ALAN D. MURDOCK, COL (DR.), USAF, MC
Consultant to the Surgeon General for Trauma
Air Force Medical Operations Agency
Lackland AFB, Texas;
Chief, Acute Care Surgery
Division of Trauma and General Surgery
UPMC Presbyterian Hospital
Pittsburgh, Pennsylvania
9: Evaluation and Treatment of the Multi-injured Trauma Patient

CLINTON K. MURRAY
Chief of Infectious Disease Service
Brooke Army Medical Center
San Antonio, Texas;
Professor of Medicine
Uniformed Services University of the Health Sciences
Bethesda, Texas
24: Chronic Osteomyelitis

GEORGE P. NANOS III, MD
CDR, U.S. Army
Navy Program Director
National Capital Consortium Hand Surgery Fellowship
Department of Orthopaedics
Walter Reed National Military Medical Center
Bethesda, Maryland
18: Soft Tissue Reconstruction
72: Amputations in Trauma

AARON NAUTH, MD
Department of Surgery
University of Toronto
St. Michael's Hospital
Toronto, Ontario, Canada
46: Trauma to the Adult Elbow and Fractures of the Distal Humerus. B: Fractures of the Distal Humerus

JOHN NEAL VI, MD
Charleston, South Carolina
35: Thoracolumbar Fractures. E: New Concepts in the Management of Thoracolumbar Fractures

SEAN E. NORK, MD
Professor
Department of Orthopaedic Surgery
Harborview Medical Center
Seattle, Washington
57: Subtrochanteric Fractures of the Femur

ARIA NOURI, MD
Division of Neurosurgery and Spine Program
Institute of Medical Science
University of Toronto
University Health Network
Toronto, Ontario, Canada
32: The Timing of Management of Spinal Cord Injuries

DANIEL P. O'CONNOR, PHD
Associate Professor of Health and Human Performance
University of Houston
Houston, Texas
25: Nonunions: Evaluation and Treatment

STEVEN A. OLSON, MD
Professor
Orthopaedic Surgery
Duke University School of Medicine
Durham, North Carolina
27: Outcome Assessment in Orthopaedic Traumatology

POLINA OSLER, MS
Harvard Medical School
Orthopedic Surgery, Spine Service
Massachusetts General Hospital
Boston, Massachusetts
35: Thoracolumbar Fractures. B: Treatment of Thoracolumbar Burst Fractures

BRETT D. OWENS, MD, LTC MC USA
Chief, Orthopaedic Surgery
Keller Army Hospital
West Point, New York
2: Global Burden of Musculoskeletal Injuries

PATRICK W. OWENS, MD
Associate Professor
Orthopaedic Surgery
University of Miami
Miami, Florida
19: Gunshot Wounds and Blast Injuries

ERIC PAGENKOPF, MD
Attending
Orthopedic Trauma
Los Angeles County + USC Medical Center
CAPT MC USN
Navy Trauma Training Center
Los Angeles, California
11: Damage Control Orthopaedic Surgery: A Strategy for the Orthopaedic Care of the Critically Injured Patient

DROR PALEY, MD, FRCSC
Director
Paley Advanced Limb Lengthening Institute
St. Mary's Medical Center
West Palm Beach, Florida
63: Malunions and Nonunions about the Knee
70: Principles of Deformity Correction

ALPESH A. PATEL, MD, FACS
Associate Professor
Department of Orthopaedic Surgery
Northwestern University
Chicago, Illinois
35: Thoracolumbar Fractures. A: Classification

ANDREW B. PEITZMAN, MD
Distinguished Professor of Surgery
Mark M. Ravitch Professor and Vice-Chair
UPMC Vice-President for Trauma and Surgical Services
UPMC Presbyterian Hospital
Pittsburgh, Pennsylvania
9: Evaluation and Treatment of the Multi-injured Trauma Patient

GEORGE A. PERDRIZET, MD, PHD, FACS
Medical Director
Wound Recovery and Hyperbaric Medicine Center
Kent Hospital
Warwick, Rhode Island
14: Medical Management of the Orthopaedic Trauma Patient. D: Substance Abuse Syndromes: Recognition, Prevention, and Treatment

EDWARD L. PESANTI
Professor of Medicine
University of Connecticut Health Center
Farmington, Connecticut
Assistant Professor of Orthopaedic Surgery
University of Connecticut Health Center
24: Chronic Osteomyelitis

MAXIMILIAN PETRI, MD
Trauma Department
Hannover Medical School (MHH)–Trauma Department
Hannover, Germany
60: Patella Fractures and Extensor Mechanism Injuries
61: Knee Dislocations and Soft Tissue Injuries

PHILIPPE PHAN, MD, FRCS(C)
Assistant Professor in Orthopedic Surgery
University of Ottawa
Orthopedic Spine and Trauma Surgeon
Department of Surgery
The Ottawa Hospital, Civic Campus
Ottawa, Ontario, Canada
35: Thoracolumbar Fractures. B: Treatment of Thoracolumbar Burst Fractures

MICHAEL S. PINZUR, MD
Professor of Orthopaedic Surgery
Loyola University Health System
Maywood, Illinois
72: Amputations in Trauma

ANDREW POLLAK, MD
The James Lawrence Kernan Professor and Chairman
Department of Orthopaedics
University of Maryland School of Medicine
Chief of Orthopaedics
University of Maryland Medical System
Baltimore, Maryland
11: Damage Control Orthopaedic Surgery: A Strategy for the Orthopaedic Care of the Critically Injured Patient

BENJAMIN K. POTTER, MD
LTC, MC, U.S. Army
Vice Chair (Research) and Associate Professor, Department of Surgery
Uniformed Services University of Health Sciences
Chief Orthopaedic Surgeon
Amputee Patient Care Program and Director,
Musculoskeletal Oncology
Department of Orthopaedics,
Walter Reed National Military Medical Center
Bethesda, Maryland
72: Amputations in Trauma

DANIEL E. PRINCE, MD, MPH
Assistant Attending Surgeon
Assistant Professor
Weill College of Medicine of Cornell University
New York, New York
63: Malunions and Nonunions about the Knee

DAVID M. PRIOR, MD
Orthopaedic Surgery Resident
Orthopaedic Surgery
Western Michigan University School of Medicine
Kalamazoo, Michigan
35: Thoracolumbar Fractures. D. Fractures of the Low Lumbar Spine

ROBERT A. PROBE, MD
Chair, Department of Orthopedic Surgery
Chair, Scott & White Board of Directors
Scott & White Healthcare
Temple, Texas
27: Outcome Assessment in Orthopaedic Traumatology

TODD E. RASMUSSEN, COL, MC, USAF
Deputy Director
U.S. Combat Casualty Care Research Program
Fort Detrick, Maryland
15: Evaluation and Treatment of Vascular Injuries

MARK C. REILLY, MD
Chief Orthopaedic Trauma Service, University Hospital, Newark
Fred F. Behrens Endowed Chair, Orthopaedic Trauma
Associate Professor
Department of Orthopaedic Surgery
Rutgers, New Jersey Medical School
Newark, New Jersey
57: Subtrochanteric Fractures of the Femur

NOAM RESHEF, MD
Orthopedic Surgeon
Orthopedics Sports services, Foot & Ankle Surgery
Ziv Medical Center
Tefat, Israel
71: Limb Salvage and Reconstruction

MARTINUS RICHTER, MD, PHD
Prof. Dr. Med.
Department for Foot and Ankle Surgery Nuremberg and Rummelsberg
Hospital Rummelsberg
Schwarzenbruck, Bavaria, Germany
67: Foot Injuries

JOHN T. RIEHL, MD
Assistant Professor
University of Louisville
Orthopaedic Surgeon
University of Louisville Hospital
Louisville, Kentucky
21: Osteoporotic Fragility Fractures

DAVID RING, MD
Director of Research
Hand Service Instructor
Orthopaedic Surgery
Harvard Medical School
Massachusetts General Hospital
Department of Orthopaedic Surgery
Boston, Massachusetts
49: Fractures and Dislocations of the Clavicle

CRAIG S. ROBERTS, MD, MBA
Professor and Chair
Department of Orthopaedic Surgery
University of Louisville School of Medicine
Louisville, Kentucky
23: Diagnosis and Treatment of Complications

HUMBERTO ROSAS, MD
Associate Professor
Department of Radiology
School of Medicine and Public Health
University of Wisconsin
Madison, Wisconsin
30: Imaging of Spinal Trauma

MELLISA ROSKOSKY, MSPH
Program Manager, Clinical Research
Athens Orthopedic Clinic
Athens, Georgia
16: Compartment Syndromes

JACK W. ROSS, MD, FSHEA
Associate Clinical Professor of Medicine
University of Connecticut School of Medicine
Chief, Divisions of Infectious Diseases, Epidemiology, HIV Programs
Hartford Hospital
Hartford, Connecticut
13: Occupational Hazards in the Treatment of Orthopaedic Trauma. B: Prevention of Occupationally Acquired Bloodborne Pathogens

MILTON LEE (CHIP) ROUTT, JR., MD
Dr. Andrew R. Burgess Endowed Chair and Professor
Department of Orthopaedic Surgery
University of Texas Health Science Center—Houston
Houston, Texas
41: Surgical Treatment of Acetabular Fractures

MICHAEL J. ROY, MD, MPH, COL. (RET.) U.S. ARMY
Director, Division of Military Internal Medicine, Department of Medicine
Uniformed Services University of the Health Sciences
Bethesda, Maryland
29: Psychological, Social, and Functional Manifestations of Orthopaedic Trauma and Traumatic Brain Injury

DAVID E. RUCHELSMAN, MD, FAAOS
Assistant Chief, Division of Hand Surgery
Clinical Assistant Professor of Orthopaedic Surgery
Newton-Wellesley Hospital/Tufts University School of Medicine
Boston, Massachusetts
42: Fractures and Dislocations of the Hand

THOMAS H. SANDERS, MD
Chief Resident, Department of Orthopaedic Surgery
MedStar Georgetown University Hospital
Washington, DC
26: Physical Impairment Ratings for Fractures

AUGUSTO SARMIENTO, MD
Professor and Chairman Emeritus
Departments of Orthopaedics
University of Miami
Miami, Florida;
University of Southern California
Los Angeles, California
6: Closed Fracture Management. H: Tibial Fractures

ADAM A. SASSOON, MD
Assistant Professor
Department of Orthopedics and Sports Medicine
University of Washington
Seattle, Washington
56: Posttraumatic Reconstruction of the Hip Joint

JASON W. SAVAGE, MD
Assistant Professor in Orthopaedic Surgery
Northwestern University Feinberg School of Medicine
Chicago, Illinois
37: Osteoporotic Spinal Fractures

THOMAS M. SCALEA, MD, FACS
The Francis X. Kelly Distinguished Professor of Trauma
Director Program-in-Trauma
University of Maryland School of Medicine
Physician-in-Chief
R Adams Cowley Shock Trauma Center
Baltimore, Maryland
11: Damage Control Orthopaedic Surgery: A Strategy for the Orthopaedic Care of the Critically Injured Patient

JOSEPH SCHATZKER CM, MD, BSC(MED), FRCS(C)
Professor Surgery (Emeritus)
University of Toronto;
Director
Mueller Institute
Sunnybrook
Toronto, Ontario, Canada
1: The History of Fracture Treatment: Maurice Edmond Müller, Internal Fixation Techniques and Hip Prostheses

LISA K. SCHRODER, BSME, MBA
Director, Orthopaedic Trauma Academic Programs
Department of Orthopaedic Surgery
University of Minnesota
Minneapolis, Minnesota;
Department of Orthopaedic Surgery
Regions Hospital
St. Paul, Minnesota
50: Scapular and Rib Fractures

CARA L. SEDNEY, MD, MA
Orthopaedics
West Virginia University
Morgantown, West Virginia
33: Craniocervical Injuries. B: Atlas Fractures and Atlantoaxial Injuries

DAVID SELIGSON, MD
Professor
Department of Orthopedic Surgery
University of Louisville School of Medicine
Louisville, Kentucky
1: The History of Fracture Treatment: Klaus Klemm and Interlocking Nailing and Local Antiobiotic Bead Chain Therapy
23: Diagnosis and Treatment of Complications

DAVID W. SHEARER, MD, MPH
Chief Resident
Department of Orthopaedic Surgery
University of California, San Francisco
San Francisco, California
3: The Challenges of Orthopaedic Trauma Care in the Developing World

RICHARD SHEPPARD, MD
Director, Orthopedic Anesthesiology
Department of Anesthesiology
Hartford Hospital
Hartford, Connecticut;
Associate Professor of Anesthesiology
John Dempsey Hospital
University of Connecticut School of Medicine
Farmington, Connecticut
14: Medical Management of the Orthopaedic Trauma Patient. A: Acute Pain Management, Regional Anesthesia Techniques, and Management of Complex Regional Pain Syndrome

MICHAEL SIMMS SHULER, MD
Hand and Upper Extremity Surgeon
Athens Orthopedic Clinic
Athens, Georgia
16: Compartment Syndromes

NICOLE SILVERSTEIN, MD, FACP
Assistant Professor
Department of Medicine
University of Connecticut
Farmington, Connecticut
14: Medical Management of the Orthopaedic Trauma Patient. B: Perioperative Assessment

CHRISTOPH SOMMER, MD
Head of Trauma and General Surgery Unit
Department of Surgery
Kantonsspital Graubünden
Chur, Switzerland
47: Fracture of the Humeral Shaft

DAVID A. SPIEGEL, MD
Pediatric Orthopaedic Surgeon
The Children's Hospital of Philadelphia;
Associate Professor of Orthopaedic Surgery
The University of Pennsylvania School of Medicine
Philadelphia, Pennsylvania;
Consultant in Orthopaedics
Hospital and Rehabilitation Centre for Disabled Children
Banepa, Nepal
3: The Challenges of Orthopaedic Trauma Care in the Developing World

ANDRE R. SPIGUEL, MD
Assistant Professor Orthopaedic Oncology
Department of Orthopaedics and Rehabilitation
University of Florida
Gainesville, Florida
20: Pathologic Fractures

CHRISTIAN SPROSS, MD
Department of Orthopaedics and Traumatology
Kantonsspital St. Gallen
Switzerland
48: Proximal Humerus Fractures and Glenohumeral Dislocations. B: Proximal Humeral Fractures and Fracture-Dislocations

ROBERT J. STEFFNER, MD
Assistant Clinical Professor
Department of Orthopaedic Surgery
University of California Davis
Sacramento, California
20: Pathologic Fractures

SCOTT P. STEINMANN, MD
Department of Orthopaedic Surgery
Mayo Clinic
Rochester, Minnesota
46: Trauma to the Adult Elbow and Fractures of the Distal Humerus. A: Trauma to the Adult Elbow

MICHAEL P. STEINMETZ, MD
Chairman
Department of Neurological Surgery
Case Western Reserve University School of Medicine
Cleveland, Ohio
31: Pathophysiology and Emergent Treatment of Spinal Cord Injury

IAIN STEVENSON, MB CHB, FRCS (TR & ORTH)
Consultant Orthopaedic and Trauma Surgeon
NHS Grampian, Aberdeen Royal Infirmary
Aberdeen, Scotland
6: Closed Fracture Management. C: Scaphoid Fractures, D: Distal Radius Fractures, G: Ankle Fracture

DANIEL J. STINNER, MD
Orthopaedic Trauma Surgeon
Department of Orthopaedics and Rehabilitation
San Antonio Military Medical Center
San Antonio, Texas
71: Limb Salvage and Reconstruction

HARLAN STOCK
Assistant Professor of Radiology
Chief of Musculoskeletal Imaging
University of Connecticut Health Center
Farmington, Connecticut
24: Chronic Osteomyelitis

MARC F. SWIONTKOWSKI, MD
Professor
Department of Orthopaedic Surgery
University of Minnesota Medical School;
CEO, TRIA Orthopaedic Center
Minneapolis, Minnesota
54: Intracapsular Hip Fractures

OLIVER TANNOUS, MD
Department of Orthopaedics
University of Maryland
Baltimore, Maryland
35: Thoracolumbar Fractures. E: New Concepts in the Management of Thoracolumbar Fractures

MARVIN TILE, CM, MD, BSC(MED), FRCS(C)
Professor Surgery (Emeritus)
University of Toronto;
Orthopaedic Surgeon
Sunnybrook HSC
Toronto, Ontario, Canada
1: The History of Fracture Treatment: Martin Allgöwer, Internal Fixation and Fracture Management

ASHISH UPADHYAY, MBBS, MS
Clinical Instructor
Department of Orthopaedic Surgery
University of Louisville;
Spine Fellow, Norton Leatherman Spine Center
Louisville, Kentucky
35: Thoracolumbar Fractures. C: Identification, Classification, Mechanism, and Treatment of Thoracolumbar Fracture-Dislocations

ALEXANDER R. VACCARO, MD, PHD
Professor and Vice Chairman
Department of Orthopaedic Surgery
Thomas Jefferson University and Hospitals
Philadelphia, Pennsylvania
34: Subaxial Cervical Spine Trauma

JAMES P. WADDELL, MD, FRCSC
Professor, Division of Orthopaedic Surgery
University of Toronto
Toronto, Ontario, Canada
6: Closed Fracture Management. A: Introduction, C: Scaphoid Fractures, D: Distal Radius Fractures, E: Humeral Shaft Fractures, F: Proximal Humerus Fractures, G: Ankle Fracture, H: Tibial Fractures

DOUGLAS WARDLAW, MB, CHB, CHM, FRCSED
Consultant Orthopaedic and Spinal Surgeon, NHS Grampian (Retired)
Honorary Professor, Robert Gordon University
Aberdeen, Scotland, United Kingdom
6: Closed Fracture Management. B: Basic Principles, I: Fractures of the Femur

J. KRISTOPHER WARE, MD, DPT, MS
Orthopaedic Surgery
University of Connecticut Health Center
Farmington, Connecticut
24: Chronic Osteomyelitis

J. TRACY WATSON, MD
Professor, Orthopaedic Surgery
Chief, Orthopaedic Trauma Service
Department of Orthopaedic Surgery
Saint Louis University School of Medicine
St. Louis, Missouri
4: Biology and Enhancement of Skeletal Repair
62: Tibial Plateau Fractures

JOSEPH C. WENKE, PHD
Manager, Regenerative Medicine Task Area
Orthopaedic Trauma Research Program
U.S. Army Institute of Surgical Research
Fort Sam Houston, Texas
17: Open Fractures

BRENT B. WIESEL, MD
Assistant Professor, Georgetown University School of Medicine
Chief, Shoulder Service, Department of Orthopedic Surgery
MedStar Georgetown University Hospital
Washington, DC
26: Physical Impairment Ratings for Fractures

SAM W. WIESEL, MD
Professor and Chair, Department of Orthopedic Surgery
MedStar Georgetown University Hospital
Washington, DC
26: Physical Impairment Ratings for Fractures

SETH K. WILLIAMS, MD
Assistant Professor
Department of Orthopedics and Rehabilitation
School of Medicine and Public Health
University of Wisconsin
Madison, Wisconsin
35: Thoracolumbar Fractures. E: New Concepts in the Management of Thoracolumbar Fractures

MARCEL WINKELMANN, MD
Trauma Department
Hannover Medical School (MHH)–Trauma Department
Hannover, Germany
40: Pelvic Ring Injuries: Parts I-III

KIRKHAM BERWICK WOOD, MD
Orthopedic Surgery
Massachusetts General Hospital
Boston, Massachusetts
35: Thoracolumbar Fractures. B: Treatment of Thoracolumbar Burst Fractures

JENNIFER WOZNICZKA, MD
Resident
Department of Orthopaedic Surgery
University of Minnesota
Minneapolis, Minnesota
5: Biomechanics of Fractures

ROBERT WYSOCKI, MD
Assistant Professor
Department of Orthopaedic Surgery
Rush University Medical Center
Chicago, Illinois
44: Fractures of the Distal Radius

VILIJAM ZDRAVKOVIC, MD
Department of Orthopaedics and Traumatology
Kantonsspital St. Gallen
Switzerland
48: Proximal Humerus Fractures and Glenohumeral Dislocations. A: Essential Principles

LEWIS G. ZIRKLE, MD
Founder and President
SIGN Fracture Care International;
Clinical Professor
University of Washington
Richland, Washington
3: The Challenges of Orthopaedic Trauma Care in the Developing World

GREGORY A. ZYCH, D.O.
Christine E. Lynn Distinguished Chair in Orthopaedic Trauma
Professor and Chief, Orthopaedic Trauma
Orthopaedics Department
Miller School of Medicine
University of Miami
Miami, Florida
19: Gunshot Wounds and Blast Injuries

Foreword

It is a great honor to write this foreword to the fifth edition of *Skeletal Trauma*. Since its introduction in 1992, *Skeletal Trauma*, through its successive editions, has become the reference of choice of orthopaedic surgeons who are involved with the diagnosis, treatment, and rehabilitation of musculoskeletal trauma patients. In the current edition, Dr. Browner and colleagues have written a text that is unmatched as a source of contemporary information for the busy surgeon.

Skeletal Trauma is superbly organized into five major sections, the first of which covers a wide range of important topics ranging from the biology of skeletal repair to closed fracture management. Subsequent book sections address spine, pelvis, upper extremity and lower extremity injuries. Within each section, chapters are expertly written by thought leaders in their fields and incorporate the best peer-reviewed literature applicable to specific orthopaedic trauma topics. The text is thoughtfully complemented by numerous high-quality line drawings, diagnostic images, and full-color clinical photographs that demonstrate not only the principles of care, but also specific surgical procedures to achieve the best possible outcome for each injury type.

As of this writing in 2014, over 52,000 Americans have been wounded in the wars in Iraq and Afghanistan. Approximately 60 to 70 percent of wounds involve the musculoskeletal system; and as such, military orthopaedic surgeons have shouldered much responsibility in both the frontline and tertiary treatment of these injuries. Providing battlefield orthopaedic care poses special challenges which are seldom confronted in civilian practice. Acutely wounded warriors must be triaged and treated in austere and often dangerous environments, undergo staged resuscitation and surgery, and endure prolonged medical evacuation, often involving multiple modes of transportation across continents or oceans. Because of advances in care, rapid medical evacuation, and personal protective equipment, many casualties with severe orthopaedic injuries have survived the wars in Iraq or Afghanistan, but would not have done so in previous wars. Treatment of combat wounds, which can be devastating in the scope of both soft-tissue and bony injury, requires a team approach that may employ hypotensive resuscitation with blood and blood products, damage-control orthopaedics, new or rediscovered methods of hemorrhage control, vacuum-assisted wound closure, and advanced reconstructive techniques for limb salvage.

To address musculoskeletal trauma that occurs on the battlefield, and analogous injuries resulting from terrorist attacks, industrial accidents, or natural disasters, this edition of *Skeletal Trauma* gives unique focus to injuries that occur in modern warfare. Although most orthopaedic surgeons practice in the civilian and not the military setting, this focus will impart a basic understanding of the injury mechanisms and treatment principles associated with battlefield trauma, as well as the military's method of echeloned care. Such knowledge will better prepare civilian orthopaedic surgeons to manage multiple, severely injured patients, and would be invaluable during a mass casualty event such as the 2013 Boston Marathon bombing. *Skeletal Trauma* will ensure that as the wars in Iraq and Afghanistan draw to a close, the legacy of the medical advances related to battlefield injuries will be inherited by those who care for severely injured patients.

Service members who have been severely wounded in action present some of the most challenging problems orthopaedic surgeons will encounter. The editors of *Skeletal Trauma* have thus included current information from military surgeons and physicians in concert with leading civilian experts to cover a number of important subjects. Contained in Section I, new information in Chapters 2, 7, 9, 11, and 12 includes relevant and related topics including injury burden, external fixation, management of the multi-trauma patient, damage control orthopaedics, and disaster management. Chapter 19, which expertly covers musculoskeletal gunshot wounds, also dedicates substantial space to management of blast-injured patients, including a discussion of dismounted complex blast injury (DCBI), a wounding pattern recently described in those severely injured in Afghanistan from improvised explosive devices (IEDs) while on foot patrol. In Section V, Chapters 71 and 72 provide leading-edge information on l imb salvage and amputation and include some battlefield perspective.

This fifth edition of *Skeletal Trauma* is an invaluable reference that has been painstakingly prepared to fit the needs of those who treat patients with musculoskeletal trauma. It is the right book at the right time. I congratulate the editors and their authors for their unerring success in bringing out the best practices to optimize patient outcomes. This book is an extraordinary accomplishment.

D. C. Covey, MD, MSc, FACS
Captain, Medical Corps, U.S. Navy (Ret.)
Clinical Professor of Orthopaedic Surgery
University of California, San Diego

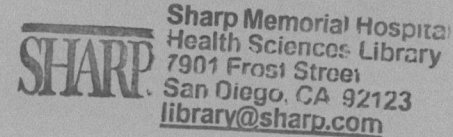

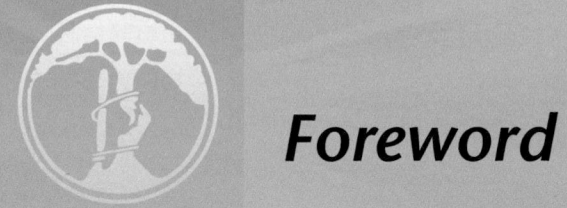

Preface

The latest edition is again dedicated to conveying comprehensive information on the basic science, diagnosis, and treatment of acute musculoskeletal injuries and posttraumatic reconstructive problems. Previous editions have focused primarily on injuries sustained in the civilian sector, but we have now expanded our scope to include in-depth coverage of injuries to wounded warriors. Sixteen active duty military surgeons and physicians from various branches of the U.S. Military have collaborated with civilian authors to cover a variety of subjects in various chapters. We have sought these contributions to educate readers on the lessons learned from modern wars and to make the text more useful to those caring for wounded warriors in conflicts around the world.

We are indebted to Col (Ret) James Ficke, MD, who served as the Military Consultant for the fifth edition. He recently retired from a distinguished 30-year career in the U.S. Army, beginning with graduation from West Point and concluding with his service as Special Advisor to the Army Surgeon General and Chairman of the Army's largest academic Department of Orthopaedics and Rehabilitation at the Brook Army Medical Center in San Antonio. Jim recently assumed the position of Chairman of the Orthopaedic Surgery Department at Johns Hopkins. Jim identified and helped recruit the most experienced military subject experts from various military branches and centers. His guidance and hands-on involvement have been invaluable in creating the fifth edition.

We were also fortunate to have Dana Curtis Covey, Captain, Medical Corps, U.S. Navy, agree to write the Foreword. A graduate of the Naval Academy, he has had a long and highly distinguished career in the Navy, with numerous deployments in wars and conflicts. He is highly decorated and winner of numerous awards, including the *Chairman of the Joint Chiefs of Staff Award for Excellence in Military Medicine* as the nation's top military physician. He is particularly proud of his multiple, lengthy deployments to Iraq and Afghanistan as a leader of Marine Corps' far-forward surgical teams responsible for saving the lives and limbs of Marines and Sailors severely wounded on the battlefield (including during the fiercest fighting in Fallujah). He is among the most revered and battle experienced U.S. Military surgeons and brings enormous perspective on the lessons learned from war.

A large number of new chapters have been added (by chapter numbers: 2. Global Burden of Musculoskeletal Injuries; 3. The Challenges of Orthopaedic Trauma Care in the Developing World; 6. Closed Fracture Management; 7. Principles and Complications of External Skeletal Fixation; 11. Damage Control Orthopaedic Surgery: A Strategy for the Orthopaedic Care of the Critically Injured Patient; 14A. Acute Pain Management, Regional Anesthesia Techniques, and Management of Complex Regional Pain Syndrome; 14B. Perioperative Assessment; 14C. Management of the Pregnant Woman; 17. Open Fractures; 19. Gunshot Wounds and Blast Injuries; 27. Outcomes Assessment in Orthopaedic Traumatology; 28. Professionalism and the Economics of Orthopaedic Trauma Care; 29. Psychological, Social and Functional Manifestations of Orthopaedic Trauma and Traumatic Brain Injury; 49. Fractures and Dislocations of the Clavicle; 50. Scapula and Rib Fractures; 51. Replantation; 71. Limb Salvage and Reconstruction). New authors have been recruited to write many chapters, and returning authors have made major revisions in their material for this edition. Half of the chapters in the upper and lower extremity were contributed by European authors who have added different perspective and shared their substantial information on recorded outcomes.

The spine section has undergone a major overhaul under the new editorial leadership of Dr. Paul A. Andersen.

The authors have reached a new level in the scholarship, clarity, and comprehensiveness in their writing. When available, the evidence base of subjects has been substantiated, including notation of level of evidence in references and discussion of meta-analyses and evidence-supported guidelines. In keeping with the tradition of the text, authors have endeavored to share their great experience in discussing the risks and benefits of alternative treatments for specific problems to guide the readers to the optimal practical management and well-illustrated surgical techniques for their individual patients.

In addition to the printed text, the content will now be available via a complete mobile e-book, accessible on a variety of devices. A new electronic format program has been utilized to allow dramatically enhanced user-friendly search and display of all components of text, figures, references, and videos. Words cannot express the impressively fast search and display capability of the Expert Consult platform–it must be experienced first-hand to allow true appreciation.

There were a number of significant changes in the editorial team since the previous edition, requiring replacement of two of the original editors. Alan Levine, who had edited the spine section since the first edition, died suddenly and prematurely. He had developed an international reputation as a master spine and tumor surgeon, educator, and scholar. In addition to his outstanding contributions as skeletal trauma editor, he served as editor in chief of the American Academy of Orthopaedic Surgeons Journal, Chairman of the AAOS Publications Committee, and Chairman of the AAOS Council on Education. Paul A. Andersen, Professor of Orthopaedic Surgery at the University of Wisconsin, and an internationally known spine surgeon, has assumed leadership of the spine section. Paul brings an emphasis on evidence-based medicine and great practical experience as a spine surgery educator to the editorial team.

Peter Trafton, who had edited the lower extremity section since the first edition, withdrew to enjoy his well-earned retirement from practice at Brown University. He is an internationally known orthopaedic trauma surgeon who has distinguished himself as a master surgeon, scholar, and educator. In addition to overseeing quality initiatives for the Orthopaedic Department at Brown, he is leading a collaborative initiative of multiple orthopaedic organizations to provide training and education for orthopedic residents at Komfo Ankone Teaching Hospital (KATH) in Kumasi, Ghana. Professor Christian Krettek, Chairman of the Department of Traumatology at the Medical School in Hannover, Germany, an internationally known orthopaedic trauma surgeon, has assumed leadership of the lower extremity section. He served as video editor of the fourth edition of *Skeletal Trauma* and brings new creative energy and European perspective to the editorial team.

We have been most fortunate that Jesse B. Jupiter, an editor since the first edition, has stayed on board. We benefit enormously from his wisdom, scholarship, and international connections.

With the current edition, we made an increased effort to coordinate with Greg Mencio and Marc Swiontkowski, the editors of *Green's Skeletal Trauma in Children*, fifth edition, the companion to the two volume adult text. Marc has been an editor since the first edition. As an internationally known expert in orthopaedic outcomes, he provided important guidance for the adult and pediatric texts. Marc has recently assumed the position of editor in chief of the *Journal of Bone and Joint Surgery*. Greg assumed the lead role held for the first four editions by Neil Green, preserving the text's base at Vanderbilt University. As an internationally known pediatric orthopaedic surgeon and current Vice President of the Pediatric Orthopaedic Society of North America, he brings enormous new energy and connections to revitalize the pediatric text.

The growing epidemic of road traffic injuries, especially in the developing countries, and the persistence of armed conflicts, civil wars, and insurgencies in many parts of the world will continue to produce many musculoskeletal injuries that require acute and reconstructive care to ensure optimal function and mobility and avoid disabling complications. I believe the material assembled here by our dedicated authors, editors, and the publisher's team will assist caregivers world wide with this continuing challenge.

Bruce D. Browner, MD, MHCM, FACS
Jesse B. Jupiter, MD
Christian Krettek, MD, FRACS, FRCSEd
Paul A. Anderson, MD

Acknowledgments

On this edition, we had the privilege of working with a talented and committed group of professionals from Elsevier, who carried on the tradition of excellence established in previous editions. We would particularly like to acknowledge Dolores Meloni, Executive Content Strategist, the driving force behind the project. We are indebted to Maureen Iannuzzi, Senior Content Development Manager, who took over when Gabriel Goodman-White, our initial Content Development Specialist, moved to another company. She tirelessly communicated with authors and editors to collect the pieces and keep the work on track, while supervising the department of content specialists. Amy Meros, a content specialist, ably assisted Maureen. Carol O'Connell, Senior Production Editor, led the production phase that converted our content to a printed text and an e-book. Steven Stave, Manager of Art and Design, and Lesley Frasier, Illustration Buyer, oversaw the wonderful cover design and illustrations. Their contributions combined with those of our authors to produce a product of which we are all justly proud.

No staff were hired by the editors for the development of the text. Again, we relied upon the hard work and dedication of our own personal staff and institutional resources. We recognize that their help was critical in helping us reach the level of excellence to which we aspired.

Bruce Browner would like to thank his academic and clinical assistants: Sue Ellen Pelletier and Carmen Propiescus at the Department of Orthopaedic Surgery, New England Musculoskeletal Institute, University of Connecticut Health Center, and his academic and clinical assistants: Susan Kohn and Jenieliz Ocasio at the Department of Orthopaedic Surgery, HHC Bone and Joint Institute at Hartford Hospital. They assisted with making phone calls to editors, authors, and the publisher during the multiple phases of development of the fifth edition.

Paul Anderson would like to thank Veronica McCann Anderson for her timely and expert review and editing of the manuscripts.

Christian Krettek would like first of all to express his strong appreciation to Dr. Med. Nael Hawi, senior resident at the Orthopaedic Trauma Department of Hannover Medical School (MHH) for his tireless efforts and pivotal role in completing this edition by numerous tasks, including proofreading manuscripts and page proofs, and communicating with the authors. Dr. Hawi's high academic work ethic, endless energy, unparalleled precision, and clear focus were absolutely outstanding.

He also would like to recognize the assistance of Mrs. Cordula Bödecker, his personal administrative assistant in the head office, who assisted him communicating with the authors, editors, and publisher during multiple phases of the development and editorial process of the fifth edition.

He would like to thank the staff of the audio-visual support team, namely Mr. Beck, Mrs. Kosmalski, and Mrs. Siefke, who were responsible for the high quality of digital images and videos in the OR, outpatient department, biomechanics lab, and other occasions.

Strong appreciation is given also to Kurt Singelmann and numerous contributors of the Hannover Videosymposium, who spent enormous time and efforts to produce videos and agreed to share their expertise and video material with the readers of *Skeletal Trauma*.

And last but not least, Dr. Krettek would like to acknowledge the enormous continuous academic, clinical, and administrative support as well as the daily inspiration of the entire staff of the Department for of Trauma and Orthopaedic of the Hannover Medical School.

Contents

SECTION TWO

Spine

Section Editor: Paul A. Anderson

Video Contents

Videos are available at the *Skeletal Trauma* collection online at https://expertconsult.inkling.com.

SECTION ONE

General Principles

EDITED BY BRUCE D. BROWNER

SECTION OUTLINE

Chapter 1

The History of Fracture Treatment

CHRISTOPHER L. COLTON

EARLY SPLINTING TECHNIQUES

Humans have never been immune from injury, and doubtless the practice of bonesetting was not unfamiliar to our most primitive forebears. Indeed, given the known skills of Neolithic humans at trepanning the skull,[49] it would be surprising if techniques of similar sophistication had not been brought to bear in the care of injuries. However, no evidence of this remains.

The earliest examples of the active management of fractures in humans were discovered at Naga-ed-Der (about 100 miles north of Luxor in Egypt) by Professor G. Elliott Smith during the Hearst Egyptian expedition of the University of California in 1903.[74] Two specimens were found of splinted extremities. One was an adolescent femur with a compound, comminuted midshaft fracture that had been splinted with four longitudinal wooden boards, each wrapped in linen bandages. A dressing pad containing blood pigment was also found at approximately the level of the fracture site. The victim is judged to have died shortly after injury, as the bones show no evidence whatsoever of any healing reaction (Fig. 1-1). The second specimen was of open fractures of a forearm, treated by similar splints, but in this case a pad of blood-stained vegetable fiber (probably obtained from the date palm) was found adherent to the upper fragment of the ulna, evidently having been pushed into the wound to stanch bleeding. Again, death appears to have occurred before any bone healing reaction had started. The Egyptians were known to be skilled at the management of fractures, and many healed specimens have been found. The majority of femoral fractures had united with shortening and deformity, but a number of well-healed forearm fractures have been discovered.

Some form of wooden splintage bandaged to the injured limb has been used from antiquity to the present day. Certainly, both Hippocrates and Celsus described in detail the splintage of fractures using wooden appliances,[54] but a fascinating account of external splintage of fractures is to be found in the work of El Zahrawi (AD 936–1013). This Arab surgeon, born in Al Zahra, the royal city 5 miles west of Cordova in Spain, was named Abu'l-Quasim Khalas Ibn'Abbas Al-Zahrawi, commonly shortened to Albucasis. In his 30th treatise, "The Surgery," he described in detail the application of two layers of bandages, starting at the fracture site and extending both up and down the limb, after reduction of the fracture. He continued:

Then put between the bandages enough soft tow or soft rags to correct the curves of the fracture, if any, otherwise put nothing in. Then wind over it another bandage and at once lay over it strong splints if the part be not swollen or effused. But if there be swelling or effusion in the part, apply something to allay the swelling and disperse the effusion. Leave it on for several days and then bind on the splint. The splint should be made of broad halves of cane cut and shaped with skill, or the splints may be made of wood used for sieves, which are made of pine, or of palm branches, or of brier or giant fennel or the like, whatever wood be at hand. Then bind over the splints another bandage just as tightly as you did the first. Then over that tie it up with cords arranged in the way we have said, that is with the pressure greatest over the site of the fracture and lessened as you move away from it. Between the splints there should be a space of not less than a finger's breadth.

It is of interest that the brother of the celebrated French surgeon Bérenger Féraud, an interpreter with the French army in Algeria, wrote in 1868 that all Arab bonesetters (*tebibs* [a tebib is an Arab medicine man, whence the modern French slang word *toubib,* meaning quack or doctor]) carried with them "sticks of *kelar,* a sort of fennel, well dried and of extreme lightness, which are used as splints." Albucasis then went on to describe various forms of plaster that may be used as an alternative, particularly for women and children, recommending "mill dust, that is the fine flour that sticks to the walls of a mill as the grindstone moves. Pound it as it is, without sieving, with egg white to a medium consistency, then use." He suggested as an alternative plaster a mixture of various gums, including gum mastic, acacia, and the root of *mughath (Glossostemon bruguieri),* pounded fine with clay of Armenia or Asia Minor and mixed with water of tamarisk or with egg white.[76]

In 1517, Gersdorf[25] beautifully illustrated a novel method of binding wooden splints, using ligatures around the assembled splint that are tightened by twisting them with cannulated wooden toggles, with a wire then passed down the hollow centers of the toggles to prevent them from untwisting (Fig. 1-2). In this book, he also illustrated the use of an extension apparatus for overcoming overriding of the fractures of the bones, although similar machines had been in use for centuries according to the descriptions of Galen, Celsus, and Paulus Aegineta.[54]

Gersdorf's technique of tightening a circumferential splint ligature was plagiarized by Benjamin Gooch,[26] who in 1767 described what must be regarded as the first functional brace (Fig. 1-3), designed as it was to return the worker to labor before the fracture had consolidated. Gooch fashioned shape splints for various anatomic sites; these consisted of longitudinal strips of wood stuck to an underlying sheet of leather that could then be wrapped around the limb and held in place with ligatures and cannulated toggles. I recollect Gooch splintage still being used for temporary immobilization of injured limbs by ambulance crews as late as the 1960s. Gooch's are perhaps the most sophisticated wooden splints ever devised.

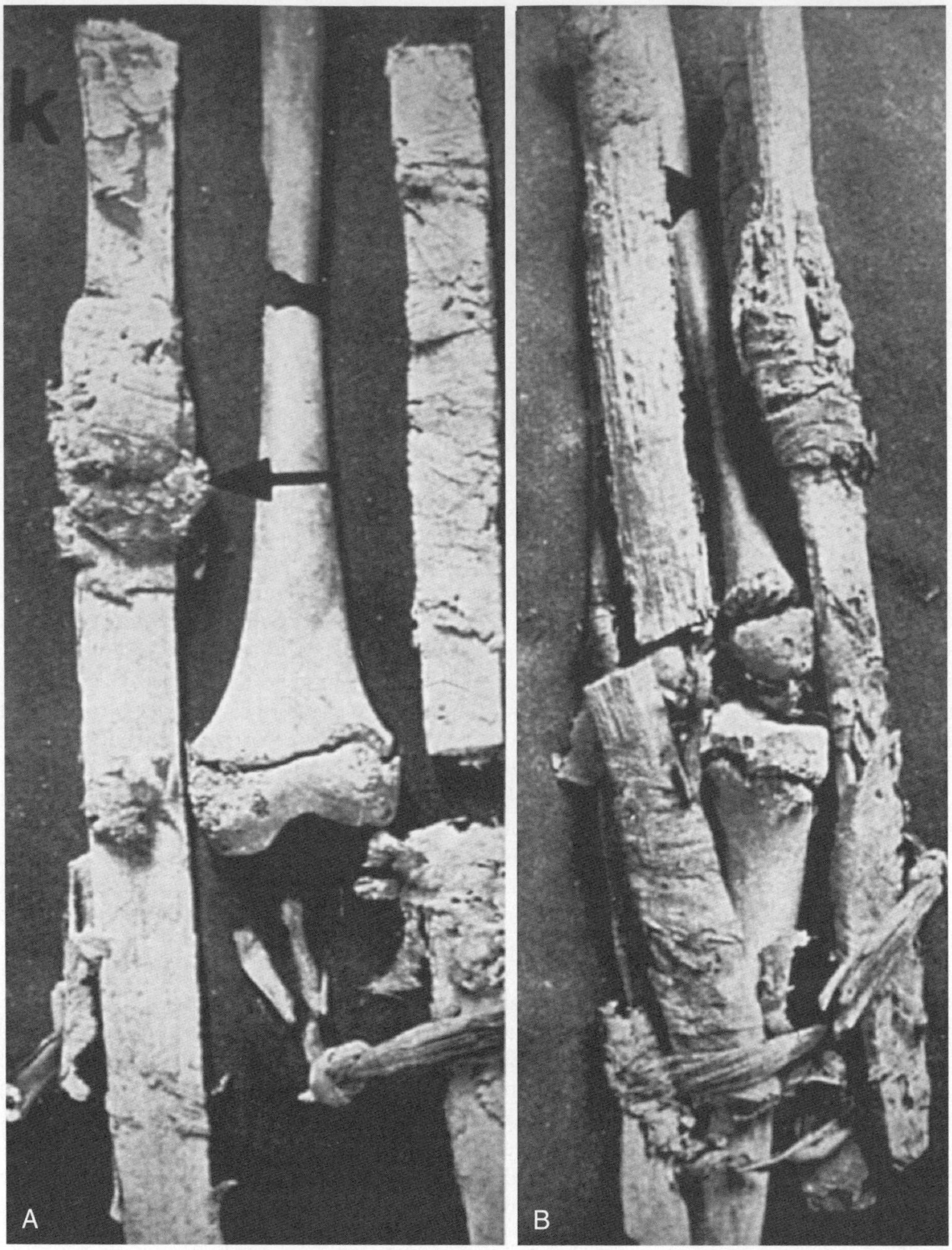

Figure 1-1. **A** and **B,** Specimen of a fracture of an adolescent femur from circa 300 BC, excavated at Naga-ed-Der in 1903. This injury was an open fracture, and the absence of any callus (*arrow* in **A**) indicates early death.

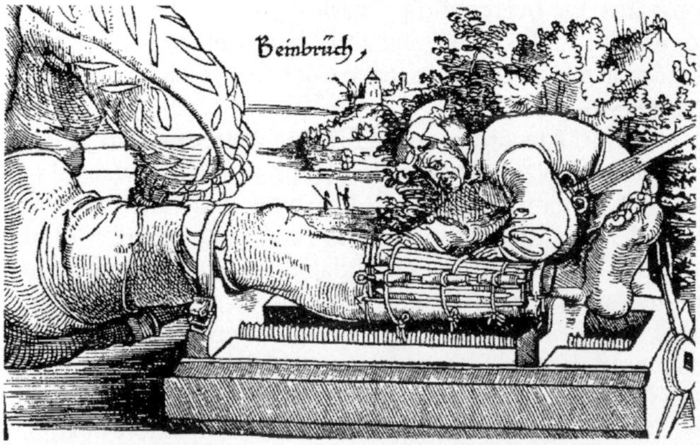

Figure 1-2. Illustration of wooden splintage from Gersdorf (1517). Note the cannulated toggles used to tighten the bindings.

The 19th century literature abounds with descriptions of many types of wooden fracture apparatus, none of which is as carefully constructed or apparently efficient as those of Gooch.

The use of willow board splints for the treatment of tibial shaft fractures and Colles' fractures in modern times has been described in great detail by Shang T'ien-Yu and colleagues[72] in a fascinating description of the integration of modern and traditional Chinese medicine in the treatment of fractures. Amerasinghe and Veerasingham continued to use shaped bamboo splints, held in place by circumferential rope ligatures, in the functional bracing of tibial fractures in Sri Lanka (Fig. 1-4).[1] They reported 88% of their patients to be weight bearing and freely mobile by 10 weeks, with a 95% union rate, and less than half an inch of shortening in 85% of patients. The Liston wooden board splint for fractures of the femoral

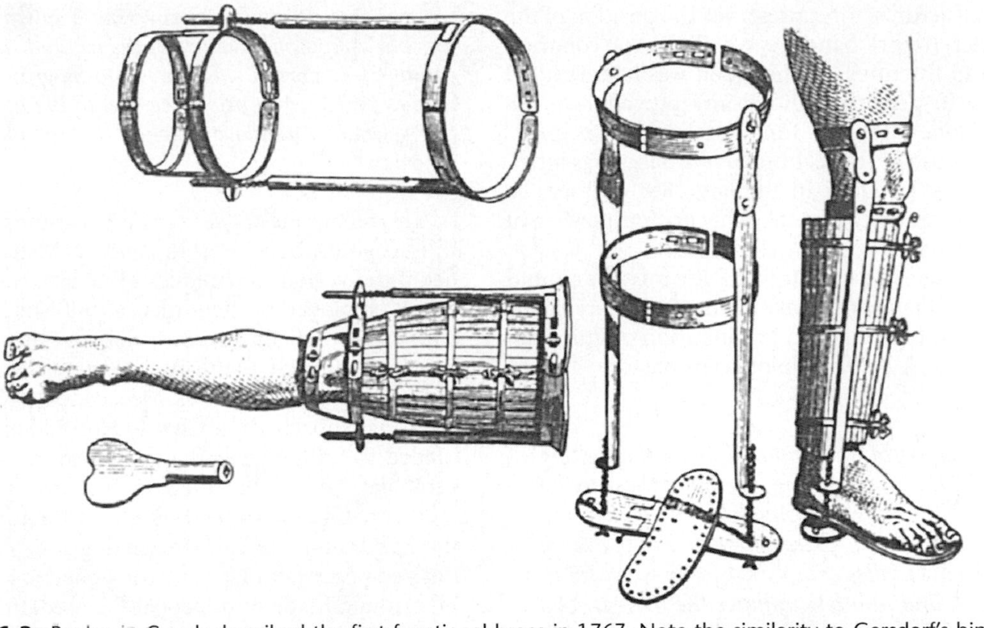

Figure 1-3. Benjamin Gooch described the first functional brace in 1767. Note the similarity to Gersdorf's bindings.

shaft is currently in use in one institution in Scotland for the management of this injury in children.

PRECURSORS OF THE PLASTER BANDAGE

As indicated previously, El Zahrawi, probably drawing from the work of Paulus Aegineta, described the use of both clay gum mixtures and flour and egg white for casting materials. In AD 860, the Arab physician Rhazes Athuriscus wrote, "But if thou make thine apparatus with lime and white of egg it will be much handsomer and still more useful. In fact it will become as hard as stone and will not need to be removed until the healing is complete."[3]

William Cheselden (1688–1752), the famous English surgeon and anatomist, as a schoolboy sustained an elbow fracture that was treated in this manner. In his book *Anatomy of the Human Body,* he recorded, "I thought of a much better bandage which I had learned from Mr. Cowper, a bonesetter at Leicester, who set and cured a fracture of my own cubit when I was a boy at school. His way was, after putting the limb in a proper posture, to wrap it up in rags dipped in the whites of eggs and a little wheat flour mixed. This drying grew stiff and kept the limb in good posture. And I think there is no way

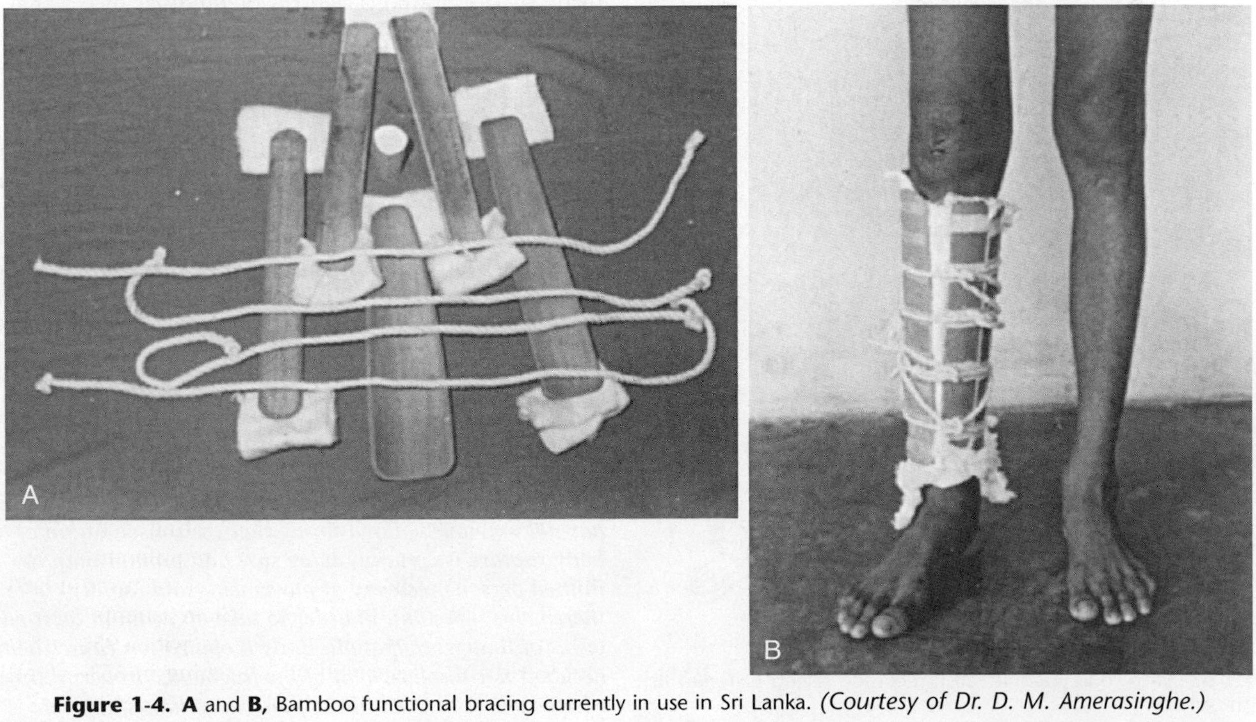

Figure 1-4. A and **B,** Bamboo functional bracing currently in use in Sri Lanka. *(Courtesy of Dr. D. M. Amerasinghe.)*

better than this in fractures, for it preserves the position of the limb without strict [tight] bandage which is the common cause of mischief in fractures."[55] Cheselden was later reputed to have been able to perform a lithotomy procedure in 68 seconds; it would appear that his functional result was excellent. A more precise use of the technique of Rhazes was introduced into France by Le Dran in the late 18th century; he stiffened his bandage with egg white, vinegar, and powder of Armenian clay or plaster.[80]

The technique of pouring a plaster-of-Paris mixture around an injured limb would appear to have been used in Arabia for many centuries and was brought to the attention of European practitioners by Eaton, a British diplomat in Bassora, Turkey. In 1798 he wrote:

I saw in the eastern parts of the Empire a method of setting bones practised, which appears to me worthy of the attention of surgeons in Europe. It is by inclosing [sic] the broken limb, after the bones are put in their places, in a case of plaster of Paris (or gypsum) which takes exactly the form of the limb without any pressure and in a few minutes the mass is solid and strong [Fig. 1-5]. This substance may be easily cut with a knife and removed and replaced with another. When the swelling subsides, [and] the cavity is too large for the limb, a hole or holes being left, liquid gypsum plaster may be poured in which will perfectly fill up the void and exactly fit the limb. A hole may be made at first by placing oiled cork or a bit of wood against any part where it is required and when the plaster is set it is to be removed. There is nothing in gypsum injurious if it be free from lime. It will soon become hard and light and the limb may be bathed with spirits which will penetrate through the covering. I saw a case of a most terrible compound fracture of the leg and thigh by the fall of a cannon. The person was seated on the ground and the plaster case extended from below the heel to the upper part of his thigh, where a bandage fastened into the plaster went round his body.[22]

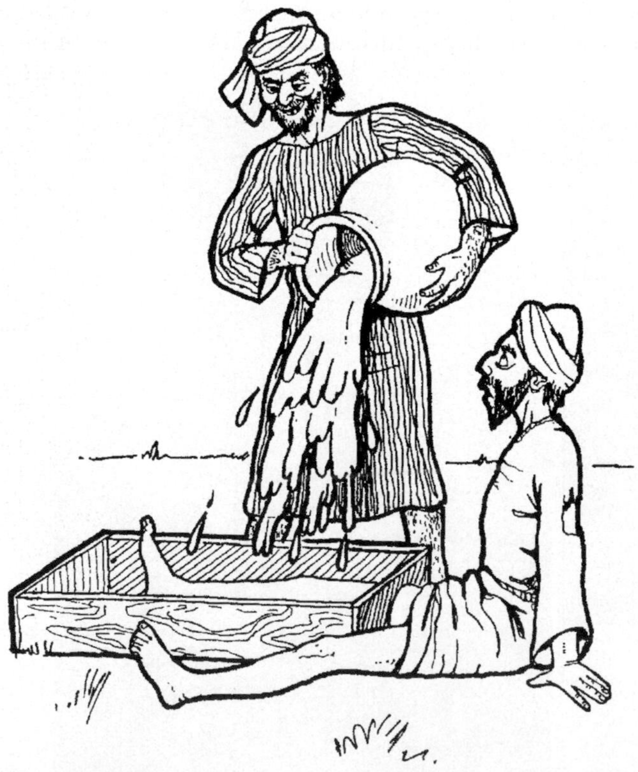

Figure 1-5. Plâtre coulé such as Eaton recorded seeing in Turkey in the 18th century.

This technique of *plâtre coulé* was enthusiastically embraced in Europe in the early 19th century. Malgaigne[52] recorded in detail the various techniques of its use, stating that he found it first employed by Hendriksz at the Nosocomium Chirurgicum of Groningen in 1814. Shortly afterward Hubenthal,[38] believing himself to be its inventor, described *plâtre coulé* in the *Nouveau Journal de Médecine.* In 1828, Keyl, working with Dieffenbach at the Charity Hospital in Berlin, finally succeeded in calling general attention to it. Although the Berlin surgeons applied the method only to fractures of the leg, Hubenthal had described its use in fractures of the forearm, the hand, and the clavicle, mixing the plaster powder with unsized paper (similar to blotting paper). He encased the limb in a trough made of pasteboard, closedat the top and bottom with toweling, and first poured in the mixture to encase only the posterior half of the limb. After this posterior cast was allowed to set, the edges were smoothed, notched, and then oiled so that a second anterior cast could be created by applying the paste to the front of the limb, thus ending up with two halves of a cast, which could be bandaged together, yet easily separated for wound inspection or to relieve any tension.[51] Malgaigne himself was not keen on *plâtre coulé* and after having problems with swelling within a rigid cast, albeit incomplete over the crest of the tibia, he abandoned the technique in favor of albuminated and starched bandages of the type recommended by Seutin—bandage amidonné.[71]

A great variety of other apparatuses have been devised over the centuries for the management of fractures, notably the copper limb cuirasse described by Heister[32] and what Malgaigne called "the great machine of La Faye." The latter was made of tin and consisted of longitudinal pieces that were hinged together so that it could be laid flat beneath the limb and then wrapped around. It was described as confining "at once the pelvis, thigh, leg and foot, hence it ensured complete immobility." Bonnet of Lyons went one stage further by producing an apparatus for the management of fractures of the femur that enveloped both legs, the pelvis, and the trunk up to the axillae.[10] The great disadvantage of all these extensive and heavy forms of immobilization of the limb was that the patient was largely confined to bed during the whole period of fracture healing. This disadvantage was particularly emphasized by Seutin,[55] who, in recommending his bandage amidonné, or starched bandage, wrote:

It has not yet been well understood that complete immobility of the body, whilst being recommended by authors as an adjunct to other curative methods, is truly but a last resort which one would be better to avoid than to prescribe. One has not previously dared to say that the consolidation of the bony rupture is certainly more sure and prompt than the injured person's recovery of movements and (ability) to forget thereby his affliction, in order to take up again at least part of his ordinary occupation. Early mobilization causes neither accident nor displacement of the fragments. In permitting the patient to distract himself and take himself out into the fresh air, instead of remaining nailed to his bed, it has the happiest influence on the formation and consolidation of callus.

Again we see the roots of the concept of functional bracing. Seutin showed a man with a light starched bandage on his leg, the limb suspended by a strap around his neck, and walking with crutches.

In the first half of the 19th century, battle lines were drawn between the European surgeons who prescribed total immobilization and those who followed Seutin's *déambulation* regimen, and much intellectual effort was wastefully expended in fruitless argument. Seutin's emphasis on the importance of joint motion was also appreciated by others. In 1875 Sir James Paget wrote, "With rest too long maintained the joint becomes stiff and weak, even though there be no morbid process in it; and this mischief is increased if the joint hath been too long bandaged." A little later, Lucas-Championnière[50] wrote:

The immobilisation of the members, which was dogma not open for discussion in the treatment of fractures and as well articular lesions, has been practised with such contentment by the authors of the immovable apparatuses, that we threw ourselves with abandon into all forms of immobilisation. It was forbidden even to discuss such immobilisation and to criticise it in the name of healthy physiology. When I attacked, at the Society of Surgery, this forced immobilisation, I was called by Verneuil an "ankylophobe" *and I remained practically alone in protesting against these practises, which are so contrary to the interests of the injured and the ill. … Absolute immobilisation is not a favourable condition for bony repair. … [A] certain quantity of movement, regulated movement, is the best condition for this process of repair.*

He then described animal experiments that confirm this view and went so far as to recommend massage of the injured limb to produce some degree of movement between the fragments. He was particularly vitriolic in his condemnation of prolonged immobilization of children and became the great champion of early and graduated controlled mobilization, not only to achieve union of the fracture but also to prevent edema, muscle atrophy, and joint stiffness, later to be christened *fracture disease.*

THE PLASTER BANDAGE AND ITS DERIVATIVES

The battle of minds between the mobilizers and the immobilizers was neither won nor lost but rather forgotten with the advent of the plaster-of-Paris bandage. In Holland in 1852, Antonius Mathijsen (1805–1878) published a new method for the application of plaster in fractures.[53] As a military surgeon, he had been seeking an immobilizing bandage that would permit the safe transport of patients with gunshot wounds to specialized treatment centers. He sought a bandage that could be used at once, would become hard in minutes, could be applied so as to give the surgeon access to the wound, was adaptable to the form of the extremity, would not be damaged by wound discharge or humidity, and was neither too heavy nor too expensive. His exact technique was described by van Assen and Meyerding[2] as follows:

He cut pieces of double folded unbleached cotton or linen to fit the part to be immobilized. Then the pieces were fixed and held in position by woollen thread or pins. The dry plaster which was spread between the layers remained two finger breadths within the edges of the cloth. The extremity was then placed on the bandage, which was moistened with water. Next the edges of the bandage were pulled over so that they overlapped one another and they were held by pins. When an opening in the bandage was necessary, a piece of cotton wool the size of the desired opening was placed between the compresses so that this area remained free of plaster. In cases in which it was found necessary to enlarge the cast, enlargement could be achieved by the application of cotton bandages, four inches wide, rubbed with plaster and moistened.

Mathijsen introduced his plaster bandage in 1876 at the Centennial Exhibition in Philadelphia at the invitation of his friend Dr. M. C. Gori. The use of plaster-of-Paris bandages for the formation of fracture casts became widespread after Mathijsen's death and replaced most other forms of splintage.

Although the fire of the intellectual contest between the mobilizers and the immobilizers was reduced to mere embers, it was not extinguished, and the early functional concepts of Gooch, Seutin, Paget, Lucas-Championnière, and many others continued for decades to be regarded by surgical orthodoxy as heretical. In Britain, the great advocate of rest—enforced, prolonged, and uninterrupted—in the management of skeletal disorders, both traumatic and nontraumatic, was Hugh Owen Thomas (Fig. 1-6), who came from a long line of unqualified bonesetters residing in the Isle of Anglesey. Hugh Thomas's father, Evan Thomas, left his home and agricultural background to work in a foundry in Liverpool. His native skills as a bonesetter rapidly became legendary, and he opened consulting rooms in Liverpool, developing an extensive practice. His eldest son, Hugh Owen, broke with family tradition and qualified in medicine in 1857. His attempt at a partnership with his father failed, and he set himself up as a general practitioner in the slums of Liverpool, where he worked for 32 years, reputedly taking only 6 days of vacation. He died in 1891 at the age of 57.[77]

There cannot be an orthopaedic surgeon in the world who is not familiar with the Thomas splint, still in current use in many centers throughout the world in the management of fractures of the femur, although it was originally designed to assist in the management of tuberculous disease of the knee joint (Fig. 1-7). As discussed later, the use of this splint in World War I saved many lives. Not the least of the contributions of this industrious, single-minded, chain-smoking eccentric was to fire his nephew with enthusiasm for orthopaedic surgery. Robert Jones, later to be knighted, practiced with his uncle Hugh for many years in Liverpool before becoming one of the best known orthopaedic surgeons in the English-speaking world. Hugh Owen Thomas and Robert Jones were the two men to whom Watson Jones dedicated his classical work *Fractures and Joint Injuries,* writing of them, "They whose work cannot die, whose influence lives after them, whose disciples perpetuate and multiply their gifts to humanity, are truly immortal." Watson Jones remained greatly influenced by Hugh Owen Thomas's belief in enforced, uninterrupted, and prolonged rest, and in the preface to the fourth edition of his book,[81] he described one of its chapters as

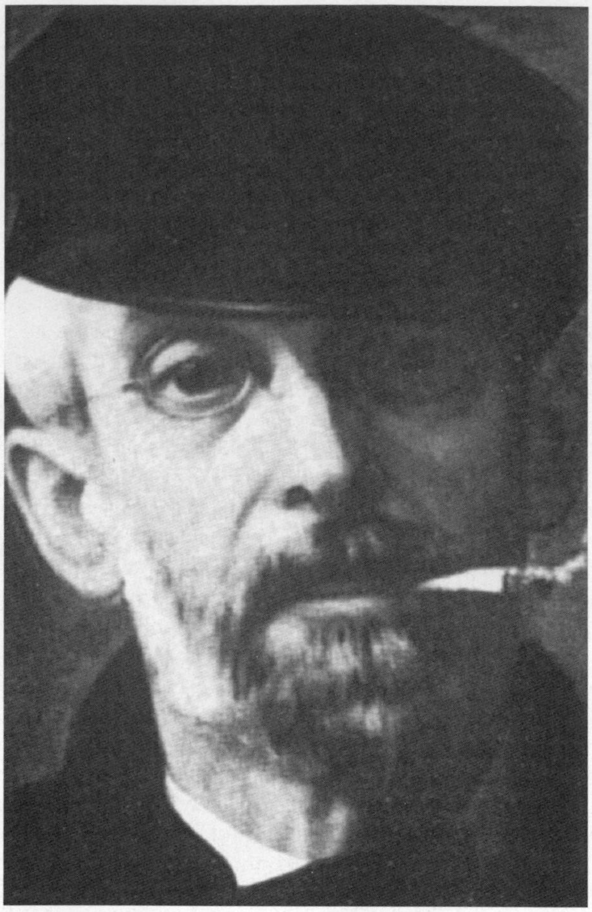

Figure 1-6. Hugh Owen Thomas (1834–1891), the father of British orthopaedics. *(Courtesy of Prof. L. Klenerman, Department of Orthopaedic Surgery, University of Liverpool.)*

... a vigorous attack upon the almost universally accepted belief that contact compression, lag screws, slotted plates, compression clamps, and early weight bearing promote the union of fractures. I do not accept a word of it. Forcible compression of bone is pathological rather than physiological and it avails in the treatment of fractures only insofar as it promotes immobility and protects from shear. In believing this and denying the view that is held so widely, I reiterate the observations of Hugh Owen Thomas. Moreover, I believe that gaps between the fragments of a fractured bone are always filled if immobility is complete. ... I still believe firmly that, apart from interposition of muscle and periosteum, the sole important cause of nonunion is inadequate immobilization.

TRACTION

Although longitudinal traction of the limb to overcome the overriding of fracture fragments had been described as early as the writings of Galen (AD 130–200), in which he described his own extension apparatus, or *glossocomium* (Fig. 1-8), this traction was immediately discontinued once splintage had been applied. The use of continuous traction in the management of diaphyseal fractures seems to have appeared around the middle of the 19th century, although Guy de Chauliac (1300 to 1367) wrote in *Chirurgia Magna,* "After the application of splints, I attach to the foot a mass of lead as a weight, taking care to pass the cord which supports the weight over a small pulley in such a manner that it shall pull on the leg in a horizontal direction *(Ad pedum ligo pondus plumbi transeundo chordam super parvampolegeam; itaque tenebit tibiam in sua longitudinae).*"[27]

Whereas Sir Astley Cooper in his celebrated treatise on dislocations and fractures of the joints illustrated the method

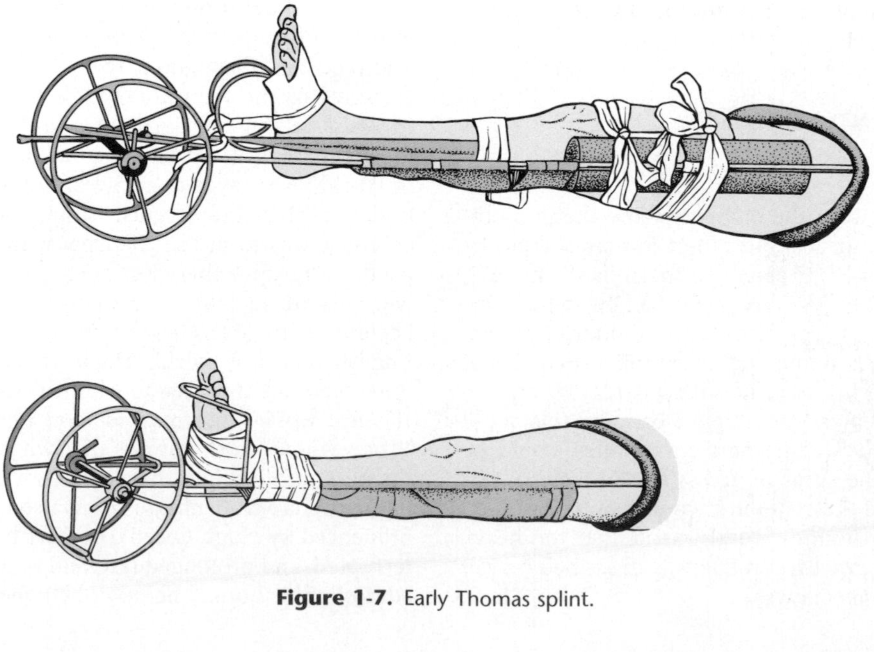

Figure 1-7. Early Thomas splint.

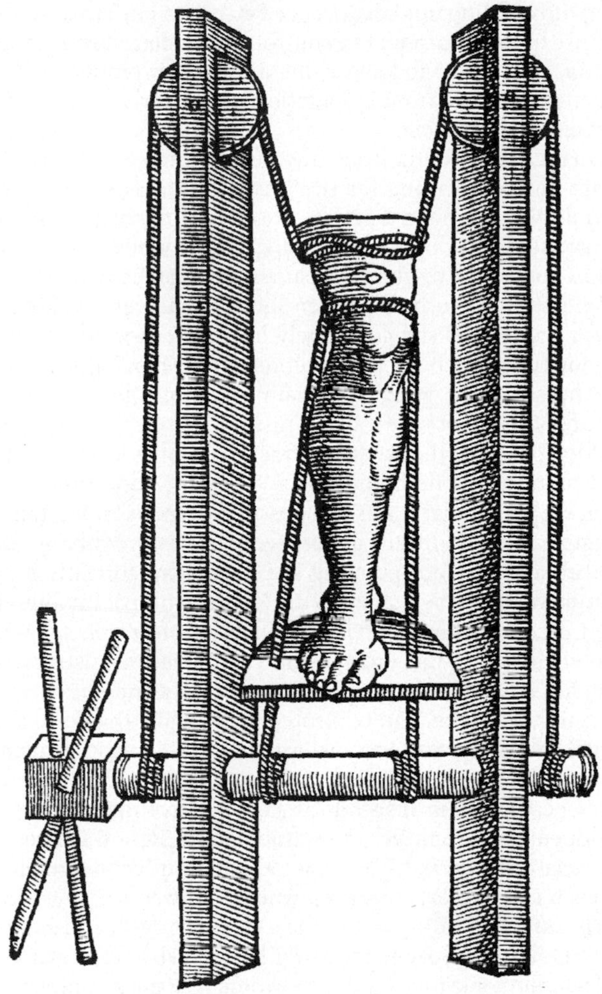

Figure 1-8. The glossocomium, here illustrated from the works of Ambroise Paré (1564).

of treating simple fractures of the femur on a double inclined plane with a wooden splint strapped to the side of the thigh, there is no mention in his work of the use of traction.[17] On the other hand, in his book on fractures and dislocations published in 1890, Albert Hoffa of Wurzburg (where Roentgen discovered x-rays) liberally illustrated the use of traction for many types of fractures—not only of the femur in adults and children but also of the humerus.[35] Straight arm traction for supracondylar and intercondylar fractures of the distal humerus recently so in vogue was clearly described and illustrated by Helferich in 1906 (Fig. 1-9).[33]

Certainly one of the earliest accounts of the use of continuous skin traction in the management of fractures must be that of Dr. Josiah Crosby of New Hampshire. He described the application of "two strips of fresh spread English adhesive plaster, one on either side of the leg, wide enough to cover at least half of the diameter of the limb from above the knee to the malleolar processes." Over these he laid a firm spiral bandage before applying weight to the lower ends of the adhesive straps. He recorded the use of this method in a fracture of the femur, an open fracture of the tibia, and, surprisingly, two cases of fracture of the clavicle in 2-year-old children. The technique of Dr. Crosby was illustrated in detail by Hamilton in his treatise on military surgery.[29] Billroth, describing his experiences between 1869 and 1870, gave the alternatives of plaster-of-Paris bandages or extension in the management of fractures of the shaft of the femur. He stated, "On the whole, I far prefer extension by means of ordinary strapping. This I apply generally on Volkmann's plan."[7] It is interesting to note that in the early descriptions of traction for the management of fractures of the femoral shaft, when no other form of splintage was used, union was usually said to have been consolidated by 5 or 6 weeks, in comparison with the 10 to 14 weeks that later came to be regarded as the average time to femoral shaft union using traction in association with external splintage.

The rapid consolidation of femoral shaft fractures was, of course, stressed by Professor George Perkins of London in the 1940s and 1950s, when he abandoned external splintage and advocated straight simple traction through an upper tibial pin and immediate mobilization of the knee, using a split bed (so-called Pyrford traction). This was in some ways a development and simplification of the traction principles outlined by R. H. Russell (who also remarked on rapid consolidation with early movement), describing his mobile traction in 1924.[67] In the same year, Dowden, speaking mainly of upper limb fractures, wrote, "The principle of early active movement in the treatment of practically all injuries and in most inflammations will assuredly be adopted before long."[21] Perkins, like Dowden and the many others before, was a great advocate of movement, both active and passive, of all the joints of the involved limb as being more important than precise skeletal form.

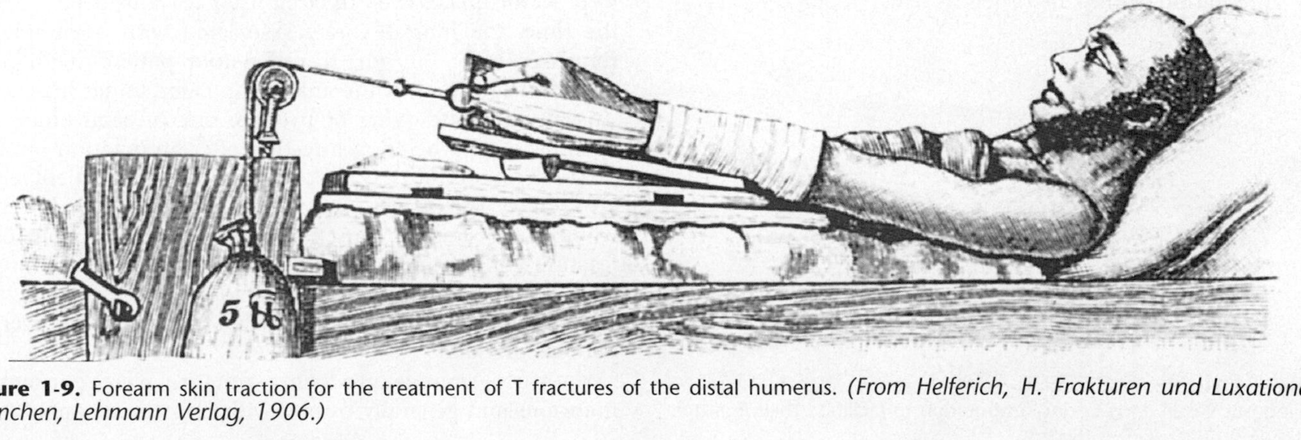

Figure 1-9. Forearm skin traction for the treatment of T fractures of the distal humerus. *(From Helferich, H. Frakturen und Luxationen. München, Lehmann Verlag, 1906.)*

FUNCTIONAL BRACING

Given that Gooch's description in 1767 of the first tibial and femoral functional braces was to remain obscure for more than two centuries, it is surprising that after the intense discussion of the technical minutiae and principles of splintage in the 19th century, there was no real modification of the "standard" plaster-of-Paris cast until the work of Sarmiento,[69] published 200 years after that of Gooch. Following experience with patellar tendon-bearing below-knee limb prostheses, Sarmiento developed a patellar tendon-bearing cast for the treatment of fractures of the tibia, applied after initial standard cast treatment had been used to permit the acute swelling to settle. This heralded the renaissance of functional bracing, and in 1970 Mooney and colleagues[56] described hinged casts for the lower limb in the management of femoral fractures treated initially with some 6 weeks of traction.

Since the mid-1970s, the development of a variety of casting materials and the use of thermoplastics in brace construction have extended the ideas of these pioneers of the 1960s and 1970s to the point where functional bracing, certainly for shaft fractures of the tibia and certain lower femoral fractures, is accepted without question as the natural sequel to early management by plaster casting or traction. The widespread use of functional bracing has liberated countless patients from prolonged hospitalization and permitted early return to function and to gainful employment.

OPEN FRACTURES

Until about 150 years ago, an open fracture was virtually synonymous with death and generally necessitated immediate amputation. Amputation itself carried with it a very high mortality rate, usually with death resulting from hemorrhage or sepsis. Until the 16th century, the traditional method of attempting to control the hemorrhage after amputation was cauterization of the wound, either with hot irons or by the application of boiling pitch. This in itself may well have caused tissue necrosis and encouraged infection and secondary hemorrhage. The famous French surgeon Ambroise Paré (1510 to 1590), who served as surgeon to the Court of Henry II and Catherine de Medici and is rightfully regarded as the father of military surgery, was in 1564 the first to describe the ligation of the bleeding vessels after amputation. He developed an instrument that he called the "crow's beak" *(bec de corbin)* for securing the vessels and pulling them out of the cut surface of the amputation stump in order to ligate them (Fig. 1-10).

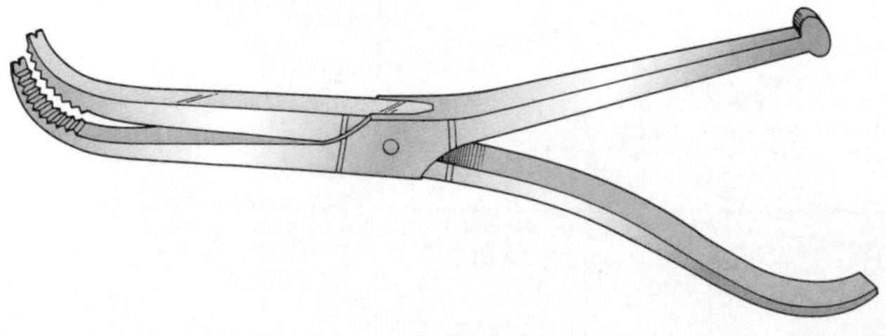

Figure 1-10. Bec de corbin—crow's beak—devised by Paré for pulling out vessel ends during amputation to facilitate their ligature.

Notwithstanding this advance, Le Petit, who in 1718 described the use of the tourniquet to control hemorrhageduring amputation,[61] is reputed to have claimed that his invention reduced the mortality rate from amputation of the lower limb from 75 percent to 25 percent.

In the history of the open fracture, Ambroise Paré[58] features again in documenting for the first time the conservation of a limb after an open fracture. He in fact described his own injury, sustained on May 4, 1561, when, while crossing the Seine on a ferry to attend a patient in another part of Paris, his horse, startled by a sudden lurch of the vessel, gave him "such a kick that she completely broke the two bones of the leg four fingers above the junction of the foot." Fearing that the horse would kick him again and not appreciating the nature of the injury, he took an instinctive step backward "but sudden falling to the earth, the fractured bones leapt outwards and ruptured the flesh, the stocking and the boot, from which I felt such pain that it was not possible for man (at least in my judgment) to endure any greater without death. My bones thus broken and my foot pointing the other way, I greatly feared that it would be necessary to cut my leg to save my life." He then described how, with a combination of prayer, splintage, and dressing of the open wound with various astringents, coupled with the regular use of soap suppositories, he survived the initial infection and by September, "finally thanks to God, I was entirely healed without limping in any way," returning to his work that month (Fig. 1-11).

Nevertheless, in insisting on conservative management of his open fracture rather than amputation, Paré was flying in the face of orthodox surgical practice, as indeed was the English surgeon Percival Pott, who in 1756 was thrown from his horse while riding in Kent Street, Southwark, and suffered a compound fracture of the lower leg. Aware of the dangers of mishandling such an injury, he would not permit himself to be moved until he had summoned his own chairmen from Westminster to bring their poles, and it is said that while lying in the January cold awaiting them, he bargained for the purchase of a door, to which his servants subsequently nailed their poles and thereby carried him on a litter to Watling Street near St. Paul's cathedral. There he was attended by an Edward Nourse, a prominent contemporary surgeon, who expressed the view that because of the gentle handling of the limb, no air had entered the wound and therefore there was a chance of preserving the leg, which otherwise was destined for amputation. Finally, success attended a long period of immobilization and convalescence.

As late as the 19th century, not all victims of open fracture were so fortunate. Even in circumstances considered ideal at the time, the mortality rate associated with open injuries remained high. Billroth[7] recorded four patients with compound dislocations of the ankle who came under his care in Zurich, with one dying of pyemia, one of septicemia, and a third of overwhelming infection after amputation for suppuration on the 36th day after injury. The fourth patient recovered. Of 93 patients with compound fractures of the lower leg whom he treated in Zurich, 46 died. Recovery from open fracture of the femur was, in Billroth's experience, so unusual that, describing the case of a woman of 23 who recovered from such an injury, he stated, "The following case of recovery is perhaps unique."

Gunshot wounds producing fracture were particularly notorious and generally treated with immediate amputation,

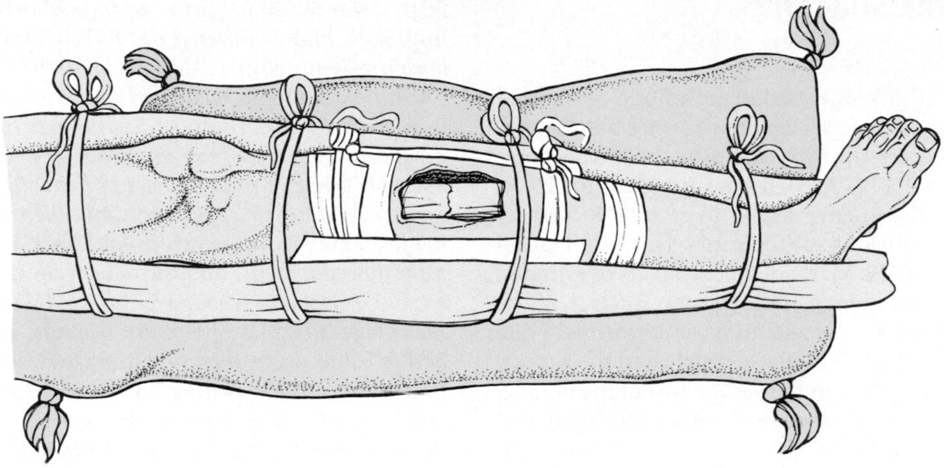

Figure 1-11. Illustration from Paré's surgical text of 1564 of his own open tibial fracture treated by splintage and open care of the wound. This is the first well-documented cure of an open limb fracture without amputation.

certainly until the early part of the 20th century. The results of this policy, however, were in certain instances quite horrifying. Wrench recorded that in the Franco-Prussian War (1870–1871), the death rate from open fracture was 41 percent, and open fractures of the knee joint carried a 77 percent mortality rate.[82] On the French side, of 13,172 amputees, some 10,006 died. On the other hand, in the American Civil War, the overall mortality rate for nearly 30,000 amputations was on the order of 26 percent, although for thigh amputations it reached 54 percent (Fig. 1-12). The difference in the mortality rates for different theaters of war around that time was probably related to the postoperative management, as very often the suppurating amputation stump was sponged daily with a solution from the same "pus bucket" used for all the patients. It has been said of that era that it was probably safer to have your leg blown off by a cannonball than amputated by a surgeon!

During World War I, gunshot wounds of the femur carried a very high mortality rate in the early years. In 1916 the death rate from gunshot wound of the femur was 80 percent in the British army. Thereafter it became policy to use the Thomas splint, with fixed traction applied via a clove hitch around the booted foot, before transportation to the hospital. Robert Jones reported in 1925 that this simple change of policy resulted in a reduction of the mortality rate to 20 percent by 1918. With progressive understanding of bacterial contamination and cross-infection after the pioneering work of Pasteur, Koch, Lister, and Semmelweis; the use of early splintage, as learned by the British forces in World War I; and the application of open-wound treatment following wound extension and excision as advocated first by Paré and later by Larrey (Napoleon's surgeon and inventor of the *ambulance*),[57,78] the scourge of the open fracture, even from a femoral gunshot wound, has been greatly reduced.

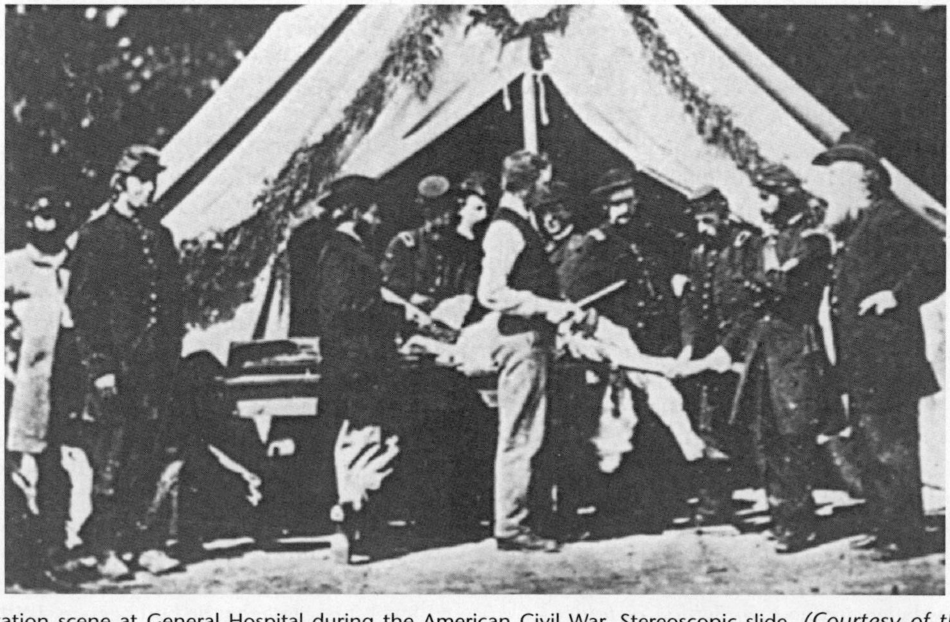

Figure 1-12. Amputation scene at General Hospital during the American Civil War. Stereoscopic slide. *(Courtesy of the Edward G. Miner Library, Rochester, New York.)*

EARLY FRACTURE SURGERY

Wire Fixation

It is generally believed that the earliest technique of internal fixation of fractures was that of ligature or wire suture and, according to Malgaigne, the first mention of the ligature dates back to the early 1770s. A. M. Icart, surgeon of the Hôtel Dieu at Castres, claimed to have seen it used with success by Lapujode and Sicre, surgeons of Toulouse. This observation came to light when, in 1775, M. Pujol accused Icart of bringing about the death of a young man with an open fracture of the humerus in whom Icart was alleged to have performed bone ligature using brass wire. In his defense, Icart cited the experience of the Toulouse surgeons in the earlier part of the decade, although denying that he himself had personally used this technique in the case in dispute.[39,63,64] In a scholarly discussion of Pujol versus Icart, Evans has called into question whether this type of operation was any more than the subject of surgical theory at that time,[24] but Icart's contention was widely accepted by so many French observers in the 19th century that it is highly probable that bone ligature was performed at least by Lapujode (if not Sicre) around 1770.

On July 31, 1827, Dr. Kearny Rodgers of New York is recorded as having performed bone suture.[31] He resected a pseudarthrosis of the humerus and, finding the bone ends to be most unstable, drilled a hole in each and passed a silver wire through to retain coaption of the bone fragments. The ends of the wire were drawn out through a cannula that remained in the wound. Although on the 16th day the cannula fell from the wound with the entire wire loop, the bones remained in their proper position and union was said to have occurred by 69 days after the operation. The patient was not allowed to leave his bed for 2 months after the operation!

In the introduction to his *Traité de l'Immobilisation Directe des Fragments Osseux dans les Fractures* (the first book ever published on internal fixation),[6] Bérenger Féraud recounted that, at the beginning of his medical career when he was an intern at the Hôtel Dieu Saint Esprit at Toulon in 1851, he was involved in the treatment of an unfortunate workman who had sustained a closed, comminuted fracture of the lower leg in falling down a staircase. Initial splintage was followed by a period of infection and suppuration, requiring several drainage procedures; eventually, after many long weeks, amputation was decided on. At the last moment, the poor patient begged to be spared the loss of his leg, so Dr. Long, Bérenger Féraud's chief, exposed the bone ends, freshened them, and held them together with three lead wire ligatures (cerclage) "as one would reunite the ends of a broken stick, and to our great astonishment then guided the patient to perfect cure without limp or shortening of the member, which for so long had appeared to be irrevocably lost." The patient survived, and the lead wires were removed 3 weeks later; the fracture united, and the workman left the hospital 105 days after his accident and resumed work 6 months after the operation. Bérenger Féraud went on to say:

> *I assisted at the operation and I bandaged with my own hands the injured for many long weeks. Can anyone understand how this extraordinary cure struck me? The strange means of producing and maintaining solid coaptation of the bony fragments by encircling them with a metallic ligature fascinated me as during my childhood I had heard tales of this technique being performed by Arab surgeons and, until then, had considered this to be a mere product of a barbaric empiricism. … In my childhood, in 1844 and 1845, I heard an old* tebib *renowned in the environs of Cherchell, in Algeria, for his erudition and his experience, recount to my father who, a surgeon impassioned with our art, avidly questioned native practitioners of French Africa, in order to sort out, from their experiences and their therapeutic means, the scientific principles, which had been passed down to them from their ancestors, amidst some of the ordinary practices of a more or less coarse empiricism. I tell you, I heard him say that in certain cases of gunshot wounds, or when a fracture had failed to unite, the ancient masters advised opening the fracture site with a cutting instrument, ligating the fragments one to another with lead or iron wire … and only to remove the wire once the fracture was consolidated.*

It therefore seems that there is some anecdotal evidence to suggest that such techniques had been used in the early part of the 19th century or even before. Bérenger Féraud himself cited the example of Lapujode and Sicre mentioned earlier. Commeiras[15] reported native Tahitian practitioners to be skilled in the open fixation of fractures using lengths of reed.

Screw Fixation

The use of screws in bone probably started around the late 1840s. Certainly in 1850, the French surgeons Cucuel and Rigaud described two cases in which screws were used in the management of fractures.[19] In the first case, a man of 64 sustained a depressed fracture of the superior part of his sternum, into which a screw was then inserted to permit traction to be applied to elevate the depressed sternal fragment into an improved position. In the second case, a distracted fracture of the olecranon, Rigaud inserted a screw into the ulna and into the displaced olecranon, reduced the fragments, and wired the two screws together *(vissage de rappel)*, thereafter leaving the arm entirely free of splintage and obtaining satisfactory union of the fracture. Rigaud also described a similar procedure for the patella. In his extraordinarily detailed and comprehensive treatise on direct immobilization of bony fragments, Bérenger Féraud made no mention of interfragmentary screw fixation, which was probably first practiced by Lambotte (see following section).

Plate Fixation

The first account of plate fixation of bone was probably the 1886 report by Hansmann of Hamburg entitled "A new method of fixation of the fragments of complicated fractures."[30] He illustrated a malleable plate, applied to the bone to span the fracture site, the end of the plate being bent through a right angle so as to project through the skin. The plate was then attached to each fragment by one or more special screws, which were constructed with long shanks that projected through the skin for ease of removal (Fig. 1-13). He recorded that the apparatus was removed approximately 4 to 8 weeks after insertion and described its use in 15 fresh fractures, 4 pseudarthroses, and 1 reconstruction of the humerus after removal of an enchondroma.

George Guthrie[28] discussed the current state of direct fixation of fractures in 1903 and quoted Estes as having described a nickel steel plate that he had been using to maintain coaption in compound fractures for many years. This plate, perforated

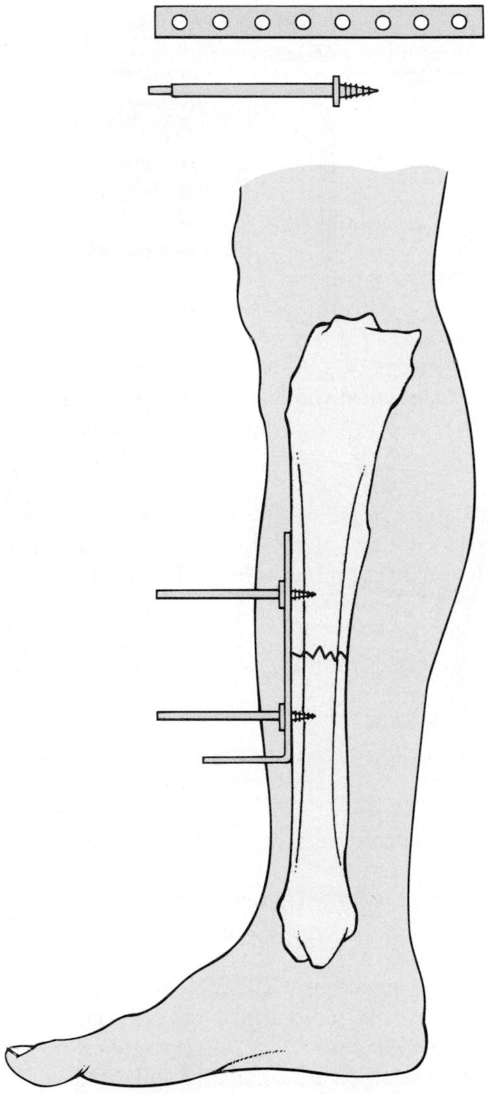

Figure 1-13. Redrawn from Hansmann's article of 1886, "A new method of fixation of the fragments of complicated fractures," the first publication on plate fixation of fractures. The bent end of the plate and the long screw shanks were left protruding through the skin to facilitate removal after union.

with six holes, was laid across the fracture, and holes were drilled into the bone to correspond to those of the plate. The plate was fixed to the bone by ivory pegs, which protruded from the wound. Removal was accomplished 3 or 4 weeks later by breaking off the pegs and withdrawing the plate through a small incision. Guthrie reported that in a recent letter Dr. Estes had said, "The little plate has given me great satisfaction and has been quite successful in St. Luke's Hospital." Guthrie also quoted Steinbach as reporting four cases of fractured tibia in which he had used a silver plate by this method and obtained good results. He removed the plate using local anesthesia. Silver was greatly favored at this time as an implant metal, as it was believed to possess antiseptic properties. Interestingly, in this article, Guthrie referred to the use of rubber gloves during surgery, seemingly antedating the reputed first use of gloves by Halstead.

The man who coined the term *osteosynthesis* was Albin Lambotte (1866 to 1955), although Bérenger Féraud referred to the restoration of bone continuity by ligature or bone suture as *synthèsisation.* It is believed, however, that by osteosynthesis Lambotte meant *stable* bone fixation rather than simply suture. Lambotte is generally regarded as the father of modern internal fixation, and in his foreword to a book commemorating the works of Lambotte, Dr. Elst briefly discussed the early attempts in the 19th century at surgical stabilization of bone and then continued, "Thus at the end of the last century, the idea was floating among surgeons. As always in the field of scientific progress, comes the right man in the right place, a genial mind who collects the items spread here and there, melts them into a solid block and forges the whole together. So did Albin Lambotte in Belgium, a pioneer of osteosynthesis."[23]

Lambotte (Fig. 1-14), the son of a professor of comparative anatomy, biology, and chemistry at the University of Brussels, was taught almost exclusively by his brother Elie, a brilliant young surgeon, who sadly died prematurely. Albin had worked under the direction of his brother at the Schaerbeek Hospital in the suburbs of Brussels and then in 1890 became assistant surgeon at the Stuyvenberg Hospital in Antwerp, rapidly progressing to become the head of the surgical department. From 1900, he tackled the surgical treatment of fractures with great enthusiasm and much innovation. He manufactured most of his early instruments and implants in

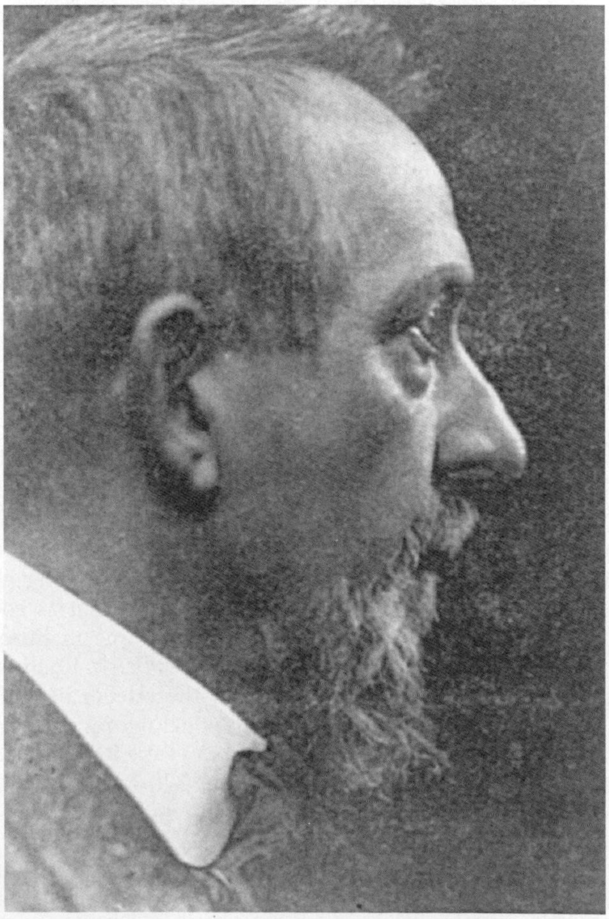

Figure 1-14. Albin Lambotte (1866–1955), the father of osteosynthesis. *(Courtesy of la Société Belge de Chirurgie Orthopédique et de Traumatologie.)*

his own workshop, developing not only plates and screws for rigid bone fixation in a variety of materials but also an external fixation device similar in principle to the ones in use today. He met with much intellectual opposition, but his excellent results were persuasive. In 1908, he reported 35 patients who had made a complete recovery after plate fixation of the femur. His classical book on the surgical treatment of fractures was published in 1913.[42] His legendary surgical skill was the product not only of a keen intellect but also of his extraordinary manual dexterity, which was also channeled into his great interest in music. He became a skilled violinist, but this was not enough for him, and he subsequently trained as a lute maker. He, in fact, made 182 violins and his name is listed in Vanne's *Dictionnaire Universel des Luthiers.* Elst related the following anecdote as an indication of Lambotte's manual skills:

One day Lambotte was in Paris staying at the Hôtel Louvois, at that time, and even nowadays, the Belgian headquarters in Paris. One morning he was on his way to the Avenue de l'Opéra, accompanied by a young colleague who was the one who told me the story. As he made his way through the old narrow streets, lined with windows and workshops belonging to every type of craftsman, Lambotte would enter one or two, admiring each one's dexterity and set of tools and discussing their methods like an expert. All of a sudden he stopped short, gazing with marvel at the instruments of a shoemaker. The idea of a new type of forceps had struck him. Suddenly inspired, he strode quickly towards the famous manufacturer of surgical instruments, the Collin factory, neighbouring the area that he was in. With great gestures and explanations, he tried to describe the instrument he desired. It seemed as if nobody could understand him, and not being able to endure it any longer he took off his jacket and rolled up his sleeves. Before a flabbergasted audience, he began to forge, file, hammer, strike, model and so finish off the piece of iron. They were all stunned with admiration and one of them came up to him and said "I have been here for forty two years sir, and never have I seen anybody work like you." Lambotte went away deeply moved, confiding in his companion "That is the highest prize I have ever received. It moves me as much as all the academic titles."

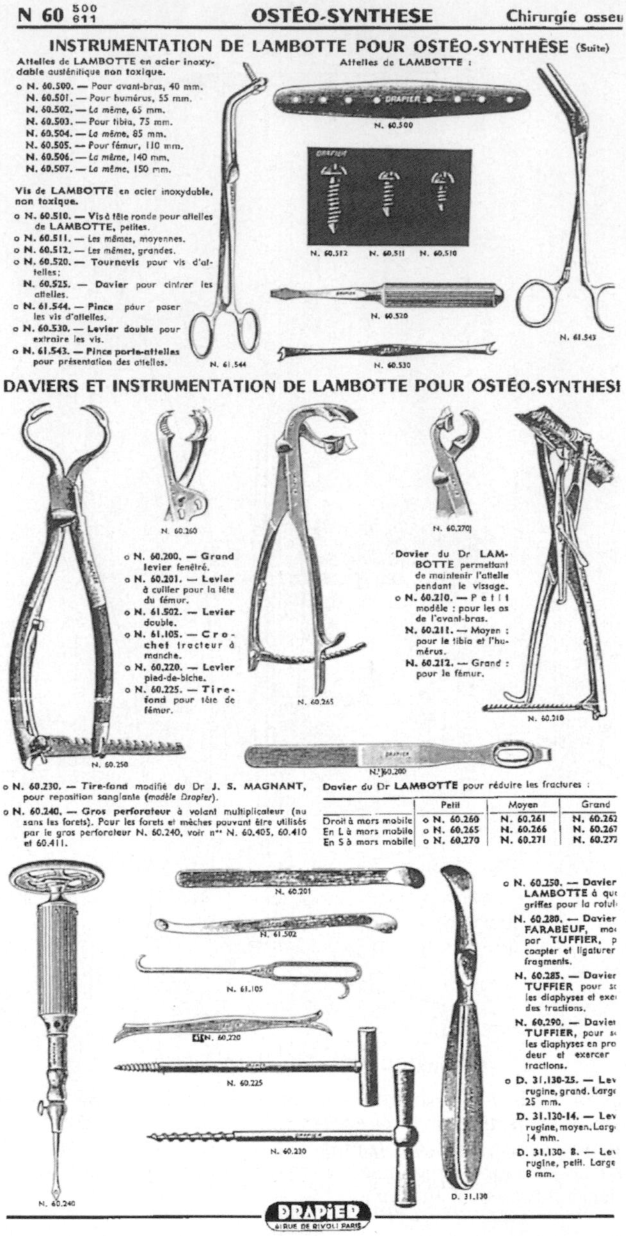

Figure 1-15. Instruments and implants designed by Lambotte featured in a surgical catalogue of Drapier (Paris) in the early 1950s.

As if these qualities were not enough, he is also recorded as being an extremely hard-working and kind man, noted for his devotion to his patients; a patron of the arts; and a great surgical teacher. Indeed, before World War I, the brothers Charles and William Mayo would take turns coming and spending several weeks in Antwerp. It is said that as soon as they disembarked, they devoted all their time in Europe to Lambotte and left only when their work in Rochester called them back. As an indication of the esteem in which he was held, among the many international figures attending his jubilee celebration in Antwerp in 1935 were René Leriche, Fred Albee, Ernest Hey Groves, and Vittorio Putti. The Lambotte instrumentarium remained in regular use until the 1950s (Fig. 1-15).

Contemporaneous with the work of Lambotte in Belgium was that of the other great pioneer of internal fixation, William Arbuthnot Lane (Fig. 1-16) of Guy's Hospital, London. The tradition in the late 19th century at this hospital was that fracture patients be admitted under the surgeon of the day and, after discharge, then be reviewed as outpatients by his assistant. Lane, working as the assistant to Clement Lucas, was most unhappy with the results of fracture management. In his biography of Lane, Layton[46] recorded:

Before Lane's time, the criteria of a good result in a fracture were indefinite and vague. They were aesthetic rather than practical. Firm union went without saying, but when a false joint, a nonunion or a weak fibrous one resulted, it was rather the patient's fault than the surgeon's. Given a firm union, the rest was an aesthetic problem, affecting the reputation of the surgeon rather than the way in which the patient could use his limb. "Pay great attention to your fracture cases" was the tradition—"with them alone the grave does not cover your mistakes."

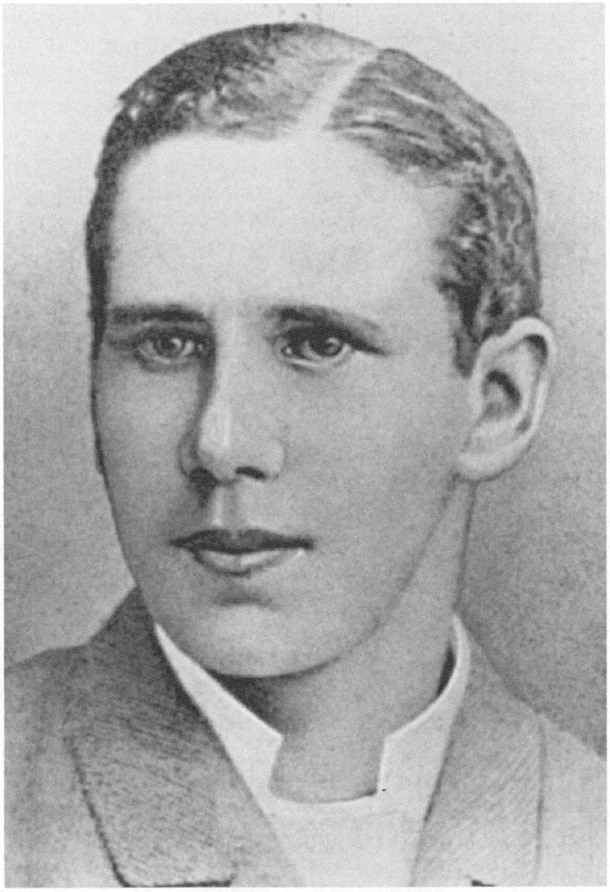

Figure 1-16. William Arbuthnot Lane (1856–1943), seen here shortly after qualifying at Guy's Hospital, London. *(From Layton, T.B. Sir William Arbuthnot Lane, Bt. Edinburgh, E. & S. Livingstone, 1956.)*

Lane had told Layton of a stevedore, who said:

Mr. Lucas thinks this is a good result. He says there is not much displacement and it looks all right. But I can't work with it. My job is carrying a sack of flour, weighing two hundredweight, up a plank from a barge to the wharfside and I can't do it. The foreman won't have me and I am still out of work.

Lane then went down to the docks and discovered that the stevedore had been telling the truth. Any slip from the plank from the barge to the wharf would have resulted in a fall onto the dock between the barge and the wharfside or between two barges. Lane observed that a man whose foot was in the slightest degree out of alignment could very easily fall. Lane thus became greatly impressed with the need for accuracy and maintenance of good reduction. Initially he started work with wires, and then in 1893 he is recorded as having used screws across a fracture site. Shortly afterward, he devised his first plate. Beginning in 1892, Lane made it his practice, whenever he could, to perform open reduction and fixation in all cases of simple fracture. This practice, however, met opposition from his chief, Mr. Lucas, and it was not until 1894, when Lucas was off work for 6 months after an attack of typhoid, that Lane had his chance to operate on a large series of simple fractures.

Although his attempts at internal fixation of compound fractures were almost universally a failure, Layton recorded that not one case of internal fixation of a simple fracture became infected during this period. During these 6 months of intensive internal fixation, Lane was using Lister's antiseptic techniques, and his dresser, Dr. Beddard, told that Lane and his associates wallowed in carbolic almost from dawn until dusk, with half of them passing black urine from the carbolic absorbed through their skins. At this time Lane insisted on his own variant of the antiseptic technique. Everyone wore long mackintoshes up to the neck, over which they applied gowns wet with carbolic or Lysol solution, and similarly the patients were draped with antiseptic towels introduced by Lane around 1889. The instruments were also soaked in Lysol, but by 1904 dry sterilization of the gowns and the instruments was Lane's routine.

Interestingly, Layton recorded the postmortem exploration of a fracture plated by Lane; the patient subsequently died of an unrelated septicemia. Layton said, "I cut down onto the bone and found this firmly joined without the throwing out of any callus around it. The plate was well in place, the screws all firmly fixed without a suspicion of any inflammation of the bone into which they had been put."[46] This surely must have been the first observation of healing without external callus formation in the presence of rigid fixation. In addition, Lane is credited with developing the nontouch technique of bone surgery and devised many instruments to enable him to hold implants without handling them directly. Of operative technique, Lane wrote:

I will now relate the several steps which are involved in an operation for simple fracture. I will do so in some detail as apart from manual dexterity and skill the whole secret of success in these operations depends on the most rigid asepsis. The very moderate degree of cleanliness that is adopted in operations generally will not suffice when a large quantity of metal is left in a wound. To guarantee success in the performance of these operations the surgeon must not touch the interior of the wound even with his gloved hand for gloves are frequently punctured, especially if it be necessary to use a moderate amount of force, and the introduction into the wound of fluid which may have been in contact with the skin for some time may render the wound septic. All swabs introduced into the wound should be held with long forceps and should not be handled in any way. The operator must not let any portion of an instrument which has been in contact with a cutaneous surface or even with his glove enter the wound. After an instrument has been used for any length of time or forcibly it should be resterilised.[45]

He then went on to describe the preparation of the skin with tincture of iodine and the use of skin toweling. By 1900 he had invented a huge variety of different-shaped plates for particular fracture problems, and in 1905 he wrote his classical work on the operative treatment of fractures, in which he illustrated both single and double plating and the use of intramedullary screw fixation for fractures of the neck of the femur.[44] In 1905 and 1906 Lambotte had also performed intramedullary screw fixation in four cases of femoral neck fracture, but this technique was not in fact new. In 1903 Guthrie quoted from Bryant's *Operative Surgery:*

Koenig operated in a case of recent fracture, making a small incision over the outer side of the trochanter major and drilled a hole through it with a metal drill in the direction of the head of the bone, applied extension to the limb to the extent necessary to overcome the deformity and then drove a long steel nail through the canal in the trochanter into the head of the bone and left it there. The limb was then immobilised and extended for 6 weeks. Good union and free motion of the joint were obtained. Cheyne, in a case of recent fracture, exposed the fragments through a longitudinal incision made over the anterior aspect of the joint, exposed the fracture, made extension and internal rotation of the limb, and with the fingers in the wound, manipulated the fragments into place. Then a small longitudinal incision was made over the outer side of the trochanter major and two canals drilled through the fragments at a distance of half an inch apart. Ivory pegs were then driven through the holes made by the drill and the limb immobilised. Good union and motion were obtained.[28]

It is understood that this procedure was in fact first suggested to Koenig by von Langenbeck, who is reputed to have treated fractures of the neck of the femur by drilling across them with a silvered drill and then leaving the drill bit in place.

Most of the screws used in plating procedures at this time were close derivatives of the traditional wood screw, with its tapered thread, although the later designs of both Lambotte and Lane were of screws with parallel threads, probably inspired by the classical publication of Sherman in 1926.[73] While stressing "the most scrupulous aseptic techniques" along the lines recommended by Lane, Sherman designed his own series of plates and also drew attention to the superior holding power of parallel threaded screws of a self-tapping, fine pitch design (Fig. 1-17). He pointed out that these had something like four times the holding power of a wood or carpenter's screw. He also introduced the use of corrosion-resistant vanadium steel. In addition, he emphasized particularly that the fixation should be firm enough to permit early functional rehabilitation. In describing his postoperative regimen for femoral fracture fixation, he recommended the following:

Immediately following the operation, the leg is placed in a Thomas' splint, flexed by the use of the Pierson attachment and then swung from a Balkan frame. Plaster is never used. The clips are removed on the fourth day and passive movements of the knee joint begun on the third or fourth day and continued daily. With immobilization of the fracture by transfixion screws, active and passive motion can be freely indulged in without any danger whatsoever of disturbing the position. ... Early mobilization is the most valuable adjunct in the postoperative treatment and should be instituted within the first few days. Great care should be taken not to permit weight bearing until the union is firm and callus hard.

Sherman reported a series of 78 cases of plating of the femoral shaft with only one death (caused by a pulmonary embolism 2 days after operation), no amputations, and no cases of nonunion; in only two patients was it necessary to remove the plates and screws because of infection, both nonetheless ending in an excellent functional result after treatment by immediate wound débridement and intermittent irrigation of the cavity with 0.5% sodium hypochlorite. He also cited the reported experience of Hitzrot, who had plated approximately

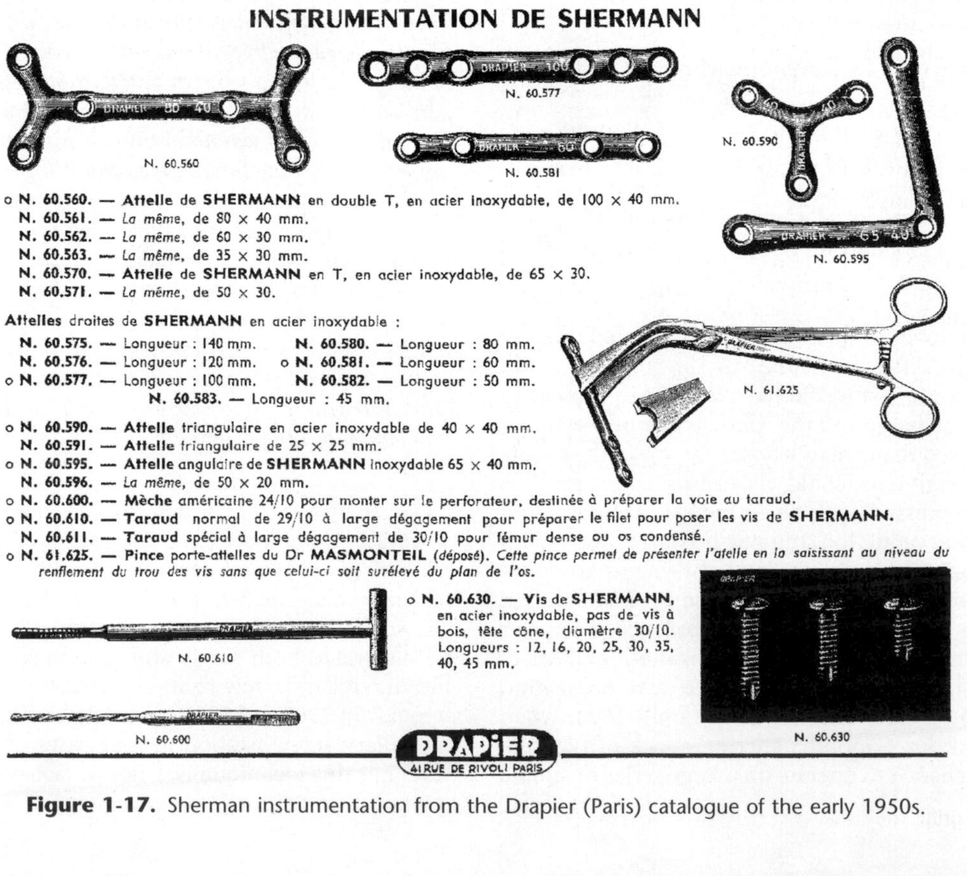

Figure 1-17. Sherman instrumentation from the Drapier (Paris) catalogue of the early 1950s.

100 cases of femoral fracture, with one death and only two infections; in the remainder there were no nonunions, no stiff knees, no plates needed to be removed, and "no appreciable changes in function or anatomy. . . ."[34]

Although now superseded by superior implant design, the Sherman plate is still in current use in hospitals throughout the world. In the 1930s and 1940s, a great variety of plate designs, some bizarre, were reported but with no great conceptual innovations. The so-called slotted plated splint of Egger, designed to hold the fracture fragments in alignment while allowing them to slide toward each other under the influence of weight bearing and muscle force, was neither new nor predictably successful: Lambotte had described, and later abandoned, a slotted plate as early as 1907. It was indeed the work of Danis in the 1940s that heralded the modern era of internal fixation, as will be discussed further on.

EXTERNAL FIXATION

Traditionally, the first external fixation device was the *pointe métallique* conceived by Malgaigne in 1840 and subsequently documented in 1843 in the *Journal de Chirurgie*.[5] This apparatus consisted of a hemicircular metal arc that could be strapped around the limb in such a manner that a finger screw, passing through a slot in the arc, could be positioned over any projecting fragment threatening the overlying skin, the screw then being tightened to press the fragment into a position of reduction. Although this apparatus and modifications of it, such as those of Roux, Ollier, and Valette, gained such a prominent place in contemporary surgery that the chapter on their use in the treatise of Bérenger Féraud occupies 126 pages, it is probably incorrect to regard it as an external fixation device in that it simply pressed one of the fragments into place but did not in itself result in any stability of the fracture.

Nevertheless, Malgaigne still retains the credit for the design of the first external fixator, for in 1843 he also described his *griffe métallique,* or metal claw, which consisted of two pairs of curved points, each pair attached to a metal plate, one plate sliding within grooves on the other and the two components being capable of approximation using a turnbuckle type of screw (Fig. 1-18). This device was designed for use on distracted fractures of the patella, and it was commonly perceived that Malgaigne proposed that the metal points were driven into the bony fragments of the patella in order to approximate them. This, in fact, is incorrect. Malgaigne's concept was that the metal points would engage in the aponeurotic substance of the quadriceps and patellar tendons and thereby obtain purchase in this tough tissue alongside the bone. This concept becomes evident from reading the discussion of Cucuel and Rigaud in which they say, "M. Malgaigne has recommended several years ago a pair of claws to maintain the fragments of the patella, but his claws were only supposed to press upon the fragments. I have gone further. I have driven the claws just inside the substance of the patella and have maintained the fragments, thus hooked, using two *vis de rappel*."[19] The *vis de rappel* was in fact the technique of inserting a screw into each fragment and then binding these screws together with twine as Rigaud described for the olecranon, as mentioned previously. Thus, the metal claw device of Malgaigne became a true external fixator. It is interesting to note in later publications[61] that this device was also used indirectly to approximate fragments of the patella by drawing together molded gutta percha splints (Fig. 1-19).

An ingenious modification of Malgaigne's metal claw was proposed in 1852 by Chassin[13] for use on displaced fractures of the clavicle. It consisted of two pairs of points of claws, smaller than but similar in design to the Malgaigne device, but also incorporating two finger screws that could, in addition, be advanced down on the fragments to correct anteroposterior displacements (Fig. 1-20). These additional pointed screws were admitted by Chassin to be inspired by the other device of Malgaigne, *la pointe métallique*. In describing this device in his treatise, Bérenger Féraud gave a glimpse of his vision of the future, saying, "Could one not say by varying the form of the claws, surgeons would be able to apply them to a great quantity of bones of the skeleton and I am persuaded that

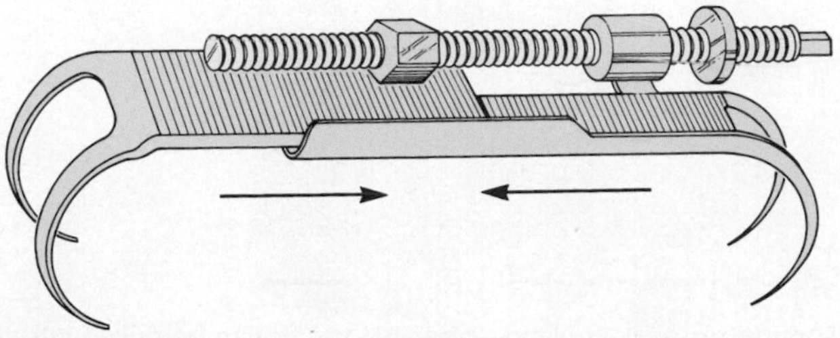

Figure 1-18. The griffe métallique, or claw, of Malgaigne (1843).

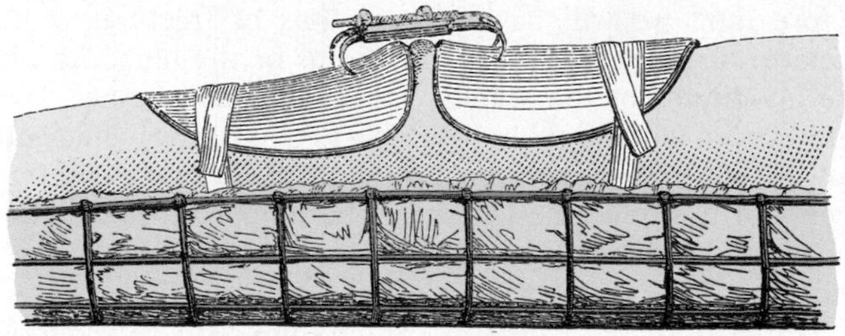

Figure 1-19. The Malgaigne claw device (1870), here used to control gutta percha splints for a fractured patella.

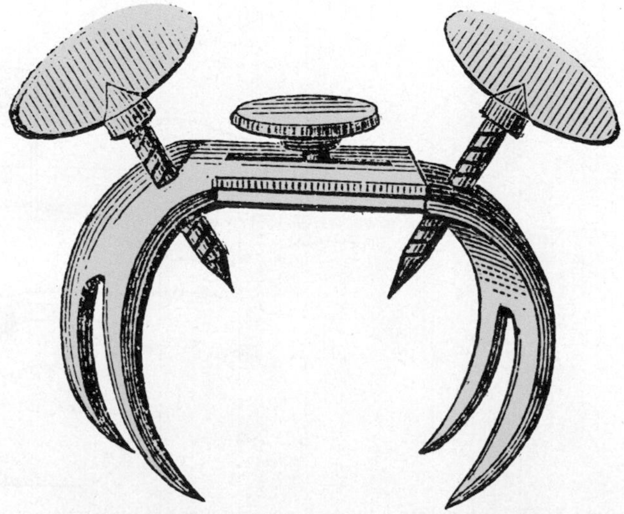

Figure 1-20. Chassin's clavicular fixator (1852).

before long we will have observations of fractures of the metacarpus, the metatarsus, the radius or the ulna, the ribs, the apophyses of the scapula treated in this manner. Who knows even if one would not be able to make claws sufficiently powerful, whilst remaining narrow enough, to maintain fragments of the tibia, the femur, or the humerus." Was he not indeed foreseeing the development in the 20th century of the widespread use of external fixation?

Hitherto, these devices had simply punctured the surface of the bone, and it was a British surgeon at the West London Hospital, Mr. Keetley,[40] who first described an external fixation device deliberately implanted into the full diameter of the bone. In 1801, Benjamin Bell wrote that "an effectual method of securing oblique fractures in the bones of the extremities and especially of the thigh bone, is perhaps one of the greatest desiderata of modern surgery. In all ages the difficulty of this has been confessedly great and frequent lameness produced by shortened limbs arising from this cause evidently shows that we are still deficient in our branch of practice."[4]

Inspired by these words, Keetley produced a device to hold the femur out to length in cases of oblique fracture. "A carefully purified pin of thickly plated steel, made to enter through a puncture in the skin, cleansed with equal care" was passed through drill holes, one in each main fragment, and then the two horizontal arms of each device, suitably notched along the edges, were united by twists of wire, the whole then being dressed with a wrapping of iodoform gauze (Fig. 1-21). This device obviously inspired Chalier, who described his *crampon extensible*, an apparatus very similar in principle but perhaps a little more sophisticated in design.[12] Something approaching the type of external fixation device with which we are today familiar was documented in 1897 by Dr. Clayton Parkhill of Denver, Colorado (Fig. 1-22). He recounted that, in 1894, he devised a new method of immobilization of bones, initially for the treatment of a young man with a pseudarthrosis of the humerus following a gunshot wound 11 months previously.[59] He described the device (Fig. 1-23) as

... a steel clamp made up of separable pieces in order to secure easy and accurate adjustment. It is heavily plated with silver in order to secure the antiseptic action of that metal. Clamps of different sizes are made to correspond with the bone upon which they are used; the largest sizes for the femur, the intermediate sizes for the humerus and tibia, the smallest sizes for radius, ulna, fibula and clavicle. The instrument consists essentially of four screws, or shafts. On these are cut threads at the lower end and also near the upper end. The extreme upper end, however, is made square so that the screw may be governed by a clock key. Two sets of wing plates are attached to these screws, a shorter pair corresponding to the inner screws and a longer pair to the outer. Each is attached to its screws by two nuts, one above the plate and the other below for accuracy of adjustment. When in position, one wing plate overlies the other in each half of the instrument. When ready to be clamped these plates lie side by side. They are fastened together by a steel clamp with a screw at either end.

In 1898, he recorded the use of his device in 14 cases, mainly of pseudarthrosis or malunion of the femur, humerus, forearm, and tibia, although there was one case of a refracture of a previously united patella treated by immediate application of the Parkhill clamp.[60] He claimed that union had been secured in every case in which the clamp had been employed, the clamp was easy to use and prevented motion between the fragments, the screws inserted into the bone stimulated the production of callus, no secondary operation was necessary, and after removal nothing was left in the tissues "that might reduce their vitality or lead to pain and infection."

It was only a few years later, across the Atlantic, on April 24, 1902, that Albin Lambotte first used his own external fixation device. This device was fairly primitive, consisting of pins screwed into the main fragments of a comminuted fracture of the femur, two above and two below, with the pins then clamped together by sandwiching them between two heavy metal plates bolted together. Subsequently, he devised a more sophisticated type of external fixator in which the protruding ends of the screws were bolted to adjustable clamps linked with a heavy external bar (Fig. 1-24). Lambotte recorded the use of his external fixator in many sites, including the clavicle and the first metacarpal.

Over the next few decades a number of devices were described, two of which were particularly notable for their ingenuity. In 1919, Crile[18] described a method of maintaining the reduction of femoral fragments that consisted of (1) a peg

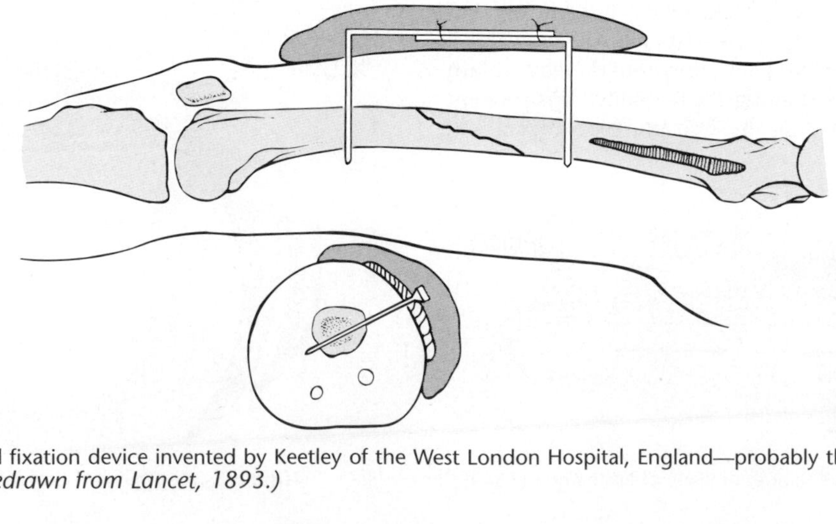

Figure 1-21. The external fixation device invented by Keetley of the West London Hospital, England—probably the first to be drilled into the substance of the bone. *(Redrawn from Lancet, 1893.)*

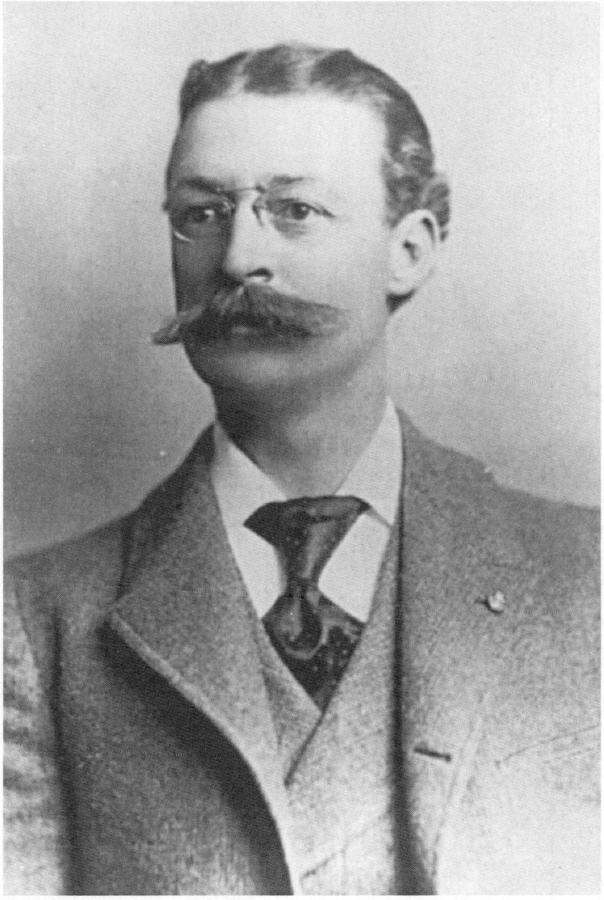

Figure 1-22. Dr. Clayton Parkhill of Denver, Colorado. *(Courtesy of Dr. Walter W. Jones and the Denver County Medical Society.)*

driven into the neck of the femur via the outer face of the greater trochanter, this peg bearing externally a metal sphere; (2) a metallic caliper bearing double points that were driven into the condyles of the distal femur that also bore a metal sphere to form part of a ball joint; and (3) an external linking device with a universal joint at each end capable of being clamped onto the metal spheres and also capable itself of extension via a lengthening screw (Fig. 1-25). He described its use in only one case, that of a gunshot wound of the femur sustained by a young soldier in 1918. This wound had been particularly contaminated and, using his device after a period of initial traction with a Thomas splint, Crile succeeded in gaining control of the soft tissue infection and securing early union of the fracture. The soldier was discharged to England 9 weeks after injury following removal of the apparatus. In 1931, Conn[16] described an articulated external linkage device that consisted of two Duralumin slotted plates linked in the center by a lockable ball-and-socket joint. Half pins were then driven into the bone fragments, two above the fracture and two below, with the pins then bolted to the slotted plates and the fracture adjusted at the universal joint before locking it with a steel bolt. He reported 20 cases with no delay in union and emphasized that the early motion of the joints of the limb, permitted by his device, had allowed prompt return to function. Conn also emphasized scrupulous pin tract care, recommending daily removal of dried serum and application of alcohol.

Hitherto, all external fixation devices had relied on half pins and a single external linkage device. The first fracture apparatus using transfixion pins with a bilateral frame was that of Pitkin and Blackfield.[62] In the 1930s and 1940s, Anderson of Seattle experimented with a great variety of external fixation configurations, enclosing the whole of the apparatus in plaster casts. He emphasized the benefits of early weight bearing and joint mobilization, but contrary to the advice of Conn, he recommended that wounds should not be dressed or disturbed "even though there is present some discharge and odour." His ideas were by no means universally accepted, and indeed in World War II, the advice given to American army surgeons working in the European theater was that "the use of Steinmann pins incorporated in plaster of Paris or the use of metallic external fixation splints leads to gross infection or ulceration in a high percentage of cases. This method of treatment is not to be employed in the Third Army."[14]

In Switzerland, Raoul Hoffmann of Geneva was developing his own system of external fixation, the early results of which he published in 1938.[36] Although many devices had been invented for external fixation and the literature abounded with reports of series of cases treated in this manner, it was not until the 1960s that, building on the groundwork of Hoffman, both Burny and Bourgois[11] and Vidal and co-workers[79] started to outline the biomechanical principles on which external fixation was based. This led the way to the universal acceptance of this method of fracture management. An interesting by-product of improved external fixation has been the opportunity for surgical lengthening of bones, although it has to be pointed out that this was first described in 1921 by Vittorio Putti, who used a transfixion device.[65]

INTRAMEDULLARY FIXATION

As previously discussed, pioneers such as von Langenbeck, Koenig, Cheyne, Lambotte, and Lane had all used intramedullary screw fixation in the management of fractures of the neck

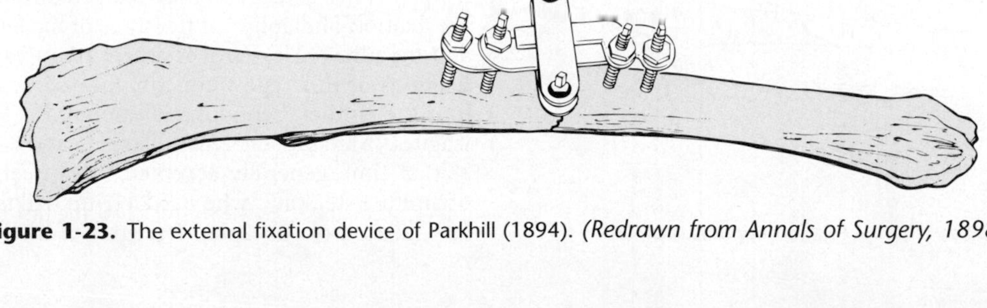

Figure 1-23. The external fixation device of Parkhill (1894). *(Redrawn from Annals of Surgery, 1898.)*

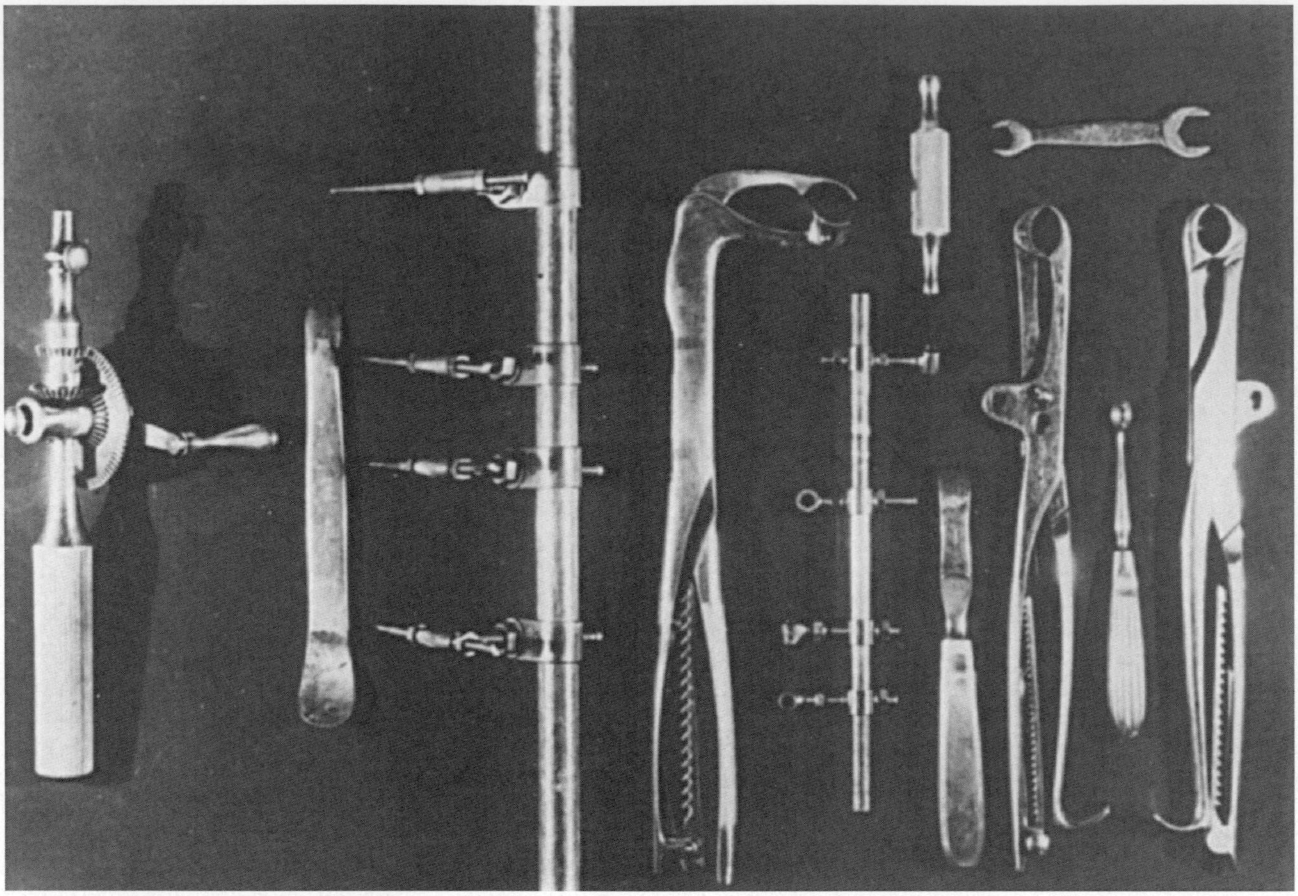

Figure 1-24. Some of the instruments of Lambotte in the collection of the University Hospital of Ghent, Belgium, including a Lambotte fixateur externé.

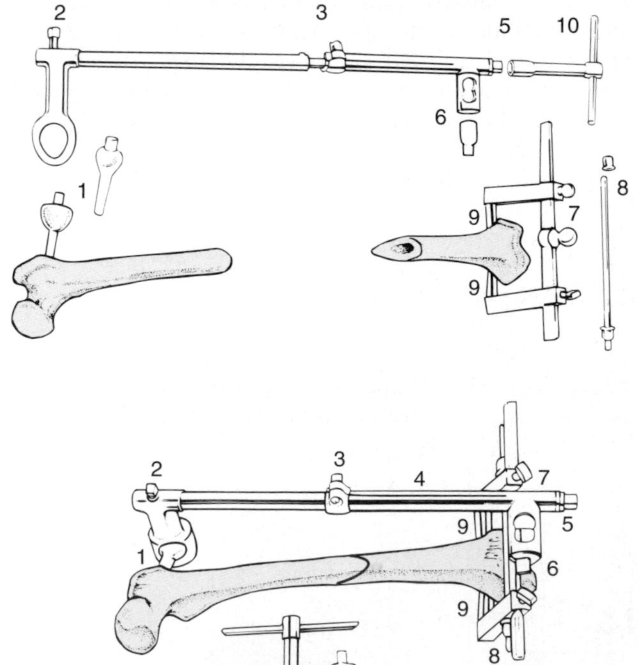

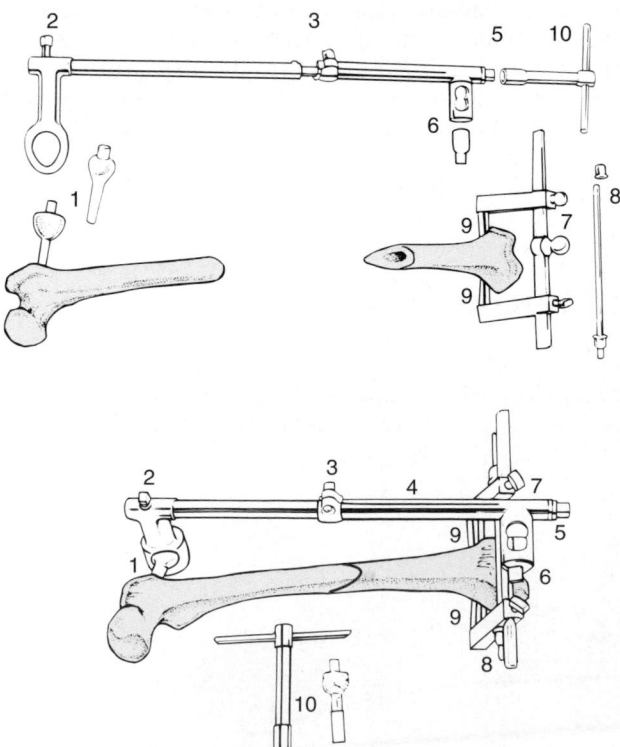

Figure 1-25. The external fixation apparatus of Crile.

of the femur. In addition, there are a number of reported instances of intramedullary devices in the neck of the femur being used for the management of nonunion, including the extensive operation of Gillette, who used the transtrochanteric approach to perform an intracapsular fixation of ununited femoral neck fractures using intramedullary bone pegs.[27] Curtis used a drill bit—as, reputedly, had Langenbeck—in the neck of the femur, and Charles Thompson used silver nails in 1899.[7] Lambotte also recorded the use of a long intramedullary screw in the management of a displaced fracture of the neck of the humerus in 1906.

In the late 19th century, attempts were made to secure fixation of fractures using intramedullary ivory pegs, and Bircher is credited with their first use in 1886.[8] Short intramedullary devices of beef bone and of human bone were also used by Hoglund.[37] Toward the end of the first decade of the century, Ernest Hey Groves, of Bristol, England, was using massive three- and four-flanged intramedullary nails for the fixation of diaphyseal fractures of the femur, the humerus, and the ulna.[66] Hey Groves's early attempts at intramedullary fixations of this type were complicated by infection, earning him the epithet "septic Ernie" among his West Country colleagues. Metallic intramedullary fixation of bone was not at that time generally accepted. In the late 1920s the work of Smith-Peterson,[75] who used a trifin nail for the intramedullary fixation of subcapital fractures of the femur, represented a great step forward in the management of what has since been referred to as the *unsolved fracture,* and that remained the standard management for this type of injury for some 40 years.

The use of stout wires and thin solid rods in the intramedullary cavities of long bones was recommended by Lambrinudi in 1940.[43] This technique was further developed in the United States by the brothers Rush,[68] who subsequently developed a system of flexible nails, still in occasional use.

The concept of a long metallic intramedullary device that gripped the endosteal surface of the bone—so-called elastic nailing—was the brainchild of Gerhardt Küntscher working in collaboration with Professor Fischer and the engineer Ernst Pohl at Kiel University in Germany in the 1930s. Küntscher originally used a V-shaped nail but then changed to a nail with a cloverleaf cross section for greater strength and designed to follow any guide pin more faithfully. Küntscher published his first book on intramedullary nailing at the end of World War II. Although it was written in 1942, the illustrations for it were destroyed in the air raids on Leipzig, so the book was not published until 1945.[41] For reasons that are not entirely clear, this outstanding German surgeon was virtually banished to Lapland from 1943 until the end of the European war. He was dispatched as head of the medical office at the German Military Surgical Hospital in Kemi, northern Finland. It is interesting to note that he departed Kemi in something of a hurry in September 1944 by air and left behind him a huge stock of intramedullary nails that became available for the Finnish surgeons to use.[48]

Küntscher was a brilliant technical surgeon, and his results, being so impressive, caused a somewhat overenthusiastic adoption of intramedullary nailing in Europe in the early years after World War II. According to Lindholm, this was reflected in the comments of the leading European trauma surgeon, Professor Lorenz Böhler of Vienna (Fig. 1-26). In 1944, Böhler[9] said:

Küntscher in his publication has briefly, thoroughly and with clarity described the techniques and indications for closed marrow nailing of fresh uncomplicated fractures of the thigh, lower leg and upper arm. He has also pointed out how to perform nailing of fresh, complicated, inveterate and nonhealed fractures. It has been an enormous surprise compared with our experiences to see a man with such a serious femoral fracture walk without a plaster cast or any bandage with reasonably moving joints only fourteen days after the accident.

A year later, he wrote in the preface to the next edition of his book,

Later experience has revealed that the risks with marrow nailing are much greater than first predicted. We therefore use it as a rule only in femoral fractures. ... Marrow nailing of other long bones which I have also recommended is shown by long term follow ups often to be more deleterious than profitable.

Britain appeared somewhat slow to adopt the teachings of Küntscher, possibly as a result of the influence of Hey Groves's early experiments with metallic intramedullary fixation. The January 3, 1948, issue of *Lancet* contained a somewhat flippant and puerile commentary by a "peripatetic correspondent" on the techniques of Küntscher, in which Lorenz Böhler, by that time advocating caution in relation to intramedullary nailing, was described as the "Moses of the Orthopaedic Sinai"! It is not surprising that the author chose to remain anonymous. In 1950, Le Vay, of London, published an interesting account of a visit to Küntscher's clinic, but in summing up his general impressions of Küntscher's technique, he wrote:

It was clear that Küntscher disliked extensive open bone operations or any disturbance of the periosteum and he stated

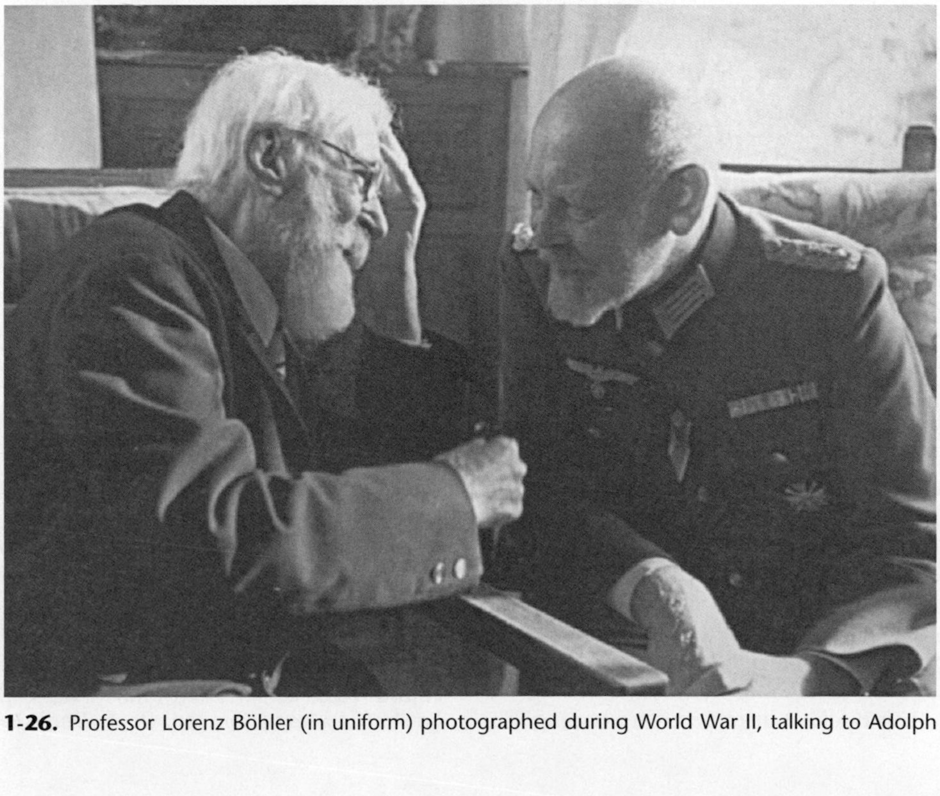

Figure 1-26. Professor Lorenz Böhler (in uniform) photographed during World War II, talking to Adolph Lorenz.

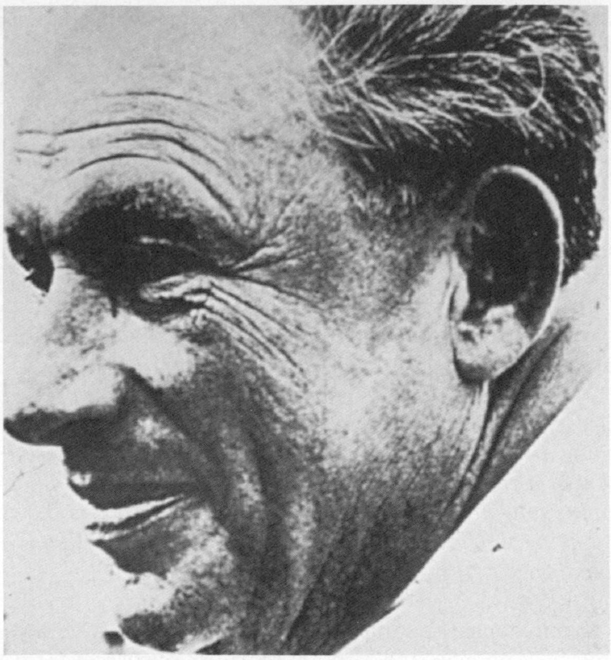

Figure 1-27. Gerhardt Küntscher (1900–1972), the great German pioneer of intramedullary nailing.

that every such intervention delayed healing. He believed that the advantage of closed nailing lay in the avoidance of such disturbance and the fact that surgical intervention could be limited. All his procedures reflected this attitude: refusal to expose a simple fracture for nailing, avoidance of bone grafting operations, dislike of plates and screws and his very limited approach for arthrodesis of the knee joint. One was bound to conclude that such methods were evolved under the pressure of circumstances—the shortage of skilled nurses, the lack of penicillin, the need for immediate fixation without transfer, and above all the total lack of certainty as to the duration of postoperative stay in hospital determined by the doubtful number of hospital beds that would be available. A virtue was made of necessity.[47]

Sadly, such smug complacency and self-satisfaction were not totally uncharacteristic of the British approach to innovation in fracture surgery at that time. In contrast, Milton Silverman in the *Saturday Evening Post* in 1955 said that Küntscher's invention was the most significant medical advance to come out of Germany since the discovery of sulfonamide. Küntscher developed interlocking femoral and tibial nails, an intramedullary bone saw for endosteal osteotomy, an expanding nail for the distal tibia, the "signal arm" nail for trochanteric fractures, cannulated flexible powered intramedullary reamers, and an intramedullary nail to apply compression across fracture sites. All this was done in collaboration with his engineer, Ernst Pohl, and his lifetime technical assistant, Gerhardt Breske, whom I had the great fortune to visit in his home in 1985. Herr Breske told me that Küntscher was a great lover of life: he swam every day, he enjoyed humor and parties and was a great practical joker, but never married, according to Herr Breske, because "he was far too busy." Gerhardt Küntscher (Fig. 1-27) died in 1972 at his desk, working on yet a further edition of his book on intramedullary nailing. He was found slumped over his final manuscript by Dr. Wolfgang Wolfers, chief of surgery at the St. Franziskus Hospital of Flensberg, where from 1965 onward Küntscher had worked as a guest surgeon.

The pioneering work of Küntscher was taken further by modifications of design and technique made by the AO group (see following section), and the distillation of this great experience resulted in the work in the 1960s and 1970s of Klemm, Schellmann, Grosse, and Kempf in the development of the current generation of interlocking nailing systems. Aside from this mainstream of development of intramedullary nailing following on the work of Küntscher, there have been a multitude of different designs of intramedullary fixation devices, such as those of Soeur, Westborne, Hansen and Street, Schneider, and Huckstep. The only other device to have achieved anything like widespread acceptance, however, has been that of Zickel, which incorporates at its upper end a trifin nail to secure purchase in the proximal femur in the management of fractures in the high subtrochanteric region.

ROBERT DANIS AND THE DEVELOPMENT OF THE AO GROUP

Robert Danis (1880–1962) (Fig. 1-28) must be regarded as the father of modern osteosynthesis. Graduating from the

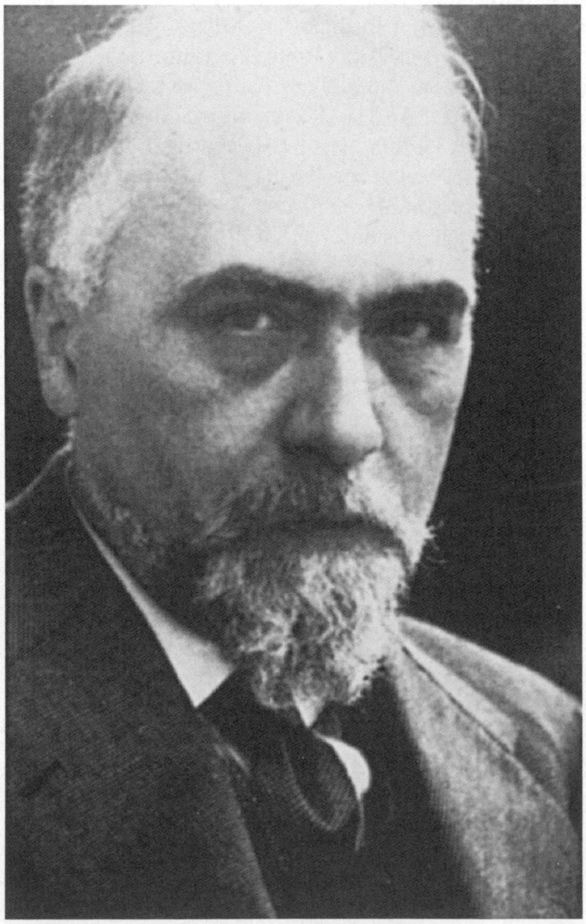

Figure 1-28. Robert Danis (1880–1962), the only known photograph. *(Courtesy of his son, Dr. A. Danis.)*

University of Brussels in 1904, he practiced as a general surgeon, his early interests being in thoracic and vascular surgery. He became professor of theoretical and practical surgery at the University of Brussels in 1921 and while there developed a great interest in internal fixation of fractures. Although there is no direct evidence, one cannot help but feel that he must have been profoundly influenced by the mobilizers—Seutin, Paget, Lucas-Championnière, Lambotte, Lane, and Sherman, to mention but a few—in developing his concepts of immediate stable internal fixation to permit functional rehabilitation. His vast experience in this field was brought together in his monumental publication *Théorie et Pratique de l'Ostéosynthèse.*[20] In the first section of this book on the aims of osteosynthesis, he wrote that an osteosynthesis is not entirely satisfactory unless it attains the three following objectives:

1. The possibility of immediate and active mobilization of the muscles of the region and of the neighbouring joints
2. Complete restoration of the bone to its original form
3. The *soudure per primam* (primary bone healing) of the bony fragments without the formation of apparent callus

Danis devised numerous techniques of osteosynthesis based principally on interfragmentary compression, using screws and a device that he called his *coapteur,* which was basically a plate designed to produce axial compression between two main bone fragments (Fig. 1-29). It would appear from his writings that Danis's primary aim was to produce fracture stabilization that was so rigid that he could ignore the broken bone and preserve the function of the other parts of the injured limb. In achieving such sound stabilization of the fracture by anatomic reduction and interfragmentary compression, he also produced, possibly by serendipity, the biomechanical and anatomic environment that permitted the bone to heal by direct remodeling of the cortical bone, without external callus. Having observed this type of healing, which he called *soudure autogène* (self-welding), he took this as an indication that his osteosynthesis had achieved its primary objective. The other side of this coin, however, was that if callus did appear, it was an indication that he had failed to produce the environment of stability that he had wished. He cannot initially have set out to produce direct bone healing before he had personally observed it, so he seems finally to have turned an observation of a secondary effect into the third aim of osteosynthesis as outlined previously, later causing some confusion of attitudes to callus. It is interesting to note, however, that Danis was not the first to observe healing of a diaphyseal fracture without external callus, as this was recorded by Layton in one of Arbuthnot Lane's cases.

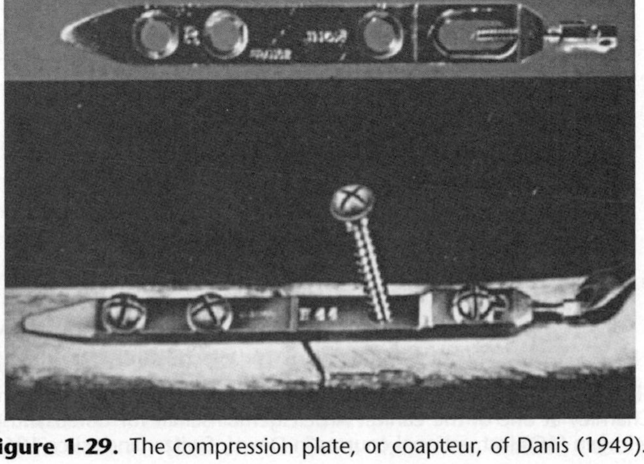

Figure 1-29. The compression plate, or coapteur, of Danis (1949).

In the first section of his book, in discussing direct bone healing, Danis made the prophetic statement, "This soudure autogène which occurs as discretely as in the case of an incomplete fissure fracture certainly merits experimental study to establish in detail what are the modifications brought about by an ideal osteosynthesis of the phenomena of consolidation."

Robert Danis could not have realized how comprehensively this suggestion would be taken up or the profound influence that it would have on the evolution of the surgical management of fractures over the ensuing 40 years.

On March 1, 1950, a young Swiss surgeon, Dr. Maurice Müller, who had read Danis's work, paid the great surgeon a visit in Brussels. This visit left such an impression on young Dr. Müller, to whom Robert Danis presented an autographed copy of his book, that the young Swiss returned to his homeland determined to embrace and develop the principles of the ideal osteosynthesis, as outlined by Danis, and to investigate the scientific basis for his observations. Over the next few years, Müller inspired a number of close colleagues to share his passion for the improvement of techniques for the internal fixation of fractures (Fig. 1-30), gathering around himself particularly Hans Willenegger of Liestal, Robert Schneider of Grosshöchstetten, and subsequently Martin Allgöwer of Chur, who together laid the intellectual and indeed practical groundwork for a momentous gathering in the Kantonsspital of Chur on March 15 to 17, 1958. The other guests at this meeting were Bandi, Baumann, Eckmann, Guggenbühl, Hunzicker, Molo, Nicole, Ott, Patry, Schär, and Stähli. Over the 3 days, a number of scientific papers on osteosynthesis were presented, and the assembled surgeons formed a study group to look into all aspects of internal fixation—*Arbeitsgemeinschaft für Osteosynthesefragen,* or AO. This was indeed a very active group that built on Danis's work in an industrious and productive way.

There were basically three channels of activity. First, a laboratory for experimental surgery was set up in Davos, Switzerland, initially under the direction of Martin Allgöwer and subsequently Herbert Fleisch, who was succeeded by the current director, Stefan Perren, in 1967. These workers, in collaboration with Robert Schenk, professor of anatomy at the University of Bern, instituted, and have since continued, an ever-expanding experimental program that early on clearly defined the exact process of direct bone healing and the influence of skeletal stability on the pattern of bone union, laying the foundation for our modern understanding of bone healing in various mechanical environments. Second, the group also set out, in collaboration with metallurgists and engineers in Switzerland, to devise a system of implants and instruments to apply the biomechanical principles emerging from their investigations and so enable them to produce the skeletal stability necessary to achieve the objectives enunciated by Danis. Third, they decided to document their clinical experience, and a center was set up in Bern, which continues to the present day with the documentation of osteosyntheses from all over the world.

positions. He was very concerned about not being able to acquire an orthopaedic position, when a friend suggested he meet with Professor Robert Judet. He did this out of desperation, without any hope of obtaining a position. The meeting with Judet was very brief. Professor Judet asked Letournel for his letters of recommendation, of which he had none, but Letournel indicated to him his sincere desire to obtain Judet's training position. Judet told him that he had a 6-month opening the following year. The 6-month position lasted 12 months, and Letournel then became Judet's assistant in his private clinic and advanced to associate professor and professor in 1970. He did not leave Judet until Judet's retirement in 1978. Letournel then became head of the Department of Orthopaedic Surgery at the Centre Medico-Chirurgie de la Port de Choisy in southeastern Paris. He remained there until his retirement from academic medicine in October 1993. He subsequently went into private practice at the Villa Medicis, Courbevoie, France, a suburb of Paris.

It was during his time at Choisy that physicians from North America had their greatest contact with Professeur Letournel. The importance of his work, inspired and begun by Robert Judet, was not widely recognized until the 1980s. Despite this long delay in acceptance and recognition, North America was actually one of the first areas to understand and adopt his techniques, which was a fact he certainly recognized and appreciated through his continued contact with us.

An intelligent and creative surgeon is typically able to contribute only a few components of new discoveries during the course of his or her career, but Emile Letournel accomplished much more. He completely revolutionized the way we conceptualize and treat acetabular fractures. Judet recognized problems with nonoperative treatment of acetabular fractures and inspired Letournel to begin the work that would define the surgical anatomy of the acetabulum, the pathologic anatomy of fresh fractures, and the radiographic interpretation to define these injuries. Following this, he developed surgical approaches. First, Judet combined the Kocher and Langenbeck approaches to make the Kocher-Langenbeck. Later, Letournel developed the ilioinguinal and finally the iliofemoral approach. Techniques of reduction as well as internal fixation were developed. Finally, the radiographic, clinical, and statistical documentation of immediate and long-term results of the surgical treatment became a lifelong passion of Letournel.

Letournel was committed to the idea of creating a comprehensive instructional course that taught the surgical treatment of fractures of the acetabulum and pelvis. Although he had been received so positively in North America, he felt he remained incompletely recognized in France. Therefore, the first course in 1984 was held in Paris but with faculty from North America and England, and he conducted the course in English. Letournel's Paris course set the standard and educational model for acetabulum and pelvis courses to follow. In all, there were nine courses consisting of lectures with intense study of radiographs. Surgical technique was taught with lectures, plastic bones, and live surgery, and there was always a day at the historic Paris anatomy institute, the Fer à Moulin. Every course included a black-tie banquet, always with the same fine musicians and Letournel singing "La Prune" and, if the spirit was right, the "Marseillaise." His Paris meetings culminated in the May 1993 first international symposium on the results of the surgical treatment of fractures of the acetabulum. His radiographic description and classification system, which was originally established in 1960 and by this time was well established worldwide, was used throughout the symposium for clear understanding of the statistical results.

Professeur Emile Letournel died relatively suddenly after an illness of only 2 months. Up to this time, he maintained his busy surgical schedule, traveled, and taught. We, his pupils and patients throughout the world, are fortunate to have enjoyed his great persona and contributions.

KLAUS KLEMM AND INTERLOCKING NAILING AND LOCAL ANTIBIOTIC BEAD CHAIN THERAPY

David Seligson

Dr. Klaus Klemm (1932–2001): Who was he, and why remember him in a book about skeletal trauma?

Dr. Klaus Klemm (Figs. 1-33 and 1-34) developed two important techniques for fracture care—interlocking nailing and local antibiotic bead chain therapy. These advances are appreciated by thousands of injured patients who benefit from his ideas. Klemm always said that his third great passion after interlocking nails and bead chains was chocolate, but it was really his wife, Dr. Brigitte Winter-Klemm. Let me share with you some of my memories of Dr. Klemm and look more into his story so you will understand his importance to those in traumatology whom he influenced.

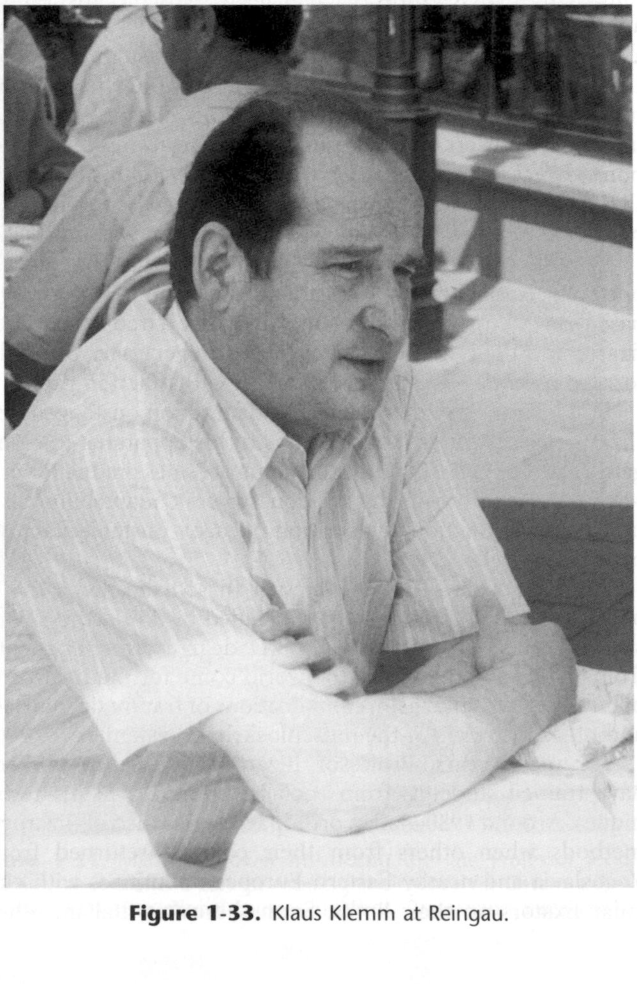

Figure 1-33. Klaus Klemm at Reingau.

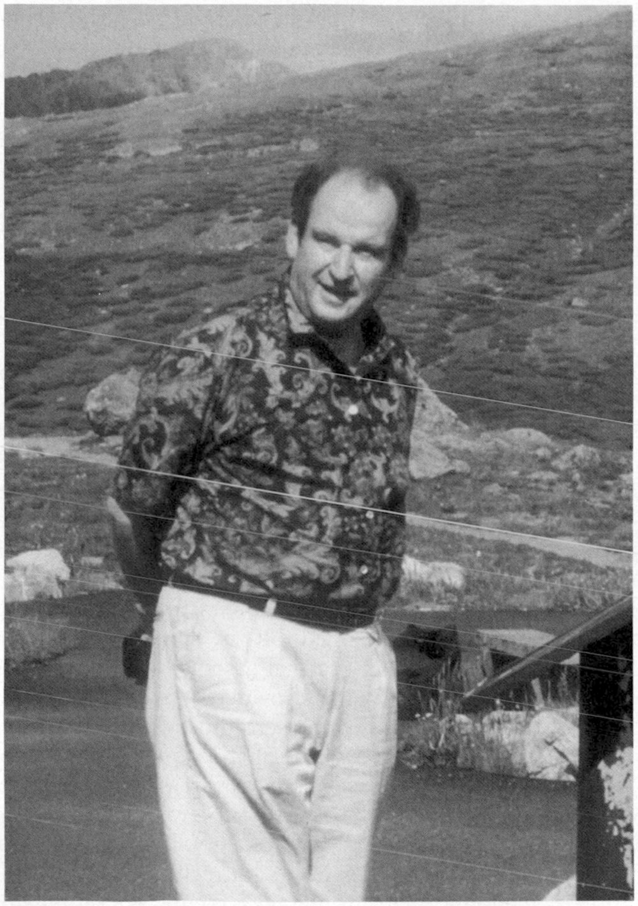

Figure 1-34. Klaus Klemm at Grant's Pass.

Klaus Klemm was born into a comfortable Frankfurt am Main family on May 19, 1932. He spent some of World War II as part of a youth group at a rail station in the Black Forest. He entered medical school in Frankfurt/Main in 1952, took a semester in Freiburg, and finished his medical degree in 1958. He then went to the Northern Westchester Hospital in Mount Kisco, New York, from 1958 to 1960 and returned to Germany, where he was licensed as a physician in 1962. Next, he took a position as an assistant to Professor Junghans in the new Workman's Hospital (BG) Frankfurt. At the BG, he was part of the new Septic Unit. From 1966 to 1969, he took his training in Surgery at St. Markus Hospital, Frankfurt/Main, and became Oberarzt and Chief of the Septic Unit at BG/Frankfurt first under Prof. Junghans and later with Prof. Contzen and finally until his retirement in 1999 under the direction of his student, Professor Börner.

Therefore, Dr. Klemm trained during the confusion of postwar Germany, spoke good English because of his 2 years in Westchester County, and accepted the task of treating bone infection with limited resources in a rebuilding country. Conventional treatment for osteomyelitis was implant removal, bed rest, suction drainage, and long courses of intravenous antibiotics. Klemm pioneered interlocking nailing as a method for fracture stabilization, and antibiotic implants as a way to provide ambulatory antibacterial therapy. Indeed, he corresponded with Küntscher about the "Detensor" and was advised not to use the term interlocking nailing but went ahead anyway, working with W. D. Schellmann to make a practical system for intramedullary locked nailing.

Antibiotic bead chains evolved from antibiotic bone cement implants. The bead chains have been commercially available in Europe since 1978 but were never, to Klaus's frustration, approved by the U.S. Food and Drug Administration (FDA). It was ironic in those days in the 1980s to visit with Klemm in the U.S. military hospital down the Friedberger Landstraße from the BG. The Americans were trying to educate Germans in basic hygiene such as handwashing and were treating femur fractures in cast braces.

Klemm was not a great speaker, nor did he write a great deal. One learned from Klaus by being around him. He operated frequently, and saw his patients personally. If you spent time with him, you always picked up tips such as the "free hand" method for placing locking screws or how to take a bone graft from the proximal tibia. Klemm always included his guests either at dinner at Claudio's, a restaurant near his home on the Marbachweg, or at home or perhaps for an evening with his team at his retreat in Eichelsachsen. At one such evening, I asked Guy Jenny how long one could leave antibiotic bead chains in a patient. Dr. Jenny replied, "I don't really know, my first chains are still in place after twenty years."

Klemm was a great supporter of the Gerhard Küntscher Society and its Secretary for more than a decade. Though quintessentially German at a time when it was not fashionable to be nationalistic, he nurtured connections throughout Europe and the United States. However, his relationship with the BG became more problematic as his career grew toward retirement. After all, the visitors to the clinic came to see Klaus, not the Chief. Furthermore, the development of competing nail systems did not help matters. At his retirement, we all gathered again in Frankfurt/Main at the Römer. It was a magical evening. Many of the younger colleagues present had served in menial roles during the years of American occupation. Here in the refurbished Ratskellar in the basement, the beer flowed, his friends and family were there, everyone toasted Klaus, and the old German songs rang out.

Retirement was not kind to Klemm. Klaus developed symptomatic lumbar spondylosis. He had back surgery. The site became infected. Ironically, the most innovative surgeon for the treatment of bone infection died of sepsis in the intensive care unit at the BG, where he had worked for three decades.

MAURICE EDMOND MÜLLER, INTERNAL FIXATION TECHNIQUES AND HIP PROSTHESES

Joseph Schatzker

Maurice Müller was born on March 28, 1918, in Biel on the shores of the Bielersee, which is a beautiful corner of the world where the Jura Mountains meet the water. While attending high school, Müller was very active in rowing. Because of his small size and light weight, he was always the coxswain. Another member of the crew was a tall youth named Robert Schneider. The two were friends but had no idea that their friendship would someday contribute to a revolution in trauma and orthopaedic surgery.

During a holiday in the mountains, after Müller finished high school, he chanced upon an old text on magic tricks. At the end of the holiday, Müller mesmerized the mountain folk with his wizardry, and they thought that because of his dark complexion and piercing eyes, he surely must be a disciple of the devil. During his long career, Müller used magic many times to entertain and break the ice at social and professional gatherings.

Surgical training in Switzerland in the 1940s was not organized, and every trainee had to arrange his own training and experience. In 1945, Müller saw an ad in the newspaper for a surgical position in Ethiopia. The war had isolated Switzerland, and the prospect of travel was enticing. When Müller returned from Ethiopia 2 years later, he was a self-taught surgeon who had become a technical wizard.

After a junior residency at the Balgrist, a bastion of conservative orthopaedic surgery in Zurich, Müller began to travel and visit famous surgeons in Europe. While in The Netherlands on a 6-month fellowship with Van Ness, an organizational genius, from whom Müller learned how to organize surgical departments, Müller traveled on weekends to visit other surgeons. On one such visit to Belgium, he met Robert Danis, who introduced Müller to the concepts of bone healing by means of absolute stability achieved by compression. Despite the short visit, Müller saw enough to alter his concept of bone surgery and saw a future for the use of lag screws and *coapteurs* or compression plates whose use made subsequent plaster immobilization no longer necessary. Immediate mobility was possible, and the bone healed while the soft tissue was recovering and the joints were regaining a full range of motion.

In 1952, Müller became chief resident of surgery in Fribourg, Switzerland, and immediately put to test his new and developing concepts of surgery. He surgically treated many fractures with implants he had developed and without the use of plaster immobilization, and achieved spectacular results.

Like all the young men in Switzerland at that time, Müller had compulsory military service for about 3 weeks annually. By 1952, Müller had risen through the ranks to head of a surgical military unit, and his old friend Robert Schneider, who was now the surgeon in chief of a regional hospital in Grosshoechstetten, was a member of Müller's unit. The reunion of these two old friends was to have great significance. Schneider was so impressed with the ideas of his young colleague that he not only invited Müller to do surgery on difficult cases in his hospital, but he began to introduce him to his friends who were chiefs in their own district hospitals in the canton of Bern. Müller began to operate in the hospitals of his friends on challenging cases and in this way developed a group of highly motivated, trained, and enthusiastic surgeons and supporters. On November 6, 1958, this surgical group founded the Swiss Arbeitsgemeinschaft für Osteosynthesefragen (AO), which is the Swiss association for the study of problems of internal fixation. The Swiss AO soon set about to change the whole world of bone surgery.

Müller was the inventive genius of the group and together with Robert Mathys, a mechanic, began in 1957 to develop a new set of implants and instruments for the purpose of internal fixation. In 1960, at the first AO course held in Davos, Switzerland, the AO introduced the participating surgeons and the world to their radically new concepts of absolute stability and immediate mobilization as well as to their completely novel set of implants and instruments.

From the very beginning, the AO understood the importance of documentation and research, and with their own funds, in 1959 in Davos, the members of AO Switzerland established a center for documentation and a center for research. Education and the Davos courses became extremely important as a means of training other surgeons to avoid misuse and surgical errors. In the AO courses, Müller pioneered the teaching of fracture repair on preserved human bones with simulated fracture patterns. In this way, the AO group became not only the pioneers of new bone surgery but also of radical new ways of educating surgical colleagues.

Müller was not only an inventive genius and superb organizer and teacher, but he was also a visionary. Müller realized that he could not establish a new school of surgery alone—he needed a team. The Swiss AO became his team. With von Rechenberg, an accountant, Müller created Synthes AG Chur, which became the commercial arm of the Swiss AO. Müller then magnanimously donated all his intellectual property to Synthes AG Chur, thus allowing Synthes AG Chur to enter into a business relationship with the producers of their implants and instruments, Mathys and then Straumann, who were charged with the manufacture and distribution of the AO products. The doctors remained fully in charge of all medical matters. For the exclusivity of manufacture and distribution under their trademark, "Synthes," owned by Synthes AG Chur, the producers paid a royalty on each implant and instrument sold. Synthes AG Chur was thus able to fund the teaching, documentation, development, and research activities of the Swiss AO, which could operate without any outside funding. To guarantee the high quality and safety of the AO instruments and implants, Müller formed a technical commission and remained the chair of the AO technical commission (AOTK) for 20 years.

Müller made his mark not only in the AO and trauma surgery but also in orthopaedics in general. In 1960, Müller was appointed the surgeon in chief of the largest trauma and orthopaedic department in the hospital of St. Gallen. Under his leadership, the department and hospital blossomed. His inventive genius did not rest. In February 1961, Müller designed and implanted the first total hip in Europe. Soon the hospital in St. Gallen became an orthopaedic mecca.

In 1963, Müller received further recognition and was appointed professor and head of the department of orthopaedics and trauma at the University of Bern, a position he did not assume until 1967.

To finance further teaching, research, and education, in 1964, Müller established Protek, a firm that sold all the new total joint implants and instruments that he continued to develop. In 1967, he also established the Foundation Protek, which in 1974, became the Maurice E. Müller (MEM) Foundation of Switzerland. Like Synthes AG Chur for AO, the MEM Foundation held the trademark "Protek," and the company Protek had to pay a royalty to the MEM Foundation for each total joint and instrument it sold. The MEM Foundation soon became financially responsible for many of the Müller innovations and research activities that followed. Müller introduced novel surgical teaching by finding a way to transmit images from the operating room onto a large screen for the surgical audience, making it possible for each surgeon to enter into direct contact with the operating surgeon. His new surgical innovations and novel methods of teaching made the Bernese total joint courses world famous, and Bern became an orthopaedic mecca.

Müller did not limit his activities to Bern. He became a founding member of the International Hip Society in 1979 and subsequently its president until 1982. In 1975, he became extremely active in SICOT and became its president from 1981 to 1984. From 1988 to 1990, he chaired the SICOT committee for documentation and evaluation, which expanded his work in evidence-based medicine, a field in which he was an active pioneer since chairing the first AO documentation center in Davos in 1959.

Müller became the honorary member of many orthopaedic and trauma societies and became the recipient of 10 honorary doctorates from universities around the world. He was showered with many surgical prizes and distinctions. In 1988, together with Martin Allgöwer and Hans Willenegger, Müller received the highest Swiss award, the Marcel Benoist prize, for his contributions to orthopaedic and trauma surgery (see Fig. 1-30).

Müller was not only inventive but also philanthropic. His generosity reached outside of Switzerland. In Spain, he established a daughter foundation, the MEM Foundation of Spain, which was chaired by Professor Raphael Orozco.

In North America, he established the ME Müller Foundation of North America, which was chaired by Professor Joseph Schatzker. The North American ME Müller Foundation is still active and has made it possible for many North American surgeons to be educated in European hip concepts and surgical techniques. In 1988, Müller endowed the ME Müller professorship in orthopaedic surgery at Harvard Medical School in Boston, and in 1990, he endowed the chair of orthopaedic surgery at McGill University of Medicine in Montreal, Canada. In 1992, he endowed a program of documentation and evaluation in Toronto, Canada, which continued research in evidence-based medicine for years. One of the early pioneers of evidence-based medicine, Müller was the chair of the AO commission for documentation. He was also responsible for major progress in the classification of fractures, and in 1990, he published with his coauthors Koch, Nazarian, and Schatzker, the Comprehensive Classification of Fractures, which was adopted by the Swiss AO and subsequently by OTA, and has become the universally accepted basis of trauma documentation.

Toward the end of his active life as an orthopaedic surgeon, Müller turned his attention to the humanities and left Switzerland a major legacy in the form of the Klee Art Museum in Bern designed by Renzo Piano. He used the funds from the sale of the firm Protek to Sulzer to fund the building and the initial operation of this unique cultural center.

In 2002, SICOT awarded Maurice Edmond Müller the "Orthopaedic Surgeon of the Twentieth Century," a title which he justly deserved.

MARTIN ALLGÖWER, INTERNAL FIXATION AND FRACTURE MANAGEMENT

Marvin Tile

Martin Allgöwer was one of the master surgeons of the twentieth century. His most lasting and well-known contribution, along with his Swiss colleagues, Maurice Müller, Hans Willenegger, and others, was to lead the revolution in fracture care by the Swiss AO (or Association for the Study of Internal Fixation [ASIF]). Allgöwer was a general surgeon and contributed in many other areas of medicine, through his research and clinical endeavors, especially burns.

Allgöwer was born on May 5, 1917, in St. Gallen, Switzerland. He studied medicine at the University of Basel in Switzerland, graduating in 1942 during the Second World War. He became a captain in the Swiss Medical Corp during the Second World War, which interrupted his training. He spent 2 years in the tissue culture laboratory at CIBA, a pharmaceutical company in Basel. At that time, he developed his interest in surgical research and produced his doctoral thesis in 1944, "Occurrence, Nature and Relevance of Sulfonamide Antagonists (Inhibitors) in the Body." He also worked in cancer treatment. He befriended Ernest Frei, who would later play a role in the development of the AO Laboratory for Experimental Surgery in Davos.

He left Switzerland on a research fellowship from the University of Texas Medical School in Galveston, a leading center for burn research and treatment, to study with Professors Blocker and Pomerat. After completing his training in Galveston, he visited other world-renowned burn centers, mainly in the United States.

In 1952, he returned to the University of Basel to work with Dr. Hans Willenegger, one of the other pioneers of the AO. In 1953, he wrote his post doctoral thesis, "The Cellular Basis of Wound Repair." At the time, he was working on single nucleus monocytes, and this research was one of the precursors of our current stem cell research.

In 1956, he became chief surgeon at the Canton Regional Hospital in Chur, Switzerland, where, by his own admission, he really had little knowledge of the treatment of fractures. He himself had suffered a fracture of the tibia during military service, treated with cerclage fixation, a plaster cast followed by pulmonary embolism. In Chur, he was faced with a large volume of ski injuries and recognized that better treatment options were essential to improve the outcomes of those fractures.

In 1957, he met Maurice Müller. He had invited Müller to come to Chur to discuss skeletal trauma and to help with a complex fracture. He immediately recognized that the future of fracture care was not long-term immobilization in plaster casts, but a new approach, which included what would become the AO principles of anatomic reduction, stable fixation, and immediate rehabilitation. Stable internal fixation with screws replaced cerclage wires as the treatment of choice for lower extremity fractures in Chur.

On November 6, 1958, in Biel, Switzerland, the AO organization was founded. The leaders at the time were Maurice Müller, Martin Allgöwer, Hans Willenegger, and others. Müller was the innovator; Allgöwer, the organizer and researcher; and Willenegger, the teaching missionary. Together, they left a lasting legacy in fracture and trauma management.

With his continual research interest, Allgöwer found an unused tuberculosis sanitorium in Davos and suggested that it become a center for musculoskeletal trauma research; thus, he founded in 1959, the Laboratory for Experimental Surgery in Davos. He was helped in this endeavor by his colleague Ernest Frei, and was supported by the AO surgeons. Herbert Fleisch became the first director. Robert Schenk performed groundbreaking research on fracture healing under stable fixation.

In 1963, Stephan Perrin became director of the laboratory in Davos. His biomechanical studies on stable internal fixation of fractures clearly placed fracture care on a scientific basis. The center of AO activities shifted to Davos, where the first AO course on internal fixation of fractures was held in 1960. More than 50,000 surgeons and operating room (OR) personnel have trained in the AO courses in Davos.

Allgöwer made Davos his second home. He was instrumental in the international spread of AO principles and methods. He was president of AO International from 1983 to 1988. Eventually in 1992, most AO activity moved to the new AO Centrum in Davos, which he championed.

Martin coauthored the original *AO Principles Book* in 1963 and the first AO manual in 1969 with Müller and Willenegger. He was a prolific writer, with many publications and book chapters.

In 1967, he was appointed chair of the department of surgery at the University of Basel, where he remained until 1984. From 1976 to 1978, he was president of the Swiss Society for Surgery, working closely with general and orthopaedic surgeons to amalgamate all surgeons in the Union of Swiss Surgical Societies. From 1979 to 1981, he was president of the Society Internationale de Chirgurie (SIC/ISS) and subsequently became their Secretary-General. He was a driving force in the founding of the AO Foundation, now the governing body of the AO and was its inaugural president from 1984 to 1992, stepping down at the opening of the AO Center in Davos.

He won many honors in his career. In 1988, the founders of the AO including Allgöwer, Müller, Bandi, Schneider, and Willenegger were awarded the Marcel Benoist Prize, also known as the Swiss Nobel Prize, for their contributions to fracture and trauma care.

The AO needed the leadership of Müller with his sharp innovative mind, and the missionary zeal of Willenegger, teacher and traveler, but also essential were the organization skills, the devotion to research and education, and the clinical skills of Allgöwer for the AO to succeed.

Allgöwer was a master surgeon. His handling of soft tissues in trauma and fracture work was legendary. He passed this along to his many residents and colleagues and was an excellent mentor. He was a gifted teacher and showed great leadership qualities. He had charm, charisma, and a good sense of humor. He was a skilled powder skier and was an exceptional pilot.

It was through his leadership and that of his colleagues that eventually the AO principles and methods, which at first were not accepted, became conventional wisdom. As with all conventional wisdom, the AO principles themselves have undergone an evolution, which he accepted. Many of the basic principles are still valid today; especially with respect to articular fractures. The principle of anatomic reduction has changed for diaphyseal fractures, except for the radius, where it is still essential.

The lasting legacy, which is stable internal fixation and early rehabilitation without external casts or splints, remains and has contributed to improved function following severe fractures. Also pioneered was early fracture stabilization in polytrauma care. Allgöwer was in the forefront of AO education in manual skills courses and laboratories, another important legacy in learning.

I followed Martin Allgöwer as president of the AO Foundation in 1992, working closely with him. It soon became obvious to me how his great leadership qualities had thrust the AO into the forefront of trauma care. He was a great teacher, mentor, leader, and a gifted general surgeon. His contributions to surgery in his many areas of expertise are unrivalled in the twentieth century. He remained intellectually active even to his ninetieth birthday. He died on October 27, 2007, but his legacy lives on.

SUMMARY

Christopher L. Colton

As technology advances, so do the severity and frequency of traumatic insult, and the demand for ever-increasing skill on the part of the fracture surgeon grows likewise. It is only by the study of the history of our surgical forebears and by keeping in mind how they have striven, often in the face of fierce criticism, to achieve the apparently unattainable that young surgeons will continue to be inspired to emulate them and so carry forward the progress they have achieved.

Any consideration of the history of 5000 years of endeavor, confined of necessity within the strictures of a publication such as this, is perforce eclectic. Nevertheless, in deciding to highlight the achievements of some, I have not in any way set out to minimize the pioneering work of those whose activities have not been specifically detailed in this overview, and with respect to these necessary omissions I ask the reader's indulgence.

The complete References list is available online at https://expertconsult.inkling.com.

Chapter 2

Global Burden of Musculoskeletal Injuries

KAVI BHALLA • BRETT D. OWENS • RENAN C. CASTILLO

Injuries are a leading cause of death and disability around the world. In 2010, injuries killed 5.1 million people globally, corresponding to a rate of 73.6 per 100,000 people. Figure 2-1, *A* shows the relative distribution of global deaths, from communicable diseases (Group A, in *red*), noncommunicable diseases (Group B, in *blue*), and injuries (Group C, in *green*) in 2010. The area each box represents is proportional to the associated mortality. Of the 52.8 million people who died in 2010, almost 10% died due to an injury (Group C, Fig. 2-1, *A*). In addition to deaths, nonfatal injuries result in substantial disability. Public health researchers use disability-adjusted life years (DALYs) lost (Box 2-1), to quantify the total public health burden of ill health. DALYs provide a comparable measure of the health loss due to fatal and nonfatal diseases and injuries. Figure 2-1, *B* shows the relative distribution of global DALYs, from communicable diseases (group A, in *red*), noncommunicable diseases (Group B, in *blue*), and injuries (Group C, in *green*) in 2010. The area each box represents is proportional to the associated burden of disability. In 2010, 11.2% of the global DALYs lost from all causes were due to injuries (Group C, Figure 2-1, *B*).

Over the past two decades, global population health is in the midst of a transition away from communicable, maternal, neonatal, and nutritious disorders (Group A causes) and toward noncommunicable diseases and injuries. While the number of deaths from Group A causes declined by 17% from 1990 to 2010, deaths from injuries in that period rose by 24%. The extent of this global health transition varies across global regions. While only 6.3% of the health burden in developed regions now is due to Group A causes, in developing regions these causes currently account for 40.2% of the burden. However, despite the shifts in communicable causes, injuries are a major threat even in the poorest regions of the world. For example, in sub-Saharan Africa, injuries account for 7.8% of the health burden, which is only a little less than Western Europe (9.1%).

Globally, 3 of the top 25 leading causes of years of healthy life lost (measured in DALYs lost) are due to injuries, including road injuries (ranks tenth), self-harm (ranks eighteenth), and falls (ranks nineteenth) (Fig. 2-2). Two other major drivers of disability, low back pain (ranks seventh) and other musculoskeletal (ranks twenty-third) are also likely to reflect primarily injury and trauma. However, the rankings can vary dramatically across different regions. For example, road injury is a top five cause of DALYs lost in seven global regions, including second overall in Andean Latin America. Falls and self-harm are top five causes of DALYs lost in Central Europe and the high-income Asia–Pacific regions, respectively. Low back pain, which we believe has primarily an injury etiology, is a top five cause of DALYs lost in 11 regions of the world, although it tends to rank lower in sub-Saharan Africa.

CAUSES OF INJURY

Road traffic crashes kill 1.33 million people annually and result in 77 million DALYs lost. They are the eighth leading cause of death, eighth leading cause of life years lost, and the tenth leading cause of DALYs lost globally. In 2010, road injuries killed more people than tuberculosis and malaria, two diseases that have been a central focus of the global health agenda. Road injury deaths have grown by 46% since 1990 (rates grew by 12%). Road traffic crashes are the leading cause of injury deaths, accounting for more than a quarter of all injury deaths (Fig. 2-3).

Violence, self-inflicted and interpersonal, together killed another 1.33 million people in 2010. Intentional self-harm was the thirteenth leading cause of death among all causes, killing 0.88 million people. It is the second leading cause of injury deaths, accounting for 17% of injury deaths. Interpersonal violence (homicide) killed 0.45 million people in 2010, accounting for 9% of injury deaths. Although total homicides grew by 35% since 1990, this was slower than the rate of population growth during this period.

Falls were the third leading cause of injury deaths, resulting in 0.54 million global deaths in 2010, 11% of all injury deaths. Deaths from falls have grown by 55%, and death rates grew by 18% since 1990. These trends likely reflect the increasing mean age of the global population.

GEOGRAPHIC AND DEMOGRAPHIC DISTRIBUTION OF INJURY BURDEN

Most injury deaths occur among young adults. In contrast, global injury related disability is greatest in middle age (Fig. 2-4, *A*), while the rate of injury related disability is greatest in the elderly (Fig. 2-4, *B*). Injuries are much more common among men than women, with the notable exception of fire deaths. In 2010, the overall injury death rate and the injury health burden (i.e., DALYs lost) among men were over twice that among women. Road traffic crashes are the leading cause of injury death and disability up to the age range of 40 to 44 years. Among older adults, falls emerge as the leading cause of injury deaths and disability.

Injury rates vary substantially across different world regions (Fig. 2-5). In general, low- and middle-income regions have higher injury rates than high-income regions. The 10 least safe

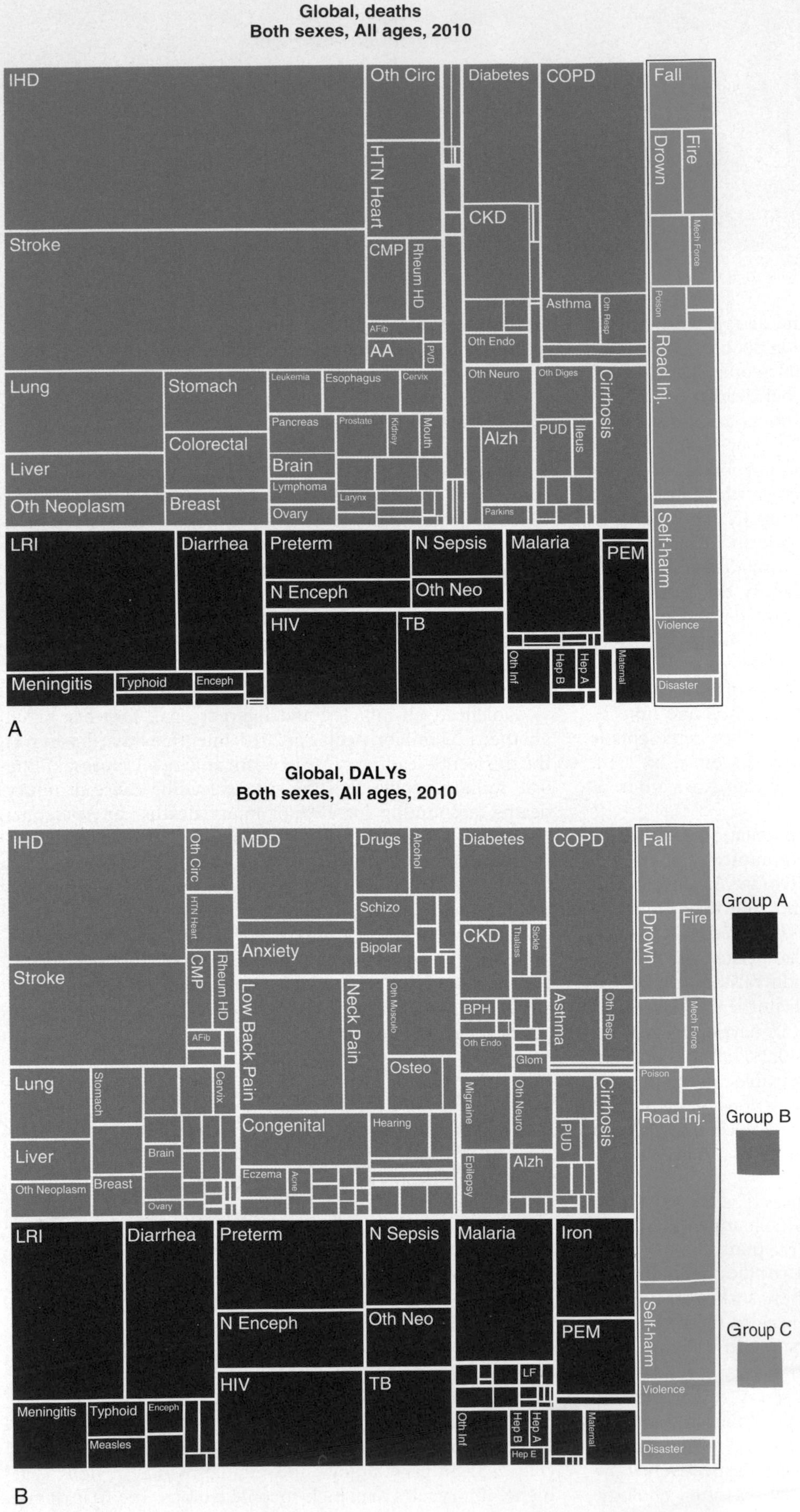

Figure 2-1. Relative distribution of global deaths, (**A**), and DALYs, (**B**), from communicable diseases *(red)*, noncommunicable diseases *(blue)*, and injuries *(green)* in 2010. The area each box represents is proportional to the health burden. *AA,* Aortic aneurysm; *AFib,* atrial fibrillation; *Alzh,* Alzheimer disease; *CKD,* chronic kidney disease; *CMP,* cardiomyopathy; *COPD,* chronic obstructive pulmonary disease; *Glom,* acute glomerulonephritis; *HD,* heart disease; *Hep,* hepatitis; *HIV,* human immunodeficiency virus; *HTN,* hypertension; *IHD,* ischemic heart disease; *LRI,* lower respiratory infection; *MDD,* major depressive disorder; *Oth,* other; *Oth Endo,* other endocrine; *PEM,* protein-energy malnutrition; *PUD,* peptic ulcer disease; *Rheum HD,* rheumatic heart disease; *TB,* tuberculosis.

BOX 2-1 *What Is the Global Burden of Disease Study?*

The statistical estimates presented in this chapter are from the Global Burden of Disease, Injuries, and Risk Factors (GBD) Project. In 1991, the World Bank commissioned the first GBD study to develop a comprehensive and comparable assessment of the burden of 107 diseases and injuries and 10 selected risk factors for the world and eight major regions.[1] The findings represented a major improvement in global knowledge of population health metrics and proved to be influential in shaping the global health priorities of international health and development agencies. The study also stimulated numerous national burden-of-disease analyses that have informed national debates on health policy over the last two decades.

The current revision of the study, GBD 2010[2-5] is a comprehensive update of the original study and presents estimates for 291 diseases and injuries, 67 risk factors, and 1160 sequelae (nonfatal health consequences) disaggregated by sex and 20 age groups for 21 regions covering the entire globe. The study is a collaboration of hundreds of researchers around the world, led by the Institute for Health Metrics and Evaluation at the University of Washington and a consortium of several other institutions including: Harvard University, Imperial College London, Johns Hopkins University, University of Queensland, University of Tokyo, and the World Health Organization.

Diseases and injuries result in either premature death or life lived with ill health. GBD aims to quantify the gap between the ideal of a population that lives a full life in full health and the reality. GBD uses the following concepts to measure this health burden:

- **Years of Life Lost (YLL):** This is the number of years of life lost because of premature death. It is calculated by multiplying the number of deaths at each age by a standard life expectancy at that age.
- **Years of Life with Disability (YLD):** This is number of years of life that are lived with short-term or long-term health loss weighted by the magnitude of the disability due to the sequelae of diseases and injuries.
- **Disability-Adjusted Life Year (DALY):** This is the main summary measure of population health used in GBD to quantify health loss. DALYs provide a metric that allows comparison of health loss across different diseases and injuries. They are calculated as the sum of YLLs and YLDs. Thus they are a measure of the number of years of healthy life that are lost due to death and nonfatal illness or impairment.

	Global	High-income Asia Pacific	Western Europe	Australasia	High-income North America	Central Europe	Southern Latin America	Eastern Europe	East Asia	Tropical Latin America	Central Latin America	Southeast Asia	Central Asia	Andean Latin America	North Africa and Middle East	Caribbean	South Asia	Oceania	Southern Sub-Saharan Africa	Eastern Sub-Saharan Africa	Central Sub-Saharan Africa	Western Sub-Saharan Africa
Ischemic heart disease	1	3	1	1	1	1	1	1	2	1	2	3	1	3	1	2	4	5	15	21	19	20
Lower respiratory infections	2	7	21	27	21	17	6	13	15	7	6	4	2	1	5	4	1	1	2	3	4	2
Stroke	3	2	3	5	7	2	2	2	1	4	11	1	3	11	2	3	12	14	7	16	14	15
Diarrheal diseases	4	46	52	53	46	76	43	48	47	25	14	8	17	8	11	8	3	4	3	4	2	3
HIV/AIDS	5	108	59	87	34	72	33	3	39	11	13	13	31	15	57	9	17	9	1	1	5	4
Malaria	6	160	159	155	158	160	165	161	167	144	154	27	160	141	68	60	44	7	22	2	1	1
Low back pain	7	1	2	2	3	3	4	4	4	3	7	7	6	5	4	13	11	13	13	17	22	13
Preterm birth complications	8	58	43	28	25	35	11	35	28	9	9	11	8	6	8	11	2	6	6	5	6	7
COPD	9	18	7	3	2	7	7	9	3	10	16	10	11	16	13	22	5	18	9	20	20	22
Road injury	10	15	12	10	9	8	5	6	5	5	4	5	5	2	6	10	10	15	14	11	12	9
Major depressive disorder	11	12	4	4	5	6	3	5	8	6	5	6	7	4	3	7	14	12	10	13	17	19
Neonatal encephalopathy	12	84	66	50	54	65	40	40	24	20	20	12	4	9	18	15	6	19	12	8	10	10
Tuberculosis	13	42	107	122	123	54	64	17	37	44	44	2	15	21	33	17	7	3	4	7	7	12
Diabetes	14	10	10	15	8	9	10	15	9	8	3	9	12	14	9	6	16	2	8	27	28	26
Iron deficiency anemia	15	40	85	35	117	28	27	29	32	18	18	14	13	7	10	5	9	20	11	12	11	11
Neonatal sepsis	16	119	120	111	100	114	51	81	132	29	30	35	54	18	22	14	8	24	29	9	13	5
Congenital anomalies	17	39	34	26	29	32	12	25	16	12	10	16	10	10	7	16	15	17	17	18	8	17
Self-harm	18	5	16	18	14	11	14	7	13	28	25	29	14	31	39	33	13	27	27	31	35	67
Falls	19	11	6	7	15	5	17	14	10	24	28	21	20	27	19	20	20	31	40	32	31	21
Protein-energy malnutrition	20	112	118	128	116	120	78	122	98	59	33	49	68	35	36	32	18	21	35	6	3	6
Neck pain	21	9	9	9	10	14	9	19	11	15	17	19	18	17	16	23	27	33	24	29	32	30
Lung cancer	22	6	5	8	4	4	15	10	6	30	38	24	28	47	28	26	47	58	43	92	73	95
Other musculoskeletal	23	4	8	6	6	13	8	16	14	14	15	22	19	19	21	24	30	26	26	34	33	35
Cirrhosis	24	17	19	36	16	10	16	11	21	19	12	15	9	20	15	34	22	16	37	30	27	25
Meningitis	25	90	101	91	91	80	59	77	73	51	45	36	33	37	29	29	21	8	23	10	9	8

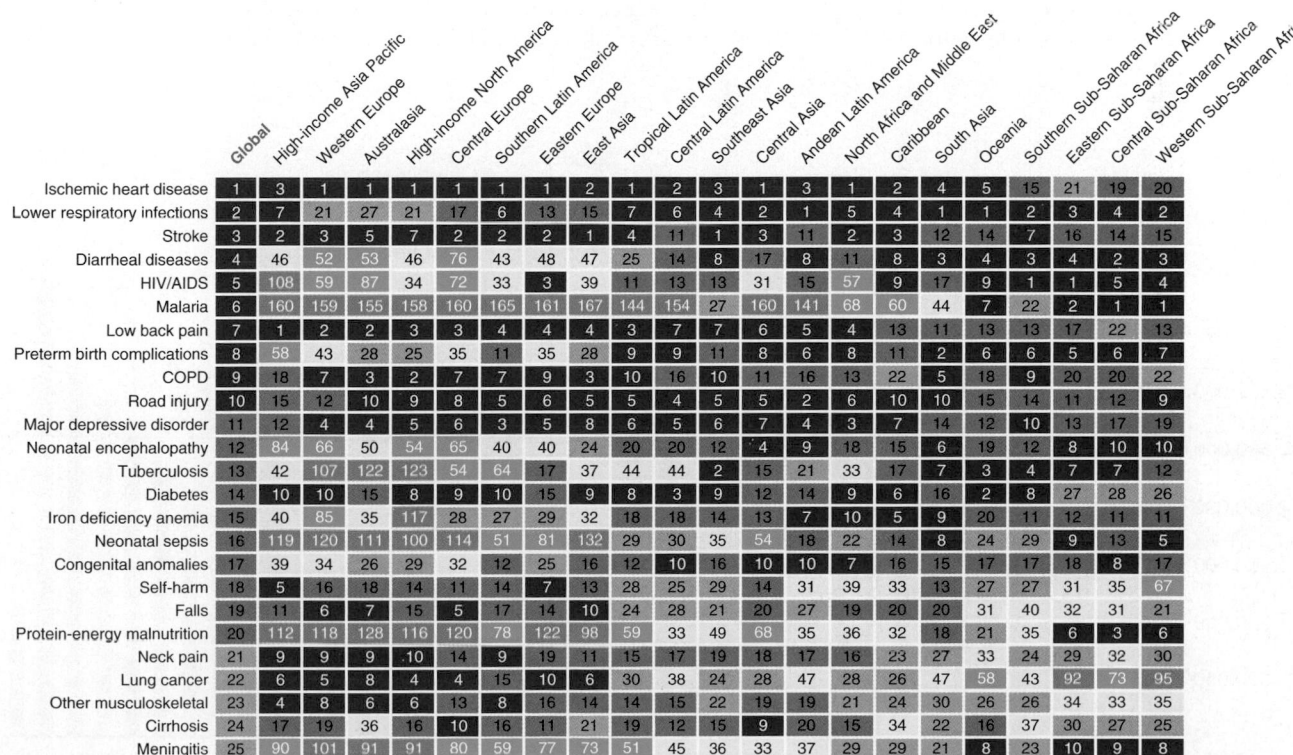

Figure 2-2. Heat map showing the top 25 global causes of years of healthy life lost (disability-adjusted life years) and their ranking in different regions in 2010. Cell color identifies ranking range (e.g., ranks 1-10 are shown in *red,* and ranks 100+ in *blue*). *AIDS,* Acquired immunodeficiency deficiency syndrome; *COPD,* chronic obstructive pulmonary disease; *HIV,* human immunodeficiency virus.

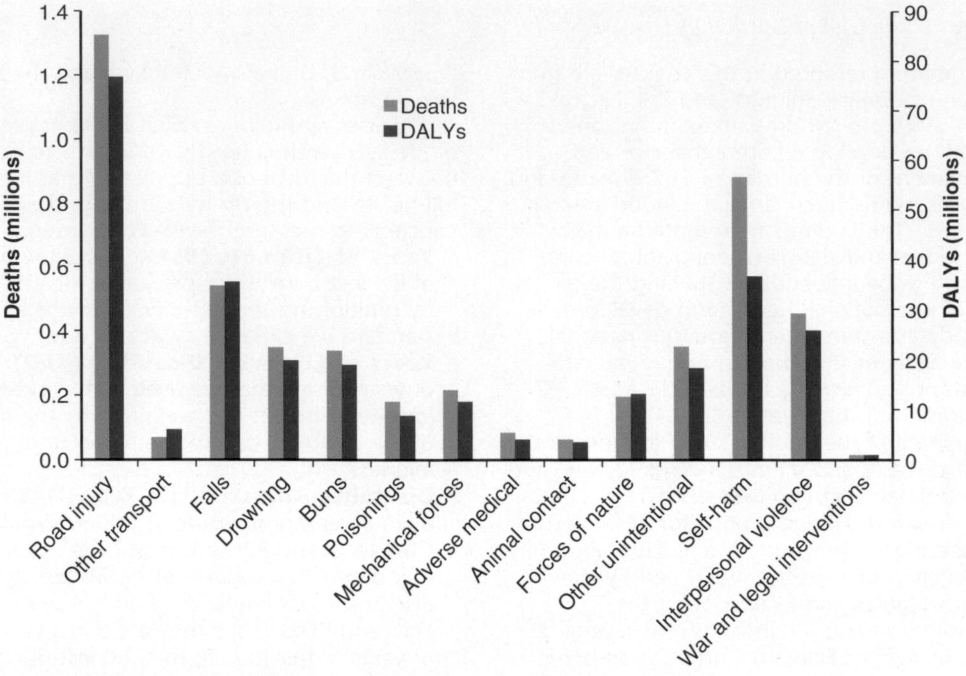

Figure 2-3. Global deaths and disability-adjusted life years (DALYs) from various external causes of injuries, 2010.

regions (i.e., regions with the highest injury death rates) are all low- or middle-income regions. Three of the five safest regions are high-income regions. In 2010, the Caribbean had the highest injury disability rate globally, dramatically exceeding the rate from injuries in other regions. This was primarily due to the 2010 Haiti earthquake, which resulted in approximately 195,000 deaths (448 deaths per 100,000 people) and approximately 200 years of life with disability (YLD) per 100,000 people. This illustrates the impact that a major natural disaster has on population health statistics.

In 2010, there were 35.1 million nonfatal injuries that would have warranted hospital admission if the victims had access to medical care (Fig. 2-6). In addition, there were 312.1 million nonfatal injuries that would have required outpatient care at a medical facility if the victims had access to medical care. Despite the large number of injuries warranting

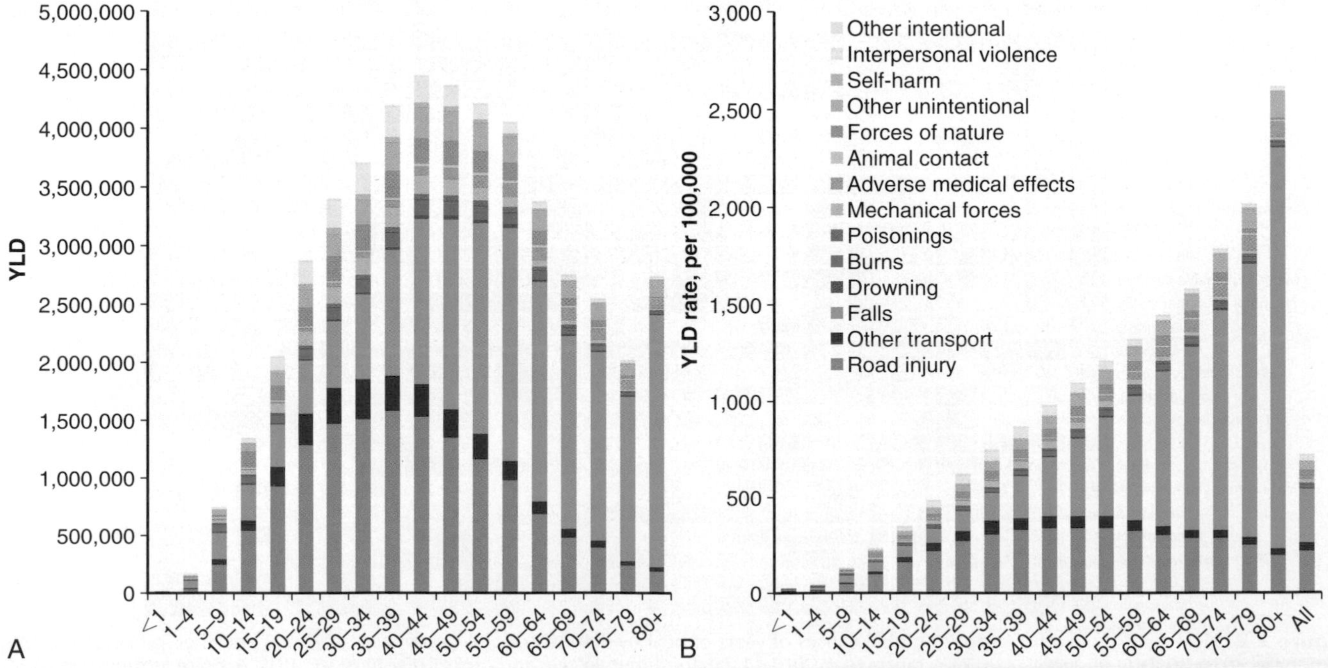

Figure 2-4. Age distribution of global years of life with disability (YLD), (**A**), and YLD rates, (**B**), in 2010.

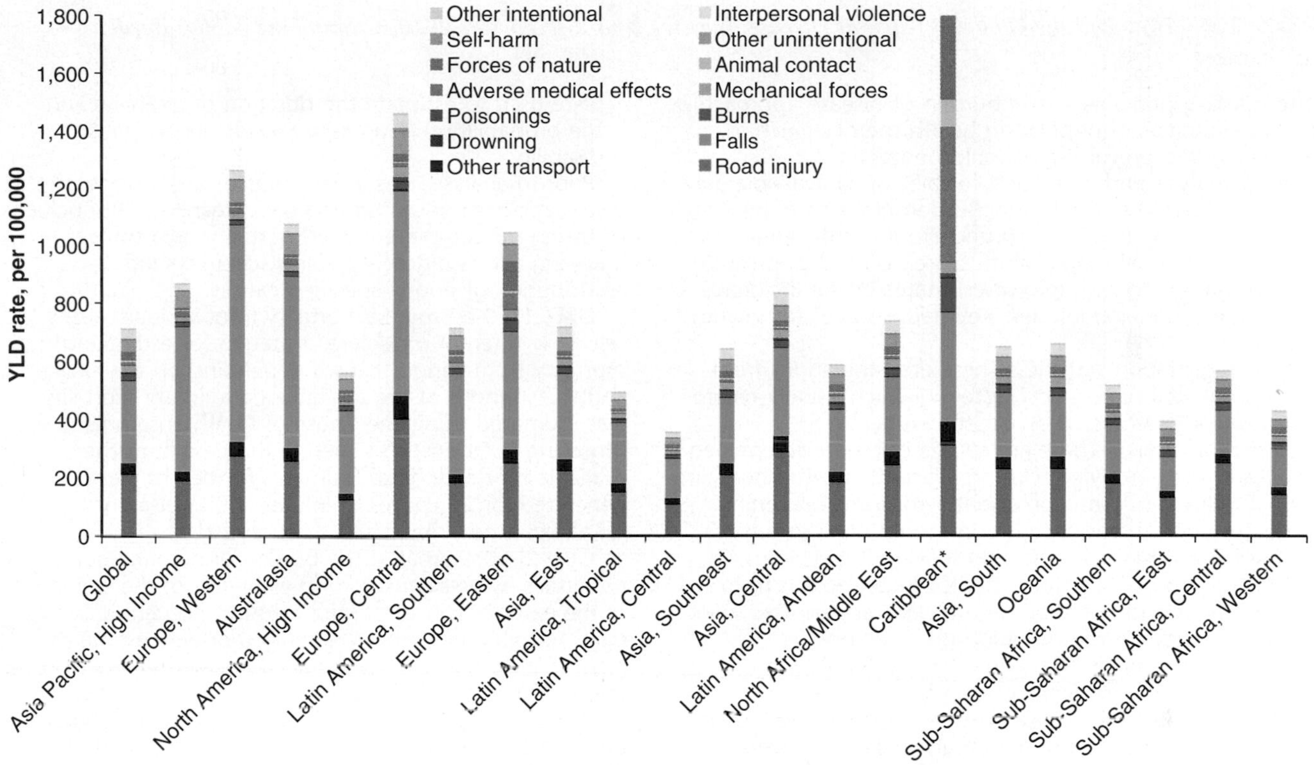

Figure 2-5. Regional rates of years of life with disability (YLD) (rate per 100,000) due to injuries in 2010.

outpatient care, these are relatively less severe and only contribute 3% of the total health loss (YLD) because of the much smaller disability per event.

In contrast to deaths, the leading cause of nonfatal injuries are falls, accounting for 13.5 million severe injuries (i.e., warranting admission), 38% of all severe injuries, and 43% of the burden of nonfatal injuries. Road injuries are responsible for another 9.2 million severe injuries, 26% of all severe injuries, and 30% of the burden of nonfatal injuries. Thus, together, road injuries and falls account for almost three-fourths of the burden of severe nonfatal injuries.

ESTIMATING THE BURDEN OF MUSCULOSKELETAL INJURY

Despite the availability of global data about injuries in general, estimates of the global burden of musculoskeletal injuries can

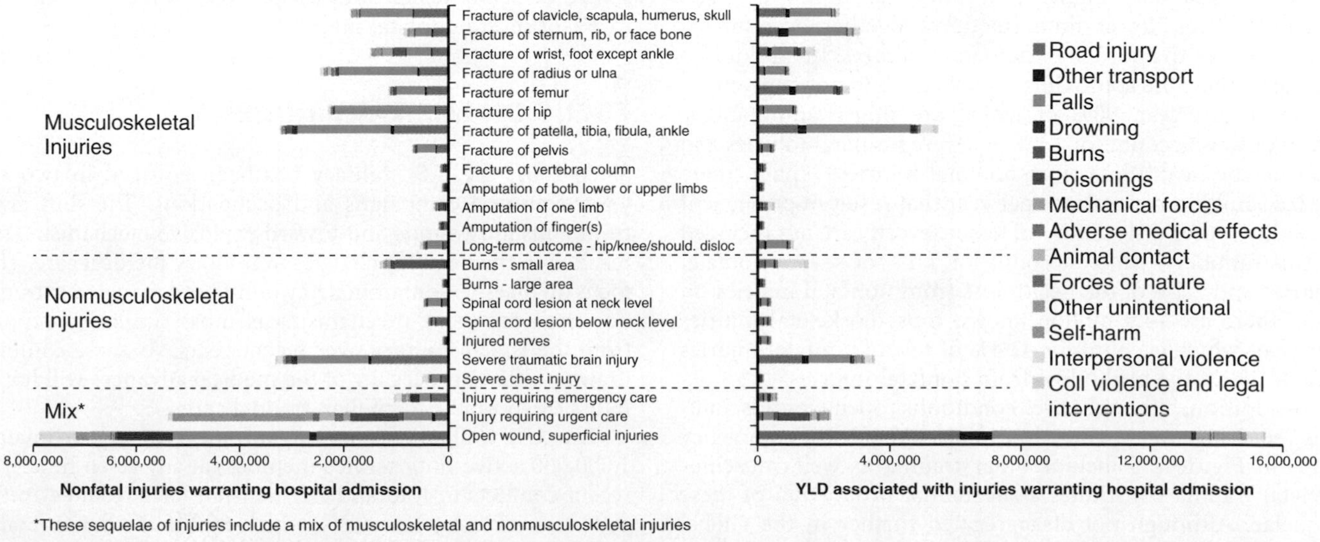

Figure 2-6. Incidence of severe nonfatal injuries warranting hospital admission and the associated burden measured in years lived with disability.

BOX 2-2 *How Did the Global Burden of Disease, Injuries, and Risk Factors 2010 Estimate the Global Burden of Disease?*

The guiding principle of the burden of disease approach is that estimates of population health metrics (such as incidence and prevalence) should be generated after careful analysis and correction for bias of all available data sources. Therefore, the Global Burden of Disease, Injuries and Risk Factors (GBD) 2010 undertook a substantial effort to access all empirical measurements of population health that could help inform estimates of the incidence of fatal and nonfatal injuries. Key data sources for injuries included:

- Vital registration statistics: These are tabulations from national vital registration systems, which usually record causes of death listed on death certificates.
- Verbal autopsies: These are causes of death determined by a trained interviewer using a structured questionnaire that collects information about symptoms preceding death. Such surveillance is commonly done in regions that do not have reliable vital registration systems.
- Mortuary/burial registers: Medico-legal records from mortuaries and burial permit offices were another key source of data for information-poor regions.
- Household surveys: These were a key source for estimating the incidence of nonfatal injuries.
- Hospital databases: Large hospital registries were used as a key source of information about the sequelae resulting from injuries.
- Prospective studies of disability outcome: The results from studies that follow up victims after an injury event were used to estimate the duration of disability and the probability that an injury results in permanent disability.

Prior to analysis, these data sources are subjected to a systematic harmonization and data cleaning. This includes adjusting for completeness of mortality data sources, mapping across different coding schemes, and reattribution of poorly specified causes.

GBD 2010 estimated mortality from various causes using six different modeling strategies for estimating mortality from various causes depending on the cause and the strength of the available data. Injury mortality was estimated using the Cause of Death Ensemble Modeling (CODEm) to generate the best fit to the available mortality data. Estimates for deaths were generated for 22 causes of injuries, 40 age-sex groups, for all countries from 1980 through 2010.

GBD 2010 estimated the burden of nonfatal outcomes of injuries by first constructing estimates of the incidence of the external causes of injuries using household survey data, hospital data, and the injury mortality estimates. Next, the incidence of external causes was mapped to the incidence of sequelae using hospital data. Next, prevalence of injuries was estimated using durations and proportions of cases that experience long-term disability. YLD were computed by applying disability weights.

only be inferred (Box 2-2). With the notable exceptions of burns and traumatic brain injury, most sequelae of injuries relate to musculoskeletal trauma (see Fig. 2-6). Fractures result in 13.9 million severe nonfatal injuries, 40% of all nonfatal injuries, and account for 40% of the health burden (YLD) of nonfatal injuries. Almost one third of this burden (31%) is due to fractures of the patella, tibia, fibula, and ankle. Femur fractures, which only account for 6% of severe nonfatal injuries, nevertheless account for 15% of the burden because of the substantially higher morbidity per injury of these fractures. Thus, lower limb fractures together account for almost half of the burden of nonfatal fractures. In addition to fractures, there are approximately 0.49 million nonfatal amputations every year, 90% of which are finger amputations. Amputations account for 1.4% of severe nonfatal injuries and 1.5% of the health loss from nonfatal injuries. Finally, there are 0.51 million dislocations per year that result in permanent disability (other dislocations of lesser severity are not included in this number), which account for 1.4% of severe nonfatal injuries and 2.2% of the health loss from nonfatal injuries. In total, there are 14.9 million known musculoskeletal injuries per year, which account for 42.4% of severe nonfatal injuries and 43.2% of the health loss from nonfatal injuries.

In addition, although three conditions (open wounds, injuries requiring urgent care, and injuries requiring emergency care) in Figure 2-6 include other trauma as well, musculoskeletal trauma constitutes a substantial proportion of these sequelae. Although not disaggregated further in the Global Burden of Disease, Injuries and Risk Factors (GBD) 2010 report, the injuries classified to open wounds and superficial injuries, which alone constitutes more than one third of the health burden (34%), includes dislocations with short-term disability, sprains and strains of ligaments, contusions, and injuries of muscles and tendons. Data regarding the burden of injury in the United States[6] shows that these types of nonfracture injuries (open wounds, sprains/strains, contusions, and dislocations) amount to roughly half of the hospitalizations resulting from fractures. If this proportion were assumed to apply globally, it would result in an estimate of 22.4 million severe musculoskeletal injuries per year, which account for 71.1% of severe nonfatal injuries.

FOCUS ON MILITARY INJURIES

Since 2001, the U.S. military has been engaged in two extended ground campaigns and occupations. The shift away from gunshot wounds and toward explosive mechanisms has resulted in the need for changes in military medical care. This focus on massive contaminated wounds and mangled extremities from explosive mechanisms is most similar to reports from the Israeli military over recent years. As these conflicts draw to a close, the legacy of the medical advances will hopefully be exportable to civilian trauma care.

The U.S. military is an organization of approximately 1,000,000 active-duty service members at any given time. The recent conflicts in Iraq and Afghanistan have resulted in the activation of many reservists, which makes the denominator for injuries somewhat confusing. However, recent reports have illuminated the burden of musculoskeletal injuries that result from peacetime operations and training as well as combat operations.

Musculoskeletal (MSK) injuries comprise the majority of all injuries to personnel deployed to a war zone. The injuries sustained as the result of direct enemy contact are classified as battle injuries, and early reports using the Joint Theater Trauma Registry (JTTR) suggested that MSK wounds are 55% of all wounds, which is consistent with prior wars. However, the biggest difference noted was the mechanism of injury, with wounds resulting from explosive blasts (i.e., improvised explosive devices [IEDs]) predominating in contrast to previous conflicts, which saw more wounds from small-arms fire.[7]

The same authors further described the MSK wounds in this cohort,[8] and found that of 3575 battle injury wounds evaluated, 53% were penetrating soft-tissue wounds, while 26% were fractures. This last finding was noted to be consistent with previous wars that had records available.

Fractures were evenly distributed between the upper and lower extremities (50%-50%). Among the upper extremity fractures, the hand comprised the greatest proportion of injuries (36%). In the lower extremity, 48% of fractures were of the tibia or fibula, which is concerning given the thin soft tissue envelope in this region. A total of 82% of all fractures were open, highlighting the importance of orthopaedic surgical and wound care.

The same group performed a cost-utilization analysis performed using billing data,[9] and found that while MSK wounds accounted for only 54% of all wounds, they also consumed 65% of all inpatient care costs as well as 64% of all disability costs (see Fig. 2-1). Contrary to popular belief, MSK injuries and conditions represented approximately twice the proportion of head and neck injuries, healthcare resource utilization, and disability costs when compared to head and neck injuries.

An examination of the rates of repeat hospitalization in this cohort found a similar trend.[10] Extremity injuries accounted for 64% of all hospital readmissions, 66% of inpatient days, and 67% of all costs.

Subsequent work by Belmont and colleagues followed a brigade combat team (approximately 4000 soldiers) during a 15-month deployment to Iraq during the "Surge" in 2007, a time with some of the heaviest fighting in that war.[11] This removed some of the selection bias seen in the JTTR and other single-center studies; however, the overall wounding patterns were confirmed.[12] Further analysis of this cohort showed that in addition to the battle injuries, the nonbattle injuries had an even larger burden of disease and injury. There were 167 MSK battle injuries, 62 of which were medically evacuated from theater, compared with 667 MSK nonbattle injuries of which 57 were evacuated.[13]

And on return from theater, 19% of the cohort received orthopaedic consultation and 4% an orthopaedic surgical procedure for nonemergent MSK injuries that were treated conservatively in theater.[13,14] The anterior cruciate ligament disruption and first-time shoulder dislocation incidence rates from noncombat injuries are nearly five times greater than that of the civilian population and similar to the endemic rates found in the nondeployed military population,[15] and is indicative of the daily rigors of the combat environment. Further examination of the previously cited brigade combat team service members who completed a combat deployment revealed that 19% had an orthopaedic surgical consultation on return and 4% required an orthopaedic surgical procedure, with greater than 50% of these involving the knee or shoulder.

This work on MSK nonbattle injuries shows that disease and nonbattle injuries are an even greater problem affecting the readiness of soldiers than combat wounds. These nonbattle injuries have received relatively little attention in the literature and certainly in the press; however, the impact of these injuries is tremendous.

Even in a peacetime military, these nonbattle injuries are endemic. In a database study of nondeployed service members in 2006, Hauret and colleagues reported 743,547 MSK conditions, which is a rate of 628/1000 person-years. This study did not even report on the approximately 1,000,000 MSK injuries coded using the 800 International Classification of Diseases, Ninth Revision (ICD-9) series.[16] Other studies focusing on a particular pathologic process suggest that sprains of major joints occur at a rate that is an order of magnitude greater than the reported rates in the civilian populations. This has been reported for ankle sprains,[17] shoulder dislocations,[18] patella dislocations,[19] and knee anterior cruciate ligament tears.[15]

MSK injuries are endemic in the military population. This holds true across the spectrum of injuries, from combat wounds on the battlefield to joint sprains sustained during training. Study of this unique population can have an impact on both military readiness as well as the care of injured civilians.

REFERENCES

1. Murray CJ, Lopez AD: *The global burden of disease: a comprehensive assessment of mortality and disability from diseases, injuries, and risk factors in 1990 and projected to 2020*, Cambridge, MA, 1996, Harvard University Press.
2. Multiple Authors: Global and regional mortality from 235 causes of death for 20 age groups in 1990 and 2010: a systematic analysis for the Global Burden of Disease Study 2010. *Lancet* 2012 Dec 13(380):2095–2128, 2012a.
3. Multiple Authors: Years lived with disability (YLDs) for 1160 sequelae of 289 diseases and injuries, 1990–2010: a systematic analysis for the Global Burden of Disease Study 2010. *Lancet* 2012 Dec 13(380):2163–2196, 2012b.
4. Multiple Authors: Disability-adjusted life years (DALYs) for 291 diseases and injuries in 21 regions, 1990–2010: a systematic analysis for the Global Burden of Disease Study 2010. *Lancet* 2012 Dec 13(380):2197–2223, 2012c.
5. Multiple Authors: Common values in assessing health outcomes from disease and injury: disability weights measurement study for the Global Burden of Disease Study 2010. *Lancet* 2012 Dec 13(380):2129–2143, 2012d.
6. United States Bone and Joint Initiative: *The Burden of musculoskeletal diseases in the United States*, ed 2, Rosemont, IL, 2011, American Academy of Orthopaedic Surgeons.
7. Owens BD, Kragh JF Jr, Wenke JC, et al: Combat wounds in operation Iraqi Freedom and operation Enduring Freedom. *J Trauma* 64:295–299, 2008.
8. Owens BD, Kragh JF Jr, Macaitis J, et al: Characterization of extremity wounds in Operation Iraqi Freedom and Operation Enduring Freedom. *J Orthop Trauma* 21:254–257, 2007.
9. Masini BD, Waterman SM, Wenke JC, et al: Resource utilization and disability outcome assessment of combat casualties from Operation Iraqi Freedom and Operation Enduring Freedom. *J Orthop Trauma* 23:261–266, 2009.
10. Masini BD, Owens BD, Hsu JR, et al: Rehospitalization after combat injury. *J Trauma* 71:S98–S102, 2011.
11. Belmont PJ Jr, Goodman GP, Zacchilli M, et al: Incidence and epidemiology of combat injuries sustained during "the surge" portion of operation Iraqi Freedom by a U.S. Army brigade combat team. *J Trauma* 68:204–210, 2010.

12. Belmont PJ Jr, Thomas D, Goodman GP, et al: Combat musculoskeletal wounds in a US Army Brigade Combat Team during operation Iraqi Freedom. *J Trauma* 71:E1–E7, 2010.
13. Belmont PJ Jr, Goodman GP, Waterman B, et al: Disease and nonbattle injuries sustained by a U.S. Army Brigade Combat Team during Operation Iraqi Freedom. *Mil Med* 175:469–476, 2010.
14. Goodman GP, Schoenfeld AJ, Owens BD, et al: Non-emergent orthopaedic injuries sustained by soldiers in Operation Iraqi Freedom. *J Bone Joint Surg Am* 94:728–735, 2012.
15. Owens BD, Mountcastle SB, Dunn WR, et al: Incidence of anterior cruciate ligament injury among active duty U.S. military servicemen and servicewomen. *Mil Med* 172:90–91, 2007.
16. Hauret KG, Taylor BJ, Clemmons NS, et al: Frequency and causes of nonbattle injuries air evacuated from Operations Iraqi Freedom and Enduring Freedom, U.S. Army, 2001-2006. *Am J Prev Med* 38:S94–S107, 2010.
17. Owens BD, Dawson L, Burks R, et al: Incidence of shoulder dislocation in the United States military: demographic considerations from a high-risk population. *J Bone Joint Surg Am* 91:791–796, 2009.
18. Hsiao M, Owens BD, Burks R, et al: Incidence of acute traumatic patellar dislocation among active-duty United States military service members. *Am J Sports Med* 38:1997–2004, 2010.
19. Waterman BR, Owens BD, Davey S, et al: The epidemiology of ankle sprains in the United States. *J Bone Joint Surg Am* 92:2279–2284, 2010.

Chapter 3

The Challenges of Orthopaedic Trauma Care in the Developing World

RICHARD A. GOSSELIN • CHARLES N. MOCK • MANJUL JOSHIPURA • DAVID A. SPIEGEL • DAVID W. SHEARER • LEWIS G. ZIRKLE • R. RICHARD COUGHLIN

INTRODUCTION

This chapter proposes an overview of the challenges in meeting the increasing needs for trauma care in low- and middle-income countries (LMICs). The epidemiologic aspects of the burden of injuries are discussed elsewhere in this book (see Chapter 2), as well as nonsurgical management of fractures (see Chapter 6) so a special effort was made to keep overlaps to a minimum. Topics addressed include systematic approach to trauma care, barriers to access, resources, education, the role of the World Health Organization (WHO), management of common pediatric and adult injuries, with special mention of the Surgical Implant Generation Network (SIGN) system, and different avenues for orthopaedic volunteerism.

For most high-income country (HIC) surgeons, trauma care is synonymous with surgical treatment. This is not the case for LMICs: Most trauma care, at least initially, is provided in the informal sector (traditional healers, bone setters, nurses, pharmacists, etc.), and most of the care provided in the formal sector is conservative (i.e., nonsurgical). The benefits of appropriate surgical over conservative management, in appropriate environments, are well documented for many orthopaedic injuries, starting with this textbook. For myriad reasons detailed below, this is too often unavailable in resource-poor settings, where results of conservative treatment are standard of care. The worldwide increases in economic development, life expectancy, and motorization translate into an epidemiologic transition from communicable diseases to noncommunicable diseases and injuries (GBD 2010).[1] There is proportionally less premature death and more life lived with disability. The burden of injuries is disproportionally shouldered by LMICs: The 2013 WHO report on global road safety showed that 94% of all traffic deaths and 90% of disability related to road traffic injuries (RTIs) occur in LMICs.[2] Estimates are that RTIs alone killed more than 1,250,000 people in 2010, permanently disabled the same number, and temporarily disabled between 10 and 50 times more. An aging population comes with an increase in "insufficiency fractures" and degenerative joint disease (DJD) and inflammatory arthropathies (IAs). All these combine to create a "perfect orthopaedic storm," and resources to manage it are woefully lagging behind. The following sections will discuss and analyze the necessary determinants to best meet these daunting challenges.

IMPROVING TRAUMA CARE SYSTEMWIDE GLOBALLY: THE WORLD HEALTH ORGANIZATION'S ESSENTIAL TRAUMA CARE PROJECT

Background

Injury has become a huge global health problem. Each year more than 5 million people die from motor vehicle crashes, violence, and other forms of injury. Ninety percent of these injury deaths occur in LMICs. In addition to the need for improvements in injury prevention, such as road safety, there is a need for improvements in trauma care globally. One study showed significant disparities in outcome after injury among countries at different economic levels. Case fatality rates for serious injuries (Injury Severity Score > 9) rose from 35% in high-income Seattle, Washington, to 55% in middle-income Monterrey, Mexico, to 63% in low-income Kumasi, Ghana.[3] Thus, mortality rates for the seriously injured are nearly twice as high in low-income settings as in high-income settings. If we could eliminate these disparities and bring injury case fatality rates in LMICs down from their current high rates to the rates in high-income countries, we could potentially save 2,000,000 lives per year.[4]

Many millions more people are left with temporary or permanent disabilities from their injuries. One of the leading causes of injury-related disability is extremity injury. One study from Ghana showed that the vast majority (78%) of injury related disability is due to extremity injuries, in comparison to a higher proportion of disability from more-difficult-to-treat neurologic injuries in HICs.[5] Disabilities from such extremity injuries should be readily amenable to improvements in orthopaedic care and rehabilitation.

These discrepancies in outcome are due to several types of problems, such as deficiencies in human resources (skills, training, staffing) and physical resources (equipment, supplies). Improving these resources is often hampered by financial restrictions, with many countries having only small sums per capita per year to spend on health. Despite these barriers, many committed individuals and their institutions have been making notable progress, often working against considerable odds. A few brief examples are presented in the next section.

Case Studies of Individual Institutions

In the prehospital setting, an increased number of ambulance stations (to allow more rapid dispatch) decreased the response times to reach injured victims in Mexico. Improved training, in the form of more regular use of in-service courses, led to improved process of care in the field. The net result was a decrease in mortality from 8.2% to 4.7% among transported trauma patients.[6,7]

In the hospital setting, regular use of continuing medical education for trauma care (in the form of the Advanced Trauma Life Support Course) led to significant improvements in the use of appropriate treatments for severely injured patients in Trinidad. The net result was a decrease in the mortality of such seriously injured patients at the main hospital caring for injured patients in Trinidad, from 67% to 34%.[8,9]

In Thailand, the main trauma hospital in Khon Kaen instituted a basic trauma quality improvement program. This program identified a high rate of medically preventable deaths and several correctable problems, such as inadequate resuscitation for shock, delayed surgery for head injuries, and problems with record keeping and communications. Low-cost corrective action was instituted to target these problems, including improved communication within the hospital by use of radios, better supervision of junior doctors through increased senior staffing in the emergency department at peak times, and improved reporting on and monitoring of trauma cases. These improvements resulted in a decrease in mortality among all admitted trauma patients from 6.1% to 4.4%.[10]

In terms of orthopaedic care, one hospital in Malawi instituted a protocol for open fractures that emphasized primary external fixation, scheduled sequential débridement, coverage of exposed bone through local muscle flaps, controlled secondary healing, and early mobilization, all low-cost techniques that could be practiced well in the local circumstances and within the economic resources available. They reported recovery of normal function in 80% of patients, functional results similar to those from HICs.[11,12]

These are obviously just a few brief examples. Many of the readers of this textbook likely have similar success stories to report on from their own institutions. The question now is how to build on such individual institution experiences and make more progress globally.

Global Efforts to Improve Trauma Care

There are several potential avenues to pursue to promote improvements in trauma care globally, such as through international professional societies. Another avenue that has been increasingly influential but which many clinicians are not as familiar with is WHO. In this section, we highlight some of the work being done on trauma care by WHO.

In the past 10 years, WHO's Department of Violence and Injury Prevention and Disability published two sets of policy recommendations, primarily aimed for ministries of health. Prehospital Trauma Care Systems[13] gives recommendations on ways to institute or improve formal ambulance services (i.e., emergency medical services [EMS]). It also addresses steps that can be taken in areas where such formal ambulance systems are not affordable or feasible. This includes such efforts as building on existing, informal systems of prehospital transport and care, such as by providing training (and where appropriate providing equipment) and better organizing those members of society who are already providing prehospital first aid, such as fire service, police, commercial drivers, or other members of the lay public.

TABLE 3-1 *ESSENTIAL TRAUMA CARE SERVICES*

- Obstructed airways are opened and maintained before hypoxia leads to death or permanent disability.
- Impaired breathing is supported until the injured person is able to breathe adequately without assistance.
- Pneumothorax and hemothorax are promptly recognized and relieved.
- Bleeding (external or internal) is promptly stopped.
- Shock is recognized and treated with intravenous (IV) fluid replacement before irreversible consequences occur.
- The consequences of traumatic brain injury are lessened by timely decompression of space-occupying lesions and by prevention of secondary brain injury.
- Intestinal and other abdominal injuries are promptly recognized and repaired.
- Potentially disabling extremity injuries are corrected.
- Potentially unstable spinal cord injuries are recognized and managed appropriately, including early immobilization.
- The consequences to the individual of injuries that result in physical impairment are minimized by appropriate rehabilitative services.
- Medications for the above services and for the minimization of pain are readily available when needed.

Source: *From Mock CN, Lormand JD, Goosen J, et al: Guidelines for essential trauma care. Geneva, World Health Organization, 2004.*

In terms of care at hospitals and clinics, WHO worked collaboratively with the International Society of Surgery and other partners to create the Guidelines for Essential Trauma Care.[14] The goal of this project was to set reasonable, affordable, minimum standards for trauma care services worldwide and to define the resources needed to actually provide these services even in the poorest parts of the poorest countries. In part, this publication sought to do for trauma care globally what the Committee on Trauma (COT) of the American College of Surgeons (ACS) has done for trauma care in North America with its Resources for Optimal Care of the Injured Patient.[15] However, the recommendations were oriented for countries that had only ten to hundreds of dollars per capita to spend for health, versus thousands of dollars per capita in HICs.

The Guidelines for Essential Trauma Care lays out 11 core essential services that every injured person should realistically be able to receive (Table 3-1). The International Society of Surgery has endorsed these as the "Rights of the Injured."[16,17]

To assure the availability of these services, the Guidelines for Essential Trauma Care delineate 260 individual items of human resources (skills, training, staffing) and physical resources (equipment and supplies) that should be in place at the range of healthcare facilities globally, going from small rural clinics, to small hospitals, to large hospitals, to tertiary centers. Items are designed as either essential, meaning they are applicable in countries at all economic levels, or designated as desirable, referring to those that are more costly, and more applicable in middle-income circumstances or in larger hospitals in low-income countries. These resource recommendations were intended to be a flexible matrix, to be adjusted based on the circumstances of the particular country. Addressed in these 260 items is the spectrum of trauma care, including initial resuscitation, definitive care of injuries to all body regions, and longer term rehabilitation. Orthopaedic issues are addressed in several sections of these recommendations, including extremity injury, spinal injury, and rehabilitation.

General examples of what these recommendations are trying to promote, first looking at low-income circumstances as in most of Africa and much of Asia are below:

A. Rural clinics caring for the injured should have capabilities for rapid basic first aid, which many do not. It is important to note that in rural areas of low-income countries, much of care of the injured, even seriously injured, does occur in such small rural facilities.
B. Smaller hospitals (such as those staffed by general practitioners) should have capabilities for placement of chest tubes, airway maintenance, and certain minimum blood transfusion capabilities, which many do not have.
C. Larger hospitals, including tertiary care centers, should have capabilities for endotracheal intubation on an emergency basis (which is problematic for many) and basic trauma quality improvement programs, which very few have.
D. Similar recommendations pertain to middle-income countries. However, there is greater emphasis on the resource items categorized as "desirable" given the higher level of resources available.[12,16-18]

The Guidelines for Essential Trauma Care were intended to be part planning guide for individual hospitals and clinics and for ministries of health and part advocacy statement to be used by whoever wishes to promote improvements in trauma care in their area. Through both of these mechanisms, it was hoped that the Guidelines would serve as a catalyst to promote real, on-the-ground improvements in trauma care globally. Although much more does need to be done, there has been considerable progress in implementing the Guidelines. The Guidelines have received high-level political endorsement from a wide range of individual country professional groups, including the Ghana Medical Society, the Academy of Traumatology (India), and the Mexican Association for the Medicine and Surgery of Trauma, among others.[19] They have been used in developing national health policy in Colombia, Mexico, Sri Lanka, and Vietnam.[10,19]

The Guidelines have also been the basis for systemwide needs assessments in several countries, providing for the first time an internationally applicable metric for countries at all levels to use to assess their hospitals and trauma systems.[20-24] These needs assessments give some idea of priorities for ways in which trauma care can be strengthened cost-effectively and systematically. These assessments have addressed orthopaedic care. Selected items of relevance to orthopaedics from these assessments are included in Table 3-2. In terms of human resources, large hospitals were fairly well staffed by fully trained orthopaedic surgeons, except in Africa, where general surgeons did much of the orthopaedic work. At small hospitals, only those in better-resourced Mexico had partial coverage by orthopedists. At other smaller hospitals, either general surgeons or general practitioners provided care for orthopaedic injuries, with this level of hospital being solely staffed by general practitioners at the hospitals evaluated in Ghana.

With nonspecialists providing much of the orthopaedic and other trauma care, continuing education courses are an important opportunity to strengthen such care. All four countries had such courses available, such as Advanced Trauma Life Support (ATLS) in Mexico, National Trauma Management Course (NTMC) in India, or other similar locally developed courses in the other countries. However, coverage by such courses was suboptimal. In small hospitals, far less than 50% of frontline trauma care providers (e.g., doctors working in the emergency department [ED] or surgeons taking trauma call) had such training. Even in large hospitals, in most countries, less than 50% of frontline trauma care providers had such training. The situation for continuing education for nurses was even lower (see Table 3-2).

Capabilities for rehabilitation were particularly deficient. Ratings showed significant deficiencies in the availability of human resources for rehabilitation, whether fully trained physician specialists or other providers such as physical therapists (PTs), were considered. PT coverage was especially limited in availability at small hospitals (see Table 3-2).

In terms of physical resources for care of extremity injuries, the main essential items for orthopaedic trauma care were fairly well supplied at big hospitals. Portable radiography was limited. Capabilities at small hospitals were much more limited. It should be pointed out that the ratings pertain to the level of care that would be expected for *that* level, not for the highest level. Hence, these are the ratings compared to the essential trauma care standard for small hospitals, not large. Related to the shortages of human resources for rehabilitation, availability of prosthesis for amputees was extremely limited in all circumstances (see Table 3-2).

Many times the problems with availability of physical resources were not the presence or absence of the equipment, but periods of inactivity while waiting for repairs, lack of supplies (such as film), or requirements for payment in advance before receiving services, which limited the availability of diagnostic tests to all who needed them. There were several instances in which mismatch of human and physical resources decreased availability of some services. For example, in Ghana, one large hospital had an image intensifier (C-arm). However, there were no staff trained to use it and the machine lay idle. In India, several small hospitals had radiography machines and trained staff. However, the facilities were greatly limited in the number of plates (films) which they received each month. Thus many persons needing radiographs could not receive them. Many such problems could be easily remedied cost-effectively by better organization and planning.[12,24]

In all countries and at all levels, there was a dearth of administrative functions to monitor and assure the availability of trauma care, including trauma registries and trauma quality improvement programs.

In addition to pointing out opportunities for affordable and sustainable improvements in trauma care capabilities, these needs assessments have served as a stimulus for action. For example, a needs assessment conducted in the network of healthcare facilities managed by the Hanoi Health Department in Vietnam showed multiple deficiencies in low-cost but important items of human training and physical resources. These items were addressed by improved organization and planning, with no additional budgetary allotment for trauma care. Repeat assessments every 2 to 3 years since that time have documented steady improvement in availability of both skills levels and physical resources.[10,21]

Further details of the development and implementation of the Guidelines for Essential Trauma Care and the related Essential Trauma Care Project are available on the WHO

TABLE 3-2 *RESOURCES FOR MANAGEMENT OF ORTHOPAEDIC INJURIES AT 49 HOSPITALS IN FOUR COUNTRIES (GHANA, VIETNAM, INDIA, AND MEXICO)*

	Small Hospital				Large Hospital			
	G	V	I	M	G	V	I	M
Number of facilities evaluated	8	8	14	4	2	5	1	7
Human resources: acute care								
Nurse in emergency department	2	3	2	2	2	3	3	2
Doctor for emergency call*	2	3	3	3	3	3	3	3
General surgeon*	1	2	1	2	2	3	3	3
Orthopaedic surgeon*	0	0	0	2	0	3	3	3
CE course for doctors†	1	1	0	1	1	1	1	2
CE course for nurses‡	0	1	0	1	0	1	0	1
Physical resources: extremity injury								
Skeletal traction	1	1	0	1	2	3	3	3
External fixation	0	1	0	1	1	3	3	2
Internal fixation	0	2	0	1	1	3	3	2
X-ray	1	2	2	3	2	3	3	3
Portable x-ray	1	0	0	1	2	1	2	3
Image intensification	0	0	0	0	0	1	1	1
Limb prosthetics	0	0	0	0	0	0	0	1
Physical resources: spinal injury								
Operative capabilities for spine management	NA	NA	NA	NA	0	1	1	3
Physical resources: wound care								
Skin grafting	1	2	1	2	2	3	3	3
Tetanus prophylaxis (toxoid and antiserum)	3	3	3	3	3	3	3	3
Human resources: rehabilitation								
Specialized rehabilitative nursing	NA	NA	NA	NA	0	1	0	2
Physical therapy	1	1	0	1	1	3	1	2
Physical medicine and rehabilitation specialist	NA	NA	NA	NA	0	2	1	2
Administrative functions								
Trauma-related quality improvement program	NA	NA	NA	NA	0	0	0	0
Trauma cases integrated into broader quality improvement programs	0	2	0	1	1	2	1	1
Trauma registry with severity adjustment	NA	NA	NA	NA	0	0	0	0

Adequacy of resource based on Guidelines for Essential Trauma Care assessed as:
NA (not applicable for that level);
0 (absent);
1 (inadequate, available to less than 50% of those who need it);
2 (partly adequate, available to greater than 50%, but not everyone who needs it);
3 (adequate, available to virtually everyone who needs it).

Facility descriptions:

- Small hospital: in Africa called district, in India called community health center. Usually doing some type of surgery, but with more limited range of specialist. Usually with around 50–200 beds.
- Large hospital: provincial, regional, with at least one or more category of specialist, usually >200 beds. But not including tertiary care centers.

Data from Arreola-Risa C, Mock C, Vega Rivera F, et al: Evaluating trauma care capabilities in Mexico with the World Health Organization's Guidelines for Essential Trauma Care, Pan Am J Public Health 19: 94–103, 2006; Mock CN, Nguyen S, Quansah R, et al: Evaluation of trauma care capabilities in four countries using the WHO-IATSIC Guidelines for Essential Trauma Care, World J Surg 30:946–956, 2006; Nguyen S, Mock CN: Improvements in trauma care capabilities in Vietnam through use of the WHO-IATSIC Guidelines for Essential Trauma Care, Int J Inj Contr Saf Promot 13:125–127, 2006; Nguyen TS, Nguyen HT, Nguyen THT, et al: Assessment of the status of resources for essential trauma care in Hanoi and Khanh Hoa, Vietnam, Injury 38:1014–1022, 2007; Quansah R, Mock CN, Abantanga F: Status of trauma care in Ghana, Ghana Med J 38:149–152, 2004.

CE, Continuing education; *G*, Ghana; *I*, India; *M*, Mexico; *NA*, not applicable; *V*, Vietnam.

*Available 24 hours per day, 7 days per week in hospital or promptly available on call from home.

†CE course on trauma care, such as Advanced Trauma Life Support, National Trauma Management Course, or local equivalent: ideal is that all doctors who provide first-line trauma care in emergency department and all general surgeons who provide trauma care are credentialed in such an in-service training course.

‡CE course on trauma care, such as Trauma Nursing Core Course or local equivalent: ideal is that all nurses who provide first-line trauma care in emergency department are credentialed in such an in-service training course.

website (www.who.int/violence_injury_prevention/services/en/ and www.who.int/violence_injury_prevention/services/traumacare/en/index.html).

THE ROLE OF THE WORLD HEALTH ORGANIZATION: THE WORLD HEALTH ASSEMBLY RESOLUTION ON TRAUMA AND EMERGENCY CARE SERVICES AND THE CREATION OF THE GLOBAL ALLIANCE FOR CARE OF THE INJURED

In an effort to promote greater implementation of improvements in trauma care, two additional actions have been taken: adoption of World Health Assembly Resolution 60.22 and creation of the Global Alliance for Care of the Injured.

In 2007, the World Health Assembly (WHA) adopted a resolution on trauma and emergency care services: WHA 60.22 "Health Systems: Emergency Care Systems." The WHA is the governing board of the WHO. It consists of the ministers of health of all 194 member states. Its resolutions direct WHO's activities and carry considerable influence on policies in individual countries, as well as actions of nongovernmental organizations (NGOs) and funders.

WHA Resolution 60.22 called on governments to improve care for victims of injury and other medical emergencies and listed 10 actions that governments could take to achieve this, including things such as identifying a core set of trauma services and developing methods to assure and document that such services are provided to all who need them (recommendations directly from the Guidelines for Essential Trauma Care).

This WHA resolution was probably the single greatest expression of support for trauma care from governments worldwide. WHA resolutions carry a lot of weight in orienting WHO's own activities. However, they are taken up variably by country governments. They are most useful if concerned individuals and organizations use a resolution to advocate for and promote its recommendations. In this regard, readers are referred to a recent publication,[60] which gives some suggestions about how the resolution can be used to promote increased political support for trauma care within country governments and to lobby for increased funding. It also contains the full text of the WHA resolution.

In 2012, WHO founded the Global Alliance for Care of the Injured, in collaboration with a number of other stakeholders. These include a number of international professional societies, NGOs, and country governments. The Global Alliance is primarily oriented toward promoting advocacy for increased attention to trauma care. Further information on the Global Alliance and ways in which to become involved with it can be found at the WHO website on violence and injury prevention (www.who.int/violence_injury_prevention/services/gaci/en/).

There are many examples of successful innovative programs and efforts improving trauma care at individual hospitals in LMICs. There is a need to expand on what is being done and make more sustained progress globally. The WHO's Guidelines for Essential Trauma Care represents a method to accomplish this by providing for the first time an internationally applicable metric for countries to use to evaluate and monitor resources for trauma care in their hospitals and systemwide. Further, WHA Resolution 60.22 on trauma and emergency care services provides high-level political endorsement for improvements in trauma care globally. Likewise, the creation of the WHO Global Alliance for Care of the Injured provides an avenue for increased political advocacy for increased attention to and investment in trauma care. Orthopedists and other trauma care clinicians can effectively use all of these in their own efforts to promote systemwide improvements in trauma care in the areas where they work.[25]

In addition to the technical aspects, trauma care must be viewed within broader societal and economic considerations. Although much can be improved in trauma care by better organization, planning, and training, more extensive improvements are hampered by poverty. Most countries can spend only very little on health. In addition specific policies of international organizations compound the problem. For example, World Trade Organization rules keep many medicines unaffordable for the average person in the world. World Bank and International Monetary Fund policies often dictate restrictions on how much some governments can spend on healthcare as part of loan repayment conditions. Some African countries spend more on repaying debt than they do on healthcare.

Care of the injured would be strengthened by measures that would allow greater funding of the health sector, including many measures currently being discussed, such as debt relief, relaxation of restrictions on health sector financing, and requiring World Trauma Organization proceedings and rulemaking to be open and democratic, which they currently are not. In addition to our own technical work, we as individuals and as societies of professionals, need to be aware of and address these bigger global economic issues.[26,27]

BARRIERS TO ACCESS

Only a fraction of the population in LMICs will ever receive treatment from a trained orthopaedic surgeon. Gross deficiencies in the availability, utilization, and/or quality of orthopaedic services result in an enormous burden of disability in LMICs, and the magnitude has yet to be quantified using existing health metrics.[28-33] The barriers to accessing care for orthopaedic injuries are complex, often overlap, and relate to both an individual's willingness to seek medical attention and the ability of the health system to provide timely, effective, safe, and affordable services. The relative importance of individual barriers will, of course, depend on the local context. Improving the delivery of musculoskeletal trauma care services will require a multidisciplinary, multisectoral effort aimed at eliminating these barriers by educating patients and their families and also addressing deficiencies at the level of the health system. Strong advocacy efforts, including the mobilization of key stakeholders and civil society, will be required to influence decision makers.

The definition of "access" has been debated, and several authors have attempted to describe it.[34-37] McIntyre and colleagues suggested that access be viewed as a multidimensional concept based on the interaction of individuals and the health system, and defined access based on availability (spatial access), affordability (financial access), and acceptability (cultural access).[36] Obrist and colleagues suggested availability, affordability, acceptability, accessibility, and adequacy, highlighting the importance of the quality of services.[35] A systematic review concerning barriers to surgical care suggested that these be grouped according to (1) social/cultural, (2) financial, and (3) structural.[38] The authors emphasized the importance of cultural factors, and stressed the need to overcome financial and geographic accessibility.

From a practical standpoint, barriers may be characterized based on the individual and the health system, which resonates with a health system framework promoted by WHO. This focuses on the interrelationship between people (demand) and six system "building blocks" (supply) including (1) governance, (2) service delivery, (3) human resources, (4) medicines and technologies, (5) financing, and (6) information.[39] Table 3-3 illustrates a host of barriers according to this scheme, as well as measures that may be considered to address these barriers.

Factors which lead a patient and/or his or her family to use health services have received less attention than system-level barriers. In the absence of formal medical services, a sizeable percentage of the rural population in LMICs likely prefer to have their injured cared for by traditional healers and bonesetters for a variety of reasons. Out-of-pocket expenses commonly serve as a deterrent to using formal health services, and thousands of families in LMICs are pushed below the poverty line each year because of unforeseen healthcare costs. In some settings there may be a fear of hospitals or of receiving surgical care. These issues can only be addressed by first studying perceptions concerning injuries and facilities-based care within the local communities, and then engaging the community in discussions and perhaps educational programs. Another solution may be to engage the traditional practitioners, gain a better understanding of their treatment methods, and then work with them to develop the system for service delivery. Any such efforts will fall short of expectations unless quality services are available to the public.

On the health system side, with regard to governance, few countries have included surgical care in their national health plans, and we estimate that few countries have developed, implemented, and monitored the policies and regulations to support the provision of trauma care services. As such, mandates at the local, regional, and global levels should be sought to promote and enforce such standards. Political support will be required to move the agenda forward, and this may also be viewed as a barrier.[40] Shiffman has developed a conceptual framework to explain why certain global health issues receive attention and others do not, based on (1) the power of the actors, (2) the power of ideas portraying the issue (frames), (3) the political contexts in which the actors operate, and (4)

TABLE 3-3 *BARRIERS TO THE DELIVERY OF ORTHOPAEDIC CARE*

Barriers				**Possible Solutions**
Demand side	Patient and family	Culture and/or religious beliefs	• Negative social stigma to certain conditions • Fear of hospitals or of surgical care • Perceived severity of condition • Influence of family and/or friends • Preference for traditional healers • Illiteracy or lower educational level	• Educational programs at community level to enhance awareness of selected health conditions, promote early referral, increase acceptance of formal medical services • Work with community leaders, including religious leaders, to enhance educational programs
		Financial	• Direct costs of treatment including transportation • Indirect costs (time off from work)	• Develop insurance programs (risk pooling) • Public-private partnerships • Partnership with nongovernmental organizations (NGOs) or global health initiatives
		Geographic	Distance Terrain Season and weather Mechanism of transportation	• Improve road infrastructure and mechanisms for transportation • Improve distribution of health facilities
Supply side	Health system	Governance	Policies	• Incorporate emergency and essential surgical care into national health plan
			Monitoring and oversight Lack of trauma care guidelines	• Consider implementing World Health Organization (WHO) Guidelines for Essential Trauma Care
		Service delivery	Infrastructure	• Investment in facilities
			Physical resources and supplies	• Investment in operating costs
			Mechanisms for transport and referral	• Develop and implement guidelines for referral • Establish communication links between facilities at different tiers of health system
			Convenience or hours of business	• Establish 24-hour services for trauma care

TABLE 3-3 ***BARRIERS TO THE DELIVERY OF ORTHOPAEDIC CARE*** (Continued)

Barriers		**Possible Solutions**
Human resources	Number of providers	• Task shifting • Include musculoskeletal surgical care in undergraduate and nonsurgical postgraduate training • Orthopaedic training programs • Regional orthopaedic educational opportunities • Specialist outreach • Surgical camps and mobile clinics • Educational programs for traditional practitioners to enhance skills and define indications for referral
	Distribution of providers	• Incentives for rural service • Formal linkage between levels within health system • Develop partnerships between academic institutions and rural facilities
	Education of providers or quality of service	• Telemedicine • Develop partnerships between academic institutions and rural facilities
	Gender	• More female providers in selected regions
	Job dissatisfaction	• Better remuneration • Opportunities for professional advancement • Continuing medical education • Better living conditions • Better opportunities for family (e.g., education of children)
Medicines and technology	Lack of essential equipment and supplies	• Promote and enforce standards for availability of equipment and supplies at each tier within health system
Health information system (HIS)	Inadequate data on orthopaedic burden of disease and epidemiology	• Develop and incorporate surgical metrics • Quality improvement (QI) initiatives
	Lack of monitoring (disease burden, service availability, outcomes)	• Incorporate monitoring into health information systems (HISs) • Use Global Information System (GIS) technology
Financing	Inadequate government expenditure on health	• Develop insurance programs Public-private partnerships • Partnership with NGOs or global health initiatives

the nature of the issue itself.[41,42] Insufficient data concerning the burden of musculoskeletal injuries, and a lack of metrics to capture the burden, precludes our ability to document the magnitude of the problem and capture the attention of decision makers and health planners. The global surgical community has been fragmented, and no single body has emerged to push an initiative to achieve universal access to essential surgical and trauma care. Musculoskeletal injuries are diverse, and fall within the larger initiative of trauma care, making it difficult to find a way to "frame" the issue. While the millennium development goals may be viewed as an excellent policy window, and improvements in musculoskeletal trauma care would certainly impact those goals related to alleviating poverty, maternal health, and child health, the window has yet to be captured.

Recognizing the importance of injury prevention, service delivery remains the cornerstone of musculoskeletal trauma care services. This requires an organized system including prehospital care, in-hospital care, and rehabilitation. Mechanisms for communication, transportation, and referral between tiers of the health system are critical. While healthcare programming over the past few decades has focused on "vertical" or disease-specific initiatives (human immunodeficiency virus (HIV)/acquired immunodeficiency syndrome (AIDS), tuberculosis, maternal health, etc.), improvements in health indicators have been realized but have often come at the expense of overall health system function. This has led to renewed interest in "horizontal" programming, efforts aimed at strengthening the health system, and promotion of universal access to extend services to the more remote and marginalized segments of a population. While surgical care has traditionally been neglected by the public health community because of the perception that it is resource intensive, costly, and benefits only a fraction of the population, evidence is amassing to refute these perceptions. As such, a worthy goal is to provide universal access to a package of "essential" musculoskeletal trauma care. These services are priority interventions that address conditions with the largest public health burden, are highly successful, and are cost-effective.[43] Essential surgical care, including trauma care, certainly resonates with the concepts of horizontal programming and health systems strengthening. The question, of course, is how they can be integrated into health systems. Specific interventions for musculoskeletal injuries will vary depending on the local context, but should likely include irrigation and débridement for open fractures, the closed treatment of common fractures and dislocations, skeletal traction, fasciotomy, and amputation. The use of more sophisticated treatments and/or technologies may be appropriate at secondary or tertiary referral facilities, depending on the local resources. WHO has developed guidelines to assist health planners with prehospital care and trauma care guidelines[13,14] and also developed a basic training package for the delivery of surgical and anesthetic services for the primary referral level of district hospital.[44-46] These materials serve as a starting point and can be augmented by other educational programs and training materials. Strengthening the delivery of services will require improvements in the availability of skilled providers, and also the provision of adequate infrastructure and physical resources to allow practitioners to care for patients. Mechanisms for financing must be available to support the delivery of services and minimize out of pocket expenses for patients. Recognizing that the development of insurance programs would be desirable, innovative financing solutions that are contextually relevant will need to be pursued such as public-private partnerships, or partnering with NGOs and/or global health initiatives. For example, stakeholders interested in maternal and child health might be interested in strengthening care for the injured to help reach those millennium development goals relating to child and maternal health.

Deficiencies in human resources have received the greatest attention in the literature, and relate to not only the absolute number of trained surgical providers, but also their distribution. The few surgeons tend to be located at tertiary centers in major cities, leaving most of the population without access to a trained surgical provider. Reasons cited for the problems with distribution include inadequate resources to deliver services, poor remuneration, few opportunities for continuing medical education and for career advancement, and limited opportunities for other family members, including education for their children. A sizeable number of patients will be treated by traditional healers. Strategies to address this human resource crisis have included the training of general surgeons, medical doctors, and/or paraprofessionals to provide surgical care (task shifting). Orthopaedic clinical officers (OCOs) care for the majority of orthopaedic problems in rural Malawi[47,48] and surgically trained paraprofessionals are active in several other countries in sub-Saharan Africa including Uganda and Mozambique. Surgeons from resource-rich countries may also contribute to the education and training of health providers caring for orthopaedic patients.

Even if caregivers have the appropriate knowledge and skills, they must have the resources, or medicines and technologies, to use their training. A host of studies have identified gross deficiencies in the availability of essential surgical services at the district hospital level in LMICs, including infrastructure and physical resources and supplies, in addition to human resources.[29-33,38,49-53] One report noted the similarities between modern-day facilities in LMICs and hospitals at the time of the U.S. Civil War.[54] Having a qualified surgical provider is hardly enough; he or she must have safe anesthesia, the basic equipment required to care for the injured, and the ability to adequately monitor the patient whether or not a surgical procedure is required.

Finally, the health information system (HIS) is responsible for data collection and analysis, as well as the dissemination of information to inform allocation of resources and the delivery of services. There is limited information on the burden of musculoskeletal injuries in LMICs, their economic impact, and on the efficacy and cost-effectiveness of interventions aimed at reducing the burden. Such knowledge is required to assess the burden of disease and unmet need for trauma care, the educational requirements for caregivers, the quality of service delivery, the impact of programs to strengthen the delivery of trauma care, and others. Research must be supported,[55] and monitoring and evaluation frameworks can be used to inform decision making, resource allocation, and track progress with health system interventions such as the integration of essential surgical care.

EDUCATION

With the increasing awareness of the enormous burden of injury and the stark disparity between developed and developing countries, recent initiatives have been established in an attempt to mitigate the impact. Through education and training of basic trauma care and principles, knowledge and skills can be transferred at the undergraduate, medical school, and postgraduate levels. To that end, professional societies and independent NGOs have been established targeting various aspects of education in trauma care in developing nations.

Among the more prominent professional societies is the International Association for Trauma Surgery and Intensive Care (IATSIC), an affiliate of the International Surgical Society (ISS).[56] The IATSIC was established in 1989 with a primary purpose of facilitating communication and education for the care of the injured. The educational component includes local courses known as the Definitive Surgical Trauma Care (DSTC) course, which attempts to teach principles similar to the ACS ATLS adapted for low-resource environments. The IATSIC has also worked with WHO in the development of Guidelines for Essential Trauma Care, which help to establish a basic standard for human and material resources for trauma care systems in LMICs.[57]

NGOs have been similarly established to address the educational needs for trauma care in developing countries. A prime example is the Primary Trauma Care Foundation (PTCF). Established in 1996, the PTCF seeks to teach trauma care principles through locally based courses.[58] Their curriculum includes a free trauma care manual for teaching, which has been used for courses in more than 60 countries worldwide. Notably, each 2-day course is followed by a 1-day instructor course, which aims to empower local practitioners to spread knowledge within their communities.

Through the continuing education provided by these organizations, they help not only to maintain skills but also impact new knowledge, challenge old dogma, and develop best practices for each context and region. Furthermore, these courses target not only doctors and nurses, but also other key personnel such as community health workers, hospital personnel, and potential first responders who can be better prepared to meet the challenge of the growing burden of trauma. Successful training programs for lay first responders are well documented.[59] Other programs have focused on the training of nonphysician "orthopaedic technicians" and their contribution to trauma care in many under-resourced countries cannot be overstated.[60]

There has also been recently an increased interest in "global health" in academic circles of many HICs. Global health is now an area of focus of many U.S. universities: Harvard, Johns Hopkins, University of Utah, and the University of California, San Francisco (UCSF) to name a few. The benefits of bilateral academic partnerships are also well documented.[61] The capacity for international collaboration has become a criteria for an increasing number of students at all levels in their selection of an institution.[62] Some institutions, such as UCSF, offer global health programs at master's or doctorate levels. Others, such as UCSF's Institute for Global Orthopaedics and Traumatology (IGOT) offer fellowships at the undergraduate and graduate levels. Many surgical programs across the country now offer optional surgical rotations in resource-poor countries, as well as visiting fellowships for national trainees. This is also true of some professional associations, such as the American Academy of Orthopaedic Surgeons (AAOS), through their international committee, organizations, such as Orthopaedics Overseas, and volunteer programs.

All these opportunities are gaining momentum because it is now widely accepted that training and teaching are much more likely to have a sustainable impact than activities focused on delivery of care.

PEDIATRIC TRAUMA (MANAGEMENT OF COMMON INJURIES)

While the principles of management for pediatric fractures and dislocations have been covered in detail in other sections of this text, several important differences must be acknowledged when planning treatment for the same injuries presenting for care in LMICs. An image intensifier is rarely available to help assist with closed reduction or to facilitate minimally invasive treatment strategies such as percutaneous fixation or closed intramedullary nailing. Implants are often unavailable or must be purchased by families from the market. Due to deficiencies in access to medical care, a subset of patients present days to weeks (or months) after their injury (Fig. 3-1, *A–H*). The treatment must be individualized in these circumstances, recognizing that solutions are more complex, costly, and less likely to achieve a suitable outcome. While a subset of fractures will require open surgical treatment to achieve the best results, for example, displaced intraarticular fractures or open fractures, wound sepsis is a significant risk when open procedures are performed in environments with questionable sterility.

Fortunately, the majority of pediatric fractures presenting acutely are amenable to nonoperative management, and traction is available in most environments. An understanding of the mechanism of injury is essential to guide closed reduction, and meticulous casting technique is required. It is important to recognize the remodeling potential based on the patient's age and the location and plane of motion of the deformity. Most remodeling is due to asymmetric physial growth, with the remainder from appositional bone growth in the concavity of the deformity, with concomitant resorption of bone on the convexity. Displaced physial fractures carry a significant risk of growth disturbance, and require follow-up to identify partial or complete physial arrest. Manipulation (or remanipulation) after 7 to 10 days after the injury should be avoided

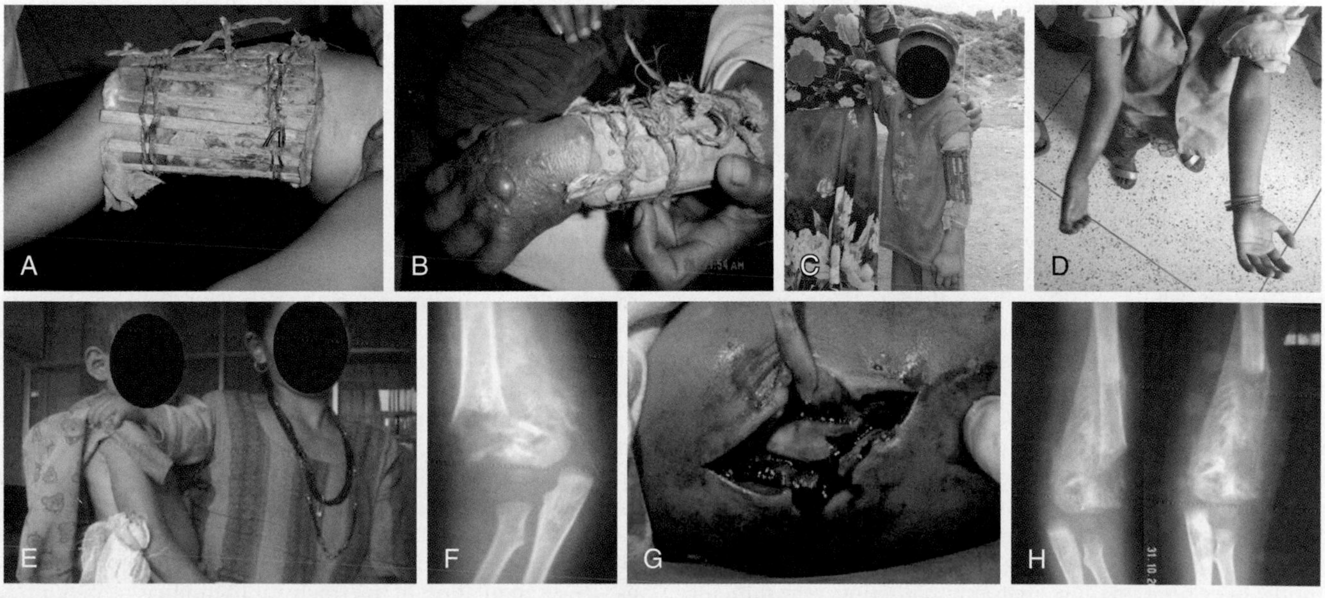

Figure 3-1. Patients often seek traditional healers when injured, and fractures are often splinted with bamboo or other devices (**A–C**), which may on occasion be complicated by compartment syndrome (**D**). This child presented with an infection following an untreated open supracondylar fracture (**E** and **F**) and was treated by débridement and splinting (**G** and **H**). *(Courtesy of the Hospital and Rehabilitation Centre for Disabled Children, Banepa, Nepal.)*

due to the risk of iatrogenic physial damage. In circumstances where patients are delayed in presentation and have significant growth remaining, it is best to wait until the fracture has healed and remodeled, reserving corrective osteotomy for that subset of cases with unacceptable deformities or loss of function. When future growth is of no concern, remanipulation or open realignment can be performed as little or no remodeling can be expected.

The management of neglected fractures and dislocations is challenging and must be individualized. Treatment decisions are based on the resources available locally, as well as the opportunities for rehabilitation and follow-up. The most appropriate strategy depends on the time since injury, individual characteristics of the fracture, patients' current level of symptoms, and anticipated function in the future. We will briefly outline the principles of management for selected injuries, which have received attention in the medical literature, recognizing that the same principles may be applied in other circumstances. The results following treatment of neglected injuries may be inferior to those presenting acutely, however it is possible to improve the patients' symptoms and function in the majority of cases.

The management of neglected, displaced supracondylar humerus fractures can be quite challenging in the absence of an image intensifier when patients present days to weeks following the injury.[63,64] One can expect some excellent remodeling of translation and some remodeling of sagittal plane malalignment. Little remodeling will occur in the coronal plane. When an image intensifier is available, it is likely that closed reduction and percutaneous fixation can be achieved up until approximately 5 to 7 days following injury. Traction has also been reported to be successful in cases between 1 and 3 weeks following injury, although a subset of cases healed in some varus.[63] After this time, options include open reduction, or allowing the fracture to heal and performing an osteotomy at a later time. Caution should be observed in performing any open surgery during the period of greatest inflammation, anecdotally between approximately 7 days and 4 weeks, given the risk of stiffness and heterotopic bone formation. This has led to the suggestion that treatment should be delayed, and osteotomy performed after complete healing. One study from Thailand has suggested that an early corrective osteotomy, after the period of heightened inflammation, may result in adequate outcomes. Patients with a healed but malaligned fracture will require an osteotomy, most commonly for cubitus varus, and a variety of techniques have been described. Some displaced fractures will heal with adequate coronal alignment; however, posterior translation of the distal fragment results in impingement, which blocks elbow flexion. Removal of an anterior bone block may improve or restore flexion in selected cases (Fig. 3-2). Alternatively, an osteotomy can be performed to realign the fracture and restore range of motion.

Neglected lateral condyle fractures may result in pain, and progressive valgus deformity with or without tardy ulnar nerve palsy.[65-67] Treatment options include observation, fixation, and bone grafting to achieve union, often in a stable but nonanatomic position, and distal humeral osteotomy with ulnar nerve transposition (Fig. 3-3). The fracture surfaces remodel over time, making anatomic reduction very difficult, and fractures that are displaced significantly are very difficult to mobilize without extensive soft tissue stripping, which might result in avascular necrosis and persistent nonunion. Care should be taken to avoid posterior dissection. A lateral approach can be used to expose the nonunion anteriorly, and the fracture surfaces can be curetted prior to fixation. Local bone graft has been used, and fixation is achieved in a position that maximizes range of motion, often in a nonanatomic position.

Chronic Monteggia lesions present with a variety of symptoms including pain, decreased range of motion, instability or popping sensation, a deformity, and even a posterior interosseous nerve palsy.[68,69] Adaptive changes including enlargement of the radial head may be observed and may preclude achieving a stable articulation. Typically, the ulna is shortened because of either a malunited fracture or plastic deformation, and restoration of ulnar length is critical to facilitate a stable reduction of the radial head. Reconstruction most commonly involves realignment of the ulna along with open reduction of the radial head with annular ligament reconstruction using the triceps fascia (Bell–Tawse), forearm fascia, or by a free tendon or fascial graft (Fig. 3-4). A Kirschner wire (K-wire) is commonly placed across the radiocapitellar joint for temporary fixation (2 weeks). Excision of the radial head may be considered for symptomatic relief in cases where reconstruction is not feasible.

Neglected elbow dislocations typically present with loss of motion, pain, and significant limitations in function.[70-72] If the patient is asymptomatic and has a functional range of motion, observation is the best option. For those with chronic symptoms, several options are available. The technique reported most frequently has been an open reduction, which may be performed via posterior approach, or medial and lateral approaches. The ulnar nerve should be isolated and protected. Barriers to reduction include soft tissue contracture, scar tissue within the joint, new bone formation, and periarticular calcification. The articular cartilage is often softened, which may make defining the plane in between fibrous tissue and articular cartilage difficult. Once the barriers to reduction are removed, a large K-wire has been used between the olecranon and the distal humerus for 2 weeks, after which range-of-motion exercises are started. Most authors have advocated a V-Y lengthening of the triceps, and in most cases, stable reduction could be maintained. Range of motion is typically improved, but reduced in comparison with the contralateral elbow. Patients with a coexisting fracture seem to have a less favorable outcome in comparison with those sustaining an isolated dislocation. The use of an external fixator, usually in concert with open surgical procedures, has also been reported.[73] Options for salvage include excisional arthroplasty, prosthetic replacement, or arthrodesis. It remains unclear which of these options offers the best long-term results, given the limited number of cases in the literature and the absence of prosthetic technologies and the environment where these neglected injuries are encountered most frequently.

The treatment of neglected femoral shaft fractures typically involves restoration of both length and alignment, and the specific treatment depends on the duration between injury and treatment.[74,75] Contractures within the soft tissues develop rapidly, and restoration of length may be a challenge. Limb shortening is caused by both overriding a fracture fragment as well as angulation of the fracture. The injury is encountered during the early phases of healing, and osteoclasis may be performed by closed, percutaneous, or open techniques. Traction can then be applied, and used as either definitive

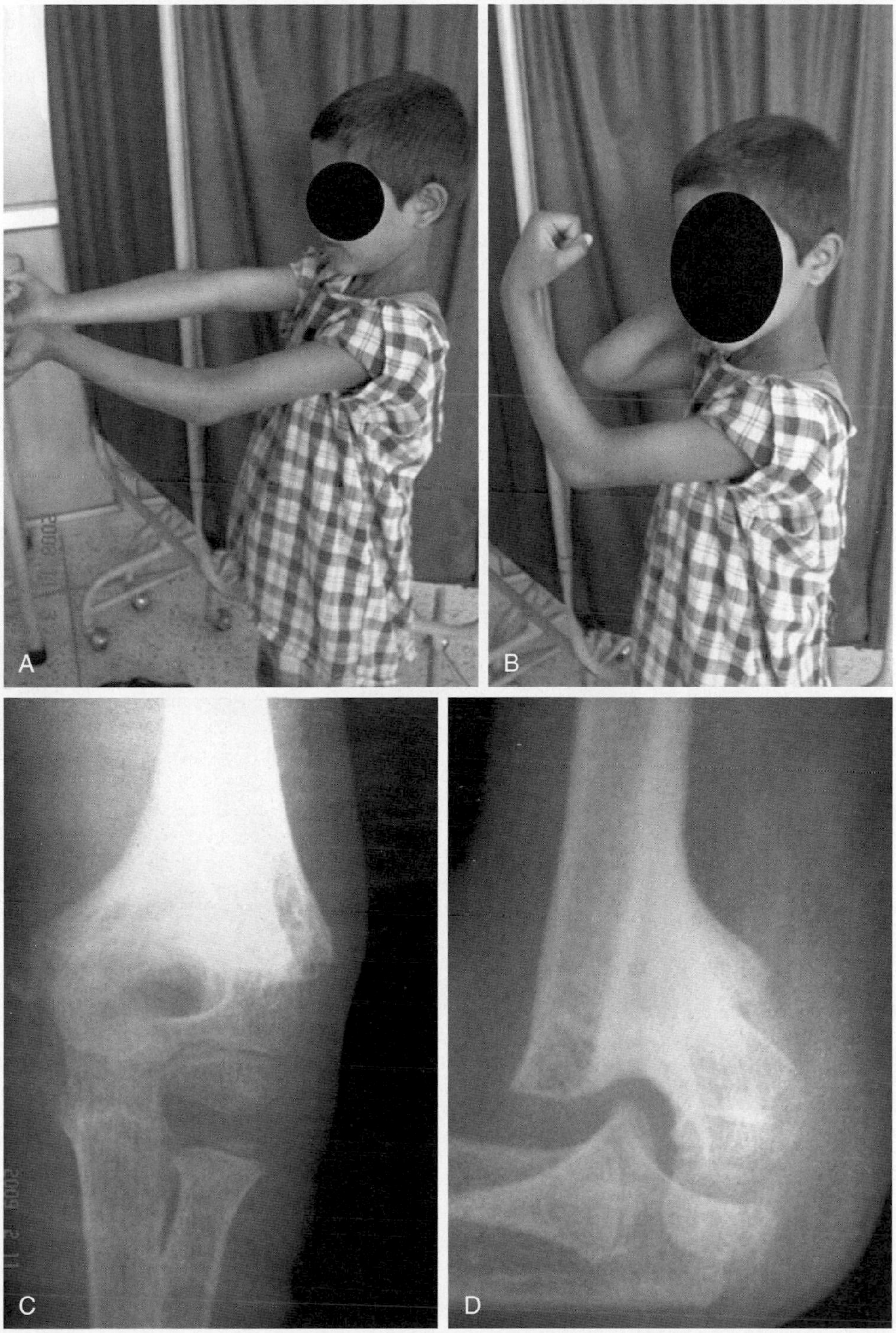

Figure 3-2. This child had a neglected supracondylar fracture with flexion block due to bony impingement (**A** and **B**) and was treated by resection of the bony prominence (**C** and **D**) to restore motion. *(Courtesy of the Hospital and Rehabilitation Centre for Disabled Children, Banepa, Nepal.)*

treatment or as a prelude to open reduction and either intramedullary fixation or plating. There appears to be an increased risk of neurovascular complications when acute lengthening of more than 4 cm is accomplished. Some authors have favored acute shortening and fixation, as an alternative to staged approach to treatment. Most of the available literature has concerned results, and has involved open reduction, acute shortening, and intramedullary fixation. Some authors have used iliac crest bone grafting. At a later time, after the fracture is healed, a realignment osteotomy is required for treatment.

Neglected femoral neck fractures are extremely rare in children, and there is only one report that we are aware of in the literature.[76] In this study, patients were treated by valgus intertrochanteric osteotomy, and the authors used preoperative traction when there was more than 4 cm of shortening. The intertrochanteric osteotomy typically heals before the femoral

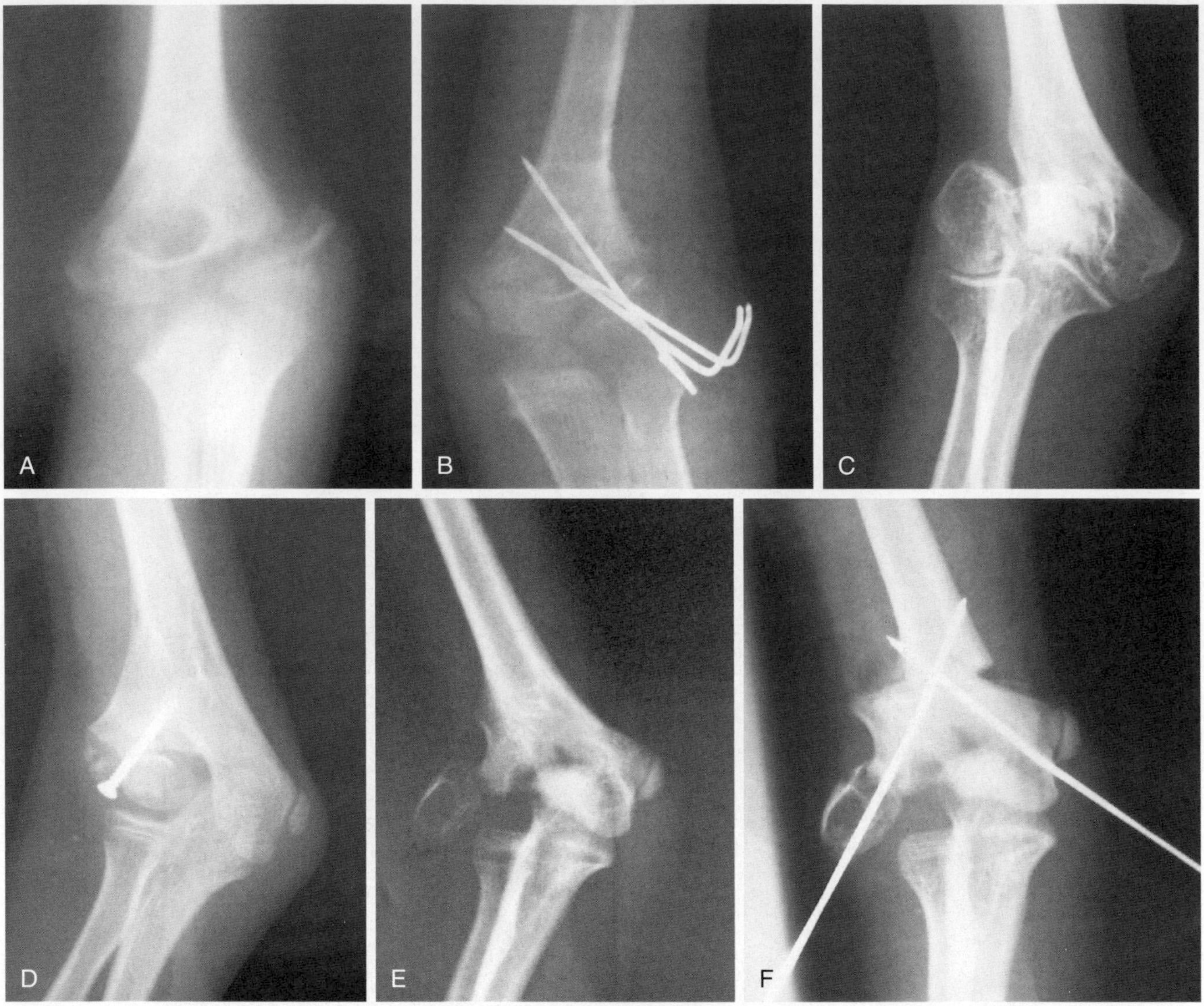

Figure 3-3. Although neglected lateral condyle fractures without significant displacement may be treated by delayed open reduction and grafting, with near anatomic restoration (**A** and **B**), the goal for those with significant displacement and shortening is a stable union in a non-anatomic position (**C** and **D**). Patients with significant valgus with or without tardy ulnar nerve palsy often require osteotomy for realignment (**E** and **F**). *(Courtesy of the Hospital and Rehabilitation Centre for Disabled Children, Banepa, Nepal.)*

neck fracture. In young adults, Roshan and Ram reviewed 22 studies from the literature, found that adequate results were achieved in 35% to 80% with an osteotomy and internal fixation, with or without bone grafting.[77]

Traumatic hip dislocations are relatively rare in children, and usually occur as a result of low energy injuries. In older children and adolescents, these usually result from higher energy mechanisms, and are more frequently associated with other musculoskeletal injuries including acetabular fractures. Options for treatment include observation, the heavy traction method,[78] open reduction with or without femoral shortening,[79,80] and salvage procedures such as pelvic support osteotomy, arthrodesis, or joint replacement (when available). The limited information in the literature in the pediatric age group suggests that open reduction with or without femoral shortening may be the most reasonable initial treatment for symptomatic patients (Fig. 3-5). A concentric reduction can be achieved in most, and while avascular necrosis is common, this does not seem to impact the results at early to midrange follow-up. Symptomatic relief was observed with improvement in range of motion, and a stable articulation was restored in the majority of cases. Even if the results deteriorate over time, the need for salvage strategies is delayed.

ADULT TRAUMA

As is true for children, many of adult trauma patients in LMICs are first treated by nondoctors: traditional healers, bonesetters, nurses, all with different levels of knowledge and experience, and varying degrees of outcomes.[81] Depending on availability, accessibility and affordability, some will be treated conservatively by general doctors, some conservatively or surgically by general surgeons, a very few by a formally trained local orthopaedic surgeon, and an extreme few by a

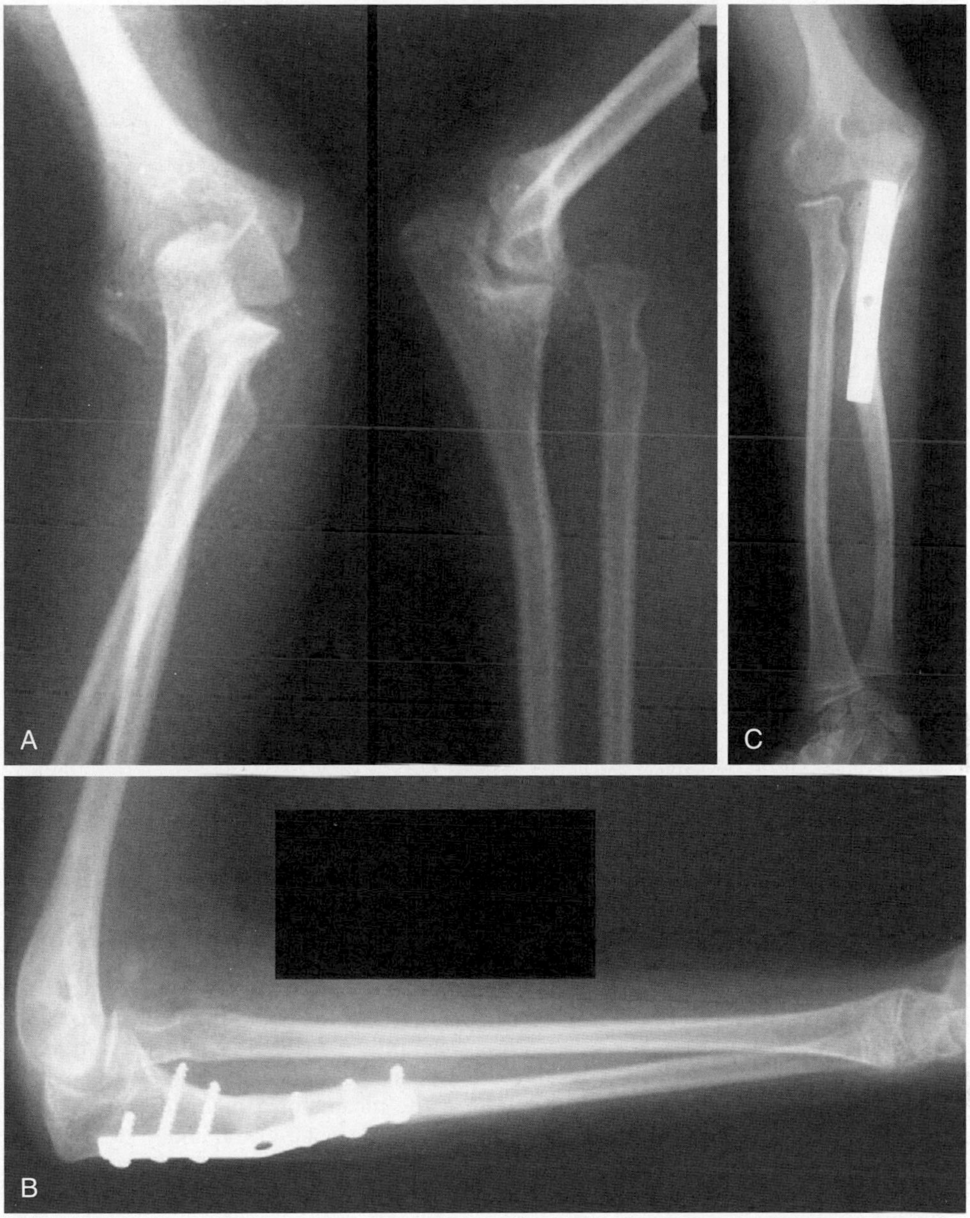

Figure 3-4. Neglected Monteggia lesion treated by ulnar osteotomy to restore length and alignment, and open reduction of the radial head with reconstruction of the annular ligament. *(Courtesy of the Hospital and Rehabilitation Centre for Disabled Children, Banepa, Nepal.)*

visiting volunteer. Those who make it "up the ladder" are not always completely truthful with their history, for fear of not being treated. Time since injury is often underestimated, sometimes grossly: A surgeon would probably not have attempted a closed reduction of a 3-day-old shoulder dislocation had he known it was in fact 3 months! Patients may also deny recent illnesses, increasing anesthesia risks, particularly for children.

Another common pitfall has to do with inadequate imaging. Plain radiographs are very often the only diagnostic tools available. They are often of poor quality, do not show both ends of the bones, or are not sharp enough to assess all fracture lines. It is not uncommon for the surgeon to make disagreeable discoveries on postoperative films. Because usually patients have to pay for tests and treatments, the initial admission radiograph is often the only one available, and fracture fragments have often since displaced. The initial radiograph of a simple transverse femur fracture in a muscular young male may look quite "benign," but reduction and fixation after 4 weeks of bed rest without traction may prove more challenging than one anticipated. The same is true for hip fractures.

Spinal Injuries

The incidence of spine fractures is increasing with the number of RTIs. Specialized spinal centers are almost nonexistent in LMICs. When associated with spinal cord injuries, the midterm prognosis is almost uniformly poor, most patients dying from septic complications from bladder and lung infections or pressure sores.[82] Unstable fractures without neurologic deficit are usually treated with postural reduction or traction, and bed rest if displaced, bed rest and precautions

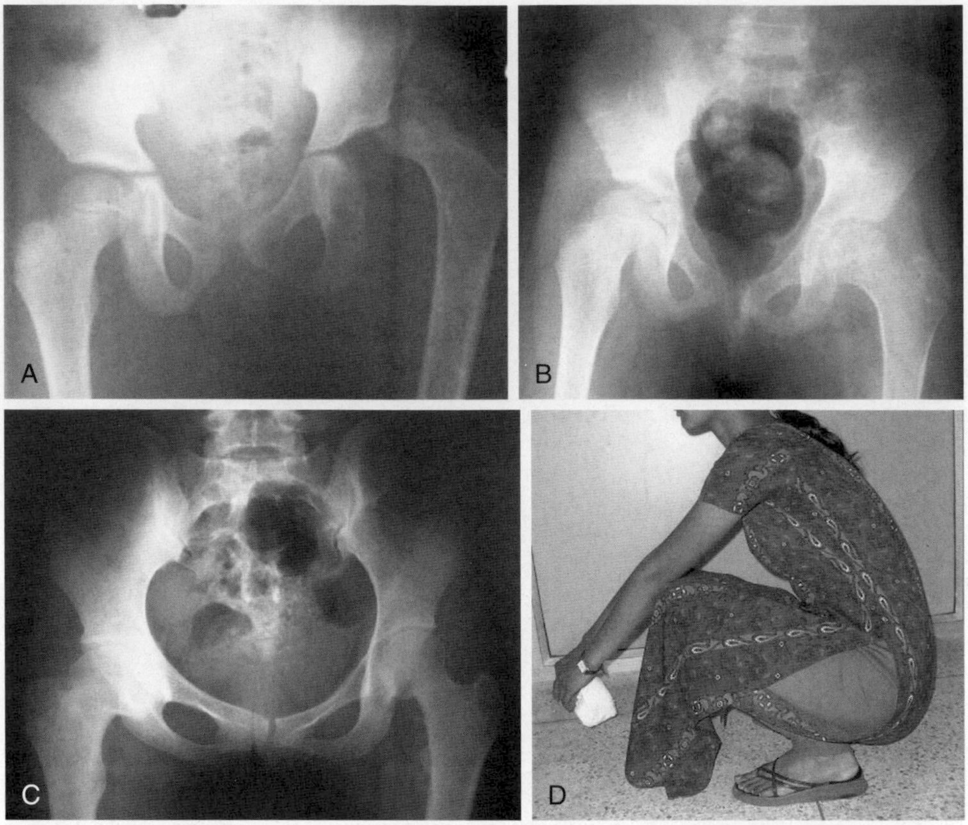

Figure 3-5. Neglected hip dislocation treated by open reduction (**A** and **B**). A second case demonstrated evidence of avascular necrosis but was asymptomatic with a functional range of motion (**C** and **D**). *(Courtesy of the Hospital and Rehabilitation Centre for Disabled Children, Banepa, Nepal.)*

only if undisplaced. In general, spinal surgery is well beyond the normal capacities of most sites.

Cervical Spine

Most displaced fractures can be gradually reduced in skeletal traction, if Gardner–Wells tongs or halos are available. Incorporating the halo in a jacket at 4 to 6 weeks, or fashioning a plaster Minerva at 6 weeks will further protect healing for an additional 6 weeks. Unfortunately, semirigid or soft collars are often the only orthotics available.

Thoracolumbar Spine (TLS)

Postural reduction of displaced unstable fracture of the TLS with bumps, rolls, or bed modifications are usually very poorly tolerated. Bed rest, log rolling, and pressure sore prevention are usually all that can be done. Prefabricated thoracolumbar spinal orthoses (TLSOs) or corsets are usually not available, so a thoracolumbar (TL) cast can be done at 4 to 6 weeks, often incorporating one hip in extension for the lower lumbar fractures.

Normal sensation is an obvious prerequisite to any kind of casting treatment.

Pelvic and Acetabular Fractures

Pelvic fractures vary greatly in severity. The more severe injuries are commonly associated with lesions to the lumbo-sacral plexus, the iliac veins and/or arteries, and the lower urinary tract.[83] A thorough neurovascular examination is mandatory and needs to be recorded in the chart. It is also mandatory to examine the perineum for wounds and to do a rectal examination to feel for protruding bony spikes or a high-riding prostate in the male. Inability to void in a conscious patient, especially if a distended bladder is palpable, if there is blood at the meatus or a high-riding prostate; these are all highly suggestive of a urethral injury. A retrograde urethrogram with any available contrast material is a quick and easy procedure to confirm the diagnosis. A cystostomy should be performed without any attempt at retrograde catheterization. Macroscopic hematuria is suggestive of a bladder injury, but is also common at 48 to 72 hours when the fracture hematoma is suffusing through the intact bladder wall.

Sophisticated pelvic imaging is rarely available and a plain antero-posterior (AP) pelvic radiograph is often all that is done[84] (Fig. 3-6). Inlet and outlet views may help for a more accurate diagnosis, but iliac and obturator oblique views are painful and should be done only if surgical treatment is seriously considered. Clinical examination is thus even more important to assess stability. The sacroiliac areas must always be examined and palpated. Significant bruising or pain should raise suspicion that the posterior sacroiliac ligamentous complex may be involved. Latero-lateral compression and push-pull maneuvers, with anesthesia if necessary, will add valuable information when the radiograph is "borderline."

Pelvic Ring Injuries

Treatment is directly related to the degree of instability, itself based on the integrity of the posterior sacroiliac ligamentous complex, and the Buchholz classification is the simplest.[85]

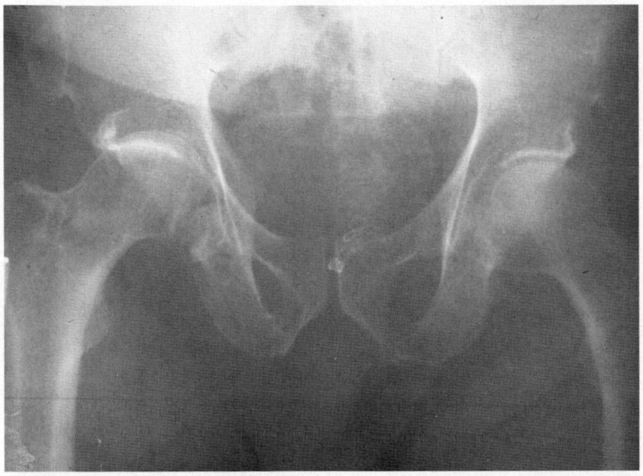

Figure 3-6. Anterior-posterior (AP) pelvis radiograph 3 weeks after right hip injury. There appears to be a fracture of the posterior wall, of the inferior part of the femoral head and possibly a nondisplaced transverse fracture of the acetabulum. Shenton's line is preserved, but the head/dome relationship is definitely abnormal. Oblique views would be helpful. Surgical exploration is indicated, even without a computed tomography (CT) scan.

Stable fractures (type 1) such as avulsions or rami fractures are treated symptomatically with mobilization and weight bearing as tolerated. Rotationally unstable but vertically stable fractures (type 2), such as open book or lateral compression patterns, are still relatively stable. Displaced open book patterns with widening of the symphysis can be treated by postural reduction with the patient lying mostly on one side or the other. There are no indications for pelvic slings. Longitudinal traction may provide comfort initially. Patients should be allowed to mobilize in bed according to pain and to start ambulating on the intact side when active sitting in bed is painless. Vertically unstable fractures (type 3) are truly unstable in all planes. Keep in mind that the residual displacement on the initial AP radiograph may significantly underestimate the amount of initial displacement, as suggested by associated findings such as fractures of the lower lumbar transverse processes or avulsion of the ischial spine or the lateral border of the sacrum.[86] These vertical patterns will usually displace further if the patient is allowed to sit or bear weight before it is "sticky," usually at 2 to 4 weeks, so skeletal traction is recommended for the duration of the bed rest period. Weight bearing should start progressively after 6 weeks.

Fresh fractures of the pelvic ring may present with hemodynamic instability that does not respond to fluid resuscitation. As blood availability is often an issue, and embolization almost never available, the threshold for external fixation may actually be lower than in resource-rich environments. A pelvic wrap is an excellent initial compression technique, but rarely tolerated for more than 24 hours.[87] It buys enough time to prepare for formal external fixation in the operating room, safely done with an open technique. Although rarely the tool of choice for reduction and fixation of the pelvic ring disruption, it will still allow earlier mobilization of the patient in and out of bed. Unfortunately, more often than not, external fixation becomes the definitive treatment of the fracture.[88] In austere environments, internal fixation can be either difficult (anything anterior) or very difficult (anything posterior), and best left to expert hands working in ideal surgical environments.

Acetabular Fractures

These are rare injuries, usually managed by specially trained pelvic surgeons in highly developed countries. Posterior wall fractures with an unstable or incongruous hip after reduction of the posteriorly dislocated hip are best managed with open reduction and internal fixation (ORIF) when the surgeon is skilled and confident, and the necessary instruments and implants are available. If internal fixation is not possible, the joint should still be explored and cleaned, and the fracture treated in traction, usually with an "airplane" cast at the ankle to maintain external rotation. All other fractures are usually treated with longitudinal skeletal traction for 4 to 6 weeks, and no weight bearing for an additional 6 weeks. The only exception is the both-column fracture with "neocongruency," treated with bed rest only.[89] There is no indication for cervicotrochanteric lateral traction using devices such as T-handled corkscrews, as still commonly seen for "central fracture-dislocations." They are difficult to insert properly, especially without fluoroscopy, confine the patient to the supine position, uniformly get quickly "soupy," and are of no proven value.

Lower Extremity Injuries

As with everything else in LMICs, conservative management of lower extremity (LE) injuries has long been the gold standard, but there is a definite trend toward an "orthopaedic transition" to increased surgical treatment and internal fixation. Still, many patients present late, or have to wait prolonged periods (sometimes months) before their treatment. This combines with the usual lack of intraoperative imaging to make ORIF in such environments even more challenging.

Hip Dislocations

It is not always easy to distinguish clinically between a posterior hip dislocation, a hip fracture, or a fracture-dislocation, but a good AP pelvis radiograph should be diagnostic. Closed reduction of a fresh posterior or anterior hip dislocation should be achieved with adequate anesthesia. A postreduction AP pelvis radiograph showing also the opposite hip is essential to confirm the reduction is concentric and symmetrical. An interposed fragment will show an aspherical, incongruous, or asymmetrical joint line, and no computed tomography (CT) scan is necessary to make the decision for an open reduction. If a closed reduction is more difficult than it should be, it is likely the duration has been underestimated. When more than a week out, or when the duration is uncertain, one should be prepared for an open reduction. Postreduction stability is assessed while the patient is still under anesthesia, and the "safe zone" determined. This will determine further treatment: from nothing to skeletal traction with derotation bar for 3 to 4 weeks. Long-standing dislocations usually present with shortening, the need for some kind of walking aid, and no or mild pain. Surgical treatment is rarely indicated, but if pain is still significant, options include a Girdlestone arthroplasty (even more functionally disabling) or a staged reduction: extensive soft tissue releases with 2 to 3 weeks of skeletal traction and repeat surgery. This restores length but at the risk of avascular necrosis (AVN).[90] Replacement arthroplasty is rarely a possibility.

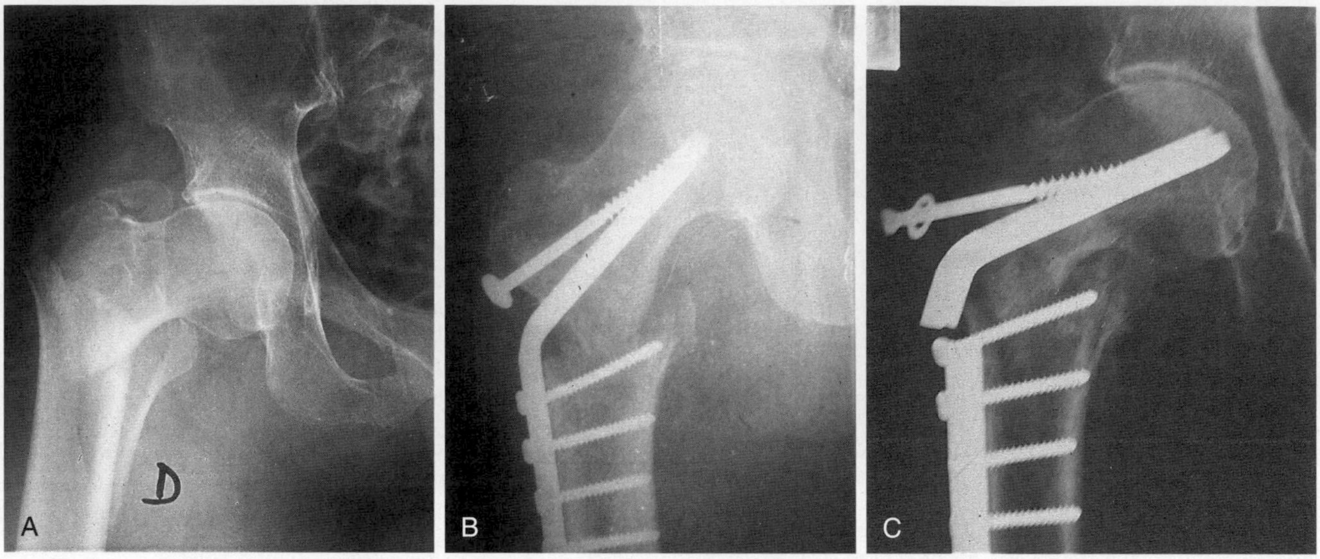

Figure 3-7. A, Comminuted intertrochanteric fracture, with a big lesser trochanteric fragment. **B,** The lesser trochanteric was reduced and fixed, the distal fragment medialized according to the Dimon-Hughston technique, but fixation was done with a nonsliding device, defeating the purpose of the medialization. **C,** The hardware lost its race against bone healing and failed.

Hip Fractures

Femoral neck, pertrochanteric, and peritrochanteric fractures remain the "problem" fractures in LMICs. As the world is aging, their incidence is steadily increasing.[91,92] They afflict mostly the elderly, who often have associated comorbidities and higher anesthetic risks. Standard surgical care in HICs involves early internal fixation, using fluoroscopy, or prosthetic replacement. In LMICs to this day, lack of access to skilled providers, properly equipped facilities, and/or affordable implants have left prolonged skeletal traction as the most common treatment, with its known morbidity: pressure sores, deep vein thrombosis, stiffness, atrophy, pin tract infection, malunion, or nonunion. Where surgery is not an option, traction should be discontinued in the elderly as soon as pain is tolerable, usually within 2 to 3 weeks. Malunion with shortening and/or malrotation, and nonunion, especially if painless, are less dangerous complications than those related to prolonged bed rest.

Where surgical treatment is possible, it is definitely the best option, particularly for younger patients. Keep in mind that the appearance on the admission radiograph might not reflect the situation at the time of surgery. This is particularly important where no fluoroscopy is available. Where it is available, closed reduction, even on a radiolucid table only, and percutaneous pinning or fixation with a dynamic hip screw or cervicotrochanteric nail is done in a standard fashion for fractures of the femoral neck or intertrochanteric area. Where there is no fluoroscopy, a wider exposure is needed for intertrochanteric fractures for adequate reduction and "semi-blind" fixation, "feeling" the neck over the anterior capsule, and slowly advancing the drill bit in a push-pull fashion to ensure one is still "in bone." Rigidity of the fixation is assessed clinically. Even if the reduction is not perfectly anatomical, a rigid fixation will yield better functional outcomes than traction, provided the fracture heals (Fig. 3-7). Femoral neck fractures should be internally fixed in the younger patient, which often means an open reduction, preferably through an anterior approach. Elderly patients are best treated with prosthetic replacement, a more "definitive" procedure, but if hemiarthroplasty is not an option, rigid internal fixation is still preferable to traction. Where the SIGN system is used, the hip construct is usually available, as discussed later.

Femoral Shaft Fractures

This is a common orthopaedic injury, on the rise with the increase in high-energy motorized crashes. Skeletal traction remains the most common treatment in LMICs, although the capacity for internal fixation is steadily increasing. All volunteer orthopaedists should familiarize themselves with the lost art of skeletal traction, and forgotten gems, such as Charnley's *Closed Treatment of Common Fractures* or Byrne's *Traction Handbook* should be mandatory predeployment readings.[93,94] Access to and affordability of trained surgeons and implants remain the biggest barriers to internal fixation in these austere environments. SIGN surgeons in numerous centers around the world are trying to circumvent these obstacles, as discussed later. Even then, late presentation or protracted preoperative hospital stay, with or without traction, present added technical challenges. Generalized lack of fluoroscopy makes open reduction mandatory in almost all cases. It is not uncommon to find an irreducible shortening of the bone, requiring trimming of the ends of the fragments. Antegrade or retrograde intramedullary (IM) nailing, preferably interlocked, or plates and screws are used for internal fixation. Tourniquets can rarely be used, and these open procedures can lose quite a bit of blood, so availability of blood for transfusion if needed is a wise precaution. Malunions, nonunions, or previous hardware failure are not rare, and require open management (Fig. 3-8).

Knee Injuries

As for every other joint, particularly weight-bearing ones, ORIF is the best treatment for displaced intraarticular fractures. Late presentation of malunions of tibial plateau or femoral condyles most often already show signs of posttraumatic DJD, and joint replacement (rarely an option) or arthrodesis may be all one can offer. Fresh patella fractures of

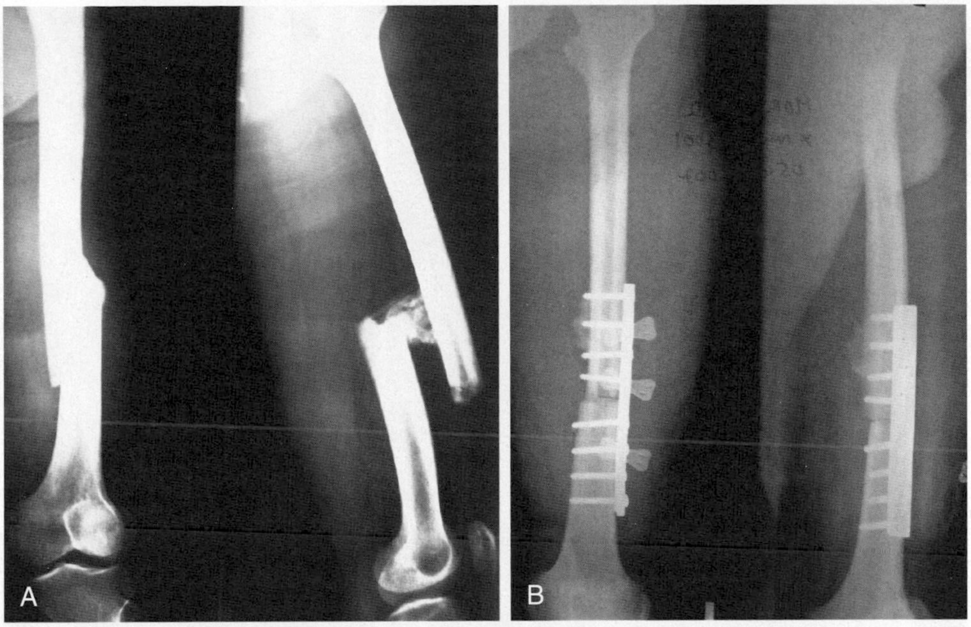

Figure 3-8. A, A 5-month-old malunion of a femoral shaft fracture treated in traction for 8 weeks. The patient was full weight bearing, but unhappy with the shortening. The overall alignment is acceptable in both planes. **B,** Internal fixation with plate and screws. Only very minimal shortening of both ends was necessary.

extensor mechanism disruptions require minimal means for repair. Chronic disruptions are still worthwhile repairing, even if it means excising a displaced patellar pole, as some loss of motion is a good trade-off for instability. The vast majority of other soft tissue injuries around the knee are treated conservatively, with functional results depending on the availability of rehabilitation and orthotics. Fresh dislocations can be managed by closed reduction, casting, and careful observation for signs of vascular complications. It is important the reduction is as anatomical as possible, and transarticular pinning with two big Steinmann pins may be necessary if the postreduction radiographs in cast show some residual displacement in any plane. The pins can be removed at 6 weeks (Fig. 3-9). Again here, better be stiff than unstable. On occasion, a neglected dislocation may be seen, with or without distal sequelae of partial or even complete compartment syndrome. An open reduction is sometimes possible, but much more commonly, a shortening and fusion is necessary, eventually allowing full weight bearing on a "peg-leg." Sophisticated arthroscopic or even open ligamentous reconstructions are rarely feasible, and results are often disappointing for lack of good postoperative rehabilitation.

Tibia-Fibula Fractures

This is the most common long bone fracture. The developing world is seeing a very rapid increase in the use of motorbikes, and open tib-fib fractures have become the scourge in these parts of the world. Maintaining acceptable alignment while achieving sound and stable wound coverage without underlying infection are the goals of the initial treatment. Windowed casts, pins and plaster, or external fixation are all useful techniques to maintain length and alignment, and provide access to the wound, which may eventually need a split-thickness skin graft or a local rotation flap for coverage. When the wound coverage is stable, conversion to a short-leg patellar tendon-bearing (PTB; Sarmiento) type cast is the preferred method to achieve bone healing. Bone loss, malunions, or nonunions may require delayed reconstruction procedures including internal fixation or bone transport.

Nonsurgical management of closed, displaced, or nondisplaced tibial shaft fractures is now almost never seen in HICs. Yet it remains the cornerstone in LMICs, and the volunteer surgeon should be comfortable with the techniques of closed reduction, molded casting, and cast wedging if necessary. Techniques for all possible casts are widely available on YouTube. An initial above-knee cast can usually be replaced at 4 to 6 weeks with a PTB-type of weight-bearing cast, depending on fracture pattern. Internal fixation of closed tibial shaft fractures is gaining universal popularity. The theoretical benefits of closed IM nailing, where available and safe, can outweigh its potential risks, but closed management is a time-honored technique that is still very successful for most fractures.[95]

Foot and Ankle Injuries

There is no doubt that ORIF of a fresh displaced ankle fracture will give the best functional results. Closed reduction and a well-molded non–weight-bearing above-knee cast can be a very successful "second best," if anatomical reduction is achieved and maintained. Timely radiograph follow-up and patient compliance are necessary, and secondary displacement can be managed with cast wedging or repeat closed reduction as needed. Unfortunately, many fractures present late and anatomical reduction cannot be achieved by closed means. Open reduction can still be attempted, but if no hardware is available, the talus can at least be centered under the tibial plafond, and temporarily stabilized with a retrograde calcaneotalotibial Steinmann pinning, removed at 6 to 8 weeks.

Displaced hind-foot and mid-foot fracture-dislocations usually have a poor functional outcome. When ORIF is not possible, closed reduction and pinning of some calcaneal fractures (Essex-Lopresti) may give better hind-foot contours,

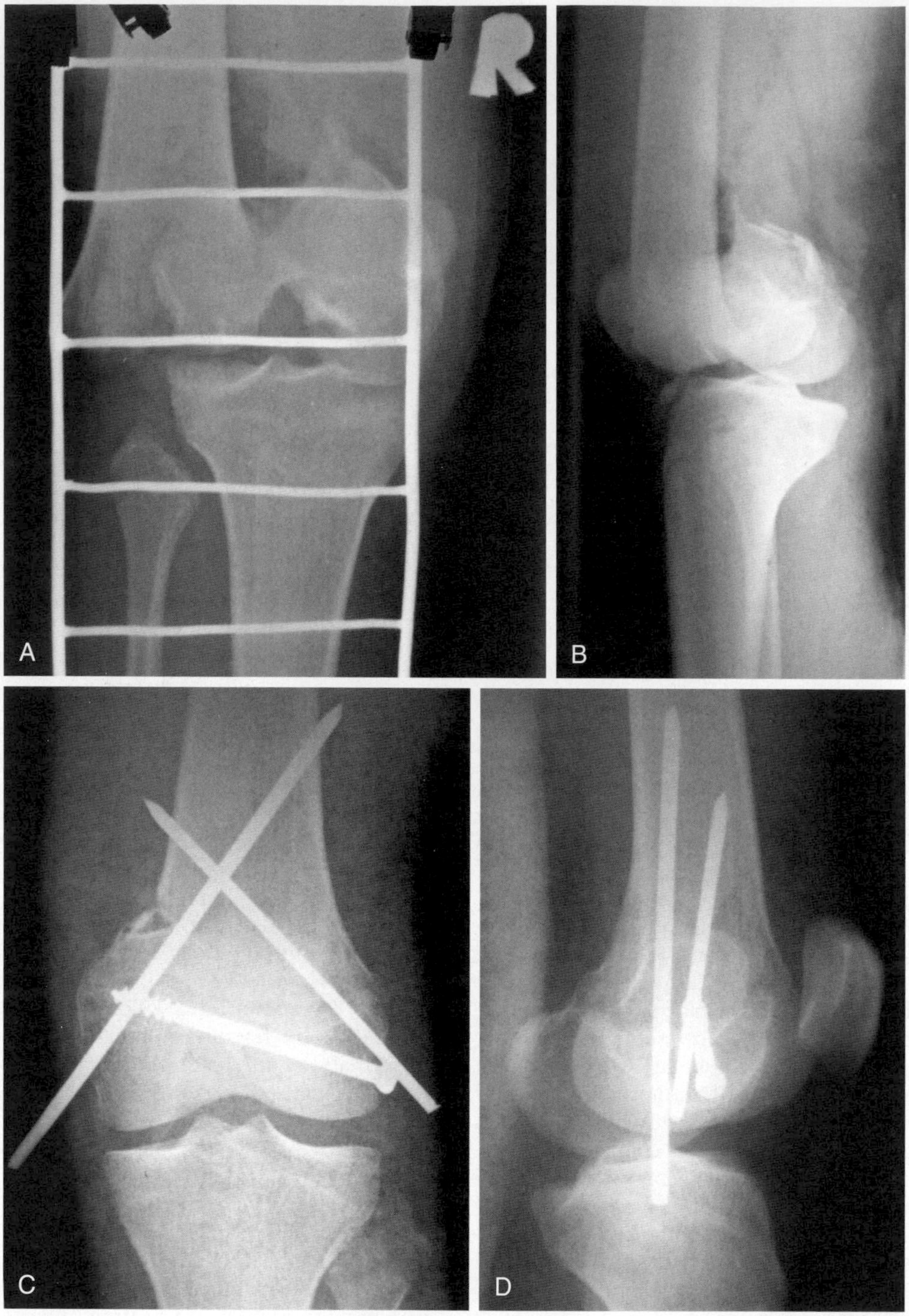

Figure 3-9. A and **B,** Anterior-posterior (AP) and lateral views of displaced T-type supracondylar and intercondylar fracture of distal femur. **C** and **D,** After open reduction and internal fixation of the articular component with one lag screw, and fixation of the supracondylar component with two crossed Steinmann pins. Obviously this is not rigid and needs additional protection with a non–weight-bearing long leg cast. The pins can be removed at 6 to 8 weeks.

making shoe wear easier. K-wires are available almost everywhere, so even without fluoroscopy, closed or open reduction of displaced or unstable fractures-dislocations of the mid-foot, such as Lisfranc's, or metatarsal fractures or metatarsophalangeal dislocations is indicated.

Upper Extremity Injuries

Because they do not involve weight bearing, many upper extremity (UE) injuries go untreated or present late.

Shoulder Injuries

The vast majority of clavicle or scapula fractures, and acromioclavicular (AC) joint separations are managed conservatively in LMICs, with sling and swath, or figure-of-8 bandages, with usually good functional results. Fresh shoulder fracture-dislocations are usually easily reduced with sedation. Displaced fractures of the proximal humerus are ideally rigidly internally fixed and mobilized early, but nonrigid fixation with tension-band techniques or even plain suturing of displaced tuberosities, and immobilization for 3 to 4 weeks, can yield good functional results also.

Humeral Shaft Fractures

An initial sugar tong or coaptation splint, from the top of the shoulder, over the flexed elbow to the axilla is the usual management of a fresh humeral shaft fracture in LMICs. It can be replaced with a clamshell "Chinese splint" at 3 to 4 weeks until consolidated.[96] Hanging casts are poorly tolerated, and patient compliance is often less than ideal. Internal fixation with IM nails or plates and screws, where available, can be done for acute injuries, but is certainly more indicated for delayed unions and nonunions, with or without bone graft, taking great care not to ensure the radial nerve. Malunions are much better tolerated than in the LE and rarely require surgical treatment.

Elbow Injuries

When anatomical reduction and fixation of displaced fractures of the distal humerus is not possible, transolecranon traction for 2 to 3 weeks and early mobilization ("bag of bones" technique) can yield acceptable functional results, particularly in low-demand elderly patients. Displaced radial/neck fractures can be repaired or excised. Displaced olecranon fractures can usually be repaired because K-wires and metal wires are usually available. Double- or triple-braiding a big #2 or #5 nonresorbable suture can be used if 18- or 22-gauge wires are not available.[97]

Forearm Injuries

Here again, when the gold standard of ORIF for fresh injuries cannot be met, the only alternative is a very well molded long arm cast with the forearm in supination for fractures of the proximal quarter, of the radius, in pronation for fractures of the distal quarter and in neutral position for fractures of the middle half.[98] So-called alignment rodding can be achieved with long K-wires, stacked if necessary, Steinmann pins, Ender nails, or small Rush rods, antegrade from the tip of the olecranon, and retrograde from the radial styloid.[99] It requires opening the fracture sites, and does not provide rigid fixation, but significantly adds to stability when an acceptable closed reduction cannot be achieved or is too unstable. The long arm cast can usually be converted at 3 weeks or so to a well-molded Munster-type of below-elbow cast (Fig. 3-10) that allows flexion and extension but blocks prosupination.

Hand and Wrist

Closed management of fresh displaced distal radius fractures, with reduction after hematoma block and below-elbow well-molded casting is the norm. As radiographs are often of poor quality, a high index of suspicion is necessary to systematically look for carpal injuries, ordering special views if in doubt. Chronic painful wrist conditions can often be treated with a wrist arthrodesis, a relatively simple procedure with very good functional results. Significant posttraumatic ulnar plus variance should be addressed with ulnar shortening, keeping excision of the distal ulna (Darrach procedure) as a last resort because of poor functional results, and persistent weakness and pain.

Open hand injuries from assault with blades or industrial injuries are common.[100] Mangled hands almost always look worse than they are. The initial débridement should be as conservative as possible, especially for the thumb. Repeated débridements, amputations "a minima," coverage with grafts or abdominal flaps can yield surprisingly good functional results, even if not cosmetically the most pleasing. Patients are resourceful and will be grateful for any preserved function. In these environments, UE prostheses are almost always only for cosmetic purposes.

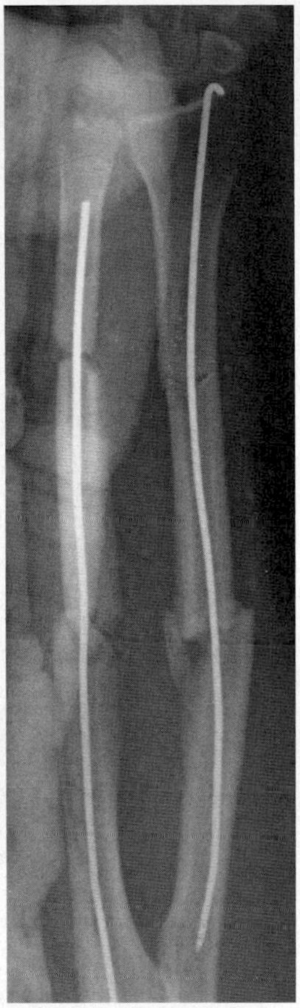

Figure 3-10. So-called alignment rodding with two K-wires of segmental fractures of both bones of the forearm. This would be protected in an above-elbow cast for 3 weeks, replaced with a Munster-type of cast for another 3 to 6 weeks.

AMPUTATIONS

Amputations may be indicated for the curative or palliative treatment of injuries, tumors, congenital deformities, or chronic infections (Fig. 3-11). Amputation is not a technique, it is a process: Postsurgical stump care, prosthetic fitting, physical therapy, psychosocial rehabilitation are all key elements.[101] In each society all over the world, amputations come with some personal, familial, and societal repercussions. In some societies, patients actually prefer death to amputation. The consent for amputations is often given by someone else than the patient himself: parents, guardians of mentally challenged adults, but also husband, clan elder, or military commander. There is nothing more frustrating for a volunteer than to see a potentially life-saving amputation refused by a third party (Fig. 3-12). Disposal of body parts is another issue not to be taken lightly, even for the smallest nubbin of an extra toe: They may go to the pathology department, in other places, they go

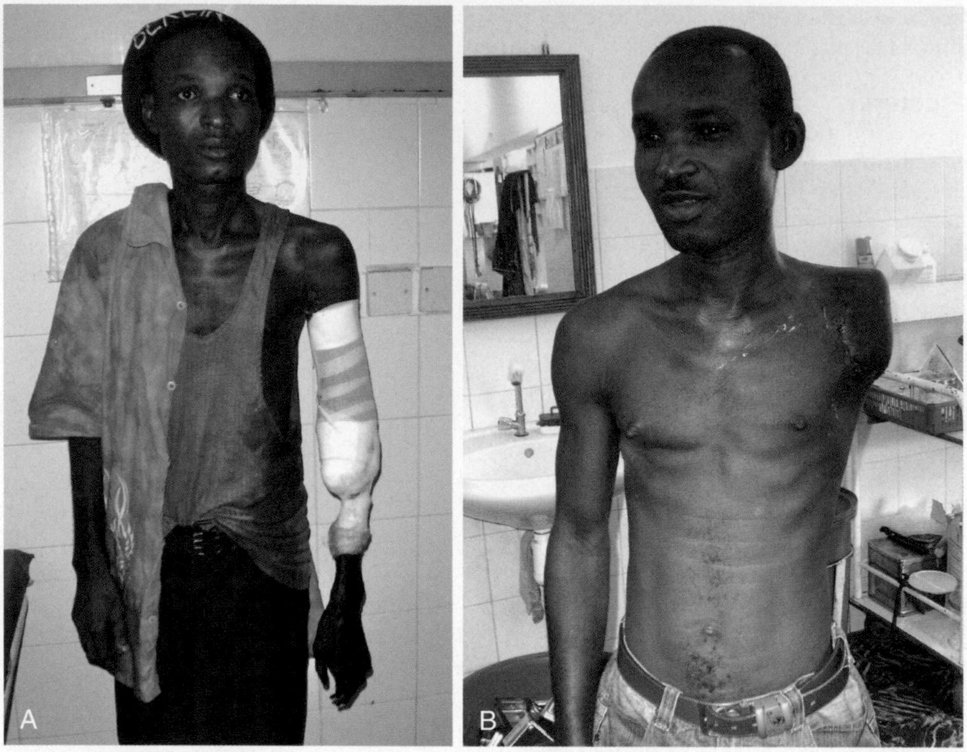

Figure 3-11. A, Patient presented several weeks after an open left forearm fracture treated with splint and herbs by a traditional healer. The distal limb is completely mummified, the proximal limb is grossly infected with draining lymph nodes in the axilla. The patient is septic, emaciated, and came requesting an amputation. **B,** An open shoulder disarticulation was performed, with delayed primary closure at 7 days, and this is the appearance at 2 months. The patient has no pain and is gaining weight.

directly to the incinerator, in others, they leave with family members to be buried or even preserved. The volunteer surgeon needs to be acutely aware and respectful of all these considerations. As for everywhere else, photographic documentation and, if possible, a documented second opinion are important additions to the patient's chart.

The surgeon needs also to be well aware of the local prosthetic and rehabilitation capacities. In many LMICs, NGOs such as Handicap International, the International Committee of the Red Cross (ICRC), Mercy Ships, and others provide prosthetic services. Whenever possible, the prosthetic specialist should be involved in the planning of an elective amputation. In general, basic, sturdy but simple prosthetic components are available, ideally made locally out of local materials. End-bearing prostheses, such as necessary for knee or ankle disarticulations, are almost never available, so amputations are through femur or tibia. Amputations below the ankle should strive to keep an end-bearing stump, and techniques preserving the heel pad, with a calcaneotibial fusion (Boyd) are encouraged. They give good functional results, even without a prosthesis (Fig. 3-13). Upper extremity prostheses are either purely cosmetic or provide very minimal function (hooks, paddle, Ys, etc.). The general rule is to keep as many joints as possible and make the terminal segment as long as possible. A wrist disarticulation is preferable to a mid-forearm amputation, a short proximal forearm amputation is still much preferable to an elbow disarticulation.

The goals of a well-padded, balanced, sensate, and painless stump are not always met and stump revision surgery may be indicated for neuromas, chronic wounds, or fitting problems (Fig. 3-14). If at all possible, the proximal joint should be protected while trying to achieve these goals.

AVENUES FOR ORTHOPAEDIC VOLUNTEERISM

Orthopaedic volunteerism falls into one of three categories that are not mutually exclusive: service provision, teaching and training, and disaster (natural or human-made) relief, which usually present a unique combination of mass casualties and austere environment. Prospective volunteers will be attracted to one or the other depending on time availability and personal preference and motivation. They are most likely to face unfamiliar (to them) presentation of familiar problems (neglected trauma, infections) and familiar presentation of unfamiliar (to them) conditions (polio, tuberculosis [TB], rickets). Both will challenge their judgment, skills, and knowledge, but also provide opportunities to care for patients in need and share information and experience with local colleagues.

Service provision missions involve direct patient care, with or without formal capacity building. They are usually short (<2 weeks) and the main focus is surgical output. To be successful, they require a strong partnership with local providers who are eager to participate and learn, even if only by osmosis, as they are providing screening and follow-up. The challenges are in the organization logistics, adaptation to local environment, meeting said and unsaid expectations, avoiding political missteps with minimal information, and the dreaded long-distance management of complications. In terms of trauma,

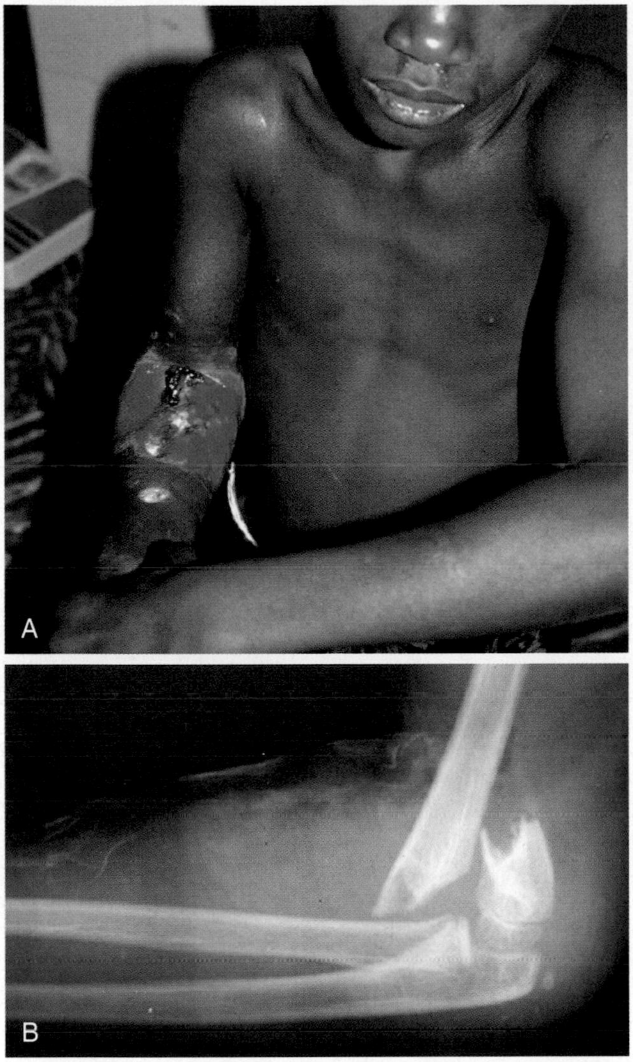

Figure 3-12. This 7-year-old young girl sustained an open type 3 right supracondylar humerus fracture approximately 3 weeks before being seen, initially treated by the traditional healer. The wound is infected, the bone is exposed, and there is ample pus drainage from the arm. She is septic, with painful axillary nodes. The father refused the proposed above-elbow amputation and brought her back to their village. She died 2 weeks later.

the volunteer will likely see cases of neglected trauma such as malunion, nonunion, chronic dislocations, or nerve injuries, and the occasional fresh injury presenting in the ED or lingering in traction or in a cast on the hospital wards. Surgical treatment, as mentioned before, needs to be appropriate: avoiding high-risk procedures, particularly when blood procurement is an issue, use of locally available implants, avoiding staged procedures where the burden of continuation of care falls on the shoulders of the national colleagues, and not using imported implants unless the ancillary equipment necessary to remove them are available after the volunteer's departure.

Teaching and Training: These programs are more likely to have a sustainable impact on the orthopaedic community and their patients. Volunteers are most often part of a long-standing relationship between their organization and the host institution, usually a university-affiliated hospital. The volunteer is incorporated in the established curriculum cycle, in addition to every teaching opportunity that presents itself in the course of the normal daily orthopaedic activity: on ward rounds, in the ED, and in the operating rooms. These assignments are usually longer: 2 to 6 weeks, which gives more time for volunteers to familiarize themselves with the normal orthopaedic routines and challenges faced by their local counterparts. The volunteer usually both follows and precedes another volunteer, so some form of continuity is present. Exposure to fresh as well as neglected trauma is guaranteed, and management skills are put to the test. Organizations such as Health Volunteers Overseas (HVO) and Orthopaedics Overseas (OO) have been active for decades now, and continue to grow each year, a testimony to both the sustainability of their long-term partnerships and the growing interest for international orthopaedic volunteerism.

Disaster relief has recently become very enticing to volunteers. The devastating 2010 earthquake in Haiti struck close to home, and brought an unprecedented response from the American medical community in general, and orthopaedic community in particular, and proved that disaster relief is, and should be, a specialized field in itself. Initial chaos is unavoidable in a catastrophe of this magnitude. The initial response requires coordination and collaboration between many different actors: military, government, NGOs, academic institutions, and all their equivalents in the afflicted host nation.

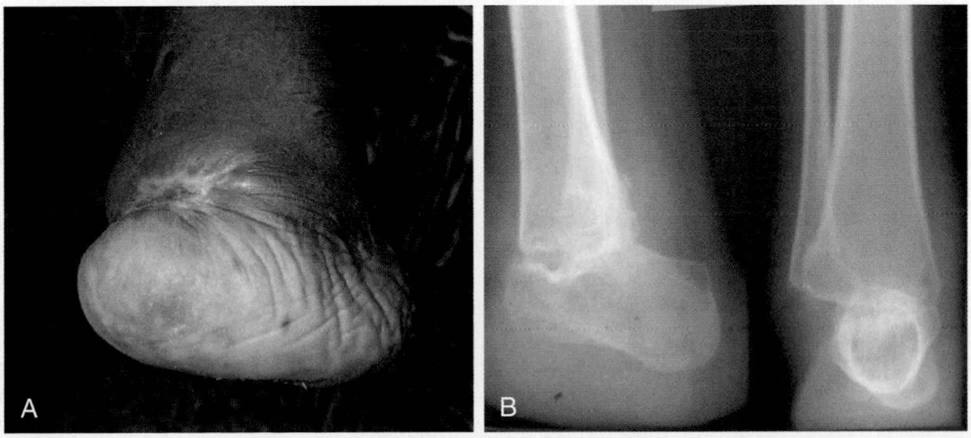

Figure 3-13. Appearance of a healed Boyd amputation with a sound tibiocalcaneal fusion. This is an end-bearing stump, and many patients go without even a shoe lift.

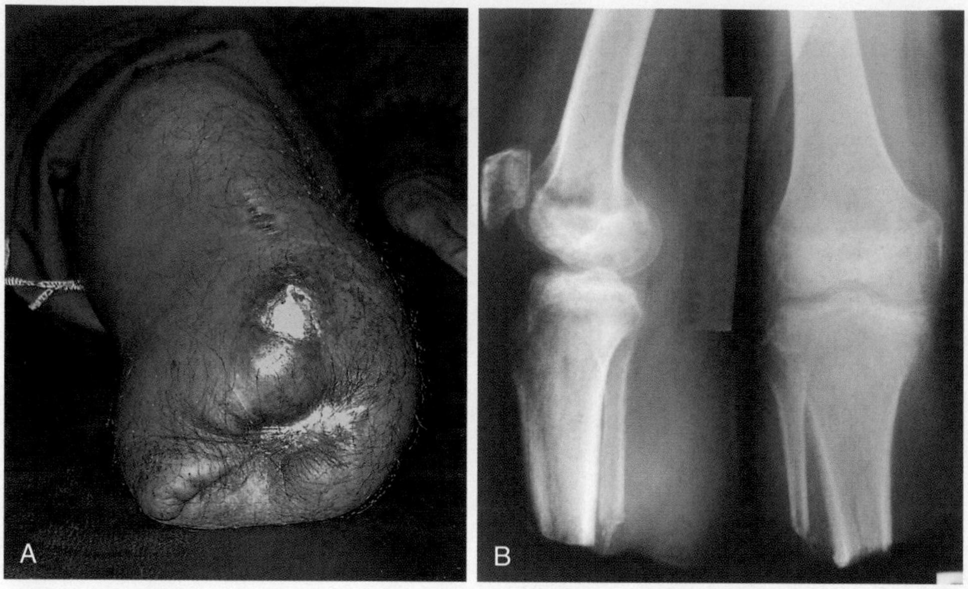

Figure 3-14. Chronic wound over the tip of the tibial stump of a below-knee amputation. The stump is not covered, the distal tibia has been cut slightly obliquely, and the anterior crest has not been beveled. The patient cannot use a prosthesis, and this will require revision.

Establishing chain of command, security, communications, water and sanitation, food and shelter, and reliable power supply all take priority over the actual provision of medical care. The volunteer orthopedist needs to understand that wound management is the critical activity for the first 1 to 2 weeks. Other critical issues will include patient identification, proper translation for informed consent and adequate charting capacity for documentation of procedures and treatment plans. "Real" orthopaedic surgery can begin only after a safe surgical environment, including reliable power and water supply, have been secured, often only after the second week. Definitive management of orthopaedic injuries will be achieved over the following weeks and months, with waves of volunteers replacing each other, and with the renewed capacity of the local medical practitioners. It cannot be overemphasized that orthopaedic volunteers should come as accredited members of accredited organizations, after proper training, not as the dreaded solitary unsolicited volunteer (SUV). To that effect, a collaborative effort between the AAOS, OTA, POSNA, and SOMOS has developed a disaster preparedness course (DPC) that is mandatory for volunteer preparation and accreditation, and has been well received so far.

Earthquake is the natural disaster that causes the most musculoskeletal (MSK) injuries. Open fractures, crush injuries, closed fractures from falls or direct impact are common, and amputation is unfortunately an all too common outcome, particularly in mass casualties situations, with late presentation. Other natural disasters such as hurricanes, tornadoes, tsunamis, volcano eruptions, avalanches, or mudslides can all be devastating, but rarely create a high burden of MSK injuries. Conflicts (human-caused disasters) and the so-called chronic emergencies share chaos and austere environments and their challenges with natural disasters, and some of the overall management principles. But MSK wounds from various weapons and those seen in natural disasters have a very different physiopathology. Their management is a stand-alone subspecialty, handled by trained military surgeons for military personnel, and a few specialized organizations such as the International Committee of the Red Cross (ICRC), Médecins Sans Frontières (MSF [Doctors Without Borders]) or the national organizations such as Merlin in the United Kingdom, Emergency in Italy, Médecins du Monde (MDM) in France, or the International Medical Corps (IMC) in the United States, for civilian victims. Interested volunteers are offered appropriate training before deployment. A certain level of comfort with different degrees of insecurity is a mandatory prerequisite. The management of orthopaedic injuries usually follows basic, safe, conservative, time-proven protocols for each organization.

THE SURGICAL IMPLANT GENERATION NETWORK INTRAMEDULLARY NAIL SYSTEM

Introduction

Background

As stated earlier, one of the main barriers to surgical care is the high cost of orthopaedic implants, which are paid for out-of-pocket by patients in most developing settings despite the fact that other hospital costs may be covered by government health insurance programs. For patients who seek and have access to formal medical care, skeletal traction may be the only affordable option. This can lead to prolonged immobilization with consequences for both health and financial well-being. In other cases a cheaper implant that is either poorly manufactured or not ideally suited for the fracture pattern is selected leading to worse outcome. Even where modern implants are available, the lack of working C-arm and intermittent electrical supply make many modern implants inappropriate. Through these mechanisms, implant availability has a significant impact on global disparities in the quality of fracture care.

SIGN was founded in 1999 as a nonprofit organization to address the need for low-cost fracture implants specifically intended for use in low-resource environments. The company designs and manufactures an interlocking IM nail system that is donated to hospitals in developing countries. In addition to supplying implants, education is at the foundation of SIGN's mission. With more than 5000 SIGN surgeons in developing countries, knowledge flows in a two-way exchange between SIGN, its volunteers, and surgeons across the globe. This is facilitated electronically by email, the Internet, technique manuals, and conferences as well as visits by US SIGN surgeons to developing countries that are often part of an exchange that allows SIGN surgeons to visit US medical centers.

Design Features

The SIGN nail was designed as a stainless steel tibia nail with 9-degree proximal bend, 1.5-degree distal bend and no arc of radius. An external jig allows the placement of both proximal and distal interlocking screws without fluoroscopic guidance. Because no other IM implants were readily available, surgeons in developing countries expanded the indications for SIGN nailing to fractures of the tibia, femur, and humerus. More recently, the SIGN nail has been used for knee and hind-foot arthrodesis. The same implants and instruments are used for all applications.

In contrast to most contemporary cannulated nail systems, the SIGN nail is a solid nail, which has the advantage of improved mechanical stability even when smaller diameter nails are used.[102] In addition, solid nails have shown greater resistance to infection in animal models.[103] All reaming is performed using hand reamers. The 7- to 9-mm reamers are sharp at the end and the 10- to 14-mm reamers have blunt ends. This allows the surgeon to feel the reamer as it progresses down the canal. The blunt-tipped reamers can be used to measure the length of the nail and determine if the reamer is in the canal, which is important in the absence of C-arm. An additional advantage of hand reaming is that bone can easily be recovered from the flutes of the reamer and placed at the fracture site if open reduction is performed. It also avoids the complication of thermal necrosis from excessive reaming.[104]

Proximally, the nail has one static locking hole and one slot for dynamic locking. Distally, the nail has two dynamic locking slots. The slots facilitate placement of the interlocking screws and allow dynamic compression to promote healing. The screws have threads on both ends with a wide tapered end on the near side. There are no threads in the middle so the screw can bear the forces of distraction and compression within the slot. The proximal and distal interlocking slots are found using a long jig and a slot-finding system described later in the chapter (Fig. 3-15). The system and training emphasize the importance of the tactile sense of the surgeon.

Innovation

SIGN is making a constant effort to continue innovating both to improve on existing implants and develop novel surgical tools. For example, a distraction device that uses bone-holding clamps rather than Schanz pins was developed to assist in regaining length in delayed fractures and maintain a provisional reduction during nailing. Drill covers with sterilizable chucks were designed for use with household carpentry drills because fully sterilizable drills are not affordable for many surgeons. These efforts are potentiated by the growing network of SIGN surgeons that has created a cooperative environment that stimulates innovation. These ideas and other research are shared at an annual conference at the SIGN headquarters in Richland, Washington.

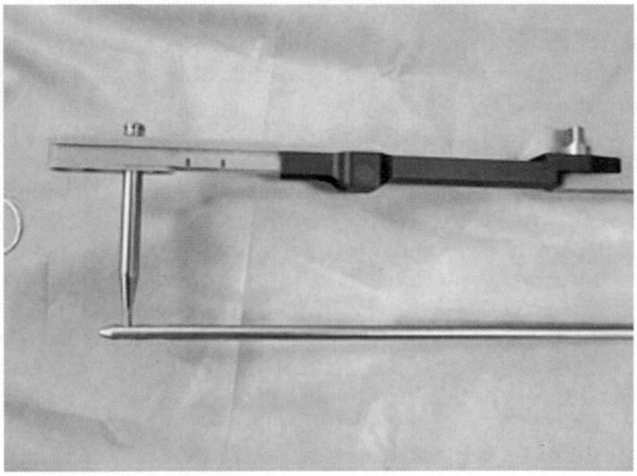

Figure 3-15. The target arm acts as an external jig to allow placement of the distal interlocking screw. *(Courtesy of Surgical Implant Generation Network.)*

Outcomes

There have been several published studies evaluating the outcomes of SIGN nailing. Among the first was by Shah and colleagues, who reported 32 patients with open tibial shaft fractures treated with débridement and primary medullary nailing using the SIGN nail in Nepal.[105] In their consecutive series, there were two superficial infections (6.4%), one deep infection (3.2%), and one nonunion (3.2%). Ikem and colleagues subsequently published a series of 40 patients with fractures of the tibia, femur, and humerus treated with SIGN nailing in Nigeria. The average time to union was 3 months with the only reported complication a case of screw loosening.[106] Most recently, Sekimpi and colleagues published the largest series of 50 patients with femoral shaft fractures treated with SIGN nailing.[107] In their series from Uganda, there were two dynamizations for delayed union (4%), two missed interlocking screws (4%), one superficial infection (2%), one deep infection (2%), and one hardware removal (2%). There are several other small published[108,109] and unpublished series that have been presented at the annual SIGN conference.

In addition to published studies, SIGN maintains an online database of all surgeries that records basic demographic data, characteristics of the injury and surgery, implant specifications as well as clinical follow-up data. The database is used both for inventory purposes and to provide feedback to surgeons who submit each postoperative radiograph. More recently the database has been used as a research tool. The first publication in 2009 reported data from more than 26,000 patients treated with SIGN implants for femoral and tibial shaft fractures, all from countries classified as low- or middle-income by WHO.[110] The rate of reoperation for infection reported was 1.3% and 1.9% for closed femur and tibia fractures, respectively, and 5.3% and 6.5% for open femur and tibia fractures, respectively. A more recent publication by Young and colleagues included 34,361 tibial and femoral fractures from the SIGN database. The overall infection rate was 0.7% for femoral fractures and 1.2% for tibial fractures; however, if the denominator were modified such that only patients with documented follow-up were included, infection rates were 3.5% and 7.3% for femoral and tibial fractures, respectively.[111] In a follow-up study by the same authors, the risk factors for infection included fracture of the tibia, open fractures, lack of preoperative antibiotics, and surgery for nonunion.[112] The primary limitation of all studies using the SIGN database is a follow-up rate below 20%; however, the follow-up rate has steadily improved over time with greater emphasis on the importance of clinical research.

Another important consideration is the cost-effectiveness of SIGN nailing given the resource constraints and large burden of disease that must be treated. Gosselin and colleagues showed that skeletal traction for femoral shaft fractures in Cambodia costs $1107 per patient compared to $888 for SIGN nailing.[113] The results suggest that surgical treatment is both more effective and less costly than nonoperative management with skeletal traction.

Surgical Technique

Interlocking Screw Placement

Distal interlocking is accomplished easily and efficiently without C-arms using the target arm and slot finders. Longitudinal orientation of the slot is determined by the target arm, while rotational orientation is aided by three different SIGN slot finders. Prior to inserting the nail, the target arm and nail are assembled on the back table, taking care to ensure that the target arm and slots are aligned. The target arm is removed for nail insertion, then reattached after the nail has been inserted to the desired depth and the surgeon is ready for interlocking. Throughout the process of interlocking, the surgeon or an assistant should ensure that the reduction is maintained.

The interlocking incision is marked by placing the alignment pin through the target arm. After making a skin incision and dissecting bluntly down to bone, the cannula is placed flush with near cortex. The drill guide is placed, and the near cortex is drilled. The larger drill guide is then used for the step drill, which enlarges the hole in the near cortex and is designed to lock into the slot in the nail, providing a firm end point if successful. In hard bone, the hole may have to be enlarged using the broach. The solid slot finder is inserted after the step drill. If the slot finder successfully engages the interlocking slot, it will allow 10 to 15 degrees of rotation, known as the "SIGN feel." At this point, the solid slot finder is replaced with the cannulated slot finder, which acts as a guide to drill through the interlocking slot through the far cortex. The screw length is determined with a depth gauge measured off the cannula, and the interlocking screw is inserted. Screw placement can be checked by attempting to rotate the nail, which should be fixed relative to the distal fragment if interlocking is successful.

An important concept to understand is the effect of deflection of the nail that can occur with forceful insertion. Bending of the nail leads to malalignment between the target arm and the interlocking slots (Fig. 3-16). Typically, the target arm will direct the cannula posterior to the tibia and anterior to the femur because of the orientation of the isthmus relative to the entry site. In these cases, the sequence described above using the target arm and cannula will not be successful because of bending of the nail. When this occurs, the surgeon should first check the reduction to ensure it has been maintained. If the reduction is lost after the near cortex is drilled, the longitudinal relationship between the target arm and interlocking slot will be lost. Assuming the reduction is maintained, the cap screw connecting the proximal and distal target arm should be loosened to allow the target arm to move over the bone. A pilot hole is drilled and enlarged using the step drill. If the solid slot finder does not enter the slot in the nail, the target arm is removed and the curved slot finder is placed into the hole while simultaneously rotating the nail to identify the slot. Longitudinal orientation is guided by the target arm while rotational orientation must be compensated for by rotating the nail. Once the curved slot finder enters the slot, place the cannulated slot finder and drill the far cortex. The interlocking screw is then inserted.

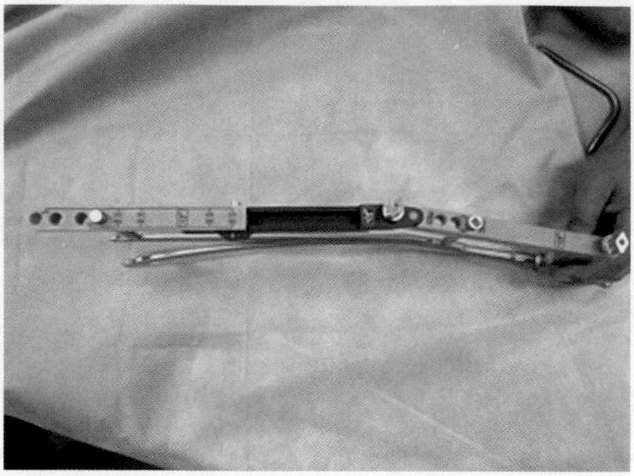

Figure 3-16. Effect of deformation of the nail on alignment of the target arm with the distal interlocking hole. If the nail is inserted forcefully into a curved canal, there will be mismatch between the target arm and the distal interlocking slot. *(Courtesy of Surgical Implant Generation Network.)*

Prior to attempting to place a second screw, an alignment pin can be placed through the target arm into the first interlocking screw head. This will hold the target arm in proper alignment with the interlocking slots to facilitate placement of the second screw. Two screws are usually necessary in the metaphysis because of weaker bone. If the surgeon elects to use one screw, we recommend using the slot nearest the fracture. The fracture can be compressed after the distal interlocking screws have been placed.

The proximal interlocking screws are placed using the target arm for guidance. The slot finders are not necessary. After placing the cannula on bone, both cortices are drilled at once using the drill guide. The near cortex is enlarged with the step drill, and the appropriate-length interlocking screw is inserted.

Fin Nail

The fin nail is an alternative to distal interlocking that uses a static configuration of the distal end to engage the femoral canal. We initially hypothesized that ideal fixation would be achieved by placing the fin in the isthmus, and comminuted, unstable fracture patterns should be avoided because the fin does not provide sufficient longitudinal stability. Nonetheless, there are many successful cases documented in the SIGN database where a fin nail was placed engaging in the metaphysis in a comminuted fracture. This may be explained, in part, by computer modeling, which has shown the straight nail in a curved canal leads to three-point fixation causing the distal end of the fin to engage against one side of the canal

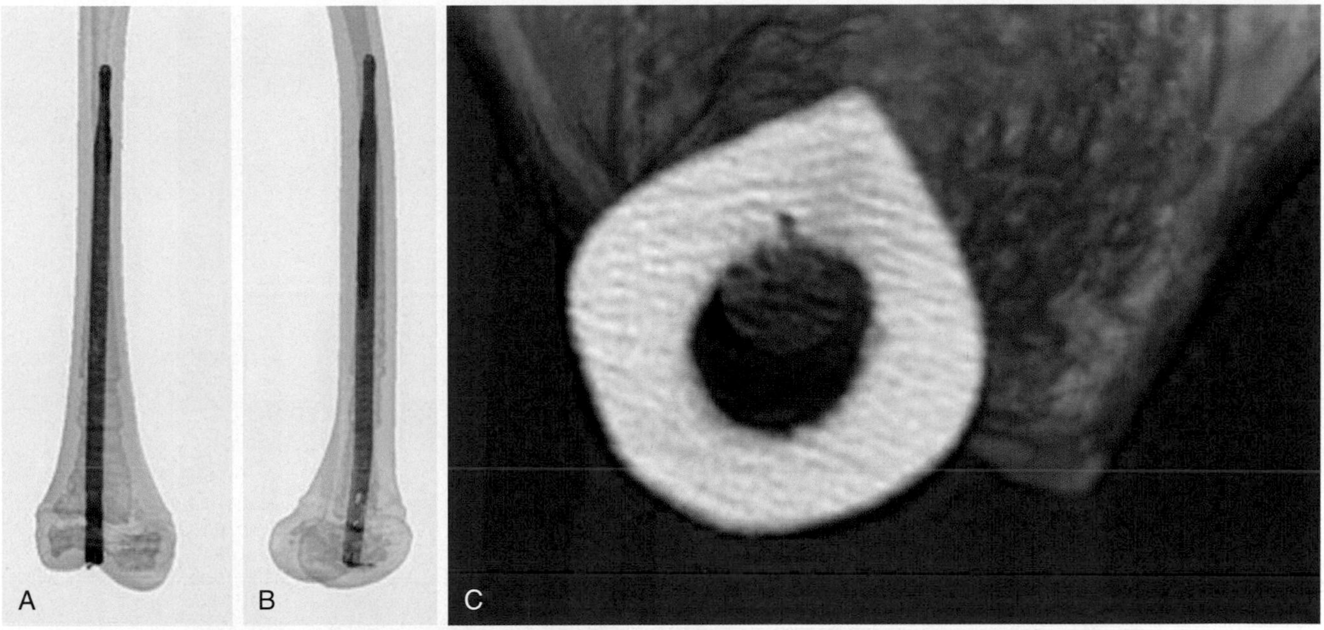

Figure 3-17. The fin nail is typically used in stable fracture patterns in which the fin can engage the isthmus of the canal for rotational stability. **A** and **B,** A common application is a distal femoral fracture treated using retrograde technique. **C,** The fin uses a distal flare to achieve an interference fit in the canal. *(Courtesy of Surgical Implant Generation Network.)*

(Fig. 3-17). This has allowed successful treatment of unstable fractures using the fin even when fixation in the isthmus is not possible.

The fin nail has been used commonly in the femur using antegrade and retrograde approaches as well as in the humerus. While less common, it can be used to treat tibial fractures successfully as well. A key advantage of the fin is the ease and speed with which it can be inserted, which may be particularly important in the polytrauma patient. The nail and interlocking screws can be placed in less than 20 minutes by an experienced SIGN surgeon.

The insertion technique for the fin is similar to the standard SIGN nail except that reaming follows a more specific sequence. After reaming until chatter, the final reamer is inserted only to the beginning of the fin configuration, leaving the remaining portion underreamed. This allows improved press-fit when the fin nail is placed. The proximal interlocking screws are placed using the target arm as described for the standard nail.

Tibial Nail Technique

Design Features. With a 9-degree proximal bend and 1.5-degree distal bend without an arc of radius, the SIGN nail is well suited for treating tibia fractures. The distal interlocking slots allow for fixation near the subchondral bone in distal fractures. The small distal bend was designed to facilitate distal interlocking screws using the slot finder, but it has the added benefit of enhancing feedback as the surgeon rotates the nail during advancement down the canal.

Incision and Bone Entrance. As with other tibial nails, the approach is made either through the center of the patellar tendon or at its medial or lateral borders depending on surgeon preference. In our experience, splitting the tendon is the most reliable approach for achieving a favorable start site. Planning the incision is facilitated by flexing the knee, which makes palpating the tendon easier. After the incision is made, a curved awl is used to make the entrance in the tibia. The awl should be directed anteriorly to avoid having the reamers pass through the fracture site posterior to the distal fragment.

Reduction. Closed reduction of middle- and distal-third tibial fractures without the C-arm is usually possible with 7 of 10 injuries. The knee is placed in 90 degrees of knee flexion either by hanging the leg off the edge of the table or placing a bump made from sterile gowns under the knee. If open reduction is needed, we recommend using an anterior incision lateral to the tibial crest with elevation of the anterior compartment. If the fracture has telescoped, be sure to observe for compartment syndrome after the tibia has been brought out to length.

Fractures of the proximal tibia require special attention as malalignment has been reported in up to 84% of cases.[114] A useful technique is to place the leg in the "figure 4" position, which prevents valgus deformity and allows pressure to be placed on the proximal fragment for reduction during reaming and nail insertion. If pressure is placed distal to the fracture, the deformity is accentuated and the nail will not pass into the distal fragment. Blocking screws may be used to prevent the nail from taking an undesirable path through the canal by inserting a screw across the canal in the aberrant path prior to reaming.[115] Typically, an anterior-to-posterior screw placed laterally in the proximal fragment and/or a medial-to-lateral screw placed posteriorly in the proximal fragment will prevent the common valgus and apex-anterior deformities, respectively. If the proximal fragment is displaced posterior to the distal fragment, correction of the alignment is more difficult and open reduction may be necessary. In these cases, pressure on the proximal fragment will accentuate the translational deformity. Once the reduction is obtained, placing the foot on the table gives counterpressure for stabilization of the fracture fragments during reaming.

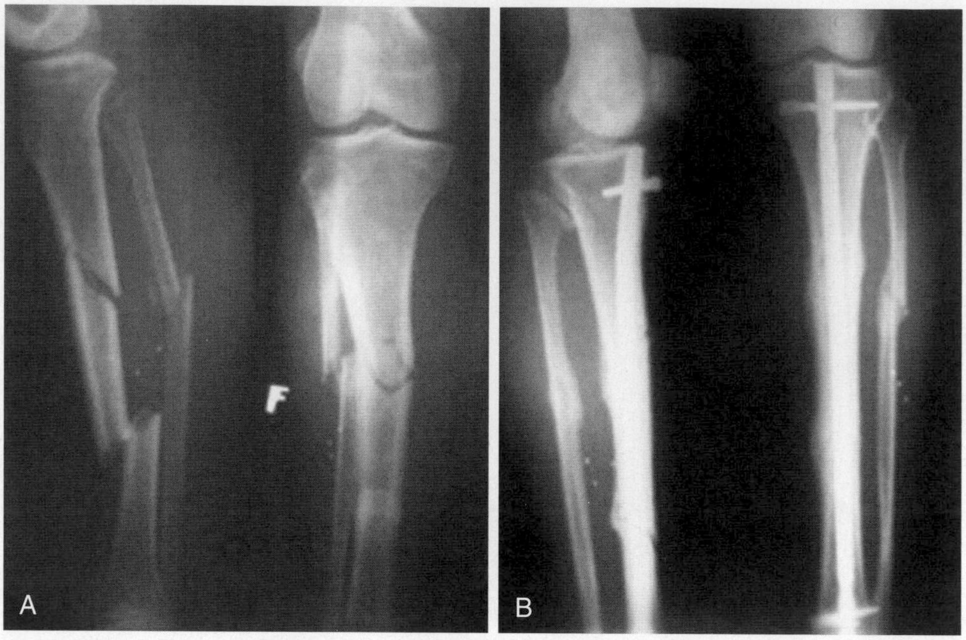

Figure 3-18. The first Surgical Implant Generation Network (SIGN) nail used for a tibial shaft fracture. *(Courtesy of Surgical Implant Generation Network.)*

Reaming. Typically, knee flexion of at least 110 degrees is necessary for placement of reamers and insertion of the nail.

Reduction must be maintained during reaming and nail insertion. The SIGN system uses semirigid hand reamers, which help the surgeon feel whether the reamer is in the canal using tactile sense without a C-arm. This is important if attempting a closed reduction because the reamer cannot be visualized crossing the fracture site. In cases where closed reduction is not possible, the bone from the flutes of the reamer is placed at the fracture site. We recommend a nail diameter 1 to 2 mm smaller than the reamer that causes cortical "chatter" for 360 degrees of rotation along 4 to 6 cm of the canal. The nail length can be determined by pushing the blunt-nosed reamer until it stops at the subchondral bone and measuring the length from the markings on the reamer shaft.

Nail Insertion. The tissue protector is used to keep the nail off the skin as it enters the bone. The nail is usually pushed in by hand without the use of a mallet. If a mallet is used, a rhythm is developed using two light taps and a 10-degree twist as the nail progresses down the canal. The nail is left 1 to 2 mm proud above the proximal tibia to add stability, particularly in proximal fractures. Forceful insertion of the nail should be avoided, as it may cause difficulty with distal interlocking.

Placement of Interlocking Screws. Interlocking screws are placed using the technique described earlier in the chapter. Distal interlocks are placed first using the target arm and slot finders. Proximal interlocks are placed using the target arm alone. We recommend two distal screws if the fracture is comminuted or located in the distal third (Fig. 3-18).

Femoral Nail Technique

Introduction. The SIGN nail was first adapted from tibial nailing for use in the femur to treat floating knee injuries using the retrograde approach. The antegrade nailing technique was later performed successfully by innovative SIGN surgeons. Postoperative knee stiffness was initially a concern with use of the retrograde approach. However, these concerns were mitigated after a study showed no loss of knee flexion using a postoperative protocol involving knee manipulation at the conclusion of the surgery and a postoperative home exercise program. The choice between antegrade and retrograde approach is therefore primarily based on the location of the fracture and surgeon preference.

To consider the retrograde approach, it should be confirmed preoperatively that there is at least 60 degrees of knee flexion. In the case of a very distal fracture in a patient with a long-standing knee extension contracture, we suggest removing the medial one-third of the patellar tendon from the attachment at the tibia tubercle. This tendon slip can be repaired at the end of the procedure.

Reduction. Open reduction is usually necessary for femur fractures if a C-arm is not available. The fracture site is palpated and the incision made through the skin and tensor fascia lata. In many cases a fracture fragment has penetrated the muscle and blunt dissection through the resultant tract will lead directly to the fracture site. This tract is then widened for additional exposure. If there are no defects in the vastus lateralis, a periosteal elevator is used to spread the muscle fibers and enter the fracture site. Cutting across muscle fibers should be avoided, and perforating vessels can be coagulated before damage and bleeding occur. Once the fracture site is localized, the incision is extended appropriately as needed. The bone ends should be prepared sequentially by removing any callus, scar, or hematoma that may impede reduction. Once both fracture fragments have been prepared, reduction may be accomplished using one of several methods:

1. If the fragments are telescoped 1 cm or less after traction is applied, a periosteal elevator can be placed between the fragments to lever them into a reduced position.

2. If the fragments are telescoped more than 1 cm, the fracture fragments can be flexed to bring one cortex into apposition, then slowly extended by an assistant to achieve the reduction.
3. If shortening is too severe to achieve either of these methods, a distraction device may be used. Distraction requires patience because achieving adequate length requires gradual relaxation and tearing of muscle fibers, which may require several minutes. In some cases, tight bands of quadriceps fascia can be released to facilitate the restoration of anatomic length.

After a provisional reduction is obtained, the rotational alignment should be assessed by palpating the linea aspera on each side of the fracture. Although this may be more difficult when the fracture is comminuted, proper alignment can still be achieved using the linea aspera as a guide. In our experience, open reduction avoids many of the problems with rotational malalignment experienced with closed nailing, where malrotation of greater than 15 degrees has been reported in 28% to 56% of cases.[116]

Antegrade Nail Technique. For the antegrade approach, the lateral position is preferred for ease of exposure. After reduction, an oblique incision is made along the axis of the fibers of the gluteus maximus. The tip of the trochanter is palpated and the gluteus fascia incised. Blunt dissection through the muscle fibers extends to the gluteus medius muscle and fascia, which inserts into the greater trochanter. In the absence of a C-arm, the start site is identified using palpation. The desired start site is at the tip of the greater trochanter at the junction of the middle and posterior thirds. This is achieved by palpating the anterior and posterior borders of the trochanter and making a fascial incision over the gluteus medius at the intended start site. A curved awl is inserted through the fascial incision to make a hole at the tip of the trochanter. After the entrance is made, the canal is sequentially reamed using the hand reamers until chatter occurs. The diameter of the nail selected is 2 mm smaller than the reamer that causes chatter. The bone from the flutes of the reamer is saved for placement at the fracture site. If additional bone graft is needed, a curette can be used to harvest bone from the metaphysis through the entrance hole. In some cases, reaming of the canal is done through the fracture site separately for the proximal and distal fragments into the metaphysis. In these cases reaming proximally to create the entrance hole is not advisable because the SIGN nail is a trochanteric nail, not a piriformis nail. If the fracture is old and has bony ingrowth into the canal, it may be necessary to over-ream by 3 mm at the fracture site before nail insertion.

The length of the nail is determined preoperatively using a template of the plain radiograph or by holding the reamer over the thigh and measuring from bony landmarks. During nail insertion, use the tissue protector to keep the nail from contacting the skin. Ideally the nail is inserted by hand with gentle rotation, which improves tactile feedback. If a mallet is used, we recommend striking the locking bolt with two light taps followed by a 10-degree twist of the L-handle in a rhythm as the nail progresses down the canal. Leaving the nail 3 mm above the cortical bone at the tip of the greater trochanter improves stability of the nail in the proximal fragment (Fig. 3-19). It is crucial that an assistant maintains the reduction using bone clamps during nail insertion. If the fracture slips after the hole in the near cortex is made for interlocking, reduction must be regained or it will be impossible to find the

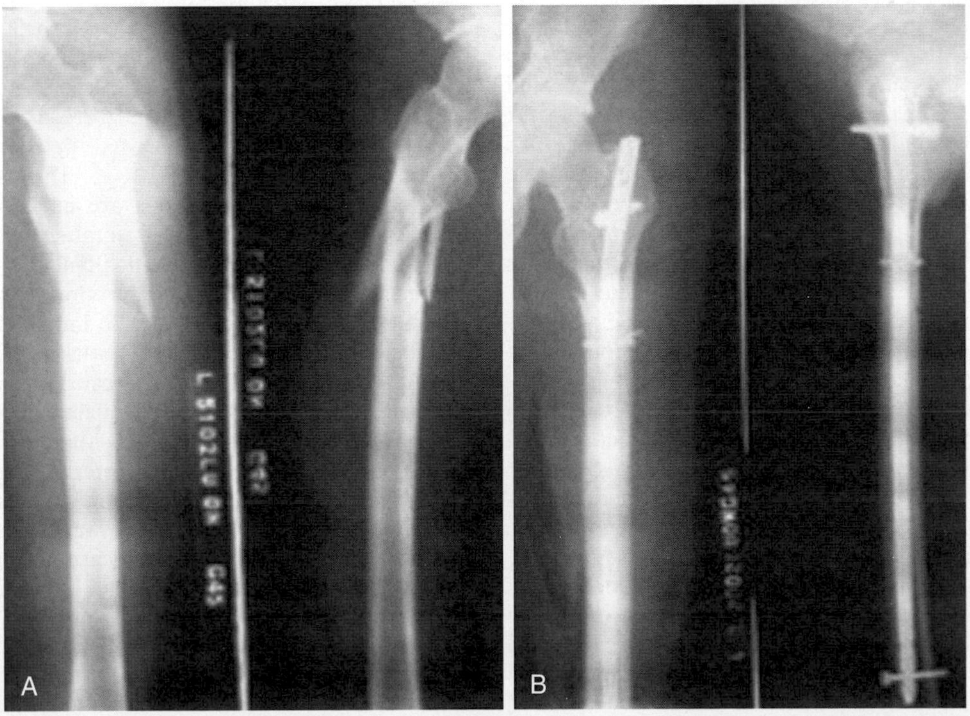

Figure 3-19. The first Surgical Implant Generation Network (SIGN) antegrade femur nail done by Dr. Han Khoi Quang in Vietnam. *(Courtesy of Surgical Implant Generation Network.)*

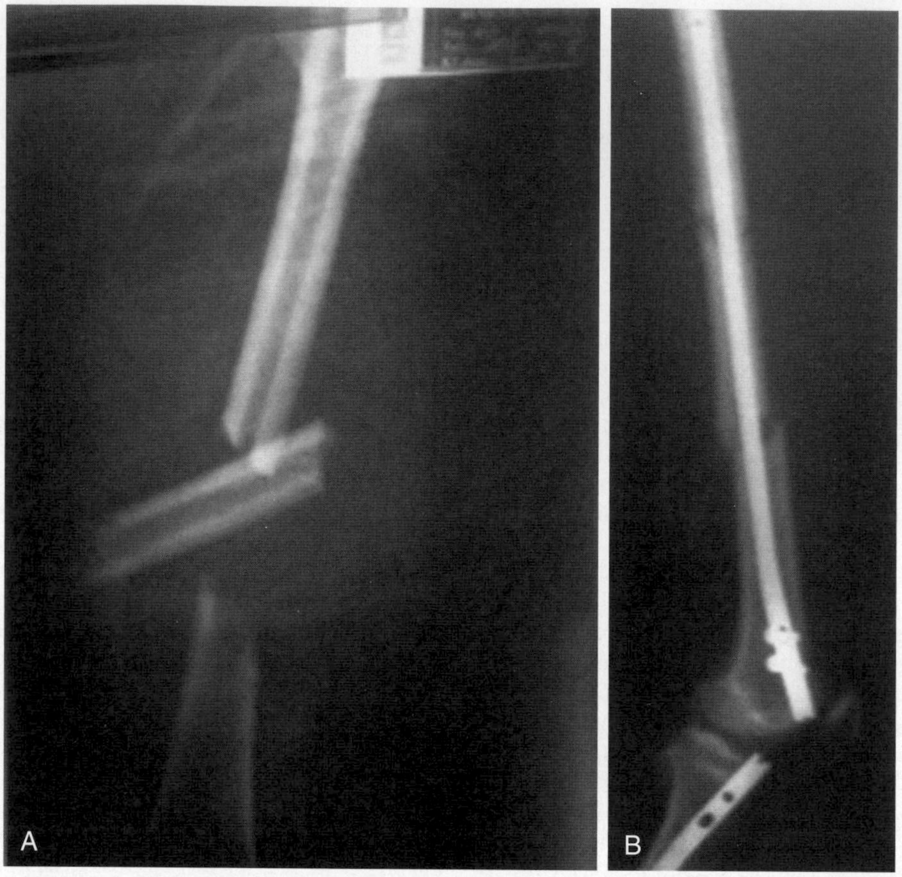

Figure 3-20. The first use of Surgical Implant Generation Network (SIGN) in the femur—a retrograde femoral nail in the setting of a floating knee injury in Vietnam. *(Courtesy of Surgical Implant Generation Network.)*

slot. Having an assistant apply countertraction facilitates nail insertion and helps to maintain the reduction.

Retrograde Nail Technique. The retrograde approach is performed with the patient in the supine position. Closed reduction without a C-arm may be successful for distal femur fractures treated within 1 week of injury. Open reduction is performed prior to entering the knee unless there is intraarticular involvement that requires exposure of the joint for reduction. If so, it is necessary to open the knee joint to judge reduction of the intraarticular fracture. If the fracture is intraarticular and involves the metaphysis, the medial parapatellar incision is extended proximally through the quadriceps tendon. This incision is used for total knee replacement surgery and provides excellent fracture reduction.

After reduction is obtained, an incision is made medial to the patellar tendon. A window is taken out of the fat pad and the femoral notch is exposed. A curved awl is inserted slightly anterior to the posterior cruciate ligament attachment. Counterpressure is applied to maintain fracture reduction while creating the start site, reaming, and insertion of the nail. The surgeon should orient the direction of reamers and nail by observing the direction of the fracture site. The end of the nail should not rest at the lesser trochanter or within 6 mm distal where the stress in the femur is highest. We have experienced several peri-implant fractures due to stress concentration at the end of the nail or the slot for the interlocking screw if the nail ends in this area. A blocking screw can be used to direct the nail from the metaphysis to the diaphysis in selected fractures. To ensure the appropriate depth of nail insertion, the ring on the stem should rest on the medial articular cartilage, which is easily palpated. This will leave the nail resting just below the articular cartilage (Fig. 3-20).

Hip Fractures

Background. Hip fractures are increasing in developing countries due to an increased number of road traffic injuries in younger patients and an aging population with osteoporosis suffering low-energy falls. Options for operative treatment are limited by economics and lack of implants that can be safely implanted without a C-arm. Initially SIGN surgeons were using the standard SIGN nail because it was the only implant available. Although this was adequate for some fractures, especially subtrochanteric fractures with a large enough proximal fragment to accommodate two interlocking screws, it became apparent that a dedicated hip implant was needed for more proximal patterns. The SIGN Hip Construct (SHC) was designed to address this need, bearing in mind the following criteria:

- No C-arm necessary
- Ability to treat both stable and unstable fractures
- No large holes in the lateral trochanteric wall
- Modularity to allow stabilization of different fractures
- Ability to stabilize combined hip and femoral shaft fractures

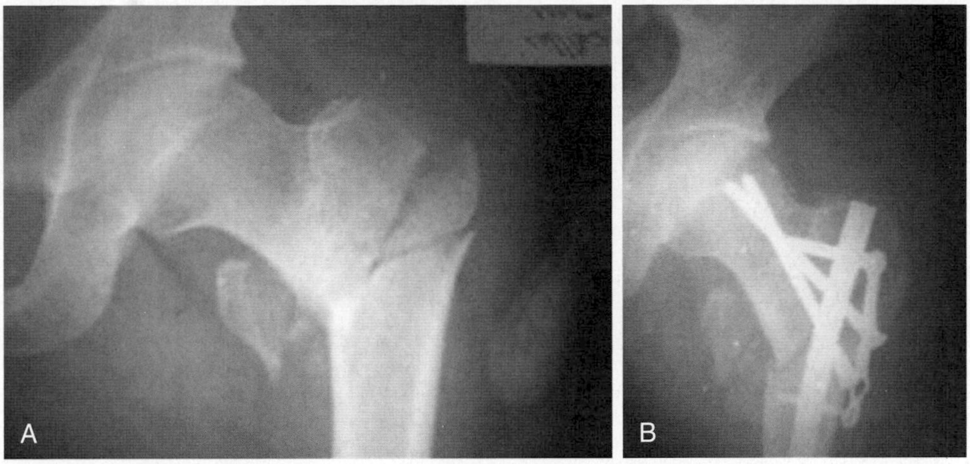

Figure 3-21. Surgical Implant Generation Network (SIGN) Hip Construct used to fix a four-part intertrochanteric fracture. The lateral plate is used in this case to address the unstable lateral wall. *(Courtesy of Surgical Implant Generation Network.)*

- Ability to apply intraoperative compression of the fracture site

The load to failure and fatigue to failure bench testing on the hip implant revealed the following:

- Distal interlocking screws for the nail are necessary.
- The proximal bend of the nail must be decreased to 6 degrees to rotate the nail and allow the interlocking screw to enter the femoral head.
- Threads on both ends of the compression screws provide additional stability.
- In fracture patterns involving the lateral trochanteric wall, a specialized plate connecting the interlocking screw to a bicortical screw distal to the fracture improves the stability of the construct.

The Surgical Implant Generation Network Hip Construct Technique. Prior to surgery a template of the unaffected hip determines the length and angle of the compression screws and proper length of the nail if there is a femoral shaft fracture. The patient is placed in the lateral position. A lateral approach to the proximal femur is performed extending from the vastus ridge distally for 4 cm. The vastus lateralis is incised. A finger placed under the anterior vastus lateralis allows palpation of the fracture site both anteriorly and inferiorly, which guides reduction using traction and rotation by an assistant. Intertrochanteric fractures can be successfully reduced using this technique up to 4 weeks after the injury. The quality of the reduction is the most important factor in determining the final stability of the construct.

After reduction is obtained, a 3.5-mm hole is placed in the anterolateral femoral shaft 1 cm below the vastus ridge and enlarged using the step drill. The screw hole broach is used to chamfer the hole to the proper angle prior to inserting the pilot drill to create a path for the compression screws into the femoral head. The pilot drill is a handheld drill bit designed to provide the surgeon with maximum tactile feedback as it progresses into the femoral head. The screw length can be measured from markings on the pilot drill. The compression screw is inserted while the reduction is maintained by the assistant. Once the screw is in place, the reduction is generally stable enough to allow placement of the SHC nail and interlocking screws.

The SHC nail is introduced through the tip of the trochanter with the target arm attached using the same technique as the standard SIGN nail. We have observed that putting the target arm in the same plane as the posterior femoral shaft roughly approximates anteversion for placement of the proximal interlocking screw. If there is a fracture in the lateral trochanteric wall, the interlocking screw is inserted through a plate that is attached distal to the fracture with a bicortical screw (Fig. 3-21). We believe placing the plate such that the distal screw is anterior to the nail helps prevent external rotation deformity.

The posterior compression screw is placed after the nail is inserted using the same technique as the anterior compression screw. The surgeon must not allow the holes for the compression screws to be less than 2 cm apart or for either screw to be located below the lesser trochanter to avoid a stress riser. The two compression screws or the interlocking screw may strike each other as they enter the femoral head. In this situation partially remove the interlocking screw and allow the compression screws to be inserted. At that point, the interlocking screw can be replaced.

In reviewing the patients who were treated with the SHC using this technique, it was found that the majority of reductions were maintained between radiographs immediately postoperatively and during later follow-up. However, this assessment is limited by the quality and consistency of available radiographs. The technique has a demonstrable learning curve with the quality of reduction and hardware placement improving with experience.

KEY REFERENCES

4. Mock CN, Joshipura M, Arreola-Risa C, et al: An estimate of the number of lives that could be saved through improvements in trauma care globally. *World J Surg* 36:959–963, 2012.
12. Mock C, Cherian M: The global burden of musculoskeletal injuries: Challenges and solutions. *Clin Orthop Relat Res* 466:2306–2316, 2008.
18. Mock CN: Strengthening care for the injured globally: 2010 Fitts oration. *J Trauma* 70:1307–1316, 2011.
25. Mock C, Arafat R, Chadbunchachai W, et al: What World Health Assembly Resolution 60.22 means to those who care for the injured. *World J Surg* 32:1636–1642, 2008.

28. Spiegel DA, Gosselin RA, Coughlin RR, et al: The burden of musculoskeletal injury in low and middle-income countries: challenges and opportunities. *J Bone Joint Surg Am* 90:915–923, 2008.
38. Grimes CE, Bowman KG, Dodgion CM, et al: Systematic review of barriers to surgical care in low-income and middle-income countries. *World J Surg* 35:941–950, 2011.
93. Charnley J: *The closed treatment of common fractures*, ed 4, London, 2004, Greenwich Medical Media.
94. Byrne T: Zimmer traction handbook. Available at: <http://www.zimmer.com/content/pdf/en-US/zimmer_traction_handbook.pdf>. Accessed July 24, 2013.
101. Smith DG, Michael JW, Bowker JH, editors: *Atlas of amputations and limb deficiencies*, ed 3, Rosemont, IL, 2004, American Academy of Orthopaedic Surgeons.
113. Gosselin RA, Heitto M, Zirkle L: Cost-effectiveness of replacing skeletal traction by interlocked intramedullary nailing for femoral shaft fractures in a provincial trauma hospital in Cambodia. *Int Orthop* 33:1445–1448, 2009.

The complete References list is available online at https://expertconsult.inkling.com.

Chapter 4

Biology and Enhancement of Skeletal Repair

J. TRACY WATSON

INTRODUCTION

The last 10 years has seen the rapid advancement of fracture fixation devices and surgical techniques. The development of preshaped locking plates in concert with minimally invasive surgical exposures has revolutionized the trauma surgeon's ability to treat complex periarticular injuries. Percutaneous instrumentation, the refinement of insertion portals, and the development of blocking screw techniques has expanded the range of intramedullary (IM) nailing from midshaft injuries to the articular margins. Likewise, the arena of orthobiologics has seen tremendous technological advancements in biomaterials and biologics in an attempt to avoid the perceived morbidity associated with the harvest of autogenous iliac crest bone graft (AICBG). Multiple materials have become available to enhance fracture healing through a myriad of biologic pathways. The purpose of this chapter is to review the basic fund of knowledge on the topic of bone graft substitutes. Currently available adjuvants for *approved* clinical use will be discussed. As well, the current levels of evidence in supporting the use of these various materials will be reviewed.

BIOLOGY OF GRAFT SUBSTITUTES

The biology of bone grafts and their substitutes is appreciated from an understanding of the bone formation processes of osteogenesis, osteoinduction, and osteoconduction.[1-5]

Graft osteogenesis: This is the ability of cellular elements within a donor graft, which survive transplantation, to synthesize new bone at the recipient site. Osteogenesis can occur in two ways. Surface osteoblasts can survive the transplantation by receiving nutrition through diffusion at the recipient site, and then proliferate to form more living bone tissue. There is more surface area in cancellous graft, and thus it has more potential for surviving cells than a cortical graft. Likewise the transplantation of marrow elements alone has demonstrated this ability to survive and form bone.

These transplanted cells or circulating pluripotential cells must have the appropriate substrate to attach to, or become attached to, once the cells have localized to the site of defect or injury. This substrate site for cellular attachment has to have the appropriate three-dimensional architecture to allow for these cells to proliferate. Subsequently, these cells then use this substrate as a scaffolding through which to build bone. This three-dimensional process involves vascular proliferation and ingrowth of capillaries along the open spaces in the substrate and thus the porosity of these materials is critical. Attachment is then followed by the differentiation of cells into bone-forming cells types, and the production and remodeling of bone then proceeds.[2,3,5]

Graft osteoconduction: A major category of available graft substitutes for defect management intervention is to provide a lattice-like substrate material that will facilitate the attachment and proliferation of osteoblastic cellular elements.

Graft osteoinduction: As all skeletal tissues evolve from mesenchyme, undifferentiated mesenchymal cells make a genetic commitment to a particular cellular lineage early in the developmental or repair process.[6] In the case of repair, some stimulus must signal the undifferentiated mesenchymal cells to differentiate along a chondro-osteogenic pathway. Prior to this differentiation into an osteogenic lineage, these cells are affected by multiple factors that provide chemotactic and mitogenic stimuli to these cells. This process is jump-started by graft-derived growth factors, such as transforming growth factor-*ß*, insulin-like growth factors 1 and 2, platelet-derived growth factor, and others. They influence these cells to migrate, attach, and multiply at the locale that provides a competent osteoconductive substrate as a site of cellular attachment.[7] This phenomenon, known as *osteoinduction,* is defined as "a process that supports the mitogenesis of undifferentiated mesenchymal cells leading to the formation of osteoprogenitor cells with the capacity to form new bone."[8-10] Thus, any material that induces this process could be considered to be osteoinductive.

The concept of osteoinductive new bone formation is realized through the active recruitment of host mesenchymal stem cells (MSCs) from the surrounding tissue, which differentiate into bone-forming osteoblasts. This process is facilitated by the presence of growth factors within the graft, principally bone morphogenic proteins.

Marshall R. Urist described the induction principle in the 1960s.[8] The concept of bone matrix—demineralized bone matrix (DBM)—is that this material contains properties that can induce de novo new bone formation when implanted into an extraskeletal site. It should be noted, however, this response is seen in animal models but has not been demonstrated in humans.

Urist and his colleagues soon identified a protein that they named *bone morphogenetic protein* (BMP).[8,10] Other molecules were soon identified and helped to characterize an entire family of osteoinductive molecules.[11] This family of specific factors now contains at least 15 BMPs and is part of the larger transforming growth factor-β (TGF-β) superfamily of molecules.

TABLE 4-1 *AVAILABLE FRACTURE HEALING ADJUVANTS WITH THEIR INHERENT PROPERTIES*

	Osteoconductive Scaffold	Osteoinductive Growth Factors	Osteogenic Living Cells
Synthetic Ca^{+} ceramics	•		
Marrow concentrates			•
Bone morphogenic protein (BMP)		•	
Autograft	•	•	•
Platelet-rich concentrates		Osteopromotive indirect cellular effect No intracellular transcription	
Banked demineralized bone matrix (DBM)	•	•	

Protein extracts derived from bone can initiate the process that begins with cartilage formation and ends in de novo bone formation. The critical components of this extract, BMPs, which direct cartilage and bone formation as well as the constitutive elements supplied by the animal during this process, have long remained unclear. Amino acid sequence has been derived from a highly purified preparation of BMP from bovine bone. Now, human complementary DNA clones corresponding to three polypeptides present in this BMP preparation have been isolated, and expressions of the recombinant human proteins have been obtained.[9,10]

Each of the three (BMP-1, BMP-2A, and BMP-3) appears to be independently capable of inducing the formation of cartilage in vivo. Two of the encoded proteins (BMP-2A and BMP-3) are new members of the TGF-β supergene family, while the third, BMP-1, appears to be a novel regulatory molecule. BMP factors can be synthesized by recombinant gene technology or derived from autologous bone, allogeneic bone, or from DBM.[9,10,12]

DBM is allogenic bone that has undergone the acid extraction of the mineralized extracellular matrix of the allograft bone. In theory, the noncollagenous proteins, including osteoinductive proteins such as the BMPs, remain viable while the structural portion of the allograft has been removed.[13]

All bone graft and bone-graft-substitute materials can be described through these three processes. While fresh autologous graft has the capability of supporting new bone growth by all three mechanisms, it may not be necessary for a bone graft replacement material to have all three properties inherent in that material in order to be clinically efficacious (Table 4-1). When inductive molecules are locally delivered on a scaffold, ultimately, MSCs are attracted to that site and are capable of reproducibly inducing new bone formation provided minimal concentration and dose thresholds are met. In some clinical studies, osteoinductive agents have been shown to potentially perform superiorly compared to conductive materials alone.

When bone marrow aspirate (viable stem cells) is applied to an osteoconductive scaffold, these cells are still reliant on the local mechanical and biological inductive signals to ultimately form bone. Similarly, osteoconductive materials work well when filling noncritical size defects that would normally heal easily without any additional adjuvants added. However, in more challenging critical-size defects, all three types of these materials are necessary as an adjunct in order to achieve efficacy equivalent to autograft.[2,3,14]

STAGES OF BONE GRAFT INCORPORATION

Bone grafts and bone graft substitutes incorporate via a well-defined pathway that can be divided into five distinct stages of host response, with the duration of each phase depending on the type of graft or adjuvant material used.[2,3,14,15]

Stage 1: Initial injury and hemorrhage: Initiates the pathway with the degranulation of platelets at the site of injury.

Stage 2: Inflammation: Under the influence of many active cytokines that are produced at the site of injury. These cause migration of cells to the site of injury.

Stage 3: Vascular proliferation and ingrowth. Under the influence of many cytokines invading capillaries bring perivascular tissue with mesenchymal cells that can differentiate into osteoprogenitor cell lines. A competent conductive substrate is required for this process to occur. This vascular invasion can be significantly inhibited by nonsteroidal antiinflammatory medications, which will inhibit this process and thus alter the fracture healing pathway.

Stage 4: The fourth stage consists of osteoclastic resorption of the avascular (dead) bone graft lamellae and simultaneous production of new bone matrix by osteoblasts.

Stage 5: In the final stage, the newly formed bone is remodeled and reoriented based on the mechanical environment of the host site.

Orthobiologic interventions have been specifically designed to target these stages to achieve a specific effect. Each broad category of intervention will be discussed in terms of the desired effect these material have on the specific stage of graft incorporation. The gold standard and prime material that all others are compared to is AICBG.

AUTOGENOUS ILIAC CREST BONE GRAFT

Fresh cancellous autograft provides the quickest and most reliable type of bone graft. Its open structure allows rapid revascularization; a 5-mm graft may be totally revascularized in 20 to 25 days. These grafts depend on ingrowth of host vessels and perform best in well-vascularized beds. The large surface area of harvested autograft allows for survival of numerous graft cells. It is estimated that approximately 30 mL of graft can be reliably harvested from an anterior iliac crest.[16] However, many other sites of harvest have been described, differing only in the amount of graft obtained from each harvest site (see Table 4-1). Recent literature has demonstrated histologic differences between iliac crest and tibial bone graft, suggesting superiority of iliac crest in terms of osteogenic and hematopoietic progenitor cell content.[17] Studies document success rates approaching 100% for subcritical-size defects (1- to 2-cm defects) requiring 20 mL or less of autograft.[9,18]

There are many issues regarding AICBG because of limited quantity available, and the reported rates of postoperative pain from the graft harvest site.[19,20] Substantial rates of complications related to the harvest site have been reported.[17,19] It has been thought that this technique is restricted to short defects, in the range of 4 to 6 cm. Numerous studies report favorable union results for critical-size defects up to 4 cm. However, in many of these studies, multiple graft procedures were required to achieve solid union.[18,21-23]

The ability to obtain substantial amounts of autogenous graft material would appear as an advantage for the treatment of critical-sized defects. The reamer-irrigator-aspirator (RIA; Synthes, Paoli, PA) offers a technique to achieve substantial amounts of graft volumes for the treatment of larger segmental defects. The medullary canal of the femur or tibia is reamed with a device designed to collect the reamings and deliver them for potential grafting procedures.[24,25] Variable amounts of harvested graft with this technique have been reported in the literature and range from 30 to 90 mL. A recent comparison between a historical control group using anterior iliac harvesting (40 patients) versus a study group using femoral shaft RIA harvesting (41 patients) documented on average 25 to 75 mL of harvested RIA graft (average = 40.3 mL).[24] The authors reported a favorable union rate with RIA bone grafting (37 of 41 patients) versus AICBG (32 of 40 patients), although not statistically significant. There were significantly lower postoperative harvest site pain scores from the RIA group versus the AICBG group at 48 hours, 48 hours to 3 months, and greater than 3 months (P = 0.001, 0.001, and 0.004, respectively). There were a total of two complications related to the graft harvest site in the RIA group (one perforation of the distal anterior femoral cortex treated conservatively and one excessive reaming of the femoral neck treated with prophylactic cannulated screws) versus 12 harvest site complications in the AICBG group (3 infections, 1 hematoma, and 8 patients with numbness).

This study has several limitations including the concurrent use of BMP-2 in most cases. This somewhat limits the ability to draw strong conclusions regarding the relative efficacy of RIA bone graft versus AICBG from this study.[24]

A recent study reported on the treatment of 20 bone defects ranging from 2 to 14.5 cm (average = 6.6 cm) using RIA bone graft. Eighteen of the 20 patients were initially treated with an antibiotic cement spacer using the Masquelet technique[26-29] (Fig. 4-1). The average graft volume obtained using the RIA was 64 mL. Seventeen of 20 bone defects ultimately healed, although 7 of these required repeat surgery. The authors reported no significant complications related to the bone graft harvest site[19,30] (see Fig. 4-1).

Numerous basic science studies have demonstrated the biologic potential of RIA bone graft. Investigators have documented elevated amounts of osteoinductive growth factors[31-35] and osteoprogenitor and endothelial progenitor cell types compared to AICBG. The RIA filtrate contains large numbers of MSCs that could potentially be extracted without enzymatic digestion and used for bone repair without prior cell expansion. Medullary autograft cells harvested using RIA are viable and osteogenic. Cell viability and osteogenic potential were similar between bone grafts obtained from both the RIA system and the iliac crest.[36]

Elevated levels of fibroblast growth factor-α (FGF-α), platelet-derived growth factor (PDGF), insulinlike growth factor-1 (IGF-1), TGF-β_1, and BMP-2 were measured in the reaming debris as compared to iliac crest curetting's. However, vascular endothelial growth factor (VEGF) and FGF-β were significantly lower in the reaming debris than from iliac crest samples. In comparing platelet-rich plasma (PRP) and platelet-poor plasma (PPP), all detectable growth factors, except IGF-1, were enhanced in the PRP. In the reaming irrigation FGF-α (no measurable value in the PRP) and FGF-β were higher, but VEGF, PDGF, IGF-1, TGF-β_1, and BMP-2 were lower compared to PRP. BMP-4 was not measurable in any sample. The bony reaming debris is a rich source of growth factors with a content comparable to that from iliac crest. The irrigation fluid from the reaming also contains growth factors. Although the early evidence regarding RIA bone grafting is encouraging, there is currently a lack of high-level comparative evidence.

OSTEOCONDUCTIVE GRAFT SUBSTITUTES

There is considerable interest in creating osteoconductive matrices using nonbiological porous structures implanted into or adjacent to bone. The host substrate must mimic the cancellous bony architecture and have very specific surface kinetics to facilitate the migration, attachment, and proliferation of MSCs, which then differentiate into osteoprogenitor cells (augmentation of stages 2 and 3 of graft incorporation). Broad categories of these materials are available and, in general, are classified as calcium ceramics. These include the specific materials of calcium sulfate, calcium phosphate, synthetic tricalcium phosphate as well as β-tricalcium phosphate, and coralline hydroxyapatite (HA).

The history of bioceramics dates back to 1892 with the use of calcium sulfate for space-occupying lesions. Calcium sulfate has the distinction of being the alternative that is both one of the simplest as well as that which has the longest clinical history as a synthetic bone graft material—spanning more than 100 years.[37]

The original material was plaster of Paris, which is noninflammatory and nonreactive and encouraged bone healing in a contained lesion. Peltier took commercial-grade plaster of Paris, which was then mixed with water, poured into molds made of wax paper or aluminum foil, and then allowed to set, forming small pellets or columns. He performed a series of bone defect studies in dogs to determine the role these materials had in the ability to heal these defects.[38] From his experiments, he determined that the plaster of Paris itself does not stimulate osteogenesis. Its chief effect was found to be a mechanical one of preventing the collapse of the periosteal tube and favoring regeneration. In this way the material provided a supportive scaffolding.[38-40] There is no doubt, however, that subperiosteal resections in which plaster of Paris columns were inserted regenerated, in whole or in part, more frequently than was the case in subperiosteal resections alone.

Subsequently, coralline HA was reported for similar lesions followed by other ceramics. All of these bone graft substitutes

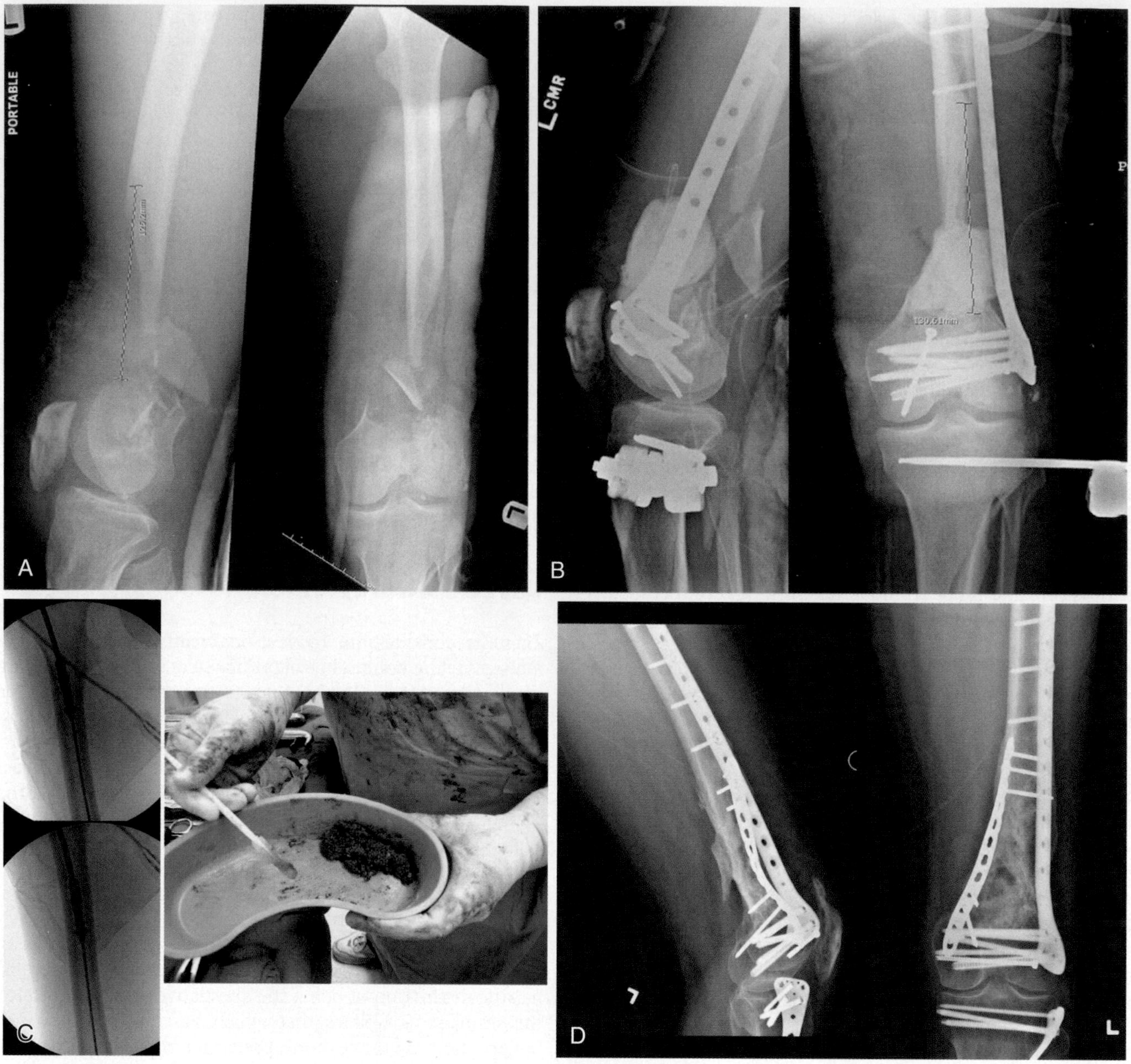

Figure 4-1. A, Open distal femoral shaft fracture with 13-cm segmental defect. **B,** Fracture underwent multiple débridements with eventual placement of a large antibiotic spacer into the skeletal defect with stabilization using a plate and spanning external fixator. **C,** After complete soft tissue healing had been accomplished, and the development of an enveloping psuedomembrane surrounding the antibiotic cement spacer to form (Masquelet technique), massive autografting was carried out. The reamer-irrigator-aspirator (RIA) was used to harvest a substantial amount of graft from the contralateral femur. The spacer was carefully removed leaving the psuedomembrane intact grafting into the well-defined space spanning the defect. **D,** Complete healing of the defect at approximately 6 months after grafting.

have the advantage of being nonimmunogenic, noninflammatory, in an unlimited supply, and packaged sterile.

Calcium Sulfate Substitutes

Calcium sulfate was one of the first orthobiologic materials to be used commercially as a bone graft substitute. Calcium sulfate has a crystalline-independent rate of incorporation and is very consistent in terms of dissolution and incorporation. The crystalline structure is consistent throughout a whole range of materials, with a constant rate of osteointegration. In contrast to calcium phosphate, calcium sulfate behaves as a true salt, that is, if it egresses into the joint, it quickly dissolves into sulfate and calcium ions and is then absorbed into the synovium. This resorption mechanism involves a fluid exchange mechanism and may promote excessive drainage if used in wounds with questionable soft tissue coverage or integrity. A low but consistent complication rate, specifically serous drainage from the wound as the calcium sulfate absorbs, has been reported. This complication is higher when the material is used in higher volumes (greater than 20 mL) or in subcutaneous bones (tibia, ulna).[41]

This may cause a potential increase in osmotic load at the site of implantation. Therefore, to avoid subsequent drainage at the graft site, the calcium sulfate product should be reserved for situations with adequate blood supply and competent soft tissue coverage. Additionally, this material should be used in a contained defect only.[42] Studies document that implanted calcium sulfate pellets in contact with joint synovial fluid are at risk for resorption without any significant bony healing response.[43] If calcium sulfate pellets are to be implanted in periarticular locations, complete bony containment is necessary.[44]

Calcium sulfate hemihydrate has been used for many years as a self-setting biomaterial due to its good setting properties. The fairly rapid degradation rate of these materials, which occurs in 3 to 4 months, was once viewed as an advantage.[45] However, as these materials began to be used to support articular subchondral surfaces in cases of periarticular plateau and pilon fractures, this rapid degradation becomes a distinct disadvantage.[46] Transition to full weight bearing occurs normally at 3 to 4 months after surgery, and many cases of late articular collapse have been subsequently reported due to this rapid incorporation with the simultaneous loss of articular support.[21,47] Additionally, this material demonstrates rapid loss in its mechanical compressive strength following implantation, when compared to the phosphate ceramics.

This combination of rapid degradation rate, speedy loss of compressive strength, and lack of bioactivity have currently limited its application for bone defect management.[37] Three case series examining the use of calcium sulfate for the treatment of bone nonunion revealed a significant failure rate, suggesting that this material, used in isolation, is not optimal to promote union in that setting.[41,48]

The current best use of this material appears to be that of a carrier for adjuvant antibiotics as a treatment for osteomyelitis. The characteristics regarding rapid resorption and degradation are now advantageous for delivering high-dose antibiotics. McKee and colleagues demonstrated results for the treatment of chronic osteomyelitis and infected nonunions, using an antibiotic-impregnated calcium sulfate pellet. He felt that this was equivalent to standard surgical therapy in eradicating infection and reducing the number of subsequent surgical procedures necessary.[49,50]

There is level I and II evidence (one randomized trial, one case-control study, one prospective cohort study) that antibiotic-impregnated bioabsorbable calcium sulphate has the potential to reduce the number of procedures and surgical morbidity associated with the surgical treatment of chronic osteomyelitis and infected nonunion while maintaining a high rate of infection eradication. Calcium sulphate remains an inexpensive, safe, reliable bone-void filler that can also serve as an absorbable delivery vehicle for antibiotics or other compounds.[49,50]

Calcium Phospate Substitutes

Calcium phosphate substitutes are osteoconductive, but they are not osteoinductive unless growth factors, BMPs, or other osteoinductive substances are added to create a composite graft. Calcium phosphate is available in a variety of forms and products, including ceramics, powders, and cements. Ceramics are highly crystalline structures created by heating nonmetallic mineral salts at temperatures greater than 1000° C, a process known as *sintering*. These phosphate materials have variable rates of osteointegration based on their crystalline size and stoichiometry.[1]

Hydroxyapatite

Synthetic HA is a crystalline calcium phosphate osteoconductive bone substitute that is also manufactured as a ceramic through a sintering process. This material was some of the first available to be used clinically as a bone graft substitute. Porous HA (Interpore 500) was formed by conversion of the *Porites goniopora* coral exoskeleton, with pores averaging 600 μm and pore interconnections averaging 260 μm in diameter.[1,21]

Clinical studies with this material used for augmentation of tibial plateau fractures were successful when used with internal fixation. No significant radiographic or clinical differences were appreciated between those patients that were randomized to have the defect filled with either autogenous bone or porous HA.[51]

The investigators felt that a major drawback of the material was that the rate of incorporation was very slow. The appositional process of incorporation of the implant was confirmed by the finding that only 66.5% of the surface of the Interpore 500 was covered with bone ingrowth at 12 months. Thus, a relatively long incorporation time was documented.[51-53]

Other investigators studied the ability of this material to act as a conductive substrate and determine the effectiveness of coralline HA as a bone graft substitute for lumbar spine fusion when used in combination with bone marrow, or when mixed with autogenous bone graft (ABG), or combined with an osteoinductive material (BMP).[54] The data indicated that coralline HA with bone marrow was not an acceptable bone graft substitute used alone for posterolateral spine fusion when compared to autograft.

When combined with AICBG, coralline HA served as a graft extender yielding results comparable to those obtained with autograft alone.[51] In addition, coralline HA served as an excellent carrier for the bovine osteoinductive bone protein extract yielding superior results to those obtained with autograft or bone marrow.[54] As with other characteristics of these materials, the rates of osteoinduction were greatest when a porous architecture was maintained.[55,56] Animal studies have suggested that HA may have some osteoinductive properties in addition to its osteoconductive capabilities.[1-3,57,58]

The crystalline structure dictates the rate of osteointegration. These materials integrate via a cell-mediated response, and the pore structure found in these materials serves as sites for cellular attachment. This porosity makes these materials very brittle with minimal tensile strength.[59] Because of these material properties, and concerns regarding very slow bone formation, HA used alone is not commonly used as an osteoconductive bone substitute at this time.

The porosity of these materials is the primary factor in determining the ability to foster ingrowth and osteointegration. No osseous ingrowth occurs with pore sizes of 15 to 40 μm. Osteoid formation requires minimum pore sizes of 100 μm, with pore sizes of 300 to 500 μm reported to be ideal for osseous ingrowth.[60] Some authors, however, have reported that pore size may be less critical than the presence of interconnecting pores for osseous ingrowth. Interconnecting pores prevent the formation of blind alleys, which are associated with low oxygen tension; low oxygen tension prevents osteoprogenitor cells from differentiating into osteoblasts.[1,61]

Highly porous interconnected materials have abundant sites available for cellular interactions, which help these materials osteointegrate faster. This is accompanied by a corresponding decrease in the compressive strength afforded. If the material is designed with minimal porosity, the rate of osteointegration will be prolonged because of the paucity of cellular interactions. The corresponding compressive strength will also be very high. As noted, their ability to provide structural support is dependent on the degree of porosity inherent in each unique material that can be highly manipulated.[1,21] These materials have the advantage of incorporating at a slower rate than calcium sulfate materials. They increase bone formation by providing an osteoconductive matrix for host osteogenic cells to create bone under the influence of host osteoinductive factors shores.

Tricalcium Phosphate

Tricalcium phosphate (TCP) is a commonly available resorbable ceramic. It can be obtained in block, granular, powder, or putty form. Coralline ceramics are formed by thermochemically treating coral with ammonium phosphate, leaving TCP with a structure and porosity that is similar to that of cancellous bone.

TCP is less brittle and has a faster resorption rate than HA because of the increased porosity. Animal studies demonstrated that 95% of calcium phosphate is resorbed in 26 to 86 weeks.[62,63] This is much faster when compared to the previous HA reported rates of osteointegration.

TCP and HA have been combined into a biphasic calcium phosphate composite that has a faster resorption rate than pure HA. In a clinical study using a composite graft, a mixture of porous beads composed of 60% HA and 40% TCP ceramic and fibrillar collagen was used as a graft substitute and combined with autogenous bone marrow. Collagraft (Zimmer and Collagen Corporation) was randomized against cancellous iliac crest autografts in the treatment of long bone fractures. This material appeared to function as well as autogenous graft when used in the treatment of acute long bone fractures.[64]

Calcium phosphate can also be manufactured as cement, by adding an aqueous solution to dissolve the calcium, which is followed by a precipitation reaction in which the calcium phosphate crystals grow and the cement hardens. The primary advantage of cements over blocks, granules, or powders is the ability to custom-fill defects[21,47] and produce increased compressive strength. However, cement can be extruded beyond the boundaries of the fracture, potentially damaging the surrounding tissue. This is especially problematic if these materials extrude into a joint cavity following repair of a subchondral defect such as a tibial plateau. This presents a potential disadvantage of these phosphate materials, as they will not dissolve if they happen to migrate into the joint.[65] The ability of calcium phosphate bone substitutes to act as a bone-void filler has been documented in multiple preclinical animal studies and biomechanical and human case series.[66]

One such representative biomechanical study evaluated the fatigue strength of calcium phosphate–augmented repairs versus ABG repairs for lateral tibia plateau fractures. Reproducible split-depression fractures were simulated and repaired with each specimen randomly assigned to either calcium phosphate or ABG as augmentation. Calcium phosphate–augmented repairs subsided less and were more stiff during the fatigue loading than were ABG repairs at the 70,000, 140,000, and 210,000 cycle intervals ($P < 0.03$). The authors concluded that the calcium phosphate repairs had significantly higher fatigue strength and ultimate load than ABG repairs and may serve to increase the immediate weight-bearing capabilities of the repaired plateaus in clinical practice.[67]

A large clinical retrospective case series reviewed 43 patients with traumatic bone defects or nonunions treated. Defects of the femur, tibia, calcaneus, humerus, ulna, or radius had treatment augmented with TCP. Ninety percent of the fractures and 85% of the nonunions had united at the time of follow-up, average of 12 months. The authors concluded that TCP was a useful substitute for cancellous[68] bone if the local biology provided a suitable blood supply. This was deemed necessary to provide competent cells and circulating inductive factors.

The use of injectable bone calcium phosphate cements offers the opportunity to support the reduced joint surface without open bone grafting. This is a valuable adjuvant, as less invasive fixation approaches are becoming widely accepted and the ability to limit the exposures for grafting and subchondral defect augmentation would also be a valuable tool. Jubel and colleagues evaluated the clinical and radiologic outcomes of an injectable calcium phosphate material (Norian SRS) used for tibial plateau fractures. The time interval from surgery to partial weight bearing was 3.7 weeks. The results demonstrated that this material can be successfully used to fill metaphyseal bone defects in tibial plateau fractures. The clinical and radiologic results were comparable to those of fractures treated with autologous bone graft. The high compression strength allows early full weight bearing without the risk of secondary loss of reduction. Soft tissue reactions due to the cement were not observed.[69] However, on all radiographs taken 36 months after the operation, the phosphate cement block was still visible indicating a very slow rate of osteointegration, which may be of some concern to some clinicians. Once the transition to full weight bearing has been achieved, it would be desirable to have the material almost completely integrated. There are newer phosphate materials now available that have shorter times to complete osteointegration as these crystalline structures can be manipulated accordingly.

In a critical study by Russell and colleagues, the efficacy of a bioresorbable calcium phosphate cement was compared with standard autogenous iliac bone grafting in a multicenter, prospective, randomized study for the treatment of these osseous defects.[70] Randomization to treatment with calcium phosphate cement (82 fractures) or autogenous iliac bone graft (38 fractures) occurred at the time of surgery. There was a significantly ($P = 0.009$) higher rate of articular subsidence during the 3- to 12-month follow-up period in the bone graft group. The bioresorbable calcium phosphate cement used in this study appeared to be a better choice, at least in terms of the prevention of subsidence, than autogenous iliac bone graft for the treatment of subarticular defects associated with unstable tibial plateau fractures.

Many studies have specifically evaluated these materials as bone graft substitutes in the management of subchondral bone defects associated with tibial plateau fractures. A meta-analysis study compared calcium phosphate cement substitutes directly to these other conductive substrate materials used for plateau augmentation: HA granules, calcium sulphate, bioactive glass, TCP, DBM, allografts, autografts, and xenografts.[71] Fracture healing was uneventful in more than 90% of the cases over the variable time period of the meta-analysis. Secondary collapse of the knee joint surface ≥2 mm was highest in the biological substitutes group, 8.6% (allograft,

DBM, autograft, and xenograft). This is similar to the results noted by Russell in his randomized study comparing autologous iliac bone graft (AIBG) to calcium phosphate cement. Late collapse was less in the HA-treated group, 5.4%, and the material that had the least subsidence was the calcium phosphate cement group. 3.7%. The group that experienced the highest rate of subsidence was the calcium sulfate cases, 11.1%.[72] This is consistent with the rapid dissolution time and relative biomechanical properties of this material discussed previously in this chapter.

The recorded incidence of primary surgical site and donor site infection (3.6%) was not statistically significantly different among all the grafting groups. However, donor site-related pain was reported up to 12 months following AIBG harvest. Shorter total operative time, greater tolerance of early weight bearing, and improved early functional outcomes within the first year after surgery were noted in the studies reporting on the use of injectable calcium phosphate cements. Despite a lack of good quality randomized controlled trials, there is arguably sufficient evidence supporting the use of bone graft substitutes in the clinical setting of depressed plateau fractures.[69,71,72]

These materials have also been extensively used for the augmentation of distal radius fractures. Zimmermann and colleagues evaluated patients treated with cement augmentation 2 years after the surgery. The authors concluded that the use of injectable calcium phosphate cement (Norian SRS) to supplement pin and screw fixation was effective in maintaining the reduction of unstable intraarticular distal radius fractures in osteoporotic patients and provided superior functional outcomes at 2 years after the surgery compared to percutaneous pinning alone.[73] With the widespread use of locked plating for these injuries, the efficacy of these materials for use in this situation must be questioned. A recent randomized study sought to determine whether augmentation of volar locking-plate fixation with calcium phosphate bone cement had any benefit over volar locking-plate fixation alone in an elderly patient population with unstable distal radial fractures.[74] The two groups were comparable with regard to age, sex, fracture type, injury mechanism, and bone mineral density. No significant differences were observed between the groups with regard to the clinical outcomes at the 3- or 12-month follow-up examination. No significant intergroup differences in radiographic outcomes were observed at 1-year follow-up.

The authors concluded that augmentation of metaphyseal defects with calcium phosphate bone cement after volar locking-plate fixation offered no benefit over volar locking-plate fixation alone in elderly patients with an unstable distal radial fracture. This highlights the point that with the improved biomechanics that locked plating provides, prospective studies are required to determine the role of these conductive substrates when they are combined with locked plating techniques.[75]

The treatment of intraarticular calcaneal fractures is commonplace in busy trauma practices. Although open reduction and fixation are favored by many authors, increased risk of soft tissue complications makes this method of treatment a challenge. Again the value of an injectable, minimally invasive material to augment posterior facet elevation would be valuable. Wee and colleagues documented in a recent clinical study the safe use of an injectable calcium phosphate cement to augment standard plate fixation of calcaneal fractures. A total of 10 patients with 12 displaced intraarticular calcaneal fractures underwent this method of treatment. Full weight bearing was started at 1 month postoperatively, and no cases demonstrated loss of reduction. The authors felt that the early results with stabilization and augmentation were encouraging.[76]

In a similar study Eisner and colleagues compared patients treated surgically with and without injectable carbonated apatite cement. In the cement group, full weight bearing on the affected extremity was regained at an average of 4 weeks postoperatively. During the study period of 3 years, only a slight decrease in the density of the peripheral zones of the cement block was observed (again referring to the relatively long integration time with these first- and second-generation materials). Complete resorption and remodeling of the bone cement were not complete at 3 years.[77]

These findings should be temporized by the results of an earlier study by Schildhauer and colleagues, who reported on a series of 36 joint depression–type calcaneal fractures treated by internal fixation augmented with calcium phosphate cement.[78] Patients began to bear weight as early as 3 weeks after the surgery without loss of reduction, and no significant difference in functional outcome scores between patients with early versus late weight bearing. Of concern, however, was a finding of an 11% infection rate. The majority of infections occurred in smokers. In spite of the infection rate, the authors concluded that cement augmentation of the fixation for joint-depression calcaneal fractures allowed earlier weight bearing with no change in postoperative outcomes.

Proximal humeral fracture augmentation has also been reported. Reinforcement with calcium phosphate cement in the treatment of proximal humeral fractures with locked plates decreased fracture settling and significantly decreased intraarticular screw penetration and helped to prevent varus deformation in clinical series. Augmentation was able to decrease the tendency for subsequent superior screw cutout from the humeral in biomechanical studies.[79,80]

Civinini and colleagues reported on the results of the treatment in patients with early-stage osteonecrosis of the femoral head (ONFH) that underwent core decompression, injection of autologous bone marrow concentrate, and the use of a composite injectable bone substitute calcium sulfate and tricalcium phosphate as a mechanical supplementation associated with decompression.[81]

At final follow-up, the mean hip scores increased from 68 points preoperatively to 86 points postoperatively, and radiographic improvement occurred in 29 hips (78.4%). The overall clinical success rate of the procedure was 86.5%. The authors felt that backfilling the defect with an injectable bioceramic for the treatment of early stages of ONFH helped to relieve hip pain and prevent the progression of ONFH in the majority of the cases.[81]

Rouvillain reported on the clinical, radiologic, and histologic findings following high tibial valgus osteotomy (HTVO) augmenting the distraction osteotomy with a micro-macroporous biphasic calcium phosphate wedge. This is one of the first studies to examine the results by histologic analysis of the graft incorporation.[82]

Forty-three knees underwent clinical and radiologic follow-up at days 1, 90, and 365 to evaluate consolidation and bone substitute interfaces. Biopsies were obtained at least 1 year after implantation from 10 patients who requested plate removal. Radiographic consolidation was observed in 98% of patients with no late collapse noted. Histology confirmed normal bony architecture with trabecular and/or dense lamellar bone growth throughout the wedge implants. Radiographs and microcomputed tomography (CT) scan revealed a well-organized, mineralized structure in the newly formed bone. This study confirmed that using medial biphasic calcium phosphate (MBCP) wedges in combination with locked plates offered a simple, safe, and fast surgical technique for HTVO.[82]

Early results have demonstrated that augmentation of femoral neck and intertrochanteric hip fractures with calcium phosphate cement is feasible, with no substantial increase in complications.[83,84]

A recent meta-analysis was undertaken to evaluate this concept of hip fracture augmentation and came to differing conclusions: 411 studies were identified, of which 22 met the rigorous inclusion criteria, comprising 12 experimental and 10 clinical reports. The clinical studies were evaluated with regard to their levels of evidence. Only four were prospective and randomized. Polymethylmethacrylate (PMMA) and calcium phosphate cements increased the primary stability of the implant-bone construct in all experimental and clinical studies. In randomized, controlled studies, augmentation of intracapsular fractures of the neck of the femur with calcium-phosphate cement was associated with poor long-term results. There was a lack of data on the long-term outcome for trochanteric fractures. Because there were only a few, randomized, controlled studies, there is currently poor evidence for the use of any orthobiologic bone cement in the treatment of fractures of the hip and it should not be undertaken.[85]

Investigators continue to manipulate these calcium phosphate substrates in an attempt to find the optimal resorption/incorporation rate with the optimal strength ratios maintained. No authors of human studies have been able to clearly demonstrate the actual resorption rate of calcium phosphate cement (Figs. 4-2 and 4-3). However, the creation of macropores can significantly improve the resorption rate of these materials. This increased degradation is associated with almost complete bone replacement. Animal studies have shown that up to 80% of the cement is resorbed at 10 weeks, with resorption and replacement with bone continuing for as long as 30 weeks.[86,87] This process occurs by dissolution as well as by osteoclast resorption. Biomaterials depicted a significant increase in bone content, when compared to ABG, concerning bone regeneration at the same time period.[88]

The lack of osteoprogenitor cells and osteoinductive potential of calcium-based bone substitutes has led to the development of composite grafts in an attempt to accelerate bone formation. A composite graft is created by adding an osteoinductive factor to an osteoconductive calcium phosphate matrix to theoretically increase bone formation. Many clinical series use composite ceramic grafts combining the scaffolding properties of TCP materials with biological elements to stimulate cell proliferation and differentiation.[89]

As previously mentioned, the incorporation times of some of these materials can be prolonged because of a number of factors. In an attempt to improve the incorporation and integration characteristics, investigators combined ultraporous β-TCP synthetic graft material (Vitoss Bone Graft Substitute, Orthovita) with bone marrow aspirates, with the hypothesis that bone marrow aspirate speeds incorporation of the bone graft substitute. The study prospectively examined healing of cavitary defects filled with TCP versus TCP and bone marrow (BM) aspirate (TCP/BM). While significant improvements in radiographic parameters were observed in both TCP groups over 2 years of follow-up, the addition of BM was not found to provide any significant benefit.[90] This highlights the need for comparative data to determine the effectiveness of just randomly combining these adjuvants.

In an effort to improve the performance of calcium phosphate materials, many investigators are manipulating the materials themselves in an attempt to improve the incorporation characteristics or the osteoinductive capabilities of these materials. The inherent osteoinductivity of silicate-substituted calcium phosphate materials was investigated in a sheep muscle pouch study.

Silicate substitution had a significant effect on the formation of bone both within the implant and on the implant surface during the study period. The formation of bone within muscle during the 12-week period showed both silicate-substituted calcium phosphate and stoichiometric calcium phosphate to be osteoinductive in this model. Silicate substitution significantly increased the amount of bone that formed and the amount of bone attached to the implant surface. New bone formation occurred through an intramembranous process within the implant structure.[91] This material manipulation continues to be the focus of great research interest at this time in attempt to develop materials that have *both* inductive and conductive properties within the same material.

DEMINERALIZED BONE MATRIX

DBM is formed by acid extraction of the mineralized extracellular matrix of allograft bone. It contains type I collagen, noncollagenous proteins, and osteoinductive growth factors,[92] including BMPs and other inductive factors found in the TGF-β group of proteins. As noted earlier, the TGF-β superfamily includes a number of factors in addition to BMPs. The factors that are known to be osteoinductive are BMPs, growth differentiation factors (GDFs), and possibly $TGF\text{-}\beta_1$, $TGF\text{-}\beta_2$, and $TGF\text{-}\beta_3$.[93] DBM is highly osteoconductive because of its particulate nature and presents a large surface area and three-dimensional architecture to serve as a site of cellular attachment.[94,95] Thus, when DBM is implanted in an animal, all of these factors potentially work in combination to produce the observed osteogenic response.

DBM is, strictly speaking, allogeneic bone tissue. In theory, the noncollagenous proteins, including osteoinductive proteins such as the BMPs remain viable. However, because the true test of osteoinductivity is whether a material that has been implanted in a nonosseous site forms bone, the inability of allograft bone to do this in human patients argues against allograft bone having substantial osteoinductive activity. DBM has been shown to produce this effect in animal studies,[96-98] but it too has never demonstrated this effect in human patients. The relative quantities of BMPs in DBMs are low, in the order of 1×10^{-9} g of BMP per gram of DBM. The osteoinductive variability has been found not only across different DBM products but also among production lots from the same DBM formulation.[99] Bae and colleagues demonstrated that there is higher variability in the concentration of BMPs among different lots of the *same* DBM formulation than among different DBM formulations. Each individual lot has a different osteoinductive capacity that can vary considerably among

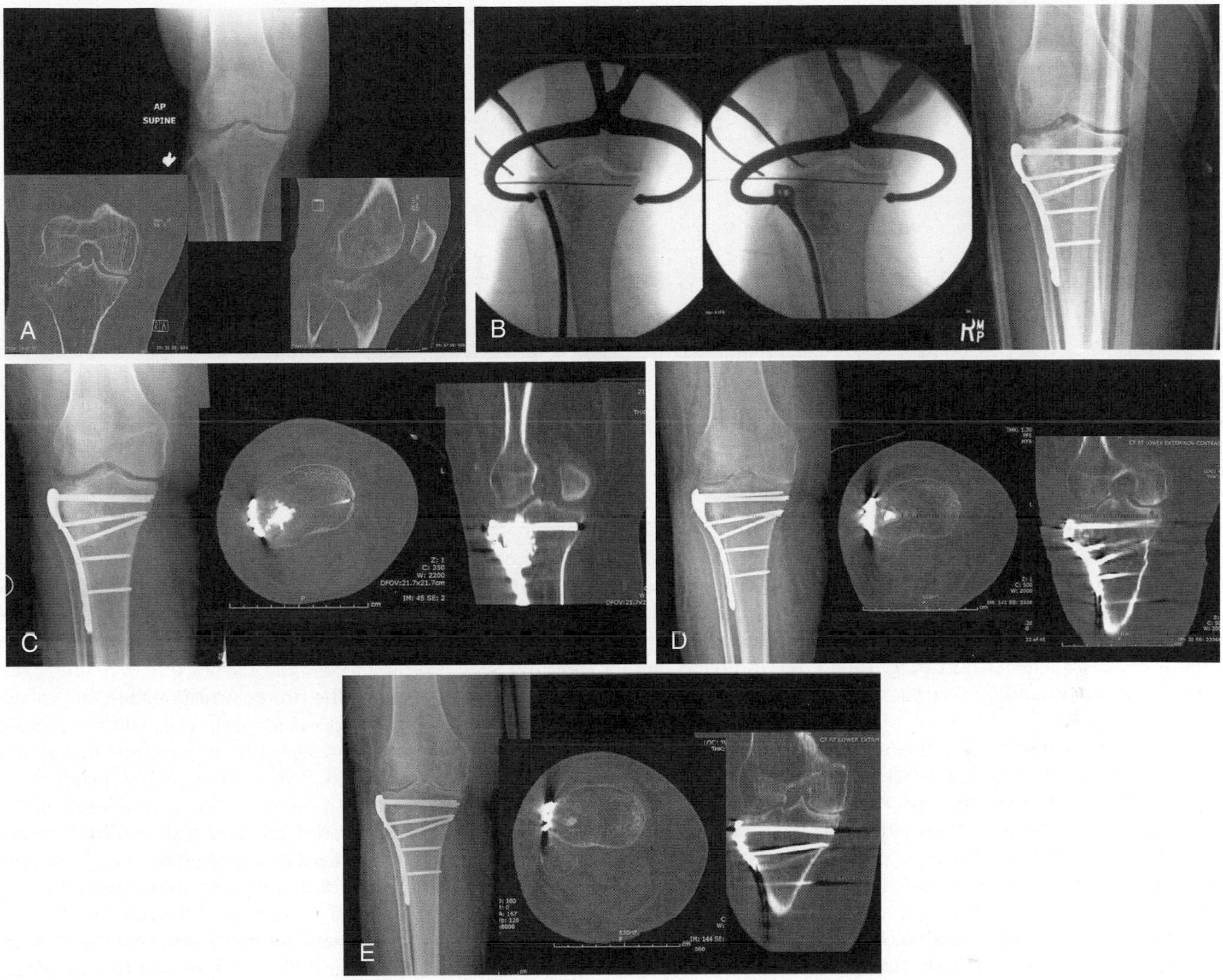

Figure 4-2. A, Split depression tibial plateau fracture. Computed tomography (CT) scans demonstrate significant lateral compartment articular impaction and comminution. **B,** Lateral articular surface was elevated and the subchondral defect grafted with a particulate calcium-phosphate-sulfate composite osteoconductive bone-void filler to help maintain articular reconstruction *(left).* To fill all cancellous voids, an injectable form of the same material was injected, and following a short set period, the plate and screw construct was applied, drilling directly through the material *(center).* This particulate material allows instrumentation immediately after the initial set time without degradation of the resulting crystalline structure of the material. Final fixation radiograph demonstrating reconstructed surface with large void filled with the conductive substrate. Note a small particulate piece of material has egressed into joint. Because of the particulate material properties, this small amount dissolved in the synovial fluid environment and was absorbed without any harmful articular sequela *(right).* **C,** Sequential images and CT scan to document osseous incorporation of material over time. Initial postoperative radiograph and CT scan showing material in place with articular reduction maintained and supported by the material. **D,** Three-month postoperative images. Articular surface reduction remains intact. Calcium ceramic is noted to be much smaller with enveloping bone around the material noted. **E,** Six-month postoperative images. With most of the material osteointegrated, the articular reduction has been maintained and the patient has advanced to full weight bearing at approximately 2.5 months.

different donors. This variability questions the reliability of DBM products and, possibly, their efficacy in providing consistent osteoinduction.[100]

Prior investigations have shown that the osteoinductive potential can vary widely, with influence from both donor and processing sources. There appears to be sex-related differences in donor DBM. DBM derived from female donors appears to have significantly greater concentrations of BMP-2 and BMP-7 than that derived from male donors ($P = 0.0257$ and 0.0245, respectively). There was no significant correlation between donor age and the levels of any of the measured BMPs in a study evaluating BMP levels in commercially available DBM preparations.[101] The presence of other growth factors found in DBM has also been evaluated.[102] Wildemann and colleagues attempted to quantify the activity and presence of eight growth factors important for bone healing in multiple different "off-the-shelf" DBM formulations, which are already in human use. Differences between the products were seen in total protein content and the absolute growth factor values. The type of the growth factors found in these preparations was almost comparable between the materials. FGF and BMP-4 were not detectable in any analyzed sample. BMP-2 revealed the highest concentration extractable from the samples without a significant difference between the three DBM formulations.

In general, all the materials had variable concentrations of TGF-β_1, FGF-α, IGF-1, and PDGF. No differences were

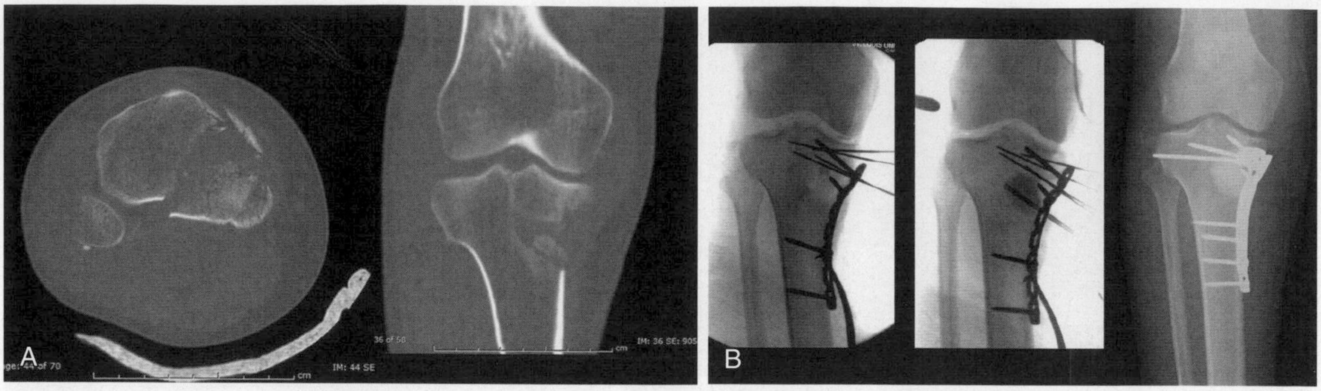

Figure 4-3. A, Computed tomography (CT) images demonstrating significant metaphyseal defect following a crushing injury to the medial tibial plateau. **B,** At the time of definitive fixation, a percutaneous injection of a calcium ceramic was completed, completely filling the metaphyseal defect and supplying articular support in conjunction with the fixation hardware. Plain radiograph at 3 months demonstrates minimal incorporation of the material. This material was selected for its longer integration time period to help maintain the metaphyseal region past the transition to full weight bearing.

accessed for VEGF. This and other similar studies highlight the differences in the growth factor concentrations between the individual materials, independent of the product formulation. As well, there is evidence of differential potencies of each available growth factor within individual DBM preparations, based on the individual manufacturer and manufacturing process.[13]

There are numerous DBM formulations based on refinements of the manufacturing process. They are available as freeze-dried powder, granules, gel, putty, or strips. They have also been developed as combination products with other materials such as allogeneic bone chips and calcium sulfate granules. There is now evidence of differential potencies of DBM preparations based on the manufacturer and manufacturing process.[13] Sterile processing of the bone may also affect the protein effectiveness of these materials. Some tissue banks harvest and process the DBM under "sterile" conditions whereas other manufacturers sterilize the DBM after processing. Gamma irradiation is frequently used to sterilize implanted devices but has limitations when used on biologically active materials and composites.

Studies indicate that if the DBM is irradiated prior to the addition of any aqueous carrier, the activity of DBM in the dry state remains relatively stable with only a small loss of activity. Composites of DBM with a carrier such as lecithin, to which no water has been added, lose activity at approximately the same rate as DBM in the dry form. In composites that contain water, the loss of activity occurs even at much lower levels of radiation exposure. Osteoinductivity of DBM decreased with the increase of gamma-irradiation dose at ambient temperature, whereas no decrease occurred when treated with gamma irradiation at low temperature. However, the hydrated DBM showed diminishing osteoinductivity after 6-month storage at ambient conditions, whereas the DBMs in dry form retained their osteoinductivity after the 6-month storage. The findings in this study indicate that DBM and demineralized bone matrix/acellular dermal matrix (DBM/AM) composites could retain their osteoinductivity when they are in dry configuration and are irradiated at low temperature (–40° C to –70° C).[103]

Gamma irradiation does not change cell attachment to the DBM matrix but has an influence on both stem cell and osteoprecursor cell proliferation rates. Because of the limitations imposed by radiation, it seems most practical to handle DBM aseptically throughout the procedures of compositing pastes, putties, or suspensions, and only if necessary, exposing bone components to radiation sterilization prior to mixing.[103,104]

In addition, many of the proteins responsible for "turning on" the differentiation process for stem cells will not function if damaged, and protein preservation is therefore important in the delivery of DBM and BMPs. Some DBM products are lyophilized and mixed with carrier at the time of implantation, while others are prehydrated or premixed and could potentially remain on the shelf for a long period of time.[105] If precise control of conditions is not maintained, many proteins might be susceptible to chemical and physical degradation.[106]

Ethylene oxide as a means for sterilization of DBM is used by some manufacturers and has been shown to attenuate its osteoinductive potential.[107] Exposure of DBM to ethylene oxide for the duration required to kill most common bacterial pathogens results in a marked reduction of its osteoinductivity most likely due to destruction of BMPs and other inductive factors.[108] The effect of ethylene oxide has been shown to be dose dependent.[108]

It is clear that processing and sterilization techniques have significant effects on DBM viability. With this in mind, clinicians should be aware of how these factors influence the efficacy of each particular DBM product that they may choose to use in each clinical application.

The shelf life of the product may also vary with the specific carrier, which may or may not affect the overall activity of the product. All available in vitro assays evaluate the DBM without the carrier added by the manufacturers. Carriers include glycerol (Grafton DBM, Osteotech, Inc., Eatontown, NJ), synthetic polymer (Dynagraft, GenSci OrthoBiologics, Inc., Irvine, CA), porcine gel (Osteofil, Regeneration Technologies, Inc., Alachua, FL), and carboxymethylcellulose (Allomatrix Injectable Putty, Wright Medical Technology, Inc., Arlington, TN). DBM is also available in a particulate powder form that has no carrier material present. This form is useful to admix to other materials such as iliac aspirate or autograft and platelet gels (Fig. 4-4).

Bioactivity can be measured by in vivo assays (which measure de novo bone formation and alkaline phosphatase

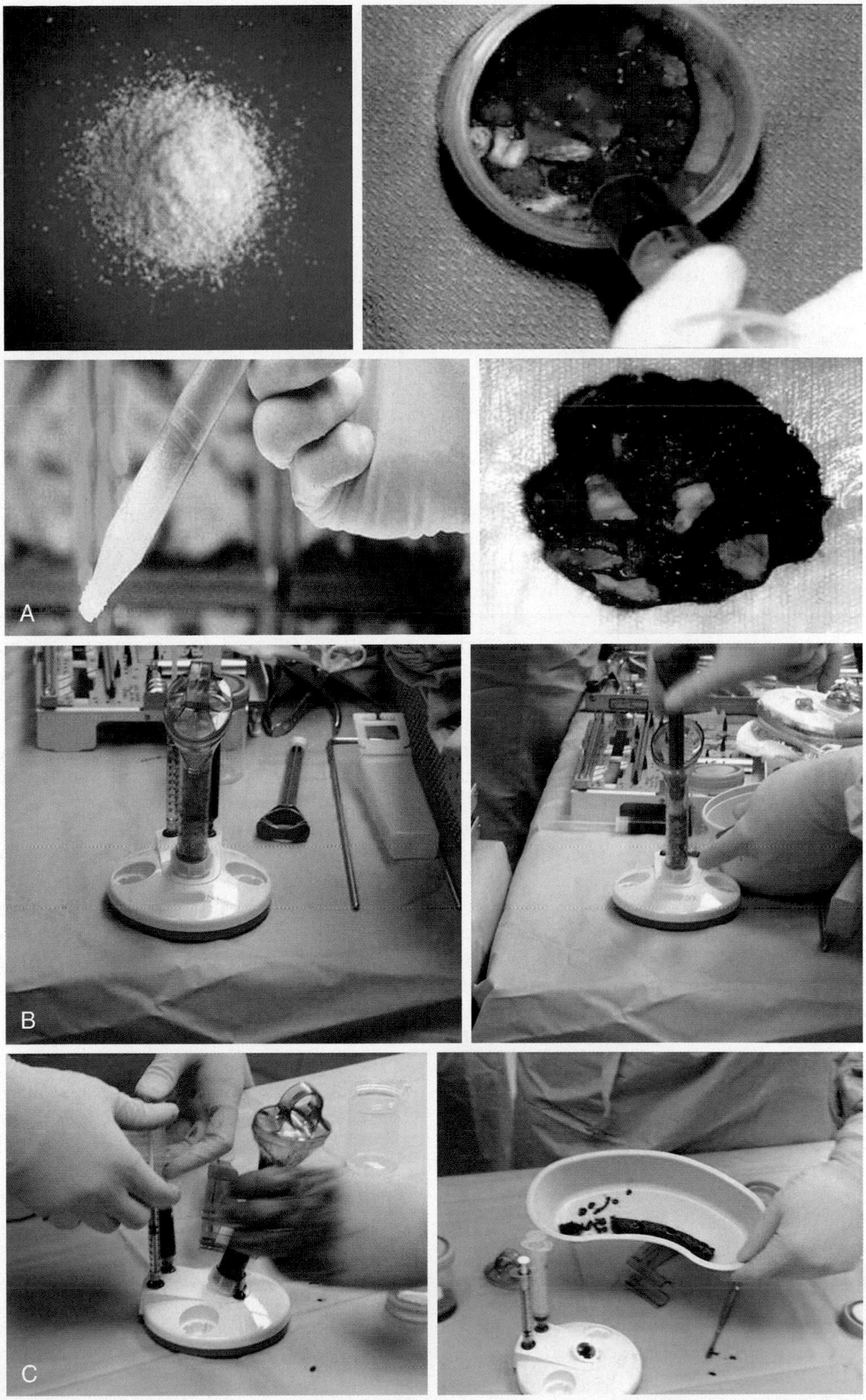

Figure 4-4. A, Demineralized bone matrix (DBM) can be delivered in many forms. Particulate DBM is a powder without any carrier *(top left)*. A DBM composite putty is infiltrated with a carrier that allows the material to be applied directly or injected *(bottom left)*. Demineralized cancellous chips can be infiltrated with concentrated marrow or platelet concentrate as seen here *(right)*. **B,** A graft chamber is filled with particulate DBM as well as demineralized cancellous chips. This chamber is then loaded with other adjuvants to facilitate delivery of the DBM graft. **C,** This graft chamber was injected with concentrated marrow elements. This allowed delivery of a graft with significant conductive properties with interconnecting pores and presenting a tremendous surface area (DBM) as a site for potential marrow cellular attachment.

levels) and in vitro assays (which measure stimulation of human osteoblast culture).[109-111]

Only a few tissue banks use an in vivo model to measure the bioactivity of the final DBM product with the carrier. A study by Han and colleagues evaluated the effects of moisture from water-based carriers and the storage temperatures on osteoinductivity of known DBM products. This was done to evaluate these materials with regard to shelf life in an operating room. In a dry state, without a carrier, DBM can preserve its osteoinductive activity when temperatures reached 65° C (149° F), but in the presence of moisture, (carrier substances) the activity decreases with incubation time. Nearly 90% of the DBM activity is lost when maintained for 5 weeks at 65° C (149° F).[105]

While the preclinical data are impressive for DBM forming de novo bone in lesser animal models,[98] the human clinical data are deficient with only isolated case reports and uncontrolled retrospective reviews. These level 3 and 4 studies suggest the potential therapeutic effects of DBM.[112] The maxilla-craniofacial field published the bulk of the literature documenting successful reconstruction of complex deformities using DBM alone as a bone graft substitute.[113-115] Reported success rates for mandibular and maxillary reconstructions are consistently more than 90%.

One of the first clinical series was published by Tiedeman and colleagues. They reported on an uncontrolled case series of 48 patients in whom DBM had been used in conjunction with BM for the treatment of skeletal injuries. Thirty-nine patients were available for follow-up, and 30 of them demonstrated healing.[116] These results were encouraging; however, because there was no control group, the role of DBM in patients who demonstrated healing remains unknown. Unfortunately, most clinical series combined DBM with other adjuvants and, as noted earlier, the singular effectiveness of DBM alone is difficult to elucidate.

Two separate investigators evaluated the effectiveness of combining DBM with BM aspirate for the treatment of acute long bone fractures and nonunions. Wilkins and colleagues treated 66 patients with 69 "stiff" nonunions with a prospective protocol. The only therapeutic intervention was the percutaneous administration of a mixture of autologous BM and allograft DBM on an outpatient basis. Sixty-one of the percutaneous treatments (88%) resulted in union (level III evidence), however, there was no comparative control group other than historic controls with which to compare the effectiveness of this composite graft.[117]

Lindsey studied the effectiveness of a composite graft consisting of DBM putty (Grafton DBM) and aspirated BM for treating long bone acute fractures.[118] Patients were randomized to treatment with either the DBM putty composite or iliac crest autograft, with a minimum of 12 months of radiographic follow-up. Ninety percent of DBM patients achieved full bone formation compared to 75% of autograft patients ($P = 0.41$). Additionally, all DBM patients were healed compared with 63% of autograft patients ($P = 0.07$). Both of these studies suggest that DBM putty enriched with BM may be comparable to autograft for treating long bone fractures and nonunions.

However, in the case of acute fractures, the number of patients in each group was 10 or less, and although this was a randomized prospective trial (level I evidence), the numbers are too small to draw definitive conclusions regarding this composite graft option. Despite these limitations, both of these studies suggest that DBM putty enriched with BM may be comparable to autograft for treating long bone fractures and nonunions. This option offers the distinct advantages of decreased morbidity, reduced costs, and shorter hospital stay compared to AICBG.[117]

There is only one level 1 randomized prospective study in humans available, evaluating the use of DBM as a solitary graft material. This study used DBM alone to treat a standardized critical-sized fibular defect, grafted using only DBM (positive control) compared to a similar defect with no graft applied negative (untreated) controls.[119]

This was the first phase of a study done in conjunction with a prospective, randomized double-blind study in 24 patients undergoing high tibial osteotomy to evaluate the effectiveness of human recombinant osteogenic protein (OP-1) on a type I collagen carrier in a critically sized fibular defect (phase II). The results of phase I established the critically sized nature of the defect. In the defect group with no graft augmentation, no bony changes were observed while nonunion resulted in all of these defects. In the group grafted with DBM, formation of new bone was visible from 6 weeks onward with many defects undergoing complete healing. The results of the second phase showed no significant formation of new bone in the presence of collagen graft alone, while in the OP-1 group, all patients except one showed formation of new bone from 6 weeks onward. This study demonstrated that both DBM and OP-1 exhibited osteogenic activity in a validated critically sized human defect.

In a similar study, Hierholzer and colleagues attempted to evaluate the healing of humeral shaft nonunions using a consistent surgical protocol but compared the use of two different types of bone graft: autologous iliac crest bone graft and DBM in a consecutive retrospective cohort series.[120] Forty-five patients were treated with AICBG and 33 grafted with DBM only. Union was noted clinically and radiographically in 100% of the 45 patients treated with autologous bone graft and 97% (32) of the 33 patients treated with DBM (not significant evidence). The overall functional outcome did not differ between the groups; however, 20 (44%) of the autologous bone graft recipients had donor site morbidity, including prolonged pain in the majority and a superficial infection requiring irrigation and débridement in 1 patient. These results demonstrated that consistent healing could be achieved with commercially available DBM alone (level III evidence).

Augmentation of spinal fusion appears to be the most frequent application of DBM. In the more challenging environment, such as posterolateral spine fusion, multiple formulations and combinations have been used.[121] Significant differences exist between the various forms of DBM in their ability to generate spine fusion in animal models. This must be considered when analyzing the data from human studies.

In a side-by-side comparative study, a total of 120 patients underwent posterolateral spine fusion with pedicle screw fixation and bone grafting. Iliac crest autograft was implanted on one side of the spine and a Grafton DBM/autograft composite was implanted on the contralateral side in the same patient. The bone graft mass was fused in 42 cases (52%) on the Grafton DBM side and in 44 cases (54%) on the autograft side. The authors concluded from this level III study that DBM can extend a smaller quantity of autograft than is normally required to achieve a solid spinal arthrodesis. Consequently, a reduced amount of harvested autograft may be required, potentially diminishing the risk and severity of donor site complications.[122]

Thus, the use of DBM as a bone graft extender appears to be a viable indication for its use.

In a larger 2-year prospective study, a randomized clinical trial compared the outcomes of Grafton DBM combined with local bone, with that of iliac crest bone graft (ICBG) in a single-level instrumented posterior lumbar fusion. Patients were randomly assigned (2 : 1) to receive Grafton DBM with local bone or autologous ICBG.

At 2-year follow-up, subjects who were randomized to Grafton DBM and local bone achieved an 86% overall fusion rate versus 92% (ICBG) ($P = 1.0$, not significant evidence) and improvements in clinical outcomes that were comparable with those in the ICBG group.[123] There was a statistically significant greater mean intraoperative blood loss in the ICBG group than in the Grafton group ($P < 0.0031$).

A recent comprehensive meta-analysis reviewed the use of DBM for spinal fusion series. Articles were critically examined and compared according to study design, DBM type, outcomes, and results. The primary outcome of interest was fusion rate. Secondary outcomes included the Oswestry Disability Index, SF-36 survey, Odom's criteria, visual analog scale (VAS), neurologic pain score, Japanese Orthopedic Association myelopathy score, Neck Disability and Ishihara Curvature indices, and pseudarthrosis and surgical failure rates. The majority of human clinical trials report high fusion rates when DBM is employed as a graft extender or a graft enhancer. Few prospective randomized controlled trials have been performed comparing DBM to autologous ICBG in spine fusion.[124]

Although many animal and human studies demonstrate comparable efficacy of DBM when combined with autograft or compared to autograft alone, additional high level of evidence studies are required to clearly define the indications for its use in spine fusion surgeries and the appropriate patient population that will benefit from DBM.

PATIENT-DERIVED CELLULAR THERAPIES

Current orthobiologic strategies have progressed from an approach based primarily on biomaterials to a cell- and tissue-based approach that includes understanding of cell sourcing and bioactive stimuli. New options include methods for harvest and transplantation of tissue-forming cells, combined with bioactive scaffold matrix materials, and delivery of bioactive molecules that allow these stem and progenitor cells to differentiate into the appropriate cell lineage for specific tissue repair.[125,126] Available cell-based strategies include targeting local cells with use of scaffolds or bioactive factors, transplantation of autogenous connective tissue progenitor cells derived from BM or other tissues, and the use of autologous growth factors obtained from the patient's own platelets.

Marrow Aspirate

The critical component necessary to all bone formation is the ability to provide viable osteoprogenitor cells. BM is a plentiful source of musculoskeletal stem cells, but the cells can also be found in periosteum, cartilage, muscle, fat, and vascular pericytes.[127] Connective tissue progenitors describe the population of stem cells and progenitors that are actively engaging in proliferation and differentiation into connective tissue. A BM aspirate has a high concentration of connective tissue progenitors. One milliliter of iliac aspirate contains approximately 40 million nucleated cells, 1500 of which are connective tissue progenitors.[126]

Historic Perspective

Connelly's work with unfractionated BM aspirate was instrumental in stimulating clinical interest for using marrow as an adjunct graft material for fracture and nonunion healing. His initial clinical series used autologous marrow injection to stimulate healing in 20 ununited tibial fractures over a 5-year period. His injections were combined with either the use of a cast (10 patients) or a Lottes nail (10 patients).[128] The two failures were in the cast treatment group. BM injection was as effective as past open autologous grafting but with considerably fewer disadvantages. These early results were not duplicated by others, but did stimulate researchers to document enhanced bone healing through the use of marrow cell–based strategies in vitro and in animal studies.

Connolly continued to investigate the effects of concentrating marrow by centrifugation in a rabbit nonunion model. The results with centrifugation were superior to those with unprocessed marrow. And thus the concept of a threshold level of cells necessary for osteogenesis to occur in ectopic sites was promulgated.[128-130]

Current Methodology

The failures and low rates of healing associated with the use of unfractionated BM may reflect the paucity of osteoprogenitor cells present in the mature marrow aspirate. Even in a normal adult only 36 to 55 of every million nucleated BM cells will undergo osteogenic differentiation.[127] Because osseous regeneration is dependent on the number of cells available to participate in bone synthesis, patients with fewer local cellular precursors will typically have a poorer healing response leading to potential nonunion. As greater volumes of BM are harvested from the iliac crest, the concentration of osteoprogenitor cells decreases because the sample undergoes considerable dilution with peripheral blood.

The aspiration technique is very specific in order to maximize the number of effective progenitor cells per unit volume.[131] Muschler and colleagues studied this issue and determined that no more than 2 mL of blood should be aspirated from any given area in the iliac crest to avoid dilution with peripheral blood[127] (Fig. 4-5). On the basis of these data, a selective retention (filtration) system was developed that has the ability to concentrate progenitor cells three to four times and load them onto an allograft substrate for delivery.[132]

Other sites of harvest for marrow aspirate have been assessed to determine if there is variability of the quality of cells obtained compared to the results of aspirate from the iliac crest.[133] A comparative study harvested BM aspirates from the ipsilateral anterior iliac crest, distal tibial metaphysis, and calcaneal body all from the same patients. The samples were then centrifuged to obtain a concentrate of nucleated cells, which were plated and grown in cell culture. The anatomic locations were compared between the 40 patients enrolled in the study. Clinical parameters (including sex, age, tobacco use, body mass index, and diabetes) were assessed as possible predictors of osteoblastic progenitor cell yield. BM aspirate collected from the iliac crest had a higher mean concentration of osteoblastic progenitor cells compared with the distal tibia or the

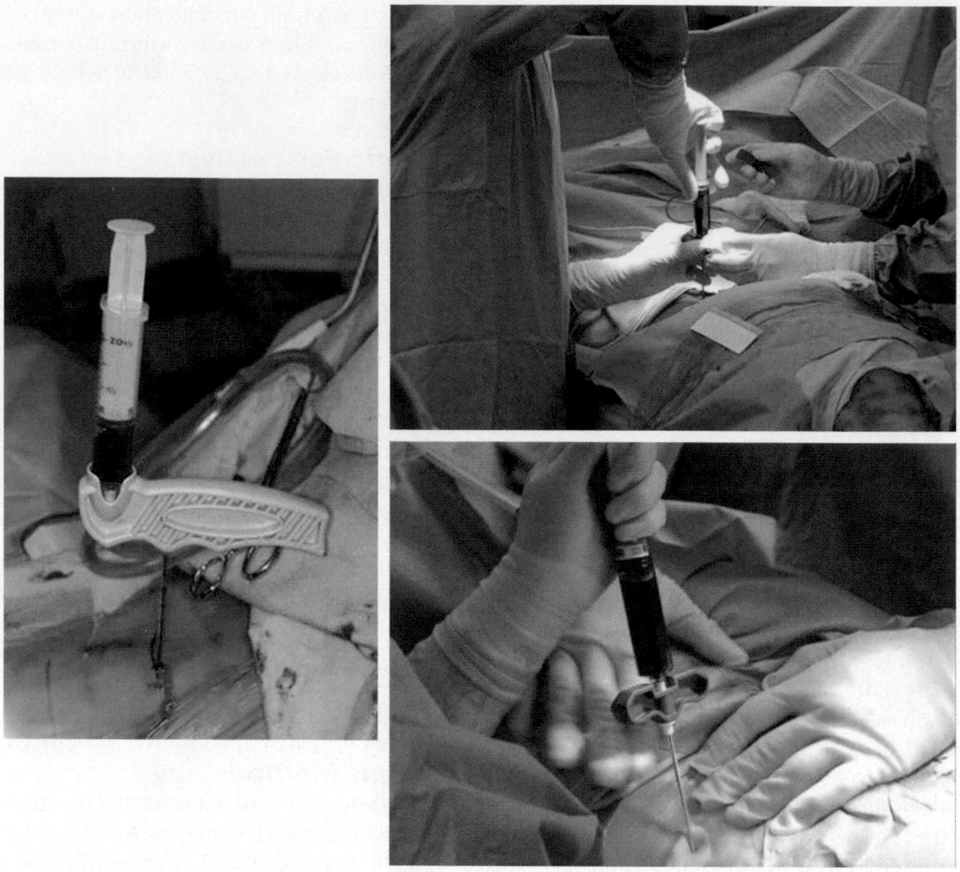

Figure 4-5. Many devices are available for marrow harvest. These all have large-bore needles with multiple side ports and differing handle types to facilitate correct aspiration technique; 3 to 4 cc should be aspirated at any one location and as a single aspirate. The needle should be slowly withdrawn, rotated, and reoriented to aspirate from a different location. Many aspiration syringes available can be locked into position after small quantities are aspirated. This permits needle repositioning without losing the suction of the plunger. Following needle repositioning, the plunger can be unlocked and additional aspirate obtained.

calcaneus ($P = 0.0001$). There was no significant difference in concentration between the tibia and the calcaneus ($P = 0.063$). Age, sex, tobacco use, and diabetes were not predictive of osteoblastic progenitor cell yield.[133]

Similar comparisons evaluated aspirates of vertebral body marrow compared to matched controls from the iliac crest of the same patient. Vertebral body aspirates demonstrated comparable or greater concentrations of progenitor cells compared with matched controls from the iliac crest. The concentration of osteogenic progenitor cells was, on the average, 71% higher in the vertebral aspirates than in the paired iliac crest samples ($P = 0.05$).[133,134]

However, the concentration and yield of colony-forming connective-tissue progenitors is greater when aspirate is obtained from the posterior crest compared with the anterior iliac crest. It has also been found that the biologic potential of the cells derived from both of these sites appears to be comparable.[135]

Cellularity of BM has been found to decrease with age and for women.[126,136] Surprisingly, there appears to be no relationship between smoking status and marrow cellularity, cellular prevalence, or cellular numbers. Studies have found that tobacco use is not associated with a change in prevalence of osteogenic progenitor cells in BM, or their intrinsic biologic capacity to undergo early osteoblastic differentiation.[126]

Preclinical Substantiation

Many investigators reported enhanced bone healing through the use of cell-based strategies in vitro and in multiple preclinical animal studies. In addition to the rabbit model that Connolly used to evaluate the beneficial effects of cellular concentration, a similar study was performed using a canine tibial nonunion model. Distraction gaps were maintained with external fixators and were treated with either a bone graft of concentrated marrow aspirate, or DBM, or a composite graft of both materials.[137] A separate group treated with autograft was used as the control group. Use of the combination of DBM and marrow concentrate (composite graft) yielded results that were superior to DBM or aspirate groups alone. The results of the composite graft were similar to those in the autograft group.

The concept of composite grafts combining marrow elements with other conductive and or inductive substrates has become a major area of interest based on the early results documenting the superiority of composite grafts compared to grafting with marrow aspirates alone. The ability to load cells into an osteoconductive substrate with a microporous structure provides the cells with a potentially stable and well-vascularized environment.[138] In this situation, most of these cells will differentiate into osteoblasts, whereas in sites that are mechanically unstable and less well vascularized, the cells tend to become chondrocytes.[139] If conditions are not right for the optimal differentiation of these MSCs into bone or cartilage cells, they will differentiate along a default pathway and become fibroblasts[140]; when this occurs, nonunion results. Thus, the emphasis on providing the optimal conditions for these composite grafts.

Bruder and colleagues evaluated BM combined with a porous TCP cylinder in a canine nonunion model stabilized with plates. Use of the composite graft demonstrated results that were superior to those of treatment with the ceramic cylinders alone, which resulted in only modest bone formation.[141]

Bruder continued to investigate marrow elements in a composite graft using a selective retention filtration strategy to concentrate marrow elements. In a canine model, selective retention cellular aspirate concentrates were mixed with DBM and were found to be equivalent to autograft in their ability to repair critical-size defects.[142] Additional studies using the concept of cellular concentrates enriching a DBM carrier matrix in a canine spine fusion model demonstrated similar results. The selective cellular concentration process allows the number of connective tissue progenitors to be increased three- to fourfold.

In a canine study by Muschler and colleagues, enriched aspirate composite DBM grafts delivered a mean of 2.3 times more cells and approximately 5.6 times more progenitors than DBM mixed with simple unconcentrated BM. A union score, quantitative CT, and mechanical testing results all demonstrated the use of the selective-retention-enriched bone DBM to be superior to the use of bone DBM alone and DBM plus unconcentrated marrow.[132]

Composite grafts have also been devised using cellular elements in addition to osteoinductive proteins. Lane and colleagues investigated the potential of combining BM cells with recombinant human BMP (rhBMP-2) in a rat femoral defect model.[143] This combination was superior to either rhBMP-2 or marrow cells by themselves as well as to treatment with syngeneic bone grafting. The authors believed that this represented a synergistic effect of the two materials and emphasized the importance of growth factors being present.

Animal models have been used to evaluate composite grafts that incorporate all three components, that is, cellular concentrate, a conductive substrate, and inductive proteins in varying combinations. A preclinical defect study evaluated a sheep tibial defect treated with HA combined with either rhBMP-7 or BM compared to autograft application.[134] Treatment with the composite grafts yielded results that were as good as those in an autograft control group and were superior to those in either a void group or a group treated with HA alone.

With the vast improvements in limb salvage techniques, the reconstruction of large defects in humans has become more commonplace and has historically relied on autograft bone grafts. Limiting factors include availability of graft material, comorbidity, and insufficient integration into the damaged bone. Complex animal models now routinely evaluate hard and soft tissue scaffoldings in combination with a multitude of inductive materials as well as applied cellular concentrates in an attempt to determine the optimum cocktail that can compare to the gold standard of AICBG for the treatment of segmental defects.[144-146]

Clinical Application of Marrow Elements

The use of marrow elements has been used clinically to augment bone healing with variable results. Most of the early series involved the simple aspiration and injection of iliac crest aspirates as noted previously in this chapter documenting the work of Connelly.[128-130,147] He was one of first surgeons to report on the use of BM aspirate as a clinical alternative to autograft (level IV evidence). Other early case studies or series document results for simple marrow injections. These studies were primarily single or multiple surgeons with no historic or case-matched controls (level IV evidence). These studies include Garg et al., who reported good results in his series of 20 patients treated with BM injection[148] for long bone nonunion. Healey et al. successfully treated nonunions in a group of eight children with cancer by simply injecting BM aspirate.[149] Wientroub et al. reported on the use of autologous marrow to improve the effectiveness of allografts in 23 children.[150] And finally, Goel et al. sequentially injected 3 to 5 mL of aspirated BM directly into the nonunion site. Multiple iliac crest aspirations were performed until a maximum of 15 mL of marrow was injected. Clinical and radiologic bone union occurred in 15 out of 20 patients (75%).[151]

These studies were performed without the benefit of our current knowledge regarding appropriate aspiration techniques, the advantage of cellular concentrates, or the use of composite grafting methods, yet meaningful results were achieved.

In spite of the encouraging preclinical and rudimentary clinical studies, the use of these grafts as a substitute have not enjoyed widespread use. This may be due to a host of reasons, such as (1) the variability resulting from inconsistent and incorrect aspiration techniques and faulty instrumentation necessary to achieve consistent aspirates; (2) low osteoprogenitor content of these insufficient aspirates; and (3) the combination of these aspirates with suboptimal scaffolding materials.[152]

Contemporary clinical series have demonstrated excellent results when the above factors have been attended to. Studies that use correct aspiration and concentration methodologies as well as adhere to using appropriate documented composite grafting techniques do document the value of marrow aspirates for graft substitution.

The use of bone marrow aspirate (BMAC) in conjunction with specific osteoconductive substrates appears to be a suitable substitution for AICBG when used in specific situations. Multiple level IV studies have documented the effectiveness of this modality for a variety of indications. It has been used primarily for defect management found in posttraumatic long bone defects and acetabular bone defects discovered during revision total hip arthroplasty.[153-155]

A new area of clinical use for BMAC is for the treatment of avascular necrosis (AVN) of the femoral head, as results have been seen following grafting using BMAC with a variety of carrier matrices.[156,157]

Hernigou and colleagues reported on 60 patients with noninfected nonunion who had undergone BM aspiration from both iliac crests. These aspirates were then concentrated using a centrifuge technique to achieve a baseline number of colony-forming units (CFUs) present in the composite graft to be injected into the nonunion site.

He demonstrated complete healing in 53 of the 60 patients. Those patients contained >1500 progenitors/cm^3 and an

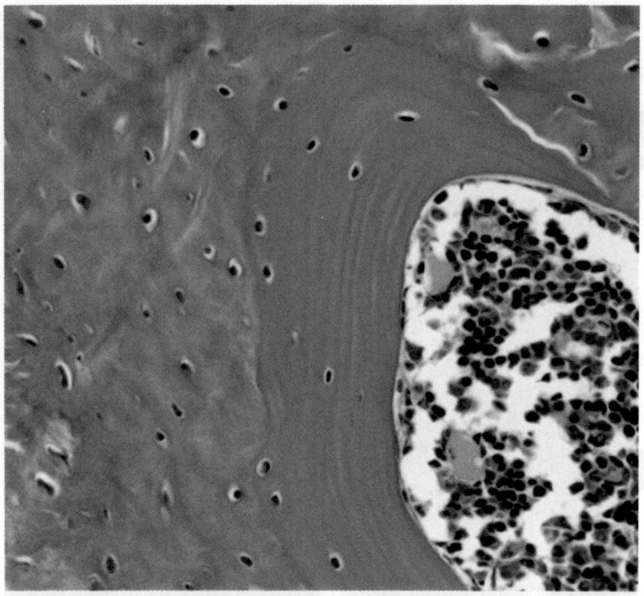

Figure 5-22. Remodeling of woven bone results in the organized structure of lamellar bone.

bone. As discussed later, weaker woven bone compensates by producing more material and placing it further from the center as demonstrated with typical callus formation. Remodeling into more streamlined lamellar bone provides economy of material, with lower weight, while increasing resistance to the loads applied during activities.

While this chapter focuses primarily on bone properties and relation to fracture propensity and healing, the soft tissues surrounding bone have unique material properties as well. For example, tendons, which are composed primarily of collagen fibers surrounded by a sheath, are stronger per area than muscle and have the same tensile strength as bone.[6] Tendons transmit the large forces generated by the muscle to the bone to create movement.[6] A tendon stress-strain curve (Fig. 5-23) exhibits some unique characteristics. There is an initial "toe region" that corresponds with the straightening of a slight crimp in the fibers, sometimes referred to as *fiber recruitment*. After the toe region, there is the standard linear region, but beyond this region, collagen fibers fail unpredictably.[6]

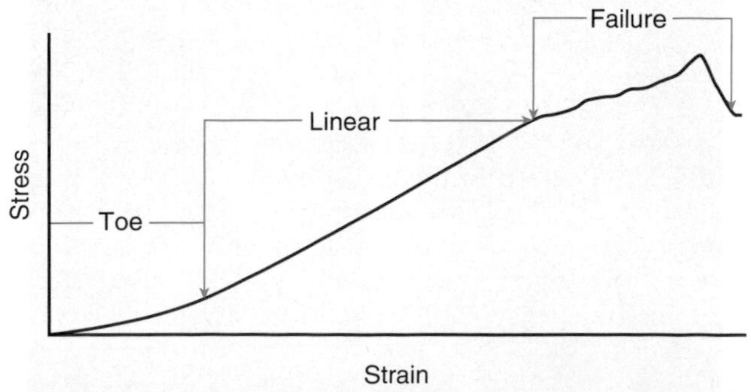

Figure 5-23. A stress-strain curve from a tendon differs from the traditional stress-strain curve caused by the initial straightening of the fibers, called the *toe region*. *(Redrawn from Annual Review of Biomedical Engineering, Volume 6, © 2004 by Annual Reviews,* www.annualreviews.org.*)*

TABLE 5-3 *ANISOTROPIC MATERIAL PROPERTIES FOR HUMAN CORTICAL BONE**

Loading Direction	Modulus (GPa)
Longitudinal	17.0
Transverse	11.5
Shear	3.3

*In comparison, moduli for common isotropic materials used in orthopaedic implants are stainless steel, 207 GPa; titanium alloys, 127 GPa; bone cement, 2.8 GPa; ultrahigh molecular weight polyethylene, 1.4 GPa.
Mean values from Reilly DT, Burstein AH: The elastic and ultimate properties of compact bone tissue, J Biomech 8(6):393–405, 1975.

Cortical Bone Properties and Microstructure

Cortical bone is the strong, dense bone that lines the outer surface of long bones. Cortical bone consists of layers called *lamellae,* which are mineralized collagen fibers. These mineralized collagen fibers provide structure to the bone and the lamellar tissue layers are 3 to 7 μm thick.[7] The collagen fibers are parallel within each layer, but the orientation varies in the adjacent layers. In certain cortical bone, the lamellae wrap in layers around a canal to form a Haversian system, as outlined in previous chapters.

The structure of cortical bone, especially in the diaphysis of long bones, provides load-bearing support. The mechanical properties of cortical bone change depending on the orientation of the loading. As described earlier in this chapter, an anisotropic material, like bone, defines a material where the properties vary and are direction dependent. In contrast, an isotropic material is one where the properties remain constant in all orientations. A common example of an anisotropic material is wood, which is easier to splinter along its grain than against it.

The anisotropic properties of bone are demonstrated in bench testing in the laboratory. In the longitudinal direction the elastic modulus is 17 to 19 GPa and ultimate strength is 100 to 150 MPa, but only 8 to 10 GPa and 9 to 11 MPa in the transverse direction.[3] Tables 5-3 and 5-4 highlight these direction-dependent differences seen in bone.

Material properties of cortical bone are also dependent on the rate at which the bone is loaded. Materials such as bone whose stress-strain characteristics are dependent on the applied strain rate are termed *viscoelastic* or *time-dependent* materials. However, as noted previously, the strain rate

TABLE 5-4 *ULTIMATE STRENGTH VALUES FOR HUMAN FEMORAL CORTICAL BONE*

Ultimate Loading Mode	Strength (MPa)*
Longitudinal	
Tension	135 (15.6)
Compression	205 (17.3)
Shear	71 (2.6)
Transverse	
Tension	53 (10.7)
Compression	131 (20.7)

*Standard deviations in parentheses.
Mean values from Reilly DT, Burstein AH: The elastic and ultimate properties of compact bone tissue, J Biomech 8(6):393–405, 1975.

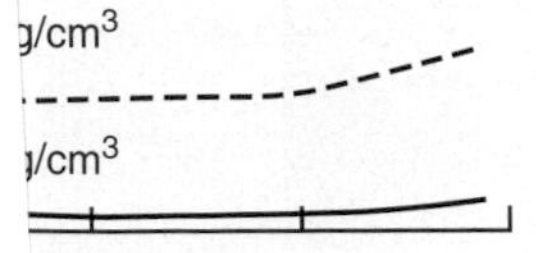

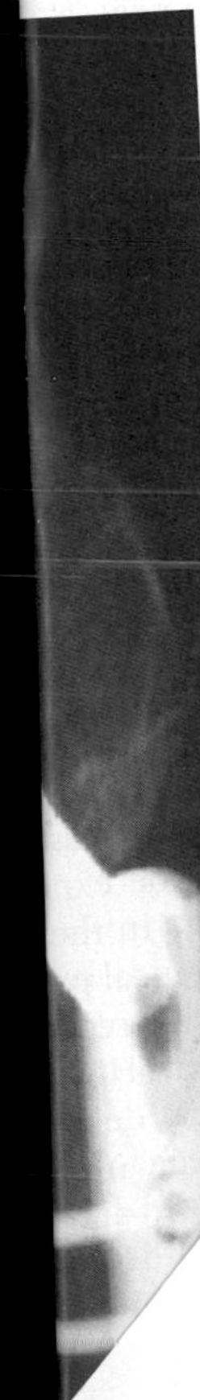

shape and its apparent mechanical properties.[15] Overall, bone mass and bone strength in humans peaks around age 30 to 35 years. Up until this age, more bone formation is occurring than bone resorption, resulting in a net increase in bone. After this age, bone resorption begins to predominate, governed by factors such as hormones, sex, activity, and disease. It is important for teenagers and young adults (particularly females) to build up a large bone mass during their peak years for bone accrual.

Age-related changes in bone include reduced toughness and increased brittleness, because of changes to the collagen matrix, less mineralization, and change in structure with fewer trabeculae and less connectivity.[10] Fracture can occur with lower loads as one ages, because of the net bone loss and reduced mechanical properties. Furthermore, as bone becomes more brittle, it is less able to absorb energy and also more prone to fracture.

Traditionally, bone loss and subsequent fracture risk is a concern with menopause in women, from a sex-steroid deficiency, and later in men, from age-related factors. This traditional understanding of bone loss fits well with cortical bone loss through time. Studies of cortical bone loss have shown that significant loss does not occur until midlife for women and is correlated with menopause and estrogen deficiency.[16] In men, cortical bone loss occurred with age beginning with a small amount of loss in young adulthood and increasing at a faster rate later in life.[16] However, in trabecular bone, bone loss varies from the traditional theory. Quantitative studies of trabecular bone morphology document that the thickness of trabeculae decreases while the spacing between trabeculae increases. There are surprisingly few fundamental differences in trabecular bone between the sexes other than that bone is lost faster in females between the ages of 50 and 85 years. Both males and females had loss of trabecular bone that began in young adulthood.[16] This began as early as the third decade for women and the fourth decade for men. There is an acceleration of bone loss that occurs in both men and women. In women, this corresponds to menopause, but men also have an acceleration of bone loss around age 65 years, which is thought to be caused by the decrease in sex steroid levels as well.[17] These age-related morphological changes significantly reduce the strength of vertebrae, the proximal femur, and other bones, contributing to the observed increased fracture incidence in the elderly.

At the tissue level, several age-related changes in the material properties of femoral cortical bone have been demonstrated. With bone tissue specifically, the tissue elastic modulus has been shown to decline 0% to 2% per decade, while ultimate strength decreases 2% to 5%, and ultimate strain 6% per decade[18] (Fig. 5-25). The energy required to fracture through bone, which is the area under the stress-strain curve, decreases with aging bone, making it more prone to fracture. Since the elastic modulus does not decrease as much, the energy to failure is predominantly reduced by age-related decreases in ultimate strain. Thus, with aging, the bone behaves more like a brittle material, and the capacity of bone to absorb the energy and resist fracture propagation from a traumatic event decreases.

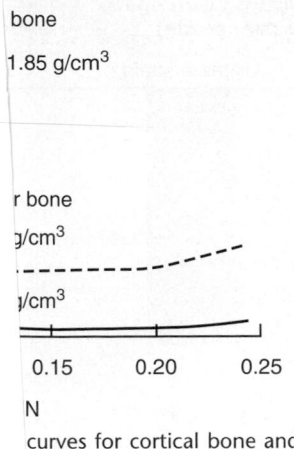

Studies of skeletal aging typically focus on bone density and often do not consider the overall geometry and distribution of bone tissue.[19] In a study of femoral density and geometry of thousands of men and women, a loss of bone density was

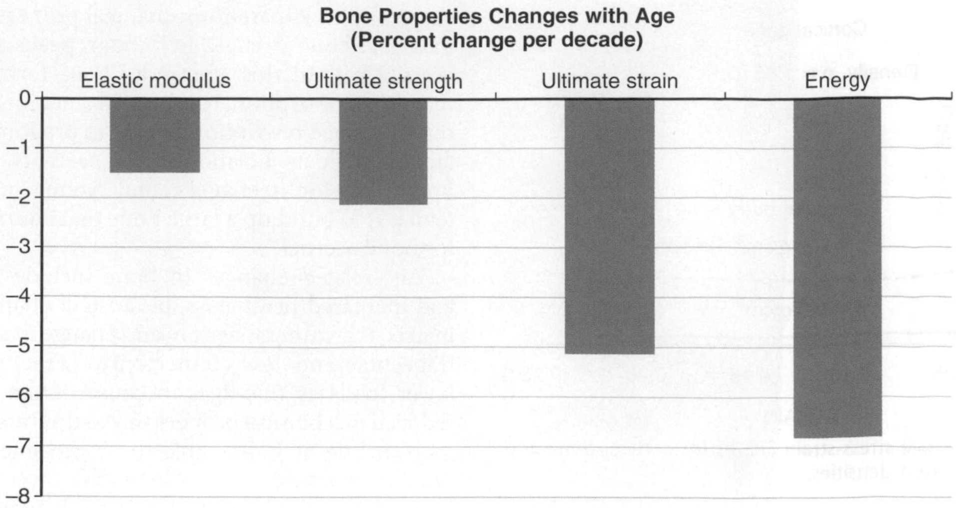

Figure 5-25. The graph demonstrates that large decreases of ultimate strain and toughness are seen with aging per decade, brittle bone. Elastic modulus and ultimate stress also decrease with time, but the relative changes are smaller over time.

clearly seen in both sexes, in both the femoral neck and in the diaphysis. In addition, the femurs expanded in periosteal diameter, but the cortical thickness decreased.

Age-related changes are not restricted to changes in the material and structural properties of bone mineral. Age-related changes in bone occur in collagen, as well as the mineral component of bone. Collagen changes with age reduce a bone's energy absorption capability. These are also implicated as a factor in increased fracture risk in older patients.[20]

Osteoporosis

A discussion of aging bone is not complete without a discussion of osteoporosis. Osteoporosis is a disease that results in deterioration of bone structure and low bone mass (Fig. 5-26). It is defined as a lumbar density that is 2.5 or more standard deviations less than mean peak bone mass of a healthy 25-year-old as measured by the T-score. Osteoporosis can increase the number of atraumatic fractures and the severity of traumatic fractures.

The changes seen with osteoporosis affect the skeletal long bones in a similar fashion. There is a loss of cortical bone, but the overall diameter of long bones remains the same. In osteoporosis, the ratio of trabecular to cortical bone is increased.[21] Additionally, there is an overall loss of trabecular bone that affects strength and ability for adequate fixation negatively (Fig. 5-27).

Common fracture sites include hip fractures, distal radius fractures, and vertebral fractures. Fracture healing depends on multiple factors including fracture location and severity, as well as patient factors, such as age and nutritional status. It is unclear from the literature whether osteoporotic fractures themselves heal more slowly. Animal models have demonstrated decreased fracture healing with increasing age,[21] but these models do not assess the complex relationship between fracture healing and osteoporosis. One common theme, however, is that osteoporotic fractures have an increased failure rate of implant fixation. They present unique fixation challenge from a biomechanics standpoint. Poor bone stock can result in inadequate fixation often from lack of adequate purchase.

More orthopaedic surgeons are working primary care physicians to address and prevent fractures through routine laboratory testing vitamin D, complete blood count, nutrition, and tory values to address the preventable cause fractures. Referring patients with fragility frac

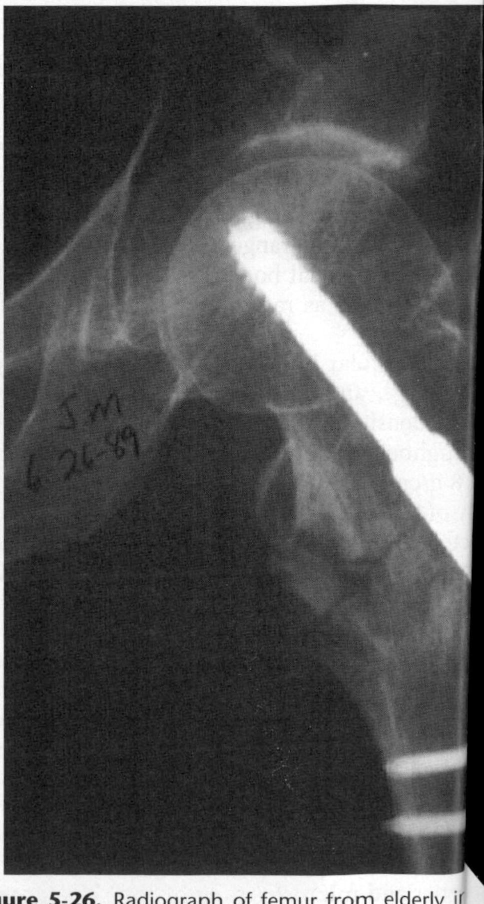

Figure 5-26. Radiograph of femur from elderly ir strating osteoporotic (osteopenic) appearance.

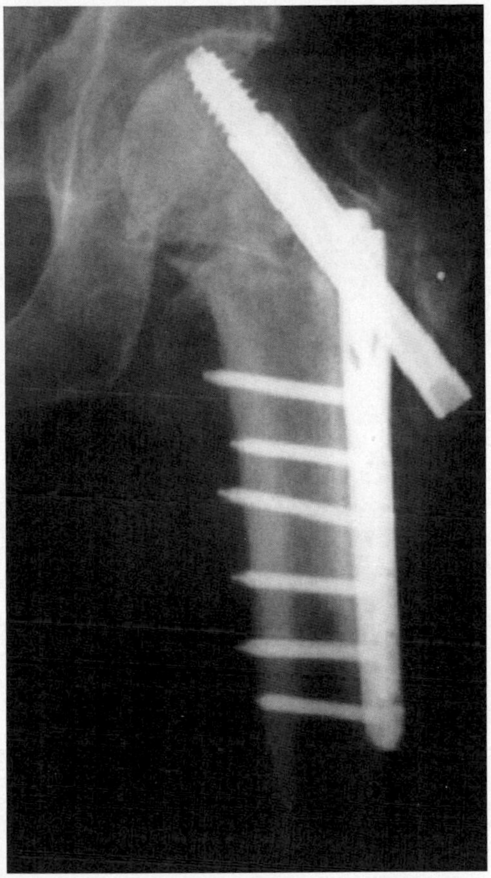

Figure 5-27. Radiograph of failure of fracture fixation in osteoporotic bone.

primary care physicians can help to prevent subsequent fragility fractures.

Both osteoporotic and age-related fragility fracture mechanisms are discussed in more detail in the "Osteoporosis and Age-Related Fracture" section.

STRUCTURAL PROPERTIES AND LOADING MODES

Structural properties incorporate information on both the material (represented by factors such as Young's or elastic modulus, ultimate strength) and the shape of an object. Including measures of the complex shape of a bone and distribution of the material within that shape allows consideration of not just the quality of the material or tissue, but where it is placed. For example, knowledge of structural properties allows mechanists to understand, for example, why bone strength is increased in individuals with a larger outer diameter (but same cortical thickness). Note that this process (enlarging diameter while maintaining cortical thickness) occurs in aging or in fracture callus formation (enlarging diameter with weaker woven bone).

How is the shape of the bone described? Engineers approximate irregular shapes (such as bones) as amalgams of common shapes for which they have developed general formulas. For a long bone, a circular cylinder approximates its shape. For a fracture fixation plate, a rectangular prism approximates its shape.

This section explores the concepts and implications of shapes and structural properties of objects, and also discusses consequences of applying force or torque to these structures.

Definition (Area Moment of Inertia)

The area moment of inertia *(I)* is simply a mathematical expression for the shape of a structure (and its resistance to acceleration; however, that is not critical for the purposes of this chapter). The moment of inertia takes into account several factors. It incorporates the presence of voids (such as screw holes) and flat or curved surfaces and solid or hollow interiors (such as medullary canals). There are equations to calculate the moment of inertia for standard shapes, and approximations for common anatomic shapes, as shown in Figure 5-28. *The common theme is that the moment of inertia is large if the bulk of the material is far from the center (femur) and small if the bulk of the material is near the center (phalanx).* Simply put, the moment of inertia is a tool to differentiate the ability of different shapes to resist deformation and fracture.

Cylinder (Long Bone, Intramedullary Nail, Screw)

The cylinder is a common shape of both long bones and the hardware used to stabilize their fractured parts. The moment of inertia of a cylinder is based on its transverse cross section, a circle. The equation to represent the moment of inertia for a circle is comprised simply of the circle's diameter to the fourth power, multiplied by the appropriate constant. This means that material located at a larger diameter will have disproportionately more effect (to the fourth power) than material located near the center. Note that a solid interior of a cross section retains material that does not contribute substantially to the overall moment of inertia. This is because it is in the interior and, hence, is represented by a smaller diameter. It is disproportionately the material on the periphery (larger diameter) that determines the object's moment of inertia. Table 5-5 shows that increasing the diameter five times, from 1 to 5 cm, results in a moment of inertia that

Circle

$$I_r = I_y = \frac{1}{4}\pi r^4$$

$$Jo = \frac{1}{2}\pi r^4$$

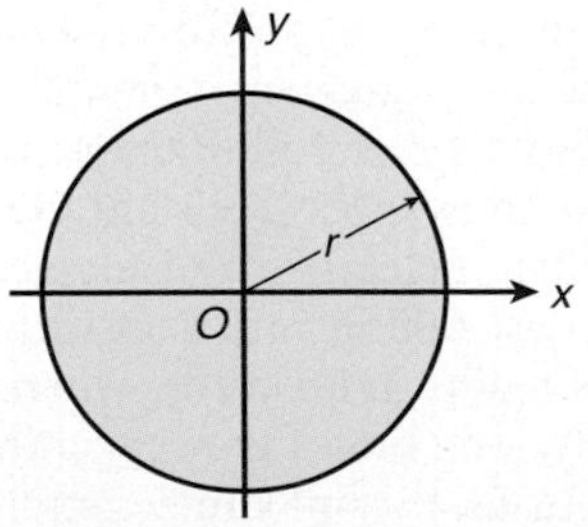

Rectangular prism

$$I_x = \frac{1}{12}m(b^2 + c^2)$$

$$I_y = \frac{1}{12}m(c^2 + a^2)$$

$$I_z = \frac{1}{12}m(a^2 + b^2)$$

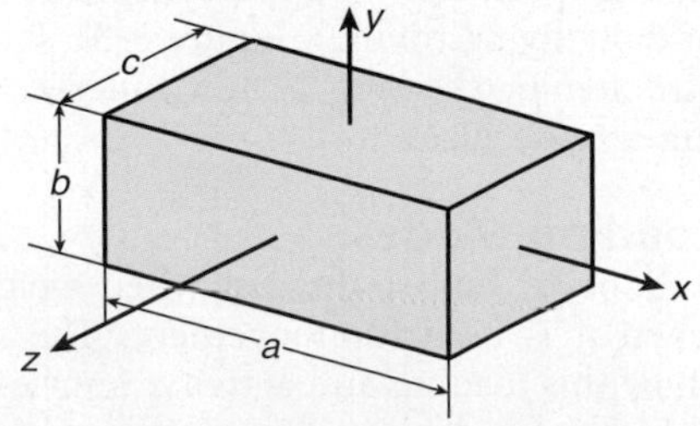

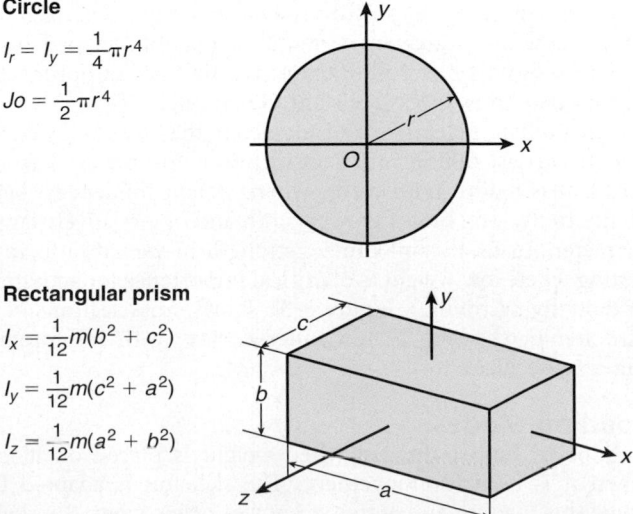

Figure 5-28. Equations to describe the shape of a circle and rectangular prism, by defining the moment of inertia. *(From Higdon A, Olson E, Stiles W, Weese J, Riley, W: Mechanics of materials, ed 3, New York, 1976, Wiley.)*

TABLE 5-5 *MOMENT OF INERTIA CHANGES WITH INCREASED BONE DIAMETER*

Bone Diameter (*d*) (cm)	Fourth Power of *d* (cm^4)	Moment of Inertia—Solid (cm^4)	Moment of Inertia—Hollow (cm^4)
1	1	0.049	−0.0031 = 0.046
2	32	1.57	−0.049 = 1.52
3	81	3.98	−0.062 = 3.92
4	256	12.6	−1.57 = 11.03
5	625	30.7	−7.67 = 23.0
5×	625×	625×	500×

increases by 625 times, from 0.049 to 30.7. If that cylinder were hollow, the void removes the least mechanically advantageous material (near the center, smaller diameter). Because least mechanically useful material is removed, hollow cylinders (with inner diameter half of outer diameter) still have a markedly increasing moment of inertia, by 500 times, from 0.046 to 23 cm^4.

Rectangle (Plate) and Optimization (I Beam, External Fixator)

In industrial design, there is often a trade-off between the weight of an item (material cost or fuel efficiency) and its strength. One example is a bicycle tube, where aluminum frames have larger diameter tubes than steel frames. This allows the bicycle to be made from a lighter material (aluminum), yet maintain the same strength. It accomplishes this by increasing the tube's moment of inertia to reach equivalent structural modulus with steel. Figure 5-29 shows tube shapes for various bicycle frame designs and materials.

Another example is an I beam. This shape forms the basis of many bridges and buildings because it provides a favorable weight-to-strength ratio. The "I" shape places material far from the center (top and bottom of the "I"), which gives it a larger moment of inertia for equivalent weight. Figure 5-30 shows how an equivalent amount of material shaped in a rectangle has a smaller moment of inertia than an optimized I beam and, thus, is less resistant to bending.

The human skeleton is well adapted to the loads and weight that it carries, taking into consideration the material from which it is made. With birds, where weight influences their ability to fly, long bones are very thin and of a relatively large diameter. Again, this maximizes strength-to-weight ratio, in a setting where low weight is of critical importance for activities of daily living (flying). Figure 5-31 shows cross sections of a bird femur, showing a thin outer cortex (with reinforcing inner trabeculae).

Loading Modes

A bone or limb is loaded when weight is placed on it, or when it is used for movement. The skeleton is adapted to allow this loading and activity; injuries occur when the skeleton is placed in an unaccustomed position, or when it is struck by an outside load. Then, following fixation to stabilize a fracture, the device itself needs to resist loads placed upon it. Understanding the loading that caused a fracture assists

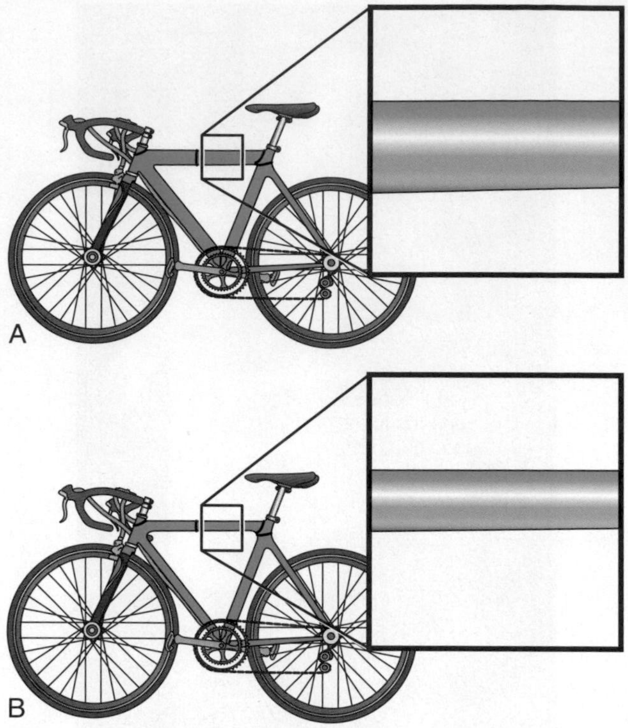

Figure 5-29. Bicycle frames with aluminum (**A**) and steel (**B**) tubes. Aluminum is about a third as dense as steel, and what it lacks in inherent stiffness can be made up by forming the tubes into stronger structures. *(From Bicycling Magazine, April 2013, p 48,* www.bicycling.com.*)*

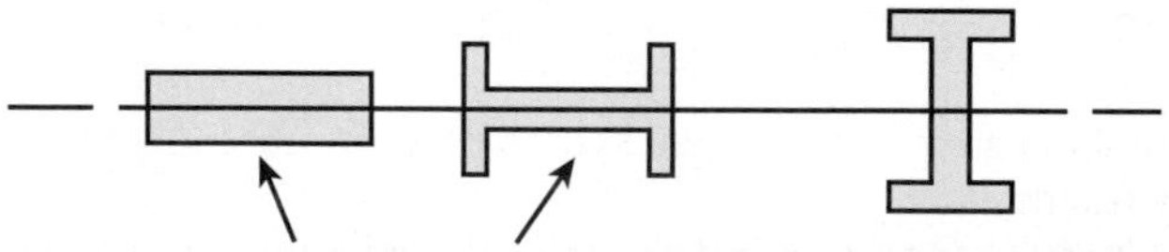

Figure 5-30. The image shows how an equivalent amount of material shaped in a rectangle has a smaller moment of inertia than an I beam, and thus is less resistant to bending.

in maneuvers to reduce it back to its undisplaced configuration. Knowledge of loading leading to a particular fracture also provides information regarding which loads a stabilization device needs to resist. Fortunately, characteristic fracture patterns occur due to separate loading modes, as discussed in the following sections (Fig. 5-32).

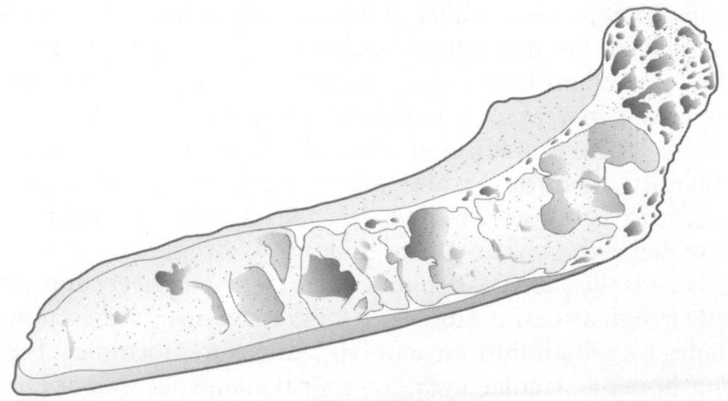

Figure 5-31. Cross section of bird femur, showing the thin cortex and the supporting interior trabeculae.

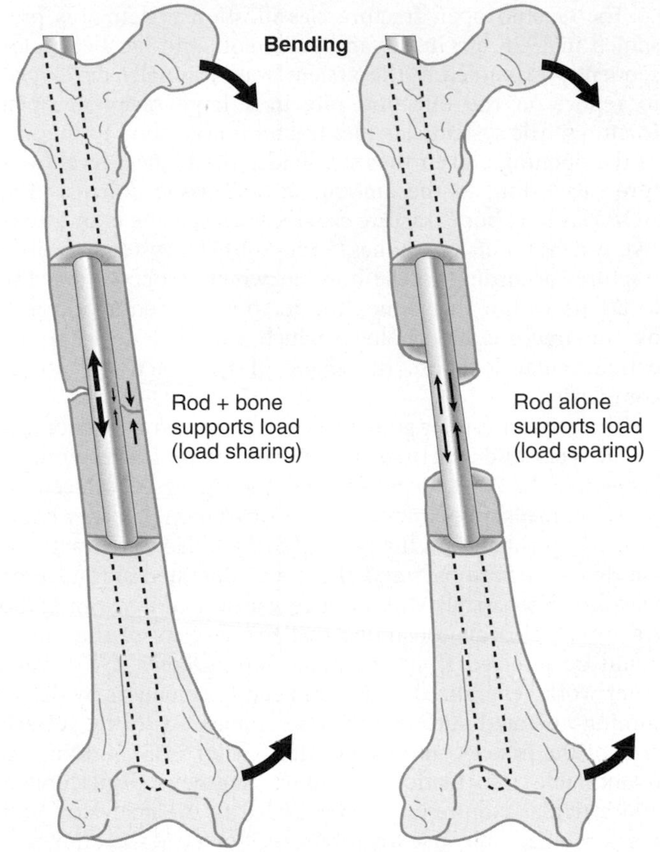

Figure 5-32. Loading the femur and other long bones during locomotion and activities of daily living induces a combination of loads. In the example of a femur, bending induces compression on the medial cortex and tension on the lateral cortex.

Tension/Compression and Shear

When loaded in tension, diaphyseal bone normally fractures because of tensile stresses along a plane that is approximately perpendicular to the direction of loading. When loaded in compression, a bone will typically fail along planes that are oblique to the bone's long axis. With compressive loads, high shear stresses develop along oblique planes that are oriented at roughly 45 degrees from the long axis. These maximum shear stresses are approximately one-half the applied compressive stress. However, because the shear strength of cortical bone is much less than the compressive strength (see Table 5-3), fracture occurs along the oblique plane of maximum shear. Thus, compressive failures of bone occur along planes of maximum shear stress, whereas tensile fractures occur along planes of maximum tensile stress.

Bending

When a bone is subjected to bending, high tensile stresses develop on the convex side, while high compressive stresses develop on the concave side. The resulting fracture pattern is consistent with that observed during axial compressive and tensile loading of whole bones. A transverse fracture surface occurs on the tensile side, whereas an oblique fracture surface is found on the compressive side. Two fracture surfaces commonly occur on the compressive side, creating a loose wedge of bone that is sometimes referred to as a "butterfly" fragment (Fig. 5-33).

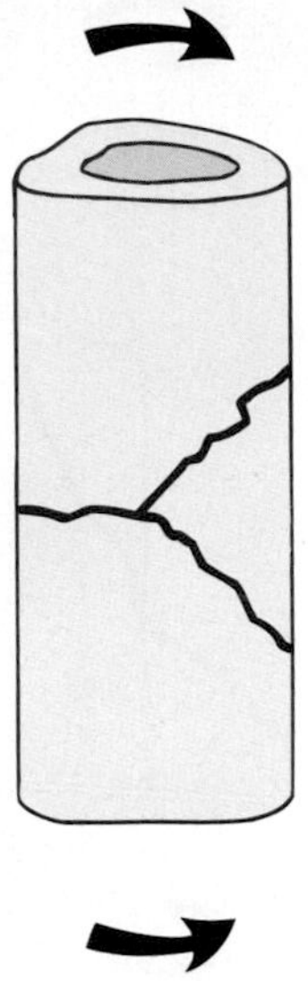

Figure 5-33. A characteristic fracture typically found for bones loaded to failure with "pure" bending-loading modes.

Torsion

The fracture pattern is more complex when a bone is subject to torsion. Fractures usually begin at a small defect at the bone surface and then the crack follows a spiral pattern through the bone along planes of high tensile stress. The final fracture surface appears as an oblique spiral that characterizes it as a torsion fracture (Fig. 5-34).

Loading Experienced by the Skeleton

The ratio of load-bearing capacity over load-bearing requirement is frequently termed the *safety factor*. The inverse of this ratio has been termed the *factor of risk for fracture*. For loads approximating the midstance phase of gait, the average load-bearing capacity of mature and osteoporotic human femurs averages around 9000 N (2000 lb) with a standard deviation of around 3000 N.[22] Peak loads at the hip joint have been recorded to be as high as 3 to 5 times body weight during high-demand activities such as stair-climbing, and even more for vigorous jumping in professional basketball players. Knee joint loads of 2 to 2.5 times body weight are routine.[23] Therefore, a 600 N (140 lb) individual who applies 5 times body weight to his or her femur has a femoral load-bearing capacity from less than 1 to 5 times as strong as needed, depending on the properties of the femur. For the tibia, axial loads while walking are estimated to be 3 to 6 times body weight,[24] and the greatest bending moment applied during restricted weight-bearing is estimated to be about 79 newton-meter in men.[25]

Clinical Examples of Combined Loading

The fracture patterns discussed for idealized loading conditions are consistent with some fractures seen clinically. However, with many traumatic loading conditions, bone is

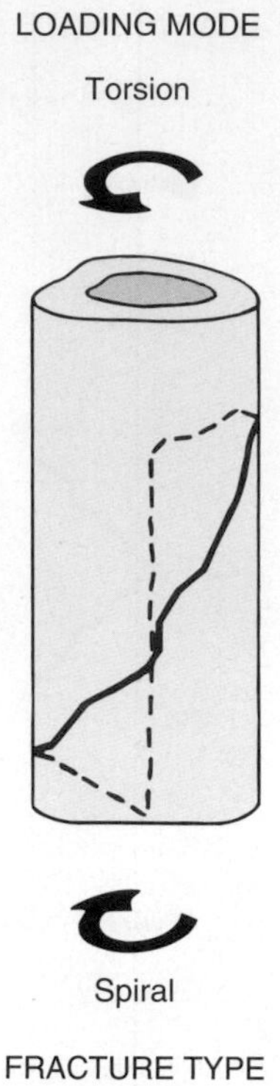

Figure 5-34. A characteristic fracture typically found for bones loaded to failure with "pure" torsion-loading modes.

subject to a combination of axial, bending, and torsional loading, and the resulting fracture patterns can be complex combinations of the preceding patterns. Additionally, high loading rates often result in additional comminution of the fracture caused by the branching and propagation of numerous fracture planes. Also, as discussed previously, through viscoelastic effects, bone may tolerate higher loads if the loads are applied rapidly,[26] although the ability of bone to absorb energy may not change with loading rate. In addition, fractures can occur owing to a single load that is greater than the load-bearing capacity of the bone (ultimate strength).

Repeated application of a variety of accumulated loads smaller than the ultimate failure load can fatigue the bone, resulting in the accumulation of microcracks in the bone, and can eventually lead to failure.[27] Fatigue failures of bone are common in military training and in athletes. If the loading is stopped or sufficiently reduced before gross failure of the bone, then each microcrack will be repaired through direct cortical remodeling.

Fracture Severity Quantification

There are many ways to differentiate fractures. Most commonly, fracture classification schemes are used for this purpose. From a clinical practice and research standpoint, the goal of fracture classification is to more systematically establish the best treatment options for different fracture presentations. Fracture classification can also provide insight into the loading mechanism that caused the fracture and provides a valuable tool for orthopaedic researchers seeking to understand complications and long-term outcomes following surgery. Two common fracture classifications systems are the Gustilo-Anderson and Arbeitsgemeinschaft für Osteosynthesefragen (AO)/Orthopaedic Trauma Association (OTA).

The Gustilo open fracture classification system was presented in 1976 by Gustilo and Anderson, and has been subsequently expanded.[28] The system was originally developed to report on the infection rate in a large series of open fractures. The system classifies fractures according to the size of the opening and further subdivides the highest-level fractures according to the amount of soft tissue damage. The AO/OTA long bone fracture classification scheme is an extensive system for all long bones.[29] The AO/OTA system classifies fractures according to the bone in which it occurs and the locations within that bone. The fracture is then subdivided by the fracture morphology, which can include intra- or extraarticular location, the shape of the fracture, and its complexity.

These systems offer guidelines to segregate fractures of different types and severities; however, they are still essentially subjective. In 2004, Beardsley and colleagues introduced an objective measure of fracture severity based on objective engineering mechanics. In that work, bovine tibiae were fractured via drop-tower impact and the newly liberated surface area was shown to correlate to the energy absorbed in creating the fracture.[30] This demonstrated that the severity of the injury could be inferred from computed tomography (CT) scans. Later work generalized and automated this analysis by determining liberated surface area via comparison to the surface area of the intact contralateral limb[31] (Fig. 5-35). Additional quantifiable information including fragment displacement and articular comminution was added to the analysis,[32] and the combined objective fracture severity metric was shown to be predictive of osteoarthritis development in tibial plafond fractures[31] (Fig. 5-36).

Fractures Associated with Particular Diseases and Conditions

There are several groups in whom fractures are prevalent and for whom prevention may be possible if fracture mechanisms and the patients at greatest risk can be identified. One group is the growing elderly population in which age-related fractures are prevalent. Another group is cancer patients with metastatic bone disease in which prophylactic stabilization of impending fractures may increase the patients' quality of life. A third group are patients with fractures that occur due to altered load conditions from an adjacent implant (periprosthetic) or due to distal and proximal implants in the same bone (interprosthetic). The next few sections will discuss the fracture risk and methods for predicting fracture risk due to aging and metastatic bone lesions.

Osteoporosis and Age-Related Fractures

The epidemiology of age-related fractures suggests a relation between osteoporosis and increased fracture risk, and the risk factors associated with hip fractures have been the subject of much research. The effects of age and gender have been documented, but these factors are confounded by comorbid conditions and an increased propensity for falls in the elderly.[33] Fractures related to osteoporosis are commonly associated with falls, and the frequency of falls increases with age. This increase is partially associated with comorbid conditions and associated medications. Additionally, falls are more common in elderly women than men, and fracture rates are also greater in women than men.[34] Common sites for fall-related fractures are the proximal femur and distal forearm. Vertebral fractures

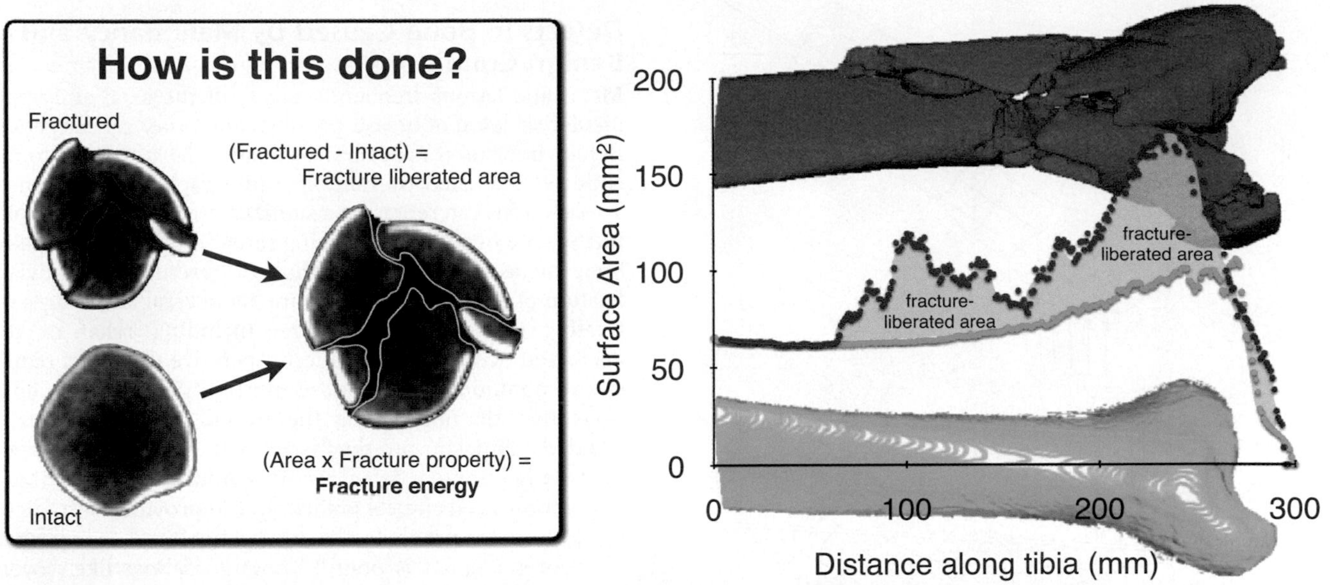

Figure 5-35. The amount of energy leading to a fracture is calculated by comparing the intact surface area to the contralateral surface area. *(From Anderson DD, Marsh JL, Brown TD. The pathomechanical etiology of post-traumatic osteoarthritis following intraarticular fractures, Iowa Orthop J 31:1–20, 2011.)*

are also frequently associated with traumatic loading such as backward falls, although relatively nontraumatic vertebral fractures may be much more common than nontraumatic femoral fractures.

When age- and sex-specific incidence rates are compared for all major fractures of different skeletal regions, considerable variability is observed. This may in part be due to varying proportions of cortical and trabecular bone at different sites and to the difference in pattern of bone loss of these two types.[35] The type and direction of loads during a fall (Fig. 5-37) are quite different from the loads during activities of daily living. Because the femur is adapted to support activities of daily living, it may be particularly sensitive to the abnormal loads during a fall. These factors emphasize both the complex interactions that occur between age-related bone loss and skeletal trauma and the need for improved understanding of the biomechanics of fracture risk in specific skeletal sites. Reduced skeletal resistance to trauma and the increased propensity for falling are cofactors in determining hip fracture risk. This leads to the conclusion that both bone loss and trauma are necessary, but not independently sufficient, causes of age-related hip fractures.

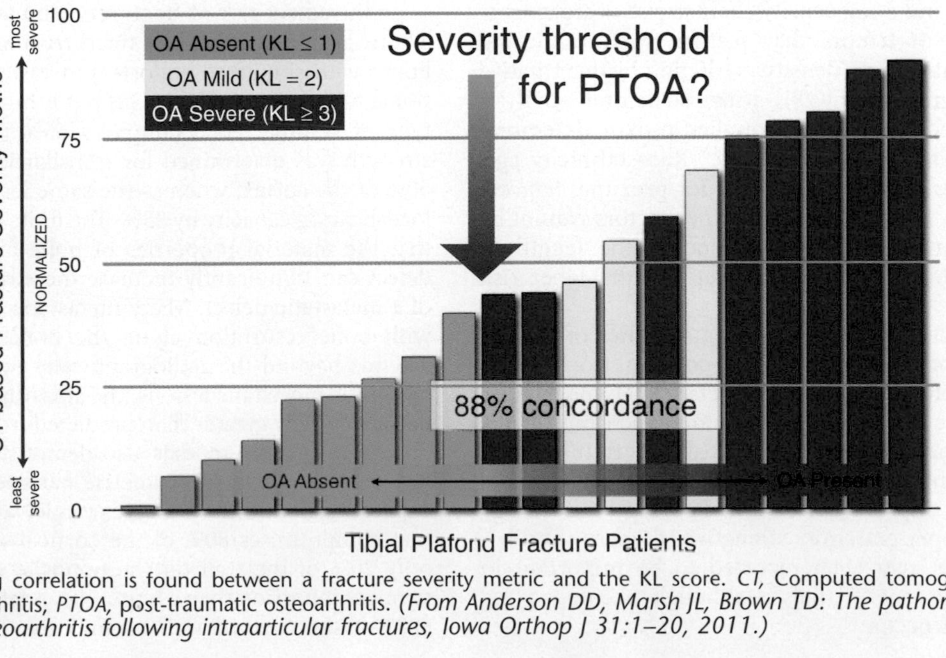

Figure 5-36. A strong correlation is found between a fracture severity metric and the KL score. *CT,* Computed tomography; *KL,* Kellgren-Lawrence; *OA,* osteoarthritis; *PTOA,* post-traumatic osteoarthritis. *(From Anderson DD, Marsh JL, Brown TD: The pathomechanical etiology of post-traumatic osteoarthritis following intraarticular fractures, Iowa Orthop J 31:1–20, 2011.)*

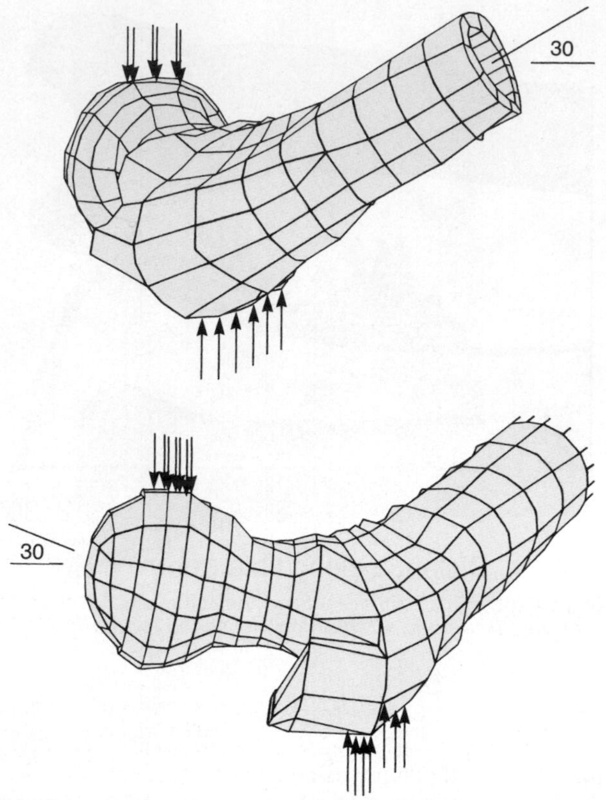

Figure 5-37. Contact loads at the femoral head and greater trochanter representing a fall to the side. *(Adapted from Lotz JC: Doctoral dissertation, Massachusetts Institute of Technology, Cambridge, MA, 1988.)*

Fractures of the proximal femur are a significant public health problem and a major cause of mortality and morbidity among the elderly,[36] and attempts to reduce the incidence of age-related hip fractures have primarily focused on preventing or inhibiting excessive bone loss associated with osteoporosis. Specific anatomic and bone density characteristics are emerging as signatures of femurs that sustain fractures during falls.[18,37,38] Combining bone density prediction by quantitative computed tomography (QCT) with structural analysis through bone-specific FEA can predict proximal femoral strength for different fall configurations.[39] Race, ethnicity, age, and sex differences have been reported for proximal femoral strength, although lifestyle, diet, and other factors cannot be ruled out.[40-42] Femoral geometry, including the length of femoral neck moment arm, are associated with higher risk of fracture.[43]

More recent data indicates that characteristics of the fall (including direction of fall and landing position, trochanteric soft tissue, as well as flooring characteristics) may be as important as bone loss.[44-46] Strategies to reduce injury due to falls range from neuromuscular, balance training and recovery (including martial arts techniques), method of falling, as well as hip protectors and flooring with energy absorption.[46-51] Upper extremity strength and energy absorption capability has also been reported to be important in mitigating fracture due to falls,[52] although accompanying wrist fracture can occur.

Defects in Bone Caused by Malignancy and Benign Conditions

Metastatic lesions frequently occur in the axial and appendicular skeleton of breast, prostate, and other cancer patients. Benign bone tumors occur in as many as 33% of asymptomatic children evaluated by random radiographs of long bones.[53] These lesions can represent a significant fracture risk. Approximately 5% of patients receiving radiation therapy for painful bone metastases suffer a pathologic fracture.[54] Prophylactic fixation of an impending fracture has several advantages over treating a pathologic fracture, including relief of pain, decreased hospital stay, reduced operative difficulty, reduced risk of nonunion, and reduced morbidity. Conversely, operations that do not reduce the overall morbidity must be avoided. Clinicians are thus faced with the task of determining whether or not a defect requires prophylactic stabilization. Commonly used clinical guidelines can provide contradictory indications for prophylactic stabilization, and the specificity of these guidelines is poor.[55] These guidelines likely overestimate the risk of pathologic fracture.[56] There are many aspects of metastatic and benign defect geometry and material properties that determine the structural consequences of the lesion. In common sites of osseous metastases, such as the proximal femur, even experienced orthopaedic oncologists cannot predict the strength reduction caused by the defect from radiographs or from qualitative observation of CT examinations.[57]

Numerous laboratory research studies have been reported that specifically address the structural consequences of metastatic defects in axial and appendicular skeleton.[55,57,58] In general, these studies demonstrate that finite element models and other analytical methods can be used to account for bone density and geometry and predict the structural consequences of metastatic lesions in bone. In all experiments, good agreement was found between the computer model predictions and actual measurements of strength reductions because of the defects.

Existing guidelines for determining when to prophylactically stabilize long bones with metastatic lesions can overestimate the actual risk of fracture in some cases[56] but can place a bone at significant risk of fracture in others. The strength of bones with simulated endosteal metastatic defects is proportional to defect size (Fig. 5-38) but is highly dependent on the type of loading. For example, a 65% reduction in bending strength was determined for transcortical lesions destroying 50% of the cortex, whereas the same lesion reduces torsional load-bearing capacity by 85%. The finite element models show that the material properties of bone along the border of a defect can significantly increase the structural consequences of a metastatic defect. Many metastatic lesions are associated with bone resorption along the border of the lesion that extends beyond the radiographically evident lysis. Thus, for osteolytic metastatic lesions, the structural consequences may be significantly greater than predicted from plain radiographs. The finite element models also demonstrated that for endosteal defects, a critical geometric parameter is the minimum cortical-wall thickness. For example, an asymmetric defect that compromises 80% of the cortical wall at one point but only 20% of the wall on the opposite side will be only 2% stronger in torsion than a bone with a defect that compromises 80% of the cortical wall around the entire circumference.

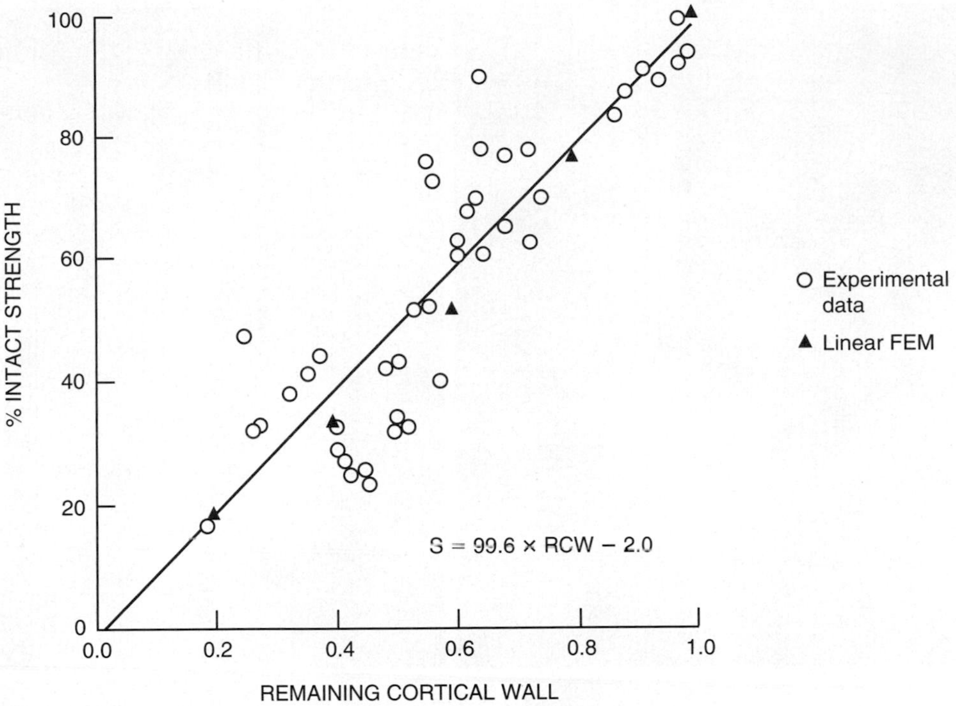

Figure 5-38. Percentage of intact bone bending strength as a function of endosteal defect size. Endosteal defect size is expressed as the ratio of reduced wall thickness to intact cortical wall thickness. Both experimental and analytical results are shown. *FEM,* Finite element model; *RCW,* remaining cortical wall; *S,* percent of intact strength. *(Adapted from Hipp JA, McBroom RJ, Cheal EJ, et al: Structural consequences of endosteal metastatic lesions in long bones, J Orthop Res 76:828–837, 1989.)*

Femoral neck lesions can reduce fracture strength by nearly 50%,[59] and the medial location has the largest reduction in axial strength, followed by anterior and posterior locations.[60] The method to provide prophylactic stabilization often suggests an IM device. In one study evaluating torsional stiffness and strength of various clinically based lesions, retrograde IM nails were as good as or better than plates for providing stability and involved less soft tissue stripping.[61,62] A small series of three cases of tumor progression in soft tissues adjacent to IM nail insertion suggests that copious irrigation and postoperative surveillance be considered.[63]

Imaging is important to fully evaluate the extent of lesions. Even biplanar radiographs will fail to detect critical geometric parameters if the critical defect geometry is not aligned with respect to the radiographic planes. In a retrospective study of 516 metastatic breast lesions using anteroposterior radiographs, Keene and colleagues[64] could not establish a geometric criterion for lesions at risk of fracture, perhaps because critical geometric parameters were missed using plain radiographs. Results of ex vivo experiments with simulated defects suggest that CT scans at small consecutive scan intervals could facilitate evaluation of the fracture risk due to metastatic or benign lesions.

Strength reductions due to long bone or vertebral defects can be determined from CT data using relatively simple engineering models.[55,58,64] These CT-based measurements require placing a phantom under the patient during the examination so that CT attenuation data can be converted to bone density. Known relations between bone density and bone modulus are then used to convert the bone density data to modulus. For each cross section through the bone, the product of area and modulus is summed over the entire cross section, excluding posterior elements. The lowest axial rigidity of all cross sections was linearly related to the measured failure load, and predicted almost 90% of the variability in the measured failure loads in a laboratory study.[66] In a similar study using the same CT-based technique, a one-to-one correspondence between measured and predicted failure load was found, although this study looked at a wider range of defect locations and was able to predict only 74% of the variation in measured failure loads.[65]

In a clinical study, the CT-based rigidity of a bone with a benign defect has been shown to be significantly more sensitive and specific to pathologic fracture than criteria based on defect size.[55] In this study, the rigidity of a bone with a benign lesion was normalized to corresponding sections through the contralateral bone. A combination of the minimum bending and torsional rigidities calculated from the CT data provided was 100% sensitive and 94% specific in distinguishing between the 18 patients who sustained a pathologic fracture and the 18 patients with nonfracture. In contrast, radiograph-based criteria were 28% to 83% sensitive and 6% to 78% specific.

Implant-Related Bone Fracture: Periprosthetic and Interprosthetic Fractures

If a hip fracture occurs in a patient with a stemmed revision femoral component of a knee replacement, a further sequela that needs to be avoided is an interprosthetic fracture between the implant stabilizing this hip fracture and the stemmed femoral component (Fig. 5-39). Clinically, external plating of the entire span of the femur has been shown to provide reliable results for treatment of a periprosthetic fracture without further sequelae such as plate pull-off or fracture destabilization.[67-69]

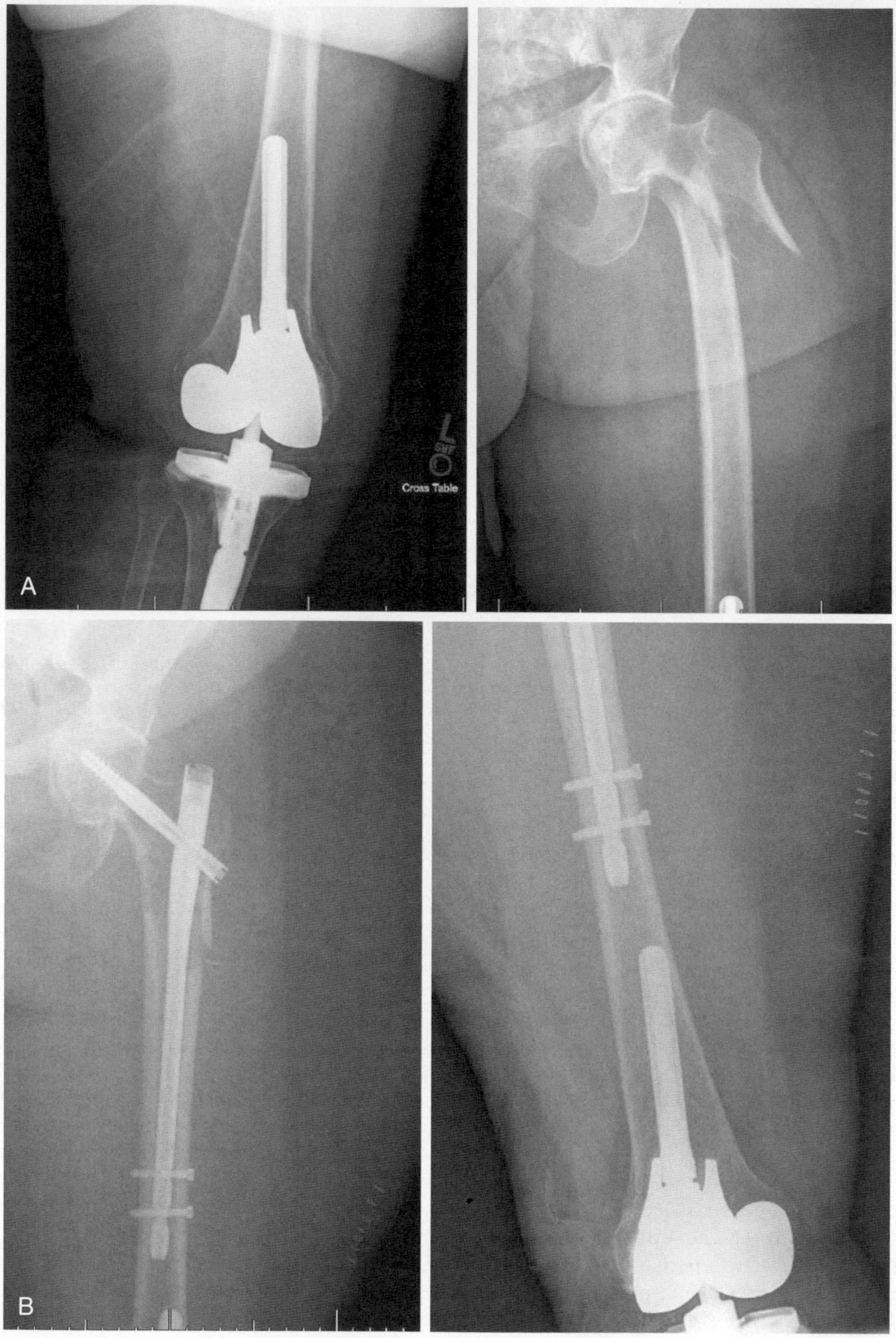

Figure 5-39. A and **B,** Subtrochanteric fracture with ipsilateral stemmed total knee arthroplasty. Treated with intramedullary fixation, which can increase forces on bone between the implants and put it at risk for refracture.

One numerical FEA evaluating the role of gap size and cortex thickness[70] found the major influence in stress at the stem tip is cortex thickness rather than the size of the gap between the two stem tips (Table 5-6). For example, in that study, for a 3-mm cortex with gaps ranging from 1 to 85 mm (round tip), the strains only ranged from 192 to 197 MPa, whereas for a thicker 7-mm cortex the stresses were all reduced to approximately one-fourth (58.1 to 59.6 MPa). Stems that were modeled as loose had significantly increased strains compared to stems that were modeled as well fixed. This study would support attention paid to loose stems, and minimal further reaming (to maintain cortex thickness); however, note that clinical results do not fully reflect these findings of insensitivity to gap length. An experimental study found that

TABLE 5-6 *PEAK TENSILE STRESSES BETWEEN TWO INTRAMEDULLARY STEMS WITH INCREASING GAP DISTANCES*

Stress at Tip (MPa)	Size of Gap between Stem Tips				
	Control	*1 mm**	*10 mm**	*35 mm**	*85 mm**
3-mm cortex	203.7	192.0	197.7	197.4	193.0
5-mm cortex	101.2	99.4	99.0	97.7	96.7
7-mm cortex	60.0	59.6	58.5	58.8	58.1

*Round stem tip; well-fixed.
Adapted from Iesaka K, Kummer FJ, Di Cesare PE: Stress risers between two ipsilateral intramedullary stems: a finite-element and biomechanical analysis, J Arthroplasty 20(3):386–391, 2005.

stronger constructs were those where IM implants were "kissing" or where an overlapping plate extended past the fracture zone.[71]

Guidelines for minimum interprosthetic distance for periprosthetic fractures (and to prevent interprosthetic fractures) need further studies in order to develop robust recommendations.

Stress Shielding

Compression plates require anatomic reduction and absolute stability of fixation. This type of plating technique promotes direct bone healing by osteons crossing the fracture line. A complication of this type of rigid fixation was concern for refracture caused by weakened, osteopenic bone from underneath the plates due to stress shielding (Figs. 5-40 and 5-41).

Refracture is always a concern after fracture fixation, whether operative or nonoperative techniques were employed. Refracture rates have been studied in the pediatric population, with refracture rates in the forearm of 5%.[72] Although pediatric fractures heal and remodel rapidly, there is an initial stage where the bone is not at its original strength and is at risk for refracture. Proximal- and middle-third forearm fractures, were found to be at higher risk as well as a fracture line that was still visible at the radius.[72]

FRACTURE HEALING

From a biomechanical perspective, fracture healing is a process that restores the strength and stiffness of bone. Fracture healing depends on the overall intrinsic stability of the fracture fragments and the dimensions of the fracture gap. Additionally, there are biologic components to fracture healing that are addressed in greater detail in previous chapters. In any case, there needs to be enough mechanical stability, whether that is due to the nature of the fracture or assisted by immobilization or implant fixation, to allow the biologic process to be completed.[17]

Fracture healing can evolve through direct primary bone healing, where absolute stability is achieved or through secondary bone healing. Direct healing occurs in fractures where anatomic reduction with more rigid fixation is achieved. When immobilization is less rigid, such as in casts or IM fixation, secondary bone healing occurs, with repair through callus formation.

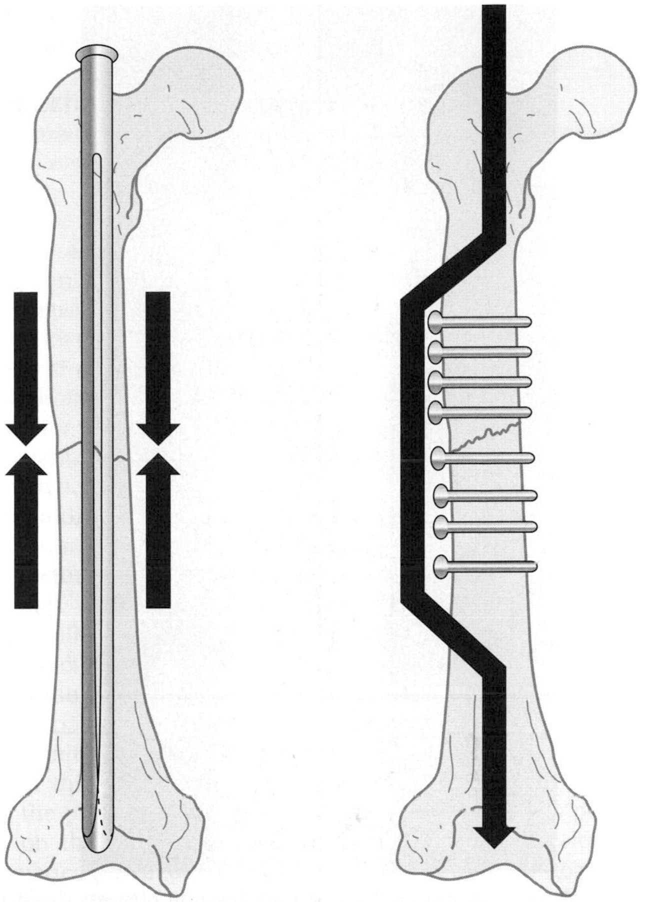

Figure 5-40. Stress shielding can occur underneath a fracture stabilization plate because of the stress-bypass effect. Intramedullary nails continue to have circumferential load across the fracture site, through the cortex.

In direct healing, small gaps are filled with woven bone through a process called *gap healing*. This is followed by direct cortical reconstruction. This process occurs in fractures with minimal comminution and rigid fixation.

Secondary bone healing differs from primary bone healing in that bony callus is formed. This process results from less rigid immobilization, such as casting or IM fixation. This type of bone healing occurs in four general steps: inflammation, callus differentiation, ossification, and remodeling. After a fracture occurs, the disruption of blood vessels form a hematoma and mesenchymal stem cells trigger the initial formation of fracture callus releasing growth factors.[73,74] Fracture callus begins as a soft substance made of fibrous tissue, fibrocartilage, and hyaline cartilage. Eventually, the cartilage is replaced by new bone through endochondral ossification where callus is converted into woven bone. Bone callus growth begins at the periphery of the fracture site where strain is the lowest.[75] Over time, remodeling of the disorganized immature woven bone to mature bone occurs. This time course varies with fracture type, location, and severity (Fig. 5-42).

Healing by Callus Formation—Biomechanical Considerations

In contrast to direct cortical healing, fracture healing by callus formation typically involves resorption of fracture surfaces along with prolific woven bone formation originating

TABLE 5-7 *MATERIAL PROPERTIES FOR ORTHOPAEDIC FRACTURE FIXATION DEVICES*

Material	Loading Direction	Elastic Modulus (MPa)	Ultimate Strength (MPa)
Meniscus	Compression	0.1–0.6	NA
Articular cartilage	Compression	0.3–1.0	NA
Intervertebral disc	Tension	0.5	0.3
Articular cartilage	Tension	3–6	5–10
Trabecular bone	Compression	10–150	1–10
Meniscus	Tension	50–150	1–4
Ligaments	Tension	300	40
Tendons	Tension	300–600	40–60
Ultrahigh-molecular-weight polyethylene	Compression	400–1200	40
Cortical bone	Compression	18,000	200
Stainless steel	Tension	110,000	490–1400
Titanium	Tension	200,000	550

NA, Not applicable.
(Source: Caffrey JP, Sah RL: Biomechanics of musculoskeletal tissues. In: O'Keefe R, Jacobs JJ, Chu CR, Einhorn TA, editors: Orthopaedic basic science: foundations of clinical practice, ed 4, Rosemont, IL, 2013, American Academy of Orthopaedic Surgeons.)

Nonoperative Treatment, Casting and Splinting, Traction

Without intervention, bone undergoes the fracture stabilization process as just described, with surrounding muscles and soft tissue providing some stability for the fracture site. With splinting or casting techniques, pressure is applied through the stiff materials of the splint, and reduces movement at the fracture. Proper molding can direct bone alignment by exerting pressure on the surrounding soft tissues.

Clubfoot casting well illustrates how pressure exerted by a well-molded cast can slowly correct a deformity. The Ponseti method first corrects cavus by aligning the first ray, followed by subsequent manipulation and lateral pressure to correct forefoot adduction and varus of the heel, and finally dorsiflexion (Fig. 5-46).

Material selection in casting is important just as it is in internal fixation. Plaster has been traditionally used and has the advantage of being more moldable and pliable. Disadvantages of plaster include a low strength-to-weight ratio, which results in thicker casts to achieve the same stability as synthetic material. Synthetic fiberglass materials are lightweight, strong, and more radiolucent allowing for better imaging. They are more difficult to mold and may result in pressure areas on the soft tissues more readily than plaster casts.

Using biomechanical principles, three-point fixation is used once reduction is obtained to maintain alignment. As the image demonstrates (Fig. 5-47), each of the three forces is needed to hold reduction.

Various studies have looked at the shape of casts and their role in maintaining alignment. Well-fitting casts have been found to have an optimal sagittal-to-coronal ratio of 0.7, creating an oval-shaped cast, not a circle.[77] Figure 5-48 demonstrates ideal casting technique.

There is a limit to a cast's ability to shape bone. For example, a cast that is too tight in combination with swelling from acute trauma can lead to compartment syndrome with the cast acting like a tourniquet.[77] Soft tissue breakdown is also a concern in casting, especially in patients with neuromuscular disorders, resulting in spasticity, or in those with sensation abnormalities, such as peripheral neuropathy from diabetes.

Surgical Fixation—Biomechanical Considerations

Many fractures require surgical reduction for adequate alignment or more stability than can be provided by casting. Generally, devices such as external fixators and IM nails provide relative stability, and allow interfragmentary movement, which can stimulate callus formation. The various types of fixation and their biomechanical considerations are listed in the following subsections.

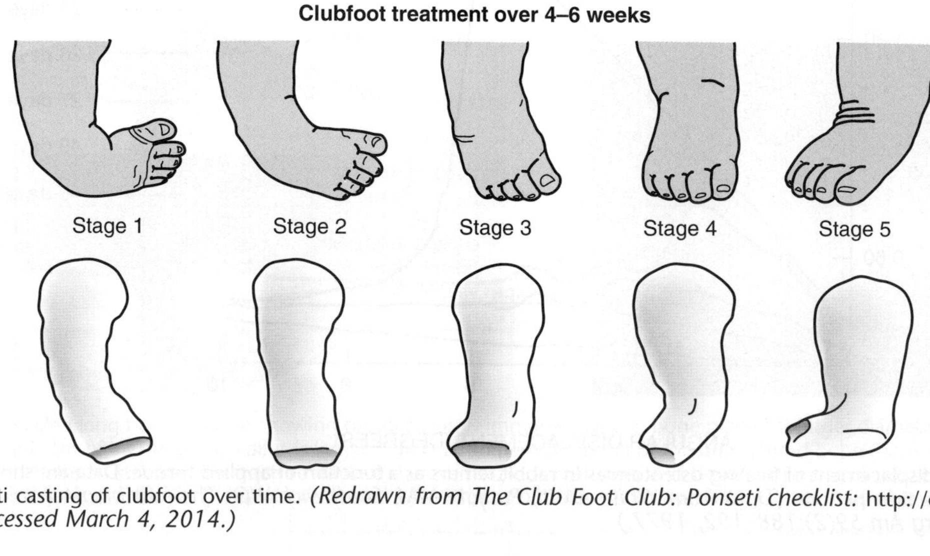

Figure 5-46. Ponseti casting of clubfoot over time. *(Redrawn from The Club Foot Club: Ponseti checklist:* http://clubfootclub.org/about/ponseti-checklist. *Accessed March 4, 2014.)*

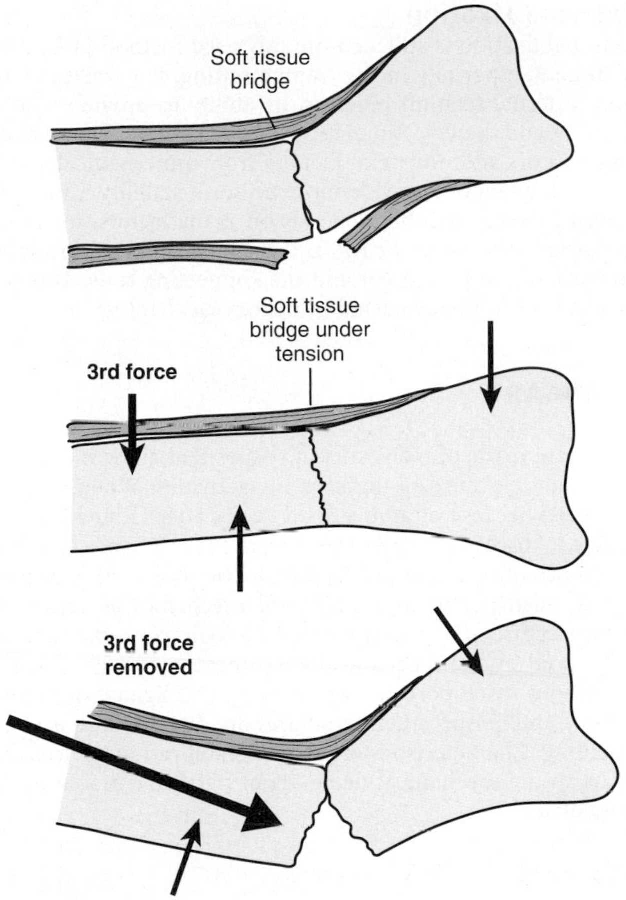

Figure 5-47. Three-point fixation diagram. *(Redrawn from Rockwood CA Jr, Green DP, Bucholz RW, Heckman JD: Rockwood and Green's fractures in adults, ed 4, Baltimore, MD, 1996, Lippincott Williams & Wilkins, Fig. 1-45, p. 35.)*

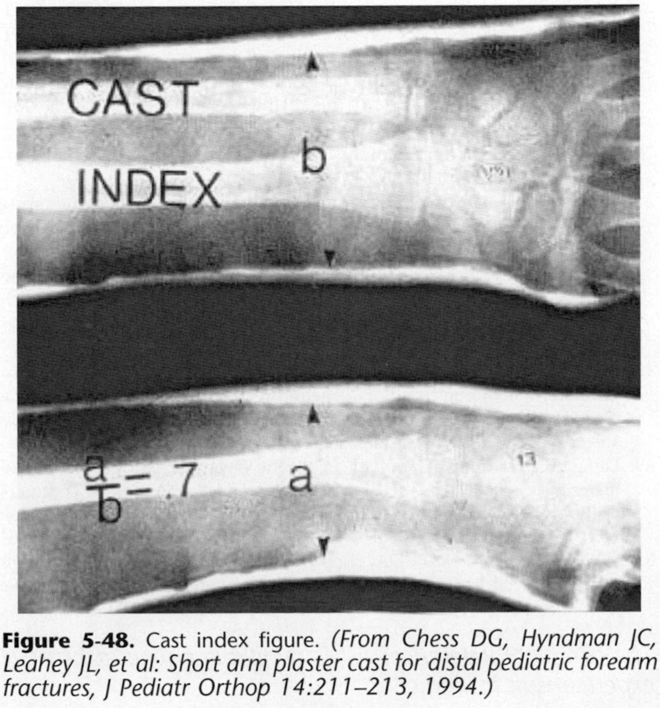

Figure 5-48. Cast index figure. *(From Chess DG, Hyndman JC, Leahey JL, et al: Short arm plaster cast for distal pediatric forearm fractures, J Pediatr Orthop 14:211–213, 1994.)*

Intramedullary Rods

IM rods are a method of fracture fixation that provide relative stability, allow for some motion at the fracture fragments, resulting in secondary fracture healing with callus formation that results in fracture healing.

IM rods act as internal splints, and rod design is dependent on the rod-to-bone interaction and the structural properties of the rod, including material properties, such as shape and diameter.[78,79]

As described previously, physiologic loading within bone consists of a combination of compression, tension, and torsion. Traditional slotted nails were designed to increase contact stress and friction between the nail and wall. These nails had stability against bending moments and shear forces perpendicular to the long axis, but were unstable when torque was applied. Greater stability to torsional moments was provided by the introduction of locked IM nails. Screws proximally and distally are used and the physiologic loads are transmitted through the ends. Screws experience four-point loads (Fig. 5-49). Screws experience significantly higher forces if the screw is closer to the fracture or where there is not cortical contact at the fracture site.

Rod diameter changes the rigidity of the construct. In a solid nail, bending rigidity is proportional to the nail diameter to the third power and torsional rigidity to the fourth power.[79] The general cross-sectional shape of IM rods is very similar, so there is typically little variation between devices with regard to this. IM reaming also changes the rigidity with bending and torsion as reaming allows for larger diameter to be used and increases the contact area between the rod and bone.

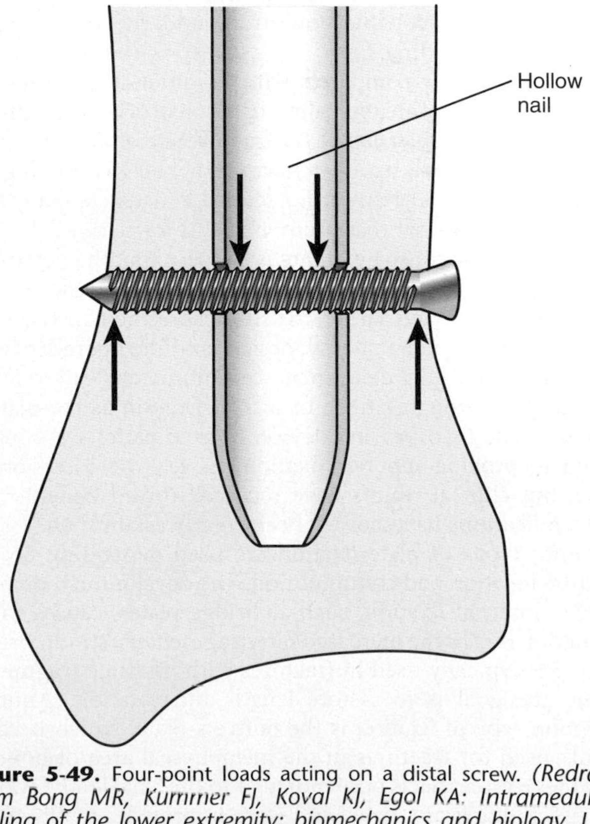

Figure 5-49. Four-point loads acting on a distal screw. *(Redrawn from Bong MR, Kummer FJ, Koval KJ, Egol KA: Intramedullary nailing of the lower extremity: biomechanics and biology, J Am Acad Orthop Surg 15:97–106, 2007.)*

One of the advantages of IM rod fixation of fractures over traditional plate fixation is early weight-bearing and mobilization. Specifically, femoral fractures fixed with interlocked nails can withstand greater than four times body weight before failure. Previous biomechanical studies[80] have shown that rods with a 12-mm diameter or greater and two distal locking bolts can withstand normal weight-bearing forces even in fractures without bony contact. In fractures with bony contact, smaller diameter nails or only one distal locking bolt supported normal weight-bearing forces.

Plate Fixation

There are various methods of plate fixation available. The choice depends on the fracture location, degree of comminution, and surgical goals. The bone and plate share the load, and the interface between the two affects the mechanical environment of fracture healing.

There are many properties of a plate construct that affect fracture healing. The stiffness of the construct is one of the important factors in determining fracture healing by affecting fracture-site motion. As noted earlier, stiffness is determined by material, thickness of the plate, and other factors (and is calculated by dividing a load that is applied by the displacement). Bending stiffness is proportional to the third power of thickness of the plate. The properties of the bone work in conjunction with the plate properties. Bone that is weaker, from osteoporosis for example, increases the load sharing of the plate.

Compression plates require anatomic reduction and absolute stability of fixation. This type of plating technique promotes direct bone healing by osteons crossing the fracture line. A complication of this type of rigid fixation was concern for weakened, osteopenic bone from underneath the plates due to stress shielding.

Locked plating compared with traditional compression plate constructions are typically stiffer constructs. The stiffness of locking plate constructs at the fracture site of the far cortex, opposite of the plate, has been measured to be 10 times higher, 833 N/mm to 2100 N/mm, for locked constructs compared with external fixators that promote callus formation.[81]

With a stiffer construct, there is concern that the decreased intrafragmentary motion may lead to increased risk of nonunion. As mentioned earlier, the stiffness of the construct has to do both with plate material, design, and the operative techniques used. Healing deficiencies can ultimately lead to hardware failure through fatigue or loss of fixation as the plate is then the sole load-bearing device. Locked plates were introduced to provide superior fixation in weak or osteoporotic bone, but clinical results have reported mixed benefits and their indications have not yet been clearly established.[82]

Other types of plate fixation are used depending on the fracture location and comminution. The development of more flexible internal fixation, such as bridge plates, causes callus formation due to the increased interfragmentary strain. Bridge plating is typically used in fractures with multiple fragments, where the goal is to restore length and rotation. Another common type of fixation is the buttress plate, which is commonly used for fractures in the metaphyseal area of bone. It provides a force that is perpendicular to the axial load. Overall, plate techniques are varied and work to provide stability until bony healing occurs.

External Fixation

External fixation is still a commonly used method of fracture treatment, especially in the trauma setting. For fracture fixation, external fixation relies on its ability to provide relative stability, and thereby stimulate callus formation. In comparing ring fixators and unilateral fixators from a mechanical standpoint, ring fixators provide more uniform stability. Unilateral external fixator stability depends on many factors, including the distance between the rod and the bone and the placement and size of pin placement and the connecting rods. This will be outlined in further detail in upcoming chapters.

SUMMARY

Bones are made of material and shapes that allow movement and loading occurring under many activities. When they are fractured because of an overload event, after fatigue loading, or due to disease, an understanding of the mechanics involved is important to guide proper treatment choice. This chapter has detailed pertinent concepts of mechanics as related to bone fracture, and has presented biologic concepts that are influenced by the mechanical environment. Specific fracture conditions (osteoporosis, defects due to malignant or benign tumors and periprosthetic fracture) are discussed, as is stress shielding. Characteristics of fracture stabilization devices that relate to the mechanical demands of particular fractures are presented.

KEY REFERENCES

The level of evidence (LOE) is determined according to the criteria provided in the preface.

8. Carter DC, Hayes W: Bone compressive strength: the influence of density and strain rate. *Science* 194(4270):1174–1176, 1976. doi: 10.1126/science.996549. LOE V
9. Bayraktar HH, Morgan EF, Niebur GL, et al: Comparison of the elastic and yield properties of human femoral trabecular and cortical bone tissue. *J Biomech* 37(1):27–35, 2004. LOE V
12. Kreider JM, Goldstein SA: Trabecular bone mechanical properties in patients with fragility fractures. *Clin Orthop Relat Res* 467(8):1955–1963, 2009. doi: 10.1007/s11999-009-0751-8; 10.1007/s11999-009-0751-8. LOE V
13. Hernandez CJ, Keaveny TM: A biomechanical perspective on bone quality. *Bone* 39(6):1173–1181, 2006. doi: 10.1016/j.bone.2006.06.001. LOE V
20. Burr DB: The contribution of the organic matrix to bone's material properties. *Bone* 31(1):8–11, 2002. LOE V
24. Taylor WR, Heller MO, Bergmann G, et al: Tibio-femoral loading during human gait and stair climbing. *J Orthop Res* 22(3):625–632, 2004. doi: 10.1016/j.orthres.2003.09.003. LOE V
32. Anderson DD, Mosqueda T, Thomas T, et al: Quantifying tibial plafond fracture severity: absorbed energy and fragment displacement agree with clinical rank ordering. *J Orthop Res* 26(8):1046–1052, 2008. doi: 10.1002/jor.20550. LOE V
42. Meta M, Lu Y, Keyak JH, et al: Young-elderly differences in bone density, geometry and strength indices depend on proximal femur sub-region: a cross sectional study in Caucasian-American women. *Bone* 39(1):152–158, 2006. doi: 10.1016/j.bone.2005.11.020. LOE V
49. Laing AC, Feldman F, Jalili M, et al: The effects of pad geometry and material properties on the biomechanical effectiveness of 26 commercially available hip protectors. *J Biomech* 44(15):2627–2635, 2011. doi: 10.1016/j.jbiomech.2011.08.016; 10.1016/j.jbiomech.2011.08.016. LOE V
55. Snyder BD, Hauser-Kara DA, Hipp JA, et al: Predicting fracture through benign skeletal lesions with quantitative computed tomography. *J Bone Joint Surg Am* 88(1):55–70, 2006. doi: 10.2106/JBJS.D.02600. LOE V

The complete References list is available online at https://expertconsult.inkling.com.

Chapter 6

Closed Fracture Management

6A Introduction

JAMES P. WADDELL

INTRODUCTION

Nonoperative management of fractures is presumably as old as humankind. One would therefore anticipate that as part of the evolutionary biology of humans that there would be an intrinsic ability for fractures to heal without surgical interference. Over centuries this has been demonstrated to be the case; fractures, left to their own devices, will heal and, even more importantly, this healing process is expedited by active use of the injured limb.

There has been an increasing tendency to treat surgically those fractures that might equally effectively be treated without open reduction and internal fixation. The reasons for this are multiple including more convenience for the patient and the surgeon, enjoyment for the surgeon (not the patient!), advertising by implant companies, and financial compensation for both surgeons and hospitals.

Although the surgical treatment by means of reduction and fixation of certain fracture types undoubtedly brings an added benefit to the patient, there are many fractures in which this is not the case. In a number of randomized clinical trials, the surgical treatment for common fractures has been proven to be no more effective than the nonsurgical treatment but at considerably greater expense to the system in terms of providing care. The common fracture-dislocation studies include fractures of the distal radius,[1] fractures of the humeral shaft, fractures of the proximal humerus,[2] fractures of the surgical neck of the humerus[3] or acromioclavicular dislocations,[4,5] fractures of the calcaneus,[6] and some ankle fractures.[7]

In the era of evidence-based medicine, it is perplexing and a bit disheartening to find that surgical procedures are routinely performed that do not bring benefit to the patient. Although this is not unique to fracture surgery or indeed to orthopaedics in general, it is an activity that should concern the thinking orthopaedic surgeon.

The nonsurgical management of fractures is technically demanding, time consuming, and requires more diligence then surgical treatment. Recognizing the benefits to the patient, however, makes it mandatory that every fracture that can be managed without surgery with an equal or better outcome to those treated by surgery should be considered for the nonsurgical option. Unfortunately, because of the increasing tendency to surgical treatment for virtually all fractures that could be managed nonoperatively, the ability to reduce, splint, and rehabilitate these fractures and the patients in whom they occur is becoming increasingly rare as the skill required atrophies by lack of use and training.

In North America and Europe, as well as parts of Asia, surgeons and patients have the luxury of opting for surgical or nonsurgical care. In many areas of the world, the so-called low- and middle-income countries (LMICs), the option for surgical management is frequently not available. Under these circumstances, nonsurgical management is the norm even for fractures that might better be treated by reduction and fixation. The ability to carry out good nonsurgical treatment in order to minimize patient disability is therefore imperative, and strategies to address fractures that would be routinely treated by reduction and fixation in the North American or European environment must be managed without fracture implants.

This chapter is being written so that there is a reference for the routine nonoperative management of fractures that do well with conservative treatment as well as to review the nonsurgical management of fractures that might ordinarily be treated by surgery were that option available. We have divided the section into upper and lower limbs addressing specifically the management of fractures of the scaphoid, distal radius, humeral shaft, and proximal humerus. All of these fractures are common, many of them can be treated in a very satisfactory fashion without surgery, and there is ample evidence to suggest that the outcome for nonsurgical management equals the results obtained by reduction and fixation.

In the lower limb, we focused on fractures of the ankle, many of which can be managed without surgery and added two special sections, one on the tibia and one on the femur.

The functional treatment of tibial shaft fractures results in a very high incidence of fracture union with excellent residual function. Its great advantage, of course, is the absence of infection and absence of complications related to fixation, such as nonunion, hardware failure, and anterior knee pain. The program for functional management of tibia fractures is rigorous, but if followed appropriately, excellent results can be anticipated without the expense or inconvenience of surgery.

The section on femoral shaft fractures will be of particular interest to those surgeons who do not have routine access to image intensification and intramedullary nailing. Treatment of femoral shaft fractures by means of traction is arduous for both the patient and the surgeon, but if done correctly, a very satisfactory outcome can be achieved in the great majority of patients.

We do not advocate nonsurgical treatment for those fractures that are best treated by surgery. What we do advocate is nonsurgical treatment for those fractures that do well when treated without surgery providing the treatment is appropriate and done correctly; as well, we hope to assist those surgeons and their patients who do not have access to routine surgical care.

I asked a number of individuals to write on these topics based on their interest and expertise. I think they did an excellent job in bringing together the disparate parts of nonsurgical management; their subjects are well referenced and amply illustrated.

In addition, the video that accompanies this text is very clear in detailing methods of reduction, splint application, and the application of traction.

I hope you enjoy this chapter.

REFERENCES

The level of evidence (LOE) is determined according to the criteria provided in the preface.

1. Arora R, Lutz M, Deml C, et al: A Prospective randomized trial comparing nonoperative treatment with volar locking plate fixation for displaced and unstable distal radial fractures in patients sixty-five years of age and older. *J Bone Joint Surg Am* 93:2146–2153, 2011. LOE II
2. Fjalestad T, Hole M, Hovden I, et al: Surgical treatment with an angular stable plate for complex displaced proximal humerus fractures in elderly patients: a randomized controlled trial. *J Orthop Trauma* 26(2):98–106, 2012.
3. Boons HW, Goosen JH, van Grinsven S, et al: Hemiarthroplasty for humeral four-part fractures for patients 65 years and older. *Clin Orthop Relat Res* 470:3483–3491, 2012. LOE II
4. McKee MD, Pelet S, Vicente MR: Operative versus nonoperative treatment of acute dislocations of the acromioclavicular joint: results of a multicenter randomized, prospective clinical trial. Canadian Orthopaedic Trauma Society—Proceedings of the Orthopaedic Trauma Association Annual Meeting, Minneapolis, MN, 2012. LOE II
5. Li X, Ma R, Bedi A, et al: Current concepts review—management of acromioclavicular joint injuries. *J Bone Joint Surg Am* 96:73–84, 2014. LOE II
6. Agren PH, Wretenberg P, Sayed-Noor AS: Operative versus nonoperative treatment of displaced intra-articular calcaneal fractures: a prospective, randomized, controlled multicenter trial. *J Bone Joint Surg Am* 95:1351–1357, 2013. LOE II
7. Sanders DW, Tieszer C, Corbett B: Operative versus nonoperative treatment of unstable lateral malleolar fractures: a randomized multicenter trial. *J Orthop Trauma* 26(3):129–134, 2012. LOE II

6B Basic Principles

DOUGLAS WARDLAW

In the developed countries of the Western world, there is sadly a real risk that the skills required for the conservative management of fractures and fracture bracing will be lost. This is partly attributable to the increasing costs of inpatient care, so that in many instances, conservative management costs money, partly because it is true for most surgeons that internal fixation is fun and partly because many aspects of conservative management of fractures are delegated very often to persons of inappropriate experience or expertise. The purpose of this chapter is to attempt to redress the balance and to provide a sound theoretical and practical basis for the closed treatment of fractures.

The resources available in different hospitals throughout the world vary enormously, both in the availability of inpatient hospital facilities and medical and paramedical personnel and in the equipment for fracture treatment available to them. It should never be forgotten that the surgeon in charge of the patient's care is responsible for his or her total management and for the supervision of medical and paramedical staff to whom he or she delegates.

The three principles of fracture treatment are:

1. Reduction
2. Maintenance of reduction throughout the treatment period
3. Promotion of functional recovery

Reduction involves restoring the position of the fractured fragments as close to normal anatomy as possible. It is essential to restore normal alignment, length, rotation, and lateral shift as far as possible. The best possible position of the fracture should be obtained at the first manipulation[1,2] and the method of maintenance of reduction chosen to ensure that reduction will be maintained throughout the treatment period. Suitable exercises should be commenced as early as possible and increased in a graded fashion as healing takes place to promote the optimum recovery of function in the shortest possible time.[3] In a nutshell, the object of treatment is to restore the injured part to normal function as soon as possible with the best cosmetic result.

The management of acute fracture, the biology of fracture healing, and the biomechanical and physiologic management of the injury have to be understood and considered together. A fracture is not an isolated injury and cannot occur without concomitant soft tissue injury of varying degrees. The mechanism of injury and the degree of force applied to cause the injury are roughly proportional to the severity of the injury. In general, the more severe the injury, the greater the damage to soft tissue and bone, the greater the fracture hematoma, and the greater the damage to the blood supply. When the fracture occurs, a fracture hematoma is formed with swelling of the limb. The degree of swelling is related to the severity of the fracture and amount of soft tissue injury, and this will in turn relate to the severity of displacement of the fracture. In open fractures, the injury is compounded by loss of the blood of the hematoma as well as the risk of infection. There is splinting of the damaged bone or joint with muscle spasm. After definitive treatment is carried out, there is rapid development of inactivation atrophy of muscles and absorption of the fracture hematoma; to the naked eye, gross muscle wasting takes place. At 2 to 3 weeks, the fracture hematoma has largely resolved. All of the tissues involved in the fracture hematoma become involved in the concomitant granulation tissue and scar formation. The hematoma in relation to the fracture subsequently forms callus, and as early as 3 weeks, flecks of calcification may be seen on radiographs. At this stage, the fracture is "sticky." The degree of inherent stability in a fracture varies. Fractures through cancellous bone and long oblique fractures of the diaphysis of long bones have a fairly high degree of stability at this stage. Short oblique or transverse fractures of the diaphysis may allow a degree of angulatory displacement to occur with significant shortening or overriding taking place. There will be some stability to axial loading, with reduced and "hitched" transverse fractures being very stable to axial loading. As healing progresses stability, of course, increases.

The treatment of a fracture should not be considered in isolation. Rather, fracture treatment should be properly planned so that the full program of fracture management should be considered from the start along with concomitant injuries and thought through to the full rehabilitation of the patient. With this in mind, the ideal combinations of treatment may be undertaken. For instance, some fractures might be best dealt with by internal fixation, such as those adjacent to or involving joints, but others are treated nonoperatively. Any combination of nonoperative treatment, external fixation, or internal fixation may be used. Multiple injuries may be treated nonoperatively with minimal complications, and fracture bracing enhances the management of these injuries during the recovery phase.[4-7]

FRACTURE REDUCTION AND MAINTENANCE OF REDUCTION

I have studiously avoided the word "immobilization" for the conservative management of fractures. Immobilization in the real sense of the word does not take place. The only way one can truly immobilize a fracture is by rigid internal fixation. A fracture within a cast is subjected to the action of muscles attached to the fractured bone and whose actions pass across the fracture. They subject the fracture to recurrent stresses and movement. Provided only axial loading takes place and that angulatory rotational and shear stresses are minimized, the fracture will usually progress to union.[7,8]

There are four recognized methods of reducing and maintaining reduction of fractures:

1. Manipulative reduction and plaster
2. Manipulative reduction and continuous traction
3. Manipulative reduction and external fixation
4. Operative reduction and internal fixation

Under certain circumstances, operative reduction may be used with plaster, traction, or external fixation to maintain reduction.

In general, closed reduction may be used for closed fractures, and operative reduction may be used for open fractures. The reason is that the soft tissue injury in compound fractures requires exploration by wound excision, often an extension to the main wound, to properly explore and excise the wound, and it seems logical in doing so to obtain an anatomic reduction of the fracture if possible. Perhaps the most common situation when this form of management could be used is in a tibial fracture. If the fracture is transverse or stable on reduction, the wound may be closed and plaster immobilization used. If, however, the fracture is grossly unstable, external fixation may be applied, anatomic reduction obtained, and then the wound closed. As with many tibial fractures, it may be found that the wound cannot be closed, and secondary closure or skin grafting may be necessary.

It must always be remembered that a limb is a functioning unit. The skeleton is the framework on which that function is based, and it depends on mobile joints, the activity of muscles and nerves, and an adequate blood supply. The object of fracture treatment is to restore the skeletal framework to as near normal as is possible after injury, thereby restoring a stable anatomic base on which the limb may function. Fracture treatment should be thought of therefore in three phases: phase 1, primary treatment; phase 2, definitive treatment; and phase 3, rehabilitation.

Phase 1 involves the initial treatment of reduction and fixation with plaster, traction, external fixation, or internal fixation followed by a period of rest and elevation to allow swelling and pain to subside. As far as possible within the limitations of treatment, early movement is encouraged to prevent the inevitable muscle wasting that occurs in the fractured limb and to minimize adhesion formation in relation to the area of the trauma and adjacent joints. This also promotes recovery of the blood supply and venous and lymphatic return by the action of the muscle pump.

Phase 2 commences with the application of a definitive cast or fracture brace after primary treatment by traction, cast, external fixation, or internal fixation. This should be applied in most cases between 10 days to 4 weeks to allow rehabilitation and more active use of the injured part, thus promoting recovery of function of muscle and nonimmobilized joints. Fracture bracing as far as possible does not immobilize joints and therefore allows a more complete recovery of muscle and joint function during this stage in recovery.

Phase 3, the phase of rehabilitation, commences with active mobilization after the application of a fracture brace and external or internal fixation of fractures. However, in patients treated by prolonged immobilization in a plaster cast or continuous traction until fracture union occurs, rehabilitation then commences. Very often a fairly long period of physiotherapy and exercise is needed to mobilize very stiff joints and build up wasted muscles and osteoporotic bones.

MANIPULATIVE REDUCTION

A famous orthopaedic surgeon once described manipulative reduction as "a little bit of this, and a little bit of that." This, to say the least, is a gross oversimplification. It is essential to understand the pathologic anatomy of the fracture. For a fracture to become displaced, it requires either comminution of bone or periosteal damage to occur (or both of these things). The force required to reduce the fracture and the direction in which the force is to be applied depend on many factors. The simplest fractures to reduce are often comminuted fractures, but because of the nature of the fracture, they are inherently unstable. Oblique fractures of long bones are caused by a rotational force transmitted along the axis of the limb, and they often result in the spiking of the soft tissues by the sharp ends of the fragments. This inevitably leads to muscle interposition, and it is often impossible to bring about disimpaction completely. Transverse fractures occur because of a force applied at right angles to the diaphysis and are potentially cheapness have not been bettered by any of the modern bandages. The properties of plaster of Paris were known in ancient Egypt, India, and Arabia, where it was first used for building. The *Oxford English Dictionary* states that the first reference to the term *plaster of Paris* was in a poem written in 1462 and that the name is derived from the material first prepared from the gypsums of Montmartre, Paris. During the early part of the 1800s throughout Europe and North America, the use of plaster of Paris became widespread. In 1816, it was being applied by Hubenthal mixed with ground-up blotting paper, and in 1828, Kayel and Kluge used it by pouring it around a limb placed in a box. In Europe in 1852, Matthysen used bandages smeared with plaster of Paris, and in 1894, Holst-Korsch was still using plaster directly applied to the skin, and in the United States, Samuel St. John applied a layer of cotton wool next to the skin and recommended splitting the cast in acute fractures.[15,16]

Management of Acute Fractures

The modern synthetic materials have no place in the management of acute fractures, and plaster of Paris remains the material of choice. The type of cast to be applied and the method of application depend on the severity of injury. A layer of cotton wool or synthetic padding that comes in rolled bandages of 4- or 6-in widths should be first applied to the limb below each cast. An injury caused by minimal trauma such as an undisplaced transverse fracture of the tibia with a small amount of swelling associated with it can have a snug cast applied early on. One layer of padding with at least two layers around the malleoli, heel, and foot may be used and a toe-to-groin cast applied with the knee in 10 to 20 degrees of flexion and the foot in a plantigrade position. On the other hand, a very severe injury or a crush injury with a lot of soft tissue damage and reactionary swelling should be treated in a cast with at least three layers of wool padding, and in addition, if there is a high degree of anxiety regarding the circulation, the cast should be split instantly from top to bottom, including the wool padding so that the skin is visible. This is especially important in compound fractures in which the wool may become blood soaked. When the blood dries, the wool then becomes rigid and may produce a tourniquet effect. Alternatively, a plaster slab can be used. This is made of eight to 12 layers of plaster depending on the size of the patient and wide enough to pass around the limb approximately half to two-thirds circumference. It is laid over the wool padding and bandaged in position using usually a fine mesh bandage. Again, in compound fractures, it may be necessary to cut it longitudinally anteriorly from top to bottom. Always remember it is more important to apply extra padding over bony prominences such as the malleoli, heel, and foot and the head and neck of the fibula than around the muscular parts of the limb.

For the application of a definitive cast, only stockinette or one layer of wool padding may be used with appropriate padding over bony prominences. The usual casting positions are as shown in Figure 6B-2.

The definitive stages of applying a below-knee cast are shown in Figure 6B-3. Clearly, the limb must be supported in whatever way is necessary to maintain the position of the fracture during application of the cast. For a definitive cast, a layer of stockinette is first applied and will hold any necessary dressings in position (Fig. 6B-3, *A*). Wool is then applied from the metatarsophalangeal joints of the toes to the head of fibula, with an extra layer of wool applied around the malleoli, heel, and foot The casting material is then applied starting at the narrowest point in the limb to avoid drift of the bandage, and it is rolled firmly onto the contours of the limb to ensure snug contact and without applying undue pressure (Fig. 6B-3, *B*). It is rolled on in such a way counting the layers applied so that even layers of bandage are applied from the top of the cast to the bottom of the cast. For the fiberglass materials, usually two lengths of 10- or 15-mm bandage are enough to complete a cast. If plaster of Paris is used, which is the cheapest material per bandage, probably four to six bandages will be required for the average below-knee cast. It is important after application of each bandage to work the resin or the plaster of Paris through the bandage by smoothing it all the way up and down with the flat of the hand. This must be done when the material is still soft before curing or hardening of the material takes place.

Before the last layer of bandage is put on, the stockinette is folded back to make a nice padded, rounded edge to the bandage, and in doing so, the casting material can be rolled back to the appropriate level. The bottom end of the cast should be obliquely shaped, covering the metatarsal heads and the sole of the foot and allowing free movement of all the toes. The upper end of the cast should finish just below the knee, allowing free knee movement (Fig. 6B-3, *C*). It is essential at all stages of the process to hold the relative positions of the foot and leg in a plantigrade position, which is the position of function for walking. If the exact position is not maintained throughout the process and at some point the position of the ankle has to be changed, then folds or tucks will appear in the wool or the bandage itself, which will create high-pressure areas within the cast and may well cause cast sores. In plaster of Paris casts, it is important to remember that the strength of the cast is in the crystal lattice, which builds up during the hardening process. If any molding or changing of position of the cast is carried out while this is happening, then this will not allow a strong crystal lattice to build up, and a weakened cast will result.

Application of Three-Point Loading Techniques

In certain fractures such as bimalleolar or lateral malleolar ankle fractures with lateral talar shift, and Colles fractures, a three-point loading technique may be used to maintain fracture position.[9,16] Both of these fractures are liable to redisplacement as the swelling goes down and the cast becomes loose and can be avoided by three-point loading. To do this, one applies a full cast quickly with the help of a colleague. While the plaster is still in the creamy state, using the flat of one's hand and avoiding the application of local pressure over bony prominence, three-point loading may be applied to the upper and midpoints of the cast and over either the lower end of radius[16] or lateral malleolar areas (Fig. 6B-4). The loading built into the cast ensures that as the swelling subsides, sufficient loading remains to maintain the fracture position. This has been proven to be a viable technique in the case of Colles fractures while at the same time leaving the wrist free to move.[17]

Postreduction Management of Acute Fractures

Elevation and early mobilization are of utmost importance. Elevation is done to reduce the possibility of further swelling

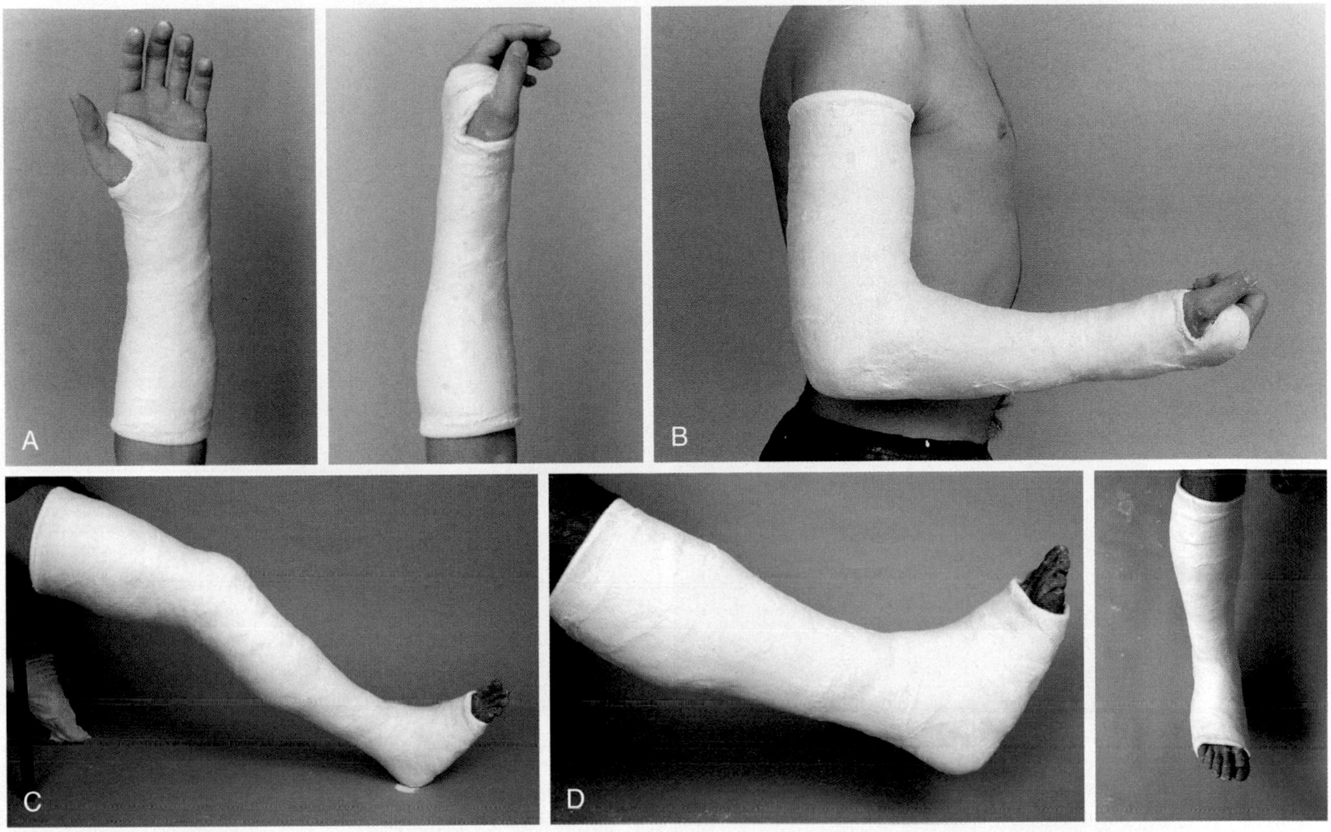

Figure 6B-2. A, Forearm cast for treatment of injuries or fractures to the forearm and wrist. It extends from the metacarpal heads to below the elbow. The plaster must not reach beyond the distal palmar crease (two views). **B,** Long arm cast for immobilization of the elbow and treatment of fractures around the elbow and of the forearm. The elbow is at 90 degrees, the wrist is in slight dorsiflexion, and the forearm is in the appropriate position of pronation/supination (one view). **C,** Long leg cast for treatment of fractures and injuries around the knee and fractures of the tibia and ankle. The knee is in 10 to 15 degrees of flexion with the foot plantigrade, that is, sole of foot at 90 degrees to the front of leg (one view). **D,** Below-knee cast for treatment of injuries of the ankle and foot. On the sole, the plaster must go beyond the metatarsal heads, and for a walking cast, the foot must be plantigrade (two views).

and enhance the dissipation of swelling already present. Early active movements must be encouraged not only in the injured limb itself but also the patient as a whole. He or she must be reassured that early movement is not harmful and is instead beneficial to the healing processes and in doing so helps reduce swelling and prevent joint stiffness.

In all patients, after application of a cast, it is essential in the first 24 hours to make the necessary checks of the circulation. For minor fractures, the patient should be advised to see a doctor or nurse the morning after or return to the emergency department (ED) to have the circulation and the cast checked. It is customary in most EDs for patients to be given instructions with them (Fig. 6B-5). These are sometimes attached to the cast in a position in which they can read them; these instructions give general advice regarding the cast. When patients are kept in the hospital for elevation and there is a genuine worry regarding circulation, then the circulation should be checked as often as is necessary for 24 to 48 hours. Adequate levels of analgesia should be given to control pain and in doing so will encourage activity.

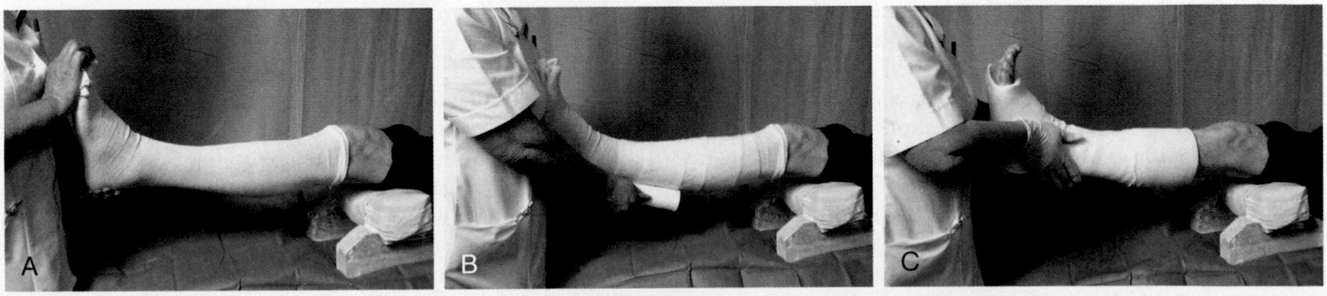

Figure 6B-3. A, Leg with stockinette applied. Wool is then applied around the head of fibula to protect the popliteal nerve and around the malleoli, heel, and foot as far as the metatarsal heads. **B,** Material is rolled on starting at the narrowest part of the limb. **C,** A finishing layer with stockinette folded back at the appropriate level to cover rough edges.

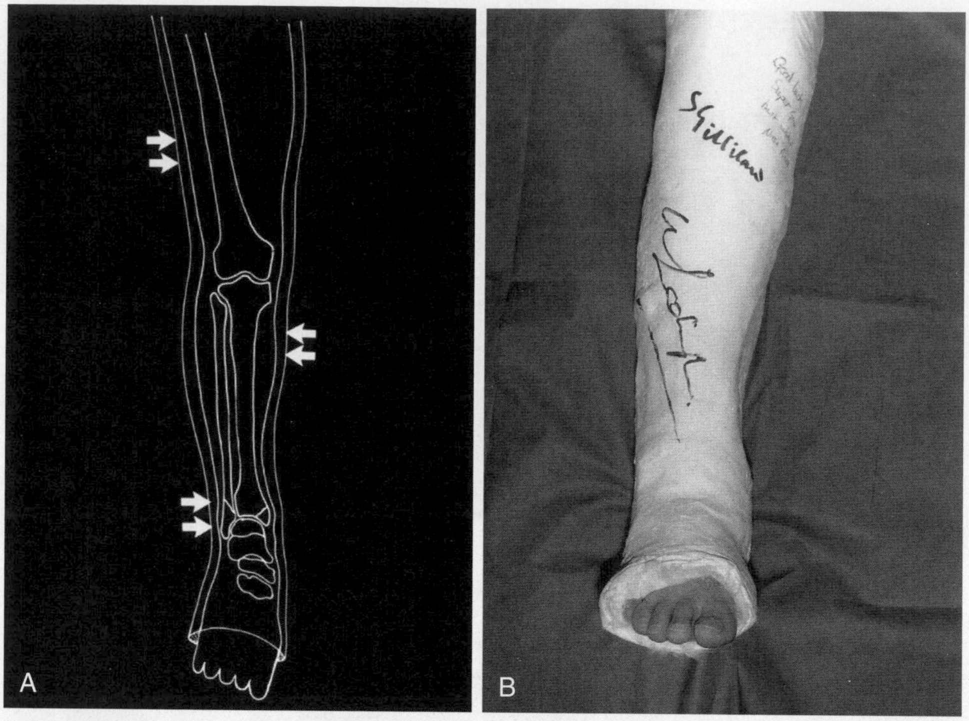

Figure 6B-4. **A,** Diagrammatic presentation of three-point loading in a long leg cast. **B,** Long leg cast with built-in loading. This is applied with appropriate layers of plaster wool applied the whole length of the cast from the toes to the groin. Plaster is then applied from the groin to two-thirds of the way down the leg and allowed to harden. More plaster is then applied overlapping the hardened cast at the join from the knee to the toes. As this portion of the cast hardens, three-point loading is applied using the flat of the hand at the mid or upper calf level and flat of the other hand at the ankle level. It is possible to apply loading with the foot held in a plantigrade position, remembering to avoid high pressure over the bony prominence of the lateral malleolus.

Wedging of Casts

Fracture angulation may be corrected by wedging the cast. The timing of wedging is important; in general, it is better to obtain the optimum fracture position as early as possible. However, wedging of unstable fractures may simply cause displacement and require remanipulation. On the other hand, if one waits until the fracture hematoma has clotted and early organization has taken place at 2 to 3 weeks, then significant displacement is unlikely to occur. Alternatively, the angulation may be corrected during the application of a definitive cast.

Accurate wedging is carried out by dividing the cast two-thirds of its circumference on the concave or inner angle of the fracture and then opening up the cast.[18] This is done by lining up a piece of paper or a T-square with the distal fragment and keeping the piece of paper parallel with it, mark a point on the convex side of the cast and the concave side of the cast at the fracture level. The piece of paper is reversed, aligned with the proximal fragment and the mark on the cast on the concavity of the fracture and another mark made on the cast outline opposite. Two points will result on the cast outline on the convex side of the fracture. A measurement of this is the amount by which the cast should be opened (Fig. 6B-6). It is the author's experience that if these measurements are taken, then very accurate correction of the angulation takes place (see Fig. 6B-6). The cast should be finished by filling the wedge with a piece of plaster or material cut to the size of the wedge and laid into the space filling it completely. The standard method of wedging is to open the wedge, cut a block of wood of appropriate size, and insert it into the wedge to hold it open while a check radiograph is taken. If a block of wood is present, this should be removed, and the cast finished off as discussed. Finally, one or two plaster bandages are wrapped around this to complete the cast. If this procedure is used, then a very strong and durable cast is produced.

If angulation is present in both AP and lateral planes, then the position of the wedge "hinge" should be rotated so that it lies opposite the true convexity of the fracture angle. The amount to which the wedge should be open is then calculated from the AP and lateral radiographs as described earlier and the opening calculated according to the degree of rotation.

Walking Casts

Gait analysis of walking casts has demonstrated that a normal gait pattern is present in patients with below-knee walking casts with the foot in a plantigrade position, that is, with the flat surface of the foot or cast at 90 degrees to the front of the leg. The foot in any other position will lead to an abnormal gait pattern. Therefore, for the patient to recover a normal walking pattern after injury, it is essential that a walking cast has the foot applied in a plantigrade position. There are many appliances available on the market; many of them produce an abnormal gait pattern because they are too thick and elevate the fractured limb higher than the patient's normal shoe, or they are simply unnatural. A simple walking cast shoe such as the Aberdeen boot is ideal (Fig. 6B-7). The action of walking in a below-knee cast tends to cause breakdown of the heel and sole of the cast because these areas are subjected to recurrent impact forces and are areas of high stress. In addition, because the heel and sole are on the convexity of the ankle, the cast is thinner in this area. The sole and heel of the cast may therefore

Do ....

- ✓ Move joints not held in your cast as much as possible. This will stop them becoming stiff.
- ✓ Use your limb for light activities (e.g., partial or touch weight bearing for lower limb and doing up buttons, eating etc for upper limb)
- ✓ Raise your limb when resting.
- ✓ Use a waterproof "protector" for bathing.
- ✓ Telephone the Accident & Emergency Department if you have any of the following:
  - your cast feels too loose or too tight
  - your fingers become cold, numb or bluish in color for more than 30 to 60 minutes
  - you have pins and needles in your fingers
  - you have an increase in pain
  - you drop any object inside your cast
  - your cast softens, cracks, or splits

Don't ....

- x Get your cast wet
- x Use plastic bags or bin liners when bathing or showering
- x Insert any objects such as knitting needles or pencils under your cast

Figure 6B-5. Patients' plaster instructions (general).

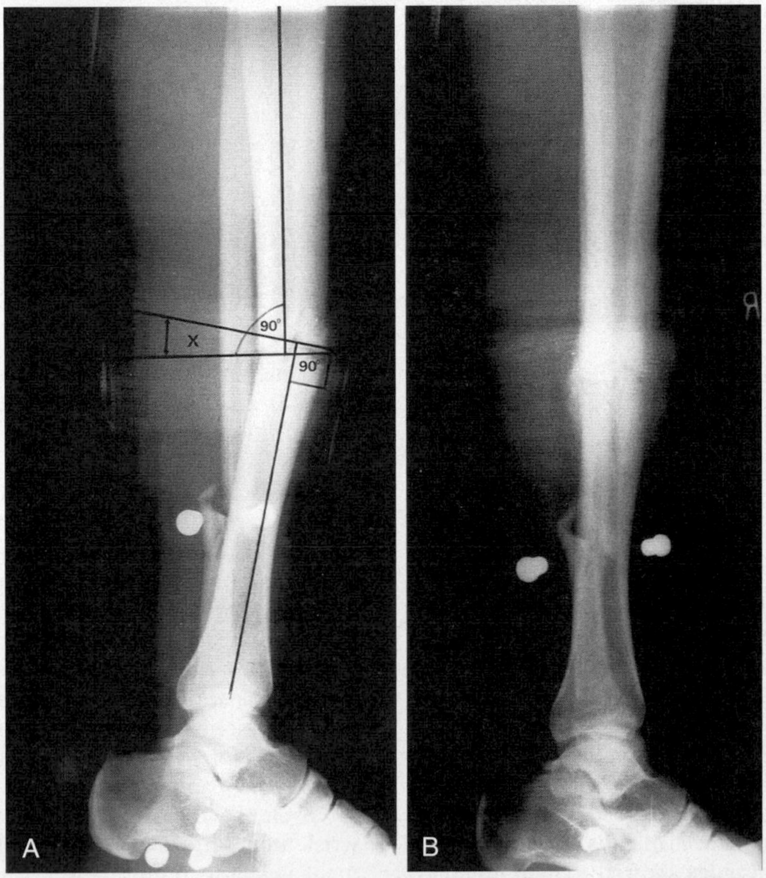

Figure 6B-6. Wedging of a cast by calculation from the radiograph (**A**) and the correction obtained (**B**).

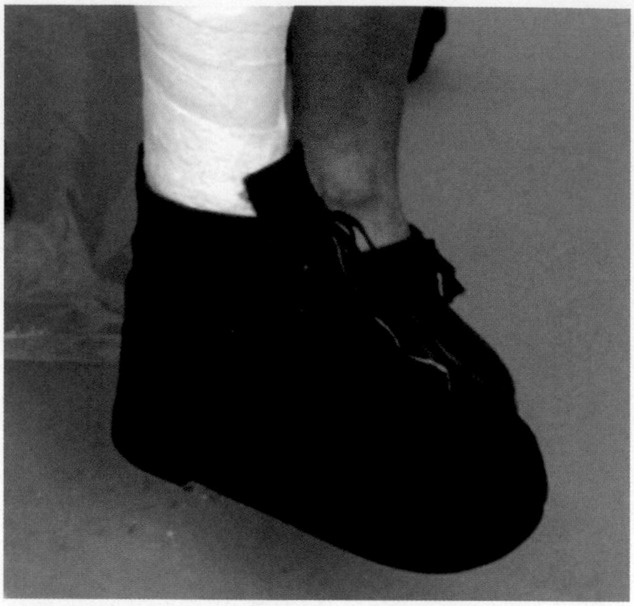

Figure 6B-7. Aberdeen boot. Water-resistant material in an upper with a thin sole of nonslip material.

be strengthened with a slab of an appropriate casting material, and this can also be extended to above the ankle, which is also sometimes an area of cast breakdown. In addition, one-fourth Plastazote is a useful buffer to apply over the area of the sole and heel to help absorb the impact of walking.

KEY REFERENCES

The level of evidence (LOE) is determined according to the criteria provided in the preface.

1. Wardlaw D: Cast bracing in practice: a two year study in Aberdeen. *Injury* 12(3):213–218, 1980b. LOE III
5. Connolly JF, King P: Closed reduction and early cast brace ambulation in the treatment of femoral fractures. Part I: an in vivo quantitative analysis of immobilization in skeletal traction and a cast-brace. *J Bone Joint Surg Am* 55:1559–1580, 1973. LOE II
6. Connolly JF, Dehne E, Lafollette B: Closed reduction and early cast-brace ambulation in the treatment of femoral fractures. Part II: results in 143 fractures. *J Bone Joint Surg Am* 55:1581–1599, 1973. LOE II
7. Wardlaw D: *A clinical and biomechanical study of cast brace treatment of fractures of the femoral shaft*, Master of Surgery Thesis, 1980a, University of Edinburgh. LOE II
8. Wardlaw D, McLauchlan J, Pratt DJ, et al: A biomechanical study of cast brace treatment of femoral shaft fractures. *J Bone Joint Surg Br* 63:7–11, 1981. LOE III

The complete References list is available online at https://expertconsult.inkling.com.

6C Scaphoid Fractures

IAIN STEVENSON • JAMES P. WADDELL

The following video is included with this chapter and may be viewed at https://expertconsult.inkling.com:
6C-1. Scaphoid cast.

INCIDENCE AND DEMOGRAPHICS

Scaphoid fractures are the most common bone of the carpus to be fractured and occur most frequently in young men (85%) between the ages of 18 and 35. Wolf's study used a public database of acute injuries within the United States and found that there is a male preponderance with 66.4% versus 33.6% females.[1] Hove's series showed 225 of 330 total scaphoid fractures to have occurred in males, which is a predominance of 82%.[2] Van Tassel and colleagues showed a male predominance of 66.4% but nearly one-third of scaphoid injuries occurred in girls and women.[3] This higher incidence in females, which was found in comparison to previous studies, was postulated to be perhaps caused by an increase in participation in organized sports. The typical mechanism of injury is a fall on outstretched hand (FOOSH) with experimental studies showing extreme dorsiflexion (greater than 95 degrees) coupled with compressive force to the radial side of the wrist can result in fracture of the scaphoid. Also some researchers believe a fall backward with the hand directed anteriorly is most likely to result in extreme dorsiflexion of the wrist.[4] These falls of relatively low energy make up the majority of scaphoid fracture mechanisms.

Other mechanisms of injury would include any high-energy trauma involving the wrist, and more rarely, a direct blow to the scaphoid can also result in fracture. Historically, this was described as a "crank-handle kickback," which because of the high forces involved, often resulted in displaced oblique or unstable scaphoid fractures.

Given the important role of the scaphoids in hand and wrist function, prompt diagnosis and appropriate management is key in minimizing potential complications, such as nonunion, avascular necrosis, and subsequent osteoarthritis with or without development of a scaphoid nonunion advanced collapse (SNAC) and dorsiflexed intercalated segment instability (DISI) or volar intercalated segment instability (VISI) deformities. Typically the mechanism of injury and patient type will lead the clinician to have a high index of suspicion.

CLINICAL EXAMINATION

Thereafter, a thorough clinical examination should involve examination of the upper limb including elbow, palpation of the bony landmarks around the wrist and hand paying particular attention to tenderness elicited on palpation of the anatomic snuffbox. The boundaries of the anatomic snuffbox are posteriorly the tendon of extensor pollicis longus and anteriorly the tendons of extensor pollicis brevis and abductor pollicis longus.

The proximal border is the styloid process of the distal radius and the distal border by the apex of the tendons giving the anatomic snuffbox an isosceles-triangle shape. Snuffbox tenderness is frequently taught as a clear sign of scaphoid fracture, but although it has a high sensitivity, it has been shown to have a relatively low specificity in diagnosing scaphoid fractures.[5-7]

General examination may reveal bruising, or an effusion and tenderness on palpation of the scaphoid tubercle is highly suggestive of scaphoid fracture. Radial deviation of the wrist alters the scaphoid position so that the tubercle becomes prominent on the radial side of the volar wrist crease allowing for palpation.[8]

Other clinical tests include the scaphoid compression test, which Chen found to have great sensitivity and specificity in diagnosis of scaphoid fracture.[9] Studies performed in other institutions have shown poorer specificity.[10,11]

The scaphoid compression test is performed by holding the thumb of the affected wrist in one hand while stabilizing the forearm with the other hand. A compressive force is applied with pain providing a positive result.[9]

Forced deviation maneuvers of the wrist should probably be avoided as they will more than likely result in pain in the acute setting while yielding little clinical information.

RADIOLOGIC EXAMINATION

After a thorough careful examination, plain radiographs should be performed. In most institutions, this will include four views of the wrist. These should be (1) a posterior-anterior view with the wrist in ulnar deviation, (2) a true lateral, (3) a semipronated oblique, and (4) a scaphoid view with the wrist pronated in ulnar deviation with the x-ray beam 25 degrees off vertical directed cephalad.

Leslie and Dickson reported that, in a series of 222 scaphoid fractures, 98% were visible on radiograph film at first examination. The remaining 2% became visible after 2 weeks.[12] Other authors reported less optimistic figures—as low as 84% visible on first examination.[13,14]

The key is to get one clear view profiling the trabeculae of the scaphoid, which can then be thoroughly examined. On older standard radiographs, some surgeons advocated the use of a magnifying glass to examine the trabeculae, but most images can be now be manipulated digitally. The scaphoid fat strip (SFS) is a radiolucent stripe adjacent to the radial side of the scaphoid and can be displaced in the presence of a fracture.[15-17] Radial convexity or obliquity of the SFS are considered pathognomonic of a fracture similar to the posterior fat pad sign of the elbow.

Clenched-fist views can be used if suspicion of a scapholunate injury exists. The intrascaphoid angle is the intersection of two lines drawn perpendicular to the diameters of the proximal and distal poles. Amadio and colleagues used a trispiral computed tomography (CT) scan and two techniques to delineate abnormal values of more than 45 degrees.[18] Bain and coworkers described that the height-to-length ratio of the scaphoid was the most reproducible way of measuring the humpback deformity that could be used to indicate collapse. The height-to-length ratio should average less than 0.65. A greater ratio indicates collapse of the scaphoid.[19]

Four bony parameters that suggest displacement are translation, gap, angulation, and rotation. Conventionally, a fracture is considered displaced if the gap is 1 mm or more.[20]

On occasion, in the acute phase, up to 25% of scaphoid fractures can be radiographically occult. Patients with clinical mechanisms of injury and clinical examination findings suggestive of scaphoid fracture are normally placed in cast immobilization and brought back for either repeat radiographs or further, more specialized imaging. At 2 weeks, when repeat radiographs are performed, radiographs may show bone resorption at the fracture sight making the nondisplaced fracture more visible. If the fracture shows signs of having displaced, then it declares itself as unstable and potentially suitable for operative fixation.

An international survey of hospital practices revealed marked inconsistency in acute scaphoid imaging protocols. The authors believed this is probably caused by various factors but also attributed it to a deficiency in scientific evidence on the matter.[21] A recent meta-analysis by Zhong-Gang and colleagues investigated imaging modalities used in diagnosing scaphoid fractures. A systematic review and meta-analysis was performed that assessed and compared the available imaging modalities. These included bone scintigraphy, magnetic resonance imaging (MRI), and CT. They found that bone scintigraphy and MRI have equal sensitivity and high diagnostic value for excluding scaphoid fractures; however, MRI is more specific and better for confirming scaphoid fracture.[22]

CLASSIFICATION AND FRACTURE INCIDENCE

In general, the fracture of the waist is the most common of scaphoid fractures (70%) with distal pole fractures at 10% to 20%, proximal pole fractures at 5%, and tubercle fractures at 5%.[23] Bindra studied cadaveric scaphoid with CT scanning and found that the bone is most dense at the proximal pole, where the trabeculae are the thickest and are more tightly packed, whereas the trabeculae in the waist are thinnest and sparsely distributed.[24]

Classification systems should be reproducible, aid in decision making regarding treatment, and give information on prognosis. The Herbert classification has been shown to have good interobserver reliability and reproducibility as well as helping to determine treatment.[25,26] The classification system attempts to define stable and unstable fractures, with Herbert type A being an acute stable fracture and Herbert type B being an unstable fracture.

Stable fractures include fractures of the tubercle and incomplete fractures of the waist. These fractures can potentially be

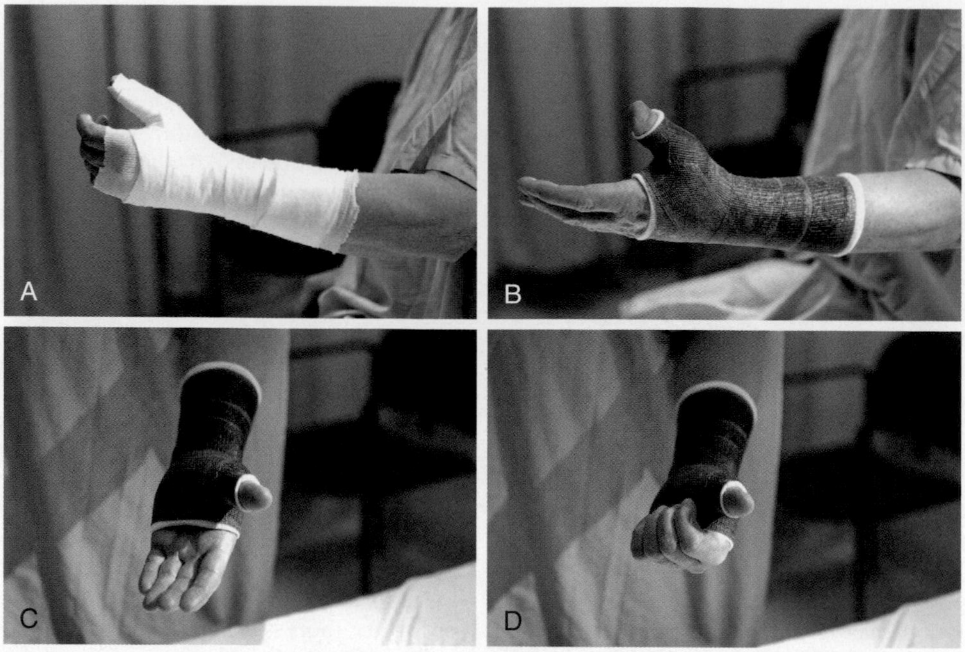

Figure 6C-1. **A,** Stockinette and cast paper for scaphoid cast. Notice that the metacarpals are free and the thumb is wrapped up to the interphalangeal (IP) joint. **B,** Lateral view showing the finished cast. **C,** The IP joint of the thumb is free; metacarpal-phalangeal joints of the fingers are free. **D,** Note full finger flexion.

treated conservatively, which will be discussed further in the following section; the unstable fractures normally require surgical intervention.

TREATMENT OPTIONS

Operation versus Conservative Treatment

Displaced fractures of the scaphoid have a four times higher risk than undisplaced fractures when treated in a cast, and patients should be made aware of this. Nonunion is more likely if the patient is treated in a cast. Factors contributing to nonunion include displacement greater than 1 mm, delay in diagnosis and immobilization greater than 4 weeks, location at the waist or proximal pole, and a history of smoking.[27]

Minimally Displaced and Undisplaced

Evidence suggests that percutaneous fixation may result in faster union rates by approximately 5 weeks and an earlier return to work and sport by approximately 7 weeks over cast treatment.[28] This difference is not seen when comparing casting with open reduction and internal fixation (ORIF). Cast treatment has a slightly higher nonunion rate than ORIF, which has to be balanced against an approximate 30% minor complication rate.

Manual workers require significantly longer times off work than nonmanual workers regardless of the treatment type, although one study showed that they did return to work sooner after ORIF than after cast.[29] The majority of these injuries can be managed in a cast with good results with operative treatment reserved for delayed presentation greater than 4 weeks, most manual workers, and high-level athletes.[30]

CAST TREATMENT

Before radiographs were invented, fracture of the scaphoid was poorly understood and difficult to manage. In the early 1900s, treatment consisted of brief splintage followed by massage and early mobilization. The poor results of this technique led to development of different types of immobilization. From 1925 to 1941, Bohler used a simple back slab leaving the thumb free, and then from 1942, included the thumb. By 1954, he had treated 734 fractures, and of the 580 available for review, only 4% failed to unite.[31]

This drastic increase in union and decrease in morbidity, as well as the observation by Bohler and others that nonunion is more common when treatment is delayed, led to many favoring conservative management of scaphoid fractures.

The observation of very low nonunion rates following immobilization alone has not been universal and led to a variety of cast types being used by different surgeons. Soto-Hall found in cadaveric studies that any movement of the interphalangeal joint of the thumb led to a definite change in fracture fragment position. He felt this could be eliminated by immobilization of the thumb up to the base of the thumb nail and reported 95% union rates using this method[32] (Fig. 6C-1).

It is difficult to establish exactly when inclusion of the thumb became known as a "scaphoid cast" and the belief that the thumb should be immobilized is yet to be definitely shown by a study. Given the relatively low rate of nonunion in scaphoid fractures, a study demonstrating significantly increased union rates would have to have large numbers and be rigorously designed.

In their study, Clay and colleagues found union rates to be roughly equivalent when comparing thumb immobilization with a Colles cast and concluded that for "fresh, undisplaced fractures of the waist of the scaphoid, the simpler Colles cast would appear to be equally as effective."[33]

Despite this, it remains a controversial matter, and many surgeons tend to err on the side of caution in immobilizing the thumb and using below-elbow casts, as convincing evidence of the benefit of above-elbow cast has not been shown.

A recent meta-analysis by Alshryda and colleagues examined this topic. They found that only one trial compared Colles cast versus scaphoid cast. The trial recruited 291 patients and showed no significant difference between the two groups.[34]

Two studies compared above-elbow versus below-elbow casts and had insufficient data for meta-analysis. There was no statistical difference in the union rate, complication rate, or time to union.[35,36]

One study investigated the position of the wrist in a Colles cast and found that there was not a significant difference in union rate. They found there were more complications and less grip strength in the flexed wrist group but that these differences do not reach statistical significance.[37]

Only one study was identified that examined the use of adjunct ultrasound treatment with standard scaphoid cast and found no difference in union rate but that the ultrasound group had a significantly shorter time to union by approximately 19 days.[38]

A recent study by Hannemann and coworkers, investigating the use of pulsed electric magnetic fields in the treatment of scaphoid fractures, showed no benefit in their use with similar union rates and times to union in the control group.[39]

CONCLUSION

The authors advocate nonsurgical treatment for nondisplaced fractures of the scaphoid. Minimally displaced transverse fractures of the waist of the scaphoid may be treated closed or with reduction and fixation. This should be decided on an individual basis with the patient in terms of the patient's expectations, tolerance for surgery and its complications, and functional demands of the patient's wrist. Displaced scaphoid fractures, scaphoid fractures associated with subluxations, and/or dislocations of other carpal bones and delayed presentations of scaphoid fractures longer than 4 weeks should, as a general rule, be treated surgically.

KEY REFERENCES

The level of evidence (LOE) is determined according to the criteria provided in the preface.

5. Rhemrev SJ, Ootes D, Beeres FJ, et al: Current methods of diagnosis and treatment of scaphoid fractures. *Int J Emerg Med* 4(1):4, 2011. LOE III
10. Waeckerle JF: A prospective study identifying the sensitivity of radiographic findings and the efficacy of clinical findings in carpal navicular fractures. *Ann Emerg Med* 16(7):21–25, 1987. LOE II
22. Zhong-Gang Y, Jian-Bing Z, Shi-Lian K, et al: Diagnosing suspected scaphoid fractures: a systematic review and meta-analysis. *Clin Orthop Relat Res* 468:723–734, 2010. LOE III
26. Herbert TJ, Fisher WE: Management of the fractured scaphoid using a new bone screw. *J Bone Joint Surg Br* 66:114–123, 1984. LOE IV
27. Haisman JM, Rohde RS, Weiland AJ, et al: Acute fractures of the scaphoid. *J Bone Joint Surg Am* 88:2750–2758, 2006. LOE III
28. McQueen MM, Gelbke MK, Wakefield A, et al: Percutaneous screw fixation versus conservative treatment for fractures of the waist of the scaphoid: a prospective randomised study. *J Bone Joint Surg Br* 90:66–71, 2008. LOE II
30. Modi CS, Nancoo T, Powers D, et al: Operative versus nonoperative treatment of acute undisplaced and minimally displaced scaphoid waist fractures—a systematic review. *Injury* 40(3):268–273, 2009. LOE III
36. Alho A, Kankaanpaa U: Management of fractured scaphoid bone. A prospective study of 100 fractures. *Acta Orthop Scand* 46(5):737–743, 1975. LOE IV

The complete References list is available online at https://expertconsult.inkling.com.

6D Distal Radius Fractures

IAIN STEVENSON • JAMES P. WADDELL

The following video is included with this chapter and may be viewed at https://expertconsult.inkling.com:
6D-1. Distal radius cast.

DEMOGRAPHICS

Distal radius fractures are one of the most common fractures with more than 640,000 cases reported in 2001 in the United States alone.[1] The annual incidence of distal radial fractures in the U.S. population older than 65 years of age has been reported to be 57 to 100 per 10,000.[2-4] The exact reason for the current trend toward increasing incidence is not fully understood but among other factors, includes an aging population with less sedentary pastimes.

The overall impact on society of this large number of patients with fractures of the distal radius is direct and indirect. The cost of medical care from assessment through conservative or operative treatment and all the costs that entails would be considered direct costs. For example, in 2007, Medicare paid $170 million in distal radius fracture–related payments. Perhaps even more important to consider would be the indirect costs of decreased school or work attendance, loss of work hours, loss of independence, need for care, and potential lasting disability.

Lack of homogeneous coding and databases at all hospitals treating these fractures makes the true number of these fractures difficult to estimate with the true number being potentially much larger than that just mentioned.[1]

Distal radius fractures can affect anyone of any age but their incidence falls into three main age groups: children and adolescents, young adults, and the elderly. Gender and ethnicity can also play a part in determining risk.[1]

Demographic studies have shown that distal radius fractures account for 1.5% to 2.5% of all emergency department attendances.[5]

One study showed that 32% of all fractures seen in women older than the age of 35 years are of the distal radius and that distal radius fractures can account for up to 18% of all fractures in the over-65-years age group.[1] It has also been shown that the overall lifetime risk of a distal radius fracture is 15% for women and 2% for men.[6,7]

CLINICAL ASSESSMENT

As with any musculoskeletal injury, initial assessment should focus on the Advanced Trauma Life Support (ATLS) guidelines, and subsequent history and examination should be tailored according to the findings of the primary and secondary survey. Special consideration should be given to certain patient subgroups regarding the mechanism of injury, for example, in the pediatric population to exclude nonaccidental injury (NAI) and in the elderly population to determine the underlying reason for the fall.

The mechanism of injury also allows the clinician to begin to build a picture of the underlying bone quality and injury to the surrounding tissues, both of which may alter the treatment strategy.

Once a full history and assessment have been made, if an obvious deformity is noted, then at the least, the limb should be splinted after analgesia and potentially manipulated depending on the circumstances. Rings and other jewelry should be removed. Careful neurovascular examination should be performed and if any abnormality is found, it should be carefully documented and emergent treatment should be undertaken to reduce the fracture and address the neurovascular compromise.

Open fractures should be treated as per local protocol with wound irrigation, photography, dressing, tetanus prophylaxis, and intravenous antibiotic administration. Special attention should be paid to farmyard injuries and aquatic injuries, which may require special antibiotics on the advice of the microbiologist.

RADIOLOGIC ASSESSMENT

Accurate and appropriate radiographs and their interpretation can play a large part in providing surgeons with information on which to base their treatment plans.

Normal radiographic evaluation of the distal radius should include a posterior-anterior (PA) and true lateral projection. Also a modified lateral view with the beam angled 10 degrees proximally should be performed to assess fracture reduction and provide more detail about the articular surface.[8]

PA radiograph allows assessment of the radial styloid, articular surface of the distal radius, proximal and distal carpal row, distal radioulnar joint, and distal ulna.

A true lateral projection is essential for basing further management. Occasionally, radiographic technicians can place the arm in extremes of pronation or supination; simply superimposing the radius on the ulna can result in an oblique view of the articular surface. A simple method to avoid this is to use the relative position of the pisiform to the distal pole of the scaphoid as the reference for judging the quality of the lateral radiograph—the "scaphopisocapitate alignment criterion."[9] On a true lateral radiograph, the pisiform should overlap the distal pole of the scaphoid. If the pisiform is positioned dorsal to the distal pole, then the forearm is in relative pronation, and if the pisiform is volar, then the forearm is supinated.[9]

In a standard view, the radiograph is perpendicular to the shaft. Because the radial inclination of the ulnar two-thirds of the articular surface is 10 degrees, this results in an oblique view of the joint surface on standard lateral radiograph. The 10-degree lateral tilt projection allows more accurate assessment of the articular surface, identification of the apical ridges of the dorsal and volar rims, and the teardrop. Basic parameters measured on the lateral radiograph would be volar tilt, carpal alignment, and cortical integrity. On the PA view, standard assessment would include radial height, inclination, ulnar variance, and assessment of the visible carpi.[8]

NORMAL PARAMETERS

See Table 6D-1 for the normal parameters, as described by Medoff and colleagues in 2005.[8,10]

HOW MUCH DEFORMITY IS ACCEPTABLE IN ADULTS

As will be repeated throughout this chapter, a wide variety of literature exists regarding this matter but few papers can convincingly demonstrate a link between degrees of malunion and decreased function, increased pain, or long-term risk of arthrosis.

Short and coworkers have shown an increase of 18% to 42% of forces borne by the distal ulna with a relative shortening of as little as 2.5 mm. As the radius shortens relative to the ulna,

TABLE 6D-1 ***NORMAL PARAMETERS OF DISTAL RADIUS***

	Radial Inclination (degrees)	Ulnar Variance (mm)	Volar Tilt (degrees)
Average	23.6 ± 2.5	11.6 ± 1.6	11.2 ± 4.6
Men	22.5 ± 2.1	−0.6 ± 1.0	10.2 ± 3.2
Women	24.7 ± 2.5	−0.6 ± 0.8	12.2 ± 5.6

Source: *From Medoff RJ: Essential radiographic evaluation for distal radius fractures, Hand Clin 21:279–288, 2005; Feipel V, Rinnen D, Rooze M: Posterior-anterior radiography of the wrist. Normal database of carpal measurements, Surg Radiol Anat 20:221–226, 1998.*

the triangular fibrocartilage complex (TFCC) becomes tighter, and this can lead to pain at the distal radial ulnar joint (DRUJ) and decrease forearm rotation.[11]

Shortening of 6 to 8 mm can cause ulnar impingement on the triquetrum or extreme ulnar border of the lunate. Bronstein and colleagues found 10 mm of shortening resulted in a mean 47% loss of pronation and 29% loss of supination. The DRUJ was effectively locked by ulnocarpal abutment at 15 mm of shortening.[12]

It could be argued that there is a general agreement that shortening of greater than 5 mm is associated with poorer outcomes.[13]

Dorsal angulation is very commonly observed in distal radial malunions, but despite this, there appears to be widespread differences of opinion about what constitutes an acceptable value. As angulation increases, the load increases from volar-radial to dorsal-ulnar. In a cadaveric study, Short and colleagues demonstrated that the load through the distal ulna increased from 21% at 10 degrees of volar tilt to 67% at 45 degrees of dorsal tilt. At 30 degrees of dorsal tilt, 50% of the load was borne by the ulna.[11]

Miyake and coworkers concluded that osteotomy to address abnormal wrist loading should be conducted when dorsal angulation exceeds beyond 20 degrees.[14]

Lafontaine and colleagues identified several risk factors associated with secondary fracture displacement despite a satisfactory initial reduction. These included the presence of dorsal tilt greater than 20 degrees, comminution, intraarticular involvement, an associated fracture of the ulna, and age older than 60 years.[15]

Graham defined acceptable parameters of the distal radius as ulnar variance of less than 5 mm compared with contralateral wrist, radial inclination on the PA radiograph greater than 15 degrees, and tilt measured on the lateral radiograph as between 15 degrees dorsal and 20 degrees volar.[16]

Relatively recent American Academy of Orthopaedic Surgeons (AAOS) guidelines state acceptable figures of less than 5 mm of radial shortening at the DRUJ compared with the contralateral side, radial inclination more than 15 degrees on PA radiographs, sagittal tilt on the lateral projection between 15 degrees dorsal tilt and 20 degrees volar tilt, intraarticular step-off or gap of less than 2 mm, and articular incongruity less than 2 mm of the sigmoid notch of the distal radius.

TREATMENT

In the majority of cases (as described in the next paragraphs), a well-executed closed reduction using analgesia with or without sedation as per local protocols and skill levels is nearly always indicated. Adequate analgesia should be administered in a controlled and safe manner prior to attempts at reduction and casting. Analgesia can range from nitrous oxide, routine oral analgesia, local anesthetic hematoma block, Bier block, conscious sedation, or general anesthetic. The best technique for reducing a fracture is to replicate the deformity, apply traction, and then manipulate it into appropriate position. A well-molded cast with three-point molding should be applied and radiographs in the cast obtained (Fig. 6D-1; see video 6D-1). The authors repeat radiographs at 1 week and at 2 weeks to assess for displacement. They then reassess the patient at 6 weeks for removal of the cast and obtain radiographs plus offer referral to physical therapy for rehabilitation if clinically indicated.

Young Patients

Buckle fractures are a very common type of fracture seen in the skeletally immature patient. They are extraarticular, inherently stable, and at low risk of displacement. Debate has occurred over the years as to the optimal treatment for these types of fracture and Williams and colleagues performed a prospective trial on casting versus splinting. They showed a clear trend favoring splints over cast for almost every measure.[17] Plint and coworkers found children treated with a removable splint had better physical functioning and less difficulty with activities than those treated with a cast.[18]

Forward and colleagues reviewed 106 patients who had sustained a fracture of their distal radius when younger than 40 years old, with a mean follow-up of 38 years. They found radiologic evidence of osteoarthritis in 68% of patients who had sustained an intraarticular fracture of the distal radius but that Disabilities of the Arm, Shoulder, and Hand (DASH) scores were similar to population norms and that subjective function using the Patient Evaluation Measure was impaired by less than 10%.[19]

In distal radial fractures in the pediatric patient, Noonan and coworkers described the acceptable degree of deformity for conservative treatment. In fractures at any level in children younger than 9 years old, complete displacement, 15 degrees of angulation, and 45 degrees of malrotation are acceptable.[20]

In children 9 years or older, 30 degrees of malrotation is acceptable, with 10 degrees of angulation for proximal fractures and 15 degrees for more distal fractures. Complete bayonet apposition is acceptable, especially for distal radial fractures, as long as angulation does not exceed 20 degrees and 2 years of growth remains.[20]

Operative intervention is indicated when the fracture is open or when acceptable alignment cannot be achieved or maintained. Distal radius fractures treated conservatively can be adequately treated in a below-elbow cast.[21]

Generally with distal radial fractures, radiographs should be taken for the first 2 weeks at weekly intervals to check for displacement and the wrist protected for 6 weeks in total.

Elderly Patients

Relatively recent research has shown that many distal radius fractures in the elderly may be treated nonoperatively even after loss of initially obtained reduction.

Arora and colleagues found that there was no difference at 12 months in terms of range of motion (ROM), pain, or subjective outcomes when comparing patients older than age 65 years who had been randomized either to volar locking plate or conservative treatment with cast.[22] Similarly Egol and coworkers compared patients older than age 65 years who had failed closed reduction and either received surgery or continued cast immobilization. Grip strength and radiographic parameters were significantly better in the operatively treated group at 1 year, but these parameters did not correlate with subjective outcomes.[23]

In an effort to answer whether an initial attempt at closed reduction is always necessary, Neidenbach and coworkers looked at patients at a mean age of 62 years who were treated conservatively either with or without attempts at closed

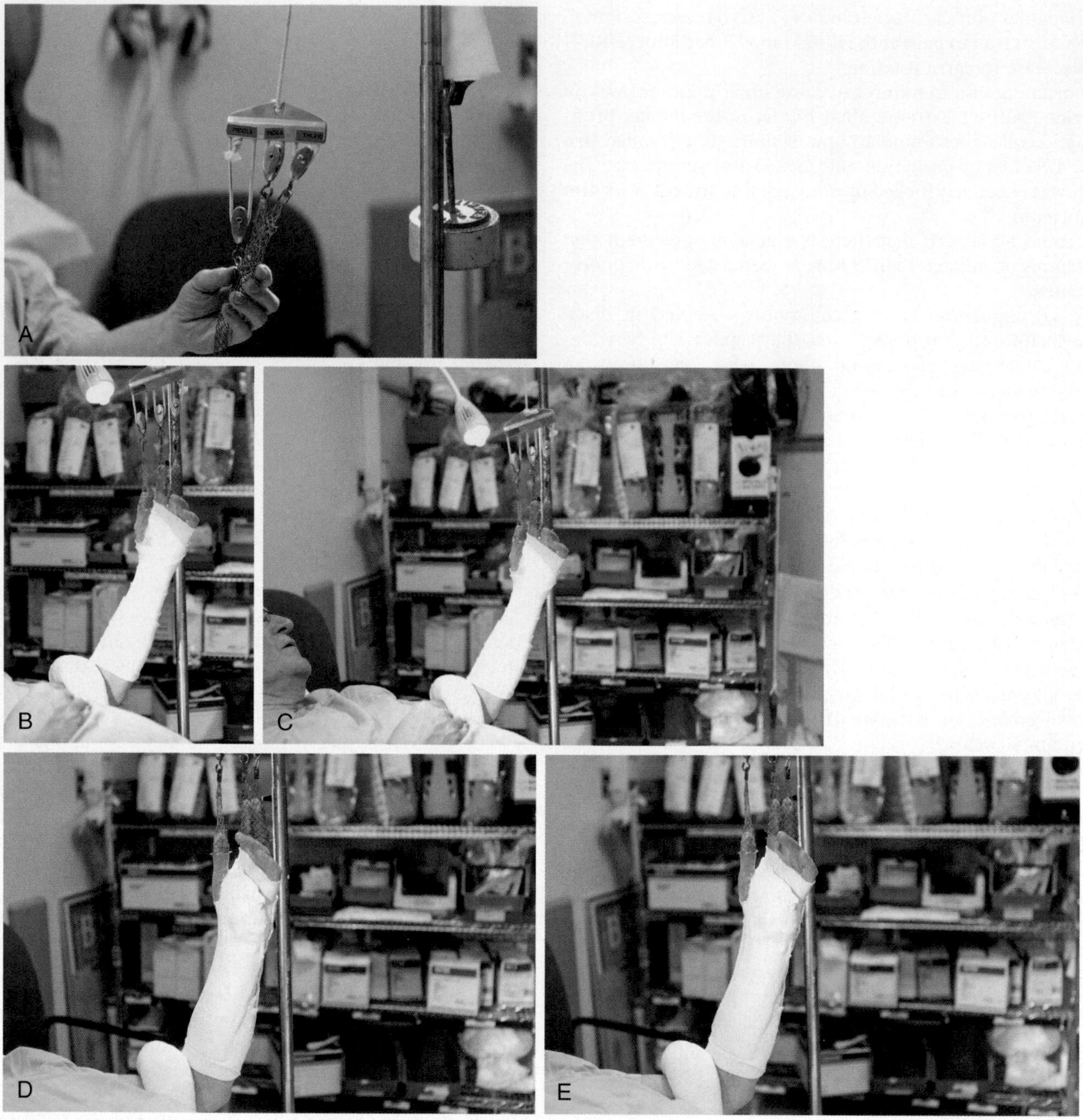

Figure 6D-1. A, Note finger traps: These are used to help obtain and maintain reduction. They allow the application of plaster without the need of an assistant. **B** and **C,** Note the thumb, index, and middle fingers in the finger traps. A counterweight of 2.3 kg (5 lb) is applied to the arm just above the elbow. Stockinette is applied to the forearm prior to inserting the fingers in the finger traps. Cast paper is then applied. Overall view of the appearance of the forearm: Note the finger traps maintain ulnar deviation of the wrist. **D,** Volar plaster slab is applied over the stockinette and cast paper. **E,** A dorsal slab is applied ensuring that there is an open space along the ulnar border of the forearm.

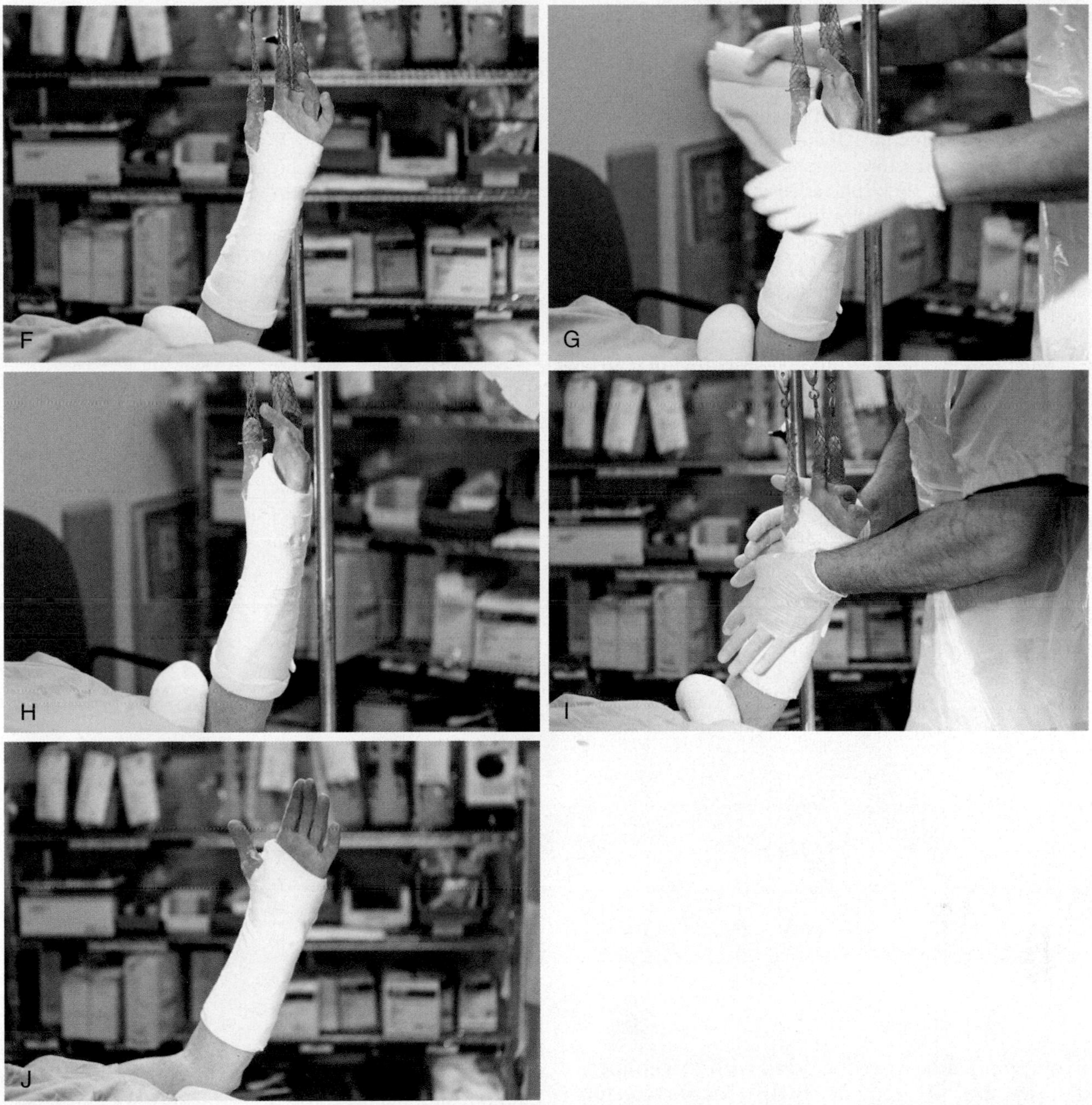

Figure 6D-1, cont'd. F, The slabs are held in place with a nonelastic gauze bandage. **G,** Slabs are then covered with a 4-inch flannel bandage. **H,** Note the space on the ulnar side of the forearm between the plaster slabs, which allows for easy relief of the cast should swelling occur. **I,** With the reduction maintained in the finger traps, molding occurs: Note the palmar molding hand is over the proximal fragment and the dorsal molding hand is over the distal fragment. **J,** The finished immobilization. Note the thumb and fingers are free to promote hand use.

reduction before casting. All patients attained a "successful level of activity in their daily life regardless of treatment."[24] Beumer and McQueen found a lack of benefit to closed reduction in the old and frail individual with 53 out of 60 patients with distal radius fractures treated by closed reduction subsequently losing the reduction. There was no correlation with initial displacement fracture classification and final radiographic appearance.[25] They concluded that reduction of fractures of the distal radius is of minimal value in the very old and frail, dependent, or demented patient. Perhaps closed reduction is not always necessary but further higher powered studies are required before we would necessarily recommend this treatment.

A 21-center multicenter study in North America led by the Mayo Clinic aims to look at unstable wrist fractures in the elderly patient and compare closed reduction plus pinning, external fixation with or without percutaneous pinning, and volar plating with closed reduction and immobilization, but this trial is currently in the enrollment phase.

Despite the ever-increasing number of publications based on varying treatments for distal radius fractures, a recent Cochrane Collaboration could not find enough evidence to support a particular definitive treatment for any given fracture type, so at present, we would suggest treating all patients on an individual basis taking the available evidence and personal circumstances into consideration.

KEY REFERENCES

The level of evidence (LOE) is determined according to the criteria provided in the preface.

2. Singer BR, McLauchlan GJ, Robinson CM, et al: Epidemiology of fractures in 15,000 adults: the influence of age and gender. *J Bone Joint Surg Br* 80:243–248, 1998. LOE III
4. Vogt MT, Cauley JA, Tomaino MM, et al: Distal radius fractures in older women: a 10 year follow-up study of descriptive characteristics and risk factors: the study of osteoporotic fractures. *J Am Geriatr Soc* 50:97–103, 2001. LOE III
8. Medoff RJ: Essential radiographic evaluation for distal radius fractures. *Hand Clin* 21:279–288, 2005. LOE IV
15. Lafontaine M, Delince P, Hardy D, et al: Instability of fractures of the lower end of the radius: apropos of a series of 167 cases. *Acta Orthop Belg* 55:203–216, 1989. LOE III
22. Arora R, Gabl M, Gschwentner M, et al: A comparative study of clinical and radiologic outcomes of unstable Colles type distal radius fractures in patients older than 70 years: nonoperative treatment versus volar locking plating. *J Orthop Trauma* 23:237–242, 2009. LOE II
23. Egol KA, Walsh M, Romo-Cardoso S, et al: Distal radial fractures in the elderly: operative compared with nonoperative treatment. *J Bone Joint Surg Am* 92(9):1851–1857, 2010. LOE III

The complete References list is available online at https://expertconsult.inkling.com.

6E Humeral Shaft Fractures

ASHESH KUMAR • JAMES P. WADDELL

The following videos are included with this chapter and may be viewed at https://expertconsult.inkling.com:
6E-1. Sugar-tong splint.
6E-2. Sugar-tong cast.
6E-3. Application of the fracture brace.

INTRODUCTION

Conservative treatment of humeral shaft fractures has been discussed in surgical textbooks since the beginning of recorded medical history. Indeed, reduction maneuvers and bandaging are discussed in records dated to before 1600 BC.[1] Today, conservative management of humeral shaft fractures by functional bracing remains the cornerstone of treatment modalities.[2] There is a well-established history of success with a high rate of union as well as acceptable functional results.

In North America, humeral diaphyseal fractures represent 1% to 5% of all fractures and occur more than 70,000 times a year.[3] Fractures of the midshaft account for 20% of all fractures of the humerus.[4] There is a well-documented bimodal distribution with the first peak occurring in young males between the ages of 21 and 30 years. A second peak is seen among older females between the ages of 60 and 80 years.[5]

Fractures of the humeral midshaft have a high propensity to heal with few limitations on functionality. This region is well enveloped in muscle, which contributes a rich vascular supply. The upper arm is easily splinted and can remain non–weight-bearing for the duration of treatment. While rare, complications of conservative management do occur. These include nonunion, malunion, persistent radial nerve deficits, loss of motion due to adhesive capsulitis, and transient shoulder subluxation. Unfavorable body habitus has been shown to increase the risk of varus malunion. Morbid obesity and large pendulous breasts are examples of body habitus features that may provide challenges to functional brace treatment of humeral shaft fractures, and evidence exists that these may be better treated by operative means.[6] Skin maceration is another important potential complication from brace wear and thus daily hygiene with careful observation of the skin under the brace should be stressed throughout treatment.[7]

Humeral diaphyseal fractures tolerate a wide degree of angular, axial, and rotational malunion with little effect on functional significance.[8-12] This is largely due to the unique biomechanics of the glenohumeral (GH) joint, which impart an exceptional range of motion in many planes. The freedom of motion about the shoulder joint coupled with the wide range of motion of the hinged elbow joint allows for this tolerance of malunion. Guidelines for an acceptable reduction when treating by conservative means include less than 3 cm of bayonet apposition; less than 20 degrees of anterior angulation; less than 30 degrees of varus angulation; and less than 30 degrees of rotational deformity.[13-15]

TREATMENT

Sarmiento and coworkers introduced the concept of functional bracing to humeral shaft fractures in 1977 after good results with this technique in tibial, femoral, forearm, and wrist fractures. Their initial report of 51 patients revealed excellent outcomes with little morbidity.[10] Other investigators confirmed a high rate of union with few complications.[15-19] Treatment of humeral shaft fractures using a functional brace is currently the gold standard and has replaced all other forms of bracing.[2]

Indeed, the advantages of functional bracing are numerous and include ease of application, adjustability, allowance of shoulder and elbow motion, low cost, reproducible results, and reliability. Although complications do exist, there are few reported when associated with this technique. However, functional bracing of humeral shaft fractures is an involved process. It is an active therapeutic modality that under ideal circumstances has dedicated participation by the patient as well as thorough supervision by the treatment team.

The technique of functional bracing rests on three main principles. First, active muscle contraction surrounding the fracture works to correct rotation and angulation. With respect to a fractured humeral diaphysis, the triceps, brachialis, and biceps undergo a coiling of their fibers after the injury as the bone fragments rotate. During active muscle contraction, the fibers recoil and then self-correct the malrotation.[20] Sarmiento and colleagues hypothesized that motion at the fracture site is an important factor in osteogenesis through the release of a cascade of favorable events including increased vascularity, piezoelectric potentials, and local thermal and chemical changes. The milieu of factors favorable to fracture healing is maintained by the local activation of muscles around the area of fracture.[20-24] Additionally, in those cases of transient inferior GH subluxation, the early voluntary contraction of biceps and triceps, which attach proximally on scapula and distally on humeral diaphysis, helps to restore congruity of the GH joint. Second, the "hydraulic effect" of soft tissue compression by the fracture brace assists in aligning fracture fragments. Circular compression of the muscle compartment around the fracture serves as an "inner splint." Third, a fracture brace makes use of the beneficial effect of gravity on fracture alignment.[10,15,17,25-29]

There are a number of options for initial immobilization of the injured extremity in the emergency room. The most commonly used splinting methods are the hanging arm cast and the coaptation splint (Video 6E-1). Other less commonly employed but still useful alternatives, depending on materials available, can include abduction casting and bracing, sling and swathe, longarm cast, shoulder spica cast, and Velpeau dressings. The goals of initial splinting are to provide protection of the injured extremity and pain control while providing non-circumferential support to allow room for increasing limb girth caused by swelling. Typically, these can be left on for 5 to 10 days (Figs. 6E-1 through 6E-4, and Video 6E-2).

During the initial immobilization phase, patients are encouraged to immediately perform daily active and passive exercises of elbow, wrist, and fingers to avoid stiffness of these uninjured joints. Once the acute pain and swelling subsides, a functional brace can then be applied. The functional brace consists of two prefabricated polypropylene sleeves held together with adjustable Velcro straps. A cuff and collar sling can also be used during this period to further enhance comfort of the injured limb. Minor reduction maneuvers of the fracture can be performed during initial application of the brace (Figs. 6E-5 through 6E-7).

It is critical that patients are instructed in proper removal and application of the brace as daily self-care is paramount.

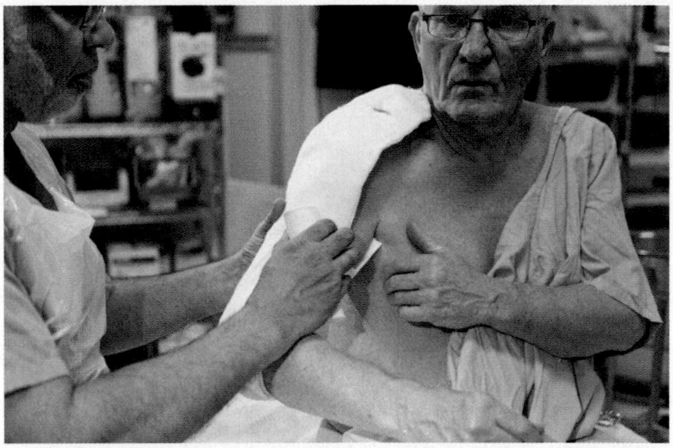

Figure 6E-1. The slab is measured and then cut. Note the end of the slab just fits under the axilla (not too high into the axilla). It comes around the elbow up over the lateral aspect of the arm and over the top of the shoulder. Note the small hole cut in the top of the slab for application of the collar and cuff sling.

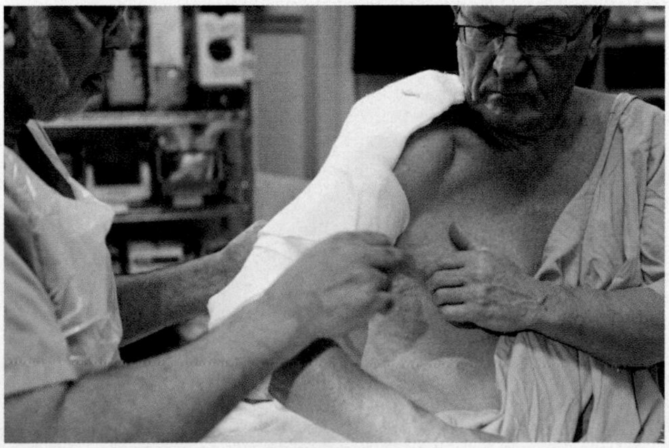

Figure 6E-2. The slab is then wrapped snugly with a flannel bandage around the arm ensuring adequate padding of the axilla and around the elbow.

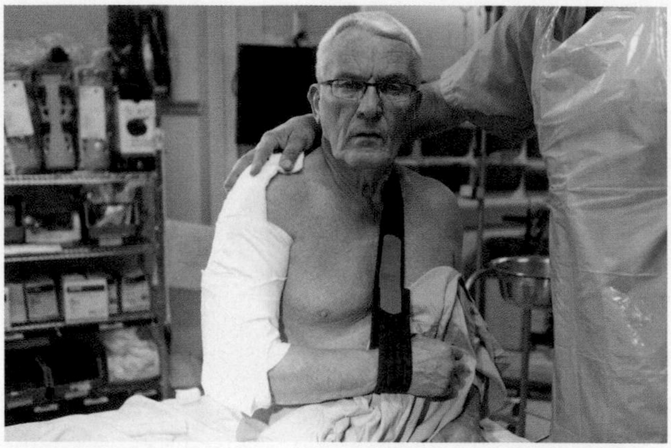

Figure 6E-3. The completed bandage; note the elbow is maintained at a right angle, the axilla is appropriately padded, and the slab extends over the top of the shoulder. The collar and cuff sling is placed about the wrist to maintain the elbow in 90 degrees of flexion.

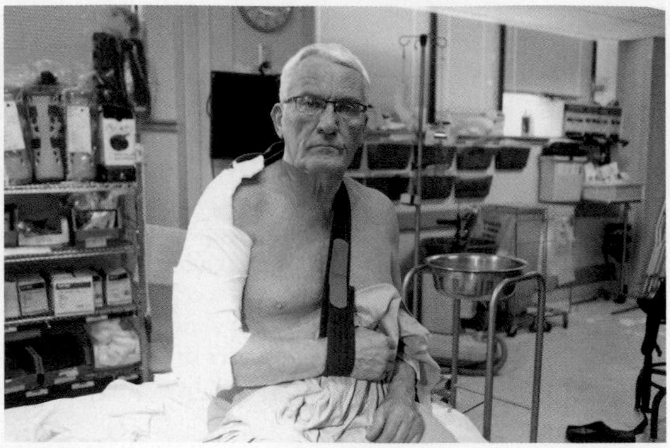

Figure 6E-4. The collar and cuff sling is then attached to the top of the slab to maintain the slab over the top of the shoulder, maintaining the humerus in appropriate position.

Patients must understand how to adjust and tighten the Velcro straps to account for changes in the girth of the arm caused by soft tissue edema and muscle atrophy. It is recommended that adjustments be done several times daily if necessary. Often one finds the sleeve of the brace may slip distally, especially in large conically shaped arms. In these cases, an option for a shoulder harness exists to prevent the sleeve from slipping.

Once bracing has begun, patients are instructed to immediately perform passive pendulum exercises with the elbow in full extension. If a cuff and collar is used, then it should be removed several times a day for these exercises. Use of the cuff and collar while walking may be discontinued once the patient has achieved full extension of the elbow. The cuff and collar may still be used while the patient is recumbent for comfort if necessary. We typically limit our patients with respect to active elevation and abduction until the fracture is clinically stable to prevent the development of a varus deformity. Instructing our patients not to lean on the elbow of the injured arm can also prevent potential varus angulation. This can be especially challenging in those who are wheelchair bound. At this time, we typically instruct patients to increase the frequency and intensity of elbow (active and passive) and shoulder (passive flexion) exercises.

Only once clinical and radiographic union is confirmed can fracture brace treatment be safely discontinued. Clinical healing may be deduced by the absence of pain and motion at fracture site. Radiographic healing is demonstrated by the formation of visible callus at the fracture site (Video 6E-3).

Outcomes

Most studies reveal that functional bracing is in fact associated with a loss of range of motion about the shoulder and elbow. External rotation, flexion, and abduction are limited in 10% to 30% of patients, whereas loss of elbow range of motion occurs in approximately 10% of patients.[2,10,30] The incidence of nonunion is likely dependent on the fracture pattern and the location of the fracture in the diaphysis. Identifying these subtypes may play a role in nonoperative versus operative decision making. The incidence of nonunion is higher with simple fracture patterns (Orthopaedic Trauma Association [OTA] type A). Many studies have found a higher rate of nonunion in displaced middle- and distal-third fracture as well as those with transverse fracture patterns.* Conversely, nonunions in type B or C fractures are extremely rare.[2,32,33] However, the evidence can be conflicting. Pehlivan showed that young adults with isolated and closed distal humeral fractures are also good candidates for functional bracing.[28] A total of 21 distal-third humeral shaft fractures were treated with a brace

*References 2, 3, 7, 25, 31, 32.

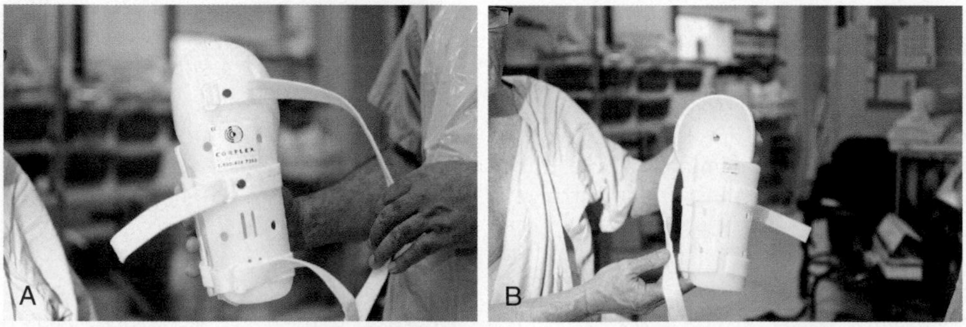

Figure 6E-5. A, This is a commercially available humeral fracture brace. These are widely available; if not, they can be readily manufactured with local materials. **B,** The longer side goes on the lateral aspect of the arm and the shorter side on the medial aspect.

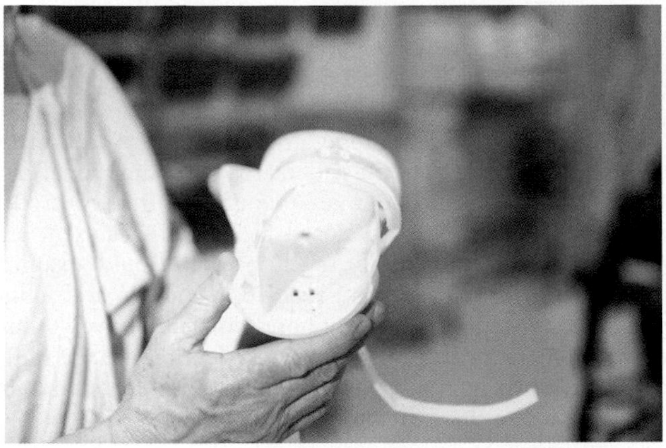

Figure 6E-6. The interior of the brace is smooth without prominence.

with an average time to union of 12 weeks. The union rate was 100% and limitations on shoulder abduction and external rotation were minimal.

Sarmiento and coworkers reported a follow-up to the initial report of 1977 and were able to follow 620 fractures out of a total of 922 enrolled in the study.[7] The investigators confirmed a high rate of union with a nonunion rate of less than 2% for closed fractures and 6% for open fractures. Overall, patients were reported as having excellent outcomes with 60% having full shoulder range of motion and 76% having full elbow range of motion at the time the brace was discontinued. Furthermore, they found that significant degrees of deformity could be well corrected with functional bracing. In their study, almost 90% of 565 fractures for which final radiographs were available healed with angular deformities of less than 16 degrees with most of these within 5 to 10 degrees of anatomic alignment. However, one weakness of the study often cited is that minimal functional outcome data was collected. For example, elbow range of motion was only recorded for 301 out of the 922 patients enrolled.

Recent studies challenged some of the findings of Sarmiento and colleagues as they have not been able to replicate their results. There are a number of possible reasons. First, Sarmiento and associates lost many patients to follow-up, suggesting a positive selection bias. Second, the rigorous protocol of treatment proposed is difficult to replicate and most investigators feel that a lack of patient compliance may contribute to their inferior results. Third, and most important, newer studies are incorporating the use of patient-reported outcome measurement tools. It is possible the patient perspective may paint a different picture of outcome than the traditional surgeon-reported outcomes.

Koch and colleagues reported an 87% union rate in a retrospective review of 67 fractures treated nonoperatively.[2] In this study, only 52% of patients achieved excellent outcomes as measured by their surgeons. Excellent was defined as normal symmetric range of motion of shoulder and elbow with no pain. Similarly, Ekholm and coworkers reported a 90% overall union rate again with approximately 50% of patients reporting they were not fully recovered after closed treatment using the Short Musculoskeletal Functional Assessment (SMFA) tool to assess their musculoskeletal functional status.[33] The incidence of radial nerve palsy in both studies was about 10%, which is consistent in the literature.[7,10,34,35]

Interestingly, in a retrospective review, Rutgers and Ring found a higher incidence of nonunion in proximal-third humeral shaft fractures with a long oblique fracture pattern.[36] Their overall reported union rate was 90% matching other studies; however, 29% of the fractures in the proximal diaphysis failed to heal. They postulated that the pull of the deltoid on the proximal fragment tends to allow soft tissue interposition into the fracture site thereby creating the conditions for nonunion. These results were similar to a study by Toivanen and coworkers in which almost half of the fractures in the proximal-third diaphysis failed to heal.[14]

Overall, the current literature is unable to provide a definitive answer as to whether operative or nonoperative treatment results in different clinical outcomes. In a retrospective study, Mahabier and colleagues found no difference between time to union, rates of delayed union, and development of radial nerve palsies between fractures treated operatively versus those treated nonoperatively.[37] However, the study was limited by a lack of statistical power because of the wide variation in fracture subtypes in both the nonoperative and operative groups. The inherent lack of randomization with respect to the choice of operative versus nonoperative intervention implies that decisions were made at the surgeon's discretion. As such, the study provides a good example of how much of the decision making is colored by the surgeon's experience and personal philosophy and may account for wide variations in treatment approaches between regions and institutions.

Controversies

The traditional belief that nonoperatively treated patients do uniformly well is being challenged in current times. Part of this comes from surgeons' increasing operative experience and

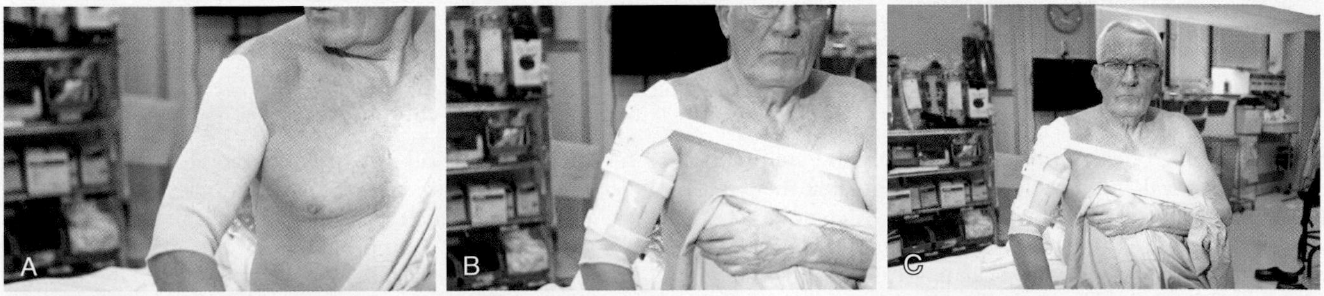

Figure 6E-7. A, A stockinette is applied to the arm. It is cut on a bias on the superior border to accommodate the axilla. **B** and **C,** The brace is then applied. The two lower straps are tightened to maintain constant tension on the brace; the top strap passes under the opposite axilla and merely has to be sufficiently snug to prevent the brace migrating distally.

their access to newer technologies. The development of intramedullary and rotationally stable implants and the success of conventional plate osteosynthesis led Schittko to claim that operative intervention for these fractures should be the gold standard.[38] Surgeons may also be increasingly less tolerant of the labor involved in treating these injuries nonoperatively and of what constitutes an acceptable level of deformity. Furthermore, recent studies that assess patient-reported functional outcomes have shown a permanent loss of motion.[2,33] Finally, elevated rates of nonunion found among specific fracture patterns, including simple transverse fractures with little bony surface area for apposition and proximal-third oblique patterns, may further shift the pendulum toward operative management.[2,14,25,31-33,36]

CONCLUSION

We maintain that conservative management by functional bracing of humeral midshaft fractures is an appropriate treatment modality when done with proper oversight and patient instruction. It must be underscored that many communities have varying degrees of access to health care and resources for surgical management including adequate postoperative care. Widely differing economic climates can further contribute to lack of access. There is a cost benefit to nonoperative treatment of humeral shaft fractures. A low nonunion rate, diminished need for hospitalization, and a relatively short recovery period all contribute. Patient illness may also preclude surgical management. Overall surgeons must maintain their fund of knowledge of appropriate conservative care and not forget the long and successful history of fracture brace treatment for these injuries.

A large part of the decision-making tree rests on understanding the balance between surgical risk and benefit. The patient-related benefits of surgical management include early full motion, rapid return to work, and pain control. Indeed, surgical treatment can result in improved fracture reduction, more stable fixation, and easier and less painful mobilization. However, these are offset by surgical risks. Iatrogenic radial nerve palsy, infection, bleeding, delayed union, nonunion, shoulder impingement, reoperation, and anesthetic risk can all be potentially more devastating than the original injury.

Overall, there are few studies that are able to report on long-term follow-up of nonoperative treatment. Additionally, few studies provide data on patient-reported functional outcomes. In our opinion, a large-scale randomized controlled trial is needed to compare closed functional treatment and operative treatment. Ideally, such a trial would examine patient-reported and surgeon-reported shoulder and elbow function, time to union, rates of nonunion and delayed union, residual malalignment, infection rates, development of radial nerve palsies, pain scores, and track those patients who are able to return to their previous level of work.

KEY REFERENCES

The level of evidence (LOE) is determined according to the criteria provided in the preface.

2. Koch P: The results of functional (Sarmiento) bracing of humeral shaft fractures. *J Shoulder Elbow Surg* 11(2):143–150, 2002. doi: 10.1067/mse.2002.121634. LOE IV
3. Ekholm R, Adami J, Tidermark J, et al: Fractures of the shaft of the humerus. An epidemiological study of 401 fractures. *J Bone Joint Surg Br* 88(11):1469–1473, 2006. doi: 10.1302/0301-620X.88B11.17634. LOE III
7. Sarmiento A, Zagorski JB, Zych GA, et al: Functional bracing for the treatment of fractures of the humeral diaphysis. *J Bone Joint Surg Am* 82(4):478–486, 2000. LOE III
16. Sharma VK, Jain AK, Gupta RK, et al: Non-operative treatment of fractures of the humeral shaft: a comparative study. *J Indian Med Assoc* 89(6):157–160, 1991. LOE II
31. Sarmiento A, Waddell JP, Latta LL: Diaphyseal humeral fractures: treatment options. *Instr Course Lect* 51:257–269, 2002. LOE IV
32. Denard A, Richards JE, Obremskey WT, et al: Outcome of nonoperative vs operative treatment of humeral shaft fractures: a retrospective study of 213 patients. *Orthopedics* 33(8):2010. doi: 10.3928/01477447-20100625-16. LOE III
37. Mahabier KC, Vogels LMM, Punt BJ, et al: Humeral shaft fractures: Retrospective results of non-operative and operative treatment of 186 patients. *Injury* 44(4):427–430, 2013. doi: 10.1016/j.injury.2012.08.003. LOE III

The complete References list is available online at https://expertconsult.inkling.com.

6F Proximal Humerus Fractures

ASHESH KUMAR • JAMES P. WADDELL

There are detailed descriptions of reduction and splinting of proximal humeral fractures dating back greater than three millennia found in surgical texts from both Ancient Egypt and Greece.[1a] Today, proximal humeral fractures account for up to 5% of all fractures treated.[1] Most can be treated nonoperatively and are nondisplaced or minimally displaced two-part fractures, which account for 50% to 80% of all proximal humeral fractures.[2-7] Conversely three- and four-part fractures account for only 15% of all proximal humeral fractures. Seventy percent of these are seen in patients older than 60 years of age, and 50% of such fractures are seen in those older than 70 years of age.[1] Comorbid conditions predispose elderly adults to low-energy falls, which account for the dominant mechanism of injury in this population. Such comorbid conditions include poor vision, balance problems, loss of protective reflexes, and polypharmacy. Furthermore, poor bone

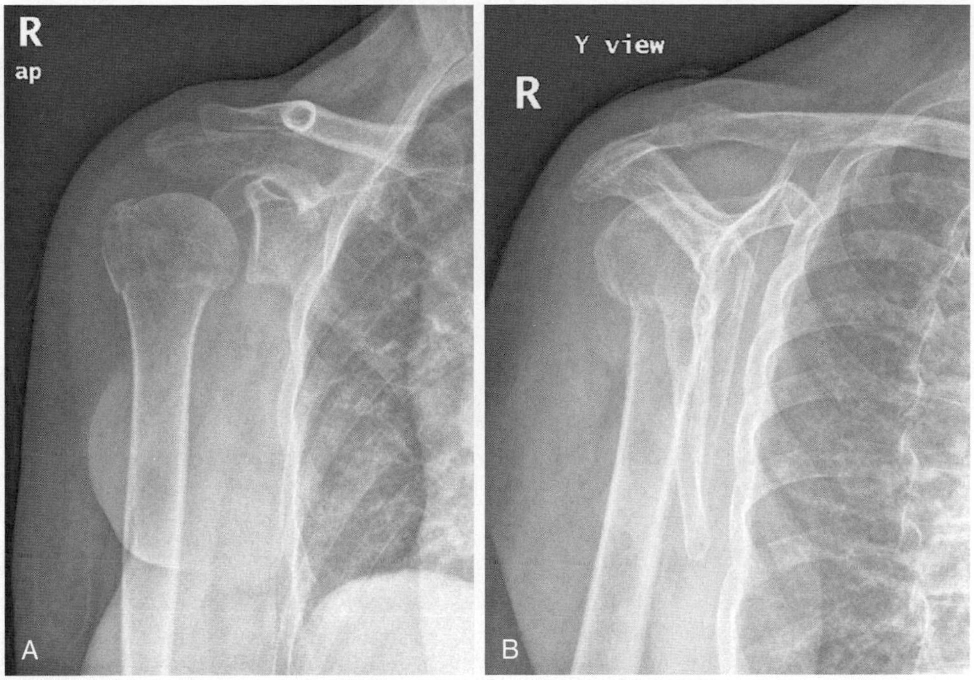

Figure 6F-1. **A,** Anterior-posterior radiograph demonstrating a comminuted fracture of the proximal humerus. **B,** Transscapular lateral or "Y" view demonstrating minimal fracture displacement and no evidence of dislocation or subluxation.

quality in the elderly population accounts for a greater severity of injury with more complex fracture patterns despite little mechanical insult. With a growing elderly population, the rate of proximal humeral fractures has increased by an average of 13% per year between 1970 and 2002.[1,8-11] By 2030, the number of proximal humeral fractures in the elderly population is expected to triple.[5]

The effect of proximal humeral fractures on patients can be tremendous. Patients are often left with the inability to care for themselves at the most fundamental level. Dressing, bathing, toileting, feeding, and even the ability to leave the house may all be affected. Previously independent patients can become quite dependent, and the period of dependence may last for several months. Approximately 6 months to 1 year can lapse before good or very good recovery is seen and results are better with nondisplaced than displaced fractures.[2,4,12-18]

Treating orthopaedic surgeons should have a thorough understanding of this common problem. However, heterogeneity among studies and treatment algorithms exists. These differences manifest at all levels of the therapeutic chain. The importance given to patient-related factors such as age, functional demand, and comorbid conditions varies among surgeons. There is also variability in standard imaging protocols for diagnosis, splinting options for initial immobilization, and rehabilitation regimens. Variability exists among surgeons, institutions, and regions.[19-21] Also, there is controversy regarding surgical versus conservative management of three- and four-part proximal humeral fractures.[22] Consequently, there is a need for a clear evidence-based consensus on how to manage these challenging fractures. Understanding the natural history of conservative treatment is important for establishing a baseline for which to compare the usefulness of emerging operative technologies.

DIAGNOSIS

Our treatment algorithm starts with good-quality radiographs (Fig. 6F-1). We use a trauma series that includes a true anterior-posterior (AP) and a scapular Y view perpendicular and parallel to the plane of the scapula, respectively. An axillary lateral view is also taken to assess the reduction of the humeral head within the glenoid. If radiographs are insufficient to understand the fracture morphology and identify all the components of the fracture, then a computed tomography (CT) scan is indicated. A CT scan can further aid in the diagnosis by giving information regarding fracture morphology, bone stock of the humeral head and tuberosities, degree of comminution, size of the fragments amenable to fixation, and the length of the posteromedial metaphyseal extension.

Proper imaging allows the determination of both fracture displacement and angulation. Both are helpful in deciding if nonoperative treatment is appropriate. Neer has previously described acceptable displacement to be 1 cm and acceptable angulation to be 45 degrees.[23] Clinical or fluoroscopic image intensification can be used to determine the stability of the head and shaft. If the head and shaft move as a single unit, then the fracture is deemed impacted and thus stable. If there is significant motion between the head and shaft, then the fracture is deemed unstable.

Stable fractures respond well to short-term immobilization to allow time for swelling and pain to resolve. Although unstable fractures are often treated operatively, the decision to operate must take into account other patient factors. Displaced fractures in patients in whom surgery may not be warranted include elderly, low demand, uncooperative because of mental illness or substance abuse, significant comorbid conditions, and patients with active infections elsewhere. This group of patients with unstable fractures can still be treated

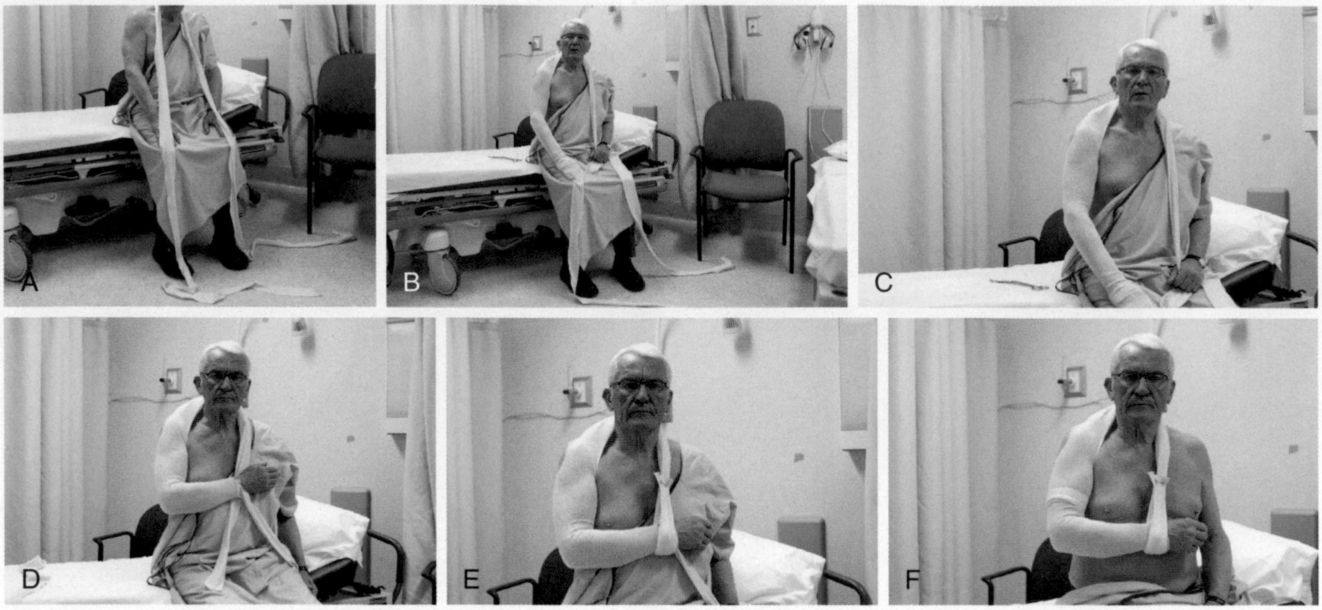

Figure 6F-2. **A,** A Velpeau dressing made with stockinette begins with approximately 8 feet of stockinette. **B,** The injured arm is placed into the stockinette through a small opening made halfway through its length. **C** and **D,** The stockinette is then filled with a roll of soft material and brought over the opposite shoulder, and the excess stockinette distal to the forearm is removed. **E,** The short end of the stockinette that has been looped over the opposite shoulder is then brought around the wrist and pinned to itself to support the forearm. **F,** The stockinette distal to the forearm is then brought around the patient's chest and looped around the arm and pinned to itself. This dressing provides excellent mobilization for the proximal humerus, prevents posterior movement of the arm, and supports the forearm.

nonoperatively. However, they often require a prolonged period of immobilization ranging from 2 to 4 weeks.

INITIAL IMMOBILIZATION

The goal of initial immobilization is to provide mechanical support. Supporting the fracture acutely prevents fracture displacement and promotes fracture consolidation while pain and swelling resolve. Short-term immobilization can take on a variety of forms. Splinting options include but are not limited to the broad arm sling, collar and cuff, sling and swath, shoulder immobilizer, Gilchrist bandage, and the shoulder abduction cushion. There is limited evidence for the superiority of one type of immobilization device over another. In 1993, Rommens and colleagues compared the Desault bandage with the Gilchrist bandage in 28 patients with proximal humerus fractures. There was no effect on fracture healing or functional outcome. However, the Gilchrist bandage appeared to cause less pain and skin irritation. In our opinion, there is not enough evidence to advocate for one sling over another as long as the goal of providing mechanical support is adhered to. Our preferred splinting methods include a simple collar and cuff or a Velpeau sling, both of which are shown in Figure 6F-2.

REHABILITATION

Historically, what was considered the adequate time for the initial period of immobilization varied anywhere from a few days to more than 3 weeks. Before the 1990s, recommendations were based on clinical experience and uncontrolled case studies.[15,17,24-28] Since then, controlled clinical trials that examine when to begin mobilization of the injured arm have emerged and continue to be a topic of interest today.

The goal of rehabilitation is to restore a patient's functional range of motion and strength to levels that closely approximate the patient's preinjury status. As stated, regimens vary among surgeons, institutions, regions, and patient's personal resources. The recommended duration of immobilization, timing of first physiotherapy session, intensity and frequency of sessions, and setting for therapy be it home or hospital or private center all play into this heterogeneity.[29]

Prolonged immobilization is frequently complicated by shoulder stiffness and thus poorer outcomes. At our institution, we emphasize self-performed early movement exercises after a short course of immobilization to ameliorate loss of function as shown in Figure 6F-3. Rehabilitation generally follows two stages. Passive and assisted range of motion exercises are followed by progressive resistance exercises.

Brostrom hypothesized that mobilizing patients immediately after sustaining a proximal humeral fracture results in faster recovery of functional mobility.[17] His brief report of 97 proximal humeral fractures found good or excellent results in 59 fractures treated with immediate passive mobilization on the fourth day after injury and active range of motion initiated 9 to 11 days after injury. Brostrom graded range of motion on a 100-point scale with good outcomes having a score of 75 or greater.

Recent studies have supported Brostrom's historical findings.[12,30] Hodgson performed a prospective randomized controlled trial (RCT) examining 86 minimally displaced two-part proximal humeral fractures comparing two rehabilitation regimens. Immediate physiotherapy within 1 week of injury was undertaken in one group and compared with a conventional 3-week period of immobilization in the other group.

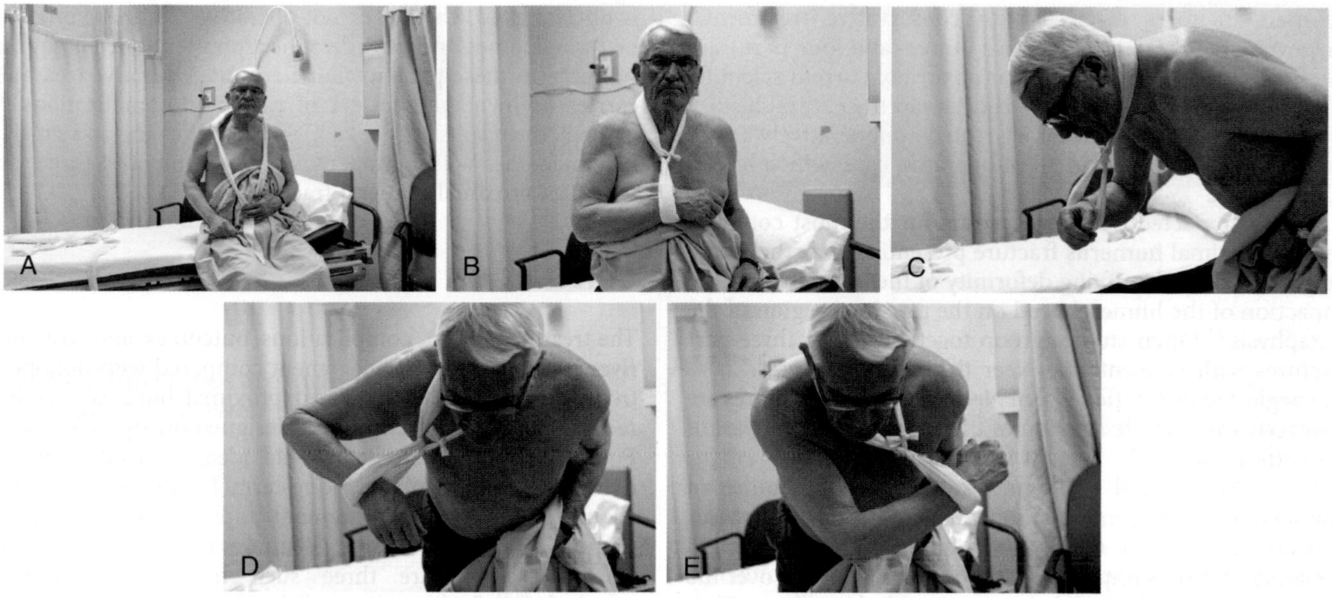

Figure 6F-3. **A,** Collar and cuff sling. Approximately a 3-foot length of stockinette is cut and padded with a rolled bandage. **B,** The two ends of stockinette are tied together, and a second rolled bandage is placed within the stockinette at the wrist. The stockinette is tied to itself to provide a sling to support the wrist. **C** to **E,** Using the collar and cuff sling it is possible to carry out pendular exercises as well as abduction exercises of the shoulder.

This study found better shoulder function in the group of patients mobilized immediately at the 8- and 16-week follow-up visits as measured by the Constant score. However, a statistical difference between the groups disappeared by 52 weeks. Importantly, patients who were immediately mobilized also reported less pain over the course of their treatment.

Hodgson and colleagues' results were supported by an earlier study performed by Kristiansen and colleagues in 1989.[13] This study was a prospective RCT that randomly allocated 85 patients with proximal humeral fractures to start mobilization exercises at 1 week or 3 weeks. Using a modified Neer's score,[23,31] they found that patients mobilized early had statistically significant better scores of overall shoulder function largely as a result of a reduction in their sensation of pain over the first 3 months. The effect disappeared after 6 months, and both groups continued with similar outcomes over the 2-year duration of the study.

Most recently, Lefevre-Colau and colleagues performed a single-institution RCT in 2007.[14] Seventy-four patients with impacted proximal humeral fractures were randomized to either early versus conventional mobilization regimens. Those in the early group began movement exercises within 72 hours of injury while those in the conventional group were immobilized for 3 weeks. Both groups were evaluated, and the Constant score was recorded at 3 months serving as the primary outcome measure. Secondary outcomes measured were reduction in pain intensity and differences in active and passive range of motion compared with the uninjured shoulder. The results echo previous studies in that patients in the early mobilization group had significantly better Constant scores, reduction in pain intensity, and superior mobilization early during the course of treatment. However, as in the previous study, statistical significance between the two groups disappeared after 6 months.

Lefevre-Colau and colleagues pooled their data with other studies, including those previously described to examine the safety of early mobilization. Both fracture nonunion and fracture displacement were considered. Studies that evaluated a conventional regimen of 3 weeks of fracture immobilization reported four patients out of a total of 373 with either a nonunion or fracture displacement requiring surgical intervention.[4,6,14,28] Studies that evaluated early mobilization within 1 week of injury failed to find a single case of nonunion or fracture displacement out of a total of 165 patients.[12,14,30] The authors concede that these proportions are not statistically different when assessed with the Fisher exact test ($P = 0.32$).

Overall, it appears that early mobilization reduces the subjective experience of pain early in the course of treatment. However, the outcomes between early and late mobilizers seem to equalize after a period of 6 months to 1 year. The data suggest that longer periods of immobilization for more complicated fractures may not worsen the final outcome and thus may be an appropriate treatment option for those patients who are not suitable surgical candidates because of medical comorbid conditions.

However, currently there is insufficient evidence to definitively state when to begin rehabilitation. In a Cochrane database systematic review, Handoll and Ollivere explain the difficulties and dangers of trying to establish a general consensus for treatment with small, single-institution trials.[32] Furthermore, trial heterogeneity prohibits the pooling of results in a meaningful manner. The need for large-scale and high-quality clinical trials with robust methodology is apparent.

NONOPERATIVE TREATMENT OUTCOMES

There is interest in identifying subgroups of proximal humeral fractures that can be successfully managed nonoperatively. It is generally agreed that nondisplaced and minimally displaced

RADIOGRAPHIC EVALUATION

Radiographs of the ankle should be sought, and at minimum, should include AP lateral and mortise views.[7] A variety of other views can be sought as clinically necessary, but these views are essential. In some cases, additional stress views and/or contralateral comparison views of the uninjured side may be indicated. The mortise view is taken with the ankle in approximately 10 to 15 degrees of internal rotation. Brandser and colleagues showed that ideally all three projections should be used as using only two missed a small but significant number of ankle and foot fractures.[7]

A variety of radiologic parameters exist, which have to be carefully assessed by the clinician to detect fractures. On the mortise view, these include medial and superomedial clear space, talar tilt, talofibular line, and talocrural angle.

Talar tilt is measured by drawing a line parallel to the articular surface of the distal tibia and a line parallel with the articular surface of the talus. These lines should be parallel. The talocrural angle is formed by a line drawn parallel to the articular surface of the distal tibia and aligning the connecting tips of both malleoli (intermalleolar line). This angle should normally be between 8 and 15 degrees.

Classification Systems

A variety of ankle fracture classifications exist, including the Danis-Weber, Lauge-Hansen, and Arbeitsgemeinschaft für Osteosynthesefragen (AO)/Orthopaedic Trauma Association (OTA) systems.

The Lauge-Hansen classification system was devised in 1950 and was based on the position of the foot and the deforming force at the time of injury.[8,9] The study used cadaveric ankles with feet fixed to boards. By subjecting the specimens to different stresses, they established four basic types of ankle injury: pronation–abduction, pronation–eversion, supination–adduction, and supination–internal rotation. The first term relates to the position of the foot at the time of the injury and the second to the deforming force.

The Danis-Weber classification system relates to the level of the fibular fracture with regard to the level of the ankle joint or syndesmosis. Fractures below the syndesmosis are deemed Weber A, fractures at the level of the syndesmosis are deemed Weber B, and fractures above the syndesmosis are deemed Weber C.[10,11]

Determining Stability

Historically, determining if an ankle fracture has been unstable has been an important factor in predicting whether the patient and fracture require surgery. Fractures of the lateral malleolar tip (Weber A equivalents) would be treated nonoperatively; Weber C would be determined as probably unstable and treated surgically in the majority of cases; and bimalleolar fractures would be deemed by definition unstable. More difficulty and therefore interest has focused on Weber B type unimalleolar fractures and how to classify a fracture as stable or unstable. Burwell and Charnley found that 80% of lateral malleolar fractures had no medial involvement.[12] Classically, medial tenderness, swelling, and bruising or ecchymosis was suggested as an indicator for instability in lateral malleolar fractures without medial fracture. Relatively recent papers have proven the validity in using stability as a criterion for fixation.[13,14] Many of these criteria measure the medial clear space on radiographs before and, if necessary, after stress testing. The medial clear space is measured from the superior-medial aspect of the talus to the superior-medial corner of the plafond on a mortise radiograph and is used to evaluate the deep deltoid ligament indirectly.

Pankovich suggested that a medial clear space of greater than 3 mm implied deep deltoid disruption.[15] Harper felt that 5 mm was the upper limit of normal for the medial clear space.[16] Recent evidence suggests that the normal medial clear space averages 2.7 mm, with the vast majority of people falling between 1.7 and 3.7 mm.[17] Therefore, we conclude that 4 mm and below could be considered normal. We routinely would recommend a control radiograph of the patient's contralateral unaffected ankle if in doubt.

Biomechanical studies have shown that with a displaced fibular fracture and intact deep deltoid and syndesmosis ligament, the ankle can resist horizontal forces and the talus does not translate with the fibula.[18] In a bid to quantify if medial damage can be predicted by clinical findings, McConnell and colleagues reported their study on 138 Weber type B supination–external rotation (SER) type ankle injuries detailing clinical findings and performing stress radiographs.[19] They correlated their findings and defined a positive stress examination as having a medial clear space of greater than 4 mm. They found tenderness as a clinical sign to have a positive predictive value of 56% and negative predictive value of 69%. Swelling only occurred in 24%, 35%, and 69% of SER type II, stress-positive SER type IV, and SER type IV fractures respectively. Ecchymosis was found to be the worst predictor of instability.[19]

The gravity stress test has been shown to be as sensitive as the manual stress test[20] but can be uncomfortable for the patient, and DeAngelis and colleagues believe the stress–external rotation radiograph is at least as sensitive and more comfortable.

These findings were validated by DeAngelis and coworkers in their study of 55 Weber B fractures[21]; 23.6% of patients with medial tenderness had stable stress examinations, whereas 18.2% of patients with no medial tenderness had positive stress examinations. Schuberth and colleagues examined the deltoid arthroscopically after clinical examination in a similar patient subset and found a high false-positive for deltoid incompetence in patients with similar findings.[22]

Medial-sided tenderness as a measure of deltoid incompetence had a sensitivity of 57%, specificity of 59%, positive predictive value of 50%, and negative predictive value of 66%.

Koval and colleagues published a preliminary report showing in their study there was a small subset of patients with 5 mm or more medial clear space who did not have deep deltoid complete disruption after magnetic resonance imaging (MRI) evaluation and who fared well with nonoperative intervention.[23] Thus, they concluded, more work is needed to identify these patients without MRI.

Therefore, we would conclude that a Weber B type fracture with a stress test of less than 5 mm medial clear space could be deemed stable and treated conservatively.

Certain subgroups of patients need to be considered separately when deciding on operative or conservative management for an ankle fracture. Smokers, diabetic patients, elderly patients, and children are discussed briefly in the following sections.

SMOKERS

Patients' status with regard to whether they smoke or not should be ascertained. This may impact their treatment choice with regards to operative versus nonoperative treatment, if fixation is favored, what type of anaesthetic should be used, and subsequent fixation techniques.

A recent paper suggested the odds ratio (OR) for smokers developing any postoperative complication compared with nonsmokers to be 1.9. The OR for smokers having a deep infection was 6.0 and a superficial infection as 1.7. This along with other factors should be taken into consideration when deciding on definitive management for a patient's ankle fracture.[24]

ELDERLY PATIENTS

Historically, surgical treatment of the ankle fracture in the elderly patient was anecdotally associated with high complication rates. Several more recent studies investigated this with reasonable numbers and found complication rates to be comparable to that of a younger patient subgroup.[25] Therefore, they advocate not using age alone as a determining factor in whether or not to operate. The goals of management, however, may be different in the elder patient who may have multiple medical comorbidities, decreased ambulatory status, poor skin quality, and so forth, which must be taken into consideration. Factors such as mental status and ability to comply with postoperative rehabilitation must also be considered. The goal of avoiding longer term posttraumatic osteoarthritis of the ankle in younger patients may be superseded by the benefits of early mobilization, avoidance of complications associated with either anesthesia, prolonged bed rest, or hospital stay.

TREATMENT

General

Serial radiographs should be performed after application of the plaster to ensure adequate reduction of the fracture and then at 1 week and 2 weeks to assess for fracture displacement. The ankle should remain in a cast for 6 weeks and then weight-bearing and physical therapy should commence.

Special Techniques

Treatment consists of identifying the fracture and considering the soft tissues, reducing the fracture if necessary, and stabilizing it to allow the soft tissue swelling to subside and the bones to unite (Figs. 6G-1 through 6G-10). This involves application of a plaster of Paris cast in the majority of cases needing manipulation and a lightweight fiberglass cast in cases of minimal displacement or swelling.

Once the decision has been taken to treat an ankle fracture conservatively, then there are several options available to the clinician, depending on the fracture type, soft tissues, and patient-dependent factors.

In young patients with stable ankle fractures, we routinely place them into plaster of Paris in a well-fitting molded cast for 6 weeks (Video 6G-2). They would have check radiographs at 1 week and 2 weeks to assess for displacement and then would have the plaster removed at 6 weeks. On occasion, once the initial swelling subsides, the plaster becomes looser fitting and, therefore, can be changed to a more snug fit at approximately 2 weeks.

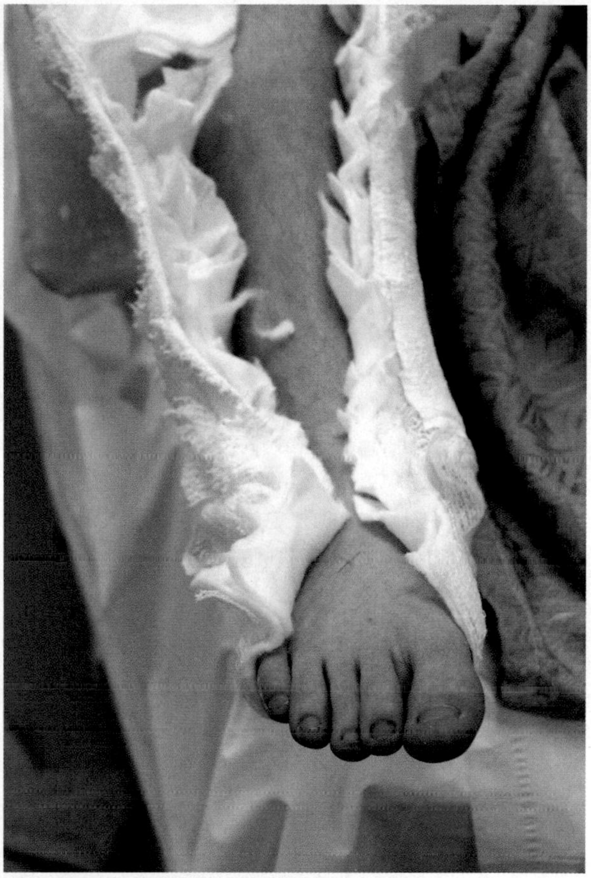

Figure 6G-1. Emergency room stirrup splint split prior to removal.

Thereafter, they would be assessed by a physical therapist and start a standardized rehabilitation program focusing on range of motion, proprioception, and then strengthening exercises.

In some circumstances, additional fixation may be necessary in situations where definitive open reduction and internal fixation is not suitable or possible but plaster alone is not deemed sufficient.

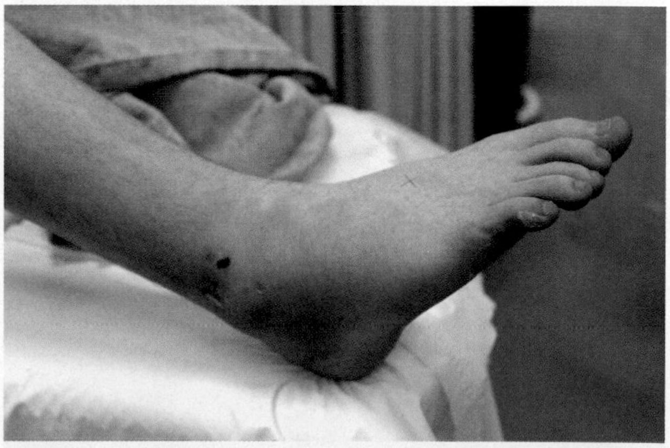

Figure 6G-2. Splint removed. Note fracture blister on the lateral aspect of the ankle.

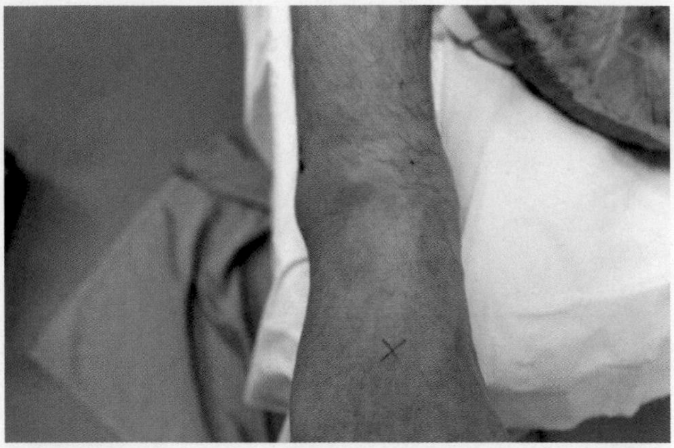

Figure 6G-3. Anterior-posterior (AP) view of the ankle demonstrating displacement.

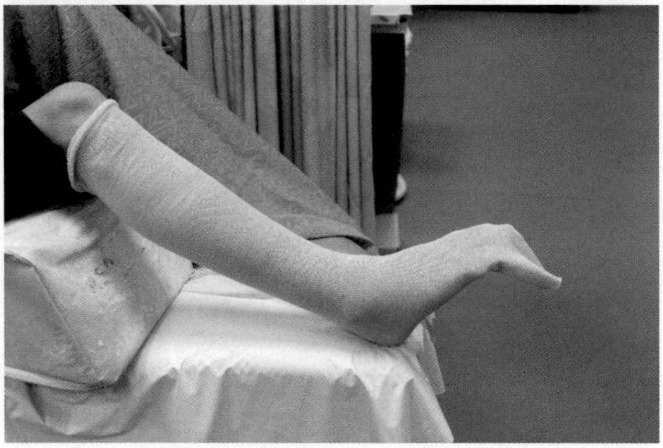

Figure 6G-4. Stockinette applied.

In these situations, the options could be external fixation with a standard construct. We use a delta frame construct with a Hoffmann External Fixation System. A pin is also placed into the base of the first metatarsal to keep the ankle neutral and prevent plantar flexion to aid stability. In grossly unstable fractures with posterior subluxation, placement of the pin into the talar head can provide stability and has not been associated with avascular necrosis of the talus.

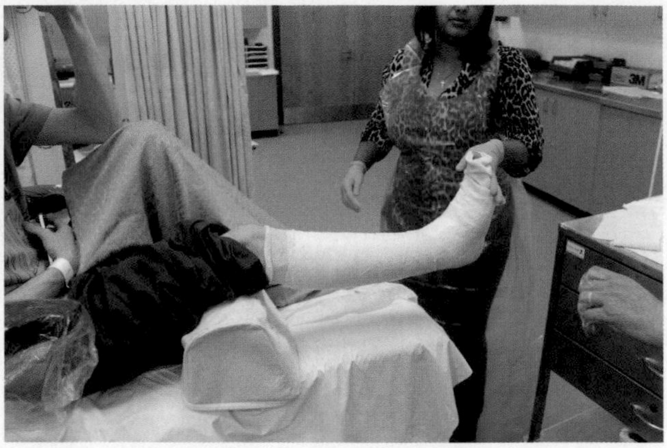

Figure 6G-6. Leg is now held by the toes. The knee remains flexed with the bolster thus relaxing the gastrocnemii. The weight of the leg helps reduce any posterior subluxation of the talus.

Other techniques include the use of Steinmann pins, which can be transcalcaneal as well as transtibial.[26,27]

Richards and others describe a reproducible technique of incorporating two Steinmann pins into plaster. One pin is placed in a transtibial position and one is placed through the calcaneus. The plaster is then applied as usual and the ankle held in the appropriate position while the mold is applied and the cast dries.[28]

Long Term

Relatively few long-term studies exist on conservative treatment of ankle fractures. Kristensen and Hansen showed little functional difference between supination inversion type II injuries treated conservatively and operatively.[29] Again a recent Cochrane review revealed insufficient evidence to support one rehabilitation regimen over another.

CONCLUSION

An approach to ankle fractures based on patient characteristics, fracture type, patient expectations, and the orthopaedist's surgical skill should be developed. The great majority of low-velocity, minimally displaced ankle fractures can be treated

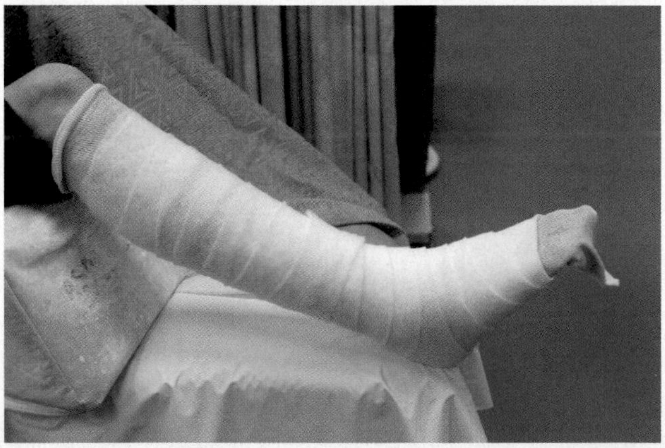

Figure 6G-5. Cast paper applied.

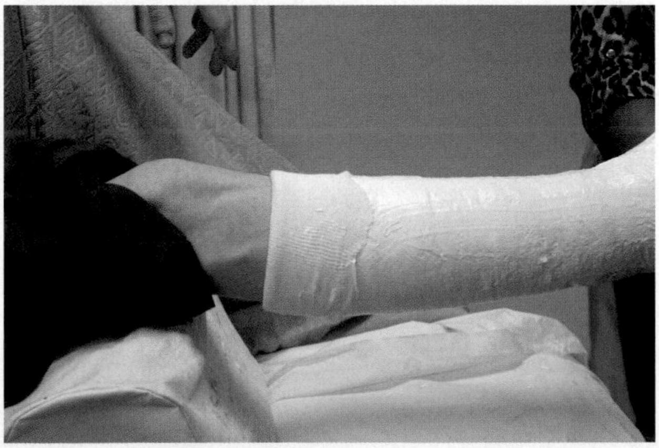

Figure 6G-7. Rolls of plaster applied over the cast paper.

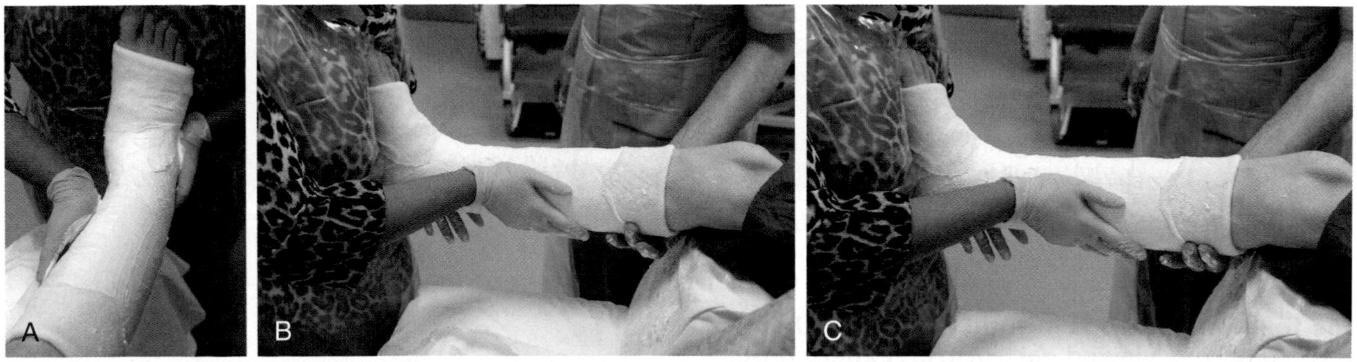

Figure 6G-8. **A** through **C,** Molding of the plaster. Note the lateral hand is on the distal fragment and the medial hand is on the proximal fragment producing a varus mold to maintain the reduction of the fracture.

without surgery, and we advocate this as the primary approach for these patients. High-velocity ankle fractures, ankle fractures associated with marked instability, or fractures in patients with potential high demand for lower limb function should be considered for surgical treatment. Patient-specific factors are extremely important when selecting treatment for ankle fractures. Bone quality, fracture type, condition of the overlying skin, and comorbid conditions, such as diabetes and peripheral vascular disease, are all important in what should be recommended to the patient for the best outcome. In ankle fractures, possibly more than any other fracture, treating the patient rather than the radiograph is the key to success.

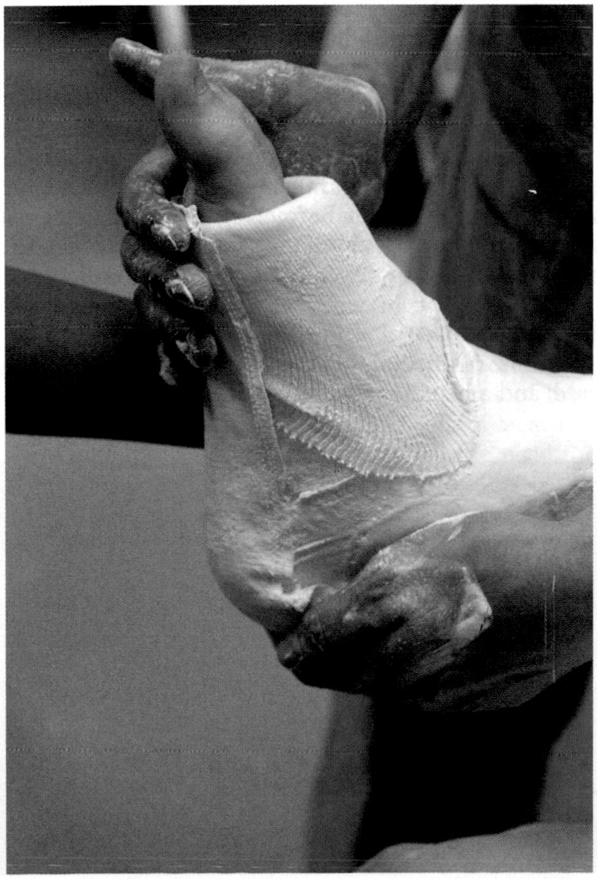

Figure 6G-9. Additional plaster is applied on the plantar surface in order to reinforce the cast.

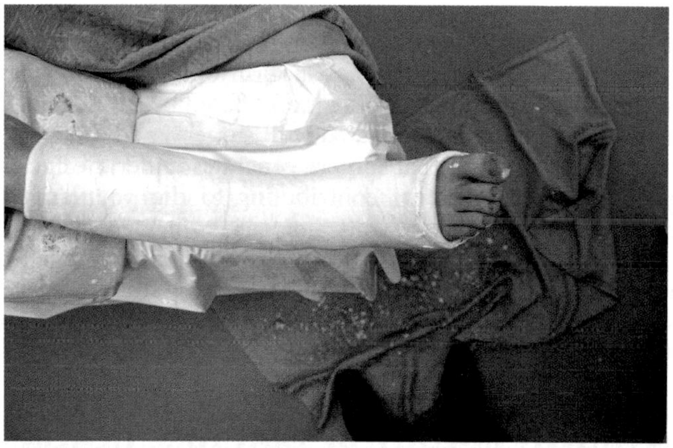

Figure 6G-10. The final appearance of the cast. Note that the stockinette has been finished off with plaster both around the toes and below the knee. Note the smooth contour of the plaster and the well-molded cast.

KEY REFERENCES

The level of evidence (LOE) is determined according to the criteria provided in the preface.

6. Stiell I, Wells G, Laupacis A, et al: Multicentre trial to introduce the Ottawa ankle rules for use of radiography in acute ankle injuries. Multicentre Ankle Rule Study Group. *BMJ* 311(7005):594–597, 1995. LOE II
13. Pakarinen HJ, Flinkkil TE, Ohtonen PP, et al: Stability criteria for non-operative ankle fracture management. *Foot Ankle Int* 32(2):141–147, 2011. LOE III
14. Michelson JD, Magid D, McHale K: Clinical utility of a stability-based ankle fracture classification system. *J Orthop Trauma* 21(5):307–315, 2007. LOE IV
20. Michelson MD, Varner KE, Checcone M: Diagnosing deltoid ligament injury in ankle fractures: The gravity stress view. *Clin Orthop Relat Res* 387:178–182, 2001.
23. Koval KJ, Egol KA, Cheung Y, et al: Does a positive ankle stress test indicate the need for operative treatment after lateral malleolus fracture? A preliminary report. *J Orthop Trauma* 21(7):449–455, 2007. LOE III
25. Vioreanu M, Brophy S, Dudeney S, et al: Displaced ankle fractures in the geriatric population: operative or non-operative treatment. *Foot Ankle Surg* 13:10–14, 2007. LOE II
29. Kristensen KD, Hansen T: Closed treatment of ankle fractures: stage II supination-eversion fractures followed for 20 years. *Acta Orthop Scand* 56:107–109, 1985. LOE III

The complete References list is available online at https://expertconsult.inkling.com.

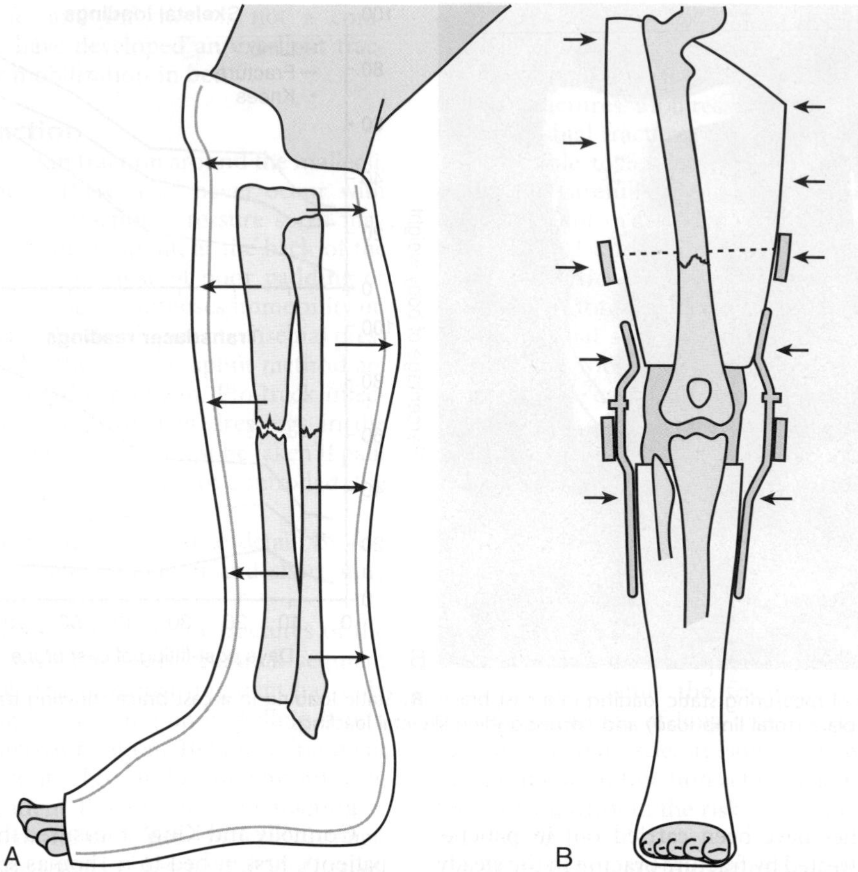

Figure 6I-4. Forces at the skin–cast interface in tibial bracing (**A**) and in femoral bracing (**B**).

fracture bracing in both static studies[40] and dynamic studies[42] and by intracast pressure studies[46] (see Fig. 6I-4). This is contrary to a suggestion of Meggit and colleagues,[41] who described a femoral fracture brace treating lower third fractures as "an anti-buckling hinged tube" preventing the development of lateral angulation. Hardy and Baddeley[47] measured the pressures generated in the thigh muscle and at the skin–cast interface in a normal subject wearing a cast brace. The pressures increased during muscle contraction and were highest under the ischial seat. Hardy[48] measured the pressures at the skin cast interface in patients with similar findings and suggested that during muscle contraction, there was an increased stabilizing effect on the fracture. This probably also serves to increase the venous and lymphatic return and will be beneficial for the circulation.

The development of angulation within a cast brace has been very carefully studied. The tendency to angulation is undoubtedly greater in middle and upper third fractures. It may be seen in postapplication check radiographs of the fracture in the brace. It is present either because angulation was allowed to develop and was present as the brace was applied or the brace was not a snug fit, and after release of traction, the extra space within the brace was taken up by the limb settling into the brace with shortening and angulation. The idea that the brace becomes loose after a period of time is quite wrong. The measurement of thigh volume within a fracture brace has been carried out using magnetic resonance imaging (MRI) and demonstrated that limb volume does not change throughout the period of fracture treatment.[42] MRI showed that the quality of muscle improved as recovery of function progressed. Therefore, limb volume does not change, and provided the brace is a snug fit, angulation does not occur. Experience with hip hinges showed that holding the hip in abduction using a hip hinge required a very large force and was quite impractical in reality. Therefore, a hip hinge may control alignment because it tends to pull the brace proximally on the conical shaped thigh, creating a snug fit. Some patients with upper third fractures have pain on mobilization. This occurs because the short section of the brace around the proximal fragment does not control rotation well. Application of a hip hinge attached to a pelvic band in a neutral position controls or abolishes this pain.

The recovery of muscle function in an unselected series of femoral shaft fractures treated by fracture bracing was shown to be equal to a series treated by closed intramedullary nailing[49] and significantly superior to a selected series treated by open nailing.[50] This shows that direct operative treatment on a fracture causes permanent muscle damage and adhesion formation, significantly affecting its function.

Two cases in which refracture of a fractured tibia occurred in a fracture brace showed that in both cases, poor proximal rotatory control had been imparted on the fracture because of poor brace fitting. A study was made of the properly applied upper section of a tibial fracture brace. This showed that in full extension to 30 degrees of flexion, 63% of a torsional load applied to the foot was resisted; at 60 degrees of flexion, this decreased to 13%. The implications of these findings are that during the stance phase of gait, significant resistance to torsional forces is imparted by the proximal section of the brace because during stance, normally the limb does not flex beyond much more than 20 degrees. Finally, Svend-Hansen and colleagues[51] showed that there was no difference in the load beneath the foot in a subject wearing three different casts: a below-knee cast, a Sarmiento-type patellar tendon bearing (PTB) brace, and a long leg cast with the knee in 20 degrees of flexion, indicating that the PTB portion did not significantly off-load the fracture.

Thus in lower limb fracture bracing the fracture brace acts to provide the functional environment for fracture healing where the brace controls alignment and minimizes rotatory and angulatory forces. There is a feedback mechanism from the fracture site to the patient's central nervous system which controls the degree of longitudinal stress through the fracture depending on the degree of union. As union progresses the patient is able to gradually increase weight-bearing on the limb, until at union of the fracture, full weight-bearing in the brace can be achieved.

Application Procedure for Femoral Fracture Bracing

The patient is transferred from bed to the fracture cast table and seated on a low plinth to allow easy access around the back of the thigh for application of the brace. At this stage, the traction cords are removed, and with the leg still resting on Thomas splint, the skeletal traction is removed from the tibia. Dressings are applied to the pin sites, and a fracture cast sock is rolled on. Double stockinette may be used with a piece of tubigrip at the knee to control edema. Further short pieces of stockinette are positioned above and below the knee and at the upper end of the thigh so that when the bandage has been rolled on, these can be folded back, creating a rounded edge. One 5-inch-wide polyurethane-impregnated fiberglass bandage is adequate for the average thigh. The upper thigh portion of the cast should be molded into a quadrilateral shape (Fig. 6I-5), either using the flat of one's hands or using a plastic quadrilateral brim (Fig. 6I-6) to create the molding (Fig. 6I-7). During this procedure, the assistant supports the knee in the most comfortable position of knee flexion with one hand, and

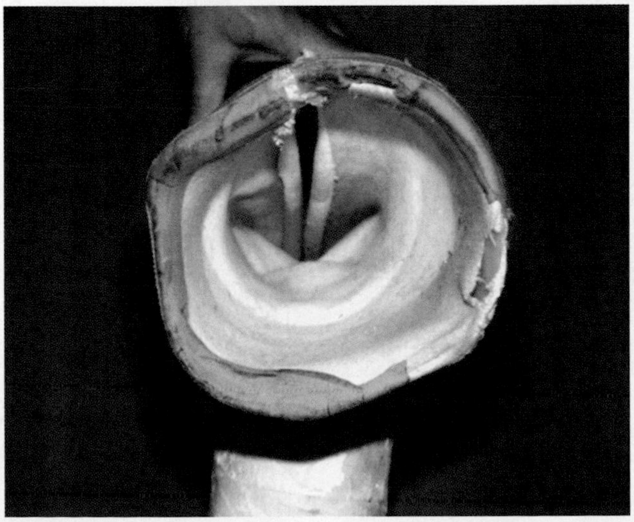

Figure 6I-5. Molding looking down through the brim of a cast brace after removal.

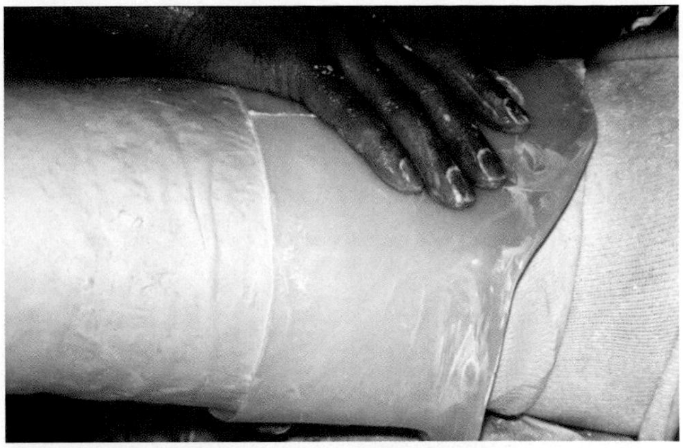

Figure 6I-6. Plastic brim used to create quadrilateral top to the thigh portion of the femoral brace.

with the other hand gripping the leg above the ankle, applies gentle traction. As the thigh portion is hardening, the operator molds the thigh with an anterior bow. The below-knee portion of the cast is then applied, again with the knee held in the most comfortable position of knee flexion and the foot in a plantigrade position in the same way as a below-knee cast. The leg is then rested over a pillow or pillows with the knee in 20 to 30 degrees of flexion. This ensures that the patella is pointing forward and makes it easy for the knee hinges to be aligned correctly. As an aid, a cross is marked in the center of the patella (see Fig. 6I-8), and the transverse axis should be opposite the adductor tubercle (Fig. 6I-8). Metal hinges are preferred to plastic ones because they bend freely in a fixed axis, ensuring that flexion occurs only at the knee (Fig. 6I-9). If the hinges are not parallel or in the same axis as the knee, then on flexion, shearing stress is applied to the hinge attachments to the plaster, causing them to loosen.[52] Plastic ones are considered easier to apply but require more effort for the patient to overcome their resistance in knee flexion, and they often balloon outward under the weight of the thigh portion of the cast, causing this to lose its snug fit. This may allow the fracture to angulate. The hinges are best aligned using a jig after bending the metal arms with plate benders to allow 1 cm or half an inch gap from the knee itself (Fig. 6I-10). They are aligned at right angles to the long axis of the tibia at the level of the adductor tubercle two-thirds of the way from front to

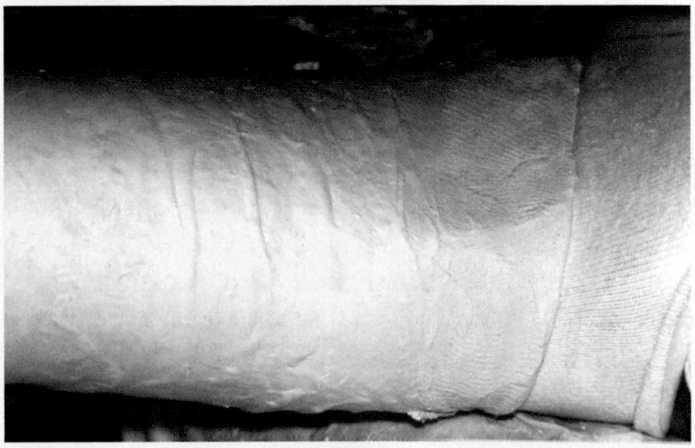

Figure 6I-7. Molding of the upper thigh cast produced by plastic brim.

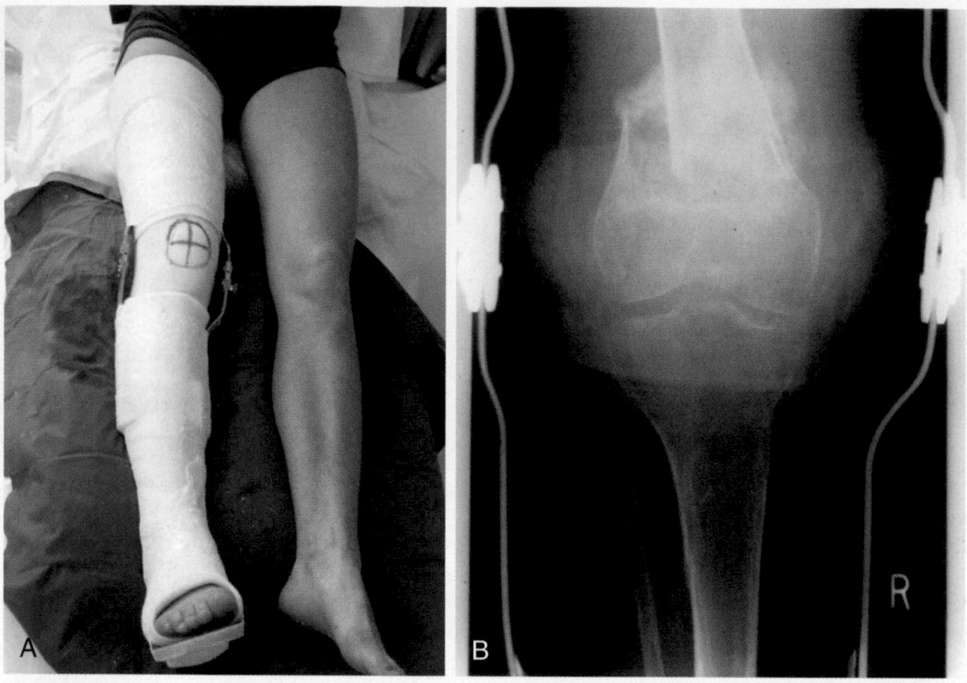

Figure 61-8. A, A cross is drawn on the patella to aid centering of the knee hinges. **B,** A radiograph demonstrates the hinges centered opposite the adductor tubercle.

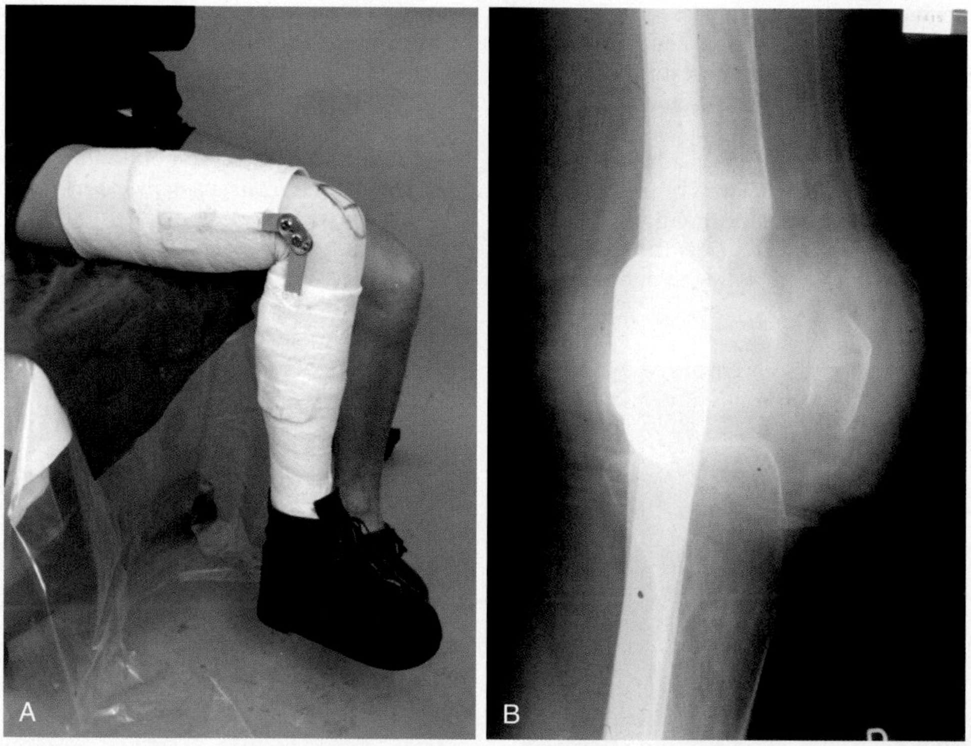

Figure 61-9. A, Knee flexion occurs in the axis of the knee. **B,** Lateral radiograph showing the centering of the hinges opposite the level of the adductor tubercle two-thirds of the way from anterior to posterior.

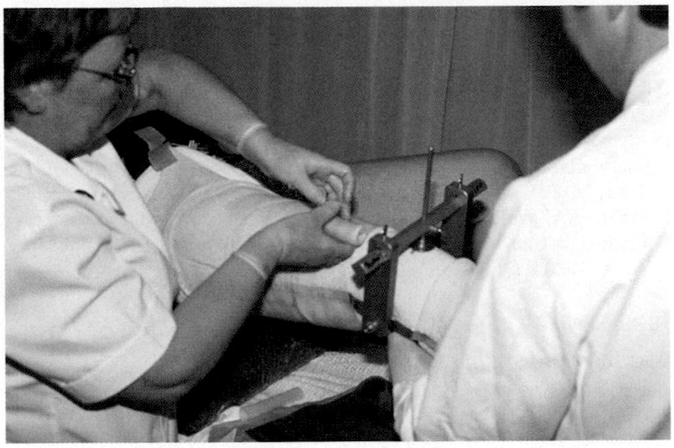

Figure 6I-10. A jig attached to the hinges is used to aid alignment to the knee.

back of the knee. They may be held in position with Jubilee clips while further rolls of bandage are applied over the flanges to fix the hinges in position. The back of the lower part of the cast and sole may be strengthened with a slab of material, and often a Plastazote sole is used to act as a buffer. Immobilizing the foot does not lead to ankle stiffness.[33] The patient can immediately begin mobilizing after the plaster is fully hardened (Fig. 6I-11). If the fracture is in the upper third of the shaft, it is best to hold the leg in abduction during application to relax the pull of the abductor muscles, which tend to pull the upper fragment, causing lateral angulation of the fracture. Finally, a hip hinge is applied to provide further rotator stability to the proximal fragment. It should be aligned with the hinge axis just above and anterior to the greater trochanter (Fig. 6I-12, *A*) and will allow only flexion and extension of the hip, which are adequate for ambulation (Fig. 6I-12, *B*).

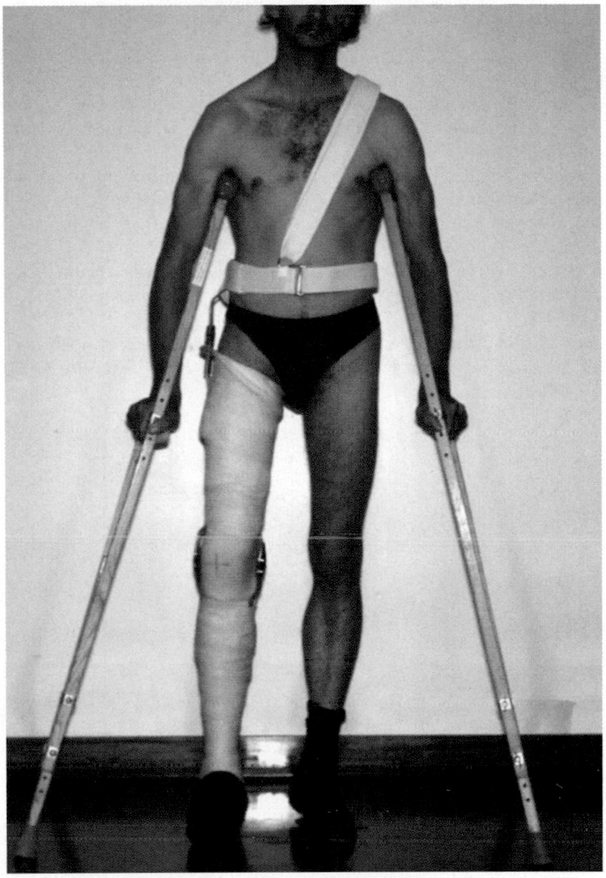

Figure 6I-11. Patient ambulating with crutches. This patient has an upper third fracture with a hip hinge.

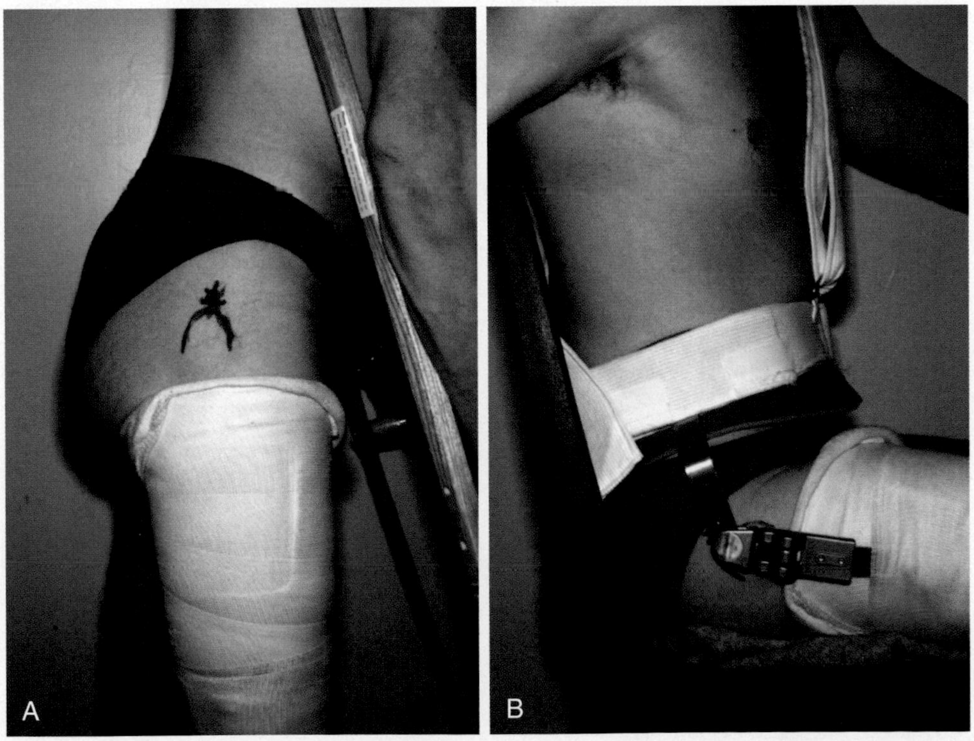

Figure 6I-12. **A,** Center of axis for the hip hinge. **B,** The hinge in position.

KEY REFERENCES

The level of evidence (LOE) is determined according to the criteria provided in the preface.

17. Ricker HA, Bajema SL, Bagg RJ: Modification of the Thomas' splint with Pearson attachment for balanced suspension. *J Bone Joint Surg Am* 53:787–790, 1971. LOE III
19. Patterson FP: Results of conservative treatment of fracture of the shaft of the femur. *J Bone Joint Surg Br* 43:611, 1961. LOE III
21. Wardlaw D: The cast brace treatment of femoral shaft fractures. *J Bone Joint Surg Br* 59:411–416, 1977. LOE III
25. Dehne E, Metz CW, Deffer PA, et al: Non operative treatment of the fractured tibia by immediate weight bearing. *J Trauma* 1:514–535, 1961. LOE III
28. Brown PW, Urban JG: Early weight-bearing treatment of open fractures of the tibia. An end-result study of 63 cases. *J Bone Joint Surg Am* 51(1): 59–75, 1969. LOE III
32. Dehne E: The weight-bearing principle in treatment of lower extremity fractures, 1885-1972. *J Trauma* 12:539–540, 1972. LOE IV
36. Sarmiento A: A functional below-the-knee brace for tibial fractures. A report on its use in 135 cases. *J Bone Joint Surg Am* 52:259–311, 1970. LOE III
41. Meggit BF, Juett DA, Smith JD: Cast bracing for fractures of the femoral shaft: a biomechanical and clinical study. *J Bone Joint Surg Br* 63:12–23, 1981. LOE III
44. White AA, Wolfe JW, Panjabi MM, et al: Rigid fixation versus cyclical loading in the management of experimental fractures. *Orthop Transl* 4:356, 1980. LOE II

The complete References list is available online at https://expertconsult.inkling.com.

Chapter 7

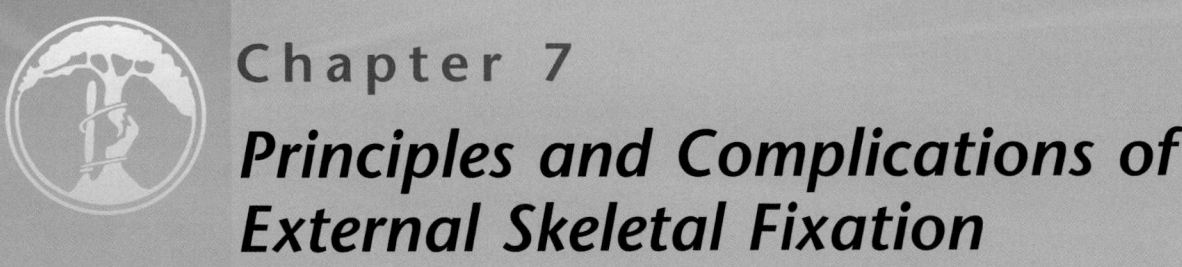

Principles and Complications of External Skeletal Fixation

STUART A. GREEN

Additional videos related to the subject of this chapter are available from the Medizinische Hochschule Hannover collection. The following video is included with this chapter and may be viewed at https://expertconsult.inkling.com:

7-1. The modular technique of applying external fixation.

7-2. Taylor Spatial Frame.

HISTORICAL BACKGROUND

Early Fixators

The external fixator was invented 12 years before the plaster cast. In 1846, Jean Francois Malgaigne devised an ingenious mechanism consisting of a clamp that approximated four transcutaneous metal prongs to reduce and maintain patellar fractures[1] (Fig. 7-1). In the 160 years since Malgaigne's invention, many other external fixation systems have been introduced. Among the best known are the Parkhill bone clamp (1897),[2] Lambotte's monolateral external fixator (1902),[3] Roger Anderson's 1934 fixation system,[4] the 1937 Stader apparatus—originally developed for managing fractures in large dogs[5]—and the external fixator of Swiss physician Raoul Hoffmann (1938)[6] (Fig. 7-2).

Several of these devices saw use during the Second World War. Toward the end of that cataclysm, however, the high incidence of complications associated with external fixation became apparent. The major disadvantages noted by a military commission who studied the matter included nerve and vessel injuries by pins, the presence of soft tissue infections at the pin sites, the possibility of ring sequestra and osteomyelitis, and the danger of delayed union or nonunion. Other surgeons were distressed by the mechanical difficulty associated with external fixators, as well as by the prospect of converting a closed fracture to an open fracture.[2] As a consequence, by 1950 most American orthopaedic surgeons were not using mechanical fixators although the pins-in-plaster technique was used for special problems, such as unstable wrist fractures[7] and displaced fractures of the tibia and fibula.[8]

In Europe, conversely, clinical research on external skeletal fixation continued throughout the years during and following World War II. Raoul Hoffmann improved his device, providing a stronger universal joint and an enlarged pin-gripper that held the pins more securely. Charnley, of England, presented his concept of compression arthrodesis of the major joints,[9] using a rather simple skeletal fixator that provided continuous compression of cancellous surfaces of the joint to be fused. In time, the Arbeitsgemeinschaft für Osteosynthesefragen (AO) group of Switzerland modified Charnley's device to more pins in his frame configuration.[10]

Also in France during the 1960s, Jacques Vidal and coworkers used Hoffmann's equipment but designed a quadrilateral frame to provide rigid stabilization of complex fracture problems and septic pseudarthroses under treatment[11] (Fig. 7-3, *A*).

Fixators for Limb Lengthening

External fixators specifically designed for limb lengthening began to appear after W. V. Anderson developed an apparatus that employed full transcutaneous pins connected to threaded bars.[12] The device permitted gradual distraction of an osteotomized bone. Heinz Wagner,[13] working in Germany, modified Anderson's concept even further, substituting half-pins for Anderson's full pins, while employing a universal distraction bar that patients could lengthen themselves (Fig. 7-3, *B*). These pioneers accurately recorded the incidence of complications with their techniques, some of which are unique to limb lengthening.[14]

In Russia, external fixation as a modality for fracture treatment remained viable in the period subsequent to World War II. Surgeons in that country focused attention on ring-type fixators that were connected to the bone by thin transfixion wires tensioned by special wire-gripping clamps. While these fixators were quite cumbersome, some contained ingenious geared articulations that permitted precise displacement of the rings in any of three planes independently.

Circular Fixators

In 1951, Dr. Gavriil A. Ilizarov of Kurgan in the former Soviet Union developed the first model of his transfixion-wire circular fixator, which is still used today[15] (Fig. 7-3, *C*). Other Soviet surgeons subsequently designed similar devices, some with geared couplers that allowed gradual repositioning of bone fragments. Within a few years, Ilizarov discovered that bone would form in a widening distraction gap under appropriate conditions of stability, delay, and distraction.[16] His observations and subsequent clinical research revolutionized deformity correction and limb salvage surgery and contributed to a revived worldwide interest in circular external fixation.[17]

Ilizarov's apparatus consists of separate components that can be assembled into an unlimited number of different configurations that allow a surgeon to perform:

The percutaneous treatment of all closed metaphyseal and diaphyseal fractures as well as many epiphyseal fractures

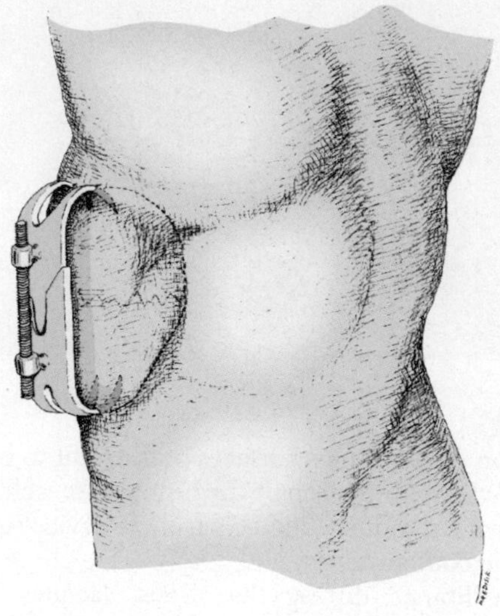

Figure 7-1. Malgaigne's 1846 external fixator for patellar fractures.

The repair of extensive defects of bone, nerve, vessel, and soft tissues without the need for grafting—and in one operative stage
Bone thickening for cosmetic and functional reasons
The percutaneous one-stage treatment of congenital or traumatic pseudarthroses
Limb lengthening or growth retardation by distraction epiphysiolysis or other methods
The correction of long bone and joint deformities, including resistant and relapsed clubfeet
The percutaneous elimination of joint contractures
The treatment of various arthroses by osteotomy and repositioning of the articular surfaces
Percutaneous joint arthrodesis
Elongating arthrodesis—a method of fusing major joints without concomitant limb shortening
The filling in of solitary bone cysts and other such lesions
The treatment of septic nonunion by the favorable effect on infected bone of stimulating bone healing

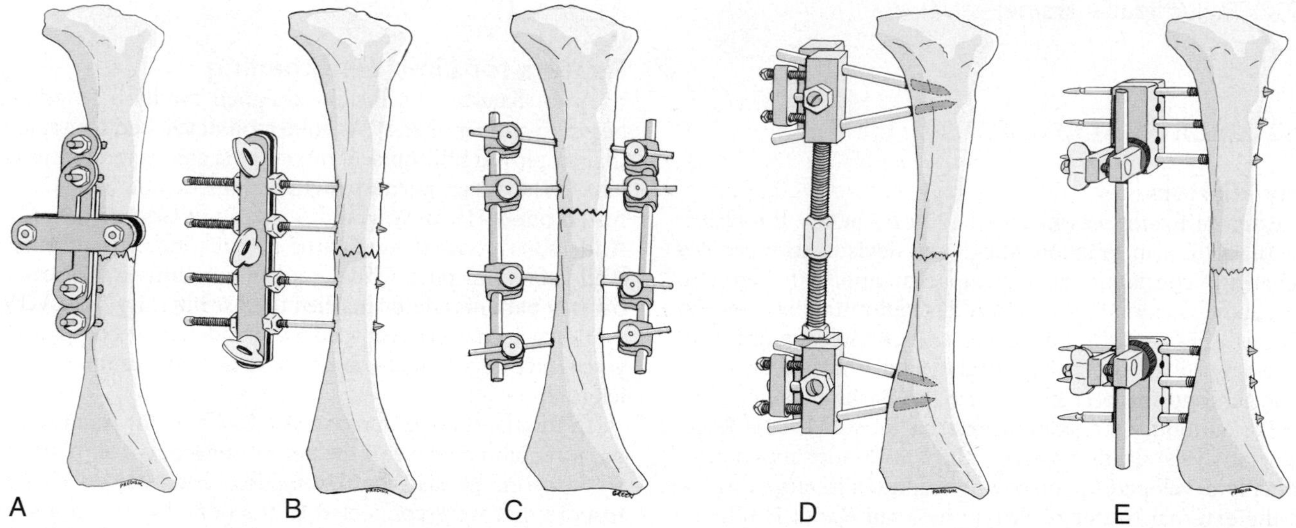

Figure 7-2. Historic external fixators. **A,** Parkhill bone clamp. **B,** Lambotte fixator. **C,** Anderson apparatus. **D,** Stader apparatus. **E,** Hoffmann fixator.

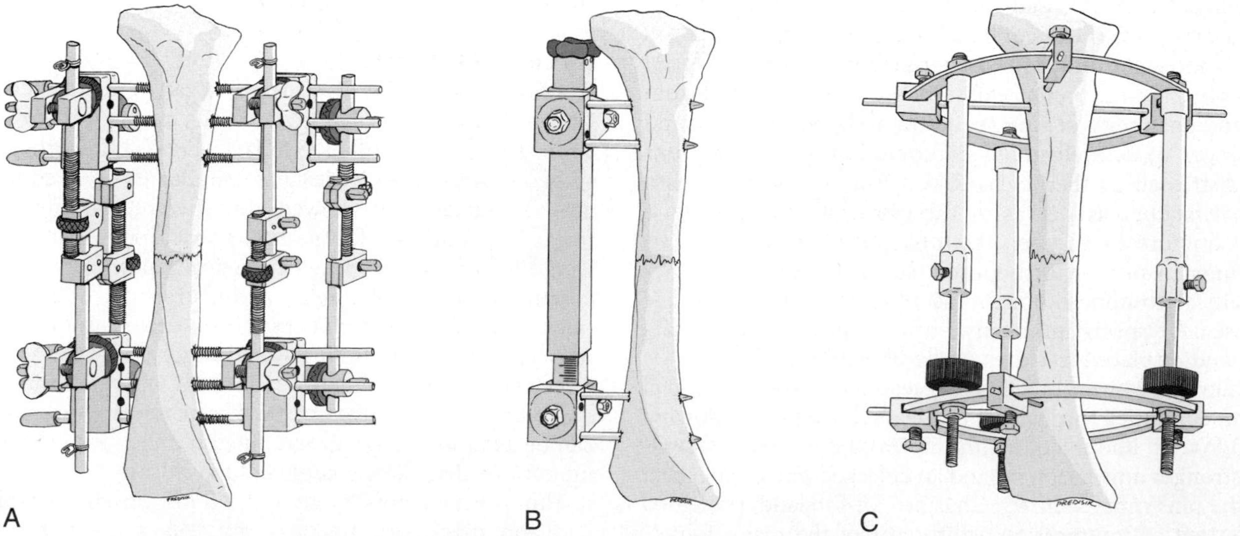

Figure 7-3. Modern external fixators. **A,** Vidal quadrilateral frame. **B,** Wagner limb lengthener. **C,** Ilizarov apparatus.

- The filling of osteomyelitic cavities by the gradual collapsing of one cavity wall
- The lengthening of amputation stumps
- Management of hypoplasia of the mandible and similar conditions
- The ability to overcome certain occlusive vascular diseases without bypass grafting
- The correction of achondroplastic and other forms of dwarfism

An American orthopaedist, David Fischer, visited Moscow in 1975 where he obtained several different Soviet circular external fixators. After applying these frames to his own patients, he became concerned with the problems of frame instability associated with transfixion wires, as well as the perceived weight of the circular frames he tried. Thereafter, Fischer developed a circular fixator, which attached to bone via full pins and half-pins.[18] The entire system was originally fabricated from titanium—a lightweight, yet strong metal. In general, he noted fewer pin-site infections when his device was mounted with titanium pins instead of steel implants. Moreover, when titanium pin-site sepsis did occur, the reaction was more benign appearing, with far less cellulitis and soft tissue reaction than was commonly observed with steel pins.

North American orthopaedic surgeons, exposed to Ilizarov's methods by Italian practitioners in the mid-1980s, modified Ilizarov's technique. Among the most useful of these improvements has been the fabrication of rings and plates of the Ilizarov apparatus from radiolucent carbon fiber. This material, while more expensive than steel, is substantially lighter and thus popular with the patients.

At Rancho Los Amigos Medical Center, the author and his coworkers began using titanium half-pins (in place of steel wires) to secure Ilizarov's circular fixator to long bones requiring either limb lengthening or deformity correction.[19] In this manner, the adaptability of the circular device was retained, but the problem of muscle impalement and transfixion was reduced, especially in bones such as the ulna or tibia that have large subcutaneous surfaces. In certain anatomic locations, however, wire mounts still appeared superior to pin mountings—especially in the juxtaarticular regions where cancellous bone predominates. For more substantial fragments that include both the articular and metaphyseal regions, combinations of pins and wires have proven successful for mounting circular external skeletal fixation.[20]

Several new fixator configurations have been devised specifically for applications that require anchorage in cancellous bone at one end of the frame and cortical bone on the other. These fixators, which are often referred to as *hybrid designs*, usually combine an Ilizarov-type ring with an AO-type tubular bar. The tensioned wires are secured to the ring (which surrounds the cancellous portion of the bone) while the bar connects to half-pins in the cortical bone.

Ring fixators have a distinct advantage over unilateral or bilateral devices because the apparatus—especially Ilizarov's device—permits a surgeon to gradually reposition fracture fragments (or osseous fragments following osteotomy) with respect to each other in three-dimensional space. To match this capability, several new unilateral fixators incorporate geared articulations that permit the controlled movement of one pin-gripper with respect to the others.

Fixators for Severe Trauma

One modern concept of care for severe polytrauma starts with the application of a simple external fixator for preliminary stabilization of each seriously injured limb, followed by more definitive reconstruction later on.[21] The goal of most surgeons who apply a fixator for the temporary stabilization of a limb is to convert from external fixation to internal fixation, usually an intramedullary nail. The concept is discussed at length later in the section, "Using the Atlas for Damage Control Orthopaedics."

While a number of protocols have been recommended to reduce the likelihood of such an infection, one promising concept has been the development of a "pinless" external skeletal fixator by the AO group. With this device, a spring-loaded pair of pins that resemble ice tongs, which grip the cortex but do not penetrate into the endosteal surface, secures bone fragments. In this manner, the medullary canal is (in theory, at least) free of microbial contamination. Time will tell if such an invention reduces the incidence of implant sepsis when an intramedullary nail replaces an external fixator.

A complete understanding of the ideal milieu for rapid fracture healing has yet to be ascertained. Around the world, pioneering clinicians and researchers are using fixators to study the influence of stability, distraction, and compression on fracture healing and regenerate new bone formation. The results of these studies will certainly advance the clinical applications of both internal fixation and external fixation, and improve fracture care in general.

When trauma surgeons discovered in the mid-1980s that open fractures could safely be treated with intramedullary nails, it appeared that external fixation's role in orthopaedic surgery would be greatly diminished. Ilizarov's discovery of distraction osteogenesis, however, has rendered the prediction of external fixation's demise premature indeed. Fixators have become an important part of deformity correction, especially where limb elongation is a concomitant requirement. For this reason, worldwide use of external skeletal fixation is on the rise again, as it was before World War II and again in the 1970s and early 1980s.

Computerized Correction

In the 1990s, Dr. Charles Taylor—codeveloper of the Russell-Taylor intramedullary nail—realized that the reduction of a displaced bone fragment (or correction of a deformity) could be accomplished by mathematically defining the path a bone fragment travels as it moves from its displaced position to its corrected position.[22] Using an ingenious design, Taylor connected rings of an Ilizarov-type circular fixator to each other with six struts, each of which could be independently lengthened or shortened (Fig. 7-4). In this way, the relationship between the rings can be altered in a precise manner, modifying the relationship of the rings—and their attached bone fragments—to each other.[22]

After measuring the precise displacement of the bone fragments and the relationship between the fragments and their respective rings, the data are fed into a computer that has been programmed to determine the pathway to reduction in all planes—angulation, rotation, shortening, and translation.[23] Moreover, the computer program outputs a schedule of strut length changes needed to effect the reduction at whatever predetermined speed is needed for both safety and efficacy. The system, called the Taylor Spatial Frame, is

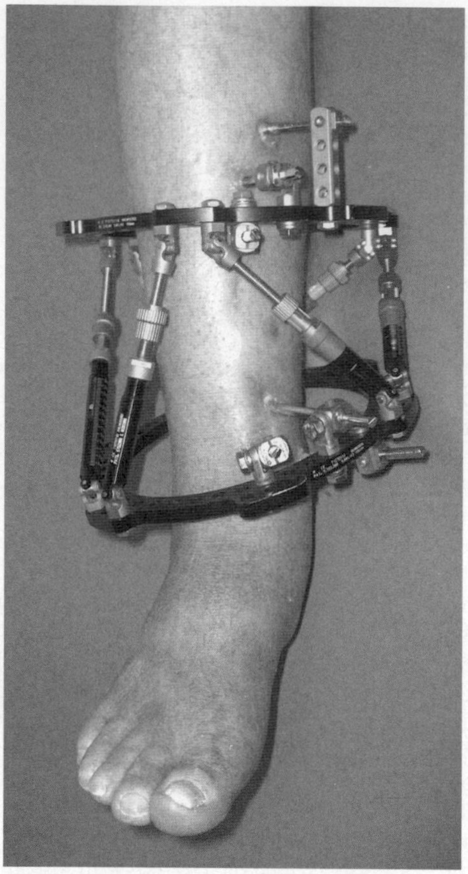

Figure 7-4. **The Taylor Spatial Frame.** Six adjustable struts control the relationship between the two rings, one of which must be mounted orthogonal to either the proximal or distal fragment. All deformity and mounting parameters are fed into a computer, which calculates the strut length changes needed to restore the displaced fragment to anatomic alignment.

quite popular with surgeons who have become familiar with its use.[24]

Combined Internal and External Fixation

Certain additional developments have occurred since the last edition of this book. External fixation is now frequently combined with internal fixation to reduce the total time and external fixation frame.[25-27] This strategy not only reduces patient discomfort and problems with activities of daily living, but also reduces the incidence of pin tract infections, which rises slowly but steadily during the time a fixator is in place. This evolution started with lengthening over an intramedullary nail, a strategy devised in the Baltimore protocol by Paley and coworkers,[28] whereby an intramedullary nail is inserted into a bone following osteotomy for limb elongation. During the same operative session, an external fixator is applied to the limb with care to avoid contact or even close proximity of the transosseous implants with the intramedullary implant. This requires careful fluoroscopy-controlled pin or wire insertion.

Typically, pins or wires are inserted from the posterior to the implant in the femur and tibia, although anterior placement is also acceptable.

The strategy is particularly appealing to patients who can have the fixator removed and transverse locking screws inserted into the limb as soon as the distraction phase of the treatment protocol has been completed. Thereafter, ordinary weight-bearing, usually with ambulatory aid support to protect the implant, continues until the regenerate bone forms around the implant.

Two comparable strategies have evolved in recent years, both coming from the group at the Hospital for Special Surgery in New York.[29,30] The first is lengthening and then nailing, a strategy that starts out with a typical Ilizarov-type lengthening that would consist of either a classic ring fixator or a modified ring fixator, such as the Taylor Spatial Frame (particularly if there is concomitant deformity correction), or even a multilateral fixator. Once the deformity is fully corrected and the bone is straight, with early regenerate formation in the distraction gap, an intramedullary nail is inserted and secured with transverse locking screws, and the fixator is removed. Obviously, the transcutaneous transosseous implants must be inserted in a place far enough away from the anticipated medullary canal passage of the nail to prevent contamination by microbes in the pin or wire tract.[29,30]

Another strategy from the same facility involves the use of external skeletal fixation to achieve length, followed by the use of a plate and screws to shorten the fixator time once the final position of the bone has been achieved.[29] The advent of locking plates makes such a strategy possible, because the plate often has to span a zone where the regenerate new bone is very weak, sometimes only a wispy shadow, thus requiring a particularly strong and stable plate and screw fixation (Video 7-1).

Fixator-Assisted Nailing

With certain kinds of periarticular osteotomies, such as a high tibial osteotomy or distal femoral osteotomy, precise control of the osseous fragments is essential to a successful outcome. Where internal fixation, particularly intramedullary fixation, is employed to secure the fragments, it is helpful to use a temporary external skeletal fixator for alignment after osteotomy, but before inserting the definitive implant. In this case, as with lengthening over a nail, or lengthening and then nailing, the transcutaneous transosseous implants must be situated in a way that does not block placement of the definitive hardware. However, unlike situations where the fixator will be left on for some protracted period of time, temporary application of a fixator in the operating room for alignment purposes does not risk implant-site sepsis where the transcutaneous pins or wires come in contact with the definitive implants. Therefore, the technique is particularly appealing where precision is required.

External Skeletal Fixation in the Future

Profound changes in implant technology will soon cause a paradigm shift in the use of external skeletal fixation. Self-lengthening intramedullary nails will stimulate the change. Initially, such devices used mechanical methods to elongate. Specifically, a ratchet mechanism within the device caused the implant to lengthen when the proximal portion of the nail was rotated with respect to the distal portion. Three nails using this strategy, the Bliskunov, the Albizzia, and the intramedullary skeletal kinetic distractor (ISKD),[31] all had the same drawbacks. Because these implants elongated with limb rotation, they would sometimes lengthen too fast, particularly if the patient was too active with the device in place.[32,33] Conversely, if the distraction proceeded too slowly, early hardening of the regenerate new bone would prevent counterrotation of the fragments, necessitating a return trip to the operating room for osteotomy of the regenerate.[34]

The second generation of self-lengthening nails uses internal rotating components and threaded spindles to motor the elongation. In one case, the Fitbone, an electric motor energized through a subcutaneous induction coil powers the lengthening.[35,36] A rotating magnet, responding to external magnetic fields, elongates both the Phenix and the Precice intramedullary nails. The devices are so new, that a body of literature does not exist yet that supports their use.

These self-lengthening implants allow gradual limb elongation without the use of bulky external skeletal fixation. Likewise, the absence of transcutaneous implants associated with fixators greatly reduces patient discomfort with internal lengthening devices. Moreover, pin tract infections are a thing of the past with self-lengthening nails.

At present, none of the internal lengthening implants can achieve active deformity correction as part of the elongation process. However, a new strategy combining wedge resection and deformity correction (often stabilized with plates and screws) with a self-lengthening nail will eliminate the use of external skeletal fixation for substantial limb deformities. Instead, the deformity will be corrected and secured with internal fixation until the fragments unite. Thereafter, a self-lengthening nail will restore limb length.

Alternatively, implants are being developed that consist of bone plates containing self-lengthening mechanisms, permitting both deformity correction and limb elongation with one operation. While the cost of such implants may limit their use to the more affluent nations, the ability to simultaneously lengthen and realign a limb without the use of external skeletal fixation is clearly appealing.

What then will be the role of external skeletal fixation when such devices become available? Certainly, damage-control orthopaedics employing temporizing fixators will continue as a strategy for initial trauma management.[31] Likewise, fixator-assisted surgery will continue to play a role where precise correction of a deformity before applying any internal fixation plate or intramedullary nail is required.

A bewildering variety of fixators possessing ingenious articulations and pin-grippers are currently available. Surgical appliance manufacturers continue to add new components and fixator frames to the marketplace at a steady pace, even as the demand for external fixators may diminish in the future. The devices vary considerably in configuration and in technique of frame assembly. The feature common to all fixators, however, is that they are attached to the human body with pins or wires that penetrate the skin and affix to bone. The complications associated with transcutaneous pins are thus common to all past, present, and future fixators, regardless of design or construction. Reducing pin-site sepsis will, more than any other measure, ensure the continued development of external skeletal fixation.

FIXATOR TERMINOLOGY

Pin: The term pin refers to that portion of the fixator that penetrates the skin and soft tissues and attaches to bone. In the European literature, pins are sometimes referred to as *screws* or *nails* (the distinction resting perhaps on the presence or absence of threads).

Full pin: A full pin is one that protrudes through the skin and soft tissues on both sides of the limb. Such pins are sometimes referred to as *transfixion* pins or *through-and-through* pins.

Half-pins: A half-pin is one that penetrates the skin and soft tissues on one side of the limb only and that penetrates bone but does not emerge on the other side of the limb. When inserted, such pins are supposed to penetrate both cortices of the bone but not much beyond the second cortex.

Wire: A thin transosseous implant, usually less than 2 mm in diameter, which is not stiff enough to provide stability to a fixator-bone configuration until tensioned and bolted to the fixator. For this reason, most wires must penetrate the entire limb and be secured to the fixator at both ends.

Olive wire: A wire with a bead somewhere along its length, which prevents the wire from being pulled through the bone. An olive wire can be employed to pull bone fragments into position or to enhance stability of the bone-fixator configuration.

Pin-gripper: The device that holds the pin to the rest of the fixator.

Bar: A part of the apparatus that connects the pin-grippers. Bars may be solid or hollow, smooth or threaded, and they may incorporate a compression-distraction apparatus in their structure.

Ring: A circular bar (or modified bar) that attaches to pin-grippers in a plane that is usually perpendicular to the long axis of the limb. The rings may or may not completely encircle the limb. (Incomplete circles are called *half-rings.*) The rings must be connected to each other by bars to create a fixator configuration.

Articulations: A device that connects one bar to another (or a bar to a ring). Some articulations consist of universal joints or hinges, but most do not.

Frame Configuration

Throughout this chapter, frame configuration terminology modified from Chao and coworkers[37] will be used (Fig. 7-5).

Unilateral: The unilateral frame is one that employs one bar connecting two or more pin-gripping clamps, which are attached to half-pins. It is the simplest configuration. This category includes Parkhill's original bone clamp, Lambotte's external fixator, and the apparatuses devised by Stader, Hoffmann, and Wagner.

Bilateral: A bilateral frame is one that employs a rigid bar on both sides of the limb, connected to full pins that transfix the bone. Roger Anderson's external skeletal fixator was of bilateral design.

Bi- or multiplanar: A frame is one that employs pins in two (or more) planes for increased stability.

Ring: A ring fixator is one that uses transverse bars that completely encircle the limb. Pins transfix the limb and connect to the rings in various locations. Additional bars, as noted earlier, connect the rings to each other. Russian investigators have been using these fixators for many years.

Half-ring: A half-ring fixator is one employing bars that incompletely encircle the limb in a manner similar to the ring fixator.

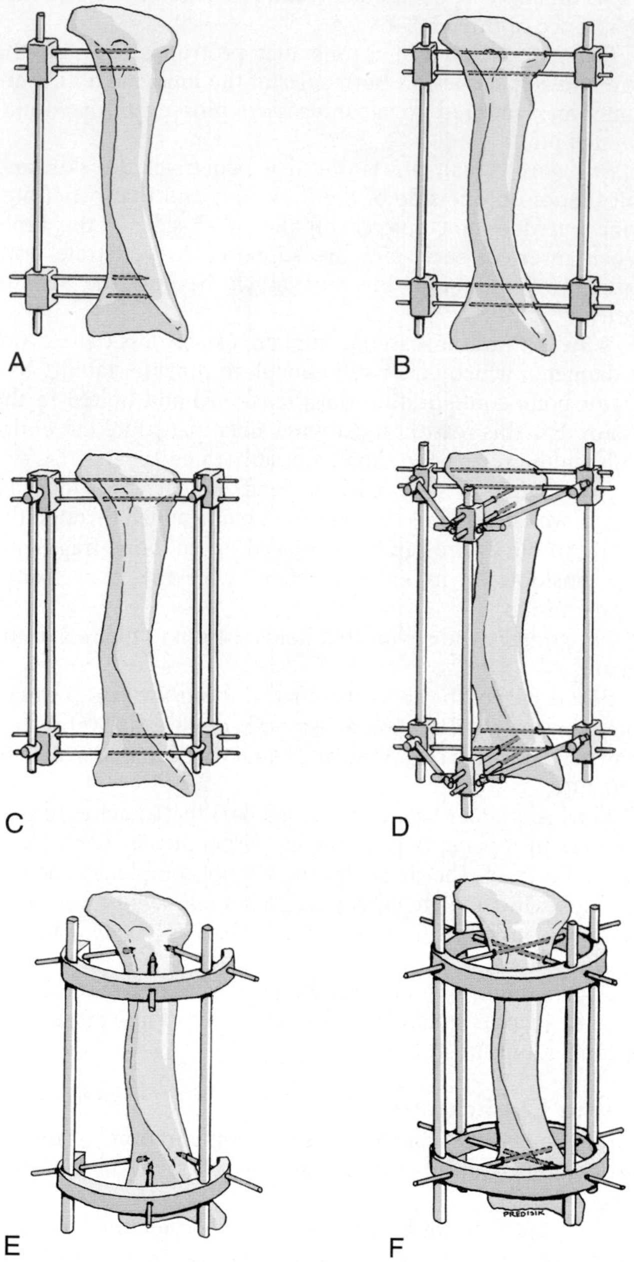

Figure 7-5. Basic fixator configurations. **A,** Unilateral. **B,** Bilateral. **C,** Multiplanar (quadrilateral). **D,** Multiplanar (delta configuration). **E,** Ring fixator. **F,** Hybrid fixator.

Prefabricated Fixators

External fixation systems in which a manufacturer prefabricates the components can be divided into two broad categories: those with fixed configurations and those with variable configurations.

Fixed configuration: These external fixation frames are characterized by a relatively fixed, but usually adjustable, spatial configuration that dictates the position, direction, or number of transcutaneous pins.

Variable configuration: The variable configuration fixator systems are similar to each other in that they consist of many separate components that can be assembled into any spatial configuration as dictated by the nature of the musculoskeletal problem. Precise pin position is generally required only with the individual pins within a cluster (those held by the same pin gripping clamp).

Improvised Fixators

This category comprises systems of external fracture management where transcutaneous pins are connected to an unsolidified substance that hardens within a few minutes after being applied. The classic pins-in-plaster technique, methylmethacrylate external pin fixation, and epoxy-filled tube systems belong in this group. These systems permit unlimited pin positions, but they lack adjustability and preclude compression or distraction.

PROBLEMS, OBSTACLES, AND COMPLICATIONS

The application of an external skeletal fixator, especially one that involves the slow repositioning of bone fragments, is different from most other surgical procedures because the "operation" does not end when the patient leaves the operating room (OR). Instead, the procedure stretches out over many months, with many clinic visits needed to follow the progress of the bone fragments. As will be evident from the following discussion, pin tract infections, numbness from nerve stretching, delayed union, deviation of mechanical axis during elongation, and numerous other difficulties occur during a typical case. To call all of these challenging events "complications" leads to the conclusion that external fixator applications have a 500% complication rate. Many practitioners who do large numbers of fixator applications use a scheme of analysis popularized by Paley that includes problems, obstacles, and complications.[38] Problems in this paradigm are those difficulties that are correctable in the clinic, often by either a modification of the mounting parameters or a prescription medication. Obstacles are those difficulties that require a return trip to the OR for correction, including repeat osteotomy for premature consolidation, pin or wire replacement for sepsis or loosening, or even a bone graft for tardy bone healing. True complications in this scheme are the permanent sequelae of treatment that adversely compromise the outcome. This includes permanent nerve injury, persistent infection, failure to obtain union, and so forth. This three-level perspective more correctly describes the entire external fixation encounter and allows comparison to other methods of treatment.

NERVE AND VESSEL INJURY

Introduction

Reports of serious neurovascular injury from fixator pins and wires are surprisingly uncommon. In fact, workers reporting large series of external skeletal fixator applications usually note the absence of a significant nerve or vascular injury. However, they are not unheard of, and descriptions of such injuries do appear from time to time in reports dealing with external skeletal fixation.[39,40]

Vessel Injuries

When vascular injuries do occur, they sometimes present in a most peculiar way.[41] A pin directed at a vessel will usually push

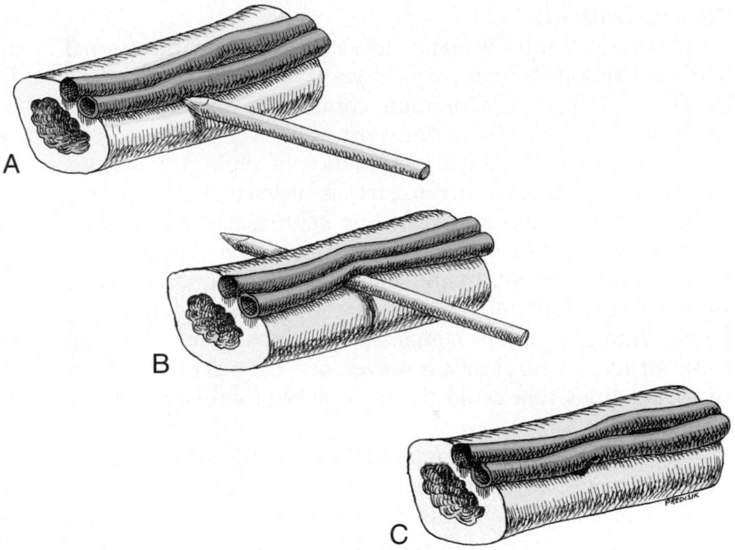

Figure 7-6. A, A pin or wire directed at a vessel will often push the structure to the side. **B,** A vessel resting on an implant may erode and bleed 2 or more weeks after implant insertion. **C,** Alternatively, bleeding may occur at the time of implant removal.

it to the side without transecting it[42] (Fig. 7-6, *A*). As time passes, the vessel, resting against the pin, develops an erosion in its wall. As a result, the patient may suddenly experience bleeding from the implant hole quite some time after fixator application[43] (Fig. 7-6, *B*). Alternatively, the pin may create a hole in the side of a vessel, which does not become apparent until the pin is removed. Excessive bleeding through the pinhole may occur[44] (Fig. 7-6, *C*), or a false aneurysm may develop in the soft tissues. If the vessel wall necrosis involves an adjacent artery and vein, an arteriovenous fistula may be created shortly after pin removal.

Reports describing serious distal vascular compromise following pin insertion are also rare, perhaps because collateral circulation is usually adequate to sustain the limb. In those few cases where a limb becomes ischemic after pin or wire insertion, severe trauma usually preceded fixator application, suggesting loss of collaterals.

One location in particular may be subject to frequent yet undetected neurovascular injury—the distal lateral tibial surface. In that location, Raimbeau and coworkers[45] analyzed damage to the anterior tibial artery caused by transcutaneous pins. They performed arteriograms on cadaver limbs and determined that the region of the tibia between the lower end of the third quarter and the upper end of the fourth quarter is a danger zone for transfixion pin placement because the anterior tibial artery and deep peroneal nerve lay directly on the tibia's periosteum (Fig. 7-7).

Compartment Syndrome

On rare occasions, external fixation pins have been blamed for causing anterior tibial compartment syndrome.[42,46,47] Raimbeau and his associates also measured tissue pressures in the anterior compartment after insertion of transcutaneous pins.[45] They determined that the intracompartmental pressure was not significantly elevated after insertion of one transfixion pin, but it more than doubled when a second pin was inserted. Insertion of a third pin did not significantly raise the pressure any higher. Thus, they identified two vascular syndromes associated with pin fixation of the lower leg. The first, interference with the distal circulation of the anterior tibial artery, is quite rare because adequate collateral circulation is usually present. The second, anterior compartment syndrome, may also be due to partial occlusion of the anterior tibial artery combined with the increased compartment pressure associated with transfixion pins.

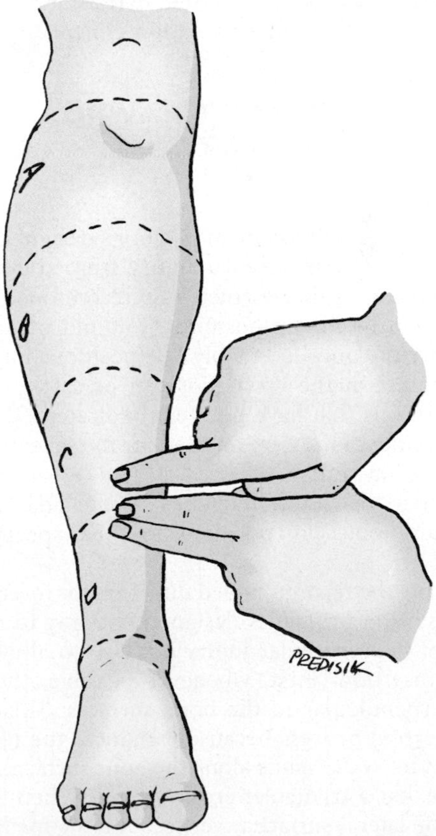

Figure 7-7. The danger zone for implants is one fingerbreadth above and two fingerbreadths below the junction of the third and fourth quarter of the tibia where the anterior artery and deep peroneal nerve lay directly on the bone's lateral surface.

Nerve Injuries

Acute transection of a major nerve is unlikely with external skeletal fixation. Nerves may, however, be nicked during the course of pin insertion, or, more commonly, stretched during limb lengthening or bone transport.[39,40]

In spite of the relative infrequency of reports of serious neurovascular injury, great care is nevertheless required during pin insertion so that major neurovascular structures are not stretched or damaged. I recommend a skin incision, with observation of major neurovascular bundles, when pins are inserted into certain anatomic areas, such as the lateral humerus or proximal radius. Instead of exposing these structures surgically, however, one can select pin placement positions that avoid the possibility of damage to these structures.

Two difficulties are encountered during pin or wire insertion that could lead to a nerve or vessel injury. First, the surgeon is occasionally unsure of the precise position of a major nerve or vessel with respect to the bone at the level of the limb selected for implant insertion. This confusion arises from the surgeon's orientation to the local anatomy, which usually considers the position of a nerve or vessel in its *longitudinal* relationship to surgical exposure. Indeed, surgical exposures are purposefully parallel to both the bone and the neurovascular structures in each anatomic region. Second, it is frequently difficult to assess the exact depth to which a pin has penetrated into the bone. This may seem surprising, considering how easy it is to "feel" when a drill bit penetrates the opposite side of a bone during drilling. Nevertheless, because the pin is threaded, there is enough resistance to forward progress to make depth determination difficult.

IMPLANT PLACEMENT TO AVOID NEUROVASCULAR INJURY

Introduction

An atlas showing pin placement positions designed to reduce the likelihood of neurovascular injury from transcutaneous implants appears in this chapter.[41] By recommending pin or wire placement in certain positions, I do not mean to imply that these are the only acceptably safe positions for insertion. At many points in the limb, pins can be safely inserted in several directions that have not been indicated. The descriptions of these positions were omitted for the sake of simplicity and clarity of illustration.

With experience (and reference to the atlas), surgeons will find additional pin positions to solve specific clinical problems.

In selecting the recommended direction for inserting a pin, I followed several principles designed not only to reduce the incidence of neurovascular injury but also to allow easy, yet solid, pin insertion. First, whenever possible, the pins are inserted perpendicular to the bone surfaces. This facilitates the pin insertion process because it reduces the tendency of the pinpoint to "walk" (slide along the bone surface). The tibia, for example, has a triangular cross section. When the patient is supine, the lateral surface is vertical and the medial surface is oblique. Full pins are more easily inserted from lateral to medial because of this anatomic feature.

Second, pin directions should cross the center of the medullary canal to engage both cortices. When widely separated cortices are engaged by a pin, the tendency of the pin to wobble and loosen is reduced and maximum stability of pin fixation is achieved.

Third, pin insertion into dense bony ridges is to be avoided wherever possible. Drilling into very dense cortical bone with hand tools is tedious and frustrating, tempting the surgeon to try to overcome the resistance by pushing harder and drilling faster, which increases thermal injury to bone and consequently the likelihood of pinhole sepsis.

Fourth, pin positions should have a margin of safety on the opposite side of the bone. A pin is considered "safe" if it passes through the bone and emerges from the opposite side of the limb without encountering a major neurovascular structure. Such pins are illustrated as full (through-and-through) pins, although wires or half-pins could, of course, be safely inserted from either direction.

A pin is labeled "caution" if a major nerve or vascular structure is located on the opposite side of the bone at a distance equal to or greater than the diameter of the bone itself. In this respect, the designation refers only to half-pin placement. A full pin may be labeled caution if the direction or angle of pin insertion is critical to avoid neurovascular injury.

A pin is labeled "danger" if a major neurovascular structure is between one-half and one bone diameter away from the bone on its opposite side. It is wise to insert such pins under radiographic or fluoroscopic control. A pin is also considered a danger pin if it must be inserted adjacent to a neurovascular structure on the near side of the bone. Generally this requires open pin insertion—a longitudinal incision to identify the location of the structure prior to pin insertion.

Pin placement is measured in degrees, rotating around the bone from anterior to posterior, with the center of the bone always presumed to be the center of pin placement. Thus, the direct anterior position is considered to be 0 degrees, and the direct posterior position is considered to be 180 degrees. Pin placement from directly lateral to directly medial is considered to be 90 degrees lateral and a pin placed from directly medial to directly lateral is considered to be 90 degrees medial. In the forearm where there are two bones available for pin placement, the pin position for each is noted separately. The limb must be in the anatomic position during pin insertion if the atlas is to be used correctly. The humerus should be in neutral rotation, and the forearm supinated to correlate with the location of the anatomic structures indicated.

I recommend image intensification fluoroscopy for pin or wire insertion. The correct assessment of the position and depth of the pin can best be determined if the pin is seen in its true lateral projection. (In the true lateral projection of the pin, the central beam of the x-ray tube must be perpendicular to the pin itself.) At times, there is a tendency by surgeons to judge pin position through use of an oblique projection because a true lateral projection of the pins is difficult to obtain when the patient is supine on a large operating table. The surgeon may have to use considerable ingenuity to position a limb for fluoroscopy with a C-arm image intensifier. It may be necessary, for example, to rotate the limb 45 degrees or more, while rotating the C-arm in the opposite direction in order to obtain a true lateral projection. To determine the exact location of a pin within a bone, it is necessary to direct the central beam of the x-ray tube along the pin itself. A perfect axial projection of the pin will result in a small circular image equal to the diameter of the pin. In this manner, the position of the pin relative to the cortices can be determined. If roentgenograms, rather than fluoroscopy are used, the initial evaluation can be obtained after the first pin is inserted to the presumed proper depth. Before the roentgenogram is taken, it is safer to be too shallow than too deep. If a pin is inserted too deeply, there is the obvious danger to neurovascular structures. Also, "backing out" a pin reduces its fixation in bone. When the depth of the first pin is satisfactory, additional pins of the same length can be inserted to the same depth. This strategy for pin insertion can also be employed to reduce x-ray exposure to the OR personnel when image intensification fluoroscopy is used. Only a brief exposure is necessary to determine the position and depth of the first pin. Thereafter, pins can be inserted to the same depth without checking the progress of each pin individually.

The cross section atlas in this book was specifically created to aid the surgeon in the OR. Proper orientation of the cross-sectional diagrams to a patient on the operating table depends on the location of easily palpable landmarks. Each limb section in the atlas is treated in an identical manner. Each anatomic area is divided into four equal zones. Palpable bony landmarks identify the upper and lower limits of each anatomic area under consideration.

In the thigh, the proximal bony landmark is the lateral prominence of the greater trochanter of the femur; the distal landmark is the lateral prominence of the lateral epicondyle of the femur.

In the lower leg section, the proximal landmark is the medial tibial joint line; the distal landmark is the medial prominence of the medial malleolus.

In the upper arm, the proximal landmark is the lateral prominence of the greater tuberosity of the humerus, which is one thumb's width below the lateral tip of the acromion process. Distally, the landmark is the lateral epicondyle of the humerus.

In the forearm, the proximal landmark is the lateral prominence of the radial head, which is one thumb's width distal to the lateral epicondyle of the humerus. The distal landmark is the lateral prominence of the radial styloid process.

Technique of Identifying Landmarks

Each limb segment in the atlas is divided into four zones which are labeled A, B, C, and D, with A proximal and D distal (Fig. 7-8). The zones approximate, but are not exactly, the quarters of each limb segment. The atlas illustrates cross-sectional anatomy in the top, middle, and bottom of each zone. Key diagrams on each plate orient the reader to the zones illustrated. For purposes of clarity, bones, nerves, arteries, and veins have been emphasized in relief. Muscle planes are indicated, but the muscle masses themselves are not labeled. Small cutaneous nerves, veins, and muscular branches of arteries have been omitted. Major arteries are shown with one vein even if they are usually accompanied by two venae comitantes. In the forearm, deep veins have been omitted completely. Some neurovascular structures are emphasized by making them slightly larger than natural size.

Many structures are labeled only once on each page, rather than on each slice. Mental reconstruction of the zone will fill in labels on the unlabeled slices. Unfortunately, some anatomic features are not easily presented in cross-sectional views. These are the transverse vessels and nerves that wind around the bone at one level. Furthermore, the atlas plates do not take into account variations in anatomy that can occur at any level. For these reasons, the atlas illustrations must be considered schematic, rather than representational (Figs. 7-9 through 7-27).

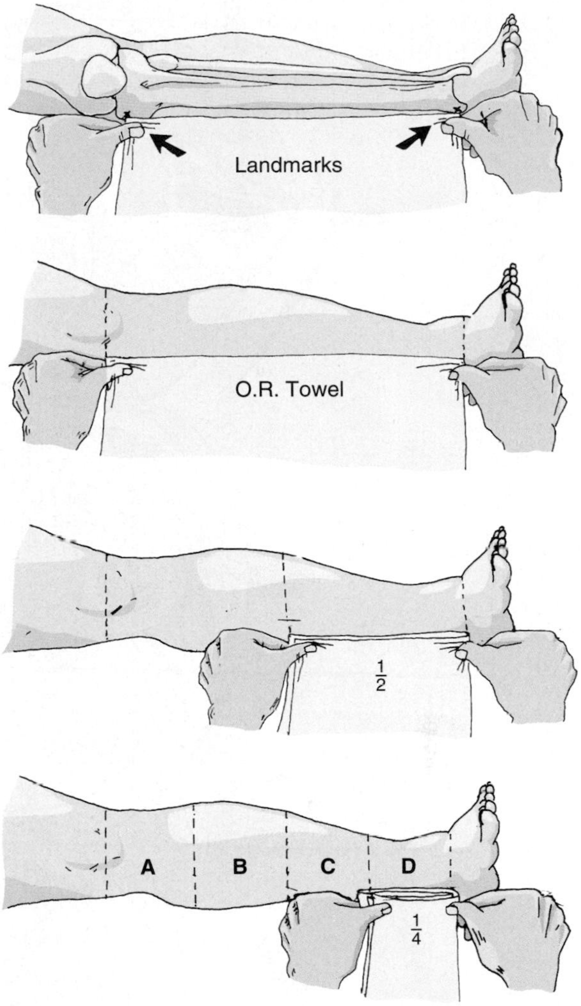

Figure 7-8. To mark the zones, stretch a surgical towel between the proximal and distal landmarks described in the text and mark the position of the landmarks on the towel with a surgical pen. Fold the towel so that the marks touch each other and mark the midpoint of the fold. Lay the towel against the limb again and mark the midpoint on the limb using the towel as a guide. In this manner, the limb section will be divided in half. Repeat the procedure and find the midpoint of each half, thus dividing the limb segment into four equal zones.

PIN TRACT INFECTION

Introduction

Pin tract infection has always been the principal drawback to the use of external fixation. Unfortunately, preliminary communications announcing the development of new fixators rarely take note of this complication. Subsequent reports of external fixator applications, however, provide evidence that the pin tract infections continue to plague the devices.[48-52] One

Text continued on p. 204

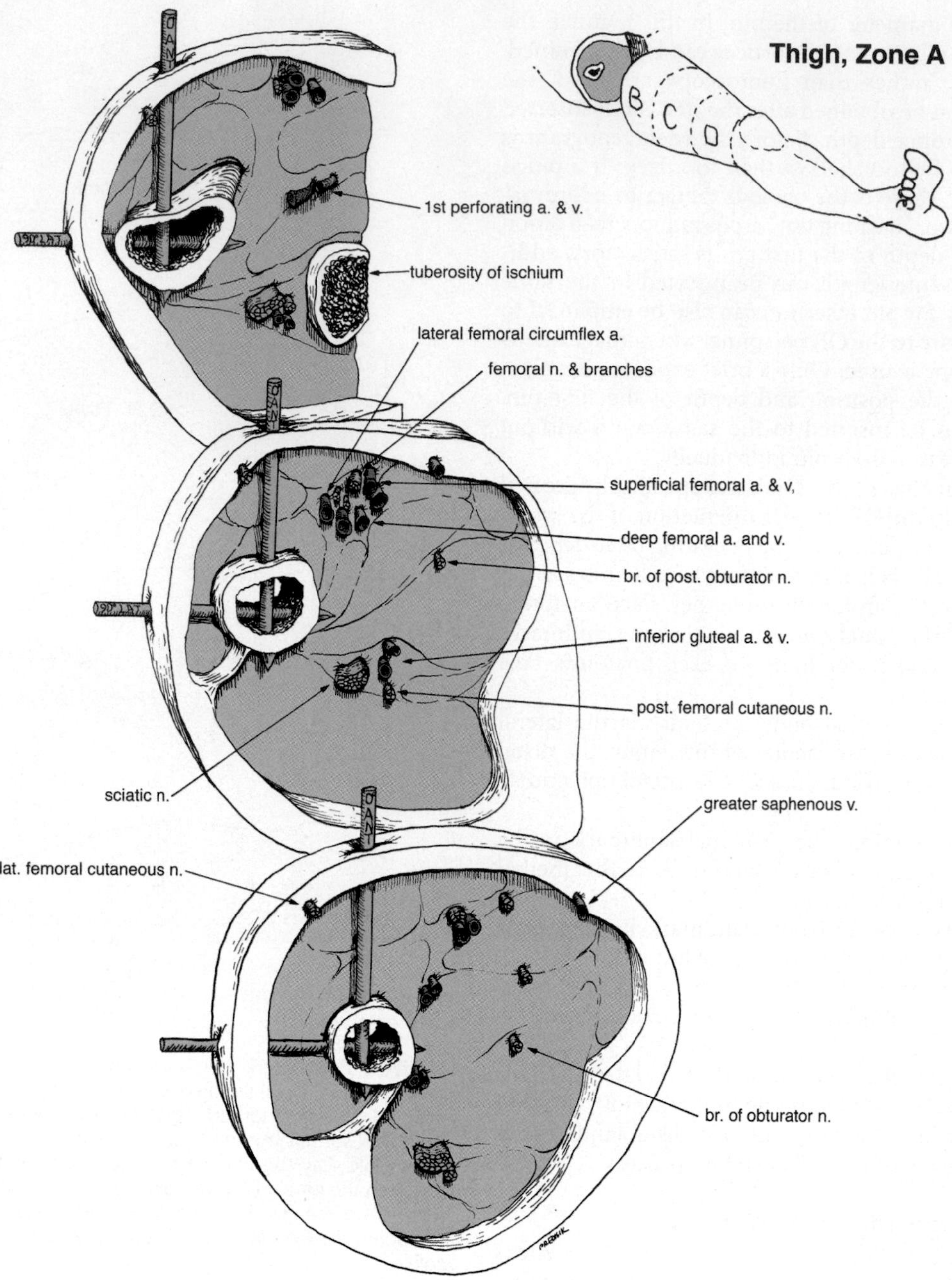

Figure 7-9. Thigh Zone A. Anatomic Considerations

1. The femoral shaft is quite lateral in the proximal thigh.
2. The sciatic nerve remains posteromedial to the femur throughout zone A.
3. The deep femoral artery comes to lie medial to the femur in the lower end of zone A, separated from it by the origin of the vastus medialis muscle, but only one-half bone width away.
4. The lateral femoral cutaneous nerve is in line with the lateral cortex of the femur.
5. The lateral femoral circumflex artery winds around the lateral cortex of the femur at the base of the greater trochanter.

Pin Placement

1. Half-pin insertion from the 90-degree lateral position can be done with caution in the upper two-thirds of zone A, and with extreme caution in lower zone A.
2. With care, and image intensification control, additional pin insertion can be obtained throughout a wide range in the upper portion of this zone.

a., Artery; *br.*, branch; *lat.*, lateral; *n.*, nerve; *post.*, posterior; *v.*, vein.

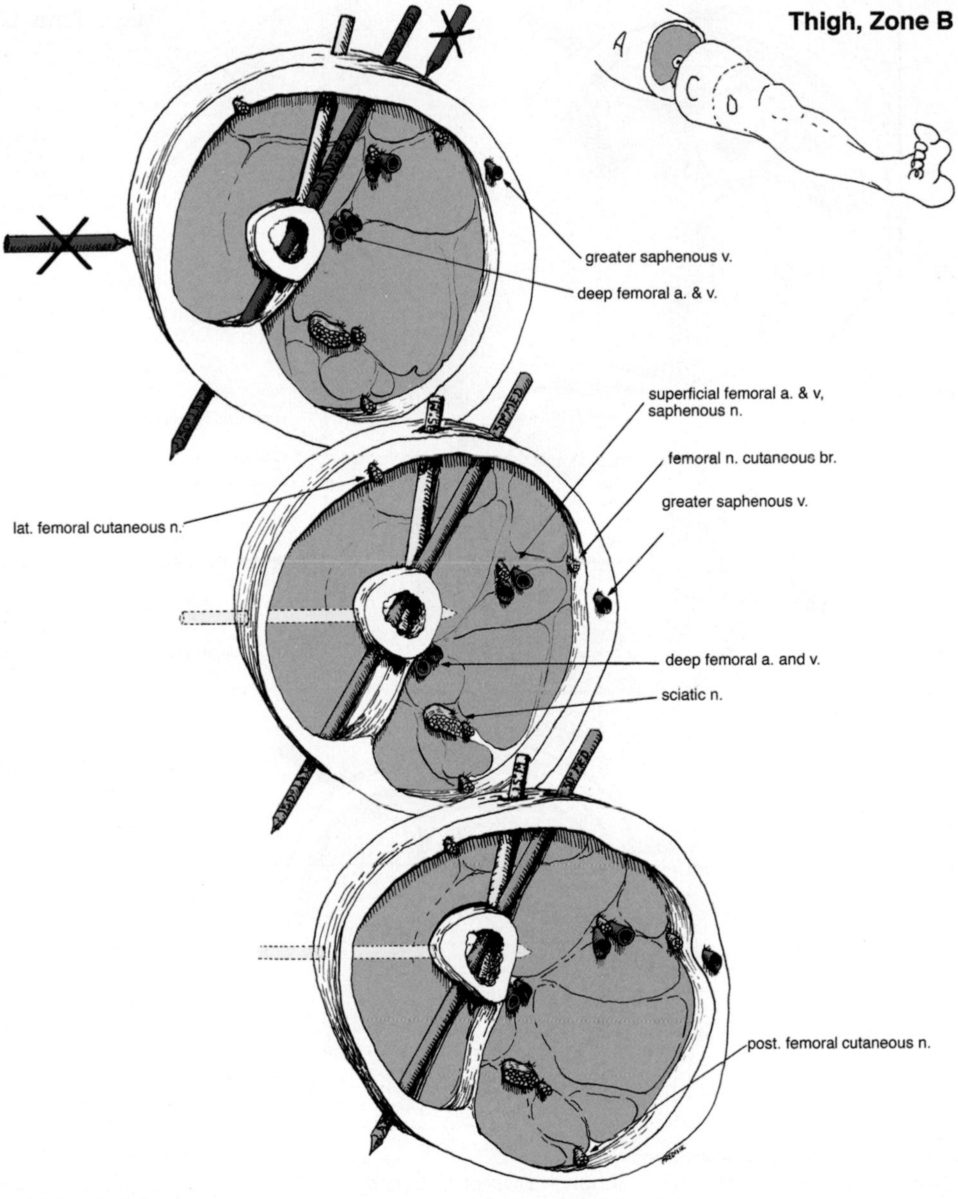

Figure 7-10. Thigh Zone B. Anatomic Considerations
1. The femur is laterally placed throughout zone B.
2. The sciatic nerve is posteromedial to the femur, separated by one bone diameter.
3. The superficial femoral artery crosses the coronal plane of the femur between zone B and zone C.
4. The deep femoral artery and vein are medial to the femur in proximal zone B and posterior to the femur in distal zone B.
5. The lateral femoral cutaneous nerve is anterior to the femur.

Pin Placement
1. Extreme caution is necessary in proximal zone B with 30-degree medial placement, because the superficial and deep femoral vessels are in a straight line and can both be injured with a pin or wire placed too far medially.
2. Additional half-pins may be placed in other directions, but keep in mind the intimate association of the deep femoral vessels to the shaft of the femur.

a., Artery; *br.*, branch; *lat.*, lateral; *n.*, nerve; *post.*, posterior; *v.*, vein.

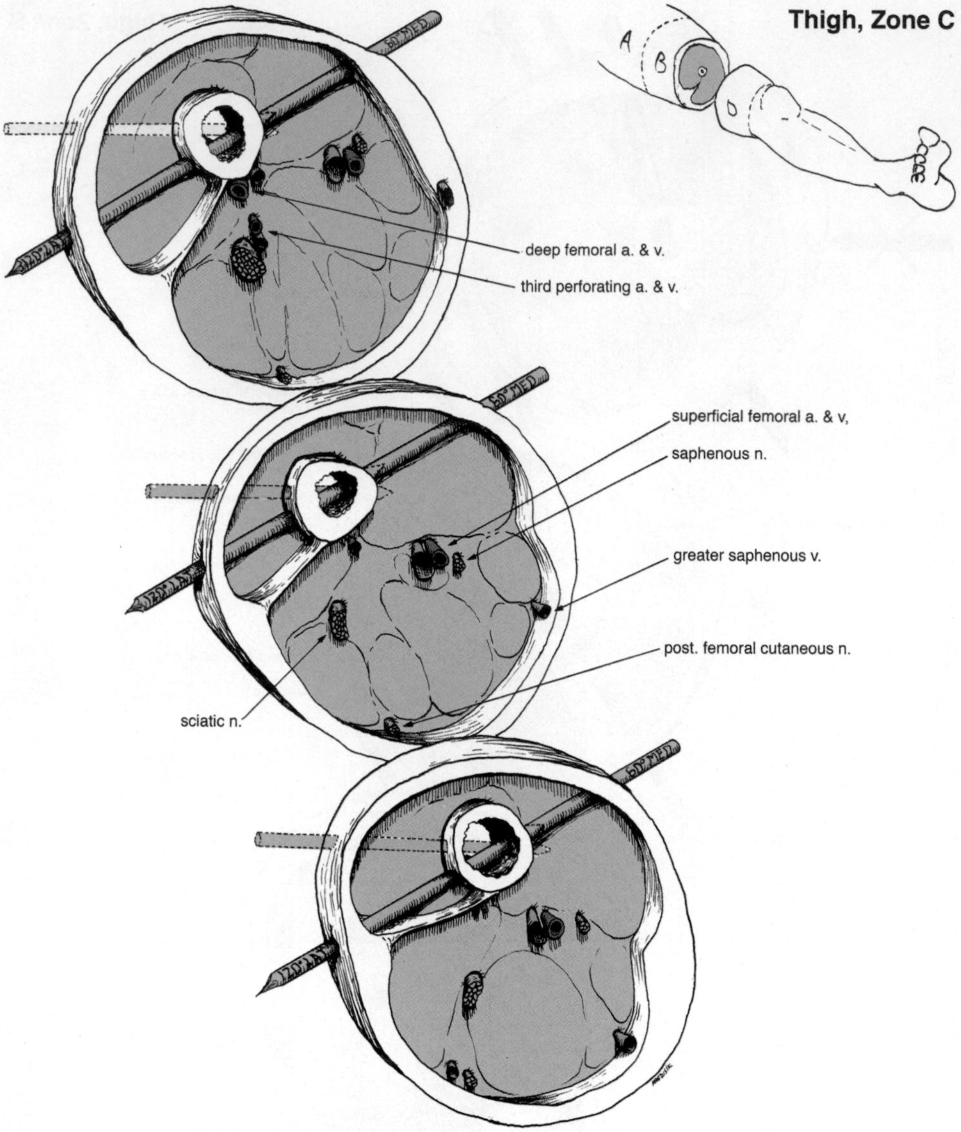

Figure 7-11. **Thigh Zone C.** Anatomic Considerations
1. The femur is more centrally placed on cross section, although anteriorly situated.
2. The sciatic nerve passes from medial to lateral behind the femur, approximately one bone width away.
3. The superficial femoral artery passes the coronal plane of the femur in zone C and is posterior to the bone at the lower end of this zone.
4. The deep femoral artery and vein are adjacent to the posterior surface of the femur, but terminate at the lower end of zone C.

Pin Placement
1. Wires, full pins, or half-pins can be inserted from the 60-degree medial or 120-degree lateral position.
2. Half-pins can be cautiously inserted from the 0-degree anterior position in distal zone C because the deep femoral artery and vein are no longer present (not shown).
3. Wires, full pins, or half-pins can also be inserted 90 degrees medial or 90 degrees lateral in distal zone C.

a., Artery; *n.,* nerve; *post.,* posterior; *v.,* vein.

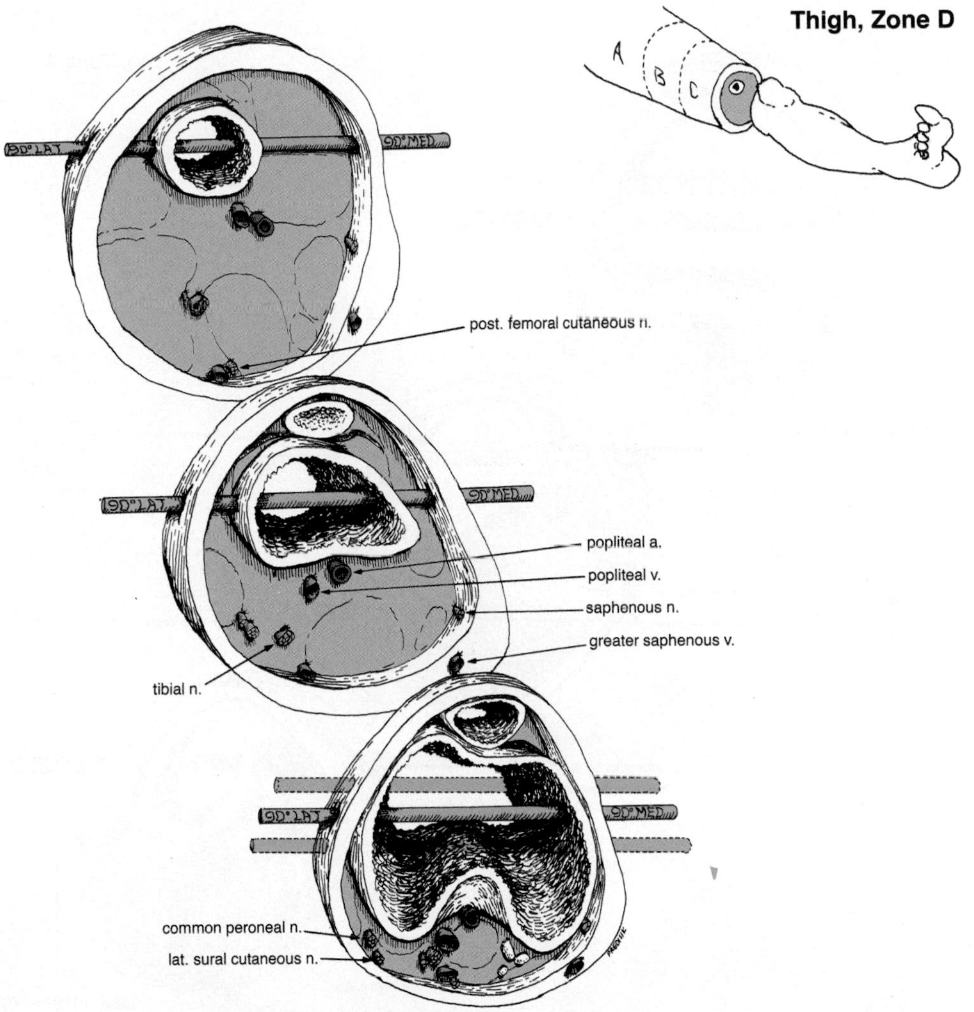

Figure 7-12. **Thigh Zone D.** Anatomic Considerations

1. The femur is an anterior structure until the flair of the condyles.
2. The sciatic nerve is posterior to the femur in proximal zone D crossing to the lateral side while dividing into the tibial and peroneal divisions.
3. The femoral artery becomes the popliteal artery and with the popliteal vein, is immediately posterior to the femur in zone D.
4. The synovial cavity of the knee joint enlarges to encompass the anterior half of the femur immediately above the joint line.

Pin Placement

1. Wires, full pins, or half-pins from 90 degrees medial or 90 degrees lateral are safe.
2. Half-pins from the 90-degree lateral position have the additional advantage of not transfixing the vastus medialis muscle.
3. At the level of the epicondyles, the synovial cavity is present anteriorly and posteriorly, leaving only 1 inch of extrasynovial bone. Three or four pins may be placed close to each other in a transverse plane through the bone at this level, although if four pins are placed, the most posterior pin may pass through the synovial cavity.

a., Artery; *br.,* branch; *lat.,* lateral; *n.,* nerve; *post.,* posterior; *v.,* vein.

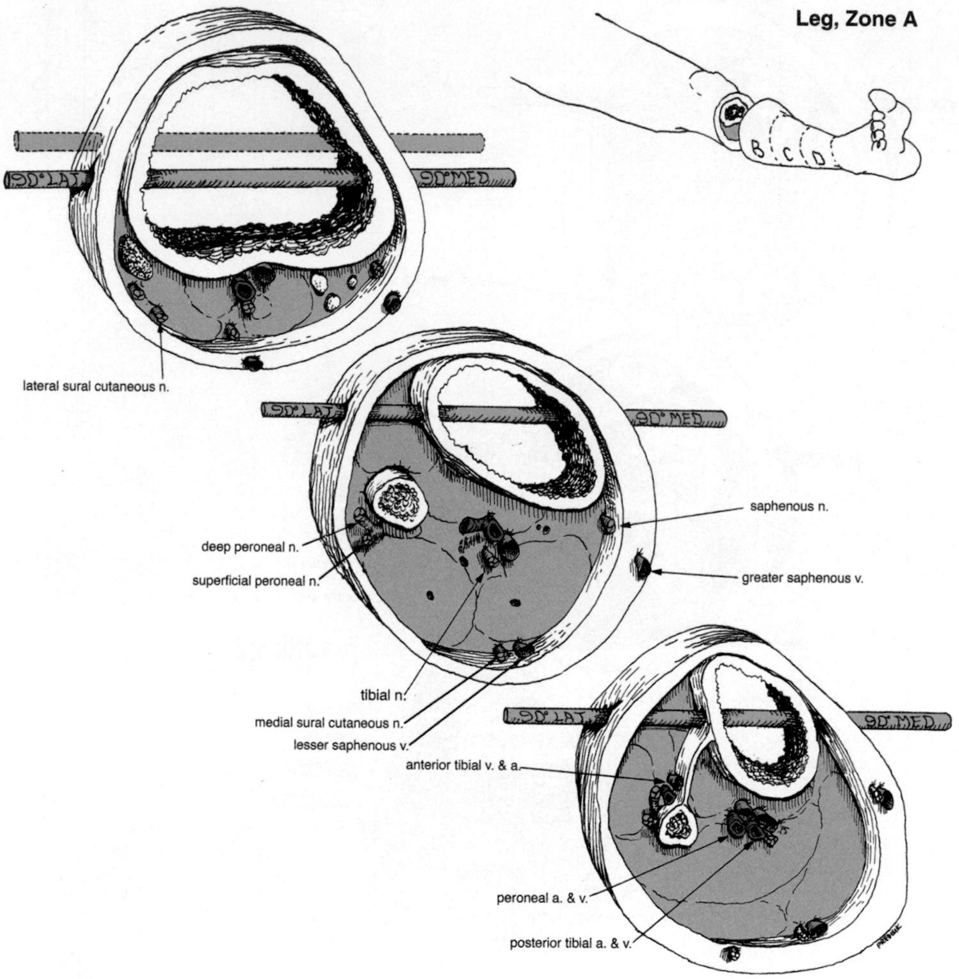

Figure 7-13. Leg, Zone A. Anatomic Considerations
1. The shape of the tibia changes rapidly through this zone.
2. The popliteal artery is posterior to the tibia where it divides into its terminal branches.
3. The superficial and deep peroneal nerves are lateral to the fibula as they wind around the fibular neck.
4. The saphenous nerve and greater saphenous vein are posterior to the tibia on the medial side of the limb.
5. In distal zone A, the anterior tibial artery is on the anterior surface of the interosseous membrane and the peroneal and posterior tibial arteries are posterior to the tibia, accompanied by their associated veins.

Pin Placement
1. Wires and full pins (or half-pins) can be placed in the 90-degree medial to 90-degree lateral direction throughout zone A.
2. Pins can be placed parallel to the joint line (and to each other) through the condyles of the tibia in proximal zone A.

a., Artery; *n.*, nerve; *v.*, vein.

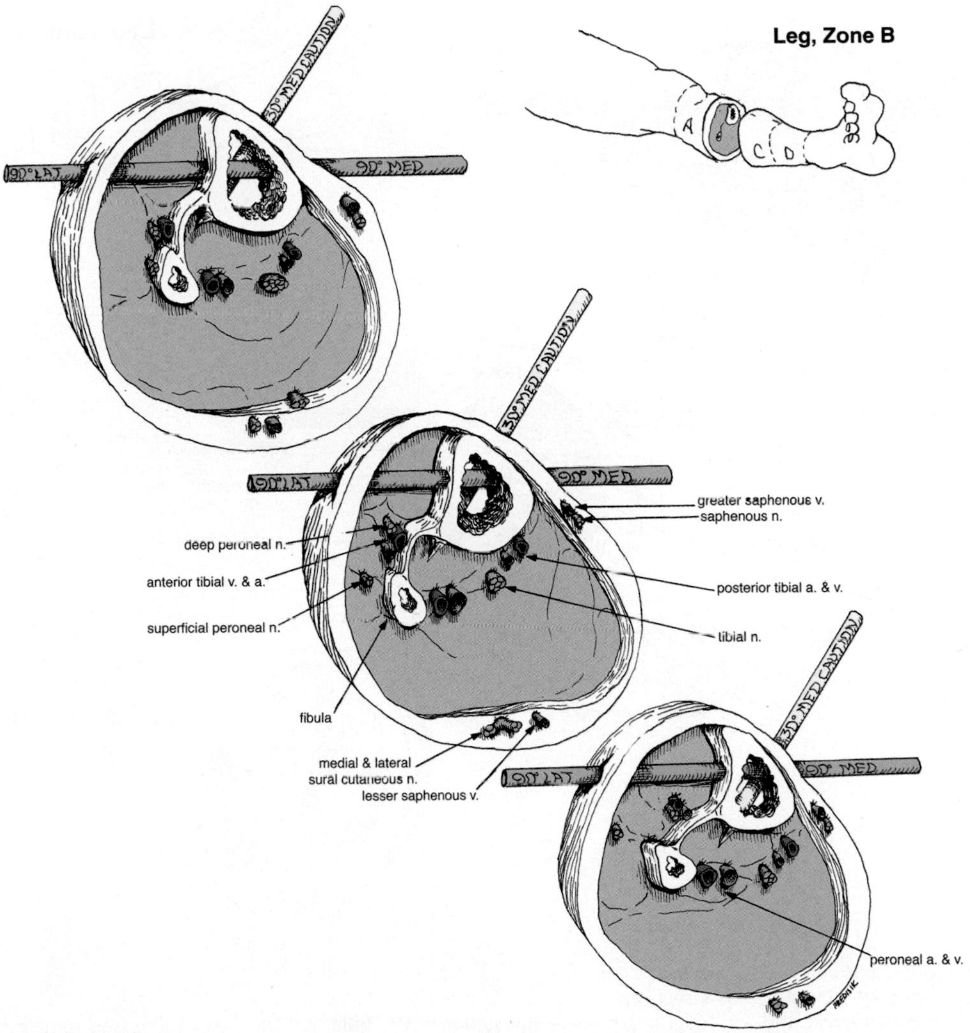

Figure 7-14. Leg, Zone B. Anatomic Considerations

1. The tibia has a triangular cross section throughout zone B, with the lateral surface relatively vertical, and the medial surface oblique.
2. The posterior tibial vessels, the tibial nerve, and the peroneal vessels maintain a constant relationship throughout zone B with respect to the posterior surface of the tibia and the medial surface of the fibula.
3. The anterior tibial artery and vein, and the deep peroneal nerve, lie on the anterior surface of the interosseous membrane in zone B, traversing from the anterior ridge of the fibula toward the lateral ridge of the tibia.

Pin Placement

1. Wires, full pins, or half-pins can be inserted from 90 degrees lateral or 90 degrees medial.
2. Half-pins can be inserted with caution from the 30-degree medial (or 45-degree medial) position perpendicular to the oblique medial surface of the tibia.

The tip of the pin will penetrate the tibialis posterior muscle. Bear in mind the relationship of the peroneal artery and vein, adjacent to the medial corner of the fibula.

a., Artery; *n.,* nerve; *v.,* vein.

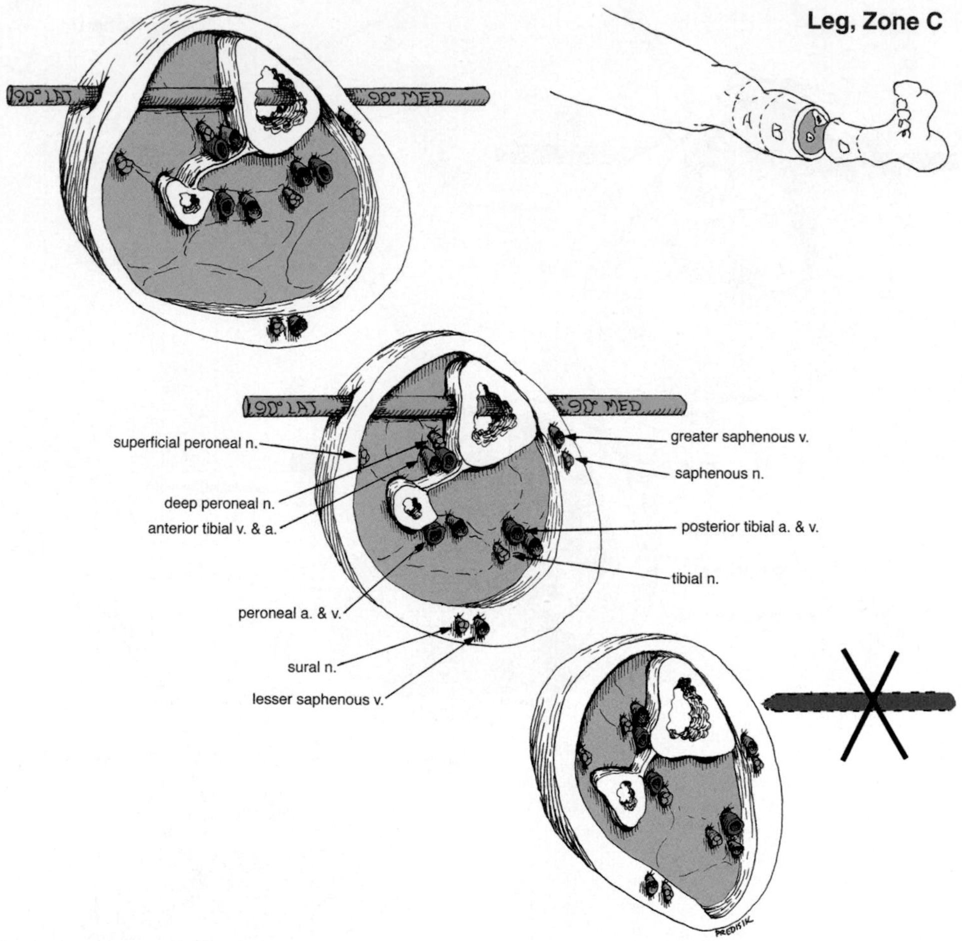

Figure 7-15. Leg, Zone C. Anatomic Considerations

1. The tibia retains its distinctive triangular cross section.
2. The posterior tibial artery and vein and the tibial nerve remain posterior to the tibia and the peroneal vessels remain slightly medial to the fibula.
3. The anterior tibial artery and vein and the deep peroneal nerve have completed their traverse of interosseous membrane and are adjacent to the posterolateral corner of the tibia throughout zone C. These structures begin to traverse the lateral surface of the tibia in distal zone C.
4. The saphenous nerve and greater saphenous vein are located at the posteromedial corner of the tibia in the subcutaneous tissue.

Pin Placement

1. In the upper part of zone C, wires, full pins, or half-pins can be safely placed from the 90-degree medial or 90-degree lateral direction.
2. Half-pins are difficult to place into the oblique medial surface of the tibia in zone C, because of the intimate relationship of the anterior tibial vessels to the bone. A 0-degree half-pin would be safe in distal zone C, but it is technically difficult to place because of the obliquity and thickness of the bone.
3. In distal zone C, pin placement from the 90-degree lateral or 90-degree medial position can endanger the anterior tibial artery and deep peroneal nerve.

a., Artery; *n.*, nerve; *v.*, vein.

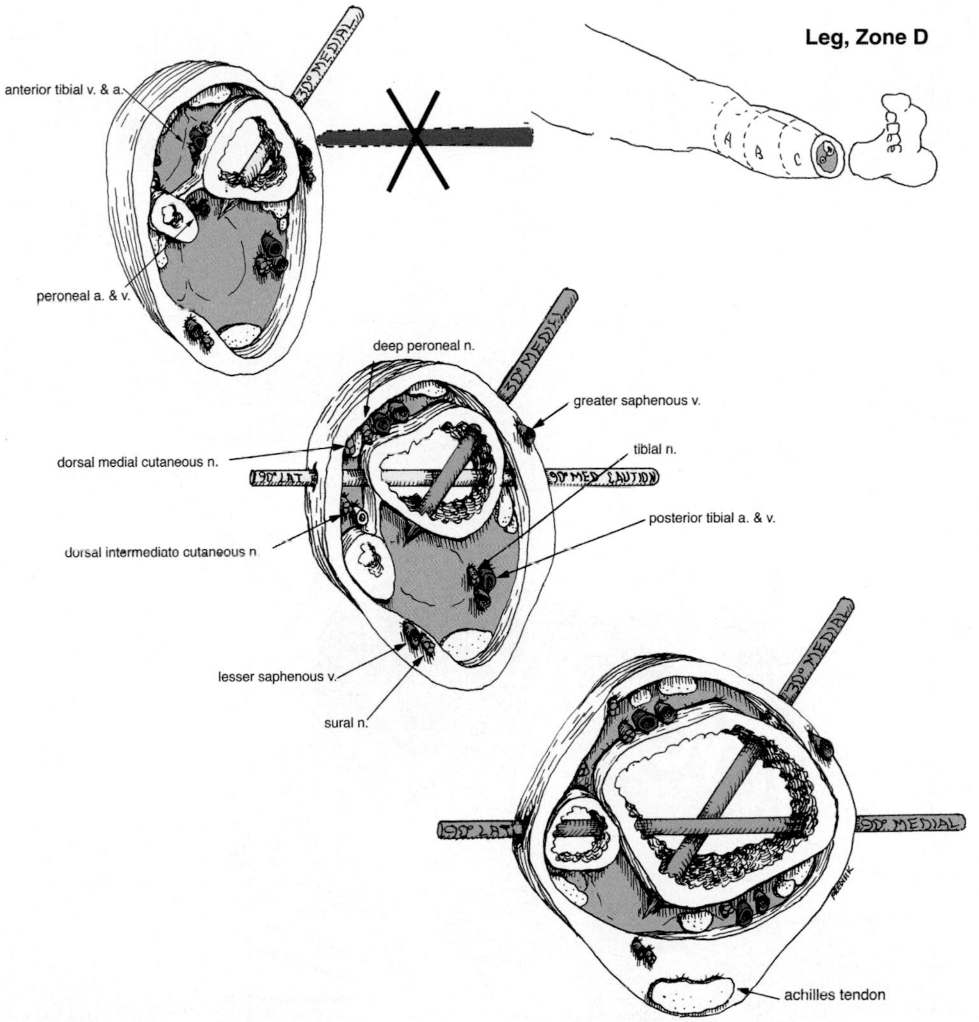

Figure 7-16. Leg, Zone D. Anatomic Considerations

1. The posterior tibial artery and vein and the tibial nerve remain posterior to the tibia, traversing medially as they approach the ankle joint.
2. The anterior tibial artery and vein, and the deep peroneal nerve, are on the lateral surface of the tibia in proximal zone D. They lie on the anterior surface of the tibia in distal zone D.
3. The saphenous nerve and greater saphenous vein are on the medial side of the tibia throughout zone D.
4. The superficial peroneal nerve has divided into its terminal branches in this zone.

Pin Placement

1. Half-pins can be placed from the 30-degree medial position into the subcutaneous portion of the tibia.
2. Wire, or full-pin, placement from the 90-degree medial and 90-degree lateral directions can be accomplished in the distal two-thirds of zone D.
3. Wire, full pin, or half-pin placement from 90 degrees medial or 90 degrees lateral can endanger the anterior tibial artery and deep peroneal nerve in the proximal one-third of zone D.

a., Artery; *n.*, nerve; *v.*, vein.

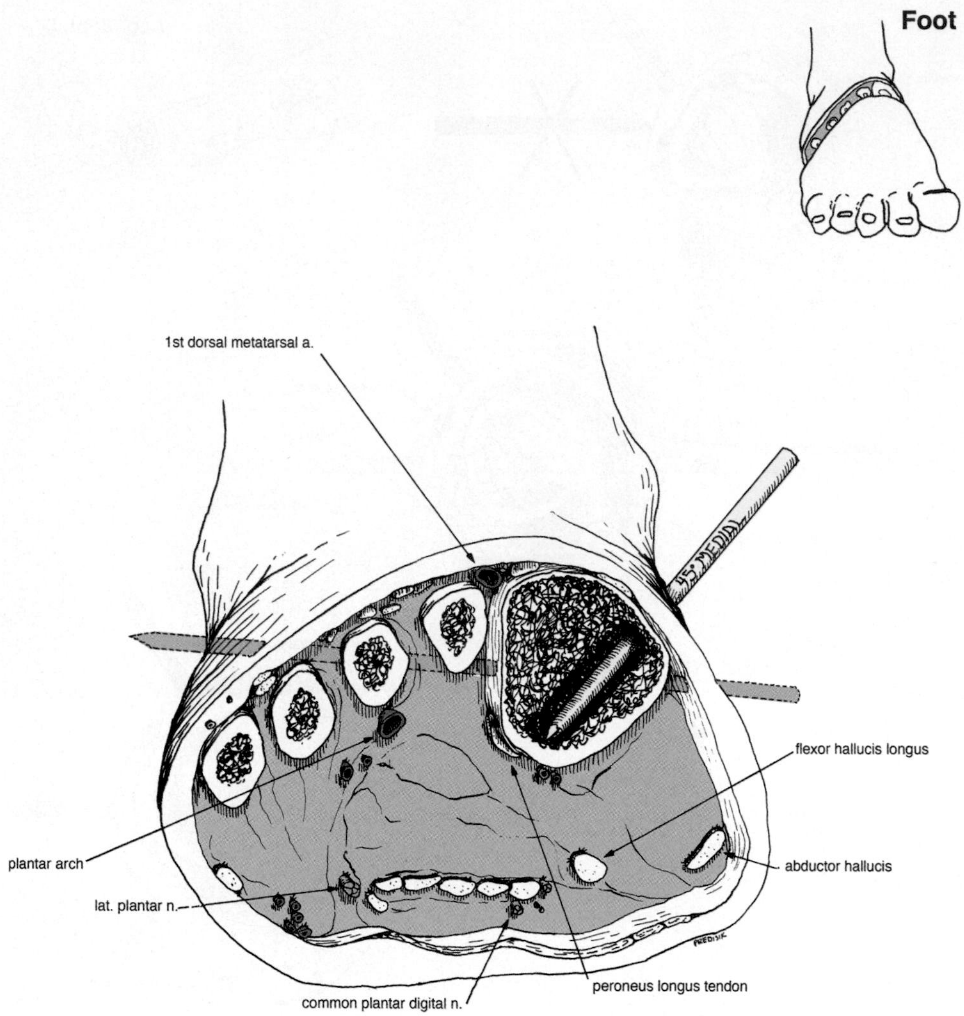

Figure 7-17. Foot. Anatomic Considerations

1. Cross section through the metatarsals demonstrates the curvature of the transverse metatarsal arch.
2. The dorsalis pedis artery is between the first and second metatarsal shafts.
3. The plantar arterial arch is crossing beneath the third metatarsal shaft at the level illustrated.
4. The flexor hallucis brevis tendon is adjacent to the lateral inferior surface of the first metatarsal shaft.

Pin Placement

1. A wire, full pin, or half-pin can be inserted from the 90-degree medial position into the first metatarsal shaft. It will penetrate one or perhaps two other metatarsal shafts but cannot transfix all of them.
2. A 45-degree medial half-pin can be inserted into the first metatarsal.
3. Other half-pin positions can be safely used into the metatarsal bones, including a 90-degree lateral pin into the fifth metatarsal shaft (not shown).

a., Artery; *lat.,* lateral; *n.,* nerve.

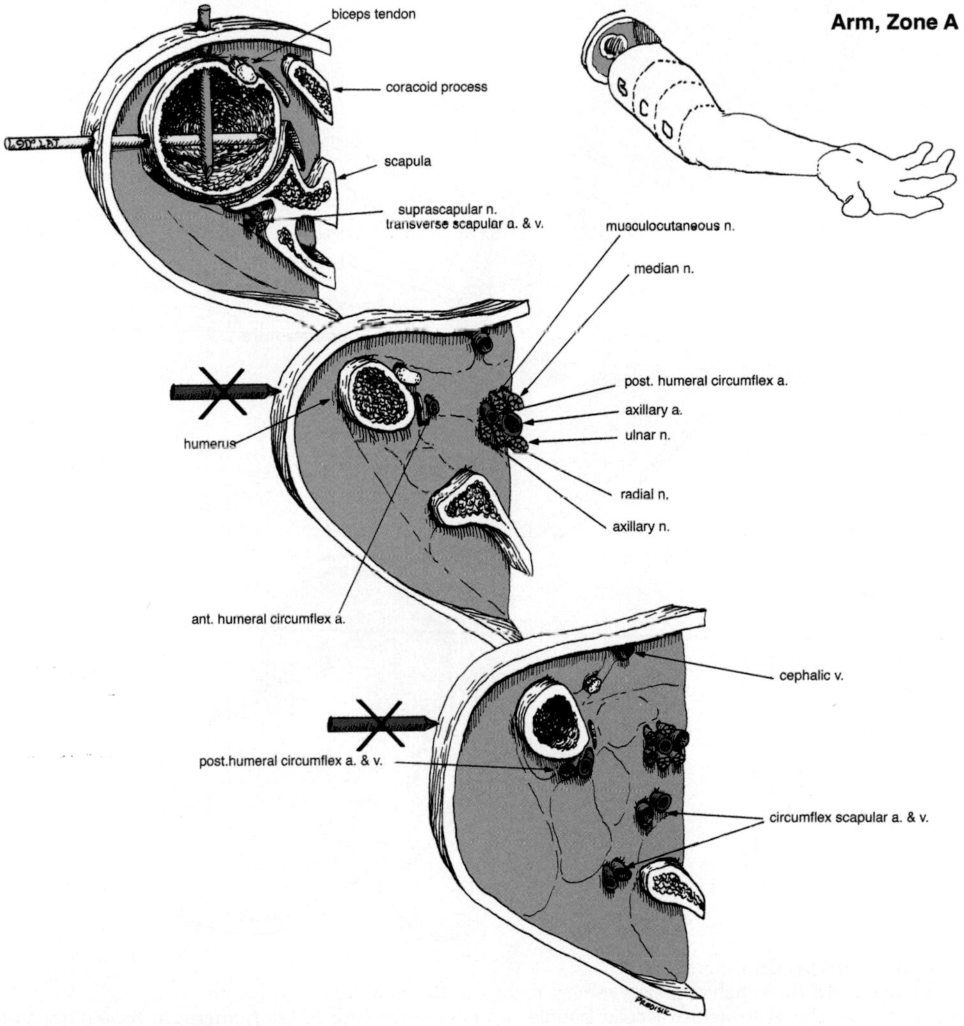

Figure 7-18. Arm, Zone A. Anatomic Considerations

1. The humeral head is largely intrasynovial, being surrounded by a joint cavity medially and posteriorly and by the subacromial bursa anteriorly.
2. The main neurovascular bundle containing the brachial plexus is medial to the humerus, separated from it by a distance equal to the width of the bone.
3. The anterior and posterior humeral circumflex vessels surround the upper humerus slightly below the surgical neck, accompanied by the axillary nerve.

Pin Placement

1. Half-pins may be cautiously placed in the 90-degreee lateral position.
2. Half-pins can be inserted into the humeral head from 0 degrees anterior around laterally to the 90-degree lateral position, if the tip of the pin does not penetrate the opposite cortex of the humeral head.
3. Below the level of the surgical neck of the humerus, pin placement may endanger the humeral circumflex vessels and the axillary nerve.
4. Below the anatomic neck of the humerus, half-pins can be placed from the 90-degree lateral position (not shown).

a., Artery; *ant.*, anterior; *n.*, nerve; *post.*, posterior; *v.*, vein.

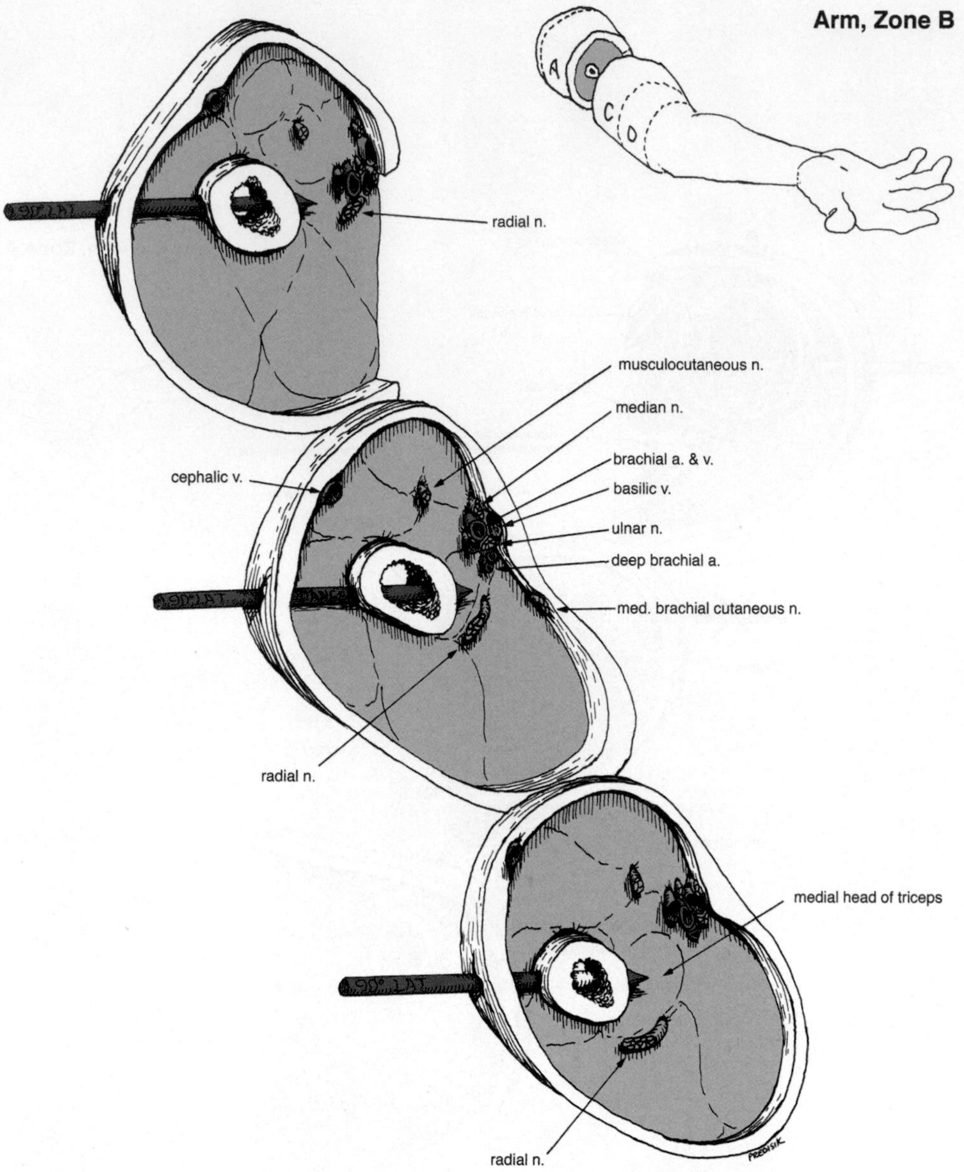

Figure 7-19. Arm, Zone B. Anatomic Considerations

1. The brachial artery and veins and the brachial plexus remain medial to the humerus in this zone.
2. The radial nerve separates from the main neurovascular bundle and passes posterior to the humerus in zone B, separated from the bone by the medial head of the triceps.
3. The musculocutaneous nerve and cephalic vein are anterior to the humerus in zone B.

Pin Placement

1. Half-pins from 90 degrees lateral must be accomplished with caution in mid-zone B because of the position of the radial nerve medial to the humerus.

a., Artery; *med.*, medial; *n.*, nerve; *v.*, vein.

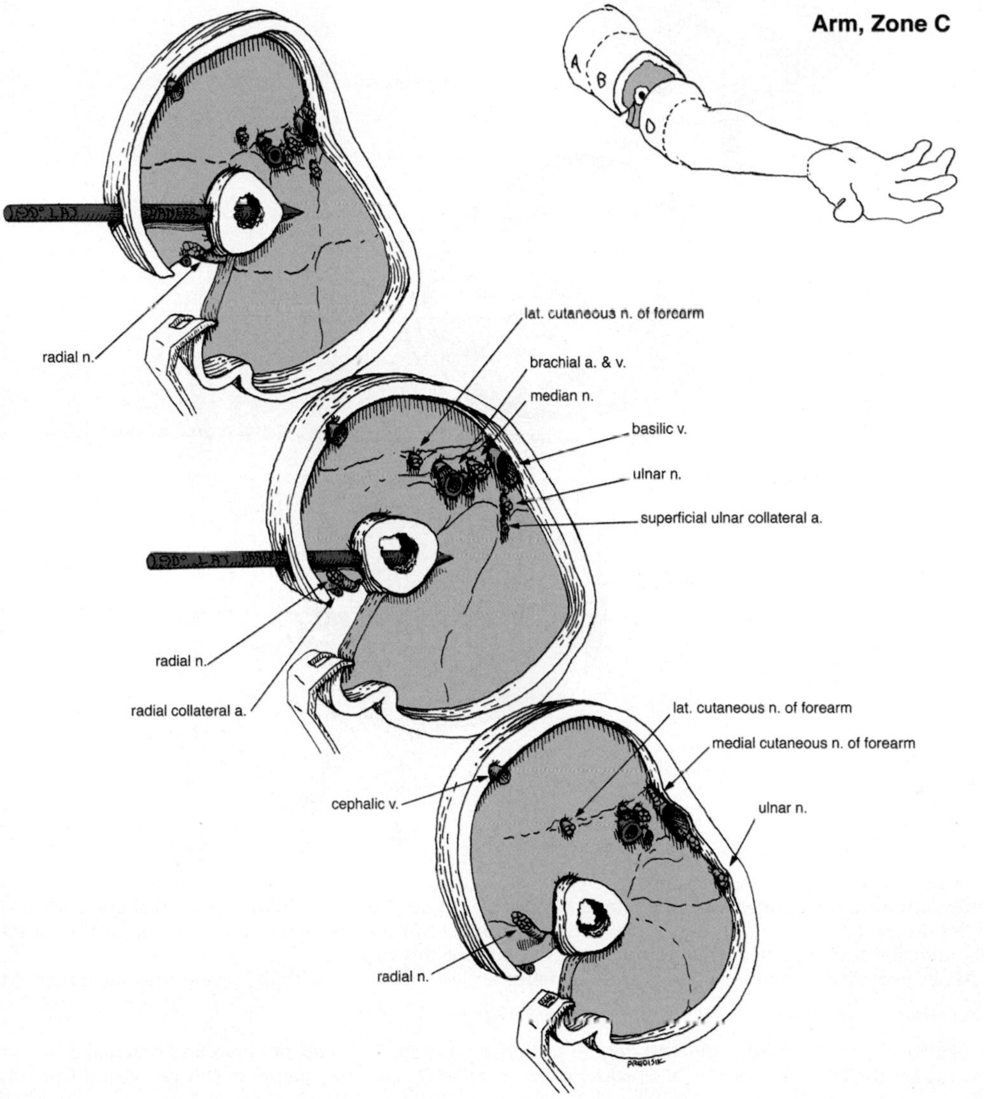

Figure 7-20. Arm, Zone C. Anatomic Considerations

1. The radial nerve winds around the lateral side of the shaft of the humerus in contact with the bone.
2. The brachial artery, veins, and branches of the brachial plexus remain medial to the humeral shaft. The ulnar nerve separates from the main neurovascular bundle in this zone.
3. The musculocutaneous nerve becomes the lateral cutaneous nerve of the forearm and remains anterior to the humerus.

Pin Placement

1. Half-pins should only be placed in the 90-degree lateral position in the humerus with direct observation of the radial nerve through a surgical exposure.

a., Artery; *lat.*, lateral; *n.*, nerve; *v.*, vein.

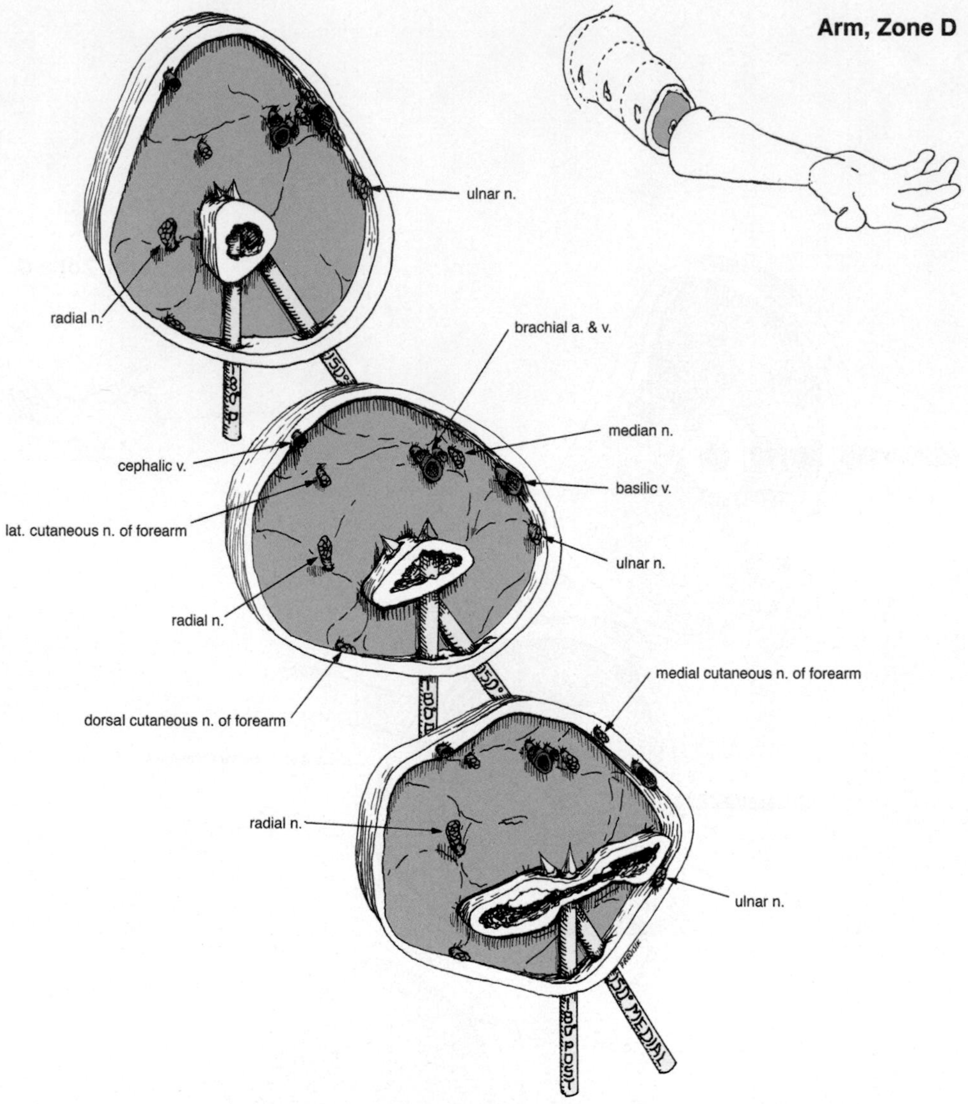

Figure 7-21. Arm, Zone D. Anatomic Considerations

1. The distal humerus flattens and is rotated with the lateral epicondyle 30 degrees posterior to the medial epicondyle.
2. The radial nerve lies on the lateral side of the radius in proximal zone D but is anterior to it in the distal portion of the zone.
3. The median nerve remains anterior and medial to the bone throughout this zone.
4. The ulnar nerve passes posterior to the plane of the distal humerus and lies in contact with the posteromedial corner of the bone immediately above the elbow.

Pin Placement

1. Half-pins can be placed with caution from the 180-degree posterior position. The median nerve and brachial artery are separated from the shaft of the humerus by the thickness of the brachialis muscle in zone D. Likewise, half-pins can be placed from the 150-degree medial position.
2. Half-pins, full pins, or wires can be placed from the lateral epicondyle into the medial epicondyle. Unfortunately, the proximity of the ulnar nerve to the medial epicondyle of the humerus makes pin placement in this position somewhat dangerous. It is recommended that the ulnar nerve be exposed for transepicondylar wire or placement.

a., Artery; *lat.*, lateral; *n.*, nerve; *v.*, vein.

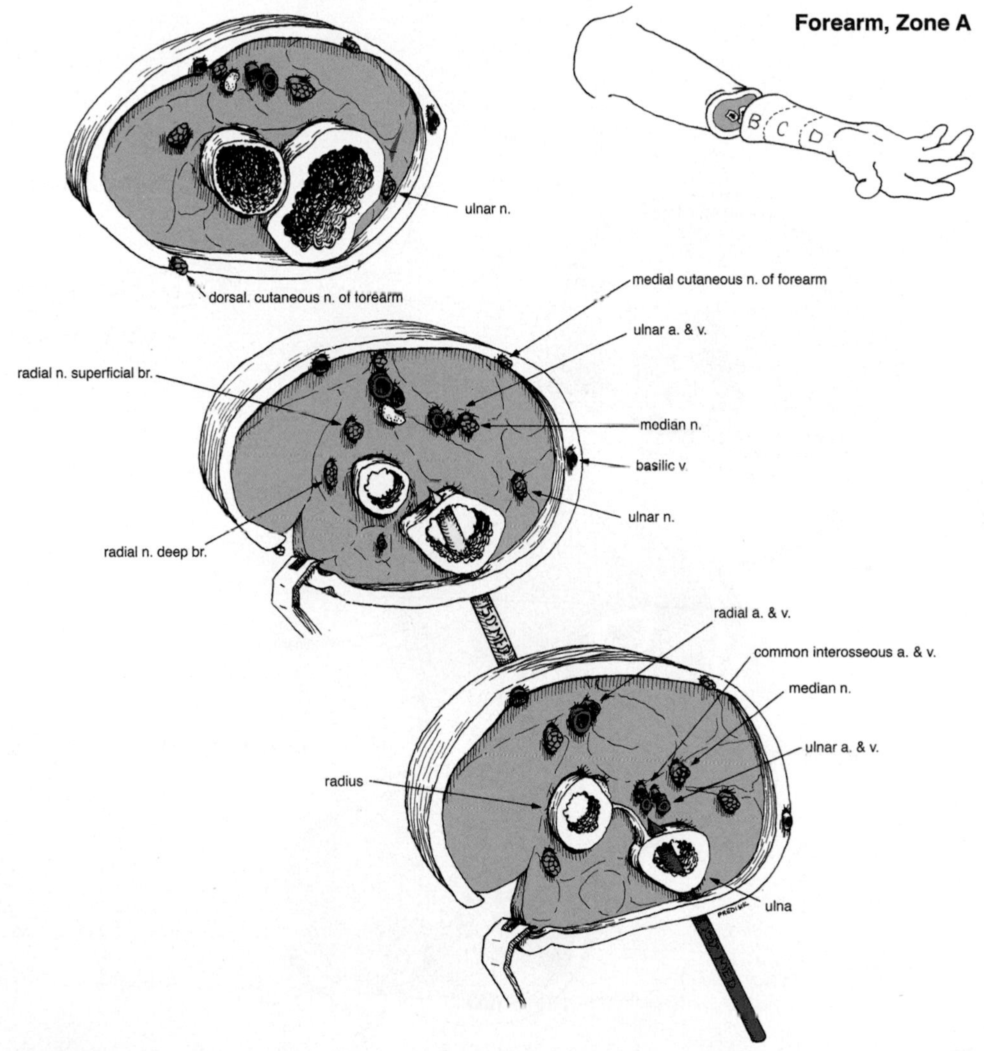

Figure 7-22. Forearm, Zone A. Anatomic Considerations

1. The deep branch of the radial nerve winds around the lateral side of the humerus within the substance of the supinator muscle.
2. The brachial artery divides into its terminal branches (the common interosseous artery and the ulnar artery) in zone A; they are anterior to the proximal ulna in distally.

Pin Placement

1. Half-pins can be inserted into the proximal ulna from the 150-degree medial direction. Image intensification fluoroscopy is recommended. Cross-wires can be placed in the proximal ulna posterior to the ulnar nerve.
2. Pin placement into the proximal radius is dangerous because of the location of the deep branch of the radial nerve. If it is necessary to stabilize the proximal radius with external fixation, it is wise to identify this structure surgically before pin insertion.
3. In distal zone A, pins may be placed into the ulna from the 150-degree lateral position (not shown).

a., Artery; *br.*, branch; *n.*, nerve; *v.*, vein.

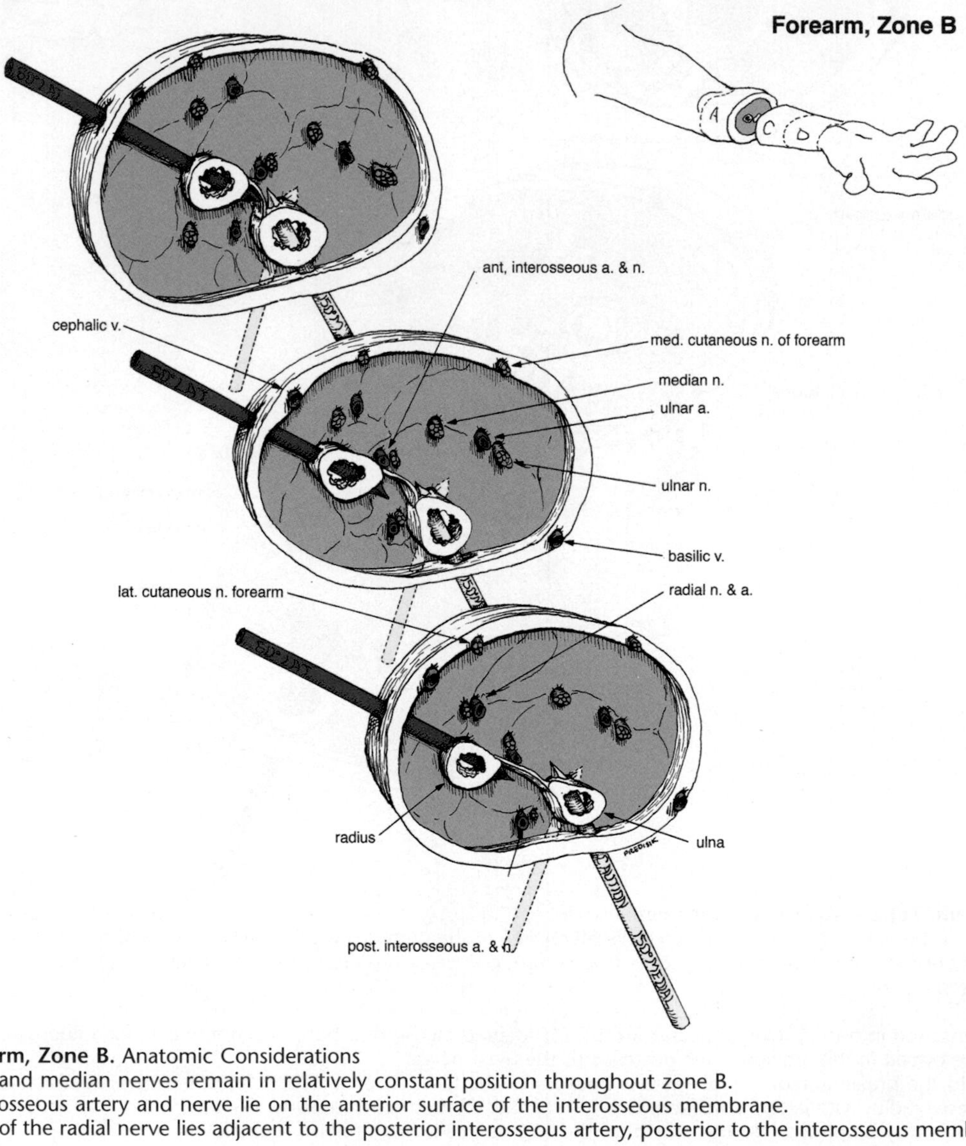

Figure 7-23. Forearm, Zone B. Anatomic Considerations

1. The radial, ulnar, and median nerves remain in relatively constant position throughout zone B.
2. The anterior interosseous artery and nerve lie on the anterior surface of the interosseous membrane.
3. The deep branch of the radial nerve lies adjacent to the posterior interosseous artery, posterior to the interosseous membrane and separated from it by muscle.

Pin Placement

1. Half-pins can be inserted into the ulna from the 150-degree medial position. Depth can be assessed with fluoroscopy.
2. Half-pins can be inserted (employing considerable caution) into the radius via the 60-degree lateral position. As with half-pin insertion into the ulna, fluoroscopy control is recommended.

a., Artery; *ant.*, anterior; *lat.*, lateral; *med.*, medial; *n.*, nerve; *post.*, posterior; *v.*, vein.

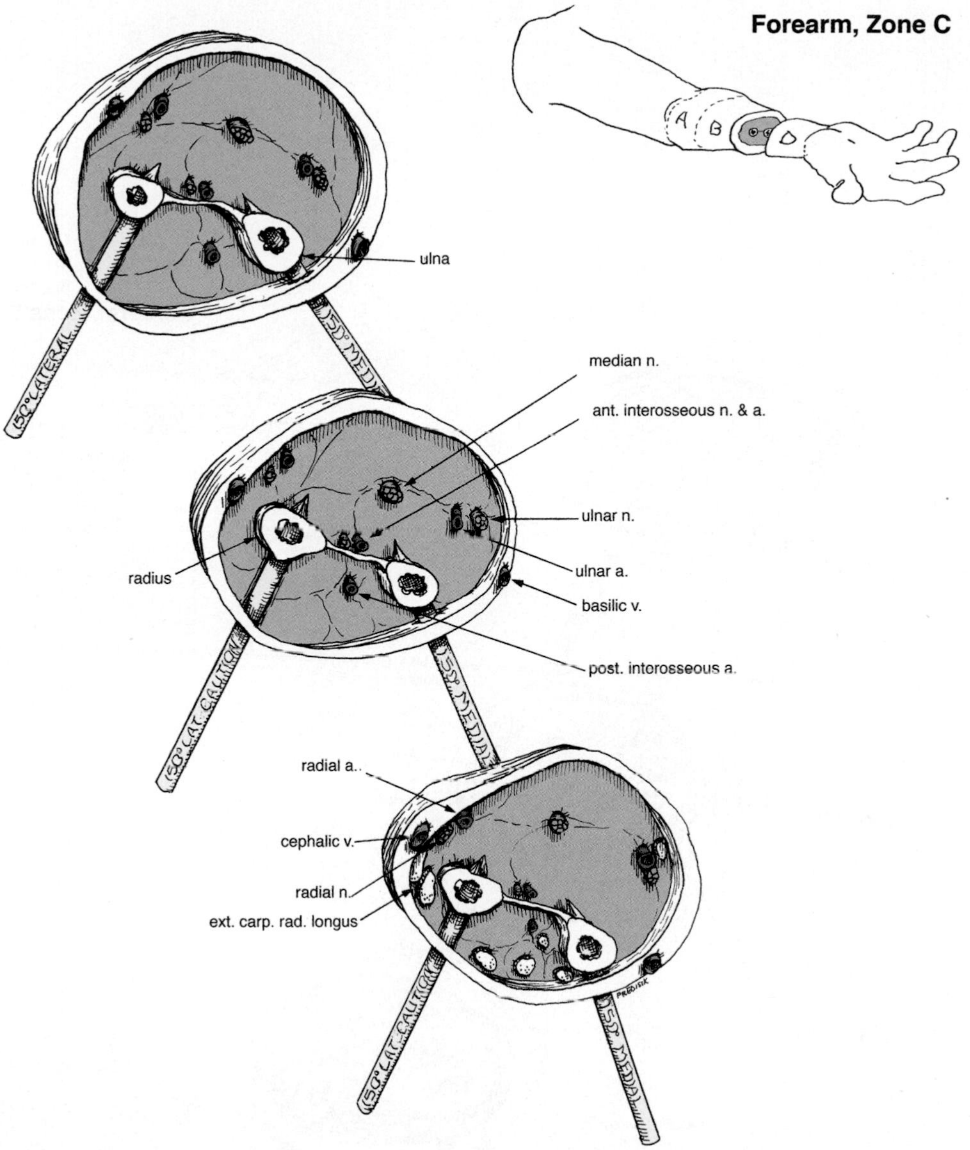

Figure 7-24. Forearm, Zone C. Anatomic Considerations

1. The superficial branch of the radial nerve and radial artery are anterior to the radius in zone C, becoming more lateral and superficial in the distal part of this zone.
2. The median nerve remains in the middle of the forearm, surrounded by muscle.
3. The ulnar nerve and ulnar artery remain anteromedial to the ulna throughout zone C.

Pin Placement

1. Half-pins may be placed into the ulna with caution from the 150-degree medial direction. In fact, half-pins may be inserted into the ulna from the 180-degree posterior position and the 150-degree lateral position as well, being mindful of the position of the extensor tendon as illustrated in distal zone C.
2. Half-pins may be placed into the radius from the 150-degree lateral position. Pins may also be placed into the radius from the 180-degree posterior position if care is taken to avoid impalement of extensor tendons.

a., Artery; *ant.,* anterior; *ext. carp. rad.,* extensor carpi radialis; *lat.,* lateral; *n.,* nerve; *post.,* posterior; *v.,* vein.

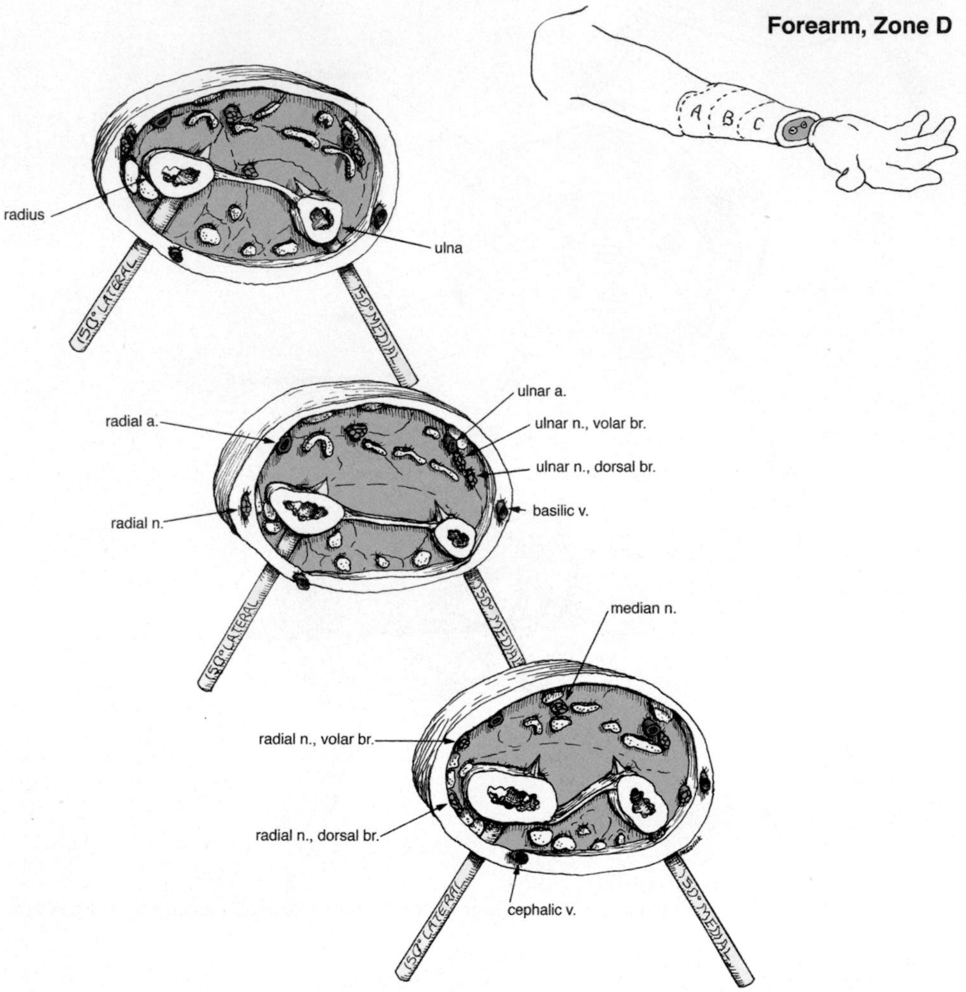

Figure 7-25. Forearm, Zone D. Anatomic Considerations
1. The radius and ulna are posteriorly located in the cross section of the forearm.
2. The radial nerve is lateral to the shaft of the radius, dividing into dorsal and volar branches in zone D.
3. The median nerve remains within the volar muscle mass.
4. The ulnar nerve divides into dorsal and volar branches, the dorsal branch passing to the posterior aspect of the distal forearm.
5. The extensor and flexor muscles become tendinous in zone D.
Pin Placement
1. Half-pins may be inserted with caution from the 150-degree medial direction into the ulna.
2. Half-pins may be placed into the distal radius from the 150-degree lateral direction. Note the relative position of the extensor tendons.
a., Artery; *br.,* branch; *n.,* nerve; *v.,* vein.

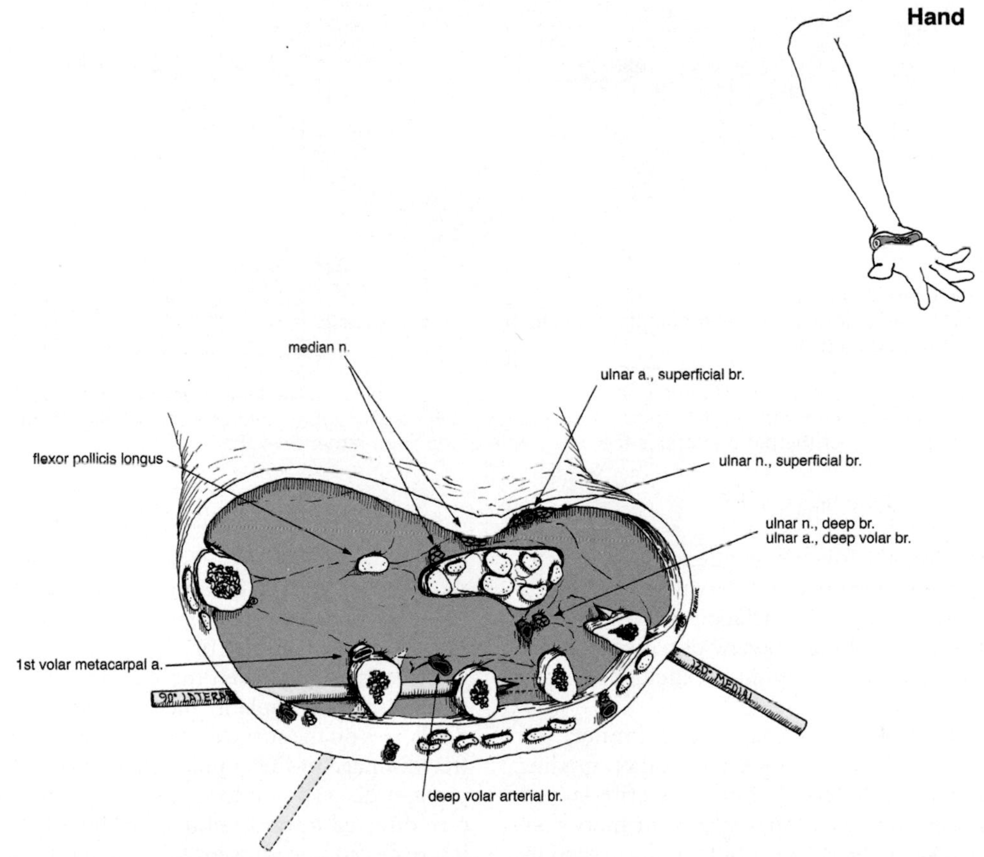

Figure 7-26. **Hand.** Anatomic Considerations

1. Cross section through the metacarpal shafts demonstrates the close relationship of the radialis indicis artery to the volar surface of the second metacarpal.
2. The palmar metacarpal artery to the second web space is adjacent to the radial volar surface of the third metacarpal shaft.
3. The ulnar artery and deep branch of the ulnar nerve are volar to the fourth metacarpal shaft, separated from it by muscle, a distance equal to the width of the bone.

Pin Placement

1. Wire, full-pin, or half-pin placement from the 90-degree lateral position can be safely passed through the shafts of the second, third, and fourth metacarpals. Extensor tendon impalement may occur as the pin passes through the skin on the medial side of the dorsum of the hand. The oblique lateral surface of the second metacarpal makes pin insertion difficult because the tip of the pin tends to slide on the bone.
2. Half-pin insertion into the second metacarpal from the 150-degree lateral position can be safely accomplished if done carefully.
3. Half-pin placement into the fifth metacarpal shaft from the 120-degree medial position can be done with caution, although the curved surface of the bone makes pin insertion difficult.

a., Artery; *br.*, branch; *n.*, nerve.

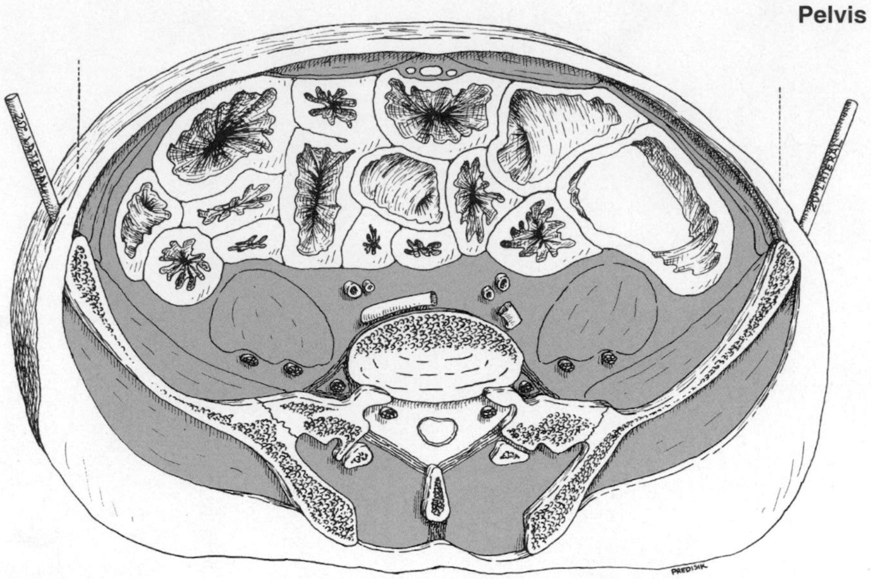

Figure 7-27. Anatomic Considerations
1. The ilium's inner table is separated from the abdominal contents by the iliacus muscle.
2. The iliac wings are concaved medially.

Pin Placement
1. Half-pins can be inserted along the iliac crest aiming at either the sciatic notch or sacroiliac joint from the 20-degree lateral position.
2. Full-pin placement from the anterior inferior iliac spine to the posterior inferior iliac spine requires a special alignment guide.
3. Pin placement is safer if the tip of the pin penetrates the outer table of the ilium rather than the inner table.

problem in determining the overall incidence of pin tract infections is that different authors use different sets of criteria to define pin tract infection. This variance is present even within a single institution, making a review of patients' charts an inaccurate procedure for determining the incidence of pin tract sepsis.

For this reason, the concept of "major" and "minor" pin tract infection was introduced, followed by other grading systems using numbers or letters. Using such criteria, just about every patient wearing an external fixator for more than a few weeks can expect at least one implant-site infection, something that must be kept in mind when informing a patient about a planned fixator application.

Pathophysiology of Pin- or Wire-Site Sepsis

Fluid Secretion

A metallic pin—or most hard foreign substances for that matter—when inserted into the body's tissues will provoke the development of a membrane separating the foreign material from the adjacent tissues. If relative motion is present between the foreign material and the local tissues, a bursal membrane usually forms to secrete lubricating fluid. With a transcutaneous pin, however, the bursal fluid becomes contaminated with microorganisms through the pinhole. Nevertheless, the contamination presents no special problem as long as the pinhole drains freely to the outside. Pinholes become infected when the delicate balance between the patient's natural defenses and the bacteria's infective capability changes. This alteration can result from (1) the development of an abscess (closed space) around the pin; (2) the presence of necrotic tissue in the pinhole, which can become the focus of sepsis; and (3) the presence of excessive motion between a pin and adjacent tissues, which increases fluid production.

Abscess Formation

As noted earlier, the fluid formed around the pin by the local tissues drains to the external surface and is contaminated with microorganisms in the process. The amount of fluid may be limited, especially when there is no motion between the soft tissues and the implant, such as over the anterior tibia. The fluid dries on the surface, forming a crust. If this crust restricts free drainage of the contaminated bursal fluid by sealing the pinhole, deep abscess formation may result. Thus, frequent pin care directed toward removal of the crust from the pin–skin interface reduces pin sepsis.

Skin Necrosis

Necrosis of the skin will occur if the tension (or compression) produced by the pin interferes with the circulation of the local subdermal capillary plexus. Plastic surgeons are mindful of this principle when transposing skin flaps; trauma surgeons using transcutaneous pins for external skeletal fixation must also keep it in mind. Skin tension can occur immediately after implant insertion or whenever a change in alignment or length is made. Skin can also be pinched between pins or wires if they are too close together.

Heat Injury

Thermal damage to skin and soft tissues occurs when a high-speed drill bit becomes hot while passing through hard cortical bone, burning tissue as it emerges from the opposite side of a bone. Avoid heat buildup by using a stop/start drilling rhythm and irrigating the drill sleeve while drilling (Fig. 7-28).

Deep Soft Tissue Necrosis

Necrosis of deeper soft tissues develops when tissues are compressed by an implant after it has been inserted. Such tension

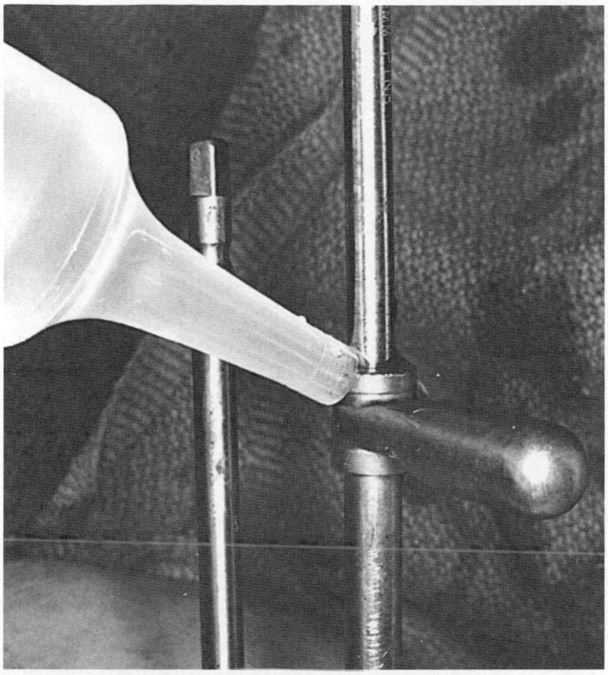

Figure 7-28. Irrigate the drill bit while drilling to cool it.

occurs in the anterior compartment of the lower leg if a pin pushes the anterior compartment musculature posteriorly. (It is far wiser to transfix the muscle by pushing the pin straight in, thereby avoiding undue tension.) Necrosis may also be produced if soft tissue "winds up" around a spinning implant or drill bit. (This can best be prevented by the use of a sleeve for both drilling and pin insertion.) Smooth wires will not likely wind up soft tissues, although a spinning bayonet point might do so (Fig. 7-29).

Bone Necrosis

Necrosis of bone can occur with the heat generated from drilling. Damage to osteocytes occurs after exposure to temperatures of 55° C (131° F) for 1 minute or more. Indeed, the mechanical properties of cortical bone change when exposed to temperatures of 50° C (122° F) or more.[53-55] The best way to prevent heat buildup is to predrill bone holes with a sharp drill bit, cooled with irrigation fluid, followed by the hand insertion of the implant.

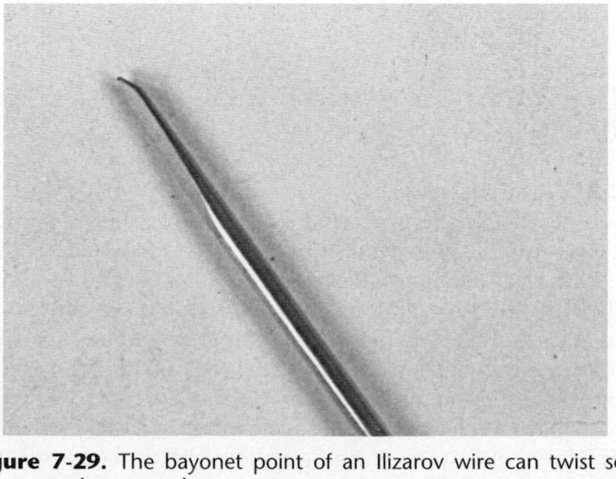

Figure 7-29. The bayonet point of an Ilizarov wire can twist soft tissue, causing necrosis.

Because each pinhole provides a continuous portal of entry for bacteria into the bone, heat-damaged bone is more likely to become a focus of chronic infection than is normal bone.

Excessive bone pressure—due to compression of a frame—may cause necrosis of osseous tissue at the pin–bone interface. The pressure reduces local bone circulation, resulting in death of osteocytes; necrotic bone may become the focus of a chronic infection.

Motion

Relative motion between a pin and adjacent tissues contributes to pinhole sepsis. As far as the microenvironment of the pinhole is concerned, it makes little difference whether the pin is moving with respect to the tissue or the tissue is sliding back and forth along the pin. The effect is the same, which is relative motion between soft tissue and a contaminated foreign body (the pin). Reduction of motion at the pin–tissue interface decreases the incidence of pin tract infections. (The low incidence of pin tract infections in reported series of fractures managed with pins-in-plaster is due, no doubt, to skin immobilization by the plaster cast.)

The Pin–Skin Interface

Wherever possible, reduce motion between the pin and soft tissues by selecting areas for pin insertion that avoids muscle transfixion. Further reduction in soft tissue/implant motion can be accomplished by wrapping the pins with a bulky wad of gauze dressing between the skin and the fixator.

Recognizing that implant-site sepsis usually starts at the pin–skin interface (rather than the pin–bone interface) has led some researchers and clinicians to try to reduce the infection rate associated with external fixation by coating the shaft of pins and wires with a known bacterial inhibitor, specifically, silver or tobramycin.[56-60]

Silver-based antiseptics are being employed in everything from neonatal eye drops to burn ointments. While initial experimental studies suggested that silver coating of pins could reduce infections in vitro[60] and in a sheep iliac crest model,[57] subsequent human trial revealed no difference in infection rate.[56] Moreover, the presence of free silver in the serum of patients in the silver-coated pin group caused the researchers to terminate the study and recommend against the continued use of such implants, effectively eliminating further development with such devices.[58]

The effectiveness of the antibiotic tobramycin against both staphylococci and gram-negative rods suggested that local application of the medication might reduce pin-site sepsis for transcutaneous implants. Unfortunately, tobramycin cannot be coated directly onto metallic pins with any predictable elution, so tobramycin-impregnated methylmethacrylate pin sleeves were developed[59] employing the antibiotic-cement combination used for total joint replacement or formed into beads for the treatment of osteomyelitis. As with silver coatings, the tobramycin-acrylic sleeves failed to deliver the expected benefit. Indeed, it seemed to some clinicians that the infection rate increased when tobramycin sleeves were used. A reasonable explanation for this observation is the tobramycin is eluted from the surface of the pins for a very limited amount of time, with antimicrobial levels surrounding tissue dropping off rapidly after a few days following implantation.

While the initial high concentration of tobramycin may sterilize a closed space like a cavitary osteomyelitis or a joint replacement, a pin sleeve, constantly exposed to fresh bacteria on the skin surface, may function as a contaminated foreign body perpetuating the infection once the antibiotic has leached out of the cement.

The Pin–Bone Interface

Pin loosening contributes to the development of pin tract infections. Perren, Schatzker and colleagues,[61,62] and others[51,63] studied the pathophysiology of loosening hardware within bone. They noted that bone resorption and subsequent implant loosening results from cyclic (rather than constant) pressure at the bone–metal interface. Once a pin becomes loose, pin–tissue interface motion will promote sepsis in a manner consistent with mechanisms already described.[51]

Employing only threaded pins can decrease motion at the pin–bone interface. If properly inserted, they will not slip back and forth in the bone as will smooth pins. Threaded pins, especially tapered threaded pins, should not be "backed out" once they are inserted, as they tend to loosen more quickly thereafter.

Another way to reduce cyclic pin motion is to increase the stability (stiffness) of the fixator configuration. Briggs and Chao[64] and others[65-71] determined that fixator stiffness can be increased by (1) increasing the number of pins; (2) increasing the distance between the pins within each pin cluster; (3) applying pins closer to the fracture site; and (4) incorporating pins that are mechanically stiff into the fixator.

The problem of fixator stability becomes critical if one or more loose pins must be removed for sepsis. Loosening of the remaining pins may occur as the overall stiffness of the frame configuration decreases. These difficulties can be avoided in the first place if a sufficient number of pins are inserted to allow removal of one or more pins without affecting the integrity of the fixation. As Naden puts it, it is "better to add a pin than to have one too few."[72]

Certain recent developments have helped reduce the incidence of pin tract infections caused by loosening, including the use of titanium—rather than steel—pins, and hydroxyapatite (HA)-coated threads (usually applied to steel pins).

The use of pins made from a titanium alloy rather than stainless steel results in a reduction in implant-site sepsis (as observed with other orthopaedic implant systems, including total joint implants and intramedullary nails).[73] The toxic effect of steel on cellular function may be related to the elution of certain metallic ions—perhaps nickel or chromium—from the implant's surface. Titanium pins reduce the incidence of pin tract infections by about 50%.[74] Moreover, it has been noted that when implant-site infections do occur around titanium pins, the problem stays localized to the immediate environment around the implant. Extensive cellulitis that extends for many centimeters around the pinhole (a common phenomenon when stainless steel pins are employed) occurs rarely, if at all, with titanium implants.

The only drawback to the use of titanium pins (aside from their higher cost) is their reduced stiffness when compared to stainless steel pins. While in some situations, such flexibility might be desirable, most surgeons prefer stiff fixator-pin-bone configurations, especially when bone fragments must be moved by the fixator to correct deformities. For this reason, researchers and manufacturers searched for a way to retain stainless steel's stiffness yet reduce the likelihood of implant loosening. The result was HA-coated threads of stainless steel pins.[55,75,76]

HA, the mineral of bone, is applied via an expensive but reliable ion-plasma coating technique to the surface of stainless steel pins to permit osteointegration of the patient's bone with the implant to reduce loosening. In a 1997 prospective randomized study using a sheep model,[75] Italian researchers found that local pin-site osseous rarefaction was significantly lower—and extraction torque significantly higher—when HA-coated pins were compared to uncoated pins. Five years later, German researchers conducted a similar project with human patients, comparing titanium pins to HA-coated pins.[76] They found a fourfold difference in extraction torque in the coated-pin group, and a marked reduction in pin-site sepsis as well.

Conversely, Pizà and coworkers in Spain compared HA-coated pins to uncoated pins in a group of patients undergoing limb elongation for stature increase.[77] Although they found a 20-fold decrease in pin loosening in the coated-pin patients, the incidence of pin-site sepsis did not differ between the two groups.

Thus, it appears that HA coating on pins, whether studied in animals or human, significantly reduces implant-site loosening but may not decrease pin-site sepsis, except perhaps in those situations where the infection is associated with osteolysis and loose pins.

In our own clinical experience, the osteointegration associated with either HA-coated steel pins or biologically inert titanium pins makes it almost impossible to remove threaded external fixation pins from cortical bone in awake patients. Injecting local anesthetic into or around the pin site does not help reduce the intolerable pain associated with trying to break loose an osteointegrated pin; instead, general anesthesia is used for fixator removal when bone ingrowth pins have been used.

Clearly, modern technology has improved the longevity of external fixation with threaded implants, diminishing both late loosening and those infections associated with osteolysis and diminished fixation. However, as previously mentioned, early soft tissue pin- or wire-site sepsis has not responded favorably to antibiotic- or antiseptic-coated implants. Instead, surgeons must resort to the time-honored methods of eliminating tissue necrosis at the time of pin or wire insertion, as well as those techniques that stabilize the implant–skin interface once the device is in place.

STRATEGIES TO REDUCE IMPLANT-SITE SEPSIS

Fixator Selection

The selection of the appropriate fixator construct is particularly important. In general, the configuration should be quite stiff. This feature alone will do much to prevent pin sepsis.[51,77] When dealing with a chronic bone infection or an extensively contaminated wound, the fixation frame should be capable of extraordinary rigidity. If the orthopaedic problem is less complex and the application short term, a less rigid configuration will do. If planning a secondary surgery while the fixator is in place, select a frame configuration with the contemplated procedure in mind. If comminution of fracture fragments is present, the frame should permit control of intermediate fragments. Because it is better to insert pins through intact skin, the fixator should permit pin placement to be dictated by the nature of the injury rather than by the configuration of the frame.

Pin Selection

Smooth pins: Smooth pins should not be used for external skeletal fixation. They create two holes in the bone but do not offer the advantage of "screwed-in" bone fixation. The unfortunate experience with the Stader and Anderson devices in the 1940s was due, I believe, to insufficient fixation with smooth pins.

Threaded pins: Both cylindrical and tapered-thread pins are available with or without the HA coating.[63] Most knowledgeable surgeons prefer the coated pins, although there is no clear consensus about which thread shape works best. Some pins are both self-drilling and self-tapping, but such implants have fallen out of favor with most surgeons, who prefer to predrill each pin site.

Pin and Wire Insertion Considerations

Fracture Alignment

Align the fracture as precisely as possible prior to pin insertion. An unaligned fracture will create undue skin tension (a source of possible necrosis) by the skin on the concave side of the fracture deformity when the fracture is reduced. The pins or wires may also pinch the skin on the convex side of the fracture deformity, creating additional skin necrosis. Moreover, some fixators require precise alignment of rotation at the fracture site before pin insertion because the frame does not permit correction of axial malalignment once the pins are in place.

Predrilling

Inserting a self-drilling stainless steel pin into the tibia of a young healthy adult male can be an exercise in frustration for the surgeon. After drilling for a while and making no headway, there is a tendency to push harder and turn the drill faster. Heat (from drilling) increases the microhardness of bone, making progress difficult.[53] To make matters worse, the cuttings (chaff) from the drilling of bone have no place to go because the pin contains no fluting (groove). The chaff also increases friction, making the drilling even more difficult. Friction created by these factors increases the temperature of the pinpoint until it is too hot to touch when it emerges from the opposite side of the limb. It is easier (and safer) if the surgeon predrills cortical bone through a drill sleeve before pin insertion. A sharp drill bit will penetrate bone more easily than will a pointed pin because the fluting of the drill bit permits the chaff to be carried away from the worksite, reducing friction and also the amount of effort required of the surgeon.

When drilling, stop the drill every few seconds to allow the cutting tip to cool. The heat generated by drilling not only damages the bone, but also "work hardens" osseous tissue, which then resists further advancement. A worthwhile practice is to irrigate the drill bit to cool it and conduct heat away from the tip.

If much resistance is encountered during drilling, check the drill-bit tip between your fingertips for excessive temperature. If the tip cannot be comfortably held for 15 or 20 seconds, do not leave an implant in the bone hole, as there will be necrotic (thermally injured) bone in communication with the pin's bacteriologic environment—a setup for chronic osteomyelitis. Instead, insert the pin (wire) elsewhere. Likewise, the bone in the drill bit's flutes should be white, never black or brown, which are signs of burnt bone (Fig. 7-30).

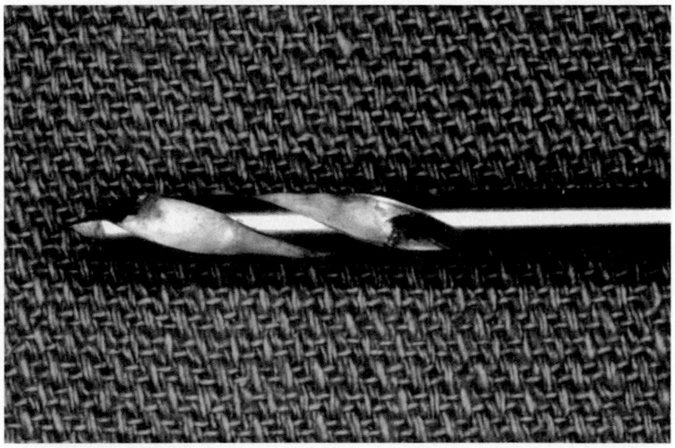

Figure 7-30. Bone in the flutes of a drill bit should be creamy white in color. Any brown or black spots on the bone's surface indicate that the bone was burned during drilling. Such a bone hole should never be used for external pin or wire fixation, since the risk of osteomyelitis is high.

Pin Insertion

Use a manual handle for pin insertion, which should be accomplished through the drill sleeve. Avoid overinsertion.

Inserting Transfixion Wires

As with pins, avoid tissue necrosis when inserting wires, which can be caused by either wrapping up of tissues, excessive tension, or thermal injury from heat buildup during drilling.

With transfixion wires, a spinning bayonet point may wind up soft tissues, causing necrosis. Therefore, push transfixion wires straight through the tissue to bone before turning on the drill. If the wire misses the bone, withdraw it completely and reinsert it rather than redirecting it within the limb's tissues.

When inserting transfixion wires into bone with a power drill, the dense cortical bone, by offering substantial resistance to the wire point's progress, may cause heat buildup, which hardens the bone even more, resisting additional progress of the wire point. For this reason, stop the drill every few seconds with a stop–start action to advance a wire slowly through hard osseous tissue

When inserting a transfixion wire with a motorized chuck, wire flexibility may, at times, cause the wire to bend, reducing accuracy of placement. For this reason, whenever inserting a wire, manually grasp the wire close to its tip to stabilize it. Since a spinning wire can wrap up surgical gloves, hold the wire with a wet gauze pad.

As soon as a transfixion wire's point penetrates a bone's far cortex, do not continue drilling since the spinning wire tip might damage tissues on the limb's opposite side. Instead, grasp the wire with pliers and hit the pliers with a mallet to drive the wire through (Fig. 7-31).

A most important principle when using any transfixion implant: If the tip of a wire (or pin) emerges from the opposite

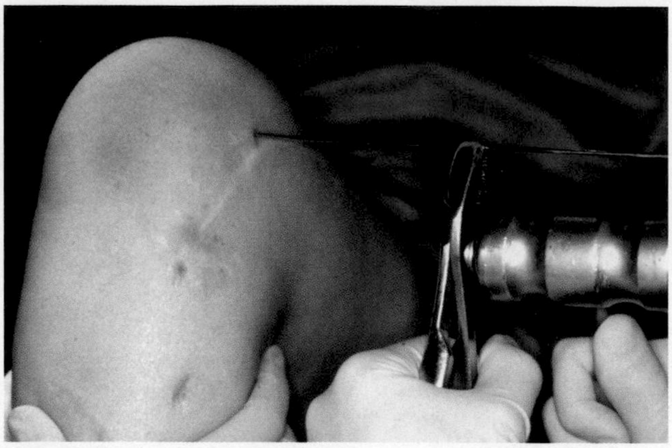

Figure 7-31. Use a mallet to drive a wire through soft tissues on the opposite side of the limb, thereby reducing the risk that a spinning bayonet pit will damage soft tissues.

side of a limb either smoking, or too hot to be comfortably held between the surgeon's fingertips, the wire should be withdrawn, cooled, and reinserted elsewhere.

Implant–Skin Interface Management

After inserting a wire or pin, but before attaching it to the frame, check the skin interface for evidence of tissue tension while the limb is in its most functional position—that is, with the knee extended, the ankle at neutral, and so forth. Interface tension will create a ridge of skin on one side of a wire or pin. Incise the ridge to enlarge the skin hole around either a transosseous pin or an olive wire. Close the enlarged hole with a nylon suture (if necessary) on the side of the wire opposite the released ridge.

When the ridge of skin is adjacent to a smooth wire, slowly withdraw the wire (with pliers and a mallet) until its tip drops below the skin surface. Allow the skin to shift to a more neutral location and advance the wire again until it passes through the skin in an improved position (Fig. 7-32).

If the interface tension exists on the insertion side of a limb, snap off the wire's blunt end obliquely to create a point and advance the wire to just below the skin surface by the pliers–mallet method on the limb's far side. Tap the wire back through the skin after making a position adjustment.

With either transfixion wires or pins, check the range of motion to make sure that no undo tension occurs during the anticipated movement required while the fixator is on the limb. If necessary, an implant should be reinserted if movement of an adjacent joint causes skin tension.

Certain important techniques of transfixion-wire insertion ensure maximum functional limb use and joint mobility:

- Avoid impalement of tendons.
- Avoid (whenever possible) transfixing synovium.
- Penetrate muscles at their maximum functional length.

This last rule—critically important for a successful long-term application—means that the position of a nearby joint must change as a pin or wire passes through the flexor and extensor muscle groups. For example, when inserting a wire into the lower leg, plantarflex the foot when transfixing the anterior compartment, invert the foot when inserting wires into the peroneal muscles, and dorsiflex the foot during triceps surae impalement.

Frame Assembly

Frame assembly can be extremely time consuming if the surgeon is not familiar with the technical details necessary for constructing the proper spatial configuration of the fixator. It is important to practice frame assembly prior to surgery. A piece of wood or synthetic bone can be used. Learn the correct names for the components, asking for them as one would ask for any surgical instrument. The OR personnel will quickly learn the names of the components if they are expected to hand them to the surgeon.

Once the frame is assembled, skeletal alignment should be evaluated with roentgenograms or fluoroscopy. Some projections will be difficult to interpret because of the presence of radiopaque components of the fixator. If this occurs, oblique projections can be obtained of both limbs (for purposes of comparison). If alignment is unsatisfactory, the entire frame should be loosened, and a manual correction of the limb carried out. The frame should not be used to correct malalignment of a fracture by compressing the convex, and distracting the concave, side of the fracture deformity.

Pin Care Routine

As noted earlier, it makes little difference to the pinhole microflora whether the pin is moving in the soft tissues or the tissue is sliding along the pin; the effect is the same, which is relative motion between the tissue and a contaminated foreign body. Reduction of soft tissue motion around the pinhole can be accomplished by forming a bulky wad of gauze dressing wrapped around the pin to completely fill the space between the skin and the fixator. This controls sliding of the skin when the limb swells, following ambulation or activity.

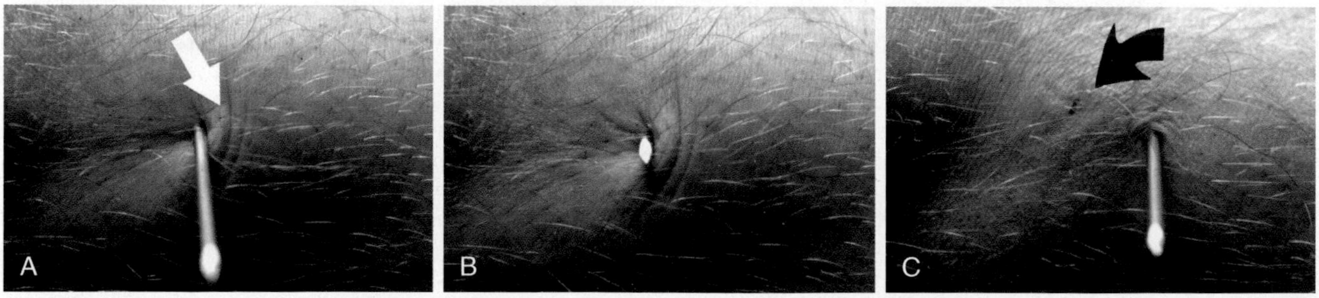

Figure 7-32. **A,** A wire can cause skin tension as it emerges *(white arrow)*. **B,** Withdrawing a wire causes skin tension and allows the skin to shift to a more neutral position. **C,** Push the wire forward through the skin in the new location with a mallet and pliers. The *black arrow* points to the original wire position in the skin.

The question of daily pin care stirs much controversy among workers in the field of external skeletal fixation. My routine for pin care consists of daily cleansing of the pins and surrounding skin with a soapy solution, using small swabs or applicator sticks. If the patient is reasonably agile, he or she can wash around the pins with soap and water in the shower. This is followed by application of an antibiotic ointment (Neosporin or Bactroban), and then a bulky wrap—as described earlier—to control the space between the skin and the fixator.

In spite of diligent efforts, however, some pins will become septic. Furthermore, pin tract infection, at times, seems to occur when least expected. A most carefully placed, thoroughly released, and well-managed pinhole may become infected while others in the same patient do not. Nevertheless, close adherence to the principles outlined in this chapter will do much to control the factors primarily associated with pinhole sepsis.

Ambulatory Aids

Because implant loosening is associated with sepsis, efforts should be focused on reducing cyclic stresses at the implant–bone interface. Such stresses occur with unprotected weight-bearing in lower extremity applications. Therefore, do not permit patients to ambulate with a fixator in place without supplementary ambulatory aids such as crutches (until the bone consolidates). The reason for this is obvious. The external fixator serves as an exterior skeleton when there is no continuity of bone following a fracture. The mechanical stresses of weight-bearing are transferred from the bone to the fixator at the implant–bone interface. The implants, being flexible, will transmit cyclic pressure associated with ambulation to the bone. This results in bone resorption and subsequent implant loosening. For this reason, unprotected early weight-bearing with an external skeletal fixator on the lower extremity should be discouraged.

Dealing with Pinhole Problems

If the patient presents with evidence of pinhole sepsis following application of an external skeletal fixator, the surgeon should make every effort to resolve the problem. Initial management consists of rest with elevation of the affected limb. The frequency of cleansing around the pinhole should be increased. I may enlarge the skin hole by infiltrating the skin around the pin with a local anesthetic, and then insert a size 11 blade into the skin adjacent to the pin. I also start the patient on oral antistaphylococcal antibiotics. If these measures fail to promptly relieve the problem, the pin clamp should be opened slightly and the pin checked for loosening by wiggling it. If the pin is loose—or if the maneuver produces pain—the pin should be removed. If removal of the loose pin affects the stability of the fixator, a new pin must be inserted in another location. The pinhole should be curetted with a small curette after a septic pin is removed. If, however, an infected pin is securely fastened to the bone, the patient should be admitted to the hospital for a brief course of parenteral antibiotics, bed rest, and a deep incision and drainage of the soft tissues around the pinhole. Antibiotic therapy can be guided by cultures of the implant site. If the septic process is not resolved by these actions, the involved pin should be removed and replaced with a new one in a different position. If the infection does not involve the bone, drainage should stop in a few days. If draining persists, there is a significant probability that the patient has developed a chronic implant-hole infection, which will require curettage and perhaps even more extensive care.

FIXATOR-ASSOCIATED PROBLEMS

Introduction

It is a rare individual indeed who happily wears an external skeletal fixator. Patient-related problems caused by the frame are pressure necrosis of the skin and undue or excessive pain. Pin or wire breakage may occur while a fixator is in place, causing distress to the patient and his or her surgeon. Disruption of the patient's lifestyle and psychosocial problems associated with external skeletal fixation, generally related to long-term application combined with protracted hospitalization, may occur.

Pressure Necrosis

Continuous contact with the frame or one of its components will cause intense burning pain for several hours, followed by ischemic necrosis of the tissues being compressed. This usually leads to an infection and a worsening of the fixator experience of all concerned.

The amount of clearance required between the skin and the fixator varies from region to region. In the upper extremity, and in lower extremity applications where there is bone immediately under the subcutaneous tissues (as in the pretibial region of the leg), two fingerbreadths between the skin and the fixator is sufficient. Three or more fingerbreadths are required over most soft tissue areas in the lower extremity where there is muscle between subcutaneous tissue and bone.

If limb swelling is anticipated, additional clearance will be necessary. Often more than three fingerbreadths are required in the lateral aspect of the thigh in an obese patient, because the soft tissues there bulge laterally when the patient is lying down. When applying an external fixator to the pelvis, 10 to 15 cm clearance must be left for the abdomen, so the patient can sit up. It is important to fill the space between the skin and the fixator with a bulky gauze wrap, to prevent excessive motion between the skin and the implants.

Broken Components

Occasionally, pins break while the fixator is on a patient. Chao and colleagues[78] observed that static stresses on the pins of a fixator applied without compression are 70 times greater than the stresses on the pins of a fixator applied with compression because of the overall fixator stability made by the bone being compressed. Thus, compression of the fracture site should be achieved if at all possible.

Disruption of Lifestyle

When applying an external fixator, the surgeon should consider the logistical problems associated with wearing the frame. Cover the sharp ends of pins and wires with plastic protectors. (Some manufacturers provide protectors with their fixation systems, but they are easy to fabricate from intravenous [IV] tubing.)

Pins and wires should not interfere with the function of the opposite limb. When applying a fixator to the upper extremity, do not inhibit the arm from adducting to the side of the body, if possible. In femoral applications, the frame should not occupy the area medial to the upper thigh for reasons of personal hygiene and comfort. In general, fixators should not be applied around the posterior thigh area, which would force the patient to lie prone for the entire time the fixator frame is in place.

Fixator frames have a tendency to loosen while they are on the patient. At each clinic or office visit, check the patient's frame and tighten if necessary. Loosening tends to occur where the fixator components meet at right angles. Compression or distraction, if necessary, should be carried out in a systematic fashion, that is, symmetrical length adjustments done at each visit. It is important to check for pin loosening, especially if evidence of pin tract sepsis or pain is present when the patient is evaluated.

PAIN

Pain following application of an external skeletal fixator is to be expected during the postoperative period and thereafter. The pain is usually well tolerated but excessive or undue pain requires evaluation and management.

Postoperative Pain

External fixation, like any surgical procedure, can be expected to produce pain postoperatively. The pain is usually appropriate to the nature of the problem for which the fixator was initially applied; for example, one can anticipate as much postoperative pain from the application of a tibial external fixator as would result from the use of internal fixation for the same injury. The patient's personality and pain tolerance threshold also determine the level of pain experienced and, consequently, the quantity of analgesics necessary for pain control. Patients with considerable drug experience seem to require more narcotic medication for relief than do other patients.

Pain around implant sites following surgery, while significant, is usually overshadowed by the operative site symptoms. However, if pain around an implant predominates among the early postoperative complaints, inspect the site. Occasionally, pressure from these dressings against the skin can produce discomfort, not unlike the pressure from a snug-fitting cast. The patient often complains of burning and can usually specify the implant causing the problem.

Skin and soft tissue tension occurs with shifting of a mobile tissue area impaled by transcutaneous implants. As with a too tight bulky wrap, tension on the skin at the implant site produces pain or a burning sensation.

Pain While the Fixator Is in Place

Ordinarily, the pain associated with a fixator diminishes to a tolerable level within 1 week after frame application. However, it is not unusual for patients, including those who are quite stoical, to describe a *continuous dull ache* requiring codeine or a similar analgesic medication for control during the entire time the fixator is in place. In some individuals, these symptoms vary with activity levels, being greatest when the patient is ambulatory and relieved by rest.

When the patient is permitted to ambulate in the fixator without supplementary aids (such as crutches), the problem is worse. For this reason (and to prevent pin loosening), supplementary ambulation aids are recommended whenever a lower extremity fixator is applied. The aids should be continued until the fixator is removed.

Excessive or *undue pain* may develop during the time the fixator is in place. This symptom is most distressing to the patient and should be investigated. At times, the patient may describe pain starting at a particular implant and radiating proximally or distally, suggesting nerve compression. The sensation may be continuous or intermittent and may be related to the position of the limb. Any pin that produces significant radiating pain should be removed because the involved pin may be putting pressure on a sensitive nerve.

Pain on Pin Removal

Patients who have had a very unpleasant pin removal experience seem to remember the event years later, even when other aspects of the fixator application have long been forgotten. A general anesthetic is usually needed for removal of a modern fixator that is securely integrated into the bone.

Persistent Pain after Fixator Removal

Pain following pin removal usually falls into one of the following categories: (1) bone pain associated with bone hole sepsis; (2) neurogenic pain resulting from persistent nerve irritation; and (3) pain associated with a healing fracture. Other causes of postfixator pain include the usual problems that occur in the posttrauma period. These include joint pain associated with restriction of motion and malalignment of the joint surfaces.

Bone Pain

Persistent bone pain localized over the pinhole and lasting more than 3 or 4 days after an external fixator is removed is unusual. If it does occur and is associated with persistent inflammation or drainage, expect a chronic implant-site infection to develop. Pain at the site can also occur after the hole has sealed over and the limb is quiescent. The patient may describe episodes of recurrent pain, sometimes accompanied by redness and swelling, which may subside spontaneously or after a brief course of oral antibiotics. However, if left untreated, a pathologic fracture can occur through the pin site as the cavity expands.

Neurogenic Pain

Chronic pain from nerve irritation should subside with the passage of time unless caused by limb lengthening or deformity correction. In such cases (which are rare in posttrauma reconstruction but fairly common in limb elongation for congenital deformities), a release of a band of tissue compressing the nerve may be necessary.

Pain Associated with Fracture Healing

Pain associated with fracture healing localized to the site of injury is similar to that seen with other modalities of treatment and usually subsides as the fracture consolidates. Solid union in a position of malalignment sometimes causes a dull ache that lasts for many years.

Psychological Problems

Many patients, toward the end of their treatment program, are anxious to have the fixator removed, even if no complications or problems developed while the fixator was in place. Professor Jacques Vidal and his associates found numerous socioeconomic and psychological effects of long-term treatment in an external skeletal fixator—including a sense of estrangement from their families, concerns about their ability to make a living, and fear of amputation.[79] Their patients were plagued with anxieties and many had suicidal thoughts at one time or another. Alcohol and drug consumption increased while in fixation. The incidence of these problems reflected the recently described posttraumatic stress disorders and depression symptoms that often accompany severe trauma. However, the prolonged nature of an external fixator application usually makes a bad situation worse.

Thus, viewed objectively, patients endure protracted hospitalization, psychological duress, disruption of their personal lives, and significant personality changes for the preservation of a dysfunctional limb. Professional psychological counseling may help.

The surgeon has the responsibility to prepare the patient for fixator application. It is worthwhile to tell the patient that pin tract infections are *likely to* occur. They should be told that one or more pins will probably have to be changed during the course of therapy, and that the procedure will probably require general anesthesia. These odds may be a bit higher than the actual likelihood of another anesthetic for pin management, but no harm is done by preparing the patient for the worst and hoping for the best.

PRINCIPLES UNIQUE TO THE ILIZAROV METHOD

Introduction

In acute traumatology, external fixator applications tend to be static: After application, the surgeon tightens the device's interconnecting hinges and the apparatus remains unchanged until removal. Once Ilizarov discovered bone's capacity to form new osseous tissue in a widening distraction gap, however, the indications for external fixation expanded, with limb lengthening and correction of deformities (both congenital and acquired) now being routinely treated with fixator frames.[15,80-85] To the familiar complications of external fixation—implant-site sepsis, nerve and vessel injury, inhibition of function, failure to obtain union—were added an entirely new set of problems related to moving bone fragments and regenerating bone formation. Moreover, the common complications of fixators tend to become more troublesome when the apparatus is employed for limb lengthening because tension on the soft tissues at the implant–skin interface during elongation increases the likelihood of ischemia and subsequent necrosis of dermal tissues, a setup for infection.

A limb's deep soft tissue structures—especially thick fascial sheets, such as the interosseous membranes of the forearm and lower leg and the thigh's linea aspera—resist stretching, even when performed slowly over weeks or months. This, in turn, can cause angulation of the lengthening bone segment or contractures of adjacent joints. If the contractures are not addressed while elongation continues, the joints can sublux or even dislocate completely.[86] The author is aware of cases of thigh lengthening for proximal focal femoral deficiency, for example, where both the hip and knee dislocated during treatment, a worrisome and difficult-to-correct combination.

Likewise, along with the typical difficulties encountered while trying to obtain union of fractures treated with external fixation, the creation of a long column of newly formed regenerate bone by the Ilizarov method presents a set of problems unique to that tissue, including failure of ossification, bending while in fixation, and fracture after fixator removal.

Because posttrauma reconstruction usually involves *restoration* of a limb to its original dimensions, one would expect fewer problems than might be encountered when lengthening a congenitally short limb because the injured limb was, after all, once of normal length. This is not always the case: Deep muscle trauma and secondary scarring results in tissue as resistant to stretching as natural fascial bands, or even more so. Likewise, protracted unsuccessful trauma care often leads to severe joint contractures before fixator application. Indeed, the equipment may be used solely to overcome posttrauma joint contractures. Needless to say, attempting to restore limb length, even of only a few centimeters, in a limb that already has a stiff posttrauma equinus or knee contracture is a challenging ordeal for both the surgeon as the patient.

Additionally, our capacity to create a column of new bone of substantial length has enabled surgeons to rebuild limbs that otherwise would have been unsalvageable. The treatment strategy in such cases usually involves intercalary bone transport, a technique that includes internal bone elongation. The moving bone fragment must, of necessity, be secured to a mobile component of the fixator, which slowly pulls the fragment from its original position to its "docked" position on the other side of the original gap (Fig. 7-33). In doing so, the wires securing the fragment to the frame cut through the skin and deeper tissues by a process that involves tissue necrosis and sloughing along the implant's path, with healing, one hopes, on the trailing side. Thus, in spite of advances in pin fixation attributable to HA coating, pin-site infections are still a problem, especially when bone fragments are in motion. Therefore, meticulous attention to the principle outlined earlier in this chapter is even more important for fixator applications involving moving bone segments than it is for frames applied for static purposes (see Fig. 7-33).

Because this volume deals with trauma to the musculoskeletal system and its consequences, the following considerations apply to those situations in which bone fragments move with respect to each other, either for restitution of limb length and alignment, or for filling in a defect created by traumatic loss of osseous tissue.

Treatment Principles for Nonunions and Malunions

One fundamental difference between treating a nonunion and a healed malunion is that with a nonunion, the site of any deformity correction (if needed) has been predetermined for the surgeon, as the correction must usually be made through the nonunion site.

If the nonunion is transverse (perpendicular to the bone's longitudinal axis), compression with either external (or internal) fixation will stimulate union. Many nonunions, however, are oblique, and often combined with malalignment of the bone fragments in angulation, rotation, displacement (of the mechanical axes), and shortening. When any or all of these deformities are associated with a nonunion, circular external fixation permits the surgeon to gradually correct all deformities, either simultaneously or in succession. With simple angular displacements, a hinged fixator will prove sufficient to solve the geometric problem, but for more complex

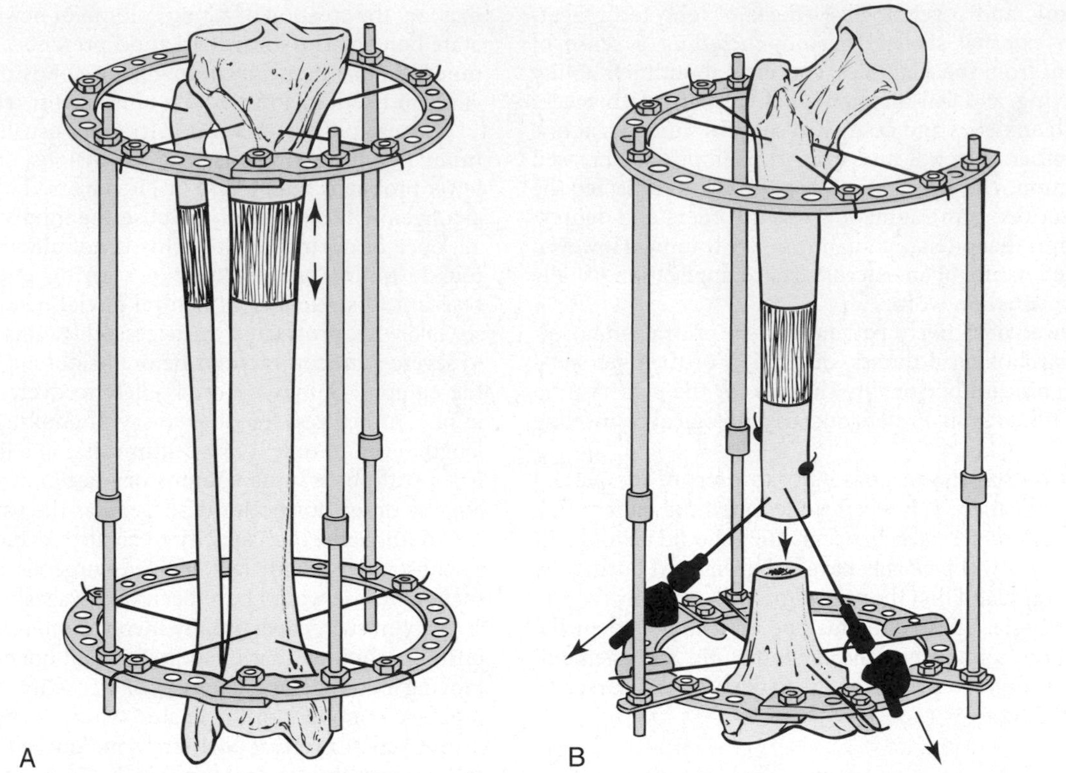

Figure 7-33. The Ilizarov method can be employed to elongate a shortened limb (**A**) or to overcome a skeletal defect (**B**).

malalignment involving multiple planes, the Taylor Spatial Frame, although rather expensive, has proven invaluable. A surgeon interested in employing this modality should attend a workshop on its use because many parameters of the deformity and frame configuration must be accurately determined and entered into a proprietary computer program, which produces a prescription for frame adjustment that the patient uses to lengthen or shorten the frame's struts.

When an infection is present at the nonunion site, the surgeon should thoroughly débride the infected bone—while stabilizing the limb in an external fixator—thereby converting the problem of an infected nonunion to an uninfected nonunion. Reconstruction of the limb following débridement usually involves intercalary bone transport if the débridement has resulted in any substantial loss of bone tissue and a segmental skeletal defect.

Segmental Skeletal Defects

Segmental defects may be due to either bone loss at the time of trauma, removal of nonviable fragments at initial débridement, or the result of resection of a tumor or necrotic infected bone. When a segmental defect is present, any angulation, rotation, translation, or combination of displacements can easily be corrected through the soft tissues at the level of the defect. For this reason, circular frames designed to deal with segmental defects are usually rather simple; the configuration is tubular, with the connecting rods of the frame parallel to each other and to the bone's biomechanical axis.

A skeletal defect can be overcome by Ilizarov's bone transport method (Fig. 7-34). The bone ends must be matched to fit at final docking of the intercalary fragment with the target fragment. The target site is often bone grafted to hasten healing. With very large defects, it may be possible to perform two corticotomies, and move the resulting bone fragments toward each other.

To eliminate the defect, make a corticotomy through healthy bone at some distance from the defect; thereafter, the intercalary segment between the defect and the corticotomy is pulled through the tissues until the defect is closed and new bone forms in the distraction zone. The fragments should be perfectly aligned with the longitudinal elements of the fixator. If this is not achieved, the transported fragment will not meet up with the target fragment.

If the defect is smaller than 1.5 cm, it is possible to compress the defect acutely (after appropriate débridement) and lengthen the bone through a corticotomy elsewhere.

It is unwise to acutely close a skeletal defect that is more than 1.5 cm, as the redundant soft tissues surrounding the defect tend to bulge out when the fragments are brought together, creating an unsightly appearance to the leg and kinking of both lymphatic and venous drainage. As this redundant skin is trapped between the wires, it cannot contribute to lengthening of the limb through another section of the bone. Therefore, the patient is left with a peculiar-looking limb with bulky redundant tissues at one level and tight, stretched skin at another. With this problem in mind, when dealing with a segmental defect of more than 1.5 cm, it is better to leave the soft tissues at length, and eliminate the defect by gradual transport of the intermediate segment.

A segment of bone can be pulled through a limb with (1) a transport ring and cross wires or pins or (2) with oblique directional wires.

A transport ring and an attached pair of crossed wires or pins is the most stable way to pull a bone fragment through

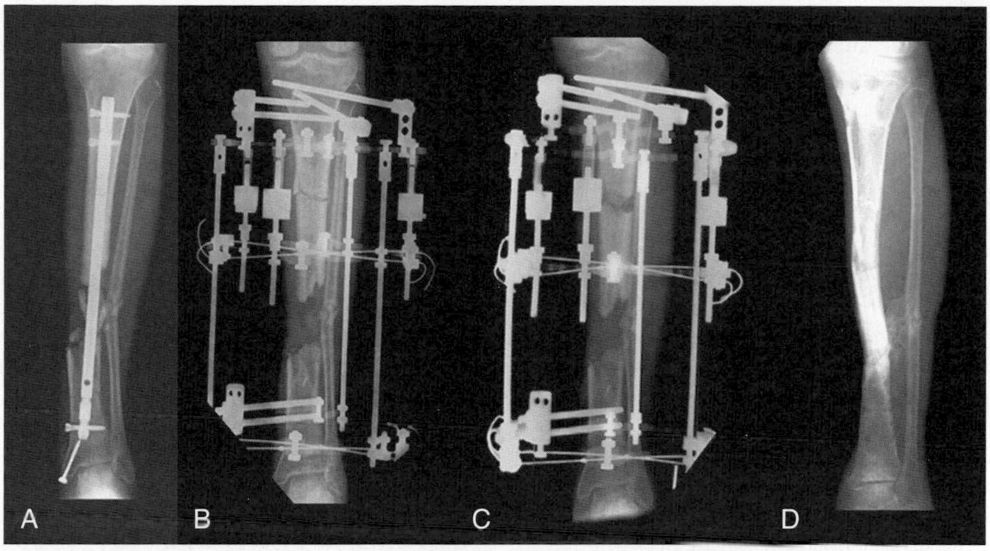

Figure 7-34. Infected intramedullary nail treated with débridement and bone transport. **A,** Initial presentation. **B,** At surgery, following removal of nail, débridement of nonviable bone and proximal corticotomy. **C,** During bone transport. Note the widening distraction gap and the narrowing defect. **D,** Oblique view demonstration cancellous autograft to create a tibiofibular synostosis.

tissue. Unfortunately, the wires cut through the skin and soft tissues as the ring and its attached bone segment move through the limb. At the end of bone transport, however, the crossed transport wires enhance compression at the point of contact between the intermediate fragment and the target fragment.

When oblique directional wires are used to move a bone segment through a limb, there is far less cutting of tissues, because the wires start out nearly parallel to the limb's axis. Unfortunately, such oblique wires often do not provide enough pressure at the end of bone transport to ensure stable interfragmentary compression between the intermediate fragment and the target fragment. For this reason, a surgeon using oblique directional wires must often insert a pair of crossed wires (connected to a ring) into the intermediate fragment at the end of bone transport to enhance compression at the point of contact. In such a case, the patient would require a second operation to insert the supplementary compression wires.

Joint Mobility

Intensive physiotherapy is also necessary to prevent the joint contractures and subluxations associated with limb elongation and the correction of deformities. Even if the fixator is applied to deal with a fracture or a nonunion—conditions not ordinarily associated with stretching of tissues—irritation of muscles impaled by pins or wires can lead to restriction of joint mobility. Thus, physical therapy has an important place in the management of all patients in external fixation.

Whenever bone fragments are moved with respect to one another, soft tissues are placed under tension: the greater the movement, the greater the tension. For this reason, it is important for the surgeon to consider every Ilizarov fixator application that involves movement of bone fragments as a form of limb lengthening, even if the extremity does not end up longer as a result of the procedure.

The important elements of every postoperative physical therapy treatment plan designed to prevent deformities and contractures include elastic splinting, passive stretching, active use of the limb, and appropriate nighttime positioning.

Stretching

Passive muscle stretching is another essential measure designed to prevent contractures. The physical therapist must teach patients and family members how to stretch the calf, the hamstrings, and other muscle groups. At least 2 or 3 hours a day should be devoted to this activity, especially in cases involving substantial lengthening. In fact, the greater the anticipated elongation, the more time per day must be devoted to passive muscle stretching.

Interestingly, active muscle exercises do not help much in preventing contractures. For example, active dorsiflexion of the ankle is not nearly as effective as passive stretching of the calf musculature in limiting equinus contractures.

Contractures

Contractures can occur, of course, whenever a fixator is applied, especially if the movement of muscles and joints is inhibited, either by the implants, muscle impalement, or pain. The most serious contractures develop, however, when bone segments are moved with respect to each other—especially during limb lengthening. Fortunately for the traumatologist, contractures associated with external fixation for the treatment of acute fracture, nonunions, or malunion almost never proceed to subluxation or frank dislocation. When joint contractures do occur, however, they can prove quite stiff and resistant to correction by simple means (such as Achilles tendon lengthening).

Limb Positioning

Proper limb positioning during the night is one of the most important prophylactic measures available during limb elongation or bone fragment movement. The 7 or 8 hours a patient spends in bed may be the most important hours of the day for a patient wearing an external fixator. During that time, joints allowed to fall into suboptimal positions will resist correction during daylight. A lower extremity that is permitted to rest with the foot in equinus and the knee flexed will likely develop a problem at both joints. A support behind the heel (rather than under the knee) forces the knee into neutral position. Likewise, dynamic or static supports of the ankle should be used at all times during bone elongation.

Functional Limb Use

Ambulation and upper extremity use not only promote ossification of the regenerate, but also help prevent contractures, subluxations, and dislocations. Weight-bearing, for example, serves as a means of passive calf muscle stretching while maintaining tone and stimulating circulation in the limb. Eating, hair combing, gymnastics, dance therapy, and other similar activities are also useful adjuncts to therapy. The rhythmic movements involved with swimming, cycling, and walking are among the best therapeutic exercises available.

Regenerate Healing and Maturation

Frame stiffness may have to change throughout the course of treatment. Initially, a fixator must be rigid enough to hold the fragments and the proper position, yet flexible enough to allow axial dynamization during loading. Additionally, an overly stiff frame may cause osteoporosis between the proximal and distal mounting clusters as the frame bypasses the bone's weight-bearing function. In the final stages of healing, individual longitudinal elements can be loosened completely or even removed. Likewise, individual pin- or wire-gripping clamps can be released in sequence permitting greater and greater load on the bone. Before removing the frame, it is wise to allow the patient to walk around for a few days with the transosseous implants in place, but no load sharing by the fixator. Ilizarov calls this final period of consolidation "training the regenerate."[87]

There is evidence that tardy regenerate ossification responds to certain physical stimuli, including ultrasound and electromagnetic stimulation, which speed maturation of the newly forming bone.[88-91] It is best to use such modalities after reaching the limb ultimate length or axis correction, lest premature ossification stop the process before reaching the goal. Bone grafting of the regenerated region is rarely necessary. Slow ossification can almost always be traced to limited ambulation or inhibited functional use of the limb.

With bone transport procedures, the "docking site" where the moving intercalary fragment of bone meets the target fragment, tardy bone healing frequently occurs. This happens because the advancing edge of the intercalary fragment becomes progressively dysvascular as it is pulled through the tissues and away from its blood supply. In Russia, Ilizarov's group routinely freshens up the bone ends about 1 cm before docking by returning the patient to the OR for curettage of bone ends about to make contact with each other. In the United States, surgeons will often preemptively apply a fresh autogenous bone graft to the docking site shortly after contact between the bone ends is established (see Fig. 7-34, *D*). This may lead to a few too many grafting operations, as some docking without grafting does result in union, especially if the spike of one fragment impales the medullary cavity of the other.

Toward the end of treatment, test the limb manually. The bone should feel quite solid, resisting deflection in any plane. I usually have the patient test the stability of the limb by standing on it. He or she should report no difference in the sense of stability, compared to having the frame secured. I require the patient to walk around for a week with the pins or wires and rings still connected to the limb, but with no longitudinal connecting rods or struts in place. Most often, patients prefer crutches for assisted ambulation during this period of time.

Post-Ilizarov Management

After the frame is removed, it should not be necessary to apply a splint, orthosis, or cast to the patient's limb, although this is commonly done by surgeons who remove fixators before radiographic studies show solid cortical bone on three sides of the regenerate. As Ilizarov once told me, "physiotherapy should be finished the day the fixator comes off."

By following the principles outlined in this chapter for both Ilizarov and standard external skeletal fixator applications, a surgeon will reduce the incidence of problems that might lead to an unpleasant experience for both patient and practitioner.

EXTERNAL FIXATORS AS NONUNION MACHINES

External fixators have been condemned as nonunion machines because it seems that so many patients in trauma frames fail to heal their fractures (Fig. 7-35). There are several reasons for this observation: first, fixators are applied to the most severe fractures, those with a natural propensity toward nonunion; second, with so-called spanning external fixators, weight-bearing or functional use is either very difficult or precluded altogether. And third, patients are transferred (often for insurance reasons) to surgeons not familiar with the original treatment plan leaving a patient in a sort of therapeutic limbo.

When applying an external fixator to an acute injury, reduction of bone fragments must be as accurate as with internal plate fixation if the frame is to remain on the limb during the entire treatment protocol. Suboptimal reduction might be acceptable with a temporizing fixator when the surgeon plans to soon remove the device and employ internal fixation as the

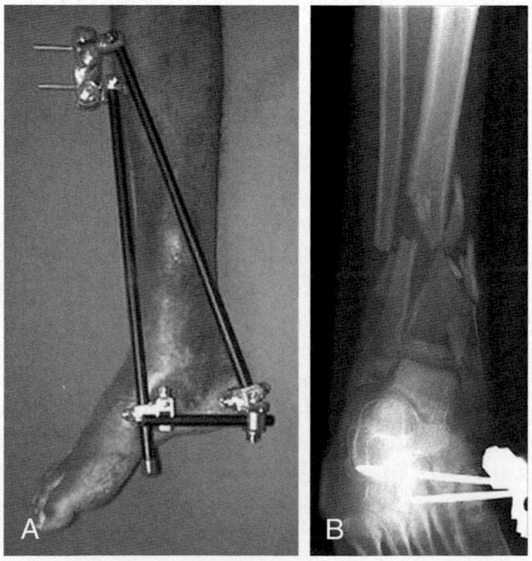

Figure 7-35. Patient placed in external fixator spanning the region of injury. **A,** The frame was left in place for 6 months without further treatment. **B,** Established nonunion with severe disuse osteopenia and not a molecule of osteogenesis.

definitive form of stabilization. However, bear in mind that the best laid plans of mice and men often go astray. Patients are transferred after accidents to facilities where a new caregiver may not be comfortable with the plan of the first surgeon, and decides to continue the patient in the fixator. The suboptimal alignment then becomes the basis for tardy healing or results in a malnonunion requiring a difficult reconstruction effort. It is far better to strive for optimal alignment when the frame is first applied (unless circumstances preclude the time required to achieve this goal), and then deal with any subsequent tardy union by bone grafting the troublesome region without the need for realignment. Indeed, early bone grafting is the hallmark of a well-thought-out treatment plan wherein the surgeon recognizes the worrisome nature of the fracture pattern at the time of injury and prepares to bone graft the limb within the first 6 to 8 weeks after the injury.

EXTERNAL FIXATORS FOR DAMAGE CONTROL ORTHOPAEDICS

Introduction

An abundant body of trauma care literature has confirmed that certain strategies of initial management of severely injured extremities reduce the likelihood of serious complications, while simultaneously enhancing the probability that the patient's functional outcome will be the best possible under the circumstances.[92]

One of these strategies involves early coverage of exposed tissues, either by delayed primary closure if enough local soft tissue is available, or coverage with transposed or transplanted soft tissue flaps. Even though centuries of civilian and wartime experience have taught us the danger of primary closure over devitalized muscle, bone, and adjacent soft tissues, we have also learned that prolonged exposure of any type of tissue to the atmosphere invites microorganisms to move in and establish long-term residence.[93]

A second strategy involves delayed definitive repair of displaced fractures, with the goal of restoring fragments to their original anatomic relationships without excessive devitalization caused by soft tissue dissection.[94] Reduction and internal fixation of fractures, regardless how carefully accomplished, causes reactive swelling of tissues. If such engorgement is superimposed on the swelling caused by the original traumatic injury, wound closure without tension becomes difficult; excessive traction of tight soft tissues frequently leads to incision breakdown, necrotic wound edges, exposed hardware, bone, tendons, and soft tissues.

Waiting 7 to 14 days for swelling to diminish after a traumatic injury before performing an open reduction and internal fixation has become a hallmark of thoughtful musculoskeletal trauma management.[95] While the early healing during the 1- or 2-week waiting period may make reduction of cancellous fracture fragments a bit more challenging (compared to the ease with which fresh fracture fragments can be pushed around), the trade-off yields substantial reductions in postsurgical wound dehiscence and, thus, a lower risk of infection.[37]

Third, unstable fractures, especially those associated with significant soft tissue damage, benefit from mechanical stabilization as soon as possible after injury. As patients are moved around acute care facilities, on and off radiograph, computed tomography (CT), and magnetic resonance imaging (MRI) tables, to and from the operating suite, and into and out of the intensive care unit, jiggling of fracture fragments is not only intensely painful, but also macerates and may even kill marginally viable soft tissues and especially skin of questionable vascularity. Likewise, blood clots are disturbed by undue tissue motion, and bleeding may resume after too much movement. Finally, delicate surgical repairs of vascular injuries are easily torn apart when limbs flop around after surgery.

Fourth, surgeons often find it difficult to judge soft tissue viability immediately after a catastrophic injury. At times, tissues we thought were dead may truly be so, whereas in other wounds, marginal soft tissue may survive unexpectedly. A "second look" return to the OR by patient and surgeon 24 to 48 hours after an injury is often the best way to judge the viability of tissue remaining in the wound.[94,96,97]

The goal of limb stabilization in this context permits return trips to the OR for repeated débridement without disruptive manipulation of fracture fragments, a potential source of further soft tissue injury.

With these objectives in mind, the concept of temporary spanning external fixators has evolved.[97] During fixator application, precluding transcutaneous implants near the region when subsequent internal fixation is planned eliminates the risk of pin- or wire-site sepsis contaminating the operative field of the open reduction and internal fixation surgery (Fig. 7-36).

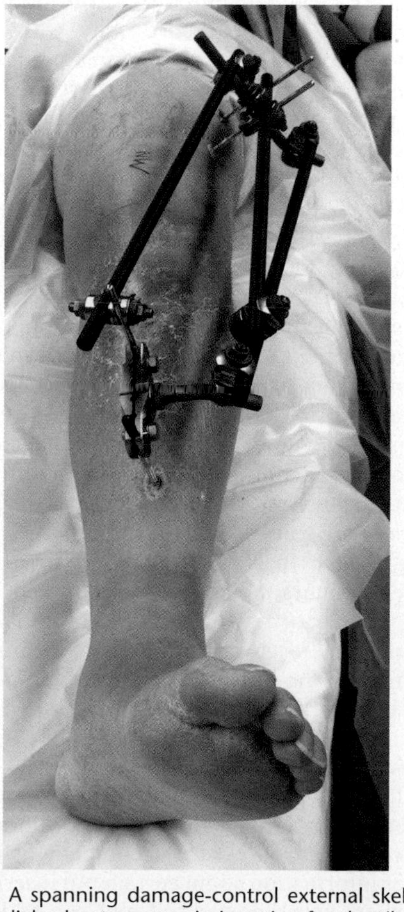

Figure 7-36. A spanning damage-control external skeletal fixation. Notice the medial subcutaneous pin insertion for the tibia and lateral pin placement for the femur.

When the zone of injury scheduled for definitive internal fixation is limited to the middiaphyseal region of a long bone, spanning external fixation can often be applied to the same bone, with external fixation limited to the ends of that same bone. This would be the ideal situation because freedom of movement of the adjacent joints would not be inhibited during the period of temporary external fixation. Indeed, in such cases, it is also possible to convert a temporary external fixator to a more permanent one and dispense with internal fixation altogether.

More commonly, however, joint involvement accompanies injuries that lead surgeons to apply spanning external skeletal fixation: Either the fracture lines of the diaphysis extend into the joint, or the joint itself may be severely damaged. In either event, applying a temporizing external fixator stabilizes the osseous and soft tissues, preventing further damage and reducing pain.

The Temporary Fixator

When an external skeletal fixator is used as a temporizing device, the frame configuration need not be as sturdy as would be required for a more definitive application.[96,98] As a general rule, patients who are so severely injured as to require a temporizing external skeletal fixator as an early step in a protracted therapeutic strategy are rarely capable of getting up out of bed and walking around with a fixator in place on a lower extremity. Likewise, for upper extremity applications, such individuals will not soon be bowling or playing basketball.

Under the circumstances, temporizing external fixators usually consist of two half-pins secured to bone proximally, and two more half-pins inserted distally, with one or more longitudinal rods connecting the proximal pin group with the distal pin group. Typically, universal joint articulations connect one rod to another when spanning a substantial distance.[98]

Pin-gripping clamps, typically incorporating universal joints, completed the configuration. In many cases, one multihole pin clamp is used for each pin cluster, although from a mechanical perspective, spreading out the pins in each fragment, and securing each pin to its connecting rod with its own pin-gripper, creates a more stable mounting.[96]

Specific strategies for timing of frame application, initial and subsequent wound débridement procedures, soft tissue management, antibiotic prophylaxis, anticoagulation, and other general principles of trauma care are covered in detail elsewhere in this volume. Likewise, operative techniques for the reduction in fixation of fractures and dislocations are described in chapters organized by anatomic regions.

This section will emphasize concepts common to all fixator applications used as part of damage control orthopaedics, whereby the configuration should be mounted in a manner that affords access to the wound for additional therapeutic measures and, wherever possible, allows definitive fixation without increasing the risk of deep sepsis caused by an earlier pin-site infection.

Military Applications

Because military surgeons may be forced by circumstances to apply temporizing external skeletal fixators without the benefit of a fluoroscopic control,[99-102] the accompanying cross section atlas includes information about certain pin insertion sites and directions where half-pins and full pins can be inserted with low risk to nearby nerves, muscles, and tendons.

The Drill Sleeve

Regardless of the availability or lack thereof of sophisticated OR equipment, whenever threaded implants are used for external skeletal fixation, a drill sleeve should be employed for pin insertion. Ideally, predrilling the bone hole with a sharp drill bit is desirable but not absolutely necessary if the implant itself has a cutting tip and flutes to carry away the bone dust generated while the hole is being made. Even in this situation, however, where no high-speed drill bit is used, a drill sleeve is essential. Without a sleeve, drill bits and, to a somewhat lesser extent, threaded pins wrap up soft tissues during insertion. This action strips the tissues from their blood supply, creating necrotic material in the implant site, necessary pablum for microorganisms.

Indeed, the single measure that increased acceptance of external skeletal fixation by orthopaedics surgeons in the third quarter of the twentieth century was the introduction of the drill sleeve. Before that, septic pin sites were the hallmark of external fixator applications.

Conversion to Permanent External Fixation

In some situations, primarily related to wound care logistics, a temporizing fixator is on a limb far longer than originally anticipated. In some cases, such a fixator may even be transformed into a definitive fracture care device. Although it is certainly possible to remove a temporary external fixator and apply a more permanent configuration with new transcutaneous implants, it is certainly more elegant to plan for such a conversion in advance.

Often times, experience with similar fracture patterns and soft tissue wounding allows a more experienced surgeon to recognize that definitive internal fixation may not be possible in a given situation. With this in mind, the location, number, and material properties of the implants would certainly differ from those contemplated for short-term applications.

Choice of Implants

A substantial reduction in pin-site sepsis occurred when titanium pins were introduced. Osseous integration at the pin–bone interface reduced early implant loosening, a precursor to pin-site sepsis. Likewise, coating a pin's threads with an osteoconductive substance, specifically calcium HA, regardless of the metal, further diminished the incidence of implant site sepsis.[76,103-106]

Each advance in the external fixation pin technology appears to enhance the potential longevity of a fixator application. However, every improvement seems to increase the cost of the transcutaneous implants.

For temporizing external fixation, where device removal is expected 2 or 3 weeks after mounting, costly transcutaneous pins are not necessary, since the benefit of titanium pins or coated pins does not become a critical factor in reducing pin-site sepsis unless the frame is on for several months.

Therefore, when applying a temporizing external skeletal fixator, low-cost stainless steel pins will do.

Reducing Costs from Inventory Control

A potential way of lowering the cost of a temporary external skeletal fixator is to reduce inventory by having only a limited number of implant sizes available.

For adult applications, as one would expect in a military field hospital, 6-mm-diameter pins are far more rigid, and thus more stable, than 5-mm pins. Stiffness of the material is proportional to the 4th power of diameter, so the extra millimeter provided by thicker pins enhances the stability of the overall configuration and reduces the need for more than two transosseous implants per segment.

Likewise, a pin with a 30-mm thread length, when used in an adult, can transverse the medullary canal and engage both cortices of the femur and tibia and even the calcaneus with hardly any threads protruding from the far cortex.

Implant Depth

For most upper extremity applications, especially those where the fixator application is short term, 5-mm-diameter pins are adequate, and a thread length of 20 mm will prove satisfactory for virtually all upper extremity applications.

Modern external skeletal fixation pins are manufactured from the bar stock. During the fabrication process, threads are cut into the bar so that the exterior diameter of the threads is the same as the exterior diameter of the pin. (Typically, the core diameter of the threads are about a millimeter smaller than the exterior diameter.) This feature precludes overinserting the pin because the implant will not advance in the bone once the threads have bottomed out. Ideally, when a threaded pin is fully inserted, a few millimeters of the implant should stick out the far side of the bone because the first two or three turns of the thread are of smaller diameter than the rest (or incorporate cutting flutes) and, thus, do not grip the bone very well, if at all.

Using the Atlas for Damage Control Orthopaedics

The pin locations and the directions in the accompanying cross-sectional atlas have been selected to allow for safe pin insertion even if the threads protrude beyond the far cortex.

Thus, if a pin in the atlas is designated "safe," (indicated by *green* color) it can usually be driven all the way through the limb and out the opposite side without risk of nerve or vessel injury, provided that the location and direction are as indicated.

In the accompanying atlas, when a nerve, vessel, or tendon is on the opposite side of the limb from pin insertion, but the distance exceeds one bone diameter, the level and direction of insertion is designated "caution" (indicated by *yellow* color). And if any nerve, muscle, or tendon on the opposite side of the limb from pin insertion is less than one bone diameter on the opposite side of the limb from insertion, the level and direction of implant insertion is designated "danger" (indicated by *red* color).

When a direction of insertion is designated "safe," a full pin can be used in place of a half-pin in such locations when more stability and additional fixation is needed on the opposite side of the extremity. Bear in mind, however, that when a threaded pin is driven through soft tissue without a drill sleeve, wrapping up of soft tissues can cause significant problems. While drill sleeves are widely used in conjunction with pin insertion on the near side of the limb, no such sleeves exist to protect soft tissues on the limb's far side. To overcome such concerns, special centrally threaded pins (with smooth shafts on both sides of the threads) were developed in the 1970s. Unfortunately, they are rarely, if ever, used nowadays, and may not be available except on special order.

When external fixators are applied in damage control orthopaedics, full pins (through-and-through) are virtually never employed; half-pins serve well in virtually all anatomic locations.[94,96-98]

Danger Regions for Percutaneous Pins Inserted without Fluoroscopy

As mentioned earlier, forward field hospitals in combat situations often lack fluoroscope capabilities, so military surgeons were wondering about the safety of "blind" insertion into lower extremities (i.e., half-pin insertion without the use of fluoroscopy). Topp and colleagues,[107] working at the Brooke Army Medical Center, used cadaveric lower extremities to assess the accuracy and safety of fixator application under such trying circumstances. They concluded that if military surgeons confined their pin insertion locations and directions to certain safe corridors, the likelihood of significant nerve or vessel injuries caused by the pins were within acceptable limits, considering the nature of the casualties being treated. Moreover, they learned that surgeons with greater experience with external fixation were less likely to overpenetrate very much past the far cortex during pin insertion.[107]

As a general principle, whether inserting external fixation pins or wires with or without fluoroscopy, certain nerve or vessel structures are at risk regardless of the method used to secure the frame to the bone. In several locations, a nerve or vessel lies directly on the surface of a bone where it is easily injured. In other instances, nerves or vessels traverse a limb perpendicular or oblique to its longitudinal axis, making it vulnerable to injury. The following structures our particular importance in this regard.

Deep to the femur, however, laying along its posteromedial side, is located the deep femoral artery, a structure that provides transverse feeder vessels to the thigh muscles. More importantly, the superficial femoral artery, in the mid-thigh, is one of bone diameter away from the femur in its coronal plane. A surgeon inserting pins into the lateral cortex of the femur should avoid overpenetration, a possible source of true or false aneurysms, both of which have been created by external fixation pins and wires. Limiting thread length to 25 or 30 mm should prevent damage to these structures, for reasons explained earlier.

Femur

The entire shaft of the femur is generally safe for pin insertion from lateral to medial in the coronal plane of the body. The lateral femoral cutaneous nerve, which traverses obliquely from front to back in the upper lateral thigh, is easily pushed out of the way when a trocar and sleeve is used for pin insertion.

In the middle of the thigh, between zones B and C, the superficial femoral artery crosses the coronal plane of the limb one bone diameter medial to the femur. The deep femoral artery and veins lie adjacent to the posterior-medial corner of the femur in the lower part of zone B, but this has not been a clinical problem, perhaps because the vessels are behind the coronal plane of the bone (Fig. 7-37).

At times, surgeons insert pins into the femur in the anterior to posterior direction, impaling the rectus femoris as they do so. While the anterior to posterior direction is generally safe (because the sciatic nerve is more than one bone diameter away from the femur), transfixing the rectus femoris

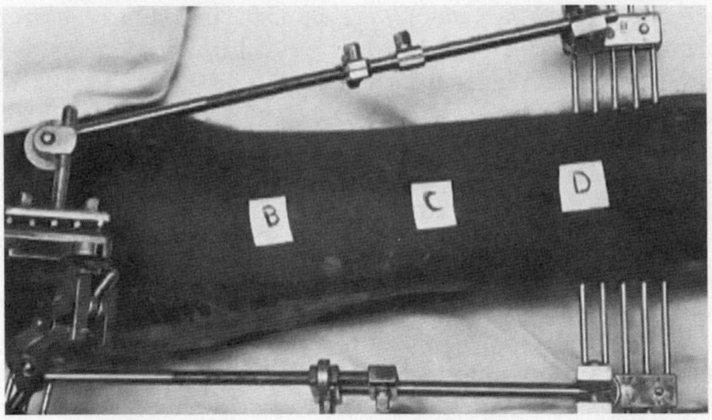

Figure 7-37. Half-pins can be safely inserted from front to back (taking care not to overpenetrate past the bone) to most of the femur. However, quadriceps impalement is undesirable. Coronal plane pins can safely be inserted in most regions of the thigh as shown in zone D here.

eliminates knee flexion. While this may be desirable in damage control orthopaedics, especially when the distal femur or upper tibia are shattered, there is risk that the central part of the quadriceps muscle will adhere to the bone if the fixator is left in place for too long. It often happens that a well-thought-out sequence of therapeutic interventions may be interrupted because the patient is transported to a different facility under the care of different doctors. Alternatively, problems pop up during treatment that makes it necessary for the surgeon to leave the external fixation device on the limb for longer than originally anticipated. Weeks sometimes stretch into months. Patients lay around in extended-care facilities waiting for insurance issues or scheduling considerations, or some other delay in prompt conversion from external fixation to internal fixation, resulting in protracted time in the frame.

The best way to prevent quadriceps binding to the front of the femur is to apply pins, even those that are used temporarily, from the lateral side in the coronal plane or even aiming slightly anteriorly from slightly posteriorly (to avoid impaling the deep femoral artery).

Typically, applying the fixator from the lateral side of the femur and extending the configuration to the tibia means that some kind of articulation and intercalary bar must be used to get from the outer side of the femur to the inner side of the tibia. This is because most tibial mountings for damage control orthopaedics occur from the medial side of the bone where the osseous surface is the subcutaneous.

Tibia

The entire anterior-medial subcutaneous surface of the tibia seems ideal for external fixation pin insertion, even without the use of fluoroscopy. Having said that, the natural tendency is to insert the pin perpendicular to the flat surface of the tibia. This approach is generally safe if the surgeon is careful about depth on the opposite side of the bone. In most locations, a 30-mm thread length that cannot overpenetrate is quite safe. Throughout the lower leg, the neurovascular structures at risk are generally a bone diameter away from the far surface of the tibia. An even safer direction, except for one location, is to insert the pins in the coronal plane, something that can be accomplished from either the medial or the lateral side of the bone (Fig. 7-38). Of course, inserting pins on the lateral side of the bone in the coronal plane means that the implants must cross the muscles of the anterior compartment, thereby limiting ankle motion if this is desired. Inserting pins from the medial side, although perhaps a bit more difficult because of interference with the opposite limb during the surgery, is remarkably safe. In fact, even if the pin passes through into the limb and sticks out from both sides, no neurovascular structures are likely to be injured, with one exception. As mentioned earlier, at the junction of the third and fourth quarters of the tibia (zones C and D), the anterior tibial artery and deep peroneal nerve rest directly on the lateral surface of the tibia and, thus, could be injured by a coronal pin (Fig. 7-39).

These neurovascular structures traverse obliquely from posterior to anterior and cannot easily slide out of the way when a pin passes nearby because of their tight attachment to the bone. Fortunately, most of the innervation of the deep peroneal nerve has already happened by the time the nerve is so distal in the limb. However, loss of nerve function at this level results in a patch of hypesthesia in the dorsal webspace between the hallux and the second toe. Motor function of the peroneal nerve controls the small extensor muscles on the dorsum of the foot. The anterior tibial artery is one of three vessels supplying the foot; it terminates as the dorsalis pedis artery. Thus, it is not critically important unless the other two vessels (the posterior tibial artery and the peroneal artery) have been damaged.

Pins inserted into the crest of the tibia directed from front to back, while seemingly simple and safe pose an unusual risk: a ring sequestrum and osteomyelitis. The anterior tibial cortices are particularly dense and, thus, can be overheated

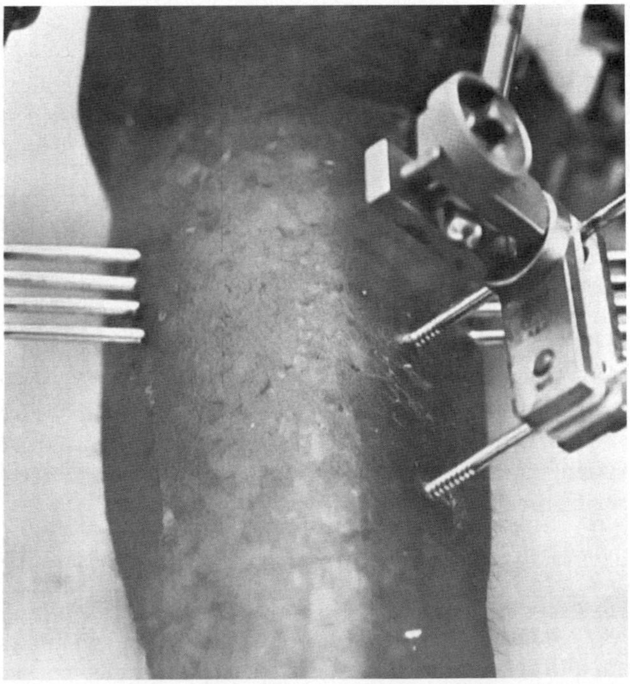

Figure 7-38. Half-pins or full pins can be inserted in the coronal plane through most of the tibia except at the junction of the third and fourth quarters (lower zone C and upper zone D) where the anterior tibial artery and deep peroneal nerve crosses the coronal plane of the tibia on the lateral surface of the bone. With control of depth, half-pins can be inserted throughout the tibia perpendicular to the subcutaneous surface.

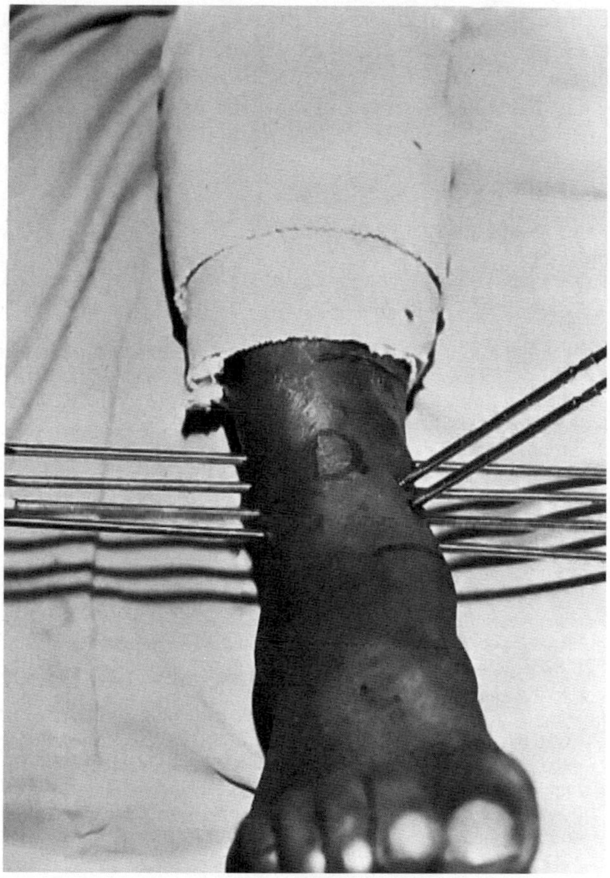

Figure 7-39. As with the proximal tibia, full pins and half-pins can be inserted in the coronal plane of the bone below the crossing point of the anterior tibial artery in deep peroneal nerve. Likewise, throughout the tibia, half-pins can be inserted perpendicular to the medial subcutaneous surface.

during drilling, causing necrosis of the bone around the pinhole, a sure setup for future infection.

Humerus

With respect to the humerus, the radial nerve is the primary danger structure because of its intimate contact with first the medial and then the posterior surface of the bone. This occurs in the upper half of the upper arm (and zones A and B). In the third quarter of the upper arm (zone C), the radial nerve moves away from the bone but is, unfortunately, directly in the lateral position with respect to the humerus and, thus, can be easily injured when the pin is screwed into the bone from the lateral side. Fortunately, the nerve can be palpated as a thick, oblique, ropey structure in the soft tissues and thus pushed either forward or backward at the time of insertion. Moreover, insertion is recommended in this region with visualization of the nerve.

There are, however, safe locations in the humerus although they are not often recognized. Pins can be inserted from front to back rather safely in the humeral head. Lateral to medial insertion in this direction risks overpenetration and the damage of the glenoid. This occurs because the bone is cancellous in this region and, thus, there is no firm cortex to stop the advancement of the pin, even one that is not threaded beyond 30 or 40 mm.

The axillary nerve, which innervates the deltoid muscle, sits on the deep surface of that structure, wrapping around the upper end of the humerus about a hand's breadth below the lateral edge of the acromion process. Proximal to the axillary nerve, the humeral head can serve as a fixation point for the upper end of a temporizing fixator. Implants can be inserted from front to back, from lateral to medial, and even from posterior to anterior. Bear in mind, however, that overpenetration of a laterally placed implant will end up in the glenoid surface of the scapula.

In the distal humerus, surprisingly, posterior to anterior insertion is reasonable. The brachial artery and median nerve are protected by the thickness of the brachialis muscle, which is at least as thick as the distal humerus (Fig. 7-40). However, as the distal humerus approaches the olecranon fossa, the bone thins out considerably making fixation difficult. In this region, no more than a 20-mm thread length should be used.

Forearm

In the forearm, the radius is a dangerous bone for pin insertion because, like the humerus, the radial nerve wraps around the proximal end. Damage control orthopaedics using external skeletal fixation is usually applied in cases of severe limb trauma. Once the radius is fractured, the biceps muscle often spins the proximal fragment into supination while the remaining portion of the bone follows the rotation of the palm and hand. This makes the exact position of the deep branch of the radial nerve difficult to ascertain (Fig. 7-41).

Distally, the superficial radial nerves can be easily injured when inserting pins in this region. For this reason, a small open incision with the section down to the bone will ensure protection of these sensitive structures.

The radius becomes progressively more superficial in the distal forearm, where pins can easily be inserted into the bone,

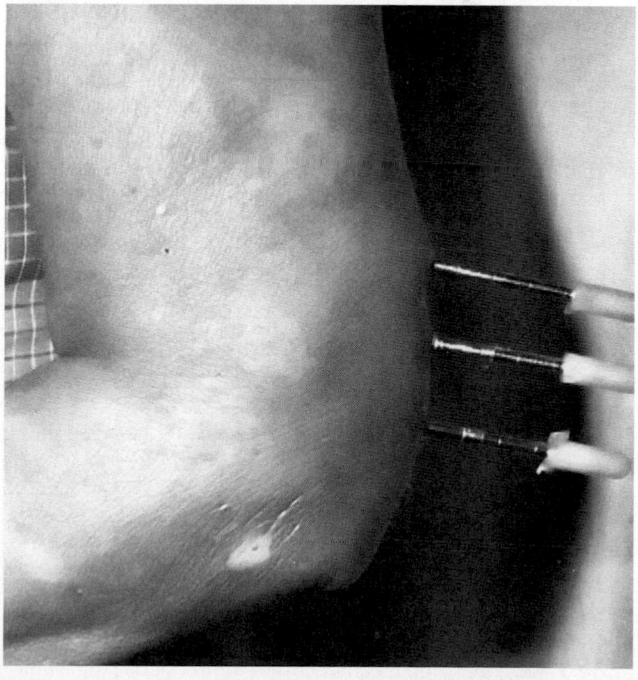

Figure 7-40. Taking care not to overpenetrate, half-pins can be inserted from posterior to anterior in the distal humerus.

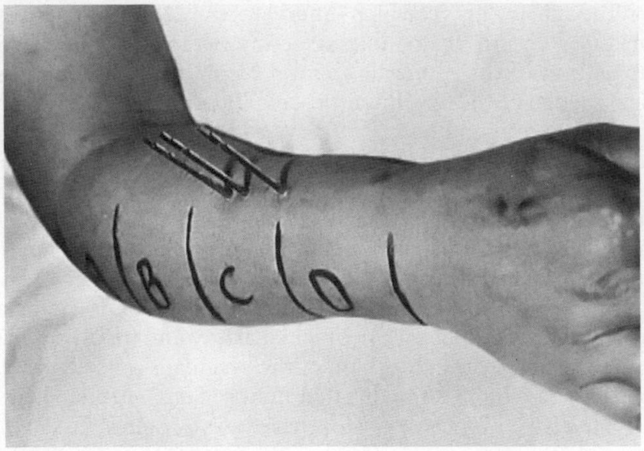

Figure 7-41. Half-pin insertion into the radius is risky without fluoroscopy and precise control of depth and direction.

although it is wise to make a small incision and expose the bone directly to best avoid damage to superficial branch of the radial nerve.

The ulna, like the tibia, has an extensive subcutaneous surface. With depth control and the thread length of no more than 20 mm, pins can safely be inserted throughout the length of the bone from the posterior medial direction; with a bit of care, an open insertion technique can be used about an inch proximal to the ulna styloid process where the superficial branch of the ulnar nerve wraps around the medial side of the forearm to supply the skin on the ulna half of the back of the hand and little finger and adjacent side of the ring finger (Fig. 7-42).

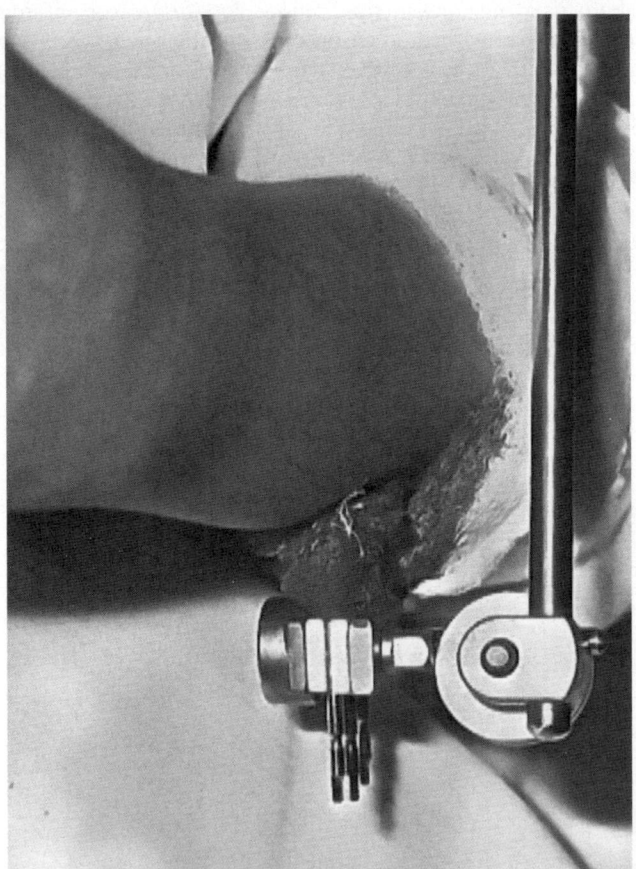

Figure 7-42. The half-pin can be inserted throughout the length of the subcutaneous surface of the ulna, except at the point where the dorsal branch of the ulnar nerve wraps around the bone medially.

KEY REFERENCES

The level of evidence (LOE) is determined according to the criteria provided in the preface.

24. Rozbruch SR, Segal K, Ilizarov S, et al: Does the Taylor Spatial Frame accurately correct tibial deformities? *Clin Orthop Relat Res* 468:1352–1361, 2010. LOE III
25. Bilen FE, Kocaoglu M, Eralp L, et al: Fixator-assisted nailing and consecutive lengthening over an intramedullary nail for the correction of tibial deformity. *J Bone Joint Surg Br* 92:146–152, 2010. LOE IV
26. Kim H, Lee SK, Kim KI, et al: Tibial lengthening using a reamed type intramedullary nail and an Ilizarov external fixator. *Int Orthop* 33:835–841, 2009. LOE III
29. Harbacheuski R, Fragomen AT, Rozbruch SR: Does lengthening and then plating (LAP) shorten duration of external fixation? *Clin Orthop Relat Res* 470(6):1771–1781, 2012. LOE III
30. Rozbruch SR, Kleinman D, Fragomen AT, et al: Limb lengthening and then insertion of an intramedullary nail: a case-matched comparison. *Clin Orthop Relat Res* 466(12):2923–2932, 2008. LOE III
32. Hankemeier S, Gösling T, Pape HC, et al: Limb lengthening with the Intramedullary Skeletal Kinetic Distractor (ISKD). *Oper Orthop Traumatol* 17(1):79–101, 2005. LOE III
33. Wang K, Edwards E: Intramedullary skeletal kinetic distractor in the treatment of leg length discrepancy—a review of 16 cases and analysis of complications. *J Orthop Trauma* 26(9):e138–e144, 2012. LOE III
34. Mahboubian S, Seah M, Fragomen AT, et al: Femoral lengthening with lengthening over a nail has fewer complications than intramedullary skeletal kinetic distraction. *Clin Orthop Relat Res* 470(4):1221–1231, 2012. LOE III
35. Baumgart R: The reverse planning method for lengthening of the lower limb using a straight intramedullary nail with or without deformity correction. A new method. *Oper Orthop Traumatol* 21(2):221–233, 2009. LOE V
37. Bluman EM, Ficke JR, Covey DC: War wounds of the foot and ankle: causes, characteristics, and initial management. *Foot Ankle Clin* 15:1–15, 2010. LOE V
74. Green SA, Harris NL, Wall DM, et al: The Rancho mounting technique for the Ilizarov method: a preliminary report. *Clin Orthop Relat Res* 280:104–116, 1992. LOE III
95. Possley DR, Burns TC, Stinner DJ, et al: Temporary external fixation is safe in a combat environment. *J Trauma* 69(1s):s135–s139, 2010. LOE IV
96. Carroll EA, Koman LA: External fixation and temporary stabilization of femoral and tibial trauma. *J Surg Orthop Adv* 20(1):74–81, 2011. LOE III
98. Pallister I, Tong A, Vannet N, et al: The diamond frame: a simple and reliable construct for damage control resuscitation for femoral and knee spanning external fixation. *Ann R Coll Surg Engl* 95(6):443, 2013. LOE V
99. Beltran MJ, Collinge CA, Patzkowski JC, et al: The safe zone for external fixator pins in the femur. *J Orthop Trauma* 26(11):643–647, 2012. LOE V
100. Gordon WT, Grijalva S, Potter BK: Damage control and austere environment external fixation: techniques for the civilian provider. *J Surg Orthop Adv* 21(1):22–31, 2012. LOE III
101. Mathieu L, Bazile F, Barthelemy R, et al: Damage control orthopaedics in the context of battlefield injuries: the use of temporary external fixation on combat trauma soldiers. *Orthop Traumatol Surg Res* 97(8):852–859, 2011. LOE IV
102. Miranda MA: Skeletal stabilization in the severely injured limb: fixation techniques compatible with soft tissue trauma. *Tech Orthop* 27(4):236–239, 2012. LOE V
106. Saithna A: The influence of hydroxyapatite coating of external fixator pins on pin loosening and pin track infection: a systematic review. *Injury* 41(2):128–132, 2010. LOE IV

The complete References list is available online at https://expertconsult.inkling.com.

Chapter 8

Principles of Internal Fixation

MATT L. GRAVES

Additional videos related to the subject of this chapter are available from the Medizinische Hochschule Hannover collection. The following videos are included with this chapter and may be viewed at https://expertconsult.inkling.com:

8-1. Reduction technique—surgical strategy.

8-2. Intraoperative three-dimensional imaging (ISO-C).

INTRODUCTION

Conservative management of fractures has limitations. Traction, splintage, and casting are limited in their capacity to restore form and function. The fundamental purpose of the skeleton is to provide structure to the body and create attachment points for muscles, tendons, and ligaments, thereby enabling joints to move. When the form of the skeleton is disrupted, the function of the skeleton is affected. In the mid-1900s, the functional limitations of conservative management became known as "fracture disease." Fracture disease consisted of skin ulceration, muscle atrophy, joint stiffness, and disuse osteopenia. The recognition of this problem propelled a search for solutions.

A battle ensued regarding the optimal treatment of fractures. Early proponents of internal fixation struggled to create generalizability of technique and therefore outcome. Complications of internal fixation—infection, wound healing problems, fixation failure—seemed more egregious than the limitations of conservative management. It was not until the late 1950s that a small group of surgeons leaned into the problem with a systematic approach that included documentation, education, and research.[1] They established a culture that prioritized the adherence to fundamental basic principles of operative fracture care. They partnered with industry to set standards for implant quality and instrument design. They were selective in the surgeons who were allowed use of the equipment, requiring a priori study of the basic principles under the tutelage of a limited group of experts. They exhibited a precise documentation of case variables in an effort to determine what affected outcome. They followed a path of purposeful, repeated application of a method with a view toward perfecting the craft and a willingness to evolve patterns of thought. A paradigm shift ensued. Internal fixation of fractures became the standard rather than the exception. These principles, although modified, are still in use today on a much broader scope. Although fracture care has improved, failure to acknowledge and follow these basic principles is still leading to treatment disasters.

PLAN OF ATTACK AND HOW TO USE THIS CHAPTER

This purpose of this chapter is twofold: (1) to provide a review of the basic principles of fracture care with an emphasis on the "why" and (2) to assist in the application of these principles to particular cases with a focus on the "how." Although we will concentrate on the general rather than the specific, these general principles should prepare the surgeon to treat specific fractures all over the body. While the individual fracture chapters will make assumptions about your preexisting level of knowledge, this one will not do so. I will make an attempt to introduce the basic language of internal fixation and try to focus on the big ideas rather than the details and exceptions (which can be found in the individual fracture chapters later in the book). The basis of what will be presented represents information that was studied and systematically promoted by the Arbeitsgemeinschaft für Osteosynthesefragen (AO) group over the last 50 years in osteosynthesis manuals and courses.[1] Whereas this is the basis, elaboration based on other material and personal experience will be included when deemed beneficial.

The system of fracture care can be simplified into a summary flowchart (Fig. 8-1). The system can be thought of as an exercise in preoperative planning or proactive failure analysis. Every solution should include a conception of how to obviate failure in all its possible manifestations. In this chapter, we will walk through the different steps in the flowchart and spend time understanding how each step relates to prevention of failure in fracture care. Each step is actually a labyrinth within itself and could provide for a lifetime of study, but this is not required and will be resisted in order to establish a simple applicable framework for preoperative and intraoperative decision making. For the system to provide the desired result of successful fracture care, the steps must remain in context, as this provides limits. To clarify, the steps are separate but interdependent and must all be respected for a winning outcome. Within each section, there will be clinical examples to aid in the application of the basic principles. At the end of each section, you will note summary statements to ensure the important points are fleshed out from many different perspectives (it is often said that we do not truly understand something until we hear it in a particular way).

When you feel superior to the material, be warned and remember this quotation from one of the greatest thinkers of our time: "If you can't explain it simply, you don't understand it well enough."[1a] Reflect on the errors in your practice. Associate your failures with disregard for the basic principles of fracture care. Commit yourself to this language and these principles. See the improvement in patient care.

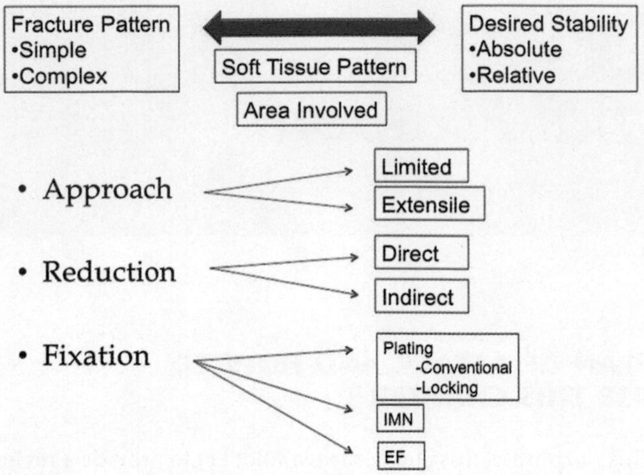

Figure 8-1. Summary flowchart of the system of fracture care. The process moves from an evaluation of the fracture pattern toward a decision regarding desired construct stability. Once this choice is made, further decision points required include surgical exposure, reduction method, and fixation choice. Each decision box will be covered in detail during this chapter with the exception of external fixation (which is covered in Chapter 7). Although we will separately cover the individual parts, the system must be considered as an integrated whole for successful fracture management. *EF,* External fixation; *IMN,* intramedullary nail.

FRACTURE PATTERN

Five things should be gleaned from every injury radiograph. These can be subsumed under the heading of fracture pattern but extend far beyond that simple title. Observational skills vary greatly among those treating fractures. Interestingly, one of the things thought to be associated with expertise is pattern recognition.[2] When you see an expert digest an injury radiograph, you realize how much information is available in the most limited of studies. Seeing these five things should help improve pattern recognition.

Fracture Pattern = Law of Conservation of Energy

First, the fracture pattern is the radiographic representation of the Law of Conservation of Energy. The total amount of energy in an isolated system remains constant over time. To clarify, there is a significant amount of energy associated with the fractures that we take care of. This energy is conserved through the accident, but changes forms. The representation of the energy is evident by viewing the injury films and the injured part. Specific types of forces create specific types of fractures.[3,4] Figure 8-2 is a common picture of fracture mechanics. Without reading the figure legend, draw which fracture pattern is expected from each force. Chapter 5, "Biomechanics of Fracture," provides more facts, laws, and specifics. In this chapter, we will focus more on why.

A force is an influence on a structure (e.g., skeleton) that tends to produce motion or deformation. There are a limited number of forces that the skeleton sees. These include compression, tension, and shear (Fig. 8-3).[5] Of note, commonly described forces of bending and torsion are more specific types that can be subsumed under the main categories of compression, tension, and shear. A compressive force is perpendicular and inward relative to the surface of an object. A tensile force is perpendicular and outward relative to the surface of an object. A bending force occurs in many forms (e.g., two-, three-, and four-point, and cantilever) and can be "simplified" into tensile and compressive components. The surfaces or molecules in an object subjected to bending are seeing a tensile or compressive force (this fact can be conceptually useful when you are considering which side of an injury is likely to have the purest fracture interdigitation or least damaged soft tissue). A shear force acts parallel or tangential to the surface of an object. A torsion force is a specific type of shear that consists of a twisting or rotation around an axis in an object.

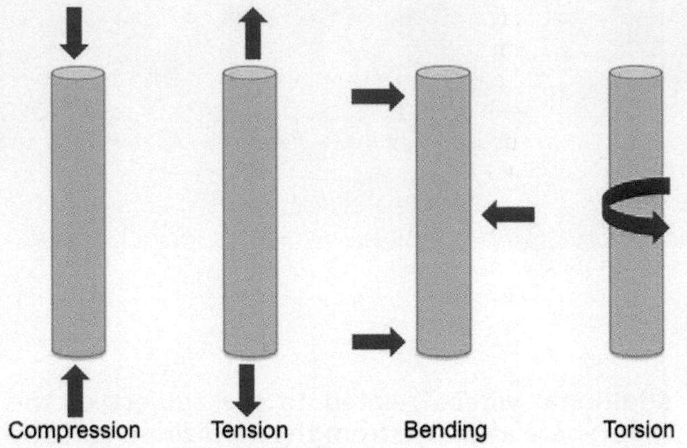

Figure 8-2. Characteristic fracture patterns in long bones occur with pure loading modes. Compression creates diaphyseal failure that is typically oblique to the long bone axis. Tension creates a failure mode that is perpendicular to the axis of loading (e.g., transverse fracture pattern). Bending loads are a combination of compression and tension loads. A transverse pattern is noted on the tension side and transitions into an oblique fracture on the compressive side. A butterfly fragment, when present, is noted on the compression side. Torsion creates spiral fracture patterns.

Why does it matter whether you know that a torsional force leads to a spiral fracture pattern? Just associating the deforming force with the pattern provides little. Understanding the character of that pattern provides a great deal. Simple patterns (transverse, oblique, spiral) are typically thought to be lower energy than their butterfly, comminuted, and segmental counterparts. This lower energy designation assists with predicting the complication profile and expected outcome when counseling the patient preoperatively.[4,6]

More importantly, associating the fracture pattern with the amount of absorbed energy helps provide your margin and guide your decision making. Surgery is a controlled form of

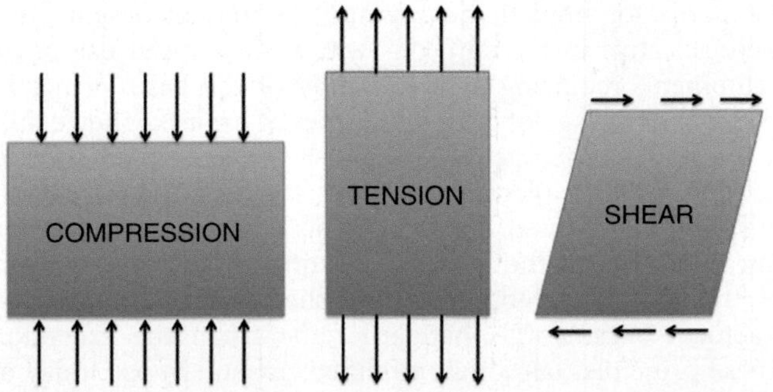

Figure 8-3. Three fundamental force components acting on bone are compression, tension, and shear. Bending and torsion are subsumed under these three fundamental forces.

energy transfer. Energy transfer is cumulative. If you start with a fracture pattern that signifies a large amount of energy, you should realize that the energy imparted via your surgical intervention must be limited and/or delayed. This is not a license for percutaneous malreductions, but rather a warning shot that signifies potential danger for early invasive intervention.[7,8] Highly comminuted diaphyseal and metaphyseal fractures demand an atraumatic surgical technique (irrespective of the chosen implant). It is well known at this point that the biologic cost of restoring every single piece to anatomic alignment is not worth the benefit.

Fracture Pattern Reveals the Intrinsic Stability of the Bone after Reduction

Second, the fracture pattern predicts the intrinsic stability of the bone after reduction. This has utility both in deciding whether or not a fracture can be successfully treated conservatively and in understanding the ultimate stability of the construct. This in turn determines the safety of physiologic loading. The specialized vocabulary is increasing, so it is important to unpack new words as we proceed. We should begin with stability, construct, and physiologic load.

Stability has many definitions. As it relates to fracture care principles, stability is defined as the amount of motion between fracture fragments when a construct is placed under physiologic load.[1] A construct is a structure that is built by a combination of implant and bone. A physiologic load is typically felt to be functional aftercare or motion of a joint rather than weight-bearing. To bring this together, the fracture pattern as noted on the injury film clarifies how stable the bone would be on its own after being reduced but prior to being fixed (i.e., intrinsic stability). Certain fracture patterns are clearly length-unstable even after acceptable reductions (e.g., comminuted pattern). If length restoration and maintenance is important in the care of that fracture, then operative techniques become necessary (i.e., it cannot be treated conservatively). When operative treatment is chosen for an intrinsically unstable pattern, then the type of instability should be clearly defined and the method of fixation should rationally follow. During the treatment period, the implant will be loaded almost exclusively until it can be protected by fracture healing, which creates some intrinsic stability. As fracture care is a race between fracture healing and implant failure, this issue deserves more detailed attention and will be covered many more times in this chapter.

Fracture Pattern Characterizes the Unbalanced Forces That Create Displacement and Subsequent Deformity

Third, the fracture pattern on injury films characterizes the unbalanced forces in the equation. Newton's third law states that for an object to remain at rest, there must be an equal and opposite reaction for every action. When there is an unbalanced force, an object is not at rest. Think of this in terms of fracture treatment. The surgeon desires to restore anatomy via reduction and to maintain that reduction until fracture healing with an implant. The goal, therefore, is to characterize unbalanced forces and then balance them. Structures obey the laws of nature; therefore, the desires of the surgeon must correspond with basic physics. Internal forces and external loads act on fracture fixation constructs.[5] Any fixation construct has a limited number of load cycles prior to failure. By considering these forces and loads, it is possible to design a fixation construct that minimizes failure potential. To reiterate, unbalanced forces create displacement and subsequent deformity and these forces must be characterized and the plan for fracture treatment must include specific resistance to them. When this is unclear, the unbalanced forces win. This is why malunion and nonunion radiographs typically resemble the injury films with hardware or implant/bone junction failure (Fig. 8-4).

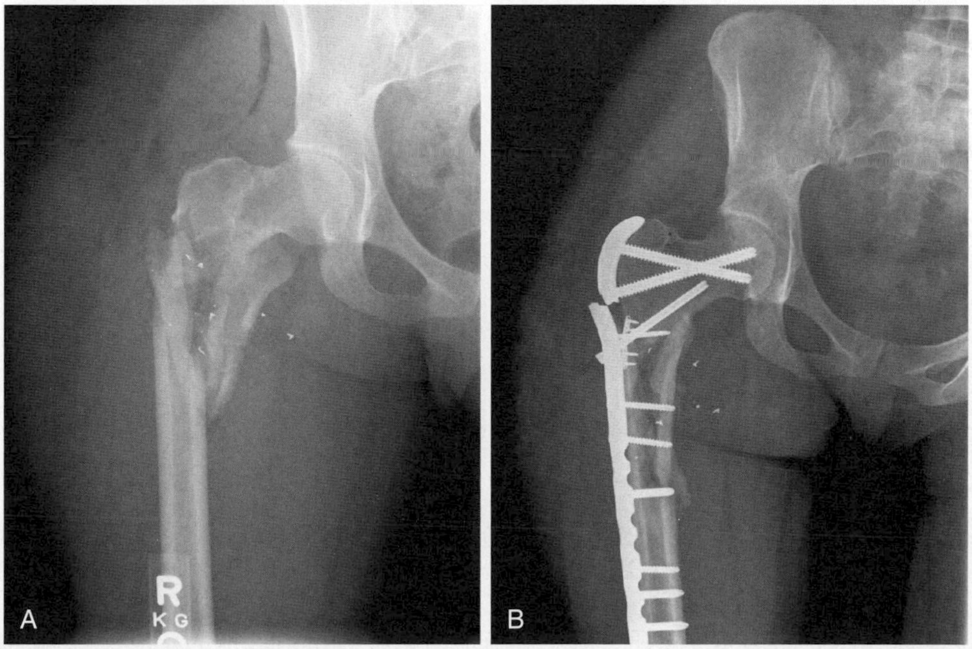

Figure 8-4. A, Anterior-posterior (AP) injury radiograph of subtrochanteric fracture with varus coronal plane displacement. **B,** AP failure radiograph once again revealing varus displacement. If you want to know what your failure films will most likely look like, take the injury films and draw in broken hardware or intact hardware with implant/bone junction failure.

Fracture Pattern Predicts Expected Soft Tissue Damage

Fourth, the fracture pattern on the injury films predicts the expected soft tissue injury, both from a general and a specific sense.[9] From a general sense, high-energy fracture patterns are typically associated with high-energy soft tissue patterns. As previously noted, high-energy soft tissue patterns forebode danger when early invasive surgical approaches are chosen. This is why multiple historical publications have shown a higher rate of wound healing problems and delayed union and nonunion with complex fracture patterns.[4] High-energy radiographs portend more vascular compromise to fracture fragments and skin, thereby naturally leading to longer healing times and more complications.

From a specific sense, this pattern recognition becomes even more valuable, especially in areas of the body where fractures and ligamentous injuries are often combined. Let us step up the level of discussion to complex knee injuries. Bicondylar tibial plateau fractures have recently been shown to have variable medial plateau injury patterns.[10,11] One of the most common medial plateau injury patterns consists of the anteromedial plateau remaining attached to the tibial diaphysis and the posteromedial plateau being separated (Fig. 8-5). The posteromedial plateau is a functional correlate for the posteromedial corner of the knee. The posteromedial corner of the knee is the secondary stabilizer against anterior translation of the tibia (the primary stabilizer being the anterior cruciate ligament [ACL]).[12] It logically follows, that when tibial eminence fractures are also present in this fracture pattern (and leave the ACL dysfunctional), the instability pattern is different (the primary and secondary stabilizers now being gone). Look closely at which relationships are maintained on the lateral image.[13] This finding is available on the injury films via pattern recognition and may guide surgical decision making, if noticed.

Now consider medial plateau fracture-dislocations in which the lateral plateau maintains continuity to the tibial diaphysis. While they may fall within the same category, there are broad differentiations.[14] Look closely at Figure 8-6. Both are medial plateau fractures. The lateral plateau maintains continuity to the tibial diaphysis in both patterns. This is where the similarities end. The first pattern exhibits lateral condylar widening, centrolateral articular impaction, shortening, and a variable medial plateau fracture pattern. The second pattern exhibits medial plateau articular impaction and varus hinge instability with avulsion of the lateral capsule, lateral collateral ligament, and biceps femoris. These injuries are treated differently. Fracture pattern recognition allows for the prediction of expected soft tissue damage. This can be the difference between success and failure in operative treatment.

Fracture Pattern Defines Expected Mode of Healing

Fifth and most important of all, fracture pattern on injury films defines the expected mode of healing. Ignoring this leads to disastrous consequences for the patient and the surgeon. This important point will be elaborated on throughout many other portions of this chapter, as it must be considered throughout the flowchart diagram (see Fig. 8-1). After all, the goal of operative fracture care is restoration of function through reduction, fixation, and healing. Without healing, it is impossible to reach this goal.

This labyrinth of fracture healing reaches very deep, and Chapter 4 in this volume will provide many details about

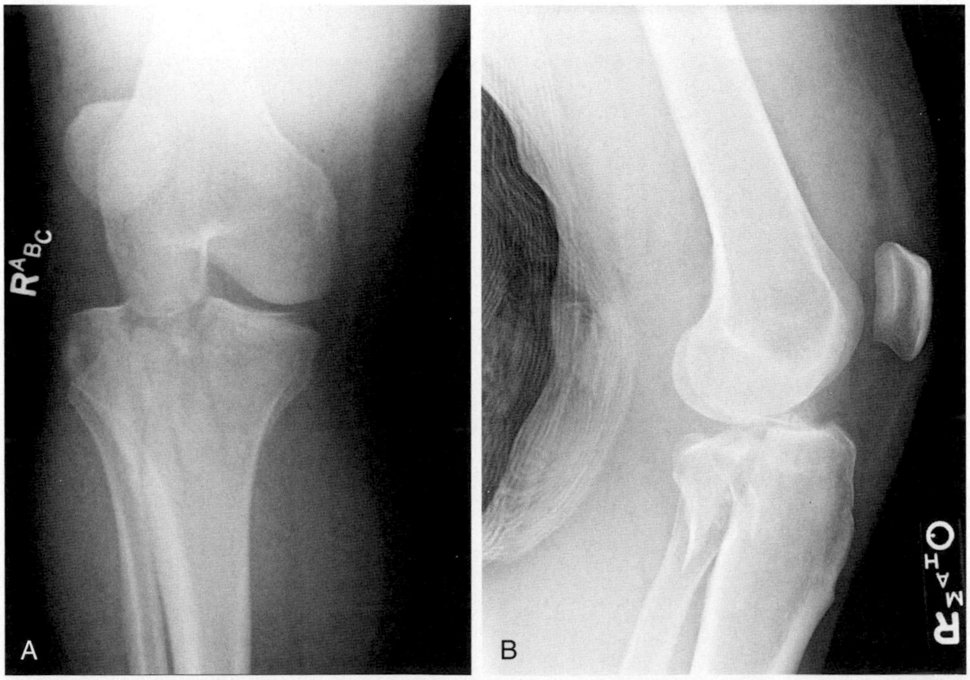

Figure 8-5. Anteroposterior (**A**) and lateral (**B**) views of a bicondylar tibial plateau fracture in which the medial-sided injury consists of a posteromedial fragment. Anterior translation of the tibial shaft (which is connected to the anteromedial fragment) is noted on the lateral radiograph. Primary and secondary stabilizers of the shaft against anterior translation are absent secondary to tibial eminence injuries and a dysfunctional posteromedial corner injury.

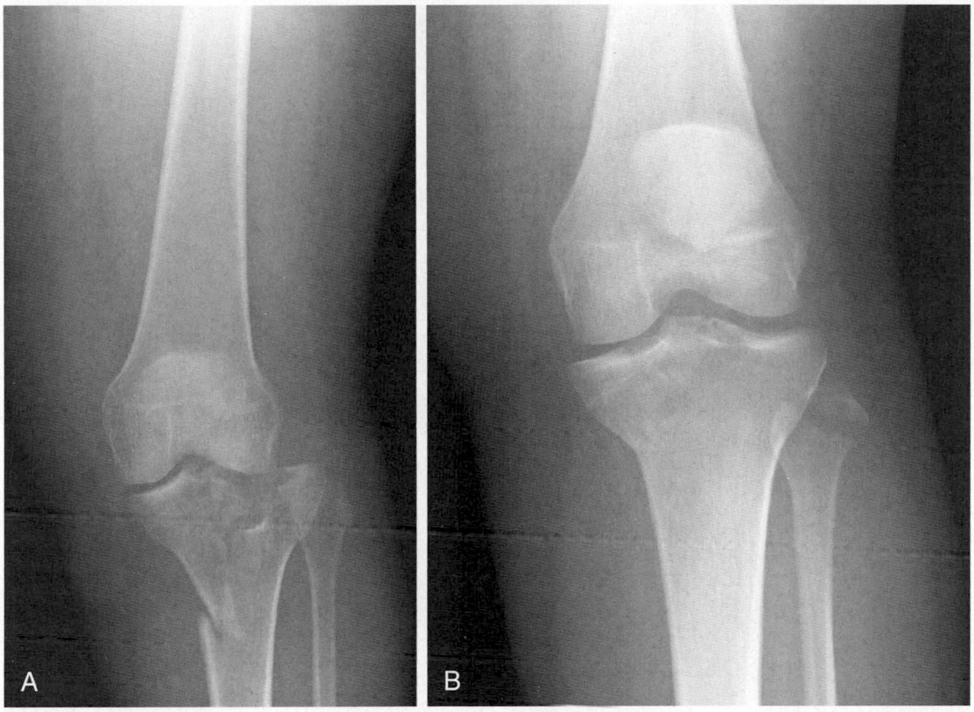

Figure 8-6. Medial plateau fractures with varying injury patterns, which indicate different soft tissue injuries. **A,** Medial tibial plateau fracture-dislocation revealing lateral condylar widening, centrolateral articular impaction, and shortening. **B,** Medial plateau fracture revealing medial articular impaction and varus hinge instability with avulsion of the lateral capsule, lateral collateral ligament, and biceps femoris.

"Biology and Enhancement of Skeletal Repair." Let us step away from the details and look at the basic principles of fracture healing through a few examples. Look closely at Figure 8-7. The articular fracture patterns can be ignored at this point (we will cover them in more detail in another section, but suffice it to say that every articular fracture pattern should be anatomically reduced, compressed when possible, and heal via primary bone healing). Both injury films reveal supracondylar femur fractures. The metaphyseal fracture patterns are very different. One is a simple oblique fracture pattern, whereas the other is complex (comminuted). How does this affect your operative decision making? To adequately answer this question, we need to cover more vocabulary and get further along the flowchart. Refer back to this question after you finish the "Desired Stability" section of the chapter.

Speaking of Fracture Patterns

- "That pilon fracture pattern appears extremely complex. It is surprising that the surgeon used an extensile approach this early in the injury period. Adding that much additional energy to the injury that early likely factored into the current wound healing complications that we are seeing."
- "That tibial fracture pattern is very comminuted. I know that if I choose operative treatment, my implant will be load bearing rather than load sharing. I should be careful with the soft tissue to ensure early healing, which will provide implant protection."
- "The vertical medial malleolar fracture with medial gutter impaction is the result of compression rather than tension. I wonder why the surgeon attempted to use a tension band construct for fixation. It doesn't seem that it logically balances the unbalanced forces."
- "This fracture occurred secondary to bending based on the radiographic pattern. Notice how the soft tissue damage reflects the position of the fulcrum. I should be more careful with the soft tissue on that side of the injury. It appears crushed."

SOFT TISSUE PATTERN

You have likely heard the expressions that a fracture is a soft tissue injury with a broken bone inside or that operative fracture care is more like gardening than carpentry work. The underlying message in these expressions is that the soft tissue injury must take precedence over the osseous injury. You cannot effectively and consistently treat fractures while ignoring soft tissue injuries. The most drastic complications of fracture care are typically defined by the soft tissue envelope rather than the fracture itself. So how do you prioritize the soft tissue in fracture care? Consider four ways.

Recognize the Severity of the Soft Tissue Injury Preoperatively

We previously covered the idea that the fracture pattern predicts the expected soft tissue injury. This is a solid general principle to follow, but does have exceptions (e.g., the transverse fracture with a crush impact injury). It is always necessary to closely evaluate the soft tissue envelope in addition to spending time dissecting the injury films. Soft tissue injury takes different forms: contusions, abrasions, blisters, lacerations, avulsions, degloving (closed and open), and crush.[9] These are all different manifestations of energy transfer. Each affects surgical decision making, both with respect to timing and placement of operative approaches. Open fracture

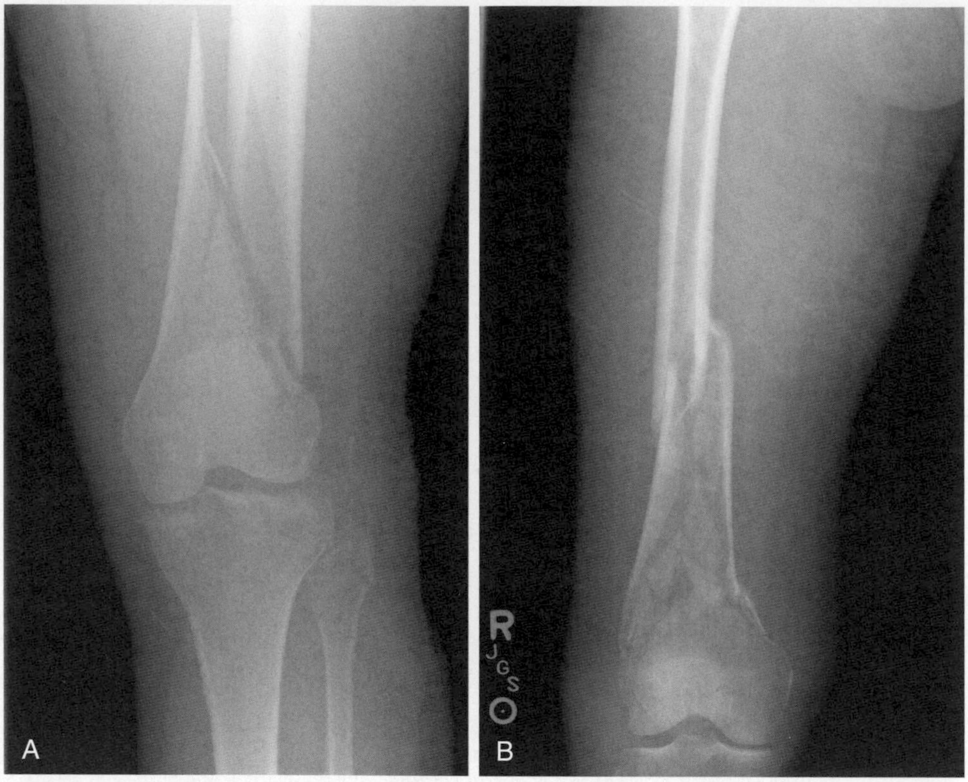

Figure 8-7. Supracondylar femur fractures with varying metaphyseal fracture patterns. **A,** Simple metaphyseal fracture pattern. **B,** Complex metaphyseal fracture pattern.

management will be covered in detail in Chapter 17 of this volume. Let us focus on the most commonly used closed fracture classification system.

Fractures with Soft Tissue Injuries is a classic publication from 1984 in which editors Tscherne and Gotzen defined a soft tissue classification of closed fractures that is still referenced today.[9] The key point of the classification scheme is that increased energy levels are represented by higher grades of injury. These grades of injury provide an understanding of prognosis and guide decision making. Grade 0 closed fractures represent injuries that are caused by indirect violence and reveal negligible soft tissue damage. The corresponding fracture pattern is typically of simple configuration (e.g., torsion fractures in skiers). These injuries can be treated in many ways and the margin for error is high. Grade I closed fractures represent soft tissue injuries created by fragment pressure from within the soft tissue envelope. The fracture pattern itself is typically mild to moderately severe (e.g., pronation abduction fracture-dislocations of the ankle in which the fractured margin of the medial malleolus creates an abrasion or contusion on the medial skin of the ankle). This soft tissue injury must be respected with early reduction of the displacement to limit further soft tissue damage. Any surgical approach in the area of damaged tissue must be done with extra care. A delay in definitive surgical treatment in the injured region may be necessary. Grade II closed fractures represent soft tissue injuries created by direct external pressure or violence. Deep, contaminated abrasions with local skin or muscle contusion are often associated with moderate to severe fracture patterns (e.g., segmental tibial shaft fractures caused by bumper injuries). Impending compartment syndrome must be ruled out or emergently treated if present. These injuries have a high propensity for soft tissue complications and must be treated with the utmost respect. Grade III closed fractures round out the closed fracture classification scheme. The skin is extensively contused or crushed, the muscle damage may be severe, and the fracture configuration is severe (e.g., multifragmentary or comminuted tibial shaft fractures caused by crushing mechanism). Closed fractures that are associated with major vascular injuries, subcutaneous avulsions and degloving, and established compartment syndrome are included in this grade III category. Treatment of these injuries is challenging and may lead to the need for soft tissue coverage procedures. Recognition of this at the beginning is important in setting realistic expectations preoperatively.

Modify Surgical Plans Based on Soft Tissue Injury Pattern

Surgical plans are created based on the fracture pattern as recognized through the injury films. Plans should incorporate the desired surgical incision; but a surgical incision is a means to an end in fracture care. The desired ends include visualization of the fracture, preparation of the bone ends, reduction of the fracture, and fixation of the fracture. These ends need to be accomplished in the absence of wound healing complications. Unfortunately, the desired approach to optimize visualization, reduction, and fixation may not be safely possible. This is where modification of the surgical plan based on the soft tissue pattern becomes necessary. Decisions need to be

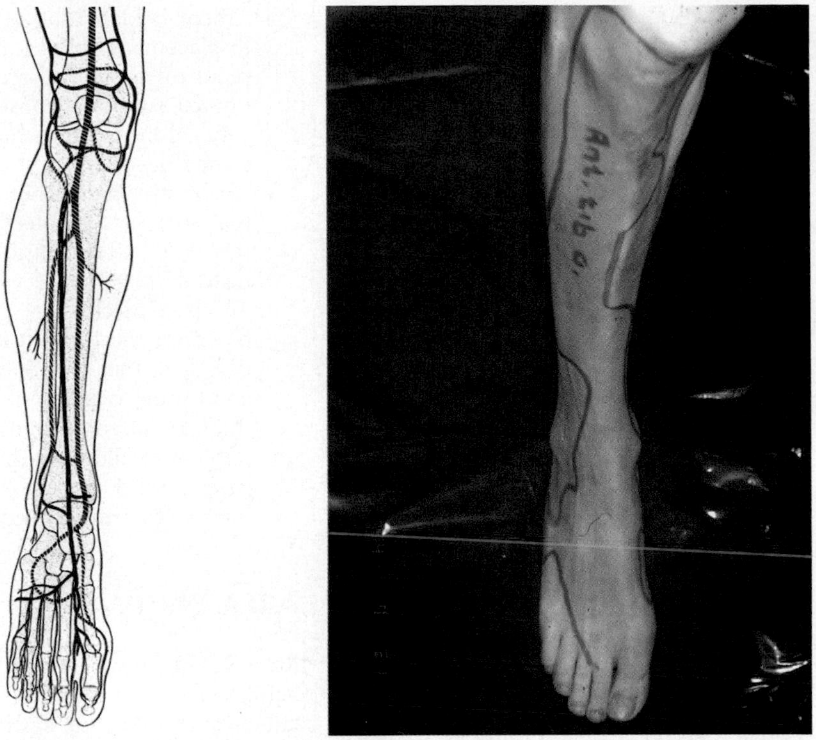

Figure 8-8. Angiosome of the anterior tibial artery. The diagram reveals the typical vascular anatomy of the lower limb. The picture reveals the vascular territory that is supplied by the anterior tibial artery. *(Source: From Attinger C: Vascular anatomy of the foot and ankle, Oper Tech Plast Reconstr Surg 4:183, 1997.)*

made by balancing desires with requirements. Every choice comes with a compromise. Choosing where to make incisions requires a familiarity with the zones of blood supply to the skin.[15] Moving away from ideal mechanical locations to stabilize a fracture requires a familiarity with methods to empower a fracture fixation construct.[16-18] Let us take time to cover these issues next.

Familiarize Yourself with the Concept of Angiosomes

One way to optimize care is by familiarizing yourself with the concept of angiosomes. An angiosome is a composite block of tissue including deep tissue and overlying skin supplied by a named source artery (Fig. 8-8).[15] It is likely that this concept will be covered in detail in Chapter 18, "Soft Tissue Reconstruction." Comprehensive articles are available in plastic surgery journals that orthopaedic surgeons may not often read.[15,19] Rather than focusing on comprehensive details, let us review a specific example and see how knowledge of angiosomes may affect surgical decision making.

Tibial pilon fractures are complex injuries to treat, primarily because of soft tissue complications.[20] It is an accepted fact that potential soft tissue complications drive surgical decision making. Some of the early results of immediate internal fixation were disastrous. Wound healing complications and infection led to unacceptable outcomes such as amputation. Some surgeons have chosen to avoid soft tissue complications by limiting surgical incisions.[21] The compromise with this approach is limited access to the articular surface for reduction and the necessity of prolonged external fixator frame duration. Others have moved toward staging surgical treatment (e.g., starting with external fixation to realign the limb while waiting for soft tissue recovery prior to proceeding with definitive care).[7,8] This staging has allowed for safer surgical incisions with the benefit of more direct access to the articular surface for reduction. When the decision is made to proceed with definitive internal fixation, care must be taken to choose the optimal surgical approach. The optimal surgical approach is based on the reduction strategy and the mechanics of instability (i.e., consider where you need to be to see, clean, reduce, and stabilize the fracture). This optimal surgical approach should take into account the angiosomes of the ankle and presence of vascular compromise. This is necessary because soft tissue complications occur even in the presence of staged treatment. It has been shown that a large percentage of tibial pilon fractures are associated with irregular arterial flow.[22] It is logical that making incisions in areas of compromised arterial flow can lead to soft tissue healing problems. Understanding the angiosomes should assist in limiting these complications. In the leg and ankle, large cutaneous vessels arise primarily from the deep fascia around the perimeter of muscles. Most tissues are crossed by two or more angiosomes, receiving supply from each.[19] Junctional zones between angiosomes are the danger areas. The primary junctional zone in the ankle is around the medial face of the tibia. The skin in this area is supplied almost exclusively by the anterior tibial artery (Fig. 8-9). When this artery is compromised, it follows that surgical incisions in this region can be problematic. It just so happens that this is the most likely area for surgical incision breakdown in tibial pilon fracture treatment (Fig. 8-10). Recognizing anterior tibial artery compromise preoperatively could logically mitigate some of these complications.

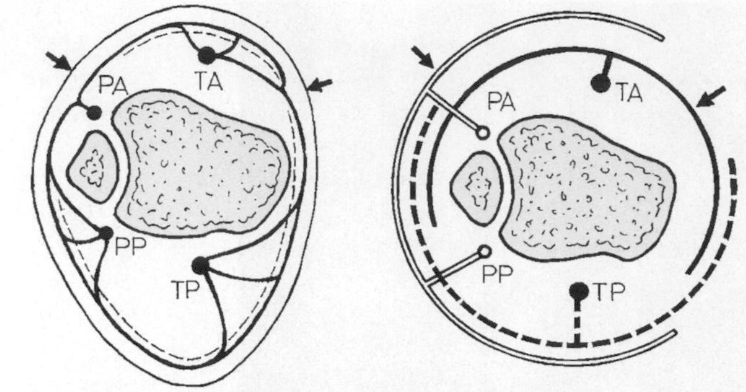

Figure 8-9. The arterial blood supply to the distal tibial metaphysis is shown in an axial section on the *left*. The *arrows* represent standard anteromedial and anterolateral surgical approaches to this area. The diagram to the *right* represents the arterial blood supply to the skin in this same region. Overlapping areas are noted, except along the anteromedial surface of the tibia. This is a critical junctional zone that is supplied only by the anterior tibial artery. It logically follows that surgical approaches in this area in the face of an anterior tibial artery injury would be more dangerous. *PA,* Anterior peroneal artery; *PP,* posterior peroneal artery; *TA,* anterior tibial artery; *TP,* posterior tibial artery. *(Source: From Heim U: The pilon tibial fracture: classification, surgical techniques, results, in which it was modified from Aubry P, Fievé J (1984) Vascularisation osseuse et cutanée du quart inférieur de jambe, Rev Chir Orthop 70:596, 1995.)*

Empower Fracture Fixation Constructs

There are times when the soft tissue pattern drives the placement of fixation to less than ideal mechanical locations. Let us consider a different scenario. Potential soft tissue compromise comes in different forms. Sometimes it is a direct result of the injury. Other times it is just a consequence of normal anatomy. Consider the patella or the olecranon. Both locations are subcutaneous. Hardware prominence is a documented issue at both sites.[23,24] Most implants are designed to serve as tension bands in these locations. The concept of a tension band will receive more attention under the "Fixation" heading in the flowchart, but let us start with the basics. A tension band is a torque converter applied to the tension surface of an eccentrically loaded bone.[1] To clarify, the implant (whether a wire or plate or suture) must be applied to the tension surface of the bone (the one that sees stretching). The tension surface of the olecranon or the patella is the subcutaneous surface (dorsal for the olecranon, anterior for the patella). Subcutaneous implants are associated with prominence and irritation of the overlying skin. It is tempting to move the implant from the tension surface to one that has more soft tissue coverage (e.g., the medial or lateral surface of the patella or olecranon). Doing so satisfies the desire to limit implant prominence but comes at a cost. The implant is no longer in the correct mechanical position to serve as a tension band. Either the construct must be empowered or the postoperative protocol must be modified (so that the implant sees less load until some healing occurs and it is protected). Failure to do so may lead to construct failure (Fig. 8-11).

Speaking of the Soft Tissue Pattern

- "Fracture blisters are already developing around the ankle. That is a sign that the soft tissue is not ready for an extensile approach and additional surgical trauma."
- "There is blanching of the skin secondary to fragment displacement in this tongue-type calcaneus fracture. That requires immediate attention and possibly even a very limited surgical exposure, despite the fact that delayed surgical treatment (when soft tissue swelling decreases) is standard."
- "No matter how atraumatic my soft tissue dissection in that area, it is a watershed zone that is already compromised. I better consider alternative surgical exposures instead."
- The best mechanical position for that implant is clear based on the injury films. Unfortunately, a surgical approach to that area does not allow for joint visualization and I want to anatomically reduce the articular surface. I think I will compromise the mechanical position of the implant to allow for the benefit of better articular exposure. Next I need to consider how to empower that implant to prevent mechanical failure."

AREA INVOLVED

Refer to the flowchart and review the concepts of "Fracture Pattern" and "Soft Tissue Pattern" as they relate to proactive failure analysis in the system of fracture care. Now we will move to the heading of "Area Involved." To understand this heading, it is necessary to review the aims of the AO method (Fig. 8-12).[1]

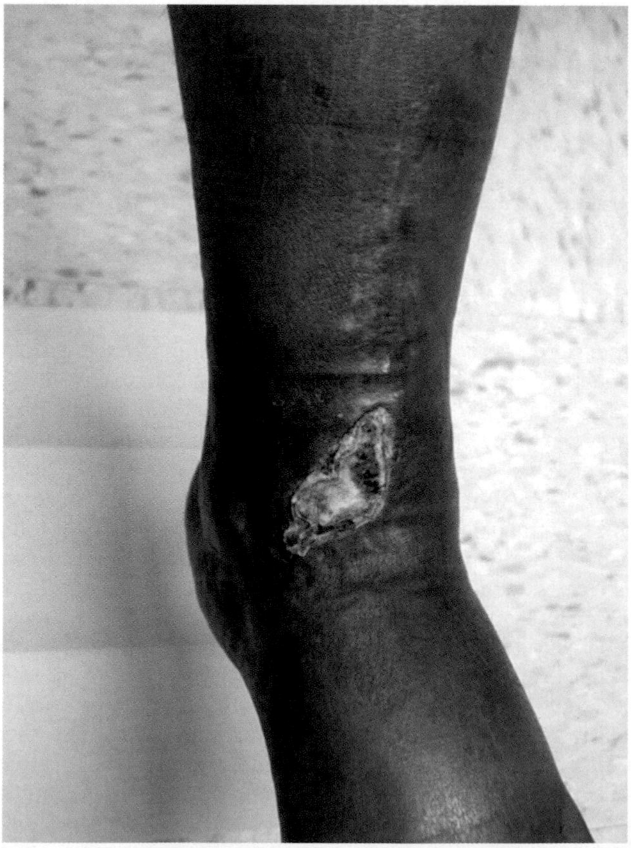

Figure 8-10. Tibial pilon fracture wound healing complication associated with anteromedial approach. Note the location of the healing problem is in the junctional area that is provided blood supply by the anterior tibial artery.

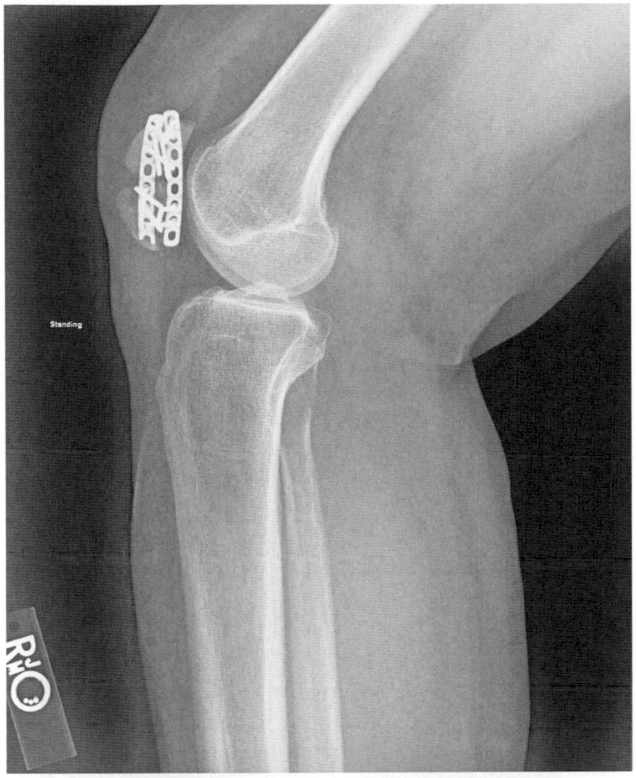

Figure 8-11. Patella fracture treated with implants placed away from the tension surface. The patella is loaded both in tension (as the quadriceps contract and pull the proximal piece away from the remainder) and in bending (as the fulcrum of the trochlea causes apex anterior bending forces). Implants placed away from the tension surface are mechanically challenged to resist bending.

Two important aims of the AO method include (1) the anatomic reduction of the fracture fragments and (2) preservation of the blood supply to the fracture fragments and the soft tissue by means of atraumatic surgery. We should strive to meet these aims while realizing the two create a conflict. We have previously discussed the idea that the quality of a reduction is inversely related to the ability of the surgeon to maintain the blood supply to fracture fragments and soft tissue. To clarify, it is not difficult to enact an anatomic reduction if you remove all the soft tissue from the fracture fragments through a poorly executed extensile exposure; unfortunately, this leaves the fracture fragments avascular and creates healing challenges. Similarly, it is not hard to maintain nearly all the blood supply to fracture fragments and enact a malreduction; unfortunately, the fracture will heal in a non-anatomic position. Neither of these is acceptable. It follows that the compromise should be to enact the quality of reduction required for each specific injury as atraumatically as possible. This means that there is a hierarchy of reduction mandates that should be understood. Thankfully, this hierarchy can be divided into the well-defined segments of the bone, specifically the articular surface (epiphysis), the metaphysis, and the diaphysis. Let us cover each one individually and see how the location of the fracture (i.e., area involved) aids us in making decisions about fracture care.

Articular Surface

The articular surface (epiphysis) mandates an anatomic reduction of all articular fragments. As a general rule, open approaches are generally required to enact an anatomic articular reduction. It is accepted that more damage to the blood supply is likely to occur with the open approach, but the desire is still to limit that as much as possible. The articular cartilage has three functions: (1) to distribute forces evenly, (2) to provide a near-frictionless motion surface, and (3) to serve as a shock absorber during loading.[1] When the articular surface is displaced, it cannot optimally serve these functions. Displacement occurs in two primary forms: (1) articular incongruence and (2) articular malalignment. *Articular incongruence* is defined as the inability of the joint surfaces to coincide when superimposed. *Articular malalignment* is defined as an incorrect relationship between the articular surface and the axis of the limb (i.e., rather than the ankle joint surface being perpendicular to the weight-bearing axis and parallel to the floor with loading, it is crooked).

Displacement leads to two primary dysfunctions: (1) point loading and (2) joint instability. One of the few mathematical formulas that is useful in the operating room is Stress = Force/Area. When joint stress is kept at a reasonable level, the articular cartilage remains healthy.[25] To maintain joint stress at a reasonable level, it is important to distribute the joint forces over large areas. This occurs in an anatomically reduced joint with balanced forces. When the area for force distribution is limited (e.g., a malreduced articular fracture that creates point loading), the stress increases and joint degradation occurs. A simple analogy is watching a lady walk on soft ground with two different types of shoes: a stiletto and a flat. The stiletto concentrates her body weight into a smaller area, increasing the stress and causing her heel to sink into the soft ground. In contrast, the flat would distribute her body weight over a larger area, decreasing the stress and allowing her to walk without sinking. The same thing is occurring at the articular surface level, but instead of sinking, the cartilage in the point-loaded area just degenerates.[26]

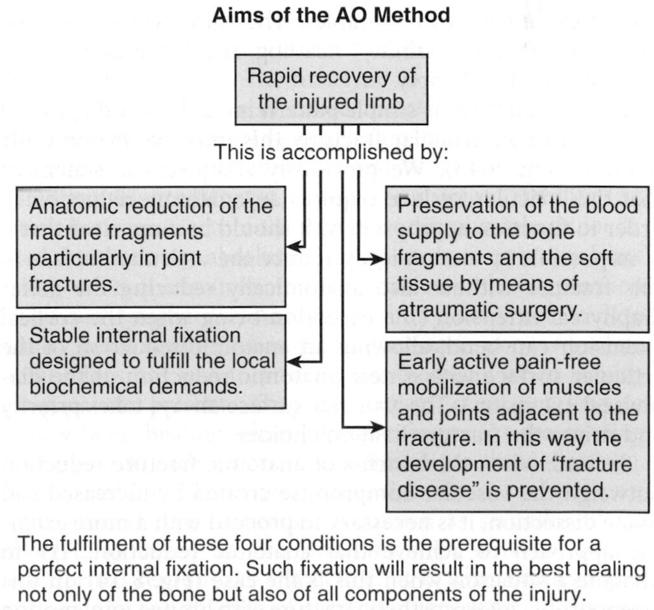

Figure 8-12. The aims of the Arbeitsgemeinschaft für Osteosynthesefragen (AO) method. *(Source: From Müller ME, Allgöwer M, Schneider R, Willenegger H: Manual of internal fixation: techniques recommended by the AO-ASIF group, Berlin/Heidelberg/New York, 1991, Springer-Verlag, p 1.)*

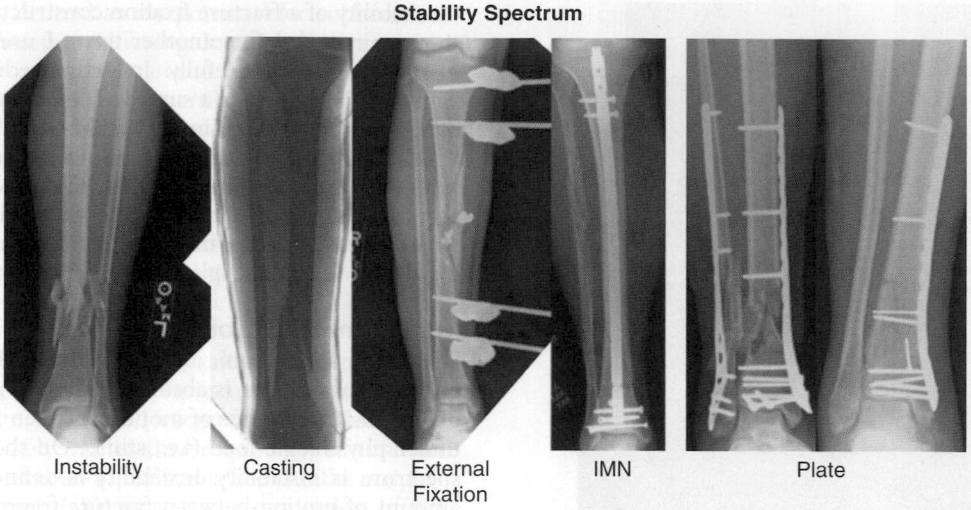

Figure 8-15. Spectrum of stability is noted with constructs used in tibia fracture treatment. Instability is noted at the *far left* with a complex tibia fracture with no support. With loading, this fracture would displace and not return to its original position. Relative stability is noted in the *middle* images with casting, external fixation, intramedullary rodding, and bridge plating. With loading, these constructs should produce micromotion to induce callus formation for secondary healing. Absolute stability is noted with neutralization plating and independent lag screws on the *far right*. With loading, no motion should occur. This construct relies on primary bone healing as no induction of callus formation through motion can occur.

maintains the reduction but allows motion between fracture fragments.[1] Relative stability does not lead to secondary bone healing when extreme gaps are present. Relative stability does not lead to secondary bone healing when no motion is occurring between fracture fragments (i.e., stiff construct). Relative stability may not lead to secondary bone healing when excessive motion is occurring between fracture fragments (i.e., flimsy construct). If healing does occur in this situation, it will be in an unacceptable alignment with a loss of the reduction (Fig. 8-16).

The second reason that the choice of stability matters is that it defines the time point when functional recovery can begin. Remember the goal of fracture treatment (and the AO method) is rapid recovery of the injured limb through an appropriate reduction, stable fixation, preservation of the blood supply, and early active pain-free mobilization. Both absolute stability and relative stability can accomplish this goal, but instability

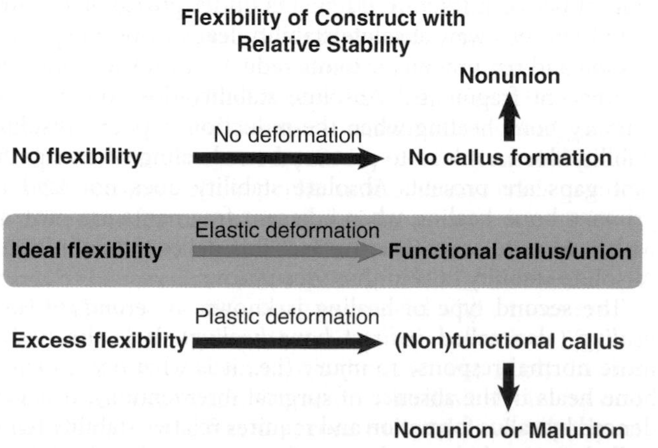

Figure 8-16. Relative stability requires the golden mean of flexibility to achieve healing while preventing plastic deformation. Both too little and too much flexibility lead to problems.

cannot. As you move toward the extremes of construct flexibility, it becomes harder to mobilize joints. The addition of immobilization after fracture fixation is less than ideal for achieving an early functional recovery.

Absolute Stability

Now let us focus more on absolute stability by discussing the indications and requirements. You should recognize the clear overlap between the different headings on the flowchart at this point, especially the ones that we have already covered (fracture pattern, soft tissue pattern, and area involved). Absolute stability is indicated for all intraarticular fractures and some metaphyseal and diaphyseal fractures. Regardless of the complexity of an intraarticular fracture pattern, absolute stability is indicated. Anatomic restoration of all articular fragments is required. This is required because the goal is to reestablish congruence between the two opposing surfaces of the joint in order to distribute forces over the largest area possible. This minimizes joint stress and improves articular cartilage health. Healing of articular fragments with hyaline cartilage occurs best in the presence of anatomic reduction and compression.[31] Rarely, intercalary osteochondral fragments will be missing (e.g., severe open fractures with joint surface loss). This is the only exception to the rule. In this rare scenario, compression of the peripheral articular cartilage fragments may constrain the joint and alter the ability to achieve congruence with the opposing articular surface (i.e., the other side of the joint). Once again, this is a rare and very complicated situation. It requires the maintenance of overall joint surface width and/or depth, and eliminates the ability to achieve compression between the peripheral joint surface fragments. Absolute stability is indicated for some metaphyseal and diaphyseal fractures, but only when the fracture pattern is simple; even then, absolute stability is not always indicated. For example, simple metaphyseal and diaphyseal fracture patterns can be successfully treated with relative stability. The best example of this scenario is the use of an intramedullary rod to treat a simple pattern tibial or femoral shaft fracture. By the nature of its mechanics, the intramedullary rod creates relative stability (controlled motion between fracture fragments under physiologic load). Another example of this scenario is the use of a plate to bridge simple pattern tibial or femoral shaft fractures. Although this is not considered ideal, it can be successful with a clear understanding of construct flexibility. When is it reasonable to treat simple pattern metaphyseal and diaphyseal fracture patterns with absolute stability? Remember the two scenarios previously mentioned. First, when there is simple pattern metaphyseal/diaphyseal extension of an articular fracture, this must be anatomically reduced. It must be anatomically reduced and treated with absolute stability in order to ensure the articular surface reduction is anatomic and remains anatomic until healing. Second, when the benefits of anatomic fracture reduction outweigh the vascular compromise created by increased soft tissue dissection, it is necessary to proceed with a more extensile approach to achieve that anatomic reduction. Consider the interprosthetic fracture with the stiff joint above and below the fracture. The decision can be made to optimize the mechanical environment by anatomically reducing the fracture and compressing it to achieve absolute stability. Here the decision is made to protect the metal by creating a more load-sharing environment. Once again, the biology must be maintained through biologically friendly exposures, atraumatic reduction techniques, and tissue-sparing implant placement. It should be clear that the requirements for absolute stability include an anatomic reduction, interfragmentary compression, and biologic techniques.

Let us spend more time with what has been called the hallmark of absolute stability, namely compression. Compression is the act of pressing surfaces together. The primary purpose of compression is to create friction between the opposing surfaces via fracture interdigitation. Remember the definition of absolute stability is the absence of motion between fracture fragments under physiologic load. As a fracture is subjected to different types of load, the amount of friction between the surfaces of the fragments acts to prevent motion between the surfaces. This friction provides intrinsic stability to the reduced bone and thereby protects the implants by unloading them. This allows the implant to serve more efficiently in a load-sharing environment and win the race between fracture healing and implant failure.[32] An implant in this scenario is less dependent on early fracture healing to protect it from reaching its load cycle limit and failing.

Compression can be divided into different categories. Let us first consider the difference between axial compression and transaxial compression. In this setting, axial is defined as along the axis of the limb. Ideally, compression is applied perpendicular to the orientation of the fracture. If applied in any direction other than perpendicular, some of the compression is lost to shear (force along the surface of the fracture rather than perpendicular to the surface of the fracture). A simple way to envision this is to consider the concept of a vector. A vector is a geometric entity that has both a magnitude and a direction. A resultant vector can be broken down into its component vectors. The magnitude in this scenario is the amount of force that is being created. The direction is the orientation of application of that force. Look closely at Figure 8-17. The force of compression is in a less than ideal direction. Because of the orientation of the fracture surfaces, a substantial amount of shear is introduced. When shear is created, it is both inefficient for compression and harmful to the reduction of the fracture (i.e., may displace an anatomically reduced fracture).

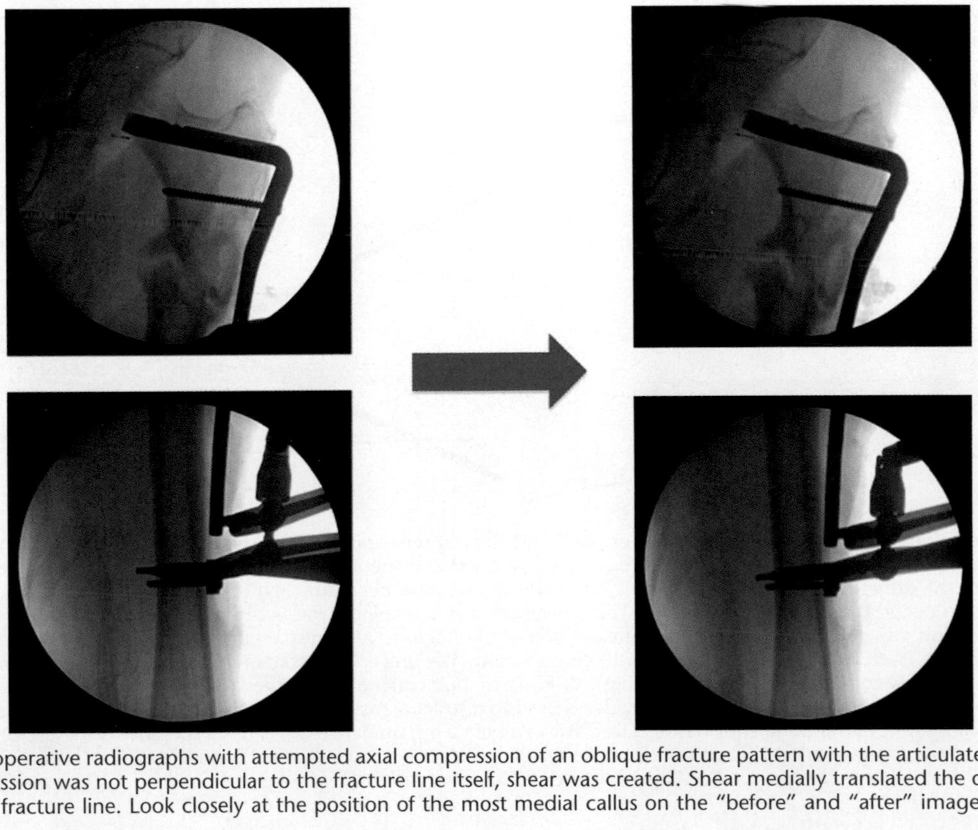

Figure 8-17. Intraoperative radiographs with attempted axial compression of an oblique fracture pattern with the articulated tensioning device. Because the compression was not perpendicular to the fracture line itself, shear was created. Shear medially translated the distal fragment along the obliquity of the fracture line. Look closely at the position of the most medial callus on the "before" and "after" images.

Following this vector concept, axial compression would be best used when the fracture is nearly perpendicular to the long axis of the bone. The fracture pattern that would be most perpendicular to the long axis of the bone would be a transversely oriented fracture.

Many different tools and implant design modifications have been created to assist with axial compression. These tools are designed to be used primarily with plate osteosynthesis. They were created primarily to achieve preload. *Preload* is defined as tensioning an implant and reciprocally compressing the bone or fracture surfaces, before the patient actively subjects the implant to load.[1,18] A logical way to approach this is through an abbreviated review of plate hole design. By understanding how and why the design of plate holes has changed over time, it allows you to reason through methods of axial compression.[33] More time will be spent describing the differences in plate holes later under the "Fixation" heading in the flowchart.

The earliest plate holes were round and slightly larger than the outer diameter of the screw shaft but smaller than the head of the screw. This required screws to be placed perpendicular to the orientation of the hole in order to fit through and seat into the hole. At this point in history, any compression that could be achieved across a fracture needed to be done outside of the plate itself. For example, compression could be achieved by loading the limb manually or by placing a clamp along the axis of the limb, which does not work very well if you think of clamp application for a transversely oriented fracture. Special plates were designed that contained a compression screw device at the end of the plate (e.g., the Danis coapteur). Alternatively, devices were created that could temporarily attach to a plate in order to enact compression, and then be removed (e.g., the articulated tensioning device). Alternative options included using the universal distractor in compression or using a Verbrugge clamp attached to a single hole in the plate and a screw outside of the plate (Fig. 8-18). As every choice necessarily comes with a compromise, design continued to evolve. The compromises made with each of the previously listed devices were increased surgical exposure, equipment, and surgical time. This led to the development of a modified plate hole that allowed for compression with the plate–screw relationship alone (i.e., no longer requiring an additional device). It seems that two plate holes were being simultaneously designed to function in this manner. The first was present on the Bagby plate.[34] The second was present on the AO plate, and became known as the dynamic compression unit (DCU).[35] It was found on a plate termed the dynamic compression plate (DCP). It consisted of an oblong hole, which was the combination of an inclined and transverse cylinder (Fig. 8-19). The plate was first attached to one side of

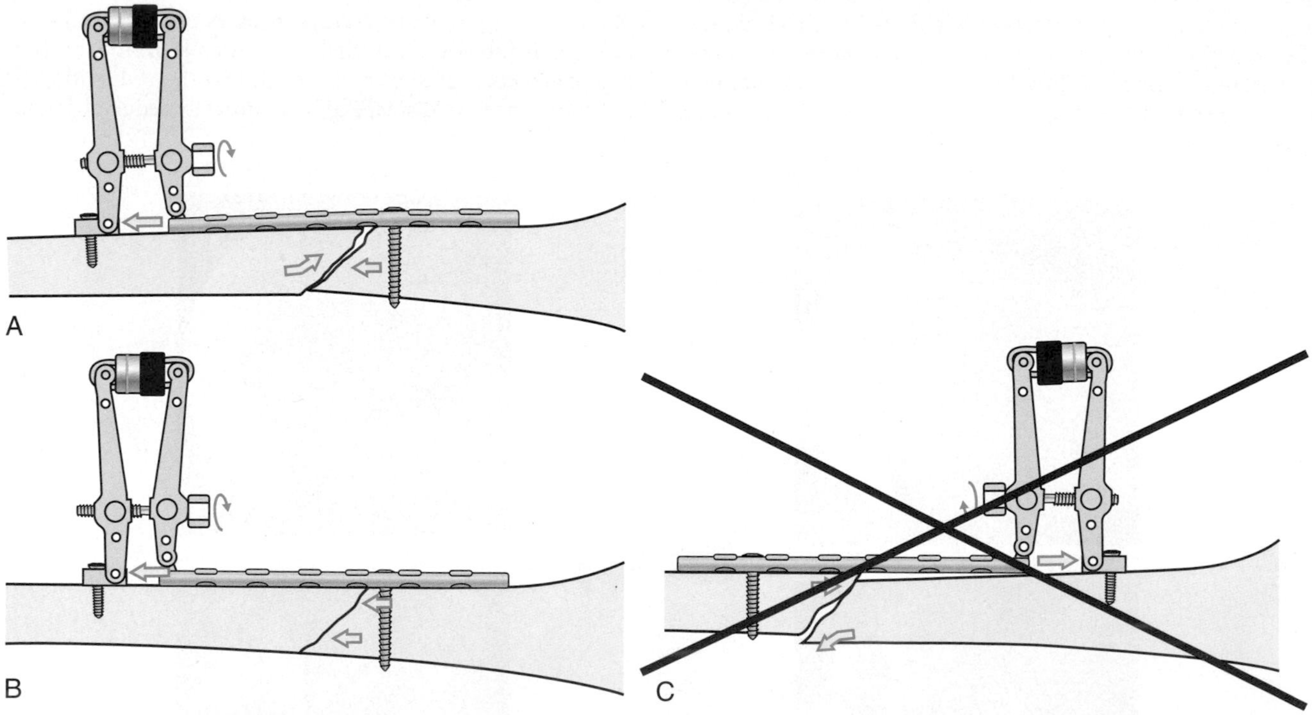

Figure 8-18. Examples of compression tools and devices. **A–C,** Articulated tensioning device. Note the same concept previously covered in Figure 8-17. Compression along an obliquity can be detrimental to reduction if the axilla created by the plate and bone is not in the position to capture the spike of the other fragment. In this example, the plate should have been attached to the other fragment first, such that compression into the axilla could occur. **D–F,** Universal distractor. This device consists of a spindle rod, a carriage, and nuts that allow for either compression or distraction through attachment to Schanz pins on each side of the fracture. After distraction, the fracture ends can be aligned, followed by compression across the fracture through reversing the force created by the universal distractor into compression (i.e., moving the other nut against the carriage, which is connected to the Schanz pin). **G–H,** Push–pull concept using the lamina spreader and a Verbrugge clamp. The plate is attached to one side of the fracture. A lamina spreader is used to distract across the fracture site via an independent screw placed outside of the plate. Once realignment of the bone ends has occurred with Weber clamp guidance, the lamina spreader is traded for a Verbrugge clamp, which then compresses the fracture using the same independent screw. *(Redrawn from Rüedi TP, Buckley RE, Morgan CG: AO principles of fracture management, vol 1, ed 2, expanded edition, Thieme, 2007, Switzerland, Figure 3.1.1-7a-b, p 170; Figure 3.1.1-4 a-c, p 175; Figure 3.2.17a-c, p 241.)*

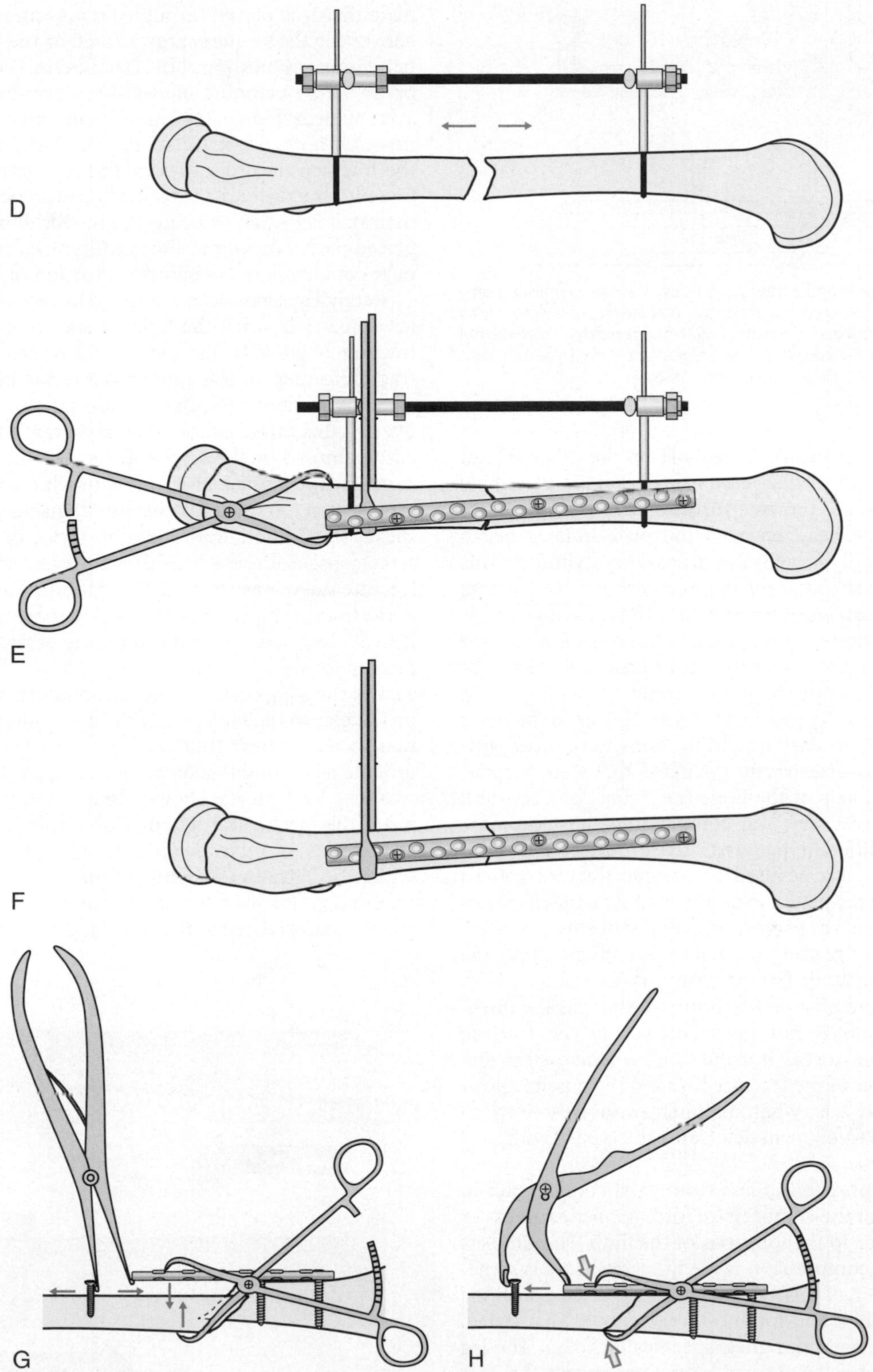

Figure 8-18, cont'd

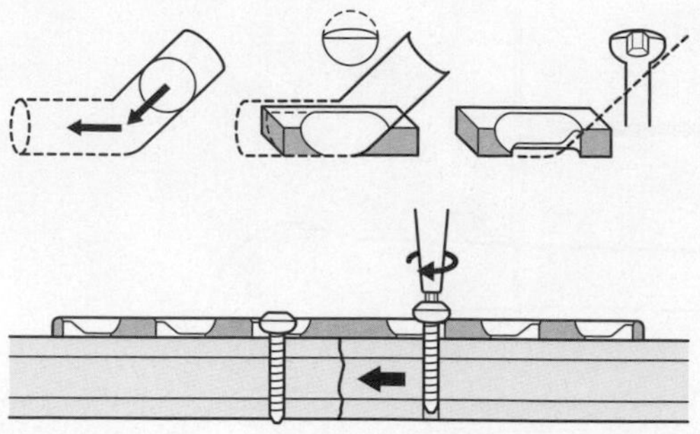

Figure 8-19. The modified screw hole known as the dynamic compression unit (DCU) allowed for eccentric placement of a screw into a plate to create a compressive effect without requiring an external device. This concept is based on a carpenter's principle, but was technically improved to limit parasitized forces.

the fracture with a screw. A screw hole on the other side of the fracture was then drilled eccentrically in the plate hole (i.e., toward the side of the hole furthest away from the fracture). As the screw head engaged the plate hole, it began to move horizontally down the transverse cylinder. This movement created a compressive force between the fracture ends by moving one relative to the other. The advantage of this plate hole design modification is that compression no longer required additional devices, exposure, or time. The disadvantage was that the compression that could be achieved was limited compared to the previously used devices. Remember that these devices and design modifications were most optimally used in transverse fracture patterns that were perpendicular to the long axis of the bone (i.e., axial compression); but fracture patterns vary and compression must be more generalizable to different patterns. These devices and plate hole modifications can be used in oblique fracture pattern variants, assuming the plate can be attached such that it creates an axilla to prevent shear from creating deformity. Review Figure 8-20 without reading the figure legend and apply the concept of a vector. Both fracture patterns are oblique. Both see the same compressive vector. Both see shear as the direction of compression is not perpendicular to the fracture surface. Which one works? It should be becoming clear that both the orientation of the fracture line and the possible position of the implant (i.e., what anatomic surface the implant can be placed onto safely) will determine the type of compression that you choose.

Transaxial compression differs from axial compression in that the direction of the compressive force applied is across or more perpendicular to the long axis of the limb. The simplest form of transaxial compression is the lag screw. This is somewhat of a misnomer, as any type of screw can accomplish the lag principle. It is first and foremost a technique. That stated, some screws have been designed specifically to lag. The lag principle states that a screw thread must not engage the near cortex but must engage the far cortex. To simplify, a hole is drilled in the near cortex and the medullary bone until reaching the fracture site that is larger than the outer diameter of the screw. The remaining medullary bone and the far cortex are drilled to create a hole that is smaller than the outer diameter of the screw (typically the same diameter as the core of the screw). This creates a glide hole in which the screw has no purchase and a thread hole in which the screw gains optimal purchase. As the head of the screw impacts the near cortex (or plate that it is placed through), it acts as a torque converter, converting the torque energy created by the operator's rotating hand into compression at the fracture site (Fig. 8-21).[36] Careful preoperative planning allows the screw to be placed in an atraumatic fashion with minimal soft tissue/vascular compromise. Of note, the screw should be placed near the center of the fragment in order to prevent propagation of the fracture line into the drill hole (this may need to be modified if more than one lag screw is being used). Additionally, it should be placed perpendicular to the fracture itself such that it creates pure compression through the direction of the vector.

Rarely lag screws can be placed as the sole fixation. This is indicated only when the fracture sees minimal load and the fracture length is at least twice the diameter of the bone at the fracture center. In this rare scenario, the lag screws must be carefully positioned such that more than one can be placed. Even in this rare scenario, it is important to consider the stability afforded by the screws alone. The lag screw is compromised by the limited lever arm with which it works. This lever arm is often too small to resist functional loads of bending and shear.[1] In addition, it provides no factor of safety.[37] If the lag screw loosens, there is little else to prevent displacement of the fracture fragments. To complicate things further, the obliquity of the fracture line is rarely parallel to the long axis of the bone; hence, the perfect position of the lag screw is rarely perpendicular to the long axis of the bone. As the bone is loaded axially, shearing occurs along the obliquity. Screws placed perpendicular to the long axis of the bone are in a better orientation to resist shear (but rarely in the correct orientation to provide pure compression across a fracture). Because of these reasons, the lag screw should almost always be protected by a plate (the mechanical function of which is termed a *neutralization plate* or *protection plate*). This will be covered further under the "Fixation" heading of the flowchart.

Another form of transaxial compression occurs when a plate is first attached to the acute angle of an oblique fracture.

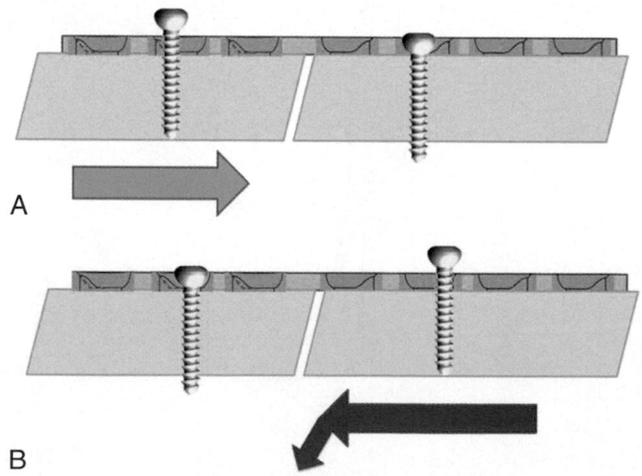

Figure 8-20. Oblique fracture patterns subjected to compression with plate application. **A,** Attaching the plate to the side that creates an obtuse angle creates an axilla such that compression prevents shear by trapping the fragment. **B,** Attaching the plate to the side that creates an acute angle fails to create an axilla such that compression leads to shear along the surface of the obliquity. This is the reason that both the fracture orientation and the surface of bone that normally accepts a plate are important in defining the mechanics of your fixation device.

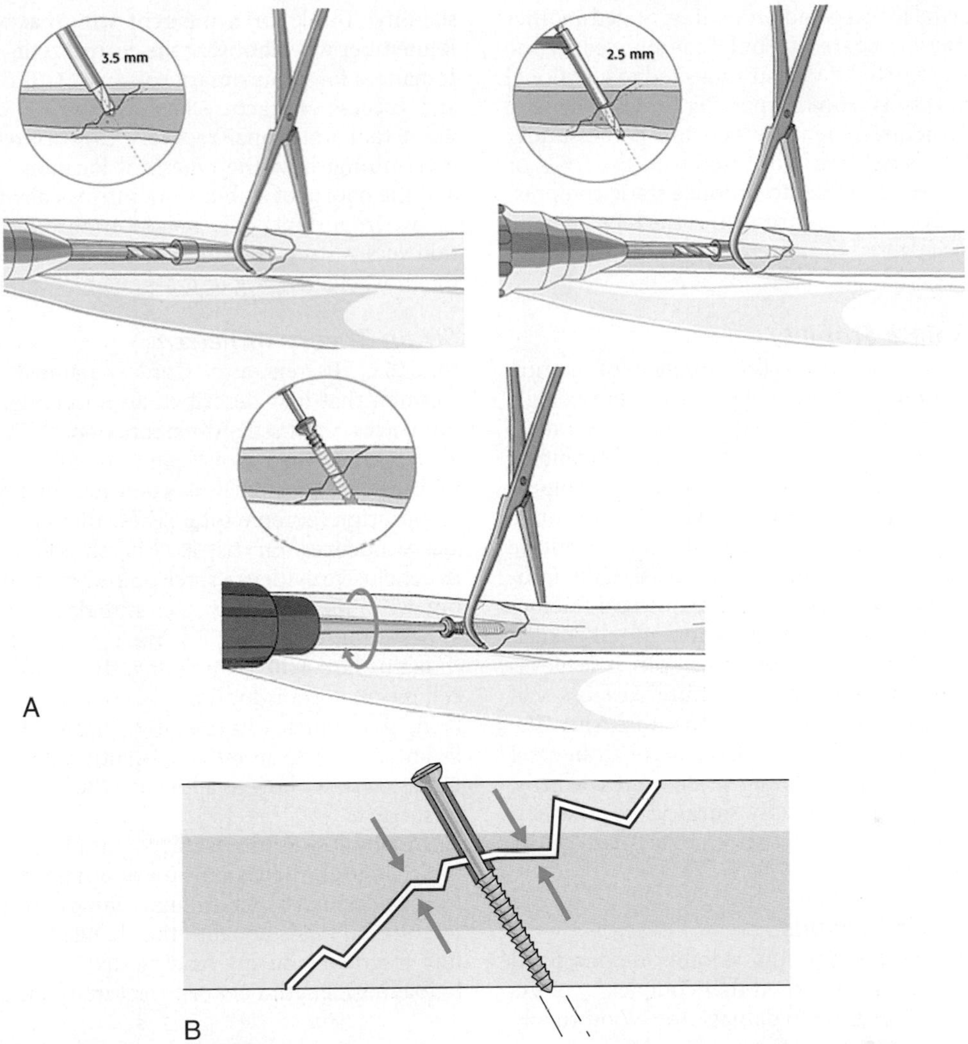

Figure 8-21. Lag screw placement by technique. **A,** The fracture is anatomically reduced and held in compression via a pointed reduction clamp. A small fragment lag screw is then placed by technique. The glide hole (which is approximately the size of the outer diameter of the screw) is first drilled. The drill guide is then inserted into the glide hole. The far cortex hole (which is approximately the size of the inner diameter of the screw) is then drilled. **B,** Lag screw placement by design. The screw is partially threaded. Only the screw threads contact the bone in the drilled hole, thereby creating the same effect as though a glide hole had been drilled. *(Source:* ***A,*** *Redrawn from Heim D, Luria S, Mosheiff R, Weil Y: Forearm shaft 22-A2.1: lag screw and plate fixation, AO Foundation, AO Surgery Reference. Available at:* https://www2.aofoundation.org/wps/portal/surgery?showPage=redfix&bone=Radius&segment=Shaft&classification=22-A2.1&treatment=&method=Lag%20screw%20and%20plate%20fixation&implantstype=&approach=&redfix_url=1325866239919&Language=en; ***B,*** *Redrawn from Rüedi TP, Buckley RE, Morgan CG: AO principles of fracture management, vol 1, ed 2, expanded edition, Switzerland, 2007, Thieme, Figure 3.2.1-4, p 160.)*

In this scenario, attempting to create compression along the axis of the bone will lead to uncontrolled shear and displacement of the reduction. This is commonly necessary in the proximal femur but can be used in other areas of the skeleton as well. Review Figure 8-17 once again. In this example, it was necessary to attach the plate first to the acute angle of the fracture (because of the design of the implant itself). Attempting to create compression along the axis of the bone with an articulated tensioning device led to shear, which created shortening and medial translation of the distal segment along the plane of the fracture.[1] Recognizing this problem led to the decision to place a conventional screw through the plate distal to the fracture. This conventional screw application created compression across the axis of the fracture (transaxial) by pulling the distal fragment toward the plate, thereby compressing the distal side of the oblique fracture to the proximal side.[32]

To review, compression can be divided into different categories. We have just distinguished axial compression from transaxial compression and described the different tools and techniques used with each. Now let us differentiate between static compression and dynamic compression. Static compression is that which is applied at the time of the surgical intervention. Once applied, it remains virtually unaltered (in reality, it decreases over time as the law of entropy states that all systems in the universe move from a position of order to one of disorder). Examples of static compression include all the axial and transaxial compression scenarios that we have previously discussed. Dynamic compression differs from static compression in that postoperative functional use of the limb leads to periodic partial loading and unloading. Stated another way, the fracture fragments are not only compressed by the preload of the implant (static), but also subjected to additional compression, which results from harnessing forces generated at the level of the fracture when the skeleton comes under physiologic load. This is not to be confused with the DCU or DCP, both of which were designed to produce static compression. An example of dynamic compression is the tension band concept. This will be covered in more detail under the "Fixation" heading.

Summary of Absolute Stability

In summary, absolute stability is the absence of motion between fracture fragments when subjected to physiologic load. It is always indicated for articular fractures, regardless of the fracture pattern. It is almost never indicated for complex metaphyseal and diaphyseal fracture patterns (as the compromise to the blood supply required to enact the anatomic reduction of every small fragment outweighs the advantage of anatomically reducing each piece). It is occasionally indicated for simple pattern metaphyseal and diaphyseal fracture patterns. It requires the perfect restoration of all loaded fracture fragments back into anatomic position. It achieves load sharing through compression of fracture surfaces that interdigitate and increase friction at the fracture site. The compression can be achieved through axial or transaxial means. It leads to primary bone healing when done correctly. This necessitates biologically friendly surgical approaches, reduction techniques, and implant placement. That can be difficult.

Speaking of Absolute Stability

- "I would like to achieve absolute stability of this tibial shaft fracture, but I am concerned that complexity of the fracture pattern will lead me to damage the blood supply to the fragments too much while trying to obtain an anatomic reduction."
- "This oblique metaphyseal tibial fracture orientation is from proximal lateral to distal medial. I am planning on using a medial plate. If I attach it distally first, I should be able to compress with the plate without creating displacement through shear."
- "That ulnar shaft fracture orientation is transverse. I would love to use a lag screw, but I don't see how that would be possible. I better choose an axial compression technique instead."
- "I have anatomically reduced this humeral shaft fracture and compressed the fracture with independent lag screws. I better protect these lag screws with a plate, since they have difficulty resisting loading all by themselves."

Relative Stability

At this point, let us shift our attention away from absolute stability and toward relative stability. Once again this is a decision that is made prior to surgery. Relative stability is defined as controlled motion of fracture fragments under physiologic loading conditions.[1] Indications for relative stability include most metaphyseal and diaphyseal fractures (excluding the two previously covered caveats). Epiphyseal or articular fractures are never appropriate for relative stability. Complex fracture patterns are ideal for relative stability. Simple fracture patterns are amenable to relative stability, but less than ideal for relative stability. Think for a moment why this would be the case. Remember why choosing the correct type of stability matters. It matters for two primary reasons: (1) It determines the type and success of fracture healing, and (2) it defines the time point that functional recovery can begin.[38] Let us focus on determining how the type (not location) of fracture pattern and the choice of stability are intrinsically linked. This teeters on two important concepts: (1) strain and (2) stress concentration versus stress distribution. Let us start with the one that is the most challenging to grasp, namely strain.

Strain Theory of Perren

In 1977, Perren and Cordey penned a manuscript in German that first described an interpretation of mechanical influences on tissue differentiation.[39] This became known as the Strain Theory of Perren. In 1980, a second manuscript by the same authors was published in English. Within this manuscript, Perren wrote: "These thoughts about the mechanical influences on tissue differentiation are not intended as conclusive evidence since precise data are still not available, but we hope that they will stimulate thought and provide a basis for discussion."[40] More than 30 years later, these thoughts are still stimulating discussion and research on cell mechanotransduction. As importantly, this theory is still being manipulated in operative theaters all around the world in an attempt to more consistently achieve fracture healing. Let us consider how to apply this theory in a practical manner in surgery.

In physics, strain is a magnitude of deformation. It is the change in the dimension of a deformed objected during loading divided by its original dimension. When translated to fracture care, it is equal to the change in length between fracture fragments during loading divided by the original (prior to loading) length between fracture fragments.

$$\text{Strain} = \Delta\ \text{Length}/\text{Length}$$

Most of you reading this chapter are not mechanical engineers or physics wizards. In light of that, just for a moment, I would like to trade perfect accuracy of mechanical terms for understanding. Stated the most useful way in terms of fracture care, strain is the motion that occurs between fracture fragments during loading divided by the resting distance between the same fracture fragments after fixation.

$$\text{Strain} = \frac{\text{Magnitude of Displacement between Fragments during Loading}}{\text{Total Resting Distance between Fragments after Stabilization}}$$

This is a formula that we all can work with. You really only need to remember this formula and one detail to be able to manipulate strain to your advantage in the operating room. The detail is that a low strain environment leads to bone formation (i.e., healing).[38,41] You already know that primary bone healing occurs in the absence of motion (absolute stability) and secondary bone healing occurs with controlled motion (relative stability). Let us take some time to consider three different scenarios to see how this works.

In scenario 1 (Fig. 8-22, *A*), we have a complex metadiaphyseal fracture pattern. We know that a complex

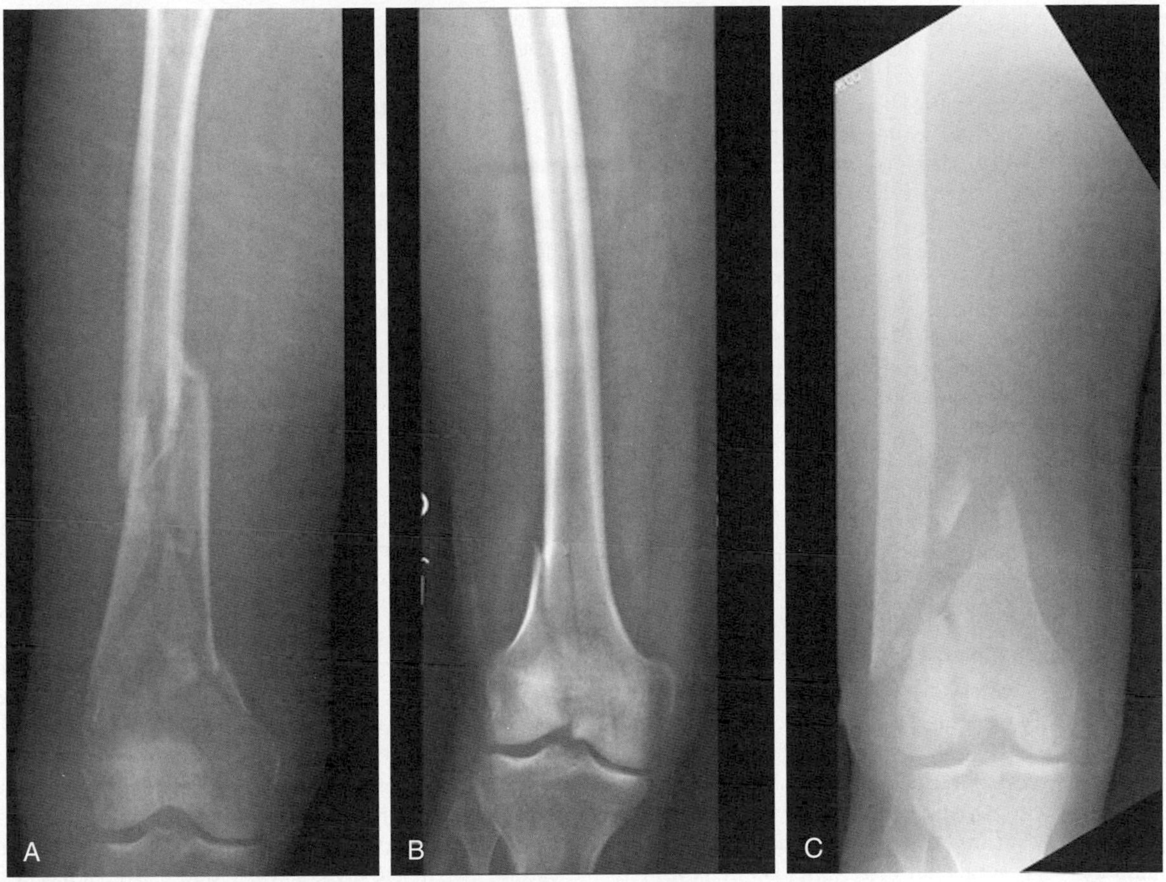

Figure 8-22. Fracture pattern affects strain. This must be considered when creating a fixation montage. The type of stability that will be present should be decided at the beginning in the preoperative plan and is based partly on the fracture pattern as noted. **A,** Complex metaphyseal fracture pattern noted in a supracondylar femur fracture. **B,** Simple articular split noted in medial femoral condyle fracture. **C,** Simple metaphyseal pattern in supracondylar femur fracture.

metadiaphyseal fracture pattern is an indication for relative stability and that relative stability provides controlled motion of fracture fragments under physiologic load. We know that restoring the relationship between the joint surface and the diaphysis is all that is necessary. Stated another way, reducing every single fracture fragment anatomically would be both unnecessary and counterproductive (i.e., it would require excessive soft tissue stripping and thereby lead to avascular fragments). Restoring length, alignment, and rotation rather than the perfect anatomic restoration of every fragment is preferred. We know that this can be accomplished with many different types of implants. Let us refer to the formula:

$$\text{Strain} = \frac{\text{Magnitude of Displacement between Fragments during Loading}}{\text{Total Resting Distance between Fragments after Stabilization}}$$

The total resting distance between all fracture fragments is a large number (as it always is with comminuted, multifragmentary fractures because of the cumulative distance between so many different fragments). When a large number is in the denominator of a fraction, then the overall value is likely to be a low number (because it is impossible to create so much motion that the numerator will be high enough to make the overall value high); therefore, the strain is likely to be low. Low strain leads to bone healing. It is hard to lose in this scenario. This is one of the easiest fracture patterns to treat successfully, despite the fact that it is broken into many pieces.

In scenario 2 (see Fig. 8-22, *B*), we have a simple articular fracture pattern. We know that any type of articular fracture pattern is an indication for absolute stability and that absolute stability is defined as no motion between fracture fragments under physiologic load. Anatomic restoration of the fracture fragments is required. Interfragmentary compression is important. Let us refer to the formula:

$$\text{Strain} = \frac{\text{Magnitude of Displacement between Fragments during Loading}}{\text{Total Resting Distance between Fragments after Stabilization}}$$

The total resting distance between fracture fragments is going to be very low (as the two fragments are compressed together in anatomic position). That means the denominator is small. Reaching a low strain in this scenario requires virtually no motion between fragments. Thankfully, that is what absolute stability provides. Using absolute stability for the treatment of simple fracture patterns requires the surgical skill to anatomically reduce the fracture with a biologically friendly technique. Assuming you possess it that day, it is hard to lose in this scenario.

In scenario 3 (Fig. 8-22, *C*), we have a simple metaphyseal fracture pattern. We know that metaphyseal fracture patterns do not have to be anatomically reduced like articular fractures. All that is required from a reduction standpoint is the restoration of the relationship between the articular surface and the diaphysis. We are left with a choice. Do we choose absolute stability and anatomically reduce the simple metaphyseal fracture pattern? If we make that choice, we know that we can reach a low strain environment and achieve primary bone healing just as we did in scenario 2. Or, do we choose relative stability instead, as perfect restoration of all fragments is not required? Certainly that is a temptation because it would allow us to do less soft tissue dissection and a more biologically friendly surgical approach. This is where it gets interesting. Let us refer to the formula:

$$\text{Strain} = \frac{\text{Magnitude of Displacement between Fragments during Loading}}{\text{Total Resting Distance between Fragments after Stabilization}}$$

If we choose relative stability and accept a near-anatomic (but imperfect) reduction, then the distance between fracture fragments (and therefore the denominator) is low. We have already stated that when the denominator is a small value, then to reach a low strain, the motion (numerator) with loading must be very small, almost nonexistent. Unfortunately, if we create a stiff construct and reach that small denominator, then we cannot achieve primary bone healing (because the fracture fragments are gapped so direct remodeling cannot occur). But we know that secondary bone healing requires a certain amount of flexibility in order to induce callus formation (remember relative stability is defined as controlled motion between fracture fragments under physiologic loading, not no motion). This controlled motion is not optional. It is necessary. Tissue differentiation into callus formation (bone healing) will not occur without it. We have a problem. Based on the strain theory and a previous publication by Perren, one option is to create a malreduction in order to increase the size of the denominator.[42] This is less than ideal because our goal of fracture care is to restore both form and function. The other solution flies in the face of the strain theory but can work. In this solution, we can keep the gap width small and make the construct more flexible in order to achieve enough motion to induce callus formation. You should recognize that even though this can work, it does not fit well into the strain theory formula, as the strain is actually a higher number. This is where the theory breaks down and has come into question.

Remember it is a theory, and while important, still has holes. How much motion is enough to induce callus but not too much (such that fibrous tissue is formed)? How do we successfully treat simple pattern femoral and tibial diaphyseal fractures with relative stability through intramedullary rodding? While it is important to understand the strain theory and apply it intraoperatively, it is also important to realize that we are making macromanipulations in an attempt to influence the microscopic environment without a clear gauge to tell us when we are correct. This is akin to measuring in millimeters, marking with chalk, and cutting with an axe. The attempt is important, but still imperfect.

Stress Distribution versus Stress Concentration

Let us move to a simpler topic that is much easier to understand and explain. Although strain is mainly concerned with the fracture site (motion and distance), stress distribution versus concentration is mainly concerned with the implant. This is best described with an analogy. Pick up a pen or pencil and subject it to three-point bending. First do it by putting your thumbs together in the middle of the pen and your hands toward the ends of the pen. Bending the pen in this manner concentrates or focuses stress on the small section of pen between your thumbs. It is likely that if you tried hard enough, you could break the pen by concentrating stress on that small area between your thumbs. Now take the pen and place your thumbs toward the periphery (close to the rest of your hands) and bend it again. Bending the pen in this manner distributes or apportions or shares the stress over the length of the pen between your two thumbs. It is likely that you can see a bowing of the pen. It will be much harder to break it in this manner, because the stress is being distributed over such a large distance. Now imagine that your pen is a bone and your thumbs represent screws that you place intraoperatively either near to or far away from the fracture. When screws are placed close to each side of a fracture, this concentrates stress on the plate. The plate has natural stress risers in the form of screw holes. This is where an implant typically fails when loaded in bending in this manner (Fig. 8-23). That is not to say that an implant cannot fail when stress is distributed over a larger area (Fig. 8-24). This is just a much more infrequent scenario. We should strive intraoperatively to distribute stress rather than concentrate it whenever possible.

Summary of Relative Stability

In summary, relative stability is defined as the controlled motion of fracture fragments under physiologic load. It is never indicated for articular fractures. It is indicated for all complex metaphyseal and diaphyseal fracture patterns, and some simple pattern metaphyseal and diaphyseal fracture patterns. It does not require the perfect restoration of all fracture fragments back into anatomic position. It does require a restoration of the relationships between the joint above and the joint below the fracture. It leads to secondary bone healing when done correctly. This necessitates an understanding of the Strain Theory of Perren as well as the concept of stress distribution versus stress concentration. Remember that motion is necessary for secondary bone formation, and therefore for fracture healing when relative stability is chosen. Refer to Figure 8-16 to review the graphic depiction of how variations in flexibility affect the ability of the surgeon to be successful when using relative stability.

Speaking of Relative Stability

- "That metaphyseal distal tibial fracture has a simple oblique fracture pattern. If I am going to choose relative stability and plating, I better consider how to ensure there will be enough motion to induce callus formation."
- "Those postoperative radiographs show a nonanatomic reduction of a simple pattern fracture that was fixed with locking screws right next to each side of the fracture. Some would call that a nonunion machine. The fracture

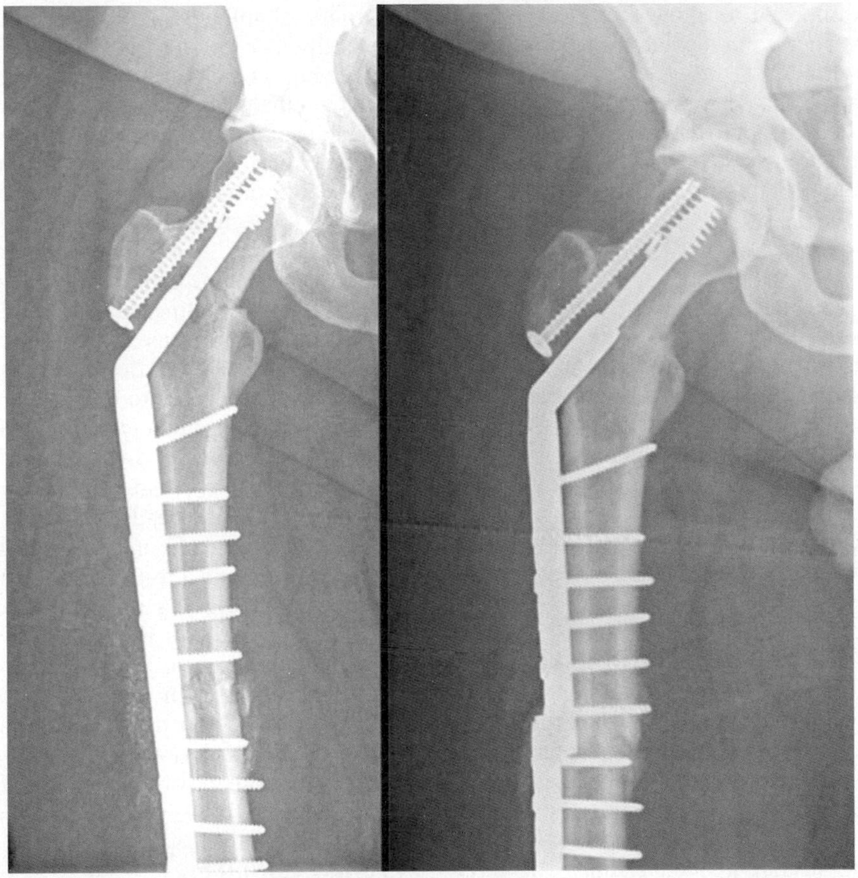

Figure 8-23. Stress concentration is noted between the two screws that were placed very close to the fracture on each side of the construct. Failure occurs in this location.

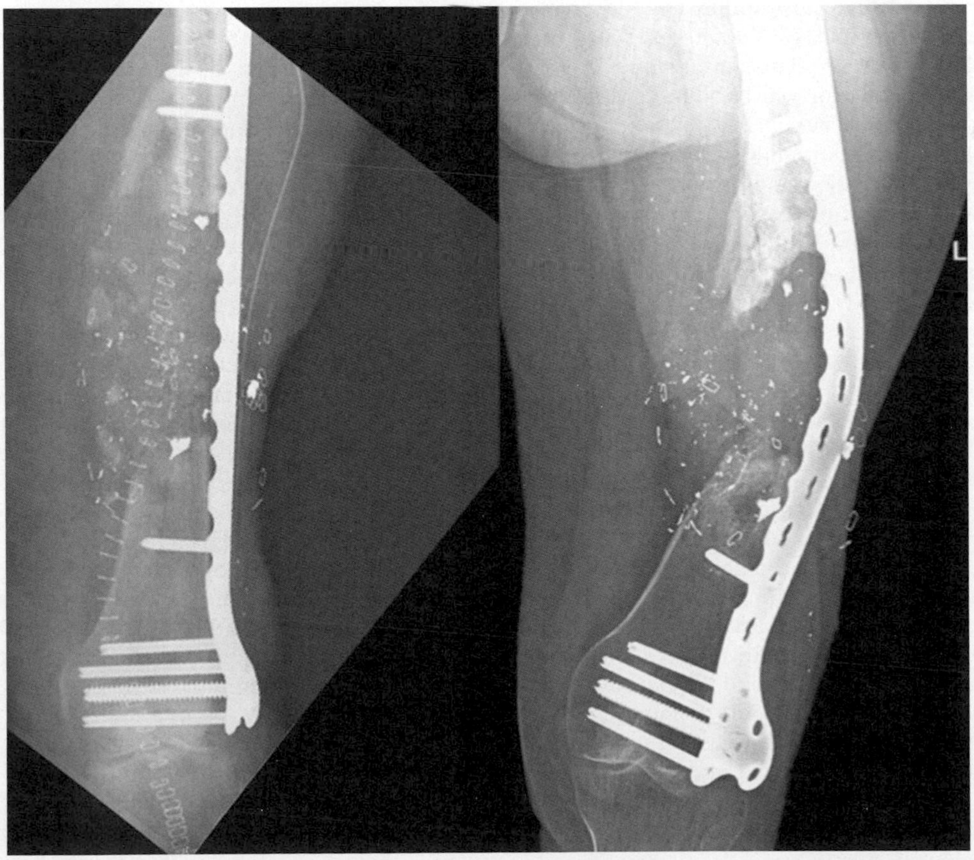

Figure 8-24. Stress distribution is noted over the large segment of bone loss that was grafted. Note the bowing of the plate over the distributed area of stress.

is not well enough apposed to allow for primary bone healing and the construct is not flexible enough to induce callus."

- "Using a thin plate for that comminuted femoral shaft fracture is not a good idea. Sure we want motion to occur in an effort to achieve relative stability, but we are hoping for elastic deformation, not plastic deformation."

APPROACH

The approach portion of the flowchart will include two primary topics. The first is intraoperative positioning. The second is the actual surgical exposure. Covering the exposure without the positioning leaves out a key portion of the surgical procedure. It is this portion that defines which exposures are even possible. It is this same portion that defines the relationship of gravity to the fracture reduction. Just as important, this portion confers risk from the outset to the patient's physiologic status and pressure/stretch-sensitive areas. Let us start with intraoperative positioning.

Intraoperative Positioning and Patient Safety

The goal of surgical positioning is to provide access to the proposed surgical site(s), while preventing position-related complications. All perioperative team members are responsible for patient safety through shared decision making and teamwork. Attention during this portion of the procedure is not just important for ensuring ideal access to the fracture. It is also important in preventing surgical-related claims. The three most common intraoperative positions used in orthopaedic trauma care include the supine position, the prone position, and the lateral position. The most common complications associated with intraoperative positioning include pressure ulcers and peripheral neuropathies.[43-45] Rarer and more severe complications include vascular-related events such as acute compartment syndrome and cortical blindness. Risk factors that are thought to predispose patients to positioning-related complications include diabetes mellitus, peripheral vascular disease, end-stage renal disease, malnutrition, advanced age, immune system compromise, preexisting contractures, both cachexia and obesity, body temperature control problems, and prolonged surgical times.[43] Let us consider the three most common positions individually and focus on common complications and safety-related measures to prevent them.

Supine Position

The supine position is the most common position for operative fracture care. It is the optimal position for addressing airway patency, gas exchange, and vascular access problems. It places common lines, tubes, and drains in standard orientation. Gravity is directed toward the dorsal recumbent portions of the patient and pressure points are dorsal osseous prominences. Stretch points are apex anterior. The most cranial pressure point is the occiput and postoperative alopecia is most commonly preceded by localized swelling and pain in this area in the immediate postoperative period. Pressure-reducing materials and pressure repositioning are recommended for prolonged procedures. Notifying the anesthesiologist when prolonged operative times are expected and periodic assessment as needed may help decrease the incidence of this problem. Cranial stretch points include the cervical spine, and anatomic alignment should be maintained while protecting the occiput.

Moving caudally, arm position is next with pressure points noted in the scapular and thoracic vertebrae (in cachectic patients) and olecranon/cubital tunnel area. Stretch points are noted primarily at the brachial plexus and antecubital fossa. Current recommendations include limiting arm abduction to less than 90 degrees and preventing both shoulder and elbow hyperextension.[43-45] The use of appropriately padded armboards at the same level as the table height limits brachial plexus stretch. Limiting contralateral head rotation is also recommended for the same reason. Forearm position should be supination or neutral to decrease pressure on the ulnar nerve. If the decision is made to tuck the arms at the side, then the forearm should remain in neutral position with care to protect against pressure to the ulnar nerve.[44]

Lower extremity pressure points include the sacrum, ischial tuberosities, fibular heads, and calcanei. Padding is recommended if pressure is noted around the fibular head. Any semi-circumferential restraints (such as restraint belts) should be placed while being mindful of anterior pressure points (e.g., anterior superior iliac spine and lateral femoral cutaneous nerve, fibular head and common peroneal nerve). In the supine position with the legs supported, stretch points only occur with hip or knee flexion contractures. In these instances, it is recommended to prevent stretch past what is comfortable preoperatively to limit the risk of femoral and sciatic neuropathy.

Prone Position

The prone position provides dorsal access and logically reverses the common pressure points and direction of stretch. It is the most limiting addressing airway patency, gas exchange, and vascular access problems; therefore, it requires a pause point preoperatively to ensure the trauma patient can be safely placed in this position. Cranial pressure points include the face, eyes, and chin primarily. Cervical alignment should be maintained while protecting these areas and the endotracheal tube.

The chest, abdomen, and pelvis are suspended from the table with rolls that extend from the anterior shoulder area to the iliac crests. This suspension allows for chest wall excursion and decreases intraabdominal pressure. Morbid obesity and macromastia create special challenges for pressure relief. Care should be taken to avoid excessive pressure on the anterior clavicle, areolar, anterior superior iliac spine, and femoral nerve areas. When placed in anatomic alignment, the spine will reveal the normal cervical and lumbar lordosis and thoracic kyphosis with respect to the tabletop.[45]

The arms should be placed at less than 90 degrees of abduction with the elbows flexed and forearms pronated. Abducting greater than 90 degrees is felt to increase the risk of stretching the plexus across the coracoid process and glenohumeral joint; alternatively, some prefer tucking and padding the arms at the side in the prone position.[44] Below the waist, pressure points include the patella and dorsal surface of the foot. Pressure-relieving positioning aids, such as gel donuts and rolls, are recommended.[45]

Lateral Decubitus Position

The lateral decubitus (also called *lateral recumbent*) position provides access to both anterior and posterior structures in a single surgical position, often at the cost of compromising ideal access to both. The position is typically named by the down side (e.g., right lateral decubitus position consists of the right side being dependent and the left facing upward). The lateral aspect of the dependent side is primarily at risk of pressure ulceration, whereas the nondependent side risks traction injuries.[43]

Starting cranially, the lateral aspect of the face and the ear are at risk. Pressure must be limited in these areas while maintaining horizontal cervical alignment to the bed. A chest roll should be placed distal to the axilla to elevate the shoulder from the bed, relieve pressure on the dependent arm, and allow chest motion with respiration. The misnomer of axillary role can be dangerous when formal teaching is not provided to ensure the correct position of this role is accomplished. Placing the role in the axilla theoretically increases the potential for compression-induced brachial plexopathies postoperatively. The arm is positioned in front of the patient with the elbow flexed (hand toward face) or extended. Flexion of the elbow provides the advantages of moving the dependent arm further away from the radiographic field on elbow procedures, but hyperflexion should be avoided to prevent stretching of the ulnar nerve in the cubital tunnel. The forearm is placed in neutral or supinated position. The nondependent arm is suspended on a positioning device or pillow in a relaxed position. Lateral position is maintained through the use of a beanbag or alternative lateral positioning device. The dependent lower extremity is flexed slightly at the hip and knee (to protect the femoral and sciatic nerves, respectively) with padding beneath the fibular head for protection of the peroneal nerve and beneath the lateral malleolus for ulcer prevention. A positioning device or pillow should be placed between the legs to relieve pressure and maintain neutral adduction.[43-45]

Special Considerations: Hemilithotomy and Perineal Post

Special considerations include the use of hemilithotomy position and the use of a perineal post. The hemilithotomy position is sometimes used to improve radiographic visualization for lower extremity procedures by flexing the nonoperative hip out of the way of the fluoroscopy beam. Unique risks in this position include compartment syndrome, femoral nerve compression beneath the inguinal ligament (controversial), and peroneal nerve compression at the fibular head against the well leg holder. If this position is chosen, care should be taken to carefully position the extremity, limit hip flexion and abduction, choose well-leg holders that focus pressure toward the foot and ankle region rather than the popliteal fossa region, and relieve pressure around the fibular head.[43-46]

The perineal post is a device used to maintain the position of the pelvis when traction is applied to the lower extremity for reduction maneuvers. It has been associated with perineal necrosis and pudendal nerve palsy.[44,47-50] When using the post, care should be taken to pad the post for pressure relief, protect the genitals from compression, limit sustained traction to reasonable amounts, and release traction as soon as possible. If prolonged traction is required, periods of pressure relief should be systematically incorporated into the surgical procedure. When the post is used, postoperative evaluation should include a discussion about sensation in the genital region.

Surgical Exposure

A surgical exposure is a means to an end in fracture care. Historically, the desired ends of the exposure included visualization of all fracture fragments, preparation of the bone ends, reduction of the fracture, and fixation of the fracture.[51] All of these ends were accomplished ideally through what came to be known as an extensile exposure. "Exposure that will vie effectively with the 'great arsenal of chance' must be a match for every shift, and therefore have a range, *extensile*, like the tongue of a chameleon to reach where it requires."[52] Extensile had a particular meaning. It meant that the exposure could be stretched out or extended to include the majority of the bone. Almost all of the classic extensile exposures in Henry's book exploited an internervous plane. An internervous plane is a plane between two muscles that are innervated by different nerves. Exploiting these planes allows the surgeon to enact a wide exposure along the length of the muscles without denervating them; therefore, these exposures allowed for the desired ends mentioned earlier. It is important to note why the desired ends were so desired. Initially it was felt that all fractures, whether simple or complex in pattern, should be anatomically reduced and compressed. Absolute stability was not just the standard but also the only choice; however, achieving absolute stability was challenging in more complex patterns. It became clearer that the compromise of stripping more soft tissue from the bone was not worth the advantage of anatomic reconstruction of all fragments (for all fracture sites). Both wound healing complications and fracture nonunions were noted. The common thread between these complications was a vascular disruption, on the one hand, to the soft tissue envelope and, on the other hand, to the bone.[1]

With the recognition of these problems, osteosynthesis evolved. If you have not yet done so, it is now important to separate the steps of fracture treatment in your head. Refer again to the flowchart (see Fig. 8-1). Precise language is required. The surgical exposure is different than the quality of reduction or reduction techniques as well as the choice of fixation. Although certain combinations of these commonly recur, different combinations of exposure, reduction technique, and fixation methods may be used. To clarify, the surgeon historically chose absolute stability, extensile surgical exposures, direct reduction techniques, and conventional screw-plate osteosynthesis. When one of these choices changes, other choices may change with it (but do not have to do so). Reviewing the evolution of osteosynthesis will clarify what is meant by this.

In the latter half of last century, it became clear that the combination of absolute stability, extensile surgical exposures, direct reduction techniques, and conventional screw-plate osteosynthesis was less than ideal in all circumstances. Damage to fracture vascularity was secondary to both poor decision making and marginal surgical technique. The end result was an unacceptable incidence of nonunions and wound healing problems.[42] Change was necessary. Changes were first made to techniques of reduction. While attention to soft tissue dissection was considered essential from early on, the license for direct reduction techniques was a slippery slope. Indirect reduction techniques were developed (this will be covered in more detail under the heading "Reduction" in the flowchart). Indirect reduction consists of the "blind" repositioning of fracture fragments through manipulation with distraction. This intimates lack of direct visualization of all the fracture lines, thereby mandating less soft tissue dissection and an improved vascular environment for bone healing. Intraoperatively, this can be accomplished, and was first recommended to be accomplished, while still using the plate as a compression device.[18] Indirect reduction techniques were successful. Intramedullary nail development and use were simultaneously occurring with the improvements in plate osteosynthesis. Consistent fracture healing was noted with intramedullary nails through callus formation. Plates subsequently began to be used as "internal splints" rather than instruments of compression.[53] This mimicked the mechanical function of an intramedullary nail. Image intensifiers and portable fluoroscopy units became more prevalent. This improvement in visualization (radiographically rather than through direct vision) enabled reduction quality to remain acceptable and generalizable. It additionally enabled surgical exposures to decrease in length and breadth. Relative stability was born and led to a tidal wave of additional changes. This tidal wave included a large volume of resources being placed toward implant and instrument design. Like all choices, this one came with compromises.

Let us first consider the advantages afforded through the popularity of relative stability. Remember the previous desired ends of a surgical exposure: visualization of the fracture fragments, preparation of the bone ends, reduction of the fracture, and fixation of the fracture. All of these were initially afforded through an extensile exposure. Consider how each of these ends changed with the acceptance of relative stability. Remember that the ideal indication for relative stability is a complex pattern metaphyseal or diaphyseal fracture. First, rather than the perfect anatomic repositioning of every fragment (as in absolute stability), relative stability accepted the restoration of the relationships between the joint above and the joint below the fracture. This meant it was no longer necessary to visualize every fracture fragment. Second, rather than the anatomic compression of fracture fragments to each other (as in absolute stability), relative stability allowed for bridging or bypassing the zone of comminution. This meant it was no longer necessary to prepare the bone ends. Third, rather than direct visualization of all the fracture fragments to ensure a reduction (as was typical of absolute stability), relative stability allowed for imperfect restoration of relationships that did not require visualization of all the fragments, but rather could be accomplished via radiographic visualization. As noted, this was greatly aided by the evolution of image intensifiers and portable intraoperative fluoroscopy units. Reduction of the fracture no longer required the extensile approach. New instruments were designed and older instruments were used differently to enact the reduction. Radiographic interpretation skills advanced. Finally, rather than the direct visualization of implant placement to assist with attaching compression devices or using compression through the plate, relative stability allowed for noncompression-type fixation to occur. This negated the need for an extensile exposure for implant placement. New instruments were developed that made percutaneous plate and screw insertion easier (e.g., aiming arms, targeting guides). Wound healing complications logically decreased.

The advantages should be clear; the implications may not be. Now let us consider the compromises that developed through the popularity of relative stability and minimally invasive approaches. Although these compromises could be grouped in many different ways, we will do so with the following: educational challenges, implant expense, and radiation exposure.

Let us first consider the significant educational challenges that arose with the advent of relative stability and minimally invasive techniques. It has been written that safety in surgery depends on knowledge of anatomy and technical skill, one being useless without the other.[54] Knowledge of anatomy traditionally involved a clear understanding of superficial and deep dissection planes. Surgically relevant anatomy included cutaneous landmarks, origins and insertions of muscles (including the station of the entire course of muscles within the dissection zone), and internervous planes. As with any knowledge that is useful, it required application and repetition to achieve success. As minimally invasive procedures gained popularity, surgical exposures became more limited in size. Conventional extensile exposures have been used less and less, leading to a deficit in application and repetition in many training programs. Knowledge of cross-sectional anatomy has become paramount in understanding danger zones for fixation based on limited working portals.

Technical skill traditionally involved soft tissue handling, clamp placement, and implant application within the zone of injury (as defined by absolute stability). Practice with direct reduction techniques was a consistent part of training. Repetition was high secondary to using the same techniques for both articular and extraarticular fracture locations. Technical skill also involved achieving compression of the fracture fragments, thereby unloading the implants. This should not be underemphasized as the natural laws of statics and dynamics have not changed. Fracture compression represented the ideal situation mechanically for a plate, which is load sharing rather than pure load bearing. In addition to a focus on compression mechanics, plate contouring was a necessary part of training, leading to a required understanding of normal osseous lines and curves and an ability to work metal.

These educational challenges continue to outpace our ability to instruct and learn. Minimally invasive exposures, indirect reduction techniques, radiographic understanding of reduction criteria, and spanning fixation mechanics are now necessary parts of many training programs. The historical advantages of and indications for extensile exposures, direct reduction techniques, and compression fixation mechanics are still relevant. Because of this, it is incumbent on the educators to broaden teaching platforms and the students to recognize personal limitations and have a respectful view of history.

A second implication of the rising popularity of relative stability and minimally invasive fixation is implant expense. Minimally invasive surgical exposures were designed during the time of conventional implants and instruments. It became clear that to reach the potential of minimally invasive fixation, changes were necessary to improve the effectiveness, efficiency, and generalizability of the procedures. Research and technological development were poured into the problem. Research and development are not free. The solution for many problems naturally came at the cost of increased expense. Integrating precontoured implants, insertion handles, percutaneous aiming arms, and locking points of fixation improved efficiency and generalizability but came with an increased implant cost.

A third implication of the rising popularity of relative stability and minimally invasive fixation is radiation exposure.

This will be more completely covered in Chapter 13A, "Optimal and Safe Use of C-Arm X-Ray Fluoroscopy Units." As direct visualization of fracture reductions gave way to radiographic visualization, radiation exposure naturally increased. Indiscriminate use of fluoroscopy poses dangers to both the surgeon and the patient. Education in this area is necessarily being incorporated into trauma course offerings and residency training curricula.

Speaking of the Surgical Approach

- "My patient came back to his six-week follow-up visit complaining of occipital alopecia. I think I remember him complaining of swelling in that area of his head postoperatively. I really need to start communicating better with anesthesia when prolonged procedures are expected, to ensure that repositioning is systematized."
- "I operated on his tibia but postoperative complaints were centered around numbness in the ulnar part of his hand. I'm not sure about arm position during the surgery. I really didn't pay attention prior to draping."
- "I will be taking this patient to surgery tomorrow for fixation of his forearm fracture. The radial arterial line cannot be in this location. It should be moved preoperatively to prevent surgical delays."
- "I don't understand how that failed so quickly. I guess I should have considered loading the bone so that it would protect the plate. I could have done that without anatomically reducing all the fragments. It only takes a few points of contact to help protect the implant."
- "I find it interesting that my hospital is giving me such a hard time about implant costs. I have never really thought about it. I guess I should take time to consider the options."
- "For the longest time I have associated limited exposures, indirect reduction techniques, relative stability, and locking fixation, without considering that they don't always have to go together."

REDUCTION: DIRECT VERSUS INDIRECT

Form has been related to function in many different disciplines. Orthopaedic trauma is no exception. The act of reduction is the restoration of the form of the injured bone. In order to discuss reduction, let us first begin with a common vocabulary. There is a distinction between the quality of a reduction and the method of a reduction. Let us start with reduction quality.

Quality of Reduction

When differentiating quality, three terms are commonly used: anatomic reduction, functional reduction, and malreduction. An anatomic reduction is defined as the perfect restoration of every fracture fragment. Each fracture line is precisely reduced. This is generally accomplished via visualization of each fracture line. As previously noted, it is encouraged in articular fractures for logical mechanical reasons. A functional reduction is the restoration of length, alignment, and rotation between the proximal and distal segments without the precise realignment of each fragment. Stated another way, it includes the restoration of anatomic alignment (relationship of articular surface to limb axis) without the anatomic restoration of each individual fragment. This is generally accomplished in the absence of visualization of each fracture line. As previously noted, it is generally accepted in diaphyseal and metaphyseal fractures. A malreduction is defined as an inadequate restoration of a fracture. In an articular fracture, this would mean lack of precise restoration of every fragment. In an extraarticular fracture, this would mean lack of realignment of the articular surface to the limb axis.

Method of Reduction

Different than the quality of reduction—but linked to it—is the method of reduction. Two specific reduction methods have been defined. Direct reduction is defined as the repositioning of bone fragments individually under direct vision. Indirect reduction is defined as the "blind" repositioning of bone fragments through manipulation with distraction. "Blind" refers to the fact that the entirety of the fracture line being reduced is not visualized.

AO Philosophy and Inherent Conflict

The aims of the AO method are fourfold and include (1) fracture reduction and fixation to restore anatomic relationships, (2) preservation of the blood supply to soft tissues and bone by careful handling and gentle reduction techniques, (3) stability by fixation or splintage, as the personality of the fracture and the injury requires, and (4) early and safe mobilization of the part and the patient.[1] The first two aims create an inherent conflict. It is generally accepted that the quality of a reduction is inversely related to the surgeon's ability to maintain the blood supply to fracture fragments. To clarify, it is not challenging to exact a precise reduction if no soft tissue is obstructing visualization or pulling on the fragments being reduced. Similarly, it is not challenging to maintain nearly all vascularity to fracture fragments if the surgeon accepts a malreduction.

The solution to this conflict is to enact the quality of reduction that is required for each specific injury as atraumatically as possible. To do that, we must understand the reduction requirements. As previously noted, these differ based on the part of the bone that is fractured. There is a hierarchy of reduction mandates that should be understood. Thankfully this hierarchy can be divided into the well-defined segments of the bone, specifically the articular surface (epiphysis), the metaphysis, and the diaphysis. This has been covered in detail under the "Area Involved" heading in the flowchart. Please refer back to this portion of the chapter for a refresher if required. Now that the quality of the reduction requirement for each area of the bone is clearer, let us focus on how to achieve it, with particular emphasis on the instruments and techniques used in the direct and indirect reduction methods. You will note that many of the instruments and techniques will overlap, with the primary difference in technique being the surgical exposure.

Direct Reduction: Instruments and Techniques

Direct reduction is the repositioning of bone fragments individually under direct vision. As such, the instruments and techniques have been designed and developed to be accomplished through extensile approaches. The instruments have varying footprints on the bone itself, ranging from limited damage to more extensive damage. The more damaging instruments should be used only after the less-damaging ones have failed, if at all. Regardless of which instrument is chosen, careful soft tissue handling with minimal periosteal stripping is required. It is important to remember that direct reduction techniques are not a license for aggressive soft tissue handling. If anything, the decision to proceed with direct reduction techniques should lead the surgeon to take even more care to maintain vascularity to fracture fragments. Remember that the trauma insult is cumulative and includes both the injury and the iatrogenic footprint. With the understanding that an extensile exposure has more potential to damage fracture fragment vascularity, it is logical that direct reduction instruments would be handled with more care.

The instruments used for direct reduction can be divided into two basic categories: (1) those that do not maintain the reduction once obtained and (2) those that do maintain the reduction once obtained. Instruments that do not maintain the reduction once obtained typically (but not always) allow for greater degrees of freedom of motion. These include instruments such as the hook, joystick (with or without drill guides), elevator, spiked pusher, and tamp. Those that do maintain the reduction once obtained are typically more challenging to accurately place, secondary to the precision required to enact the perfect vector of reduction. These primarily consist of different types of clamps. Let us consider each type of instrument used for direct reduction with a surgical example of how each is used.

Surgical hooks are designed primarily for probing and pulling but can be used to manipulate fragments rotationally and even in pushing. Hook dimensions vary widely and the sizes chosen intraoperatively are typically based on the size of the fragment being manipulated and the amount of force required (Fig. 8-25). Handles of hooks vary in form and are typically either straight, curved, or T shaped, the latter varieties providing for more force transmission through improved grip. The terminal bend or curvature is typically at least 135 degrees in order to prevent slippage from the fragment being manipulated.[55] Slippage can be decreased and the vector of force varied through drilling appropriately sized holes into the fragment in order to seat the tip (assuming safe access for drilling to the desired point of application of the tip). Hook tips can be blunt or sharp. Any form of hook—especially the sharp-tipped ones—is dangerous to the patient and surgeon if care and precision are not used during application. Placing great force on a hook as a means of reduction is generally not advised.

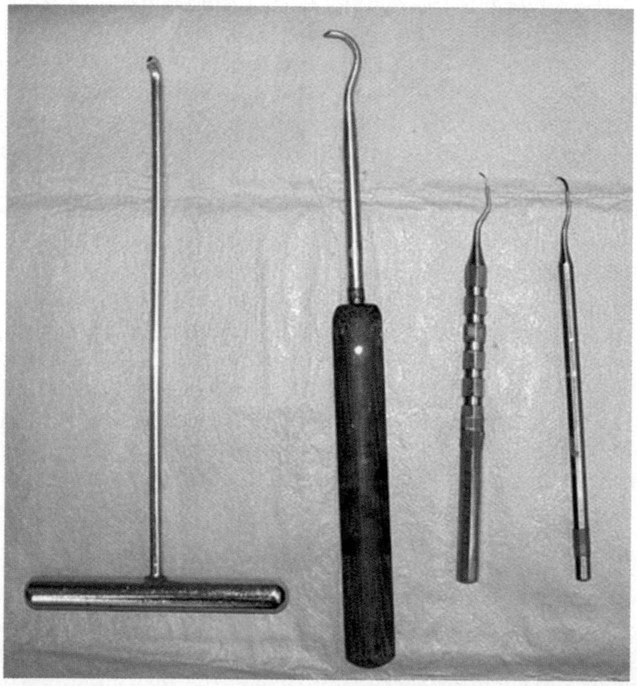

Figure 8-25. Surgical hook-type instruments used in reduction. The T-handle bone hook is shown next to the wooden handle shoulder hook and two sizes of dental picks. The size of the hook needed typically corresponds to the size of the fragment manipulated and the force required.

Names of the hooks vary based on the size of the instrument. Dental picks are the smallest type of hook used commonly in orthopaedic trauma. These vary in size both in the dimensions of the hook and the handle. Dental picks typically have straight handles with round, square, hexagonal, or octagonal profiles, the latter improving digital contact.[55] They are best used in the manipulation of small articular or cortical fragments. Shoulder hooks are intermediate in size. These typically have larger terminal ends and larger handles. The handles of these are typically straight and fit in the palm. They are primarily used for intermediate-sized fragments and are rarely useful for articular fragments. Bone hooks are the largest of those commonly used in orthopaedic trauma. These have large terminal ends and vary in handle form from straight to curved. They are primarily used for larger-sized fragments, such as diaphyseal manipulation. Both shoulder and bone hooks can be carefully used through more minimally invasive approaches in association with traction (more as an indirect reduction technique).

The joystick takes many forms in orthopaedic trauma (Fig. 8-26). Either a Kirschner wire or a Schanz pin can be used as a joystick. The size of the joystick chosen is determined by the size of the fragment to be manipulated and the amount of force to be applied. Larger core diameter sizes are chosen when the bending and rotational forces are going to be significant (as core diameter is directly related to bending and torsional strength). Joystick tips can be either smooth or threaded. Smooth tips may allow for improved insertion into the adjacent fragment with less pushing away of that fragment. Threaded tips improve the pullout resistance of the joystick. Joysticks are inserted into the bone to allow for pushing, pulling, and rotational forces. Based on which type and what degree of force is expected, an appropriate joystick design can be chosen. When combined with an appropriately sized drill guide, precision can be improved. The drill guide is especially useful when rotation and pushing are desired.

The elevator was primarily designed as a probe or soft tissue dissector, but can be used alternatively in fracture reduction (Fig. 8-27).[55] The ends are most commonly blunt and defined by width. The handles are straight and defined by both length and width. The smaller elevators useful in fracture reduction are often of the Freer variety. Freer elevators are typically double ended with a central circular cross-sectional handle. These instruments can be used inside of a joint surface to prevent over-reduction of articular fragments that are being pushed from the opposite side. Alternatively, the end of the elevator can be bent approximately 90 degrees in order to allow the surgeon to push a fragment with a broader surface area of contact (similar use to a tamp).

The spike pusher (Fig. 8-28) was designed for pushing, and typically, the pushing of larger fragments. It found its greatest

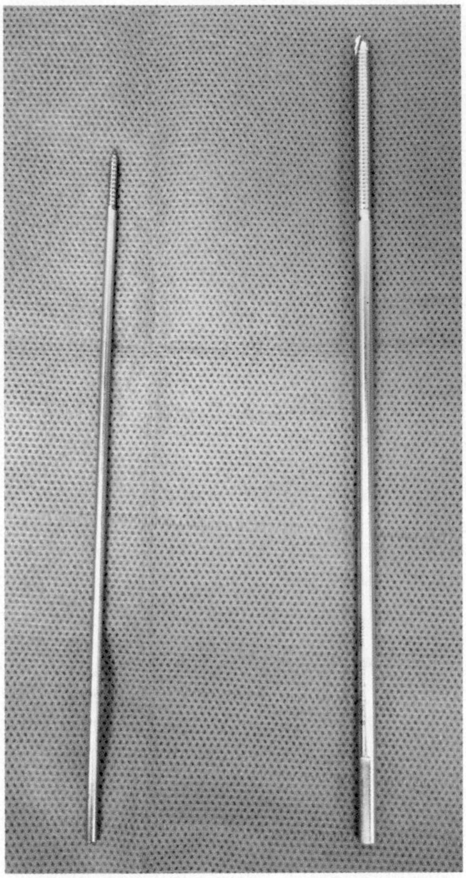

Figure 8-26. Joysticks used in reduction. Note varied sizes. To the left is a 2.5-mm threaded Kirschner wire. To the right is a 5.0-mm Schanz pin. The decision between the two would depend on the size of the fragment to be manipulated and the force required.

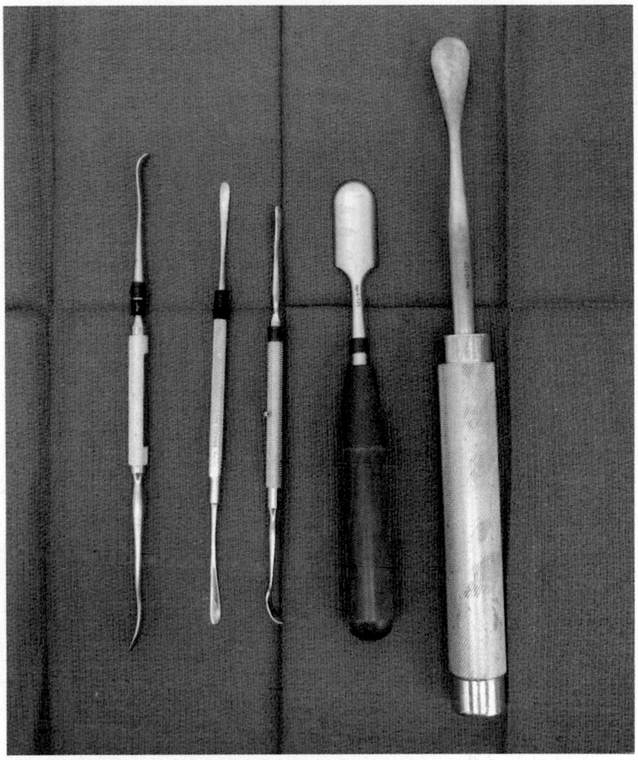

Figure 8-27. Probes used in reduction. Note the wide variability in probe size. Understanding the details of the instrument design helps the surgeon in deciding which to use.

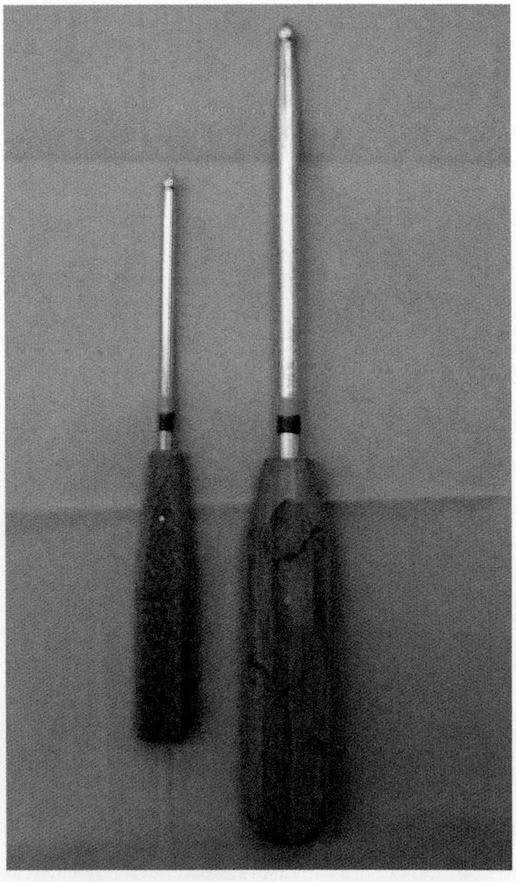

Figure 8-28. Spike pushers used in reduction.

use in the pelvis, but is also used at times in the larger bones of the lower extremity. Spike pushers occasionally have an associated ball just proximal to the spike. The ball serves two purposes: (1) It increases surface contact area, thereby distributing force if the spike pushes through the fragment being manipulated, and (2) it serves as an attachment point for a larger footing, which increases contact area even more. Pushers are often used in conjunction with hooks placed on the adjacent fragment (Fig. 8-29).

The tamp was also designed for pushing and has three basic design parts for modification: the handle, the shaft, and the tip. Current tamp designs often allow for interchangeable parts, thereby limiting instrument number (Fig. 8-30). The handle varies little and is typically designed to fit into the surgeon's palm and be struck with a mallet. The shaft of a tamp can be straight, curved, or offset, allowing use in multiple situations. The tip is typically flat to distribute forces but varies in shape from cylindrical, square, or rectangular. Tamps are commonly used for the reduction of depressed osteochondral fragments by pushing the fragments through the metaphysis in tibial plateau fractures.

Clamps are some of the most common reduction instruments and are able to maintain a reduction once it is obtained. With well-planned executions, clamps can occasionally remain in place during plate or rod application. In basic form, clamps consist of two arms, which are crossed and connected by a

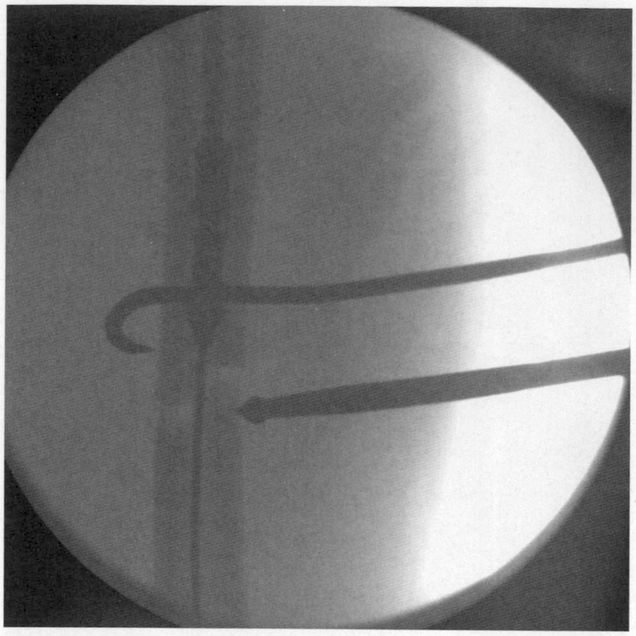

Figure 8-29. Intraoperative radiograph of the reduction of a simple pattern femoral shaft fracture with the combined use of a hook and a spike pusher. The reamer is noted inside the intramedullary canal.

pivot at the center of the crossing. This generates many possible permutations as each clamp has two jaws, two handles, a pivot, and a locking mechanism.[55] Jaws have many variations in size and form, ranging from standard curved points to more complex parts that attach to screws. The form of the jaws determines the size of the iatrogenic footprint on the bone (e.g., point to point clamps create a limited footprint while serrated jaws damage more of the periosteum). The size of the footprint is directly related to force distribution and ease of

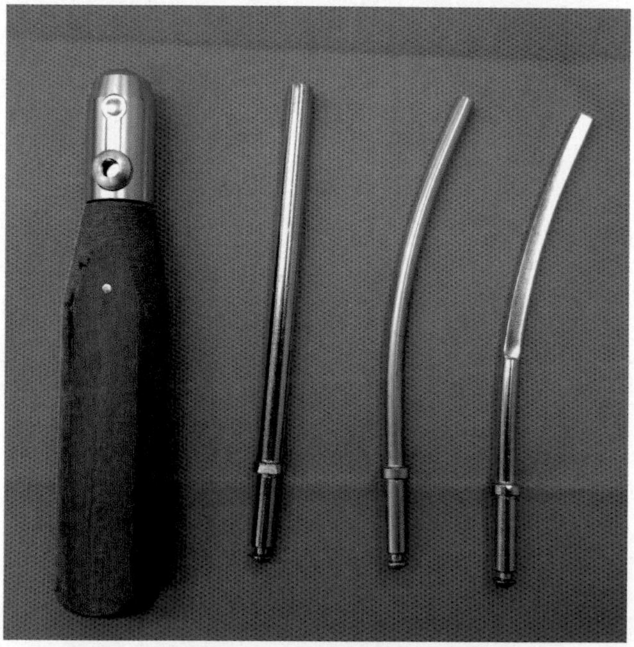

Figure 8-30. Tamps in a modular system. Each tamp can be placed inside the wooden handle.

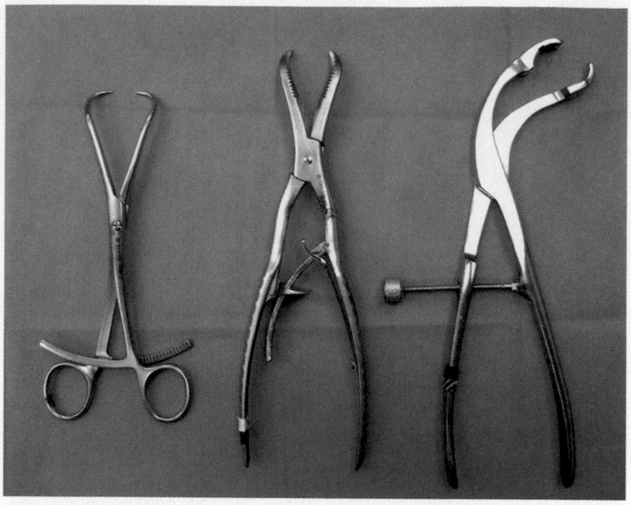

Figure 8-31. Clamps with different locking mechanisms. Each locking mechanism has advantages and disadvantages.

use. A small footprint such as a point focuses force and therefore concentrates stress, but has the tendency to slip, as frictional forces are less than what can be obtained with more aggressive jaws with larger surface area of contact. Handles can be in line or offset, the offset allowing for both better visualization (by removing the hand from the field of view) and occasionally better accommodation of the relevant surgical anatomy. The pivots or joints can be permanent or can be taken apart, the latter allowing for improved sterilization and independent jaw placement. The locking mechanism maintains the compression that is created by pulling the handles together. Ratcheting mechanisms are most common. They have the advantage of allowing unlocking of the ratchet for more independent jaw placement and a wider jaw-to-jaw span. Disadvantages include gross influence by pivot loosening, fixed points of compression strength defined by the distance between teeth, and increased difficulty unlocking the ratchet with single-hand use. Speed-lock mechanisms use a threaded spindle and nut configuration (similar to a worm drive) for locking. Disadvantages include more difficult single-hand use when disengaging or engaging the spindle and horn. Advantages include more precise modulation of compression and ease of loosening and tightening when the spindle is engaged. Commonly used clamps in orthopaedic trauma are shown in Figure 8-31. Look at the differences in the different clamp parts and review the advantages and disadvantages of each type based on the parts.

Indirect Reduction: Instruments and Techniques

Indirect reduction is the "blind" repositioning of bone fragments, often by manipulation outside of the zone of injury. As such, the instruments and techniques have been designed and developed to be accomplished through more limited approaches. This is not always the case, as indirect reduction techniques were first popularized through extensile approaches. Many of the same instruments listed earlier are used for indirect reduction techniques, the primary difference being the lack of direct visualization of all fracture lines. Indirect reduction techniques are most commonly applied to achieve functional reductions (restoration of length, alignment, and rotation without precise repositioning of each fragment). They are most commonly used in the setting of relative stability but can be combined with compression (and were originally intended to do so). Because of the limited visualization inherent in indirect reduction techniques, a clear understanding of radiographic reduction criteria is essential. Because of the limited application of direct forces to each fragment, a reliance on distraction is imperative. Remember that distraction by itself cannot reduce impacted articular fragments. For fragments to reduce with distraction, soft tissue connections to the fragments are obligatory (impacted osteochondral fragments often have no soft tissue connections). It is important to remember that indirect reduction techniques are not a license for malreduction. If anything, the decision to proceed with indirect reduction techniques should lead the surgeon to take even more care to ensure radiographic alignment is restored. There is a significant learning curve associated with the successful application of these techniques. Let us review some of the instruments and techniques in more detail.

The external fixator is a device that can be used both as a definitive or temporizing fixation tool as well as a reduction tool; let us consider its use as a reduction tool. The external fixator is a versatile reduction tool, and can be used for reduction with both plate osteosynthesis and intramedullary rod placement. The basic external fixator set consists of three parts: (1) pins that insert into the bone, (2) clamps that attach to the pins, and (3) bars that connect clamps and therefore major bone fragments. External fixator sets come in different sizes, each appropriate to certain ranges of bone size. Pins must be placed in safe zones defined by a knowledge of the cross-sectional anatomy. Clamps come in two basic varieties: those that attach pins to bars and those that attach bars to bars. Bars vary in length and are the primary determinants of the vector of reduction. Pulling on an extremity restores length along the axis of the bar orientation. Coronal and sagittal plane translation and angulation can be modified by loosening the attachment of clamp to the pin(s) and pushing or pulling on the pin(s) prior to retightening the clamp. Additional changes in these planes can be accomplished by adding pins and clamps to bars that are already in place. These pins should be placed in the desired orientation of additional pushing or pulling. Rotational changes are more challenging and somewhat dependent on the system chosen. Some clamps do not allow for rotational changes, therefore mandating the appropriate rotational alignment prior to pin placement. Others have ball joints that will allow for minor rotational changes even after clamp placement. Knowledge of the external fixator system in your hospital is an important part of preoperative planning.

The universal distractor has similar utility to the external fixator. It also can be used during plate osteosynthesis and intramedullary rod placement (Fig. 8-32). It provides the advantage of more potential force application but the disadvantages of less versatility and added weight. The basic universal distractor consists of six parts: (1) pins that insert into the bone, (2) holding sleeves that slide over the pins, (3) a threaded spindle, (4) spindle nuts, (5) A cotter pin that inserts into a hole in the threaded spindle, and (6) a sliding carriage that moves along the spindle rod while driven by the spindle nuts.[1] Distractors vary in size, allowing application for use in large- and medium-sized bones. Universal distractors are remarkably powerful, allowing for the creation of forces that can bend both the pins and the spindle rod. They are commonly used both for the restoration of length and overdistraction to allow for visualization into joints. Overdistraction takes advantage of the basic mechanical principle that distracting outside of the neutral (center) axis of the bone leads to angular forces. By virtue of its placement, the device typically distracts from the side of the pin placement, allowing for an angular force, the apex of which is on the side of the distractor.

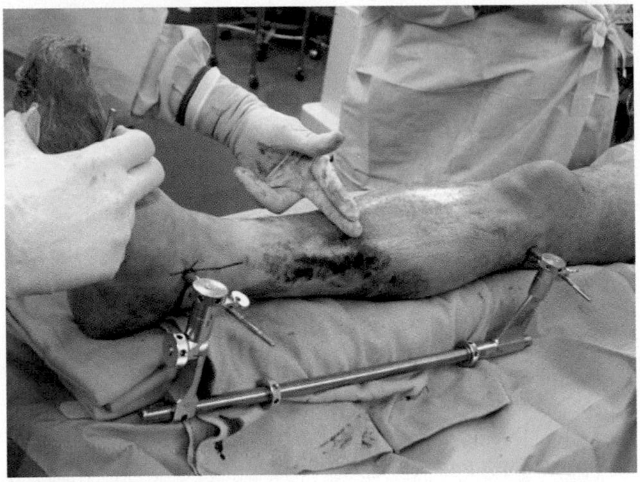

Figure 8-32. Using the universal distractor as a reduction tool prior to intramedullary rodding. The pins must be placed outside of the path of the rod. The hand reveals the location of the center of the fracture zone. Note severe soft tissue compromise. Indirect reduction techniques help prevent further damage to the soft tissues in the zone of injury.

A fracture bed is a commonly used indirect reduction tool in lower extremity applications (Fig. 8-33). A distal portion of the extremity is attached to either skeletal or skin/boot traction. Manipulation of the distal portion through this attachment allows for realignment of some fracture patterns. Occasionally additional percutaneous reduction tools such as

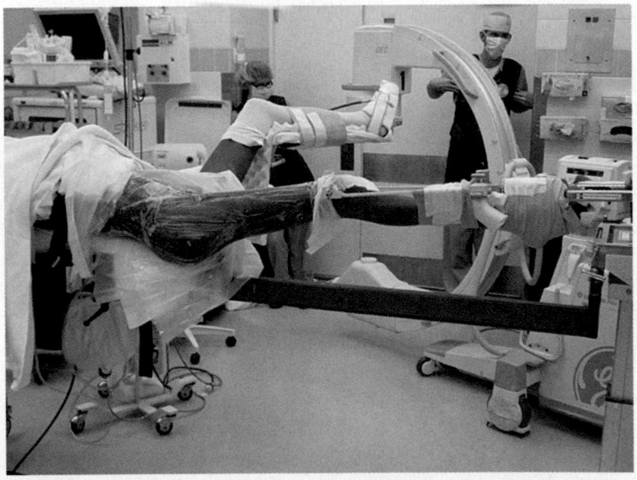

Figure 8-33. Traction table setup in the supine position for femoral shaft fracture treatment. Reduction is being achieved through distal femoral traction with pin connection to the traction arm of the table.

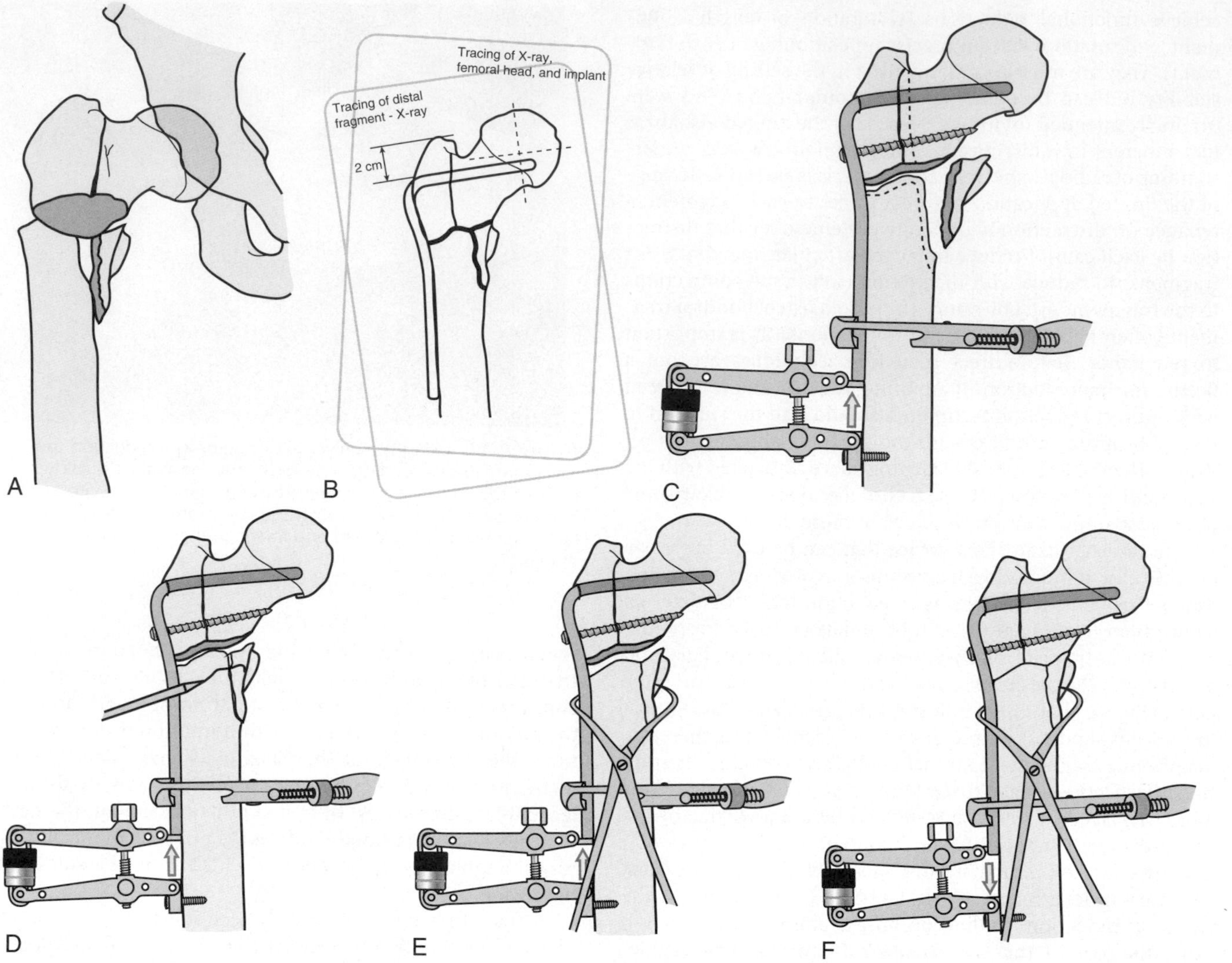

Figure 8-34. Using a precontoured plate as a reduction tool in the proximal femur with the assistance of an articulated tensioning device. A preoperative plan is created based on the contralateral side. The precontoured plate (an angled blade plate in this example) is attached to the proximal segment in a specific position that is determined through the preoperative plan. Distraction using the articulated tensioning device is accomplished. The Verbrugge clamp helps prevent the plate from pulling off of the bone with distraction. Fragments are teased back into alignment with a dental pick and compressed transaxially using a pointed reduction clamp. The ATD is then placed in compression, and the fracture ends are loaded axially. A load-sharing construct has been created. *(Source: Redrawn from Mast J, Jakob R, Ganz R: Planning and reduction technique in fracture surgery, Berlin/Heidelberg/New York, 1989, Springer-Verlag, Figure 3.34, parts a, m, q, r–t.)*

spike pushers, hooks, or joysticks are used in conjunction for finer control of the reduction. The advantage of a fracture table is that it can take the place of an assistant if the reduction can be achieved prior to the surgeon scrubbing into the case. If this is not possible, then an unscrubbed knowledgeable assistant can assist with fracture manipulation after the case has begun. Disadvantages of the fracture table include the time associated with setup, the potential for perineal post issues (pudendal nerve palsy or perineal necrosis) from sustained traction, well-leg issues (compartment syndrome), and the constraint placed on total movement of the limb.[46,47,50]

Precontoured plates can serve as powerful and elegant indirect reduction tools.[18] This technique is associated with a learning curve and demands attention to detail. It requires a clear understanding of the anatomic axes of the extremity, accurate plate application to the periarticular segment, and dedicated preoperative planning for consistent success. With this technique, the surgeon defines the appropriate positioning of the plate on the periarticular segment based on preoperative planning. The preoperative planning includes a review of how and where the implant was designed to fit from a general standpoint, and how the particular patient's anatomy correlates with the population average. The plate is then carefully applied to the periarticular segment and the act of bringing the plate to the other segment enacts a reduction. This can be accomplished with an articulated tensioning device (Fig. 8-34). Alternatively, it is often used in conjunction with a push-pull screw, another technique of indirect reduction. A plate-holding clamp is loosely placed, provisionally connecting the plate to the nonarticular segment. A screw is then placed distal or proximal to the plate (depending on the location of the bone being treated). A lamina spreader can be placed with one arm abutting the end of the plate and the other abutting the screw. Distraction occurs through spreading. Once distraction is completed, intercalary fragments can be teased back into alignment with instruments such as dental picks and clamps. If desired, the lamina spreader can then be exchanged for a Verbrugge clamp to create compression of the fracture and tensioning of the implant. Alternatively, an articulated tensioning device can be used in the same manner as the Verbrugge clamp.

Direct and Indirect Reduction: Summary

Direct and indirect reductions are methods of reducing fracture displacement. While not the same as the quality of the reduction, they are closely linked. Direct reduction is the repositioning of bone fragments individually under direct vision. It is indicated for some simple fracture patterns in the diaphysis and metaphysis and any fracture pattern that involves the articular surface. It demands an atraumatic surgical technique. It is meant to accomplish an anatomic reduction. Indirect reduction is the "blind" repositioning of bone fragments by the application of corrective force at a distance from the fracture. It is indicated for some simple and all complex fractures patterns in the diaphysis and metaphysis. It is almost never indicated for articular fractures. It was originally described to be used through extensile approaches but is now commonly used in minimally invasive surgery. It demands a clear understanding of radiographic anatomy. It is most commonly meant to achieve a reduction in length, alignment, and rotation, but not a precise reduction of each fragment.

Speaking of Direct and Indirect Reduction

- "The articular component of this supracondylar femur fracture with intercondylar extension is complex. Even if it were a simple pattern, I would still choose direct reduction techniques so that I could be certain that I had achieved an anatomic reduction."
- "The metaphyseal component of this supracondylar femur fracture with intercondylar extension is complex too. I am going to plan for indirect reduction techniques by using a precontoured plate as a reduction tool and using an external fixator to help with length and alignment."
- "I have chosen to use direct reduction techniques for this simple pattern metaphyseal distal tibia fracture. In light of that, I am going to be even more careful to ensure that I am protective of the blood supply to fragments."
- "I have chosen to use indirect reduction techniques for this comminuted metaphyseal distal tibia fracture. In light of that, I am going to make sure I understand the relationship of the articular surface to the anatomic axis in the coronal and sagittal planes. I think I will take radiographs of the contralateral side to ensure that I have restored his anatomy. I am also going to check his contralateral rotation. The relationship of his tibial tubercle to his foot should help with that. Those clinical and radiographic keys will be important since I won't be able to see all the fracture lines."
- "Why would you choose direct reduction techniques with relative stability? Those two don't commonly mix very well."
- "The soft tissue pattern for this distal tibia fracture is a Tscherne grade II. I feel pretty comfortable that direct reduction techniques don't make sense acutely. If I need to use those, I should stage his treatment to allow the soft tissues to recover. Even if I am careful with the soft tissues, they are still showing signs of significant injury, and the approach required for direct reduction techniques will damage them more."

FIXATION

Recall the aims of the AO method: (1) fracture reduction and fixation to restore anatomic relationships, (2) preservation of the blood supply to soft tissues and bone by careful handling and gentle reduction techniques, (3) stability by fixation or splintage, as the personality of the fracture and the injury requires, and (4) early and safe mobilization of the part and the patient.[1] In fracture surgery, the surgeon attempts to restore stability to a limb in an effort to allow for early functional use. In essence, the surgeon is taking something unstable (the fractured limb) and making it stable by creating a construct. A construct is a structure that consists of the combination of implant and bone.

Five primary types of implants are used in orthopaedic surgery for the creation of constructs: wires, screws, plates, intramedullary rods, and external fixators. External fixators were covered in Chapter 7, "Principles and Complications of External Fixation." Let us consider the others separately along with the devices required to insert them; but before spending time focusing on the metal used in the fixation construct, it is important to consider three important points. First, it is critical to separate the properties of the implant from the properties of the bone-implant construct. There will always be a weak point in a construct. It is often not the implant. Stated another way, modifying the properties of an implant must address the point of construct weakness to be successful. For example, choosing a material of maximum ultimate strength with little flexibility will concentrate stresses to the bone and overcome bone of marginal quality, potentially leading to construct failure that manifests not as plate failure but rather as interface (bone) failure. Similarly, modifying the dimensions of an implant in the area unlikely to fail will likely not improve construct stability. Consider increasing the diameter of an intramedullary rod to treat a metaphyseal fracture. The weak point in that construct is found in the relationship of the interlocking screw to the intramedullary rod and metaphyseal bone. Increasing nail diameter does nothing to affect this relationship. Second, using biomechanical studies to guide intraoperative decision making must be thoughtful. The mechanical data must be relevant to the expected failure mode of the bone-implant construct. The magnitude of the load and the direction of application must be logical. For example, a mechanical study that shows implant superiority in bending must be relevant to the situation present intraoperatively. The failure point may not be the one revealed in the study; rather, it may be an entirely different failure mode that was not explicitly tested. For example, using information from locked plating applications in a proximal femoral gap model that focuses on plate failure in bending may not address torsional screw loosening failures noted in practice. Third—and most important—you must remember, these are only pieces of metal. You are the one with the brain. Do not try to make them defy the laws of physics. They cannot, and your patient will lose.

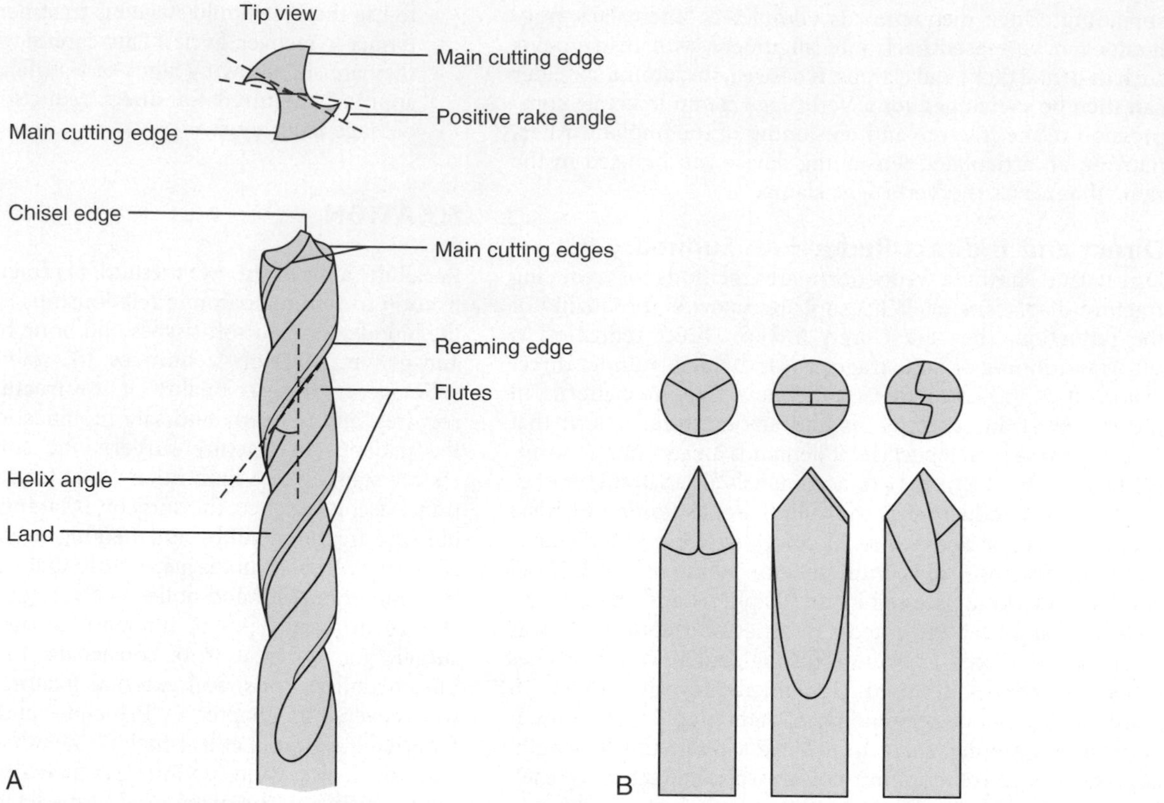

Figure 8-35. A, Design of a drill bit. **B,** Design of a wire tip. Refer to the text for a detailed description of the labeled parts. *(Source: **B**, Data from Natali C, Ingle P, Dowell J: Orthopaedic bone drills: can they be improved? J Bone Joint Surg Br 78(3):357–362, 1996.)*

Wires and Pins

In orthopaedic surgery, wires and pins are cylindrical pieces of metal of varying sizes and lengths with sharp points. The differentiating factor between a wire and a pin is size. Wires are smaller. Pins are larger. At what size a wire becomes a pin is hard to ascertain, and probably not very important. The eponyms given to these devices are of historical interest and are held over from the time in which these devices were used for axial traction primarily. Fritz Steinmann (1872–1932) was a Swiss surgeon who improved the technique of axial traction by moving the force from the skin directly to the bone. His initial idea was to use a sharp-tipped pin to pierce the skin and bone in the transverse axis. At this point in time, the pins were inserted with a hammer, and therefore needed to be of sufficient diameter to resist bending during insertion; hence, Steinmann pins were of large diameter. With the development of the electric drill, smaller diameter wires could be inserted and then tensioned after insertion to allow for axial traction.[56] Martin Kirschner (1879–1942) was a German surgeon who popularized this concept using 0.7- to 1.5-mm diameter piano wires and instruments required to achieve tension.[57] Without the tensioning device, the smaller diameter Kirschner wire would be unable to transmit adequate force for lower extremity long bone traction.

Currently, Kirschner wires and Steinmann pins are used for many different applications apart from axial traction. Three additional common applications include (1) single fragment fixation points in multiplanar external fixation, (2) transfragment fixation wires for both provisional and definitive fixation, and (3) intrafocal fixation wires in which one fragment is abutted and the other is skewered. As the pins become larger and are given specialized shaft flexibility and sled-runner tips, they serve as elastic intramedullary nails.

Wire and pin tips generally have a three-sided or four-sided cutting trocar point or a two-sided cutting diamond point (Fig. 8-35). The wire tip is an important factor in insertion technique. The typical ideal is to require as little thrust force, torque, and temperature elevation as possible. The tip should resist walking along the cortex.[58] It would additionally resist deflection when encountering a dense substance such as the cortex. This equates to improved drilling efficiency (less surgeon pushing effort, less wire buckling, and improved wire direction control), while limiting thermal damage to surrounding bone. Tips with a larger rake angle clear more of the bone surface, decreasing the tendency to walk along the cortex and increasing the ability to place at angles.[59,60] Although the trocar tip is preferred to the diamond tip for the larger rake angle, it has no means to clear debris on insertion. In light of this, some wire tips have also been designed with drill tip and flute characteristics[61] (e.g., Medin tip; see Fig. 8-35, *B*).

Wires and pins can be smooth, terminally threaded, or centrally threaded. A smooth tip and shaft have the propensity to migrate, leading to potentially severe complications.[62,63] One of the proposed advantages of threading is limiting this migration potential; however, the threading comes at the cost of weakening the wire, potentially making breakage more common on insertion or extraction. It logically follows that very small diameter wires cannot be safely threaded. Threading also establishes the need to insert with clockwise drill revolutions and remove with counterclockwise drill revolutions (i.e., reverse). Changes in direction can be more challenging as the wire advances along the thread revolution. In addition, feeling changes in bone density is difficult, often requiring more fluoroscopic assistance to ensure correct length of insertion.

Speaking of Wires and Pins

- "I would like to oscillate the drill during wire insertion to protect the soft tissues, but the decision to use a threaded wire is preventing that technique."
- "This wire is generating a large amount of heat upon insertion. I guess a drill tip and flutes do make a difference. Maybe wires were not a good choice for provisional fixation devices in light of the density of the cortex in this region. Please irrigate the insertion point."
- "I feel the need to leave in the smooth tip wires that I had used for provisional fixation. I am concerned that removing them could potentially allow for a loss of reduction. In light of that, I am going to try to prevent migration through bending the tip and tamping it into the cortex. I am also going to pay close attention to wire position on all the follow-up radiographs. The wires may require removal if they begin to migrate."
- "I am going to drill with a wire instead of a drill bit for this bicortical medial malleolar screw. I am concerned that the drill bit will skive off the endosteum and walk up the intramedullary canal instead of penetrating the cortex. Since the wire doesn't have flutes, it should be stiffer and less likely to do so."

Screws, Drill Bits, Taps, and Screwdrivers

Screw Functions

At the most basic level, a screw is a mechanical device that consists of an inclined plane wrapped around a core. As mechanical devices, screws have six primary functions: (1) positioning screws, (2) lag screws, (3) fixation screws, (4) locking screws, (5) interlocking screws, and (6) Poller screws. Let us consider each function individually.

Positioning screws secure stability while maintaining a fixed relationship between the fragments being joined together. This screw is used in the absence of a plate or a washer. The drill hole size in both the near and far cortex is approximately equivalent to the inner diameter of the screw. Tightening of the screw head creates compression but maintains a fixed distance relationship between both fragments that it connects.

Lag screws have the potential to alter the relationship of the fragments that they are connecting, for better or worse. Lag screws can be inserted by technique or by design (see Fig. 8-21). To clarify, for lag screw insertion by technique, the near cortex drill hole is approximately equivalent to the outer diameter of the screw (gliding hole) but the far cortex drill hole is approximately equivalent to the inner diameter of the screw. The screw subsequently glides through the near cortex hole and achieves fixation in the far cortex hole, thereby creating compression perpendicular to the axis of insertion. If the axis of insertion is perpendicular to the reduced fracture, this compressive force is translated into an anatomic reduction in compression. If the compressive force is not perpendicular to the fracture, then shear is induced and the reduction that was achieved prior to screw placement can be lost. Lag screws by design (rather than technique) are partially threaded. The shaft component of the screw is smooth and the terminal portion is threaded. The threaded portion should be past the fracture line for appropriate effect. If it crosses the fracture line, the compressive function of the screw across the fracture is lost, rather creating internal strain in the screw between the near cortex and the fracture.[1]

A fixation screw is placed through a plate or washer and has an effect similar to a lag screw at the plate or washer interface to the bone. The plate hole is larger than the screw thread but smaller than the screw head. When the screw head impacts the plate, it creates friction between the plate and washer and bone, imparting stability in a conventional construct.

A locking screw is also placed through a plate, but maintains the relationship between the plate and the bone rather than creating friction. In this way it acts as a positioning screw, but it relies on a different mode of stability. A locking screw attaches to a plate, becoming a single unit. It does so through different manufacturing methods, such as threading the plate hole and screw head. By doing so, it creates what is known as a *fixed-angle device*. An analogous fixed-angle device is an angled blade plate (Fig. 8-36). The angled blade plate is a single piece of metal with a bend that separates the portion that goes into the bone (blade) and the portion that sits outside of the bone (plate). The plate portion has holes for the placement of conventional screws. The angled blade plate is fixed-angle only at the bend in the plate. The relationship of the conventional screws to the plate is not fixed angle. Notice the difference. Conventional screws are placed through the holes in the angled blade plate and confer stability through friction; however, the blade that inserts into the bone is stable with respect to the plate because it is a single piece of metal that cannot change without breaking. The locking screws act in a similar way. By locking to the plate, they become in essence a single piece of metal that cannot change without breaking. This is a generalization or oversimplification as an interface is present in locked plating and loosening is rarely observed in clinical practice; that stated, the principle remains solid. Because the locking screws lock to the plate, they do not create friction, change the alignment between bone fragments, or change the alignment between the plate and the bone.[64,65]

An interlocking screw is placed through the bone and through holes in an intramedullary rod. The primary function of an interlocking screw is to resist length and rotational changes at the fracture site. It is not designed to create compression between fragments but rather to resist bending forces. This is logical because it is loaded primarily in four-point bending as extremity loading leads to motion of the intramedullary nail in the canal. This motion loads the screw in bending with the points of fixation being at the near and far cortex and the area of contact between the screw and intramedullary nail.

A Poller or blocking screw is placed adjacent to an intramedullary rod to serve as an intramedullary cortex.[66] By doing so, it is able to perform two functions: (1) modify the path of the intramedullary rod (which has the capacity to change fracture alignment), and (2) improve the stability of the bone-implant construct in metaphyseal rodding by making it more like diaphyseal rodding (where the rod contacts the endosteum conferring stability outside of that imparted by the interlocking screws). This concept will be covered in more detail in the "Intramedullary Nail or Rod" section.

As realized at this point, the ability of a screw to function in any of these mechanical applications is defined by the

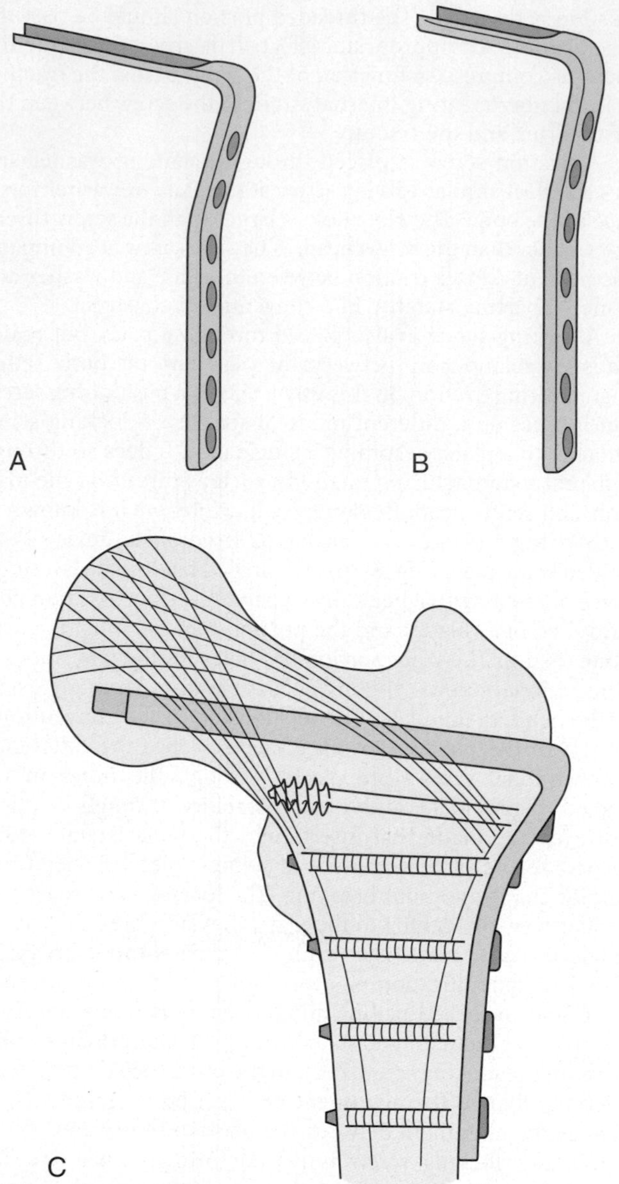

Figure 8-36. The 95-degree blade plate. **A,** T profile. **B,** U profile. **C,** Use of a blade plate in proximal femoral fixation, as for subtrochanteric fractures. Note placement of the tip of the blade at the intersection of the primary compressive and the primary tensile trabeculae. *(Source:* ***A*** *and* ***B,*** *Redrawn from Synthes Equipment Ordering Manual, Paoli, PA, Synthes USA, 1992.)*

design of the screw. Screw design is varied in the four parts of the screw: the head, the inner diameter, the outer diameter (including the thread design), and the tip (Fig. 8-37).[5,36] Each part has a specific form that is designed to assist with insertion and removal as well as to resist failure. As with any choice, compromises occur when one design feature is maximized at the expense of another. It follows that thoughtful screw design is based on the expectation of loading and the primary function of the screw.

Screw Parts: Head

The screw head has two main functions. It first acts to transmit the torque applied through the turning of the fingers or forearm. It second acts as a stop to limit the degree of insertion and to distribute forces over its surface area. In doing so, it either provides friction or locks into a plate. In a conventional screw (nonlocking application), the stop prevents further translational motion of the screw and transforms the torque into tension in the screw and compression of the bone. This creates compression between the undersurface of the screw/plate and bone interface and yields a frictional force that defines the stability afforded by a conventional screw. The shape of a screw head is differentiated by the top and bottom portion of the head. For example, the top portion of a bone screw head is most commonly either flat, oval, or round. Assuming perpendicular placement to the screw hole, the flatter-shaped heads limit screw prominence. This limits irritation of structures that glide over the area. All other design features held constant, the trade-off for a flatter head is typically a shallower screw recess, which can have the effect of increasing cam-out during insertion (slipping of the screwdriver out of the head). The undersurface of the screw head is also termed the countersink. The countersink is typically either conical or hemispherical. A screw with a conical undersurface is designed to be inserted in the center portion of a hole and perpendicular to the hole. If inserted in any other direction, the countersink does not adapt well to the surface it impacts and creates point loading and stress concentration. This has the potential to propagate a fracture line. A screw with a hemispherical undersurface is designed to allow for insertion at an angle other than perpendicular to the hole. The rounded undersurface improves force transmission to whatever it impacts by providing a more congruent fit, distributing forces over a larger area, thereby limiting focal stress.[36] A unique and more recent modification of the screw undersurface is found in threading the screw head itself. This has been used as a mechanism to lock a screw into a plate. The screw recess is another important design feature of the screw head. Common bone screw head recesses are either hexagonal, cruciate, or star in shape. The recess is designed to create a firm engagement with the screwdriver head. This improves the efficiency of torque transmission and decreases the incidence of screw head recess stripping, screwdriver slippage, and cam-out of the screwdriver head from the screw recess. Typically the more surface area of contact provided, the more effective the torque transmission and the less likely a screwdriver head is to slip out of the screw recess.[67,68] An increase in surface area is provided by altering the shape of the contact points, including the depth of the recess and the shape of the points of contact. The compromise created by increasing the complexity of the shape of the points of contact is noticed when the surgeon must localize a screw recess without direct visualization (e.g., in percutaneous screw insertion once the screw is deep to the skin or in screw removal).

Screw Parts: Inner Diameter

The inner diameter of a screw is also termed the minor or core diameter. The inner diameter of a screw has many important functions in preventing failure. First, the inner diameter defines the size of the hole that must be drilled for screw insertion. This is especially important in screw removal, as the hole left in the bone acts as a stress riser to potentiate postoperative fracture through screw holes. Empty screw holes in bone provide areas of stress concentration in bone that are 1.6 times greater than in surrounding bone when torsional stresses

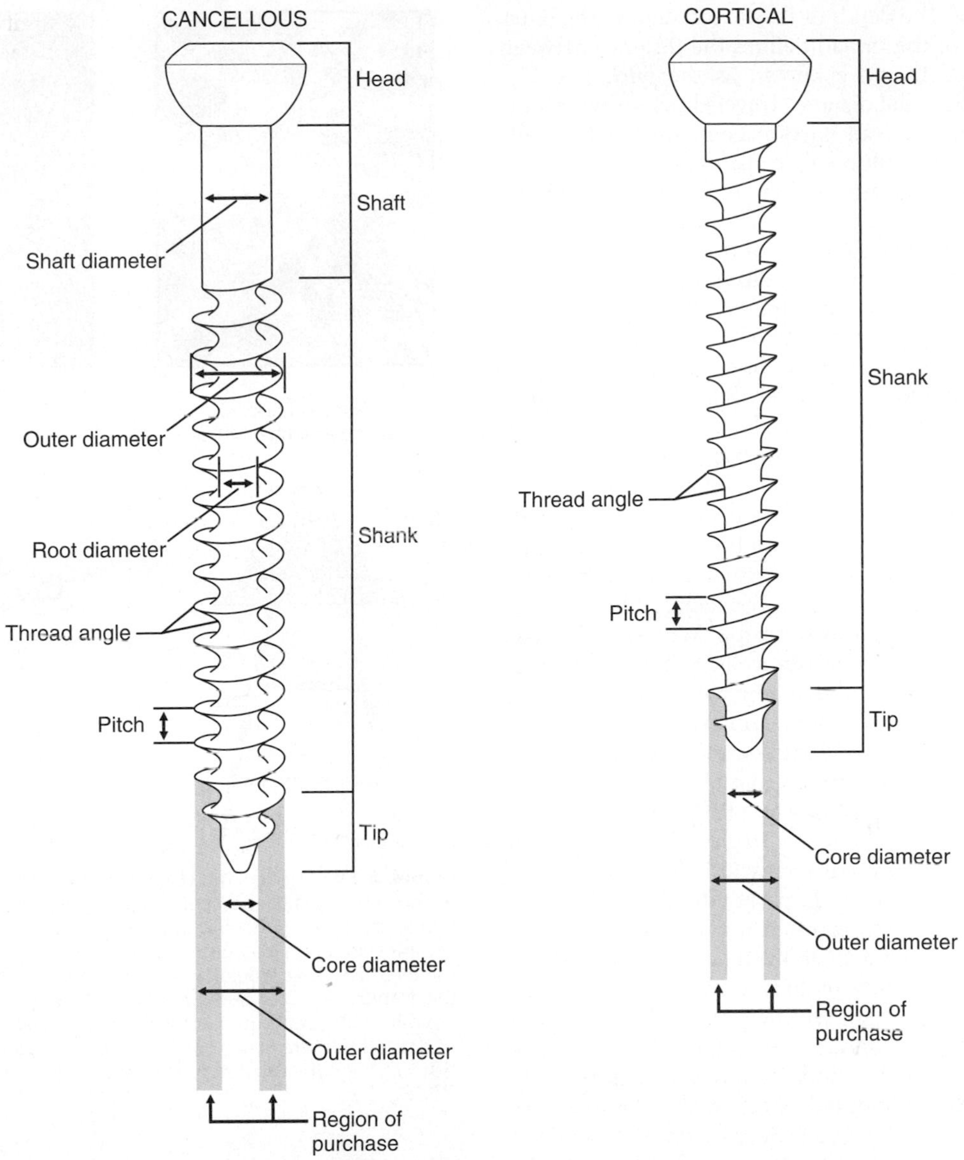

Figure 8-37. The parts of a screw. See the text for details regarding the different labeled parts.

are applied.[69] Although these screw holes are visible on radiographs long after screw removal, the holes are filled with dense woven bone in approximately 4 weeks, limiting the stress concentrating effect. The second important function of the inner diameter in preventing failure is that it defines the bending and shear strength of the screw. In situations where screws are loaded primarily in bending and shear, the design goal often revolves around maximizing the core diameter. The bending strength is a function of the moment of inertia. The moment of inertia varies based on the cross-sectional dimensions of the object. These terms are not important in the operating theater. Practical application only requires remembering that material farthest away from the center of an object is most important in defining the strength of that object.[5] When material is distributed farther from the center, then the object is better able to resist bending in that direction. This is especially important in cannulation and plate design, and will be covered in more detail in those areas. For now, consider the similar design features of an interlocking screw for an intramedullary rod and the locking screw for a locked plating construct. These screws are known to be loaded primarily in bending and torsion and should therefore be designed to primarily resist those failure stresses. This is accomplished by maximizing the core diameters of these screws.

The distance between the screw head and the first thread is part of the core diameter. It is often termed the *run out* of the screw.[36] This portion represents a location of stress concentration secondary to the abrupt change in shape and presence of corners. When screw failure occurs during insertion by torque overload, it most commonly occurs at this point in the screw. When screw failure occurs in bending or shear, it also commonly occurs in this area, partly because of the stress riser, but also because of the concentrated loading at this motion interface adjacent to the plate and near cortex.

Screw Parts: Outer Diameter

The outer diameter of the screw is also termed the *major diameter* or *thread diameter.* The thread shape varies primarily in depth and shape. The depth of the thread defines the outer diameter. The coil of the thread defines the distance between successive threads, otherwise known as the *pitch* (see Fig. 8-37). The lead is the axial distance traveled per screw revolution. In most cases, the lead is equivalent to the pitch. This varies if the screw has multiple threads. In that case, the lead is equal to the pitch times the number of threads. For example, a triple-threaded screw will travel three times the pitch in one revolution. The primary design goal of the thread diameter is to maximize resistance to pullout failure. Pullout strength is dependent on many things, including (1) the length of screw engaged in the bone, (2) the quality of the bone engaged, (3) the number of threads engaging the bone (pitch), (4) the difference between the inner and outer diameter of the screw, and (5) the size of the hole drilled in the bone.[5,70] Notice again the importance of the bone in defining bone implant construct failure. That stated, in terms of screw design features, the outer diameter of the screw is the most important factor in determining pullout resistance. Stated another way, when other factors remain stable, using a screw with a larger outer diameter will equate to improved pullout resistance.

So why do all screws not look the same? Why would screws not be designed to maximize resistance to all types of failure? The answer lies in the trade-off that is created by manipulating specific screw design features and the difference between cancellous and cortical bone. To clarify, screws fail in two basic ways: (1) bending and shear forces that break the screw and thereby decrease construct stability and (2) pullout forces that loosen the connection of the screw to the plate and thereby decrease construct stability. (In reality, this is more complex as forces are not distributed only perpendicular and parallel to the screw. The complexity is important and fascinating but only complicates the discussion and will not be addressed. For a more in-depth study of how pullout strength may not be the ideal choice for screw design, see the work of Ricci and colleagues.[71]) The first failure mode (bending or shear failure) is resisted by maximizing the inner diameter of a screw. The second failure mode (pullout failure) is resisted by maximizing the outer diameter of a screw. So why do all screws not have a large inner diameter and a large outer diameter? This would logically resist both failure modes. The difference can be seen in the microarchitecture of bone and how this relates to pullout strength (Fig. 8-38). In cortical bone, the area of the bone that confers the greatest resistance to pullout is the cortex itself, not the intramedullary canal. The cortex consists of tightly packed trabeculae that are consistently in contact with the screw threads at the outer diameter. Because of this, the inner diameter can be maximized as well to confer improved bending resistance to the screw. In cancellous bone, the area that confers the greatest resistance to pullout is the intramedullary portion (as cortical bone is extremely thin at the metaphyseal and epiphyseal level). The intramedullary portion consists of loosely packed trabeculae that may or may not contact the screw threads at the outer diameter. Because of this, the design of the screw represents an attempt to capture contact with as many trabeculae as possible, understanding that they may not be at the periphery or outer diameter of the screw. In this sense, a sacrifice is made by marginalizing the inner diameter of the screw in order to have more trabecular contact area with the thread. This screw design sacrifices bending resistance in favor of improved pullout strength.

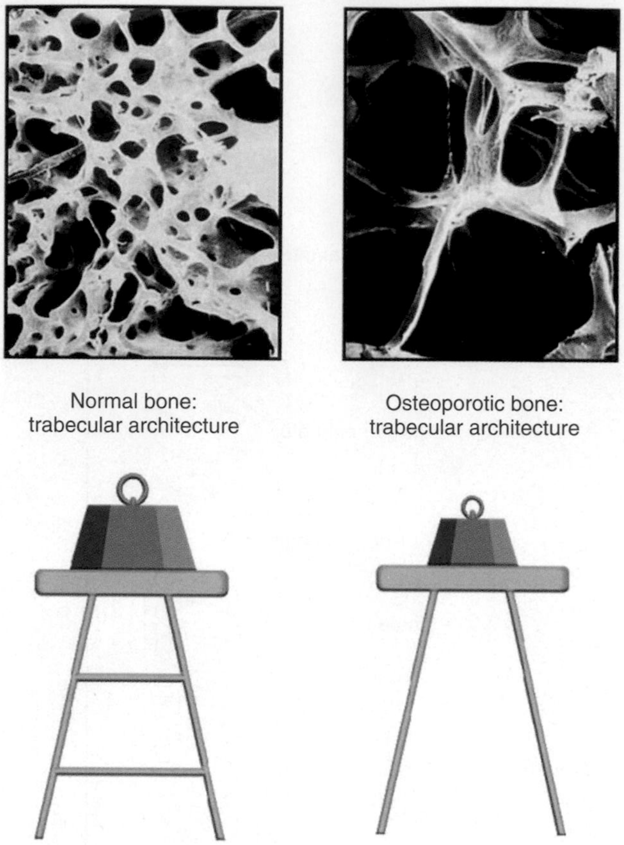

Figure 8-38. Microarchitecture of bone. The improved microarchitecture of normal bone could logically support more load as represented by the weight. By analogy, the ability of a screw to create compression in bone can be inferred from this image as well. Imagine the interfaces that would be present between the screw threads and the trabeculae. This also helps explain why cancellous screws are designed differently than cortical screws. *(Source: From Brandi ML: Microarchitecture, the key to bone quality, Rheumatology 48(Suppl 4): iv3–8, 2009; Figure 3, p iv5. © Maria Luisa Brandi, 2009.)*

With the advent of locked plating, the resistance to pullout changed forms. When multiple locking screws are engaging a segment at different angles, then pullout strength is maximized. The shear cylinder no longer is defined by the number of trabeculae in contact with the bone at the outer diameter; rather, it is now defined by all the bone present between the screws as well. Screws are no longer acting individually with the potential to loosen one at a time, but now are acting in concert as a single fixation unit (Fig. 8-39).

Screw Parts: Tip

The tip of the screw does not contribute as significantly to the bending, torsional, or pullout strength of the screw. It does contribute to the efficiency of insertion. Screws with self-tapping tips are now commonplace. This was not always the case. The term *self-tapping screw* refers to a screw that is inserted into a predrilled hole without prior tapping of threads into the hole. This was opposed for some time secondary to four primary reasons: (1) the force required for insertion and the inefficiency of force transmission; (2) the risk of insertional torque required for insertion overcoming the torsional strength of the screw leading to screw breakage; (3) the

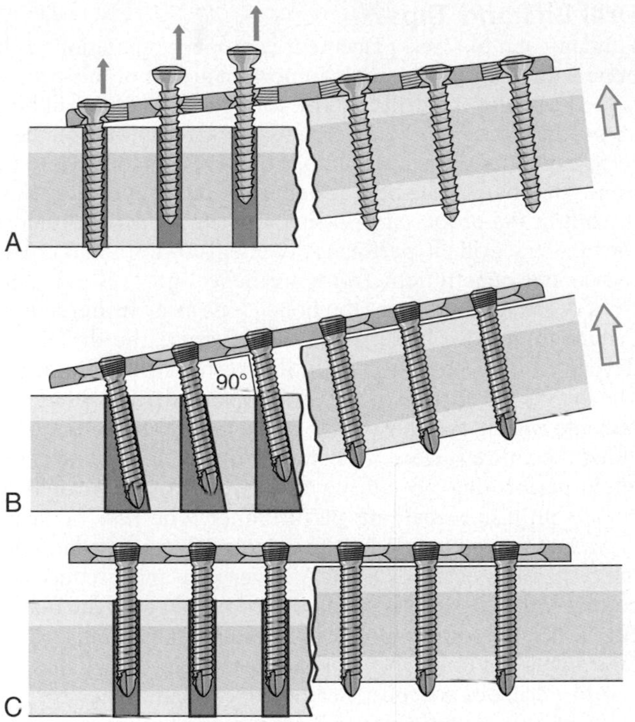

Figure 8-39. Pull-out resistance. Note how this differs between conventional screws in **A** and locking screws in **B** and **C.** Note also how the direction of loading plays a part in implant failure. With conventional screw placement, each screw can independently loosen. The *arrow* represents the small amount of force required to accomplish this. With locking screw placement, screws act as single fixation unit. When loaded in the same direction as the conventional construct, more load is required to reach failure. Despite this advantage, when locking screws are loaded in the direction of screw placement, failure occurs more easily through the removal of less bone (see **C**). This helps explain why variable angle locking mechanisms could be mechanically advantageous. With locking screws angled in different directions, it would be impossible to pull out along the axis of all the screws (as they are placed in different axes).

potential for the force required for screw insertion to interfere with the accuracy of insertion, leading to a missed hole in the far cortex and potential fracture of the cortex during insertion; and (4) the concern that the cutting flutes on the self-tapping screws would decrease pullout strength if left in the far cortex (i.e., the cutting flutes have fewer screw threads to engage the far cortex).[72,73] The introduction of self-tapping screws provided one primary clinical advantage: improved time efficiency of insertion by decreasing the number of steps required (eliminating tapping). After significant research, the decision was made to accept the self-tapping screw as modifying other design features allowed it to perform comparably to the non–self-tapping screw with the added convenience of eliminating the tapping step.[72] Other screw tip designs of note include the self-drilling, self-tapping screw (which eliminates another step, is commonly cannulated to ensure accuracy of placement, and should only be used in less dense bone) and the trocar tip (which has both manufacturing and self-centering advantages but does not efficiently clear debris during insertion) (Fig. 8-40).[72]

Screw Types

Now that screw functions and screw parts have been clarified, let us spend some time describing the common names given to screws. As in plate design, the function of a screw is often different than the name given to the screw. Stated another way, screws of many different names can serve the same mechanical function. Similarly, a screw with a single name can serve many different mechanical functions. Historically, screw names are commonly defined by the outer diameter of the threads (e.g., 3.5-mm screw, 4.5-mm screw, etc.), the length of the screw, the presence or absence of cannulation, the extent of threading (e.g., fully threaded or partially threaded), whether or not they are self-tapping, and whether they are designed primarily for use in a particular area.[1] Size, length, cannulation, and the extent of threading are self-explanatory. We have already discussed the difference in self-tapping and non–self-tapping screws. All that is left to cover are the names given to screws used in particular areas.

Cortical screws are designed to be used in cortical bone. As previously noted, this means the trabecular architecture is typically dense, and the screw design can maximize core diameter at the expense of limiting the difference between the inner and outer diameter of the screw. Cancellous screws are designed to be used in cancellous bone. This means the trabecular architecture is less dense, and the screw design maximizes pullout strength in ways other than just maximizing outer diameter. This compromises the bending strength of the screw by limiting the core diameter. Malleolar screws were originally designed for fixation of medial malleolar fractures. They are partially threaded screws (to lag by design) with trephine tips that allow them to cut their own path in cancellous bone.[74] These are less commonly used now secondary to the large size of the screw heads and the hardware irritation that this creates in a subcutaneous location. Shaft screws are partially threaded cortical screws that were designed to be used as lag screws through a plate in diaphyseal bone. The shaft diameter is equal to the outer diameter of the screw thread, differentiating them from other more commonly used partially threaded screws. The logic behind this screw design reflects the interplay between plate holes and screws. It was noted that the use of a fully threaded screw placed obliquely through a plate hole led to a 50% loss of compression because of indentation within the cortical bone of the gliding hole. The

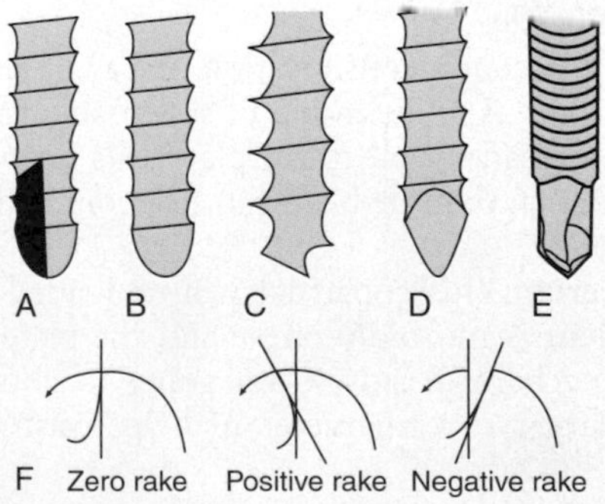

Figure 8-40. Differences in screw tip profiles are noted graphically. **A,** Self-tapping screw. **B,** Non-self-tapping screw. Note the absence of flutes to clear bone debris. **C,** A corkscrew tip seen in some cancellous screws. **D,** A trocar tip (compare to Fig. 8-35 that shows an end-on view of wire tips). **E,** A self-drilling, self-tapping tip seen in some Schanz screw designs. *(Source: Redrawn and modified from Perren SM, Cordey J, Baumgart F, Rahn BA, Schatzker J: Technical and biomechanical aspects of screws used for bone surgery, Injury Int J Orthop Trauma 2:31–48, 1992.)*

smooth shank of this screw did not engage the near cortex and the sliding of the larger smooth shank in the gliding hole prevented motion of the screw in a direction other than along its longitudinal axis during tightening.[74] These are also less commonly used in current practice, likely just from an inventory reduction standpoint.

Screw Function Revisited

After reviewing the different parts of the screw and the design modifications to resist the common failure modes, it is worthwhile to think practically about when to apply the different screw functions. Let us first consider the ones that are applied primarily with plates (conventional and locking screws). The utility of a conventional screw is defined by the quality of bone into which it is inserted. Remember the bone implant construct is different than the implant itself. Conventional screws achieve stability by creating friction. This friction is created between fracture surfaces as well as between the plate and the bone. The frictional force is dependent on the screw stretching or the bone compressing. When the head impacts the cortex or plate, it stops, and any further insertional torque is transformed into compression through this tensile effect. It is this insertional torque that creates the friction upon which the construct stability relies. If the patient load overcomes the frictional force created by the screw, then the construct fails. It follows that in situations where the frictional force is marginal (e.g., osteoporotic bone), conventional screw application is often met with failure of the bone implant construct. The mechanical functions of position screws, lag screws, and fixation screws are chosen when the bone is of adequate quality to allow for reasonable friction. When this is not possible, locking screw application has value. This is the general indication for the use of locking screws: when the patient load is expected to overcome the frictional forces that can be exerted by the conventional screws. The specific indications for locked plating will be covered in depth under the locked plating section below.

Speaking of Screws

- "I am concerned that I cannot place this screw perpendicular to the fracture. Rather than placing it in lag mode and risking a loss of reduction, I am going to accept the compression that the clamp is providing and place it in position mode."
- "This is a subcutaneous location. If I angle my screw trajectory, there is a likelihood of soft tissue irritation from the screw head. I will try to place this perpendicular to the plate such that the head can seat completely and limit prominence."
- "I feel certain this construct will be loaded in bending. The patient is morbidly obese and the plate is eccentric to the mechanical axis. I am going to choose a screw with a larger core diameter to help resist the bending load."
- "This interlocking screw design looks remarkably similar to the locking screw design. Clearly the inner diameter is maximized in both cases in order to empower the device in resisting bending and shear rather than pullout."
- "This screw is taking forever to insert. It is not advancing very far with each rotation of my forearm. It must be because it is a single lead screw that has a small pitch."

Drill Bits and Taps

Fundamental to screw placement is proper preparation of the bone with drilling. The most important aspect of this process is the design of the drill bit. The configuration of a drill bit is shown in Figure 8-35 (adjacent to the wire tip figure) and is relatively simple. The central tip is the first area to bite into the bone. The sharper the tip, the better the bite and the less skive or shift in the proposed drill site. The *cutting edge,* located at the tip of the drill bit, performs the actual cutting and is crucial to efficient penetration. *Flutes* are helical grooves along the sides of the bit that direct the bone chips away from the hole. Failure to remove bone debris could cause the drill bit to deviate from its intended path, decreasing drilling accuracy. The *land* is the surface of the bit between adjacent flutes. The *reaming edge* is the sharp edge of the helical flutes that runs along the entire surface, clearing the drill hole of bone debris while performing no cutting function. Disruption of these edges diminishes reaming performance. The *rake* or *helical angle* is the angle made by the leading edge of the land and the center axis of the drill bit. A larger rake angle reduces the cutting forces regardless of the direction in which the bone is cut. This angle can be positive, negative, or neutral. Positive rake angles cut only when rotated clockwise.

Most drill bits are constructed with two flutes; they are used with rotary-powered drills and are provided in standard fracture fixation sets. To limit drilling damage to the soft tissues adjacent to bone, an attachment has been developed that converts a drill's action from rotary to oscillating drive. With the oscillating drive, there is less tendency for the drill bit to damage neighboring soft tissue. An oscillating drill bit can be placed on skin and will not cut it because of the skin's elasticity. A three-fluted drill bit has been developed for use with oscillating drill attachments. To work effectively, a two-fluted drill bit must rotate beyond 180 degrees. Because the excursion of the oscillating device is less than 180 degrees, a three-fluted drill bit must be used to achieve cutting. This drill bit also provides an added advantage when drilling on an oblique angle. Although the oscillating three-fluted drill bit may be safer for soft tissue, the two-fluted rotary drill bit cuts through bone more efficiently and is used more commonly.

Drilling into bone is different from drilling into wood because bone is a living tissue. The process of drilling in bone must minimize physiologic damage. Jacob and Berry determined the optimal drill bit design and method for bone drilling. They found that the cutting forces are higher at lower rotational speeds and suggested a physiologic bone drilling method that includes the following: (1) bone drill bits with positive rake angles between 20 and 35 degrees; (2) a point on the drill to avoid walking (skiving); (3) high torque and relatively low drill speeds (750 to 1250 rpm) to take advantage of a decrease in flow stress of the material; (4) continuous, copious irrigation to reduce friction-induced thermal bone necrosis; (5) reflection of the periosteum to prevent bone chips from being forced under the tissue, clogging the drill flutes; (6) drill flutes that are steep enough to remove chips at any rake angle; (7) sharp and axially true drill bits to decrease the amount of retained bone dust; and (8) drilling of the thread hole exactly in the direction in which the screw is to be inserted for accuracy and strength.[75] These techniques reduce local bone damage significantly.

Most drill bits are constructed with high-carbon stainless steel and are heat-processed for increased hardness. Damaged

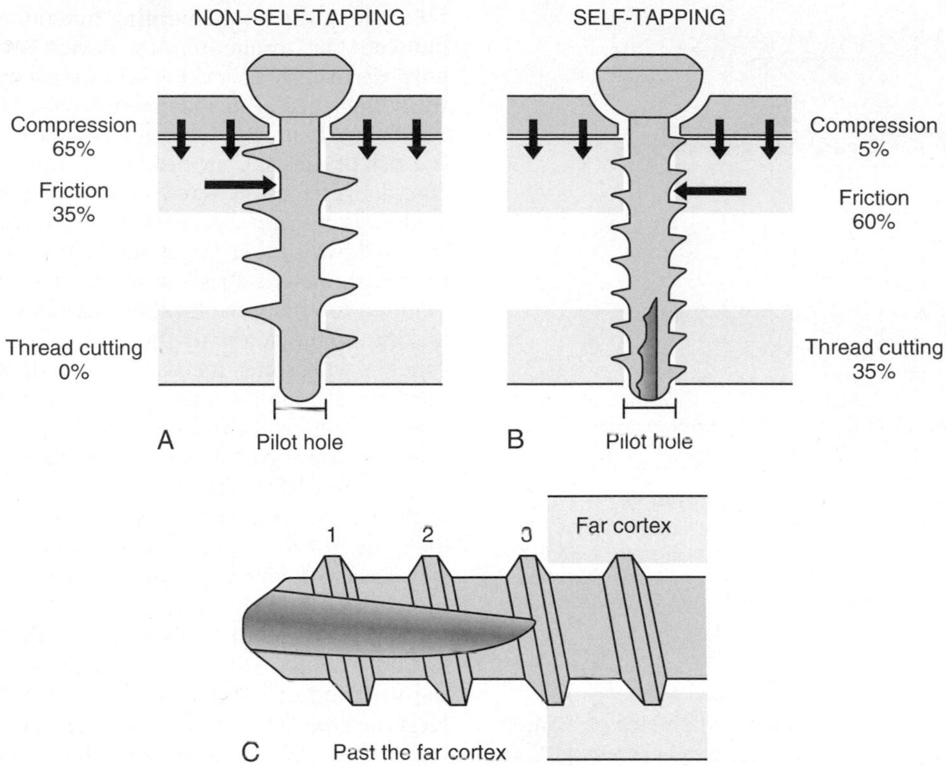

Figure 8-41. Tapping limits the amount of parasitized forces during screw insertion. **A** and **B,** Note the figures that reveal the percentages of screw insertion force that are lost to friction and used for thread cutting. Although the non-self-tapping screw would be considered a more efficient instrument, it does not lead to more efficient screw insertion (in light of the additional step required). **C,** The amount of screw tip that was originally recommended to extend past the far cortex in order to have full thread engagement (i.e., not lose any engagement secondary to the flutes incorporated into the self-tapping screw).

or dull bits decrease drilling efficiency significantly and may cause local trauma to bone. A damaged drill bit can increase drilling time by a factor of 35.[75a] Damage is frequently caused by contact with other metal (plate or drill sleeve). The Arbeitsgemeinschaft für Osteosynthesefragen/American Society for Internal Fixation (AO/ASIF) recommends certain procedures to decrease drill bit damage. The first is to drill only bone. Pohler found that drilling of 110 bone cortices had a negligible effect on the bit itself. The second is to always use the drill guide. This minimizes bending, which is the leading cause of drill failure. The drill guide or sleeve should be of correct size; an excessively large guide results in a larger hole because of wobbling of the drill. The third recommendation is to start the drill only after the drill bit has been inserted into the drill guide. This technique limits contact with the drill guide and consequent damage to the cutting and reaming edges. These recommendations combined with the defined physiologic bone drilling method limit local damage to bone and result in optimal holes for screw fixation.

Most standard fracture fixation sets provide specific drill bits that are used to drill, tap, and glide holes appropriate for all screws contained in the set. Drill bits are named by their diameter and, because they should always be used with soft tissue protective sleeves, they have both a total and an effective length, the latter being the portion of the bit that extends past the drill sleeve and is responsible for cutting. The diameters of drill bits correspond to specific screws in the fracture fixation set. Generally, the size of the drill bit used to make the pilot hole for the screw threads is 0.1 to 0.2 mm larger than the core diameter of the corresponding screw. The size of the drill bit used to make glide holes is the same size as the diameter of the shaft of a shaft screw or the outer diameter of a fully threaded cortical screw. The cutting edge of the bit is at its tip; it should always be protected and should frequently be examined for flaws.

Taps are designed to cut threads in bone that resemble exactly the profile of the corresponding screw thread. The process of tapping facilitates insertion and enables the screw to bite deeper into the bone. This allows the torque applied to the screw to be used for generating compressive force instead of being dissipated by friction and cutting of threads (Fig. 8-41). Tapping also removes additional material from the hole, thereby enlarging it. The screw pullout strength depends on the material density. The larger hole created by the tap does not decrease pullout strength in cortical bone because of its density; in less dense trabecular or osteopenic bone, the larger hole has a progressively larger effect and can decrease pullout strength by as much as 30%.[75b]

Taps are threaded throughout their length and increase gradually in height up to the desired thread depth. A flute extends from the tip through the first 10 threads to facilitate clearing of bone debris, which can collect and jam the tap (Fig. 8-42). Proper technique calls for two clockwise and one counterclockwise turn to facilitate bone chip removal. The entire far cortex should always be tapped, because screw pullout strength increases substantially with full cortical purchase. The tap size, which corresponds to its outer diameter, should be the same as the outer diameter of the screw. For example,

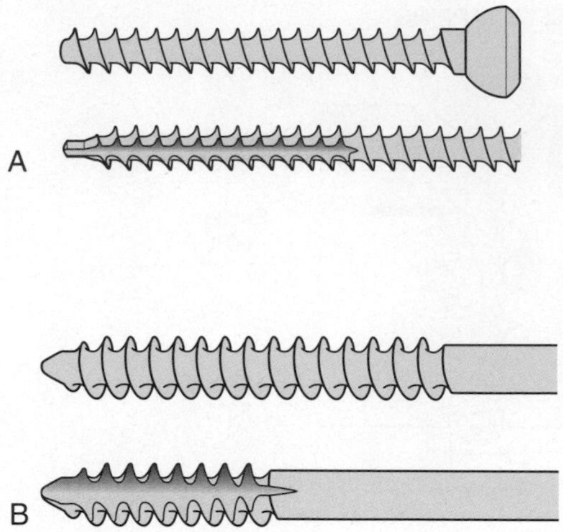

Figure 8-42. Taps and their corresponding screws. **A,** The size of the tap should be consistent with the outer diameter of the screw to be used. For example, if using a 4.5-mm cortical screw (which has an outer diameter of approximately 4.5 mm), the tap size should be 4.5 mm. **B,** A 6.5-mm cancellous screw uses a corresponding 6.5-mm tap.

a 4.5-mm cortical screw has an outside diameter of 4.5 mm and uses a 4.5-mm tap; a 6.5-mm cancellous screw with an outside diameter of 6.5 mm uses a 6.5-mm tap.

Speaking of Drills and Taps

- "I feel like I am having to push excessively for this drill to advance. That is affecting my ability to maintain the desired drilling direction. I should try a new drill bit because this one must be dull."
- "I am struggling to maintain my starting point with the drill. Do we have a drill bit of the same size with a sharper point?"
- "I know this is a self-tapping screw, but it is small diameter and the cortex is dense. Maybe I should tap to ensure the screw doesn't break upon insertion from torsional overload."

Screwdrivers

Screwdrivers are simple handheld mechanical devices designed for manual screw insertion. Screwdrivers can be single piece or modular. They consist of three primary parts: the handle, the shaft, and the tip.

The handle has two basic functions: (1) to conform to the palm or fingers and (2) to translate forearm or hand torque to the screwdriver shaft. Standard handles are made of slip-resistant material and take varying shapes. As a handle becomes larger in diameter, it allows for increased torque transmission by increasing the moment arm of the mechanical device. This is especially notable in the T-shaped handles, which sacrifice feel for power. Some of the current handles incorporate ratcheting, where the screwdriver shaft is locked to the handle for clockwise rotation, but unlocked for counterclockwise rotation. This locking can be reversed for screw removal. One of the most important modifications of the handle is the torque-limiting device. This mechanical device is often fashioned to fit inside the handle, unfortunately creating a heavier handle and an unbalanced screwdriver. The increased weight and lack of screwdriver balance limit feel. Fortunately, the torque-limiting function eliminates the need for feel. The torque-limiting device serves one important purpose: to ensure a locking screw is adequately but not excessively tightened. This may seem trivial, but it is actually very important. If smaller locking screws are overtightened, there is a risk of shearing the head off of the screw. Remember the core diameter of the screw defines its resistance to torsional load, so as the screw becomes smaller, its resistance to torsional load follows suit. If larger locking screws are inadequately tightened, there is a risk of not reaching the level of stability required to satisfy the locking mechanism (i.e., maintain the locking of the screw to the plate). There is the additional concern with softer metals that overtightening could create mechanical bonding of the screw to the plate, making removal very challenging.[76] Knowing why the torque limiter is present is an important part of understanding the screwdriver.

The screwdriver shaft transmits the torque from the handle to the tip. The primary variation in the shaft is related to the diameter. Smaller diameter shafts allow for improved surgeon feel. To clarify, when conventional screws are used, the insertional torque needs to be optimized. The right amount of compression should be created, but the screw head should not be stripped. This is often a delicate balance. Because of the variation in bone quality among patients and anatomic locations, the optimal insertional torque cannot be standardized.[77] This is why a torque-limiting screwdriver is not typically used in conventional screw application.[40] The feeling of screw purchase (the perception that the screw is getting tighter rather than stripping) is best assessed empirically. This means it is subject to user variability, which seems to be affected by the volume of experience.[78] This feeling of screw purchase is an important skill to develop for two reasons: (1) inadequate insertional torque will lead to slippage between the conventional plate and bone and construct instability, and (2) overtightening leads to screw stripping and screw recess failure. In addition, torque tests have shown that once screw recess failure occurs, additional attempts at insertion or removal will only produce 50% of the original maximum torque.[67] Because the failure most commonly occurs through permanent deformation of the walls of the screw socket, changing screwdrivers does little to help. Stated another way, once the screw head is stripped, it is challenging to remove the screw. The feeling of screw purchase should be maximized. From the design side, it can be educated by smaller diameter screwdriver shafts that provide more feedback prior to screw stripping.

The screwdriver tip is the male end that accommodates the female recess of whichever screw head design was chosen. As previously noted, hexagonal, cruciate, and star-drive tips are most commonly used in orthopaedic trauma. Ensuring the tip is in good condition is one of the best ways to prevent the screw head stripping that occurs from irregular points of contact between the driver tip and the screw recess.

Speaking of Screwdrivers

- "I am not going to use this torque-limiter. I know that I will achieve enough force upon insertion to lock the screw to the plate. Hmmm. I think the screw just broke. What is the purpose of that torque-limiter again?"
- "This screwdriver keeps stripping the screw head recess. It must have rounded edges. Time for a new screwdriver."

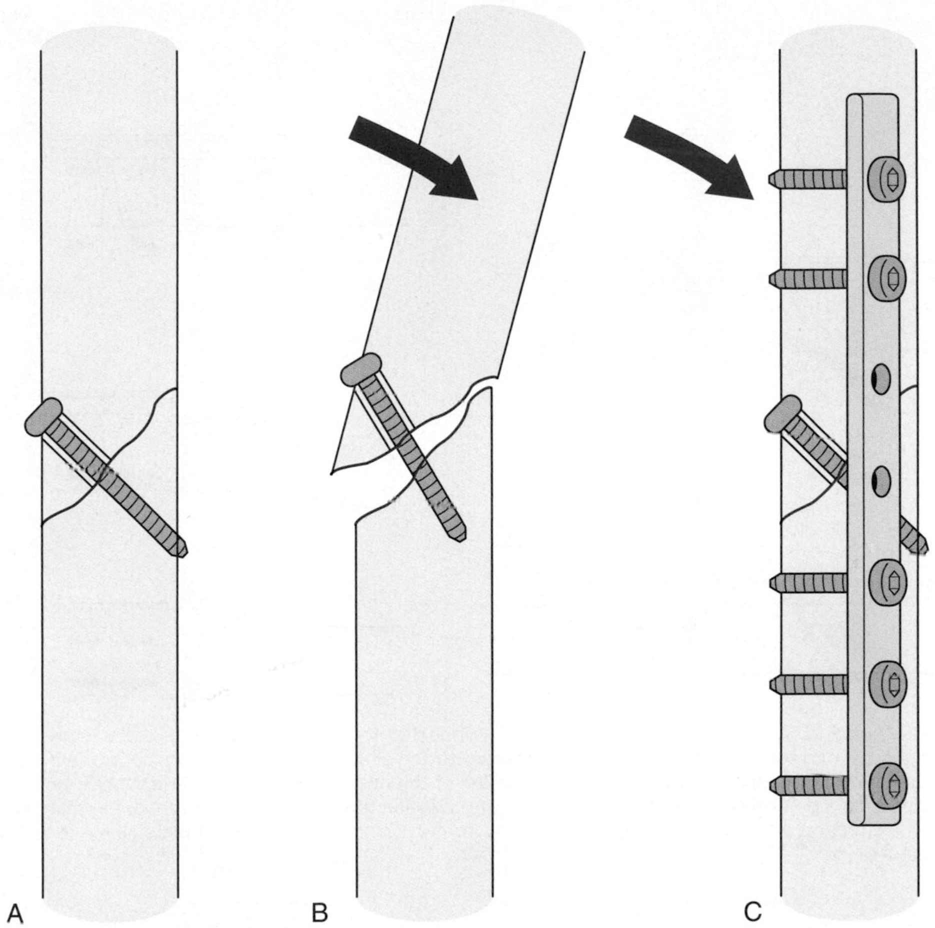

Figure 8-43. Neutralization or protection plate. The mechanical purpose of this type of plate is to protect an independent lag screw from bending and torsional forces.

- "You just said the screw is stripped. Do you mean you have lost the feeling of screw purchase or you have head recess failure? The two have very different fixes."
- "The insertional torque seems tremendous. Do we have a screwdriver with a larger handle?"

Plate

In orthopaedic trauma surgery, a plate is a thin sheet of metal or other material that is most commonly used to fasten pieces of bone together. A plate is defined both by its function and by its name. The function is the biomechanical purpose of the plate. The name typically refers to the plate shape or plate design. It is important to differentiate between the function and the name. One plate design can be used to achieve a number of different mechanical functions. Similarly, many different plate designs can be used to achieve the same mechanical function. Stated most simplistically, a plate is just an implant. The surgeon defines how it is to be used.

Mechanical Function

Plates have six basic mechanical functions: (1) neutralization, (2) compression, (3) tension band, (4) buttress, (5) bridge, and (6) locked internal fixator.[1] The first four are commonly identified with conditions of absolute stability. The fifth is noted in conditions of relative stability. The sixth can be found in either, but is most often associated with relative stability. Let us consider each mechanical function individually.

Neutralization Plating

A neutralization plate is also called a protection plate. The mechanical function of this plate is to protect a lag screw from bending and torsional forces; for this reason, a plate is not serving in neutralization mode unless a lag screw is present. As previously noted, lag screws are the fundamental instruments of achieving compression; but, as stand-alone implants, they rarely function adequately to maintain construct stability until healing (Fig. 8-43).[74] Neutralization plates are placed after the lag screw has compressed an anatomically reduced fracture. They are typically placed through extensile approaches in the setting of direct reduction techniques; however, this is not always the case. They are typically used when the lag screw has been placed independently of the plate rather than through the plate. When the lag screw is placed through the plate, the plate is typically deemed a compression plate, and the lag screw is placed after the plate is used to compress the fracture. This means that the orientation of the fracture line and possible position of the plate will typically determine whether a plate is used in compression or neutralization mode. To clarify, when the plate can be placed such that the obtuse angle of the fracture can first be connected to the plate, and

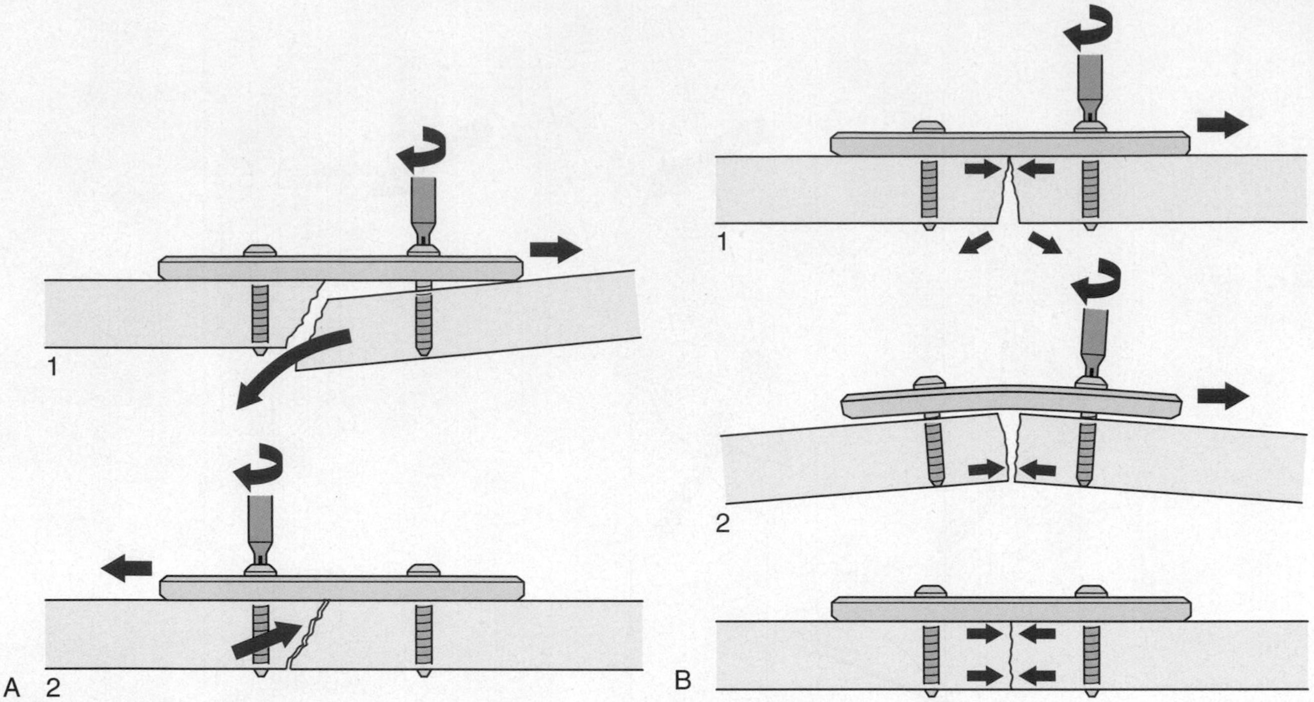

Figure 8-44. Compression plating. **A,** The plate should be initially connected to the obtuse angle of the fracture such that the acute angle can be compressed into the created axilla. When the plate is connected to the acute angle first, sliding along the fracture obliquity can potentially lead to loss of compression and reduction. **B,** Compression outside of the neutral axis (i.e., center axis) of a bone creates an angular force that has the potential to induce a deformity. When compressing a transverse fracture, there is the potential to create compression immediately adjacent to the plate and distraction at the far cortex. To prevent this from occurring, prebending a plate allows it to place compression across the entire width of a fracture.

the acute angle of the fracture can be compressed into the axilla created by the plate and bone, then compression plate application is typically chosen rather than neutralization plate application (Fig. 8-44). This is because a lag screw placed through the plate is able to achieve superior fixation than one placed outside of the plate. Screws in neutralization plates can be either conventional, locking, or a combination of the two. These plates can be used in many different areas of the skeleton.

Compression Plating

The mechanical function of a compression plate is to compress a fracture. Compression creates interdigitation of fracture surfaces and maximizes friction at the fracture site. This leads to a load-sharing bone-implant construct and protects the implant. It requires a simple fracture pattern (typically oblique or transverse). In transverse fracture patterns, lag screws are nearly impossible to place perpendicular to the plane of the fracture, making the compression plate application the logical choice. In oblique fracture patterns, the decision between compression or neutralization plate application is based on the orientation of the obliquity and the space available for plate placement. Attempting to connect the plate to the acute angle of the fracture prior to compression creates a problem. Because an axilla is not created by the plate and bone, compression leads to shearing along the obliquity of the fracture (see Fig. 8-44).

A compression plate requires undercontouring in order to achieve symmetric compression across the fracture gap. To clarify, anytime an implant or instrument is used in compression outside of the neutral axis (center axis) of the bone, then it also creates a bending force. This bending force is manifested by eccentric compression, whereby the cortex adjacent to the plate is compressed, but the cortex far from the plate sees tension and therefore opens slightly (see Fig. 8-44). This degree of opening is dependent on the amount of compression that is eccentrically generated. Compression can be achieved through an external compression device (e.g., an articulated tensioning device) or through eccentric placement of a screw in an inclined plane hole (Fig. 8-45). Undercontouring of the plate accommodates for this eccentric compression and allows for more symmetric compression to be achieved across the entire fracture plane.[74]

Tension Band Plating

The mechanical function of a tension band plate is torque conversion. It acts as a torque converter applied to the tension surface of an eccentrically loaded bone. This is a simple phrase to memorize, but a more challenging concept to understand without a background in engineering. Let us break down the different parts of the definition to achieve an understanding of what this means, rather than attempting to memorize the phrase. The understanding will allow for appropriate application of the concept in the operating theater.

It is first important to understand what is meant by eccentric loading and tension. We have previously covered the concept that compression outside of the neutral axis of the bone leads to bending. We covered this as it related to compression plating. Plates are not placed in the neutral axis of the bone. This would require placement inside of the

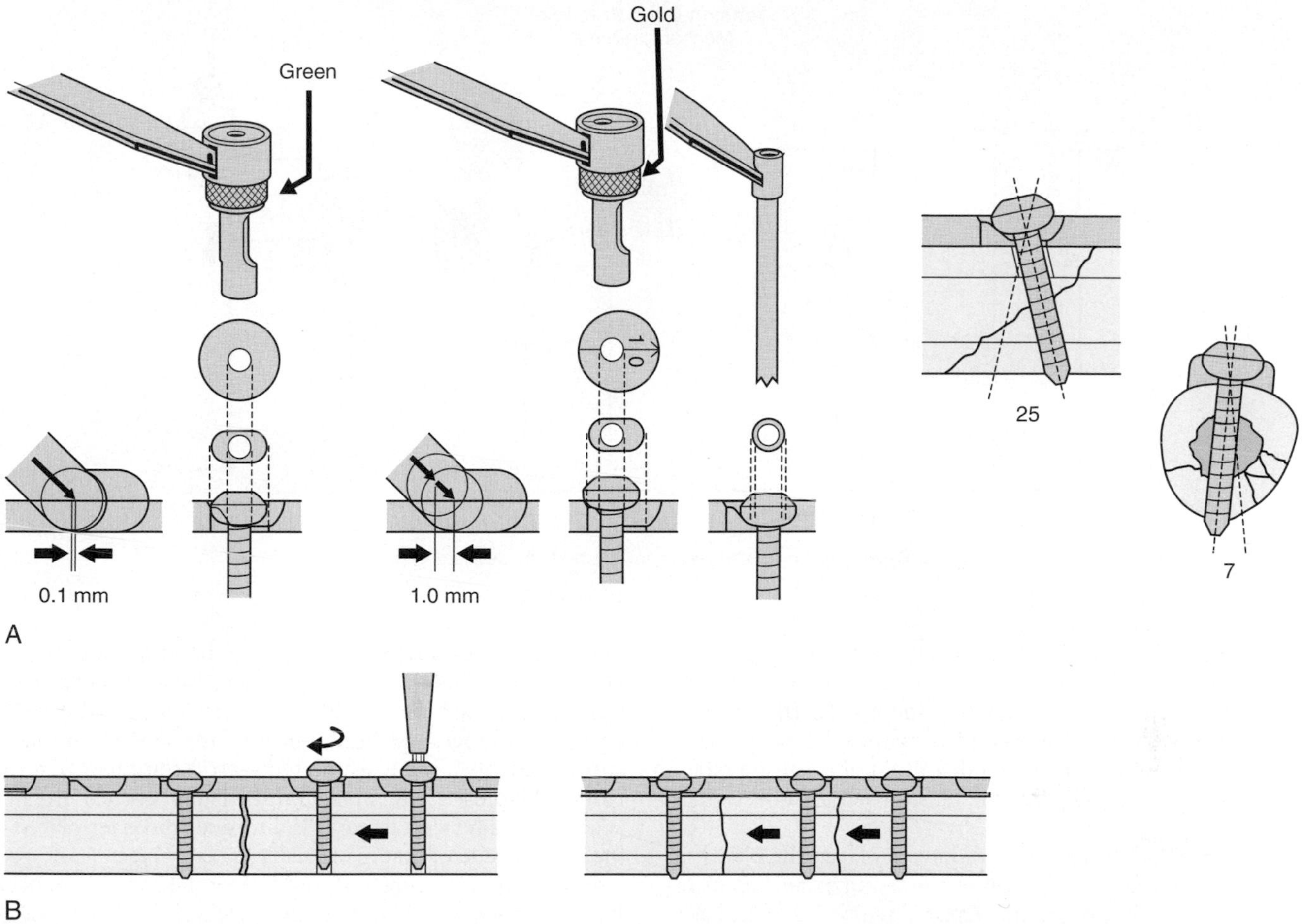

Figure 8-45. Compression plating using the dynamic compression unit plate hole. This took advantage of an old carpenter's principle: When a screw is eccentrically positioned in a plate hole, the inclined surface of the screw hits the edge of the plate, creating displacement perpendicular to the long axis of the screw

intramedullary canal. They are placed eccentrically on the bone or on a cortex outside of the neutral axis.

A load is an external force that influences a body and tends to produce motion.[5] Loads are defined by the direction in which they are employed. The loads create stress within the structure. There are three principal stresses that are seen by structures: tension, compression, and shear (refer again to Fig. 8-3). This is the case because any potential stress within a structure can always be described as a combination of the three principal stresses. When the stress is a pulling apart, it is called *tension.* When the stress is a pushing together, it is called *compression.* When the stress is a sliding, it is called *shear.* Remaining faithful to engineering nomenclature is important, but not when it prevents the surgeon from applying the basic principles in the operating theater. Because of this, for a moment we will simplify concepts to enhance understanding.

A simple diagram that is useful when thinking about forces on bone is seen in Figure 8-2. Compression, tension, and shear have already been defined and are simple to understand. Bending occurs when forces are applied to a structure perpendicular to the surface. Bending takes many forms based on the location of the force and any fixed points (fulcrums) that are present (e.g., three-point, four-point, cantilever, etc.). Torsion is a form of twisting, turning, or rotation. It is most simply thought of in terms of twisting around a center of rotation (similar to bending around a fulcrum).

Take a moment to review Figure 8-46. The figure is an illustration of the tension band concept. At the far left of the illustration is a platform that sits on a base. The two are connected by springs on each side. Note the hooks on the left side of the platform and base. Now transition to the right in the illustration. A weight is placed centrally (not eccentrically) on top of the platform. The springs are compressed symmetrically, both seeing an equal amount of force because the weight is centered on the platform between the springs. Now transition to the right again. The weight is now placed to the right side of the platform. It is in an eccentric location rather than being centered on the platform. Notice the difference in the forces seen by the springs. The spring on the right is compressed, while the spring on the left is stretched. Stated another way, the spring on the right is experiencing compression, while the spring on the right is experiencing tension. This is what happens with a torsional or bending force. This is why there are three principal stresses (compression, tension, and shear). The torsional force experienced by the platform can be broken down into compression and tension in the object, and therefore is not required to be a separate principle stress. Now move to the far right in the illustration. The weight is still placed eccentrically to the right of the platform; but the springs

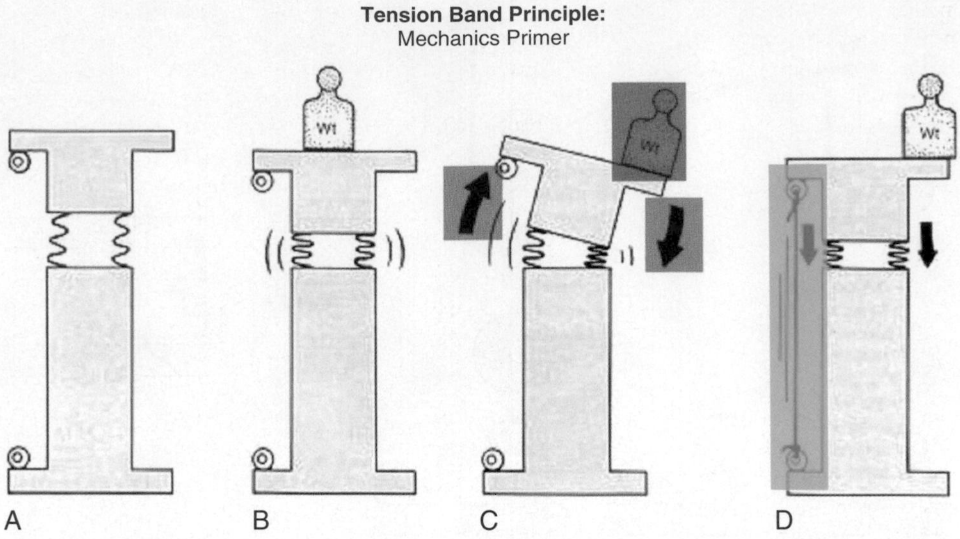

Figure 8-46. Tension band concept. See text for detailed explanation.

look different. Once again, the springs are both seeing compression and appear to be symmetrically compressed. The difference lies in the string connecting the hooks. The string is acting as a tension band. It is converting torque into symmetric compression. Remember the definition of a tension band: a torque converter applied to the tension side of an eccentrically loaded object.

Now move to Figure 8-47. We have replaced the platform and base with a femur. The top of the femur is analogous to the platform. The bottom of the femur is analogous to the base. The medial cortex is analogous to the right spring. The lateral cortex is analogous to the left spring. Now move to the right in the illustration. When a load is placed centrally directly above the anatomic axis of the femur (the center of the intramedullary canal), the medial and lateral cortex see a symmetric compressive force. But the femur is a bent bone (i.e., it has a neck and a head). Body weight is not distributed above the anatomic axis of the bone; rather, it is distributed above the femoral head (eccentric to the anatomic axis). Now the medial cortex sees compression, while the lateral cortex sees tension. The femur is experiencing torque or bending, just like the platform that was eccentrically loaded. Now move to the far right in the illustration. Body weight is still placed eccentrically over the femoral head; but now the medial and lateral cortices are once again seeing symmetric compressive forces. Notice the presence of a plate on the lateral cortex. The plate is acting as a tension band. It is a torque converter placed on the tension side of an eccentrically loaded object.

Now move to Figure 8-48 and feel torque conversion occur. Like the person in the diagram, place your right hand on the top of your head. Feel the torque or bending that your neck experiences. It is seeing compression on the right side and tension on the left side. Now interlace your hands on top of your head. Your neck should now feel symmetrically compressed. Your left hand is acting as a tension band. It is a torque converter placed on the tension side of an eccentrically loaded object. As you pull harder with your right hand, you feel increasing symmetric compression of your neck. Release

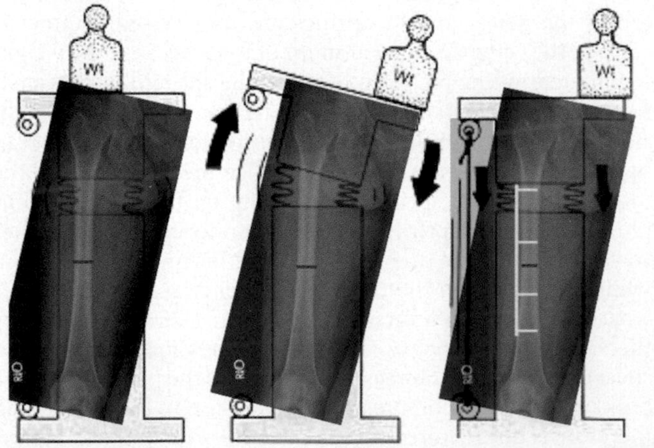

Figure 8-47. Tension band concept applied using a femoral shaft fracture as a model.

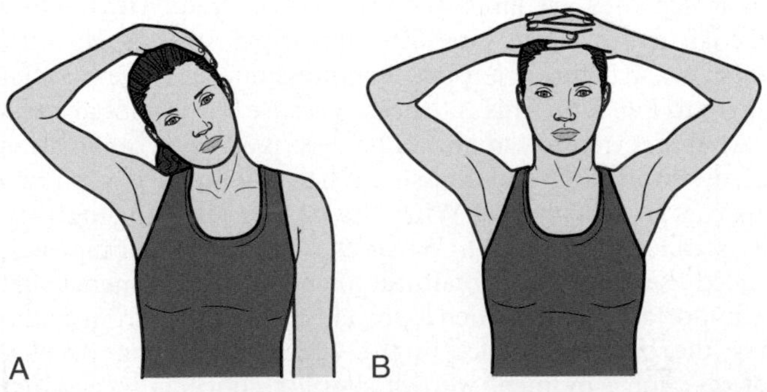

Figure 8-48. Mechanical concept of a tension band understood via interlacing hands on head. **A,** If you place your right hand on your head and pull, it creates a bending force, with compression along the right side of your neck and tension along the left side. **B,** If you interlace your left hand with your right, then pulling with the right hand will no longer result in bending, but rather in pure compression along the axis of your neck. *(Source: Redrawn from Salvadori M:* The art of construction: projects and principles for beginning engineers and architects, *Chicago, 1990, Chicago Review Press, Figure 10-12a and b, p 83; drawings by Saralinda Hooker and Christopher Ragus, 1979, ed 1.)*

your hands and consider how this applies to tension band application in common areas of the body. Let us use the olecranon for illustration. Put your right hand back on top of your head. Your right hand is acting as the triceps. Your head is the olecranon tip fragment. It is being pulled away from the remainder of the ulna and bent over the trochlea. Now interlace your hands again on top of your head. Your left hand is acting as a dorsally applied plate or figure-of-8 wire. As you pull with your right hand (triceps contraction), your neck just feels more and more compression (dynamic fracture site compression).

Now that the concept makes sense, let us consider how it fails. Tension band application has four prerequisites in order to function appropriately. First, the fractured bone must be eccentrically loaded. If no torque is present, then a torque converter does not make sense. Bent bones are eccentrically loaded. Bones that move around a fulcrum are eccentrically loaded. When closely viewing radiographic displacement, it becomes apparent that tension banding is an option in many areas of the body. Second, the implant must be placed on the tension side of the fractured bone. If it is placed on the compressive side, when the bone is loaded, the tension side will continue to gap open. Third, the bone must be able to withstand compressive force. Tension banding is based on the concept of dynamic compression. If the bone cannot withstand compression, the concept cannot work. Fourth (and similar to the third prerequisite), the far cortex must be intact or reconstructed. If this is not the case, then the plate is acting not as a tension band, but more akin to a bridge plate, which will be covered later. Successful treatment can still occur, but it relies on early callus formation on the side far from the plate to prevent implant failure.

Buttress Plating

In architecture, a buttress is defined as a projecting support built against the wall of a structure (Fig. 8-49). Understanding why they became necessary helps you to understand the mechanical purpose of buttress plating. Roofs on buildings are generally valued. One of the problems associated with sloped roofing, however, is the lateral thrust created by the roofs. This thrust was traditionally supported by the walls of the building. As windows became more and more valued, wall thickness became an aesthetic detraction. Windows are less pleasing when centered within thick walls. As wall thickness decreased, the lateral thrust of the roof needed to be counteracted in another way to prevent the walls from collapsing beneath the outward thrust of the roof. The buttress was a solution.

The function of a buttress plate is analogous to the function of architectural buttresses. Consider a split depression lateral tibial plateau fracture (see Fig. 8-49). The lateral femoral condyle wants to fall into the depressed hole in the lateral plateau. As it does so, it creates further condylar widening. The lateral femoral condyle is acting as the roof and creating the axial and lateral thrust. The lateral tibial cortex is acting as the thin wall. The depressed hole is acting as the empty space to the inside of the wall. A buttress is needed. The buttress plate resists the axial load and lateral thrust of the lateral femoral condyle by applying a force that counteracts the deforming forces. This should take you back to the fundamental purpose of an implant and the surgeon's onus to recognize and characterize the deforming forces. Unbalanced forces create displacement and subsequent deformity. These forces must be characterized, and the plan for correction must include specific resistance to them. Implants are placed with logical purpose: to counteract the specific deforming forces until healing is accomplished. When implants are placed without this explicit purpose, then failure is more likely to occur.

A buttress plate supports the fractured bone in the area of the metaphyseal deficiency. It prevents the deforming forces created by the opposing bone by compressive forces that are applied perpendicular to the deformity. It must be firmly anchored to the main fragment (diaphyseal portion) and must

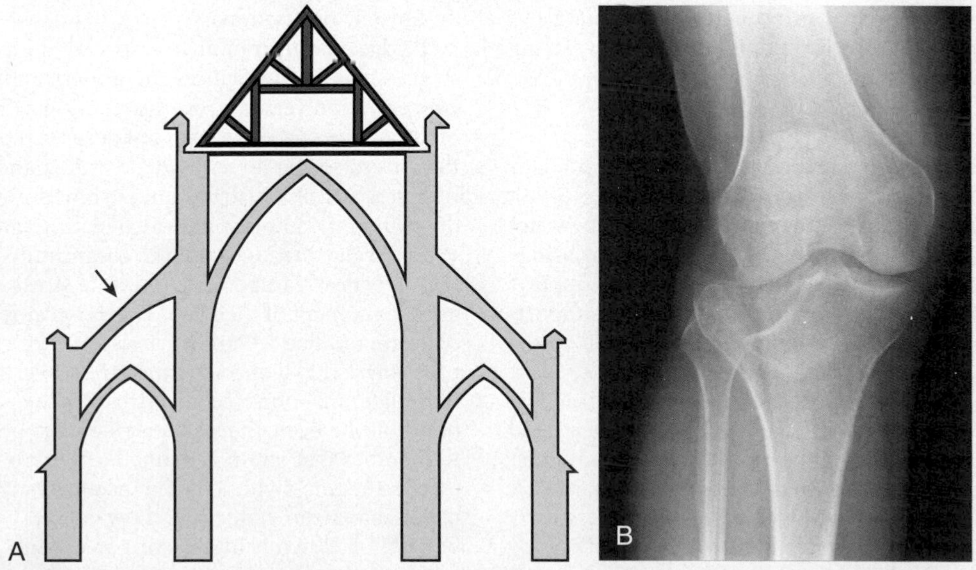

Figure 8-49. A, Architectural example of a buttress. The *arrow* represents the flying buttress. This buttress is preventing collapse of the walls through the weight of the roof. **B,** Example of an injury film revealing a lateral tibial plateau split depression fracture. Collapse of the lateral wall (cortex) has occurred with the roof (lateral femoral condyle) falling into the defect created. Application of a buttress implant (with a force vector similar to the buttress in the architectural example), will prevent collapse after the joint surface is restored.

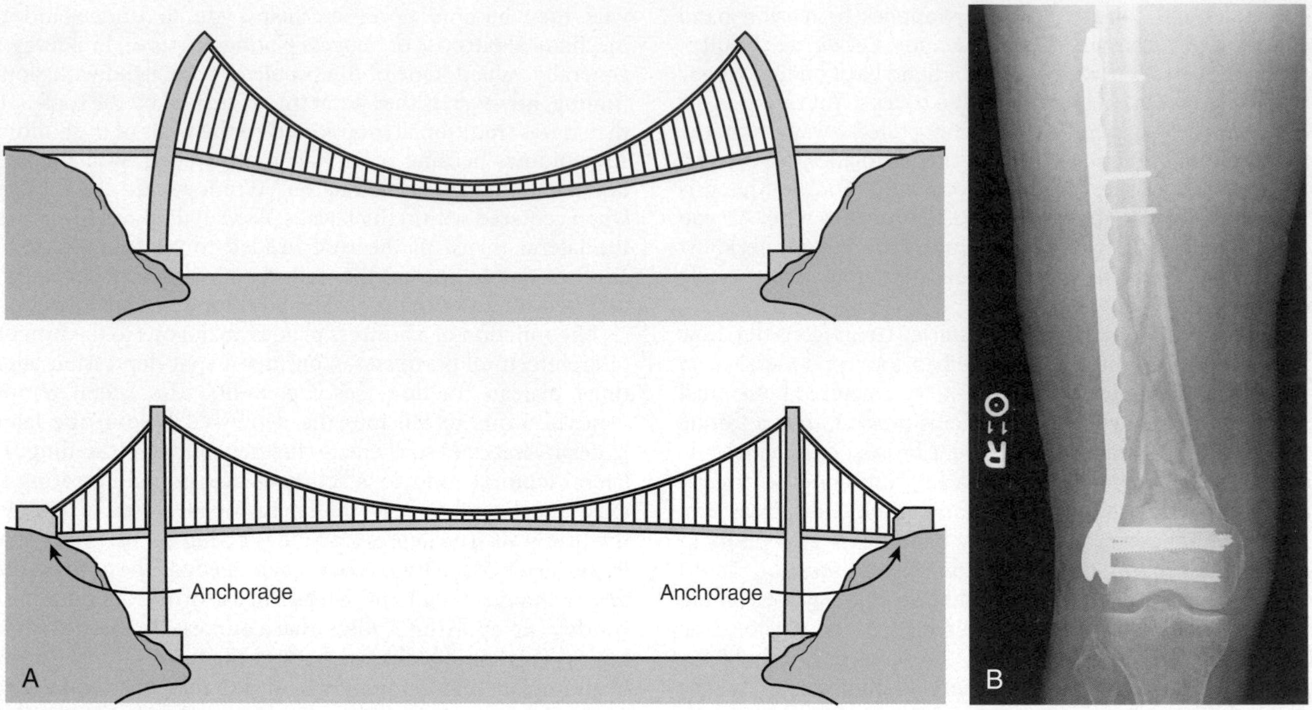

Figure 8-50. **A,** Architectural example of a bridge. **B,** Example of an injury film revealing a comminuted supracondylar femur fracture with bridge plate application. Anchorage points in the bridge are located on either side of the water. This prevents loading collapse. The same is noted in fracture care.

be intimately contoured to the underlying metaphyseal portion. Screws are inserted initially in the central portion of the implant and then peripherally. This helps to ensure an intimate fit at the apex of the fracture in the metaphyseal region.[74] In light of these requirements, buttress plates should be relatively malleable in order to autocontour to individual variabilities in anatomy via conventional screw application. For this reason, buttress plates placed with only locking screws are both counterintuitive and excessively expensive. Locking screws do not change the relationship between the plate and the bone; so if an intimate relationship is not present, placing a locking screw will not change it.

Bridge Plating

A bridge is a mechanical structure that carries a road or path across an obstacle such as a body of water (Fig. 8-50). It is a load-bearing structure. To clarify, the water is not assisting in load transfer across the bridge. Only the bridge and its supports are ensuring safe passage. These supports are built on something other than the water. The supports take advantage of the stability provided on each side of the obstacle.

A bridge plate is analogous to a bridge over water (see Fig. 8-50). The plate is load bearing. There is no assistance in load transfer by the broken pieces of bone that are spanned. Fracture treatment is a race between bone healing and hardware failure. As such, the plate is in danger of failure, unless early healing occurs away from the plate surface, preferably along the far cortex (remember the concept of moment of inertia). The supports of a bridge plate are the screws that are placed into the segments proximal and distal to the zone of comminution. These supports are stressed substantially in bending and torsion. If the supports are conventional screws, then the frictional force created by screw insertion must be greater than the patient loading in order to resist failure. Conventional screws are perfectly appropriate for bridge plating when placed in bone of acceptable quality. When conventional screws are placed in bone of marginal quality, then the patient load can overcome the frictional force created by the screws, leading to failure of the bridge plate. This is why bridge plating of osteoporotic bone is most often done with locking screws, which do not rely on friction.

Bridge plating requires a special understanding of construct stability. It requires an understanding of both stress concentration versus stress distribution as well as strain. Both of these were covered earlier but deserve repeating. Remember that stress equals force divided by area and stress concentration versus stress distribution is something we refer to when describing the implant in bridge plating (among other times). When bridge plating is used in comminuted fracture patterns, then it is nearly impossible to create stress concentration over a small segment of the plate. This is because many holes of the plate are unfilled when they are spanning a comminuted fracture zone. This distributes the stress over a large segment of the plate (as opposed to stress being concentrated over one hole or even the plate segment in between two holes). Remember that strain is defined as the motion between fracture fragments divided by the distance between fracture fragments after the reduction. Low strain environments form bone.[40,41,79] When bridge plating is used in comminuted fracture patterns, then a low strain environment is nearly guaranteed. This is because the construct created has some degree of flexibility (motion) and there are many fracture gaps (equating to a large denominator and appropriate strain). Realize that the examples provided earlier were in reference to a comminuted fracture pattern. As previously noted, attempting bridge plating in simple fracture patterns can be problematic (review the strain section again if this is unclear).

There is another point about bridge plating and construct stability that should be emphasized. Bridge plating creates a load-bearing construct until some degree of fracture healing occurs. This means it is important to optimize the stability of the plate and screw construct. In simple terms, this can be accomplished via using long plates and spreading out screws in each segment. Suggested guidelines have been provided for this.[80] The plate-to-span ratio has been defined as the total length of the plate compared to the length of the plate that spans the zone of comminution. Current recommendations are to use a plate of three to four times the length of the zone of comminution. Plate screw density has been defined as the total number of screws placed in the plate relative to the total number of holes available in the plate. Current recommendations are to use a screw density of 0.5 or less, meaning fewer than half of the available screw holes are used. It should be noted that these are empirical values and not based on perfect science.[81] It should also be noted that these values were described for the internal fixator (simply defined as a plate with all screws placed in locking mode). While the recommendations can logically be transferred to conventional plating, some biomechanical data are available for this application. This testing was completed in a fracture gap model using polyurethane foam.[82] Torsional strength was primarily correlated with the number of screws per segment, whereas bending strength was primarily correlated with plate length and screw spacing. Basic recommendations from this for bridge plating would be to use longer plates and more than two screws per segment. Realize that the number of screws per segment relates to a concept that we rarely discuss in orthopaedic trauma surgery, despite it commonly being considered in structural engineering. The concept is known as the factor of safety. In structural engineering, expected loads are calculated and a construct is devised that covers the expected loads and provides for additional safety (an amount of safety to protect against the unexpected loads).[37] This is the same thing we are doing when we consider things such as patient compliance and expected time for healing in fracture care. It is logical that a larger factor of safety would be built into a construct when it is clear the patient will not comply with postoperative recommendations or the fracture is expected to take longer than usual to heal.

One other point should become clear about bridge plating. Because success relies on early fracture healing to offload the supports, then soft tissue technique and calcium metabolism are paramount. Avascular bone takes a prolonged time to heal. Implants have a limited number of load cycles prior to failure. Consider a coat hanger. When it is bent back and forth enough times, it will break. The same is true of the plate and screws in bridge plating. Our advantage in fracture treatment compared to civil engineering is the potential of the bone to heal and offload the implant. We must always be aware of this advantage and do things to maximize that potential. One of these things is atraumatic surgical technique. It takes on extra importance in environments where the implant is load bearing. This has led to bridge plating being synonymous with limited approaches (e.g., submuscular plating) and indirect reduction techniques. These should relatively increase the blood supply to fragments in the fracture zone and encourage secondary healing. A bridge plate does not have to be introduced through a limited approach using indirect reduction techniques; but when another technique is employed, care must be taken to ensure protection of the blood supply.

Locked Internal Fixator

Conventional plating has limitations. First, the screws and plate have an uncoupled relationship. To clarify, screws can loosen independently, thereby negating construct stability. Second, the stability afforded by conventional plating occurs through friction. Friction has some disadvantages. First, friction is dependent on the quality of the bone. This means it is hard to create stability when the bone quality is marginal. Second, friction requires compression of the plate to the bone, which damages the periosteal blood supply in the area. The decrease in the local blood supply weakens the bone, theoretically providing an increased risk of infection on implant insertion and refracture on implant removal.[83] Although these findings and the subsequent plate design changes seem logical, realize that there remains controversy regarding the relationship between necrosis and porosis.[84]

Historically, these limitations led to the development of a different type of plate that could achieve stability in the absence of ideal bone and do so without damaging the vascularity at the fracture site. This became known as a locked internal fixator. A fixator is an angular stable implant that stabilizes a fracture without touching the bone, except for connecting pins or screws.[85] It does not rely on friction to establish stability, but rather on the attachment of the screw (or pin) to the plate in a rigid fixed-angle coupling. The early fixators were external in design. The Schanz pins entered the bone at a distance from the fracture site and were coupled on the outside of the skin with bars and clamps. There were many advantages: (1) angular stability, (2) unified or coupled resistance to pullout of the screws, (3) the lack of precise implant contouring (i.e., the clamps could be moved when connecting the pins to the rods), (4) less periosteal blood supply damage, and (5) no axial preload of the construct. There were also disadvantages. One of the well-known problems with external fixators is infected pin tracts, secondary to the opening through the skin to the outside environment. Internal fixators were designed to provide similar advantages without this well-known disadvantage.[86]

Despite understanding the advantages of the locked internal fixator, it remains challenging to define the indications. There are many different ways to cover this topic. In the following, my bias will be pragmatism. To clarify, the theoretical advantages of locked internal fixators do not always translate into a clear indication for the use of a locking construct.[87] The primary reason for this difference is implant cost. There is a substantial difference between the cost of a locking construct and the cost of a nonlocking construct. On average, a locking screw costs approximately seven to eight times the amount of a conventional screw. A locking plate costs approximately three times the amount of a conventional plate. This means that the advantages of using a particular implant must be weighed against the increase in implant cost that will be absorbed by the patient, the insurance company, or the hospital. Clearer data to guide practice would be ideal. At this point in time—based on a recent review of locking plate use for extremity fractures—there are no clear guidelines for when a

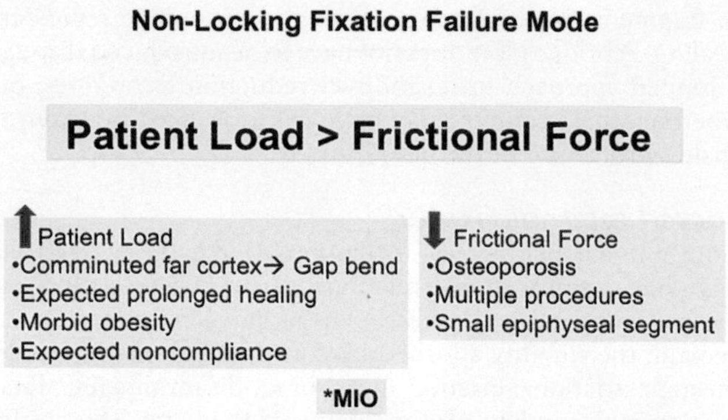
Non-Locking Fixation Failure Mode
Patient Load > Frictional Force
Patient Load
•Comminuted far cortex→ Gap bend
•Expected prolonged healing
•Morbid obesity
•Expected noncompliance
Frictional Force
•Osteoporosis
•Multiple procedures
•Small epiphyseal segment
*MIO

Figure 8-51. Indications for locked plating naturally derive from the expected failure mode of conventional plating. *MIO,* Minimally invasive osteosynthesis. *MIO does not represent an indication for locked plating based on expected failure modes of conventional plating. Rather, using locked plating in MIO has some advantages, including less precise contouring of implants and screw length choice.

locking plate will improve patient-oriented outcomes, decrease adverse events and complication, and be cost-effective as a choice.[87] Comparative studies of conventional plating to locked plating are limited. Comparisons are commonly made retrospectively to historical standards instead. Indications among locked plating studies vary, leading to challenges in pooling information. When considering the indications listed below, take time to consider the implication of the increased cost of using these implants. At this point in history, the indications for locked internal fixators should be individualized based on the economic environment within which one works and the relative benefits the technology provides.

Remember the general indication for the use of locking screws, that is, when the patient load is expected to overcome the frictional forces that can be exerted by conventional screws. The specific indications for locked plating are derived from this general indication for the use of locking screws. Using the formula for conventional screw failure (Fig. 8-51), it is possible to logically define indications for choosing locked fixation. Anything that increases the patient load or decreases the potential frictional force would be a reasonable situation to choose locked plating. Common situations that increase patient loading would include (1) comminution of the far cortex leading to gap bending, (2) expected prolonged healing times, (3) morbid obesity, and (4) expected noncompliance with postoperative weight-bearing precautions. Common situations that limit the frictional force include (1) osteoporosis, (2) history of multiple operative procedures with cavitations, and (3) small epiphyseal segmentation that limits points of fixation. Let us consider each one of these individually to unpack how locked fixation could be of benefit.

First, when a bone is subjected to eccentric loading, comminution of the far cortex creates a dangerous mechanical environment. This is a relative indication for locked plating.[88] Consider a diving board. Now consider the base of the diving board being connected to the ground with conventional screws. Jumping on the end of the platform repetitively has the potential to individually loosen each conventional screw, leading to the diving board falling into the water. This is analogous to the varus failure mode commonly seen with conventional plating of proximal femur fractures, distal femur fractures, bicondylar tibial plateau fractures, and proximal humerus fractures to name but a few. This failure mode is more common when there is no far cortex support to limit implant loading. Now consider placing the diving board over concrete rather than water and placing a block underneath the edge of the platform. It would be possible to jump on the edge of the platform repetitively without significantly stressing the screws. This is because the platform would not move, being held by the block underneath it. This is analogous to eccentric loading of a bone when the far cortex has been reconstructed or anatomically reduced. Eccentric loading has a limited effect on the conventional implant in this situation. This is analogous to the expected anatomic healing of a proximal femur fracture when the far cortex is restored and the fracture is anatomically reduced.

Second, when expected healing delays are noted preoperatively, there is a relative indication for fixation that will endure (remember factor of safety). Fracture treatment is a race between implant failure and fracture healing. When the expected duration is a marathon, care should be taken to prepare adequately. Situations that lead to healing delays include calcium metabolism abnormalities, open fractures, severe soft tissue compromise, and partial bone loss to name a few. In these situations, it may be of benefit when plating to choose the advantages of locking constructs.

Third, patient loading is increased in the setting of morbid obesity. This is basic statics and dynamics. The kinetic energy associated with loading in morbid obesity is enhanced by the high mass, which sometimes compensates for the low velocity associated with what would otherwise be considered low-energy mechanisms ($KE = 1/2MV^2$). Deforming forces must be balanced throughout the healing phase in order to ensure anatomic alignment at the end of care. Remember the different failure modes of screws and how these relate to screw design. Locking screws are designed to maximize core diameter, leading to enhanced bending and torsional screw strength. In addition, locking screws are coupled to the plate, resisting loosening and screw pullout. These aid in the resistance of failure in morbid obesity.

Fourth, expectations of patient noncompliance require forethought regarding failure prevention. While it is impossible to prevent failure in all scenarios, it is irresponsible to ignore the potential for dynamic loading postoperatively. Implants possess a limited number of load cycles prior to failure. Enhancing the factor of safety for unreliable patients is a wise decision. One of the ways this can be accomplished in plating is the application of some locking screws.

Fifth, osteoporosis decreases the frictional force that can be obtained with conventional constructs. This is the most common indication for locking fixation cited in the literature. While bone quality is not often quantitatively assessed preoperatively, the energy of the injury and the appearance of the radiographs provide some clue as to the likelihood of achieving adequate compression with conventional screws intraoperatively. Choosing a different mode of stability, namely fixed-angle coupling of screws to the plate, limits the reliance on friction and logically improves the chances of maintaining alignment.

Sixth, a history of multiple operative procedures with osseous cavitations has the potential to decrease the frictional force of conventional fixation. This is only partly secondary to the previous screw holes and cavitations, as disuse osteoporosis commonly coexists in these difficult scenarios. Locking fixation helps to compensate for an absent cortex. It cannot ensure stability, but does help to favor maintenance of alignment when compared to what would amount to unicortical conventional fixation.

Finally, fractures that consist of multiple small epiphyseal segments limit frictional force potential just by limiting the real estate available for screw engagement. In these complex scenarios, when there is a choice between reaching a segment with a single locking screw or a single nonlocking screw, it is rational to consider the utility of locking implants.

Before leaving the locked internal fixator, it is important to consider how it fits into the basic principles flowchart. Once again, refer to Figure 8-1. Locking fixation is a choice that is made by the surgeon. The choice is relatively independent of the type of stability, the choice of surgical approach, and the reduction quality and techniques. When the technology was introduced, the locked internal fixator created connections in the basic principles flowchart that have proven difficult to escape. It is useful to review the introduction of locked fixators to help understand how this occurred. Locking fixation gained popularity in the form of the Less Invasive Stabilization System (LISS; Synthes).[89] This was not the first locking plate available for use. It was the first design that established worldwide popularity. The LISS was a system that included a unicortical locking hole plate that attached to a percutaneous insertion handle and screw-targeting guide. Plates were made for the distal femur and proximal tibia. The plates had no holes for conventional screws. They were designed to be inserted through limited approaches to create relative stability through bridge plating applications after using indirect reduction techniques to restore alignment between the epiphyseal and diaphyseal segments. These were the connections that were established: limited incisions, indirect reduction techniques, relative stability, bridge plating, and locked plating. Since that time, locked plating has transitioned into a broader role. Locking holes are found on plates that also have holes designed for conventional screws. They are now designed with variable-angle fixation options (something not originally available). They come in both anatomically precontoured and generic forms for use in nearly every bone in the axial and appendicular skeleton. While they can still be used with the previously popularized connections, they can also be used in different combinations or clinical applications.[80,90] These other applications should be termed something other than locked internal fixators (e.g., locking plates used in compression plating, etc.).

In summary, conventional fixation is adequate and more cost-effective when the patient load is likely to be less than the frictional force that can be created. In all other scenarios, the use of locking implants is logical, despite the fact that it is unproven from a quality literature standpoint. Locking fixators are not a panacea. They are just another option in the surgical armamentarium, albeit a technologically advanced option. The success of fracture care relies more on the adherence to basic principles than on the selection of advanced technology.

Speaking of Plate Function

- "It looks like I fragmented this previously simple fracture pattern during a botched attempt at lag screw insertion. I am going to change my plan and go with bridge plating by removing all screws that cross the comminution zone. I do not want to leave screws crossing nonanatomically reduced fracture lines."
- "I was trying to create a tension band plating application, but am unable to reconstruct the far cortex such that it will accept load. Looks like this plate is going to bridge far cortex comminution. I can still try to load the near cortex and protect the implant though."
- "That fracture pattern is transverse. There is no way that I can use a neutralization plate. I will get the plate to function as a compression plate instead."
- "Because I wanted this plate to serve as a buttress, I placed the central screws first. Unfortunately, the vector of compression created a malreduction at the level of the joint. I better remove the screw, achieve an anatomic joint reduction again, and then place screws peripherally at the joint level prior to centrally so this does not happen again."
- "Why did you choose a locking plate with locking screws for that partial articular fracture pattern? Buttress plates are typically used with conventional screws so that they will closely conform to the contours of the bone."

Specific Design Features: Shape, Holes, and So On

To reiterate, a plate is a thin sheet of metal or other material that is most commonly used in orthopaedic surgery to fasten pieces of bone together. A plate is defined both by its function and by its name. The function is the biomechanical purpose of the plate. The name typically refers to the plate shape or plate design.[74] Different plate names were derived from the evolution of plate features. There are three primary plate features that should be considered: (1) shape, (2) surface contouring, and (3) hole design. Let us consider each one separately and review some advantages afforded by the evolution in design. Realize that these design features were simultaneously changing. Separating them helps in explaining the changes, but is somewhat artificial in light of the concurrent changes that were occurring.

Plate shape refers to the basic form of the plate. Generic plate shapes were designed to be used on many different bones in the skeleton. These generic shapes were rectangular in appearance. Surgeon contouring allowed for generic plates to be used in both flat bone applications as well as on more complex bony contours. Simple modifications of the rectangular shape included the T-shaped and L-shaped plates. While these were not perfectly anatomically contoured to fit the curves of specific bones, they did find logical applications in certain places. For example, the T-shaped and L-shaped plate designs were logically placed around periarticular areas, whereby the T or L portion was placed adjacent to the epiphysis. Because the epiphyseal component of the fracture was limited in length, that portion of the plate was designed to allow for additional screw placement outside of the centerline of screws. The goal was to allow for more balanced fixation for fractures that were closer to or included the articular surface. While generic plate shapes are still available and commonly used, anatomically precontoured plates have been designed for nearly every bone in the skeleton. This design modification allows for three specific advantages: (1) limited time required for contouring, (2) lower profile segments in periarticular areas leading to less soft tissue irritation, and (3) additional periarticular hole options leading to increased screw density.

Plate surface contouring refers to the material cutout portions noted on the surface of the plates. The original plates consisted of flat rectangles with no material cutout portions

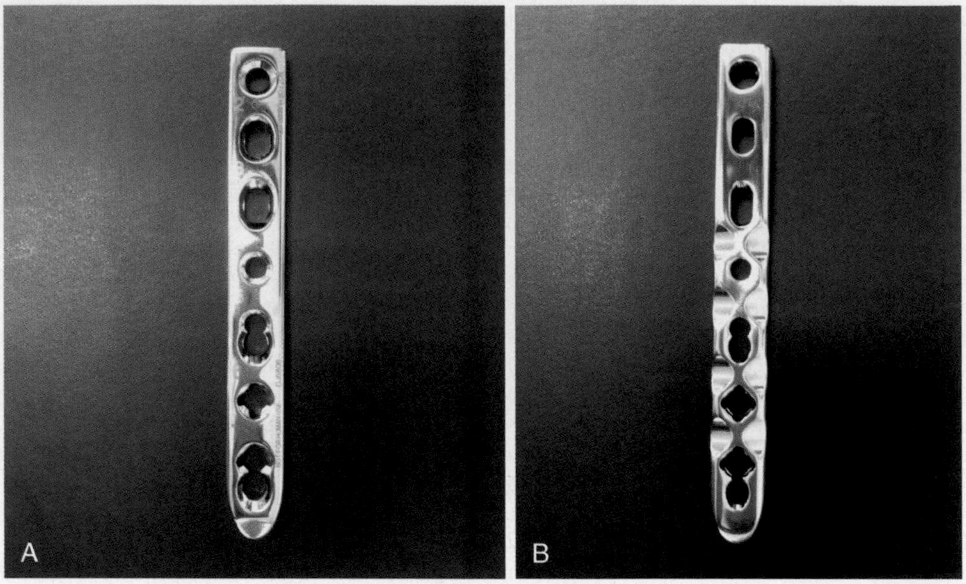

Figure 8-52. A, Plate hole design modifications. **B,** Corresponding undersurface plate hole modifications. The top hole is a conventional round hole. For the head of the screw to seat into the hole, the screw must be placed perpendicular to the hole. The undersurface of this hole reveals no material relief. The second hole is the dynamic compression unit (DCU) that was present in the dynamic compression plates (DCP Synthes). It allows for compression only in one direction (requiring a center for the plate) and the undersurface has no material relief. The third hole is found in the limited contact dynamic compression plate (LC-DCP Synthes). It is akin to a symmetric DCU that allows for compression in both directions. The undersurface has material relief, leading to less periosteal compression (i.e., limited contact) and greater screw angulation. The fourth hole is a uniaxial locking hole. Again, it requires screw placement perpendicular to the hole in the plate (similar to the original round hole), but it is threaded, allowing for threaded screw heads to lock into the plate. The fifth hole is a combination hole that combines a locking hole with a conventional compression hole. The sixth hole is a variable-angle locking hole. Only parts of the hole are threaded, allowing for threaded screw heads to lock into the hole at differing angulations. The last hole is a combination hole that consists of a variable-angle locking hole and a conventional compression hole. While this is a plate hole progression found within the implants of a single company (Synthes Holding AG), the basic design characteristics can be found across many implant company production lines. In addition, the locking mechanism presented here is not the only locking mechanism available (refer to text). *WL,* Working length.

apart from the screw holes themselves. A few challenges were encountered with this simple design.[83] First, attempts at contouring commonly led to kinking of the plate through a screw hole. This was less than ideal in that the screw holes were already serving as stress risers in the plate (hence the kinking through the holes with attempted contouring). This kinking led to improper screw seating. Second, the holes represented distinct stress risers in the plate, as the material was not distributed in a way to create continuous stiffness along the length of the plate. Third, the area of the plate in contact with the bone surface was maximized with this design. Although this was initially felt to be ideal in terms of creating friction with conventional screws, it subsequently became clear that plate contact equated to periosteal blood supply compromise. This was noticed primarily in plate removal, with avascular segments thought to increase the risk of refracture. To alleviate these three problems, material began to be taken away from the undersurface of the plate. This symmetrically distributed bending stiffness (allowing for plate contouring between the holes rather than kinking within the holes) and decreased the amount of periosteal compression (by limiting the amount of material in contact with the periosteum).[83] A correlate to this removal of material from the undersurface of the plate was removal of material from the in-line or side surface of the plate. These plates—known as *reconstruction plates*—similarly allowed for improved contouring, but in a different plane. This material cutout allowed for ease in contouring a plate on the flat (i.e., in the plane of the plate). This design change takes advantage of a physical property known as the moment of inertia (remember the earlier discussion in screw design of the inner diameter of a screw). The bending and torsional stiffness of an implant are most affected by the material farthest away from the center of the implant. When material is taken away from the undersurface of a plate, bending the plate perpendicular to its axis becomes easier. When material is taken away from the side surface of the plate, bending the plate parallel to its axis (on the flat) becomes easier. This is why reconstruction plates are commonly used in areas of complex contour (e.g., pelvis, clavicle, distal humerus). What makes the reconstruction plates easier to bend also makes them more likely to fail under smaller loads.

Plate hole design refers to the shape of the screw holes in the plate. The original screw holes were round on the top coning down to a flat undersurface (Fig. 8-52).[84] They required conventional screw placement perpendicular to the axis of the plate. A few challenges were encountered with this simple design. First, compression could not be achieved using the screw hole alone with this plate design. Compression required using either a device that was an extension of the plate (e.g., Danis coapteur), using a device that was centrally located in the plate (e.g., turnbuckle design), or using a device that was separate from but placed off the end of the plate (e.g., articulated tensioning device). These choices required either an extension of the incision required for plate placement or complex plate manufacturing and inherent mechanical property compromise. With the continued focus of achieving compression across the fracture site, plate holes changed from round to oval. This took advantage of an old carpenter's principle: When a screw is eccentrically positioned in a plate hole, the inclined surface of the screw hits the edge of the plate, creating displacement perpendicular to the long axis of the screw.[83] This further changed to a spherical geometry that allowed for a more congruent fit between the screw head and the plate in a variety of screw positions and orientations. This geometry allowed for 20 degrees of screw angulation along the long axis of the bone. The double inclined plate hole was described as the combination of an inclined and horizontal cylinder that guides the movement of a sphere (the screw undersurface). Continuing with the focus on compression, the desire to combine lag screws and a self-compressing plate led to another modification. When lag screws were placed through a plate hole at an obliquity toward the fracture, the screw head could move down the inclined plane and displace toward the fracture. This caused the threads of the screw to contact the undersurface of the plate, preventing compression. The creation of oblique undercuts on the lower side of the plate hole prevented this phenomenon from occurring (see Fig. 8-52). The oblique undercuts allowed for a further increase in range of screw angulation to 40 degrees along the long axis of the bone.[83] Additional hole modifications moved away from maximizing compression and toward creating a fixed-angle interface. Fully threaded plate holes allowed for screws with a threaded head to lock into the holes, negating the need for friction. Partially threaded plate holes allowed for variable-angle screw trajectories with fully threaded screw heads. Different modifications of the locking principle incorporated threaded caps that could fit over conventional screws to lock the screws into the plate as well as differential metal softness, allowing screws to lock into plates by cutting threads.

Speaking of Plate Design

- "I was hoping to use a precontoured plate for this malunion correction, but it doesn't fit the abnormal contours of the bone."
- "This reconstruction plate is really easy to contour along the plane of the plate. I guess that is going to make the construct less stable along that plane as well. I better make sure the bone can help support the plate."
- "This plate has material relief on the side that does not contact the bone. The purpose cannot be to limit periosteal compression. It must be to evenly distribute stiffness, limit the stress riser effect, and ease contouring."

Intramedullary Nail or Rod

Up to this point, we have placed emphasis on precise language in the description of internal fixation principles. In order to continue to do so, we must understand the history of the intramedullary nail and see how design changes have led to an altered mechanical form of stability. The name given to the device should reflect this change in stability; however, in today's parlance, it commonly does not. After covering the form of stability provided by the intramedullary device, we will move to cover general design features that are present by describing the different parts of the device. Following this, we will cover the basic steps that are necessary for the insertion of an intramedullary rod in any long bone.

Mechanical Form of Stability

In carpentry, a nail is a mechanical device that takes the form of a metal spike with a shaft that is bookended by a broad flat head and a sharp tip. It is most commonly inserted into wood as a fastening device to attach one piece to another. It achieves its mechanical function by a term known as elastic impingement or elastic locking. To clarify, the nail is hammered through two pieces of wood, which have elastic properties. The wood fibers expand temporarily, but then attempt to return to their original state. This expansion and return creates and maintains the fastening effect afforded by the nail. The construct (nail plus pieces of wood) loses stability in a number of different ways. If a pilot hole similar to the nail diameter is drilled for the nail prior to insertion, then the nail no longer provides the same degree of elastic impingement, because wood fibers have been removed and the fit is no longer elastic. It may still keep the pieces together if gravity is favorable, but rotation of the pieces of wood around the nail is possible. The pieces can even glide apart along the axis of the nail if the connection is stressed. If the wood is excessively brittle, then inserting the nail may lead to fragmentation and fracture propagation, which are parasitic to the elastic forces. If the two pieces of wood have differing mechanical properties (e.g., one is rotten and the other is not), then the fastening effect is limited by the elastic forces that can be created in the rotten piece.

The original Küntscher design for fracture fixation functioned as an intramedullary nail. It did so based on the design of the implant and the technique of insertion. Staying with the analogy of a carpenter's nail and wood, the intramedullary nail was the carpenter's nail and the bone fragments were the wood pieces. There was one distinct difference. The elastic expansion was not occurring in the bone as it did in the wood. It was occurring in the nail itself. The original Küntscher nail was slotted along its length and had a conical tip. When inserted, the nail diameter decreased through the slot closing down. As it attempted to expand, it created elastic impingement, which afforded stability (Fig. 8-53).[91] Indications for nonlocked, slotted intramedullary nail use were dependent on the location and the type of the fracture.[92] This was necessary because construct stability was a function of both the implant and the bone. The goal was to create a load-sharing environment. The device functioned as an internal gliding splint.

Stability in bending was provided by the tight connection between the bone and the nail (elastic impingement) and the relationship of the bone pieces (reduction). Imagine attempting to bend a carpenter's nail that was connecting two pieces of wood. The bending forces would be absorbed by the contact between the pieces of wood and by the nail itself. If the pieces of wood and contact were both of good quality, then bending forces would be easily resisted. If one of the pieces of wood was rotten, the nail would begin to wallow around in that piece, and stability would be compromised. If the contact between the two pieces of wood was limited (e.g., there was space between the two pieces that the nail spanned), then the nail would be the only thing absorbing the bending forces until the two pieces impacted.

Stability in rotation was provided primarily by the reduced fracture. There was some stability afforded by elastic impingement (imagine the friction that must be overcome when attempting to rotate one piece of wood around a nail). This stability was a function of the area of contact between the nail and the intramedullary canal and the tightness of fit. As elastic impingement forces faded, the fracture ends could move with respect to each other. The fracture configuration

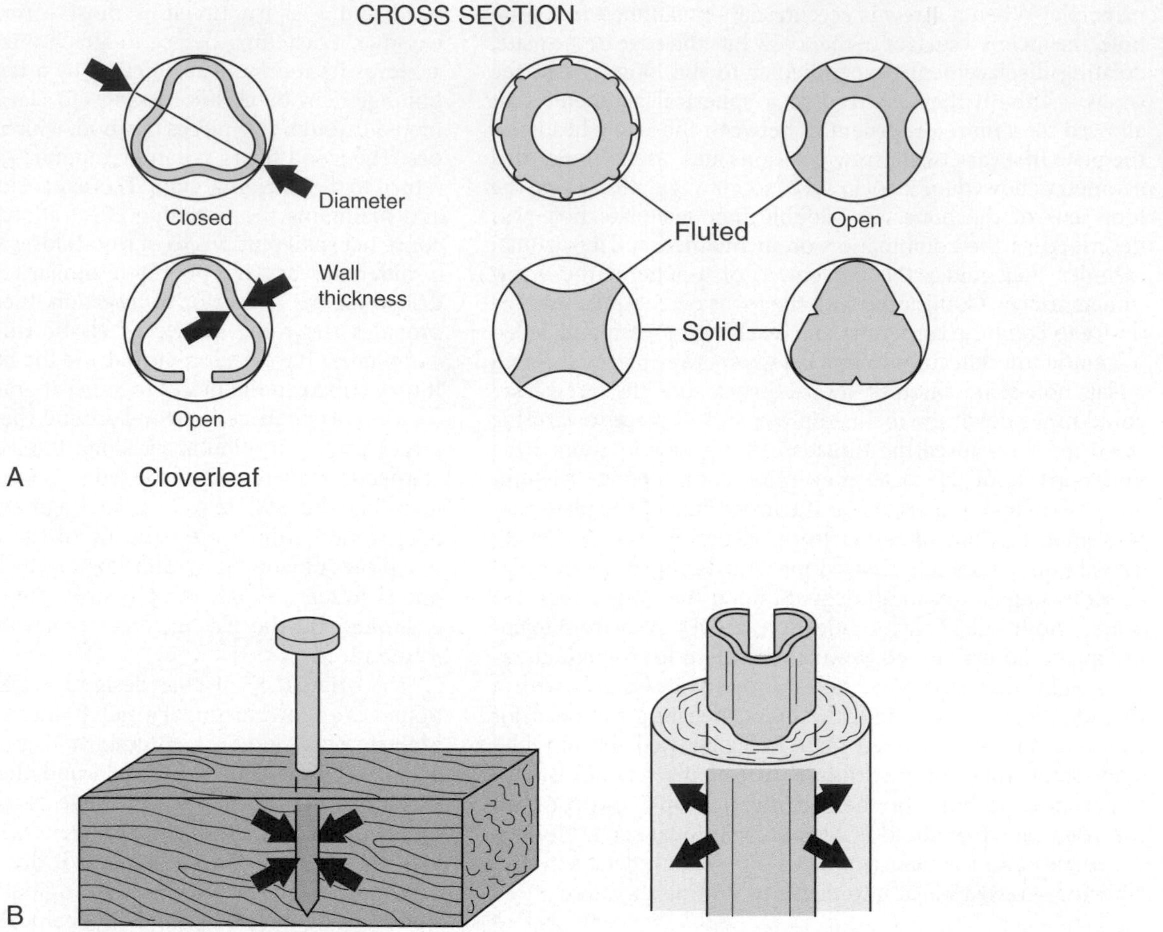

Figure 8-53. Intramedullary nail design and function. **A,** The cross-sectional designs of multiple intramedullary nails are revealed. The first differentiation noted is between open section (slotted) and closed section nails. Both of these are cloverleaf in cross section. The second differentiation is noted between cannulated and solid nails. Within this differentiation includes multiple different cross-sectional shapes. Flutes are marked. These assisted in improving torsional control (less important now that interlocking is available). **B,** The mechanism of elastic impingement is represented in a carpenter's nail and a slotted nail in bone. *(Source:* ***A,*** *Image redrawn from Bechtold JE, Kyle RF, Perren SM. In Browner BD, Edwards CC, editors: The science and practice of intramedullary nailing, ed 2, Baltimore, 1996, Williams & Wilkins;* ***B,*** *Image reproduced from Street DM. In Browner BD, Edwards CC, editors: The science and practice of intramedullary nailing, ed 2, Baltimore, 1996, Williams & Wilkins.)*

and reduction prevented this. Imagine attempting to rotate two pieces of wood with oblique edges that were connected by a carpenter's nail. The obliquity of the edges affords stability against rotation of the pieces.

Stability in length was also provided primarily by the reduced fracture. Elastic impingement once again afforded some mechanical stability. Once the elastic impingement began to fade, the reduced fracture determined length stability. Consider two pieces of wood with rotten surfaces. When the two are pushed together, the surfaces collapse until stability is reached through healthier parts of the wood coming into contact. This is analogous to a comminuted fracture gap.

It should now be obvious that with the original Küntscher nail design, the mechanical device was analogous to a carpenter's nail. The construct stability could be manipulated based on the size of the nail, but was highly dependent on the location and configuration of the fracture. With simple diaphyseal fracture patterns, the load-sharing environment that was created allowed for excellent fracture stability. Intrinsic stability was afforded by the reduced fracture even after elastic impingement forces faded. With simple metaphyseal fracture patterns, stability became an issue because the nail had minimal elastic impingement forces in the shorter metaphyseal segment. In that segment, the nail was contacting soft metaphyseal bone rather than the harder endosteal bone of the diaphysis. The elastic forces that could be created in the metaphyseal segment were parasitized by the marginal quality of the bone (similar to using a carpenter's nail in rotten wood). With complex diaphyseal fracture patterns, the load-sharing environment was compromised because the tube of bone was not intact at the level of the fracture. Load sharing could not occur until sliding allowed for intact portions of the tube to impact. The consequence of this was shortening and limb length inequality. To compensate for this, additional implants, such as cerclage wires, were used to reconstruct the tube of bone in comminuted zones in an attempt to regain some intrinsic stability.[93] The results were variable.

As the design of the intramedullary device and the technique of insertion changed, so did the mechanical form of stability afforded. Let us move ahead many years to more current intramedullary device designs. The majority of devices are now closed-section rather than slotted. This means that minimal elastic impingement is being afforded by any compression/expansion effect of the implant shape. A common technique to ease insertion is intramedullary reaming. This increases the area of contact by equalizing the diameter of the canal over a larger distance. It also is akin to drilling a hole prior to inserting a carpenter's nail; it limits potential for elastic impingement. The majority of devices today have holes drilled through the proximal and distal ends for the placement of interlocking screws. These interlocking screws (also termed *bolts*) provide the construct with length and rotational stability that is somewhat independent of the bone at the fracture site. They do so through creating fixed contact points proximal and distal to the fracture between the intramedullary device and the intact segments of bone. This both limits dependence on fracture location and configuration and makes the intramedullary device load bearing when limited osseous contact is present at the fracture site itself. In doing so, it limits shortening but transfers stress to the bone/intramedullary device/interlocking screw junctions. In terms of mechanical stability, this intramedullary device is functioning more as a connecting rod than a nail, hence the more appropriate nomenclature of intramedullary rod for currently used intramedullary devices.

Speaking of an Intramedullary Rod

- "It seems that an intramedullary screw functions like an unlocked rod. I better be careful to use it only for axially stable fracture patterns."
- "I guess it makes sense that the average intramedullary nail diameter has decreased. It is not really functioning like a nail anymore. Maybe I should limit reaming based on chatter in light of that."
- "Using an intramedullary rod for metaphyseal fracture patterns is very different than diaphyseal fracture patterns. The rod really doesn't provide as much resistance to bending in the canal of the metaphysis. The stick in the bucket analogy makes more sense now."

General Design Features

Similar to a screw or a plate, the intramedullary rod has general design features that help to determine its function. These are relatively consistent across all lines of intramedullary rods (both location-specific lines and company lines). Let us break the intramedullary rod down into its component parts and evaluate how changes in the design of these parts create changes in the insertion and function of the rod. It is first necessary to define the parts. The proximal end is the portion of the rod that extends from the proximal tip to the end of the interlocking screw holes. The central portion of the rod extends from the end of the proximal interlocking screw holes to the beginning of the distal interlocking screw holes. The distal portion of the rod is the portion that extends from the beginning of the distal interlocking screw holes through the tip of the rod.

Proximal End. The proximal end of an intramedullary rod has two important design features. The first is the point of connection to the insertion device. The point of connection commonly has both an external notched portion and internal threaded portion. The external notched portion helps to ensure the appropriate seating of the insertion device into the rod. It is often accompanied by alterations in shape of the proximal end of the device (e.g., slopes or angled surfaces). These alterations in shape improve contact area and often help to prevent inappropriate connection between the insertion device and the proximal end of the rod (e.g., backwards connection such that the bow or bend of the rod is in nonanatomic position or the interlocking screw targeting device is oriented from the wrong side of the bone). The internal threaded portion varies in diameter and length. This is important because it prevents one single insertion or extraction device from perfectly threading into every manufacturer's rod. The end of the insertion/extraction device is made to act as a screw that inserts into the female receptacle of the proximal end of the rod. It forms a tight connection that allows for improved force transmission in the presence of axial insertion or extraction forces. When tight contact does not occur, problems arise. These problems include parasitized forces in insertion and extraction and errant targeting of the interlocking screws through the interlocking holes. These problems can arise either from a loosening of the connecting device during insertion/extraction, from fracture of either the proximal end of the rod or the connecting device, or from a compromised fit between the connecting device and the rod (i.e., using a universal device for extraction that does not perfectly thread into the receptacle in the rod).

The second important design feature of the proximal end of the rod is the interlocking holes. The diameter of the interlocking holes defines the necessary diameter of the proximal end of the rod. To simplify, an interlocking hole creates a stress riser in the rod. If the decision is made during implant design to create an interlocking screw of large diameter, then the proximal portion of the rod must be able to mechanically compensate for the size of the interlocking screw. For example, consider the head element that is used in a cephalomedullary rod such as an intramedullary hip screw. The head element is typically larger than the standard interlocking screws that are placed at the distal end of the rod. This is by design because large bending forces are transferred to the head element and the resistance to these bending forces is largely determined by the core diameter of the head element (analogous to screw design discussed earlier). As the head element becomes larger in diameter, then the interlocking hole in the proximal end of the rod must also become larger to accommodate the head element. Larger holes create more significant stress risers in the rod. For this reason, a larger proximal diameter of the rod is necessary. Of interest, it should be understood that the stress riser is also used to the advantage of the designer. Most cephalomedullary rods are designed such that failure will occur through this hole rather than through breaking of the head element. The reason for this is obvious if you have ever tried to remove a broken head element. The degree of difficulty can be high and the amount of bone destruction can be great. While removing a broken cephalomedullary rod is not easy either, it is felt to be easier and less damaging than removing a broken head element.

The number of interlocking screw holes and spacing between them also differs among rods used in different locations and rods from different manufacturers used in the same location. Remember that with the changing mechanical function of the device, less emphasis is placed on the endosteal contact of the rod with the bone and more emphasis is placed on the interlocking screw/rod/bone junctions. As the design of the intramedullary device changed from a nail to a rod, so did the indications. Whereas simple diaphyseal fracture patterns were the previous norm, both complex diaphyseal fracture patterns and metaphyseal fracture patterns became more commonplace indications. As the indications expanded, there was a desire to push the interlocking screw holes to a more extreme position (closer to the ends of the rod). Remember that in these situations, the mechanical stability of the construct is largely dependent on the interlocking screw relationship with the rod and the bone.[94,95] To empower this relationship, a few design modifications have occurred. First, the number of interlocking screw options has increased. Second, the orientation of interlocking screw options has increased. Third, the relationship of the interlocking screw to the rod has been modified. In some instances, the interlocking screws "lock" into the rod through different manufacturing techniques. This locking decreases interlocking screw toggle and decreases the risk of interlocking screw backout (a less common form of interlocking screw failure).

The shape of the interlocking screw hole also deserves mention. While there has been a recent design movement to empower the relationship between the interlocking screw and the rod in the form of "locking" interlocking screws, this concept of varying the tolerance between the interlocking hole and screw is far from new. Static versus dynamic locking is based on this concept. Static locking refers to a stable nonsliding interface between the interlocking screw and the intramedullary rod. It is accomplished by interlocking screw holes with minimal tolerance, such that a relatively tight fit exists between the interlocking screw and the rod. Dynamic locking refers to a controlled motion interface. This can be accomplished in two primary ways. First, the rod can be locked only on one side of the fracture. This allows for both rotational and length changes to occur at the fracture site. This form of dynamic locking is discouraged in modern long bone fracture treatment. The second form of dynamic locking is accomplished by locking on both sides of the fracture, but through different types of interlocking screw holes. On one side, an interlocking screw is placed through a hole of minimal tolerance. On the other side, the interlocking screw is placed through a hole of increased tolerance. To allow for axial compression to occur without rotation, the shape of the dynamic interlocking hole is oblong. The diameter of the interlocking screw closely fits the diameter of the hole, but the length of the hole is much greater than the diameter. This allows for controlled impaction in the absence of rotational instability. If dynamic locking is to be used, this is the preferred form in modern practice. It should be noted that static locking is considered standard in today's practice.[96,97]

Central Portion. The central portion of the rod is the portion between the proximal and distal interlocking holes. Three important design features occur in this portion of the device. These features include the proximal bend, the central curve, and the distal bend.

The first is the proximal bend. The proximal bend has different names depending on where the device is used. The function is the same regardless of the name. The intramedullary rod is primarily contained within the intramedullary canal (hence the name). To be completely contained within the intramedullary canal, then it needs to enter at a point in line with the canal. In antegrade application, this point would be the piriformis fossa in the femur and the anterocentral portion of the articular surface of the tibial plateau for the tibia. It should be clear that using this starting point in the tibia would be less than ideal. Not only is it hard to reach with standard techniques and an intact ACL, it is also traversing an important anatomic portion of the tibial plateau. There was a desire therefore to move the starting point outside of the knee joint to a safer location; but to start outside of the anatomic axis and still reach the anatomic axis for rod placement, a bend had to be incorporated into the rod. In the tibia, this bend was named the Herzog curve. This bend is analogous to the bends found in femoral and humeral intramedullary rods. For antegrade rod insertion in the femur, the piriformis fossa can be a challenging point to reach. It is primarily challenging in patients with truncal and thigh obesity. There was a desire to alleviate starting point struggles by moving the starting point more lateral. This starting point change had a similar effect to that in the tibia, and necessitated a similar design change in the intramedullary rod. Because the starting point was outside of the anatomic axis but the rod was designed to rest in the anatomic axis, a bend was necessary. In the femur, this bend has been named the *proximal offset*.[98,99] It serves the same function as the Herzog curve, but is found in a different plane (coronal plane rather than the sagittal plane). It is in a different plane because that is the plane of movement of the starting point outside of the intramedullary canal. For antegrade rod insertion in the humerus, the rotator cuff must be traversed. There was a desire to alleviate this cuff intrusion, so the starting point changed from one in line with the anatomic axis to one more lateral (with some of the newer designs, this starting point is moving back more medial). Because the starting point was outside of the anatomic axis, but the rod was designed to sit in the anatomic axis, a bend was necessary. In the humerus, this bend was also described in terms of lateral offset and serves the same function as the Herzog curve in the tibial rod and the proximal offset found in lateral entry femoral rods.

The second design feature in the central portion of a rod is the central curve. This is most commonly noted in femoral intramedullary rods and has been termed the *radius of curvature of the rod* (Fig. 8-54).[100] It is found in the sagittal plane because this is the plane of anatomic curvature of the anterior femoral bow. The radius of curvature has received attention because it affects three primary things. It is somewhat artificial to separate these three things, as they are necessarily interrelated; but for the purposes of simplifying the explanation to understand principles, we will do so. First, the starting point and ending point of the rod are affected by the radius of curvature. Consider a straight rod with no radius of curvature inserted into an intact femur with an average anatomic anterior bow of 120 cm.[100] Unlike the coronal plane anatomic axis of the femur, the sagittal plane anatomic axis is more bowed (secondary to the sagittal plane anatomic bow of the femur). In order for the rod to be placed into the anatomic axis, it either has to bend to accommodate the bow or start and end anterior to the anatomic axis. Starting anterior places the rod in the region of the femoral neck. Ending anterior places the rod out of the anterior cortex of the distal femur in the patellofemoral joint. Neither is considered ideal application. By designing a rod with a radius of curvature that nearly matches the anterior bow, then the rod can be maintained in the anatomic axis throughout its course. This is even more important with stiffer rods that will not flex on insertion and thereby put

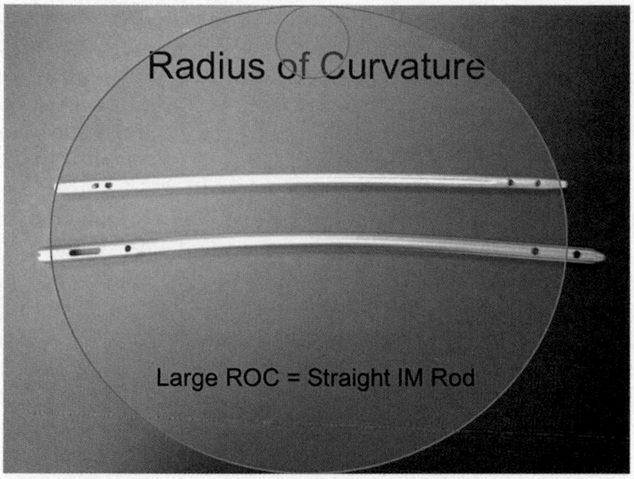

Figure 8-54. Radius of curvature of an intramedullary rod. Two rods are presented. The rod on *top* is straighter. It has a larger radius of curvature (compare to the different radii of the circles that are present). A larger circle has a larger radius. The sides of that circle are straighter than one of a smaller radius. The majority of intramedullary rods today have a radius of curvature that is larger than the sagittal plane anatomic bow of the femur. This helps in understanding how anterior cortical impingement can occur distally. *IM,* Intramedullary; *ROC,* radius of curvature.

the bone at increased risk of iatrogenic fracture. Second, the three-point bend effect of the rod is determined by the mismatch between the radius of curvature of the rod and the bow of the femur. Remember that elastic impingement is no longer prioritized with closed section rods. It is necessary to achieve stability from other mechanical forces. One that we have already discussed is the interlocking screw relationship. Another is the mismatch between the radius of curvature of the rod and the bow of the femur. This mismatch creates a three-point bend effect that helps to maintain construct stability.[100] As a side note, it is likely that this three-point bend effect was just as important as elastic impingement for stability even in the earlier devices. While the radius of curvature of more current rod designs more closely matches the anterior bow of the femur, a mismatch still exists, with the intramedullary rods being straighter (i.e., larger radius of curvature) than the average femur. Third, the insertional hoop stresses are affected by the radius of curvature and starting point. Femoral bursting is a real phenomenon.[101] It can be best understood by thinking about the function of the hoops on a wine cask (Fig. 8-55). When wine is poured into the cask, it begins to exert a centrifugal force (push the slats apart away from the center of the barrel). This centrifugal force is counteracted by hoops that are placed around the barrel. The rod is analogous to the wine. When inserted into the bone, it creates a centrifugal force causing the cortex to spread apart. This force is known as hoop stress. It is alleviated by a rod contour that matches the bone contour and by drilling a larger hole for rod insertion. It is exacerbated by starting the rod more anteriorly (see Fig. 8-55). When the rod starts more anteriorly, it must be directed more posteriorly to reach the anatomic axis. This direction causes the rod to impact against the posterior cortex of the femur. Something has to give at this point. There are two options: (1) Either the rod bends to accommodate the mismatched insertion point and entrance angle, or (2) the bone undergoes fragmentation secondary to the hoop stresses that have been created. This fragmentation is most commonly seen as fracture propagation into the proximal segment.[101]

The third design feature in the central portion of the rod is the distal bend. The distal bend is a design feature most commonly seen in tibial rods (Fig. 8-56). The distal bend typically occurs before the distal interlocking screw holes. Understanding the history of rod design allows one to understand the logic behind the distal bend; it also helps to explain how every design choice is made in the face of a compromise. As the

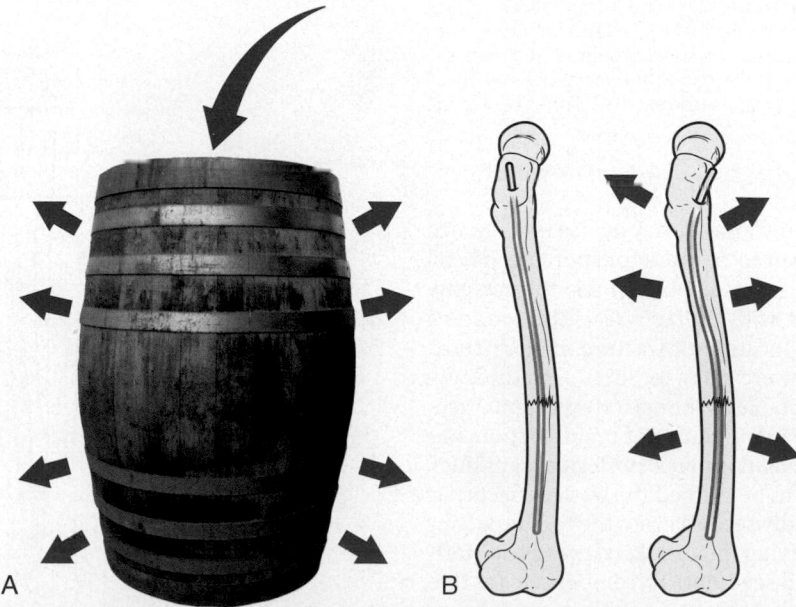

Figure 8-55. **A,** Wine cask with circumferential bands that resist centrifugal forces created by filling the cask with wine. The *arrows* represent the outward forces created by the introduction of more wine. **B,** Hoop stresses created by an intramedullary rod inserted into the femur. Note how an incorrect starting point and entrance angle require the rod to change shape within the canal of the femur. This leads to centrifugal forces (represented by the *arrows*), otherwise known as hoop stresses in the proximal femur. If the stresses are greater than the bone will allow, fragmentation or fracture propagation occur.

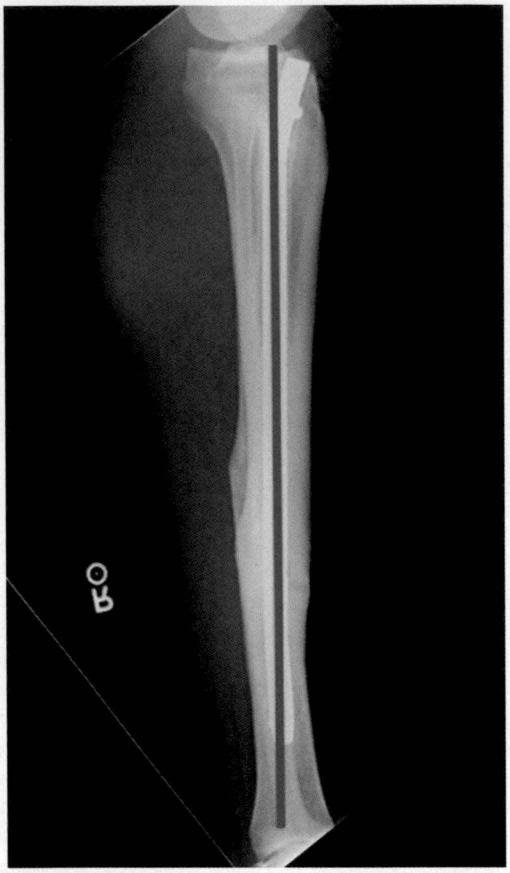

Figure 8-56. Distal bend in a tibial intramedullary rod with a small proximal Herzog curve. The *red line* is centered in the intramedullary rod. Proximally, the rod extends anterior to this line secondary to the Herzog curve. This allows the rod to have an extraarticular starting point, but still reach the anatomic axis of the bone. Distally, more rod is seen anterior to this line secondary to the distal bend that is required to centralize the rod in the anatomic axis secondary to such a small proximal bend. If endosteal healing has occurred proximal to this distal bend, it has the potential to decrease the intramedullary space available for rod extraction. Remember that each design choice comes with a consequence. Using a rod with a small proximal Herzog curve requires a distal bend to re-center the rod in the canal distally. These small proximal Herzog curves were introduced to limit the wedge effect noted in Figure 8-57.

mechanical function of the intramedullary device transitioned from a nail to a rod, it began to be used for more peripheral fractures (i.e., transitioned from diaphyseal use to metaphyseal use). The early results with metaphyseal tibial rodding were fraught with the complication of fracture malreduction. Initial malreduction rates were 60% to 80%, something we would never consider acceptable in modern surgical intervention.[102,103] While there were many causes of malreduction, one was felt to be rod design. Sagittal plane posterior translation of the distal segment came to be termed the wedge effect (Fig. 8-57). It was felt to be partially secondary to the rod impacting the posterior cortex and driving the distal segment posteriorly with respect to the proximal segment. To compensate for this, manufacturers chose two design changes. First, the Herzog curve was moved more proximally. Second, the Herzog curve was lessened (smaller angle of bend). These changes helped to contain the Herzog curve within the proximal segment and move it further away from the posterior cortex. While helping to prevent the wedge effect, it came with a compromise. With the starting point and entrance angle into the proximal segment held constant, a smaller Herzog curve led to the rod being located posteriorly at the level of the distal tibia. To compensate for this effect and return the intramedullary rod to the anatomic axis distally, an apex posterior distal bend was incorporated into the rod design (see Fig. 8-56). To understand why this matters, compare the difference in relationship of the proximal bend and the fracture to that of the distal bend and the fracture. Once healing has occurred and the decision is made to remove the rod, this difference takes on significance. The proximal bend does not have to traverse the healed fracture on extraction. The distal bend does. With any sagittal plane malalignment of the intramedullary canal or endosteal callus formation at the site of the fracture, extracting the distal bend became problematic.[104] It was so problematic, that more current tibial rod designs take care to limit the distal bend as much as possible.

Distal End. The distal portion of the rod is the portion that extends from the beginning of the distal interlocking screw holes through the tip of the rod. It has two important design features. The first is a feature previously discussed in the proximal rod discussion, namely interlocking screw holes. The concepts are exactly the same and will not be repeated. The second feature is the tip of the rod. The original design was a conical shape. The conical shape assisted with insertion and allowed the tip to act as a wedge, decreasing the distal diameter with respect to the central diameter. This assisted the nail in finding its way into the distal segment. The tip of the cone was rounded rather than sharp in order to

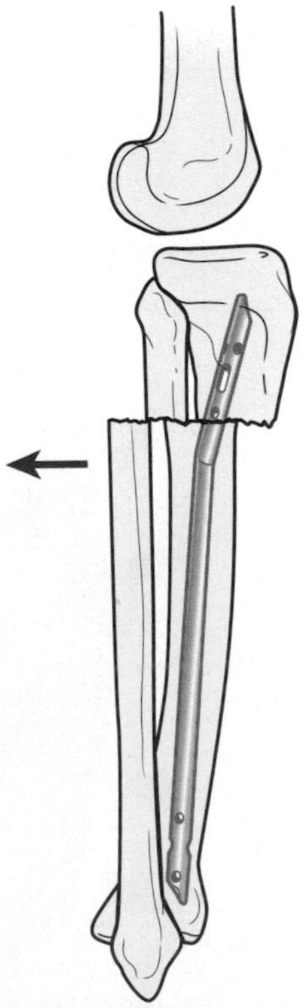

Figure 8-57. Proximal tibial rodding and the wedge effect. Contact of the Herzog curve with the posterior cortex of the distal segment led to posterior translation of that distal segment. To counteract this, smaller and more proximal Herzog curves were developed.

prevent damage to neurovascular structures if the rod inadvertently escaped from the intramedullary axis. The flute at the tip was also tightened in an effort to prevent binding of the guide pin between the nail and the cortex. The tip itself was more rounded at the leading edge to prevent binding of the cortex between the nail and the guide pin.[91] With the transition in the mechanical function from the nail to the rod, very little has changed with respect to the tip design. It is typically conical and slightly rounded in a more symmetric fashion.

Other Design Features. A few other design features deserve mention. These include cross-sectional shape, rod diameter, and cannulation.

Cross-Sectional Shape. The early intramedullary nails developed by Küntscher had a V-shaped cross-section, which allowed the sides of the nail to compress and fit tightly in the canal. The design was modified to a cloverleaf shape with a longitudinal slot running the length of the implant to increase the strength of the nail and permit insertion over a guide wire (see Fig. 8-53). As with the V-design, the two halves of the cloverleaf are compressed into the slot as the nail is driven into the medullary canal. Because the amount of compression is within the elastic zone of the nail, the nail springs open and presses on the endosteal surface, increasing the frictional contact in the medullary canal (see Fig. 8-53).[91] Conversely, having a slot running down the nail decreases the nail's torsional rigidity.[105] When the nail-bone complex is loaded, the decreased torsional rigidity permits a small amount of motion, which promotes callus formation. The decreased torsional rigidity also allows the nail to accommodate to the bone and is therefore said to be more forgiving. If the nail does not match the shape of the medullary canal exactly, an accommodative will decrease the likelihood of iatrogenic fracture. If the nail is too stiff and does not deform on insertion, the bone can shatter. The cloverleaf shape has been used extensively for decades with great success. The design has been successful because it has adequate torsional rigidity to permit fracture union but sufficient elasticity to adapt to bone anatomy on insertion.

In contrast to the slotted cloverleaf shape found in early nails, rods have been designed with no slots and a variety of other cross-sectional shapes. Removal of the slot significantly increases the torsional rigidity of the nail. This design is desirable when a small-diameter rod is used (e.g., when the medullary canal is small or its enlargement is contraindicated). Closed-section locking rods were designed for the femur to avoid excessive torsional deformation of the rod on insertion, which complicated distal screw fixation. The torsional stiffness of any implant can be increased substantially by the addition of spines that run the entire length of the nail. The curved indentation in the surface of the nail between the spines is called a *flute*. The edges of the spines can be designed to cut into the bone, increasing frictional resistance at the nail-bone interface. However, this contact can increase the difficulty of implant removal.

Diameter. The medullary canals of long bones have a narrow central region called the *isthmus*. Before reaming was developed, the diameter of intramedullary nails was limited to the narrowest diameter of the medullary cavity at the isthmus (Fig. 8-58). With reaming, larger implants can be introduced and, when compared to rods with a smaller diameter, large-diameter rods with the same cross-sectional shape are stiffer and stronger. In practice, the relationship between diameter and strength is not linear. The rod stiffness can be kept constant by changing the wall thickness. For example, a 12-mm-diameter rod has a wall thickness of 1.2 mm while for 14- and 16-mm rods, it is decreased to 1.0 mm.

Cannulation. The final nail construction characteristic is the core geometry. A hollow-core, or cannulated, rod allows insertion of the nail over a guide wire. In general, a curved-tip guide wire can be maneuvered across a displaced fracture site more easily than a solid intramedullary nail. Another advantage of the cannulated rod may be a reduction in intramedullary pressure. Haas and coworkers found a 42% increase in compartment pressures when introducing a solid rod, compared with 1.6% for a cannulated rod.[106] One reported disadvantage of cannulation is the potential space for harboring bacteria. Although noted to be the case in an animal model, transition of this finding to human fracture management should be done with caution.[107]

Speaking of Intramedullary Rod Design

- "This rod has a proximal bend but the anatomic axis doesn't. I better understand how that bend was designed to relate to the starting point and entrance angle; otherwise, I will create a malreduction."
- "Since this fracture pattern is metaphyseal, I should choose an intramedullary rod with multiple interlocking options. The number and orientation of interlocking screws will be even more important in determining my construct stability than if it were a diaphyseal fracture."
- "We have to remove the tibial rod in an effort to clear the intramedullary osteomyelitis. It looks like it has a distal bend. This could be trouble since the fracture has healed and the canal looks narrowed around the area of healing."
- "I want to use a long cephalomedullary rod for this osteoporotic pertrochanteric fracture. I should be careful to ensure the radius of curvature comes close to matching the anterior bow of the femur. The difference between the two will not be absorbed at the fracture since it is so proximal. That means this rod could end very anteriorly once it reaches the distal femur."

STEPS OF INTRAMEDULLARY RODDING

Now that the common design features of an intramedullary rod are known, the common steps of insertion warrant attention. These steps are consistent regardless of which bone is being rodded and which manufacturer's system is being used. They are generic steps that are defined only by the concept of inserting a rod into a fractured tube of bone. To simplify the discussion, the terms will be used with respect to antegrade rodding. The same steps apply to retrograde rodding, but the location terms would be reversed (i.e., proximal vs. distal, etc.). The steps include (1) starting point and entrance angle into the proximal segment, (2) reduction of the fracture, (3) reaming (if chosen), (4) entrance angle into and ending point in the distal segment, and (5) interlocking screw insertion. Let us take time with each step individually to better understand how each is important and how the sequence occasionally varies.

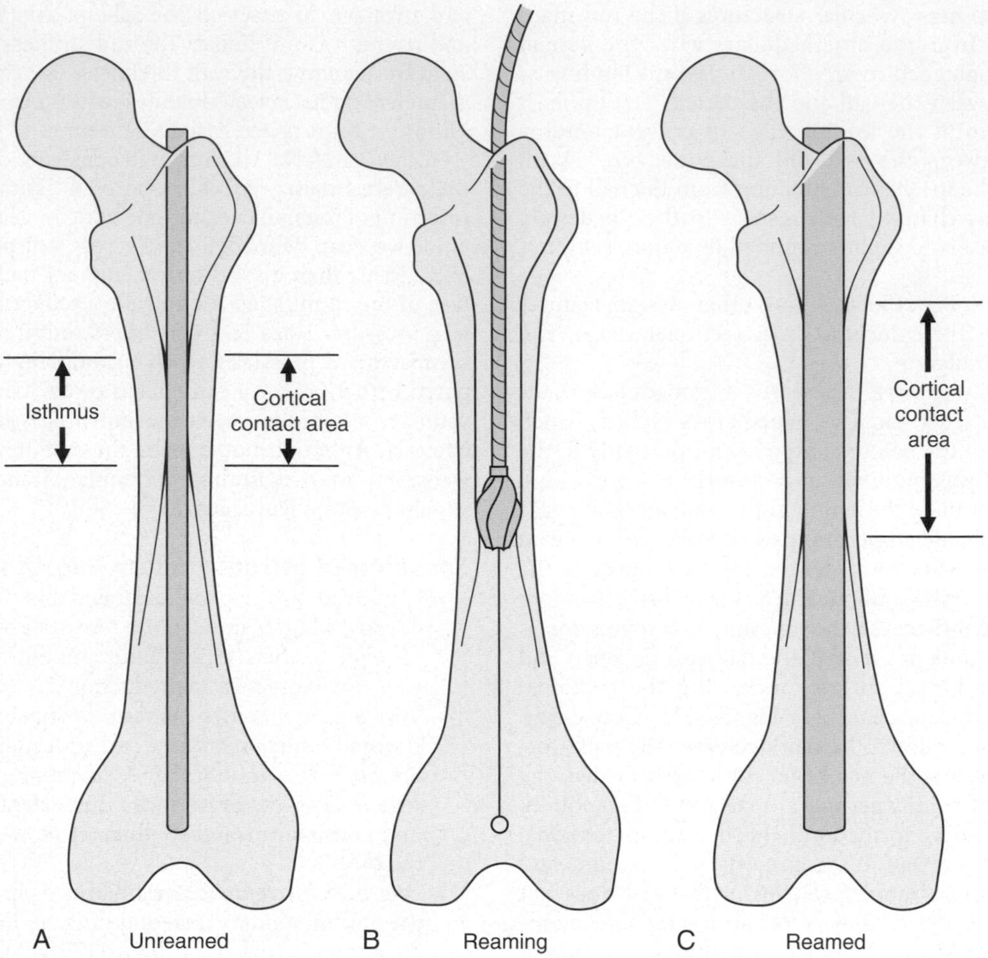

Figure 8-58. The effect of reaming on cortical contact area. **A,** The isthmus is the narrowest portion of the intramedullary canal of the femur. Without reaming, the isthmus limits the size of the nail to be placed and the area of cortical contact with the nail. **B,** Reaming widens and lengthens the isthmic portion of the intramedullary canal. **C,** After reaming, a larger diameter nail may be placed and greater cortical contact area achieved.

Starting Point and Entrance Angle into the Proximal Segment

Listing starting point and entrance angle as a single step is purposeful; splitting this step into two separate parts is as well. The starting point is commonly discussed and as a concept well understood. It refers to the point at which the rod starts in the proximal segment. It is defined by the starting wire and opening reamer. The entrance angle refers to the angle at which the rod enters the segment. These two are separated because it is possible to choose an excellent starting point and a poor entrance angle.[102] Similarly, it is possible to choose a poor starting point and an appropriate entrance angle. Accomplishing the first step appropriately requires both the starting point and the entrance angle to be correct. Let us diagrammatically represent the two parts of this single step (Fig. 8-59). Both the starting point and the entrance angle are defined by the implant that is being used. The implant design is dependent upon two things: (1) The safe zone for entrance into the bone, and (2) the beginning point of the anatomic axis. These two are not always the same. For example, in tibial rod insertion, the beginning point of the anatomic axis is in the articular surface of the tibial plateau. This is not considered a safe zone for entrance. Because of this, the optimal starting point was moved outside of the anatomic axis and the implant incorporated a proximal bend. It is important to understand the design of the implant in order to know what starting point and entrance angle is required.[98] The part of the implant that defines the starting point and entrance angle is the proximal bend. To clarify, if a piriformis start femoral rod design is chosen, there will be no proximal bend. The starting point is the piriformis fossa. The entrance angle is straight into the anatomic axis. If a starting point other than the piriformis fossa is chosen, then getting into the intramedullary canal will require an entrance angle that is out of line with the anatomic axis. This creates a mismatch between the design of the rod and the shape of the bone, which leads to hoop stresses and potential fragmentation of the proximal segment.

Starting point and entrance angle errors lead to three common problems. First, the starting point can damage important structures when placed in a poor location. For example, if the starting point of a tibial rod is placed too laterally, it has the potential to damage the anterolateral articular surface.[108] If the starting point of a retrograde femoral nail is placed too anteriorly, it has the potential to damage cartilage in the patellofemoral joint.[109-111] Second, a mismatch between the starting point/entrance angle and the proximal bend in the

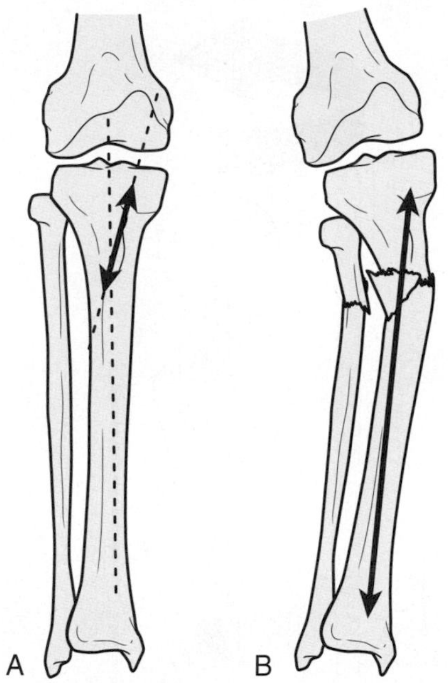

Figure 8-59. Starting point and entrance angle diagram. This concept was introduced after it was noted that intramedullary rodding led to a high malreduction rate for proximal fractures. One cannot just consider the starting point. The entrance angle is equally important. This is a mechanical concept and can be applied to other bones. For example, starting lateral to the piriformis fossa and entering with a medial entrance angle leads to a varus deformity of the proximal femur. It can also be applied to the same bone in a different plane. For example, starting anteriorly and aiming far posterior in the tibia leads to an apex anterior sagittal plane deformity with tibial rodding. *(Source: Redrawn from Freedman EL, Johnson EE: Radiographic analysis of tibial fracture malalignment following intramedullary nailing, Clin Orthop Relat Res (315):25–33, June 1995.)*

implant can lead to a malreduction of the fracture.[98,102] For example, it a tibial nail is started too medially, it requires a laterally oriented entrance angle to reach the anatomic axis. When the rod is inserted into the distal segment, this imparts a valgus deformity to the fracture (see Fig. 8-59). This is one of the reasons that proximal tibial fracture rodding through a medial parapatellar starting point has been deemed problematic. Similarly, consider proximal femoral rodding using a piriformis entry rod. If the starting point in the coronal plane is lateral to the piriformis fossa (i.e., on the greater trochanter), then a medially based entrance angle is required to reach the anatomic axis. When the rod is inserted into the distal segment, this imparts a varus deformity. Third, a mismatch between the starting point/entrance angle and the proximal bend in the implant can lead to proximal propagation of the fracture secondary to hoop stresses. For example, if a piriformis start rod is inserted too anteriorly, it requires a posteriorly oriented entrance angle. The rod then impacts the posterior cortex and something has to give.[101] Either the rod bends creating internal strain or the bone breaks (Fig. 8-60, *B*).

Reduction of the Fracture

Reduction of the fracture is required prior to insertion of the rod (and prior to reaming across the fracture site if reaming is chosen). Reduction can be accomplished in either an open or closed manner (the defining difference between open and closed rodding) and with direct or indirect reduction techniques. The quality of reduction typically chosen is the restoration of length, alignment, and rotation between the proximal and distal segments rather than precise repositioning of every fracture fragment. This time point in the sequence of steps of intramedullary rodding is the latest that reduction should occur. It should not occur after the reamer is passed across the fracture. It may, however, be necessary to enact a reduction prior to achieving an appropriate starting point and entrance angle into the proximal segment. To clarify, a subtrochanteric fracture commonly presents with proximal fragment displacements of flexion, abduction, and external rotation. Without improving the reduction of the proximal segment in this scenario, it is impossible to achieve a safe and accurate starting point and entrance angle. Attempting to do so is hampered by the iliac wing in the coronal plane and by the sciatic nerve in the sagittal plane. This means that restoring more normal alignment of the proximal segment is necessary prior to achieving a starting point and entrance angle into that segment. It does not mean that the fracture must be perfectly reduced at this point. In fact, at times it is useful to over-reduce the proximal fragment (e.g., increase adduction past neutral) in order to gain access to the starting point. There is a caveat: Care must be taken not to ream across a malreduced fracture with the opening reamer in this setting.

Reaming (If Chosen)

Küntscher initially attempted intramedullary fixation of fractures with implants that were designed to fit within the normal medullary canal. Dissatisfied with the high rates of malunion, nonunion, and implant failure obtained with these small-diameter nails, he developed the technique of reaming to enlarge the intramedullary canal.[112] This method produced a more uniform canal diameter and increased the potential surface area for contact between the implant and the endosteum. Increased contact facilitated better alignment of the fracture fragments and enhanced the rotational stability of fracture fixation. Additionally, larger canal diameters permitted insertion of larger nails with greater stiffness and fatigue strength. The successful use of larger diameter intramedullary nails paved the way for the production of rods containing holes through which interlocking screws could be inserted.

To enlarge the medullary canal, reamers are passed within the bone. They were developed for industry to precisely size and finish an already existing hole without removing large amounts of material. They have a larger caliber than drill bits because their main purpose is to enlarge an already existing hole. Reamers are designed to be end cutting, side cutting, or both. The tip design of most reamers is a truncated cone called a *chamfer.* The *chamfer angle* is the angle between the central axis of the reamer and the cutting edge at its end. With end-cutting reamers, the majority of the cutting is accomplished by the chamfer. Additional flutes are added along the sides of the reamer to increase the cutting surface and distribute the force more evenly. If additional relief or angle is added to the land (the area between the flutes), it provides for a longitudinal cutting edge. This change permits an increase in accuracy but weakens the cutting edge. If cutting is performed primarily by the longitudinal edges, the reamer is said to be side cutting. Generally, end-cutting reamers are used only for the initial passes. An end-cutting reamer has the potential to cut eccentrically when reaming across displaced fractures because it

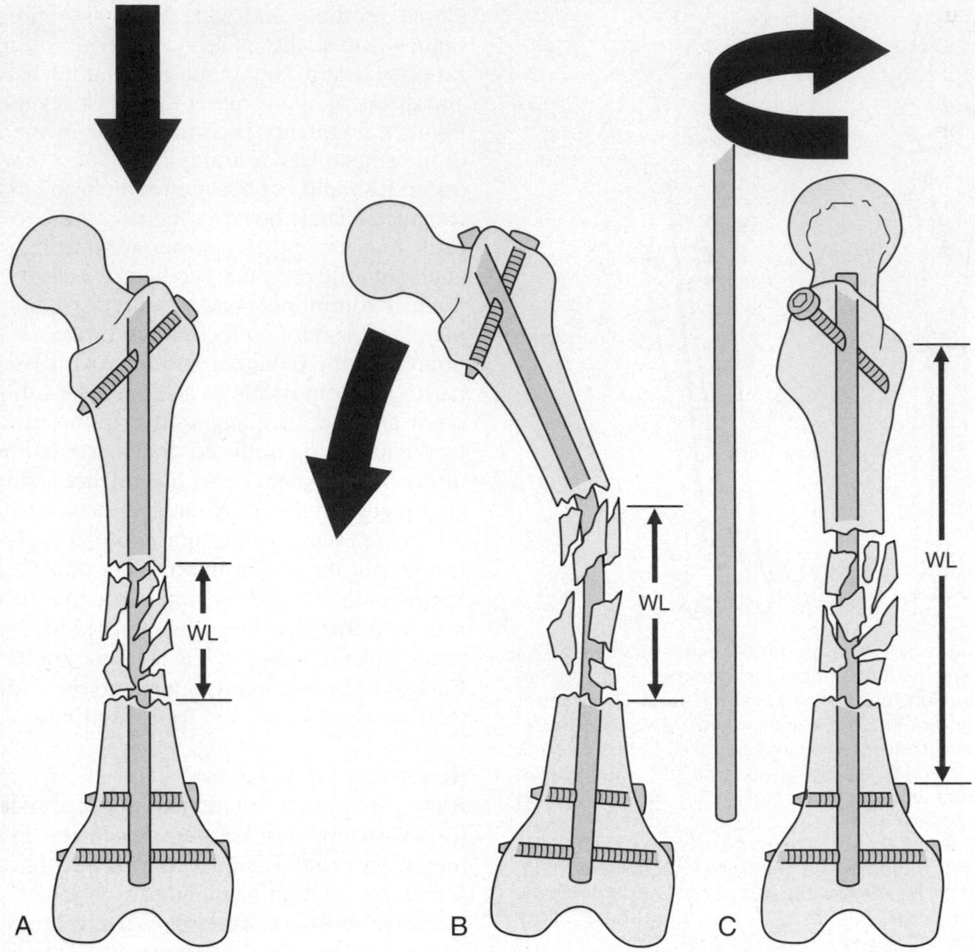

Figure 8-60. Working length for an intramedullary rod. Note the differences depending on the force applied. The working length refers to the point of stability above and below the fracture zone. **A,** With axial loading, the rod deflects slightly and contacts the endosteum just above and below the fracture zone. **B,** With bending, the rod deflects and again contacts the endosteum just above and below the fracture zone. **C,** With torsional loading, the rod twists but the points of contact are at the interlocking screw sites. This means that the same rod in the same bone has different working lengths which depend on directional loading. Compare this definition of intramedullary rod working lengths to the definitions of working length used for screws and plates seen in Figure 8-64. *WL,* Working length.

cuts its own path. Most reamers used for orthopaedic applications are side cutting.

The process of reaming is relatively straightforward. A small-diameter reamer head is selected, and then heads of gradually increasing size are used until the desired medullary canal diameter is reached. The reamer's speed of rotation is usually two-thirds of the speed used for drilling. *Chatter* is uneven cutting that causes vibration of the reamer head, which can lead to reamer dullness or damage. Chatter is reduced with slower rotational speeds. Reamers used for orthopaedic applications are of variable design; manufacturers attempt to maximize size and strength of reamers while minimizing physiologic damage.

The process of reaming causes an increase in medullary pressure and an elevation in cortical temperature. The former has been linked to an increase in extruded marrow products and the latter to cortical and medullary vascular damage. Design modifications can decrease the amount of physiologic stress sustained. Three main parts of a reamer apparatus influence the amounts of pressure and temperature generated: the reamer head, which is responsible for the actual cutting; the reamer shaft, which is usually flexible and drives the reamer head; and the bulb tip, which is the diameter inside the reamer head connection to the shaft. These components require space in the medullary canal and form a gap with the endosteal cortex. The reamer system acts like a piston and increases pressure in the relatively closed environment of a long bone.

Temperature increases during reaming have been reported to occur in stepwise increments with the successive use of larger diameter reamers. It was also reported that blunt reamers produce significantly greater temperature increases than sharp reamers do.[74] Several factors contribute to the elevation in bone temperature, including the presence or absence of flutes in the reamer head. Deep flutes that clear large amounts of bone attenuate the rise in bone temperature, whereas reamers with shallow or no flutes lead to greater increases in temperature. Sharp cutting edges and slow advancement of the reamer head decrease the rise in temperature. Blood flow to the area reduces the overall temperature increase through conductive heat transfer.

Destruction of the medullary contents by reaming has both local and systemic consequences. Reaming obliterates the remaining medullary blood supply after injury. This vascular system reconstitutes in 2 to 3 weeks.[112a] Disruption of the medullary blood supply and intracortical intravasation of medullary fat during reaming result in necrosis of a variable amount of endosteal bone. If the medullary canal becomes infected before the bone is revascularized, the entire area of dead bone can become involved and act as a sequestrum in continuity. The long bones of adults contain primarily fatty marrow, with a large reserve of hematopoietic tissue in the marrow cavities of flat bones. Therefore, destruction of marrow during reaming does not produce anemia, apart from that created through blood loss into the soft tissues. During medullary reaming, a communication is temporarily created between the marrow cavity and the intravascular space. Use of reamers in the medullary space is somewhat like the insertion of a piston into a rigid cylinder. Exceedingly high canal pressures during medullary broaching before insertion of a femoral total hip component have been found in animals and humans.[112b] Unlike the total joint broach, the medullary reamers used to prepare the canal before nail insertion are cannulated. This difference may offer some decompression of the pressure in the distal canal, but the communication is partially occluded by the guide wire and the pressurized marrow contents. Sampling of femoral vein blood during intramedullary reaming of the femur reveals embolization of fat and tissue thromboplastin. In the early days of reamed intramedullary nailing, there was great concern regarding the danger of death from fat embolization syndrome and shock. Although reamed nailing does result in embolization of marrow contents into the pulmonary circulation, this process is well tolerated if the patient has had adequate fluid resuscitation and receives appropriate hemodynamic and ventilatory support during surgery.[112b]

In addition to obliterating the soft tissue in the marrow space, reaming shaves cancellous and cortical bone from the inner aspect of the cortex. This mixture of finely morcellized bone and marrow elements has excellent osteoinductive and osteoconductive potential. The rich osseous autograft is delivered by the increased interosseous pressure and by mechanical action of the reamer directly into the fracture site. In the open nailing technique, this material is exuded during reaming, but it can be collected and applied to the surface of the bone at the fracture site after the wound is irrigated, but before wound closure.

Entrance Angle into and Ending Point in the Distal Segment

Analogous to the connection between starting point and entrance angle into the proximal segment, this step of the intramedullary rodding procedure helps to establish whether a reduction is maintained. The entrance angle and ending point in the distal segment are similarly connected but somewhat independent of each other. To clarify, it is possible to enter the distal segment at an inappropriate angle and end in the center of the anatomic axis. This can occur when the entrance angle occurs at a point at which the rod does not contact the endosteum. Ideally, both the entrance angle and the ending point are correct and centered in the anatomic axis. If one is slightly compromised, it should be the ending point in order to prioritize the fracture reduction.

Interlocking Screw Insertion

As previously noted, the primary form of axial plane stability (rotation and length) with current intramedullary rod systems is the interlocking screw. At the portion of the rod that is closest to the insertion device, these screws are typically percutaneously targeted via a guide. At the portion of the rod farthest away from the insertion device, these are most commonly placed via a free-hand technique that takes advantage of intraoperative fluoroscopy. Radiation exposure is the compromise for this choice. Forays into different techniques to limit fluoroscopy have been numerous. The attempt to create a mechanical guide that functions similar to the one at the insertion end of the device has been fraught with the complication of errant targeting. The reason for the errant targeting is the deformation of the intramedullary rod within the canal secondary to flexibility inherent in the system and the mismatch between the shape of the rod and the intramedullary canal.[113] Alternative means of interlocking targeting include laser-assisted interlocking and electromagnetic navigation systems.[114,115] One of the issues with specialized interlocking systems is that they are not generalizable across implants manufactured by different companies. Regardless of which form of interlocking is chosen, it is important to choose the correct size drill bit and screw. Choosing screws with a smaller core diameter than recommended leads to increased ease of insertion, but compromised mechanical characteristics. Remember the tolerance between the interlocking screw size and hole size is standardized based on the implant of choice. Some systems have correspondingly larger interlocking screws (and hole sizes) based on the diameter of the intramedullary rod used. This is advantageous in that screws of larger core diameter are more resistant to bending; however, not recognizing this change can lead to insertion of a smaller screw into a hole designed for a larger screw. This will increase the slope in the system and potentiates change in fracture alignment postoperatively through construct loading.

Working Length Revisited

Bone healing after intramedullary rodding will occur if the motion at the fracture site falls within an acceptable range. The exact specifications of this motion are not known, but it has been observed that small amounts of motion promote callus formation while excessive motion delays union (remember Perren's Strain Theory). Fracture motion results from loading in bending and torsion. The amount of motion that occurs at the fracture site is described in part by the concept of working length. The working length is the portion of the nail that is unsupported by bone under forces of bending or torsion (see Fig. 8-60). The unsupported length of nail differs in bending and in torsion.[115a,115b]

In bending, the major bone fragments come into contact with the nail, and therefore, the unsupported length is the distance between the proximal and the distal fracture fragments, the fracture gap or comminution. In other words, it is the portion of the fixation that is not supported by bone, where the nail can bend independently. As the bone heals, this distance decreases. In torsion, the major bone fragments do not stabilize the nail. Because reamed nails are inserted with space between the implant and the endosteal surface, there is limited frictional contact between the nail and the bone. As a result, the locking screws are the primary restraint to torsion, and the unsupported length in torsion extends the full distance between the two locking screws. Because the working length in torsion is the distance between the proximal and the distal points of fixation, it is always greater than the working length in bending.

Speaking of Intramedullary Rod Technique

- "Last week I malreduced a subtrochanteric fracture and a proximal humerus fracture into varus with intramedullary rodding. I think in both cases I started too lateral and aimed too medial. The only way the rod could get into the distal segment was to create a varus malreduction. Come to think of it, I guess this explains why the proximal tibial rodding also led to apex anterior angulation. I started too anterior and aimed too posterior. Same concept. Different plane."
- "I have to improve the position of the proximal segment of this subtrochanteric fracture prior to achieving a safe starting point and entrance angle. It might even be easier if the fracture is not perfectly reduced. I just have to make sure I do not ream across a malreduced fracture. Separating the steps is really helpful."
- "I think I am going to choose a piriformis start rod for that subtrochanteric fracture. It may be harder to reach the starting point compared to the trochanteric rod, but at least I don't have to match the starting point and entrance angle with the proximal bend in the rod."

CONSTRUCT STABILITY

After reading a long chapter describing the basic principles of internal fixation, it is important to have gained the ability to practically apply these concepts to fracture care. Facts about plates and intramedullary rods are important, but only achieve relevance when they are applied to improve patient outcomes. In light of this, we will spend some time putting this system to use in a discussion of construct stability.

As previously noted, a plate and a rod are mechanical devices that vary in design features but are ultimately used to allow functional aftercare while maintaining a fracture reduction through the healing process. They are one single component of a construct. The construct is the surgeon-built structure that consists of the combination of implant and bone. Stability is the amount of motion between fracture fragments when the construct is placed under physiologic load. Construct stability is relevant primarily because fracture care is a race between fracture healing and hardware failure. The surgeon's goal is to win the race. Winning the race requires optimizing the environment for fracture healing while minimizing the chances of hardware failure. Optimizing the fracture-healing environment includes using biologically friendly surgical techniques, addressing the patient comorbidities, and considering bone metabolism. Limiting hardware failure includes optimizing construct stability and limiting postoperative patient loading (when needed).

Construct stability is not defined solely by the size of the plate or rod or the number of screws placed in each fragment. It consists of four main components that should be considered in the preoperative planning process for any fracture. These four components include (1) bone quality, (2) fracture pattern, (3) implant characteristics, and (4) surgical technique. If you think of these four components as additive and the ultimate sum as a constant, then intraoperative decision making can follow a logical path. When one or more of the components is marginalized, the others must be maximized to reach the same sum. This is why answering the common question of how many screws are required is iterative rather than constant. Let us consider the interplay of these four components in fracture care.

First, the quality of bone plays an important role in construct stability.[116,117] It does so for two primary reasons. The quality of bone defines the quality of the docking site for whatever implant that is chosen. Marginal bone quality compromises the docking site. When this is the case, alternative modes of stability must be considered. Conventional screw fixation is dependent on frictional forces created by screw elongation and bone compression. When high compressive forces are not possible, then either locking fixation should be considered or alternative materials must be placed in the bone to change the compressive characteristics (e.g., graft, cement, etc.). The quality of the bone also defines the ability of the bone to share load with the implant. Poor bone may not be able to achieve adequate load sharing. This necessitates either spreading the load over a larger area of the bone (and thereby distributing stress) or consigning the construct to a load-bearing function. An example of spreading the load over a larger area would be choosing a rod that takes advantage of some endosteal contact rather than relying on fixed points of screw/plate/bone cortical interfaces. An example of consigning the construct to load bearing would be bridging a fracture rather than attempting a compression application. In both scenarios, the fracture pattern, implant, and surgical technique take on greater significance in the ultimate construct stability.

Second, the fracture pattern plays an important role in construct stability. Simple fracture patterns allow for anatomic reconstruction, thereby restoring some intrinsic stability to the bone itself. This logically protects the implant from loading through providing the potential for a load-sharing environment. Complex fracture patterns often negate the potential for anatomic reconstruction, as the amount of soft tissue dissection (and therefore fracture fragment blood supply damage) required may outweigh the benefit of precise coaptation. As the complexity of fracture patterns increases, the bone quality, implant, and surgical technique take on greater significance in construct stability.

Third, the implant chosen plays a large role in construct stability, as does the technique with which it is applied. The implant receives the greatest attention, but is only one part of the equation. Plate length and screw density are frequent questions at fracture courses. The answers have changed over time, but the simple fact is that one standard answer is inadequate. Thought should be given to each fracture, while keeping the rules of fracture care and some basic principles in mind. With the evolution of implant and instrument design, these principles are easier than ever to apply, but unfortunately commonly forgotten. Four principles to remember are load sharing, balanced fixation, maximized working lengths, and substitution as required. Let us take each one separately.

Load sharing should be prioritized when possible. It limits the amount of metal required (by protecting the amount of metal that is present). It allows for the use of implants with shorter working lengths and fewer points of bone contact. Load sharing is not associated only with intramedullary rodding (Fig. 8-61). Load sharing is created by things other than just an anatomic reduction and compression. Consider the hat on hook analogy for femoral neck fracture fixation or the valgus osteotomy for femoral neck nonunion management (Fig. 8-62).[17,25] Manipulating the mechanical environment just

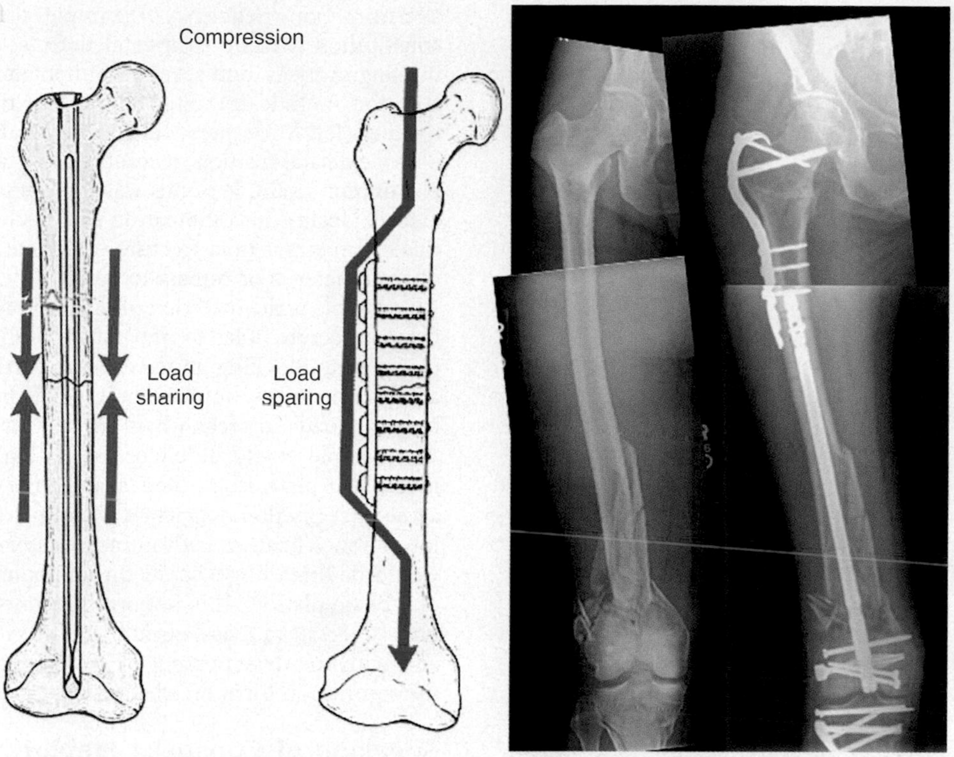

Figure 8-61. Load sharing versus load bearing. Traditionally, intramedullary nails have been described as load sharing and plates have been described as load bearing. Prior to interlocking screw development, intramedullary nails were required to share load with the bone until stable impaction occurred. With the advent of interlocking screws and the changing mechanical function from a nail to a rod, the implant became load bearing or load sharing based on the fracture configuration. Bridging across comminution with a statically locked intramedullary rod is a load-bearing function. Plate application can be load sharing. When compression is achieved across a simple pattern fracture, then the reduced fracture is sharing load with the implant. Note the fracture to the *right* of the image. The intramedullary rod is load bearing and the proximal femoral plate is load sharing.

requires a basic understanding of statics and dynamics and thought. We all possess a physical intuition of structural principles through our daily experience. It should be applied intraoperatively.

Balanced fixation is both aesthetically pleasing and mechanically optimal. In diaphyseal fractures, this is a simple enough concept. Implants should be equal in length and number on each side of the fracture (Fig. 8-63). In metaphyseal fractures, this is eased by implants designed with extra plate holes in the epiphyseal region. A useful analogy is to consider the seesaw. The fulcrum is the center of the fracture; the children on each end are the sum of your fixation. Normal-size children symmetrically placed on the seesaw provide balance in diaphyseal fixation. In metaphyseal fixation, sometimes you need the fat kid. Because the distance the kid sits away from the fulcrum is limited by the length of the epiphyseal fragment, the kid must be bigger to balance the length of the proximal fixation. Limiting the length of the diaphyseal fixation is not the answer; empowering the epiphyseal fixation is.

The concept of working length can be confusing secondary to varying definitions in the literature. In intramedullary rodding, it is the distance between implant/bone points of contact in the proximal and distal segments and differs based

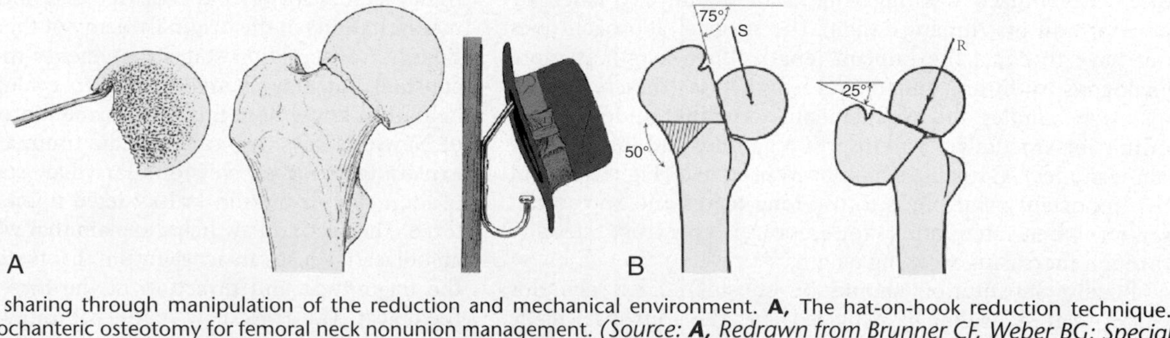

Figure 8-62. Load sharing through manipulation of the reduction and mechanical environment. **A,** The hat-on-hook reduction technique. **B,** The valgus intertrochanteric osteotomy for femoral neck nonunion management. *(Source:* ***A,*** *Redrawn from Brunner CF, Weber BG: Special techniques in internal fixation, Berlin/Heidelberg/New York, 1982, Springer-Verlag;* ***B,*** *Redrawn from Pauwels F: Biomechanics of the normal and diseased hip: theoretical foundation, technique and results, Berlin/Heidelberg/New York, Springer-Verlag, 1976.)*

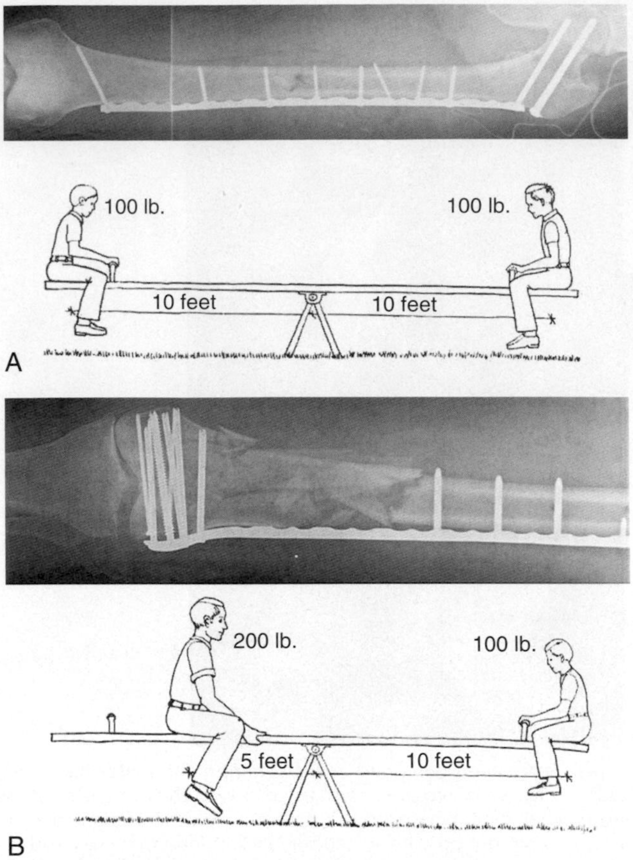

Figure 8-63. Balanced fixation. The fulcrum is the center of the fracture; the children on each end are the sum of your fixation. Normal-size children symmetrically placed on the seesaw provide balance in diaphyseal fixation. In metaphyseal fixation, sometimes you need the fat kid. Because the distance the kid sits away from the fulcrum is limited by the length of the epiphyseal fragment, the kid must be bigger to balance the length of the proximal fixation. Limiting the length of the diaphyseal fixation is not the answer; empowering the epiphyseal fixation is. *(Source: Illustrations redrawn from Salvadori M, Hooker S, Ragus C: The art of construction: projects and principles for beginning engineers and architects, Chicago, 2000, Chicago Review Press.)*

on whether torsional or bending working lengths are specified (Fig. 8-64).[5] In screw application it is the length of screw contact from the point at which it enters the cortex to the point at which it exits the cortex.[80] In plate application, it is the length of fixation in the segment proximal or distal to a fracture.[80] Maximized working lengths in plating are aided by implant and instrument design. The surgical approach does not have to equal the implant length. Plate length is more analogous to intramedullary rod length since the creation of insertion handles and percutaneous targeting guides (which mimic intramedullary nail insertion handles and interlocking screw guides). Guidelines have been provided (Fig. 8-65), but the important principle is to use long plates and spread out screws when attempting to empower construct stability through increasing working length.[64,81,82,118]

Finally, substitution should be considered in scenarios when delayed healing is expected and the implant will be cyclically stressed. Substitution creates what has been termed *artificial stability,* or the use of an implant to substitute for a structural bone deficiency.[18] Examples that lend themselves to substitution include segmental defects, severe osteoporosis, missing cortices, and severe fragmentation. Methods of substitution include framing, filling, blocking, conflicting, and locking (Jeff Mast, personal communication). Framing is the use of external fixation in combination with internal fixation. A common example of this was the use of a medial uniplanar external fixator in combination with a lateral plate for extraarticular proximal tibia fracture treatment.[119] Filling is the use of graft material or cement to nullify holes or large interstices. An example is the insertion of calcium phosphate cement into previous screw holes to prevent instability of adjacent screw placement. Blocking is the use of cortical substitution via an intramedullary implant or graft. It is used to counteract bending loads in areas where the far cortex is compromised. An example would be endosteal plating, whereby the intramedullary plate is blocked against the far cortex that has areas of segmental deficiency.[120] Conflicting is the creation of interference fixation with intraosseous implants. An example would be threading a screw through a hole created in the tip of a blade plate.[121] This not only tensions the screw on metal but also creates a truss. Locking has been previously discussed and with the development of new implants has become the most common form of substitution.

Speaking of Construct Stability

- "The amount of metal needed is dependent upon many things. Standardization should not prevent thought."
- "The injury film helps me understand the forces I am trying to resist. I am going to build my construct in light of that, with each part logically resisting the forces that are trying to create failure."
- "I expect healing to be prolonged in this case. I better build in a factor of safety into my construct so failure does not occur first."

Construct Failure

Possessing a knowledge of the end at the beginning is very useful. Most failures are predictable. The study of failure is more advanced in other construction disciplines, but has some history within orthopaedic trauma as well.[122] To systematically evaluate the etiology of failure, it is useful to break the problem down into contributing categories. Three previously defined categories include injury factors, patient factors, and surgeon factors. We will start with these and proceed to a more focused inventory of radiographic failure.

Injury Factors

Injury factors are beyond the surgeon's control. All of these are manifestations of the original energy of the injury. The Law of Energy Conservation states that energy in a system remains constant but may change forms. To evaluate an injury, it is helpful to know how this transformation occurs. Translation of Newton's laws into orthopaedic trauma language helps to explain the process. Newton's First Law states that objects in motion stay in motion unless acted upon by an unbalanced force. The Second Law helps explain that when a force acts on an object, it causes an acceleration that is predictable based on the magnitude and direction of the force and the mass of the object. The Third Law states that for every action, there is an equal but opposite reaction; but sometimes the object with the smaller mass may not be able to withstand the larger

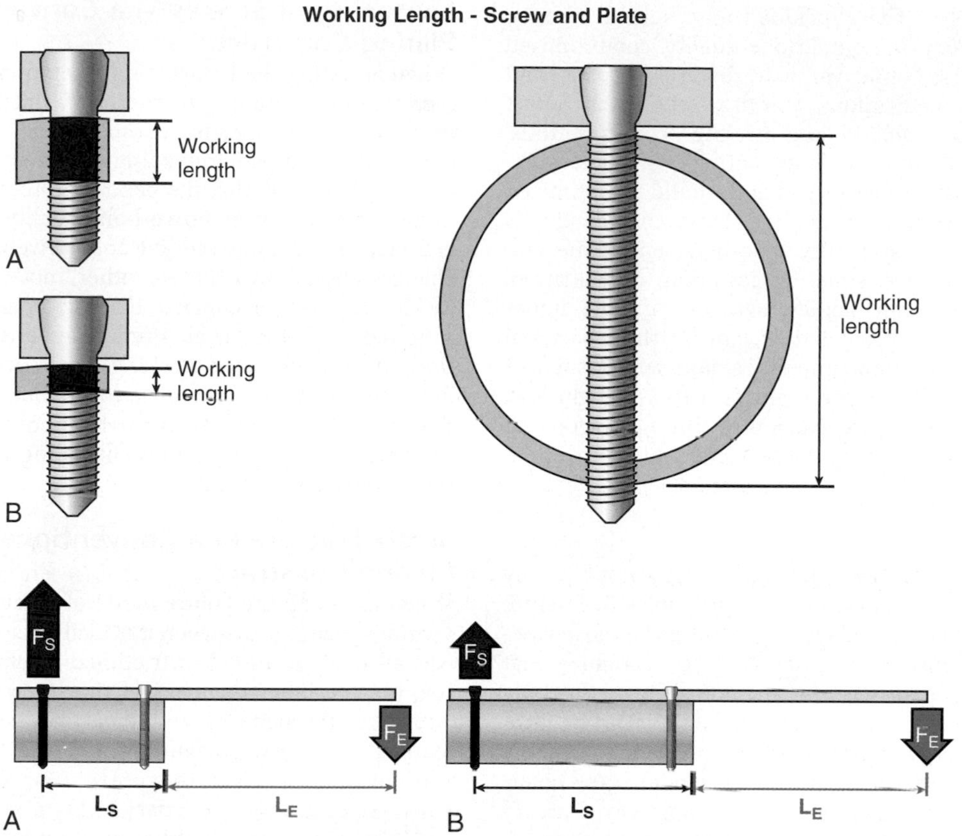

Figure 8-64. Screw and plate working length. Working length for screws is defined by the distance from which the screw enters the cortex to which it exits the cortex. For monocortical screws, this is dependent only on cortical thickness. For bicortical screws, it also depends on bone diameter. Working length for plates is defined by the distance from the first point of contact to the last point of contact in a segment of bone. F_E, External force creating a bending moment on the plate; F_S, pullout force of the screw.

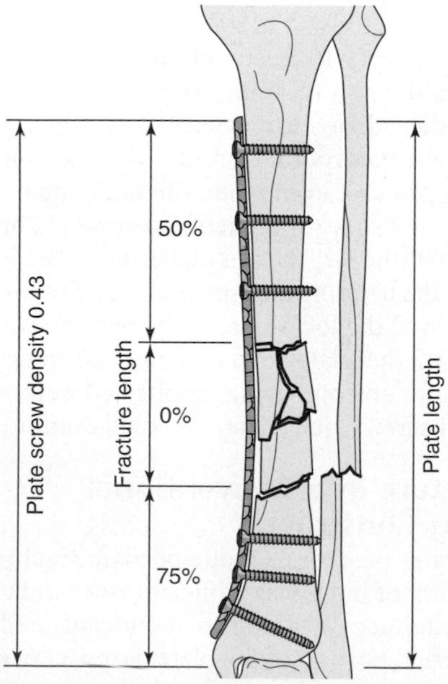

Figure 8-65. Bridge plating values to remember. Plate-to-span ratio has been defined as the total length of the plate compared to the length of the plate that spans the zone of comminution. Current recommendations are to use a plate of three to four times the length of the zone of comminution. Plate screw density has been defined as the total number of screws placed in the plate relative to the total number of holes available in the plate. Current recommendations are to use a screw density of 0.5 or less, meaning fewer than half of the available screw holes are used.

acceleration resulting from the interaction and energy is transferred to a different form. To clarify, a motorcycle that hits a reinforced brick wall will stop moving forward and the human on top will fly into the wall and absorb excess energy, overcoming the ultimate strength of his bones and soft tissue. This different form is recognizable radiographically by the complexity of the fracture pattern and the initial severity of displacement. It is recognizable clinically by the severity of soft tissue injury, the open or closed nature of the fracture, and associated neurovascular insult. All of these serve as markers for devitalization of bone fragments and the potential for a delayed healing response or a compromised healing environment. When retrospectively evaluating these injury factors in a failure scenario, information should be gleaned from a review of the original injury films and a review of the operative records or discussion with the original surgeon. Failure to invest the time to do so may prevent a clear understanding of the cause of the failure. More importantly, it places the surgeon at a disadvantage for successful reconstruction by limiting his or her understanding of the unbalanced forces that must be neutralized. When assessing these factors prior to initial treatment, decision making can be guided based on basic principles of fracture care (refer to the sections "Fracture Pattern" and "Soft Tissue Pattern").

Patient Factors

Patient factors are partially under the control of the surgeon. Some factors cannot be timely optimized but should be addressed nonetheless. These include things such as obesity, traumatic brain injury, marginal bone quality, compromised immune function, systemic vascular diseases, hepatic and renal failure, and medications and treatments that affect bone and soft tissue quality and healing (corticosteroids, immunomodulators, anticoagulants, antibiotics, prior radiation therapy, etc.). Other factors can and should be optimized to maximize the chances of success. These include things such as treatment of psychiatric disorders, endocrine and metabolic bone disorders, smoking cessation, malnutrition, visual and balance abnormalities, syncope, limited upper extremity strength for protected weight-bearing, bacterial carrier status, previous noncompliance, and family support and living situation. Discovery requires a thorough history and can be completed more efficiently through a focused failure inventory. By assessing these factors prior to initial treatment, failure prevalence can be lessened.

Surgeon Factors

Surgeon factors include the additional energy imparted by the surgeon and the violation of basic principles of fracture care. Fracture care can be challenging even for the most experienced traumatologist. It is important to recognize that even the best preoperative plans are not always effectively realized at the time of surgery. Surgery is a controlled form of trauma. The energy imparted obeys the laws of energy conservation but can be more difficult to recognize and quantify. Telltale radiographic signs of overly aggressive surgery include unusual fixation montages, implants placed in multiple planes that indicate circumferential stripping, and excessive screw density. Other common radiographic signs of basic principle violation include incorrect choice of desired stability for a given fracture (e.g., choosing absolute stability for a highly complex extraarticular fracture pattern), initial malreductions, incorrect implant type, incorrect implant sizing, imbalanced constructs, poor plate span width, irregular working lengths, screws placed across malreduced fractures, disregard of directional loading (e.g., choosing an implant that commonly fails in the mode of the original fracture displacement), and unlocked intramedullary rods. By considering these factors prior to initial treatment, most mistakes can be avoided.

Proactive Failure Analysis

The object of construct design is to either avoid destructive forces or to provide, within understood limits, sufficient resistance to them in the structure.[37] In reality, this is an educated guessing game, with the surgeon's preconceived ideas about failure driving the construct design. When considering how failure might occur, some fundamental principles can help. These principles are derived from basic mechanical principles and empirical failure observation. They are best employed in the acute fracture fixation setting in the form of proactive failure analysis. They extend directly from the previously defined concept of a construct. The construct is the surgeon-built structure that consists of the combination of implant and bone. It is not just the implant or just the bone. It is the combination of the two and how they interact. Every construct has a weak point. It is incumbent on the surgeon to consider this in a proactive failure analysis preoperatively and guard against it using basic mechanical principles. Let us clarify this concept with multiple examples.

Loosening of Screws in a Conventional Plating Construct

When assessing the failure mode of loosening of screws in a conventional plating construct, it is likely that the quality of bone was insufficient to establish a frictional force that could withstand patient loading parameters. When pullout is evident, it is likely that the bending forces exceeded the frictional force. When marginal bone quality is expected preoperatively or encountered intraoperatively, proactive design changes should incorporate other modes of stability (e.g., locking screws), or enhance the frictional forces that can be achieved (e.g., bicortical screw purchase, screw augmentation). Alternatively, the working length of the implant can be increased such that resistance to pullout is empowered. The flexibility of the implant can also be modified such that elasticity is present in the plate, thus alleviating some of the force on the plate/screw/bone interface.[80]

Screw Fracture in a Conventional Plating Construct

When assessing the failure mode of screw fracture of a conventional plating construct, it is likely that the quality of bone was adequate to establish frictional stability without loosening, but the inner diameter of the screw was insufficient to withstand the bending and shear forces created by patient loading. The screw portion that fractures is often termed the *run out of the screw*.[36] This portion represents a location of stress concentration secondary to the abrupt change in shape and presence of corners. When screw failure occurs in bending or shear, it most commonly occurs in this area, partly because of the stress riser, but also because of the concentrated loading at this motion interface adjacent to the plate and near cortex. The initial frictional forces always decrease to some degree. This is a manifestation of the law of entropy. Everything in nature is moving toward a state of decreased order. When micromotion begins to occur at the run out of the screw, this increases the risk of failure through cycling. When high bending or shear loads are expected postoperatively, design changes should incorporate screws of larger inner diameter (e.g., locking screws), even when the bone quality is adequate enough to establish strong frictional forces. This serves two purposes. First, the larger core diameter of the locking screw better resists the bending and shear forces. Second, the mechanism of action of the locking screw is antientropic. It fixes the relationship of the plate to the bone. By doing so, it limits the potential for entropy being manifested as loosening of the conventional screws (Jeff Mast, personal communication).

Plate Fracture in a Conventional or Locking Construct

When assessing the failure mode of plate fracture, it is likely that the quality of bone was sufficient to maintain the screw/plate/bone interface. By doing so, it concentrated the stress to the unsupported portion of the plate. Stress concentration was occurring over the portion of the plate that fractured. When stress concentration is felt to be present intraoperatively, design changes should incorporate removing screws adjacent to the point of instability such that the stress is distributed over a larger area in the plate. A simple way to achieve this is to consider the portion of the plate that is unsupported at the fracture site. If this portion is between two adjacent plate holes (very small distance), then care should be taken to ensure the bone does not see much load. In the forearm, this might be reasonable. In the femur, this is a dangerous practice. If the unsupported portion consists of a single plate hole between screws, then recognize the stress riser danger of the plate hole. Again care should be taken to ensure the bone does not see much load in this area. One way to accomplish this is to ensure the bone is seeing load at this fracture site, thereby protecting the plate. As the unsupported portion becomes larger (e.g., two to three plate holes), then stress distribution is occurring and safety margins are likely better in bones that see higher loads.

Bone/Screw Interface Failure in a Locking Construct

When assessing bone/screw interface failure in a locking construct, it is likely that the rigid interface of the locking construct overwhelmed the marginal quality of the bone in that region. To clarify, the locked fixator acts as a single beam. In doing so, it does not allow motion at any of the plate/screw interfaces. This concentrates stress in the plate itself and in the bone/screw interfaces. The plate is typically more able to withstand the stress than a bone/screw interface that relies on marginal bone. The end result is that the screws wallow around in the marginal bone, creating bone/screw interface failure. This is a complicated problem without a clear mechanical solution at the point of this publication (this assumes a load-sharing environment cannot be created by fracture reduction). While modifying plate material seems logical (i.e., choosing a more flexible plate material such as titanium rather than stainless steel), it has not been clearly borne out in clinical practice as advantageous.[123] Modifying plate thickness also seems logical, but minor thickness modifications are not available and major modifications (such as choosing a small fragment implant rather than a large fragment implant) are unsafe in most situations. Another proposed solution is modifying the plate/screw/bone interface through near cortical slotting, far cortical locking, or dynamic locking screw application.[124,125] These are not yet accepted as standard techniques for many reasons, but are current options to address the concern of bone/screw interface failure in a locking construct.

Interlocking Screw Fracture in an Intramedullary Rod Construct

When assessing interlocking screw fracture in an intramedullary rod construct, it is likely that the core diameter of the screw was inadequate to withstand the four-point bending load imposed by patient loading. This presents a challenging problem in light of the fact that a small tolerance typically exists between the interlocking screw hole and the outer diameter of the interlocking screw. Furthermore, interlocking screws are designed such that the core diameter is already maximized. Because of this, choosing a screw with a larger core diameter than can withstand greater bending forces is not an option. When large bending forces are predicted preoperatively based on patient size, lack of compliance, or expected delayed healing, then care should be taken to empower the interlocking screw/rod/bone relationship. Because this cannot be accomplished through using a larger interlocking screw, it should be accomplished by building in a factor of safety. Placing additional interlocking screws in a segment provides this factor of safety, such that when the one closest to the fracture fails, there are others to absorb the load and prevent alignment changes. Occasionally a change in rod diameter equates to a larger interlocking screw core diameter. If this is the case with the system being used, one should also consider this option.

Interlocking Screw Backout and Bone/Screw Interface Failure in an Intramedullary Rod Construct

Interlocking screw backout is a less common mode of failure than interlocking screw fatigue fracture, but still occurs. One of the reasons this occurs is the design of the interlocking screw itself. As previously noted, each design choice comes with an inherent compromise. Because the most common mode of mechanical failure is screw fatigue in bending, interlocking screws have been designed to primarily resist this failure mode. Choosing a screw with better resistance to pullout would necessarily compromise this bending strength. When the bone quality is so poor that this failure mode is anticipated, then the addition of multiple interlocking screws in different planes should assist in preventing screw toggle in a single plane (which leads to screw backout). Placing Poller or blocking screws adjacent to the rod also has the potential to limit the toggle that leads to backout. Alternative proactive methods include choosing rod designs that limit screw backout (e.g., threaded hole, end cap that impinges on screw) or screw designs that incorporate improved resistance to backout (e.g., locking interlocking screw).[94,95] Alternatives include screw augmentation (which is concerning in case removal is required) or even placing a similar sized locking screw through a locking plate that is fixed to the bone in that segment with additional screws. Bone/screw interface failure provides a similar picture with similar methods for resistance.

Speaking of Construct Failure

- "Well that was predictable…and not just because hindsight is 20/20. The implant chosen was not empowered to resist the expected mode of failure noted on the injury films."
- "It is difficult to understand the limits of safety until failure is encountered. I have fixed this fracture the same way ten times successfully, but now I see the forces more clearly. Next time things will be different."

PREOPERATIVE PLANNING

"Better to throw your disasters into the wastepaper basket than to consign your patients to the scrap heap" has been a proverb of one of the greatest fracture and deformity surgeons in the history of our specialty (Jeff Mast, personal communication). Stated differently, one of the major values of simulation is that it allows one to make mistakes in a consequence-free environment.[126] Preoperative planning is a mental (and sometimes physical) simulation exercise. It incorporates proactive failure analysis and establishes a forcing function that requires time and a thoughtful approach. The primary goal of this section is not to provide you with a recipe of how-to steps. That has been completed in a book that should sit in the library of every practicing fracture surgeon.[18] Rather, the primary goal is to define the different elements of preoperative planning and reveal how they are practically incorporated into an everyday routine.

The Elements of Preoperative Planning

Preoperative planning consists of three parts: (1) the desired end result, (2) the surgical tactic, and (3) the operation logistics. Since the inception of preoperative planning, these three parts have evolved, primarily because of modifications in surgical technique, a wealth of instrumentation and implants, and variations in imaging. These modifications—particularly the movement to picture archiving and communication systems (PACS)—have altered the face of preoperative planning. Let us take each one separately and review some of the changes.

The Desired End Result

As originally described, the desired end result included a tracing of the final reduction and fracture fixation construct. This tracing allowed for a direct comparison of the postoperative radiographs to the preoperative plan. The overlay technique could be used to place the preoperative tracing on top of the postoperative hard copy films in order to reflect on the insight of the plan (surgeon), the mistaken preconceived notions, and the accuracy of the psychomotor skills. This is (was) a humbling experience. Reflection is felt to be an important part of crystallizing learning. The reflection provided for a pause point, which improved future retention of information gained from that procedure. The copy of the plan provided for a source document for review when similar cases were encountered in the future.

With the popularization of digital radiography and PACS, the tracing of the final reduction and fracture fixation construct has been largely lost. Currently available systems allow for a digitized version of the plan, but something important was lost: the process of tracing. Take a moment to draw an oblique view of the bones of the foot. Now compare this to an oblique radiograph of a foot from your hospital PACS. Honestly assess your accuracy in the contour of the bones, the relationship between the bones, the relative sizing or proportions among them. Now consider treating a complex midfoot fracture-dislocation in which the contralateral extremity is also injured at that level and does not provide comparative films. How effective is your gestalt at restoring anatomy?

The process of learning osseous anatomy and radiographic correlates is not simple. We are not born with a knowledge of radiographic anatomy. Staring at radiographs is rarely enough to cement important relationships. Intensive studying is necessary. It requires discipline for details and practice with mental manipulation of three-dimensional objects into two-dimensional pictures, commonly in the setting of bone models. Tracing was and is helpful in this regard. Surprisingly, this visuospatial practice does not just improve recognition; it also improves motor skills. Visuospatial ability has been correlated with improved psychomotor control in surgical performance.[127]

The advantages of reflection and tracing are not necessarily lost in the setting of PACS. Digital images can still be printed and traced, albeit often at less than ideal magnification. The repetitive process still allows for crystallization of osseous anatomic relationships and postoperative metacognition. It still provides the potential for an improved gestalt and should arguably be incorporated into training programs in fields that commonly incorporate imaging in the diagnosis of pathoanatomy.

The Surgical Tactic

The surgical tactic portion of preoperative planning has historically included the essential kinetics of reduction and fixation.[18] The predefined surgical tactic demanded a consideration of the patient's comorbidities and existing injuries and how these affected surgical positioning. Similarly, it forced a consideration of how the chosen surgical positioning would affect the deforming forces created through gravity. It required contemplation on how the chosen surgical approach would allow for the placement of reduction instruments and fixation implants and a clarification of how reduction and fixation interacted in the limited space of the surgical field. This clarification provided a forced ordering of steps. It offered the opportunity to examine how different reduction tools could be used for the same reduction step, thereby allowing a mental rehearsal of the different options. It necessitated a consideration of which sets would be needed on the back table and which ones should be available in case the first plan was unsuccessful. It allowed for the minimization of intraoperative delays from wasted motions and illogical quick decisions.

With the advent of modifications in surgical technique and an explosion in the choices of instrumentation and implants, the surgical tactic portion of the preoperative plan has become more complex. An increased volume of operative fractures and changes in the process of implant consignment and storage have necessitated improved coordination in hospital systems. These changes also have the potential to leave the surgeon focusing on the trees and missing the forest. Zooming out and applying the basic principles of operative fracture care to each case prevent some of the problems associated with choice overload. A systematic method of approaching fracture care has been provided in this chapter. Remember and use Figure 8-1 in your preoperative planning exercise. Reviewing this system of fracture care prior to each procedure is a useful method of preventing failures that relate to breaches in the basic principles of fracture healing. After ensuring the plan adheres to the basic principles of care, creating a stepwise listing of the essential minimum necessary steps will provide a roadmap for successful surgery.

The Operation Logistics

The operation logistics portion of preoperative planning has historically been included as part of the surgical tactic, but with the increasing system complexities and communication barriers inherent in large hospitals, it has been optimized as a separate part of the plan. The operation logistics largely follow from the created surgical tactic. If the logistics are broken down based on communication couplets, the entire patient care team can efficiently focus on the needs at hand. For example, the surgeon–anesthesia communication couplet requires transmission of information such as the need for patient muscle relaxation, patient positioning, the antibiotic choice or the decision to hold preoperatively, the expected duration and blood loss of the procedure, available blood products, the history of anesthetic complications or untoward reactions, whether isolation precautions are required, and cervical spine clearance. The surgeon–operating room (OR) nurse communication couplet requires transmission of information such as the operative table of choice, patient positioning, the need for intraoperative imaging, the desire for Foley catheterization and tourniquet use, mechanical thromboembolic disease prophylaxis, and informed consent issues. The surgeon–OR technologist communication couplet requires transmission of information such as the desired sets and surgical drapes and the proposed order of steps. Take time to reflect on your personal cases that have gone poorly. Have there been instances where improvements in communication could have made a difference? Invest the time to create a reproducible and effective system of communication in your operative setting.

Speaking of Preoperative Planning

- "My circulating nurse seems frustrated because she is always chasing after things that I did not tell her we would need. It seems to be making it harder for her to do the other parts of her job. I think she has asked to be replaced."
- "I don't understand why the anesthesiologist doesn't trust me. Maybe it would help to communicate case expectations more effectively prior to the procedure."
- "My operating efficiency is mediocre. It seems like I am always waiting on things that are not there and repeating steps that could be better planned out ahead of time. I should consider preoperative planning."
- "Clearly my Gestalt was inadequate for this case. I should spend more time educating my understanding of radiographic anatomy. Maybe using the other side as a template has merit."

SUMMARY

The principles of internal fixation provide power. When combined with a knowledge of anatomy and competent psychomotor skills, they change lives. They prevent a selection bias from invalidating training. They allow for patient-specific approaches to care, while ensuring a reasonable opportunity for healing. When ignored, they almost ensure a poor result. They can and should be understood rather than memorized, applied rather than recited. It is our duty to follow them.

KEY REFERENCES

The level of evidence (LOE) is determined according to the criteria provided in the preface.

1. Rüedi TP, Buckley RE, Moran CG: *AO Principles of fracture management*, New York, 2007, Thieme.
5. Tencer AF, Johnson KD: *Biomechanics in orthopedic trauma: bone fracture and fixation*, London, 1994, Taylor & Francis.
18. Mast J, Jakob R, Ganz R: *Planning and reduction technique in fracture surgery*, Berlin, Heidelberg, New York, 1989, Springer-Verlag.
36. Thakur AJ: *The elements of fracture fixation*, ed 2, New Delhi, 2012, Elsevier India.
43. McEwen DR: Intraoperative positioning of surgical patients. *AORN J* 63(6):1059–1063, 1066–1079, quiz 1080–1086, 1996.
44. Winfree CJ, Kline DG: Intraoperative positioning nerve injuries. *Surg Neurol* 63(1):5–18, 2005. LOE V
45. American Society of Anesthesiologists Task Force on Prevention of Perioperative Peripheral Neuropathies: Practice advisory for the prevention of perioperative peripheral neuropathies: an updated report by the American Society of Anesthesiologists Task Force on prevention of perioperative peripheral neuropathies. *Anesthesiology* 114(4):741–754, 2011. LOE V
74. Müller ME, Allgöwer M, Schneider R, et al: *Manual of internal fixation: techniques recommended by the AO-ASIF group*, Berlin, Heidelberg, New York, 1991, Springer-Verlag.
80. Gautier E, Sommer C: Guidelines for the clinical application of the LCP. *Injury* 34:63–76, 2003.
83. 2007 LCDCP Design INJURY 1991 22 Supl.1 pg 1-25-2. 2007:1–25.

The complete References list is available online at https://expertconsult.inkling.com.

Chapter 9

Evaluation and Treatment of the Multi-injured Trauma Patient

ALAN D. MURDOCK • ANDREW B. PEITZMAN

INTRODUCTION

Each year civilian trauma accounts for 35 million emergency department (ED) evaluations and 1.9 million hospital discharges admissions across the United States.[1] It is the leading cause of death in individuals ages 1 to 44 years (47% of the deaths) and the third leading cause of death overall, covering all age groups with 180,811 deaths in 2011.[1] The leading mechanism of civilian injury deaths is motor vehicle crashes, 26%; firearms, 18%; poisoning, 17.8%; and falls, 11.4%.[2] Thirty percent of life-years lost are due to trauma followed by cancer (16%) and heart disease (12%).[3] The economic burden is enormous ($400 billion) in both health care costs and loss of productivity.[4]

The Department of Defense (DoD) reports U.S. deaths from Operation Enduring Freedom and Operation Iraqi Freedom, including military and DoD civilians, at 6651 with those wounded in action totaling 50,602.[5] The mechanism of military injuries is 67% penetrating, 38% blunt, and 3% burns. Leading causes of injury including battle and non–battle related, are improvised explosive device (IED), 52%; gunshot wounds, 28%; other, 13.8%; and motor vehicle crashes, 5.9%, which is in contrast to civilian injuries causes of falls, 40%; motor vehicle crashes, 28%; and firearms, 4.35%.[6,7]

The concept of a trimodal distribution of death after injury has been popularized in both civilian and military settings.[8,9] This trimodal distribution of deaths associated with civilian trauma is categorized as immediate, early, and late.[10] Immediate deaths occur as a result of brain or spinal cord injury, major vessel injury, or cardiac injury; prevention is the best approach in reducing these fatalities, particularly from the military perspective.[11,12] At the other end of the spectrum, late deaths occur several days to weeks after admission. Organ failure and sepsis are the most common cause of late deaths.[13] Fifty percent of trauma deaths occur within 12 hours of injury, and 74% die within 48 hours, emphasizing the need for expedient and definitive intervention.[14] Deaths within 1 to 24 hours after injury occur from hemorrhage in the first 6 to 12 hours and severe brain injury in the 12- to 24-hour period.[15,16] The military died-of-wounds rate (deaths that occur after reaching the first level of medical care) have also been investigated and categorized in nonsurvival (NS) and potential survival (PS).[17] The predominant mechanism of death in NS group was overwhelming traumatic brain injury (83%) and hemorrhage (16%). However, in the PS group, the percentage is reversed with hemorrhage as the leading cause of death at 80%. These data underscore the necessity for initiatives to mitigate bleeding, particularly in the prehospital environment.

A general understanding of trauma systems, prehospital care, Advanced Trauma Life Support (ATLS) assessment, and a brief overview of initial injury management are critical in the understanding of how we might mitigate injury-related complications and mortality in multi-injured trauma patients.

TRAUMA SYSTEMS

In 1966, the landmark article "Accidental Death and Disability: The Neglected Disease of Modern Society" was published by the National Academy of Sciences.[17] The publication emphasized the need for an organized approach to the treatment of injured patients. A decade later, the American College of Surgeons (ACS) Committee on Trauma published "Optimal Hospital Resources for the Care of the Seriously Injured," which became the framework for modern-day U.S. trauma systems.[18]

The Trauma Care Systems and Development Act created guidelines for the development of an inclusive trauma system integrated with the emergency medical services (EMS) system to meet the needs of acutely injured patients.[19] The objective of the system is to match the needs of patient to the most appropriate level of care through a well-organized approach of care delivery to the injured within a community. The process of designation of trauma centers as level I, II, III, or IV depends on the commitment and resources of the medical staff and administration to trauma care at facilities seeking designation. Trauma centers may be designated either by a state or regional trauma system authority or by the ACS verification process.[20] The verification process evaluates several key factors, including (1) the institutional commitment to injured patients; (2) injury volume and acuity; (3) facility layout, dedicated material, and human resources; (4) operation of the clinical trauma program; and (5) trauma performance improvement program. The relationship between the formal verification of a trauma center and the improved outcomes has been demonstrated across a number of quality indicators, including in-hospital mortality, length of stay, lethal injury complex outcomes, and resource uses.[21-23]

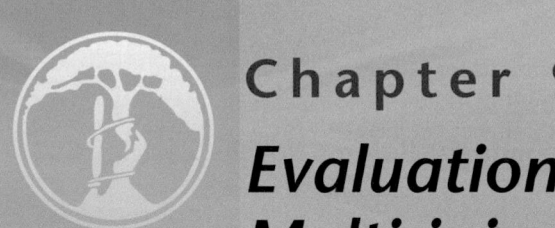

Although the development of the civilian trauma system has been closely tied to the lessons learned by the U.S. military during conflicts over the past two centuries, the U.S. military trauma system stagnated in the 1980s and was initially unprepared for the number of casualties incurred during Operations Enduring Freedom and Iraqi Freedom. The Joint Theater Trauma System (JTTS) was developed by military medical leaders to provide a systematic approach to battlefield care resulting in mitigating mortality and morbidity. The JTTS was based on U.S. civilian trauma systems with further refinement in creating a continuum of care from the battlefield care to rehabilitation through levels of care in 2004.[24] The Joint Theater Trauma Registry (JTTR), which included a comprehensive injury and outcome database, was developed to account for ongoing performance improvement and research. This database has had a significant impact on the care of wounded warriors through the development of evidence-based clinical practice guidelines.[25,26]

The general thrust of both civilian and military trauma systems is a paradigm of the right patient, right injury, right care, and right time.

PREHOSPITAL EVALUATION AND CARE

Major studies of both civilian and military trauma epidemiology suggest that the majority of deaths in injured patients occurs in the prehospital phase.[27-37] Whereas nearly 50% of civilian injury-related deaths occur within the first 12 hours, 50% of current U.S. military combat-related deaths occur within the first 6 hours. Death and late complications have been linked to the timeliness and appropriateness of early interventions, including airway management, hemorrhage control, and resuscitation. Thus, the development of prehospital treatment and resuscitation algorithms has the great potential to improve mortality and morbidity.

In every system, the goal of evaluation and treatment of a trauma patient in the field is to evaluate airway, breathing, and circulation (ABCs); provide spinal immobilization; initiate appropriate resuscitation; perform a secondary survey; properly prepare the patient for transport; and minimize the time on the scene. The specific standards or protocols are determined by the regulatory agency governing that region and local medical control.

Prehospital Personnel

The on-scene evaluation and treatment of trauma patients can be widely variable and are dependent on the level of training of the provider, local standards and protocols, and available resources. Each EMS system has a unique structure, but in general, there are four levels of providers: first responder, emergency medical technician (EMT), paramedic, and prehospital critical care provider. Prehospital critical care providers include critical care–trained paramedics, nurses, respiratory therapists, and physicians. These providers operate in ground and air transport systems.

Although local protocols often follow nationally accepted standards, there may be small variations for each specific protocol based on regional need or the local medical director's preference. In general, more densely populated areas have a greater number of EMS providers and resources. Unfortunately, as the population density decreases, EMS resources often decrease. In rural areas, there may be only one ambulance and a basic EMT team for a large geographic area.

Each level of prehospital provider has specific required training that increases in conjunction with the number and complexity of the available protocols and interventions to be performed. The U.S. Department of Transportation (DOT) establishes the National Standard Curricula (NSC) as the minimum standards for each level and recommends the range of required training hours.[38]

Prehospital and En Route Critical Care Providers

This category of provider covers a wide range of disciplines, including critical care–trained paramedics, respiratory therapists, nurses, and physicians. These providers are often required to have a certain amount of in-hospital critical care experience before joining a transport team. Commonly, they receive further training, both didactic and practical, as part of an orientation to the transport program; most advanced teams receive 2 to 6 months of training after joining the transport team.

This group of practitioners provides the highest level of care outside of the hospital setting. The assessment of a trauma patient is generally the same as done by other prehospital medics but involves more attention to detail. The interventions follow the same general principles but are often more aggressive, including intravenous (IV) fluid resuscitation and administration of analgesia. The same principles for immobilization are used, and the patient is transported to the hospital.[39]

A paradigm shift in the U.S. military during the cold war necessitated the development and heavy reliance on specialized teams of en route critical personnel. Military operations became smaller and more mobile, leading to a shift from fixed combat support hospitals to scalable deployable assets with forward surgical operations providing damage control surgery. With this new paradigm of surgical care, a gap existed in the transfer of intensive care level (ICU) of treatment in the patient who may be stable but not appropriate for the standard military aeromedical evacuation system. Some of the teams created include the U.S. Army Burn Flight Team (1950s), the U.S. Air Force (USAF) Critical Care Air Transport Team (1990s), and the USAF Acute Lung Rescue Team (2005). These specialized teams impact military care and civilian care via augmentation during disasters.

Airway Control

The first objective is to evaluate, manage, and secure the airway. Inspection of the airway for foreign bodies such as broken teeth, foodstuff, emesis, and clotted blood is essential before an artificial airway is placed. In all Basic Life Support courses, the emphasis on chin lift and jaw thrust cannot be overemphasized as the initial treatment.[40] This simple maneuver moves the tongue away from the back of the throat and in many instances reestablishes a patent airway. At this point, an oral airway may need to be placed. Appropriate size selection is essential to prevent the complication of airway obstruction. The nasopharyngeal airway may also be placed through the nasal passage into the back of the oropharynx to prevent the tongue from occluding the airway.

After this maneuver has been performed, the airway may need to be definitively controlled in patients who are unresponsive or have an altered mental status (Glasgow Coma Scale [GCS] score <8), are hemodynamically unstable, or have multiple injuries including the head and neck. Of importance remains cervical spine protection while the optimal airway is maintained, with in-line cervical spine stabilization. This maneuver minimizes iatrogenic injuries to the spine and spinal cord during the process of definitive airway control.

Prehospital endotracheal intubation remains a controversial intervention because of the success rate and amount of time required to perform the definitive airway. The EMS systems with the highest endotracheal intubations rate have very stringent requirements for certification (i.e., 20 live intubation or a minimum of 12 field intubations annually).[41] Neuromuscular blockade increases the success rate (97%), but the current use is limited to a few ground EMS systems and aeromedical agencies under direct medical control.[42]

Besides direct endotracheal intubation there are other airway adjuncts available. The use of the laryngeal mask airway (LMA) has gained popularity because of the relative ease of placement and relatively low cardiovascular stress that the patient undergoes compared with standard endotracheal intubation. It must be remembered that the LMA does not technically protect the airway from aspiration and was designed for use in spontaneously breathing patients. The LMA may be used emergently for a patient to whom a paralytic agent has been given but successful intubation has not been achieved or before the injection of the paralytic agent if mask ventilation is not adequate

The King LT is a commonly used rescue technique to manage the airway in the prehospital setting. The King LT is a single-use supraglottic airway that uses two cuffs to create a supraglottic ventilation seal at the pharynx and esophagus. It has a single ventilation port and a single valve and pilot balloon that go to both the pharyngeal balloon and the esophageal balloon. Although it is possible to insert the distal tip of the King LT directly into the trachea instead of the esophagus, its overall short length and preformed curve makes this very unlikely. Several studies have shown the King LT to have a higher rate for success for airway control in the prehospital setting compared with other supraglottic airways or endotracheal intubation.[43-45]

Whenever the decision is made to emergently secure an airway, it must be accomplished as quickly and safely as possible. Pharmacologic agents must be chosen that will allow the safe placement of an airway while minimizing the risk to the patient. The most rapidly acting agents with the shortest duration (i.e., etomidate for sedation and succinylcholine for paralysis) along with an acceptable side effect profile should be chosen. In all circumstances, the practitioner must avoid the situation in which a long-acting agent has been given and the airway cannot be intubated or ventilated with a bag mask device.

In the case of the standard rapid sequence induction, the patient should be preoxygenated, and a hypnotic agent should be given and immediately followed by the paralytic agent. Mask ventilation is not attempted (it may induce aspiration), and it is hoped that the immediate successful placement of the endotracheal tube will proceed. Proper placement is verified by auscultation of the lungs bilaterally, lack of gastric sounds with ventilation, and the presence of end-tidal carbon dioxide at the proximal end of the endotracheal tube.

Thermal injuries to the airway initially may not be symptomatic or present as hypoxia for some time after the insult. During the initial survey, documentation of singed hair, soot, or burns around the air passages should be noted. The decision may be made to secure an airway with an endotracheal tube prophylactically before significant edema and swelling may make securing the airway much more difficult.

As the anesthetic induction is begun, an assistant should apply enough pressure onto the cricoid cartilage so as to occlude the esophagus, which lies directly posterior.[46,47] It should be remembered that trauma, pain, and the use of narcotics may all delay gastric emptying. Release of cricoid pressure occurs only after proper positioning of the endotracheal tube has been verified.

Hemorrhage Control

Uncontrolled hemorrhage is the second leading cause of death in civilian trauma and the leading cause of death in military trauma.[11,14,28] Compression of hemorrhage is one of the first priorities for prehospital personnel in the care of injured patients, and on the battlefield, it takes precedence in Tactical Combat Casualty Care. When direct pressure cannot control hemorrhage, advanced maneuvers are needed, including the use of tourniquets and hemostatics as adjuncts for control.

Extremity hemorrhage is common with penetrating trauma and especially during wartime. Despite previous debate concerning the use of tourniquets in the prehospital setting, recent experience and research in combat causalities have led to a dramatic increase in the use of tourniquets. Current literature suggests that tourniquets are strongly associated with survival when applied early and have a low morbidity risk without amputations resulting solely from their application.[48-50] Although all military personnel deployed to combat are provided tourniquets with training, the use of tourniquets in the civilian prehospital setting is not common. One recent review of community experience of isolated exsanguinating extremity hemorrhage noted that more than 50% of patients who died had a bleeding site anatomically amenable to tourniquet control.[51] Based on military experience and improvements in tourniquet technology, emergency medical personnel are now being trained in the application of the tourniquet, and it is endorsed by Prehopital Trauma Life Support (PHTLS).[52] Universal acceptance, indications, and application of the use of tourniquets might benefit in disaster or mass casualty situations.[53]

The role of topical hemostatic agents in control of hemorrhage has been predominately in combat resuscitation but is becoming more common in civilian practice. The compounds in general are most useful in curtailing hemorrhage associated with broad or deep wounds, particularly in junctional areas. The ideal agent would be package ready, light weight, simple to apply, work rapidly, and control both arterial and venous bleeding.[54] Although no agent currently meets these requirements, the three most common classes include mucoadhesive agents (WoundStat, HemCon, and Celox), procoagulant supplementors (QuikClot Combat Gauze), and clotting factor concentrators (QuikClot Zeolite granular and QuikClot ACS+). All agents have shown benefit over traditional field dressings in animal models of hemorrhage.[54-57] Although these agents have demonstrated efficacy, there are some safety concerns.[58,59] Similar to tourniquet application, the use of hemostatic agents is currently limited in civilian prehospital care by scope and application compared with military use.

Resuscitation

A primary goal of prehospital providers in conjunction with airway and hemorrhage control is the restoration of perfusion. Prompt and appropriate access to intravascular space is critical, and the placement of large-bore peripheral catheters is still the standard. However, rapid access is not always easily achievable, and an alternate approach with placement of intraosseous (IO) devices has steadily increased. IO devices can be placed in children and adults in a variety of locations, but caution must be used because each IO device is specifically designed for age group (pediatric vs. adult) and specific anatomic location (sternal vs. tibia).

The traditional prehospital resuscitation treatment regimen of 2 L of crystalloid fluid to achieve a minimum systolic blood pressure of 90 mm Hg has been reduced to 1 L of crystalloid with the 9th Edition of the Advanced Trauma Life Support (ATLS) course based on growing evidence that aggressive crystalloid resuscitation may not be beneficial.[60,61] The concept of withholding resuscitation and allowing permissive hypotension with ongoing hemorrhage dates back to World War I and has been uniformly adopted in the current management of gastrointestinal (GI) hemorrhage and aortic aneurysm rupture. In selected groups of trauma patients, it has been shown to increase survival.[62,63] This concept of controlled resuscitation has already been adopted by the military with limited administration of fluids (maximum of two 500-mL boluses of Hextend a minimum of 30 minutes apart).[64] The rationale for this recommendation is based on limited resources on the battlefield and the cumulative literature regarding limited resuscitation.

The deployment of blood components and fresh whole blood in the prehospital realm is becoming more frequent, particularly with prehospital critical care providers on both rotary wing and ground transports. Currently, several air services carry packed red blood cells, and a few carry plasma.[65-69]

Tranexamic acid (TXA) is an antifibrinolytic agent that has been used since the 1960s to control bleeding from blood dyscrasias, heavy menstrual bleeding, and GI bleeding and is now also being evaluated in trauma patients as part of the resuscitation.[70] In a very large multicenter, randomized, double-blind, placebo-controlled trial, trauma patients who received TXA had a significant reduction in all-cause mortality and an overall reduction in death secondary to hemorrhage.[71] Those who benefited the most received TXA within 3 hours of injury. The military recently, in a retrospective study, compared combat-injured patients who received TXA with those who did not, demonstrating improved survival in the group that received TXA.[72] Current efforts are under way to study the use of TXA in the prehospital setting to assess if earlier administration of the drug would extend the benefits previously seen in the hospital treatment.

HOSPITAL EVALUATION AND CARE

Trauma Team

The configuration of the trauma team receiving patients is variable but includes emergency medicine physicians, nurses, allied health personnel, and the trauma surgeon as the team leader.[61] Various subspecialists in surgery, orthopedics, neurosurgery, cardiothoracic surgery, anesthesia, and pediatrics are readily available at a level I center. The receiving facility should have a dedicated area for the resuscitation of trauma patients as well as a dedicated operating room (OR) available 24 hours a day. A resuscitation room should be well equipped with devices for the warming of fluid, rapid infusers, and appropriate surgical supplies for the performance of lifesaving procedures. Permanently fixed radiographic equipment expedites the evaluation of injured patients in the resuscitation room. Staffing in the trauma room should be limited to those with experience in trauma resuscitation, and their duties should follow the guidelines outlined in the ACS Committee on Trauma Resources for Optimal Care of the Trauma Patient 2010.[20]

After the acute phase of resuscitation and operative intervention, a level I trauma facility maintains a highly trained staff of surgical intensivists. The staff provides 24-hour coverage of the intensive care unit (ICU). These patients are susceptible to complications such as sepsis, acute respiratory distress syndrome (ARDS), and multisystem organ failure, which require the technical support provided by a level I center. Intermediate care units provide intensive supervision of the patient before placement on the trauma floor, which is critical for the recovery of the patient. During this time, patients receive rehabilitation to prepare for dealing with disabilities and limitations that may have changed their lives owing to their injury. The patient's physical and emotional health is evaluated, and treatment is initiated. Patients who have sustained significant injury will have special nutritional needs, given their increased caloric demands. The patient's nutritional status is assessed by nutritional services and a recommendation made to the trauma service. As the patient nears discharge, arrangements for home needs and potential placement are made by social services and case care coordinators. The availability of and relationships with rehabilitation centers and chronic nursing facilities are essential for injured patients.

Assessing the Severity of Injury

Several scoring systems have been developed in an attempt to triage and classify patients both in the field and at the receiving hospital. Champion and coworkers have classified the scoring systems into physiologic and anatomic types.[73] The GCS for brain injury is perhaps the most widely accepted physiologic score. This scale ranges from 3 to 15, with 15 being normal. Each section, with its weighted score, is as follows: eye movement (4 points maximum), verbal response (5 points maximum), and motor response (6 points maximum) (Table 9-1). The GCS is a part of the Revised Trauma Score (RTS), which allows inferences to patient outcome as a result of these scores. This score comprises the GCS score, systolic blood pressure, and respiratory rate (Table 9-2).[74]

HOSPITAL RESUSCITATION

After the trauma patient has reached the trauma center, resuscitation is continued according to the principles of a primary, secondary, and tertiary survey as established by the ACS Committee on Trauma. The primary survey encompasses the ABCs, disability, and exposure. The goal is to identify and immediately address threats to life. The focus of the primary survey is to restore normal physiology in an unstable patient. Realize that this may require operative intervention to control hemorrhage. Thus, the primary survey is a physiologic concept and not a temporal one. The team does not move to the secondary survey until immediate threats to life have been addressed. The secondary survey involves a head-to-toe

TABLE 9-1 *GLASGOW COMA SCALE*

Response	Score
A. Eye Opening	
Spontaneous	4
To voice	3
To pain	2
None	1
B. Verbal Response	
Oriented	5
Confused	4
Inappropriate words	3
Incomprehensible sounds	2
None	1
C. Motor Response	
Obeys commands	6
Localized pain	5
Withdraw to pain	4
Flexion to pain	3
Extension to pain	2
None	1

Total points (A + B + C) = 3–15.
Adapted from Teasdale G, Jennett B: Assessment of coma and impaired consciousness. A practical scale, Lancet *2:81–84, © by The Lancet Ltd, 1974.*

TABLE 9-2 *REVISED TRAUMA SCORE*

Response	Variables	Score
A. Respiratory Rate (breaths/min)		
	10–29	4
	>29	3
	6–9	2
	1–5	1
	0	0
B. Systolic Blood Pressure (mm Hg)		
	>89	4
	76–89	3
	50–75	2
	1–49	1
	0	0
C. Glasgow Coma Scale Score Conversion		
	13–15	4
	9–12	3
	6–8	2
	4–5	1
	3	0
Revised Trauma Score = Total of A + B + C		

Adapted from Champion HR, Sacco WJ, Copes WS, et al: A revision of the Trauma Score, J Trauma *29:623–629, 1989.*

evaluation of the patient's injuries and implementation of appropriate interventions. The tertiary survey involves serial reevaluation of the patient's status during his or her hospital course. This section reviews the process of trauma resuscitation and diagnostic modalities and treatment options for specific injuries.

PRIMARY SURVEY

Airway

Airway assessment is performed immediately on arrival to the trauma bay. If the patient already has airway control with endotracheal intubation or other tube adjunct, the intervention is assessed via end-tidal CO_2 detection, breath sounds, and possible direct visualization if the patient is not appropriately responding to oxygenation or ventilation. If patient's airway is not controlled, the patient is managed as previously outlined earlier. It is critical that the patient's airway is controlled before or concurrently breathing and hemorrhage control are addressed in the primary survey.

In the rare instance when an airway cannot be obtained by the previous methods, a surgical airway may need to be created.[75] The standard emergency adult surgical airway procedure is cricothyroidotomy (Fig. 9-1). This surgical airway procedure requires a vertical incision to be made in the skin over the cricothyroid membrane followed by a transverse incision into the trachea through this membrane. An endotracheal or tracheostomy tube is then placed into the trachea and secured to provide ventilation and oxygenation. A needle cricothyroidotomy may be performed in some instances with positive-pressure ventilation as a bridge to the definitive surgical airway. This involves placing a large angiocatheter (14-gauge) through the cricothyroid membrane and ventilating with 30 to 60 pounds per square inch of pressurized oxygen. After the airway is secured, supplemental oxygen must be given to begin the process of providing adequate tissue oxygenation.

Breathing

A wide range of breathing devices is currently available. The use of SteriShields or more sophisticated mouth-to-mask breathing devices has introduced an element of safety for the resuscitator. These devices are small and are found in first responder mobile units as a standard approach to resuscitation. Some of these devices allow for supplemental oxygen to be used in the resuscitation. Hyperoxygenation is essential for cardiopulmonary stabilization and resuscitation.

At the more advanced level, the use of bag valve ventilation via an endotracheal tube provides the most effective method of oxygen delivery. Another method of ventilation is the use of portable and stationary ventilators, which have the added benefit of allowing more sophisticated control of ventilatory mechanics.

After the airway has been secured, the patient's chest, neck, and breathing pattern must be assessed. Respiratory rate, depth of respiration, use of accessory muscles, presence of abdominal breathing, chest wall symmetry, and the presence of cyanosis must all be evaluated. Life-threatening injuries causing tension pneumothorax, open pneumothorax, flail chest, or massive hemothorax are identified and treated immediately.

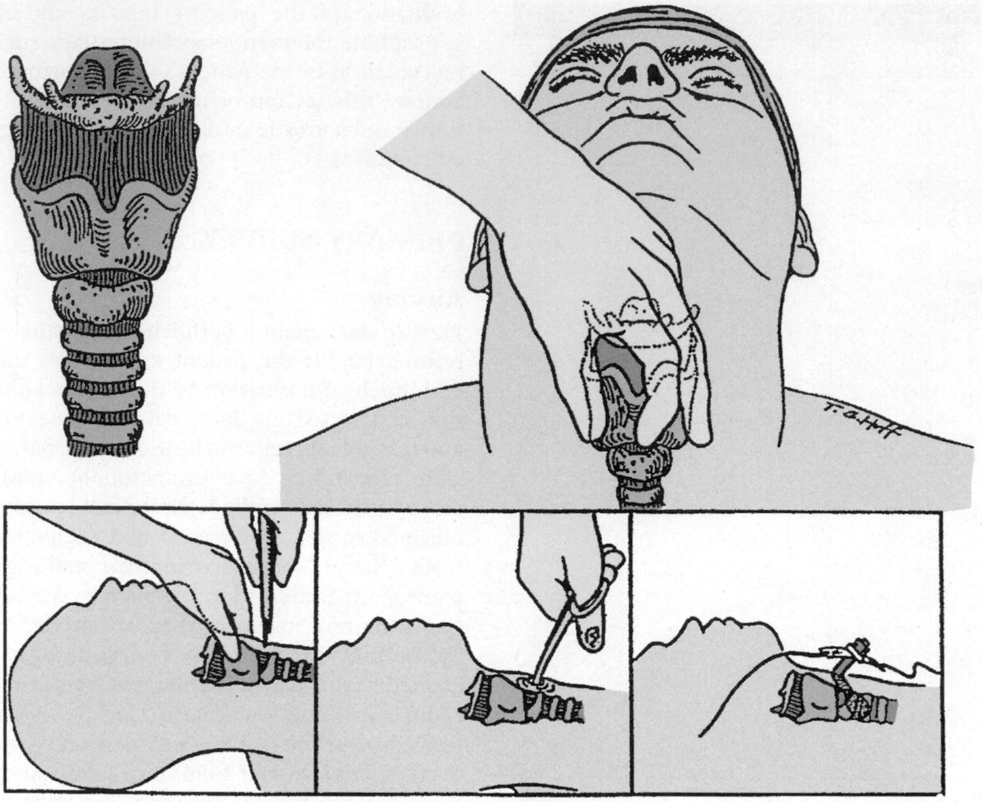

FIGURE 9-1. Technique for cricothyroidotomy.

It is imperative to remember that positive-pressure ventilation will worsen a pneumothorax unless a thoracostomy tube is placed to prevent a tension pneumothorax. Tension pneumothorax is diagnosed by the identification of decreased breath sounds (on the ipsilateral side), hyperresonance to percussion (on the ipsilateral side), respiratory distress, hypotension, tachycardia, hypoxia, and cyanosis. Less common is tracheal deviation (toward the contralateral side), and jugular vein distention may not be present in a hypovolemic patient. Emergent treatment is lifesaving and consists of a needle thoracostomy (14-gauge needle, $2\frac{1}{4}$-in length) at the second intercostal space at the midclavicular line on the affected side. This procedure is always followed by placement of a chest tube (36–40 Fr) at the fifth intercostal space anterior to the midaxillary line (Fig. 9-2).

Open pneumothorax (sucking chest wound) is initially treated with a three-sided occlusive dressing, thereby preventing a tension pneumothorax, followed by chest tube placement (36 Fr) as described. It should be noted that the chest tube should not be placed through the injury but through a separate incision. The need for intubation and surgical closure of the defect is based on the severity of the defect, associated injuries, the ability to provide adequate oxygenation, and the patient's overall condition.

Flail chest, described as more than two consecutive rib fractures with multiple fractures in each rib resulting in a loss of chest wall integrity, will result in the development of paradoxical chest wall movement and respiratory embarrassment. This condition usually is associated with underlying pulmonary contusion, which will worsen for the first 24 hours. The paradoxical chest wall movement with resulting ventilation-perfusion mismatch and pulmonary contusion leads to hypoxia. Intubation with mechanical ventilation will "splint" the flail segment and recruit alveoli, allowing more effective alveolar ventilation and more efficient oxygenation. It is essential to provide adequate analgesia to provide comfort and facilitate aggressive pulmonary toilet whether or not the patient is intubated. In some cases, placement of chest tubes may be required to prevent the development of a pneumothorax if high levels of ventilator support are needed or a hemopneumothorax already exists.

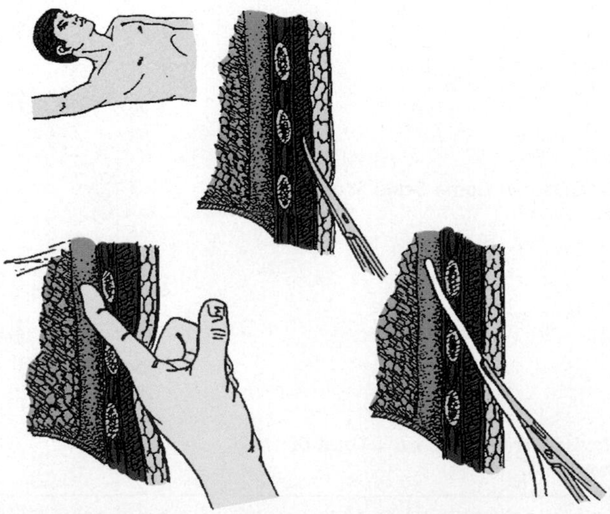

FIGURE 9-2. Technique for chest tube thoracotomy.

Massive hemothorax, described as greater than 1500 mL of blood from the injured hemithorax, more than 200 mL of blood per hour for 4 consecutive hours, or a significant retained hemothorax after chest tube placement, requires surgical intervention.

Circulation

Maintaining adequate circulation and controlling hemorrhage for the prevention or reversal of shock are of utmost importance in the resuscitation of trauma patients. Shock is defined as a compromise in circulation resulting in inadequate oxygen delivery to meet a given tissue's oxygen demand. The most common cause of shock in trauma patients is hypovolemia secondary to hemorrhage. The initial management of the patient should include establishing two IV lines (16 gauge or greater), one in each antecubital fossa vein. Central access in the form of an introducer (8.5-Fr, IV line) may be necessary for more rapid infusion of crystalloids and blood products in an unstable patient. These lines should be placed in the femoral or subclavian vein depending on the patient's injuries. Resuscitation with 1 L of lactated Ringer or normal saline solution is recommended followed by blood if indicated.[20]

If possible, rapid infusion devices, which warm all fluids, should be used. Hypothermia may be exacerbated by the infusion of room temperature or colder fluids, which in turn may hinder the normal activity of platelets and worsen the coagulopathy.

If the patient remains unstable after the infusion of 1 L of a balanced salt solution, then blood should be given.[20] The type of blood product in part depends on the urgency with which the transfusion must be given. Typed and cross-matched packed red blood cells are the product of choice, but the cross-matching process may take up to 1 hour. Type-specific packed red blood cells are the second choice; however, it takes approximately 20 minutes to perform a rapid cross-match. Universal donor O-positive or O-negative blood (for female patients of childbearing years) is usually well tolerated when given to trauma victims in severe shock. Approximately 200,000 units of O-negative are used each year in emergency situations.[76]

In the trauma patient, hemorrhage or hypovolemia is the most common cause of shock. Hemorrhagic shock has been classified as follows[20]:

Class I hemorrhage: loss of 15% of blood volume or up to 750 mL; clinical symptoms are minimal, and blood volume is restored by various intrinsic mechanisms within 24 hours

Class II hemorrhage: loss of 15% to 30% of blood volume or 750 to 1500 mL; tachycardia; tachypnea; decrease in pulse pressure; mild mental status changes

Class III hemorrhage: 30% to 40% blood loss or 1500 to 2000 mL; significant tachycardia; tachypnea; mental status changes; and decrease in systolic blood pressure

Class IV hemorrhage: greater than 40% blood loss or greater than 2000 mL; severe tachycardia; decreased pulse pressure; obtundation; or coma

Patients who have sustained minimal blood loss (<20%) require a minimal volume of fluid to stabilize their blood pressure. A 20% to 30% blood loss requires at least 2 L of a balanced salt solution, but blood may not be required. Blood loss greater than 30% usually requires blood for stabilization. Patients who stabilize initially but then become hemodynamically unstable usually have ongoing bleeding and require operative intervention.

Patients who are identified as having ongoing hemorrhage are treated with direct pressure and elevation if applicable. Hemorrhage can be obvious and external or contained in body cavities (chest, abdomen, retroperitoneum, or pelvis) or surrounding a fractured bone. Radiographs of the chest and pelvis can quickly evaluate these areas as a source of hemorrhage. Hemothorax is managed as previously described. Blood contained in the pelvis secondary to a fracture is best controlled by stabilization of the pelvis, as described in detail in this textbook. Pelvic binders, bed sheets, or operative stabilization in the resuscitation suite using external fixators helps approximate the pelvis to its original size. This decreases the volume of the pelvis and compresses the pelvic hematoma. The resultant rise in intrapelvic pressure compresses the pelvic vasculature and stops the hemorrhage. This is an excellent way to control pelvic venous hemorrhage but is not as effective for pelvic arterial bleeding. The use of pelvic angiography and embolization provides a method for identifying and treating arterial pelvic bleeding. Other contained areas of significant bleeding occur with long bone fractures. These injuries should be managed by gentle reduction and splinting to help mitigate hemorrhage.

Perhaps the most insidious and lethal of circulatory insults secondary to trauma is cardiac tamponade. Cardiac tamponade occurs more commonly with penetrating injuries and is uncommon with blunt injury. The degree of tamponade depends on the size of the defect, the rate of bleeding, and the chamber involved. Tamponade may be caused by as little as 60 to 100 mL of blood in the pericardial space. Progression from compensated to uncompensated tamponade can be sudden and severe. Cardiac tamponade should be suspected in hypotensive patients with evidence of a penetrating injury in the "danger zone," which includes the precordium, epigastrium, and superior mediastinum. Beck's triad, which includes distended neck veins, muffled heart tones, and hypotension, may be present only 10% to 40% of the time. Diagnostic options in a stable patient include a two-dimensional echocardiogram or transesophageal echocardiogram. The type of injury, presence of distended neck veins, distant heart sounds, and hypotension should raise the possibility of the diagnosis of cardiac tamponade. Definitive treatment is sternotomy or left thoracotomy (if in the ED) with repair of the cardiac injury. If surgical backup is not available and the patient is in shock, subxiphoid needle decompression of the pericardial space is an option as a temporizing maneuver (Fig. 9-3). The removal of 10 to 50 mL of blood from the pericardial space can significantly improve survival. Pericardiocentesis should be followed by emergent operative decompression and repair of underlying cardiac injury.

Disability

An initial brief neurologic evaluation should be performed to ascertain the level of consciousness and pupillary response and whether there is any gross neurologic deficit either centrally or in any of the four extremities. Any progression of a neurologic deficit may require an immediate therapeutic maneuver or operative procedure. A quick way to describe the level of consciousness is using the acronym AVPU (*a*lert, responds to *v*oice commands, responds to *p*ain, *u*nresponsive). The GCS is a more detailed assessment of the level of consciousness. Patients with a GCS score of 3 to 8 are considered to have a severe head injury and require airway control.

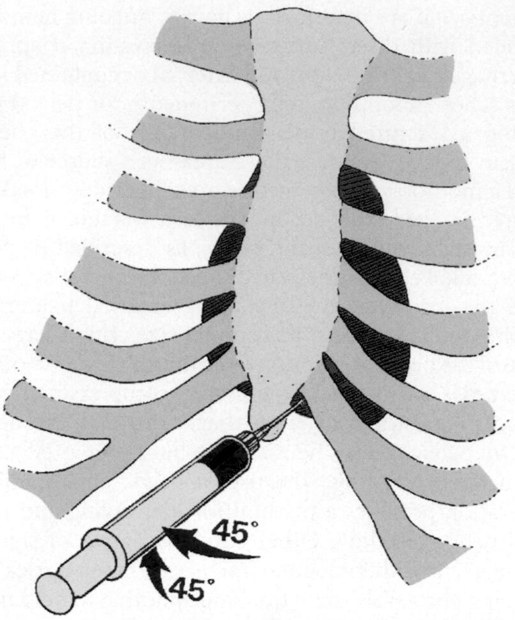

FIGURE 9-3. Pericardiocentesis. *(Adapted from Ivatury RR. In Feliciano DV, Moore EE, Mattox KL, editors:* Trauma, *ed 3, Stamford, CT, 1996, Appleton & Lange.)*

A score of 9 to 13 signifies a moderate head injury, and a score of 14 to 15 is consistent with a minor head injury. The cervical, thoracic, and lumbar spine are protected from injury by being placed on a long board with cervical spine immobilization.

Exposure and Environmental Control

A head-to-toe examination of the patient must be performed. All clothing should be removed to facilitate a complete examination. After this examination has been completed, the patient should be covered with a warm blanket for protection from hypothermia.

Patients with hypo- or hyperthermia require immediate intervention to return to normothermia. The patient should be removed from the exposure as quickly as possible. In cold exposure, gradual rewarming is preferred to avoid the potential problem of dysrhythmia. Patients with thermal burns should have any burned clothing rapidly removed to prevent further injury from continued heat transmission. It is essential to determine the type, concentration, and pH of any contaminating agent that has had contact with the patient. The agent should be removed and the area either irrigated with water or saline or neutralized. The skin should be constantly reexamined to be sure that contamination or burning is not continuing. The area is then covered with sterile dry dressings.

Hazardous materials create a special problem, not only for the victims but also for caregivers, especially in cases of radiation or chemical exposure. The most important step is developing a plan before the event. Prehospital protocols established in conjunction with receiving facilities capable of handling such emergencies are necessary to protect the staff and other noninvolved patients at that facility. These protocols should be available in the "disaster manual," which should be immediately available in the ED. Decontamination protocols are important in the initial phase of any treatment in patients who have been exposed to toxic materials. Personnel should not contaminate the ED with a patient who has been exposed to hazardous material.

As the trauma surgeon completes the primary survey and life-threatening injuries are identified and treated, a secondary survey is then initiated. In addition, the placement of a pulse oximeter, an electrocardiogram, and initiation of blood pressure monitoring provide continuous monitoring of vital signs. The resuscitation phase occurs simultaneously with primary and secondary surveys. The placement of a naso- or orogastric tube, placement of a Foley catheter, chest and pelvic radiographs, and FAST (focused assessment by sonography in trauma) are then performed.

SECONDARY SURVEY

The secondary survey begins after the primary care survey is completed. This involves a complete head-to-toe evaluation combined with definitive diagnosis and treatment of injuries. If indicated, more extensive tests such as ultrasonography, diagnostic peritoneal lavage, computed tomography (CT), angiography, and imaging of suspected bone injuries may be performed unless the patient requires immediate surgical intervention to address findings in the primary survey. The basic evaluation and management of commonly incurred injuries as well as the role of damage control surgery are discussed here.

Damage Control Surgery

Historically, a decisive operation completed in one setting had been a standard of modern surgery. In this paradigm, the injured patient is taken to the OR, all areas of injury are identified and addressed completely, and the patient is definitively closed. However, this approach led to death, either during the operation or shortly thereafter, in seriously injured patients. The concept of abbreviated surgery to address physiologic instead of anatomic parameters was termed *damage control* in 1993 specifically addressing initial laparotomy followed by intensive resuscitation.[77] The term has since been applied broadly to a surgical management philosophy and surgical techniques across multiple disciplines, including orthopaedic surgery, neurosurgery, vascular surgery, burn surgery, and emergent general surgery. Damage control surgery is usually described as stages of care, which include stage 1, control hemorrhage, limit contamination, and temporary closure; stage 2, treatment of hypothermia, correction of coagulopathy, and reversal of acidosis; and stage 3, definitive surgery, which may require multiple operations and still may not result in full establishment of normal anatomy (i.e., colostomy vs. bowel reanastomosis, external fixation vs. open reduction and internal fixation).[78,79] The damage control surgery paradigm should always be considered in the care of severely multi-injured patients.

Trauma to the Cranium

Closed head injury is a significant contributor to the morbidity and mortality associated with multitraumatized patients. It is estimated that approximately 30% to 45% of traffic fatalities involve associated head injuries.[80] The most common mechanism of injury for head trauma in adults is motor vehicle crashes followed by falls. Computed tomography is the diagnostic modality of choice.

Brain injury may be classified in terms of primary and secondary injury. Primary injury is caused by the mechanical damage that occurs at the time of insult as a result of the contact between the brain parenchyma and vascular structures and the interior of the cranium or a foreign body entering the cranium. The brain undergoes distortion from shearing forces, leading to contusions and lacerations of the parenchyma, and disruption of the arterial and venous arcades. This may result in subarachnoid hemorrhages, epidural hematomas, and subdural hematomas.

Secondary brain injury with continuing neural damage is caused by cerebral hypoxia, hypo- or hypercapnia, increased intracerebral pressure, decreased cerebral blood flow, hyperthermia, or electrolyte and acid–base abnormalities.[81] Interventions are geared toward preventing or lessening the neurologic destruction by optimizing cerebral perfusion and oxygenation. Ventriculostomy catheters may be placed to monitor intracranial pressure (ICP) and maintain pressures less than 20 mm Hg. Monitors to assess the oxygen partial pressure may be placed to assess cerebral oxygenation.[82] Hemodynamic monitors should also be placed to assist with the maintenance of adequate intravascular volume and mean arterial pressure (MAP). The ultimate goal is to maintain cerebral perfusion pressure (CPP) greater than 60 mm Hg. CPP is the difference between MAP and ICP.[83] Acid–base balance, electrolytes, and coagulopathy should be evaluated and corrected. Failure to do so may result in significant morbidity or even death.

Intracranial hematomas also cause secondary brain damage and are classified as epidural, subdural, or intracerebral. Early identification and evacuation of a significant mass lesion is critical in the management of head injury.[84,85] Epidural hematomas (EDHs) occur usually secondary to a skull fracture with subsequent laceration of the middle meningeal artery. They appear on CT scan in a characteristic lentiform or lens shape. Patients may have a classic lucid period followed by an alteration in mental status. Subdural hematomas (SDHs) occur as a result of injury to bridging veins. This type of hematoma is more common and may cause greater morbidity than epidural hematomas because of the associated cerebral contusions. They appear on CT scan as concave shapes that do not cross the midline. Causes of intracerebral hematomas include penetrating injuries, depressed skull fractures, or shearing forces sufficient enough to tear the brain parenchyma. The hematoma and accompanying cerebral edema can cause a mass that results in a shift of the cerebrum and herniation.

Neck Injury

Penetrating neck injuries account for up to 11% of deaths. To better aid in the diagnosis and treatment of neck injuries, the neck can be divided into three zones (Fig. 9-4). Zone I is inferior to the cricoid cartilage. Zone II extends from the cricoid cartilage to the angle of the jaw. Zone III is located between the angle of the mandible and the base of the skull. These anatomic regions become important in the evaluation and treatment of neck injuries. Vascular injuries in zones I and III pose difficult technical surgical challenges to obtaining proximal and distal control; therefore, it is essential to delineate the vascular structures by angiography. Treatment of injuries in these areas may require interventional radiologic techniques or open operative procedures. Zone II vascular

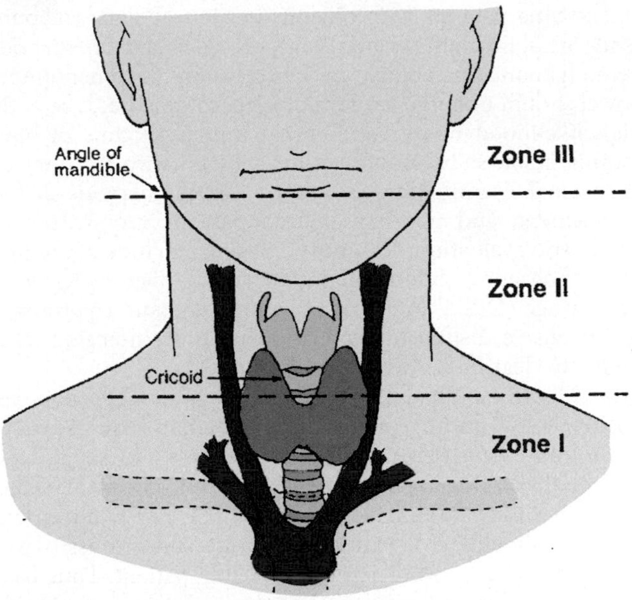

FIGURE 9-4. Monson's anatomic zones for penetrating injury to the neck. *(Adapted from Thal ER. In Feliciano DV, Moore EE, Mattox KL, editors:* Trauma, *ed 3, Stamford, CT, 1996, Appleton & Lange.)*

structures are more easily accessible and can be evaluated by CT angiography, digital angiography, or direct surgical exploration.[86-88] Injury to the cervical spine is addressed in detail in this textbook.

Thoracic Injury

Injury to the thorax results in significant morbidity and mortality.[89] Twenty-five percent of trauma deaths are primarily from chest injury, and these injuries are contributory in up to 50% of deaths. On the other hand, only 15% of chest injuries require operative intervention, and most are managed by appropriate intubation or placement of a thoracostomy tube. Injuries that require immediate lifesaving therapeutic intervention include tension pneumothorax, open pneumothorax, flail chest, massive hemothorax, or pericardial tamponade, as previously described. The use of CT, bronchoscopy, angiography, and esophagoscopy or esophagography further delineates injured structures.

Abdominal Injury

Intraabdominal injury should be suspected in any victim of a high-speed motor vehicle crash, fall from a significant height, or penetrating injury to the trunk. Up to 20% of patients with hemoperitoneum may not manifest peritoneal signs.[20] The major goal during trauma resuscitation is not to diagnose a specific intraabdominal injury but to confirm the presence of an injury and particularly need for laparotomy. The diagnosis of abdominal injury should begin with the physical examination during the secondary survey. This should include inspection, auscultation, percussion, and palpation. A rectal examination and examination of the genitalia should also be performed. A nasogastric tube and Foley catheter must be placed to aid in diagnosis of an esophagogastric or urinary tract injury.

Patients with penetrating injuries to the abdomen that violate the peritoneal cavity, especially from gunshot wounds, and trauma patients with obvious peritoneal signs (rebound tenderness, involuntary guarding), presence of a foreign body, hemodynamic instability, or evisceration of omentum or bowel should undergo exploratory laparotomy because of the high likelihood of intraabdominal injury. Victims of blunt trauma, stable stab-wound victims, patients with an equivocal abdominal examination caused by central nervous system impairment, and multiply injured patients require further diagnostic evaluation. Diagnostic options include abdominal ultrasonography, abdominal and pelvis CT, diagnostic peritoneal lavage (DPL), angiography, and diagnostic laparoscopy. An extensive diagnostic evaluation is contraindicated when there are clear indications for celiotomy.

FAST can rapidly detect the presence of hemoperitoneum. Positive FAST findings in an unstable patient require prompt laparotomy. Sensitivity of FAST is reported to range from 60% to 93%. Thus, a negative FAST result does not definitively exclude abdominal injury.[90,91] The FAST ultrasound machine should be kept in the trauma suite to assist with obtaining results rapidly in the unstable patient. Four basic areas are evaluated for fluid. The subcostal view evaluates the heart motion and pericardium. The Morrison pouch view visualizes the right upper quadrant at the interface between the liver and right kidney. The splenorenal view evaluates the left upper quadrant between the spleen and kidney. The pouch of Douglas view allows evaluation for fluid around the bladder.

The abdomen and pelvis CT provides the ability to evaluate intraperitoneal and retroperitoneal injuries. CT has sensitivity of 93% to 98%, specificity of 75% to 100%, and accuracy of 95% to 97%. Its major drawback is the low sensitivity for identifying intraperitoneal bowel or pancreatic injury.[92,93] CT is indicated in the stable patient after significant blunt mechanism of injury without indication for immediate abdominal exploration. The major disadvantage of a CT is the need to transport the patient from the trauma suite to the CT scan room; thus, it should be performed only in the hemodynamically stable patient.

DPL has sensitivity of 98% to 100%, specificity of 90% to 96%, and accuracy of 98% to 100%.[94] It is also useful in the evaluation of intraperitoneal solid and hollow viscous injury, particularly when the patient remains hypotensive and FAST findings are equivocal. The procedure may be performed in one of three ways: open, semi-open, or closed. Details of this procedure may be found in the ACS ATLS manual. Positive DPL results for blunt injury include more than 10 mL of gross blood on initial aspiration, cell count of greater than 100,000 red blood cells or greater than 500 white blood cells, or evidence of enteric contents after removal of warmed crystalloid previously instilled for the procedure.

Angiography can be both diagnostic and therapeutic. Diagnostic angiography is useful in detecting injury, defining the precise site of injury, evaluating patency of the vessel, and assessing collateral flow. Angiography may be used for therapeutic embolization, stent graft placement for arterial disruptions, pseudoaneurysms, and arteriovenous fistulas, as well as retrieval of embolized foreign objects. Transcatheter embolization has been reported to be successful in 85% to 87% of cases.[95-97]

The majority of injuries to the spleen, liver, and kidney can be managed nonoperatively, provided the patient is hemodynamically stable. Hemodynamic status is the key decision point in the decision to operate upon or observe the patient with blunt solid organ injury. Currently, 85% of blunt liver injury and 70% of blunt splenic injury can be managed nonoperatively. Not coincidentally, the majority of these injuries are low grade (grades 1–3). In general, high-grade injury (grade 4 or 5) to the spleen and liver require operative intervention because of hemodynamic instability on presentation. In a stable patient, angiography and embolization are invaluable in the management of grade 4 and 5 injuries of the liver and spleen.[96-100]

Diagnostic laparoscopy is useful in evaluating the presence of penetration of the peritoneum from penetrating injury, and it has utility in evaluating the diaphragm for injury.[101]

Retroperitoneal Injuries

The duodenum, pancreas, parts of the colon, great vessels, and urinary system are retroperitoneal structures. Injury to these organs can be missed by physical examination, FAST, and DPL but may be diagnosed with CT of the abdomen and pelvis or intraoperatively.

Three fourths of duodenal injuries are penetrating injuries, whereas the majority of pancreatic injuries are due to blunt trauma. Injuries to both organs may be diagnosed with a CT scan of the abdomen or intraoperatively. DPL with elevated amylase levels is nonspecific but can contribute to an increased level of suspicion of an injury to one of these organs. Endoscopic retrograde cholangiopancreatography is useful for evaluating injuries to the duodenum, biliary system, and pancreatic duct.[102] Remember that CT may miss as many as 50% of pancreatic injuries.[103]

When considering management options, one must separate the nature of injury according to blunt and penetrating causes of retroperitoneal hematoma. For retroperitoneal hematomas from blunt causes in hemodynamically stable patients with no other reason for exploratory celiotomy, treatment is conservative. A massive or rapidly expanding hematoma on CT scan may require an arteriogram of the abdomen and pelvis with injured vessel embolization. When exploratory celiotomy is warranted, decision making is centered on anatomic considerations based on mechanism of injury and zones of the retroperitoneum, of which there are three (Fig. 9-5). Basically, all penetrating wounds of the retroperitoneum are explored when found operatively.

Zone I extends from the diaphragm to the sacral promontory. The aorta, vena cava, proximal renal vessels, portal vein, pancreas, and duodenum are located in this area. In general, a retroperitoneal hematoma in this area should be explored for both blunt and penetrating injuries.

Zone II includes the right and left flanks and contains the kidneys, adrenal glands, suprapelvic ureters bilaterally, and hilum of the vascular pedicle to the kidney. Retroperitoneal hematomas in zone II usually do not require exploration when resulting from blunt trauma unless there is a colon injury, expanding hematoma involving Gerota fascia, or a urinoma.

Zone III is the pelvis and contains the iliac vessels, distal sigmoid colon, rectum, bladder, and distal pelvic segment of the ureters. Zone III hematomas associated with pelvic fractures and hemodynamic instability may require reduction and fixation of the pelvis to control bleeding and may require angiography, as described earlier. Nonexpanding hematomas are observed.

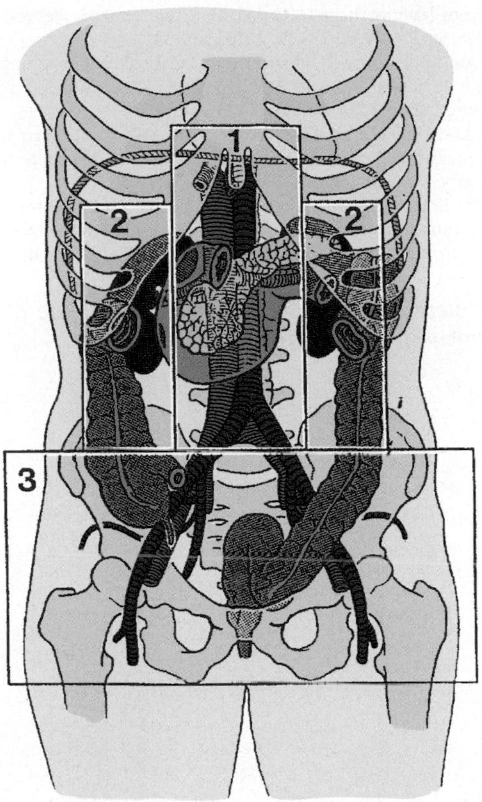

FIGURE 9-5. Anatomic zones for retroperitoneal hematomas. *(Adapted from Meyer AA, Kudsk KA, Sheldon GF. In Blaisdell FW, Trunkey DD, editors:* Abdominal trauma, *ed 2, New York, 1993, Thieme Medical Publishers.)*

Genitourinary Injuries

Hematuria in the setting of significant blunt abdominal trauma, penetrating trauma, or pelvic fractures should signal that there might be significant injury to the genitourinary tract. Placement of a Foley catheter is important during the initial resuscitation of the trauma patient. Before placement of the Foley catheter, a digital rectal examination and visual inspection of the urethral meatus, scrotum, or labia should be performed. Blood at the urethral meatus or scrotal or labial hematomas may be indicative of a pelvic fracture or urethral injury. In this case, a retrograde urethrogram must be performed in male trauma patients before Foley catheter placement to rule out a urethral injury.

Further evaluation of significant hematuria may include a cystogram with filling, voiding, and post voiding radiographs to diagnose bladder injuries. In addition, CT of the abdomen and pelvis with IV contrast may assist with the diagnosis of a renal or ureteral injury. A penetrating injury to the abdomen may warrant a "one-shot" intravenous pyelogram (IVP) in the setting of hematuria to help evaluate renal excretory function of the ipsilateral and contralateral kidney, but this is being less frequently done.

The majority of blunt injuries to the genitourinary tract do not require surgical intervention. In the event that significant disruption of the renal parenchyma, ureter, bladder, or urethra is identified, definitive treatment is warranted. Depending on the extent of the injury, treatment may range from primary repair to resection of the injured area and adequate closed suction drainage.

Musculoskeletal Injuries

Detailed management of specific bony injuries is addressed in this textbook. Fractures with significant displacement may be associated with significant soft tissue injury. For example, patients with rib, scapular, clavicular, or sternal fractures may have great vessel or cardiac injuries that may require angiography or duplex ultrasonography and possibly operative intervention. Fractures of the axial skeleton may have associated neurologic, vascular, or visceral injury that may take priority in the management scenario of a patient. Pelvic and long bone fractures may be associated with vascular injuries that result in hemorrhagic shock. Early reduction and fixation will contribute significantly to hemodynamic stabilization of the patient. The stabilization results in significant improvement in the patient's overall pulmonary status, rehabilitation, hospital course, and length of stay. With any fracture of an extremity in a trauma patient, there must be an awareness of the possibility of a compartment syndrome or vascular injury that may result in limb ischemia.

TERTIARY SURVEY

The tertiary survey consists of a repeat head-to-toe evaluation of the trauma patient along with reevaluation of available laboratory data and review of radiographic studies. Any change in the patient's condition must be promptly evaluated and treated. The most expeditious method to accomplish this task is to begin with the ABCs of the primary survey followed by the secondary survey. Any newly discovered physical findings are further investigated. Injuries often missed during earlier assessments include minor fractures, lacerations, and traumatic brain injury. Emphasis on repeated physical examinations and evaluation of newly obtained laboratory and radiology studies will continue to impact positively on patient outcome. Implementation of a standardized tertiary survey has been shown to decrease missed injuries by 36%.[104]

SUMMARY

Successful identification, resuscitation, and treatment of the multiple-injured patient require a carefully systematic, thorough approach. Special priority and attention have to be given to addressing injuries that are life threatening. After the primary survey has been completed and lifesaving interventions are initiated, a secondary survey that is designed to identify other injuries has to be rapidly performed. An appropriate management plan can be rapidly developed and implemented to minimize the risk of missed injury. Finally, a tertiary survey should be performed to detect any latent problems that present hours after the patient has been admitted to the hospital. A comprehensive, careful approach to management will afford severely injured patients the best possible outcomes.

KEY REFERENCES

The level of evidence (LOE) is determined according to the criteria provided in the preface.

11. Eastridge BJ, Mabry RL, Seguin P, et al: Death on the battlefield (2001-2011): implications for the future of combat casualty care. *J Trauma* 73(6):S431–S437, 2012. LOE IV

22. Maggio PM, Brundage SI, Hernandez-Broussard T, et al: Commitment to COT verification improves patient outcomes and financial performance. *J Trauma* 67(1):190–195, 2009. LOE IV
25. Eastridge BJ, Constanzo G, Jenkins D, et al: Impact of joint theater trauma system initiatives on battlefield injury outcomes. *Am J Surg* 198:852–857, 2009. LOE III
49. Kragh JF, Walters TJ, Baer DG, et al: Practical use of the emergency tourniquets to stop bleeding in major limb trauma. *J Trauma* 64(Suppl 2):S38–S50, 2008.
61. *American College of Surgeons COT Advanced Trauma Life Support for doctors—student course manual*, ed 9, Chicago, 2012, American College of Surgeons.
62. Bickell WH, Wall MJ, Pepe PE, et al: Immediate versus delayed fluid resuscitation for hypotensive patients with penetrating torso injuries. *N Engl J Med* 33(17):1105–1109, 1994. LOE I
71. Shakur H, Roberts I, Bautista R, et al: Effects of tranexamic acid on death, vascular occlusive events, and blood transfusion in trauma patients with significant haemorrhage (CRASH-2): a randomized, placebo-controlled trial. *Lancet* 376(9734):23–32, 2010. LOE I
72. Morrison JJ, Dubose JJ, Rasmussen TE, et al: Military application of tranexamic acid in trauma emergency resuscitation (MATTERs) study. *Arch Surg* 147(2):113–119, 2012. LOE III
77. Rotondo MF, Schwab CW, McGonigal MD, et al: Damage control: an approach for improved survival in exsanguinating penetrating abdominal injury. *J Trauma* 35(3):375, 1993. LOE IV
88. Inaba K, Branco BC, Menaker J, et al: Evaluation of multidetector computed tomography for penetrating neck injury: a prospective multicenter study. *J Trauma Acute Care Surg* 72(3):576–583, 2012. LOE II

The complete References list is available online at https://expertconsult.inkling.com.

Chapter 10

Initial Evaluation of the Spine in Trauma Patients

KEVIN L. JU • MITCHEL B. HARRIS

More than 50,000 spinal column fractures occur in the United States each year,[1] and those resulting in a spinal cord injury (SCI) can be devastating. Although we may not be able to prevent most spinal injuries from occurring, proper management of these injuries can potentially minimize any further neurologic injury and the associated morbidity and mortality. To optimize the care of trauma patients, a thorough understanding of appropriate evaluation and management algorithms, as well as the evidence behind those recommendations, is needed. This chapter reviews the principles of evaluation of spinal trauma patients.

INITIAL EVALUATION AND STABILIZATION

All trauma patients are presumed to have a spinal injury until proven otherwise, and appropriate management of these patients requires the close cooperation of multiple disciplines, including general surgery, neurosurgery, orthopaedic surgery, and critical care specialists. Vigilant adherence to spinal precautions during the initial evaluation and resuscitation is crucial to preventing further neurologic damage. SCI, especially those associated with vehicular crashes, is commonly accompanied by other injuries, including loss of consciousness (43%), fractures of the trunk or long bones (40%), head injury (18%), and pneumothorax (17%).[2] Because SCI is commonly associated with other severe and life-threatening injuries, proper protocols must be followed to ensure that the patient as a whole is cared for properly.

The initial evaluation and management of polytrauma patients starts in the field with first responders and continues en route and upon presentation to the hospital. Treatment priorities involve preserving life, then limb, and finally function. The American College of Surgeons has established Advanced Trauma Life Support (ATLS) protocols for the initial assessment, resuscitation, and stabilization of polytrauma patients.[3] These protocols are designed to systematically evaluate and identify life-threatening injuries while maintaining precautions necessary to prevent further harm to the patient. It is precisely in this type of high-pressure environment where occult spinal injuries may not be immediately recognized because the initial focus needs to be on the airway, respiratory, and circulatory systems.

All polytrauma patients should be treated as though they have sustained an unstable spinal column injury until proper evaluation has excluded an injury. In fact, up to 25% of patients with traumatic spine injuries experience further neurologic deterioration after coming under the care of medical personnel.[4] Thus, provisional stabilization and appropriate immobilization of the spine starting at the scene is crucial for preventing the onset of a neurologic injury or to avoid exacerbation of an existing neurologic injury. This entails returning the head and neck to a neutral alignment by aligning it with the long axis of the trunk and keeping the neck out of flexion or extension. The currently accepted practice is to apply a rigid cervical collar to help immobilize the cervical spine in the neutral position before extrication from the accident scene. It bears mentioning that even though the application of rigid cervical collars in trauma patients is still the standard of care, alone they may not sufficiently immobilize an unstable cervical spine and eliminate motion during transfers.[5] In the past, the accepted method for moving a patient onto and off a spine board was using the logrolling maneuver. However, recent research has shown that this technique results in significantly more cervical, thoracic, and lumbar motion than other available techniques,[6] such as the scoop stretcher,[7] straddle lift and slide, and 6 + lift and slide[8] methods. Thus, some authors recommend using one of these alternative techniques rather than logrolling when transferring trauma patients. The one exception is when a patient is found prone at the scene; he or she should be transferred directly onto a spine board using the logroll push technique.[6,9] After the patient is positioned on a flat, rigid spine board, sandbags are placed on either side of the head and neck, and the head is taped to the board to adequately immobilize the spine. Of note, children have disproportionately larger heads; therefore, elevating the trunk on padding or using special pediatric spine boards with a recessed head section is needed to prevent potentially dangerous neck flexion and possible cord compression resulting from being placed directly onto a regular adult spine board

ADVANCED TRAUMA LIFE SUPPORT

Early communication between first responders and the hospital emergency department (ED) is important to ensure that the proper personnel and resources are present as soon as the trauma patient arrives. Upon arrival, the first priority of the ATLS protocols involves initiation of the "primary survey" following the mnemonic "ABCDE," which corresponds to airway, breathing, circulation, disability (i.e., neurologic status), and exposure (i.e., completely undress the patient).

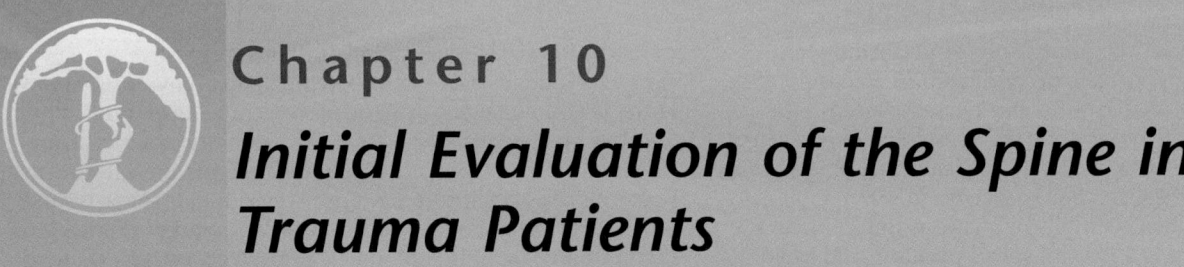

The patency of the airway is first to be assessed. In a trauma patient, this can be obstructed by blood, teeth, the tongue, maxillofacial trauma, or laryngeal injury. If the patient is able to communicate verbally, the airway is patent and most likely not in immediate jeopardy. On the other hand, if there is an obstruction, then an airway must be quickly established by removing the obstruction, intubation, or performing a cricothyroidotomy. The prevalence of cervical spine fractures in the setting of head or facial injuries has been reported to be 7% to 24%.[10-13] During the process of reestablishing a patent airway, it is important to maintain cervical spine precautions, especially if the cervical collar needs to be temporarily removed. This can be accomplished with in-line cervical stabilization, maintaining a neutral spinal position, and avoiding any flexion or extension.

After an airway is secured, the next step is to assess the ability of the patient to ventilate, a process that requires adequate function of the lungs, chest wall, and diaphragm. Tension or open pneumothorax, massive hemothorax, and paralysis can all interfere with one's respiratory function and can rapidly lead to death if not recognized and urgently addressed. The absence of respiratory effort can originate from a brainstem injury or a high cervical cord injury. The diaphragm is innervated by the phrenic nerve, which receives contributions from the third, fourth, and fifth cervical nerve roots. When evaluating the chest wall, it is important to keep in mind that the sternum–rib–costotransverse articulation acts as a physiologic buttress or "fourth column"[14]; thus, sternal fractures and multiple rib fractures in flail chest have been shown to further compromise the stability of thoracic spine fractures.[15]

As the airway and respiratory status are being evaluated, the patient's temperature, heart rate, blood pressure, and oxygen saturation should simultaneously be determined. Evaluation of the patient's circulatory and hemodynamic status includes assessing the patient's intravascular blood volume, cardiac output (via the heart rate, blood pressure, and urine output), and identifying sources of hemorrhage. In a trauma patient, hypotension (defined as a systolic blood pressure of <90 mm Hg) is presumed to be hypovolemic in origin until proven otherwise. External sources of bleeding should be controlled with direct manual pressure whenever possible, and appropriate intravenous (IV) access should be obtained. In the setting of hemodynamic instability and shock, IV access should involve at least two large-bore (minimum of 16-gauge) peripheral IV lines, preferably in the upper extremities. Initial resuscitation is with crystalloid, but if there is no improvement in end-organ perfusion (i.e., level of consciousness, urinary output, peripheral perfusion) after 2 L, packed red blood cells (universal donor blood—group O, Rh negative, if necessary), platelets, and fresh-frozen plasma should be given in a 1 : 1 : 1 ratio.[16] Of note, the finding of hypotension without tachycardia on presentation should raise clinical suspicion for neurogenic shock from a SCI above T6. Disruption of the sympathetic innervation results in unopposed vagal tone, resulting in vasodilation, decreased systemic vascular resistance, and decreased cardiac output. This form of shock, referred to as neurogenic shock, is often treated with vasopressors when the fluid challenge proves ineffective and, in severe circumstances, cardiac pacing.

Patients can lose large amounts of blood internally in the thorax, peritoneum, retroperitoneum, and thighs, so these areas demand careful examination in a hypotensive trauma patient. A hemothorax should be identifiable during the assessment of the patient's respiratory status. Peritoneal blood is commonly identified by a Focused Assessment with Sonography Test (FAST) or diagnostic peritoneal lavage (DPL). Pelvic injuries can also result in substantial blood loss into the retroperitoneal space, which may not be picked up by FAST or DPL. Physical examination findings suggestive of pelvic injury include scrotal or labial swelling and ecchymosis, blood at the urethral meatus, or perineal or genital lacerations. Provocative maneuvers to assess pelvic stability, such as compressing the iliac wings medially or applying an anterior to posterior stress against the anterior superior iliac spine, should only be performed once because these maneuvers can lead to disruption of the initial blood clot. A retrospective review of 18,644 trauma patients showed that the presence of a pelvic fracture was an independent risk factor for cervical spine injury, increasing the risk ninefold.[17] The thigh is another potential space and is capable of containing up to 4 units of blood when there is a femur fracture.[18] Femur fractures are usually the results of high-energy trauma and thus are often associated with other injuries. In fact, a multicenter retrospective review of 201 patients with femoral shaft fractures showed that 3.5% of them were also found to have concurrent thoracic or lumbar spine fractures.[19] Missing a spine injury in a patient with a femoral shaft fracture can be dangerous because the process of positioning and the traction required to place a femoral intramedullary rod could exacerbate an unstable spine injury.[19]

As part of the initial trauma evaluation, a rapid neurologic evaluation should be performed to determine the patient's level of responsiveness (Glasgow Coma Scale [GCS] score). This is based on the patient's best eye response, verbal response, and motor response to verbal commands or painful stimuli. Scores range from 3 to 15, with a GCS score of 15 corresponding to a patient that is awake, alert, appropriate, and following commands. A GCS score of 13 or 14 represents mild brain injury, a score of 9 to 12 corresponds to moderate injury, and a score of 8 or less is indicative of severe brain injury.

Finally, during the evaluation of a trauma patient, it is important to remove all clothing to perform a thorough assessment. However, it is equally important to cover up the patient again with blankets to prevent hypothermia after the assessment is completed. Even though ATLS outlines the ABCDEs of the primary survey, this is not a linear process. Rather, it is usually carried out in parallel, with the patient being undressed and vital signs and IV access being obtained while the airway, respiratory, and cardiovascular systems are being evaluated.

After the primary survey is completed and resuscitative efforts are underway, the secondary survey begins. This involves a head-to-toe examination of the head, neck, chest, abdomen, perineum, and musculoskeletal system and a complete spine and neurologic examination. With the patient still supine on the spine board, the scalp and head should be examined for any lacerations, contusions, and fractures. The eyes are assessed for pupillary size and reactivity, hemorrhage, and ocular muscle entrapment, as well as for midface stability. The anterior neck is evaluated for swelling, tracheal deviation, and subcutaneous emphysema. The entire chest is inspected for wounds and bruising, the chest cage is palpated for tenderness and flail segments, and the lungs are auscultated to confirm proper air movement and to identify a pneumothorax or hemothorax. The abdomen is examined for tenderness and peritoneal signs, but normal initial examination findings do not exclude significant intraabdominal injury. Patients with unexplained hypotension, neurologic injury, impaired sensorium, or equivocal abdominal findings are candidates for FAST, DPL, or, if hemodynamically stable, an abdomen and

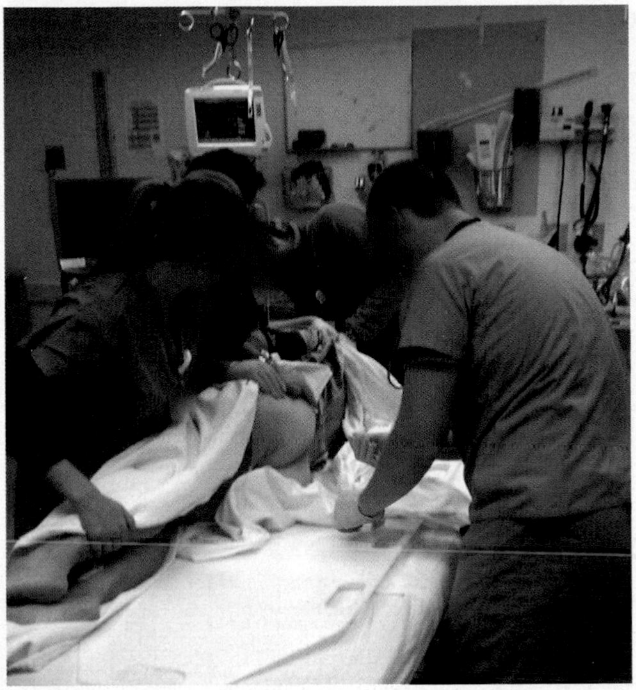

Figure 10-1. Clinical photograph showing a patient being logrolled. One assistant stabilizes the head and neck while two or three additional assistants support the patient's trunk and legs.

pelvis computed tomography (CT) scan. The perineum is examined next for lacerations, ecchymosis, and urethral bleeding. A vaginal examination should be performed in patients at risk for vaginal injury. The extremities and pelvis are then evaluated for any wounds (e.g., open fractures), deformities, and pain or tenderness with palpation or range of motion. Peripheral pulses should be assessed to identify accompanying vascular injuries and to confirm sufficient resuscitation and restoration of appropriate blood pressure.

CLASSIFICATION OF NEUROLOGIC INJURY

The spinal examination is an essential part of the comprehensive musculoskeletal examination. It is essential to replace the field collar with an appropriate rigid cervical collar. With the appropriate personnel present, the patient should be rolled onto his or her side for direct visualization, palpation, and examination of the back and spine. One assistant stabilizes the head and neck while two or three additional assistants support the patient's trunk and legs (Fig. 10-1). The examiner then inspects the back, looking for abrasions, ecchymosis, and the rare open spinal fracture. The midline spinous processes should be carefully palpated from the cervical through the lumbar spine to identify areas of tenderness, stepoffs, malalignment, and abnormal diastasis between adjacent-level spinous processes. One must also examine the perineum for sensation, rectal tone, and the presence of any gross or occult blood in the rectal vault. The bulbocavernosus reflex can also be examined to evaluate for spinal shock. The backboard is then slid out and the patient carefully rolled back onto the stretcher. After this, a complete neurologic examination should be performed.

The American Spinal Injury Association (ASIA) neurologic classification of SCI and the ASIA impairment scale (modified from the Frankel classification[20]) are useful tools for precisely mapping motor and sensory deficits to a specific spinal cord level (Fig. 10-2 and Table 10-1). Motor strength is tested bilaterally in each of five upper extremity muscle groups (Fig. 10-3) and five lower extremity muscle groups (Fig. 10-4) and graded on a scale from 0 to 5. Sensation to light touch and pinprick is tested bilaterally in each of 28 sensory dermatomes. According to ASIA definitions, the neurologic injury level in SCI is the most distal level of the spinal cord with normal motor and sensory function bilaterally. A "complete injury" (ASIA A) is one in which there is complete absence of motor and sensory function below the neurologic injury level, including the lowest sacral segment (S4–S5) (see Table 10-1). Sensation at these levels involves sensation at the anal mucocutaneous junction (Fig. 10-5) and deep anal sensation; sacral motor function requires the voluntary contraction of the external anal sphincter. "Incomplete injuries" (ASIA B–D) have partial preservation of sensory or motor function in the lower sacral segments and are associated with a greater potential for some neurologic recovery (see Table 10-1).

The examination is considered unreliable if the patient is intoxicated, obtunded, or in spinal shock. If the patient is intoxicated or unresponsive, the initial neurologic assessment involves gathering information from the first responders regarding neurologic function (i.e., witnessed voluntary extremity motion) at the scene and in transport. Careful observation of spontaneous movements and response to noxious stimuli, reflexes, and rectal tone can give some information about spinal cord function in these patients. In a patient with no voluntary movement or response to noxious stimuli, the presence of reflex arcs indicates an upper motor neuron injury; their absence implies a lower motor neuron injury. Figure 10-6 illustrates the locations of the upper and lower extremity stretch reflexes and the responsible nerve roots. Other important reflexes include the plantar reflex and anal wink. The plantar reflex is tested by firmly stroking the plantar aspect of the foot with a pointed object and observing toe movement. Flexion of the toes is normal, but extension of the great toe with splaying of the lesser toes is abnormal ("Babinski sign") and indicates an upper motor neuron lesion. The anal wink reflex is mediated by the S2 to S4 nerve roots and is elicited by stroking the skin around the anal sphincter and watching for its contraction. This reflex is abnormal if no sphincter contraction is observed.

Patients may also present in spinal shock, which is the transient physiologic depression in spinal cord function caudal to the level of injury. This usually results in 24 to 72 hours of paralysis, diminished tone, loss of sensation, and the absence of reflexes caudal to the injury level. The end of spinal shock is marked by return of the bulbocavernosus reflex mediated by the S1, S2, and S3 nerve roots. This reflex arc is tested by squeezing the glans penis or tugging on an indwelling Foley catheter and looking for contraction of the external anal sphincter (Fig. 10-7). Any significant neurologic deficits that persist after this resolution often are slow to recover if they recover at all. It should be emphasized that the neurologic assessment should be systematically repeated and updated over time as the patient's level of consciousness improves.

If the patient is alert, cooperative, and sober and there are no "distracting injuries," areas of tenderness on examination

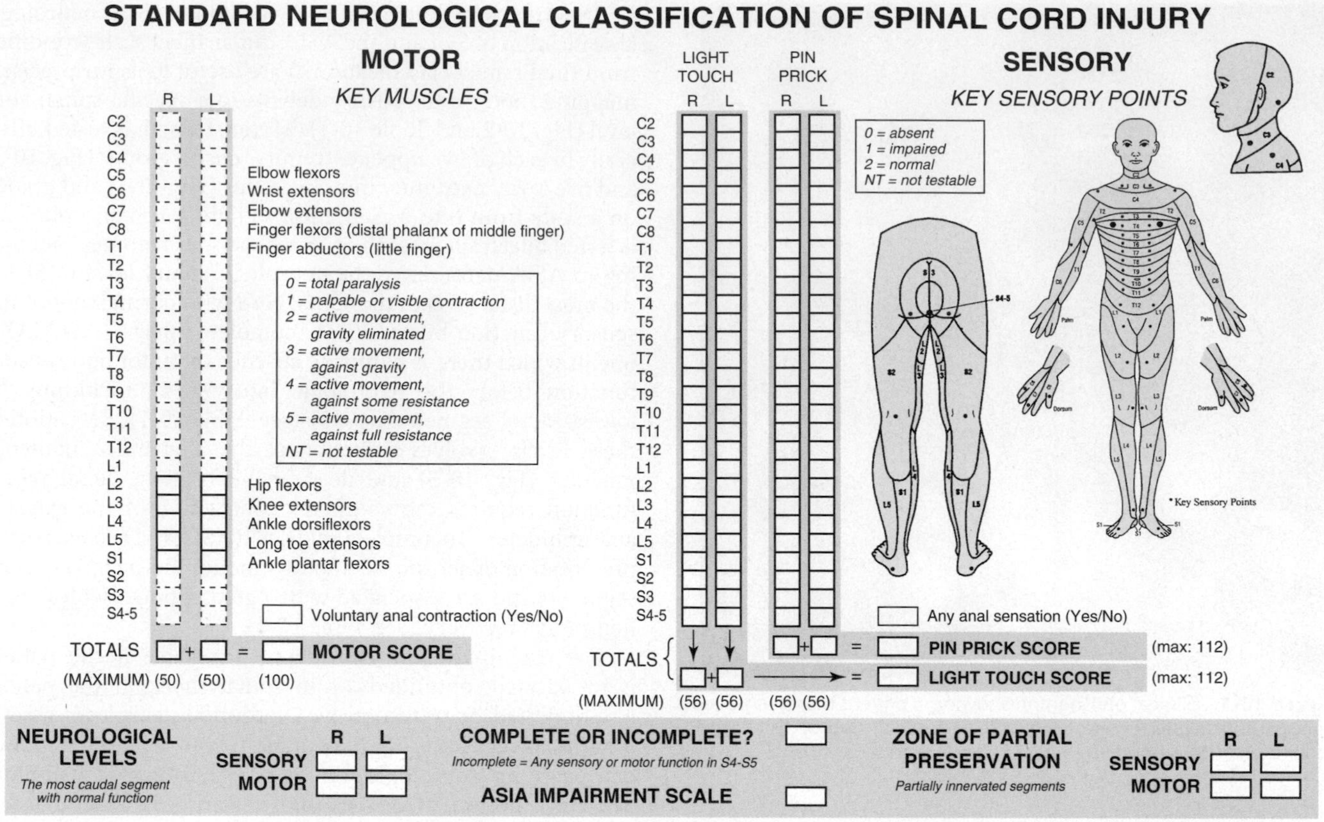

Figure 10-2. The American Spinal Injury Association (ASIA) neurologic classification of spinal cord injury and the ASIA impairment scale are useful tools for precisely mapping motor and sensory deficits to a specific spinal cord level.

can help guide further radiographic evaluation. Otherwise, one needs to maintain a high suspicion for spinal injury, and knowledge of associated injuries can help. Head, facial, or neck trauma should raise suspicion for cervical spine injury. Additionally, the presence of a pelvic fracture increases the risk of the presence of a concomitant spine injury. The presence of a "seatbelt sign," ecchymosis on the trunk from shoulder or lap belts, is associated with abdominal and thoracolumbar spine (TLS) injury, especially if only lap belts are used.[21] In fact, there is a significant correlation between flexion–distraction injuries of the TLS and intraabdominal and retroperitoneal injuries.[22,23] Importantly, if one finds an injury at one vertebral level, the entire spine needs to be imaged to evaluate for noncontiguous spinal injuries. Keenen and colleagues[24] reported a 6.4% incidence of noncontiguous spine fractures based on retrospective review of 941 patients with spine fractures. Similarly, a series of 137 pediatric patients with spine injuries at a single trauma center revealed that 7% of patients had multilevel noncontiguous spine fractures.[25]

TABLE 10-1 ***AMERICAN SPINAL INJURY ASSOCIATION IMPAIRMENT SCALE (MODIFIED FRANKEL CLASSIFICATION)***

Category	Characteristics
A	Complete: No sensory or motor function is preserved below the neurologic level, including in the lowest sacral segment (S4–S5).
B	Incomplete: Sensory but not motor function is preserved below the neurologic level and includes S4–S5.
C	Incomplete: Motor function is preserved below the neurologic level, and more than half of the key muscles below the neurologic level have a grade of 0–2.
D	Incomplete: Motor function is preserved below the neurologic level, and more than half of the key muscles below the neurologic level have a grade of 3–5.
E	Normal sensory and motor function

RADIOGRAPHIC ASSESSMENT

Radiographic examination remains an integral part of the initial polytrauma workup; however, this should never interfere with patient resuscitation. In fact, the two plain radiographs that are still consistently obtained in the trauma bay are primarily performed to assess for life-threatening injuries. These two radiographs are an anteroposterior (AP) view of the chest and pelvis. The AP chest, in addition to evaluation of the cardiac shadow and the lung fields, can identify subtle thoracic spine injuries. Special attention should be paid to vertebral body heights and their endplates, as well as the location and alignment of the spinous processes and pedicles. The AP pelvis can identify unstable pelvic injuries and help predict potential blood loss. Importantly, part of the lumbar spine and

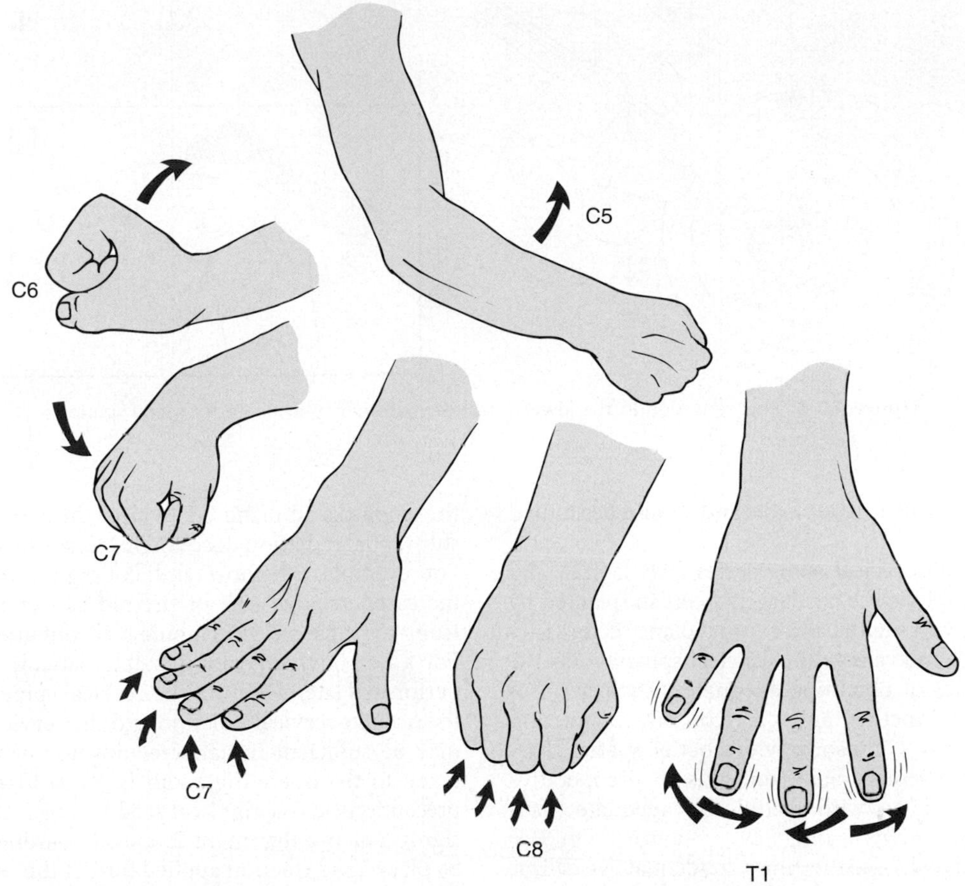

Figure 10-3. Examination of muscle groups innervated by nerve roots in the upper extremity should include elbow flexion (C5), wrist extension (C6), wrist flexion (C7), finger flexion (C8), and finger abduction (T1).

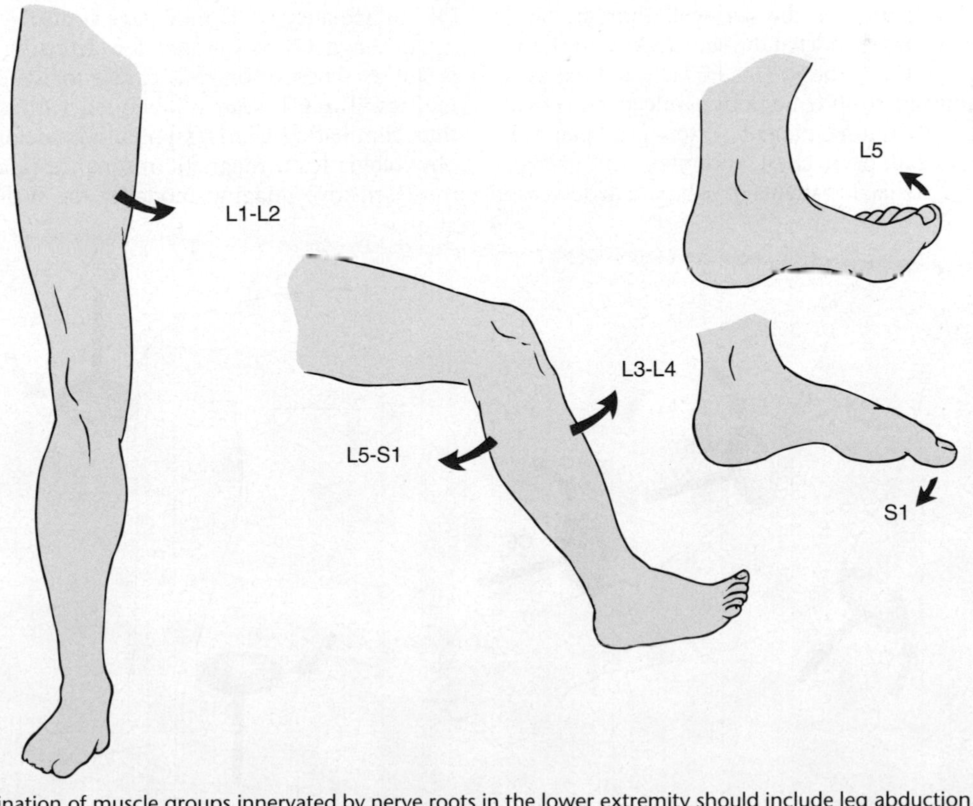

Figure 10-4. Examination of muscle groups innervated by nerve roots in the lower extremity should include leg abduction (L2), knee extension (L3), ankle dorsiflexion (L4), great toe extension (L5), and great toe flexion (S1).

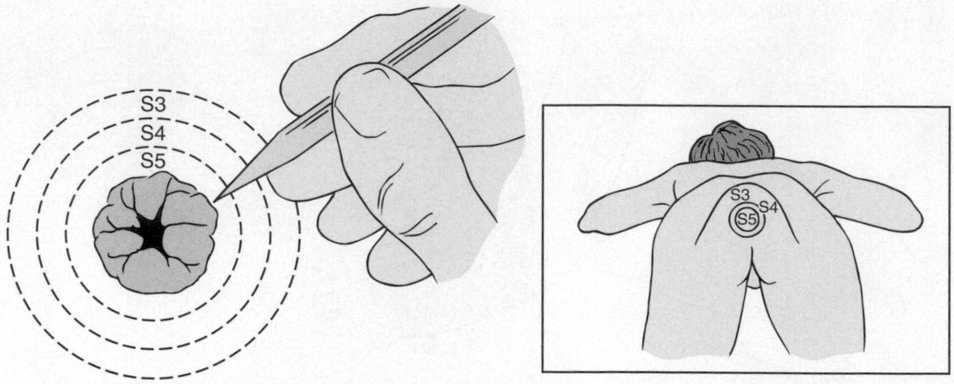

Figure 10-5. Test sensation in the lower sacral dermatomes to evaluate for sacral sparing.

lumbosacral junction will also be visible and should be studied for any anomalies.

The traditional ED cervical spine series (AP, lateral, and open-mouth odontoid views) has largely been supplanted by the use of CT scans with sagittal and coronal plane reconstructions. The use of CT to evaluate the cervical spine avoids the traditional difficulties of obtaining adequate visualization of the occipitocervical junction and cervicothoracic junction with plain radiographs. CT also provides better spatial characterization of the osseous injury and aids in preoperative planning if needed. Even with technically adequate plain radiographs, their sensitivity is only 52%,[26,27] and 36% to 61% of injuries can be missed.[28] Furthermore, inadequate visualization has been reported as being responsible for 94% of errors leading to missed or delayed diagnosis of cervical spine injuries.[29] In contrast, a retrospective review of 3537 trauma patients showed that helical multidetector CT (MDCT) identified 99.3% of all fractures of the cervical, thoracic, and lumbar spine.[30] Others have reported the sensitivity and specificity of cervical spine CT to be 98%.[26] In fact, as long as a patient can be stabilized from a hemodynamic perspective, these high-energy polytrauma patients often get "pan CT scanned" (including head, neck, chest, abdomen, and pelvis). Of note, protocols for pediatric patients have begun to decrease the emphasis on using CT to clear the cervical spine given the substantial radiation dose and increased lifetime risk of cancer. For example, Muchow and colleagues reported a lifetime increased relative risk of thyroid cancer in females of 25% from a single cervical spine CT obtained for clearance.[31] For a hemodynamically unstable patient, a technically well-performed lateral view of the cervical spine that clearly shows the occipitocervical junction and the cervicothoracic junction may be sufficient initial screening to enable a patient to be taken to the operating room (OR) as long as proper spinal precautions and a rigid cervical orthosis are maintained.[32] If significant malalignment is found, Gardner-Wells tongs can be placed and traction applied during the resuscitation period followed by further imaging and treatment after the patient is stabilized. So, in summary, the only time a plain lateral cervical spine radiograph should be obtained in the trauma bay would be in a trauma patient in extremis who is going to the OR immediately for hemorrhage control.

Although CT is tailored for detecting osseous injury, it is not as sensitive or as accurate for detecting ligamentous injuries. The CT scan is obtained with the patient supine, thus eliminating gravity's potentially deforming force under physiologic load. Magnetic resonance imaging (MRI) is the most sensitive imaging modality for evaluating soft tissues,

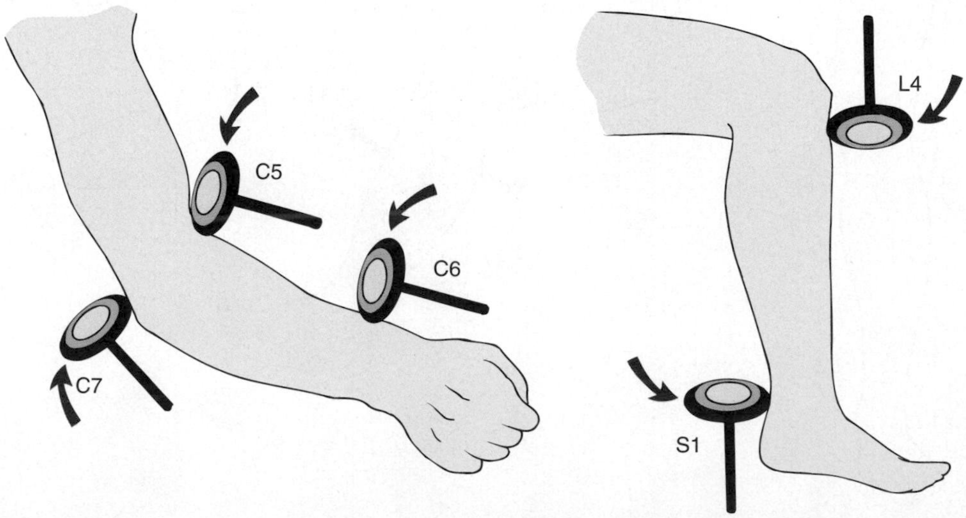

Figure 10-6. Upper and lower extremity muscle stretch reflexes and the responsible nerve roots.

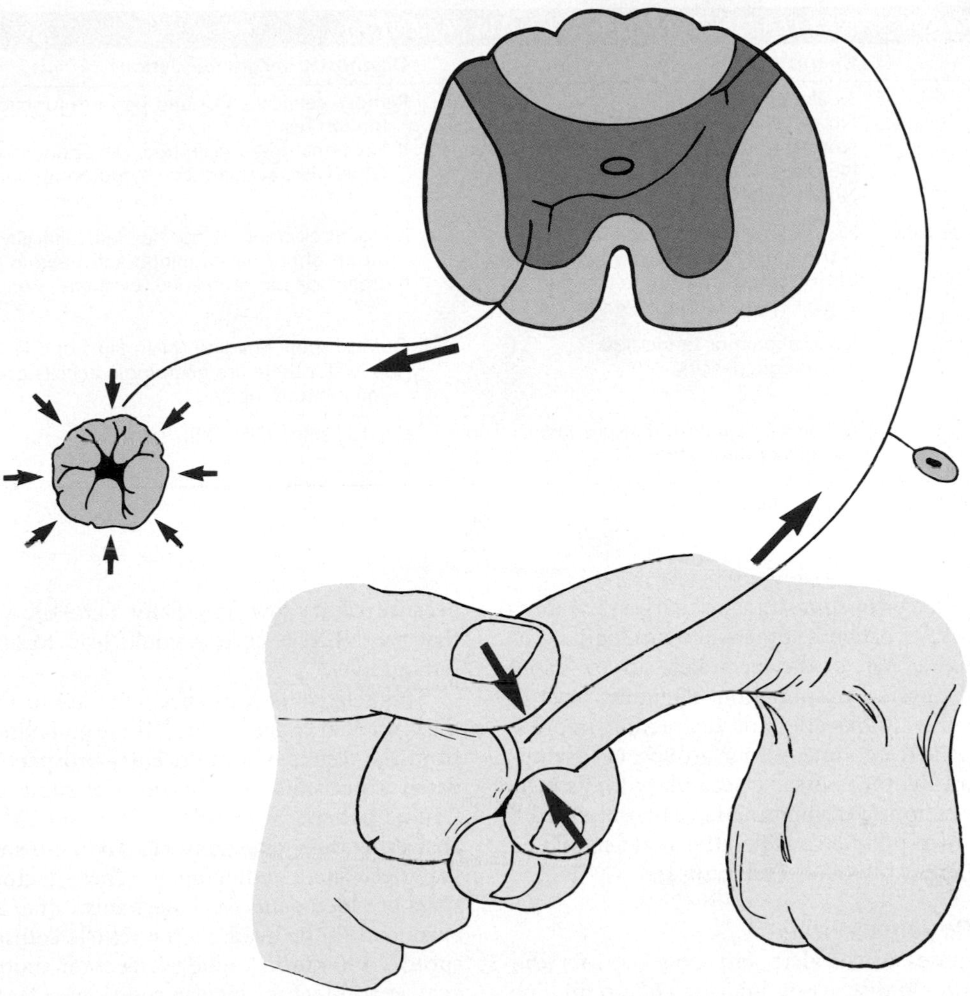

Figure 10-7. The bulbocavernosus reflex is tested by squeezing the glans penis or tugging on an indwelling Foley catheter and looking for contraction of the external anal sphincter. This reflex is mediated by the S1, S2, and S3 nerve roots.

including neural elements, ligaments, and discs. MRI can provide valuable information about spinal stability without the additional, albeit small, risk of SCI associated with physician directed flexion–extension radiographs.[33] However, not every trauma patient requires an MRI. In a prospective study of patients with isolated cervical spine fractures, MRI findings did not change the treatment plan for neurologically intact patients. However, in those with a neurologic deficit, MRI findings altered the treatment plan in 25% of patients.[34] In general, MRI should be considered for patients with suspected ligamentous injury, those whose neurologic examination is not concordant with their findings on CT, those with a progressive neurologic deficit, or those who will remain intubated or unable to participate in a credible examination for several days.

CERVICAL SPINE CLEARANCE

The goal of clearing the cervical spine is to establish that there is no cervical spine injury that would put the spinal cord at risk after the collar is removed and the patient mobilized. A total of 1% to 3% of patients with blunt trauma have cervical spine injuries.[35,36] Levi and colleagues[37] reported 24 patients who had adverse neurologic outcomes as a result of missed spinal injuries, including radiculopathy, SCIs, and even death. The most common etiology for the missed injury was insufficient imaging (58.3%) followed by misread radiographs (33.3%) and poor-quality studies (8.3%). Thus, early recognition of patients with cervical injury has the potential to prevent or limit further neurologic injury and maximize future functional recovery. On the other hand, if a patient does not possess a cervical spine injury, timely cervical spine clearance is important to minimize the complications associated with cervical collar immobilization, including bed rest immobilization, skin breakdown (especially occipital and submental pressure sores), difficulty with airway management, potentially increasing intracranial pressures, and inhibiting thorough assessment of other organ systems.[38-40] Cervical spine precautions and collar immobilization also make daily nursing tasks more difficult, including skin care, pulmonary toilet, and transfers and mobilization.[41]

Patient Classification

The first step of cervical spine clearance involves obtaining a detailed history, including the mechanism of injury, presence of any transient or persistent neurologic deficits, presence of any alcohol or drugs, and any history of spinal pathology

TABLE 10-2 *CERVICAL SPINE CLEARANCE IN BLUNT TRAUMA PATIENTS*

Category	Characteristics	Diagnostic Recommendations
Asymptomatic	Awake and alert No cervical pain or tenderness Normal neurologic examination findings No distracting injuries No intoxication	Remove cervical collar and perform functional range of motion test. If functional test is pain free, discontinue cervical restrictions. Otherwise, evaluate as a symptomatic patient.
Temporarily nonassessable	No neck pain or tenderness Normal neurologic examination findings Intoxicated or has distracting injuries Expect resolution in 24–48 hr	If urgent clearance is not needed, clinically reassess after return of normal cognition and treating distracting injuries. If urgent clearance needed, evaluate as an obtunded patient.
Symptomatic	Cervical pain or tenderness Neurologic deficits	Cervical spine imaging (plain films or CT) Also MRI if there are neurologic deficits or suspected ligamentous injury
Obtunded	Abnormal cognition that precludes reliable clinical examination	Cervical spine CT ± MRI

CT, Computed tomography; *MRI,* magnetic resonance imaging.

(ankylosing spondylitis, prior spine injury or surgery). A thorough examination of the patient's spine and neurologic status should be performed as part of the secondary survey. Based on the history and physical examination, including level of consciousness and any intoxication or distracting injuries, patients can be classified into one of four groups: (1) asymptomatic, (2) temporarily nonassessable secondary to distracting injuries or intoxication, (3) symptomatic, or (4) obtunded.[42] Each group has its own unique considerations and should be evaluated using different protocols (Table 10-2).

Asymptomatic Patients

This first group includes awake, alert, and sober patients who have no cervical pain, no distracting injuries, and no midline cervical tenderness to palpation. Distracting injuries include any significantly painful injury that interferes with the patient's ability to fully concentrate and cooperate with a clinical examination (e.g., major injury above the shoulder, thoracic or lumbar spine injury, pelvic fracture, long bone fracture, or major visceral or soft tissue injury). These patients can be cleared clinically without the need for cervical spine imaging. The cervical collar is removed, and the patient is guided through a functional range of motion that includes first demonstrating active lateral rotation of the head 45 degrees to each side followed by actively flexing and extending the neck without complaints of pain.

Several large studies, systematic reviews, and meta-analyses have focused on cervical spine clearance in this group of awake, alert, asymptomatic patients. The National Emergency X-Radiography Utilization Study (NEXUS)[43] validated a clinical protocol for cervical spine clearance in low-risk patients without the need for radiographic imaging. For a patient to be deemed low risk, the patient must be alert and have no evidence of intoxication, no painful distracting injury, no midline cervical tenderness, and no focal neurologic deficit. Following their algorithm, the injury was identified in all but eight of the 818 patients found to have a cervical spine injury. Of the eight missed injuries, only two patients had a clinically significant injury, and only one of these two patients received surgical treatment. The NEXUS criteria yielded a sensitivity of 99.0% and negative predictive value of 99.8%, indicating its usefulness in ruling out significant cervical injury. However, because of its low specificity (12.9%), there was concern that the NEXUS criteria could lead to an increased use of radiography.[44]

This relative lack of specificity led to the development of the Canadian C-spine rule.[44] These guidelines were established from the results of a multicenter prospective study that validated a decision rule for cervical spine clearance in blunt trauma patients with a GCS of 15 and stable vital signs by answering three questions: (1) Are there any high-risk factors that necessitate radiography? These factors include age 65 years or older, dangerous mechanism (fall ≥1 m or five stairs, axial load to the head, motor vehicle collision involving high speed [>100 km/hr], rollover, ejection, motorized recreational vehicle accident, or bicycle collision); (2) Are there any low-risk factors present to allow safe assessment of cervical range of motion? These factors include simple rear-end motor vehicle collision, patient sitting up in the ED, ambulatory at any time since the injury, delayed onset of neck pain, and the absence of midline cervical spine tenderness; (3) Is the patient able to actively rotate the neck 45 degrees to the left and right without pain? The Canadian C-spine rule has a 100% sensitivity, 100% negative predictive value, and 42.5% specificity.[44] In a subsequent prospective study published by Stiell and colleagues[45] comparing the clinical performance of the Canadian C-spine rule and the NEXUS criteria, the authors found that the Canadian C-spine rule would have resulted in 10% fewer radiographs being obtained. After performing a comprehensive review of the literature and subsequent meta-analysis, Anderson and colleagues[46] concluded that alert, asymptomatic patients without painful distracting injuries or evidence of intoxication can be safely cleared from cervical spine immobilization without radiographs if they are able to complete a functional range of motion test without symptoms. The pooled sensitivity was 98.1%, and negative predictive value was 99.8%. Our recommendation is that in an awake, alert, asymptomatic patient, the cervical spine can be clinically cleared using the Canadian C-spine rule or NEXUS criteria.

Temporarily Nonassessable Secondary to Distracting Injuries or Intoxication

The second group includes patients who temporarily cannot be examined reliably secondary to intoxication or the presence of a painful distracting injury, but resolution of those issues is expected within 24 to 48 hours. This group has not been well defined in the literature, so there are no good published studies focusing specifically on this group of patients. Our recommendation is that the cervical collar remain in place and the patient be clinically reexamined in 24 to 48 hours after his or her cognition improves and any painful distracting injury has been managed. If at that point the patient is asymptomatic, he or she can be managed as an asymptomatic patient (group 1) described earlier. If, on the other hand, the patient has any neck pain, tenderness, or neurologic deficits, he or she should be managed as a symptomatic patient (group 3). Finally, if more urgent cervical spine clearance is needed during the period when the patient is not reliably examinable, the patient is evaluated as if he or she were obtunded (group 4). Quite frequently, these patients have already undergone a cervical CT scan as part of the initial ED evaluation.

Symptomatic Patients

The third group consists of patients with neck pain, midline tenderness, or neurologic deficits. All of these patients require formal radiographic imaging to evaluate the cervical spine. Although MDCT has largely become the study of choice, some centers still rely on AP, lateral, and open-mouth odontoid views of the cervical spine followed by adjunctive CT if the initial radiographs are thought to be inadequate. As previously discussed, MDCT has been demonstrated to be cost effective, more efficient, and more accurate when cervical spine injuries are being considered. Additionally, these polytrauma patients are often already getting CT scans of the head, chest, abdomen, and pelvis, and including a cervical spine CT makes this even more cost effective.[42] Most authors have come to the conclusion that MDCT is more cost effective than plain films for moderate- to high-risk patients when considering the potential for disastrous complications of missed injuries.[47] Currently, MRI is not indicated as the primary modality for cervical spine clearance. However, it is useful in patients with neurologic deficits. In a prospective study of patients with isolated cervical spine fractures, MRI findings did not change the treatment plan for neurologically intact patients. However, in those with a neurologic deficit, MRI findings altered the treatment plan in 25% of patients.[34]

Obtunded Patients

The fourth group consists of patients with an altered sensorium that prevents a meaningful clinical examination. Clearance of the cervical spine in this group is controversial. Some argue that MDCT alone is adequate for cervical spine clearance, but others advocate for the use of CT and MRI or CT and a credible examination.[48] If CT alone is deemed adequate, it saves the cost of an additional MRI study, and the acquisition time for CT is less than MRI. Additionally, the cardiovascular monitoring often required in obtunded patients is more difficult with MRI because of the requirement for nonferromagnetic equipment. There is abundant published evidence supporting the use of CT alone. Harris and colleagues[49] retrospectively evaluated 367 obtunded blunt trauma patients who underwent a cervical spine CT in the emergency department. Initial CT imaging identified all clinically significant injuries and only failed to identify a minor injury in one patient. Likewise, Tomycz and colleagues[50] retrospectively analyzed 180 trauma patients with normal cervical spine CT findings, no neurologic deficits, and GCS scores of 13 or less who also underwent cervical spine MRI. Of the patients with normal CT imaging findings, 21% were found to have acute traumatic findings on MRI. However, none of these patients had an unstable injury, no patient required surgery, and none developed evidence of delayed instability. Similar results demonstrating the sensitivity of CT for unstable cervical spine injury were published by Como et al.[51] and Schuster et al.[52] Hogan and colleagues[53] retrospectively reviewed 366 obtunded patients and calculated that CT had a negative predictive value of 98.9% for ligamentous injury and 100% for unstable cervical spine injury.

On the other hand, MRI is the ideal study for evaluating soft tissues and is better than CT at identifying ligamentous injuries. The sensitivity of cervical spine CT for detecting ligamentous injury in obtunded blunt trauma patients has been reported to be only 32%.[54] Menaker and colleagues[55] evaluated 203 obtunded blunt trauma patients who had normal CTs and found that 8.9% had abnormalities on their MRI scans. Two patients required operative intervention for ligamentous injury, and an additional 14 required extended cervical collar use. Thus, they concluded that CT can miss clinically significant cervical injuries in obtunded patients and that MRI should be used for cervical spine clearance in this population. In a study in which all obtunded trauma patients underwent CT and MRI as part of a cervical spine clearance protocol, CT missed 30% of ligamentous injuries, but MRI identified all patients with abnormal CT findings. Thus, these authors argued for using both modalities to clear the cervical spine in obtunded trauma patients.[56]

Schoenfeld and colleagues[57] performed a meta-analysis in which 1550 trauma patients with negative cervical spine CT findings were subsequently evaluated with MRI. The authors found that 5% of these patients required prolonged cervical immobilization and an additional 1% required surgical stabilization. The pooled sensitivity of MRI for detecting significant injury was 100%, pooled specificity was 94%, and negative predictive value was 100%. Thus, relying on CT alone for cervical spine clearance in unexaminable patients can miss clinically significant cervical injuries, and there is a continued role for MRI. Muchow and colleagues[58] also performed a meta-analysis and reported that MRI has a 100% negative predictive value for cervical spine injury, and the authors concluded that MRI is the gold standard for excluding cervical spine injury.

Controversy remains as to whether adjunctive MRI is needed for cervical spine clearance in obtunded patients. At the very least, all obtunded trauma patients require a cervical spine CT. If the CT findings are negative, several options exist. The first is to accept that the negative CT findings indicate that there is no clinically significant cervical spine injury and to discontinue cervical collar immobilization and restrictions. The alternative is to then obtain an MRI and clear the cervical spine based on the combined findings of CT and MRI. The intermediate option is to discontinue the cervical collar in pharmacologically sedated patients while in bed but protect the cervical spine with a collar when the patients are mobilized until a thorough examination is possible.

Conclusion: Cervical Spine Clearance

In summary, there are three methods by which one can examine the cervical spine. The first is a comprehensive

TABLE 10-3 *THORACOLUMBAR SPINE CLEARANCE IN BLUNT TRAUMA PATIENTS*

Category	Characteristics	Diagnostic Recommendations
Asymptomatic and low risk	Awake and alert (GCS score = 15) Normal neurologic examination findings No thoracolumbar pain, tenderness, deformity, or ecchymosis No cervical spine fracture No intoxication or distracting injuries No high-energy mechanism (see below)	No thoracolumbar imaging needed
Symptomatic or high risk	Thoracolumbar pain or tenderness Neurologic deficits High energy mechanism (fall ≥10 ft, vehicular accident with ejection or ≥50 mph) Cervical spine fracture	Thoracolumbar CT (+ MRI if any neurologic deficits)
Not examinable	Any alteration in cognition (GCS score <15) or distracting injury that precludes reliable clinical examination	Thoracolumbar CT (+ MRI if any neurologic deficits)

CT, Computed tomography; *GCS,* Glasgow Coma Scale; *MRI,* magnetic resonance imaging.

physical examination looking for any pain, tenderness, and neurologic abnormalities, both at rest and with functional range of motion. The other two methods are cervical spine CT with sagittal and coronal reformats or MRI. As a general rule of thumb, cervical spine clearance can follow the "two thirds rule" proposed by Simon and colleagues,[48] which requires normal CT findings and either normal clinical examination or MRI findings before discontinuing the cervical collar and restrictions.

THORACOLUMBAR SPINE CLEARANCE

Whereas large multicenter prospective studies have been done on cervical spine clearance, there is less literature on the necessary imaging required for satisfactory evaluation of the TLS and its subsequent "clearance" (Table 10-3). The incidence of thoracic or lumbar spine fractures in blunt trauma patients ranges from 2% to 15%.[59,60] However, 50% of all vertebral fractures occur in the TLS.[61] Furthermore, there is a 40% to 50% incidence of neurologic deficits with TLS fractures.[62] Similar to the cervical spine, blunt trauma patients who are awake and alert and lack any back pain or tenderness do not routinely need radiologic evaluation of the TLS provided there is no suspicion of a high-energy mechanism and no spinal fracture has been identified elsewhere. Despite literature supporting the notion that TLS fracture may be asymptomatic,[63] several studies have demonstrated that physical examination in appropriate patients is highly sensitive. Terregino and colleagues[64] found that in trauma patients with normal cognition and no distracting injuries, the absence of back pain or tenderness had a 95% negative predictive value for TLS fractures. A study by Durham and colleagues[65] showed that alert trauma patients with a negative clinical examination had a 5% rate of acute injuries, but all were minor (transverse process fractures) and none required treatment. On the other hand, patients in the same study with back pain or tenderness, ecchymosis, deformity, or any neurologic deficit had a 14% incidence of acute TLS injury and a 10% incidence of injuries requiring treatment. It is important to remember that multiple studies have documented the occurrence of noncontiguous spinal fractures[24,64,66-68]; therefore, if a fracture is found in any region of the spine (e.g., the cervical spine), the entire spine requires radiographic screening.

If a reliable clinical examination is not possible, however, radiographic imaging should be obtained. Even mild alterations in cognition make the clinical assessment of back pain or tenderness difficult because 63% of patients with GCS scores of 13 or 14 did not report any back pain or tenderness despite having a thoracolumbar fracture.[61] Meldon and colleagues[66] had similar results when they studied patients with a GCS score less than 15 and no complaints of back pain or tenderness and found that 42% had a thoracolumbar fracture. In addition, concurrent major distracting injuries both decrease the sensitivity of the clinical examination of the spine and serve as a marker for the severity of the trauma. The rate of associated major injury in patients with thoracolumbar fracture ranges can be as high as 47%[61,66,69,70]; thus, patients with painful distracting injuries, especially if they are high-energy injuries, require imaging of the TLS to rule out injury.

Hsu and colleagues[67] created a diagnostic pathway for deciding which patients require thoracolumbar imaging. They recommended imaging if the patient has back pain or midline tenderness, back ecchymosis, any neurologic deficits, any cervical spine fracture, GCS scores less than 15, or a major distracting injury or if the patient is intoxicated. Patients who fell 10 ft or more or were involved in a motor vehicle or motorcycle accident with ejection or at 50 mph or faster should also have thoracolumbar imaging.[71] The authors reported a 100% sensitivity with their algorithm. Holmes and colleagues[72] and Frankel and colleagues[71] published separate prospective studies defining very similar criteria for obtaining TLS imaging, and both reported a sensitivity and negative predictive value of 100%. The limitation is that plain radiographs were used to screen for TLS fractures in those three studies. Inaba and colleagues[73] is currently the only known study that correlates physical examination findings with CT findings and showed that clinical examination had a 48% sensitivity for all TLS fractures and 79% sensitivity for clinically significant fractures (i.e., those requiring an orthotic or surgery). More studies need to be done investigating the correlation between physical examination and CT.

In terms of imaging modalities, whereas plain radiographs have a 62% sensitivity for thoracic spine fractures and 86% sensitivity for lumbar spine fractures,[74] CT has reported sensitivities that approach 100% for both thoracic and lumbar fractures.[74,75] In one study, plain radiographs missed 42% of TLS fractures, and of the 19 total fractures missed, three (15.7%) were unstable.[74] Wintermark and colleagues[76] similarly demonstrated the low sensitivity (33.3%) of plain radiographs for diagnosing unstable TLS fractures, a finding that has support in the literature.[60,77] Additional benefits of CT include an improved ability to distinguish acute from chronic fractures and significantly decreased the time to TLS clearance to around 3 hours with CT from 12 to 48 hours with initial plain films.[78] Thus, CT is currently the imaging modality of choice for identifying TLS fractures. The chest, abdomen, and pelvis CT that most polytrauma patients receive to rule out thoracic and intraabdominal injury sufficiently images the thoracic and lumbosacral spine with current MDCT scanners and processing software. Sagittal and coronal reformats should be performed on the axial images to allow for thorough examination of the TLS. Berry and colleagues[60] reported the sensitivity and specificity of CT with sagittal and coronal reformats for TLS fractures are 100% and 97%, respectively. Others have also verified the high sensitivity and specificity of CT reformats, making this the gold standard for detecting osseous injury in the TLS.[74,75] Currently, MRI is not indicated for initial TLS clearance. For blunt trauma patients, MRI should be reserved for individuals with neurologic deficits, to further evaluate CT findings for possible neurologic involvement (e.g., a burst fracture), or to further investigate the integrity of the associated ligamentous structures.[79]

CONCLUSION

All trauma patients are presumed to have a spinal injury until a comprehensive physical examination is completed. Thus, during the earliest portion of the evaluation, cervical immobilization with a rigid orthosis, supine positioning, and in-line spinal precautions should be followed at all times. The initial evaluation and management of trauma patients should follow the ATLS guidelines, which systematically evaluate and address life-threatening and then limb-threatening injuries. In the acute setting, respiratory and hemodynamic instability may take precedence over the identification and treatment of spinal and musculoskeletal injuries. However, after the airway is secured and immediate life-threatening conditions are ruled out, the spinal and neurologic examinations take high priority. In terms of cervical spine clearance, patients can be classified into four groups, each with different management protocols. An alert, sober patient who has no neck pain, no distracting injuries, and no midline cervical tenderness on palpation can be clinically cleared without cervical spine radiographs. Asking the patient to perform a functional range of motion test increases the sensitivity of all clinical testing. Patients who have an altered sensorium (e.g., intoxicated) or have painful distracting injuries are often not able to be clinically assessed at the time of presentation. However, if this condition is expected to resolve in 24 to 48 hours, the cervical collar should stay on until a reliable clinical examination can be performed. Patients complaining of neck pain, midline tenderness, or any transient or persistent neurologic deficits are symptomatic and accordingly require maintenance of cervical collar immobilization and formal protocoled radiographic evaluation. The majority of these patients should receive an MDCT of the cervical spine. Patients who are unable to undergo a credible physical examination require a cervical spine CT with sagittal and coronal reformats. If this is negative for injury, there are several options. One option is to discontinue use of the cervical collar and all spinal restrictions. If this option is endorsed, the authors recommend that in addition to the formal radiology reading, a second "set of eyes" evaluate the MDCT studies to provide further support of the benign nature of the radiographic examination. However, there are several published studies and meta-analyses demonstrating that cervical spine clearance with CT alone misses unstable cervical injuries.[48,54-58] An alternative option, with excellent support in the literature, is to obtain an MRI to aid in cervical spine clearance.[57,58]

In terms of TLS clearance, many polytrauma patients already undergo chest, abdomen, and pelvis CT scans, and the TLS can be adequately evaluated using sagittal and coronal reformats of these images. An alert, sober patient who has no back pain or tenderness, no distracting injuries, and no other spinal fractures and was not involved in a high-energy traumatic event can be clinically cleared without radiographic evaluation. However, a CT imaging of the TLS is indicated in patients with clinical symptoms, neurologic deficits, altered sensorium, distracting injuries, or high-energy mechanisms. After a spine injury is identified, the entire spine requires radiographic imaging, a spine consultation should be obtained, and surgical timing should reflect the principles of early decompression and stabilization.

KEY REFERENCES

The level of evidence (LOE) is determined according to the criteria provided in the preface.

37. Levi AD, Hurlbert RJ, Anderson P, et al: Neurologic deterioration secondary to unrecognized spinal instability following trauma–a multicenter study. *Spine (Phila Pa 1976)* 31(4):451–458, 2006. LOE IV
43. Hoffman JR, Mower WR, Wolfson AB, et al: Validity of a set of clinical criteria to rule out injury to the cervical spine in patients with blunt trauma. National Emergency X-Radiography Utilization Study Group. *N Engl J Med* 343(2):94–99, 2000. LOE I
44. Stiell IG, Wells GA, Vandemheen KL, et al: The Canadian C-spine rule for radiography in alert and stable trauma patients. *JAMA* 286(15):1841–1848, 2001. LOE I
45. Stiell IG, Clement CM, McKnight RD, et al: The Canadian C-spine rule versus the NEXUS low-risk criteria in patients with trauma. *N Engl J Med* 349(26):2510–2518, 2003. LOE I
46. Anderson PA, Muchow RD, Munoz A, et al: Clearance of the asymptomatic cervical spine: a meta-analysis. *J Orthop Trauma* 24(2):100–106, 2010. LOE I
48. Simon JB, Schoenfeld AJ, Katz JN, et al: Are "normal" multidetector computed tomographic scans sufficient to allow collar removal in the trauma patient? *J Trauma* 68(1):103–108, 2010. LOE II
49. Harris TJ, Blackmore CC, Mirza SK, et al: Clearing the cervical spine in obtunded patients. *Spine (Phila Pa 1976)* 33(14):1547–1553, 2008. LOE I
50. Tomycz ND, Chew BG, Chang YF, et al: MRI is unnecessary to clear the cervical spine in obtunded/comatose trauma patients: the four-year experience of a level I trauma center. *J Trauma* 64(5):1258–1263, 2008. LOE I
55. Menaker J, Philp A, Boswell S, et al: Computed tomography alone for cervical spine clearance in the unreliable patient–are we there yet? *J Trauma* 64(4):898–903, discussion 903–4, 2008. LOE I
57. Schoenfeld AJ, Bono CM, McGuire KJ, et al: Computed tomography alone versus computed tomography and magnetic resonance imaging in the identification of occult injuries to the cervical spine: a meta-analysis. *J Trauma* 68(1):109–113, discussion 113–4, 2010. LOE III
58. Muchow RD, Resnick DK, Abdel MP, et al: Magnetic resonance imaging (MRI) in the clearance of the cervical spine in blunt trauma: a meta-analysis. *J Trauma* 64(1):179–189, 2008. LOE III
59. Mancini DJ, Burchard KW, Pekala JS: Optimal thoracic and lumbar spine imaging for trauma: are thoracic and lumbar spine reformats always indicated? *J Trauma* 69(1):119–121, 2010. LOE IV

61. Cooper C, Dunham CM, Rodriguez A: Falls and major injuries are risk factors for thoracolumbar fractures: cognitive impairment and multiple injuries impede the detection of back pain and tenderness. *J Trauma* 38(5):692–696, 1995. LOE II
72. Holmes JF, Panacek EA, Miller PQ, et al: Prospective evaluation of criteria for obtaining thoracolumbar radiographs in trauma patients. *J Emerg Med* 24(1):1–7, 2003. LOE III
73. Inaba K, DuBose JJ, Barmparas G, et al: Clinical examination is insufficient to rule out thoracolumbar spine injuries. *J Trauma* 70(1):174–179, 2011. LOE III
79. Sixta S, Moore FO, Ditillo MF, et al: Screening for thoracolumbar spinal injuries in blunt trauma: an Eastern Association for the Surgery of Trauma practice management guideline. *J Trauma Acute Care Surg* 73(5 Suppl 4):S326–S332, 2012. LOE II

The complete References list is available online at https://expertconsult.inkling.com.

Chapter 11

Damage Control Orthopaedic Surgery: A Strategy for the Orthopaedic Care of the Critically Injured Patient

CHRISTIAAN N. MAMCZAK • ERIC PAGENKOPF • THOMAS M. SCALEA • ANDREW POLLAK

INTRODUCTION TO THE CONCEPT OF DAMAGE CONTROL ORTHOPAEDICS

The initial treatment of a femur fracture can significantly impact patient survival, as was dramatically demonstrated during World War I. In the first 2 years of that conflict, open femur fractures carried an 80% mortality rate. Remarkably, this was reduced to approximately 7% by 1918 after initiating the early, routine use of the Thomas splint, which resulted in length stable reductions and, presumably, a decrease in associated blood loss.[1,2] Long bone fractures, particularly femoral shaft fractures, can result in significant hemorrhage and liberation of marrow contents into the systemic circulation. Although the exact mechanisms continue to be elucidated, these events have the potential to adversely impact patient physiology well beyond the musculoskeletal system, particularly in multiply injured patients (MIPs). A recent combined review of the trauma registries at two level I trauma centers, which included 2027 femoral shaft fractures, revealed that femur fractures remain an independent predictor of mortality and acute respiratory distress syndrome (ARDS).[3] As a result, femur fractures have served as the model for studies examining techniques to reduce complications in MIPs.[4]

Currently, it is nearly universally accepted that early total care (ETC), defined as the definitive fixation of fractures within approximately the first 24 hours after injury, is appropriate for the vast majority of patients.[5,6] When contrasted and compared with treatment of femur fractures with prolonged traction and delayed fixation, ETC avoids the deleterious effects of prolonged recumbence and is associated with improved survival and decreased complication rates.[7-13] Some studies, however, have suggested that ETC has the opposite effect in certain subsets of the MIP population, namely those with severe pulmonary and head injuries.[14-16] For these individuals, damage control orthopaedics (DCOs)—namely, the initial treatment of fractures with provisional external fixation followed by delayed definitive fixation—has potential advantages and is commonly used (Fig. 11-1). Similar to ETC, such an approach avoids the deleterious effects of prolonged recumbence but in contrast spares the patient from the additional physiologic burden of major surgery soon after injury, particularly the embolization of fat and marrow contents associated with intramedullary instrumentation that has been associated with secondary injury to the pulmonary capillary endothelium.[17-20]

Although DCO protocols have been implemented at most trauma centers in the United States and Europe, the specific clinical indications remain unclear. Unfortunately, much of the DCO literature describes studies of limited scientific and statistical power because of the complex nature of this patient population. Difficulties in the study of these patients include their dynamic and often complicated clinical course, quantification of the impact of associated injuries, and an evolving understanding of the underlying pathophysiology of the inflammatory process. Confounding factors include multiple significant trauma care improvements in resuscitation, ventilation and intensive care unit (ICU) clinical advances that occurred concurrently with the implementation of DCO protocols, as well as potential underlying differences in the populations and geographic variation in resuscitative protocols.

In addition, the definition of DCO has gradually expanded in some studies to include non-MIP patients, further confusing the literature.[21,22] At first, the term DCO described the use of femoral external fixation in a MIP as a temporizing measure—or bridge—to allow appropriate resuscitation before the definitive procedure.[23] Over time, a change in this definition has resulted in the use of the term DCO to describe external fixation of relatively isolated extremity fractures to provide temporary stabilization, typically to allow for resolution of soft tissue swelling or local wound healing or to protect a vascular repair before definitive fracture fixation. Clearly, these patients differ dramatically from MIPs in need of systemic resuscitation to allow for safe definitive fracture treatment. It is therefore useful to adopt the term *limb damage control* (LDC), as used by Roberts and colleagues, to differentiate between these diverse patient populations and treatment strategies.[24,25] The local advantages of LDC are well documented and discussed elsewhere in this text (i.e., periarticular tibial plateau or pilon fractures). The systemic advantages of DCO are less clear.

Today's orthopedic traumatologists must be adept in evaluation of MIPs and prepared to individualize treatment strategies in a dynamic manner, often in collaboration with other trauma-related specialists. This chapter reviews the history of ETC and DCO, presents the pathophysiologic basis for DCO, and provides evidence-based practice recommendations for patients in whom ETC may be inappropriate in an effort to limit adverse systemic effects of fracture treatment.

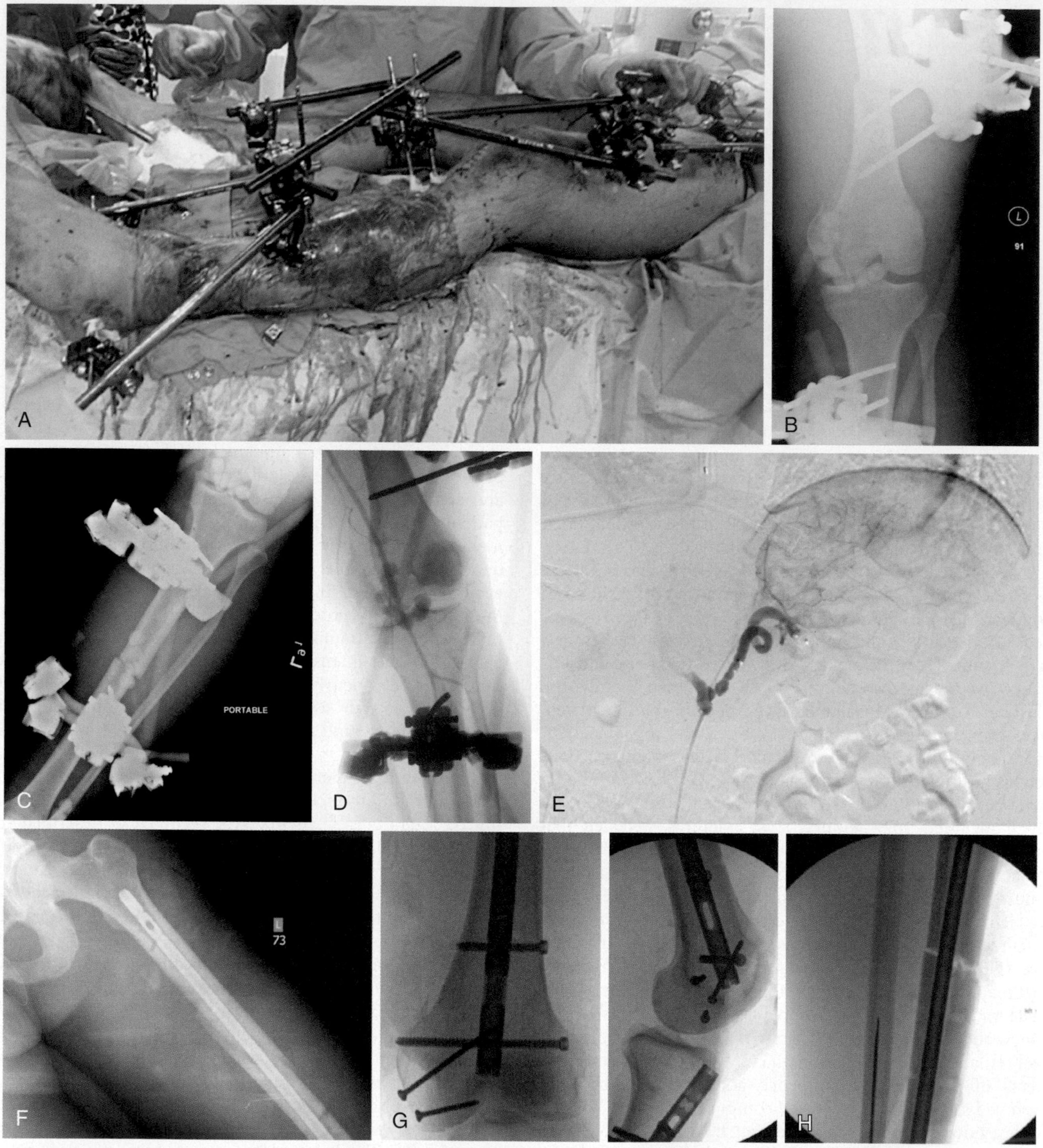

Figure 11-1. In the context of a physiologically unstable patient, damage control orthopaedics (DCO) in the form of débridement and dressing of open fractures and temporary stabilization with external fixation represents an attractive alternative to early total care. This case involved a 24-year-old motorcyclist who sustained a closed segmental femoral shaft fracture, a fracture-dislocation of the knee, and a Gustillo type III open tibia fracture. He presented hemodynamically stable but with a pulseless foot and ongoing bleeding from his open fractures. In this case, damage control consisted of urgent débridement of the open tibia fracture and open knee fracture-dislocation, implantation of antibiotic impregnated methyl-methacrylate beads into the open wounds inside bead pouches, and external fixation to stabilize the femur, knee, and tibia (**A**). Achievement of alignment and better stability resulted in clinical restoration of blood flow to the limb (**B** and **C**). He was taken to angiography after DCO for embolization of a grade IV splenic injury and evaluation of the leg (**D** and **E**). This demonstrated patency of the major vascular structures in the leg without evidence of traumatic injury. He was taken back to the operating room for eventual definitive stabilization of the femur, knee, and tibia after resolution of physiologic stability (**F** to **H**).

HISTORY OF DAMAGE CONTROL ORTHOPAEDICS VERSUS EARLY TOTAL CARE

Early termination of emergent laparotomies for penetrating trauma upon completion of lifesaving interventions was initiated by general surgeons in the 1980s. Appreciating the similarities that this approach shared with shipboard damage control efforts practiced by the U.S. Navy, Rotondo first used the term *damage control* to describe this laparotomy management tactic in 1993.[26] Maritime damage control is a shipboard doctrine applied to limit damage from a fire or other hazard to a defined area of the ship and therefore maximize the overall survivability of a damaged vessel. This is achieved by anticipating and rapidly containing the cascade of aftereffects of a potentially catastrophic initial hazard, typically fire or flooding. Simply stated, it is an effort to "keep the ship afloat."[27] With similar goals in mind for trauma patients, surgical damage control consists of three phases, as described by Feliciano and colleagues: (1) initial operative intervention for control of life-threatening bleeding and decontamination; (2) intensive care transfer for correction of the deadly triad of hypothermia, acidosis, and coagulopathy followed by (3) a return to the operating room (OR) for definitive repair of the intraabdominal injuries.[28] Better than expected survival rates have been realized with this strategy,[29] which remains popular and effective today.[30] Eventually, damage control strategies were developed for the initial treatment of extraabdominal trauma[31] to include the musculoskeletal system.[23]

In the mid-20th century, early manipulation of long bone fractures was considered unsafe.[32] Because of concerns that fracture manipulation and fixation would increase the incidence of fat emboli, these patients were considered "too sick" for surgery. Traction, prolonged bed rest, and delayed operative interventions were therefore the typical and accepted practice for long bone fractures. In 1967, Kuntscher recommended: "Do not nail immediately, but wait a few days," with special precautions for patients with multiple fractures or evidence of fat emboli.[33] Others advocated delays of up to 14 days before intervention.[34] Predictably, the consequences were severe. As noted by John Border, "traction produces an obtunded patient in the enforced supine position,"[2] which led to deleterious pulmonary effects, poor functional results,[35] and high mortality rates.[36]

In the 1980s, delayed care of femur fractures began to be supplanted by early or immediate fixation. Theorizing that fat embolization was an ongoing process that continued until fracture fixation, Riska and Myllynen of Finland, from the Arbeitsgemeinschaft für Osteosynthesefragen (AO) Foundation, first demonstrated improved outcomes with early fixation.[7] In their retrospective series, 22% of patients in the non- or late-stabilization group developed fat emboli syndrome compared with only 4.5% in the early stabilization group. With the primary goal of improving functional recovery, the AO group also actively promoted early fixation for closed fractures, considering fracture patients "too sick not to be treated surgically."[2,35,37] Such an approach was subsequently supported by multiple outcome studies (10 retrospective, one prospective), which focused on the relationship between the timing of fixation of fractures and associated morbidity or mortality.[38] Among the retrospective studies, LaDuca and colleagues extended the AO approach to open fractures using plate osteosynthesis and reported no episodes of fat emboli syndrome or cardiopulmonary failure.[11] Describing the experience of the John Border group, Seibel noted increased ICU stays with delayed stabilization of femur or acetabular fractures. Early fixation reduced the risk of complications, with the caveat, "as long as they are done correctly and in the presence of good oxygen transport and blood clotting." In contrast, traction significantly increased the cost of care and risk of multiple systems organ failure.[12] Goris and colleagues reported their experience in the Netherlands, where reductions in mortality and ARDS were realized with early plate osteosynthesis.[9] Johnson and colleagues similarly reported a fivefold increase in ARDS and mortality rate if fixation was delayed beyond 24 hours. This was most pronounced for the severely injured (Injury Severity Score [ISS] >40).[10]

The first randomized, prospective study to support early fixation of long bone fractures was conducted by Bone and colleagues at Parkland Memorial Hospital, Dallas, Texas. Eighty-three patients with femoral shaft fractures and ISS of 18 or greater were divided into early fixation (<24 hours) and late fixation (>48 hours) groups. In the 46 patients in the early fixation group, a total of 16 pulmonary complications were observed (ARDS, pulmonary embolism [PE], fat emboli syndrome, or abnormal blood gases), including only one case of ARDS. In the 37 patients in the late fixation group, 50 pulmonary complications were observed with six cases of ARDS. These results were considered a confirmation of the findings of the previous retrospective studies, and resulted in ". . . the overwhelming recommendation . . . that early stabilization of long bone fractures should be performed in multiply injured patients."[8] ETC became the standard of care, and practice patterns changed. In Border's group, the average duration for traction before fixation of femoral shaft fractures decreased from 9 to 2 days.[2] Today, the Bone study is viewed with only slightly less enthusiasm. The only statistically significant difference presented was an increase in total hospital costs for the delayed fixation group. The more clinically relevant findings exhibited by the late group—increased pulmonary complications and longer hospital and ICU stays—were merely trends that failed to reach statistical significance. In addition, the randomization process was somewhat flawed, resulting in associated pulmonary injuries in 10 of 37 patients in the delayed fixation group compared with only one of 46 in the early group.

In the 1990s, concerns were raised that in a select group of MIPs—those with severe chest injuries and hemodynamic instability—ETC, particularly intramedullary nailing (IMN) of femur fractures, could actually increase rather than decrease the incidence of ARDS or multiple organ failure (MOF).[14] ARDS and MOF are the dreaded end points of the systemic inflammatory response syndrome (SIRS), an exaggerated inflammatory response that ultimately damages organ systems that may have been uninvolved in the initial trauma. There are two inflammatory models for SIRS that are described: in the "one-hit" model, a massive initial injury and shock incite SIRS, resulting in early end-organ injury. In the "two-hit" model, an initial injury or "first hit" incites a more appropriately heightened state of SIRS that, if followed by a "second hit," can be amplified and result in late MOF.[39-41] Second hits may be from severe hemorrhage, incomplete resuscitation, infection, or major surgery.[40,42-45] Of concern for this MIP subset was the potential for the timing of fixation and/or method of fixation to act as a second hit.

The damage control concept used for truncal injuries was applied to long bone fractures under the moniker of "damage control orthopaedics" (DCO), as coined by Scalea and colleagues.[23,46] DCO is generally conducted by immobilizing a long bone or pelvic fracture with a temporizing external fixator to achieve the advantages associated with ETC (fracture stability, decreased pain, ease of nursing care,[23] improved patient positioning in the ICU,[47] decreased fat emboli[48]) while minimizing the potential adverse effects of major surgery (blood loss, hypothermia, and inflammatory system stimulation associated with medullary canal manipulation), which could serve as a second hit. After adequate resolution of physiologic stability and after the patient is no longer hypersusceptible to the second hit of intramedullary instrumentation, definitive fixation is conducted. Avoiding the consequences of an exaggerated second hit and the development of the lethal triad is the goal of DCO,[45,49] which far outweighs the major disadvantage of external fixation, which is a need for a second surgical procedure, potentially increased cost, and an increased infection risk with prolonged application.[48,50]

Identification of the subset of patients who would benefit from DCO is a continuing process, generating much controversy because indiscriminant application of DCO strategies could actually be harmful and associated with significant unnecessary expense. The generation of all-inclusive algorithms and strictly defined indications and treatment recommendations for the orthopaedic management of MIPs has proven elusive. In 2005, Rixen and colleagues reviewed 63 controlled DCO trials and failed to find a "generalized management strategy."[51] Even proponents admit that considerable clinical judgment and experience remain prerequisites to the appropriate application of DCO. Despite considerable experience, published DCO implementation rates varied dramatically among highly regarded institutions—12% at the University of Maryland's R. Adams Cowley Shock Trauma Center (2002–2005) versus 57% at Denver Health Medical Center (1993–2006) for similarly described patient populations.[52,53] Improved understanding of the inflammatory process and the importance of resuscitation are critical in better defining the appropriate DCO population.

DIAGNOSIS AND CLASSIFICATION OF THE BASIC PATHOPHYSIOLOGY AND INFLAMMATORY PROCESS IN CRITICALLY INJURED PATIENTS

The Basic Characteristics of Shock

A complex neuroinflammatory response follows injury. The precipitating causes of this are generally the combination of inadequate cellular perfusion, severe soft tissue injury, or both. Regardless, any combination of shock, defined as inadequate oxygen delivery or injured or nonviable tissue, precipitates this reaction. This reaction was first called the *ebb and flow phenomena*.[54] More recently, it has been characterized as inflammatory first and then counterinflammatory later. If there is no inflammatory response, the patient succumbs to overwhelming shock. If the inflammatory response is hyperexaggerated, organ failure typically occurs. Thus, a balance of inflammation and counterinflammation is necessary for good patient outcomes. Unfortunately, clinicians have essentially no ability to actually manipulate the inflammatory response. Many compounds have been investigated as the "silver bullet" that will modulate the inflammatory response; none has been shown to be effective.[55,56] This is likely because of the complex nature of the inflammatory response. A single compound or treatment is simply not sufficient. Even if one pathway is blocked, the body finds a way around that particular pathway.

Clinically, this complex system is manifested in one of three ways. In the first scenario, injuries and hemorrhage are recognized early, and the patient is resuscitated quickly. Although there may be complications of direct organ injury, in general, these patients do well. In the second scenario, patients present in profound shock or with multiple injuries. If resuscitation attempts are unsuccessful, these patients generally die of acute fulminant organ failure early on, generally within 24 hours. In the third scenario, resuscitation is delayed in which case organ failure usually complicates injury. The goal of early treatment is to achieve resuscitation early to avoid adverse outcomes.

Multiple organ dysfunction syndrome or MOF almost always occurs in the same order. The lungs fail first, usually within 48 to 72 hours. This is followed in sequence by renal failure and hepatic failure. Although our ability to support patients in ICUs has become greatly amplified in the past few years, in fact, the mortality rate from sequential organ failure remains quite high and largely unchanged over the years. Patients with a combination of respiratory failure, oliguric renal failure, and hepatic failure still have mortality rates that approach 80%.[57]

The Basic Principles of Resuscitation

Optimal resuscitation involves early recognition of injury and shock and then rapid restoration of circulating volume to support cardiac output and peripheral oxygen delivery. Various philosophies exist to optimally resuscitate patients. Although an in-depth discussion of these is beyond the scope of this chapter, it is probably important to articulate certain principles.

Achieving Hemostasis

Traditionally, 2 L of isotonic crystalloid was used as the initial bolus of fluid to treat patients who presented in hemorrhage shock.[58] This was both diagnostic and therapeutic and allowed classification into one of three categories, responder, transient responder, and nonresponder. However, we now realize that ongoing crystalloid resuscitation contributes to the overall proinflammatory state.

There are now two randomized prospective trials that demonstrate that raising blood pressure to normal before surgical hemostasis is obtained is of no benefit.[59,60] Raising blood pressure to normal in response to hypotension merely displaces the hemostatic clot that is formed on the injured blood vessels. Hypotension recurs, and the patient again requires resuscitation, which is often accomplished using additional crystalloid. This creates a dangerous cycle of repeated bleeding, hypotension, and dilution of coagulation factors. Hypothermia soon follows, and the mortality rate increases.

Damage control resuscitation is a treatment scheme that is used in the most severely injured patients as part of a total strategy to limit ongoing injury caused by shock.[61] This involves limited crystalloid resuscitation and permissive hypotension until surgical hemostasis has been obtained.

Crystalloid fluid is minimized, and volume replacement is achieved with a combination of packed red blood cells (PRBCs), fresh-frozen plasma, and platelets. Although the optimal ratio of red blood cells and component therapy has yet to be defined, many have espoused that this should be 1 : 1 : 1.[62] Others disagree, believing that less plasma is necessary.[63] Virtually all would agree that red blood cells, plasma, and platelets should be used as opposed to crystalloid fluid, particularly in the most severely injured patients.

Volume Replacement

After initial hemostasis has been obtained, volume replacement can be liberalized. Good data suggest that the ability to normalize lactate is the single most important prognostic feature in patients after injury.[64] However, the best method to normalize lactate is variable. Certainly, supporting cardiac output and oxygen delivery to optimally perfuse peripheral tissues seems reasonable. However, estimating the amount of intravascular volume necessary to do that can be difficult. In previous years, invasive monitoring was used to more precisely define filling pressures and cardiac output. More recently, the use of bedside echocardiography has been demonstrated to be a useful way to guide resuscitation.[65]

Optimizing Pulmonary Function

Respiratory failure after injury is relatively common. This may be due to direct concussive force injury to the lungs, as well as the inflammatory response to injury outside of the thoracic cavity and inadequacy of resuscitation. Early ARDS or respiratory insufficiency is relatively common in MIPs. The discussion around the role of bony injury complicating early respiratory failure has evolved over the years. Earlier data suggested that early total fracture care was deleterious to pulmonary function .[66] More recent data suggest that this is often not the case.[67] It is important to optimize pulmonary function and achieve normalization of lactate before proceeding with fracture stabilization, particularly intramedullary instrumentation. However, this can almost always be accomplished within a relatively short period of time, allowing fracture care to proceed safely.

Intraoperative management of hemodynamics is also an important part of the philosophy of early total fracture care. Ideally, anesthesiologists very familiar with the care of MIPs will be available. They should understand the blood loss associated with both fractures and fracture fixation. Intraoperative fluid needs may be quite impressive. Intraoperative hypotension may negatively impact the long-term outcome, particularly in patients with traumatic brain injury (TBI).[15,16,68] Thus, careful monitoring of cardiovascular performance in the OR is essential to allow early total fracture care to be a useful strategy. If an experienced anesthesiologist is not available at the time of patient presentation, initial damage control followed by definitive fracture fixation later may be wise as opposed to early total fracture care.

Early Fracture Care versus Damage Control Orthopaedics

In the case of a MIP with bony injury, decisions must be made as to when early total fracture care is appropriate as opposed to DCO. This generally involves discussions among the orthopaedic surgeons, ICU staff, and trauma surgeons. Risks and benefits of each therapeutic scheme must be weighed for every individual patient. In general, if patients are optimally resuscitated as evidenced by ability to clear lactate to normal, early total fracture care is often the wisest idea. If not, a damage control approach would be wiser.

Some specific injuries may influence the decision to proceed with ETC versus damage control. For instance, care for TBI usually involves serial physical examinations, repeat imaging, or both. Operative early total fracture care does not allow that to happen. Thus, DCO may be preferable to allow for careful monitoring of the brain injury.

The same may be true in patients with traumatic aortic injury and in patients with complex solid viscus injuries. The catecholamine swing that may be associated with IMN may increase blood pressure, negatively impacting the aortic injury. Certainly, serial physical examinations and serial hematocrits are a part of the nonoperative management of patients with blunt liver and spleen injuries.

However, in a well-functioning trauma system, many of these issues can be resolved and still allow for early total fracture care, perhaps not 12 hours after admission but within 24 hours. Repeat head computed tomography (CT) at 6 hours can be very helpful in predicting the trajectory of brain injury. Early stent grafting of traumatic aortic injuries stabilizes the aorta. A period of observation of liver and splenic injuries may often give the general surgeon sufficient comfort that definitive fracture care can proceed safely.

The decision as to whether to use early total fracture care versus DCO can be complicated. Optimal communication between all services involved is necessary to develop a cohesive plan. General surgeons must understand the important role that bony injury plays in patient outcome and the physiologic burden that comes with multiple fractures. Orthopaedic surgeons must understand the physiologic principles around resuscitation and optimization of cardiovascular performance. However, when this conversation occurs, early total fracture care is possible in the vast majority of patients, even those with significant injuries other than those to the bones.

MANAGEMENT OF THE MULTIPLY INJURED PATIENT

The Decision for Damage Control Orthopaedic Surgery

The ultimate goals of fracture treatment are to allow patient mobilization, early joint range of motion, and reconditioning therapy to achieve fracture healing and functional recovery consistent with the preinjury state. Fracture stabilization allows for a reduction in painful neurostimulation; optimizes muscle and soft tissue relationships, thereby preventing ongoing soft-tissue damage; and facilitates easier nursing care, rehabilitation, and hospital discharge. Isolated orthopaedic injuries in a patient without polytrauma are treated according to the requirements of the injury, the skill and clinical bias of the surgeon, and the characteristics of the patient. However, orthopaedic injuries in MIPs require surgeons to use a tactful reserve based on a "triage mentality." In these patients, fracture care must reflect the level of physiologic stability or instability, and orthopaedic surgeons must appropriately time and titrate interventions to enhance the patient's physiologic recovery rather than risk exacerbation of the inflammatory response by overaggressive pursuit of ETC. The management philosophy of DCO involves the use of rapid temporizing techniques and the maturation of a professional discipline necessary to avoid temptation to be overly invasive in the initial phase.

Damage control orthopaedic surgery is not for every patient with multiple fractures or every patient with multiple injuries and several fractures. Rather, it is for injured patients whose inflammatory responses will potentially be overwhelmed by further stimuli (i.e., reaming and intramedullary nail fixation of long bones, excessive surgical blood loss, and intraoperative fluid shifts). These are patients with a major constellation of injuries that have been recognized as having significant impact on the inflammatory and physiologic response. These injuries are usually associated with deranged physiology that has been difficult to correct or is undercorrected, such as hypovolemic shock, coagulopathy, or acidosis. Delayed manifestations of certain conditions such as lung or intracranial injury are also clues to deciding which patients may be better served by a damage control mode of care.

Assessment

One aim of the assessment during the initial resuscitation is to determine whether the injured patient with orthopaedic injuries can withstand ETC without overwhelming the inflammatory process.[38] Pape and colleagues have proposed classifying patients into one of four categories (grades) of relative physiologic stability based on a series of parameters including level of shock, core body temperature, degree of associated coagulopathy, and characteristics of associated injuries to other body systems.[69]

Patients who are stable according to the criteria offered by Pape and colleagues are generally able to safely undergo ETC, presuming there is ongoing monitoring of the critical parameters of physiologic stability throughout the case with reconsideration at any point if those parameters change resulting in relative instability. However, appropriate management of patients in other categories is more controversial. Most North American trauma centers use ETC much more aggressively than the criteria proposed by Pape and colleagues would indicate is appropriate. For example, using Abbreviated Injury Scale (AIS) chest of 3 or less as a marker for patients who are unstable or in extremis is wholly inconsistent with practice at most North American trauma centers. Furthermore, measurement of individual clotting factor levels, fibrinogen levels, or D-dimer levels is uncommon. Coagulopathy is initially defined as "present" or "absent" based on simpler, less effective gauges, including platelet counts and international normalized ratio. However, regardless of the specific criteria, the development of center-specific protocols for determining which patients are sufficiently stable to tolerate ETC versus those who are either borderline or unstable and therefore better suited for DCO is necessary. This determination must be based on readily available measures of injury severity, coagulopathy, shock, and body temperature. DCO is generally appropriate for patients who are not stable and will not become stable within 24 hours of the original injury.

Care for the Stable Patient (Grade I)

These patients have never been in shock and have only minor associated injuries that are not expected to further compromise physiologic stability. These patients are treated with the preferred method of care for their musculoskeletal injuries. Long bone fractures can be definitively fixed with reamed intramedullary nails or plates. The timing of the index surgery is usually in the first 24 to 36 hours, depending on OR and surgeon availability.

Care for the Borderline Patient (Grade II)

These patients are the most difficult to define and are the subjects of considerable debate within the literature on DCO.[70] In general, these patients have lower extremity fractures, especially of the femur or a pelvic ring injury. They have also sustained other severe trauma, such as pulmonary contusions or brain injuries, which have the potential to worsen. These patients often demonstrate episodes of cardiovascular instability and hypoxia. The initial response to injury and treatment may compromise the patient's ability to withstand the second surgical hit necessary for the definitive management of the orthopaedic injuries. Therefore, the borderline patient has the propensity to deteriorate and develop major complications and die. These patients require additional resuscitation, and more important, time for the severity of injuries to declare themselves before definitive surgical intervention is recommended for the musculoskeletal injury.[49,71,72]

Care for Unstable Patients (Grade III)

These patients have persistent cardiovascular instability and require ongoing resuscitation to correct the abnormal physiologic state. Major non-lifesaving procedures that would cause blood loss or major fluid shift must be avoided. These patients should undergo continued resuscitation in a controlled intensive care environment. The initial stabilization of long bone fractures can be accomplished with skeletal traction. As the patient's clinical course is better defined and more normal physiology is achieved though resuscitation, early intramedullary nailing (IMN) may be performed. If, however, the patient remains unstable, damage control using external fixation of the fractures should be considered. When necessary, these procedures can be performed at the bedside in the trauma ICU to prevent further instability from transport to and from the OR. Definitive fracture fixation should wait until there has been adequate resuscitation and physiologic stability, which may involve multiple days from the injury.

Care for Patients in Extremis (Grade IV)

These patients are the most critical and unstable after sustaining acute life-threatening injuries. Adequate resuscitation is difficult to achieve during the initial 24 hours after injury. These patients are not candidates for any major non-lifesaving surgical procedures in the first few days of hospitalization. External fixation of the long bone fractures should be considered as a bridge to definitive internal fixation. Temporary skeletal traction can be used in the acute resuscitation period but should be revised to formal external fixation if definitive fixation is expected to be significantly delayed. If the patient is in the OR for lifesaving surgery, expedited external fixation of the long bone fractures should be performed in concert with other lifesaving surgery.

Damage Control Orthopaedic Treatment Principles

Management Goals

The primary goal in the care of musculoskeletal injuries in MIPs is to limit the ongoing local and systemic injury associated with the musculoskeletal injury itself without causing a second physiologic hit in a patient who is in a hyperinflammatory state as a result of total injury load. Care is directed at resuscitation, correction of acidosis and coagulopathy, and limiting ongoing soft tissue injury associated with unstable long bone or pelvic fractures. For musculoskeletal injuries, the hierarchy of interventions follows this algorithm: (1) control extremity and pelvic hemorrhage, (2) correct ischemia (including reduction of dislocations and gross limb deformity, (3) débride contaminated traumatic wounds, (4) stabilize long bone fractures or unstable pelvic ring injuries, (5) reconstruct articular injuries, and (6) care for lesser fractures.

The revascularization of ischemic tissue occurs through fracture reduction, joint relocation, acute compartment syndrome fasciotomies, or vascular repair. Timely intervention helps to preserve functional tissue and can restore perfusion to critical tissues at risk for necrosis. Adequate surgical débridement of devitalized tissues and decontamination of open wounds minimizes the negative sequelae of the inflammatory response and decreases the risk of sepsis. Reduction and stabilization of major long bone fractures and unstable pelvic injuries reduces blood loss and transfusion requirements and minimizes ongoing soft tissue injury. The relocation of joints and the reduction and splinting of closed articular fractures helps to reduce pain and protect soft tissues until definitive fixation is physiologically appropriate.

Surgical Timing and Titration of Care

A multidisciplinary team approach is recommended for effectively coordinating resuscitation and surgical goals in MIPs. The general trauma surgeon is the "captain of the ship" and should clearly communicate the overall treatment plan, including the timing and appropriateness for surgical interventions. The decision to proceed to the OR versus the trauma ICU is dictated by the patient's physiologic recovery from trauma and response to resuscitative measures. If the patient is in the OR for lifesaving surgical procedures, communication of the immediate orthopaedic goals with the trauma team is critical. Fractures can be quickly stabilized with external fixation and contaminated wounds quickly debrided along with fasciotomies to address compartment syndrome or impending compartment syndrome as needed. When possible, simultaneous surgeries (i.e., laparotomy and extremity) should be orchestrated with prioritization of the critical procedures and reasonable end points established to limit surgical insult. Lifesaving thoracic, abdominal, pelvic, and neurosurgical procedures take precedence over extremity fracture stabilization. In critically unstable patients, DCO offers a safe and effective means to stabilize musculoskeletal injuries. It is impractical and often impossible to proceed with definitive care of long bone or complex periarticular fractures in these patients.

Teams should avoid heroic measures and know "when to quit" if a patient's condition deteriorates intraoperatively. Constant reevaluation of the patient's resuscitation and condition is critical along with communication among the trauma team, anesthesiologist, and subspecialty surgeons. Index surgeries in MIPs should be limited to 2 hours.[49] Falling core temperatures, worsening coagulopathy, unresolved or worsening base deficit, hypoxia, mixed venous desaturation, increasing peak airway pressures, and increased intracranial pressure (ICP) are all signs of imminent danger and signals that procedures should cease unless they are immediately lifesaving. At this point, the patient requires further stabilization and resuscitation in the trauma ICU. Bedside DCO, including fracture-spanning external fixation, fasciotomies, and basic wound débridement, may be necessary for patients too labile for the OR. These measures serve to bridge the gap before definitive orthopaedic surgery occurs in the OR.

External Fixation

External fixation is the workhorse of DCO and postulated to reduce the systemic inflammatory response and subsequent organ dysfunction and mortality.[23] It does require a second operation to convert to definitive fixation and possibly an increase in the rate of infection if the timeframe to conversion becomes markedly prolonged.

Although this approach may increase the final cost of care, the surgeon must decide, based on the relative risks of ETC versus staged procedures, whether or not the patient will benefit from the DCO approach. Short, simple, and relatively bloodless fracture stabilization can be achieved with external fixators. Simple frame half pin external fixation using two pins above and below each fracture segment provides excellent provisional stability for diaphyseal fractures. Joint-spanning frames achieve indirect reduction through ligamentotaxis to stabilize periarticular fractures. Complex and elaborate frames are unnecessary for DCO and prolong operative time. Self-drilling and self-tapping half-pins are time efficient and adequate for temporizing frames that bridge the gap between resuscitative fracture stabilization and later definitive fixation. These frames can be revised to increase stability or converted to definitive plate or nail fixation after adequate physiologic stabilization.

It is typically desirable for external fixators intended to achieve DCO to be applied rapidly. To accomplish rapid application, DCO frame systems typically recommend use of self-drilling pins as opposed to separately predrilling and then placing pins by hand. Separate predrilling with hand placement of pins may have the advantage of decreasing thermonecrosis at the pin site and therefore potentially prolonging purchase at the pin–bone interface.[73] Predrilling does not improve the pullout strength of pins acutely.[74] Because the pins in a DCO frame will generally be removed within 2 to 3 weeks to allow for definitive operative stabilization of the injury with internal fixation, there is minimal opportunity for them to fail secondary to generation of excessive heat on insertion. Therefore, the benefit of predrilling in terms of decreased bone necrosis is offset by the advantage of predrilling in terms of speed of application in the typical DCO circumstance.

Pelvic Stabilization and Hemodynamic Control

Pelvic ring injuries with widening or rotational or vertical displacement often require emergent, provisional stabilization to prevent hemorrhage and control hypovolemic shock. Repeat examinations to test pelvic stability should be avoided during the acute setting because the goal of pelvic stabilization is to encourage hemostasis and stabilize intrapelvic clot formation. Simple but effective temporizing means of pelvic volume control include internal rotation with taping of the lower extremities and circumferential pelvic antishock sheets or binders centered over the greater trochanters. These devices limit surgical access to the abdomen and perineum, however. Emergent laparotomy may require removal of these binders with resultant destabilization of the pelvic reduction and disruption of intrapelvic clots.

Percutaneous stabilization of the pelvis can be achieved with the pelvic C-clamp or resuscitative iliac crest pelvic external fixation. These methods can be performed rapidly at the bedside or in the OR. Pelvic external fixation techniques such as supraacetabular pin placement that are necessarily more time consuming and require significant fluoroscopic assistance should be avoided in hemodynamically unstable MIPs whenever possible. Persistent exsanguination in MIPs with unstable pelvic injuries may require a combination of external fixation, retroperitoneal packing, and angiography with embolization. In some severe injuries, emergent percutaneous screw stabilization of the sacroiliac joint may be beneficial, although this technique should be reserved for surgeons who are highly experienced with the procedure. Distortions to normal anatomy associated with wide displacement of the sacroiliac joint and the pressures of performing the procedure in the context of gross hemodynamic instability combine to markedly increase the degree of difficulty relative to more elective situations. Definitive internal fixation of the pelvis should be delayed until the patient's condition will tolerate prolonged surgery and blood loss.

Managing Other Musculoskeletal Injuries

High-energy open fractures, traumatic amputations, and acute compartment syndrome are common in MIPs. Awake examinations by the orthopaedist are not often possible because these patients are usually intubated early on in the trauma resuscitation. A low threshold for fasciotomy is recommended for patients with tense compartments in the face of high-energy fracture patterns and vascular or crush injuries. Emergent fasciotomy may be done at the bedside or in the OR. Fasciotomies in this situation should be considered as part of the damage control process. The goal is to limit the ongoing injury to the muscles within affected compartments secondary to actual or impending ischemia.

Wound contamination and necrosis associated with mangled extremities and traumatic amputations present a significant metabolic load to the MIP. A delay in treatment can intensify the systemic inflammatory response. Débridement, irrigation, and revision amputation to a stable level can be lifesaving. The decision concerning limb salvage versus amputation is especially important in critical patients. The physiologic stress and suspected systemic impact of multiple surgeries necessary to achieve limb salvage must be weighed before deciding whether or not to amputate acutely in the context of a physiologically unstable patient.

Other closed, non–long bone fractures and dislocations can be managed with provisional reduction and splinting until the patient is sufficiently stable to tolerate extended procedures. This reduction and splinting can often be done at the bedside with adequate sedation and little additional stress to the MIP. These injuries are often uncovered during secondary and tertiary examinations.

It is often tempting to proceed with acute operative stabilization of distal musculoskeletal injuries using tourniquet control to limit hemorrhage and arguing that by limiting intraoperative blood loss, there is minimal risk of worsening the acute systemic inflammatory response. There is evidence, however, that tourniquet-mediated ischemia-reperfusion is associated with pulmonary dysfunction in animal models and may increase vent days in MIPs undergoing IMN of associated femoral shaft fracture at the same operative sitting.[75-77]

Avoiding Missed Opportunities: Value of the Team Approach for Care of Multiply Injured Patients

Multiply injured patients can present with any combination of injuries to different bodily systems (e.g., intracranial, thoracoabdominal, musculoskeletal). Agreement about the basic concepts of care by each subspecialist involved in the case needs to be developed early on in the treatment plan. Clear communication among the major players (i.e., trauma, neurosurgery, and orthopaedic surgery) needs to occur throughout the course of care for a patient. Too often, DCO opportunities are missed as the trauma team brings the patient to the OR rapidly for a lifesaving procedure and then, as an afterthought, notifies the orthopaedic team of multiple suspected fractures as the patient is in transit to the trauma ICU. Débridement and external fixation equipment need to be readily available to the trauma room. Use of a radiolucent table for the emergent care of the trauma patient facilitates a smooth transition of care from the trauma team to the orthopaedic team. Arguments that patients cannot remain in the OR for an additional 20 to 30 minutes to allow for the application of an external fixator and débridement of contaminated wounds are often flawed and warrant careful consideration. The OR and the trauma ICU should be equally capable of continuing resuscitation, and resuscitation may be facilitated by wound débridement with associated extremity hemorrhage control and external fixation of long bones with associated limitation of ongoing soft tissue injury. Conversely, a blunt trauma victim who is rushed to the OR before obtaining a head CT to rule out epidural or subdural hematoma may be better served by going to CT without the delay that management of the extremity injuries might entail.

These decisions require the attention of trauma surgeons, orthopaedic surgeons, and neurosurgeons working closely together and communicating effectively with one another in an open and collegial fashion. Often the stress of the acute resuscitation makes this type of interaction more difficult and unnatural. Developing functional interpersonal relationships with other members of the trauma team in advance will likely lead to better patient care.

Conversion to Definitive Fixation

Damage control orthopaedic external fixation results in restoration of relative fracture stability. If applied appropriately, it should not burn any bridges relative to options for late conversion to definitive fixation. As the patient's general condition improves, opportunities for return trips to the OR for non-lifesaving secondary procedures will emerge. Again, clear communication of orthopaedic treatment goals with the critical care and other trauma teams is critical to avoid missing opportunities at serial débridements and conversion of temporizing fixation to appropriate internal fixation constructs.

Definitive treatment of long bone fractures with external fixation is associated with high rates of complications, including malunion, shortening, nonunion, local and regional pin-related infection, and loss of motion at joints in proximity. The conversion of external fixation to IM nail appears to be relatively safe in the femur. The timing of this event should be considered so as not to incur substantial risk of compromising the patient's recovery by secondary injury to the pulmonary capillary endothelium through reaming. The best time is when the inflammatory response has settled and the risk that a second hit will stimulate deterioration is not likely. Because monitoring the inflammatory process through assay of the mediators has not been demonstrated to be clinically functional, most surgeons wait until the inflammatory process has abated, usually 5 to 8 days after the injury. The patient must have no evidence of SIRS. A recent prospective study showed that MIPs operated on for secondary definitive surgery between days 2 and 4 have a significantly (P<0.0001) increased inflammatory response compared with those operated on between days 6 and 8.[71]

Nowotarski and colleagues reported on 59 patients with acute femoral shaft fractures treated with initial external fixation followed by staged conversion to an IM nail. The time in the external fixator averaged 7 days. All but four of the femurs were converted in a single-stage procedure. The four patients treated by a staged conversion had evidence of pin tract infections. For those cases, the external fixator was removed with curettage of the pin sites, and the patients were placed in traction to allow resolution of the pin tract infection with antibiotics. Ninety-seven percent of the fractures healed in 6 months. There was one deep infection that occurred in a patient with a type III open fracture.[48] Bhandari and colleagues conducted a meta-analysis of studies looking at the infection rates and time to union for femoral and tibial fractures treated with IMN after initial external fixation. Of the six studies of femoral fractures, the average infection rate associated with single-stage conversion of external fixation to IMN was 3.6% (95% confidence interval: 1.8%–7.4%). The duration of external fixation ranged from 7 to 15 days. Union rates averaged 98%. In the single study evaluating two-stage femoral nailing after markedly extended periods of external fixation (50 days), the incidence of infection was 40% even after a 17-day interval between procedures. Results for the nine studies evaluating the results of tibial nailing after external fixation showed a higher risk of secondary infection with rates averaging 8.6% and an 83% reduction in the risk of infection if the length of external fixation was less than 8 days. Overall, the authors concluded that more prospective studies with better controls are needed but that it appears that extended time in frames before conversion to intramedullary fixation increases the risk of infection, particularly for tibial fractures.[78]

TREATMENT OF PATIENTS WITH SEVERE THORACIC AND MUSCULOSKELETAL INJURIES: ESTABLISHING THE MODEL FOR DAMAGE CONTROL ORTHOPAEDICS

Pulmonary contusion is the most common pulmonary parenchymal consequence of blunt trauma.[79] A recent prospective study of blunt trauma patients described a pulmonary contusion incidence of 26%.[80] It has been suggested that an isolated pulmonary contusion has an associated mortality rate of 25%, which can increase to nearly 50% with the development of ARDS.[81] Injured lungs are at increased risk for secondary trauma associated with further insult, such as that secondary to the embolization of fat and marrow contents that results from intramedullary instrumentation.

In the early 1990s, two important studies evaluated the consequences of ETC in patients with chest injuries. In 1992, Pelias and colleagues retrospectively reviewed 130 consecutive patients with major blunt chest injury.[82] They were stratified according to the presence or absence of long bone fractures and timing of fixation: less than 48 hours (n = 65) versus greater than 48 hours or nonoperative treatment (n = 17). The pulmonary complication rates were essentially equivalent between the groups (27.6% early vs. 29.4% late), with no difference in mortality rate. However, in comparing patients with blunt chest trauma and long bone fractures with patients with blunt chest injury and similar ISS but without long bone fractures, a statistically significant increase in pulmonary morbidity and death was noted in the fracture group. The authors concluded that "early operative fixation did not protect against pulmonary dysfunction or death in this group of patients."

In 1993, Pape and colleagues from Hannover, Germany, raised concerns that early (<24 hours) femur fracture fixation with IMN was associated with deleterious pulmonary effects and higher mortality rates in patients with concomitant chest injuries.[67] They retrospectively reviewed 106 patients with femur fractures and an ISS of 18 or greater, splitting them into four groups based on the presence or absence of a severe chest injury and early (<24 hours) or late (>24 hours) IMN fixation. Consistent with other studies, ETC was noted to be advantageous in the non–chest-injured group. In the chest-injured group, however, they found a higher (although not statistically significant) incidence of ARDS in the early IMN group (33%) compared with the late IMN group (7.7%). They concluded that "in the presence of pulmonary injury, primary intramedullary femoral nailing causes additional pulmonary injury and may trigger ARDS." Critics of the study point to the small group size; lack of statistical significance; a higher incidence of ARDS than reported in the North American literature; and the fact that among the chest-injured patients, 29% of the early IMN group had bilateral chest injuries versus only 7.7% in the late IMN group. The magnitude of the chest injury, a factor poorly considered by the AIS scoring system, has been associated elsewhere with significant clinical importance.[83] Regardless, the findings were concerning and led to efforts to avoid early reamed IMN in this subset of patients.

Some have advocated for unreamed nailing as an alternative technique to achieve the benefits of early stabilization while decreasing the pulmonary morbidity rate associated with reaming.[84] Careful review of the literature, however, demonstrates that unreamed nailing is not associated with lower rates of ARDS or mortality.[85] Conversely, it is positively associated with increased rates of nonunion and need for reoperation. The clinical findings with respect to pulmonary outcome are consistent with animal models demonstrating that the greatest embolization of fat and marrow contents is associated with the initial opening of the intramedullary canal, a step common to both reamed and unreamed procedures.[86]

The Effect of Timing

Charash and colleagues thought that the Hannover results were contrary to their experience at the University of Tennessee and therefore conducted their own identically designed study, which was published in 1994.[87] They retrospectively reviewed 138 patients with femur fractures and an ISS of 18 or greater. In the chest-injured group, 56 patients underwent early IMN, and 25 patients underwent delayed IMN. In contrast to the Hannover experience, a statistically significant increase in pulmonary complications (pneumonia) was exhibited in the chest-injured group who underwent delayed IMN.

There was no difference in ARDS, mortality, or length of stay (LOS). Because this group also had a higher incidence of bilateral pulmonary contusions, an additional review of that subset of patients with unilateral pulmonary contusions was conducted, which showed similar statistically significant findings.

Multiple retrospective studies comparing early and late treatment of femoral shaft fractures in thoracic-injured patients were subsequently published, with similar conclusions.[88-90] In 1997, Boulanger and colleagues[88] retrospectively reviewed 68 femur fractures with chest injury treated early (<24 hours) versus 15 treated late and found no difference in pulmonary complications (ARDS, fat embolism syndrome [FES], pneumonia, PE) or MOF between groups. There was also no difference when compared with thoracic-injured patients without femur fractures, suggesting that the risk of pulmonary complications may actually be independent of fracture. In 2002, Brundage and colleagues[89] retrospectively reviewed 1362 femur fractures with chest injury treated over a 12-year period at a level I trauma center that used a protocol in which ETC was conducted for physiologically stable patients. They found that early treatment (<24 hours) resulted in lower rates of ARDS, shorter LOS, and no difference in mortality rate and concluded that chest trauma was not a contraindication to early reamed IMN. In 2011, Nahm and colleagues,[6,90] retrospectively reviewed 171 femoral shaft, neck, and intertrochanteric fractures with AIS of 3 or greater and found lower rates of sepsis and no difference in ARDS or mortality rate when comparing the 122 patients treated early (<24 hours) versus the 49 treated late.

Unfortunately, many of the retrospective studies in the DCO literature suffer from a common confounding factor. Because the patients were not randomized to early or late treatment, some underlying difference likely exists between the groups other than just the timing of fixation. In centers that routinely conduct ETC, virtually all patients who can tolerate surgery within the first 24 hours receive operations. Those that cannot for some reason (e.g., hemodynamic instability, severe acidosis, head injury, underlying medical comorbidities), become the delayed group. The underlying cause for delay may be the actual explanation for the difference in outcomes rather than the delay itself. Two other common limitations are present across many of these studies. First, most of the studies use thoracic AIS (AIS-T) as a means of comparing groups with respect to overall injury severity. Although average AIS-T is a useful means of comparing similarity of lung injuries from an anatomic perspective, it is limited in that it does not distinguish between unilateral and bilateral pulmonary injuries and between those associated with impaired ventilation and those that are not. Second, most of the studies in the literature comparing ETC with DCO do not compare or consider differences in level of resuscitation between treatment groups. It is certainly possible that inadequate resuscitation from shock predisposes to secondary injury from ETC, particularly femoral intramedullary reaming.[91]

The Effect of Reaming

The Hannover study[67] implicated not only the timing of fixation but also the method of fixation—reamed IMN—as the cause of the higher incidence of ARDS in their patients with thoracic trauma. Although not directly supported by their data, this was an understandable concern. The generation of systemic emboli by fracture manipulation and instrumentation of the medullary canal has been well described.[92,93] The high intramedullary pressures generated by reaming result in embolization of marrow contents—fat, clot, bone marrow, and inflammatory mediators—to the pulmonary vasculature. Several theories exist regarding the resulting pathologic effects, which include mechanical blockage by fat or marrow particles, pulmonary endothelial damage caused by toxic effects of fat or free fatty acids, and damage triggered by inflammatory mediators.[94] A prospective nonrandomized study was conducted by Pape and colleagues[95] to evaluate the effects of reaming on the pulmonary system. Seventeen patients with femoral shaft fractures, ISS greater than 20, and no associated head or thoracic injury underwent reamed IMN, and 14 similar patients underwent unreamed IMN. The reamed group was noted to have statistically significant decreases in oxygenation ratio (PaO_2/FiO_2) and increases in pulmonary artery pressures, which the authors believed could predispose to the development of ARDS, although no actual clinical outcomes were provided. Giannoudis and colleagues conducted a prospective study to evaluate the effects of reaming on the inflammatory system. Fifteen patients underwent reamed IMN, and 17 underwent unreamed IMN. The proinflammatory serum cytokine interleukin-6 (IL-6) and plasma elastase were significantly elevated in all patients after nailing. These markers tended to be higher in the reamed group, but the increase did not reach statistical significance. Again, no clinical outcomes for the groups were presented.[40] These results suggest that instrumentation of the femoral intramedullary canal is associated with a potential second hit to the pulmonary endothelium in the MIP. They do not confirm, however, that reamed nailing is significantly worse than unreamed nailing in terms of the effect on the pulmonary microvasculature.

In response to these studies, multiple alternatives to reamed IMN in patients with concomitant thoracic injuries were considered in an effort to protect the pulmonary microvasculature from the secondary injury during reaming despite the lack of certainty that a clinically relevant relationship actually existed. These included external fixation[18,23,96] followed by staged IMN after initial physiologic recovery (DCO), unreamed IMN,[14,67] unreamed small-diameter retrograde IMN ("damage control nailing"),[84] single-pass reaming, and use of the reamer-irrigator-aspirator (RIA) in place of standard reamers.[84,97,98]

Other studies have attempted to better define the clinical impact of reaming on the lungs. Bosse and colleagues[99] retrospectively reviewed populations at two separate level I trauma centers where femur fractures were treated acutely (within 24 hours) but with different fixation methods. Whereas the R. Adams Cowley Shock Trauma Center in Baltimore, Maryland, treated 95% of femur fractures with reamed IMN, Allegheny General Hospital in Pittsburgh treated 92% with plating over the same period. Patient characteristics between the two institutions were similar, so any difference in outcomes theoretically could have been attributed to the presence or absence of reaming. Patients with femur fractures were grouped according to the presence or absence of an associated thoracic injury, and those with major underlying medical comorbidities were excluded. Additionally, similar groups of patients at each institution with thoracic injuries but no femur or tibia fractures were compared, confirming that there were no underlying institutional differences in ARDS rates. The authors found no detectable differences in the rates of pulmonary complications (ARDS, pneumonia, PE), MOF, and mortality between the patient groups regardless of the presence or absence of a thoracic injury and regardless of the method of fixation (three of the 117 patients with thoracic injuries treated with reamed IMN developed ARDS compared with one of 104 of those treated with plating). Detrimental pulmonary effects attributable to intramedullary instrumentation were not apparent. Interestingly, the ARDS rate was highest in the groups with thoracic injury only.

In response to the disparity between the Pape and Bosse studies (both of which were retrospective), the Canadian Orthopaedic Trauma Society (COTS)[100] conducted a prospective, randomized, multicenter trial comparing clinical outcomes between 151 unreamed femur IMN and 171 reamed femoral IMN, all fixed within 24 hours of initial injury. Similar to Bosse, they found a low overall incidence of ARDS (3.7% in MIP), and no significant difference in ARDS rates between the groups (two of 151 unreamed vs. three of 171 reamed). In addition, thoracic injury, ISS, and postoperative oxygenation ratios were not found to be predictive of ARDS in this series.

The Effect of the Fracture

In 1995, Reynolds and colleagues[101] reported on the results of a retrospective review of 424 femur fractures, of which 105 occurred in patients with an ISS of 18 or greater. The statistically significant finding was a higher rate of pulmonary complications in high ISS compared with low ISS patients. The timing of fixation was not found to be predictive of pulmonary complications, which led the authors to conclude that severity of injury, not timing of fixation, was the predominant risk factor for development of pulmonary complications.

Several later studies then compared the morbidity and mortality of patients with isolated chest injuries with those with similar chest injuries but with associated femur fractures. Turchin and colleagues[102] compared groups with isolated pulmonary contusions with pulmonary contusions and early femur IMN, finding no difference in pulmonary complications or mortality rate. Similar findings were reported by Boulanger and colleagues.[88,103,104] Specifically, the rates of ARDS, MOF, and mortality associated with isolated chest injuries have not been increased as a result of early IMN of an associated femur fracture, which suggests that pulmonary complications in this population are independent of the fracture.

Current Treatment Recommendations in Cases of Severe Thoracic Injury and Musculoskeletal Injury

It is currently well accepted that ARDS and MOF result from a common, trauma-induced inflammatory pathway, which can be exacerbated by early fracture surgery in underresuscitated patients. Much of the presented literature does not directly stratify patients according to resuscitation parameters but merely by the presence of thoracic injury, femur fracture, and time of fixation. It is possible, if not likely, however, that many patients in the late fixation groups (regardless of retrospective, prospective, or randomized study design) were different in terms of resuscitation status and were thus indirectly stratified. Today, advances in ICU care and basic understanding of the inflammatory process allow more specific guidelines for the conduct of ETC than has been possible in the past.

Generally, patients with femur fractures and associated thoracic injuries should undergo definitive fixation as early as it can be safely performed. Safety for definitive fixation can be judged based on resuscitation status and cardiopulmonary parameters.[52] Helpful in this regard are the clinical parameters defining the four different clinical grades of stable, borderline, unstable, and in extremis, as per Pape and colleagues.[49] Real-time resuscitation status is well judged using serum lactate because it is not normalized by physiologic buffer systems. Even patients who appear to be hemodynamically stable may experience occult end-organ hypoperfusion (diagnosed by elevated serum bicarbonate and lactate), which is associated with increased mortality rates.[105,106] Other markers include decreased urine output, hypothermia, coagulopathy, and impaired oxygenation. In patients with chest injuries, additional clinical indicators of potential pulmonary dysfunction should be evaluated before contemplating surgical intervention. Airway pressures above 30 cm H_2O may be indicative of pulmonary interstitial fluid accumulation.[49] In the absence of evidence of impaired oxygenation—and all other parameters being appropriate—it is safe to use ETC despite the presence of a thoracic injury.

Emergent fixation of femoral shaft fractures in polytrauma patients is usually not necessary and may be dangerous. Morshed and colleagues[107] conducted a retrospective cohort review of 3069 femur fractures with ISS greater than 15 from the U.S. National Trauma Data Bank to evaluate the effect of fixation timing on mortality. The highest mortality rates were in patients fixed in less than 12 hours from injury. The authors suggested that delay in surgery past the initial 12 hours may have allowed for better resuscitation. O'Toole and colleagues[52] also documented continual improvement in sequential lactate levels in their study, in which the average time from injury to fixation was 14 hours. In the interim, application of skeletal traction provides the clinical benefits afforded by fracture reduction. Traditionally, traction pins are placed; however, a recent study documented the equivalent efficacy of cutaneous traction for provisional (<24 hours) reduction and immobilization.[108]

DAMAGE CONTROL ORTHOPAEDIC GUIDELINES FOR OTHER UNIQUE MUSCULOSKELETAL INJURIES: CLINICAL EVIDENCE BASED ON META-ANALYSIS AND SYSTEMATIC REVIEWS

Clinical Experience: Bilateral Femur Fractures

The concerns about the relative risks and benefits of ETC versus DCO for the treatment of femoral shaft fractures in polytrauma become magnified in patients with bilateral diaphyseal femur fractures. Historic rates of early mortality for these injuries have ranged from 26% to 40% with more recent studies substantially lower at 5.6%.[109,110] In patients with bilateral femur fractures, associated pulmonary and intracranial injuries are concerns for precipitous declines in lung function, cognitive impairment, and the second-hit systemic inflammatory response. Compared with unilateral femur fractures, a MIP with bilateral femur fractures often has a higher ISS, an increased risk of ARDS and pulmonary dysfunction, increased critical care requirements, and an increased hospital LOS.[111-113]

The literature describing the management of bilateral femoral shaft fractures consists of retrospective reviews from a small cases series in which various different nailing techniques and surgical timelines were used. Prospective and randomized studies are not available to guide treatment algorithms, and recommendations for care must be inferred. Certainly, the best method of avoiding pulmonary dysfunction is to prevent it from occurring or to use measures that reduce the risk of exacerbating it. Authors have expressed trepidation over the potential negative effects of fat embolization during sequential intramedullary instrumentation in patients with bilateral long bone fractures.[111] However, Bonnevialle and colleagues found that simultaneous unreamed nailing in 40 patients with bilateral femoral shaft fractures was a safe treatment pathway if PaO_2 levels and Gurd's criteria for fat embolization syndrome were appropriately monitored and managed intraoperatively. Yet in their study, 10 patients had considerable drops in the PaO_2 with two patients developing FES and two deaths.[114] In the largest cases series of 89 patients, Canada and colleagues performed bilateral reamed retrograde intramedullary nail fixation within 48 hours of injury. Despite thoracic injury in 39% and head injuries in 16% of cases, the overall incidence of ARDS and mortality rate were 14.6% and 5.6%, respectively. The authors concluded that bilateral retrograde femoral nailing is an acceptable treatment method and possibly a DCO alternative.[110]

In contrast, Zalavras and colleagues warned that thoracic injury and multiple IMN procedures were independent risk factors for respiratory failure with odds ratios of 40.6 and 25.6, respectively.[115] In an analysis of four studies describing the results of 197 patients treated for bilateral femoral shaft fractures, Stavlas and Giannoudis found these patients to be at high risk for morbidity and mortality with an average ISS of 20.6 (range, 9–75), a 4.1%, incidence of fat embolism, a 14.6% incidence of ARDS, and a 6.9% incidence of PE. The overall rate of mortality in these studies was 6%. The authors recommended consideration of damage control surgery in cases of bilateral long bone fractures, especially when systemic complications are anticipated.[116]

It goes without saying that MIPs with bilateral femoral shaft fractures are at greater risk of pulmonary complication than their counterparts with unilateral fractures. Treating surgeons must accurately define the degree of severity of injuries to other organ systems, namely the central nervous system and lungs. Patients with significant known head and chest injuries (borderline or extremis patients) may benefit from damage control external fixation or skeletal traction in cases of bilateral femur fractures. Conversion to nail or plate stabilization can be performed on a delayed basis, 5 to 7 days after injury, after the patient's medical condition has been optimized. However, prolonged intervals between DCO and definitive femoral fixation may pose a risk to further pulmonary dysfunction. The only study directly comparing primary intramedullary nail fixation with external fixation in bilateral femur fractures involves a controlled, sheep trauma model. In this study, the investigators found significantly higher pulmonary embolic loads in the nailing group ($P < 0.001$), but both treatment arms were comparable with regard to stimulation of the pulmonary inflammatory process and systemic coagulation.[117] A multicenter, prospective study comparing external fixation with intramedullary nail fixation for the acute treatment of bilateral femur fractures would be beneficial to better define treatment guidelines for borderline patients with polytrauma and bilateral femur fractures. On the contrary, patients with bilateral femur fractures and no concerning signs of respiratory compromise or head injury should undergo timely (<24 hours) reamed IMN of their fractures. The extent to which simultaneous nailing or interrupted nailing is superior is largely unknown at this time, and further studies are needed to draw conclusions.

Clinical Experience: Femoral Fracture and Head Injury

The presence of a TBI commonly and significantly impacts associated fracture treatment. In a prospective cohort of more than 1000 MIPs with orthopaedic injuries, Taeger and colleagues found 81% to have sustained an associated TBI.[118] In addition, along with blunt chest trauma, TBI is associated with high rates of morbidity and mortality. In a prospective, multicenter study from the Netherlands, Andriessen and colleagues reported 6-month mortality rates of 46% in patients with severe TBI (Glasgow Coma Scale [GCS] score <9) and 21% in patients with moderate TBI.[119]

The clinical management of a MIP with TBI is complicated by the need to prevent secondary brain injury caused by hypotension or hypoxia, influence on other organ systems, and difficulties monitoring neurologic function under anesthesia. Initial diagnostic head CTs—which may be normal or show only minimal evidence of injury—are not predictive of functional abnormalities, mandating serial clinical or imaging examinations. Stein and colleagues showed that 48% of MIPs eventually developed new or progressive lesions on serial CT scans. Of those, the majority had coagulopathies. Their results indicated that if one or more clotting parameters was abnormal, an 85% risk of progressive or secondary injury was present.[120] In addition, it appears that many of the immunologic and pro- and antiinflammatory responses known to occur after blunt injury to the torso and extremities also appear after even isolated TBI, predisposing these patients to SIRS or multiple organ dysfunction syndrome (MODS).[121] Non-neurologic organ dysfunction can be widespread but most commonly affects the respiratory system.

Traumatic brain injury is classified as primary or secondary. Whereas primary tissue injury is the result of direct mechanical trauma associated with the energy transfer of the initial traumatic event, secondary injury is caused by inadequate cerebral oxygenation after injury. Secondary injury causes additional cell destruction and can significantly degrade the potential for recovery and ultimate functional outcome. Even a single episode of hypoxia can adversely affect outcomes for all severities of head injury.[122-124] It is absolutely necessary to avoid the detrimental effects of secondary injury that makes fracture care decisions in this patient population so challenging.

Current guidelines recommend ICP monitoring and cerebral perfusion pressure (CPP)–guided therapies to avoid secondary injury.[125] Failure to maintain either parameter within appropriate limits is an important cause of unfavorable outcome in TBI.[126] CPP is calculated as the mean arterial pressure (MAP) minus ICP ($CPP = MAP - ICP$) and is dependent on ICP measurement via an intraventricular or intraparenchymal probe. Guidelines recommend maintenance of CPP greater than 60 to 80 mm Hg.[125,127] A CPP of less than 50 mm Hg, even if only transient, has been shown to be associated with poor outcomes.[128] The most common cause of low CPP is an elevated ICP. Described interventions used by neurosurgeons or neurointensivists to decrease ICP include ventriculostomy, hyperosmolar therapy, barbiturate coma, hypothermia, and decompressive craniectomy. Low CPP can also be encountered as the consequence of systemic hypotension or hypovolemia. Inadequate resuscitation or operative procedures that result in significant blood loss or major fluid shifts are common sources of systemic hypotension.

The treatment of a MIP with TBI and fractures requires coordinated multispecialty care. Several important principles guide the process. First, the injured brain has little functional reserve and a very narrow window of time during which salvage is possible.[129] Outside of emergent lifesaving procedures, priority is therefore given to neurosurgical interventions. Aggressive resuscitation (to increase MAP), reversal of coagulopathy, and treatment of the primary intracranial injury (to reduce ICP) are the initial priorities. Second, the injured brain is highly susceptible to secondary injury. CPP and cellular oxygenation are maintained by applying damage control techniques to other injuries while providing appropriate circulatory and ventilatory support. Common neurocritical care tactics include monitoring of brain oxygenation and ICP and continuous electroencephalography (to detect ischemia and seizures) as well as glycemic and thermoregulatory control. Third, the injured brain has limited reparative capacity. Musculoskeletal injuries initially "neglected" as a consequence of TBI may result in functional limitations that, if severe, can be addressed with late revision surgery. In contrast, any secondary brain injury incurred intraoperatively will likely be permanent and cannot be surgically corrected. Surgeons must therefore carefully consider the relative risks before undertaking any operative procedure for non–life-threatening or non-neurologic conditions.

There is currently no level I or II evidence to guide the management of fractures in MIPs with TBI. It appears, however, that the timing of fracture care is less important than the potential for secondary injury sustained intraoperatively. Poole and colleagues found no adverse neurologic effects in patients treated with early fixation as long as oxygen saturation was maintained greater than 90% and systolic blood pressure greater than 90 mm Hg. Pulmonary complications were associated with TBI regardless of fracture fixation timing.[130] Kalb and colleagues reported on 123 femur fractures with TBI in which 84 were treated early (<24 hours). No difference was found between the early and late groups in terms of neurologic or non-neurologic complications. Of note, despite higher intraoperative blood loss and fluid requirements in the early group, CPP was maintained at higher levels versus the late group.[131]

In a review of the trauma registry at Allegheny General Hospital, Townsend and colleagues found 61 patients with femur fractures and TBI. Of those treated within the first 2 hours of injury, 68% had an episode of intraoperative hypotension compared with only 8.3% of those treated after 24 hours, highlighting the importance of adequate initial resuscitation before operative interventions.[68] Interestingly, they reported no difference in neurologic outcomes between the groups based on the Glasgow Outcomes Scale.[132,197] All of these studies suffer from their retrospective design and therefore inherent selection bias. In addition, GCS score has not been found to be a good predictor of cognitive function, which limits the usefulness of multiple other published studies.[133]

Possibly the best current guidance for the timing of fracture care in MIPs with TBI continues to be that of Hippocrates: *Primum non nocere*—"first, do no harm." As the treating orthopaedic surgeon contemplates operative intervention, careful consideration should be given to the anticipated length of the procedure and potential blood loss, as well as an assessment of the institution's ability to provide appropriate intraoperative monitoring. Whenever possible, damage control techniques for orthopaedic injuries should be conducted concurrently with neurosurgical or lifesaving procedures. If that opportunity is missed, return to the OR for even damage control procedures may prove difficult because of the often labile and progressive nature of severe TBI. In that case, external fixation can sometimes be accomplished at the bedside in the ICU. Definitive orthopaedic care should be delayed until the potential for secondary brain injury has been diminished. Once cleared, intraoperative monitoring of ICP and brain oxygenation is recommended, and the surgeon should remain prepared for early termination or modification of the procedure should those parameters dictate.

Clinical Experience: Unstable Pelvic Ring Injury and Polytrauma

The principles of DCO are paramount in the acute management of unstable pelvic ring injuries, especially those in multiply injured trauma patients with signs of hypovolemic shock. Prehospital care and trauma bay evaluation should first focus on the principles of advanced trauma life support: airway, breathing, and circulation. In the case of patients with unstable pelvic ring injuries and exsanguinating retroperitoneal hemorrhage, the orthopaedic surgeon is a critical member of the team and decision-making algorithm. The pelvis can be viewed as an inverted cone where the volume is exponentially related to the radius (Volume = $\frac{1}{3}\pi r^2 h$). Thus, unstable pelvic ring injuries with widening of the pelvic diameter are associated with significant risk of acute blood loss and early mortality if restoration of more normal anatomy cannot be rapidly achieved. Various radiographic classification schemes have attempted to predict which patterns and mechanisms of injury lead to pelvic injuries at risk for internal hemorrhage; however, other variables such as advanced age and injury scores also suggest that the treatment of acute pelvic ring injuries should be managed on an individualized basis with serial clinical examinations and assessment of the patient's physiologic status.[134-138] Of note, repeated pelvic ring examinations are not encouraged because they may dislodge a stable clot. Only a single examination by an experienced provider is necessary. Pelvic ring injury patterns traditionally are associated with significant acute blood loss, and their specific treatment guidelines are discussed in detail in Chapter 40 on pelvic ring disruptions.

Options for management of unstable pelvic injuries are plentiful with various means employed to control pelvic volume in the acute phase. Due to variations in opinion and practice, standardized protocols do not exist and prospective, randomized studies are needed to further define the optimal treatment algorithms. Damage control measures typically focus on controlling hemorrhage through pelvic stabilization and component therapy resuscitation. Definitive fixation occurs after the patient has regained physiologic stability. Advanced Trauma Life Support guidelines recommend index resuscitations with 2 L of crystalloid followed by PRBCs and fresh-frozen plasma given at a 1 : 1 ratio.[139] Transfusions alone are not sufficient to control exsanguination in unstable pelvic injuries. Timely stabilization of the pelvis is also a critical step in the treatment pathway. Historic use of the pneumatic antishock garment fell out of favor after reports of iatrogenic compartment syndromes and subsequent extremity amputations occurred from prolonged use. More important, randomized controlled studies failed to show their efficacy in decreasing mortality rates.[140] In addition, the device was cumbersome and did not allow access to the pelvis and abdomen without deflating the pelvic compression.[141,142] Routt and colleagues described the technique of temporarily using a circumferential pelvic antishock sheet (CPAS) with surgical clamps to acutely stabilize hemodynamically unstable pelvic fractures but warned of the potential hazards of pressure ulcers and worsening sacral nerve root compression with prolonged use.[143] Routt and colleagues have expanded on the use of the CPAS to include percutaneous sacroiliac screw fixation or external fixation placed through working portals covered in sterile occlusive dressing. The authors describe using this technical trick in 35 cases of unstable pelvic ring injuries treated within the initial 72 hours from admission with only two cases of superficial skin blistering and no wound infections.[144] The use of noninvasive commercial binders has become more common because they are often used by first responders before hospital admission. Cadaveric studies show these devices work best at reducing expanded pelvic volume without overcompression when centered over the greater trochanters; however, specific guidelines for duration of use are unclear, and soft tissue breakdown remains a concern with markedly extended use.[145,146] The advantages of pelvic sheets and binders are that they represent relatively safe and noninvasive modalities to achieve compression using a simple, low-cost device.

A more invasive but effective option for pelvic ring stabilization is the pelvic C-clamp, a form of external fixation. These devices can be effectively applied within minutes through small percutaneous incisions and are not dependent on fluoroscopy. They offer direct compression at the sacroiliac region, which is mechanically advantageous in reducing open-book, posterior ring and vertically or rotationally unstable pelvic injuries. The mobile ring can be swung cranial or caudal to allow access to the abdomen or perineum without compromising the reduction. Pohlemann and colleagues demonstrated the safe application of emergent pelvic C-clamps in 43 patients with unstable pelvic ring injuries. The authors described the reliable anatomic landmark for pin insertion at the lateral aspect of the sacroiliac joint where an easily palpable "groove" is located below the iliac wing.[147] Successful variations in C-clamp pin placements have been described to allow compression vectors over the anterior aspect of the ileum for predominately anterior ring widening, as well as directly over the greater trochanters. Complications of skin breakdown, clamp displacement, loosening, and pin penetration into the pelvis have all been described.[147-150]

Resuscitative pelvic external fixation has been a longstanding and reliable method for controlling pelvic volume in hemodynamically unstable patients. Various uniplanar and multiplanar techniques exist for pin placement in the anterosuperior iliac wing, the subcristal anterior superior iliac spine (ASIS) position, and the supraacetabular or anterior inferior iliac spine (AIIS) location. Traditionally, external fixators with multiple iliac crest pins have been rapidly applied for lifesaving measures in the trauma bay without the use of fluoroscopy.[151,152] Incorrect pin placement in locations other than between the inner and outer tables by inexperienced surgeons using the anterosuperior iliac crest approach is reported to be as high as 18%.[153] Fixation pins in the subcristal ASIS and supraacetabular positions offer increasing frame stiffness and versatile access to the abdomen, but these techniques require skilled surgeons and fluoroscopic assistance. Although mechanically superior to the iliac crest frames, fluoroscopy-dependent pelvic fixation techniques are not recommended in unstable patients demonstrating signs of hypovolemic shock.[154,155]

When patients remain hemodynamically unstable after initial resuscitation plus temporizing mechanical pelvic ring stabilization, at least two options are available to effectively achieve control of pelvic hemorrhage: angiographic evaluation with embolization of sources of arterial bleeding and open perivesicular pelvic packing.

Laparotomy with pelvic packing has been widely used in the European trauma community because advocates claim this method directly addresses the majority of peripelvic bleeding that is venous in origin. Modern, minimally invasive and retroperitoneal packing techniques can be performed rapidly and potentially result in successful tamponade of life-threatening bleeding from iliac vein lacerations and cancellous pelvic fractures.[156] Pohlemann and colleagues found a reduction in mortality rate from 46% to 25% in complex pelvic injuries when a protocol using pelvic external fixation and surgical hemostasis with pelvic packing was implemented within 30 minutes of admission.[157]

However, Tötterman and colleagues described extraperitoneal pelvic packing (EPP) as a salvage procedure to control massive pelvic hemorrhage and found arterial injury present in 80% of patients when angiography was performed after EPP. Because of the high incidence of arterial injury with this technique, the authors recommend that angiography supplement EPP when patients are unstable.[158] In contrast, Cothren and colleagues found that only five of 24 patients (21%) required angioembolization after preperitoneal packing was performed for hemodynamically unstable pelvic ring injuries that did not respond to 2 units of PRBCs and pelvic stabilization.[159]

The role of angiography in hemodynamically unstable pelvic injuries continues to evolve. Because of advances in imaging, this technique tends to be favored over pelvic packing at trauma centers in the United States. In a review of 806 pelvic fractures, Agolini and coauthors determined that a small percentage of pelvic injuries actually require embolization, but in those cases, angiography performed within 3 hours of admission had a significant impact on overall survival. In their study, the most important factors influencing survival were patient age, initial hemodynamic instability, and time to embolization.[160] However, pelvic fracture patterns do not consistently correlate with the need for embolization, and determining which cases require angioembolization is still difficult. Although angiography can effectively control arterial pelvic hemorrhage, it offers little advantage for the venous bleeding inherently present in the majority of major pelvic injuries.[161,162] Despite its effectiveness, there are no reliable protocols to predict which patients require angiography, and valuable time spent waiting for embolization neglects critical venous exsanguination.[163] The ideal approach to recalcitrant pelvic hemorrhage is likely a multidisciplinary team approach in which index pelvic stabilization and hemostatic resuscitation are followed by expedited retroperitoneal packing and subsequent angiography with embolization. Further research into developing these complementary techniques into a single protocol is necessary.

Clinical Experience: Military Combat Casualty Care Lessons Learned

Lessons learned from previous wars have been integrated into the current standard of care for trauma protocols. After more than a decade of war, including the conflicts in Iraq and Afghanistan, the military trauma and orthopaedic communities have developed significant expertise and experience in the area of damage control surgery. For the past 8 years, the Extremity War Injuries Symposium, a collaboration of the American Academy of Orthopaedic Surgeons (AAOS), Orthopaedic Trauma Association (OTA), Orthopaedic Research Society (ORS), and Society of Military Orthopaedic Surgeons (SOMOS), has convened to discuss critical treatment challenges and future research priorities related to modern combat casualty care. Panels of experts from both military and civilian trauma backgrounds work together at these events to help define the most effective treatments for MIPs.

Penetrating wounds from blasting ordinance remain the most common mechanism of injury for soldiers engaged in the Global War on Terrorism; gunshot wounds, motor vehicle accidents, and blunt trauma occur to a lesser extent.[164-167] The improvised explosive device (IED) has become the defining ordinance used against U.S. and coalition troops in these conflicts, resulting in a myriad of devastating amputations and wounding patterns.[168-170] Widespread use of protective body armor and helmets has resulted in increased survival rates and an associated increased burden of extremity wounds, which are present in up to 54% of casualties.[171] Through adaptive advances in combat triage using early extremity tourniquet application to achieve hemorrhage control and early blood product transfusion, critical care nurse first responders continue to push the envelope in lowering the rate of casualties who expire from their wounds before care at a treatment facility.[172] Despite soldiers sustaining higher injury severity scores than in previous conflicts, effective advances in modern combat casualty care have led to survival rates greater than 90% and battlefield mortality rates as low as 7.5%.[172,173]

Acute hemorrhage is a significant challenge in modern combat trauma because the majority of injuries result from the penetrating blast effects of explosives in a hostile arena, often remote from advanced hospital care. In a retrospective analysis of combat victims who died of wounds (DOW), Eastridge and colleagues discovered that 51.4% of cases were potentially survivable (PS) with hemorrhage comprising 80% of those cases; truncal hemorrhage predominated (48%) followed by extremity hemorrhage (31%) and junctional hemorrhage (i.e., axillary or groin, 21%). The authors extrapolated that the overall DOW rate during the study period was 4.6%, and comparable to rates of death recorded in the National Trauma Data Bank for level I trauma centers in the United States, thereby indicating that advances in modern combat trauma care are saving lives.[174]

Effective predeployment education and the pervasive use of combat tourniquets applied shortly after injuries have dramatically reduced the number of casualties expiring from exsanguination, although these are essentially ineffective in junctional and truncal hemorrhage.[175,176] In a review of 232 casualties admitted to a downrange combat hospital with major limb trauma, Kragh and colleagues found a statistically significant survival rate when tourniquets were applied before signs of shock (prehospital) versus after (emergency department application). Four patients suffered transient neuropathy at the site of tourniquet application, but there were no amputations related to tourniquet use and no major long-term complications attributable to the tourniquet.[177] Combat tourniquet time greater than 2 hours is associated with a higher but nonsignificant number of limb fasciotomies; however, the overall benefit of early application in penetrating or open wounds justifies continued use.[178] The success of combat tourniquet protocols in improving survival rates suggests that civilian protocols using earlier and more aggressive use of tourniquets to manage extremity hemorrhage should be considered. Recent editions of textbooks for first responders and emergency medical technicians have incorporated the military philosophy of tourniquet use given the compelling combat related data, the lack of data supporting more limited indications, and the difficulties associated with design of meaningful civilian studies.[179] Military education models such as the Emergency War Surgery Course, Tactical Combat Casualty Care, and Joint Forces Combat Trauma Management Course provide valuable experience for civilian trauma training.

Traumatic amputations and nonsalvageable mangled extremities continue to be unfortunate and common problems encountered during the conflicts in Iraq and Afghanistan.[180] In a retrospective review of combat injuries, Stansbury and colleagues reported on 423 major limb amputations; 95% occurred before the evacuation out of theater and were not a result of failed limb salvage. In this series, 88% were the result of blast munitions, and 18% had more than one extremity amputated.[181] Despite valiant attempts to achieve limb salvage with DCO principles, late amputations are still a frequent secondary decision pathway for patients with chronic pain, nerve deficit, infection, soft tissue loss, and posttraumatic arthritis.[182,183] Patients with multiple extremity amputations and other associated blast-induced injuries, including complex pelvic fractures, hollow and solid organ injury, and destructive soft tissue wounds to the perineum, constitute some of the most critically injured and challenging patients from these conflicts.[184-187] Coordinated multidisciplinary team efforts along with the use of prehospital field tourniquets, rapid medevac triage, damage control resuscitation, and skilled surgeons following clinical practice guidelines have allowed patients with these extensive injuries to survive the early phase of injury where in previous wars they may not have.[188-190] Although not as common, reports from the civilian trauma literature describe similar cases of massive pelvic injuries with traumatic amputations secondary to high-speed motor vehicle accidents or pedestrians struck by trains.[191,192]

The lessons learned from the most severe combat casualty care continue to pave the way for future success in noncombat trauma. Military surgeons downrange have restricted resources and stricter guidelines while treating seriously injured war victims. Continued collaboration among civilian and military experts in the fields of trauma surgery, critical care, and orthopaedics will ensure that these lessons expand the principles of damage control surgery and advanced trauma protocols.

CONCLUSION

Today's orthopaedic traumatologist must be adept in evaluation of MIPs and prepared to individualize treatment strategies in a dynamic manner, often in collaboration with other trauma-related specialists. Early stabilization of long bone fractures offers the distinct advantage of earlier mobilization, fewer pulmonary complications, better pain management, decreased ongoing soft tissue injury, and decreased LOS. However, for some patients who are at particularly high risk because of severe associated pulmonary or neurologic trauma, inadequate resuscitation from shock, hypothermia, or coagulopathy, the risks of ETC may outweigh the benefits. In these patients, ETC, particularly instrumentation of the intramedullary canal of the femur, may result in an inflammatory second hit to a primed capillary endothelium that results in increased pulmonary capillary permeability; poorer ventilatory function; and a progressive acute lung injury that leads to ARDS, MODS, and potentially death. For these patients, DCO may be preferable to ETC with staged definitive fracture fixation completed after sufficient physiologic recovery. Because the choice to proceed with DCO results in additional operative procedures to complete fracture fixation, it is beneficial to reserve this approach for patients at highest risk for complications with use of ETC. The clinical challenge remains with identifying these at-risk patients.

KEY REFERENCES

The level of evidence (LOE) is determined according to the criteria provided in the preface.

4. Pape H-C, Giannoudis PV, Krettick C, et al: Timing of fracture fixation in multitrauma patients: the role of early total care and damage control surgery. *J Am Acad Orthop Surg* 17:541–549, 2009. LOE V
5. Pape HC, Hidebrand F, Pertschy S, et al: Changes in the management of femoral shaft fractures in polytrauma patients: from early total care to damage control orthopedic surgery. *J Trauma* 53:452–462, 2002. LOE III
8. Bone LB, Johnson KD, Weigelt J, et al: Early versus delayed stabilization of femoral fractures: a prospective randomized study. *J Bone Joint Surg Am* 71:336–340, 1989. LOE I
17. Pape HC, Grimme K, Van Griensven M, et al: Impact of intramedullary instrumentation versus damage control for femoral fractures on immunoinflammatory parameters: prospective randomized analysis by the EPOFF Study Group. *J Trauma* 55:7–13, 2003. LOE I
23. Scalea TM, Boswell SA, Scott JD, et al: External fixation as a bridge to intramedullary nailing for patients with multiple injuries and with femur fractures: damage control orthopedics. *J Trauma* 48:613–621, 2000. LOE II
38. Roberts CS, Pape HC, Jones AL, et al: Damage control orthopedics: Evolving concepts in treatment of patients who have sustained orthopedic trauma. *J Bone Joint Surg Am* 2:434–449, 2005. LOE II
40. Giannoudis PV, Smith RM, Bellamy MC, et al: Stimulation of the inflammatory system by reamed and unreamed nailing of femoral fractures: an analysis of the second hit. *J Bone Joint Surg Br* 81:356–361, 1999. LOE I
52. O'Toole RV, O'Brien M, Scalea TM, et al: Resuscitation before stabilization of femoral shaft fractures limits acute respiratory distress syndrome in patients with multiple traumatic injuries despite low use of damage control orthopedics. *J Trauma* 67:1013–1021, 2009. LOE II
99. Bosse MJ, MacKenzie EJ, Riemer BI, et al: Adult respiratory distress syndrome, pneumonia and mortality following thoracic injury and a femoral fracture treated either with intramedullary nailing with reaming or with a plate: a comparative study. *J Bone Joint Surg Am* 799-809, 1997. LOE III
107. Morshed S, Miclau T 3rd, Bembom O, et al: Delayed internal fixation of femoral shaft fracture reduces mortality among patients with multisystem trauma. *J Bone Joint Surg Am* 91:3–13, 2009. LOE II

The complete References list is available online at https://expertconsult.inkling.com.

Chapter 12

Disaster Management

CHRISTOPHER T. BORN • RYAN CALFEE • ROMAN HAYDA • TAD GERLINGER • WARREN KADRMAS • PETER GINAITT

INTRODUCTION

Disasters are large-scale destructive events that disrupt the infrastructure and normal functioning of a community. Disasters are both natural (e.g., earthquakes, tornadoes, hurricanes) and human made (e.g., industrial spills, explosions, structural collapses, terrorist attacks). Such an event presents the medical community with a large number of casualties that require rapid triage and treatment that is disproportionate to the available personnel and resources necessary for optimal care. In addition to events occurring outside of a facility, internal events that could limit a hospital's ability to deliver services must be considered. Facilities need to be able to identify services such as power and water outages, building compromises, labor disputes, and so on that may limit or threaten operations.

The increase in geopolitical acts of terrorism has changed civilian health care. Providers are now charged with having familiarity with mass casualty situations and must now understand both the pathophysiology and injury patterns produced by chemical, biologic, radiologic, nuclear, and explosive (CBRNE) devices. Civilian caregivers must learn to deliver care in a mass casualty setting with limited or compromised resources, fulfilling the basic mission of minimizing the population's morbidity and mortality. The bombing at the 2013 Boston Marathon underscores the requirement for increased education of civilians and physicians involved in a response to domestic mass casualty incidents (MCIs).

True MCIs are rare, providing little opportunity for real-time training. No formal components of medical school or residency prepare physicians for the unique demands and approaches required for the medical care of mass casualties. Thus, most medical care providers have limited training and experience in disaster management. Furthermore, disaster preparations in both community hospitals and even trauma centers are often rudimentary at best.[1,2] However, proper disaster training and planning are nearly universal in their application to actual scenarios. Regardless of the specific event, the elements of an effective disaster response are similar. This allows for an "all-hazards approach" to the development of disaster management principles, which are then easily applied. Well-defined goals of the disaster response and a clearly delineated command structure serve as the basis for efficient and effective recovery from such an event. In addition to true MCI events occurring within the community, hospitals must be aware that their capabilities could be equally challenged should regional diversions or an influx of patients unassociated with an event create a surge of volume that reaches a critical mass. This could be as basic as an influx of stable nursing home patients evacuated after an incident at their facility. The surge of stable patients would stress facility operations and require an immediate response upgrade.

DISASTER PLANNING

Effective planning is paramount to a community's ability to cope with any disaster. All hospitals and communities need well-rehearsed strategies for disaster management. It is accepted that nearly half of injured survivors from disasters reach hospitals within the first hour and that health care facilities can expect approximately 75% of victims within a 2-hour window. This rapid surge of patients can easily overwhelm hospital staff and resources without prearranged triage algorithms and organizational systems designed for such occurrences.

Disaster plans must have several elements. All levels of acute care providers and administrators should be actively involved in their design to ensure that practical aspects from all phases of the medical response are considered. Prehospital providers, emergency department (ED) nurses, physicians, surgeons, and anesthesiologists who routinely encounter lesser scale casualty situations add invaluable experience to the process. After being drafted, the plan requires the acceptance and endorsement of all involved to create a well-coordinated approach to an expectedly chaotic situation. Because all elements of a disaster cannot be predicted because of the large number of variables, disaster plans are designed to be generic and somewhat flexible. Incorporating common requirements, treatment principles, and expected barriers into disaster plans has been termed an "all-hazards approach." This eliminates the need for numerous individual plans that quickly become cumbersome and risk adding confusion and inefficiency into the disaster response. It is appropriate for disaster plans to vary by region and even by community, but they must be integrated with local and regional response organizations and facilities to ensure a collaborative approach. Hazard vulnerability analysis (HVA) refers to the formal evaluation of potential disasters with ranking or weighting of scenarios based on their relative probability of occurrence and the severity of impact. Such analysis, although based on both objective historical data and subjective educated projections, provides a basis upon which communities can begin to focus their disaster planning. Thus, hospitals in California may focus preparations on earthquakes, and those in Florida concentrate on the sequelae of hurricanes because these represent probable and highly significant foreseeable disasters. Plans should be based on injuries and lessons learned from previous disasters. Universal organizational schemes are based on predefined leadership positions. Within communities, trauma centers should provide the template for disaster planning because they possess both the staff and resources primed to respond to casualties. Finally, disaster plans are only as effective as the ability of those involved to carry out the objectives. To avoid having a false sense of security in a written plan, hospitals must continually educate staff about disaster care and practice regular disaster drills. The plan's execution can then become routine and deficiencies remedied while still in a controlled environment. Ideally, each drill is accompanied by debriefing sessions to give feedback from drill organizers to participants and includes a critical revisiting of the plan by all involved. As a requirement of the Homeland Security Exercise and Evaluation Program (HSEEP), all drills and exercises should also be followed up with a comprehensive After Action Report (AAR) archiving the overall performance and response with the goals of creating a corrective action plan to correct any areas needing improvements. Ideally, those corrections should then be integrated into a follow-up exercise to test the efficacy of the changes and make alterations as necessary.

DISASTER CLASSIFICATION

Disasters are classified in many ways with each adding to the detailed understanding of the event and its probable impact. This is primarily done by mechanism, with the broad categories of "natural" versus "human-made" events. This division is useful in that each type of disaster will pose unique challenges and produce varied injuries. Natural disasters can be further separated into geophysical events, such as earthquakes, and weather-related events, such as floods. Human-made disasters are subdivided into intentional and unintentional catastrophes.

Disasters are also described by the extent and duration of the event. "Open" and "closed" are accepted terminology for defining disaster extent. Open disasters are devastating for a large geographic area, such as the widespread flooding of the gulf coast after Hurricane Katrina in 2005. Closed disasters generally occur in well-defined and contained locations, such as the bombing of the federal building in Oklahoma City in 1995. Disaster duration is characterized as being "finite" or "ongoing." Ongoing events do not end abruptly and produce severe prolonged effects and strains on resources. Protracted military conflicts and natural disasters with extensive flooding can be considered ongoing disasters. The loss of infrastructure and increased incidence of postdisaster complications such as disease, starvation, and population displacement characterize ongoing events.

Scope of response, resource consumption, and casualty load are also used to describe mass casualty events. Understanding a disaster's response and resource requirements may help to accurately depict the disaster's impact. Classification in this sense has three levels. Level I events require only the use of local resources albeit with some strain on that health care system. These are episodes of multiple casualty events that extend beyond the normal volume of daily trauma. Level II disasters require the mobilization of additional regional assets. Level III disasters necessitate the allocation of large-scale resources, including state, federal, and international organizations.

DISASTER MANAGEMENT

Disaster management is broken down into four acknowledged categories: preparedness, response, recovery, and mitigation.[3] Each stage is important in coping with a disaster and in limiting the attendant devastation produced by the event.

Preparedness refers to making a community aware of the circumstances that have the potential for disaster creation (e.g., presence of an aging dam or a nuclear power plant) and planning on how to effectively cope should such an event occur. Plans should be developed to properly address the needs of local facilities before the impact is experienced. Additional tasks such as training personnel, purchasing equipment, engaging in interagency planning, and conducting timely mass casualty exercises must be practiced.[4]

Disaster response encompasses the basic elements of search and rescue, triage and initial stabilization, definitive medical care, and medical evacuation. These steps of the medical response must occur while the global needs for water, food, shelter, sanitation, security, communication, and disease surveillance are also addressed. The actual disaster response is expected to progress through well-defined phases. Initially, chaos predominates while care providers are alerted. Victims are struck with panic and fear. The more distant and less responsive the health care resources, the longer this phase may continue. Minimizing this phase is critical. Chaos is followed by the initial response and organization phase, heralded by the arrival of first responders. To effectively progress, strong leadership and implementation of an organizational framework are required. At this time, the scene is assessed, victims are triaged in the field, and security is established. Although important for all disasters, the principle of ensuring first responders' safety before rescue efforts commence is especially relevant when facing terrorist attacks. Terrorist tactics include "second-hit" attacks directed at responders. In October 2002, a suicide bomber in Bali, Indonesia, detonated a bomb in a busy business district, attracting people to the location from surrounding buildings. This event was then followed by a hugely destructive vehicle-based explosion in the street that became more lethal given the assembled crowd. First responders were targeted in Atlanta, Georgia, in 1997 when the bombing of a building was followed by an explosive device detonated 1 hour later in the parking lot as emergency personnel worked. This second-hit risk must be remembered when approaching all terrorist targets. Disaster scenes with unstable buildings represent another source of a "second hit," such as in the New York World Trade Center attacks in 2001 when hundreds of rescuers were lost when the towers collapsed. Additionally, in any explosive event, a high index of suspicion for a "dirty bomb" should be maintained.[5] In these blast situations, an assessment of the safety and the exposure risk of rescue personnel along with the risk of contamination of health care workers and hospital facilities must be considered before rescue efforts are initiated.

First responders must be educated about nuclear, biologic, and chemical (NBC) exposure hazards and understand that sequelae of such exposure may not be immediately apparent. Proceeding cautiously and suspecting potential NBC contamination after a blast are critical. Blasts with known biologic or chemical contaminants require appropriate protective gear for the rescuers to begin the triage efforts.[5] The administration of antidotes may be necessary in some scenarios, but the most appropriate time or place for this to commence (i.e., before or after decontamination or transfer of victims) may be difficult to assess for a given event.[5] After the scene is deemed safe for responders, site-clearing commences with both the decontamination and physical clearing of the disaster scene as well as the transport of casualties to hospitals. Recovery is the last phase and implies a return of normalcy to the area and reconstitution of the damaged infrastructure. This may be relatively rapid in a confined, finite event or may require significant time after a large natural disaster. This phase marks a transition in the focus of disaster response from crisis management toward one of consequence management. Although frequently underemphasized in disaster plans, this phase is essential for the reestablishment of the affected community. During this time, large-scale efforts to permanently replace damaged buildings, revitalize economies, or restore agricultural systems to their full predisaster production capacity are undertaken.[4]

Disaster mitigation refers to the ability to reduce the devastating effects of disasters before the actual event. Tornado warning systems or evacuations before hurricanes are two such examples. Mitigation can occur at any point in the disaster cycle.

Barriers to Effective Disaster Response

In any MCI, a small group of critically injured patients (typically, 5%–25% of the live casualties) will be contained within the larger crowd of less severe casualties. This was well demonstrated in the 1995 Oklahoma City bombing, where of 388 victims who went to local hospitals, only 72 (18.6%) required admission and seven (2%) required intubation.[6] The core mission of a hospital disaster response system is to identify these critical casualties and to provide the requisite level of trauma care that may be acceptable under the circumstances. Failure in this task may result in the misappropriation of valuable resources away from those casualties most in need. Although this task is quite manageable in daily trauma occurrences such as after motor vehicle crashes, mass casualty events add considerable complexity to attaining this goal. A key barrier is any obstacle that threatens this core mission. This includes a lack of warning, inaccessible resources, triage errors, or even a lack of disaster training. Disaster response plans must anticipate and attempt to remove these obstacles in advance in order to achieve success.

The rapid evolution of true mass casualty events poses the first key barrier. Disasters, especially the increasingly prevalent intentional attacks, may provide no warning and little lead time for hospital preparedness. Two corporate bombings in Turkey in 2003 produced 184 casualties for evaluation by a single medical center within the first hour after the incident.[7] This initial surge of patients may also place hospital facilities and personnel at risk for exposure to nuclear, biologic, or chemical toxins. After the sarin gas attacks on the Tokyo subway system in March 1995, hospital workers became victims before the toxin was even suspected. This resulted in contaminated hospitals and fewer caregivers available to provide treatment. Even with a well-rehearsed disaster plan, it takes time to organize a facility into an appropriate disaster response mode and to clear physical space for victim management. When the patient load outpaces the allotment of resources, an exponentially longer amount of time is necessary to restore the balance. Communication is critical in early alerts to allow hospitals the necessary time to decompress their EDs and prepare for the influx.

The timing of disasters can also present significant yet variable barriers. For instance, a daytime mass casualty situation may flood hospitals with victims while resources such as operating rooms (ORs) are in use and therefore are not available for immediate reallocation. Meanwhile, a nighttime MCI may be met by an understaffed response capability until additional assets are made available.

Communications are another consistent source of difficulty during disasters. Whether this equates to cellular phones ceasing to function or emergency lines being inundated with calls, backup plans for communication are critical. This may include dedicated land telephone lines, computer-based systems, or satellite connections. If communication both within and among the response teams (prehospital responders, hospital providers, incident command leaders) fails, then the entire response effort suffers severely. Effective communication also encompasses the relaying of accurate information and proper instruction to the general population through the media. This can reduce panic and the gridlocking of communication and resources of hospitals. Given the requirements of coordination and efficiency in a disaster response, the failure of communications must be prevented at all costs and proper communications for staff updates encouraged.

Another barrier in providing disaster care is human error. Beginning at the scene, less experienced first responders may tend to overtriage, in which case hospital systems will be overburdened with less severely injured patients. With larger MCIs, undertriage may occur because the injury numbers are so vast. At the hospital, the initial wave of casualties will be treated while there may still be limited knowledge about the true nature and scope of the surrounding event. This will cause early errors in resource allocation. Disaster training exercises may help minimize these mistakes because these issues should be identified if the exercise is properly performed and a good After Action Report completed. In addition, casualties often change triage categories throughout the course of the event. For this reason, each casualty must be retriaged at each level, or echelon, of care.

The overall lack of disaster preparedness by health care professionals poses a most formidable barrier. In any community, the majority of physicians are not involved in disaster training and planning, which will hinder an effective disaster response. This is evidenced by several physician surveys. Seventy-two percent (118 of 166) of nonurban physicians in Texas reported no CBRNE training. This mirrored a national survey in which only 21% of physician respondents felt prepared to treat bioterrorism victims.[2] Among trauma surgeons, only 60% understood the Incident Command System (ICS) for disasters, and fewer than 50% of respondents were prepared to manage an exposure to nerve or biologic agents.[8] Even the manual of Advanced Trauma Life Support (ATLS) mentions the basics of blast injury management on only a single page.[9] In addition to being unable to provide exposure-specific treatments, untrained physicians can impede disaster responses by adding to the number of unnecessary people around intake areas without assigned duties or knowledge of mass casualty triage. Now more than ever, it seems appropriate for all members of the health care community to become versed in the language and principles of disaster management.

Disaster Response Organization—Incident Command System

The effective response to any disaster is predicated on the coordination of many individuals, teams, and organizations. This may require concerted efforts by local agencies and medical specialists or involve added dimensions of resources dedicated from geographically distanced areas. To optimize outcomes and maximize communication and efficiency during disasters, the ICS was developed (Fig. 12-1). It provides a modular, scalable, and adaptable organizational hierarchy to manage mass casualty situations. This system of organization has proven to expedite responses in many settings even when a disaster is not being experienced. For hospitals, the responses to census control, unit openings, and other events requiring an organized approach have led to the Hospital Incident Command System (HICS).

Since its inception in the 1970s, the ICS concept has become standard practice as an organizational approach to managing temporary situations by safety professions.[10] In 1981, the ICS provided the basis for the National Interagency ICS Management System (NIIMS), which is the structural backbone for emergency responses by U.S. federal agencies.[11,12] This design was declared to be the "best practice" standard in 2004 by the Department of Homeland Security, and compliance with the ICS structure is required to receive federal disaster relief.[13]

The ICS structure is built on five major managerial tasks: command, operations, planning, logistics, and finance and administration. These are considered central to managing all disasters, with the size and scope of the situation dictating the number of individuals assigned to complete these tasks. Heading the ICS effort is the incident commander (IC). This individual is ultimately responsible for the entirety of the disaster response. As the ranking official, this person defines objectives, oversees all operations, and delegates responsibility. Up to seven officials will report to the IC.

The safety, public information, and liaison officers are the three officials who constitute the "command staff" and report directly to the IC. The safety officer is charged with assuring that appropriate protection is provided to first responders. With intentional terrorist activity on the rise, this officer must weigh response efforts with the risk of NBC contamination and the chances of a "second hit." The public information officer is the reference for updated knowledge to the media and public but is also responsible for internal communications to keep staff informed as the event progresses. The liaison officer is tasked with coordinating responses of the potentially numerous agencies and organizations involved and most importantly as the single point of contact for that command section. For HICS, an event-specific fourth position known as the "medical/technical" specialist can be added to the command section. After H1N1, it was observed that the professionals with expertise in epidemiology were not present at the command level. Such an appointment could aid the decisions of the IC during that type of event.

The "general staff" oversee the remaining core aspects of the ICS, including operations, planning, logistics, and finance. These areas are referred to as sections, and the head of each is titled a section chief. The assignment of individuals to these positions and the number of persons within each section depend on the nature and extent of the disaster encountered. In a small-scale event, the IC may personally oversee these additional activities. However, the modularity built into the ICS becomes important in larger disasters when individual section chiefs can be assigned with direct responsibility over teams at their disposal. These chiefs also report directly to the IC (see Fig. 12-1).

The planning section chief works in coordination with the IC to develop the designated response. It is this individual's job to conceptualize an effective strategy to approach the given disaster. Most important, this includes maintaining foresight

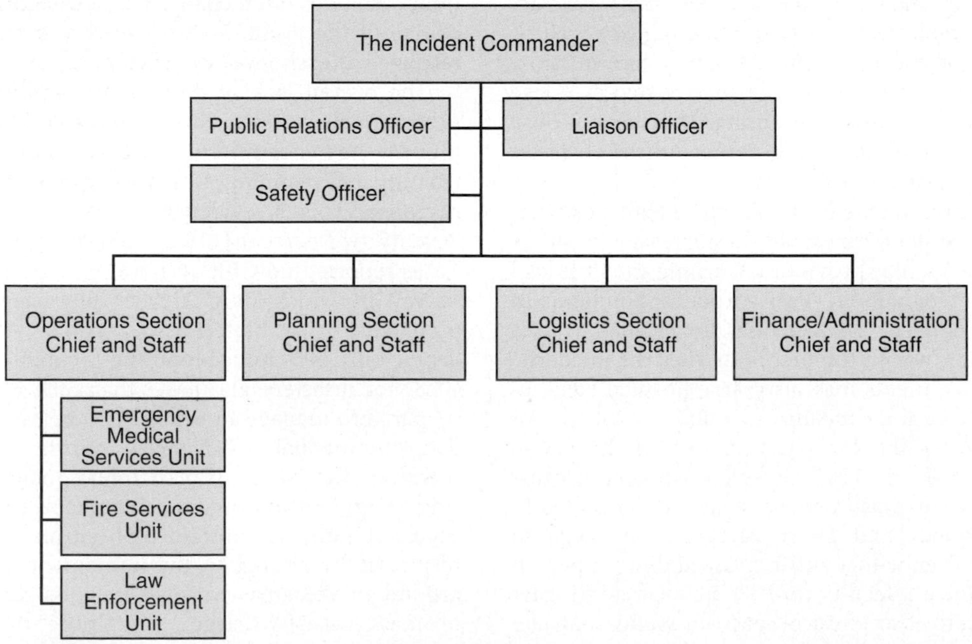

Figure 12-1. The organizational structure of the Incident Command System (ICS) demonstrates the relationship between the command staff, general staff, and section chiefs. The modular structure allows for the ICS to be expanded or contracted according to the changing needs of a disaster situation. Additional units are added as needed under the direction of each of the section chiefs.

to anticipate evolving needs and resource depletion. Meanwhile, the logistics section chief must obtain those resources and assets sufficient to perform the planned response. This includes gaining human resources, equipment, and supplies to ensure a sustainable effort. Operation section activities encompass the physical deployment of resources into the field. This includes rescue efforts, securing treatment areas, and the delivery of aid. This section chief is therefore responsible for the actual delivery of care directly to the casualties involved. The finance and administrative section chief should record and analyze the monetary cost of the disaster and the ongoing response. If a declaration of disaster is issued, this role will provide the necessary structure for Federal Emergency Management Agency (FEMA)–related reimbursements that may be very important to economic recovery.

Although the ICS is built on well-defined leadership roles as discussed, the overall function of the ICS depends on several general principles. The more rapidly the ICS is established, the quicker an effective response is mounted. To this end, the terminology, titles, and working procedures are standardized to function in any mass casualty situation. Furthermore, although the specifics of each disaster may dictate the size of the ICS and the expertise of those in charge, the overlying structure of the ICS is constant. The flexibility of the ICS is in its modularity, which permits expansion and contraction of the incident command structure as needed. The key concept dictating this fluctuating size of the ICS is one of a "manageable span of control." This equates to no one person supervising more than three to seven individuals to maintain the ability to effectively oversee the responsibility of subordinates. An additional means by which the ICS can expand when confronted with a devastating event involving significant interagency efforts is to add a unified command (UC). The UC would be composed of ICs from the primary organizations involved and allow them to coordinate efforts from a central location termed the Emergency Operations Center (EOC). This UC attempts to restore efficiency to situations where jurisdictional or functional roles of agencies overlap. Finally, all individuals involved in the response must perform within this structure. Efforts to operate outside the ICS may lead to confusion and detract from the overall coordination of efforts and reduce efficient utilization of resources.

The ICS structure has also been adapted to provide a mode of operations for hospitals facing disasters. The HICS was originally presented in 1991.[14] This system follows the ICS hierarchy, principles, and structure. Ideally, this same type of organization and distributed responsibility provides the hospital with an effective paradigm to provide organized care to casualties. The only alteration to the ICS structure in the hospital is to modify operation sections into appropriate divisions such as the medical/technical specialist, surgical, medical, intensive, and ambulatory care services. Again, the adaptable nature of this system allows for expansion of the areas most needed while preserving the universal titles and terminology to allow for easy communication with other facilities and with those involved with other phases of the disaster response such as those transporting casualties to the care facilities.

ACCIDENTAL AND HUMAN-MADE DISASTERS

Although both natural and human-made disasters produce significant morbidity and mortality, most of the detailed literature on specific injury mechanisms in mass casualty situations focuses on human-made disasters. In this age of geopolitical instability, much emphasis has been placed on the potential effects of NBC agents. The fact is that blast injury accounts for the preponderance of MCIs (Fig. 12-2). Despite this, there is significantly less awareness among physicians of how to manage blast-related injuries. In a 2004 survey of the members of the Eastern Association for the Surgery of Trauma (EAST), only 73% of the trauma surgeons queried understood the classification and pathophysiology of blast injuries.[8] As explosive munitions become an increasingly common form of civilian attack, it is critical that physicians possess basic knowledge of blast injuries and NBC agents.

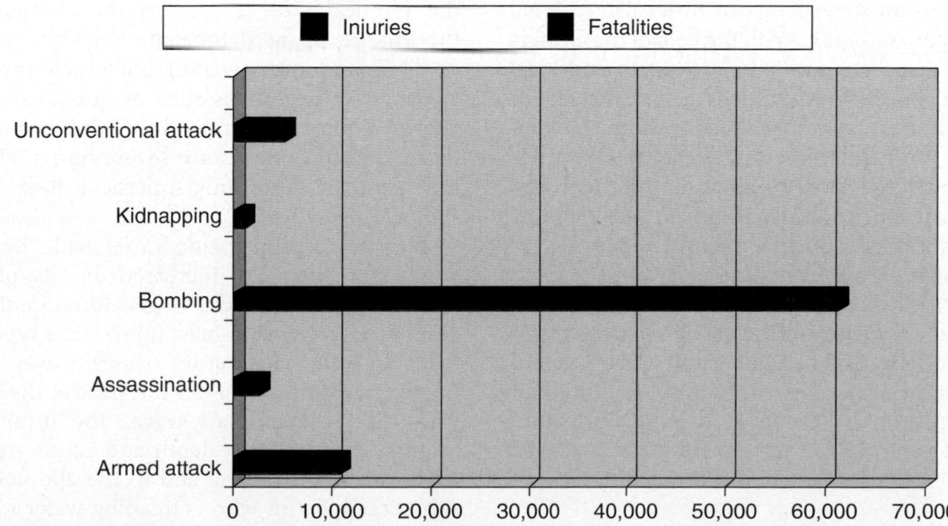

Figure 12-2. Injuries and fatalities from terrorist incidents, 1998 to 2005. Data from the RAND-MIPT Terrorism Incident Database show that bomb blast injuries account for 82% of all injuries caused by terrorists. *(Available at* www.tkb.org/incidenttacticmodule.jsp. *Accessed January 16, 2007; now defunct.)*

Nuclear and Radiologic Events

Nuclear or radiologic material may be dispersed by a detonation of a nuclear device, sabotage or meltdown of a nuclear reactor, explosion of a "dirty bomb," or a nonexplosive release of radioactive material in a public place. In approaching ionizing radiation exposure, the critical variables are time, distance, and shielding. In these situations, irradiated casualties are not radioactive themselves. Therefore, emergency trauma care may commence with life- and limb-threatening injuries being addressed without delay for radiologic decontamination. About 85% to 90% of external radiologic contamination is easily removed simply by removal of clothing.[15] Skin forms a useful protective barrier, and any decontamination technique that could traumatize the skin should be avoided. However, if open wounds are contaminated, routine débridement and delayed closure is the rule. Radioactive debris should always be removed with instruments, and the surgery may be facilitated by the use of personal dosimeters.[16] After radiation exposure has been verified, the radionuclides involved, amounts, and physical forms must be determined. It is important to be able to assess patients for exposure through the use of radiological detection devices. Without the ability to properly scan for contamination, there is no other alternative than to carry out full decontamination procedures as if they are contaminated.

The time to onset of systemic symptoms is the most important factor in determining whether significant radiation exposure has taken place. Initial symptoms include nausea, vomiting, diarrhea, skin tingling, and central nervous system (CNS) signs. If there are injuries requiring surgery, the procedures are best performed in the initial 48 hours, before exposure-induced bone marrow suppression occurs. If victims remain asymptomatic for 24 hours and show no aberration in complete blood count, particularly the lymphocyte count, they can be safely discharged.[17]

Biological Events

One of the greatest challenges of biological terrorism is the timely identification of its use. As opposed to the overt nature of explosives, biologic weaponry can be deployed covertly without immediate effects to those exposed. Instead, identification may require syndromic surveillance using local or regional health data to identify an outbreak. With the help of the Centers for Disease Control and Prevention (CDC), state and local organizations can collaborate to minimize the time needed for the detection and identification of the pathogen. Rapid biological event recognition is critical to prevent the secondary exposure of the population at large. Monitored system-level activities include school absenteeism, 911 calls, trends in sales of over-the-counter pharmaceuticals, and voluntary reporting by medical groups of apparent trends of illnesses.

The CDC has divided biological threats into groups A, B, and C. The categories are based on the ease of disease transmission, potential mortality and societal health impact, potential for inducing panic and social disruption, and the need for a specialized health response.[18] Category A sample of pathogens with the highest potential for being weaponized are listed in Table 12-1.[13,18-24]

Chemical Events

The use of sarin gas in the Tokyo subway in 1995 demonstrates the potential impact of a chemical attack. The attack, which resulted in the exposure of a number of health care providers to the neurotoxin, reinforces the importance of hospitals taking aggressive measures to preserve and protect their health care facility and resources. The most commonly used chemical agents have traditionally been pulmonary toxins with popularity among terrorists owing to their ready availability, ease of dispersal, significant clinical effects, and proven ability to disrupt and contaminate initial caregivers.

Chemical agents are categorized by their physiologic effects. The five general classes of chemical agents are nerve, blood, pulmonary, blistering (vesicants), and riot control agents. Table 12-2 summarizes the toxicity, mechanisms, clinical signs, and exposure management of common agents.[25-31]

Blast Events

Bomb detonation is the rapid chemical transformation of a solid or liquid into a gas. The gas expands radially outward as a high-pressure blast wave that exceeds the speed of sound. Air is highly compressed on the leading edge of the blast wave, creating a shock front. The body of the wave and the associated mass outward movement of ambient air (the "blast wind") follow this front (Fig. 12-3).

Under ideal conditions in an open area, the "overpressure" that results from an explosion generally follows a well-defined pressure–time curve ("Friedlander wave"). There is an initial, near-instantaneous spike in the ambient air pressure followed by a longer period of subatmospheric pressure (Fig. 12-4). The pressure–time curves are variable depending on the local topography and the presence of walls and other solid objects. The blast wave can reflect off and flow around solid surfaces. These reflected waves can be magnified by eight to nine times, causing significantly greater injury.[32,33] Blasts that occur within buildings, vehicles, or other confined spaces are more devastating and lethal because of this increased energy and slower dissipation of the complex and reflected waves.[34] The distance from the explosion's epicenter also is important because the pressure wave decays roughly proportionally to the inverse cube of the distance.[32,35]

The velocity, duration, and magnitude of the blast wave's overpressure are dependent on several factors. These include the physical size as well as the component explosive of the charge being detonated. High-energy explosives such as TNT and nitroglycerin are much more powerful than lower order explosives such as gunpowder. However, lower energy explosives can produce conflagrations with a higher thermal output that cause severe burns. High-energy explosives tend to cause only superficial flash burns on exposed skin[32] (Table 12-3).

Blast wave propagation varies with the medium through which it moves. The increased density of water allows for faster propagation and a longer duration of positive pressure. Therefore, immersion blast injuries are typically more severe. After in-water detonation, shock waves are also reflected backward off the water–air interface at the surface and admix with the incident blast wave. The resultant overpressures are greater at the 2-ft depth and cause greater injury to the lower areas of the lung and to the abdomen in the partially submerged victim who is treading water in the vertical position. A high index of suspicion should be maintained for delayed presentations of bowel injury in those injured by underwater blasts.[36]

TABLE 12-1 *POTENTIAL AGENTS OF BIOLOGICAL TERRORISM*

Agent	Route of Infection	Clinical Signs and Symptoms	Management of Exposure and Treatment
Anthrax: *Bacillus anthracis*	1. Inhalation of spores, most likely in a bioterrorism incident 2. Cutaneous 3. Gastrointestinal	1. Fever, flulike symptoms, chest discomfort in 2–42 days, severe respiratory distress 2–3 days later, death 24–36 hours later; >50% mortality 2. Black scab, dermal and lymph node involvement 3. Nausea, vomiting; abdominal pain progresses to bloody diarrhea and sepsis	Airborne precautions, decontamination of surfaces; wash exposed skin Penicillin The CDC recommends initial therapy with doxycycline or ciprofloxacin
Botulism: *Clostridium botulinum*	Foodborne illness and wound infection 1 g of botulinum toxin will kill 1 million people	Symptoms begin to show in 6–7 days from impaired acetylcholine release, resulting in cranial nerve deficits, descending skeletal musculature weakness, and paralysis	Standard precautions Ventilator support for weeks or months until patient clinically improves Trivalent equine antitoxin is available from the CDC
Viral hemorrhagic fevers: RNA viruses	Highly infectious by aerosol route from animal bites, excrement, insect vectors, and human to human	Fever, myalgias, prostration within 4–21 days, progressing to systemic inflammatory response, petechiae, bleeding, subsequent shock, and death; >50% mortality rate	Airborne and body fluids precautions Negative-pressure rooms Treatment is supportive No specific therapy
Plague: *Yersinia pestis*	Bubonic plague spread from fleas on rodents to humans Pneumonic plague spread by aerosol route from human to human	Bubonic plague, local inflammatory response at flea bite, swollen lymph nodes (buboes) in 1–3 days; if untreated, can progress to pneumonic plague Pneumonic plague, cough, fever, watery sputum, bronchopneumonia; if untreated, 100% mortality rate	Airborne and body fluids precautions Treatment is supportive Antibiotics: streptomycin, combinations of gentamicin and chloramphenicol or doxycycline and fluoroquinolone Vaccine for bubonic plague
Smallpox: variola virus	Highly infectious by aerosol route from human to human	Fever, rigors, headache, back pain, malaise in 7–17 days; vesicular and pustular rash leads to scabs and pitted scars; death occurs as a result of toxemia from viral infection	Smallpox vaccination in first week following exposure Immediate vaccination for caregivers Treatment is supportive
Tularemia: *Francisella tularensis*	Human infection from ticks, deerfly bites, contaminated animal products Inhalation from infectious aerosols	Ulceroglandular tularemia, fever, chills, headache, malaise, skin ulceration, painful adenopathy Typhoidal tularemia and pneumonic tularemia result from inhalation; symptoms include nonproductive cough and pneumonia	Standard precautions Antibiotic: gentamicin

CDC, Centers for Disease Control and Prevention.

BLAST INJURY PATHOPHYSIOLOGY

Classically, the mechanisms of injury from blast have been classified as primary, secondary, and tertiary. Quaternary, or miscellaneous, forms of injury indirectly related to the blast are now also recognized.

Primary Blast Injury

Primary blast injury (PBI) results from the high-pressure shock front and associated blast wave. Blast waves propagate through the body as stress, shock, and shear waves.[37] Stress waves are similar in speed to sound waves but have higher amplitude. Shock waves have a higher pressure and amplitude than sound waves. Shear waves are lower in velocity and longer in duration and travel in a transverse direction, producing gross distortions of tissue and organs. PBI occurs as the shock front and blast wave move through the body. The severity of injury depends on the overpressure to the bodily organs (Table 12-4). Density differences in the body's anatomic components (particularly at gas–fluid interfaces) render those components susceptible to spalling, implosion, inertial mismatches, and pressure differentials. Spalling is the forcible, explosive movement of fluid from more dense to less dense tissues such as in the lungs. Implosion relates to areas of gas that are rapidly compressed at the time of shock front impact and then rapidly reexpand after it passes, causing rebound expansion with attendant shearing and injury. Acceleration/deceleration can cause tearing of organ pedicles and mesentery when there is an inertial difference between organ structures. Unappreciated blast shock wave–related internal injuries may cause a patient to be undertriaged by prehospital responders.

TABLE 12-2 *POTENTIAL AGENTS OF CHEMICAL TERRORISM*

Agent	Toxicity and Mechanism	Clinical Signs and Symptoms	Management of Exposure and Treatment
Nerve agents GA (sarin) GV (soman) GD (cyclosarin) GS VX	Organophosphates Fatal at 1–10 mL (GA, GV, GD) or 1 drop of VX on skin Blocks acetylcholine esterase	Cholinergic crisis: salivation, lacrimation, urination, diaphoresis, GI distress, emesis Bronchorrhea: excessive airway secretions Bronchoconstriction causing respiratory distress Death from paralysis of diaphragm and respiratory muscles, essential apnea	Decontamination Respiratory support Antidotes: Atropine—anticholinergic Oxime—2-PAM-Cl reactivates acetylcholine esterase Diazepam—anticonvulsant
Blood agents Hydrogen cyanide Cyanogen chloride	Absorption Inhalation (most toxic) Ingestion Percutaneous Concentration dependent Combines with iron to inhibit cytochrome oxidase pathway	Dyspnea, tachypnea, hypertension, tachycardia, flushing (cherry red skin), vomiting, confusion, agitation, cardiac palpitation, bitter almond odor on victim Progress to arrhythmias, respiratory failure Death from inhalation within 6–8 minutes from respiratory arrest Sodium nitrate (intravenous)	Remove from exposure Antidotes: inhalation of crushed pearl of amyl nitrite (in the field)
Pulmonary agents Chlorine Phosgene	Chlorine: irritating, pungent yellow-green gas, caustic, reacts with water to form hypochlorite and hydrochloric acid Pulmonary edema, hypoxemia, respiratory failure may result Phosgene: odor of fresh-cut hay; less soluble in water, reacts over time in distal respiratory tree	Chlorine: cutaneous burning, ocular injury, respiratory irritation Phosgene: monitor at least 12–24 hours, management is expectant Phosgene: minor upper respiratory irritation, over time severe pulmonary edema and respiratory failure	Chlorine: remove from exposure, respiratory support, no antidote
Blistering agents and vesicants Mustard agents Lewisite	Mustard agents: oily, garlic-onion odor Both: exposure dependent Both cutaneous, ocular, respiratory damage Lewisite: vapor or liquid, geranium odor Lewisite: increased tissue permeability, hypovolemic shock, organ damage	Both: skin erythema, vesicles, ocular burning, respiratory eruption, potential bronchial damage, necrosis, hemorrhage Decontamination If prolonged, pancytopenia, inability to fight infection, death from respiratory failure Lewisite: immediate pain, prone to tissue necrosis, sloughing, airway obstruction Lewisite: British antilewisite skin, ophthalmic ointments	Remove from exposure Respiratory management Débride cutaneous lesions
Riot control agents	Lacrimators ("tear gas"), irritants, vomiting agents	Lacrimation, sneezing, rapid heart rate, respiratory insufficiency	Supportive, self-limiting, resolving within 15 min

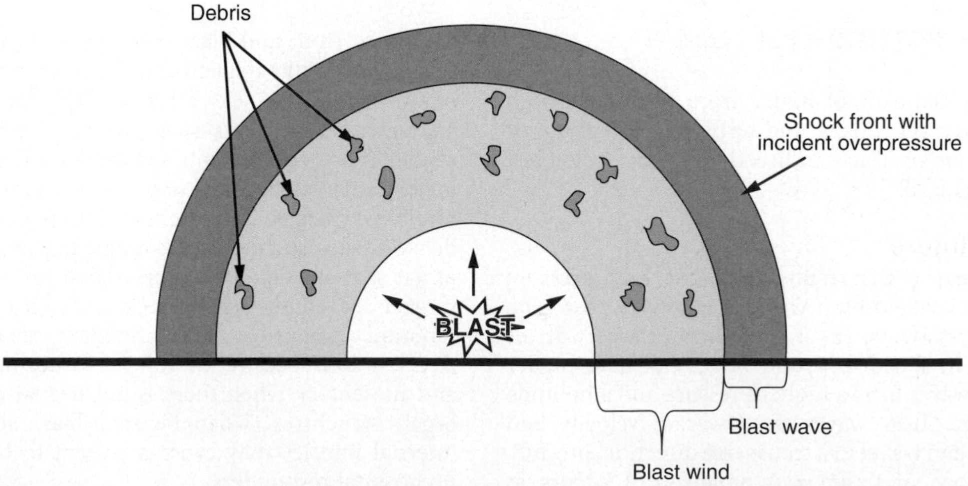

Figure 12-3. Diagram of a blast wave and associated components. *(Adapted from Hull JB: Blast: injury patterns and their recording, J Audiov Media Med 15:121–127, 1992.)*

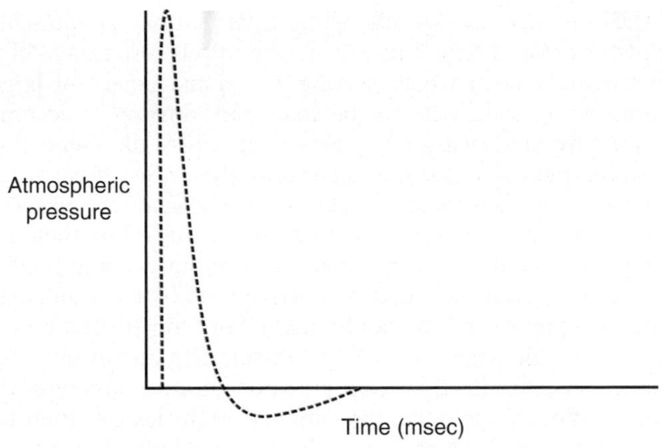

Figure 12-4. Diagram of a blast wave form.

TABLE 12-4 *VICTIM GROUPS ACCORDING TO BLAST LOADING*		
Group	**Overpressure (kPa)**	**Blast Loading**
1	<150	Minor: maximum overpressure sustained sufficient to cause ruptured tympanic membrane
2	150–350	Moderate: higher overpressure than group 1, but probably insufficient to cause primary lung damage in a significant number of casualties
3	350–550	Severe: sufficient overpressure to cause primary lung damage in a significant proportion of casualties
4	>550	Very severe: sufficient overpressure to cause severe primary lung damage with a significant incidence of death

Source: Mellor SG, Cooper GJ: Analysis of 828 servicemen killed or injured by explosion in Northern Ireland 1970–1984: the hostile action casualty system, Br J Surg 76:1006–1010, 1989.

The most susceptible organs to PBI are the ears, lungs, and gastrointestinal tract. The ears are the most sensitive organs to blast injury, and tympanic membrane rupture can be used as a marker of exposure to significant overpressure.[38,39] Tympanic injury may occur preferentially based on the orientation of the ear relative to the blast.

With enough energy exposure, severe pulmonary barotrauma can occur with disruption of the capillary–alveolar interface. Low-velocity stress waves may be the primary source of lung injury as they are reinforced by reflection off of the mediastinum. The ensuing complex pressure environment within the lung parenchyma promotes disruption of the alveolar–capillary membrane with the leakage of blood and interstitial fluid.[37,40] Emphysematous spaces can be created in addition to pneumothorax. The interstitial changes of blast lung can lead to acute respiratory distress syndrome (ARDS). Blast lung remains a common cause of fatality among initial survivors of the detonation.[40] In rare cases, air embolism of the vascular tree is thought to be the cause of sudden death.[41,42] Primary blast lung injury does not appear to stem from direct compression of the thorax but rather from coupling of the shock front into the lung tissue.[43]

As a gas-filled organ, the gastrointestinal tract is highly susceptible to primary blast effect. Injury to the mucosa may range from bruising and petechiae to frank hemorrhage and mesenteric shear injury caused by acceleration/deceleration. Solid organ laceration or rupture of the liver, spleen, and kidney in addition to late bowel perforation can also occur.[40] In the large bowel, shearing rather than stress wave propagation may be the primary mechanism of injury because the large bowel is not able to dislocate to the same degree as the small intestine.

TABLE 12-3 *EXPLOSIVE TYPES*	
High-Energy Explosive	**Low-Energy Explosive**
TNT	Pipe bomb
C-4	Gunpowder
Semtex	Pure petroleum-based bomb
Nitroglycerin	"Molotov cocktail"
Dynamite	
Ammonium nitrate fuel oil	

Other organ systems (musculoskeletal, ocular, and cardiocirculatory) have varying degrees of response to injury from primary blast.[32,44] There also is evidence that blast can lead to primary CNS injury. A variety of irregular brain wave activities may be noted by electroencephalography, including hypersynchronous, discontinuous, or irregular brain activity with increased theta activity consistent with cortical dysfunction within the first 3 days. With the variety of effects on the CNS, long-term changes may manifest as posttraumatic stress disorder (PTSD), so the term *shell shocked* may have a physiologic basis.[45]

Traumatic amputations from PBI are uncommon and are often considered a marker for a lethal injury. Blast-induced amputations primarily occur through the shaft rather than as disarticulations. Evidence suggests that these are the result of direct coupling of the blast wave into the tissues. Fracture results from axial stress to the long bone. Flailing of the extremity from the blast wind gas flow completes the amputation.[32,36]

Secondary Blast Injury

Secondary blast injury results from missiles propagated by the explosion. *Primary fragmentation* can be part of the bomb casing itself or objects intentionally imbedded into the explosive such as nails, screws, or bolts designed to inflict further wounding. Nearby objects made airborne by proximity to the explosion can become projectiles *(secondary fragmentation).* Injury from glass is the most common. If there is an expectation that a blast included radiologic materials, the imbedded shrapnel should be treated as such and proper precautions taken to minimize exposure. Without an assessment from the scene or the ED, this could go unnoticed and create additional exposure that is avoidable.

Tertiary and Quaternary Blast Injury

Tertiary blast injury stems from the victim's body being thrown as a projectile by the blast. This can result in fractures, head trauma, and other blunt injury typically seen in the survivor population. Secondary and tertiary blast injuries are the most common wounding mechanisms seen in survivors of explosive events.[36]

Quaternary blast injury represents miscellaneous blast-related injuries. These include those from structural collapse or burn secondary to the detonation. Crush, traumatic amputation, compartment syndromes, and other blunt and penetrating injuries are common sequelae of structural collapse related to the blast. Secondary fires can cause additional burns as well as smoke and dust inhalation. Victims may also be exposed to irradiation as well as toxic gas and other chemical and biologic pathogens by a "dirty bomb."

MEDICAL MANAGEMENT OF DISASTER CASUALTIES

Triage—Concept and Principles

Triage is the prioritization of patients according to injury severity and the need for immediate care. This is a familiar concept but is not often practiced given the abundance of health care resources. Triage becomes vitally important in the face of a true mass casualty event. Triage is effective only to the extent that the triage officer has a firm understanding of the nature of the injuries likely to be seen (i.e., bodily injury; biological, chemical, radiation injury), as well as comprehensive training in the unique principles of mass casualty management with limited resources. It is this knowledge base and background that determine the proper triage officer rather than a particular title. Surgeons, emergency medicine physicians, nurses, prehospital personnel, and other acute care providers all can potentially learn the skills to function in such a role. Each may possess a skill set ideal for evaluating victims of a particular disaster.

There are five widely accepted triage categories for casualties: (1) *immediate,* or the most severely injured who require urgent, lifesaving treatment; (2) *delayed,* or those who require medical treatment but are not as time sensitive; (3) *minimal,* those with minor injuries who would survive even without medical intervention (4) *expectant,* those whose extensive injuries would require time and significant resource utilization and where elevated care requirements would jeopardize the lives of many more salvageable casualties; and (5) *dead.* The acronym "ID-MED" is often used to help with remembering these. It is the approach to the expectant category that differs most markedly from that of routine medical care in developed countries. These victims, although potentially salvageable, may not receive care in the interest of applying the limited resources to an entire group of more salvageable casualties, thereby ensuring maximum preservation of lives. This runs counter to the usual civilian emergency care paradigm in which the most severely injured survivors would be selected early for immediate and exhaustive care. The definition of an expectant injury will differ with each event and should be determined early in the course of casualty management according to the victim load and anticipated resources available. When casualty influx has ceased, these expectant casualties can be reassessed in the light of remaining resources and possibly cared for at that time.[46,47]

There are numerous mass casualty triage systems in use today. One of the more widely accepted methodologies is SALT or sort, assess, lifesaving interventions, treatment/transport (Fig. 12-5). This acronym reminds responders of a systematic way in which sorting and management of large numbers of casualties can be managed. Sorting is accomplished by first seeing who can get up and walk. Generally, their injuries are minor and can be passed over. Self-evacuation is encouraged. The second level is those who can wave or make purposeful movements. The first two groups can then be assessed after those who remain still or have obvious life-threatening issues such as hemorrhage or blocked airways. Lifesaving interventions can be carried out for this last group such as hemorrhage control (e.g., tourniquet), airway opening maneuvers, needle thoracotomy, and autoinjection of antidotes. After this is done, casualties in each tier can then be reevaluated and placed into dead, expectant, immediate, delayed, or minimal categories.

The Challenge of Individual Triage

In a MCI, triage decisions must be made rapidly and aim to deliver the greatest good for the greatest number. The patterns and severity of injury produced by previous disasters serve as reference for future mass casualty events. Terrorist bombings are by far the most commonly documented mass casualty events and serve as a useful model for the practice of triage. The immediate death rate tends to be quite high, ranging from 50% to 99%. Critical injuries occur in only 5% to 25% of survivors, but late deaths among survivors generally occur in this severely injured group. The most commonly injured body systems in survivors of bombings are soft tissue and musculoskeletal, most of which are not critical and not life threatening. Most deaths among initial survivors are secondary to head, abdomen, and chest trauma. Nineteen percent of all survivors with abdominal trauma, 14% of all survivors with chest trauma, and 10% of all survivors with traumatic amputation or blast lung injury ultimately die, representing the body system injuries with the highest specific mortality rates among survivors. However, these body system injuries are found in only a small (2%–5%) percentage of all survivors because most victims with these injuries die immediately.[48] The minority of survivors with these injuries must be recognized early as having a high risk of death and be urgently attended. They often require prolonged intensive care unit (ICU) stays and significant resource utilization.

Efforts are ongoing to develop methods to improve the accuracy of field triage and optimize health care resource utilization after mass casualty disasters caused by explosions. Studies of soldiers in Iraq have demonstrated that the presence of two or more variables (sustained hypotension, three or more long bone fractures, penetrating head injury, and other fatalities sustained in the blast) is associated with increased mortality (86% vs. 20% for a single marker alone; $P = 0.015$).[49] Similarly, in 798 victims of bombings in Israel, significant associations ($P < 0.001$) with the development of blast lung were found between penetrating wounds to the head or torso, burns greater than 10% of the body surface area, and skull fractures.[50] Victims in fully confined spaces such as buses were also more likely to sustain blast lung effects. These findings are important because they provide rapid ways to identify patients who will likely require more intensive monitoring and resuscitative efforts even before the clinical manifestations of pulmonary compromise are apparent.

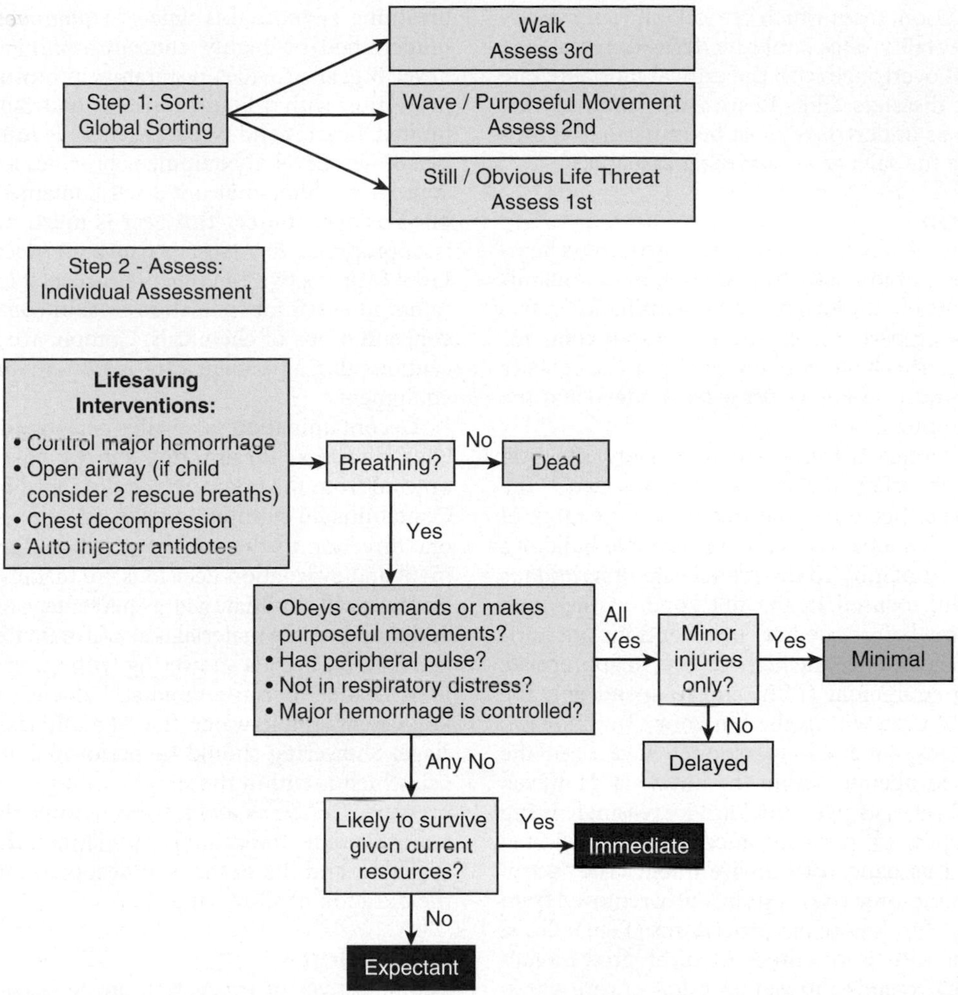

Figure 12-5. SALT mass casualty triage algorithm (sort, assess, lifesaving interventions, treatment/transport). *(Adapted from SALT mass casualty triage: concept endorsed by the American College of Emergency Physicians, American College of Surgeons Committee on Trauma, American Trauma Society, National Association of EMS Physicians, National Disaster Life Support Education Consortium, and State and Territorial Injury Prevention Directors Association, Disaster Med Public Health Prep 2(4):245–246, 2008.* www.chemm.nlm.nih.gov/salttriage.htm. *Accessed May 15, 2013.)*

Global Triage Accuracy

The accuracy of triage has a major impact on casualty outcome. *Undertriage* is the assignment of critically injured casualties needing immediate care to a delayed category. This may lead to unnecessary deaths. It can be avoided by the proper training of triage officers to recognize life-threatening problems requiring urgent treatment. *Overtriage* is the assignment to immediate care, hospitalization, or evacuation of casualties who are not critically injured, thus potentially displacing critically injured victims from necessary immediate care. In the routine practice of medicine, only errors in undertriage risks patients' well-being, so that overtriage (or erring on transporting seemingly less injured patients to hospitals to prevent missing a critical injury) is fully accepted.[51] However, in a true mass casualty disaster, overtriage is as life threatening as undertriage. The inundation by large numbers of noncritically injured patients into a system of scarce medical resources may prevent the timely detection of that small minority who need immediate care. To quantify this notion, computer modeling of a 700-bed level 1 trauma center (Ben Taub General Hospital) was challenged with the profiles of 223 urban bombing victims.[52] The analysis suggests that the global level of care suffers as the critical casualty load increases. There is a point at which the facility becomes less efficient and less able to provide care as patients continue to pile up. *Surge capacity* refers to the ability of a facility to rapidly expand its patient load capacity in response to a major public health crisis and overwhelming number of patients. For this model, a surge capacity of 4.6 critical care patients per hour using present resources was decreased to 3.8 and 2.7 patients per hour when overtriage rates of 50% and 75% were trialed. Avoidance of this situation requires extensive training of triage officers. Triage accuracy—the minimizing of both undertriage and overtriage—is thus a major prognostic factor in the medical management of all disasters.[1,48]

The *critical mortality rate* is the death rate among initial survivors expressed as a percentage of the total number of *critically injured* survivors, rather than being based on the total number of survivors, most of whom are not at risk of death.[1] The medical management of a disaster and the success of triage are best assessed by looking at critical, rather than overall, mortality, and this also allows the most accurate comparison of medical outcomes between different disasters. An analysis of 1880 survivors of 10 terrorist bombing incidents treated at one institution, from which critical injuries, overtriage, and critical mortality rates could be derived, reveals the direct correlation of overtriage with the critical mortality rate in major bombing disasters (Fig. 12-6). This confirms that overtriage as much as undertriage must be minimized in this setting to maximize the salvage of surviving casualties.[1]

Decontamination

During any mass casualty event that releases dangerous chemicals, biologic agents, or radioactivity, planning for decontamination becomes critically important. Decontamination refers to physically removing particulate, liquid, or vapor contamination from victims. This halts ongoing injury to the casualty and prevents exposure to other victims, responders, and the surrounding environment.

The concept of zones within such a casualty situation defines gradations in safety for victims and rescuers.[4] The most dangerous is the "hot zone," the area within the range of immediate danger. This area may contain unstable buildings or be in immediate proximity to the release site of hazardous materials. Efforts are focused in the hot zone on the rapid evacuation of victims before medical interventions are initiated. Responders need to have the highest level of appropriate personal protective equipment (PPE) and to spend only the necessary amount of time within the hot zone. Traditionally, HAZMAT (hazardous materials) personnel have been the responders trained to operate within the hot zone. However, emergency medical services personnel are increasingly being trained and equipped to perform medically complicated extractions within this dangerous environment. The "warm zone," although posing some risk, is sufficiently removed from the scene to allow for lifesaving procedures. Generally, a reduced amount of PPE is required. Medical professionals such as orthopaedic surgeons almost never deliver care within hot or warm zones. The "cold zone" does not pose a direct threat and is considered appropriate for providing basic medical care.

Four levels of PPE are defined by the Occupational Safety and Health Administration.[53] Level A, although being the most protective, is bulky and permits only gross motor function when in use. It includes a disposable, full-body suit, completely impervious, with a self-contained positive-pressure breathing system. This type of equipment is used for facing unidentified or highly concentrated hazardous substances. Level B gear provides respiratory protection but less surface protection with a liquid-resistant body suit. Dexterity is still limited. Level A and B gear is generally restricted to HAZMAT personnel. Level C equipment provides a respirator with the appropriate filters but not a self-contained or externally supplied oxygen source. This gear is much more functional and is appropriate for most warm zone decontamination sites. Level D protective equipment is acceptable when there is little to no potential for inhalation or skin contact with hazardous concentrations of chemicals. Compliance with universal precautions during patient care is not compromised by level D equipment.

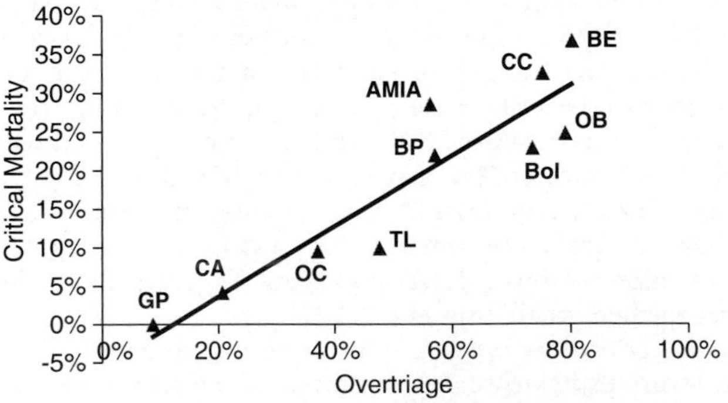

Figure 12-6. Graphic relationship between overtriage rate and critical mortality rate in 10 major terrorist bombing incidents. Linear correlation coefficient (r) = 0.92. *AMIA,* Buenos Aires; *BE,* Beirut; *Bol,* Bologna; *BP,* Birmingham pubs; *CA,* Craigavon; *CC,* Cu Chi; *GP,* Guildford pubs; *OB,* Old Bailey; *OC,* Oklahoma City; *TL,* Tower of London. *(Reprinted with permission from Frykberg, E.R. Medical management of disasters and mass casualties from terrorist bombings: how can we cope? J Trauma 53:201–212, 2002.)*

Decontamination is usually performed in the warm zone after disasters. Ideally, this should be situated uphill and upwind from the hot zone and distanced by at least 300 yards. Contaminated clothing is removed, and victims are moved in one direction to the cold zone, where further medical treatment and evacuation decisions are made. Although removing clothing will eliminate a large percentage of contaminants, any additional visible material is also atraumatically removed from the skin.[31] Copious showering with water further dilutes any toxic residue. Because rapid and efficient decontamination is key, use of simple water, free of additives, is preferred at this stage. Showering should be performed at a minimum of 60 psi, which is within the standard range for household shower pressure. Concerns about hypothermia, the specific contaminants present, the number of victims, the amount of water available, and the number of decontamination stations affect the duration of showering.

Evacuation

The objectives of evacuation are to decompress the disaster area, to improve care for the most critical casualties, and to provide specialized care to specific casualties, such as those with burns and crush injuries. "Decompressing" the disaster scene means that critically ill casualties who are consuming the most resources (supplies, casualty care space, caregiver attention) are moved to relatively resource-rich areas. Evacuation of seriously injured casualties can be made to offsite medical facilities. These can include Alternate Care Sites established by advanced hospital planning or to a facility established and operated by the Disaster Medical Assistance Teams (DMAT).[4,54,55]

In any mass casualty event, self-presenters to hospitals can be as high as 50%. For victims who are to otherwise be systematically transported by response teams, consideration should be given to the surrounding medical facilities and their respective assets. The most common tendency is to deliver a preponderance of casualties to the geographically nearest hospital. This *geographic effect* overburdens that single facility and may force providers to ration medical care at a time when other local hospitals' resources are being underutilized. To minimize this mismanagement and its associated potential morbidity and mortality, some recommend using the nearest hospital as a triage center. This would still allow for rapid evacuation of casualties from the scene but charges the nearest hospital with distributing survivors needing significant care to surrounding facilities. Conversely, extremely well-organized prehospital efforts can be made to transport equitable numbers of casualties to accepting institutions through established systems that continually monitor hospital capacities and patient tracking systems. These systems are designed to track patients from the field, through their transport to the ultimate receiving facility and provide the necessary manifests to locate these patients for follow-up by law enforcement and for critical family reunification.

The primary modes of evacuation are ground, rotary-wing aircraft, and small and large fixed-wing aircraft. Ground evacuation, although available, is inefficient; only a small number of casualties can be evacuated at once. Rotary-wing aircraft and small fixed-wing aircraft are costly and similarly inefficient in the small number of casualties evacuated. They may be better used in the disaster area for other purposes.[56] Large fixed-wing aircraft are very costly but are more efficient in allowing medical crew to manage complex multiple casualties over long distance. Large fixed-wing aircraft provide the possibility of retrograde airlift; that is, they may be used to bring in supplies to the disaster area and to evacuate casualties as they return for more supplies.[4,54]

Evacuated patients on a long-range flight are subject to stresses from the hypobaric environment—decreased partial pressure of oxygen, turbulence, vibration, temperature control, and humidity. Clinical preparation should include a systematic review of the stresses of flight and how they will apply to each casualty.[4,54-56] Consideration needs to be given to how to best address oxygen therapy, mechanical ventilation, trapped gas, decompression sickness or arterial gas embolism, casts, abdominal damage control surgery, burns, and infection control.

Oxygen supply is critical. Supplemental oxygen can be given to patients with known hypoxemia, dyspnea, and anemia. For mechanical ventilation, steps must be taken to reduce the risk of tracheal injury or endotracheal tube cuff rupture from expansion of the cuff at altitude. The air can be removed from the cuff and replaced by normal saline solution with sufficient pressure to eliminate leakage around the cuff. If the medical crew is equipped with a cuff manometer, this could be used with an air-filled cuff to monitor and adjust cuff pressure during ascent and descent.

In general, all trapped gas within the body should be evacuated before long-range evacuation by air to eliminate the risk of tissue damage from gas expansion. For pneumothorax, a functioning chest tube should be in place with a Heimlich valve in line, in case the pleural drainage unit must be disconnected for emergency exit. Recent abdominal surgery is not a contraindication to air transport, but if the casualty has an ileus, a functioning nasogastric tube must be secured and attached to suction. Obstructed middle ear and paranasal sinuses can be assessed by the casualty's response to the Valsalva maneuver. If obstruction is present, it can generally be managed by application of a topical vasoconstrictor such as oxymetazoline. Patients with decompression sickness or arterial gas embolism should not be exposed to altitudes greater than that of the origination airfield.

Patients with casts are prone to edema formation on exposure to altitude, and this risk increases with damaged tissue and reduced plasma oncotic pressure. This edema can lead to compartment syndrome inside the cast. Casts that have been in place for less than 48 to 72 hours should be bivalved before evacuation and held closed with elastic dressings if this can be done without compromising fracture stability. If this cannot be done safely, it is imperative to follow the neurovascular status of the limb closely and to be prepared to open the cast in-flight if compartment syndrome develops.[4,55]

Abdominal damage control surgery places casualties at risk for abdominal compartment syndrome with continued volume resuscitation and as edema worsens on altitude exposure. The medical crew must be prepared to monitor abdominal compartment pressures and open the abdomen if this syndrome develops. If this is not practical, patients should be transported with their abdomen open.[4,54]

Burns place patients at risk for several flight stresses, including impaired thermoregulation, increased insensible fluid loss, and difficult infection control. Blankets, sleeping bags, heat conserving dressings, or active warming devices should be used to prevent hypothermia. Wounds should be dressed immediately preflight and not undressed in flight if at all possible to reduce the risk of environmental contamination. Strong consideration should be given to performing endotracheal intubation preflight in patients with significant inhalation injury. It is difficult to monitor the airway and to perform in-flight intubation.[4,55]

Infection control is a special challenge during air evacuation. Patients with known or suspected infections requiring respiratory isolation should not be transported by air unless essential.

In all cases of medical evacuation, attention should be paid to accurate record keeping. The use of clear, concise notations and standard forms is important to prevent duplication of initial assessment efforts. Records should remain with victims at all times and provide a key tool for enhancing casualty flow in receiving institutions.

Evacuation and Echelons

Because disasters can overwhelm local medical resources, a plan for orderly movement and evacuation of patients can assist in the treatment of casualties, especially those with complex problems. Experience in Haiti and other disasters has shown that a tiered or echeloned system of care modeled on that used by the military can provide high care when the medical infrastructure has been incapacitated.

The military medical mission has evolved to provide a highly mobile and effective platform that not only has treated service members in time of conflict but has also assisted in recent international disasters. Military medical units from a number of countries were important in Haiti and other disasters. The systems that have produced unprecedented survival of war casualties have assisted in establishing medical systems and patient transport during disasters. Although the employment of military units in disasters will not exactly mimic the wartime setup, the following overview provides an understanding of concepts useful in large disasters and the evolving military-civilian cooperation in disaster care. The military medical treatment algorithm pyramid is composed of five levels, or "echelons," of care for wounded service members. Each succeeding echelon is farther away from the forward battle area and has more advanced capabilities than the previous one. Higher echelons of care possess equal treatment capabilities as those preceding it but also add new ones along the evacuation route.[57,58] Whereas minor injuries can be treated at a low echelon and personnel returned to duty, more significant wounds and those requiring longer periods of rehabilitation are evacuated to higher levels of care and potentially out of theater. The medical evacuation system coordinates available medical resources to provide injured personnel with timely and effective treatment given the geographic, security, and logistic constraints within an echelon. Entry into the medical treatment and evacuation system begins with basic first aid at the point of wounding (echelon I) and may follow with early stabilization, rapid evacuation, and critical care transport. The terminus may be definitive care provided at hospitals located in the continental United States (echelon V). In the current conflict, the goal for casualty evacuation from echelon I to II is 60 minutes, from echelon II to III is 24 hours, and echelon III to IV is 48 to 72 hours.

Echelon I

Combat casualty care begins at the unit level at the point of initial injury within the combat zone. First responders include fellow service members and service-specific medics or corpsmen if available. Self-aid and "buddy" aid is typically the first medical intervention for the wounded. Cardiopulmonary resuscitation skills, tourniquet application, shock prevention, intravenous infusion, splinting of fractures, initial care of wounds and burns, and transport of the wounded are outlined in the Soldiers Manual of Common Tasks, Level 1.[59,60] The skills necessary for self-aid and buddy care are trained at the unit level and are required before deployment to a combat zone. Level 1 echelon may include an aid station, and treatment may include restoration of the airway by a surgical procedure, use of intravenous fluids and antibiotics, and the application of splints and bandages. Patients may be either returned to duty or transported to a higher echelon of care.[59] Providers at the echelon I level may include combat medics or corpsmen, physician assistants, or even physicians based on the units involved in the operation. If the patient cannot be rapidly returned to duty, evacuation to the next echelon is at the discretion of the highest level provider. It is generally coordinated and performed by assets located at the next echelon of care. Evacuation may be to the supporting echelon II facility but may also be coordinated to the nearest echelon III facility as required by the patient's medical condition.

Echelon II

Echelon II is the first echelon at which surgical capability exists. These are supported by the Air Force, Navy, and Army forward surgical teams involved in the area of operations. These may be co-located within an Expeditionary Medical Support (Air Force EMEDS), Surgical Company (Navy), Medical Company (Army), or a ship with ORs. Additional assets may be in place such as dental, laboratory, radiography, mental health, preventive medicine, and optometry units. Care is administered by a team of physicians or physician assistants supported by appropriate medical, technical, or nursing staff. This may include basic resuscitation and stabilization as well as surgical capability, basic laboratory, limited radiography, pharmacy, and temporary holding ward facilities. Examinations and observations are in greater depth than at echelon I. Emergency procedures are applied to prevent death, loss of limb, and body functions. For patients who require more comprehensive treatment, further evacuation to a facility possessing the required treatment capability may be facilitated. This is the first echelon at which group O liquid packed red blood cells is available for transfusion.[59]

An Air Force Mobile Field Surgical Team (MFST) is a unit of the Small Portable Expeditionary Aeromedical Rapid Response (SPEARR) team (Fig. 12-7). Its five-member team consists of a general surgeon, orthopaedic surgeon, emergency medicine physician, anesthesia provider (MD or CRNA), and OR nurse or technician. It is designed to provide care for 10 major trauma patients in 48 hours, and their equipment is "man-portable" or carried by the team members. The full SPEARR team may also include a three-person Critical Care Air Transport (CCAT) team and a two-man Preventive Medicine (PM) team. The CCAT is composed of an intensive care physician (critical care, anesthesiology, or emergency medicine), and the PM team is staffed by a flight surgeon and public health officer. The complete SPEARR team is capable of 7-day operations and can provide basic primary care, postoperative care, and preventive medicine, and its equipment can be contained on a pallet-sized trailer and is not man-portable.

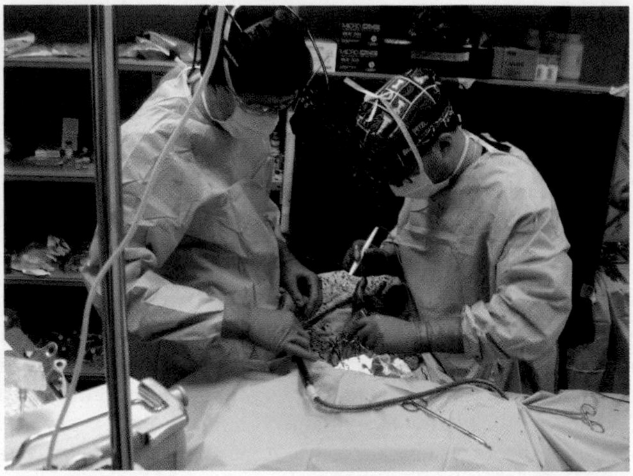

Figure 12-7. Air Force Mobile Field Surgical Team (MFST) operating in a supply closet at the American Embassy in Port-au-Prince, Haiti, January 16, 2010. *(Photo courtesy Christopher T. Born, MD.)*

The mission of the Army Forward Surgical Team (FST) is to be a rapidly deployable surgical asset for a division's forward area of operation. The FST is used in the combat zone and may be assigned one per brigade. The unit is composed of an ATLS section, OR section, and ICU section. The FST is staffed by two or three general surgeons; one or two orthopaedic surgeons; two CRNAs; an executive officer; and an officer in charge for each of the ATLS, OR, and ICU sections. The 20-member staff is completed with ATLS medics, OR technicians, and ICU LPNs. Army doctrine states that an FST is capable of providing 72 hours of emergency treatment, necessary surgery, and continuous postoperative care for 30 patients before receiving resupply. Capabilities include the ability to perform airborne and air assault insertion and the ability to maneuver with the fighting force in intrinsic vehicles. Equipment includes tents for the ATLS, OR, and ICU sections and the necessary equipment to resuscitate casualties, perform surgery, and recover postoperative patients who may require ventilator support. There is no patient holding capability within an FST.

The Navy deploys the Forward Resuscitative Surgical System (FRSS) in support of the Marine Corps. It provides one OR and two surgeons and is designed to perform resuscitative surgery for 18 patients in 48 hours before resupply. It is capable of standing alone but has no holding capability. The FRSS is frequently used with a Surgical Company, which is designed to provide surgical support for a Marine Expeditionary Force (MEF). They are normally assigned one per regiment and have a 60-bed capacity and three ORs and can hold patients for up to 72 hours.

The Navy also has ship-based echelon II capabilities. The Casualty Receiving and Treatment Ships (CRTS) are intrinsic to the Amphibious Ready Group (ARG) and contain 47 or 48 patient beds, four to six ORs, and 17 ICU beds. Troop quarters may provide up to 300 additional beds. Care is provided by Fleet Surgical Teams (FST), staffed by three or four physicians, one surgeon, one anesthesia provider, and additional support staff. Additional surgeons, to include orthopaedic and oral maxillofacial surgeons, may be assigned. Laboratory and radiography are available, and patient holding is generally limited to 3 days. CRTS may also be used in response to widespread civilian disasters such as after the earthquake in Haiti in 2010.[61]

Patients who cannot be returned to duty within 72 hours are generally evacuated to echelon III facilities. Direct transport to echelon IV is possible if the patient's condition is unlikely to allow return to duty within the echelon III evacuation policy or the medical capabilities required by the patient's condition are not available at echelon III, although this is rare.

Echelon III

Echelon III facilities offer the most advanced level of medical and surgical care within the combat zone and are geographically located in a lower level threat environment. These large hospitals are comparable to civilian trauma centers, providing triage, resuscitation, and surgical stabilization for combat casualties. This echelon's care may be the first step toward restoration of functional health compared with procedures that stabilize a condition or prolong life. It does not have the crises aspects of initial resuscitative care and can proceed with greater preparation and deliberation.[59] Although each service configures its echelon III facilities slightly differently, they all are comparably equipped and have similar capabilities. Each facility has an ED and a large patient holding capability, including postoperative care wards, inpatient wards, and ICUs. Ancillary support services include laboratory, blood bank, radiography, computed tomography (CT), pharmacy, physical therapy, and occupational therapy. Patients are either treated and returned to duty or are stabilized for further evacuation to a higher echelon of care.

The professional complement in these facilities is significant. All include general surgeons, orthopaedic surgeons, vascular surgeons, thoracic surgeons, obstetrician/gynecologists, ophthalmologists, urologists, oral surgeons, anesthesiologists, nurse anesthetists, radiologists, emergency physicians, internists, and psychiatrists or psychologists. The hospitals can be further augmented with additional specialists in fields such as neurosurgery, otolaryngology, intensive care, infectious disease, dermatology, and cardiology as necessary. Blood products available include fresh-frozen plasma; platelets; frozen group O red blood cells; and groups A, B, and O liquid cells.[59]

By doctrine, echelon III facilities are generally located far from the combat zone or near major lines of communication (harbor, airfield, large highway) to provide security for the hospital and facilitate evacuation of casualties and resupply. These facilities are designed to be mobile, but their large size requires several weeks to move, set up, and become operational. They are modular by design, allowing the medical commander to tailor the medical support to a given operation or tactical situation. Echelon III facilities may be tent hospitals or hardened facilities. Each service has units of different sizes and configurations of personnel. They involve the Air Force's Air Transportable Hospitals (ATH), the Army's Combat Support Hospital (CSH), and the Navy's Fleet Hospitals. The Navy also has two hospital ships (*USNS Mercy* and *USNS Comfort*) that can operate as an echelon III or IV facility.[62]

Before movement from echelon III to echelon IV, all patients are evaluated by an Air Force Flight Surgeon to determine stability for flight and confirm appropriate medications and treatment plans have been provided. Although electronic medical records have been developed to allow all providers within the continuum of care to access and document medical/surgical treatment provided to patients, it has been standard practice to write the surgical plan on the patient's dressing as a precautionary measure to ensure all dates and treatment plans are communicated to the next treating physician or facility.

Severely injured patients that have been stabilized are transported by Air Force Critical Care Air Transport Teams (CCATTs). These are flying ICUs composed of a critical care physician, a critical care nurse, and a respiratory therapist. The CCATT can transport critically ill casualties on ventilators, as well as continue critical care resuscitation and treatment en route to the next level of care.

Echelon IV

Echelon IV is the first level at which definitive surgical management can be provided outside the combat zone.[62] This echelon of care will provide not only Echelon III surgical capability but also further definitive therapy for patients in the recovery phase who can return to duty within the theater evacuation policy.[50] If rehabilitation and return to duty cannot be accomplished within a predetermined period of time, casualties are evacuated to an Echelon V facility.

In the current conflict, the two echelon IV facilities are Landstuhl Regional Medical Center (LRMC) and the US Military Hospital Kuwait (Navy Fleet Hospital). Virtually all of the combat-wounded casualties and severe nonhostile action–injured patients are evacuated to LRMC. At this level, all wounds are reassessed on arrival, most commonly in the OR. Wounds undergo repeat irrigation and débridement within 48 hours from the time of injury, and augmentation or alteration of skeletal fixation is performed as indicated. Because wounded patients are generally held at LRMC for no more than 3 to 5 days, definitive surgical stabilization is generally only performed for simple closed injuries when it facilitates transport.[63] However, LRMC has the capability to evaluate and treat patients for as long as necessary. Generally, if the patient could be safely returned to the combat zone within 14 days, they would remain at LRMC for care and not be evacuated back to the continental United States.

Echelon V

If the wounded cannot be returned to duty within the period of time allowed by the theater evacuation plan, they are transported to the continental United States for echelon V care. This care is convalescent, restorative, and rehabilitative and is primarily provided at military and veterans' hospitals.

It may also include civilian hospitals, as described by the National Disaster Medical System. Injured service members receive definitive care and rehabilitation with the goal of return to duty.[59]

Although any of the 59 hospitals in the Military Health System may serve as echelon V facilities, injuries may dictate more specialized care. Amputee care and rehabilitation, traumatic brain injury (TBI) evaluation and treatment, burn care, and other specific injuries are treated at few select facilities across the Department of Defense (DoD). The multisite DoD/VA Defense and Veterans Brain Injury Center (VBIC) focuses on care of TBI. It is a collaboration between the DoD, VA, and two civilian centers that is funded by DoD and includes research, education, and treatment. Defense Centers of Excellence for Psychological Health and Traumatic Brain Injury (DCoE), within VBIC, provides TBI care to wounded warriors at 19 sites.[64]

Hospital Care

After being transported to hospitals, disaster victims must be again triaged and treated according to injury severity and available resources. During the initial arrival of casualties, efforts should be made to ensure that appropriate decontamination has taken place. This may include initial evaluation bays being set up outside the facility to prevent hospital contamination. Trauma room evaluation continues to follow ATLS standards with primary surveys, first looking for life-threatening airway, breathing, or circulatory compromise. If no life- or limb-threatening injuries are identified, individual treatment then depends on the specifics of each case. Early on, when the size of the casualty load is unknown, further interventions are performed on a minimal acceptable care basis. Secondary tests and time-consuming treatments are delayed when possible until an accurate assessment of available resources is possible.

Common injury patterns include crush, environmental exposure, and dehydration. The most significant of these for the orthopaedic surgeon are crush injuries. The details of crush management are outlined in Chapter 16. Although most of the injury patterns overlap with those seen in more isolated trauma and are readily recognized and treated by surgeons, blast injuries remain an entity that are largely foreign to civilian physicians and deserve a more detailed review.

Blast Injury

After victims who have sustained PBI are identified, treatment begins with the life-sustaining measures needed for airway protection, ventilation, and circulation. Initial radiographs should include a chest radiograph. The classic "white butterfly" pattern is highly suggestive of bilateral blast lung, and free air under the diaphragm may be indicative of hollow viscus rupture.[65] In many centers, CT scanning is readily available and is the test of choice to quickly evaluate the head, chest, and abdomen.

Blast lung is a well-described entity that requires substantial respiratory support. The effects of blast lung may appear within 2 hours of injury, but signs of blast lung may appear as late as 48 hours after exposure.[66] The pulmonary compromise can be severe and potentially fatal. The chest radiographic findings and physiologic consequences are similar to those of more typical pulmonary contusion. Primary blast lung should be suspected in the presence of apnea, bradycardia, and hypotension or if patients develop dyspnea, cough, or chest pain after exposure. Avidan and colleagues reviewed the cases of 29 patients admitted to a Jerusalem trauma center following blast injury with blast lung manifestations.[67] Each had the typical hypoxia and radiographic chest infiltrates. Seven patients who were able to support their own ventilation had a PaO_2/FiO_2 above 200. Twenty-two (76%) of the victims required mechanical ventilation, and all were intubated within 2 hours of presentation. They remained intubated for a mean of 4 days. The highest required positive end-expiratory pressure support reached a maximum of 15 cm H_2O with caregivers using the minimal necessary positive-pressure ventilation for adequate oxygenation. Alternative modes of ventilation (high-frequency or nitric oxide) were also used in an attempt to minimize airway pressures. During treatment, two patients were thought to have air embolus, and one patient died of multiple organ failure. The risk of air embolism is lessened by minimizing positive-pressure ventilation, treating with supplemental oxygen, and resting in a decubitus position.[65] The supplemental oxygen is beneficial for gas exchange and allows for more efficient absorption of arterial air, which occurs when the emboli are more predominantly oxygen rather than nitrogen. Body positioning is an important consideration for these patients because remaining upright increases CNS injury, but Trendelenburg positioning has increased coronary emboli effects. If one lung has been preferentially injured in a blast, the patient should be positioned with the injured lung down in a dependent position. That will result in lower alveolar pressures with greater vascular pressures, which can lower the chances for air being forced into the bloodstream.[65] The definitive treatment for air embolism remains hyperbaric chamber therapy. Although mortality from blast lung was low in this series, other authors have reported much higher rates, with Frykberg estimating an 11% mortality rate associated with blast lung.[1]

Primary blast injury to the abdomen may cause organ edema, hemorrhage, or frank rupture and result in bleeding significant enough to cause shock. Blood pressure should be maintained with fluids without administering excess volumes, which can worsen pulmonary injury. The abdomen can be evaluated by CT scan, ultrasonography, or diagnostic peritoneal lavage (DPL). DPL is more sensitive but less specific than CT in detecting abdominal organ injury from blast.[65] As for the injured lung, treatment for abdominal blast injury is supportive until the severity or extent of the injury requires bowel resection.

Hearing loss is produced by several mechanisms with the most common being rupture of the tympanic membrane.[65] The CDC therefore recommends that all persons exposed to blast detonations be evaluated for tympanic membrane rupture, have an otologic examination, and be followed with serial audiometry.[65] Patients should have any debris removed from the external canal and have antiseptic solution irrigation. Tympanic membranes usually heal without repair if the rupture involves less than 33% of its area. Finally, victims should avoid repetitive auditory stresses because remaining in loud environments decreases the chance of regaining hearing.

Blasts also can have an impact on the ophthalmologic system. Diligent repeat examinations are required to look for globe lacerations, hypopyon, corneal ulcers, and traumatic optic nerve atrophy.[68] Ocular perforating injuries are particularly serious. In soldiers from Iraq, this type of injury was frequently grossly contaminated by a large number of small particles. Thirty-one percent of these injuries required globe excision even when eyes with minimal potential functional recovery were preserved.[69] These penetrating injuries accounted for 80% of globe excisions among 251 severe ocular injuries. The use of protective goggles in combat cannot be overemphasized.

Several aspects of open extremity wounds produced by blasts deserve special attention. First, most penetrating injuries caused by blast-driven projectiles should be considered as contaminated and survivors given appropriate antibiotics and tetanus toxoid. Open wounds from various types of shrapnel and blast debris require detailed physical and radiologic examination. Even for small entrance wounds, surgeons should maintain a low threshold for thorough débridement because deep contamination and devitalized tissue can produce highly morbid infectious complications. Second, these extremities should be thoroughly evaluated from a vascular standpoint.[70] In examinations of soldiers at Walter Reed Army Medical Center from 2001 to 2004, 107 vascular injuries were recorded with 64% resulting from explosive injuries. Remarkably, when arteriograms were ordered based solely on the injury mechanism in the absence of vascular changes on physical examination, 25% (seven of 28) were positive. Overall, two thirds of vascular injuries missed on physical examination but evident on angiography were attributable to blast. Although most occult injuries remained asymptomatic, 18% required treatment and included arteriovenous fistulas and pseudoaneurysms. The experience at Walter Reed has led to several recommendations. It seems that the physical examination is less reliable for detecting vascular injuries caused by blast than in routine civilian trauma. In the treatment of these injuries, it is important to avoid prosthetic grafts or repairs or reconstruction within contaminated zones of injury because these factors significantly increase complication rates. Most operative procedures aim to ligate expendable vessels or use autologous vein grafts for critical reconstructions. Endovascular techniques and wound vacuum-assisted closure devices have also begun to play important roles. Finally, even with ideal management, complications are expected. Forty-four percent of battlefield vascular repairs involved complications with 25% of these repairs subsequently requiring additional procedures.

Beyond emergent débridement and bony stabilization, the approach to reconstruction for high-velocity, high-energy extremity wounds has changed over time. Traditionally, these wounds underwent long-term dressing changes and immobilization. However, some surgeons now advocate for earlier definitive reconstruction and coverage. Celiköz et al. published a large experience covering 215 patients who sustained combat gunshot, missile, and land mine injuries of the lower extremity.[71] These patients were treated definitively from 1 to 3 weeks (mean, 9.3 days) after injury. After a mean of 1.9 débridement procedures, final procedures were performed. Twenty-three (10.2%) were treated with primary below-knee amputation. However, a greater number of amputations were carried out at primary hospitals on limbs not transferred to the referral center in this study. The remaining 209 defects were scheduled for simultaneous bony and soft tissue reconstruction. Soft tissue coverage consisted of 18 local muscle and 208 free muscle flaps. Associated Gustilo type III open tibia fractures or bony foot defects numbered 104 and 64, respectively. These were addressed with 106 bone grafts, 25 free fibula flaps, and 14 cases of distraction osteogenesis. Overall, the results were encouraging given the severity of injuries. All patients survived their injuries, and the success of the free flaps was 91.3%. Bony complications included early infection in 15.4%, chronic infection in 3.8%, and union difficulty in 22%. Only two late amputations were performed, and at a mean follow-up of 25 months, no patients had requested amputation secondary to functional problems or pain. Although this extensive series provides insight into aggressive treatment protocols, it is important to remember, as the authors point out, that their success is based on early, aggressive bony and soft tissue débridement and that these results are from a highly experienced referral trauma center.

Unique infectious risks are also associated with blast wounds. Reports of burn patients from blast attacks document the appearance of infected wounds and sepsis from multidrug-resistant bacteria that are novel to treating burn centers.[68] Even in the setting of private rooms, pneumonia caused by resistant bacterial strains developed in several patients in one center. Although an explosive's shrapnel and debris carry some bacteria, blast attacks are also noteworthy for increasing subsequent contamination of wounds caused by conditions at the scene or during transport to the hospital in civilian vehicles (including a garbage truck in one bombing).[68] For example, blast victims from meat and vegetable marketplaces have had an increased incidence of candidemia.[72] Furthermore, suicide bombings have been associated with the traumatic implantation of allogeneic biologic material into victims as secondary fragmentation from either the bomber or from others in proximity to the blast.[73-75] This introduces a risk of significant infectious transmission because some impaled bony fragments have tested positive for hepatitis B.[74] In response, Israel now mandates hepatitis B vaccination as part of the first-line response to suicide bombings.[76] To date, one reported transmission of the virus has occurred while bony fragments from two suicide bombers have tested positive for the virus.[74] Risk of hepatitis C and HIV inoculation may warrant screening but have not yet been reported.[68]

DISASTER EDUCATION INITIATIVES

The immediate response of U.S. Orthopaedic Surgeons to the 2010 earthquake disaster in Haiti was impressive in scale and effort but highlighted the lack of formal training and organization of volunteers responding to disasters. Most surgeons were accustomed to the well-equipped and sophisticated hospitals common in the United States. They were not prepared for the makeshift facilities of a postdisaster developing nation, nor were they well versed in the principles of security, logistics, and triage. Although many possessed the skills to treat injured patients, the nuances of providing orthopaedic care in an austere environment potentially led to decreased efficiency and possibly inappropriate care.

In response to the apparent need to train and organize U.S. orthopaedic surgeon-volunteers, the American Academy of Orthopaedic Surgeons (AAOS), in cooperation with the Orthopaedic Trauma Association (OTA), developed a Disaster Preparedness Plan that specifically included a training program, the Disaster Response Course (DRC). These two organizations have been actively involved in increasing awareness of disaster management and response among surgeons, residents, and medical students nationwide, and the events in Haiti provided the impetus to implement a comprehensive plan and training course. It is anticipated that the Core Curriculum of the OTA will also include new modules on "Principles of Disaster Management" and "Blast Injury" by 2014.[47]

The Disaster Response Course was created by the Society of Military Orthopaedic Surgeons (SOMOS), with the assistance of the OTA, customizing the Combat Extremity Surgery Course (CESC) used to prepare military surgeons for deployment to the Middle East and other areas of armed conflict. The CESC program includes modules on combat-related blast and penetrating injuries and principles of triage, security, logistics, and medical evacuation. The DRC added instruction in natural disasters and catastrophic events, medical ethics, and cultural sensitivity in an effort to prepare surgeon-volunteers for the challenges of providing orthopaedic care in the austere environment of a postdisaster area. Attending the DRC qualifies surgeons for inclusion in the AAOS Disaster Responder Registry. This registry is designed to be a central clearinghouse for organizations to select orthopaedic surgeons prepared to provide care in the wake of disaster, both foreign and domestic, and engage them in relief efforts. The curriculum is fluid and is updated to reflect recent experiences, updates in technology, and medical improvements. In addition to the didactics, the course includes a laboratory experience designed to reinforce useful clinical skills when faced with limited resource availability in the austere disaster setting.

The AAOS Disaster Preparedness Plan[77] provides a blueprint for disaster training and registration for its members. The registrant database contains information on surgeon qualifications, certifications, language skills, previous austere environment and military experience, and volunteer preferences for involvement. It is designed to allow disaster relief agencies, nongovernmental organizations, U.S. Government Department of Health and Human Services/National Disaster Medical System (NDMS), and the U.S. military medical services to rapidly identify individuals qualified and interested in serving at a time of need.

Other avenues for disaster response training and education include the National Disaster Life Support (NDLS) Basic and Advanced Courses offered by the National Disaster Life Support Foundation (NDLSF).[78] The American College of Surgeons offers a Disaster Management Emergency Preparedness (DMEP) course.[79] Furthermore, FEMA[80] conducts supplemental courses recommended for disaster responders. The FEMA Disaster Training Modules are offered online and include the Emergency Management Institute Independent Study Program Courses and the Emergency Management Institute National Incident Management System (NIMS) Courses. These training modules are required for surgeons serving on NDMS teams, although the required modules vary by team.

SUMMARY

Physicians practicing today face an increasingly unstable political world with ongoing acts of terrorism. Both civilian attacks and natural disasters have brought increased attention to disaster care. These disasters introduce risk to first responders as well as to hospital personnel that is unseen in the delivery of routine health care. Because little real-time training is available, preparation and education provide the cornerstone of any effective disaster response. The "all-hazards approach" defines the current model of generic disaster preparations, which provide uniform responses yet allow sufficient flexibility to enable adaptation to unique circumstances. It is essential that health care providers become fluent in the universal terminology of disasters as well as proper utilization of the ICS. Physicians should appreciate the changes that disasters impose on the conventional civilian approach to triage. Although MCIs are rare, their potential impact on communities or society as a whole mandate that the health care profession stand ready to deliver in the face of disasters.

ACKNOWLEDGEMENT

Joann Mead, MA
Research Assistant
Department of Orthopaedic Surgery
Brown University
Warren Alpert Medical School

KEY REFERENCES

The level of evidence (LOE) is determined according to the criteria provided in the preface.

3. U.S. Government: National Response Plan, 2005. Available at <www.dhs.gov/xnews/releases/press_release_0581.shtm> E & DA LOE V
4. Bailin MT, Beninati W, Bohanan AM, et al: Incident Command System. In Briggs SM, Brinsfield KH, editors: *Advanced disaster medical response manual for providers*, Boston, 2003, Harvard Medical International Trauma and Disaster Institute, pp 1–5, 17–26, 35–36. LOE V
8. Ciraulo DL, Frykberg ER, Feliciano DV, et al: A survey assessment of the level of preparedness for domestic terrorism and mass casualty incidents among Eastern Association for the Surgery of Trauma members. *J Trauma* 56:1033–1041, 2004. LOE II
13. Federal Emergency Management Agency (FEMA): Incident Command System. Available at <http://www.fema.gov> LOE V
53. Agency for Healthcare Research and Quality, U.S. Department of Health and Human Services: *Development of models for emergency preparedness: personal protective equipment, decontamination, isolation/quarantine, and laboratory capacity*. 27–61, Rockville, MD, 2005. LOE V
54. Grissom TE, Farmer JC: The provision of sophisticated critical care beyond the hospital: lessons from physiology and military experiences that apply to civil disaster medical response. *Crit Care Med* 33(1 Suppl): S13–S21, 2005. LOE II
55. Lhowe DW, Briggs SM: Planning for mass civilian casualties overseas: IMSuRT: International Medical/Surgical Response Teams. *Clin Orthop Relat Res* 422:109–113, 2004. LOE V
57. Levels of medical care. In Szul AC, Davis LB, Walter Reed Army Medical Center, editors: *Emergency war surgery: third United States revision*, Washington, DC, 2004, Department of the Army, pp 2.1–2.10. LOE V
61. Sechriest VF 2nd, Wing V, Walker GJ, et al: Healthcare delivery aboard US Navy hospital ships following earthquake disasters: implications for future disaster relief missions. *Am J Disaster Med* 7(4):281–294, 2012. LOE II
77. AAOS Disaster Preparedness and Response: <http://www.aaos.org/member/humanitarianprograms/disasterprep/disaster_prep_resp.asp> Accessed on August 15, 2013. LOE V
78. The National Disaster Life Support Foundation, Inc.: <http://www.ndlsf.org/> Accessed August 15, 2013. LOE V
79. Disaster Management and Emergency Preparedness (DMEP) Course: <http://www.facs.org/trauma/disaster/about.html> Accessed on August 15, 2013. LOE V
80. FEMA Training. <http://www.fema.gov/training-1> Accessed on August 15, 2013. LOE V

The complete References list is available online at https://expertconsult.inkling.com.

Chapter 13

Occupational Hazards in the Treatment of Orthopaedic Trauma

13A Optimal and Safe Use of C-Arm X-Ray Fluoroscopy Units

PETER J. MAS

INTRODUCTION

The use of fluoroscopic imaging procedures allows healthcare professionals to view the examination and procedure of the patient in real time. Modern fluoroscopic devices are greatly improved from the darkened room imaging conducted in the mid-twentieth century. The imaging system or image intensifier assembly is the fundamental component for the production of the patient image. It has grown from an approximately 6-inch-diameter image intensifier to a 12-inch-diameter device on mobile C-arm units. Stationary C-arm fluoroscopic units, such as those found in a busy radiology department, can come equipped with an 18-inch image intensifier, although it is more common to see a 15-inch intensifier (Fig. 13A-1).

The term *C-arm* was coined because of the letter C-shaped yoke of the x-ray tube-to-image intensifier geometry (Fig. 13A-2).

In addition to the x-ray production electronics, display electronics, the x-ray tube and collimation device, the C-arm unit also has an antiscatter grid, a charge-coupled device (CCD), and a video system camera to feed the image onto the display monitors. Mobile C-arm units are equipped with wheels and a steering mechanism for transport to the procedure room or operatory where it will be used.

FEATURES

The image intensifier assembly is composed of:

1. An antiscatter grid (reduces scattered x-rays entering the unit)
2. A vacuum tube with:
   a. Photoabsorptive and electroemissive surfaces
   b. Electrostatic focusing electrodes
   c. An output phosphor (CCD)
3. Light-focusing lenses, diaphragm, and video signal pickup
4. Electronic shielding
5. Lead-lined enclosure (serves as the primary x-ray barrier)

The function of each component of the image intensifier system is summarized below.

1. **Antiscatter grid:** Reduces the loss of image resolution due to scattered x-rays reaching the image intensifier (Fig. 13A-3). Scattered x-rays are those deflected from the original "straight-on" path to the image intensifier.
2. **Vacuum tube:** Made of glass or a nonferromagnetic material (Fig. 13A-4). Provides for the accelerated travel of electrons emitted from the entrance (input phosphor-to-photocathode) surfaces and directed to the output phosphor at the opposite end.
3. **Electrostatic focusing lenses:** Changing the electrical bias on these lenses will spread out (or compress) the stream of electrons coming from the photocathode surface, thereby causing a magnification (or minification) of the resultant image being captured.
4. **Output phosphor:** Produces light photons representative of the x-rays absorbed and transmitted within the patient. (Fig. 13A-5)
5. **Video signal pickup:** The image generated at the output phosphor is then viewed with the attached video system (TV camera or CCD). An Automatic Brightness Control (ABC) feedback circuit is used to drive the x-ray generator to produce more (or less) x-rays by increasing (or decreasing) the x-ray tube kVp operating potential or the x-ray tube mA current.
6. **Electronic shielding:** Used to reduce any possible distortion of the image production system from external sources of electric and magnetic fields
7. **Lead-lined enclosure:** The image intensifier system is a primary radiation barrier. X-rays do not escape out of the image intensifier back into the suite. (Figs. 13A-6 and 13A-7).

I have not given much attention to the x-ray tube itself, primarily because its purpose is limited: it either produces x-rays or not. The x-ray tube does not independently manage, manipulate, or modify the x-rays produced, but the x-ray tube housing is another matter. The tube housing (Fig. 13A-8) is a lead-lined enclosure with three important components of the x-ray generation chain in addition to the x-ray tube itself: the x-ray beam filter(s), the beam collimation (an x-ray field size-limiting device), and a thermal switch to sense overheating of the x-ray tube.

X-rays are produced when a stream of electrons are accelerated toward a high atomic (Z-number) target material, such as tungsten, functioning as the anode in an electrical circuit. The collisions of the electrons with the target results in x-rays, but approximately 99% of the collisions simply result in the heating of the target, and a thermal overload interrupt switch becomes a necessity. The tube housing also serves as a barrier against x-rays. By Food and Drug Administration (FDA)

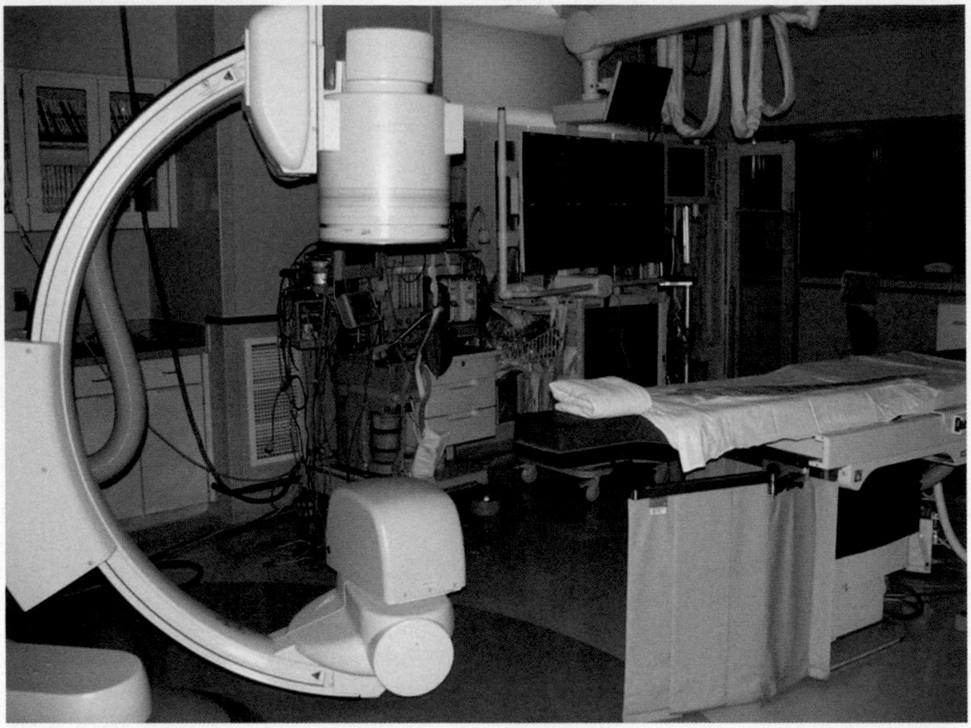

Figure 13A-1. A stationary C-arm fluoroscopic x-ray unit with a 15-inch image intensifier assembly.

regulation, the x-rays escaping the tube housing ("leakage x-rays") cannot result in a radiation exposure rate greater than 0.1 roentgen per hour, measured at 1 m from the x-ray source, when operated at its maximum kVp energy and maximum continuous mA tube current.

X-rays produced in this manner are termed "polychromatic" because they cover a wide spectrum of energies; they are not monoenergetic like gamma-ray (nuclear) sources of radiation. The addition of x-ray beam filters achieves a cleaner and higher effective energy x-ray beam profile. The insertion of aluminum metal filters will remove (filter out) the lower energy x-rays, which cause much greater (entrance-skin surface) radiation exposure to the patient and do not contribute to the creation of the diagnostic image. The higher energy x-rays continue to pass through the added aluminum filtration and reach the patient for the selective attenuation by tissues

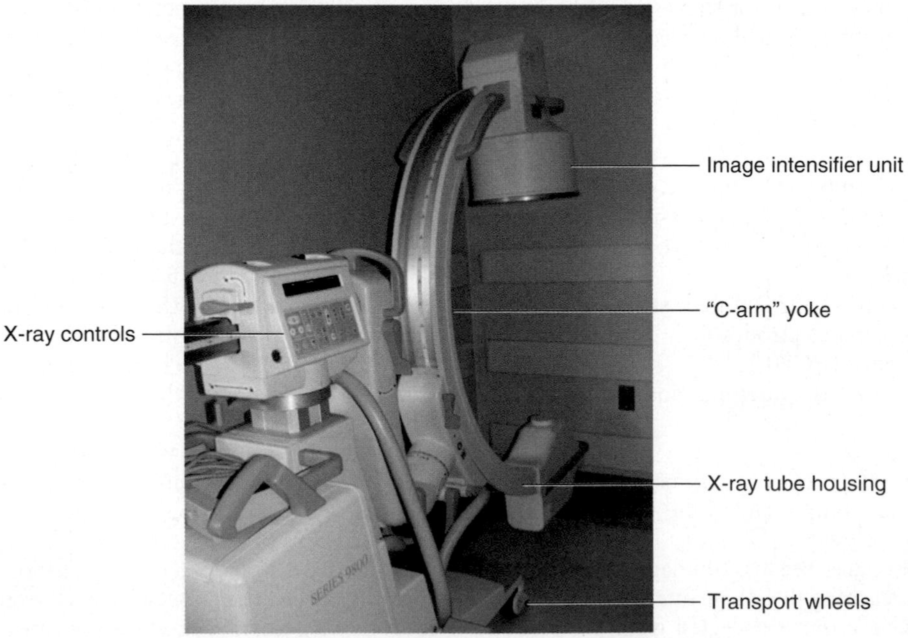

Figure 13A-2. A mobile "C-arm" unit.

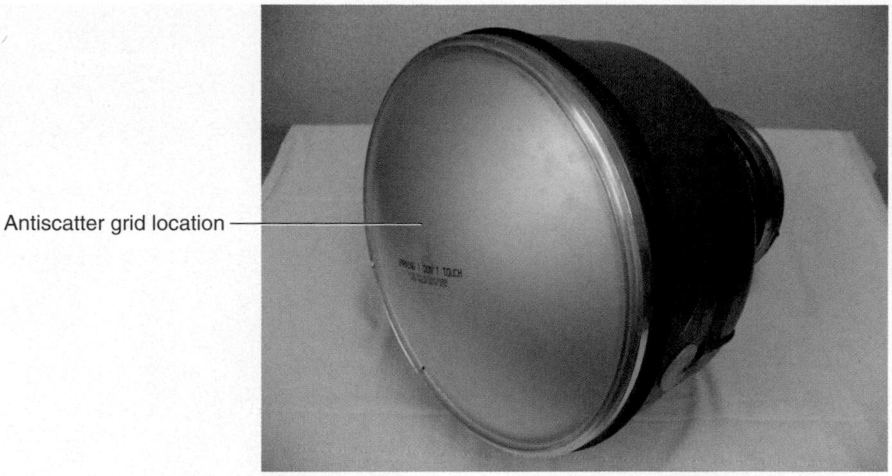

Figure 13A-3. The complete image intensifier assembly.

and anatomic structures. X-rays exiting the patient can now interact with the image intensifier input phosphor, and the imaging process commences. Higher energy x-ray imaging devices, such as computed tomography (CT) scanners, use copper metal beam filtration to essentially eliminate all low-energy x-rays.

The x-ray beam collimation component is also governed by FDA regulation. The x-ray beam can never be larger (wider) than the image intensifier diameter, and the image intensifier must be affixed to the x-ray device in such a way that it always intercepts the x-ray beam. An unattenuated, primary beam x-ray field must never extend beyond the physical size of the x-ray primary barrier that is built into the image intensifier device. In the clinical setting, such a misalignment would be comparable to standing next to a bulls-eye while the projectiles are hitting outside of the intended target. The manufacturer can place a lead diaphragm (or cone) at the x-ray tube to satisfy the beam-size limiting criteria, but physical abuse or mishandling of the unit may compromise the x-ray beam-to-image intensifier alignment.

The final components of the imaging system are the x-ray control panel (Figs. 13A-9 and 13A-10), the exposure activation switches, customarily performed via a "dead man" type foot switch (Fig. 13A-11), and the image display and recording device (Fig. 13A-12). The x-ray control panel indicates the mode of operation of the C-arm unit. Details such as the kVp beam energy, the mA tube current, the elapsed time for the procedure, the timer alarm reset, the imaging frame rate, the intensifier MAG (magnification) mode, and image display parameters are viewed and controlled at the console. Nearly every one of these has a direct bearing on the patient's (and staff) radiation exposure, which will be described in a later section.

The "dead man" foot switch is so called because you must actively depress the switch to get the x-ray beam "on." If the operator were to drop dead during the procedure, the

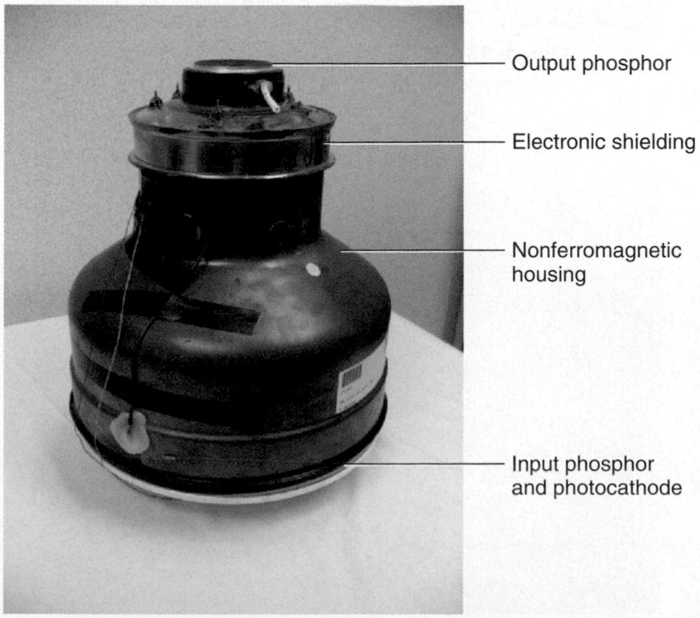

Figure 13A-4. Output phosphor electronic shielding.

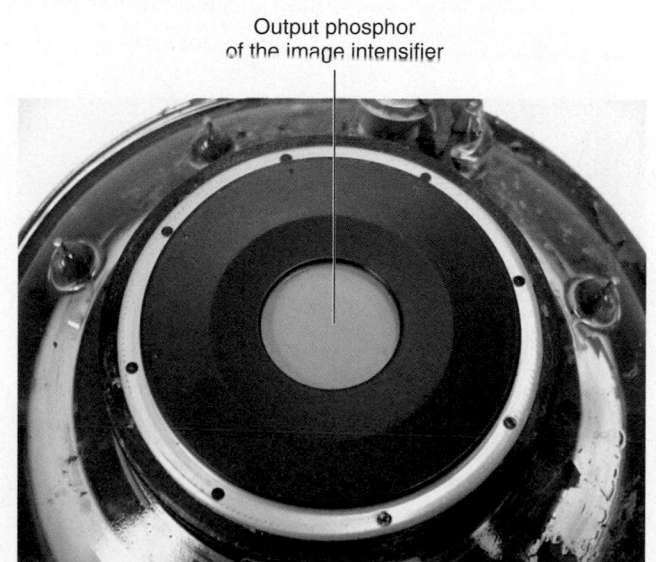

Figure 13A-5. The output phosphor of the image intensifier.

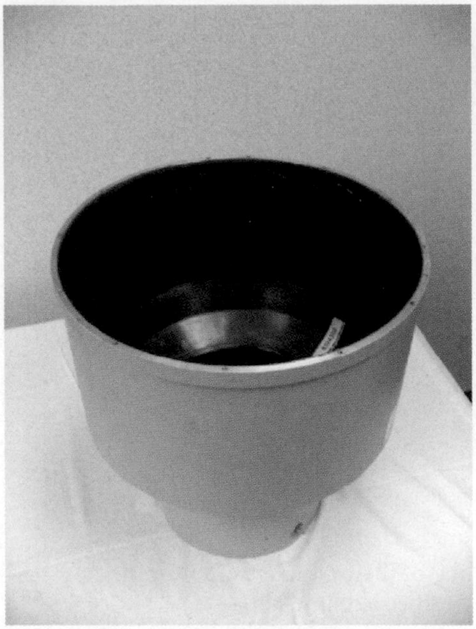

Figure 13A-6. Lead-lined housing of the image intensifier.

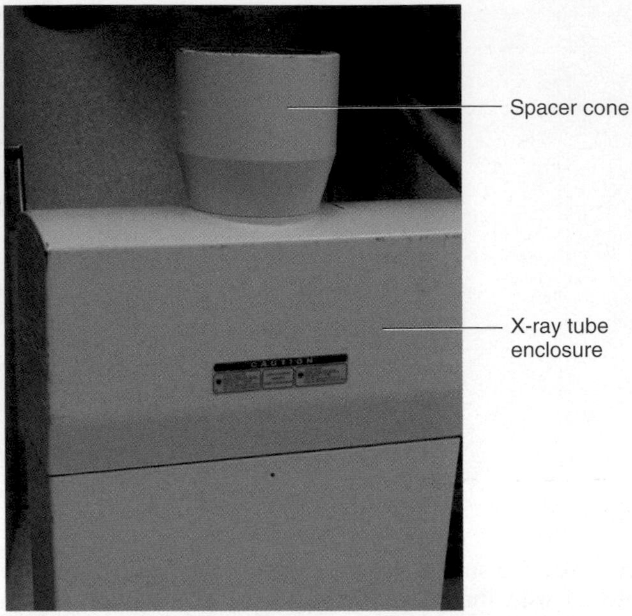

Figure 13A-8. The x-ray tube housing.

spring-loaded foot switch would return to the "off" position, the C-arm unit would drop to zero x-ray emissions, and it would again be "radiation safe." The foot switch is on a long cord for placement where most convenient to the physician or operator of the C-arm.

The image display and recording and archival device is the final leg of the diagnostic imaging process. The monitors must be of sufficient resolution and brightness to clearly display the progress of the procedure. Most C-arm units sold presently include an integrated hard drive with picture (frame) grabber hardware and software. The stored images can be called up for review and printing onto film media, but there is a finite number of images that can be stored. Depending on the hard drive capacity, that number ranges from a low of 100 to as much as 10,000, and when the storage media has been filled, the unit will write over the first image in storage and continue therefrom. The advantage of a "last image hold" frame grabber is to see the last recorded position of the device(s) you are

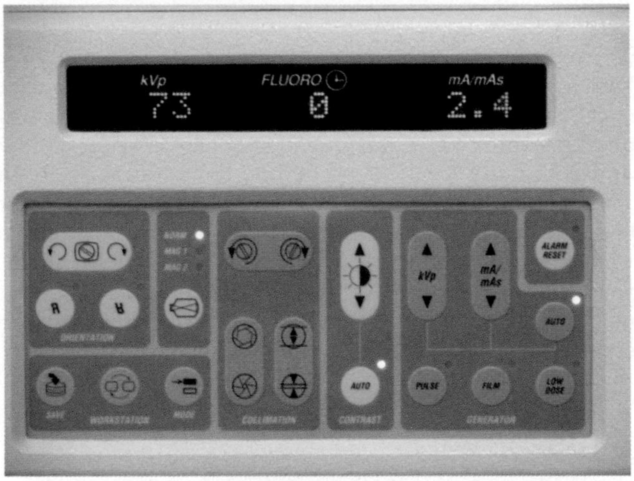

Figure 13A-9. OEC unit x-ray control panel.

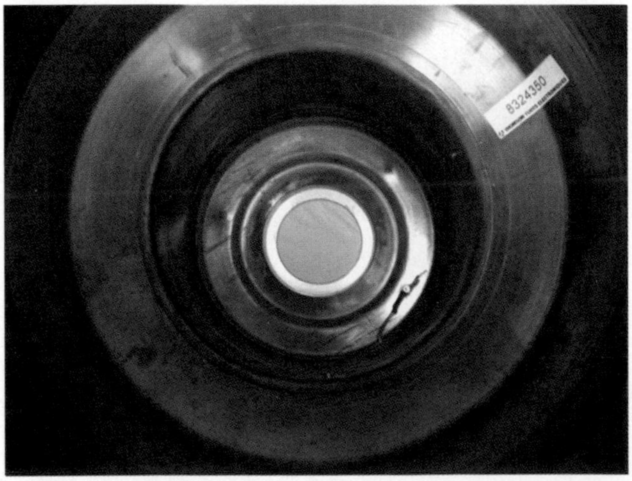

Figure 13A-7. View of the interior.

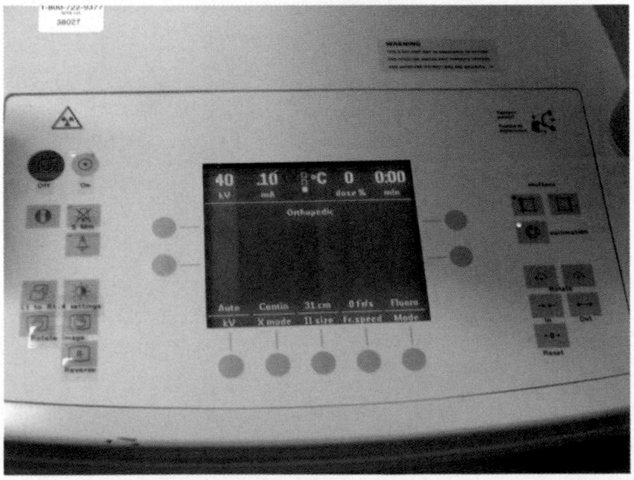

Figure 13A-10. Philips unit x-ray control panel.

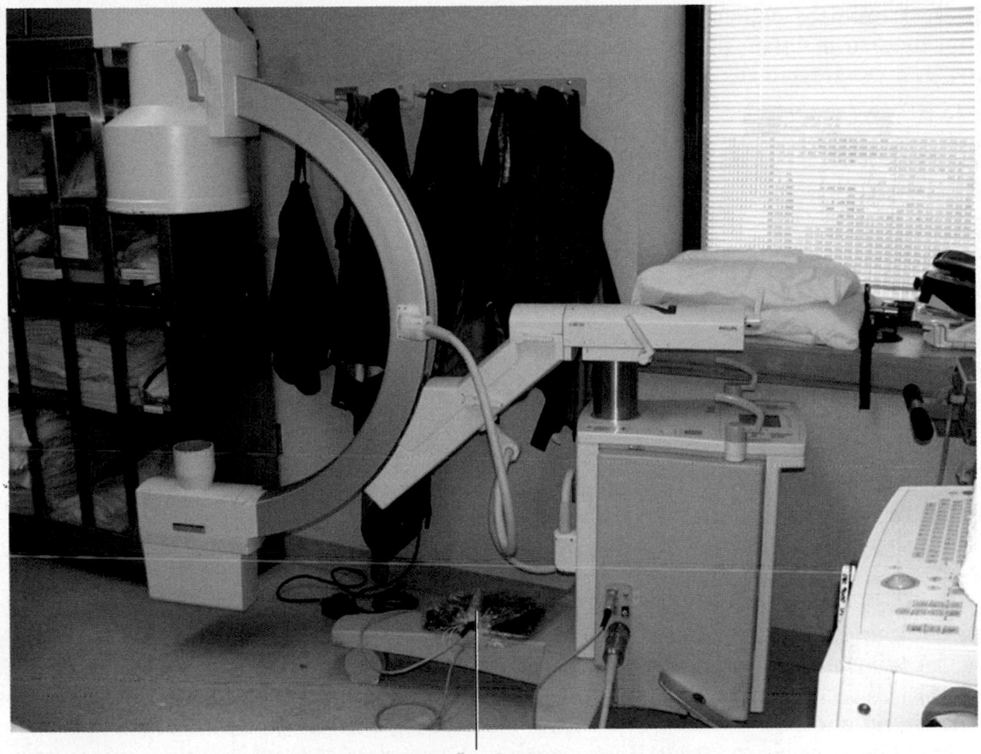

Figure 13A-11. Dead man foot switch.

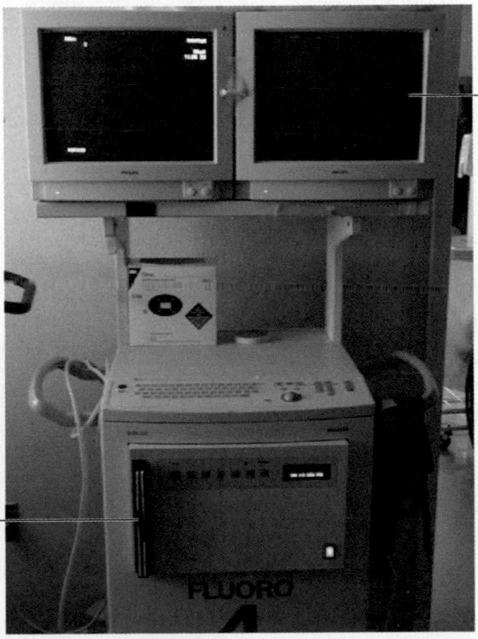

Figure 13A-12. C-arm unit display station.

manipulating or inserting into the patient on the monitors. Therefore, you do not need to maintain the x-ray beam "on" at all times to review your progress in the procedure.

REDUCTION OF RADIATION DOSE DURING C-ARM OPERATION

No two patients are exactly alike. There will be differences in size, height, weight, general shape, and anatomy, but a properly operated mobile C-arm unit will do quite well for the vast majority of cases.

Patients are routinely imaged on an operating room table, a procedure table, a stretcher, and even in a hospital bed. When you have the ability to select what surface the patient will be imaged on, it is better to select an "x-ray compatible" table surface, plus its mattress or foam padding. The designation of x-ray compatible means that the table material itself is not highly attenuating of the x-ray beam. Attenuation of the x-rays results in:

1. Loss of object contrast. The C-arm unit will be forced to operate at a higher imaging technique (greater kVp beam energy or higher mA tube current) as a result of the ABC feedback circuit. The ABC compensates for the reduced light level from the output phosphor caused by the attenuation of the x-ray beam by the table materials. The imaged object contrast (discernible shades of gray) decreases with increasing x-ray energy.
2. Greater entrance skin exposure to the patient from the increased imaging technique
3. Greater amount of scattered radiation during the procedure

The most desirable, but also expensive, surface is the carbon-fiber tabletop. It is the least attenuating because of its low atomic (Z-number) material composition.

A few words about "scattered radiation," the how and the where it occurs with a C-arm unit. How best to spatially describe the concept of scattering? I like to use the following analogy. Consider driving a car on a clear night. The headlights shine and easily illuminate the road ahead. Now picture yourself driving that same car on a foggy night. There is a "halo" or "corona" of light starting at the headlight surface and radiating outward but generally in the direction of the road surface. You have just witnessed "scattered" radiation, but in this example, the radiation is in the form of visible light that is being diffracted by the water molecules suspended in the air. X-rays can be scattered when striking air molecules, but the denser the material it interacts with, the greater the probability for scattering (and absorption) of the x-rays (Figs. 13A-13 and 13A-14).

Diagnostic imaging x-rays are a low-energy form of electromagnetic radiation. For such, the scattering of the kilovoltage x-rays is predominantly directed back *toward* the x-ray tube. In comparison, high-energy megavoltage x-rays such as those used in cancer treatment will scatter forward beyond the patient and continue in the direction of the treatment x-ray beam. From a radiation protection perspective, when the C-arm is positioned more parallel to the floor (shooting across the procedure table), personnel should not stand close to the x-ray tube. It is better to stand at the image intensifier side, where there is less scattering of the x-rays originating from the patient.

Figure 13A-13. Street lamps on a clear night.

We now move ahead to when the C-arm is brought to the patient's side while undergoing the orthopaedic procedure. The next exposure reduction step starts with the positioning of the C-arm at the patient. The single most important positioning criterion to try to adhere to is *place the image intensifier as close as possible to the patient's body* (Figs. 13A-15 and 13A-16). Use a sterile cover on the intensifier to maintain the sterility of the operatory field. In this orientation, you achieve three things in your favor:

1. Increased sensitivity to the exiting x-rays that generate the patient's image plus decreased scattered radiation because the image intensifier is a leaded barrier that has been placed nearer to the body that causes the scattering. When the intensifier is positioned closer to the patient, there is less scattering of x-rays beyond it into the room environment.
2. Increased image resolution. The improved imaging geometry will increase image sharpness, much like a hand will cast a sharper shadow the closer it gets to a wall or the floor (assuming the light is coming from overhead). Here, the hand is the object you need to "see" clearly, and the wall (or floor) is the "imaging" device.

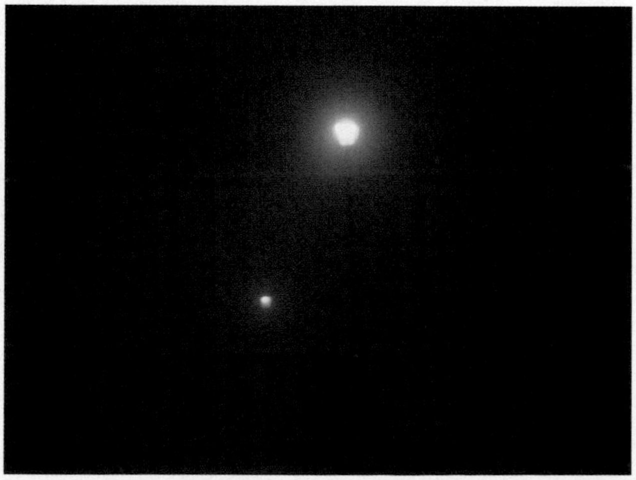

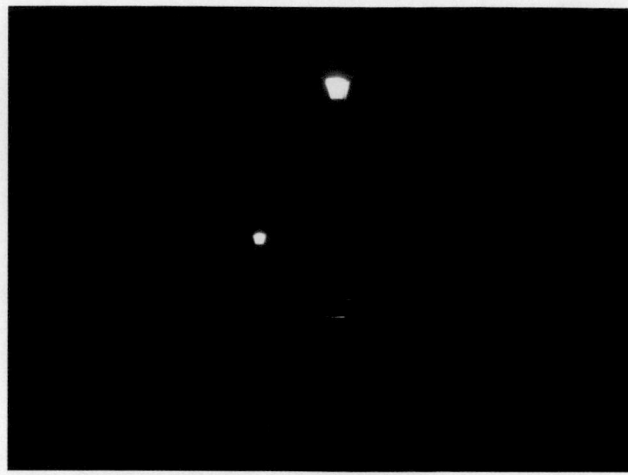

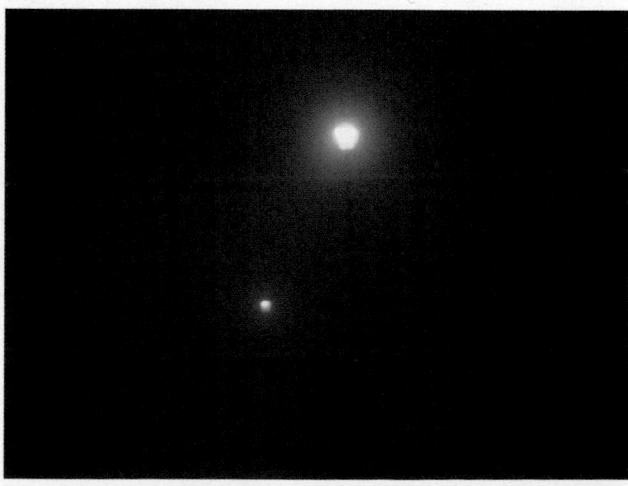

Figure 13A-14. Those same street lamps at night but with fog.

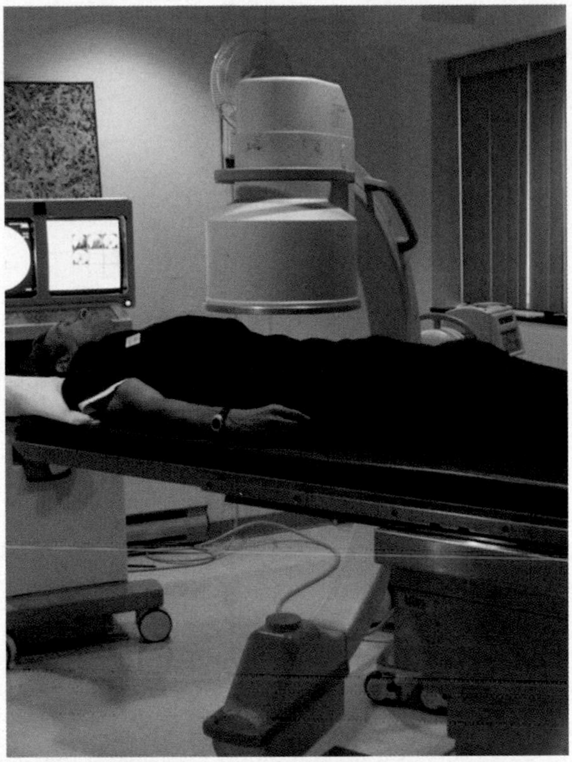

Figure 13A-15. Proper positioning, posteroanterior view.

3. Decreased entrance skin exposure at the patient because the x-ray tube is kept the farthest distance possible from the patient's skin.

Radiation intensity follows the inverse-square law: the change in intensity is proportional to the square of the distance from the source. For example, if you double (factor of 2) the distance away from the radiation source, the intensity drops by the inverse, squared product (1/2 × 1/2), which equals 1/4 (25%) of the original radiation intensity. Conversely, if you halve (1/2) the distance from a radiation source, you quadruple (4) the intensity of the exposure; this is most worrisome whenever you image in a truly lateral orientation. It is best to maintain the x-ray tube as far as possible from the patient's body surfaces and the image intensifier as close as possible. One FDA-required component of fluoroscopic imaging systems, albeit frequently removed from the C-arm, is the spacer cone (see Fig. 13A-8). The spacer cone is used to maintain a 12-inch distance from the patient's body; otherwise, very large radiation exposure rates and skin doses can be given to the patient. The FDA has publicized warnings to this effect and has identified the procedures most likely to cause conspicuous radiation damage to patients' skin. Orthopaedic surgical procedures are not on that list, but they can contribute to the deterministic (somatic) effects of skin epilation and skin erythema. For more information, go to the FDA's website at www.fda.gov/cdrh/rsnaii.html.

Today's C-arm units have the ability to magnify the area being imaged and are usually designed with two "MAG modes" of operation. Image magnification is achieved within the intensifier by changing the bias voltage on the electrostatic focusing lenses. The electron beam traveling toward the output phosphor is forced to spread out, thereby eliminating some of the signal from the periphery of the electron stream that would have struck the output phosphor. Simultaneously, the collimator assembly narrows down the field of view because less of an area of the patient is being imaged. The resultant effect is less of the image intensifier input phosphor is being irradiated; consequently, fewer electrons are released into the intensifier assembly. The process is reversed when the control panel button for "normal" viewing is pressed.

Let us look at the net effect on the production of the electron stream at the input phosphor with the following images and a bit of algebra (Figs. 13A-17 to 13A-20) for an intensifier of 12–9–6 inch viewing modes. In "normal" viewing mode, a 12-inch circular image intensifier is almost fully irradiated by the x-ray beam exiting the patient; the area (πr^2) of that surface equals 36π sq in. At MAG mode 1, the intensifier decreases to 9-in diameter and surface area drops to 20.25π sq in. At MAG mode 2, the intensifier decreases to a 6-inch diameter and surface area drops to 9π sq in. Changing the intensifier size from 12 to 9 inches has a net effect of losing

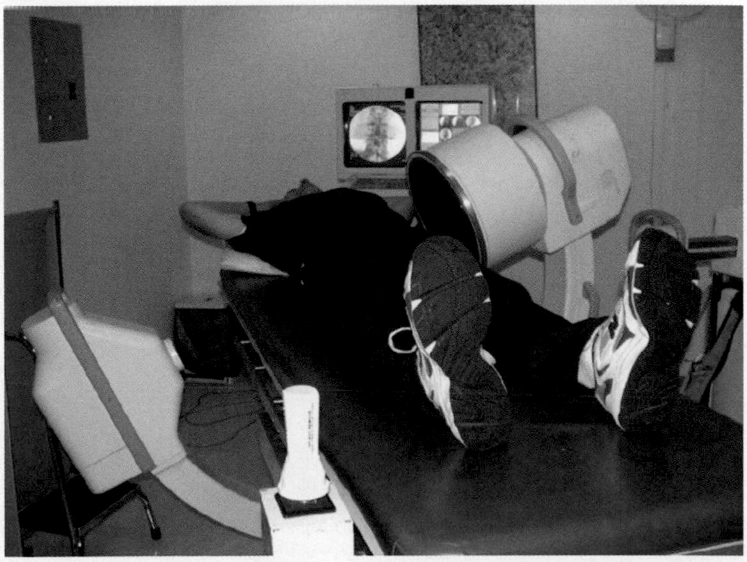

Figure 13A-16. Lateral-oblique placement of the image intensifier.

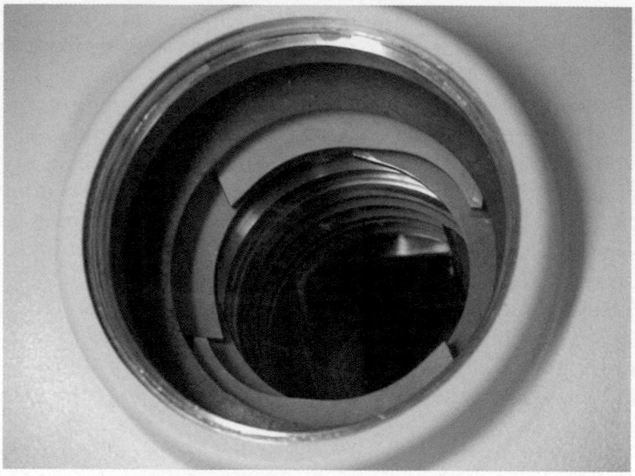

Figure 13A-17. Fully open collimation for 12-inch "normal" mode viewing.

approximately 45% of the input phosphor's imaging area. Changing the intensifier size from 12 to 6 inches has a net effect of losing approximately 75% of the input phosphor's imaging area.

The decreased input phosphor area translates directly into a decreased production of electrons inside the image intensifier. The decreased number of electrons results in decreased light production by the output phosphor. The ABC feedback circuit seeks to correct the situation by calling on the x-ray generator to increase the tube energy potential (kVp), the tube current (mA), or both. A higher energy (kVp) x-ray will cause more electrons to be released by interactions at the input phosphor. A higher tube current (mA) will increase the production of x-rays at the x-ray tube. Ultimately, a combination of these two x-ray generator adjustments will satisfy the ABC circuitry.

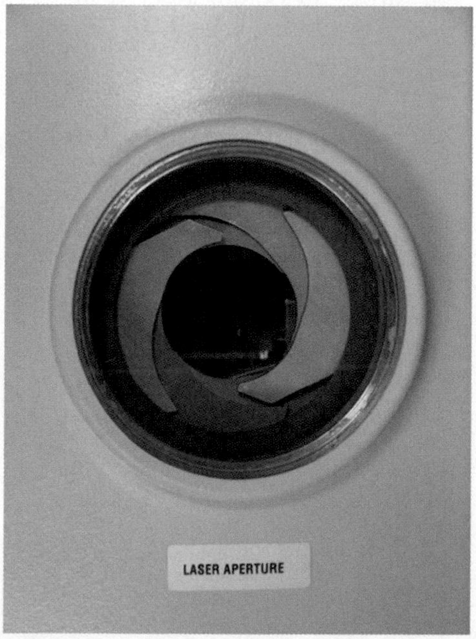

Figure 13A-18. Partially open collimation for 9-inch "MAG mode 1" viewing.

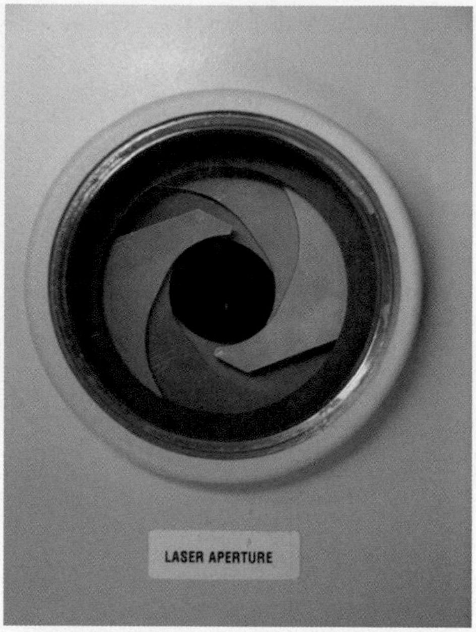

Figure 13A-19. Minimally open collimation for 6-inch "MAG mode 2" viewing.

C-arm operation in a magnification modality is one source of significant increases in the imaging techniques (kVp, mA) and will result in:

1. Increased image resolution (at high MAG mode); the patient object will appear larger allowing the viewer to see the smaller details.
2. Increased patient entrance skin exposure because the x-ray tube is operating at a higher technique. If the magnification is doubled (2×) the patient's exposure rate is quadrupled (4×).
3. Increased heat loading of the x-ray tube. The C-arm may shutdown because of overheating, particularly if performing a lengthy procedure on a larger-sized patient body.

To reduce the exposure of the patient and the personnel and to reduce the heating of the x-ray tube and increase its usable operating time, the magnification mode imaging features should be called upon *only when necessary for the task* at hand. MAG mode imaging is another tool of the C-arm but one to be used sparingly. Two other tools of the C-arm that impact image acquisition, patient exposure, and image storage are: the "high-dose rate" fluoroscopy mode and the "frame rate" pulsed fluoroscopy settings found at the control panel.

The FDA limit for the patient's skin entrance exposure rate (at tabletop) is 100 milligray (mGy) per minute (10 roentgens/min in the old terminology). Fluoroscopic examinations typically yield skin entrance exposures ranging from 10 to 100 mGy/min, with 50 mGy/min being a fair estimate for the routine, uncomplicated patient studies. An exception to the limit is the "high-dose rate" feature on fluoroscopic units, including C-arms. This feature is also known as "boost" mode and may be called into use when you encounter an extremely large patient and the normal exposure rate does not produce enough x-rays for the imaging. The high-dose rate feature can go up to 200 mGy/min (20 roentgens/min) skin entrance exposure rate, and a visible and audible alert must be produced by the imaging equipment when operated in this

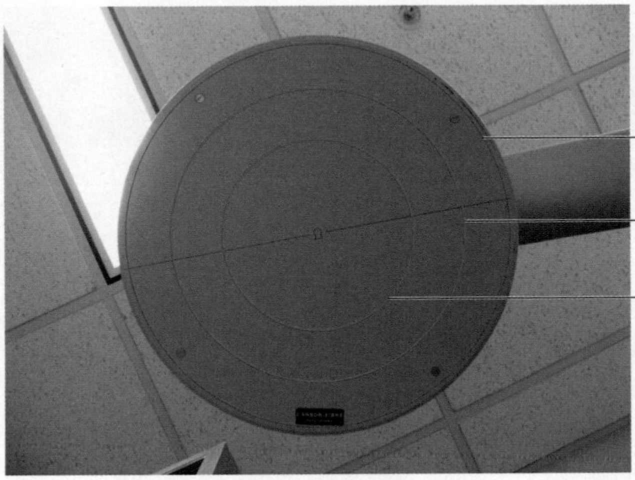

Figure 13A-20. Active viewing area for the 12–9–6 inch modes.

modality. Human skin will suffer epilation from x-rays when it has received radiation exposure as low as 1000 mGy (100 roentgens), and skin erythema occurs with 2000 mGy (200 roentgens) of exposure. These somatic effects take from 1 day to 3 weeks to become evident. You can recognize the value of having a visible and audible alert with an imaging system that can cause 200 mGy/min exposure at skin entrance; this patient may have to cope with radiation damage to the skin at little more than 5 minutes of fluoroscopy time into the procedure at this high exposure rate.

There is another alert located on C-arm devices, the elapsed fluoroscopy time warning bell. The timer routinely alarms at 4 to 5 minutes of elapsed fluoroscopy beam "on" time and has to be reset at the control panel. You can use this as a marker of your progress during the procedure and as a marker of the accrued total skin dose. If you assume 50 mGy/min (5 R/min) skin entrance exposure for a "normal-sized" patient, then 20 minutes of fluoroscopy approaches 1000 mGy.

The acquisition and recording of the fluoroscopic image can be changed at the control panel with the pulsed fluoroscopy feature. In contrast to real-time fluoroscopic images that are captured at a rate of 30 frames per second (33 msec imaging frame time), pulsed fluoroscopy operates with very short exposure times, usually 10 msec per pulse. The outcomes to using this feature are:

1. Reduced patient motion blurring in the acquired image. Picture in your mind the "frozen" and discontinuous images of dancers when a strobe light is pulsing and illuminating the dancers on a dance floor.
2. Reduced total patient and personnel exposures from the reduced amount of x-ray "beam on" time
3. Reduced heat loading of the x-ray tube target, allowing for far longer time of operation in the generation of x-rays

The exposure reduction is proportional to the decrease in the image frame rate. If you drop from 30 to 15 frames per second, you have halved (1/2) the exposures. If you further reduce to 7.5 frames per second, you are at one-fourth (1/4) of the original exposure rate. The drawback lies with the operator; he or she may not like seeing discontinuous images acquired at 15 frames per second and even less so at 7.5 frames per second.

We are accustomed to television video display of 60 frames per second, and real-time fluoroscopy was routinely performed at that imaging rate. This "watching a movie" format gives a sense of fluid motion that is lost at very low image capture rates. With fluoroscopic x-ray imaging, you must realize you are *not watching video entertainment*. You are observing the gross deposition, absorption, and transmission of radiation energy within a patient. If enough energy is imparted to parts of that living body, you may well cause the appearance of deterministic (somatic) radiation effects to the patient within a short period of time.

A lower frame rate feature is desired when the purpose is to observe the general placement of readily observed medical devices such as orthopaedic screws, electric leads, and some catheters. If you need to assess the progress of your work in a millimeter-by-millimeter fashion or you are imaging a structure with a high degree of motion, you will likely prefer 15 frames per second images.

IN SUMMARY: TO OPERATE A C-ARM AND REDUCE THE RADIATION EXPOSURE

The essential information in this chapter for the radiation safe imaging of the patient and the dose-limiting exposure to all involved staff, can be reduced to these key elemental points:

1. **Minimize** the amount of fluoroscopy "on" time. Step off the pedal whenever possible.
2. Use **"good geometry"** by positioning the patient as close to the image intensifier and as far from the x-ray tube as possible.
3. **Reduce the size** of the x-ray field (collimate) to view only the anatomical region of interest, thereby reducing the scattering of x-rays and sparing unintended body tissue(s) from the radiation.
4. **Minimize** use of MAG modes and "boost" (high dose rate) fluoroscopy.
5. Maximize your use and viewing of the **"last image hold."** If nothing has changed, rely on an image already obtained as opposed to generating more x-rays.
6. Whenever possible, select the lowest dose rate (combination of highest kV and lowest mA) **ABC setting** that gives acceptable image quality.

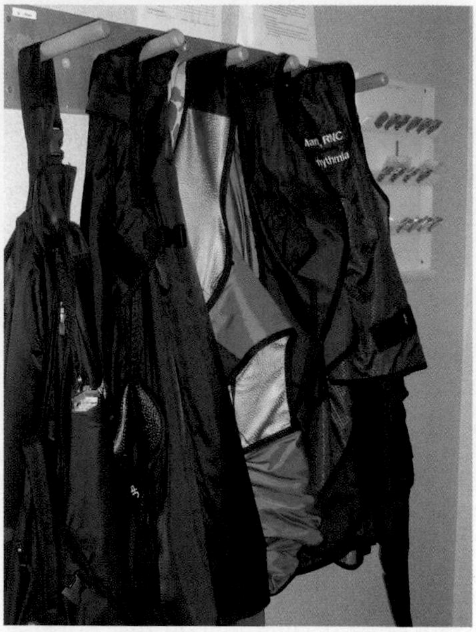

Figure 13A-21. An apron rack next to a procedure room alongside radiation dosimeters.

7. Use **pulsed fluoroscopy.** Use the lowest pulse rate and pulse width (msec) consistent with acceptable temporal resolution.
8. **Vary the x-ray tube angle** (to the extent possible) to reduce the skin dose to any one area when long fluoroscopy times (>20 min) are anticipated for a single procedure. This is especially important for the larger patient population.
9. Stand as a **far as possible** from the point where the x-ray beam enters the patient.

PROTECTION FROM RADIATION OF C-ARM EQUIPMENT WHEN IN OPERATION

The three tenets of radiation protection are:

1. **Time.** Reduce the amount of time you are exposed to radiation, and you reduce your total exposure (again, use pulsed rate fluoroscopy, use last image hold devices).
2. **Distance.** Maintain a safe distance away from the radiation source. Recall how the "inverse-square" law greatly influences the intensity of radiation with changing distance. Increase your distance away from the x-ray beam and patient whenever possible.
3. **Shielding.** When working with an x-ray source, you must wear an appropriate lead-equivalent gown of 0.35 mm lead equivalency or greater (0.25 mm lead equivalency with a mini C-arm device). To avoid cracking the shielding inside the protective garment, store these on suitable racks or laid out unfolded on a table until next use (Fig. 13A-21).

Thyroid shields and leaded glasses are optional pieces of protective equipment, but in a very busy or higher exposure environments, these may be required by your physicist or radiation safety program.

Another matter related to personnel shielding is how to ensure the quality and condition of the radiation safety protective wear for the staff, visitors, patients, and family members when using or in the presence of x-ray radiation. Or possibly

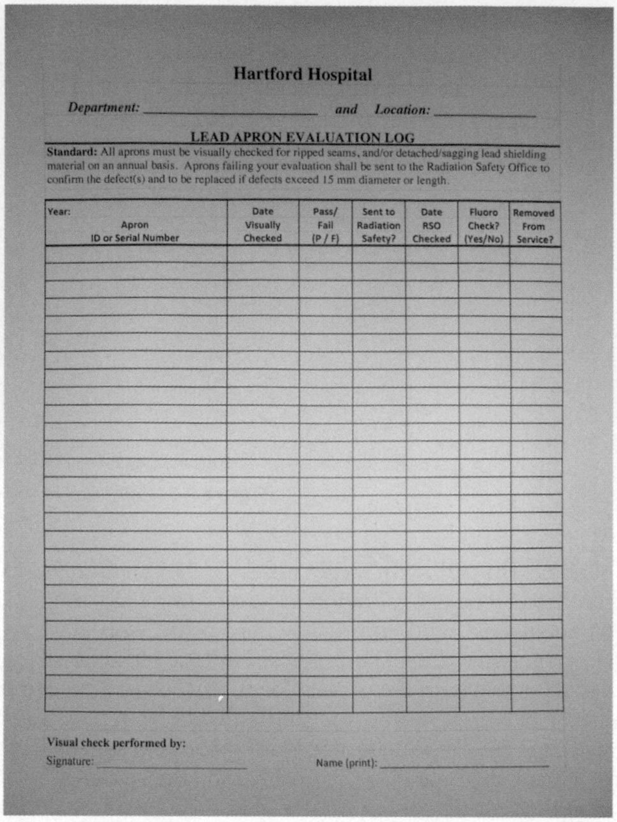

Hartford Hospital

Department: ______ *and Location:* ______

LEAD APRON EVALUATION LOG

Standard: All aprons must be visually checked for ripped seams, and/or detached/sagging lead shielding material on an annual basis. Aprons failing your evaluation shall be sent to the Radiation Safety Office to confirm the defect(s) and to be replaced if defects exceed 15 mm diameter or length.

Year: Apron ID or Serial Number	Date Visually Checked	Pass/ Fail (P / F)	Sent to Radiation Safety?	Date RSO Checked	Fluoro Check? (Yes/No)	Removed From Service?

Visual check performed by:

Signature: ______ Name (print): ______

Figure 13A-22. An inspection log for managing the leaded aprons.

how to comply with the interest of external agencies and professional organizations for the environment of care at the institution. Radiation safety programs go about these in different ways. (Fig. 13A-22). The author advocates the local (departmental) management of leaded shields and garments, with dutiful record keeping of:

- Initial x-ray inspection of a new shield by radiation safety staff
- Assignment to department inventory with unique identifier of the shield
- Yearly visual evaluation by the local user or staff (update of inventory)
- Notify the radiation safety staff if believed defective (confirm or resolve)

The use of radiation dosimeters may or may not be required. This depends on the frequency of use of C-arm units, the duration of the procedures routinely performed, and the level of radiation exposure to the staff. An assessment of the need for dosimeters and of the anticipated future x-ray workload should be conducted by the medical physics or radiation safety staff.

Generally, an imaging service that may result in the operator or exposed staff receiving more than 10% of the yearly allowable maximum radiation exposure will necessitate the use of radiation dosimeters. If used, dosimeters must be worn outside of the lead-equivalent garment (shielded apron) to be exposed to whatever levels of scattered radiation are present in the suite. Placing the dosimeter underneath the shield will keep it from being exposed, yet your head, hands, and feet are not covered by the shield and may receive a fair amount of radiation exposure from the imaging performed.

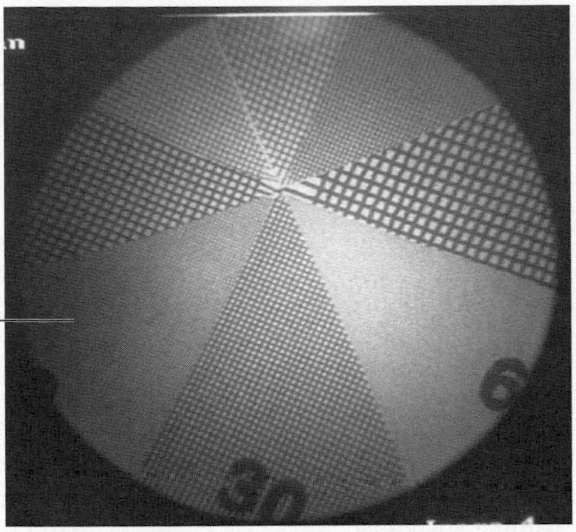

Figure 13A-23. A resolution test pattern with 3 inches of poly(methyl methacrylate) (PMMA) acrylic on the image intensifier of a mini C-arm device. The 50 lines per inch wire mesh pattern is resolved clearly.

ANNUAL INSPECTION OF C-ARM EQUIPMENT

Institutions accredited by The Joint Commission are required to perform safety inspections of radiologic equipment at least yearly. State and local governments may have the same or more stringent requirements, as well as the right to conduct public health inspections and examine the x-ray–producing equipment, the records associated with its continued use (radiologic testing), and the maintenance provided.

Hospital facilities with large radiology, nuclear medicine, and radiation oncology departments are likely to have medical physicists on board to perform the equipment inspection tasks and to ensure that patient images are of the highest quality. A preventive maintenance program will also bring to their attention any equipment that is failing to perform as intended (Fig. 13A-23). These professionals are essential elements for the safe and accurate diagnostic imaging services of the institution and are a valuable resource to the clinicians and the technologists who image patients.

BIBLIOGRAPHY

1. Bushberg JT. *The essential physics of medical imaging*, 2nd ed. Philadelphia, 2002, Lippincott Williams & Wilkins.
2. Huda W: *Review of radiological physics*, 2nd ed, Philadelphia, 2003, Lippincott Williams & Wilkins.
3. Wang J, Blackburn T: *The AAPM/RSNA physics tutorial for residents. X-Ray image intensifiers for fluoroscopy*, 2000, RSNA.
4. National Cancer Institute. *Interventional fluoroscopy. Reducing radiation risks for patients and staff*, NIH Publication No. 05-5286, March 2005.
5. The Food and Drug Administration. Publications viewed at website address; <http://www.fda.gov/cdrh/rsnaii.html>.
6. Balter S, Hopewell J, et al: Fluoroscopically guided interventional procedures: a review of radiation effects on patient's skin and hair. *Radiology* 254(2):326–341, 2010.

13B Prevention of Occupationally Acquired Bloodborne Pathogens

JACK W. ROSS • BRIAN W. COOPER • SUSAN G. MACARTHUR

The emergence of human immunodeficiency virus (HIV) during the 1980s had a profound effect on efforts to prevent occupational transmission of bloodborne infections. As of December 2001, the Centers for Disease Control and Prevention (CDC) had received reports of 57 documented cases and 138 possible cases of occupationally acquired HIV infection among healthcare personnel in the United States since reporting began in 1985.[1] In 1987, the CDC published recommendations to protect healthcare workers from exposure to bloodborne pathogens. These recommendations introduced a concept known as "universal blood and body fluid precautions," or "universal precautions." Because medical history and examination could not reliably identify all patients infected with HIV or other bloodborne pathogens, the CDC recommended that "universal precautions" be consistently used for all patients.[2] Although the CDC's recommendations were voluntarily adopted by hospitals, it was not until 1991 that the Occupational Safety and Health Administration (OSHA), urged by healthcare unions, promulgated the Bloodborne Pathogens Standard (BPS), which mandated healthcare facility compliance.[3] The OSHA Bloodborne Pathogens Standard required employers to formally establish an exposure control plan, provide education and training, institute engineering controls, provide personal protective equipment (PPE), and establish standard safety practices to assure a safe work environment. In addition, healthcare facilities were required to provide free hepatitis B vaccine or obtain a declination from employees whose work duties included contact with blood and other body fluids and to provide exposure evaluation and follow-up treatment for occupationally exposed healthcare workers. OSHA provided compliance oversight and had the administrative authority to levy substantial fines should a healthcare facility fail to adhere to the Bloodborne Pathogens Standard. Although in 1991 the OSHA Bloodborne Pathogens Standard represented a significant change, healthcare facilities have since incorporated these requirements into standard operating procedures, and today most healthcare workers could not imagine working without these basic protections.

Bloodborne infections in healthcare workers may theoretically be caused by any pathogens transmissible by blood, including syphilis, trypanosomiasis, and other bacterial or protozoan parasites. But as a practical matter, the vast majority of the infectious risks after exposure to blood and body fluids are due to bloodborne viruses, chiefly, hepatitis B virus (HBV), hepatitis C virus (HCV), and HIV.

HEPATITIS B VIRUS

Hepatitis B virus was once the most common bloodborne disease acquired by healthcare workers with blood exposure. Before the advent of hepatitis B vaccine, the CDC estimated that more than 12,000 healthcare workers per year were being infected with the HBV. Blumberg and colleagues' discovery of Australia antigen in 1967 was the first step in solving the riddle of viral "serum" hepatitis.[4] The ability to detect hepatitis B surface antigen (HBsAg) and its antibody gave epidemiologic investigators the tools necessary to discover that healthcare workers, in particular surgeons, had a high rate of infection with HBV from unprotected blood exposure.

Hepatitis B virus is an enveloped DNA virus that consists of an outer layer of glycoprotein, the HBsAg, as well as envelope lipids. The viral nucleocapsid contains the viral genome and DNA polymerase plus a protein known as core antigen. In infected liver cells, a third core-associated antigen is known as the hepatitis B e antigen (HBeAg). HBV is transmitted by exposure to blood or body fluids primarily by the percutaneous or mucous membrane route. Among the bloodborne viruses, it is the most highly communicable. Because of its route of transmission, persons are at risk from sexual exposure and vertical transmission from a pregnant woman to her fetus in addition to percutaneous exposure.

The frequency of HBV infection differs dramatically in different regions of the world. Areas of hyperendemicity, the so-called hepatitis belt, stretch from North Asia across Africa to South America. In these areas, the primary route of exposure is vertical transmission or early childhood exposure. In contrast, in the United States and Europe, sexual transmission among adults and intravenous drug use have been the chief modes of spread. Healthcare workers were found to be highly infected with HBV in the 1970s. In fact, HBV infection is likely the leading occupationally acquired illness in healthcare workers.[5]

Acute Infection

After infection, the incubation period until symptomatic illness varies from 6 weeks to 6 months, with an average of 12 weeks. It has been recognized that as many as half of the cases of HBV infection are clinically silent. In those that become symptomatic, common signs and symptoms include anorexia, low-grade fever, nausea, vomiting, and jaundice. Extrahepatic manifestations of illness include urticaria, arthritis, and arthralgias. HBsAg may be detected in serum 2 to 3 weeks before the onset of clinical illness. In uncomplicated cases, the illness resolves with clearance of the virus, clearance of HBsAg, and development of hepatitis B surface antibody, which is recognized as protective.

Chronic Disease

Chronic HBV infection is defined as persistence of HBsAg for greater than 6 months. Progression to chronic infection is higher in the pediatric age group, where 50% to 90% of children develop chronic infection.[6] In otherwise healthy adults, approximately 10% will develop chronic hepatitis B after an acute infection.

Chronic HBV infection is characterized by persistent viral replication in hepatocytes leading to an increased risk for development of cirrhosis and hepatocellular carcinoma. An estimated 15% of adult patients who develop chronic HBV infection will develop one of these complications.

Treatment

There is no treatment other than supportive therapy for acute HBV infection. Clinicians should be alert to signs of overwhelming HBV infection, which occurs in up to 1% of infected individuals. Massive hepatic necrosis may lead to hepatic coma and death. In these cases, urgent liver transplantation may be lifesaving. The therapy of chronic HBV infection is continuing to evolve. Medications such as interferon-α, the nucleoside lamivudine, and other nucleoside antiviral agents have been used with varying degrees of success. The goal of completely eliminating HBV is not achieved in a substantial number of patients who are treated for chronic HBV.

Prevention Before and After Occupational Exposure

Guidelines for the protection of healthcare workers against occupational HBV infection were updated in December 2013 in the "CDC Guidance for Evaluating Health-Care Personnel for Hepatitis B Virus Protection and for Administering Post-exposure Management."[7] The cornerstones of these guidelines are preexposure vaccination, determination of vaccine seroprotection status, and postexposure prophylaxis via passive immunity if no documented immunity.

Current U.S. hepatitis B vaccines are genetically engineered preparations that use recombinant DNA technology. The vaccine consists of recombinant HBsAg. The vaccine is highly recommended for all healthcare workers with potential blood exposure. Hepatitis B vaccine is dosed on a 0-, 1-, and 6-month schedule; however, modified schedules such as 0, 1, 2, and 12 months may also be used. The vaccine is administered by deep intramuscular injection in the deltoid region. Administration of the vaccine in fat-bearing areas such as the gluteus has been found to decrease the immunogenicity of the vaccine response. It is important to check the antibody response 1 or 2 months after receipt of the last dose of the vaccine to ensure a protective level of antibody has developed. In general, 85% to 90% of healthy individuals will develop a protective response to the vaccine. The response rates are lower for older individuals, obese individuals, and persons with chronic illness. Nonresponders to the standard three-dose series may respond to further immunization, and a number of optional follow-on immunization schedules have been recommended.[7,8]

After blood exposure such as a sharps injury in a previously unimmunized individual, the combination of vaccination and passive immunotherapy with hepatitis B immune globulin has been recommended. This combination approach is highly effective at preventing hepatitis B viral infection when the source of the response is known to be infected with HBV. Hepatitis B immune globulin is administered in a dose of 0.06 mL/kg given as a deep intramuscular injection in a large muscle group, such as the gluteal region or thigh. The initial hepatitis B vaccine dose can be given simultaneously at a separate site. It is important to follow up with the subsequent hepatitis B vaccine doses on the proper schedule.

HEPATITIS C VIRUS

By the 1950s, it was clear to investigators that the two major forms of viral hepatitis were "infectious" hepatitis, spread by fecal–oral contamination, and "serum" hepatitis, spread by blood and sexual exposure. With the discovery of hepatitis A, the main cause of "infectious" hepatitis and hepatitis B, it became clear that other agents were causing "serum" viral hepatitis. Hepatitis C was discovered in the early 1990s and found to be the major cause of so-called non-A, non-B hepatitis. HCV infection is now the most common cause of bloodborne infection in the United States. Estimates suggest that 1.0% to 1.8% of the U.S. population has been infected with HCV, depending on cohorts examined.[9,10] Indeed, hepatitis C–related chronic liver disease has become the most common indication for liver transplantation in the United States.

Hepatitis C is transmitted most efficiently by blood exposure. Sexual transmission has been reported but is less frequent. Transmission through blood transfusion, once common, has been dramatically reduced by blood donor serologic screening. It is estimated that injection drug use is the most common mode for infection with HCV in the United States.

Acute hepatitis C infection, as with other types of viral hepatitis, is often asymptomatic. Only 20% to 30% of patients develop symptoms of anorexia, malaise, and abdominal pain. Jaundice occurs in approximately 20% of those infected. The average incubation period is 6 weeks. Antibodies to HCV typically develop 8 to 12 weeks after exposure; however, some individuals remain seronegative for many months. Biochemical alterations in serum alanine aminotransferase (ALT) levels, often in a fluctuating pattern, are the most frequent abnormality found. After acute infection, 10% to 15% of individuals clear the virus without further sequelae, leaving 85% to 90% with chronic hepatitis C viral infection. Among those with chronic hepatitis C viral infection, it is estimated that 10% to 15% will develop cirrhosis over a period of many years. As with hepatitis B, hepatocellular carcinoma is associated with some cases of chronic HCV.

Healthcare workers with blood exposure are at risk for infection with HCV, although, relative to HBV, the risk is much lower. Numerous surveys of healthcare workers estimate that the seroprevalence of HCV antibodies could be similar to that in volunteer blood donors.

Screening

Antibody to HCV is commonly detected by enzyme immunoassay (EIA). This test is highly sensitive; however, false-positive results have occurred, and all positive test results should be confirmed with a more specific assay, such as a HCV RNA nucleic acid assay. Antibody tests do not distinguish between chronic hepatitis C infection and cleared HCV caused by a prior infection. HCV RNA assays can detect HCV viral presence as early as 2 weeks after acute infection. HCV RNA assays are useful in the detection of chronic infections as well as early acute disease and to monitor therapy.

Prevention of healthcare–associated HCV infection centers on prevention of sharps injuries because no vaccine or immunoglobulin has proven useful. Screening for HCV infection after a parenteral exposure is important to identify those who develop acute infection. HCV RNA assays are most useful in this setting. Serodiagnosis of HCV antibodies is less useful because of the delay in development of these antibodies. In the future, postexposure prophylaxis (PEP) may be possible with the new oral medications that are just now becoming available for the treatment of HCV infection.

HUMAN IMMUNODEFICIENCY VIRUS

Among the major transmissible bloodborne viruses that pose a potential risk to healthcare workers, it is clear that HBV and HCV make up the bulk of the risk. Although HIV accounts for substantially fewer cases of occupationally acquired infection, it elicits the most anxiety and attention from healthcare workers.

HIV, an RNA retrovirus, causes the acquired immunodeficiency syndrome (AIDS). It is called a retrovirus because of the enzyme reverse transcriptase, which reverses the usual flow of genetic information. Instead of DNA forming messenger RNA to synthesize protein, reverse transcriptase catalyzes the creation of a complementary DNA copy of the virus's RNA genes.

Upon percutaneous infection, the virus bonds to specific receptors that are chiefly found on cells engaged in host defense, such as lymphocytes and macrophages. In the skin, animal models have shown that the virus binds to dendritic cells within about 24 hours after percutaneous inoculation. The dendritic cells then migrate to regional lymphatics, where lymphocytes are subsequently infected. The virus has a particular affinity for CD4-positive lymphocytes, and its subsequent life cycle leads to the slowly progressive destruction of most CD4 lymphocytes with progressive and ever worsening immunosuppression the result. As the disease progresses, infected patients are subject to a wide variety of infections by opportunistic pathogens, chronic wasting, and a host of malignancies.

The risk for occupational infection by HIV is generally low, but given the severity of illness produced by infection with HIV, much attention has been focused on prevention of occupational HIV exposure and prevention of HIV infection after being exposed. Studies of exposed healthcare workers indicate that the risk of HIV infection after percutaneous exposure to HIV-infected blood is approximately 0.3%.[11]

The risk after mucous membrane exposure (nonpercutaneous injury) is estimated at approximately 0.09%. Although cases of occupational HIV acquisition after blood exposure on intact skin have been anecdotally recorded, the magnitude of the risk is too low to establish an estimate. The magnitude of risk for transmission of HIV after exposure depends on several factors, including the depth of injury, the presence of visible blood on the sharp instrument, the viral load in the source patient, and whether a hollow bore or solid needle transmitted the injury. During percutaneous needle-stick injury, the amount of blood transferred is reduced by glove use, leading to the recommendation for use of double gloving in high-risk settings.[12]

Exposure to a source patient with an undetectable serum viral load does not eliminate the possibility of HIV transmission or the need for postexposure prophylaxis with serial testing. Although the risk of transmission from an occupational exposure to a source patient with an undetectable serum viral load is thought to be very low, postexposure prophylaxis should still be offered. Plasma HIV RNA viral load reflects only the level of cell-free virus in the peripheral blood. The persistence of HIV in latently infected cells, despite appropriate treatment with antiretroviral agents, has been demonstrated, and such cells might transmit infection even in the absence of viremia.[13]

As of 2001, 57 healthcare workers have been reported to the CDC as being infected by HIV most likely by occupational risk. It is thought that little occult undiscovered transmission is occurring among healthcare workers. One way of indirectly assessing the risk of occupational transmission of HIV in healthcare workers is to conduct HIV seroprevalence surveys. A 1992 survey of general surgeons, obstetricians, and orthopaedic surgeons was conducted among practices in moderate to high HIV risk areas. Among the 770 physicians surveyed, only one was seropositive, and he reported nonoccupational behavioral risks.[14] Similarly, a 1991 survey found only two seropositives, both individuals who reported nonoccupational risks.[15] These studies suggest that ongoing occult transmission to surgeons is rare.

Management of Occupational Exposure to HIV

After transmission of HIV, an acute retroviral syndrome resembling a mononucleosis-like illness has been a common finding in healthcare workers who have been occupationally infected. Symptoms such as fever, myalgias, rash, pharyngitis, and adenopathy may occur a median of 25 days after exposure, with a range of 1 to 6 weeks. HIV-specific antibodies appear from 6 weeks to 4 months after exposure in infected individuals. The average interval to development of HIV-specific antibodies has been 2 months. Serodiagnosis is accomplished by routine screening EIA followed by a Western blot for confirmation if the EIA was positive. These routine antibody measurements are usually recommended to be carried out at baseline (after exposure), 6 weeks, 3 months, and 6 months. Direct detection of viral RNA by polymerase chain reaction or antigenic assays such as P24 antigen may be useful as ancillary tests to serodiagnosis, but they should not be used to routinely detect infection in exposed healthcare workers owing to the relatively high rate of false-positive results. Serologic follow-up of exposed healthcare workers should also be accompanied by follow-up counseling and expert medical evaluation.

Postexposure prophylaxis with antiviral agents has become a cornerstone of management of occupational exposure to HIV since 1996. Recommendations for the choice of antiviral agents, dose, and duration have recently been updated in September 2013 in the "Updated U.S. Public Health Service Guidelines for the Management of Occupational Exposure to Human Immunodeficiency Virus and Recommendations for Postexposure Prophylaxis."[16] Use of PEP may be appropriate in percutaneous injury or contact of mucous membrane or nonintact skin with blood, tissue, or potentially infectious body fluids. The following fluids are considered potentially infectious: cerebrospinal, synovial, pleural, peritoneal, pericardial, and amniotic fluids. Feces, nasal secretions, saliva, sputum, sweat, tears, urine, and vomitus are not considered infectious for HIV unless they are visibly bloody. The risk of HIV transmission from these latter fluids is too low to justify postexposure antiviral prophylaxis.

Antiretroviral agents used in prophylaxis should never be used as single agents. Several classes of antiviral agents are available for use as PEP, including nucleoside reverse transcriptase inhibitors, non-nucleoside reverse transcriptase inhibitors, protease inhibitors, and integrase inhibitors. Regimens containing three drugs are now the standard of care. The preferred regimen is raltegravir (Isentress), with tenofovir DF and emtricitabrine in a fixed combination tablet, Truvada. Several alternative regimens are available. The risk stratification of exposures is based on the nature of the injury and the status of the source HIV case.[16] Medication included in an HIV PEP regimen should be selected to optimize side effect and toxicity profiles with a convenient dosing schedule to encourage the healthcare worker's compliance with the regimen.[16] Most authorities recommend starting the PEP as soon as possible, preferably within hours of exposure, and continuing for 4 weeks. If the source patient is found to be HIV negative, PEP should be discontinued, and no HIV follow-up testing is indicated for the exposed healthcare provider.

These antiviral agents are potent drugs with a range of potential toxicities, including headache, nausea, bone marrow depression, diarrhea, peripheral neuropathy, rash (including Stevens-Johnson syndrome), and severe liver toxicity. Expert physicians should carefully monitor persons receiving postexposure antiviral prophylaxis. If expert consultation is not available locally, online and telephonic consultation is available via the PEPline at www.nccc.ucsf.edu/about_nccc/pepline; telephone 888-448-4911.

STRATEGIES TO PREVENT OCCUPATIONAL TRANSMISSION OF BLOODBORNE PATHOGENS

The Hospital Infection Control Practices Advisory Committee (HICPAC), convened periodically by the CDC, published guidelines that detail basic infection control strategies that can significantly reduce the risk of bloodborne and other pathogen transmission among patients and healthcare workers.[17,18] Professional surgical organizations such as the American Association of Orthopaedic Surgeons (AAOS) and the Association of Perioperative Registered Nurses (AORN), have also published specific guidelines for preventing the transmission of bloodborne pathogens. We focus here on a discussion of the screening for bloodborne pathogens, and the use of PPE and safe work practices because they are pivotal in preventing accidental exposures to blood and other body fluids.

Screening for Bloodborne Pathogens

A major prevention strategy for infectious diseases is the use of screening tests to identify infected individuals. Recognition of infection allows the use of medications to decrease the risk of transmission to others and to potentially cure the infected patient. An example of the success of this strategy is the near elimination of transfusion-associated HIV transmission in the United States. Also, routine testing of pregnant women has markedly decreased perinatal and pediatric HIV infection. Identification of infected women has allowed the use of prenatal antiretroviral therapy, the option of C-section for delivery, and the avoidance of breastfeeding post partum.

Human Immunodeficiency Virus

Guidelines are available from the CDC for the routine testing for HIV in all healthcare settings. Most providers are not aware of "Revised Recommendations for HIV Testing of Adults, Adolescents, and Pregnant Women in Healthcare Settings" published in 2006.[19] These guidelines are a departure from risk-based testing and focus on screening, testing consent, and repeat testing. Screening for HIV infection should routinely be offered to all patients age 13 to 64 years in all healthcare settings. All providers should initiate HIV testing unless the prevalence of undiagnosed HIV infection in their region has been documented to be less than 0.1%. If existing data for HIV prevalence are not available, HIV screening should be started. Annual testing is appropriate for those at high risk, including injection-drug users, commercial sex workers, men having sex with men, and heterosexuals not in monogamous relationships.[19]

The CDC recommends that all screening testing will be voluntary, with the patient given the opportunity to opt out. Written consent should not be required, and posttest counseling is optional if results are negative. Unfortunately, not all states have fully adopted these guidelines. Statutory or regulatory impediments may exist to opt-out screening, and posttest counseling may be required in some jurisdictions.[19] The possibility of legal action for failure to diagnose HIV is a concern given the success of current therapeutic regimens.

Hepatitis C Virus

In 2012, the CDC published "Recommendations for the Identification of Chronic Hepatitis C Virus Infection Among Persons Born During 1945-1965."[9] Currently, HCV infection is the leading indication for liver transplantation and a leading cause of hepatocellular carcinoma in the United States. Prior testing recommendations had limited success in identifying HCV-infected patients, and HCV is an increasing cause of morbidity and mortality. The age cohort born from 1945 to 1965 accounts for nearly 75% of Americans infected with HCV, and many of these 2.7 to 3.9 million HCV-infected patients are unaware of their infection.

Benefits of widespread HCV testing will be early identification of infected patients, linkage to care, and initiation of curative therapy. These interventions will be critical disease prevention interventions because approximately 20 new oral HCV therapeutic agents, including protease inhibitors and polymerase inhibitors, are anticipated in the next 5 years. With the first of these agents, cure rates of 70% to 90% have been reported.[20,21] The use of peginterferon for HCV therapy will soon be unnecessary for the majority of patients as additional oral agents become available.

Per CDC recommendations, all adults born from 1945 to 1965 should receive one-time testing for HCV infection without additional risk determination. Screening begins with a test for HCV antibody (anti-HCV), and if positive, confirmation with a HCV RNA nucleic acid test follows. All positive patients are referred for care initiation and HCV therapy.

Management of Bloodborne Pathogen Infected Healthcare Workers

If a healthcare provider acquires or has hepatitis B, hepatitis C, or HIV infection, comprehensive guidelines have been developed by the Society of Healthcare Epidemiology of America (SHEA) for management.[22] These guidelines emphasize the use of infection control measures and the use of virologic control for the provider. One goal is minimizing the patient's exposure to the provider's blood by avoidance of blood transfer from the provider to the patient. A second goal is individual consideration of risk from an infected provider.

Risk is assessed based on the provider's serum viral burden and the risk for bloodborne pathogen transmission in three stratified categories of healthcare-associated procedures. Other factors are frequency of injury to the provider and the infectivity of the agent present.

Expectations for monitoring the provider, for disclosure to potential patients, and for actual exposure control are well delineated. Generally, the guidelines support continued monitored practice, viral load suppression via care linkages, and no disclosure to individual patients if the first two conditions are met. The routine testing of all providers is not recommended.[22]

Personal Protective Equipment

In a surgical setting, gowns, gloves, masks, and hair coverings are worn to preserve the sterile field, but they also serve as an effective barrier against accidental blood and body fluid exposure. Healthcare facilities are required by law to provide appropriate and effective PPE to employees who can reasonably anticipate exposure to blood and other body fluids during the performance of their work duties. OSHA defines PPE as "specialized clothing or equipment worn by an employee for protection against a hazard. General work clothes (e.g., uniforms, scrubs, pants, shirts, or blouses) are not considered to be personal protective equipment."

Gloves

Gloves provide an excellent barrier to blood and body fluid exposure and represent the most common type of PPE used in healthcare. Gloves are available in a variety of sizes, styles, and textures and can be made of latex or synthetic materials. Gloves should be worn whenever exposure to blood and body fluids, excretions, secretions, nonintact skin, and mucous membranes is anticipated. Gerberding demonstrated that the volume of blood transmitted by a needlestick is reduced by 50% when the needle passes through a glove.[23] Double gloving for orthopaedic procedures is recommended by the American Academy of Orthopaedic Surgeons.[24] In addition they recommend that "during procedures where sharp instruments and devices are used, or when bone fragments are likely to be encountered, the surgeon should consider the use of reinforced or cloth gloves that offer a greater amount of protection." Although gloves are an effective barrier, small holes may go undetected; therefore, it is important to always perform a thorough handwashing when the gloves are removed.

Gowns

Surgical gowns protect healthcare workers by providing a barrier to blood and body fluids that are commonly generated during orthopaedic procedures. Gowns and aprons come in a variety of styles and are produced from a number of materials. When selecting a gown, one should consider the activity and amount of fluid likely to be encountered. Soiled gowns should be removed as promptly as possible, and hands should be washed to avoid transfer of microorganisms to other patients or environments.[17]

Masks, Eye Protection, and Face Shields

Orthopaedic surgery frequently generates spatters and splashes of blood and other body fluids owing to the use of powered tools and the types of procedures performed. To protect the mucous membranes of the eyes, nose, and mouth against potential exposures, healthcare workers must wear masks and eye protection. A variety of products are available for mucous membrane protection. Surgical masks, surgical masks with attached plastic shields, face shields, goggles, and eyeglasses with side shields can provide adequate protection against exposure. Soiled masks, eye protection, and face shields should be removed as soon as possible after the procedure, and hands should be washed to avoid transfer of microorganisms to other patients or environments. Reusable protective equipment should be cleaned with an appropriate disinfectant.

Other Personal Protective Equipment

Traditional surgical accessories such as head and shoe covering provide additional barriers against exposure to blood and body fluids during orthopaedic procedures. Hair covering is an effective barrier against spatters and splashes, and footwear such as shoe covers or tall boots protects against the wet environment that can be experienced during orthopaedic procedures. Soiled accessories should be removed as soon as possible after the procedure, and hands should be washed to avoid transfer of microorganisms to other patients or environments.

WORK PRACTICES AND ENGINEERING CONTROLS

Assuring compliance with established guidelines can pose a difficult challenge in the surgical setting. Introducing safer work practices and changing deeply engrained behaviors is a slow but necessary process. OSHA requires that all healthcare workers whose job requirements expose them to blood and other body fluids receive training on the prevention of bloodborne pathogens before they begin those responsibilities. In addition, staff should be oriented to organizational policies and procedures as well as protocols specific to the perioperative setting.

Setting Expectations

Orthopaedic surgeons must set the standard for safe behavior in the operating room and insist on vigilance and compliance by the surgical team. Because surgical team members in close proximity to each other with sharp instruments are frequently required to work with blood and body fluids, inadvertent exposures may occur. For this reason, communication among team members is especially important. If an exposure does occur, the surgeon must strongly encourage reporting of the incident as soon as feasible.

Needles and Sharps

Of the 57 healthcare workers with documented occupationally acquired HIV infection, 51 (88%) had percutaneous injuries. The circumstances varied among the 51 percutaneous injuries, with the largest proportion (41%) occurring after a procedure, 35% occurring during a procedure, and 20% occurring during disposal of sharp objects.[1] In 2001, OSHA revised the Bloodborne Pathogens Standard in response to the Needlestick Safety and Prevention Act.[25] The revised standard clarified the need for employers to select safer needle devices and to involve employees in identifying and choosing these devices. The number of safety needles and needle devices available on the market today is dizzying. New products should be periodically evaluated to determine whether they might reduce parenteral injury. Disposal of needles and other sharps into appropriately sized, puncture-resistant containers can reduce accidental exposures.

Needles are not the only sharp implements in orthopaedic surgery. For instance, the exposed end of all orthopaedic pins should be securely covered with a plastic cap or other appropriate device. The points of pins that have passed through soft tissue should be cut off. Specialized tools can cause cuts or abrasions if not handled properly.[14]

Hands-Free Technique

The traditional method of passing instruments between team members is from hand to hand. To reduce potential exposures, some propose the use of a "neutral zone" to which instruments are returned during a procedure. The neutral zone can be a tray or magnetic pad that aids in the passing of surgical instruments and suture material.

Blunted Surgical Needles

"No-touch suturing techniques should be used whenever possible. Sutures should not be tied with the suture needle in the surgeon's hand. Blunt suture needles are recommended when their use is technically feasible. Two surgeons should not suture the same wound simultaneously."[24]

REGULATED MEDICAL WASTE

During the summer of 1987, New York and New Jersey beaches were closed because syringes, blood vials, and other medical waste products repeatedly washed ashore. The public's concern about HIV/AIDS transmission prompted legislators to enact the Medical Waste Tracking Act (MWTA) of 1988.[26] The MWTA amended the Solid Waste Disposal Act and promulgated regulations on the management of infectious waste. Each state was instructed to implement a medical waste tracking program that was at least as stringent as the federal demonstration program. To protect waste handlers and the general public from inadvertent exposure, medical waste was required to be segregated from other wastes and tracked in labeled containers. The specific solid wastes that require tracking are listed in Box 13B-1, although other types may be included in specific state plans. Healthcare settings have incorporated the segregation of medical waste; however, it is unclear whether this disposal has resulted in transmission prevention.

BOX 13B-1 *Listing of Medical Wastes*

1. Cultures and stocks of infectious agents and associated biologicals, including cultures from medical and pathologic laboratories, wastes from the production of biologicals, discarded live and attenuated vaccines, and culture dishes and devices used to transfer, inoculate, and mix cultures
2. Pathologic wastes, including tissues, organs, and body parts that are removed during surgery or autopsy
3. Waste human blood and products of blood, including serum, plasma, and other blood components
4. Sharps that have been used in patient care or in medical, research, or industrial laboratories, including hypodermic needles, syringes, Pasteur pipettes, broken glass, and scalpel blades
5. Contaminated animal carcasses, body parts, and bedding of animals that were exposed to infectious agents during research, production of biologicals, or testing of pharmaceuticals
6. Wastes from surgery or autopsy that were in contact with infectious agents, including soiled dressings, sponges, drapes, lavage tubes, drainage sets, underpads, and surgical gloves
7. Laboratory wastes from medical, pathologic, pharmaceutical, or other research, commercial, or industrial laboratories that were in contact with infectious agents, including slides and coverslips, disposable gowns, laboratory coats, and aprons
8. Dialysis wastes that were in contact with the blood of patients undergoing hemodialysis, including contaminated disposable equipment and supplies such as tubing, filters, disposable sheets, towels, gloves, aprons, and laboratory coats
9. Discarded medical equipment and parts that were in contact with infectious agents
10. Biological waste and discarded materials contaminated with blood, excretion, exudates, or secretions from human beings or animals that are isolated to protect others from communicable diseases
11. Such other waste material that results from the administration of medical care to a patient by a healthcare provider and is found by the administrator to pose a threat to human health or the environment

SUMMARY

Bloodborne pathogens present an uncommon but real risk to healthcare workers. Although risk cannot be completely eliminated, implementation of basic infection control strategies is an effective way to prevent occupational transmission. Measures such as vaccination, conscientious use of PPE, strict adherence to "universal precautions," and compliance with safe work practices can further reduce the low risk of occupational bloodborne pathogen transmission. Identification of infected patients allows early treatment for the patient and reduces subsequent risks to exposed healthcare providers. Bloodborne pathogen infected healthcare workers can continue to practice in most instances if current guidelines are applied.

KEY REFERENCES

1. Do AN, Ciesielski CA, Metler RP, et al: Occupationally acquired human immunodeficiency virus (HIV) infection: national case surveillance data during 20 years of the HIV epidemic in the United States. *Infect Control Hosp Epidemiol* 24(2):82–85, 2003.
7. Centers for Disease Control and Prevention: CDC Guidance for Evaluating Health-Care Personnel for Hepatitis B Virus Protection and for Administering Postexposure Management. *MMWR* 62(RR-10):1–19, 2013.
9. Centers for Disease Control and Prevention: Recommendations for the Identification of Chronic Hepatitis C Virus Infection Among Persons Born During 1945-1965. *MMWR* 61(RR-4):1–33, 2012.
16. Kuhar DT, Henderson DK, Struble KA, et al: for the US Public Health Service Working Group. Updated US Public Health Service Guidelines for the Management of Occupational Exposure to Human Immunodeficiency Virus and Recommendations for Postexposure Prophylaxis. *Infect Control Hosp Epidemiol* 34(9):875–892, 2013.
17. Garner S: Guideline for isolation precautions in hospitals. *Infect Control Hosp Epidemiol* 17:53–80, 1996; and *J Infect Control* 24:24–52, 1996.
18. Siegal JD, Rhinehart E, Jackson M, et al, 2007 Guideline for Isolation Precautions: Preventing Transmission of Infectious Agents in Healthcare Settings. Available at: <http://www.cdc.gov/ncidod/dhqp/pdf/isolation2007.pdf>.
19. Centers for Disease Control and Prevention: Revised Recommendations for HIV Testing of Adults, Adolescents, and Pregnant Women in Health-care Settings. *MMWR* 55(RR-14):1–17, 2006.
24. American Academy of Orthopedic Surgeons. Advisory Statement: Preventing the Transmission of Bloodborne Pathogens. Available at: <http://www.aaos.org/about/papers/advistmt/1018.asp>.
26. Medical Waste Tracking Act of 1988 (H.R. 3515). 40 Code of Federal Regulations 22, 259. Mar. 24, 1989.

The complete References list is available online at https://expertconsult.inkling.com.

Chapter 14

Medical Management of the Orthopaedic Trauma Patient

14A Acute Pain Management, Regional Anesthesia Techniques, and Management of Complex Regional Pain Syndrome

RICHARD GANNON • DEAN MARIANO • DANIEL J. GIANOLI • RICHARD SHEPPARD

In 1995, the president of the American Pain Society, Dr. James Campbell, argued that pain was the "fifth vital sign" and suggested that to provide effective care, a patient's pain should be quantified and treated. In 2001, the Joint Commission on Accreditation of Healthcare Organizations (JCAHO; now The Joint Commission) recognized that "unrelieved pain has physical and psychological effects" and sought to provide care facilities with guidelines to improve access to pain assessment and management. The JCAHO guidelines sought (1) to promote respecting a patient's right to be evaluated and treated for pain, and in particular for pain to be assessed at the initial evaluation and during all clinically relevant encounters, and (2) to educate patients and their families about available pain management strategies.

The continued evolution of health care from a paternalistic model to a more consumer-based model combined with the continued growth of the Internet and various social media platforms have placed a high value on care facility services and their image. Hospital surveys such as the ones provided by Hospital Consumer Assessment of Healthcare Provider and Systems (HCAHPS) seek to provide the public with data regarding patients' perspectives on hospital care. These standardized surveys aim to obtain patients' perspectives so that consumers may have an "apples to apples" comparison of their satisfaction with local facilities. In such surveys, pain management services are evaluated with the following questions: "During this hospital stay, how often was your pain well controlled?" and "During this hospital stay, how often did the hospital staff do everything they could to help you with your pain?"

Pain is a very personal experience, and despite the best efforts on the part of health care providers, it is common for there to be a disconnect between what healthcare providers view as adequate management and what patients experience. In a study of critically ill patients,[1] 95% of surveyed house staff believed that they had achieved adequate pain control for their patients. However, 74% of patients rated their pain as being in the moderate to severe range. Recent studies have shown that pain scores do not necessarily correlate with global satisfaction ratings by patients.[2] It has been suggested that although it is important to try to obtain adequate pain control, patient satisfaction scores correlate more strongly with the patient's perception that caregivers were doing everything they could to provide pain control.[3]

As clinicians, we tend to view pain as an invaluable part of the history and physical examination that can aid in determining a diagnosis. In truth, pain is an extremely complex and dynamic process that merits special attention. Over the past 2 decades, the way clinicians approach and treat acute pain processes has undergone a dramatic evolution. It has long been recognized that a patient's exposure to noxious stimuli results in not only a stress response that can potentially increase morbidity and mortality but also a neuroendocrine response that may potentially lead to altered pain states and the development of chronic pain.[4,5] Poorly controlled pain can lead to dysfunctions in a multitude of physiologic systems. Derangements in ventilation, hemodynamics, immune response, and coagulation complicate the care of patients, especially those who are acutely injured. Ultimately, this results in delayed mobilization, rehabilitation, and discharge.[6] Given that today's society expects sophisticated and effective treatments for their pain, coupled with the fact that reimbursement is becoming increasingly linked to patient satisfaction and participation in quality assurance programs, institutions and providers must be willing to take a more customized approach to pain management.

As our understanding of pain transmission and perception continues to deepen, it is evident that a multimodal, multidisciplinary approach is better suited to provide more tailored effective pain management.

NEUROPHYSIOLOGY OF PAIN PROCESSING

"Humans'" ability to successfully navigate and survive the environment is intimately tied to our ability to process both internal and external sensory information. At its core, the ability to transduce, transmit, and process sensory information is a protective mechanism. It is a highly evolved, complex, interconnected network of neurons that allow us to perceive and react to a variety of noxious and non-noxious stimuli. Processing of sensory information in higher brain centers results in the ability to learn from the experiences so that potentially harmful exposures can be minimized in the future.

So important is our ability to sense noxious and potentially noxious stimuli that the system has extensive built-in redundancies as well as the ability to adapt. These features provide unique challenges to the clinicians who attempt to provide pain management. The redundancies and lack of a final common pathway for pain processing make it difficult to provide simple effective solutions for pain management. The plasticity of the system can reduce the effectiveness of what were once successful treatments for pain management and lead to chronic pain states. By providing a broad overview of this complex system, clinicians will be better equipped to provide effective treatment strategies.

Nociceptors and Primary Afferents

Sensory neurons are pseudounipolar and originate in the dorsal root ganglion. A single process projects from the soma and later splits. The peripheral limb goes to target structures to collect sensory information while a central process transmits sensory information to the spinal cord or brainstem. A variety of sensory neurons exist and can be classified by the diameter of their axon, the presence of myelination, and their transmission rate. As peripheral sensory axons approach their target structures, they branch to form a terminal arbor. Structures that have a high degree of spatial resolution for sensory discrimination have less branching or arborization.[7] In the periphery, sensory neurons transduce chemical, mechanical, and thermal input into electrical signals that are carried to the central nervous system (CNS). Sensory axons that transduce non-noxious stimuli can possess specialized encapsulated nerve terminals that make them efficient at responding to specific stimuli such as mechanical distortion or vibration. Sensory nerves involved in nociception tend to be unencapsulated or have free endings and can respond to a variety of stimuli (thermal, mechanical, and chemical).

When a stimulus is sufficient to evoke a response, an electrical impulse is generated. Discharge of the axon is directly related to the intensity of the stimulus. As stimulus intensity increases, the frequency of discharge increases proportionately. Low-threshold sensory neurons, such as Aβ fibers, are triggered by non-noxious stimuli. An increase in terminal discharge frequency of these fibers gives us the ability to perceive the change in stimulus. For example, non-nociceptive neurons that transduce temperature information at 30° C will increase their firing frequency as the temperature increases over a non-noxious range, resulting in the sensation of warmth. Aδ fibers are small (in diameter), myelinated neurons containing both low- and high-threshold terminals. Activation of these terminals can be initiated by non-noxious stimuli. As the stimulus intensifies, firing frequency continues to increase even when the stimulus enters an aversive range. Small unmyelinated C fibers are slow conducting and possess high-threshold terminals. Because these fibers transduce a variety of noxious stimuli such as chemical, mechanical, and thermal, they are often referred to as polymodal. When a noxious stimulus is present, high-threshold terminals from both the Aδ and C polymodal fibers are activated. Because Aδ fibers have higher conduction velocity, their activation produces sharp and focal first pain. Information carried by slowly conducting C polymodal fibers is perceived as dull, achy second pain.

In general, nociceptive neurons fall within the classification system presented. However, this is an oversimplification, and it should be noted that sensory neurons with the ability for nociception range in cell size, axon diameter, and degree of myelination. More recent efforts to find nociceptive-specific attributes have led researchers to investigate cellular markers such as protein and ion channels. To date, no particular cellular markers are exclusive to nociceptive neurons.

From a functional standpoint, nociceptors have two unique qualities. First, they have the ability to transduce and transmit noxious stimuli. Second, they have the ability to sensitize. After the application of noxious stimuli, nociceptors adapt in such a way that they become more excitable. A rise in the resting membrane potential produces a state by which less stimulation is required to produce activation. This phenomenon is referred to as *primary hyperalgesia*. Sensitization is an important process; if left unchecked, it can lead to the sensitization of higher order neurons within the CNS. Studies have shown that the alteration of ion channels that lead to sensitization are a result of the chemical milieu that develops after tissue damage. Although researchers have identified numerous chemical mediators that contribute to sensitization, it is apparent that products from the cyclooxygenase (COX) pathway play important roles. Nonsteroidal antiinflammatory drugs (NSAIDs) have been shown to be effective agents in combating primary hyperalgesia.

Central Nervous System Relay and Processing

A transverse section of the spinal cord reveals areas of white and gray matter. The white matter is an arrangement of myelinated tracts of ascending and descending axons, and the gray matter is composed of cell bodies. Cell bodies within the gray matter vary by location. The Rexed classification system divides these locations into 10 distinct laminae (Fig. 14A-1).

The central processes of the sensory neurons enter the spinal cord through the dorsal roots. These processes synapse on cell bodies located throughout the dorsal horn (laminae I–VI) as well as around the central canal (laminae X). Nociceptive neurons primarily synapse in laminae I, II, V, VI, and X. In addition to making synaptic contact at the neurons' level of entry, they may travel rostrally or caudally along Lissauer tract, reaching areas up to six spinal segments away.[8] Generally speaking, nociceptive afferents responsible for encoding information from cutaneous structures tend to localize their input in a single spinal level. Afferents originating in visceral or deep structures demonstrate collateralized branching, which enter Lissauer tract accessing distant spinal segments and a variety of laminae.[9]

As stated previously, second-order neurons located within the grey matter can vary by location. Lamina I, or the marginal zone, contains a heterogeneous group of cell bodies that form the outermost portion of the dorsal horn. This portion of the dorsal horn is highly innervated with afferent inputs that are primarily from C polymodal and Aδ fibers. Afferents from these fibers release excitatory amino acids (glutamate) and neuropeptides (substance P, calcitonin gene-related peptide) that activate cell bodies within the lamina to continue signal transduction. Projections from these second-order neurons continue to supraspinal structures such as the medulla, midbrain, and thalamus. Alternatively, they can act intrasegmentally or intersegmentally as interneurons form synapses with cell bodies in other laminae.

Lamina II, or the substantia gelatinosa, also contains a heterogeneous group of cell bodies. These cells receive direct nociceptive input from C fibers as well as indirect input from

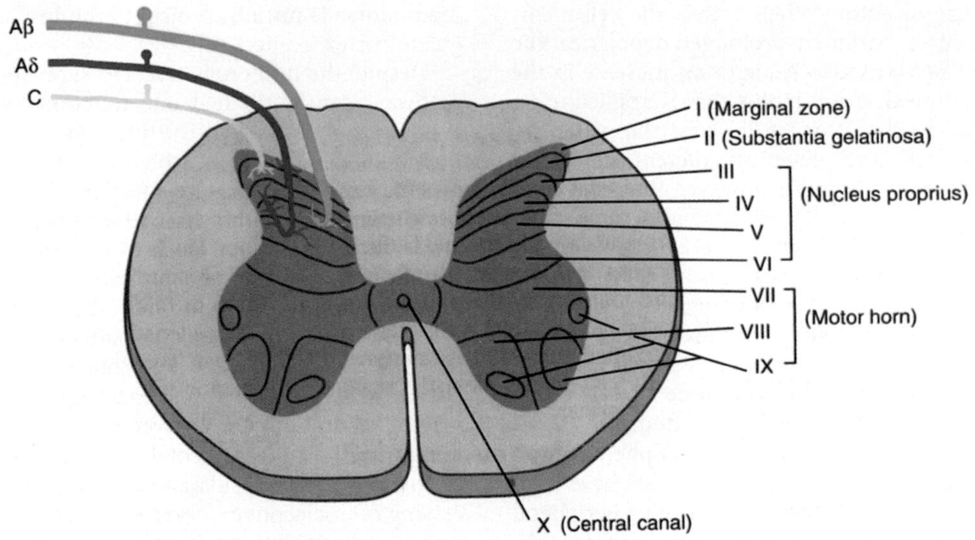

Figure 14A-1. Rexed lamina classification system.

the Aδ fibers of lamina I. In addition to primary nociceptive inputs, the cell bodies of this lamina receive serotonergic and noradrenergic connections from descending axonal projections. Although these cells have some projections to supraspinal structures, the vast majority are involved in interneuron connections with a dense network of axonal and dendritic arborizations forming axodendritic, dendrodenritic, and axoaxonic synapses. These interneurons can release inhibitory neurotransmitters, such as γ-aminobutyric acid (GABA), and their cell bodies exhibit complex responses with the ability to undergo prolonged periods of excitation or inhibition. The structure and function of these interneurons suggest that they play a significant role in the regulation of afferent signal transmission.

Laminae III, IV, and V are known collectively as the nucleus proprius. Afferent information to this area is primarily from large, highly myelinated, low-threshold Aβ fibers. Cell bodies in this lamina send their projections to overlying lamina as well as into the dorsal columns. In addition to input from low-threshold fibers, the cells of lamina V receive input from Aδ and C fibers. Dendritic extensions of these cells project throughout laminae I and II as well as to supraspinal sites, including the brainstem, thalamus, and hypothalamus.

Lamina X is an area around the central canal where cell bodies receive bilateral afferent input from mostly high-threshold (nociceptive) afferent fibers. These cells also receive afferent projections from the viscera.

In addition to differences in anatomic location, the second-order neurons display important functional differences. Functionally, second-order neurons are categorized by whether they produce excitatory responses to noxious stimuli, such as high-intensity mechanical or thermal sensory input, or innocuous stimuli such as vibration. These second-order neurons are typically described as being class 1 (excited by innocuous stimuli), class 2 (excited by both innocuous and noxious stimuli), and class 3 (excited by only noxious stimuli). Often, class 1 neurons are referred to as "low threshold," class 2 is referred to as "wide dynamic range (WDR)," and class 3 as "nociceptive specific." Class 3, or nociceptive specific, is typified by second-order neurons that exist within the superficial dorsal horn. These cells receive primary afferent input from Aδ and C fibers and are active only when the incoming stimulus is in the aversive range. As the intensity of the noxious stimulus escalates, the frequency of discharge from these second order neurons will increase. Class 2 neurons, or WDR, represent most of the second-order neurons present in the deep dorsal horn (laminae IV–VI) but they can also be found in the superficial horn (≈20%). Unlike nociceptive-specific neurons, the WDR neurons can be triggered by innocuous as well as aversive stimuli. As the intensity of the stimulus increases from non-noxious to noxious range, WDR neurons increase their frequency of discharge. WDR neurons are also referred to as "convergence" neurons because of their activation by both somatic and visceral afferents. At a given spinal level, neurons located in the nucleus proprius receive sensory information from a specific area of the body. Information from visceral structures activating the same WDR neuron that is receiving cutaneous somatic information in the nucleus proprius will be referred to that area of the body. The convergence of visceral or deep tissues (joints, bones, and muscle) with cutaneous sites on WDR neurons is the mechanism by which we experience referral patterns and referred pain. The last function that distinguishes WDR neurons from low-threshold and nociceptive-specific neurons is their ability to become sensitized. Persistent C-fiber activation of WDR neurons at a frequency greater than 0.5 Hz produces an increase in the frequency of discharge. During periods of tissue injury or ongoing inflammatory processes, repetitive C-fiber (not A-fiber) activation will result in a facilitated or sensitized state. Repeated stimulation of the WDR neurons results in prolonged partial depolarization that raises the resting membrane potential. In this state, afferent stimulation is much more likely to result in signal transmission. This phenomenon is referred to as "wind up" and has been linked to the activation of NMDA (*N*-methyl-D-aspartate) receptors. NMDA receptors are both voltage and ligand gated, and when in an open configuration, they allow for the influx of sodium and calcium. NMDA receptors that are in a closed state possess magnesium ions that intracellularly block their channels. After sustained depolarization of the cell membrane, the magnesium ion will disassociate from the receptor. When active, the cell membrane will experience an extremely prolonged depolarization. Activation of WDR neurons also leads to an increase in the receptive field, meaning that a stimulus that is applied to an area that is adjacent to the injury will cause the patient to experience pain. As mentioned previously, afferent fibers enter the spinal cord at a specific segment; however, they may send projections rostrally and caudally, synapsing in other segments via Lissauer tract. Sensitization of these distal segments produces an area of secondary hyperalgesia that is located near the site of injury. An overall reduction in threshold for these sensitized second-order neurons can lead to their activation by normally non-noxious stimuli. For example, afferent information from Aβ fibers within the zone of secondary hyperalgesia can lead to WDR neuron firing frequencies that signal painful stimulus. To prevent the central phenomenon of wind-up and secondary hyperalgesia, clinicians have tried to use preemptive analgesic strategies. The use of peripheral nerve blockade or combination pharmacotherapy (opioids, NSAIDs, and anticonvulsants) before injury can have a profound effect on reducing these hyperalgesic phenomena. Additionally, the uses of NMDA receptor antagonists such as ketamine and dextromethorphan have shown promise.

Nociceptive information relayed in the spinal cord is transmitted to distal spinal cord segments and supraspinal structures, such as the thalamus, hypothalamus, midbrain, and medulla, through long tract systems. Axons from second-order neurons in the dorsal horn travel within the white matter, forming tracts mainly in the ventrolateral quadrants and, to a lesser extent, the dorsal midline. The tracts of the ventrolateral quadrant include the spinoreticulothalamic, spinomesencephalic, spinoparabrachial, and spinothalamic projections. Cells contributing to the spinoreticulothalamic pathway originated from the deep dorsal horn and ascend to reach multiple nuclei within the reticular formation of the brainstem. These areas are involved with autonomic regulation as well as modulation of nociceptive processing. The spinomesencephalic tract is composed of axons from cell bodies within lamina I and V and project predominately to the nuclei in the midbrain. These include the periaqueductal grey, cuneiform, and collicular nuclei. With projections to the periaqueductal gray, this tract plays a role in integrating motor, autonomic, and antinociceptive responses. Projections from the spinoparabrachial tract make synaptic connections with the parabrachial region, which lies adjacent to the superior cerebellar peduncle at the junction of the pons and midbrain. The parabrachial region serves as a relay to the amygdala, ventral medial nucleus of the thalamus, and hypothalamus. Nociceptive information on this tract reaches higher brain centers that are involved with emotional and hormonal responses to pain. The spinothalamic tract plays a central role in the transmission of nociceptive information. Second-order neurons from lamina I and V send axons across the midline to the lateral spinothalamic tract, where they proceed uninterrupted to the thalamus. Information regarding the location, intensity, and duration of nociceptive stimuli is transmitted via this tract as well as the sensation of temperature. Synaptic targets of this tract include the ventrobasal thalamus, ventral medial nucleus of the thalamus, and the mediodorsalis nucleus. Information to the ventrobasal thalamus is in a strict somatotopic pattern that is preserved as it is relayed to the somatosensory cortex. The ventral medial nucleus and mediodorsalis nucleus project to the insula and anterior cingulate cortex, respectively.

Despite the numerous tracts to supraspinal structures, the pathways can be divided into functionally distinct response systems for simplicity. The first system consists of axonal projections of WDR neurons, and the second pertains to projections of nociceptive-specific neurons. WDR neurons project into the brainstem, thalamus, and hypothalamus. These neurons are able to provide not only information of stimulus intensity over a broad range, but they are also able to preserve spatial localization by their somatotopic arrangement. The nociceptive-specific pathway arises from primarily lamina I cells and encodes high-intensity stimuli. This pathway only provides information regarding location and intensity when the stimulus is in an aversive range. This group projects mainly to the ventral medial and mediodorsal nuclei before continuing to the insula and anterior cingulate cortex. Processing of nociceptive information in these supraspinal structures results in the emotional and motivational components of the pain experience.

TREATMENT OPTIONS

Advancements in pharmacotherapy and regional analgesic techniques have provided clinicians with a vast assortment of treatment options. The goal in developing any treatment strategy should be to provide a plan that is safe, simple, and efficient. Care plans should be individualized to the patient by taking into account his or her past medical history, current illness, and comprehensive physiologic function. By doing so, techniques that may potentially exacerbate already impaired functions, such as hemodynamics or ventilation, can be minimized or avoided. Ultimately, providing individualized treatment plans should help clinicians to mitigate morbidity and mortality.[10]

Opioids

Systemic opioid therapy has been used for centuries and to this day remains one of the mainstays in treating acute pain. Opioids exert their effects primarily through μ-opioid receptors. Opioids are advantageous in that they have multiple routes of delivery, vary in onset and duration, and theoretically have no analgesic ceiling. Despite these advantages, opioids are usually limited by various side effects such as nausea, vomiting, constipation, sedation, and respiratory depression. A study by Zhao and colleagues[11] suggested that administration of every 3 mg of morphine or its equivalent in a 24-hour period was associated with the development of an additional side effect or hospital-related complication.[12] Long-term administration of opioids is fraught with the potential for serious complications such as the development of tolerance, dependence, and opioid-induced hyperalgesia. Although the use of opioids remains a fundamental part of acute pain management, it should not be viewed as the only treatment available.

Patient-Controlled Analgesia

In the acute phase of pain management, the delivery of intravenous (IV) opioids by patient-controlled analgesia (PCA) systems is quite advantageous. Compared with traditional as needed (PRN) regimens, the use of PCA systems can help eliminate interpatient pharmacokinetic variances and access

TABLE 14A-1 *USUAL PATIENT-CONTROLLED ANALGESIA MEDICATIONS AND DOSES*

	Concentration	Continuous	Demand Dose	Demand Interval	4-Hour Lockout
Fentanyl	10 mcg/mL	10 mcg/hr	10 mcg	5–10 min	300 mcg
Hydromorphone	0.2 mg/mL	0.2 mg/hr	0.2 mg	6–15 min	6 mg
Morphine	1 mg/mL	1 mg/hr	1 mg	6–15 min	30 mg
Meperidine (not recommended)	10 mg/mL	10 mg/hr	10 mg	6–15 min	150 mg

delays. Deliveries by IV methods also produce more predictable drug serum levels as opposed to traditional intramuscular delivery methods. Safe and effective use of this treatment method occurs when patients adhere to self-administration of medication only when they experience pain. Violation of this premise by the patient, family members, or staff can lead to undesired complications such as oversedation or respiratory depression.[13,14] Complications related to equipment malfunction have been reported, but the vast majority of problems related to the use of PCA systems stem from user or programming errors.[13]

The initial setup of the PCA is relatively simple but requires the clinician to consider several variables. Among these variables, the clinician should select the drug to be infused, the demand dose, the lockout interval between doses, and the appropriateness of a basal infusion. Selection of these variables should be based on clinical judgment because an optimal setting for demand dose and lockout interval does not exist. After the initiation of the PCA system, its effectiveness should be assessed by reviewing visual analog pain scores with the patient as well as by interrogation of the PCA device itself. By interrogating the PCA device, the clinician can review information such as how often bolus demands were made as well as the number of doses delivered. Whereas demand dosing that is too low can result in inadequate levels of analgesia, demand doses that are too high can produce unwanted side effects such as sedation and respiratory depression.[15] Lockout intervals should be selected so that after the delivery of the demand dose, the patient has the opportunity to evaluate its effectiveness before delivering another dose. Lockout intervals that are too short can lead to stacking of boluses and increases in opioid-related side effects. Intervals that are too long can cause temporal gaps of inadequate analgesia. Opioids that are commonly used in PCAs (Table 14A-1) have onset times around 5 minutes (1–2 minutes for fentanyl) with peak effect occurring between 7 and 15 minutes (5–7 minutes for fentanyl). Based on the onset and peak time for the opioid delivered, lockout times generally vary between 5 to 10 minutes. Adjustment in the lockout interval in this range does not appear to contribute to the generation of side effects nor does it seem to change degree of analgesia.[12,15] The final element to be considered is the use of a continuous basal rate. Basal rates were initially thought to improve analgesia particularly during sleep. Studies have shown that basal infusions, even if limited to nighttime, do not improve analgesia or sleep patterns.[16-18] The routine use of basal infusions in opioid-naïve patients has been shown to result in a higher incidence of opioid-related side effects such as oversedation and respiratory depression.[16,19] Although it is not recommended that all patients receive continuous infusions, some patient populations may benefit. For example, the use of continuous infusions have been shown to improve analgesia in opioid-tolerant patients as well as children.

Studies have shown that the implementation of PCAs in postoperative settings provides superior postoperative pain control and improved patient satisfaction. Several meta-analyses comparing PCAs with traditional PRN regimens indicated that although opioid consumption was higher in the PCA group, the incidence of opioid-related side effects, with the exception of pruritus, did not differ significantly between groups.[20-22] The rate of serious complications such as respiratory depression with PCAs is less than 0.5%, but clinicians should be aware of factors that may increase this risk such as advanced age, concomitant use of sedatives, comorbid sleep apnea, and advanced pulmonary disease.

ASSESSMENT

Involving the patient in the pain assessment is crucial because the description of the patient's pain will enable the practitioner to most effectively treat the patient's pain appropriately. The use of pain scales has helped objectify a subjective phenomenon.[23] An assessment or rating of the patient's degree of sedation in conjunction with the pain scale may help avoid excessive sedation and respiratory depression.[24] Both the RASS (Richmond Agitation Sedation Scale) and the POSS (Pasero Opioid-induced Sedation Scale) have been validated as tools to assess for opioid-induced sedation.[25] Institutions use a pain scale that best suits their patient population. Examples of pain scales include numerical (0–10), descriptive (excellent–poor), faces (smiling–sad), and behavioral for cognitively impaired patients (e.g., grimacing, vocalizations, resistance to care). One of the most important questions for the patient is, "How would you describe your pain?" The importance of this question rests on the fact that if a patient has predominantly neuropathic pain (burning, muscle spasms, shooting, stabbing), then adjuvants such as anticonvulsants should be used in conjunction with opioids.[26]

Whether the patient describes mostly somatic pain (aching, throbbing) musculoskeletal pain or visceral (deep, crampy, diffuse) abdominal pain, then acetaminophen, NSAIDs, or opioids are the medications of choice.

Patients sometimes have unrealistic expectations regarding the amount of pain they will have after surgery, saying, "I want to be pain free." Patient education concerning pain management during the perioperative period is very important. The goal should be to decrease a patient's pain from excruciating to manageable. It is unrealistic for a patient to expect to have no pain or that the pain will be eliminated immediately after surgery. It is important to review with a patient during preoperative teaching all the options available for pain management during the perioperative period. For patients taking long-acting opioids before surgery, it is important for them to take a dose the morning of surgery (except Suboxone); otherwise, their pain may be more difficult to manage postoperatively.

PHARMACOTHERAPY

Nonsteroidal Antiinflammatory Drugs

Before surgery, a thorough medication history needs to be done. Medications that the patient is taking preoperatively may need to be held before surgery. Both aspirin and herbal medications need to be held for 1 week before surgery. Nonselective NSAIDs should be held for 3 to 4 days before surgery because NSAIDs cause platelet dysfunction. If an analgesic is needed, then acetaminophen or celecoxib can be used because they do not have an effect on platelet function.[27] When celecoxib (Celebrex) is part of our analgesic order set, we only give it for 3 days at doses of 200 mg once or twice per day. Doses of celecoxib, 400 to 800 mg/day, along with prolonged therapy seem to have the side effect of increased cardiovascular death.[28]

Using NSAIDs postoperatively for their antiinflammatory effect may decrease the use of postoperative opioids by 20% to 40% while maintaining the same degree of analgesia.[29-31] The NSAIDs appear to be equally effective when equivalent doses are used. The efficacy of NSAIDs may be patient specific so that if a patient fails to respond to one NSAID, a different one can be tried. It is best to give NSAIDs around the clock (ATC) rather than PRN because NSAIDs inhibit a cascade of cytokine activation. If a patient has constant pain, ATC use of NSAIDs provides more consistent and constant analgesia.

There may be a pharmacodynamic interaction between aspirin and some of the nonselective NSAIDs in terms of affecting platelet function.[32] The inhibition of platelet function is a COX-1–mediated effect. If the nonselective NSAID is given on a consistent basis or before the daily dose of aspirin, the NSAID will occupy the COX-1 site on the platelet, inhibiting the ability of the aspirin to cause an irreversible inhibition of platelet function. Nonselective NSAIDs will only temporarily impair platelet function. The COX-2–selective NSAIDs do not interfere with aspirin's effect on platelets.

Certain patients should not receive NSAIDs because of the high risk of precipitating congestive heart failure or acute renal failure.[33] Patients at risk have as preexisting conditions congestive heart failure, renal dysfunction, or liver disease with ascites.[34] Short-term use of NSAIDs (<90 days) may cause recurrent atrial fibrillation or recurrent myocardial infarction.[35,36]

Data in animals suggest that NSAIDs have an effect on bone healing.[37] It may be that short-term (<7 days), moderate-dose, and COX-2 preferential drugs have less of an effect on fracture healing. There is not enough definitive human data published to answer this question.[38-40] For patients with pain caused by acute fractures, the short-term use of NSAIDs is not detrimental, but long-term use may prevent fractures from fusing. NSAIDs can be given to hip replacement and trauma patients to prevent heterotopic ossification. Naproxen, 500 mg every 12 hours for 2 weeks, has been successful.[37]

Acetaminophen

Sometimes acetaminophen, 1 g, is given as part of a preemptive analgesic regimen and then continued postoperatively as 1 g four times a day.[41] IV acetaminophen is used in our patients who are NPO (nothing by mouth) or have impaired medication absorption. There is not a large "first-pass" effect, so the doses IV and oral are equivalent—1 g every 6 hours. If a patient weighs less than 50 kg then the IV dose is 15 mg/kg every 6 hours. It is best to give acetaminophen ATC as blood levels over 10 to 15 mcg/mL correlate with analgesia.[42] IV acetaminophen adds to opioid analgesia, is opioid sparing, and overall may decrease opioid side effects in patients.[43] Because 4 g/day is the suggested maximum daily dose of acetaminophen, other acetaminophen-containing products should be avoided. Patients may have a prolongation of the international normalized ratio when acetaminophen 4 g/day is given while they are taking warfarin.[44] Certain patients are at risk for acetaminophen hepatotoxicity if more than 4 g/day is given. Patients who are alcoholic, have liver dysfunction, or are taking enzyme-inducing medications such as rifampin or carbamazepine have a higher potential for hepatotoxicity from acetaminophen.

Opioids

Patients may be using opioids before surgery. The amount of opioid used before surgery needs to be considered when deciding what medication and what dose should be used for postoperative analgesia. If a patient is using opioids before surgery, then giving just PRN opioids for postoperative pain control may result in poor analgesia, adverse effects, overdosing or underdosing, dosing intervals that are too long, or conflicts between patients and provider willingness to give pain medication. In an effort to resolve some of these issues, PCA has become popular. With this method of administering opioids, a continuous amount of opioid may be given as well as providing the patient with access to a "demand" dose of analgesic available at a specific interval, usually every 6 to 15 minutes.[45] Currently, only morphine and meperidine are approved by the Food and Drug Administration and available in prefilled PCA syringes. We rarely use meperidine PCA because of its potential for metabolite (normeperidine) accumulation. Normeperidine accumulation, especially with renal dysfunction, may cause agitation, myoclonus, and seizures. Empty PCA syringes are available that can be filled with morphine at high concentrations, or other opioids may be used (fentanyl, hydromorphone, buprenorphine). Patients who are obese, have sleep apnea, elderly, or opioid naïve should be started on demand-only PCA. The literature suggests that demand-only dosing is just as effective and safer than continuous plus demand dosing in patients who are opioid naïve.[45]

Some patients take significant doses of opioids before surgery. If these patients are started on the "usual" doses of PCA analgesics, they will have poor pain control or opioid withdrawal. Patients using PCA can have their long-acting ATC analgesics continued, but the PCA should be used in demand mode only. These patients will require higher than usual demand dosing. Use of both the patient's own opioid and the continuous opioid from the PCA could result in side effects. What we usually do is discontinue the patient's long-acting opioid and increase the continuous dose of PCA to compensate for the long-acting opioid that has been discontinued.

Part of the education regarding PCA should include the fact that only the patient should push the demand button and

TABLE 14A-2 *OPIOID EQUIVALENT DOSES*

Chemical Class	Drug	Parenteral	Oral
Phenanthrene			
	Buprenorphine	0.3 mg	—
	Codeine	120 mg	180 mg
	Hydrocodone	—	30 mg
	Hydromorphone	2 mg	8 mg
	Levorphanol	2 mg	4 mg
	Morphine	10 mg	20–30 mg
	Oxycodone	—	20 mg
	Oxymorphone	1 mg	10 mg
Phenylpiperidine			
	Fentanyl	100 mcg	—
	Meperidine	100 mg	300 mg
Diphenylheptane			
	Methadone	1–2.5 mg	2–5 mg
Methylpentanylphenol			
	Tapentadol	—	100 mg

not the nurse or family. Allowing family members or friends to push the demand button may cause excessive sedation.

The option exists to convert all of a patient's preoperative opioids into the PCA opioid. Table 14A-2 is the opioid equivalence table that is used at Hartford Hospital. All the doses listed are equivalent to one another, both orally and parenterally. A patient's 24-hour opioid use should be totaled and converted to the equivalent opioid that will be used in the PCA. This dose should then be divided by 24 to determine the hourly continuous rate on the PCA. The demand dose is usually set at 50% to 100% of the hourly rate. Sometimes for slower onset analgesics (hydromorphone, morphine), the demand interval is set at 10 to 15 minutes to allow those analgesics to reach their peak effect before another demand dose is potentially available. Table 14A-3 lists the suggested starting doses for PCA when patients have been on long-acting opioids.

When patients are able to take oral medication, they can be switched to PRN short-acting opioids or a combination of long-acting ATC opioids plus PRN short-acting opioids. Table 14A-4 lists suggested starting doses for long-acting opioids when transitioning off of a PCA. If sustained-release oxycodone or sustained-release morphine is used, the initial doses can be given and then the PCA discontinued 2 hours later. If a fentanyl patch is used, the patch should be applied and the PCA discontinued 8 to 12 hours later. For some patients, the transition from IV opioids to oral or topical opioids is difficult. To ease the transition, the ATC oral or topical opioid is started; then the PCA is changed to demand only (after 2 or 8 hours depending on long-acting opioid) for the next 24 hours. Appropriate adjustments in the ATC opioid can be made after reviewing the next 24-hour use of the PCA demand doses. The dose conversions in Tables 14A-3 and 14A-4 are estimates, and factors such as age, trajectory for recovery, and incomplete opioid cross-tolerance need to be considered when these calculations are done.

Patients in a methadone maintenance program should always have their methadone doses confirmed by the methadone treatment facility and have their dose continued while

TABLE 14A-3 *PREOPERATIVE OPIOID CONVERSIONS*

Opioid Dose per 24 Hours	Hydromorphone	Morphine	Fentanyl
Fentanyl 25 mcg/hr Morphine SR 60–90 mg Oxycodone SR 20–40 mg	0.2 mg/mL: 30 mL Continuous: 0.3 mg/hr Demand: 0.3 mg q10min 4-hr lockout: 6 mg	1 mg/mL: 30 mL Continuous: 1.5 mg/hr Demand: 1.5 mg q10min 4-hr lockout: 30 mg	10 mcg/mL: 30 mL Continuous: 15 mcg/hr Demand: 15 mcg q10min 4-hr lockout: 300 mcg
Fentanyl 50 mcg/hr Morphine SR 120–180 mg Oxycodone SR 60–80 mg	0.5 mg/mL: 30 mL Continuous: 0.4 mg/hr Demand: 0.4 mg q15min 4-hr lockout: 10 mg	2 mg/mL: 30 mL Continuous: 2 mg/hr Demand: 2 mg q15min 4-hr lockout: 50 mg	25 mcg/mL: 30 mL Continuous: 20 mcg/hr Demand: 20 mcg q10min 4-hr lockout: 500 mcg
Fentanyl 100–125 mcg/hr Morphine SR 240–320 mg Oxycodone SR 100–160 mg	0.5 mg/mL: 30 mL Continuous: 0.6 mg/hr Demand: 0.6 mg q15min 4-hr lockout: 15 mg	3 mg/mL: 30 mL Continuous: 3 mg/hr Demand: 3 mg q15min 4-hr lockout: 75 mg	25 mcg/mL: 30 mL Continuous: 30 mcg/hr Demand: 30 mcg q10min 4-hr lockout: 750 mcg
Fentanyl 150–200 mcg/hr Morphine SR 360–480 mg Oxycodone SR 180–240 mg	1 mg/mL: 30 mL Continuous: 1 mg/hr Demand: 1 mg q15min 4 hr lockout: 20 mg	5 mg/mL: 30 mL Continuous: 5 mg/hr Demand: 5 mg q15min 4 hr lockout: 100 mg	50 mcg/mL: 30 mL Continuous: 50 mcg/hr Demand: 50 mcg q10min 4 hr lockout: 1000 mcg

q, Every.

TABLE 14A-4 *PATIENT-CONTROLLED ANALGESIA OPIOID CONVERTER*

Hydromorphone IV (mg/24 hr)	Morphine IV (mg/24 hr)	Fentanyl Patch (μg/hr)	Oxycodone SR (mg q12hr)	Morphine SR (mg q12hr)
0–7	0–35	—	—	—
8–11	36–55	25	20	30
12–16	56–80	50	30	45
17–21	81–105	75	40	60
22–26	106–130	100	60	90

IV, Intravenous; *q,* every.

hospitalized. This is to make certain that the issues of opioid withdrawal, opioid addiction, and pain management are kept separate.[46] Methadone provides little to no analgesia for patients taking this medication once daily for methadone maintenance. In fact, these patients usually have a lower than normal pain tolerance.[47] If the patient cannot be given food by mouth (NPO), the methadone should be converted to IV. The IV dose of methadone is approximately 50% of the oral dose. The total IV dose is divided so that equal amounts are given at 8- or 12-hour intervals. This is so the patient does not receive a large IV bolus of methadone as a single daily dose. Patients in a methadone maintenance program should have both a continuous and demand opioid during PCA treatment. Their initial doses should be at least 50% higher than the doses listed in Table 14A-1. Patients taking high doses of methadone will require high doses of their analgesic opioid.

Some patients may be treated with the oral film or sublingual tablets of buprenorphine–naloxone (Suboxone) instead of methadone as part of an opioid addiction program. Suboxone is strongly adherent to and is only a partial agonist at the μ-opioid receptor. The pure opioid agonists at their usual doses (e.g., morphine, hydromorphone, fentanyl) may provide some analgesia, but it may be difficult to control a patient's pain until the Suboxone has been stopped and metabolized (average half-life at least 24 hours). It is probably best to discontinue the Suboxone while aggressively treating the patient's pain and then restart the Suboxone as the patient's pain subsides.[48] Oral naltrexone is used to treat alcohol addiction. Naltrexone is a pure μ-receptor antagonist. It will block any of the opioid effects from systemically administered opioids. It should be stopped if the patient is going to have pain and require opioid analgesics. Vivitrol is an intramuscular suspension of sustained-release naltrexone, which is a full opioid antagonist. The injection is given once per month and blocks opioid effects for approximately 30 days. Using all of the nonopioid analgesics (e.g., nerve blocks, epidurals, acetaminophen, NSAIDs, ketamine, anticonvulsants) will be important. Opioid agonists–antagonists (nalbuphine, butorphanol, pentazocine) should not be given to patients taking systemic opioids, methadone maintenance, or Suboxone because analgesia will be reversed and an immediate opioid withdrawal syndrome may be precipitated. Naloxone and nalbuphine may be used to treat pruritus and nausea if a patient is receiving only epidural opioids.

Selection of Opioids

Morphine is still the gold standard for analgesia. It is available in multiple dose forms for ease of administration, including liquids (multiple concentrations), suppositories, injectable (IV, intramuscular [IM], subcutaneous [SC], epidural), immediate-release tablets, and long-acting tablets and capsules (once daily or every 8 to 12 hours). A lipid-based morphine epidural formulation is available (DepoDur) for postoperative pain that provides analgesia for 48 hours.

One drawback with morphine is the production of a metabolite, morphine-6-glucuronide. This metabolite is a more potent analgesic than morphine itself; however, it does accumulate in patients who are elderly or who have renal insufficiency. Accumulation of the metabolite can cause sedation, confusion, and respiratory depression. These adverse effects are immediately reversible with naloxone. It may take 24 to 48 hours for these adverse effects to resolve after the morphine is stopped.

Hydromorphone has become our drug of choice because of its versatility and lack of significant active metabolites at usual doses. It is especially useful in elderly patients and in patients with impaired renal function. It can be given orally (PO), IM, IV, SC, rectally, and epidurally. An oral liquid is available as well as a concentrated injection. One of the issues with hydromorphone is that it has poor oral bioavailability. There is a difference in the equipotent doses between the oral and parenteral products. Oral hydromorphone 4 mg is equipotent to approximately 1 mg of parenteral hydromorphone.

The use of meperidine has dropped dramatically owing to the availability of safer alternatives. Meperidine has a metabolite, normeperidine, that has no analgesic activity but is a potent CNS stimulant. Normeperidine accumulates especially in patients with renal insufficiency. Patients may or may not show the signs of early toxicity (agitation, delirium, myoclonus) before they have the severe toxicity, which is a generalized tonic-clonic seizure. Administration of naloxone should be avoided because it may only precipitate more seizures. A benzodiazepine will stop the seizure, and if the meperidine is stopped, the patient may not have another seizure. The half-life of normeperidine is 12 hours in patients with normal renal function. The half-life can be much longer in patients with renal insufficiency. If the meperidine is stopped, the adverse effects will decrease over the next 24 hours. If parenteral meperidine is used, the dose should be limited to at most 10 mg/kg/day (600–900 mg/day) for 48 hours in patients with normal renal function.[49] IV meperidine is still excellent for treating postoperative and amphotericin B–induced shivering. Oral meperidine is not very potent; 50 mg provides no better analgesia than 1 g of acetaminophen or an NSAID. In fact, oral meperidine generates more normeperidine owing to the first-pass effect in the gastrointestinal (GI) tract.

Fentanyl can be used as a PRN injection or in a PCA when patients develop nausea, confusion, or pruritus from other opioids. Fentanyl does not accumulate in patients with renal insufficiency and has minimally pharmacologically active metabolites. When patients are ready to stop the parenteral fentanyl, a fentanyl patch can be applied that is equal in strength to the hourly use of fentanyl that can be determined from the PCA. The patch is applied to a nonhairy area of skin and held in place for 30 seconds. This facilitates good adherence between the patch and the patient's skin. The PCA and patch are overlapped for 8 to 12 hours, and then the PCA can be stopped. Patients usually need an oral PRN short-acting opioid such as oxycodone, hydromorphone, or hydrocodone for breakthrough pain. There are available multiple transmucosal immediate-release fentanyl products and a nasal spray, but they are very expensive, and many pharmacies may not carry these items.

Oxycodone should be used cautiously in patients with renal insufficiency or receiving dialysis. Both oxycodone and metabolites accumulate, causing toxicity if doses are titrated upward too quickly or high initial doses are used. Multiple oral dose forms of oxycodone are available, including liquid, liquid concentrate, immediate-release tablets, and sustained-release tablets. OxyContin is now manufactured in an abuse-deterrent dosage form that is very difficult to crush, cut, or dissolve. Various oxycodone–acetaminophen combinations are available. Using the medication with the least amount of acetaminophen, usually 325 mg per tablet, should avoid acetaminophen toxicity. Patients should not ingest more than 4 g/d of acetaminophen on a chronic basis to avoid hepatotoxicity. Also available is an oxycodone–ibuprofen combination product (5 mg/400 mg per tablet).

Hydrocodone immediate release is not available as a standalone analgesic. It is combined with either acetaminophen or ibuprofen. A sustained-release hydrocodone, Zohydro, is now available. One of hydrocodone's metabolites is hydromorphone. Hydrocodone is safe to use in renal insufficiency. The ibuprofen dose is 200 mg per tablet; however, the amount of acetaminophen per tablet is now consistently 325 mg. A liquid formulation is available. Hydrocodone products are currently classified as controlled substance class III (CIII) narcotics, but they are being considered for a change to class II (CII) narcotics.

Tramadol as an analgesic has a dual mechanism of action. Tramadol itself inhibits the reuptake of norepinephrine and serotonin while the major metabolite, desmethyltramadol, binds to the μ-opioid receptor. Tramadol is not a controlled drug. There are two tablets; one is a 50-mg tablet, and the other is 37.5 mg combined with acetaminophen 325 mg. A sustained-release product, which is given once daily, is available in 100-, 200-, and 300-mg strengths. Slow upward titration prevents the side effects of sedation, nausea, and dizziness from being problematic. The combination of tramadol and antidepressants may cause seizures or the serotonin syndrome; however, the incidence is low.

Methadone is a unique analgesic in that it has a long half-life (at least 24 hours) and is inexpensive, and the D-stereoisomer is an NMDA receptor antagonist, which means it may have an effect on neuropathic pain. It is available as an injection (IV, IM), tablets, and liquids. Despite the long pharmacokinetic half-life, the analgesic action persists for only 6 to 8 hours, so methadone for analgesia needs to be dosed every 6 to 8 hours. When methadone is initiated, a fixed initial dose should be started and not changed for 4 to 7 days, allowing the methadone to accumulate. Patients should have short-acting opioids for breakthrough pain. What should happen after methadone is started is that over the ensuing 3 to 4 days, the use of the PRN opioids should decrease. The conversion from other opioids to methadone can be difficult. The long half-life and the equivalency change depend on the amount of daily prior opioid use. Usually the equivalency is in the range of 5% (for high-dose prior use) to 25% (for low-dose prior opioid use) of the morphine equivalent dose.

Hydroxyzine has been used as a "potentiator" of opioid analgesia for a number of years. In reality, the studies that demonstrated this effect were poorly designed as analgesic trials.[50] These studies used high doses of hydroxyzine (100 mg IM), but today the typical dose is 25 to 50 mg. It is true that hydroxyzine is an antihistamine, mild antiemetic, and sedative. It is very painful as an IM injection and has a long half-life (≈24 hours). For the most part, now we avoid using hydroxyzine so that there are fewer problems with sedation.

Opioids commonly cause side effects; however, if these are promptly recognized and treated the side effects are manageable. Nausea and vomiting should be treated with antiemetics (haloperidol, metoclopramide, prochlorperazine, promethazine), and if these side effects occur frequently during treatment, the antiemetics should be scheduled ATC. Patients will develop a tolerance to nausea and vomiting, but it may take 1 to 2 weeks. Reducing the dose of the opioid, changing the route of administration, increasing the time of infusion, or changing the opioid may all have a significant effect. Constipation is a side effect to which tolerance does not develop. Patients need to be started on a laxative that is both a softener and a stimulant. The laxatives need to be given daily so that if the patient is eating well there should be a bowel movement daily or every other day. Senokot-S, MiraLax, Amitiza, and lactulose can all be effective. An ileus can occur from opioids or surgery. For a postoperative ileus, if the patient is not taking opioids chronically, using buprenorphine may provide effective analgesia without aggravating the ileus. Buprenorphine is a partial μ-receptor agonist. It has very little effect on smooth muscle and does not cause spasm of the sphincter of Oddi. It may precipitate opioid withdrawal in patients on methadone maintenance or in patients taking opioids chronically. For analgesic use, it is available as Butrans, a sustained-release patch dosed at 5 mcg/hr, 10 mcg/hr, 15 mcg/hr, and 20 mcg/hr changed every 7 days. A 10-mcg/hr patch is equal to 30 mg of oral morphine per day or a 12-mcg/hr fentanyl patch. Buprenorphine as an injection can be given IM or IV or via PCA. The Butrans patch should be removed 24 hours before surgery so that the opioid analgesics can be most effective.

Pruritus does not necessarily indicate a true allergy unless hives and a rash accompany it. Most opioids cause histamine release, which causes pruritus. Both oral and parenteral opioids cause pruritus. It is thought that the least potent opioids (meperidine) cause more pruritus than the most potent (fentanyl). One of the treatments is to switch to a more potent opioid to relieve the pruritus. Antihistamines are somewhat effective for the pruritus.

If a patient becomes sedated, it is time to reassess the opioid therapy. Opioids cause a decrease in respiratory rate, hypoventilation, and hypoxia. They do not cause dyspnea or tachypnea. Other causes of sedation need to be ruled out such as other medications (benzodiazepines), metabolic abnormalities, and so on. Was the opioid dose titrated up too quickly? Is the patient on morphine and now has developed renal insufficiency? Is the patient elderly or opioid naïve or have a history of sleep apnea? Unless the patient is apneic, naloxone (Narcan) should be given slowly and in a low dose to avoid a rebound in pain or opioid withdrawal. Naloxone 0.4 mg (1 mL) should be mixed with 9 mL of saline with 1 to 2 mL given by IV push every 1 to 2 minutes until the patient is awake or a satisfactory respiratory rate has been achieved. Naloxone's duration of action is short (30–60 minutes), so the patient will need to be monitored carefully for a few hours.

Myoclonus is seen most often with meperidine, than with morphine, or than with hydromorphone. These involuntary, symmetrical muscle spasms occur while the patient is awake or asleep. Myoclonus occurs when the patient is being treated with high doses of opioids or the dose has been titrated up rapidly. Some adjuvants (gabapentin and pregabalin) also cause myoclonus. Sometimes the muscle spasms are painful, and other times the family is bothered by the myoclonus. Decreasing the opioid dose or switching to a different opioid (methadone) will eliminate the myoclonus. A benzodiazepine or valproic acid will effectively decrease the number or intensity of the spasms.

Neuropathic pain is sometimes difficult to identify. It is important to ask patients how they would describe their pain. Words such as burning, stabbing, shooting, aching, throbbing, and electricity-like may indicate the presence of neuropathic pain. Procedures done to bone may affect the nerves that supply the periosteum and endosteum; therefore, neuropathic pain should be considered a component of bone pain.[51] Typically, this pain is described as being opioid resistant or insensitive. What usually happens when a patient is given an opioid for this pain is that the patient has some analgesia but it is of short duration. Patients also frequently have severe side effects at low doses of opioids. These are the patients who are sedated, awaken, and ask for analgesics and then fall back asleep before the analgesic is administered. Typically, opioids alone are only fairly effective for neuropathic pain.[52,53] When opioids alone are used for neuropathic pain, patients tend to complain about poor pain control despite what we would consider adequate doses of opioid analgesics. The patient may then be labeled as an "addict" or as "drug seeking" when in reality, if an adjuvant such as gabapentin or baclofen is introduced early in therapy, the patient's pain control may be better with the combination of an opioid and gabapentin–baclofen, a "multimodal analgesia." When treating difficult neuropathic pain, multiple adjuvants may be needed, and it is best to use agents from different pharmacologic classes, for example, an anticonvulsant plus a muscle relaxant rather than an anticonvulsant plus an anticonvulsant.[54] The anticonvulsants are usually added first (gabapentin, oxcarbazepine, pregablin) because of their fast onset of action and their lack of significant drug interactions. A patient may have effective pain relief within 24 to 48 hours of initiation of therapy. If a patient has muscle spasms, opioids are not effective at relieving the spasm. Medications such as baclofen, lorazepam, and tizanidine are effective at relieving spasms. Diazepam is the classic muscle relaxant, but lorazepam will work just as well. Antidepressants are effective; however, they require a titration process, so their efficacy may be delayed. Usually when patients try an antidepressant, they respond in a shorter time and at a lower dose compared with that which is needed for an antidepressant effect. Lidocaine patch 5% (Lidoderm) is effective for topical pain syndromes. The lidocaine penetrates a few millimeters into the epidermis and dermis, so it is usually not effective for severe bone pain. The systemic blood levels are approximately one-tenth of those needed to treat an arrhythmia. Table 14A-5 lists the most commonly used adjuvants for neuropathic pain.

Appropriate and Inappropriate Use of Opioids

The use of opioid medications in the treatment of orthopaedic patients has been performed countless times for many decades. Opioids offer an effective way to reduce pain in this population and usually pose little risk of addiction. In certain circumstances, some patients do display behaviors of addiction when treated with opioids. The challenge we have as health care providers is to stop the abuse of opioids while ensuring the continued availability of these medications for patients who benefit from their use.

Approaching the use of opioid medications to treat pain should be approached like any other condition we encounter.

DIAGNOSIS AND DIFFERENTIAL

Treatable causes of pain should be identified through a history, physical examination, and testing. The treatment should be directed at the pain generator(s). Comorbid conditions need to be taken into consideration when assessing the use of opioid medications. Included in these conditions is a personal or family history of alcohol or drug abuse.[55] The presence of psychological conditions, a history of sexual abuse, and a younger age (18–45 years) are also associated with aberrant drug-related behaviors in some studies.[56]

Risk assessment screening tools are helpful for stratification of risk; however, more validation of the outcomes are needed to understand the effects on clinical outcomes. Tests that appear to have good content, face, and construct validity include the Screener and Opioid Assessment for Patient with Pain (SOAPP), Version 1; the revised SOAPP (SOAPP-R); the Opioid Intractability Risk Tool (ORT); and the Diagnosis, Intractability, Risk, Efficacy (DIRE) instrument. DIRE is clinician administered, and the others are patient self-reporting.[57]

Informed Consent

Health care providers need to thoroughly explain the entire treatment plan with the patient and the use of opioids in that complete plan. The risks and benefits associated with the use of opioids need to be understood, and issues about physical dependence, addiction, abuse, tolerance, and withdrawal need to be explored.

Abuse

Abuse is use of any substance for a nontherapeutic purpose or for what it is not prescribed.

Addiction

Addiction is a chronic neurobiologic disease characterized by impaired control over drug use, compulsive drug use, and continued drug use despite harm and because of craving.

Physical Dependence

Physical dependence is a physiologic state characterized by withdrawal symptoms if treatment is stopped or decreased abruptly. It does not equal addiction.

TABLE 14A-5 *NEUROPATHIC PAIN ADJUVANTS*

Drug	Class	Starting Dose	Dose Range	Side Effects and Comments
Amitriptyline (Elavil)	Tricyclic antidepressant	10–25 mg PO at bedtime Titrate dose up every 3 days	25–150 mg at bedtime	Sedation, anticholinergic effects, prolongation of QTc
Baclofen	Muscle relaxant	5–10 mg PO tid Titrate dose up every 2–3 days	10–30 mg tid 5 mg bid–tid with decrease in GFR or in elderly adults	Sedation, delirium, muscle weakness, withdrawal seizures
Carbamazepine (Tegretol)	Anticonvulsant	100 mg PO bid Titrate dose up every 3 days	200–600 mg bid	Sedation, SIADH, enzyme induction, bone marrow suppression; monitor serum levels for efficacy
Desipramine (Norpramin)	Tricyclic antidepressant	10–25 mg PO at bedtime Titrate dose up every 3 days	25–150 mg at bedtime	Less sedation and anticholinergic effects than amitriptyline, prolongation of QTc
Duloxetine (Cymbalta)	Antidepressant (SNRI)	20–30 mg PO daily Titrate up every 3 days	30–60 mg bid 30–60 mg daily with decrease in GFR	Nausea, insomnia, headache, diarrhea, constipation; taper off to avoid withdrawal
Gabapentin (Neurontin)	Anticonvulsant	100–300 mg PO tid. Titrate up every 24 hours	300–800 mg tid 300 mg daily or bid with decrease in GFR	Sedation, confusion, myoclonus, dizziness, diplopia, peripheral edema
Lidocaine patch 5% (Lidoderm)	Topical anesthetic	One patch daily; on for 12 hr and off for 12 hr	One to three patches per day depending on area needing analgesia, cut to fit	Skin irritation; apply to site of pain; effective for postherpetic neuralgia
Mexiletine	Antiarrhythmic	150 mg PO bid–tid Titrate up every 3 days	200–250 mg tid	Nausea, insomnia, delirium; no effect on ECG; not proarrhythmic
Oxcarbazepine (Trileptal)	Anticonvulsant	150 mg PO bid Titrate up every 2 days	150–600 mg bid 75–150 mg bid with decrease in GFR	Sedation, SIADH
Pregabalin (Lyrica)	Anticonvulsant	50 mg PO bid Titrate up every 24 hr	50–300 mg bid 25–50 mg bid–tid with decrease in GFR	Sedation, confusion, dizziness, diplopia, peripheral edema, myoclonus
Tizanidine (Zanaflex)	Muscle relaxant	2 mg PO bid–tid Titrate up every 3 days	4–8 mg tid 1–2 mg tid with decrease in GFR	Sedation, hypotension, dry mouth
Valproic acid (Depakote)	Anticonvulsant	250–500 mg PO bid Titrate up every 3 days	500 mg–1 g bid Use same dose IV	Mild sedation, tremor, increased LFT results; monitor serum level
Milnacipran (Savella)	Antidepressant (SNRI)	12.5–25 mg bid	50–100 mg bid 25–50 mg bid with ↓ in GFR	Nausea, headache, hypertension; taper off to avoid withdrawal; FDA approval for fibromyalgia

bid, Twice a day; *ECG,* electrocardiogram; *FDA,* Food and Drug Administration; *GFR,* glomerular filtration rate; *IV,* intravenous; *LFT,* liver function test; *PO,* oral; tid, three times a day; *SIADH,* syndrome of inappropriate antidiuretic hormone secretion; *SNRI,* serotonin–norepinephrine reuptake inhibitor.

Tolerance

Tolerance is a physiologic state caused by the regular use of an opioid in which increased doses are needed to maintain the same effect

Withdrawal (Abstinence)

Withdrawal is characterized by sweating, tremors, vomiting, anxiety, insomnia, and muscle pain.[58]

Opioid Agreements

Expectations and obligations of the patient and physician are understood. The plan should explain the course of treatment and the goals of therapy. It should set limits on the use of opioid therapy and expectations about follow-up care and monitoring of the therapy. It also should include indications for tapering, changing, or discontinuing opioids as part of the entire treatment plan.

INITIATION AND ASSESSMENT OF THERAPY

Opioid selection, initial dosing, and titration should be individualized according to the patient's health status, previous exposure to opioids, attainment of therapeutic goals, and predicted or observed harms.[57] The four As of opioid prescribing should be followed.[58]

Analgesia

The goal for the use of opioid medications is to decrease pain. A baseline pain score using a standard visual analog scale (VAS) or any of the other pain tracking ways is adequate. You need to use the same system every time the patient's pain is reevaluated for consistency. Failure to make progress in the reduction of pain may cause the health care provider to change, taper, or discontinue current course of treatment because of lack of efficacy.

Activity

The goal for the use of opioid medications is to improve activities of daily living and quality of life.

Adverse Effects

Side effects, including nausea, constipation, alterations in cognitive function, and respiratory depression, all need to be monitored throughout the use of opioid medications. Appropriate adjustments in the treatment algorithm may need to occur if adverse effects are not tolerated or correctable.

Aberrant Behavior

An aberrant behavior is any drug-related deviation from the medical plan. This can include unauthorized dose escalations, prescription forgery, using opioids to achieve euphoria or relief of anxiety, abnormal urine test screening results, and request for early refills or requesting refill instead of an appointment with the health care provider, to name a few.[59]

Regimens need to be tailored to the patient based on subjective, objective, and clinical findings. The goal is a stable therapeutic platform. The need for regular follow-up care to assess the outcome of therapy initiated is crucial for success. Look for warning signs of adverse effects and aberrant behavior. This will help with the rationale to continue or modify treatment.

At each visit, review the patient's diagnosis, comorbid conditions, and addictive disorders, if any. The treatment goals may need to be amended because illnesses evolve and diagnostic tests can change with time.

The management of pain in orthopaedic patients can range from the very acute to chronic, lifelong management. Maintaining safe prescribing habits, reevaluating the continued need for opioids, and monitoring the effectiveness of therapy and the possible development of aberrant behaviors are key to effective use of this class of medications.

Neuraxial Delivery Systems: Subarachnoid Injections

The delivery of opioids or local anesthetics to the intrathecal or epidural space can provide profound analgesia in patients experiencing moderate to severe acute pain. Injection of opioids into the subarachnoid space results in the selective decrease in nociceptive transmission from C polymodal and Aδ afferents with no effect on motor, sensory, or autonomic function.[60] Acting on μ and κ receptors within the spinal cord, opioids exhibit a greater affinity to C fibers than Aδ fibers, the consequence of which is a greater reduction of dull versus sharp pain.

With respect to opioids, the single biggest determinant of onset and duration is the drug's lipophilicity. Lipophilic opioids such as fentanyl are rapidly cleared from the cerebrospinal fluid (CSF), producing rapid onset but a short duration of action. Clearance from the CSF is so rapid that the primary analgesic effects of these opioids are probably produced by systemic and supraspinal mechanisms.[61] Hydrophilic (lipophobic) agents such as morphine tend to remain in the CSF after neuraxial administration, resulting in a delayed onset but extended duration of effect. Bulk flow of hydrophilic opioids within the CSF produces analgesic effects at locations that are further away from the injection site. Thus, injection of morphine into the subarachnoid space in the lumbar area can produce analgesic effects in the upper abdomen and thoracic regions. This cephalad migration may also contribute to the development of side effects commonly seen with subarachnoid injection of opioids.

Side effects from neuraxial opioids are typically dose dependent and may or may not result from interactions with specific opioid receptors. Far and away the most commonly reported side effect is the development of non–histamine release pruritus. Up to 60% of patients can experience pruritus, which is thought to develop from the activation of "itch centers" in the medulla and trigeminal nucleus.[62] Pruritus often develops in the upper thorax, neck, and face and is not associated with a rash. Patients generally respond to treatment with low-dose naloxone, nalbuphine, droperidol, or naltrexone, further supporting that histamine release is not the underlying cause.

Nausea and vomiting are other common side effects of subarachnoid opioid administration with an incidence greater than 30%.[62] The development of nausea and vomiting generally occurs within 4 hours of opioid administration in susceptible patients. Nausea and vomiting can occur in a dose-dependent fashion and primarily occur because of bulk flow and cephalad migration of opioids within the CSF.[63,64] Dispersion of opioids within the CSF results in activation of opioid receptors within the area postrema of the medulla. Other mechanisms, including the sensitization of vestibular system to motion as well as decreased gastric motility, may also play a role.[61,65] Patients who develop nausea and vomiting can be successfully treated with low-dose naloxone, transdermal scopolamine, dexamethasone, metoclopramide, or droperidol.

Urinary retention may also develop among patients receiving subarachnoid opiates. The development of this side effect does not appear to be dose dependent, and its incidence can vary widely but occurs more commonly in young males.[66] Opioid receptors activated in the sacral spinal cord (S2–S4) cause a reduction in parasympathetic outflow, leading to detrusor muscle relaxation and an increase in bladder capacity. Neuraxial administration of morphine has effects on the bladder within 15 minutes and can last as long as 16 hours.

Perhaps the most concerning side effect of subarachnoid opioids is the development of respiratory depression. Clinical studies have shown that when appropriate doses of subarachnoid opiates are given, the incidence of respiratory depression does not vary greatly from systemic administration.[62] Respiratory depression requiring intervention occurs in a dose-dependent fashion with an overall incidence of 1%. Unlike most systemic routes, subarachnoid opiates may result in both early and delayed respiratory effects.[67] Clinically relevant early respiratory depression has been linked to epidural injection of lipophilic opioids and is exceedingly rare with subarachnoid injections. Opioids such as fentanyl and sufentanil can produce respiratory depression within 2 hours of epidural injection, which is likely the result of systemic absorption. Delayed respiratory depression results from the activation of opioid receptors within the ventral medulla following the cephalad migration of hydrophilic opioids. The ventral medulla contains a large number of opioid receptors, and even small concentrations can produce significant effects.[68,69] Respiratory depression typically occurs between 6 and 12 hours after neuraxial injection of morphine but can persist up to 24 hours.[70,71] It has been suggested that patients receiving neuraxial lipophilic opioids be monitored for signs of respiratory depression for 4 to 6 hours after treatment and those receiving hydrophilic opioids (morphine) be monitored for 18 to 24 hours after their administration. The earliest signs of respiratory depression include changes in mental status as well as bradypnea with resultant hypercarbia rather than frank apnea.[72] Airway management is the initial step in treatment followed by the use of naloxone. Bolus doses in increments of 0.1 to 0.4 mg of naloxone are given until the respiratory rate recovers. This should then be followed by an infusion of naloxone at 0.5 to 5 μg/kg/hr because respiratory depression may reoccur when the initial dose of naloxone wears off.[73]

Neuraxial Delivery Systems: Continuous Epidural Catheters

The use of continuous epidural catheters has proven to be an effective tool in the management of acute pain by providing analgesia that is superior to systemic opioids.[74] Unlike the one-time neuraxial injections that provide a short duration of relief (4–6 hours for fentanyl, 24 hours for morphine, 48 hours for liposomal morphine), continuous epidural catheters can be left in situ for several days during the recovery period. Infusions can consist of local anesthetics, opioids, or a combination of both. Selection of the drug(s) to be infused should be based on the clinical needs of the patient.

Patients who experience traumatic injuries may experience pain in multiple locations on the body. When it is not possible to cover all painful areas, an epidural infusion of local anesthetic only may be appropriate. The epidural may be placed in an anatomic location that is most beneficial to the patient while secondary areas of pain are addressed through systemic opioids and multimodal pharmacology. Typically, agents such as bupivacaine or ropivacaine are selected for infusion because of their preferential sensory blockade and long duration of action. With increasing doses of local anesthetics, patients may develop unwelcomed side effects. The development of motor blockade can prevent proper assessment of peripheral nerve function, and sympathetic blockade from epidurals placed in the thoracic region can result in hypotension.

When the aforementioned side effects are undesirable, patients may benefit from opioid-only infusions. Although lipophilic agents such as fentanyl and sufentanil can be used, they are not considered ideal because several randomized clinical trials have suggested a primarily systemic rather than spinal site of action.[75] As such, infusions of lipophilic agents produce equivalent levels of analgesia and similar rates of side effects to their IV counterparts. Studies comparing epidural lipophilic opioids with IV opioids have shown either only a modest benefit with epidural administration or no difference.[75,76] Given its lack of clear benefit over parenteral routes, it makes little sense to expose the patient to the risk of epidural placement for the infusion of lipophilic opioids. On the other hand, the use of hydrophilic opioids may be useful because studies have shown better pain control with hydrophilic opioids than with traditional PRN regimens.[77] Unlike lipophilic agents, hydrophilic agents such as morphine exert their primary analgesic effect by binding to opioid receptors within the spinal cord.[75] Because of its relative lack of vascular uptake, bulk flow within the CSF allows for the distal spread of the medication. This characteristic is particularly useful when the catheter is placed at a site distant to spinal roots carrying the pertinent nociceptive information.

Continuous epidural analgesia is at its most effective when infusions that combine both local anesthetics and opioids are used. Combination therapy has been shown to provide superior analgesia and patient satisfaction compared with IV PCA usage and single-agent epidural infusions.[78,79] By combining agents, patients report improved sensory block and better dynamic pain relief. Additionally, combination infusions require less of both agents (opioids and local anesthetics) compared with epidural infusions that only contain opioids or local anesthetics.[80] This is advantageous because side effects that occur in a dose-dependent fashion are reduced. Agent selection is similar to single-agent infusions. Typical regimens use local anesthetics that are long acting and provide preferential sensory over motor blockade such as low-concentration bupivacaine or ropivacaine. Lipophilic opioids can be used because they allow for rapid titration of analgesia.[81] Although combinations that include lipophilic agents produce better analgesia than local anesthetics alone, this is probably due to primarily systemic effects.[75] The addition of hydrophilic opioids to local anesthetic infusions also improves analgesia over standard IV regimens. Although neuraxially administered hydrophilic opioids exert their primary analgesic effects at the spinal cord, their addition to local anesthetic solutions confers no additional benefit compared with local anesthetic-only solutions containing lipophilic opioids.[82,83]

In addition to providing superior analgesia to systemic opioids, the use of epidural catheters for acute pain management in perioperative settings has been associated with a reduction in morbidity and mortality.[84,85] Pain control and inhibition of sympathetic outflow aids in diminishing the stress response, which can have beneficial effects on a variety of physiologic processes. The placement of an epidural catheter in the thoracic region for pain related to chest wall injuries, thoracotomies, and upper abdominal surgical procedures has been shown to decrease the risk of pulmonary complications.[86,87] Better analgesia in these situations allows for better pulmonary toilet and use of incentive spirometry, resulting in preservation of preoperative or preinjury pulmonary function.[84] After thoracotomies or upper abdominal surgical procedures, there is impairment of diaphragmatic function. This phenomenon is due to reflex inhibition of phrenic nerve activity and does not improve with analgesia.[88] The addition of local anesthetics to thoracic epidural infusions suppresses the reflex, thereby improving pulmonary function.[89] Mitigation of the stress response by thoracic epidurals has also been shown to decrease the incidence of myocardial infarction.[90] Sympathetic blockade results in small reductions in heart rate, blood pressure, and cardiac output, thereby decreasing myocardial oxygen demand. The supply side of the equation is also altered.

Sympathetically mediated vasoconstriction at sites that are distal to preexisting coronary artery stenosis are abolished, and myocardial blood flow undergoes redistribution, resulting in improved endocardial to epicardial blood flow ratios.[91-93] Limiting a patient's exposure to opioids coupled with decreased sympathetic output has also been shown to favor the return of GI motility, improve blood flow to the bowel, and prevent the reduction of intramucosal gastric pH. The restoration of normal GI function allows for a faster return to PO intake so that nutritional goals can be met. As stated previously, patients who experience significant acute pain are subject to a significant neuroendocrine response that often leads to hypermetabolic and catabolic states. By meeting nutritional goals early, it may be possible to limit negative nitrogen balance and protein catabolism that can delay wound healing and impede patient recovery.

The use of epidural catheters provides a myriad of benefits that make it an attractive option for the management of acute pain. Although studies conflict as to whether combined local anesthetics and opioid infusions exhibit a synergistic or an additive effect, it is clear that they can improve analgesia and decrease side effects when used together.[94,95] Additionally, it has been proposed that the use of epidural analgesia may help at-risk patients from developing chronic pain syndromes. Reduction or blockade of nociceptive input into the dorsal horn may prevent the development of chronic pain states by decreasing C-fiber activation of WDR neurons, which have been linked to wind-up and central sensitization.

Despite the numerous advantages of epidural analgesia, there are potential risks to consider. Although the placement of an epidural catheter has inherent risks, the presence of an indwelling catheter represents ongoing risk to the patient. Serious complications such as epidural abscess and epidural hematoma are uncommon yet potentially devastating complications for the patient. With the introduction of low-molecular-weight heparin in North America in 1993, there was a dramatic increase in the incidence of spinal hematoma. Before this time, the incidence of spinal hematoma was estimated to be one in 220,000 for spinal techniques and one in 150,000 for epidural access. From 1993 to 1998, the frequency of spinal hematoma increased precipitously with incidences of one in 6600 for spinal techniques and one in 40,800 for epidural access. The dramatic rise in these events resulted in an increasing focus on the use of thromboprophylactic and anticoagulation medications. The American Society of Regional Anesthesia and the European Society of Anesthesiology have developed consensus statements regarding the use of hemostasis-modifying agents and the timing of neuraxial techniques (access, catheter placement, and catheter withdrawal).[96,97] These statements reflect that different agents have different pharmacokinetic properties that should be considered. In general, the consensus statements suggest that two half-lives of the medication should pass before performing neuraxial procedures. Special consideration should be taken for elderly patients and those with renal impairments.[96] The consensus statements also highlight the need for continued assessment of neurologic function and warn that patients on regimens of multiple anticoagulants are at higher risk of bleeding complications. Based on these consensus statements, most institutions have developed guidelines for the provision of neuraxial techniques. Clinicians should check with their institutions regarding their specific guidelines.

Peripheral Nerve Blocks

In the management of acute pain, it is clear that methods that provide safe and efficient analgesia can have profound effects on patient outcomes and satisfaction. The use of regional anesthetic techniques has undergone a renaissance over the past decade. In particular, the utilization of ultrasonography has given practitioners the ability to perform fast, reliable blocks. Additionally, it has provided clinicians the confidence to pursue novel techniques that confer greater selectivity and decreased motor blockade. As techniques have advanced, the implementation of indwelling peripheral nerve catheters (PNCs) has provided a means of extending the benefits of regional anesthesia.

The utilization of regional techniques has also changed the way we approach acute pain management in both civilian and war trauma patients. Under the right circumstances, simple effective blocks that do not compromise hemodynamics or respiratory function can be provided in prehospital settings to provide fast analgesia. The use of regional anesthesia in these settings should only be considered after conducting a baseline neurologic examination to rule out potential contraindications. Additionally, regional anesthesia techniques should only be used after proper stabilization of the patient and should not delay transport to higher care facilities. In France, the implementation of femoral nerve blocks has become common before transporting patients with femur fractures.[98] On the battlefield, regional anesthesia plays a vital role in providing effective analgesia in triage areas so that patients can be transported to tertiary care centers without the need for advanced airway management.[99] Victims of traumatic injuries often present with a full stomach. Additionally, they may require cervical spine stabilization from injury; it is also possible that one cannot reliably rule out injury. These circumstances place the patients at higher risk of aspiration and make it difficult for the clinician to properly secure the airway. Using regional techniques mitigates some of these risks and provides superior analgesia over systemic and oral opioids.[99]

The use of regional anesthesia is also an invaluable part of perioperative pain management. Increasing institutional demands to reduce length of stays or provide same-day discharges coupled with societal demands to provide effective pain management underscore the need for regional techniques.[100,101] Strategies that incorporate regional anesthesia combined with anesthetic management with propofol have been shown to provide rapid recovery and decrease the incidence of postoperative nausea and vomiting (PONV).[102-104] Studies also suggest that avoidance of volatile anesthetic agents has reduced incidences of unplanned admissions secondary to uncontrolled pain.[105-109]

Recent trends in regional anesthesia have seen the implementation of indwelling PNCs. As opposed to single-injection blocks that provide 12 to 24 hours of analgesia, indwelling catheters extend the benefits of the block by providing constant infusions of low-concentration local anesthetics. As opposed to epidural analgesia and IV PCA use that requires hospitalization, patients can be discharged home with PNCs in place.[110-115] This practice has been shown to be very effective for select procedures by providing superior analgesia, reducing opioid side effects, and providing high levels of patient satisfaction.[114] A meta-analysis of randomized controlled trials comparing postoperative analgesia among PNCs with opioids found PNCs to confer significant benefits. In addition to

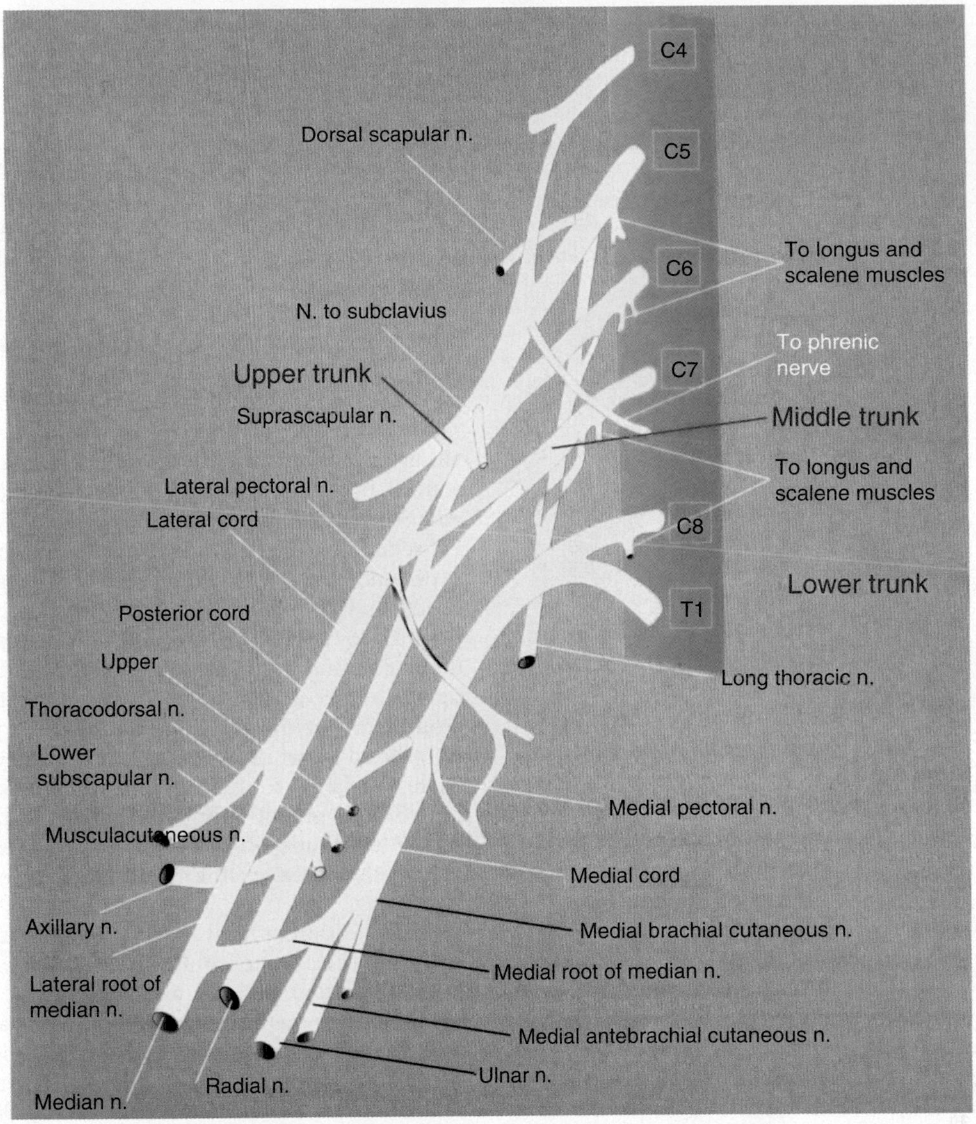

Figure 14A-2. Nervous system of the brachial plexus. *n,* Nerve.

providing superior analgesia and reduced opioid side effects, PNCs were associated with improved physical therapy, better sleep patterns, shorter lengths of stay, and better patient satisfaction.[116] Perhaps the area where PNCs have had the most dramatic impact has been in their use in the treatment of military-related traumas. Early placement of PNCs allows for improved evacuation conditions, and their continued use in tertiary care settings facilitates anesthesia and analgesia for patients who may require multiple procedures, including operations to dressing changes. Continued use throughout the recovery period aids in rehabilitation efforts. PNCs have been proven to be extremely versatile; they can be used to achieve surgical anesthesia or maintain analgesia through continuous infusions or even be temporarily stopped to assess peripheral nerve functions.

Upper Extremity Blocks

Severe acute pain of the upper extremity from surgeries or injuries can be managed by performing peripheral nerve blocks at various locations along the brachial plexus. The brachial plexus is the network of nerve fibers that is responsible for most sensory and motor function of the upper extremity. The exceptions are the spinal accessory nerve (cranial nerve XI), which innervates the trapezius, and the intercostobrachial nerve, which supplies sensation to the upper half of the medial and posterior aspect of the arm. The brachial plexus is formed by the ventral rami of the fifth to eighth cervical and the first thoracic nerves. The fourth cervical and second thoracic nerves can also make small contributions to the brachial plexus. As the brachial plexus emerges from the cervical roots in the neck through the upper extremity, it divides to form trunks, divisions, cords, and terminal branches (Fig. 14A-2). Sensory information can be interrupted at each of these locations along the plexus through the application of local anesthetics.

Interscalene Block

Halsted performed the first brachial plexus block in 1885 through direct surgical exposure by applying cocaine. It was not until the 1900s that percutaneous approaches were described.[117] In 1970, Winnie described a percutaneous approach between the anterior and middle scalene muscle at

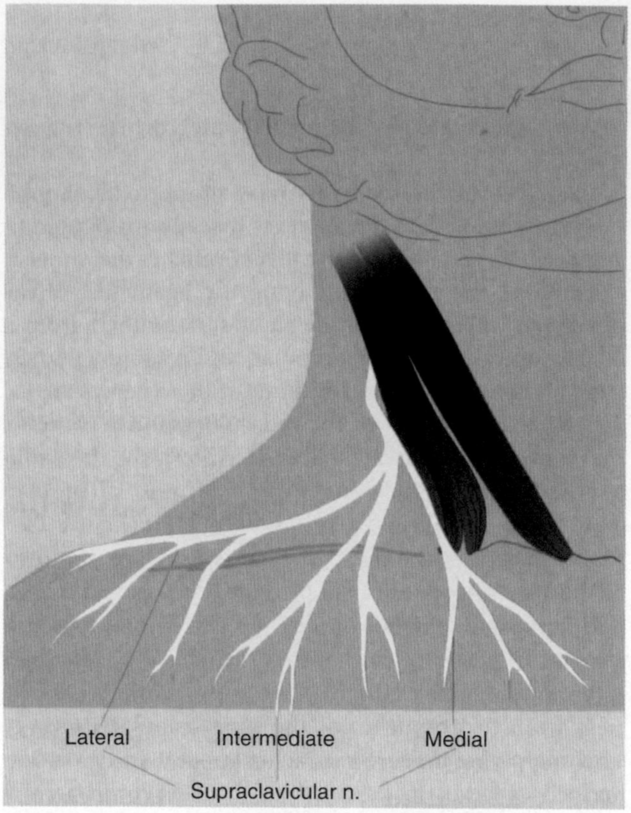

Figure 14A-3. Supraventricular nerves in the shoulder. *n,* Nerve.

the level of the cricoid cartilage that produced consistent and effective results.[118] The interscalene block (ISB) is performed at the level of the roots and trunks yielding the most proximal approach to the brachial plexus. This approach is effective in providing analgesia to the shoulder and proximal humerus from surgeries or traumatic injuries. Although the brachial plexus is responsible for all motor function of the shoulder, it is not entirely responsible for all sensory function. The cephalad–cutaneous portions of the shoulder are supplied by the supraclavicular nerves that emanate from the lower portion of the superficial cervical plexus (C3–C4) (Fig. 14A-3). The interscalene approach offers superior analgesia to the shoulder because it reliably blocks the upper (C5–C6) and middle trunk (C7) as well as the cervical plexus (C3-4). It is common for this approach to spare the lower trunk (C8–T1), thus making it unsuitable for treating acute pain in the forearm or hand.

Interscalene blocks have been used extensively for procedures involving the shoulder, demonstrating analgesia that is far superior to IV opioids. Additionally, studies have found that the use of ISB in shoulder surgeries dramatically reduces VAS pain scores as well as total opioid requirement, decreases the incidence of PONV, improves sleep patterns, shortens lengths of stay, and improves patient satisfaction.[119-124] Continuous ISBs by placement of an indwelling catheter have also been used with a high rate of success. Compared with one-time ISB injections and IV opioids for postoperative pain management, continuous blocks have demonstrated improved VAS scores, reduced opioid consumption, and improved rehabilitation.[125-128] The use of continuous interscalene catheters has also allowed previously inpatient procedures, such as total shoulder arthroplasties, to be performed in ambulatory settings. Early studies have shown that a subset of patients who do not have significant comorbidities may be eligible for same-day total shoulder arthroplasties if continuous interscalene catheters are a part of their multimodal pain management regimen.[112]

The ISB is a relatively simple procedure to perform and begins with the patient in the supine position with the head of the bed elevated to approximately 45 degrees. The patient's head is turned slightly away from the side to be blocked, and the level of the cricoid cartilage is identified. Palpating posteriorly along the lateral border of the sternocleidomastoid muscle can identify the interscalene groove. Placement of a linear, low-penetration, high-resolution ultrasound probe allows for rapid identification of the neural structures (Fig. 14A-4). The use of a nerve stimulator may also be used for either primary identification of the brachial plexus (no ultrasound) or as a method of confirmation (with ultrasound). After sterile prep and drape, the patient is typically given light IV sedation to provide anxiolysis and improve the patient experience. A 2-inch short bevel echogenic or stimulating needle is then advanced toward the brachial plexus. When the ultrasound is used, the needle is advanced "in plane" of the ultrasound beam, allowing for easier identification of the tip of the needle (Fig. 14A-5). Local anesthetic is deposited around the neural structures under direct visualization. If ultrasound is not used, the needle is advanced at a 45-degree angle in relation to the skin directed toward the contralateral nipple. The practitioner relies on evoked motor responses at low amplitude (<0.5 mA) as a means of determining the relationship between the tip of the needle and the nervous structures.

The injection of local anesthetic in the interscalene groove (between the anterior and middle scalene) invariably results in the diffusion of local anesthetic away from the groove. Although this has some advantages such as blockade of the supraclavicular nerve, it also produces some undesirable side effects. The phrenic nerve runs along the superficial surface of the anterior scalene and is blocked 100% of the time with ISB. Blockade of the phrenic nerve can be undesirable in certain patients with significant pulmonary disease. Similarly, trauma patients with pulmonary injuries or contralateral

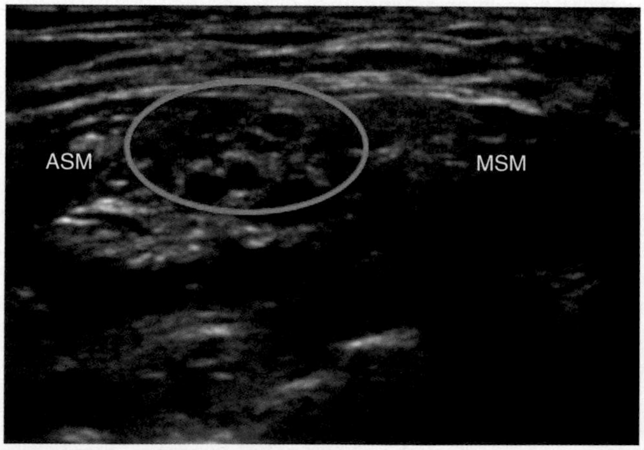

Figure 14A-4. Ultrasound image of the interscalene groove. At this level, the roots and trunks of the brachial plexus can be identified as hypoechoic structures *(circle)* lying between the anterior scalene muscle (ASM) and middle scalene muscle (MSM).

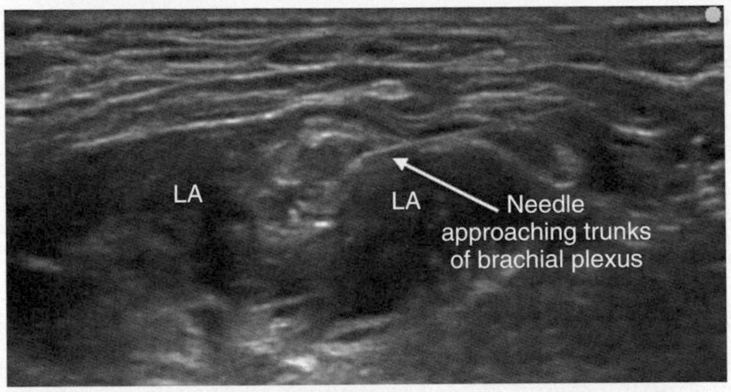

Figure 14A-5. An in-plane approach allows for direct visualization of the block needle as it approaches the trunks of the brachial plexus within the interscalene groove. The local anesthetic (LA) is hypoechoic on ultrasonography and can be seen spreading in a circumferential fashion around the nerve structures.

pneumothorax[129] are poor candidates for ISB. The effect on the phrenic nerve can last, on average, 6 hours. Interestingly, studies that have measured respiratory function in patients undergoing total shoulder repairs found that those who received continuous interscalene catheters versus opioids showed improved respiratory function at 24 and 48 hours postoperatively. The improvement in respiratory function was attributed to better analgesia, resulting in better force diaphragmatic excursion coupled with an absence of respiratory depression often caused by opioids.[130] For patients who require shoulder surgeries but are not candidates for ISB because of pulmonary concerns, it is possible to provide improved analgesia by performing a combined suprascapular and axillary block. Although this technique provides inferior analgesia than ISB for shoulder procedures, it has been shown to be more effective than PCA alone.[131]

Supraclavicular

The supraclavicular approach to the brachial plexus provides the unique opportunity to provide dense analgesia and anesthesia to most of the upper extremity. Before entering the axilla, almost all of the sensory, motor, and sympathetic innervation of the upper extremity is contained within three neural structures that lie within close proximity to one another. This allows for a rapid, dense block that does not require a high volume of local anesthetic. Kulenkampff described the first supraclavicular approach in 1911, which he reportedly performed on himself. Although his technique offered the ability to provide blockade over a vast majority of the upper extremity, it carried the inherent risk of causing pneumothorax. Kulenkampff's approach was published in 1928[132] and was widely used until the first descriptions of the axillary block were published in 1949.[133] The advent of the axillary approach eliminated the risk of pneumothorax, making it a safer choice. Over the past decade, there has been resurgence in the use of supraclavicular blocks mainly because of the use of ultrasound guidance. In experienced hands, the trunks of the brachial plexus can be easily identified as they appear lateral and superior to the subclavian artery (Fig. 14A-6). Direct visualization of the structures and advancing needle allows the block to take place quickly and safely. Although this block confers a high rate of success for procedures involving most of the upper extremity, it may not reliably cover procedures related to the shoulder. As stated previously, patients with pulmonary compromise who would not tolerate phrenic nerve blocks are not candidates for ISBs. As an alternative, supraclavicular blocks have produced moderate success. Studies indicate that the incidence of phrenic nerve blockade with the supraclavicular approach ranges from 0% to 50%. Current literature suggests that the incidence of phrenic nerve blocks is closer to 0% when ultrasound is used; use of nerve stimulator alone results in an incidence closer to 50%.[134] Failure to produce adequate coverage of the shoulder from the supraclavicular approach is due to sparing of the dorsal scapular nerve, which emanates from the root of C5, as well as the supraclavicular nerve arising from the cervical plexus (C3–C4).

To perform the block, the patient is positioned supine with the head of the bed elevated up to 45 degrees. After sterile preparation and draping of the skin, the patient is given a small amount of sedation for anxiolysis and comfort. The patient's head is turned slightly away from the side to be blocked, and a linear, low-penetration, high-resolution ultrasound probe is placed with the supraclavicular fossa. The probe is scanned in a coronal and oblique plane to optimize a transverse view of the subclavian artery and neural structures. In this region, the trunks of the brachial plexus will appear as a hypoechoic cluster of grapes lying lateral and posterior to the subclavian artery. A 2-inch echogenic or nerve-stimulating needle is advanced in plane toward the neural structures. The final needle tip position can vary slightly, but it is often advantageous to direct the needle toward the posterolateral aspect of the subclavian artery at about the 7 o'clock position. Positioning the needle at this location allows for more consistent coverage of the lower trunk and ulnar nerve (Fig. 14A-7). To avoid inadvertent puncture of the underlying pleura or subclavian artery, visualization of the needle tip is critical in performing this block.

Infraclavicular

The infraclavicular block disrupts nerve transmission at the level of the cords and divisions of the brachial plexus. Similar to the supraclavicular approach, this approach accesses the brachial plexus at a point where the neural structures are fairly compact. The first descriptions of the infraclavicular block

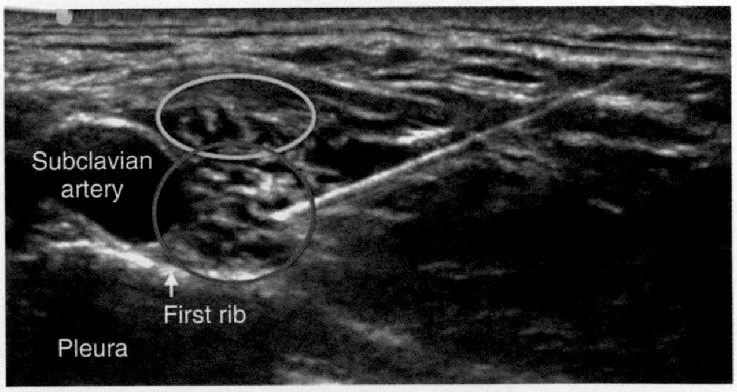

Figure 14A-6. The ultrasound probe placed in the supraclavicular fossa allows for quick identification of the brachial plexus. Above both the upper *(blue circle)* and lower trunks *(red circle)* of the brachial plexus can be easily identified. In this view, the nerve structures are hypoechoic and appear as a cluster of grapes lying superiorly and laterally to the subclavian artery. This view demonstrates that before entering the axilla, most of the nerve structures of the upper extremity lie within close proximity to each other. This allows for a single-site injection that produces anesthesia and analgesia for most of the upper extremity.

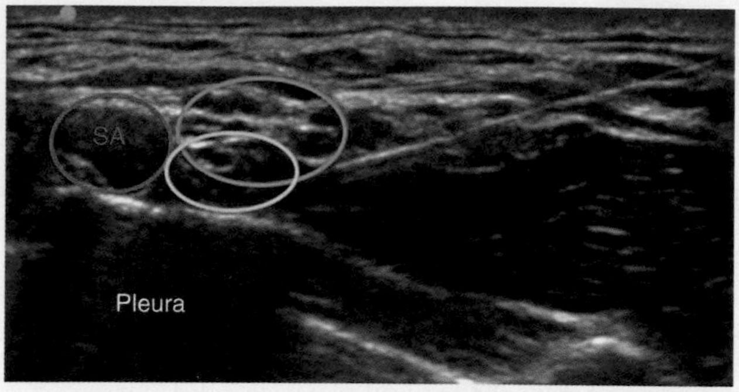

Figure 14A-7. An ultrasound-guided supraclavicular block using an in-plane technique. With the upper *(blue circle)* and lower *(grey circle)* trunks easily identified, the needle is directed toward the 5 o'clock position of the subclavian artery (SA). The initial spread of local anesthetic in this picture can be seen around the lower trunk. As the injection continues, local anesthetic will continue to surround the trunks, allowing for anesthesia and analgesia of most of the upper extremity.

were published by Bazy and colleagues in 1914.[135] The initial technique underwent numerous modifications and was only moderately used up until the 1940s. Similar to the supraclavicular block, a reduction in its popularity most likely stemmed from the increasing popularity of the axillary block. The infraclavicular block was reintroduced by Raj in 1973.[136] and later modified by Whiffler in 1981.[137] Since that time, this block has steadily increased in popularity and use.

The infraclavicular block has been shown to provide effective analgesia and anesthesia for procedures that involve the elbow, wrist, and hand.[138,139] Additionally, this approach lends itself well to the insertion of indwelling continuous catheters because they can be secured very easily to the chest wall. Positioning of the catheter on the chest wall provides stability, reducing the risk of catheter dislodgement while providing improved comfort to the patient (Fig. 14A-8). Outcome studies of infraclavicular blocks have shown improved postoperative analgesia for patients undergoing wrist and hand procedures.[140] Patients who were randomized to receive general anesthesia with volatile anesthetics, on the other hand, were more likely to have higher pain scores, longer times to ambulation, longer times to discharge, and increased admissions.[140] The use of continuous infraclavicular catheters has been shown to extend the benefits of the block by reducing pain scores while in place, reducing total opioid consumption, and minimizing opioid-related side effects.[141-143]

To perform the block, the patient is placed in the supine position with the head of the bed slightly elevated. The patient is provided a small amount of IV sedation for anxiolysis and comfort. After sterile prep and drapes are applied, a standard linear high-frequency probe is placed medial to the coracoid process and inferior to the clavicle in a parasagittal orientation. Small adjustments are made with the ultrasound until the view of the axillary vessels and cords of the brachial plexus are optimized. Below the level of the clavicle, the cord structures will appear as small, dense hyperechoic structures that are oriented around the axillary artery. The lateral cord is typically observed superolateral to the artery between the 9 and 12 o'clock positions, and the posterior cord is often identified between the 6 and 9 o'clock positions. The median cord can be harder to visualize but typically resides on the medial aspect of the artery between the 3 and 6 o'clock positions. Using an in-plane technique, a 4-inch echogenic or nerve-stimulating needle is placed inferior to the clavicle and advanced caudally. Individual identification of the cords can be achieved by nerve stimulation with subsequent deposit of local anesthetic at each site. Alternatively, to decrease block time and improve efficiency, the needle may be directed toward the posterior cord. Deposition of the

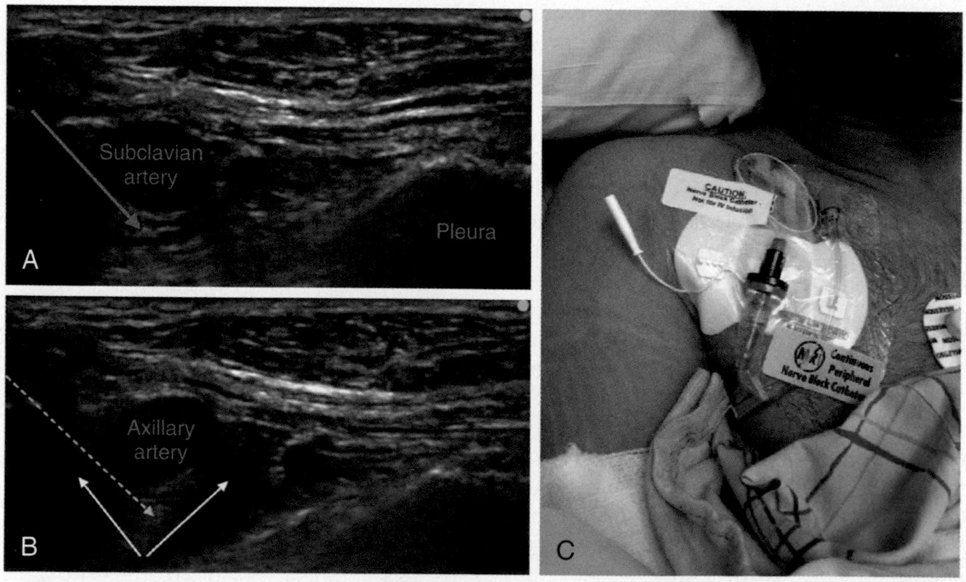

Figure 14A-8. A, The infraclavicular approach to the brachial plexus allows for blockade of the brachial plexus at the level of the cords. In this view, the cords appear as small, densely hyperechoic structures lying lateral, posterior, and medial to the axillary artery. The *arrow* signifies the desired trajectory of the block needle. **B,** With the needle placed at the 6 o'clock position, the axillary artery injection allows for circumferential spread about the artery. Spread in this distribution allows for blockade of all three cords without further manipulation of the block needle. **C,** Example of a continuous infraclavicular catheter that has been secured to the chest wall. Catheter placement at this location is less likely to migrate or dislodge than other sites (axillary) and is comfortable for the patient.

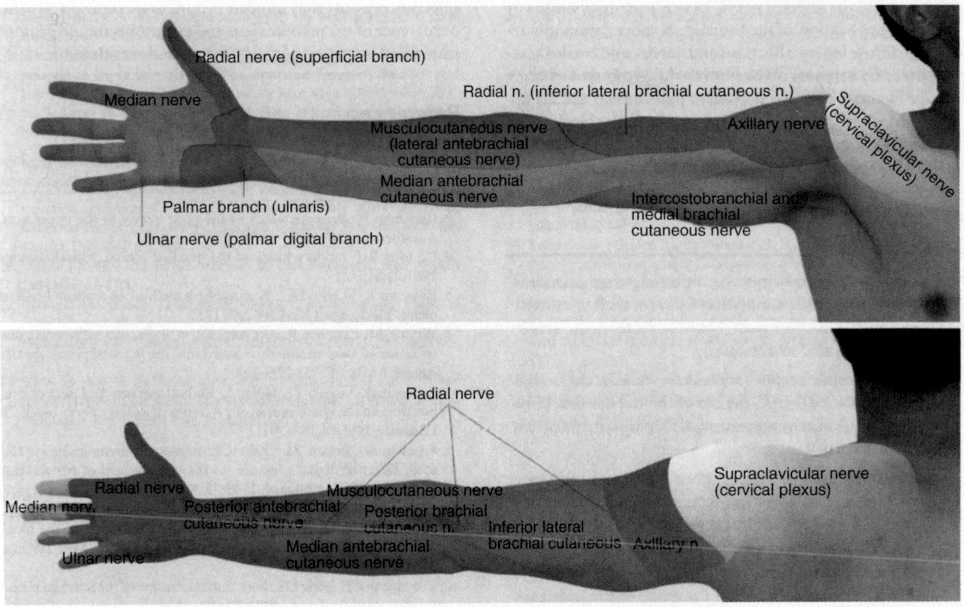

Figure 14A-9. Sensory innervation for the upper extremity.

local anesthetic posterior to the artery often results in a U-shaped spread around the artery. This distribution of local anesthetic around the artery confers successful blockade of all three cords.

Axillary

The axillary approach to the brachial plexus has been the most widely used regional technique since the late 1950s.[144,145] This has been an attractive approach to the brachial plexus because it is a relatively easy block to perform and has a low side effect profile. The goal of the axillary block is to cover the distal terminal branches of the brachial plexus, which consists of the radial, median, ulnar, and musculocutaneous nerves. Performance of this block produces analgesia and anesthesia for the distal upper extremity but may not be relied on as a sole anesthetic technique when a tourniquet is required. Coverage for cases that involve the use of an upper extremity tourniquet may require additional block supplementation of the intercostobrachial, medial brachial cutaneous, and median antebrachial cutaneous nerves (Fig. 14A-9).

As with other blocks of the brachial plexus, the axillary block has been shown to be effective in the management of acute pain. Studies have demonstrated a greater than 50% reduction in VAS scores with increased time to requested pain medication, decreased opioid consumption, and decreased opioid-related side effects.[145,146] As might be expected, benefits are discontinued with the resolution of the block. As a result, continuous indwelling catheters have been advocated. Continuous axillary catheters have been used for outpatient use with varying degrees of success.[147,148] Because of the catheter's location in the axilla, it is often difficult to maintain a clean comfortable site. Problems related to infection, failure rate, catheter kinking, and dislodgement have led clinicians to favor other sites for catheter placement (infraclavicular and supraclavicular).[149,150]

The axillary block is performed with the patient in the supine position. The patient's arm to be blocked is abducted 90 degrees, externally rotated with the elbow flexed. Although modifications using a nerve stimulating technique exist, the most common approach is a transarterial method. After sterile prep and drape, the axillary artery is palpated in its most proximal location, usually around the axillary crease. A small, thin needle is advanced toward the pulsation under constant aspiration. When bright red blood is freely aspirated, the needle is further advanced just until aspiration ceases. Half of the volume of local anesthetic to be used is injected, allowing for blockade of the radial nerve. The needle is then slowly withdrawn, again under constant aspiration. Withdrawal of the needle continues until aspiration of blood ceases. With the needle now in a medial and superficial location with respect to the artery, the remaining local anesthetic is injected for blockade of the median and ulnar nerves. This approach is fast and easy but often spares the musculocutaneous nerve, which typically leaves the neurovascular sheath at the level of the coracoid process. The musculocutaneous nerve often needs to be blocked separately and is found within the coracobrachialis muscle. More recently, ultrasound guidance has been used to deliver a fast, reliable block without having to pierce vascular structures. A linear, high-resolution ultrasound probe oriented in the transverse plane of the axillary crease allows for visualization of the vascular and neural structures. Using an in-plane approach, an echogenic or nerve-stimulating needle is advanced to each neural structure and bathed in a local anesthetic solution.

Lower Extremity Blocks

For many years, spinal and epidural infusions have been the treatment of choice for acute pain in the lower extremity from surgical procedures or injuries. Although there is no questioning the effectiveness of these techniques, the use of peripheral nerve blocks and indwelling catheters may provide more flexibility. Patients who require anticoagulation or thromboprophylactic medications may not be candidates for neuraxial procedures. Additionally, peripheral nerve blocks are not associated with the side effects commonly reported with neuraxial techniques, such as urinary retention, bilateral motor weakness, nausea and vomiting, pruritus, and respiratory depression. As the field of regional anesthesia continues to evolve, techniques that focus on providing preferential sensory blocks have the potential to radically improve pain management while facilitating early mobilization and rehabilitation. This emerging trend can be seen in the current use of adductor canal blocks, local infiltrations of anesthesia with liposomal bupivacaine, and motor-sparing knee blocks.[151]

Lumbar Plexus Blocks (Psoas Compartment Block)

The innervation of the lower extremity stems from the lumbar and sacral plexuses. The lumbar plexus is formed from the divisions of the L1–L4 nerve roots with variable contribution from T12 and give rise to peripheral nerves that innervate the anterior lower extremity (Fig. 14A-10). After leaving the intervertebral foramina, the roots of L2–L4 give rise to nerves that run within the body of the psoas muscle. The lateral femoral cutaneous and femoral nerves exist within a fascial sleeve that divides the muscle into an anterior two-thirds and posterior third. More than 50% of the time, the obturator is separated from this sheath by a muscular fold. Winnie and colleagues first described the posterior approach to the lumbar plexus in 1974.[152] and since that time, only small modifications have been made. Because of the complexity of the block, most practitioners prefer to perform a neuraxial technique, which is a proven, fast, and reliable way of providing surgical-grade anesthesia. Additionally, because of the depth of the block, as well as the possibility of entering the neuraxial space, this block should not be used as an alternative for neuraxial blocks when the patient is on anticoagulants. When done successfully, the lumbar plexus block provides anesthesia and analgesia to the lateral femoral cutaneous (L3–L4), femoral (L4–L5), and obturator (L5–S1) nerves.

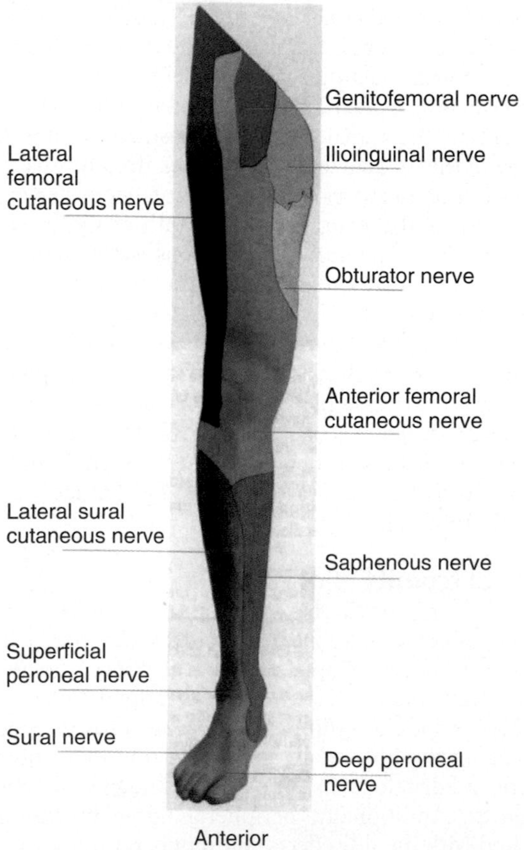

Figure 14A-10. Lower extremity innervation.

Although lumbar plexus blocks can be performed for a variety of procedures involving the lower extremity, it has been shown to be particularly useful for pain related to the hip. Studies comparing lumbar plexus blocks with general anesthesia for hip surgeries have found reductions in pain scores and opioid consumption with lumbar plexus blocks until block resolution.[153] As with other peripheral nerve blocks, the benefits of the block can be extended by the placement of a continuous catheter. When lumbar plexus catheters were compared with epidural catheters for total hip arthroplasties, the results showed that the plexus group demonstrated less motor block, quicker ambulation, and fewer complications.[154] Although data exist showing the benefit of lumbar plexus blocks in patients undergoing invasive knee procedures, it has not been shown to provide benefits beyond what can be achieved with femoral blocks.[155] Given that femoral blocks are fast and easy and present low risks, they are typically favored over lumbar plexus blocks for invasive knee procedures.

To perform the lumbar plexus block, the patient is placed in the lateral decubitus position with the side to be blocked facing upward. A line connecting the iliac crests (Tuffier line) is drawn as well as a line that connects the spinous processes of the lumbar region. The needle insertion point is located 4 cm lateral to the intersection point of the two lines. Alternatively, a line extending from the posterior superior iliac spine (PSIS) can be drawn parallel to the spinous processes. The needle is inserted at the intersection of the line from the PSIS with the Tuffier line. After sterile preparation of the skin and appropriate drape placement, the patient is given light IV sedation for anxiolysis and comfort. A 10-cm nerve-stimulating needle is inserted at an angle that is perpendicular to the skin. The needle is advanced stimulating at a current between 1.0 and 1.5 mA. Needle location is assumed to be in the right location when contraction of the quadriceps muscles occurs. When the appropriate muscle group is stimulated, the amplitude should be slowly decreased to optimize needle location. When stimulation occurs at low amplitudes (<0.4 mA), the practitioner should be concerned about the possibility of dural sleeve or epidural placement. Because this procedure has the risk of epidural or subarachnoid injection, it is suggested to carefully inject the local anesthetic in small aliquots over a 5- to 10-minute period. During the injection phase, the patient should be frequently assessed for epidural or subarachnoid spread.

Femoral

The femoral nerve block is a fast, easy block that can provide anesthesia and analgesia to the anterior thigh and medial aspect of the lower leg. The femoral nerve arises from the dorsal divisions of the anterior rami of the L2, L3, and L4 nerve roots. As the nerve emerges from the lateral border of the psoas muscle, it enters the thigh posterior to the inguinal ligament, running a course that is lateral and slightly posterior to the femoral artery. It is the nerves' relation to the femoral artery, just below the inguinal ligament, that makes it relatively easy to locate. As stated previously, this block is so basic yet

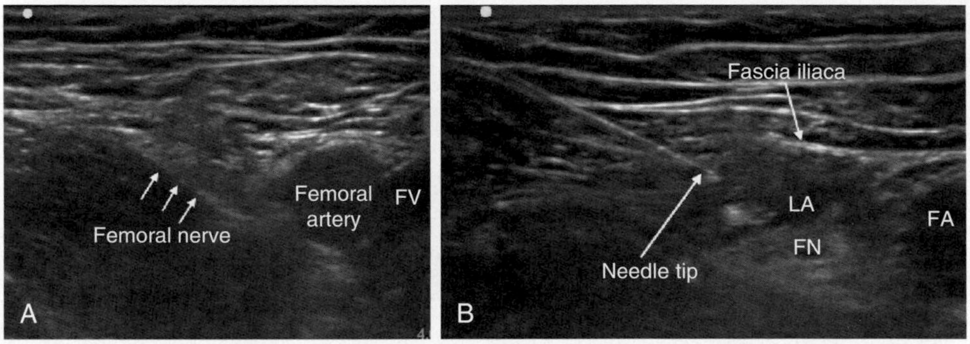

Figure 14A-11. A, View of the ultrasound anatomy in the femoral crease. The femoral nerve (FN) appears as a tear-shaped structure lateral to the femoral artery and vein (FV). The fascia lata and iliaca lie superior to the nerve. **B,** An in-plane approach to the FN allows for direct visualization of the block needle. In this image, local anesthetic (LA) can be seen surrounding the FN. The local anesthetic stays confined to an area below the fascia iliaca and fascia lata. *FA,* Femoral artery.

effective that it is even being used in prehospital settings to provide fast and effective pain management.

The femoral nerve block has been shown to provide reliable, effective analgesia for procedures or injuries of the anterior thigh and knee. When the femoral block is coupled with a sciatic block, excellent anesthesia and analgesia can be provided for invasive knee procedures. Unlike the lumbar plexus block, the femoral block fails to block the obturator nerve. As a result, a variable percentage of the population will report medial thigh pain despite evidence of adequate femoral block. Modifications of the femoral block to achieve a "three-in-one" block have produced inconsistent results. The use of indwelling femoral catheters has been shown to be advantageous in patients undergoing total knee arthroplasties. Compared with patients with IV PCA or epidural infusions, the femoral catheter patients demonstrated reduced postoperative morphine requirements, earlier ambulation, significant reductions in serious complications, and decreased lengths of hospital stay.[156-158]

To perform the femoral block, the patient is placed in the supine position, and the femoral pulse is palpated in the inguinal crease on the side to be blocked. After sterile preparation of the skin and appropriate placement of drapes, the patient is given a minimal amount of IV sedation to produce anxiolysis and comfort. A 2-inch nerve-stimulating needle is inserted just lateral to the femoral pulsation in a slightly cephalad orientation and advanced to achieve motor stimulation of the quadriceps muscles. The presence of patellar excursion indicates proper placement of the needle. The stimulating current is slowly decreased to optimize needle position. Current output between 0.3 and 0.5 mA that still produces a consistent quadriceps response suggests adequate placement of the needle. After negative aspiration, the local anesthetic is injected in 2- to 3-mL aliquots over several minutes. The use of a linear high-resolution ultrasound probe allows for the direct visualization of the femoral nerve and artery. The ultrasound probe should be placed in line with the femoral crease and scanned in a cephalad direction to optimize the view of the femoral nerve. An echogenic or nerve-stimulating needle is directed toward the femoral nerve utilizing an in-plane technique (Fig. 14A-11). The ultrasound also aids in the speed and efficiency of placing an indwelling catheter by allowing direct visualization of catheter placement next to the nerve (Fig. 14A-12).

Adductor Canal Block

Although femoral nerve blocks and continuous femoral nerve catheters have been shown to provide benefits and improved outcomes for patients undergoing total knee arthroplasties, a modification of the femoral nerve block is becoming increasingly popular. Blockade of the femoral nerve within the adductor canal allows for blockade at a location where many of the motor branches to the quadriceps muscles have already departed from the nerve. By preserving muscle strength, patients have better stability (less falls) and are able to ambulate earlier. Initial studies compared the level of muscle sparing among patients receiving either the adductor canal blocks or the traditional femoral blocks. These studies demonstrated that adductor canal blocks reduced motor strength by only 8% from baseline as opposed to 49% for femoral nerve blocks.[159] The additional quadriceps strength allowed for better stability and weight-bearing with a lower risk of patient falls. Recent studies comparing their analgesic effects have shown that adductor canal blocks produce a level of analgesia for patients undergoing total knee arthroplasties that is equivalent to femoral blocks.[160]

To perform an adductor block, the patient is placed in the supine position, and the leg to be blocked is flexed at the knee

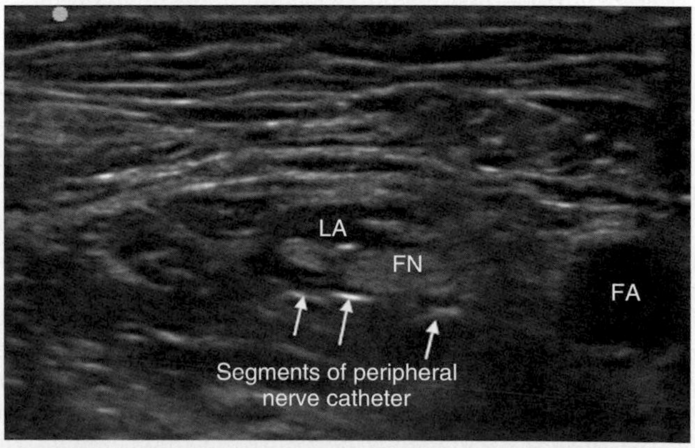

Figure 14A-12. Continuous femoral nerve catheter. In this view, a catheter that has been placed appears as bright, hyperechoic structure lying posterior to the femoral nerve (FN). Local anesthetic that has been injected through the catheter can be seen surrounding the nerve. *FA,* Femoral artery; *LA,* local anesthetic.

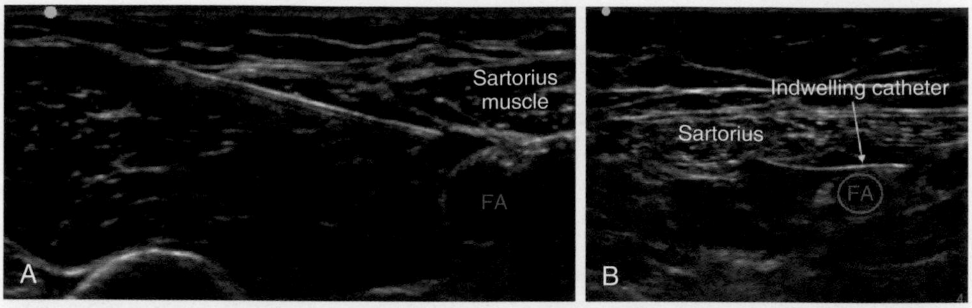

Figure 14A-13. **A,** Distal blockade of the femoral nerve within adductor canal allows for better preservation of quadriceps function while producing excellent analgesia for the knee. The position of the nerve in relation to the femoral artery (FA) within the canal can vary from medial to lateral as it travels distally within the canal. The block needle is directed toward the 12 o'clock position so that local anesthetic can be distributed on either side of the artery. When the nerve is visible, it appears as a small hyperechoic structure. **B,** In this view, a continuous catheter can be seen placed in an optimal position between the sartorius muscle and femoral artery (12 o'clock). Spread of local anesthetic can be seen medially and laterally around the artery.

and externally rotated. After the skin is prepared in a sterile fashion and the appropriate drapes are applied, the patient is given light IV sedation. A linear high-resolution ultrasound probe is placed in a transverse orientation on the medial aspect of the midthigh. In this position, the femoral artery and the roof of the canal (the sartorius muscle) can be easily identified. An echogenic 4-inch needle is advanced toward the neurovascular structures using an in-plane technique so that the tip of the needle can be visualized. The femoral nerve can vary in its location about the artery; injection of local anesthetic should be performed so that spread includes both the medial and lateral sides around the artery (Fig. 14A-13). When a catheter is used, it is optimal to thread the catheter around the 12 o'clock position on the artery to achieve perivascular spread with the infusion.

Parasacral Block

Blockade of the sciatic nerve can be very effective in the management of postoperative and acute pain syndromes associated with the posterior thigh and distal extremity below the knee. The sciatic nerve is the largest peripheral nerve in the body and measures more than 1 cm in width around its origin. It is formed from the lumbosacral plexus, which is the union of the lumbosacral trunk with the first three sacral nerves (Fig. 14A-14). The sacral plexus is formed on the anterior surface of the piriformis muscle and yields multiple collateral nerves along with the sciatic nerve, which represents its terminal ending. The sciatic nerve exits the greater sciatic notch below the piriformis and continues between the greater trochanter and ischial tuberosity. As it continues to descend in the posterior thigh, behind the adductor magnus, it eventually splits to form the tibial and common peroneal nerves.

Although there are multiple locations along the sciatic nerve where a block can take place, blockade at the parasacral plexus may offer some advantages. Mansour first described this approach in 1993,[161] and since that time, it has steadily increased in popularity. Blocks performed at the parasacral level allow for a "plexus" type of block that results in anesthesia and analgesia of the sciatic and the collateral branches, including the posterior cutaneous nerve to the thigh and to the obturator internus. Successful blockade of the sacral plexus produces analgesia for the medial aspect of the gluteus, posterior thigh, posterior knee, variable portion of the hip, and entire lower extremity below the knee with the exception of the medial cutaneous aspect, which is supplied by the saphenous nerve. Performance of a parasacral block coupled with a lumbar plexus block may provide complete anesthesia and analgesia of the lower extremity and may have clinical usefulness in patients in whom a neuraxial procedure is undesirable or contraindicated (e.g., critical aortic stenosis, difficult airway, or prior back surgery). Similar to lumbar plexus blocks, the parasacral approach should be considered a "deep" block and thus should also follow the rules for anticoagulation and thromboprophylaxis that are applied to neuraxial procedures.

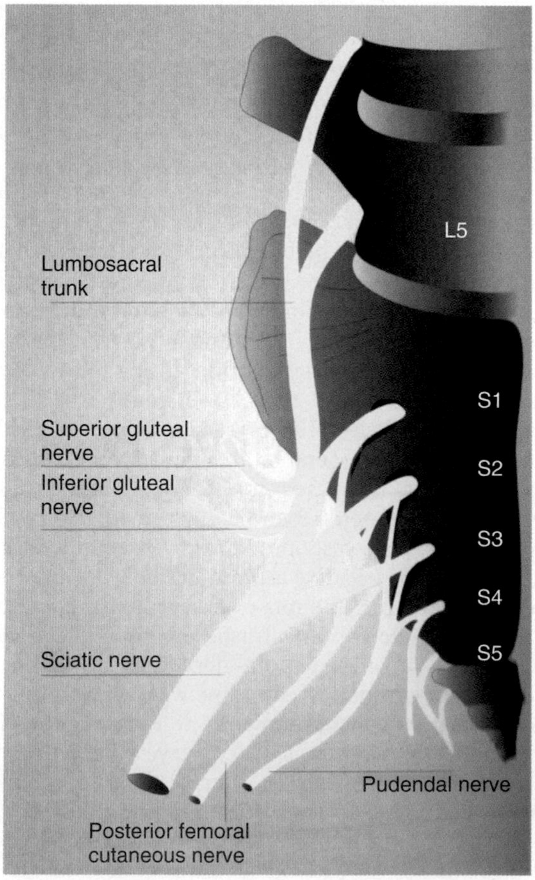

Figure 14A-14. Innervation of the sacral plexus.

It should be remembered that the contents of the pelvis lie just anterior to the plexus, and uncontrolled bleeding could result in significant harm to the patient.

To perform the parasacral block, the patient is placed in the lateral decubitus position with the side to be blocked facing upward. The knee and hip of the target extremity should be flexed. A line is drawn from the PSIS to the inferior border of the ischial tuberosity. On this line, a point measuring 6 cm from the PSIS is identified as the insertion site. The patient is given light IV sedation for anxiolysis and comfort, and the skin is carefully prepped and draped. After SC infiltration of the skin with local anesthetic, a 4- to 6-inch stimulating needle is inserted and directed perpendicular to the skin. When through the skin, the stimulator is set to 1 mA, and the needle is advanced until plantar flexion or dorsiflexion of the toes is elicited. Slowly reducing the current and making small adjustments to maintain the appropriate motor response optimizes the position of the needle tip. Generally, a motor response that is maintained below 0.4 mA indicates proper needle tip position, and local anesthetics can be incrementally injected. Ultrasound guidance may also be used to aid in block speed and accuracy, but direct visualization of nerve structures may be difficult because of body habitus and depth. When the ultrasound is used, a high-frequency, high-resolution ultrasound probe is placed transversely 8 cm lateral to the top of the gluteal fold. Body habitus and depth of structures may necessitate the use of a low-frequency, high-penetration ultrasound probe. In this position, the posterior border of the ischium (PBI) can be identified. The sacral plexus lies medial to the PBI (greater sciatic foramen) and can be accessed by using an in-plane approach. Care should be taken to visualize the tip of the needle because the inferior gluteal vessels run just medial and deep to the sacral plexus. Additionally, the peritoneum and pelvic structures that lie just anterior to the plexus can be visualized and should be avoided. Similar to other peripheral nerve blocks, a continuous indwelling catheter may be placed in this location to provide extended pain management.

Sciatic Nerve Block

As stated earlier, several locations along the course of the sciatic nerve are suitable for performing a peripheral nerve block. Pauchet described the first sciatic block in 1920[162]; however, the approach is commonly ascribed to Labat, one of Pauchet's students. This first approach is commonly referred to as the midgluteal approach and accesses the sciatic nerve at a point slightly caudad from the site of the parasacral plexus. Since the initial description of the sciatic nerve block, it has undergone many modifications, the most notable of which include the anterior approach by Beck in 1963.[163] Winnie's modification in 1975,[164] a lithotomy approach by Raj in 1975,[165] the parasacral approach by Mansour in 1993,[161] and di Benedetto's subgluteal approach in 2001.[166] There are advantages and disadvantages to each technique, and choosing among these techniques is often a function of clinical circumstance as well as the operator's familiarity with each approach. For example, whereas patients who cannot be positioned laterally may require an anterior approach, patients undergoing ambulatory procedures for the foot and ankle may benefit from a distal approach similar to the popliteal approach (see later discussion) to spare some hamstring strength. Typically, blockade of the sciatic nerve is coupled with some variation of a femoral block to provide anesthesia and analgesia for procedures involving the hip or knee. For patients with acute pain in the distal portion of the lower extremity, the sciatic block may be sufficient because it should provide coverage for the lower extremity below the knee with the exception of a small area of skin along the medial side. The use of sciatic blocks in such patient populations has been shown to be highly effective with data suggesting a decrease in VAS scores and higher patient satisfaction.[167,168] Not all approaches allow for the placement of an indwelling nerve catheter, but when used, they have been shown to improve acute pain management by reducing pain scores, decreasing opioid consumption, improving sleep patterns, and decreasing length of hospitalizations.[169-171]

To perform the classic posterior sciatic nerve block, the patient is placed in the Sims position (semiprone) with the side to be blocked facing upward. The greater trochanter and PSIS are identified, and a line is drawn to connect the two structures. At the midpoint of this line, a perpendicular line is drawn running in a caudal and medial direction measuring 4 cm. The end of this line marks the insertion point for the procedure. The patient is given a small amount of IV sedation (midazolam, fentanyl, or both), the skin over the insertion site is prepared with an antiseptic solution, and sterile drapes are applied. A 4-inch nerve-stimulating needle is inserted through the skin and advanced in a direction that is perpendicular to all planes of the skin. An initial setting of 0.7 to 1.0 mA is sufficient to produce motor responses from the gluteal muscles as well as the sciatic nerve. As the needle advances, the operator will initially see a motor response from the gluteal muscle that indicates that the needle position is too shallow. As the needle is advanced further, the gluteal response will cease, and a motor response consistent with sciatic stimulation should appear. Stimulation of the sciatic nerve can produce a motor response in the hamstrings, calf, or toes. The position of the needle in relation to the nerve is optimized by slowly decreasing the stimulating current while making small manipulations of the needle to maintain the appropriate motor response. A consistent motor response that is generated from a current of 0.2 to 0.4 mA generally indicates appropriate positioning of the needle. The local anesthetic is injected in small increments over several minutes to avoid intravascular injection. Moving distally, the sciatic nerve can be blocked using a subgluteal approach. In this approach, a line is drawn between the greater trochanter and the ischial tuberosity. From the midpoint, a perpendicular line is drawn in the caudal direction measuring 4 cm. The end of this line indicates the needle insertion point. Alternatively, the infragluteal–parabiceps approach produces sciatic blocks at a similar location. In this technique, the tendon of the biceps femoris muscle is identified and followed in a cephalad direction until it intersects with the gluteal crease (inferior border of gluteus maximus). A point just lateral to the tendon at the intersection with the crease marks the location for needle entry. The subgluteal–infragluteal technique can be performed with ultrasound guidance. In this location, the sciatic nerve is viewed as a thin, sometimes triangular, hyperechoic structure residing in the fascial plane that separates the gluteus maximus muscle from the quadratus femoris muscle. Often, visualization of the sciatic nerve can be difficult, and the use of nerve stimulation may provide a means to correlate what is observed on the ultrasound with the actual nerve structure.

When clinical circumstances dictate that a posterior approach to the sciatic nerve is not possible, the provider may elect to perform an anterior sciatic nerve block. To perform an anterior sciatic block, the patient is placed in the supine position, and a line is drawn along the inguinal crease. The femoral pulse is identified on this line and marked. The needle insertion site is determined by drawing a 4- to 5-cm line perpendicular to the inguinal crease from the femoral pulse. A 4-inch nerve-stimulating needle is oriented perpendicular to the surface and advanced dorsally. As the needle is advanced, it is common to make contact with the femur, usually the lesser trochanter. The nerve lies deep to the femur, and to facilitate advancement of the needle, the patient's foot can be externally rotated. As the femur externally rotates, the lesser trochanter will be cleared from the needle path. Stimulation of the sciatic nerve at this level produces a motor response in the calf and foot. Branches that supply the hamstrings have typically left the sciatic nerve at this level and do not represent an appropriate motor response. The depth at which the sciatic nerve is encountered is typically 8 to 12 cm. The position and the depth of the sciatic nerve from this position can often make this a difficult block to perform, and it is highly recommended that the ultrasound be used to improve efficiency and increase the likelihood of success. Using the landmarks and measurements above, an ultrasound transducer (high or low frequency depending on the patient's body habitus) is placed perpendicular to the long axis of the femur over the predetermined insertion site. A systematic survey is done to determine the position of the lesser trochanter. By scanning in both cranial and caudal directions, a widening of the femur can be observed, indicating the lesser trochanter. The sciatic nerve will appear as a hyperechoic structure deep to the adductor magnus muscle and medial (possibly deep) to the lesser trochanter. Using an in-plane technique, the needle is advanced from the lateral end of the ultrasound probe toward the nerve. This is a moderately difficult block to perform because the angle of the advancing needle is very steep, which results in reflected ultrasound waves to be directed away from the transducer. This results in a weaker signal and poor visualization of the needle.

Popliteal Block

The sciatic nerve continues down the posterior thigh and ultimately divides, forming the tibial and the common peroneal nerves. This division usually takes place in the popliteal fossa, varying 5 to 12 cm from the popliteal crease. By performing a distal sciatic block, anesthesia and analgesia can be achieved in the posterior knee and distal lower extremity while hamstring function is preserved to promote early ambulation.[172] Compared with ankle blocks, sciatic blocks in the popliteal fossa consistently produce longer durations of analgesia (1080 min vs. 690 min).[173] Additionally, the distal location allows for easy placement of a continuous catheter, and the ability to perform the block laterally obviates any concerns over patient positioning. The use of a PNC is advantageous because they have been shown to decrease opioid requirements as well as opioid-related side effects, decrease lengths of stay, reduce unexpected outpatient admissions, improve sleep patterns, and provide a high level of patient satisfaction.[169-171] For procedures that require the use of a tourniquet around the thigh, blockade of the sciatic nerve at this level may not provide sufficient coverage even coupled with a femoral block and may not be suitable as a sole anesthetic in these instances.

To perform a popliteal block, the patient is placed in the prone position. On the lateral aspect of the popliteal fossa, the tendon of the biceps femoris is identified, and on the medial side, the tendon of the semitendinosus is identified. These structures should be traced with a marking pen as they converge proximally. Next, the crease of the popliteal fossa is identified and marked. An insertion site is identified 7 to 8 cm proximal to the crease at the midpoint between the two muscle tendons. The patient can be given a small amount of IV sedation before the initiation of the block to provide anxiolysis and comfort. An antiseptic solution is then applied to the skin, and sterile drapes are placed. A 4-inch stimulating needle is advanced through the skin in a perpendicular orientation. When through the skin, the stimulator can be given an initial setting of 0.7 to 1.0 mA. The needle is then advanced, seeking motor responses commensurate with sciatic nerve stimulation (dorsiflexion or plantar flexion of the foot). The needle tip position is optimized by slowly decreasing the current while making small adjustments to maintain motor response. Consistent motor response that is achieved with currents from 0.2 to 0.4 mA generally indicates appropriate needle position. The needle is then carefully aspirated to ensure no return of blood, which may indicate intravascular placement. The local anesthetic is then injected slowly in small increments and frequently aspirated. A lateral approach can be performed when lateral or prone positioning is not possible. For this approach, the patient is in the supine position with the leg to be blocked slightly elevated so that the foot and ankle will not be hindered during evoked motor stimulus. Measuring 8 cm from the popliteal crease, the groove between the vastus lateralis and biceps femoris muscles is marked as the insertion site. A 4-inch stimulating needle is advanced, seeking a motor response in the foot to indicate proximity of the sciatic nerve. As with most blocks, the use of the ultrasound makes blocking the sciatic nerve in the popliteal region fast and efficient. Additionally, with the nerve in view, it is unnecessary to stimulate the nerve for a motor response that could be painful for patients with injuries in the lower extremity. With the patient in the lateral, prone, or supine position, a linear high-frequency, high-resolution probe is placed at the crease of the popliteal fossa, and a systematic survey is performed to identify the needle insertion point. In this position, the artery is easily identifiable with both the tibial and common peroneal nerve being visible posterior to the artery. As the ultrasound probe is moved in the cephalad direction, the tibial and common peroneal nerves can be seen moving closer to each other until they converge at the sciatic nerve (≈8 cm from popliteal crease) (Fig. 14A-15). The block needle is then inserted through the skin at the lateral edge of the transducer and guided in plane to the sciatic nerve. Alternatively, the needle can be inserted laterally between the vastus lateralis and the biceps femoris. Although this insertion site requires a longer needle pass to reach the sciatic nerve, the approach results in an orientation that is more perpendicular to the ultrasound beam. This orientation allows for better reflection of the ultrasound waves, resulting in a stronger signal and better visualization of the needle. When the needle is properly positioned, the local anesthetic is injected around the sciatic nerve to complete the block (Fig. 14A-16). Because there can be wide variations among patients in the divergence of the common peroneal and tibial nerves

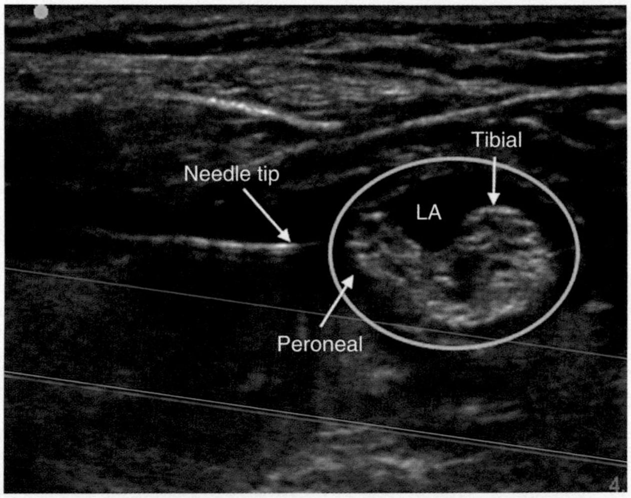

Figure 14A-15. The tibial and common peroneal nerves are easily identified by ultrasound in the popliteal crease and can be followed to their convergence by moving the ultrasound transducer proximally. This view of the sciatic nerve *(circle)* demonstrates the point at which the peroneal and common tibial nerves begin to converge.

from the sciatic nerve, ultrasound gives the practitioner the ability to visualize where this separation occurs, allowing for optimal positioning of the block needle. Additionally, it gives the practitioner the ability to provide selective blockade of either the tibial or common peroneal nerve. Certain clinical situations and surgical procedures may require periodic assessment of at risk peripheral nerves. By providing selective blocks at terminal branches that are not in question, analgesia can be improved without hindering ongoing assessment. This strategy has been used with patients undergoing total knee arthroplasties. Low-volume anesthetic selective tibial nerve blocks with femoral nerve blocks were shown to provide effective analgesia for patients having total knee arthroplasties. Although weaknesses were observed in the distribution of the peroneal nerve in some members of the study group, no patients developed complete peroneal motor block.[174]

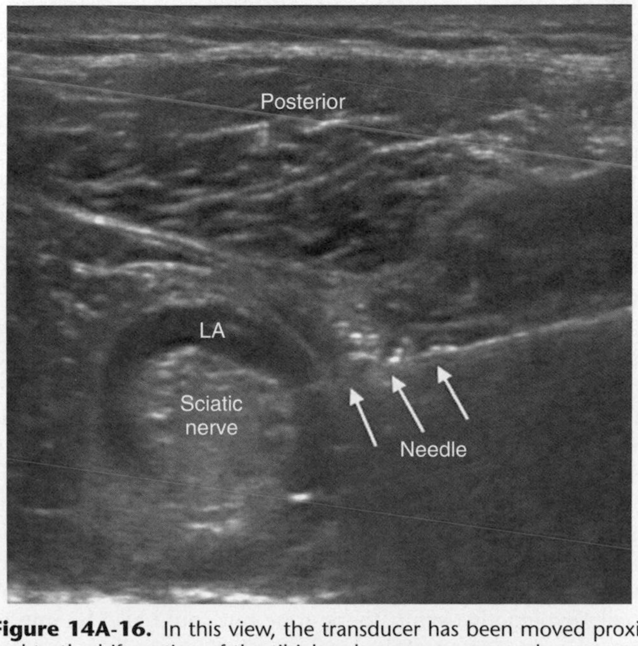

Figure 14A-16. In this view, the transducer has been moved proximal to the bifurcation of the tibial and common peroneal nerve, and the sciatic nerve appears as a single large nerve. Inserting the needle from the lateral position allows for an in-plane approach that is relatively perpendicular to the ultrasound waves. This produces a strong signal and good visualization of the block needle. Injection of local anesthetic (LA) can be seen as a hypoechoic ring that is spreading circumferentially around the nerve.

COMPLEX REGIONAL PAIN SYNDROME

Complex regional pain syndrome (CRPS) has been the subject of great debate in the pain management community for decades. The condition has evolved in both diagnostic criteria and name. In 1993, a consensus group of pain medicine experts developed the new nomenclature of CRPS for the various presenting conditions associated with the syndrome. The consensus group recommended abandoning the terms *causalgia* and *reflex sympathetic dystrophy;* however, some practitioners continue to use the former diagnosis because there are no standard minimum criteria to make the diagnosis of CRPS.

Complex regional pain syndrome is divided into two types, which are identical with respect to signs and symptoms but are classified differently according to the type of precipitating injury. Type I follows a soft tissue injury without nerve damage, and type II follows a well-defined nerve injury.

The literature describes a natural progression of symptoms over three stages.

Stage one: Pain is localized to the area of injury and is described as constant, usually burning, and moderately severe. The pain is aggravated by movement and is associated with hyperesthesia (unusually high sensitivity). Localized edema, tenderness, and muscle spasms are present. The skin in the affected area is warm, red, and dry. This stage may last for up to 6 months.

Stage two: There is a gradual decrease in pain with increasing stiffness of the joints and muscle wasting. The edema worsens and spreads to proximal areas. The skin is moist, cyanotic, and cold. Hair in the affected region is coarse. Nails can be brittle and develop ridges. Signs of atrophy usually become more prominent. This stage lasts from 3 to 6 months.

Stage three: Pain may be mild or severe. Hyperesthesia is occasionally present. This stage presents with marked trophic changes, which could progress to an irreversible degree. The skin is smooth, glossy, and drawn and can appear pale and cyanotic. The skin and muscles are atrophied. Skin temperature is lowered. The nails are brittle and ridged with lateral arching. The hair pattern is long and coarse. The patient has extreme weakness and limitations of motion. Contractions of the flexor tendons may be present.[175]

This sequence of stages is not exclusive. For example, development such as brittle nails, decreased hair growth, joint thickness, and muscle wasting are less common than previously believed. Only a small portion of patients have these changes. In all suspected cases, early intervention through treatment is recommended and may prevent a chronic and refractory condition.[176]

Risk Factors

Although risk factors are associated with developing CRPS, there is no definitive evidence that certain individuals are predisposed to develop the syndrome. Immobilization of a limb or joint for an extended period of time may increase the risk of developing CRPS. It has been proposed that a history of psychiatric illness, such as depression, anxiety, or substance abuse, may interfere with a patient's ability to cope with an injury and result in more pain and increased symptoms and disability, perhaps manifesting as CRPS. Another theory is that CRPS symptoms may be manifestations of an underlying psychiatric disorder, masking the actual disorder.[175]

Pathophysiology

The pathophysiology of CRPS is unknown. Most likely CRPS develops and is maintained by abnormalities in the peripheral nervous system and CNS. The autonomic nervous system, regional myofascial dysfunction, and psychiatric factors appear to play various roles in the development and persistence of this syndrome. These are distinct but interrelated systems; one system does not act independently of the others.

Symptomatology

Studies have shown that the symptoms reported by the patient play an important role in the diagnosis and evaluation of CRPS. However, when diagnostic criteria rely on the patient's self-reporting, questions inevitably arise about the validity of the diagnosis.

Symptoms of CRPS are located mainly in the limbs and are usually distal (hands and feet). However, CRPS has been known to affect other body parts, such as the head, and any body part that is covered by skin.

There are reported cases of CRPS symptoms spreading from the originally affected body part to other limbs or parts of the body. It is important to distinguish between true spread and the more common situation of a spreading myofascial dysfunction.

Pain associated with CRPS has been described in various ways. Most patients use adjectives such as "deep," "sharp," "sensitive," and "hot." Burning pain may be described but usually is not the most prevalent symptom. CRPS may become more symptomatic as a result of physical contact, changes in environmental temperature, and emotional stress.

Edema can occur, ranging from mild to pitting edema. Patients may describe a sense of fullness or swelling without actual physical signs of edema.

The involved body part may be hotter or colder than the opposite body part. The affected area can fluctuate in temperature within hours. Sometimes the patient reports sensing a difference in temperature, but when touched, the skin is the same temperature as the contralateral side.

The skin over the affected area can appear mottled, pale, deep purple, or red. Frequently, color changes correlate with temperature variations.

Complex regional pain syndrome can affect sudomotor activity in the affected body part, so that abnormally diffuse or decreased sweating may occur.

Patients with CRPS often describe weakness in the affected limb even though muscle testing results may be normal. Patients also report spasms, tremors, increased tone, difficulty initiating movements, difficulty holding or manipulating objects with their hands, stumbling, and tripping.

Patients with CRPS develop guarding as a protective posture and tend to avoid use of the affected body part to reduce flare-ups in pain. However, some studies suggest that there is a CNS shut-off of the limb from conscious awareness.

Patients with CRPS develop myofascial pain caused by disuse or overuse of other muscles to compensate for functional loss in the affected areas. Patients with CRPS should be thoroughly evaluated for myofascial pain and should receive appropriate physical therapy and other medical interventions.

Imaging and Testing[175]

There is no gold standard test to administer; indeed, no conclusive test is yet available, to confirm a diagnosis of CRPS. Many different techniques have been used to assist physicians in arriving at the diagnosis.

Bone demineralization has been noted in some patients. This finding may aid in the diagnosis, but such changes are not specific to CRPS. Demineralization could be caused by disuse of the limb and not by the syndrome itself. One study of bone scans showed distinctive patterns of radiotracer uptake, especially in the delayed phase of the test.

Thermography can be used to document abnormal skin temperatures.

Quantitative sudomotor axonal reflex testing (QSART) can document abnormalities in the autonomic nervous system. This is a potentially useful test, but it is not readily available and therefore has limited use.

Electromyography and nerve conduction studies can confirm the presence of peripheral nerve injury in type II CRPS. However, it is not known whether documented nerve injury has any prognostic or therapeutic relevance to CRPS.

Treatment

A multidisciplinary approach to the management of patients with CRPS is widely recommended. Treatment modalities should include medical and psychological interventions, and physical or occupational therapy. The primary goal is to achieve functional restoration for patients with CRPS. The physician leads the treatment team and attempts to provide relief from pain and symptoms through medications and procedures. The psychologist's role is to identify and treat comorbid conditions such as depression, posttraumatic stress disorder, and anxiety. The therapist's role is to organize and manage daily rehabilitative services.

Medical Therapies[177]

To date, no medications or therapy for the treatment of CRPS has been subject to a definitive controlled clinical trial and long-term clinical experience. Therefore, there is no gold standard for CRPS treatment. A classic modality is sympathetic nerve blockade, which continues to be a first-line treatment. However, the data used to support the use of sympathetic blocks in the treatment of CRPS are not derived from controlled clinic trials. The mechanism by which sympathetic blockade may act to relieve pain and symptoms is poorly understood. Relief may result from a decrease in an abnormally hyperactive sympathetic tone but could also be due to systemic absorption of the local anesthetic or spillage to adjacent nerve fibers. Neurostimulation therapies, including spinal cord and peripheral nerve stimulators, have been shown to reduce pain and symptoms in some CRPS patients. Intrathecal infusions have also been effective to relieve symptoms for some patients.

Medications currently in use include:

- Anticonvulsants such as Neurontin and Lyrica
- Calcium channel blockers
- β-blockers
- Tricyclic antidepressants
- Calcitonin
- Corticosteroids
- Clonidine
- Local anesthetic
- Opiates

CONCLUSION

Complex regional pain syndrome is a difficult syndrome to diagnose and treat. The medical community is divided on many aspects of treatment for this condition. The single agreed upon approach is to validate the patient's symptoms and to initiate a multidisciplinary treatment plan, working toward the goal of functional restoration. It is very difficult to predict the duration of treatment for CRPS. Generally, the decision as to the duration of treatment is made on a case-by-case basis. Some of the factors include the severity of the CRPS and the type or types of treatment used.

REFERENCES

The level of evidence (LOE) is determined according to the criteria provided in the preface.

1. Whipple JK, Lewis KS, Quebbeman EJ, et al: Analysis of pain management in critically ill patients. *Pharmacotherapy* 15:592–599, 1995.
2. Phillips S, Gift M, Gelot S, et al: Assessing the relationship between the level of pain control and patient satisfaction. *J Pain Res* 6:683–689, 2013.
3. Gupta A, Daigle S, Moiica J, et al: Patient perception of pain care in hospitals in the United States. *J Pain Res* 2:157–164, 2009.
4. Yaksh TL, Hua XY, Kalcheva I, et al: The spinal biology in humans and animals of pain states generated by persistent small afferent input. *Proc Natl Acad Sci USA* 96:7680–7686, 1999.
5. Omergovic M, Duric A, Muratovic N, et al: Metabolic response to trauma and stress. *Medicinski Archiv* 57:57–60, 2003.
6. Wu CL, Fleisher LA: Outcomes research in regional anesthesia and analgesia. *Anesth Analg* 91:1232–1242, 2009.
7. Johnson KO: The roles and functions of cutaneous mechanoreceptors. *Curr Opinion Neurobiol* 11:455–461, 2001.
8. Chung K, Lee WT, Carlton SM: The effects of dorsal rhizotomy and spinal cord isolation on calcitonin gene-related peptide containing terminals in the rat lumbar dorsal horn. *Neurosco Lett* 90:27–32, 1988.
9. Sugiura Y, Terui N, Hosoya Y: Difference in distribution of central terminals between visceral and somatic unmyelinated C-primary afferent fibers. *J Neurophysiol* 62:834–940, 1989.
10. Liu SS, Wu CL: Effect of postoperative analgesia on postoperative complications: a systematic update of the evidence. *Anesth Analg* 104:689–702, 2007.
11. Zhao SZ, Chung F, Hanna DB, et al: Dose-response relationship between opioid use and adverse effects after ambulatory surgery. *J Pain Symptom Manage* 28:35–46, 2004.
12. Macintyre PE: Safety and efficacy of patient-controlled analgesia. *Br J Anaesth* 87:36–46, 2001.
13. Wakerlin G, Larson CP, Jr: Spouse-controlled analgesia. *Br J Anaesth* 87:36–46, 2001.
14. Camu F, Van Aken H, Bovill JG: Postoperative analgesic effects of three demand-dose sizes of fentanyl administered by patient-controlled analgesia. *Anesth Analg* 87:890–895, 1998.
15. Ginsberg B, Gil KM, Muir M, et al: The influence of lockout intervals and drug selection on patient-controlled analgesia following gynecological surgery. *Pain* 62:95–100, 1995.
16. Smythe MA, Zak MB, O'Donnell MP, et al: Patient-controlled analgesia versus patient-controlled analgesia plus continuous infusion after hip replacement surgery. *Ann Pharmacother* 30:224–227, 1996.
17. Parker RK, Holtmann B, White PF: Patient-controlled analgesia. Does a concurrent opioid infusion improve pain management after surgery? *JAMA* 266:1947–1952, 1991.
18. Parker RK, Holtmann B, White PF: Effects of a nighttime opioid infusion with PCA therapy on patient comfort and analgesic requirements after abdominal hysterectomy. *Anesthesiology* 76:362–367, 1992.
19. Looi-Lyons LC, Chung FF, Chan VW, et al: Respiratory depression: an adverse outcome during patient controlled analgesia therapy. *J Clin Anesth* 8:151–156, 1996.
20. Walder B, Schafer M, Henzi I, et al: Efficacy and safety of patient-controlled opioid analgesia for acute postoperative pain: a quantitative systematic review. *Acta Anaesth Scand* 45:795–804, 2001.
21. Ballantyne JC, Carr DB, Chalmers TC, et al: Postoperative patient-controlled analgesia: meta-analyses of initial randomized control trials. *J Clin Anesth* 5:182–193, 1993.
22. Hudcova J, McNicol E, Quah C, et al: Patient-controlled opioid analgesia versus conventional opioid analgesia for postoperative pain. *Cochrane Database Syst Rev* (4):CD003348, 2006.
23. Gordon DB, Dahl JL, Miaskowski C, et al: American Pain Society recommendations for improving the quality of acute and cancer pain management. *Arch Intern Med* 165:1574–1580, 2005. LOE V
24. Vila H, Smith RA, Augustyniak MJ, et al: The efficacy and safety of pain management before and after implementation of hospital-wide pain management standards: is patient safety compromised by treatment based solely on numerical pain ratings? *Anesth Analg* 101:474–480, 2005. LOE III
25. Nisbet AT, Mooney-Cotter F: Comparison of selected sedation scales for reporting opioid-induced sedation assessment. *Pain Manag Nurs* 10(3): 154–164, 2009. LOE III
26. Criscuolo S, Auletta C, Lippi S, et al: Oxcarbazepine monotherapy in postherpetic neuralgia unresponsive to carbamazepine and gabapentin. *Acta Neurol Scand* 111:229–232, 2005. LOE III
27. Leese PT, Hubbard RC, Karim A, et al: Effects of celecoxib, a novel cyclooxygenase-2 inhibitor, on platelet function in healthy adults: a randomized controlled trial. *J Clin Pharmacol* 40:124–132, 2000. LOE II
28. Caldwell B, Aldington S, Weatherall M, et al: Risk of cardiovascular events and celecoxib: a systematic review meta-analysis. *J R Soc Med* 99:132–140, 2006. LOE III
29. Camu F, Beecher T, Recker DP, et al: Valdecoxib, a COX-2 specific inhibitor, is an efficacious, opioid-sparing analgesic in patients undergoing hip arthroplasty. *Am J Ther* 9:43–51, 2002. LOE II
30. Recart A, Issioui T, White P, et al: The efficacy of celecoxib premedication on postoperative pain and recovery times after ambulatory surgery: a dose-ranging study. *Anesth Analg* 96:1631–1635, 2003. LOE I
31. Rivara FP, Jurkovich GJ, Gurney JG, et al: The magnitude of actue and chronic alcohol abuse in trauma patients. *Arch Surg* 128:907–913, 1993.
32. Catella-Lawson F, Reilly MP, Kapoor SC, et al: Cyclooxygenase inhibitors and the antiplatelet effects of aspirin. *N Engl J Med* 345:1809–1817, 2001. LOE I
33. Feenstra J, Heerdink ER, Grobbee DE, et al: Association of nonsteroidal anti-inflammatory drugs with first occurrence of heart failure and with relapsing heart failure. *Arch Intern Med* 162:265–270, 2002. LOE II
34. Whelton A: Renal and related cardiovascular effects of conventional and COX-2 specific NSAIDs and non-NSAID analgesics. *Am J Ther* 7:63–74, 2000. LOE IV
35. Schjerning-Olsen AM, Fosbol EL, Lindhardsen J, et al: Duration of treatment with nonsteroidal anti-inflammatory drugs and impact on risk of death and recurrent myocardial infarction in patients with prior myocardial infarction: a nationwide cohort study. *Circulation* 123:2226–2235, 2011. LOE I
36. Schmidt M, Christiansen CF, Mehnert F, et al: Non-steroidal anti-inflammatory drug use and risk of atrial fibrillation or flutter: population based case-control study. *BMJ* 343:d3450, 2011. LOE I
37. Dahners LE, Mullis BH: Effects of nonsteroidal anti-inflammatory drugs on bone formation and soft-tissue healing. *J Am Acad Orthop Surg* 12: 139–143, 2004. LOE III
38. Boursinos LA, Karachalios L, Poultsides L, et al: Do steroids, conventional non-steroidal anti-inflammatory drugs and selective Cox-2 inhibitors adversely affect fracture healing? *J Musculoskelet Neuronal Interact* 9:44–52, 2009. LOE V
39. Li Q, Zhang Z, Cai Z: High-dose ketorolac affects adult spinal fusion. *Spine* 36:E461–E468, 2011. LOE V
40. Dodwell ER, Latorre JG, Parsini E, et al: NSAID exposure and risk of nonunion: a meta-analysis of case-control and cohort studies. *Calcif Tissue Int* 87:193–202, 2010. LOE III

41. Issioui T, Klein KW, White PF, et al: The efficacy of premedication with celecoxib and acetaminophen in preventing pain after otolaryngologic surgery. *Anesth Analg* 94:1188–1193, 2002. LOE III
42. Jarde O, Boccard E: Parenteral versus oral route increases paracetamol efficacy. *Clin Drug Invest* 14:474–481, 1997. LOE III
43. Sinatra RS, Jahr JS, Reynolds LW, et al: Efficacy and safety of single and repeated administration of 1 gram intravenous acetaminophen injection for pain management after major orthopedic surgery. *Anesthesiology* 102:822–831, 2005. LOE I
44. Mahe I, Bertrand N, Drouet L, et al: Paracetamol: a haemorrhagic risk factor in patients on warfarin. *Br J Clin Pharmacol* 59:371–374, 2005. LOE IV
45. Grass JA: Patient-controlled analgesia. *Anesth Analg* 101(5S):S44–S61, 2005. LOE V
46. Kosten TR, O'Connor PG: Management of drug and alcohol withdrawal. *N Eng J Med* 348:1786–1795, 2003. LOE V
47. Mitra S, Sinatra RS: Perioperative management of acute pain in the opioid-dependent patient. *Anesthesiology* 101:212–227, 2004. LOE III
48. Alford DP, Compton P, Samet JH, et al: Acute pain management for patients receiving maintenance methadone or buprenorphine therapy. *Ann Intern Med* 144:127–134, 2006. LOE V
49. Simopoulos TT, Smith HS, Peeters-Asdourian C, et al: Use of meperidine in patient-controlled analgesia and the development of a normeperidine toxic reaction. *Arch Surg* 137:84–88, 2002. LOE III
50. Schad RF: Hydroxyzine analgesia—fact or fantasy? *Am J Hosp Pharm* 36:1317, 1979. LOE V
51. Niv D, Gofeld M, Devor M: Causes of pain in degenerative bone and joint disease: a lesson from vertebroplasty. *Pain* 105:387–392, 2003. LOE V
52. Chen H, Lamer TJ, Rho RH, et al: Contemporary Management of Neuropathic Pain for the Primary Care Physician. *Mayo Clin Proc* 79:1533–1545, 2004. LOE V
53. Gilron I, Bailey JM, Dongsheng T, et al: Morphine, gabapentin, or their combination for neuropathic pain. *N Engl J Med* 352:1324–1334, 2005. LOE II
54. Argoff CE, Misha-Miroslav B, Belgrade MJ, et al: Consensus guidelines for diabetic peripheral neuropathic pain: treatment planning and options. *Mayo Clin Proc* 81(Suppl 4):S12–S25, 2006. LOE V
55. Fleming MF, Balousek SL, Klessig CL, et al: Substance use disorders in a primary care sample receiving daily opioid therapy. *J Pain* 8:573–582, 2007.
56. Ives TJ, Chelminski PR, Hammett-Stabler CA, et al: Predictors of opioid misuse in patients with chronic pain: a prospective cohort study. *BMC Health Serv Res* 6:46, 2006.
57. Chou R, et al: Linical Guidelines for the use of chronic opioid therapy in chronic noncancer pain. *J Pain* 10:113–130, 2009.
58. Gourlay DL, et al: Universal Precautions in pain medicine: a rational approach to the treatment of chronic pain. *Pain Med* 6(2):2005.
59. Webster LR, Dove B: Avoiding opioid abuse while managing pain, p 48.
60. Liu SS, McDonald SB: Current issues in spinal anesthesia. *Anesthesiology* 94:888–906, 2001.
61. Loper KA, Ready LB, Dorman BH: Prophylactic trans-dermal scopolamine patches reduce nausea in postoperative patients receiving epidural morphine. *Anesth Analg* 68:144–146, 1989.
62. Chaney MA: Side effects of intrathecal and epidural opioids. *Can J Anaesth* 42:891–903, 1995.
63. White MJ, Berghausen EJ, Dumont SW, et al: Side effects during continuous epidural infusion of morphine and fentanyl. *Can J Anaesth* 39:576–582, 1992.
64. Kelly MC, Carabine UA, Mirakhur RK: Intrathecal diamorphine for analgesia after caesarean section. A dose finding study and assessment of side-effects. *Anaesthesia* 53:231–237, 1998.
65. Wattwil M: Postoperative pain relief and gastrointestinal motility. *Acta Chir Scand Suppl* 550:140–145, 1989.
66. Bromage PR, Camporesi EM, Durant PA, et al: Nonrespiratory side effects of epidural morphine. *Anesth Analg* 61:490–495, 1982.
67. Katsiris S, Williams S, Leighton BL, et al: Respiratory arrest following intrathecal injection of sufentanil and bupivacaine in a parturient. *Can J Anaesth* 45:880–883, 1998.
68. Pokorski M, Grieb P, Wideman J: Opiate system influences central respiratory chemosensors. *Brain Res* 211:221–226, 1981.
69. Gregory MA, Brock-Utne JG, Bux S, et al: Morphine concentration in brain and spinal cord after sub-arachnoid morphine injection in baboons. *Anesth Analg* 64:929–932, 1985.
70. Bailey PL, Rhondeau S, Schafer PG, et al: Dose-response pharmacology of intrathecal morphine in human volunteers. *Anesthesiology* 79:49–59, 1993.
71. Kafer ER, Brown JT, Scott D, et al: Biphasic depression of ventilatory responses to CO_2 following epidural morphine. *Anesthesiology* 58:418–427, 1983.
72. Etches RC, Sandier AN, Daley WI: Respiratory depression and spinal opioids. *Can J Anaesth* 36:165–185, 1989.
73. Wang JJ, Ho ST, Tzeng JI: Comparison of intravenous nalbuphine infusion versus naloxone in the prevention of epidural morphine-related side effects. *Reg Anesth Pain Med* 23:479–484, 1998.
74. Block BM, Liu SS, Rowlingson AJ, et al: Efficacy of postoperative epidural analgesia: a meta-analysis. *JAMA* 290:2455–2463, 2003.
75. de Leon-Casaola OA, Lema MJ: Postoperative epidural opioid analgesia: what are the choices? *Anesth Analg* 83:867–875, 1996.
76. Loper KA, Ready LB, Downey M, et al: Epidural and intravenous fentanyl infusions are clinically equivalent after knee surgery. *Anesth Analg* 70:72–75, 1990.
77. Malviya S, Pandit UA, Merkel S, et al: A comparison of continuous epidural infusion and intermittent intravenous bolus doses of morphine in children undergoing selective dorsal rhizotomy. *Reg Anesth Pain Med* 24:438–443, 1999.
78. Block BM, Liu SS, Rowlingson AJ, et al: Efficacy of postoperative epidural analgesia: a meta-analysis. *JAMA* 290:2455–2463, 2003.
79. Wu CL, Cohen SR, Richman JM, et al: Efficacy of postoperative patient-controlled continuous infusion epidural analgesia versus intravenous patient-controlled analgesia with opioids: a meta-analysis. *Anesthesiology* 103:1079–1088, 2005.
80. Sitsen E, van Poorten F, van Alphen W, et al: Postoperative epidural analgesia after total knee arthroplasty with sufentanil 1mug/mL combined with ropivacaine 0.2%, ropivacaine 0.125%, or levobupivacaine 0.125%: a randomized, double-blind comparison. *Reg Anesth Pain Med* 32:475–480, 2007.
81. Wheatley RG, Schug SA, Watson D: Safety and efficacy of postoperative epidural analgesia. *Br J Anaesth* 87:47–61, 2001.
82. Ozalp G, Guner F, Kuru N, et al: Postoperative patient-controlled epidural analgesia with opioid bupivacaine mixtures. *Can J Anaesth* 45:938–942, 1998.
83. Berti M, Fanelli G, Casati A, et al: Comparison between epidural infusion of fentanyl/bupivacaine and morphine/bupivacaine after orthopaedic surgery. *Can J Anaesth* 45:545–550, 1998.
84. Liu S, Carpenter RL, Mulroy MF, et al: Intravenous versus epidural administration of hydromorphone. Effects on analgesia and recovery after radical retropubic prostatectomy. *Anesthesiology* 82:682–688, 1995.
85. Wu CL, Fleisher LA: Outcome research in regional anesthesia and analgesia. *Anesth Analg* 91:1232–1242, 2000.
86. Ballantyne JC, Carr DB, deFerranti S, et al: The comparative effects of postoperative analgesic therapies on pulmonary outcome: cumulative meta-analyses of randomized, controlled trials. *Anesth Analg* 86:598–612, 1998.
87. Rigg JR, Jamrozik K, Myles PS, et al: Epidural anaesthesia and analgesia and outcome of major surgery: a randomized trial. *Lancet* 359:1276–1282, 2002.
88. Ford G, Whitelaw W, Rosenal T, et al: Diaphragm function after upper abdominal surgery in humans. *Am Rev Respir Dis* 127:431–436, 1987.
89. Pansard JL, Mankikian B, Bertrand M, et al: Effects of thoracic extradural block on diaphragmatic electrical activity and contractility after upper abdominal surgery. *Anesthesiology* 78:63–71, 1993.
90. Rodgers A, Walker N, Schug S, et al: Reduction of postoperative mortality and morbidity with epidural or spinal anaesthesia: results from overview of randomised trials. *BMJ* 321:1493, 2000.
91. Reiz S, Balfors E, Sorenson M, et al: Coronary hemodynamic effects of general anesthesia and surgery: modification by epidural analgesia in patients with ischemic heart disease. *Reg Anesth* 7s:8–18, 1982.
92. Heusch G, Deussen A, Thamer V: Cardiac sympathetic nerve activity and progressive vasoconstriction distal to coronary stenosis: feedback aggravation of myocardial ischemia. *J Auton Nerv Syst* 13:311–326, 1985.
93. Blomberg S, Emanuelsson H, Kvist H, et al: Effects of thoracic epidural anesthesia on coronary arteries and arterioles in patients with coronary artery disease. *Anesthesiology* 73:840–847, 1990.
94. Vercauteren M, Meert TF: Isobolographic analysis of the interaction between epidural sufentanil and bupivacaine in rats. *Pharmacol Biochem Behav* 58:237–242, 1997.
95. Camann W, Abouleish A, Eisenach J, et al: Intrathecal sufentanil and epidural bupivacaine for labor analgesia: dose-response of individual agents and in combination. *Reg Anesth Pain Med* 23:457–462, 1998.

96. Gogarten W, Vandermeulen E, Van Aken H, et al: Regional anaesthesia and antithrombotic agents: recommendations of the European Society of Anaesthesiology. *Eur J Anaesthesiol* 27:999–1015, 2010.
97. Horlocker TT, Wedel DJ, Rowlingson JC, et al: Regional anesthesia in the patient receiving antithrombotic or thrombolytic therapy: American Society of Regional Anesthesia and Pain Medicine evidence-based guidelines (third edition). *Reg Anesth Pain Med* 35:64–101, 2010.
98. Telion C, Carli P: Prehospital and emergency room pain management for the adult trauma patient. Techniques in regional anesthesia and pain management. 6:10–18, 2002.
99. Buckenmaier CC, McKnight GM, Winkley KV, et al: Continuous peripheral nerve block for battlefield anesthesia and evacuation. *Reg Anesth Pain Med* 30:202–205, 2005.
100. Phillips DP, Knizner TL, Williams BA: Economics and practice management issues associated with acute pain management. *Anesthesiol Clin* 29:213–232, 2011.
101. Williams BA: Potential economic benefits of regional anesthesia for acute pain management: the need to study both inputs and outcomes. *Reg Anesth Pain Med* 31:95–99, 2006.
102. Sinclair DR, Chung F, Mezei G: Can postoperative nausea and vomiting be predicted? *Anesthesiology* 91:109–118, 1999.
103. Sneyd JR, Carr A, Byrom WD, et al: A meta-analysis of nausea and vomiting following maintenance of anaesthesia with propofol or inhalational agents. *Eur J Anaesthesiol* 15:433–445, 1998.
104. Apfel CC, Korttila K, Abdalla M, et al: A factorial trial of six interventions for the prevention of postoperative nausea and vomiting. *N Engl J Med* 350:2441–2451, 2004.
105. Williams BA, Kentor ML, Williams JP, et al: Process analysis in outpatient knee surgery: effects of regional and general anesthesia on anesthesia-controlled time. *Anesthesiology* 93:529–538, 2000.
106. Williams BA, Kentor ML, Williams JP, et al: PACU bypass after outpatient knee surgery is associated with fewer unplanned hospital admissions but more phase II nursing interventions. *Anesthesiology* 97:981–988, 2002.
107. Williams BA, Kentor ML, Vogt MT, et al: Femoral-sciatic nerve blocks for complex outpatient knee surgery are associated with less postoperative pain before same-day discharge: a review of 1200 consecutive cases from the period 1996-1999. *Anesthesiology* 98:1206–1213, 2003.
108. Williams BA, Kentor ML, Vogt MT, et al: The economics of nerve block pain management after anterior cruciate ligament reconstruction: significant hospital cost savings via associated PACU bypass and same-day discharge. *Anesthesiology* 100:697–706, 2004.
109. Kentor ML, Williams BA: Antiemetics in outpatient regional anesthesia for invasive orthopedic surgery. *Int Anesth Clin* 43:197–205, 2005.
110. Ilfeld BM, Gearan PF, Enneking FK, et al: Total hip arthroplasty as an overnight-stay procedure using an ambulatory continuous psoas compartment nerve block: a prospective feasibility study. *Reg Anesth Pain Med* 31:113–118, 2006.
111. Ilfeld BM, Gearan PF, Enneking FK, et al: Total knee arthroplasty as an overnight-stay procedure using continuous femoral nerve blocks at home: a prospective feasibility study. *Anesth Analg* 102:87–90, 2006.
112. Ilfeld BM, Wright TW, Enneking FK, et al: Total shoulder arthroplasty as an outpatient procedure using ambulatory perineural local anesthetic infusion: a pilot feasibility study. *Anesth Analg* 101:1319–1322, 2005.
113. Ilfeld BM, Wright TW, Enneking FK, et al: Total elbow arthroplasty as an outpatient procedure using a continuous infraclavicular nerve block at home: a prospective case report. *Reg Anesth Pain Med* 31:172–176, 2006.
114. Ilfeld BM, Enneking FK: Continuous peripheral nerve blocks at home: a review. *Anesth Analg* 100:1822–1833, 2005.
115. Klein SM, Evans H, Nielsen KC, et al: Peripheral nerve block techniques for ambulatory surgery. *Anesth Analg* 101:1663–1676, 2005.
116. Richman JM, Liu SS, Courpas G, et al: Does continuous peripheral nerve block provide superior pain control to opioids? A meta-analysis. *Anesth Analg* 102:248–257, 2006.
117. Etienne J: *Regional anesthesia: its application in the surgical treatment of cancer of the breast [in French]*, 1925, Faculte de Medecin de Paris.
118. Winnie AP: Interscalene brachial plexus block. *Anesth Analg* 49:455–466, 1970.
119. Al-Kaisy A, McGuire G, Chan VW, et al: Analgesic effect of interscalene block using low-dose bupivacaine for outpatient arthroscopic shoulder surgery. *Reg Anesth Pain Med* 23:469–473, 1998.
120. Brown AR, Weiss R, Greenberg C, et al: Interscalene block for shoulder arthroscopy: comparison with general anesthesia. *Arthroscopy* 9:295–300, 1993.
121. Kinnard P, Truchon R, St-Pierre A, et al: Interscalene block for pain relief after shoulder surgery. A prospective randomized study. *Clin Orthop Relat Res* 304:22–24, 1994.
122. Singelyn FJ, Lhotel L, Fabre B: Pain relief after arthroscopic shoulder surgery: a comparison of intraarticular analgesia, suprascapular nerve block, and interscalene brachial plexus block. *Anesth Analg* 99:589–592, 2004.
123. Laurila PA, Lopponen A, Kanga-Saarela T, et al: Interscalene brachial plexus block is superior to subacromial bursa block after arthroscopic shoulder surgery. *Acta Anaesthesiol Scand* 46:1031–1036, 2002.
124. Arciero RA, Taylor DC, Harrison SA, et al: Interscalene anesthesia for shoulder arthroscopy in a community-sized military hospital. *Arthroscopy* 12:715–719, 1996.
125. Ilfeld BM, Vandenborne K, Duncan PW, et al: Ambulatory continuous interscalene nerve blocks decrease the time to discharge readiness after total shoulder arthroplasty: a randomized, triple-masked, placebo-controlled study. *Anesthesiology* 105:999–1007, 2006.
126. Borgeat A, Tewes E, Viasca N, et al: Patient-controlled interscalene analgesia with ropivacaine after major shoulder surgery: PCIA vs PCA. *Br J Anaesth* 81:603–605, 1998.
127. Kean J, Wigderowitz CA, Coventry DM: Continuous interscalene infusion and single injection using levobupivacaine for analgesia after surgery of the shoulder. A double-blind, randomised controlled trial. *J Bone Joint Surg Br* 88:1173–1177, 2006.
128. Klein SM, Grant SA, Greengrass RA, et al: Interscalene brachial plexus block with a continuous catheter insertion system and a disposable infusion pump. *Anesth Analg* 91:1473–1478, 2000.
129. Urmey WF, McDonald M: Hemidiaphragmatic paresis during interscalene brachial plexus block: effects on pulmonary function and chest wall mechanics. *Anesth Analg* 74:352–357, 1992.
130. Borgeat A, Perschak H, Bird P, et al: Patient-controlled interscalene analgesia with ropivacaine 0.2% versus patient-controlled intravenous analgesia after major shoulder surgery: effects on diaphragmatic and respiratory function. *Anesthesiology* 92:102–108, 2000.
131. Lee SM, Park SE, Nam YS, et al: Analgesic effectiveness of nerve block in shoulder arthroscopy: comparison between interscalene, suprascapular and axillary nerve blocks. *Knee Surg Sports Traumatol Arthrosc* 20:2573–2578, 2012.
132. Kulenkampff D, Persky M: Brachial plexus anesthesia. Its indications, technique and dangers. *Ann Surg* 87:883–891, 1928.
133. Burnham PJ: Regional block of the great nerves of the upper arm. *Anesthesiology* 19:281–284, 1958.
134. Renes SH, Spoormans HH, Gielen MJ, et al: Hemidiaphragmatic paresis can be avoided in ultrasound-guided supraclavicular brachial plexus block. *Reg Anesth Pain Med* 34:595–599, 2009.
135. Bazy L, Pouchet V, Sourdat V, et al: *L'Anesthesie Regionale*, Paris, 1917, G Doin et Cie, pp 222–225.
136. Raj PP, Montgomery SI, Nettles D, et al: Infraclavicular brachial plexus block—a new approach. *Anesth Analg* 52:897–904, 1973.
137. Whiffler K: Coracoid block—a safe and easy technique. *Br J Anaesth* 53:845, 1981.
138. Chelly JE, Ben-David B, Williams BA, et al: Anesthesia and postoperative analgesia: outcomes following orthopedic surgery. *Orthopedics* 26:s865–s871, 2003.
139. Franco CD, Vieira ZE: 1001 subclavian perivascular brachial plexus blocks: success with a nerve stimulator. *Reg Anesth Pain Med* 25:41–46, 2000.
140. Hadzic A, Arliss J, Kerimoglu B, et al: A comparison of infraclavicular nerve block versus general anesthesia for hand and wrist day-case surgeries. *Anesthesiology* 101:127–132, 2004.
141. Ilfeld BM, Morey TE, Enneking FK: Infraclavicular perineural local anesthetic infusion: a comparison of three dosing regimens for postoperative analgesia. *Anesthesiology* 100:395–402, 2004.
142. Ilfeld BM, Morey TE, Enneking FK: Continuous infraclavicular perineural infusion with clonidine and ropivacaine compared with ropivacaine alone: a randomized, double-blinded, controlled study. *Anesth Analg* 97:706–712, 2003.
143. Ilfeld BM, Morey TE, Enneking FK: Continuous infraclavicular brachial plexus block for postoperative pain control at home: a randomized, double-blinded, placebo-controlled study. *Anesthesiology* 96:1297–1304, 2002.
144. Hadzic A, Vloka JD, Kuroda MM, et al: The practice of peripheral nerve blocks in the United States: a national survey. *Reg Anesth Pain Med* 23:241–246, 1998.
145. Klein SM, Pietrobon R, Nielsen KC, et al: Peripheral nerve blockade with long-acting local anesthetics: a survey of the Society for Ambulatory Anesthesia. *Anesth Analg* 94:71–76, 2002.

146. Chan VW, Peng PW, Kaszas Z, et al: A comparative study of general anesthesia, intravenous regional anesthesia, and axillary block for outpatient hand surgery: clinical outcome and cost analysis. *Anesth Analg* 93:1181–1184, 2001.
147. Rawal N, Allvin R, Axelsson K, et al: Patient-controlled regional analgesia (PCRA) at home: controlled comparison between bupivacaine and ropivacaine brachial plexus analgesia. *Anesthesiology* 96:1290–1296, 2002.
148. Mezzatesta JP, Scott DA, Schweitzer SA, et al: Continuous axillary brachial plexus block for postoperative pain relief. Intermittent bolus versus continuous infusion. *Reg Anesth* 22:357–362, 1997.
149. Bergman BD, Hebl JR, Kent J, et al: Neurologic complications of 405 consecutive continuous axillary catheters. *Anesth Analg* 96:247–252, 2003.
150. McGoldrick KE: Neurologic complications of 405 consecutive continuous axillary catheters. *Surv Anesthesiol* 47:234–235, 2003.
151. Egeler C, Jayakumar A, Ford S: Motor sparing knee block—description of a new technique. *Anaesthesia* 68:542–543, 2013.
152. Winnie AP, Ramamurthy S, Durani Z, et al: Plexus blocks for lower extremity surgery: new answers to old problems. *Anesthesiol Rev* 1:11–16, 1974.
153. Stevens RD, Van Gessel E, Flory N, et al: Lumbar plexus block reduces pain and blood loss associated with total hip arthroplasty. *Anesthesiology* 93:115–121, 2000.
154. Turker G, Uckunkaya N, Yavascaoglu B, et al: Comparison of the catheter-technique psoas compartment block and the epidural block for analgesia in partial hip replacement surgery. *Acta Anaesthesiol Scand* 47:30–36, 2003.
155. Kaloul I, Guay J, Cote C, et al: The posterior lumbar plexus (psoas compartment) block and the three-in-one femoral nerve block provide similar postoperative analgesia after total knee replacement. *Can J Anaesth* 51:45–51, 2004.
156. Chelly JE, Greger J, Gebhard R, et al: Continuous femoral blocks improve recovery and outcome of patients undergoing total knee arthroplasty. *J Arthroplasty* 16:436–446, 2001.
157. Capdevila X, Barthelet Y, Biboulet P, et al: Effects of perioperative analgesic technique on the surgical outcome and duration of rehabilitation after major knee surgery. *Anesthesiology* 91:8–15, 1999.
158. Singelyn FJ, Deyaert M, Pendeville E, et al: Effects of intravenous patient-controlled analgesia with morphine, continuous epidural analgesia, and continuous three-in-one block on postoperative pain and knee rehabilitation after unilateral total knee arthroplasty. *Anesth Analg* 87:88–92, 1998.
159. Jaeger P, Nielsen ZJ, Henningsen MH, et al: Adductor canal block versus femoral nerve block and quadriceps strength: a randomized, double-blind, placebo-controlled, crossover study in healthy volunteers. *Anesthesiology* 118:409–415, 2013.
160. Jaeger P, Zaric D, Fomsgaard JS, et al: Adductor canal block versus femoral nerve block for analgesia after total knee arthroplasty: a randomized, double-blind study. *Reg Anesth Pain Med* 38:526–532, 2013.
161. Mansour NY: Reevaluating the sciatic nerve block: another landmark for consideration. *Reg Anesth* 18:322–323, 1993.
162. Sherwood-Dunn B: *Regional anesthesia (Victor Pauchet's technique)*, Philadelphia, 1921, FA Davis.
163. Beck GP: Anterior approach to sciatic nerve block. *Anesthesiology* 24:222–224, 1963.
164. Winnie AP: Regional anesthesia. *Surg Clin North Am* 55:861–892, 1975.
165. Raj PP, Parks RI, Watson TD, et al: A new single-position supine approach to sciatic-femoral nerve block. *Anesth Analg* 54:489–493, 1975.
166. di Benedetto P, Bertini L, Casati A, et al: A new posterior approach to the sciatic nerve block: a prospective, randomized comparison with the classic posterior approach. *Anesth Analg* 93:1040–1044, 2001.
167. di Benedetto P, Casati A, Bertini L: Continuous subgluteus sciatic nerve block after orthopedic foot and ankle surgery: comparison of two infusion techniques. *Reg Anesth Pain Med* 27:168–172, 2002.
168. di Benedetto P, Casati A, Bertini L, et al: Postoperative analgesia with continuous sciatic nerve block after foot surgery: a prospective, randomized comparison between the popliteal and subgluteal approaches. *Anesth Analg* 94:996–1000, 2002.
169. White PF, Issioui T, Skrivanek GD, et al: The use of a continuous popliteal sciatic nerve block after surgery involving the foot and ankle: does it improve the quality of recovery? *Anesth Analg* 97:1303–1309, 2003.
170. Singelyn FJ, Aye F, Gouverneur JM: Continuous popliteal sciatic nerve block: an original technique to provide postoperative analgesia after foot surgery. *Anesth Analg* 84:383–386, 1997.
171. Ilfeld BM, Morety TE, Wang RD, et al: Continuous popliteal sciatic nerve block for postoperative pain control at home: a randomized, double-blinded, placebo-controlled study. *Anesthesiology* 97:959–965, 2002.
172. Evans H, Steele SM, Nielsen KC, et al: Peripheral nerve blocks and continuous catheter techniques. *Anesthesiol Clin North Am* 23:141–162, 2005.
173. McLeod DH, Wong DH, Claridge RJ, et al: Lateral popliteal sciatic nerve block compared with subcutaneous infiltration for analgesia following foot surgery. *Can J Anaesth* 41:673–676, 1994.
174. Sinha SK, Abrams JH, Arumugam S, et al: Femoral nerve block with selective tibial nerve block provides effective analgesia without foot drop after total knee arthroplasty: a prospective, randomized, observer-blinded study. *Anesth Analg* 115:202–206, 2012.
175. Bonica's Management of Pain, ed 3, pp 389–409.
176. Practical Pain Management, ed 3, pp 126–127.
177. Neural Blockade in Clinical Anesthesia and Management of Pain, ed 3, pp 708–709.

14B Perioperative Assessment

NICOLE SILVERSTEIN

INTRODUCTION TO PERIOPERATIVE MEDICINE

A preoperative evaluation is a comprehensive review of a patient. It is done to determine a patient's stability for surgery and how to optimize the patient's medical conditions for the proposed surgery. This may include, but is not limited to, changes in medications, suggesting preoperative tests or procedures and proposing higher levels of postoperative care. The ultimate decision to go to surgery is in the hands of the surgeon and the patient. A medical evaluation helps gather the information to limit the risks and provide knowledge for informed consent by both the surgeon and patient.

Anesthesia is an important aspect of medicine requiring knowledge of its own risks, the surgical procedures and complications, and perioperative care of the patient.

PREOPERATIVE CARDIAC RISK ASSESSMENT

One of the first areas often addressed in a preoperative evaluation is the patient's cardiac status. This includes both the patient's diagnoses and risk factors along with the risk of the proposed surgery. The American College of Cardiology (ACC) in concert with the American Heart Association (AHA) published an algorithm with their Guidelines on Perioperative Cardiovascular Evaluation and Care for Noncardiac Surgery in 2007 to help assess this risk.[1]

The first step requires determination of the urgency of the surgery. Emergent surgeries do not warrant preoperative evaluation. They are surgeries that have a high mortality rate if not immediately performed. Examples would include a ruptured appendix, infected native joint, or a cauda equina syndrome. These patients should be taken directly to the operating room with no further cardiac assessment. They should be assessed and monitored after surgery for any optimization of their medical conditions.

Once it is determined that the proposed surgery is not emergent, the patient's current cardiac condition is assessed. Specifically, one is looking to see if there are any active cardiac conditions present. These include:

1. Active decompensated heart failure.
2. Unstable angina.
3. Recent myocardial infarction defined as either an non-ST elevation or ST elevation myocardial infarction within the past month.
4. Severe valvular disease, most notably severe aortic stenosis.
5. Significant arrhythmia, such as supraventricular tachycardia, rapid atrial fibrillation or ventricular tachycardia. Rate-controlled atrial fibrillation is not considered a significant arrhythmia.

If any of these conditions are present, it is prudent that they be evaluated and treated prior to the operation. Once they have been adequately treated, then the patient should be reassessed for surgery. The risk stratification should start again.

If there are no active cardiac conditions present, then the type of surgery is determined. Surgeries are generally divided into high, intermediate, and low risk for a cardiac event. High-risk surgeries include all vascular surgeries except carotid endarterectomies and endovascular abdominal aortic aneurysm repair, surgeries with prolonged times (typically longer than 3 hours), or procedures with large blood loss or fluid shifts. High-risk surgeries have a greater than 5% chance of a perioperative cardiac event. Low-risk surgeries are typically outpatient surgeries, such as colonoscopies, endoscopies, skin biopsies, lumpectomies, and cataract surgeries with a less than 1% chance of a perioperative cardiac event. Intermediate-risk procedures follow between with a cardiac event rate of 1% to 5%. They are all other surgeries including orthopaedic surgeries in addition to abdominal, head and neck, and most urologic procedures.

Low-risk procedures do not require any further cardiac evaluation before surgery. Patients undergoing high-risk or intermediate-risk surgeries need further assessment.[2]

Most of the orthopaedic surgeries follow under the intermediate-risk category and thus would require this next step of cardiac evaluation. The ACC and AHA propose evaluation of a patient's functional capacity as their fourth step. The idea is to try and gauge the patient's cardiac reserve. This is assessed by determining the highest level of activity a patient can perform without any cardiac signs or symptoms. It is measured in metabolic equivalents. A metabolic equivalent of 1 is the ability to eat, dress, and perform basic self-care up to a level of 10 metabolic equivalents, which would be equivalent to participation in strenuous sports, such as singles tennis. Most surgeries put a strain on the heart of approximately 4 metabolic equivalents. This is equal to climbing a flight of stairs or walking on level ground at 4 mph. A patient who has a functional capacity over 4 metabolic equivalents is felt to not require any further cardiac evaluation and can proceed to surgery.

Often a patient's functional capacity is unknown because of dementia, sedation, or other causes of impaired cognition or the patient has a poor functional capacity because of a sedentary lifestyle. These patients require further evaluation by step 5, which is the determination of their clinical risk factors. The clinical risk factors have been defined differently depending on the source. The ACC/AHA has derived the Revised Cardiac Risk Index.[1]

1. Any history of ischemic heart disease
2. Any history of compensated or prior heart failure
3. Any history of cerebrovascular disease
4. Diabetes mellitus
5. Renal failure

If patients have none of these clinical risk factors, then their cardiac evaluation is complete. If they have at least three clinical risk factors and are going for a vascular (high risk) surgery, then these patients need further cardiac evaluation with cardiac stress testing. The remaining patients, with at least three risk factors going for intermediate-risk surgeries or patients with only one to two clinical risk factors irrespective of the type of surgery should only be considered for stress testing if it would affect perioperative management. This broad statement can be interpreted vastly. The idea is that these patients do not need routine cardiac evaluation but should be individually assessed for cardiac signs or symptoms. Patients exhibiting cardiac signs or symptoms that would lead the physician to order further cardiac evaluation if the patients were not going for surgery should be considered for this testing. It must be remembered that testing could lead to postponement or changing the proposed surgery. For example, a 70-year-old patient presents for preoperative evaluation for a total knee replacement. He does not have any active cardiac conditions and his functional capacity is not known. He has diabetes and a history of a stroke, thus placing him in this middle category with two clinical risk factors. Should the physician decide to do a stress test and it came out positive, the physician would be obligated to further pursue this with a cardiac catheterization. If it was determined that the patient needs angioplasty and/or a stent placement, aspirin and clopidogrel hydrogen sulfate would likely be initiated and need to continue uninterrupted for 1 year (anticoagulation is covered further in the "Medications" section). This would delay the proposed total knee arthroplasty for at least a year. The same patient with concerns of undiagnosed cardiac disease with such symptoms as dyspnea on exertion or chest pressure with ambulation could possibly be prevented from having a cardiac event perioperatively if the same stress test and angioplasty was performed. Physician knowledge of the patient and a full review of the patient's history, especially a complete review of symptoms and physical examination are essential for making this determination.

The ACC/AHA algorithm is a comprehensive tool to help in the cardiac evaluation of a patient preparing for surgery. It does not replace individual assessment of the patient and the surgery.

PULMONARY RISK ASSESSMENT

The risk of pulmonary complications is often overlooked during the preoperative evaluation. Studies have shown that pulmonary complications occur at the same rate as, if not more commonly than, cardiac complications. There is increased morbidity, mortality, length of hospital stay, and health care cost related to postoperative pulmonary complications.[3] It has even been suggested that respiratory failure may predict ill health and further complications.[4] Patients can be assessed based on their risk factors as well as the proposed surgery risk factors for these postoperative pulmonary complications. The complications typically referred to are

1. Atelectasis
2. Acute respiratory failure, which is often defined as an inability to extubate a patient after surgery or a need to reintubate
3. Pneumonia, both hospital acquired and ventilatory acquired
4. Bronchospasm
5. Asthma and chronic obstructive pulmonary disease (COPD) exacerbations

The evidence behind patient risk factors is inconsistent. There is good evidence that age older than 60 years, history of congestive heart failure, history of COPD, functional dependence, malnutrition with an albumin level lower than 3.5 mg/dL, history of obstructive sleep apnea (OSA), and pulmonary hypertension are all associated with increased postoperative pulmonary complication rates. One of the best predictors has been the American Society of Anesthesiologists (ASA) Classification. It is a five-point system ranging from a normal healthy person at ASA class I to a moribund patient as a class V. Patients with at least a class III (systemic disease that is not incapacitating) have an increased rate of postoperative pulmonary complication from 5.4% to over 11%. Less evidence exists for abnormal lung examination, smoking history, and elevated blood urea nitrogen (BUN) level, and there is unclear evidence of any association with obesity, controlled asthma, or diabetes.[5]

Smoking cessation during the acute perioperative time frame was initially felt to be detrimental to the patient. Nicotine induces an inflammatory state with increased impaired macrophages and neutrophils. Goblet cell hyperplasia causes a change in the volume and composition of mucus. There is decreased ciliary clearance and increased smooth muscle and fibrosis. The cough reflex to irritants is also suppressed. Smoking cessation causes symptoms of cough and wheezing with increased mucus production. Smokers who abstain from smoking less than 2 months have been shown to have a higher sputum volume than nonsmokers. However, there are perioperative complications associated with continued nicotine exposure. It is not an independent risk factor for major cardiac events; it is risk factor for pulmonary complications, decreased wound healing, delayed healing of fractures, and affects the requirements for anesthesia. There are nicotine withdrawal symptoms and increased risk of in-hospital mortality, rate of readmission, and length of hospital stays. A systematic review and meta-analysis of nine studies in 2011 showed that quitting smoking within 8 weeks was not associated with an increase or decrease in overall postoperative complication rate. Consensus opinion favors the benefit of smoking cessation at any point, even the perioperative time frame.[6,7]

In regard to the operation itself and postoperative pulmonary complications, there is increased risk with prolonged surgeries, surgeries close to the diaphragm, emergent surgeries, open surgeries, and surgeries under general anesthesia. There has been no proven increased risk with hip or gynecologic surgeries or epidural anesthesia.[5]

So why is pulmonary risk assessment not discussed as much as cardiac risk assessment? The answer is that no intervention has proven itself reliable in the prevention of postoperative pulmonary complications. There have been recommendations made that deep breathing exercises, incentive spirometry, continuous positive airway pressure, and selective use of nasogastric tubes may lower the risk, but not consistently nor with statistical significance. It has been shown that there is no benefit to right-heart catheterization, artificial nutrition in the form of enteral or parenteral nutrition, routine use of nasogastric tubes, preemptive use of steroids or antibiotics, routine chest radiographs, or preoperative spirometry.[4,5] The best that can be done is to identify the patient who is at increased risk of postoperative pulmonary complications and try to intervene as soon as the complication arises.

MEDICATIONS

β-Blockers

β-Blockers are a bit of a controversial topic in the perioperative arena. The idea is that noncardiac surgery increases levels of catecholamines, which in turn causes increased heart rate, blood pressure, and free fatty acid concentrations. All of which increase myocardial oxygen demand. β-Blockers are thought to attenuate the increased catecholamine levels and thus decrease myocardial consumption and ultimately decrease cardiovascular risk.[8] Numerous studies including the Atenolol Study in 1996[9] and the Bisoprolol Study in 1999[8] showed decreases in both overall mortality and cardiac death, thus concluding, "Bisoprolol reduces the perioperative incidence of death from cardiac causes and nonfatal [myocardial infarction (MI)] in high risk patients who are undergoing major vascular surgery."[8] A retrospective cohort study was done looking at patients undergoing noncardiac surgery from 2000 to 2001 at 329 hospitals in the United States.[10] The risk of in-hospital mortality with β-blocker administration was based on calculation of the revised cardiac risk index for each patient (clinical risk factors). The study authors concluded, "Perioperative beta-blocker therapy is associated with a reduced risk of in-hospital death among high risk, but not low risk, patients undergoing major noncardiac surgery. Patient safety may be enhanced by increasing the use of beta-blockers in high risk patients."[10] The MaVS study published in 2006 randomized metoprolol versus placebo for vascular surgery patients. The authors found no difference in cardiac events but an increase in bradycardia and hypotension, concluding, "Our results showed metoprolol was not effective in reducing 30 day and 6 month postoperative cardiac event rates. Prophylactic use of perioperative beta blockers in all vascular patients is not indicated."[11] Thus in 2007, the ACC published guideline recommendations for perioperative use of β-blockers. They suggested that the only class I indication for perioperative β-blockers is to continue β-blockers in all patients undergoing surgery who are already taking them and β-blockers may be given to patients undergoing vascular surgery who are at high cardiac risk (ischemia on preoperative testing).[1] Then in 2008, the Perioperative Ischemic Evaluation (POISE) trial was published. This multicenter randomized controlled trial looked at metoprolol versus placebo in patients undergoing noncardiac surgery. The results showed an overall reduction of myocardial infarction, cardiac revascularization, and clinically significant atrial fibrillation. Yet a significant excess risk of death, stroke, and clinically significant hypotension and bradycardia was found.[12] This led to the ACC publishing, in 2009, a focused update on perioperative recommendations on perioperative use of β-blockers. The only class I recommendation became that β-blockers can be continued in all patients undergoing surgery who are already taking them. The routine use of high-dose β-blockers in the absence of titration became nonuseful and possibly harmful to patients not taking β-blockers preoperatively and undergoing noncardiac surgery.[13]

In general, the recommendations for perioperative β-blockers at this time include:

1. Continue them on patients already taking them preoperatively.
2. Consider starting patients on perioperative β-blockers if their Modified Cardiac Risk Index is at least 2 (clinical risk factors).
3. Preoperative β-blockers are best started at least 2 weeks before surgery and titrated to a heart rate of 55 to 65 beats per minute.

Hyperglycemic Medications

Oral hypoglycemic medications are generally held the morning of surgery to help prevent hypoglycemia perioperatively. They can be restarted once the patient is taking adequate oral intake. There is a movement by many hospitals to discontinue all oral hypoglycemic medications in-hospital and only use insulin products to control hyperglycemia. Metformin, however, requires special consideration. The manufacturer warning lists lactic acidosis as a possible side effect of using metformin (Glucophage) during the perioperative time frame. Although it is a rare side effect, it is a dangerous one, and thus, the recommendation stands to hold metformin 48 hours before surgery and continue to hold it for 48 hours after surgery. If the decision is to restart in the hospital, lactic acidosis is increased in a patient with renal insufficiency and thus it is prudent that the creatinine be assessed prior to restarting metformin. A creatinine level of 1.4 mg/dL or greater in women or 1.5 mg/dL or greater in men prevents reinitiating metformin.[14,15]

Insulin regimens depend on the type of diabetes. An insulin-dependent (type 1) diabetic requires more coordination with an endocrinologist and care in the perioperative period to avoid diabetic ketoacidosis. Type 1 diabetic management is above the scope of this chapter. The more common type 2 or noninsulin-dependent diabetes will be addressed here. Those on oral hypoglycemics can easily follow the earlier recommendations. Those on insulin still have insulin requirements even without oral intake. The basal metabolic needs require approximately half of a patient's total daily insulin requirements without oral intake.

Some general insulin recommendations are[14,15]

1. Short-acting insulin is held the morning of surgery. Corrective doses can be given if the blood glucose levels are higher than 200 mg/dL.
2. Intermediate-acting insulin is given as one-half to two-thirds dose the night before surgery and up to one-half the morning dose the day of surgery providing the patient is expected to eat following surgery. The decision to give the morning dose relies on how likely the patient will be to eat versus the concern over sedation, nausea, or anorexia. It is often suggested that the morning dose of intermediate-acting insulin be held to avoid hypoglycemia as short-acting insulin can always be administered to prevent hyperglycemia.
3. Long-acting insulin is generally given at one-half or full dose the evening before surgery. If patients take their long-acting insulin the morning of surgery, then the same adjustments can be made. There is a lack of true consensus on what to do with long-acting insulin, as the controlled studies are still pending.

Glucocorticoids

To discuss glucocorticoid management in the perioperative period, it is essential to understand the basic pathophysiology of cortisol. The hypothalamus secretes corticotropin-releasing hormone (CRH), which causes secretion of adrenocorticotropic hormone (ACTH) from the pituitary, which stimulates the adrenal glands to secrete cortisol, hence, the hypothalamic-pituitary-adrenal (HPA) axis. Cortisol secretion is involved in metabolism of carbohydrates, lipids, and proteins, in vascular tone and endothelial integrity, in sodium and potassium management, and in antiinflammatory properties. Stress (i.e., surgery) causes a positive feedback on the HPA axis and, thus, increases CRH level and ultimately increases cortisol levels. Exogenous cortisol in the form of oral glucocorticoids imposes a negative feedback on the axis and thus prevents the increased secretion of cortisol during the time of surgical stress.[16] There have been no randomized trials illustrating the assumption that exogenous cortisol causes sufficient adrenal atrophy to prevent the generation of sufficient endogenous glucocorticoids to meet the demands of surgical stress. However, this assumption has permeated medical thinking from the early 1950s, when there were cases of adrenal insufficiency related to stopping exogenous glucocorticoid treatment perioperatively.[17,18]

The question often arises regarding which patients on exogenous glucocorticoids are at risk for postoperative adrenal insufficiency and thus need extra stress dosing of glucocorticoids. All patients who are critically ill, have primary adrenal insufficiency, or primary hypopituitary insufficiency should receive stress dose steroids prior to surgery. Identifying the patients with secondary adrenal insufficiency is more controversial. There is no one recommendation as there are no randomized clinical trials to answer the question. There is some general consensus.

- It has been found that patients on at least 15 mg of oral prednisone or its equivalent for at least 3 weeks or patients with Cushing syndrome are likely to be adrenal suppressed and thus be unable to mount an endogenous response to the stress of surgery.
- Patients on less than 5 mg of prednisone or its equivalent, less than 3 weeks of exogenous glucocorticoids or alternate-day dosing of glucocorticoids are unlikely to have had their HPA axis affected and thus need not be considered for stress dosing of steroids.[19,20]

This leaves a large gray area of those patients on exogenous steroids over 3 weeks and more than 5 mg prednisone but less than 15 mg oral prednisone. It has been suggested that some ways to possibly determine if they are suppressed may be to perform an ACTH stimulation test or check 8 AM and 4 PM cortisol levels.

Because there is such a large unclear patient population, why not just give every patient stress dose steroids? The problem remains of the large side-effect profile with cortisol. These include but are not limited to the following[20]:

1. HPA axis suppression
2. Impaired wound healing
3. Fluid retention
4. Weight gain
5. Elevated blood pressure
6. Low potassium
7. Muscle weakness
8. Diabetes exacerbation and hyperglycemia
9. Obesity
10. Cataracts
11. Personality changes
12. Increased friability of skin, blood vessels, and tissues
13. Increased risk of bleed and ulcers
14. Increased risk of fracture and avascular necrosis

The other problem is that there is emerging data that the assumption of profound HPA axis suppression may be overstated. Marik and Varon[17] completed a literature review of two randomized controlled trials and seven cohort studies looking at stress-dose steroids for secondary adrenal insufficiency. Only two patients (one in each of two cohort trials) showed any signs of hypotensive collapse postoperatively. Both of these patients had their regular home regimen held 36 to 48 hours before surgery. The authors also looked at urinary 11-hydroxycorticosteroid levels following surgery in patients treated with glucocorticoids against controls. Although the urinary levels in the corticosteroid-treated group was less than the control group, they were still sufficient to prevent signs and symptoms of secondary adrenal insufficiency.[17] More studies are needed to better define which patients are at risk for secondary adrenal insufficiency during the stress of surgery.

If it is decided that a patient is at risk for secondary adrenal insufficiency, how are stress doses of steroids given? There is no evidence-based data but only expert opinion and recommendations. The drug of choice is intravenous (IV) hydrocortisone, which gives both glucocorticoid and mineralocorticoid effects. It should begin within an hour of surgery. The initial dosing common themes include[16-20]:

1. For high-risk surgeries, patients should be started with 100 to 150 mg IV hydrocortisone at the induction of surgery.
2. For intermediate-risk surgeries, patients should be started with 50 to 75 mg IV hydrocortisone at the induction of surgery.
3. Low-risk surgeries do not have a general consensus. Recommendations include no additional stress dosing of steroids, doubling the patients' home dose, or giving 25 mg IV hydrocortisone.

Like the wide spectrum of recommendations for low-risk surgeries, how to taper the patients is also diverse. The general consensus is to taper the extra steroids over the next 2 days, but it is practitioner dependent on how this is done. It should be noted that these stress doses of hydrocortisone are given in addition to the patients' home regimens.

Antihypertensive Medications

Perioperative hypotension is always a concern, especially because anesthetic agents often lower blood pressure. Renal hypoperfusion and electrolyte abnormalities are additional considerations in recommending changes to a patients' perioperative medication regimen. There is no clear evidence on perioperative side effects for antihypertensive medications. In general, diuretics are held the morning of surgery to help prevent electrolyte abnormalities.[21] Angiotensin-converting enzyme inhibitors (ACEIs) and angiotensin receptor blockers (ARBs) are often held the morning of surgery to prevent renal hypoperfusion and, thus, postoperative renal insufficiency. They are considered beneficial in regard to cardioprotection and attenuation of the sympathetic response to surgery. However, the risk has become a bit controversial as the studies on ACEIs and ARBs given preoperatively have not shown an increased risk of postoperative renal insufficiency. They do show a profound and severe hypotension on the induction of anesthesia that lasts approximately 30 minutes. Early treatment and initiation of pressors, if necessary, has tended to avoid any sequela from the ACEI or ARB treatment.[21,22] Thus, many still hold ACEIs and ARBs on the morning of surgery. β-Blockers should be continued but may need to be switched to IV forms if the patient is unable to take oral medications preoperatively. The remaining antihypertensive medication classes are typically continued through surgery with close monitoring of blood pressure perioperatively. Oral nitrates can be switched to nitropaste if the patient is not to take pills. α-Blockers and calcium channel blockers can continue perioperatively as well.

Anticoagulation Medications[23]

Warfarin is the anticoagulant most commonly thought of during the perioperative time period. In a trauma patient, time does not allow for the slow discontinuation of its effects. In all patients, the risk of bleeding and the type of surgery needs to be weighed against the patient's own risk factors. Joint and soft tissue injections do not require any alteration of a patient's routine anticoagulation.[24] However, patients undergoing surgery need their warfarin discontinued with an international normalized ratio (INR) of 1.5 or less as the general recommendation.[24] Reversal of warfarin can be done several ways. If time allows, the medication can be discontinued 5 days before surgery and allowed to be metabolized. In geriatric trauma patients, there is not this element of time. Vitamin K or fresh-frozen plasma are other methods to more quickly reverse the anticoagulant effect. Fresh-frozen plasma works quickly but only has a half-life of approximately 4 to 6 hours and, thus, the effects of warfarin are in effect 12 to 24 hours later. Vitamin K initiation can take hours to work but has long-lasting effects and can affect the ability to anticoagulate the patient again following the surgery. The recommended dose is 1 to 2 mg oral vitamin K or 2.5 to 5 mg IV vitamin K.[25]

Bridging anticoagulation needs to be determined at this stage. Which patients need low-molecular-weight heparin (LMWH) or a heparin drip to lower their risk of a thromboembolism and which patients can safely hold their anticoagulation until after surgery?

Bridging anticoagulation is recommended for a patient with[24,25]:

1. An acute venous or arterial thromboembolism within the past 3 months
2. Atrial fibrillation with a history of a cerebrovascular event or transient ischemic event (TIA): CHADS (congestive heart failure, hypertension, age, diabetes mellitus, stroke) score 5 to 6
3. Prior recurrent venous thromboembolism
4. Mechanical mitral valve
5. Caged-ball type prosthetic heart valve
6. Recent stroke or transient ischemic attack within 6 months
7. Rheumatic heart disease
8. Severe thrombophilia

Patients with a history of antiphospholipid syndrome, particularly those who have had a thromboembolism, cancer patients, and patients with low cardiac ejection fractions should be individually considered for bridging anticoagulation.

How is it done?[21,24-26]

- Stop warfarin 5 days prior to procedure.
- Initiate LMWH (typically start the next day for simplicity but can wait until 2 to 3 days before procedure) at full treatment dose. In trauma patients, this step is not necessary.
- Stop LMWH 12 to 18 hours before the procedure. Discussion should be had with anesthesiology if considering spinal anesthesia or an epidural as they often require cessation 24 hours before surgery. Surgeries with a high risk of bleeding may require 48- to 72-hour cessation of anticoagulants.
- If bleeding is minimal, restart warfarin 12 to 24 hours after surgery.
- Restart LMWH (full dose) 12 to 24 hours after hemostasis is achieved.
- Continue LMWH until warfarin is at a therapeutic level (INR 2 to 3).
- If using unfractionated heparin (UFH), stop 4 to 6 hours before surgery and restart within 12 hours postoperatively, providing adequate hemostasis is achieved. Continue until warfarin is at a therapeutic level.

The overlap between either LMWH or a heparin drip is continued until the patient is once again therapeutic on warfarin (typically INR 2 to 3).

Other blood thinners are typically held depending on their half-life. Aspirin and clopidogrel are irreversible platelet inhibitors and thus need to be held 7 to 10 days before surgery. There are no medications to reverse these platelet effects in the trauma patient. Patients who are at moderate to high risk for cardiovascular events should have their aspirin continued perioperatively. The indication for the aspirin needs to be determined. Patients with recent coronary angioplasty or stent placement need special consideration when holding these medications.[25,27,28]

- The recommendation is that coronary angioplasty requires uninterrupted aspirin and clopidogrel for 7 to 14 days.
- Bare metal stent placement requires uninterrupted aspirin and clopidogrel for 6 to 8 weeks.
- Drug-eluding stent placement requires 6 months to 1 year of uninterrupted treatment.

Secondary prevention for strokes or peripheral artery disease may also need special consideration in consultation with their appropriate specialty to determine the risk versus benefit of holding aspirin. Nonsteroidal antiinflammatory medications are typically held 3 to 4 days before surgery.

There is no recommendation of routine use of platelet function assays or platelet transfusion if patients are on these medications.

Dabigatran is a newer anticoagulant often used for atrial fibrillation. It is a direct thrombin inhibitor with no known reversible medication. It has a relatively fast metabolism and needs approximately 24 to 48 hours' cessation before surgery. This may be extended to 1 to 2 days for major surgeries, spinal punctures, or placement of epidural catheters. It can be restarted after surgery once hemostasis has been achieved.[29]

Herbal Supplements

The area of herbal remedies and vitamin supplementation has grown vastly in the past years. Patients are often taking these additional supplements without the knowledge of the providers and often do not mention them when recalling their medication regimen. It is as important to ask patients about their over-the-counter medications as about their prescribed medications. There is a cause for safety concerns with these supplements.

Many of these herbal supplements are P450 inducers and affect the metabolism of medications. To name a few, ginkgo biloba, garlic, and ginseng have been implicated with increased bleeding risk as it is felt they can affect platelet aggregation. Echinacea can cause immunosuppression, increasing the risk of postoperative infection. Valerian has been shown to have withdrawal symptoms, and ephedra can cause hypertension, tachycardia, and even ventricular arrhythmias with halothane.[21,30] Ideally these supplements are held 7 to 10 days prior to surgery. In the geriatric trauma patient, it is essential to know the additional supplements to monitor for their potential side effects.

Other Medications

Selective serotonin reuptake inhibitors (SSRIs) have the potential to increase the risk of bleeding and serotonin syndrome with certain anesthetics. However, they have a long half-life and a withdrawal syndrome if abruptly discontinued. Trauma patients need to be monitored as 1-day cessation makes no difference in the drug levels.[21,31]

Tamoxifen and other hormone replacement medications can increase the risk of deep venous thrombosis perioperatively.[31]

Bisphosphonates have a risk of pill esophagitis if a patient is unable to sit upright and have a full glass of water following medication administration.[31]

Cholesterol-lowering agents in the hydroxymethylglutaryl coenzyme A (HMG-CoA) inhibitor family have shown some promise as antiinflammatory agents. Studies suggest that this class of medications may lower the risk of postoperative atrial fibrillation and possibly even cardiac events. A patient currently taking this class of medication should continue it throughout the perioperative time frame.[21,31]

ORDERING TESTS

Aside from the recommendations published by the ACC/AHA regarding stress testing in select patients, there is not a lot of guidance regarding which tests should be routinely ordered.

- Prothrombin time (PT)/INR should be known in patients on warfarin.
- Electrolyte and renal function should be known in patients with diabetes, renal disease, or with risk factors for abnormalities. Total bilirubin and INR are also needed to calculate the Model for End-Stage Liver Disease (MELD) score for liver patients.
- Electrocardiograms are useful in patients older than 40 years of age with a clinical risk factor or in patients older than 50 years of age if not recently performed.
- There is no need for routine chest radiography, spirometry, or blood gas levels.
- Blood counts are only needed in patients suspected to have abnormalities but are not routine.
- Routine urinalysis is not warranted unless there is concern over an abnormality irrespective of the preoperative state.
- Consider drug levels for patients on medications with narrow therapeutic windows.

DIABETES MELLITUS

Diabetes mellitus as a perioperative diagnosis warrants evaluation independently. It increases a patient's modified cardiac risk index thus increasing cardiac risk, often requires medications that need to be adjusted perioperatively, and has its own host of postoperative complications. Preoperatively, a patient should be assessed for the following:

1. What type of diabetes does the patient have and how long has the patient carried the diagnosis of diabetes?
   a. Insulin dependent
   b. Noninsulin dependent
2. What is the patient's glycated hemoglobin (hemoglobin A1C) level?
3. Does the patient have any known diabetic complications (i.e., nephropathy, neuropathy)?

From the pathophysiology standpoint, surgery puts an additional stress on the balance in a diabetic patient. Surgery and the anesthetic agents increase catecholamines, thus increasing insulin resistance and decreasing insulin secretion. Hepatic glucose production increases and peripheral glucose utilization decreases. The net effect is hyperglycemia and protein catabolism.[14]

Why is there such a concern about perioperative hyperglycemia? Hyperglycemia increases the risk of dehydration and electrolyte abnormalities. There is impaired wound healing and increased risk of infection. A retrospective observational study from the Veterans Affairs Connecticut Healthcare System was published in 2006 looking at diabetic patients undergoing noncardiac surgery. Diabetic patients with good control (glycohemoglobin <7%) had a decreased rate of infections with an adjusted odds ratio (OR) of 2.13 (*P* value, 0.007).[32] Another study in 2007 found that in general surgery patients, there was a 5.7-fold increased risk of serious postoperative infections if the blood glucose level was greater than 220 mg/dL on postoperative day 1.[33] In addition, hyperglycemic patients have prolonged hospital stays, high rates of disability after hospital discharge, increased intensive care unit (ICU) admission rates, and an increase in mortality. A case-control study from The Netherlands looked at glucose levels and mortality. The authors found that patients with glucose levels higher than 200 mg/dL had an adjusted OR of 2.1 versus an adjusted OR of 1 for nondiabetics in regard to mortality.[34]

There are some data in the literature about how to best optimize hospitalized diabetics, but it is not specific to the postoperative patient. The Normoglycaemia in Intensive Care Evaluation and Survival Using Glucose Algorithm Regulation (NICE-SUGAR) trial was a randomized study of more than 6000 patients, which evaluated intensive glucose control with target fingerstick glucose less than 110 mg/dL in comparison to conventional control with a target fingerstick glucose level less than 180 mg/dL. The trial found that the intensive control was associated with an increased ICU patient mortality. Thus the general recommendation is that the target glucose levels for noncritically ill patients should be less than 140 mg/dL with a goal of less than 180 mg/dL for critically ill patients.[35] The Randomized Study of Basal Bolus Insulin Therapy in the Inpatient Management of Patients with Type 2 Diabetes (RABBIT II) Trial in the nonsurgical patient population points toward a benefit of basal and bolus insulin over sliding-scale insulin alone for better glucose control.[33] Insulin is typically what is initiated perioperatively with many different formulas available to calculate total daily insulin requirements. For patients on insulin preoperatively, it is typically suggested to restart their home regimen postoperatively with adjustments as needed by fingerstick glucose monitoring. The question of when to restart oral hypoglycemic medications is often raised. Providing a patient is taking adequate and consistent oral intake with no signs of acute renal insufficiency or need for further surgery or radiocontrast dye, oral medications can be reinitiated. There does appear to be a growing trend in using no oral hypoglycemic medications in the hospital setting and using insulin management for better control and predictability.

OBSTRUCTIVE SLEEP APNEA

Patients are predisposed to difficulties in airway management preoperatively. There is a relationship between a diagnosis of OSA and a difficulty in intubation. Primarily, the risk is related to airway problems and postoperative pulmonary failure. Sedatives and analgesics can cause decreased pharyngeal tone and thus increase OSA. There are increases in pulmonary, cardiovascular, and postoperative complications; increased ICU admissions; and longer duration of hospital stay. Perioperative risk increases in proportion to severity of OSA. These complications can occur as late as postoperative day 3 or 4.[36]

Some clinical signs include[36]:

1. Neck circumference greater than or equal to 17 inches
2. Body mass index greater than 35 kg/m^2
3. Craniofacial abnormalities
4. Snoring
5. Observed apnea
6. Daytime hypersomnolence
7. Inability to visualize the soft palate on physical examination
8. Tonsillar hypertrophy

Several questionnaires are available to help screen as there has been some suggestion that preoperative diagnosis and treatment can lower the risk of postoperative pulmonary complications. One validated tool is STOP BANG. If a patient has two or more STOP questions positive, then there is 72% sensitivity and 33% specificity of the patient being high risk for OSA. The addition of one positive question from BANG increases the positive predicative value to 84 to 94.3 (depending on which question is positive) and to 100 if the patient has all four positive.[37]

S: Does the patient snore extremely loud?
T: Does the patient feel tired, sleepy, or fatigued during the day?
O: Does the patient have any observed apneic events?
P: Does the patient have elevated blood pressure?
B: Is the patient's BMI greater than 35 kg/m^2
A: Is the patient older than 50 years of age?
N: Is the patient's neck circumference greater than 40 cm?
G: Is the patient a male?

Patients suspected of OSA should have a formal sleep study to diagnose and manage their disease before surgery. Should surgery be delayed for suspected OSA? The American Society of Anesthesiologists Guidelines from 2006 state that patients should be screened preoperatively for OSA to have the ability to manage these patients. Sleep studies should be ordered if time allows. It may need to be a clinical diagnosis if the patient presents on the day of surgery. The surgeon and the anesthesiologist may elect to delay the surgery for testing and treatment or presumptively manage these patients as if they have OSA. This includes, but is not limited to, having the patient use their continuous positive airway pressure (CPAP) or bilevel positive airway pressure (BiPAP) machines in the recovery room, at night, or anytime they are sleeping. Postextubation supplemental oxygen should be initiated and continuous pulse oximetry monitored in those untreated. If possible, patients should be kept in nonsupine positions.[36]

LIVER DISEASE

Patients with liver disease have an increased rate of mortality and perioperative complications. Patients with acute hepatic decompensation should have their liver stabilized before surgery. There is a concern that surgery will precipitate hepatic decompensation by decreased hepatic perfusion, traction of abdominal viscera, hypotension, hypoxemia, hemorrhage, or the metabolism of drugs. It is important to evaluate all patients for their risk factors for liver disease even if they do not carry a known diagnosis. This includes a thorough history and physical examination looking for risk factors (alcohol abuse, hepatitis C or B exposure, etc.) and stigmata of liver failure (spider angiomata, gynecomastia, testicular atrophy, etc.). Laboratory investigations should be initiated to determine the degree of disease. These include a metabolic profile, complete blood count, PT, bilirubin and albumin levels, and liver enzyme levels.

Risk factors include[38]:

1. Child-Turcotte-Pugh class C
2. MELD score greater than 15
3. Age older than 70 years
4. American Society of Anesthesiologists' Classification

The American Society of Anesthesiologists' Classification system is the best predicator of mortality in the first 7 days postoperatively. After 7 days, the MELD score is the best predictor.[39] It is a logarithmic formula involving the total bilirubin, INR, and creatinine levels. A level less than 10 is considered permissible for elective surgery and 10 to 14 is considered permissible for elective surgery. A MELD score greater than 15 is considered a contraindication for elective surgery. Patients with MELD scores greater than 15 should have involvement of a gastroenterology consultant and a level greater than 20 indicates that those patients may require surgery in an institution that is prepared to care for fulminant liver failure and possibly even liver transplant.[40]

Other considerations include procedural risks. Surgeries with large blood loss have elevated risk of ischemic hepatic injury. Anesthesia can also affect liver disease. Liver disease prolongs the effects of anesthesia. Short-acting sedatives and analgesics are preferred. Benzodiazepines carry an increased risk of rare hepatotoxic reactions. The location of the surgery can cause direct liver injury as well.

Patients with a diagnosis of liver disease need to be optimized medically before surgery. This may include:

1. Vitamin K or fresh-frozen plasma if patients have elevated prothrombin times.
2. Desmopressin acetate (DDAVP) to help with platelet dysfunction and prolonged bleeding time.

3. Diuretics or paracentesis if there is large ascites.
4. Electrolyte abnormality correction. Hypokalemia and metabolic alkalosis are most common.
5. Renal function should be assessed and monitored perioperatively.
6. Nutritional support.
7. Postoperative surveillance for hepatic decompensation.

PREVENTING COMPLICATIONS

Delirium

Postoperative delirium is a common postoperative complication in the geriatric patient. It has been found in 10% to 51% of postoperative patients. It is not felt to be related to the type of anesthesia administered but is often related to a preexisting limited cognitive reserve. There is increased risk of death, prolonged hospitalization, institutionalization, and readmission to the hospital in patients with postoperative delirium.[41]

The clinical manifestations can be quite diverse. They include, but are not limited to, the following:

- Acute change in mental status, disturbed consciousness
- Impaired cognition
- Fluctuating course
- Reduced ability to focus attention
- Increased psychomotor activity (delusions, hallucinations, etc.)
- Increased sensitivity to pain

It often presents on postoperative day 1 or 2 and tends to be worse in the evening hours.

Risk factors include but are not limited to:

- Any acute physical stress (trauma included)
- Medications (polypharmacy with more than five medications)
- Cognitive impairment or dementia at baseline
- Age older than 65 years
- Dehydration
- Severe illness including hypoxia and hypotension
- Pain
- Constipation or urinary retention
- Urinary catheterization
- Vision or hearing impairment
- Immobility or physical restraints

There is little proven to prevent postoperative delirium. Attempts should be made to limit risk factors and quickly identify these patients. Postoperative delirium is not considered a normal response to surgery. An underlying cause should be sought. Management initially relies on searching for an etiology.

Initial workup includes looking for withdrawal syndromes (alcohol or benzodiazepines are most common), electrolyte abnormalities, medication side effects (benzodiazepines and anticholinergic agents), and complete blood count, urinalysis, and chest radiograph to look for infections. Depending on the clinical risk factors and the results of the patient' examination, an electrocardiogram to rule out a myocardial infarction, arterial blood gas levels looking for carbon dioxide retention or hypoxia, urine and blood cultures looking for infection, and even a computed tomography (CT) scan of the head with neurologic signs may be considered.

The treatment revolves around the underlying cause and the patient's safety. Reversal etiologies should be addressed first. Discontinue any sedative medications and treat any abnormalities found in the evaluation. Environmental interventions should be tried first. Ask family members to visit the patient for social interactions and a sense of familiarity. Objects may be brought from home, such as pictures or sentimental objects. Avoid physical restraints unless absolutely necessary for patient safety. Ensure the room is quiet and that there is normalization of the sleep cycle. Keep the lights on during the day and off at night. Attempt to limit nighttime interactions so there is no sleep deprivation. If pharmacologic treatment is required for patient safety, it should be noted that the U.S. Food and Drug Administration (FDA) has not approved any agents for the primary treatment of postoperative delirium. Haloperidol is one of the typically used medications. However, it should be noted that the FDA has issued a black box warning for haloperidol stating it is not approved for dementia-related psychosis. There is an increased mortality risk from cardiovascular or infectious causes. It is contraindicated in patients with a prolonged QTc on an electrocardiogram or in patients with a diagnosis of Parkinson or Lewy body dementia. Low doses should be initiated if using haloperidol. Other often-used agents are the benzodiazepines, most notably, lorazepam (Ativan). Lorazepam can cause a paradoxical reaction in the elderly with worsening agitation. It should primarily be considered if the patient is felt to be in alcohol or benzodiazepine withdrawal. Other antipsychotic medications are often used but have never been shown to be more effective or safe than haloperidol.[41,42] They also carry the FDA black box warning on increased mortality.

Acute Renal Failure

Postoperative acute renal failure is defined as a serum creatinine level increase of 25% to 50% within 1 week of surgery. It is considered an independent predictor of postoperative pulmonary and cardiac complications. Preoperative renal insufficiency increases the risk of postoperative renal failure.

The evaluation and treatment is the same as with any patient with acute renal insufficiency.

- Volume status should be assessed and replaced if needed.
- Perioperative hypotension should be determined.
- Sepsis should be identified.
- Heart failure should be identified and treated.
- The patient should be evaluated for nephrotoxic drugs (i.e., nonsteroidal antiinflammatories and contrast dyes) and those drugs should be discontinued.
- Urinalysis should be ordered to assess for infection or glomerulonephritis.
- Consider evaluating urine electrolytes as the fractional excretion of sodium and urea as well as urine sodium levels may be helpful in determining dehydration over an intrinsic renal complication.
- Urinary catheterization should be performed to rule out an obstructive etiology.

Attention should be paid to the metabolism of medications administered, especially narcotics and benzodiazepines to prevent additional complications.

Postoperative Fever

Epidemiologically, postoperative fever is a common finding. The magnitude of the trauma correlates to the degree of fever. It usually resolves spontaneously within 72 hours with a maximum temperature typically on postoperative day 1 and normalizes by day 4. Less than 10% of fevers within the first 48 hours of surgery are related to infection.[43] The pathophysiology is related to tissue trauma and cytokine release. Most notably the cytokines interleukin-1 (IL-1), IL-6, tumor necrosis factor-α (TNF-α), and interferon-γ (IFN-γ) are implicated.

Cytokine release

↓

Prostaglandin release from anterior hypothalamus

↓

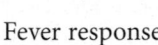

Fever response

The differential of postoperative fever is based on the timing of the fever in relation to the operation.[43]

	Time Frame
Immediate	Within hours of surgery
Acute	Within first week of surgery
Subacute	Within 1–4 weeks of surgery
Delayed	Longer than 4 weeks from surgery

The immediate time frame is within hours of the surgical procedure. Common etiologies to consider are preexisting infections, drug reactions, blood transfusion reactions, and malignant hyperthermia.

The acute time frame has the most expansive causes of postoperative fever. Within the first 48 hours of surgery, it is typically an inflammatory response to the stress of surgery as described earlier. The more invasive the surgery, the greater the inflammatory response, and the higher the potential fever spike. After postoperative day 2, infectious and noninfectious etiologies become more prominent. A common misconception is that atelectasis is the most common cause of postoperative fever. Atelectasis, however, does not cause postoperative fever. There is no association between the development of atelectasis and the finding of fever. Atelectasis causes pulmonary shunting and hypoxia.[43,44]

The management of postoperative fever involves a thorough history and physical examination looking for etiologies. Life-threatening etiologies need to be ruled out.[43]

1. Myonecrosis
2. Pulmonary embolism
3. Alcohol withdrawal
4. Bowel leak
5. Adrenal insufficiency
6. Malignant hyperthermia

In the absence of findings in the history or physical examination suggesting a particular etiology for the postoperative fever, there is no further workup necessary. Remove any catheters and intravascular lines. Review and eliminate unnecessary medications. In the first 48 hours, there is no need for routine laboratory orders or radiographs, unless the history and physical examination necessitates it. Patient comfort should be addressed with medications.

After the first 48 hours, the postinflammatory response has typically peaked, and a further evaluation for possible etiologies should be initiated. Pneumonia and urinary tract infections are common infections that cause postoperative fever in the later portion of the acute time frame.

The subacute and delayed time frames have a vast list of culprits including both infectious and noninfectious etiologies. Surgical site infections and venothromboembolism may present in the subacute patient with endocarditis and prosthetic infections in the delayed time frame. Postoperative fever should always prompt a thorough history and physical examination with further evaluation and management dictated by patient factors, surgery performed, and the postoperative time frame.

Other

Hypoxia is a common postoperative finding. There is a vast differential diagnosis including atelectasis, bronchospasm, pulmonary aspiration, anesthetic effects, pulmonary edema, pulmonary embolism, acute lung injury, and even acute respiratory distress syndrome. The workup includes a physical examination looking for signs or symptoms particular to a certain disease, chest radiograph, arterial blood gas levels, electrocardiogram, and response to supplemental oxygen. A pulmonary embolus may present as sinus tachycardia with nonspecific ST changes on electrocardiogram, new-onset atrial fibrillation, or a right bundle branch block.[45] The entire workup and management is beyond the scope of this chapter.

CONCLUSION

Geriatric trauma patients require a multidisciplinary approach to both evaluate the patients preoperatively to optimize medical conditions and choose the appropriate anesthesia and surgery and postoperatively to limit and prevent surgical and medical postoperative complications.

KEY REFERENCES

1. Fleisher LA, Beckman JA, Brown KA, et al: ACC/AHA 2007 guidelines on perioperative cardiovascular evaluation and care for noncardiac surgery. *J Am Coll Cardiol* 50(17):e159–e230, 2007.
5. Qaseem A, Snow V, Fitterman N, et al: Risk assessment for and strategies to reduce perioperative pulmonary complications for patients undergoing noncardiothoracic surgery: guidelines from the American College of Physicians. *Ann Intern Med* 144:575–580, 2006.
12. Devereaux PJ, et al; POISE Study Group: Effects of extended-release metoprolol succinate in patients undergoing non-cardiac surgery (POISE trial): a randomized controlled trial. *Lancet* 371:1839–1847, 2008.
13. American College of Cardiology Foundation, American Heart Association Task Force on Practice Guidelines: 2009 ACCF/AHA focused update on perioperative beta blockade. *J Am Coll Cardiol* 54:2102–2128, 2009.
23. Guyatt GH, Akl EA, et al: Executive Summary: Antithrombotic therapy and prevention of thrombosis (9th ed), American College of Chest Physicians evidence-based clinical practice. *Chest* 141:7S–47S, 2012.
25. Douketis JD, Berger PB, et al: The perioperative management of antithrombotic therapy: American College of Chest Physicians evidence-based clinical practice guidelines (8th ed). *Chest* 133:299S–339S, 2008.
35. NICE-SUGAR trial investigators: Intensive versus conventional glucose control in critically ill patients. *N Engl J Med* 360(13), 2009.

The complete References list is available online at https://expertconsult.inkling.com.

14C Management of the Pregnant Woman

DEBORAH FELDMAN • JOHN GREENE

INTRODUCTION

Special attention must be given to an obstetric patient who presents after trauma or is undergoing a surgical procedure. Changes in maternal hemodynamic and respiratory parameters are normal physiologic adaptations to pregnancy. In addition, the effects of medications, particularly anesthetic agents, on the fetus must be considered. For elective procedures, the optimal time for surgery is during the second trimester, although surgery can be safely performed at any time throughout the gestation.

It is important to involve an obstetrician in the management of these patients. According to a 2003 American College of Obstetricians and Gynecologists Committee Opinion, "Although there are no data to support specific recommendations regarding nonobstetric surgery and anesthesia in pregnancy, it is important for nonobstetric physicians to obtain obstetric consultation before performing nonobstetric surgery. The decision to use fetal monitoring should be individualized, and each case warrants a team approach for optimal safety of the woman and her baby."[1]

Care of the pregnant woman requires additional consideration, as there is concern for the second patient, the unborn fetus.[2-4] However, in cases of trauma or musculoskeletal emergency, initial efforts should be focused on the resuscitation and stabilization of the mother. The following are important in evaluating the gravid trauma patient:

- Evaluation of the pregnant patient should be similar to the nonpregnant patient.
- Stabilization of airway, breathing, and circulation of the mother is crucial.
- Key maternal injuries may easily be overlooked if the focus of attention becomes the fetus.
- Maintenance of appropriate maternal hemodynamic parameters is crucial for adequate fetal oxygenation in utero.
- Increasing the partial pressure of oxygen in the maternal blood will increase fetal oxygenation.

ASSESSMENT

As the patient is being stabilized, part of the assessment should be determination of the fetal gestational age and well-being. This can be accomplished fairly rapidly with the use of bedside ultrasound. Quick measurements of fetal anatomic parameters, such as the cranial biparietal diameter and length of the fetal femur, can be obtained to determine the approximate gestational age of the fetus. In addition, the ultrasound can visualize fetal cardiac activity, including the force and rate of the heartbeat.

If at all possible, attempts should be made to displace the uterus off the great vessels. Compression of the aorta and vena cava by the uterus decreases both venous return and cardiac output, which may worsen the maternal condition. This can be achieved by the following:

- Placement of the patient in a lateral position (Fig. 14C-1), or
- Placement of a wedge under the patient's hip

In pregnant patients, as in other patients, time is critical. Survival of both the mother and the fetus is more likely when shock is quickly recognized, support measures are begun, and bleeding is arrested promptly.[5]

Diagnostic testing should proceed as it would for any trauma patient. Imaging studies do not expose the fetus to levels that would cause any adverse effects. Radiation exposure from an abdominal and pelvic computed tomography (CT) scan falls below the level associated with causing any fetal anomalies or loss of the pregnancy. In addition, magnetic resonance imaging (MRI) does not produce any ionizing radiation, and there are no reports of any adverse effects to the fetus exposed in utero.[6]

PHYSIOLOGIC CHANGES IN PREGNANCY

Multiple normal physiologic changes occur in pregnancy that may affect both the assessment and management of injuries. Physiologic changes affect virtually every organ system either directly or indirectly. All of these adaptations result in an increase in the blood flow to the uterus and fetus. Indeed, the basic approach to the ABCs of initial resuscitation efforts may be altered during gestation.

Respiratory system

- Hyperventilation with increased minute ventilation
- Increased tidal volume
- Decreased lung capacity

Cardiovascular system

- Decreased blood pressure
- Increased heart rate
- Increased cardiac output
- Increased plasma volume

Blood pressure normally decreases during midpregnancy then rises back to prepregnant levels in the third trimester (after 27 weeks' gestation). This drop is because of

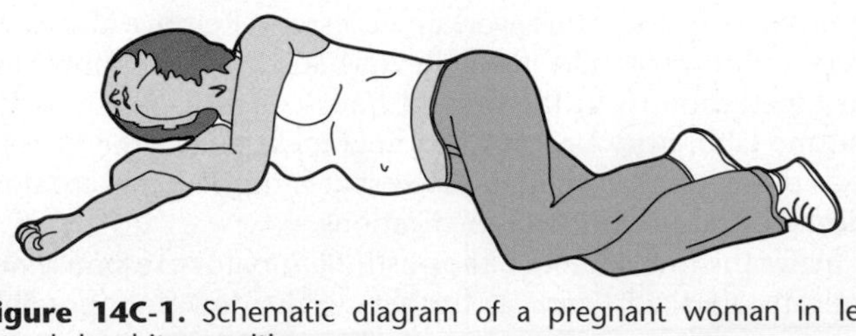

Figure 14C-1. Schematic diagram of a pregnant woman in left lateral decubitus position.

progesterone's effect on smooth muscle. There is a marked increase in cardiac output that begins in early gestation. Venous return is a key parameter in this high-output system and return from the lower extremities may be impeded in later stages of pregnancy by the enlarged uterus. This is exacerbated if the patient is in the supine position, a position commonly used in the assessment of an injured patient. If possible, examination of the patient is best carried out in the left lateral position (see Fig. 14C-1). If this is not possible, displacement of the uterus with a wedge placed under the patient to cause a lateral shift should be employed.

Another physiologic change in the pregnant patient is an increased heart rate. This increase in pulse must be kept in mind when hemodynamic assessment is made, particularly in cases of potential hemorrhage. Plasma volume also increases in pregnancy and peaks somewhere around 34 weeks of gestation. This increase is 40% to 50% above nonpregnant levels and ensures uteroplacental perfusion. Although red blood cell mass also increases in pregnancy, it does not increase to the same degree as plasma volume so there is a normal anemic state during pregnancy.

Fibrinogen levels are normally increased significantly in pregnancy, so that low or even low-normal levels should be a cause for concern in the gravid patient. The changes in the coagulation factors, in addition to increased venous stasis, result in a normal hypercoagulable state in pregnancy.

In cases of trauma, the increase in plasma volume may mask significant blood loss as the changes in pulse and blood pressures that normally occur early will be delayed because of the increased volume. Orthostatic changes and tachycardia do not typically occur until there is a loss of approximately 25% of the maternal blood volume. Vital signs may therefore be normal when significant blood loss has occurred. The fetus, however, may be experiencing hypoperfusion long before the mother manifests any signs. Larger volumes of fluid replacement will also be necessary.

Fluid replacement in these cases is often one of the first priorities. First-line therapy is crystalloid: either normal saline or lactated Ringer solution. Which specific fluid is used is not as important as replacement of adequate volume. Early and rapid fluid resuscitation should be administered even in the normotensive pregnant patient. Transfusion of blood may be crucial as this is one of the most effective ways to improve oxygen capacity and delivery to organs including the gravid uterus.

DIAGNOSTIC IMAGING IN PREGNANCY

Many imaging modalities are currently available for diagnosing various musculoskeletal injuries in pregnant women. Of these, radiographic procedures cause the most anxiety among patients and care providers because of the widespread belief that radiation exposure from a limited x-ray is enough to cause harm, or even death, to a growing fetus. In reality, most imaging studies are associated with little or no risk for fetal harm. The accepted cumulative radiation dose in pregnancy is 5 rad. According to the American College of Radiology, there is "no single diagnostic procedure which results in a radiation dose that threatens the well-being of the developing embryo and fetus."[7] The following section reviews the radiation exposure for various imaging studies, potential risks, and methods of minimizing risk in cases where imaging is needed in pregnancy.

X-RAY

Ionizing radiation is composed of high-energy photons that are capable of cell death, teratogenicity, carcinogenesis, and mutations in germ cells.[8] Data on the severity or long-term adverse genetic effects are sparse. There are animal studies that suggest that high-dose radiation (far greater than the dose used in diagnostic studies) occurring prior to implantation will likely result in early embryonic death.[8] In large doses of radiation (100–200 rad), there have been many teratogenic effects described in animals. Such large doses of radiation in pregnant humans have reportedly resulted in such abnormalities as fetal growth restriction, microcephaly, and developmental delay.[9] The fetus is most susceptible to the teratogenic effects of ionized radiation such as that due to CT between weeks 2 and 20 of embryonic life. These effects include, but are not limited to, the following:

- Microcephaly
- Microphthalmia
- Mental delay
- Growth restriction
- Cataracts
- Behavioral abnormalities

Perhaps the best human data to suggest the risk of high-dosage radiation exposure comes from atomic bomb survivors, whose fetuses carried a higher risk for central nervous system effects if exposed between 8 and 15 weeks' gestation. Mental delay in those fetuses exposed to at least 20 rad was as high as 40%, and for those exposed to 150 rad it was closer to 60%.[10] Given that there is no increased risk for anomalies, growth restriction, or spontaneous abortion at an exposure less than 5 rad, the risk for any diagnostic procedure is not increased.

The risk of carcinogenesis is also a concern for many patients undergoing radiologic procedures as well as the providers performing these tests. The actual risk for the development of cancer as a result of in utero exposure to radiation is not known. Some data suggest that a 1- to 2-rad fetal exposure may increase the risk of leukemia by a factor of 1.5 to 2.0, thereby increasing the leukemia rate from 1 in 3000 to 1 in 2000.[11]

Abdominal shielding should be performed whenever the radiographic procedure allows. The estimated fetal exposure from common radiologic studies is listed in Table 14C-1.

COMPUTED TOMOGRAPHY

The radiation dose to the fetus from a typical CT study is likely somewhere between 1 and 4 rad depending on the study and gestational age. While this is considerably higher than that of a plain radiographic study, it still falls below the accepted threshold level for induction of congenital abnormalities. The risk of carcinogenesis is similar to that of an x-ray (at a dose of 5 rad, the relative risk of childhood leukemia is 2.0). There is a risk of failed implantation within the first 2 weeks of embryonic life when the dose is greater than 10 rad. At this gestational age (often before the patient is even aware of the pregnancy), there

TABLE 14C-1 *NORMAL PHYSIOLOGIC CHANGES IN THE CARDIOVASCULAR SYSTEM DURING PREGNANCY*

Hemodynamic Measure	12 Weeks Post Partum	36-38 Weeks' Gestation	Change from Nonpregnant State
CO	4.3	6.2	+43%
HR	71	83	+17%
SVR	1530	1210	−21%
PVR	119	78	−34%
Oncotic pressure	20	18	−14%
MAP	86	90	NS
PCWP	6.3	7.5	NS
CVP	3.7	3.6	NS

CO, Cardiac output; *CVP*, central venous pressure; *HR*, heart rate; *MAP*, mean arterial pressure; *PCWP*, pulmonary capillary wedge pressure; *PVR*, peripheral vascular resistance; *SVR*, systemic vascular resistance.
Source: *Clark SL, Cotton DB, Lee W et al: Central hemodynamic assessment of normal term pregnancy, Am J Obstet Gynecol 161:1439–1442, 1989.*

is an "all or none" effect so that should the embryo survive, there are not likely to be any untoward effects.[12]

MAGNETIC RESONANCE IMAGING

MRI uses magnets that alter the energy state of hydrogen protons rather than using ionizing radiation. While a relatively new technique for diagnostic imaging in pregnancy, it is felt to be a safer alternative to nuclear imaging. In fact, MRI is often used to help diagnose fetal abnormalities. Studies of children exposed to MRI in utero at 1.5 tesla have not shown negative outcomes up to 9 years of age.[13] While there is a small amount of animal data to suggest a potential teratogenic effect of MRI in early pregnancy, no such human studies have been published.[14,15] According to the American College of Radiology, MRI is recommended in pregnancy if the "risk-benefit ratio to the patient warrants that the study be performed."[16] Results of studies evaluating potential acoustic damage to the fetus from MRI have also shown safety in this area.[17]

Use of the intravenous contrast gadolinium in conjunction with MRI has been controversial. Gadolinium crosses the placenta and is excreted by the fetal kidneys into the amniotic fluid. Animal studies of high and repeated doses of gadolinium have been shown to be teratogenic. While considered a pregnancy category C drug by the U.S. Food and Drug Administration, gadolinium is reserved for cases in pregnancy where the benefits outweigh the potential risks to the fetus (Fig. 14C-2).

NUCLEAR IMAGING

Nuclear studies are performed by combining a chemical agent with a radioisotope. These radiopharmaceuticals, once administered intravenously or orally to the patient, can localize to specific organs or cellular receptors, resulting in the ability to image the extent of a disease process in the body. In some diseases nuclear medicine studies can identify medical problems at an earlier stage than other diagnostic tests. One of the most commonly used isotopes is technetium 99m (^{99m}Tc). The fetal exposure for common scans such as brain, bone, renal, and cardiovascular is small (<0.5 rad).

The American College of Obstetricians and Gynecologists (ACOG) published the following guidelines for radiographic examination during pregnancy[10] (Table 14C-2):

1. The exposure from a single radiographic procedure does not result in harmful fetal effects. Exposure to less than 5 rads has shown no increase in the rate of fetal anomalies or spontaneous abortion. Patients should be counseled accordingly.
2. The concern regarding fetal effects of high-dose ionizing radiation should not delay or prevent medically indicated diagnostic radiographic procedures from being performed on pregnant women. Imaging procedures such as ultrasound and MRI, which are not associated with ionizing radiation, should be used in pregnancy in place of radiographic procedures when possible.
3. Radiopaque and paramagnetic contrast agents are not likely to cause fetal harm; however, they should be used only when medically necessary when the potential benefit outweighs the risk.
4. If multiple radiographs are needed in pregnancy, it may be helpful to consult with an expert in radiation dosimetry to calculate a total fetal exposure.
5. MRI and ultrasound are not associated with any harmful fetal effects.

COMMON MUSCULOSKELETAL COMPLAINTS IN PREGNANCY

Because of the normal physiologic changes that occur in pregnancy, certain musculoskeletal disorders may arise. These may

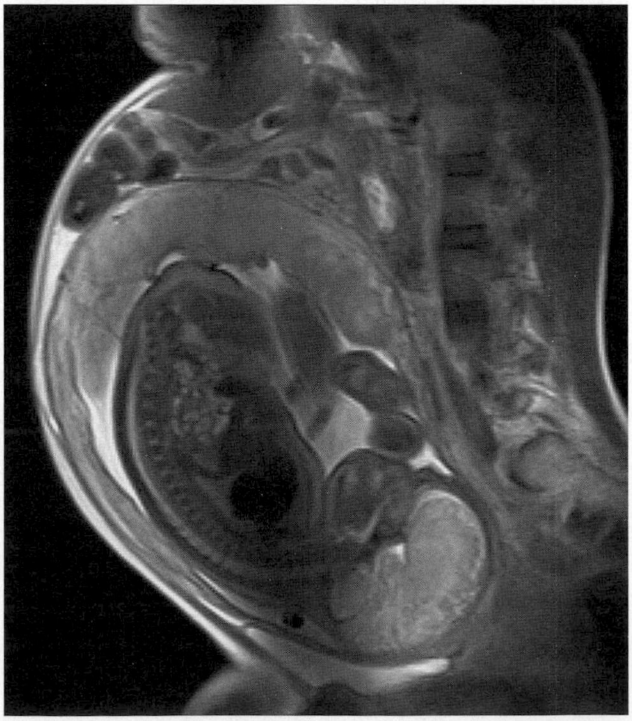

Figure 14C-2. An abdominal/pelvic magnetic resonance imaging (MRI) scan in a pregnant patient.

TABLE 14C-2 *ESTIMATED FETAL EXPOSURE FROM COMMON RADIOLOGIC PROCEDURES*

Procedure	Fetal Exposure
Chest radiograph (two views)	0.02–0.07 mrad
Abdominal film (single view)	100 mrad
Intravenous pyelogram	≥1 rad (depending on number of films)
Hip film (single view)	200 mrad
CT scan head/chest	<1 rad
CT scan abdomen and lumbar spine	3.5 rad

CT, Computed tomography.
Source: *Data from Cunningham FG, Gant NF, Leveno KJ, et al: Williams obstetrics, ed 21, New York, 2001, McGraw-Hill.*

be due to a combination of factors including progesterone-related ligament laxity, peripheral edema of the extremities including the carpal tunnel space, and an altered center of gravity as the pregnancy progresses, which may increase the likelihood of falling.

Back pain in pregnancy

- Most common musculoskeletal complaint in pregnancy
- Often due to increasing size of uterus placing pressure on lower spine
- Exaggerated lordosis of the lumbar spine in pregnancy
- Sciatic pain very common in pregnancy due to compression of the sciatic nerve by the uterus

Carpal tunnel syndrome

- Common complaint in pregnancy (affects up to 25% of pregnant women)
- More common in the third trimester
- Caused by edema in the carpal tunnel space compressing the median nerve
- Usually best treated in pregnancy with wrist splints
- Surgery not usually necessary during pregnancy as symptoms will subside post partum

Most common extremity injuries during pregnancy related to falling

- Ankle sprain (increased laxity of ligaments in pregnancy)
- Wrist sprain and fracture

In addition to the above, separation of the pubic symphysis is a rare but important musculoskeletal complication of pregnancy. Treatment is usually conservative, with pain medication as needed, physical therapy, and support with abdominal binders to decrease the pressure on the pubic bone.

FETAL MONITORING DURING NONOBSTETRIC SURGERY

During any surgical procedure in a pregnant woman, there are concerns for both the patient and the fetus. Consideration must first be made to alterations in maternal blood flow that occur during surgery. The circulation to the uteroplacental unit is not autoregulated, and the greatest impact of surgery on the fetus may come from decreased uterine blood flow and decreased oxygen content of the blood.

During the third trimester, uterine circulation represents nearly 10% of maternal cardiac output. Maternal hypotension will likely lead to decreased uterine blood flow and therefore decreased perfusion to the fetus. While medical therapy with pressors will successfully increase the maternal systemic pressure, they have little or no effect on uterine perfusion. Other maneuvers, such as intravenous fluid boluses, changing maternal position to decrease vena caval compression, or leg elevation are much more effective than medical therapy at increasing uteroplacental blood flow.

ANESTHESIA DURING PREGNANCY

Concern over the effect of inhalation anesthetic agents mainly arises in the first trimester when exposure can be associated with birth defects. While the literature is scant in this area, most experts agree that these agents are safe even in the first trimester. While elective surgery should be postponed until the second trimester or post partum, orthopaedic emergencies requiring surgical correction should proceed, as the benefit far outweighs any potential risk.

PRETERM LABOR

The risk for preterm labor is related to both gestational age and the indication for and type of surgery. The following should be considered:

- Pregnancies in the third trimester are at much higher risk for preterm contractions with or without cervical dilation compared with earlier gestational age.
- Orthopaedic surgeries not involving the maternal pelvis are much less likely to stimulate preterm labor than intra-abdominal surgeries

Moreover, abdominal surgeries and disease processes with intraperitoneal inflammation are the most likely to have postoperative courses complicated by preterm contractions and preterm labor. Both laparoscopic and open techniques have an equal incidence of preterm contractions and labor.

Treatment for such contractions, especially in the presence of cervical dilation, is performed with tocolytics. Studies show that delay of treatment of contractions after surgery can lead to preterm labor and subsequent preterm birth. While there is no general consensus on the use of prophylactic tocolytics after nonobstetric surgery during pregnancy, most studies suggest that tocolytics be used only if contractions are noted during postoperative monitoring or are appreciated by the patient.

The types of tocolytics used vary widely between medical centers. Options include magnesium sulfate (intravenous), nifedipine (oral), terbutaline (subcutaneous or oral), or indomethacin (oral). In general, these agents are equally effective in diminishing contractions when they occur postsurgically.[18,19]

TRAUMA IN PREGNANCY

Trauma is the leading nonobstetric cause of maternal mortality and affects as many as 7% of pregnancies. The most common form of trauma comes from falls or motor vehicle accidents. When compared to gestational age-matched controls, women who sustained trauma had a higher incidence of the following: spontaneous abortion, preterm labor, fetomaternal hemorrhage, abruptio placentae, and uterine rupture. Approximately 50% of fetal losses in trauma cases are due to placental abruption. Risk of abruption occurs with all placental locations, not just when the placenta has an attachment to the anterior uterine wall. While multiple studies have been unable to adequately predict adverse outcomes such as abruptio placentae and fetal loss, it is accepted that early involvement of an available obstetrician is important to evaluate both maternal and fetal well-being.

Rh_O(D) immune globulin (RhoGAM) is indicated in Rh-negative patients who have (1) vaginal bleeding, or (2) evidence of fetomaternal hemorrhage as diagnosed by a maternal Kleihauer-Betke stain test looking for fetal cells in the maternal circulation. The standard dose of Rh_O(D) immune globulin is 300 mcg, which is sufficient to cover up to 30 mL of fetal whole blood in the maternal circulation.

Direct fetal injury secondary to trauma is rare. Most of these cases result from significant maternal injury at later gestational ages. Another rare but life-threatening consequence of trauma is uterine rupture, which occurs most commonly secondary to direct abdominal injuries with substantial force.

Resuscitation of the fetus is best accomplished by resuscitation of the mother. Initial evaluation and treatment of the pregnant injured patient is identical to that of the nonpregnant injured patient, including rapid assessment of the maternal airway, breathing, and circulation, and ensuring an adequate airway avoids maternal and fetal hypoxia. In the later stages of pregnancy, the pregnant trauma patient should be placed in left lateral decubitus position with care to assess the fetus using either ultrasound or external fetal monitor.

The increased blood volume associated with pregnancy has implications in the trauma patient. Signs of blood loss, such as tachycardia and hypotension, may be delayed until the patient loses nearly 30% of her blood volume. The fetus may be experiencing hypoperfusion long before the mother manifests any signs, so early and rapid fluid resuscitation should be administered even in the pregnant patient who is normotensive.

In cases of trauma where there is isolated extremity injury, imaging with plain radiography can be safely performed with abdominal shielding. Diagnosis of musculoskeletal trauma should not be delayed because of pregnancy.

Finally, for pregnant patients in minor motor vehicle accidents (MVAs), clearance of major musculoskeletal injuries should be performed in the same manner as the nonpregnant patient. Following clearance, it is recommended that all patients beyond 23 weeks' gestation be evaluated in the delivery room for fetal and maternal assessment over the next 4 to 24 hours depending on the severity of the MVA because of the risk for placental abruption. Prior to 23 weeks, an ultrasound or Doppler auscultation of the fetal heart can be performed in the emergency room by consulting obstetric staff. If the MVA is minor, this evaluation should suffice, and the patient can be discharged to follow up with her obstetrician as an outpatient. For puncture wounds where tetanus may be a concern, vaccination with a tetanus booster is safe throughout pregnancy.

MEDICATIONS FOR USE IN MUSCULOSKELETAL INJURIES OR COMPLAINTS IN PREGNANCY

While the mainstay therapy for many musculoskeletal complaints are nonsteroidal antiinflammatory drugs (NSAIDs), in general, use of this class of drugs should be avoided in pregnancy because of the negative effect on the fetal kidneys leading to decreased fetal urine production and, therefore, decreased amniotic fluid. In addition, NSAIDs are thought to increase the risk for premature closure of the ductus arteriosus, especially if used for a prolonged period beyond 32 weeks' gestation. For those reasons, we recommend using acetaminophen for minor pain and narcotics for more severe pain. Narcotics, besides the risk for developing tolerance and thereby increasing the risk of neonatal withdrawal, are safe in pregnancy as they are not associated with any specific embryopathy or other fetal effects at normal doses for use in the short term. The use of oral steroids such as prednisone and methylprednisolone is safe in pregnancy as they do not cross the placenta in any appreciable amount. Similarly, pain control after orthopaedic surgery in pregnancy can be safely managed with epidural or intravenous patient-controlled analgesia with no significant effects on the fetus. Local anesthetic blocks for various procedures are also safe and effective in the pregnant patients.

PERIMORTEM CESAREAN DELIVERY

In very rare cases of severe trauma, it may be necessary to deliver the pregnant patient by emergency cesarean section in the emergency department. Usually these cases involve maternal cardiac arrest at a gestational age when the fetus is considered viable (24 weeks or greater). In general, the purpose of the surgery is to save the life of the unborn child when it seems clear that the mother will not survive.

While the decision for peripartum cesarean is never an easy one, it is crucial that the obstetrics team be closely involved. The following factors must be considered by the obstetrics, anesthesia, and trauma teams:

- Estimated gestational age by fundal height or expeditious ultrasound in the trauma room
- Management plan for potentially preterm infant
- Adequacy of other resuscitative efforts including chest compressions and displacement of the gravid uterus from the inferior vena cava
- Benefits of delivery in enhancing resuscitative efforts of the mother, especially in cases of severe prematurity (<28 weeks)

Small changes in maternal oxygenation can lead to dramatic changes in the fetus. Care must be taken to adequately oxygenate the pregnant woman especially in the case of a preterm infant.

In preparation for such a potential case, good communication between the first responders, emergency department (ED) staff, and obstetricians is crucial. Obstetricians and anesthesiologists should be called to the ED in anticipation of the arrival of such a patient.

If the decision is made that delivery will improve the ability to resuscitate the pregnant patient, or if saving the patient's life proves futile because of the extent of trauma, then the appropriate team should be available to perform a rapid cesarean delivery.

While there is scant data on outcomes of perimortem cesarean delivery, infant survival rates in such cases has been reported to be as high as 70%.[20] More recently, successful maternal resuscitations due to expedited delivery by cesarean have been reported.[21] The key to success in these cases is communication between all caretakers in a controlled trauma room. Fortunately, these cases are very rare.

KEY REFERENCES

The level of evidence (LOE) is determined according to the criteria provided in the preface.

10. Yamazaki JN, Schull WJ: Perinatal loss and neurologic abnormalities among children of the atomic bomb. Nagaski and Hiroshima revisited, 1949 to 1989. *JAMA* 264:622–623, 1990. LOE I
12. Chen MM, Coakley FV, Kaimal A, et al: Guidelines for computed tomography and magnetic resonance imaging use during pregnancy and lactation. *Obstet Gynecol* 112:333–340, 2008. LOE II
19. Lamont RF, Khan KS, Beattie B, et al: The quality of nifedipine studies to assess tocolytic efficacy: a systematic review. *J Perinat Med* 33:287–295, 2005. LOE I

The complete References list is available online at https://expertconsult.inkling.com.

14D Substance Abuse Syndromes: Recognition, Prevention, and Treatment

CAESAR A. ANDERSON • GEORGE A. PERDRIZET

"Whiskey claims to itself alone the exclusive office of sot-making."

—THOMAS JEFFERSON

INTRODUCTION

Substance-dependent patients are frequently hospitalized for acute care and require surgical interventions.[1,2] This section of the chapter will assist the surgeon in answering three questions:

1. Which of my patients are at risk for the development of an acute withdrawal syndrome while hospitalized?
2. How can I recognize these individuals early?
3. What can I do to prevent this medical complication from occurring?

Alcohol syndromes will be emphasized, as they are the most common and problematic substance abuse syndromes encountered in orthopaedic, trauma, and surgical patients,[3-8] because the individuals often come to acute care hospitals with injuries and illnesses that are a direct result of substance abuse. Alcohol is involved in 25% to 35% of nonfatal motor vehicle injuries and in 40% to 50% of traffic fatalities.[9] It is estimated that between 10% and 40% of such patients are alcohol dependent and therefore at risk of developing alcohol withdrawal syndrome (AWS) during their hospital stay.[10] Acutely intoxicated and injured patients have a 75% chance of having a diagnosis of chronic alcoholism.[11] The prevalent association of substance abuse and injury prompted the Eastern Association for the Surgery of Trauma (EAST) Committee on Injury Control and Violence Prevention to publish a position paper reviewing the role that alcohol and other drugs play in the care of the injured patient.[12] Approximately 8.2 million persons in the United States are dependent on alcohol and 3.5 million are dependent on illicit drugs, including stimulants (1 million) and opiates (750,000). Each year in the United States, there are approximately 85,000 deaths and $185 billion in costs related to alcohol abuse.[13] Owing to the high prevalence of substance abuse disorders, it is likely that the surgeon practicing in the acute care setting will encounter this challenging and frustrating medical condition.

A preexisting substance abuse disorder adds greatly to the risk for the development of complications following hospital admission for injury or illness.[14-16] The postoperative patient who develops an acute withdrawal syndrome will have a protracted and complicated hospital stay.[17-19] Alcohol withdrawal syndrome causes increased length of stay, morbidity, and mortality in hospitalized patients and can lead to life-threatening complications.[20] The development of delirium tremens (DTs) or acute psychoses can become life threatening.[21,22] Finally, substance abuse patients often harbor significant medical and psychiatric illnesses that must be recognized and addressed.[23,24] Chronic diseases in the form of end-organ dysfunctions secondary to the protracted nature of substance abuse are common. Cardiac, central nervous system, pulmonary, immunologic, and gastrointestinal organ dysfunction are common and further dispose these patients to a complicated postoperative and hospital course.[25,26] Many alcoholics have significant bone disease, which puts them at further risk for poor bone and wound healing.[27] Osteopenia and fractures, especially of the spine and ribs, are associated with osteoporosis. Ethanol is directly toxic to osteoblasts. Other factors contributing to bone pathology include hypogonadism, decreased calcium intake and malabsorption, increased urinary calcium excretion, decreased exercise, and altered parathyroid hormone response to hypocalcemia. Alcoholics are also at increased risk for osseous avascular necrosis.[28]

The most common substance abuse syndromes encountered in the surgical patient hospitalized for trauma are (1) alcohol intoxication, dependence, and withdrawal (40% to 50%); (2) opiate addiction and withdrawal (10%); (3) acute cocaine intoxication (5% to 10%); and (4) iatrogenic benzodiazepine withdrawal.[12,29,30]

DEFINITIONS

The term substance abuse refers to the use of alcohol or other drugs that places the individual at risk of injury, addiction, and dependence. Associated with these conditions are the related social and legal problems that often develop. To minimize confusion around disease definitions, the American Society of Addiction Medicine (ASAM) in 1990 selected and defined standard addiction terminology. A few key abuse syndrome definitions are summarized in Table 14D-1. As with most medical conditions, prevention of acute withdrawal syndromes is the primary goal of managing the hospitalized, substance-dependent patient. Prevention can happen only if the physician is attuned to the potential for the problem to occur. Risk stratification and a working knowledge of the early signs and symptoms of withdrawal are critical elements in effectively managing these cases.[31]

TABLE 14D-1 *ALCOHOL ABUSE SYNDROMES*

Syndrome	Definition
"At-risk use": drinks (no. female : no. male)*	For females, >3 drinks daily, >7 drinks weekly; for males, >4 drinks daily, >14 drinks weekly*
Abuse	Harmful use of a specific psychoactive substance
Addiction	Disease process characterized by the continued use of a specific psychoactive substance despite physical, psychological, or social harm
Tolerance	State in which an increased dose of a psychoactive substance is needed to produce a desired effect
Withdrawal	Onset of a predictable constellation of signs and symptoms following the abrupt discontinuation of, or rapid decrease in, dosage of a psychoactive substance
Delirium tremens	An acute organic brain syndrome due to alcohol withdrawal resulting in life-threatening delirium and autonomic hyperactivity
Wernicke encephalopathy	Abrupt onset of a confusional state, associated with thiamine deficiency, accompanied by unsteadiness of gait and visual disturbance
Korsakoff syndrome	Chronic memory impairment often associated with amnestic confabulation, with relative preservation of cognitive capacity

*1 Drink = 14 g ethanol = 12 oz beer = 5 oz wine = 1.5 oz spirits. Behavioral risk of developing alcohol abuse: >14 drinks/week (male), >7 drinks/week (female).

Source: *Data from American Society of Addiction Medicine, Mee-Lee M, editor: ASAM-PPC-2R: Patient placement criteria for the treatment of substance-related disorders, second edition-revised, Chevy Chase, MD, 2001, American Society of Addiction Medicine, Inc.*

BOX 14D-1 *CAGE Scoring System*

C Have you ever felt you ought to *c*ut down on your drinking?
A Have people *a*nnoyed you by criticizing your drinking?
G Have you ever felt *g*uilty about your drinking?
E Have you ever had a drink in the morning (*e*ye opener) to steady your nerves or get rid of a hangover?

Scoring: One point assigned for each "yes" response; a score of 2 is considered clinically significant for alcohol abuse risk.

RECOGNITION—ESTIMATING RISK

Who is at risk for the development of an acute withdrawal syndrome while hospitalized?

In general, any patient who has a measurable ethanol level (blood alcohol level [BAL]) and has suffered a traumatic injury is at moderate-to-high risk (40%) for harboring an alcohol abuse syndrome. A combination of a carefully elicited past medical history and a liberal policy of drug screening is recommended in all nonelective surgical patients. For nonalcohol substances, any patient with a known history of abuse or addiction or any patient with a positive urine toxicology screen is considered to be at significant risk for withdrawal or abstinence syndromes. Once recognition of a patient's substance abuse problem is made, this diagnosis should be clearly documented in the patient's medical record, and appropriate substance abuse counseling obtained.

Alcohol

The prevalence of alcohol abuse in the general population is estimated to be 5% and of alcohol dependence to be 4%.[13] Questionnaires, surveys, and scoring systems are available for grading a person's risk for AWS. The most commonly used screening tools are the AUDIT (*A*lcohol *U*se *D*isorder *I*dentification *T*est) and CAGE (*c*ut down, *a*nnoyed, *g*uilt, *e*ye-opener) questionnaires. These clinical tools are widely used in the setting of alcohol detoxification programs. The CAGE questionnaire has practical utility in the setting of acute injury and illness, as it can be administered in minutes (Box 14D-1). The literature is replete with examples of inadequate screening and recognition of alcohol abuse in acute care settings and has not changed over time.[32,33] A recent report found that alcohol-related problems were addressed by physicians in only 25% of patients admitted to a level I trauma center.[34] Table 14D-2 lists the aspects of a medical database required to accurately identify the "at risk" patient along with common screening tools, questionnaires, and their relevant scores. Surgeons typically fail to screen their patients for alcohol abuse.[35,36] Therefore, we have created the "Surgeon's Short Form," which can be used preoperatively to identify patients likely to be alcohol abusers (Table 14D-3). It has been reported that 90% of the patients at risk for alcohol abuse can be identified by establishing the

TABLE 14D-2 WHO IS AT RISK FOR ALCOHOL WITHDRAWAL SYNDROME?

Factor	Sign/Symptom
Past medical history	Abuse, withdrawal, seizures, delirium tremens, hospitalization, traumatic event with positive BAL
Social history	Previous or current family, work, or scholastic performance problems
Clinical scoring systems	CAGE ≥3 CIWA-Ar >10 Alcohol use score ≥20 Addiction severity index score ≥6
Blood alcohol level (BAL)	>150 mg/dL with clear sensorium or >300 mg/dL in any person

CAGE, Cut down, annoyed, guilt, eye-opener; *CIWA-Ar*, Clinical Institute Withdrawal Assessment for Alcohol revised scale.

presence of just two factors: (1) a positive past medical history for alcohol abuse syndromes and (2) the ingestion of alcohol within 24 hours of presentation. The presence of both these factors places the patient at moderate-to-high risk (40%–60%) for AWS during the period of abstinence imposed by hospitalization.[37]

Opiates

Opiates are naturally occurring or synthetic agents with morphine-like properties. They elicit their effect via central nervous system (CNS) receptors, causing analgesia, respiratory depression, hallucinations, sedation, miosis, bradycardia, dysphoria, and ultimately drug dependence. Patients abusing opiates have withdrawal symptoms and a high tolerance to opiate analgesics, making their postoperative management difficult. Opiate abuse accounted for 604,039 (30.8%) of the 1.96 million substance abuse treatment admissions reported to the Substance Abuse and Mental Health Services Administration (SAMHSA) Treatment Episode Data Set (TEDS) in 2010. Of these, 331,703 (16.9% of all admissions) were for a non-heroin opiate. Non-heroin opiates include methadone, codeine, hydromorphone (Dilaudid), morphine, meperidine (Demerol), opium, oxycodone, and any other drug with morphine-like effects.[22]

Tolerance, physiologic dependence, and psychological dependence on opioids usually occur after 3 weeks of daily usage.[38] The most commonly abused opiate remains heroin. Its use is only surpassed by marijuana, which was reported to be only approximately 5% higher in the most recent 2010 SAMHSA data set. The relative risk for abuse of opiates and other drugs is variable and poorly understood. The variables are attributable to genetic, environmental, or combined factors. It is important to note that outside of stereotypical notions, many patients, especially the injured, are at risk of drug and opiate abuse, adding to the difficulty in screening and subsequent management. Regardless of an individual patient's results of a urine toxicology screen, the clinician must remain alert for the possibility of opiate abuse. Multiple factors exist that prevent drug screening from being completely reliable in the preoperative patient, including dose ingested, time interval from last dosing, innate host metabolism, associated medical comorbidities, and the presence of polysubstance abuse. Several drug screening scales exist; however, most are complex and too cumbersome for applicability on a busy orthopaedic service. The most reliable indicator for assessing opiate abuse risk, aside from a thorough history and physical examination, is the presence of certain key signs and symptoms. Aside from signs and symptoms, the presence of infectious diseases (human immunodeficiency virus [HIV], hepatitis B and C, sexually transmitted diseases, and tuberculosis) should also raise the suspicion of possible opiate abuse.[31]

TABLE 14D-3 PREOPERATIVE INTERVIEW—SURGEON'S SHORT FORM

Questions to Ask	Risk of Alcohol Dependence*
1. Have you ever had† a drinking problem?	Yes = 70%, no = unclear implications
2. Have you had any alcohol in the past 24 hours or a positive blood alcohol level?‡	Yes plus no.1 = 90%

*Male gender and age >30 years further increases risk.
†Past tense is used, as patient is more likely to be truthful.
‡Any level of ethanol indicates the patient has recently consumed ethanol.

Cocaine

Cocaine, a derivative of the *Erythroxylum coca* plant, is often used in combination with heroin. It is well absorbed from snorting, smoking, or injection. Fatalities from seizures, respiratory paralysis, and cardiac arrhythmias can occur.[39] The lipid solubility of cocaine is quite high. Brain concentrations can be elevated up to 10 times that of plasma, making it extremely addictive. The National Survey on Drug Use and Health (2003) found 35 million Americans older than 12 years have reported using cocaine at least once, with 8 million of these reported to have used cocaine in crack form. In 2011, there were 670,000 persons aged 12 or older who had used cocaine for the first time within the past 12 months; this averages to approximately 1800 initiates per day. The annual number of cocaine initiates declined from 1.0 million in 2002 to 670,000 in 2011. The number of initiates of crack cocaine declined during this period from 337,000 to 76,000.

Cocaine-related emergency department (ED) visits increased by 78% from 1990 to 1994 and by 33% as of 2002. Cocaine abuse was reported to be second only to alcohol abuse. It was the most frequently reported substance associated with drug abuse death by 2003 medical examiners and coroners.

Recognizing patients at risk for the development of cocaine withdrawal is an important consideration in the management of the hospitalized patient. Like opiate screening, there are no clear indicators for accurately assessing risk of withdrawal. Cocaine stimulates dopaminergic release, increased sympathetic tone, blockade of serotonin reuptake, and local anesthesia as a result of neuronal sodium current inhibition.[40] Intense vasospasms leading to myocardial ischemia in patients with well-perfused coronary arteries have been reported.[41] Profound CNS effects also can occur, leading to ischemic or hemorrhagic stroke, confusion, violent behavior, and seizures. The seizures associated with cocaine abuse are typically self-limited and may occur on the very first exposure, because cocaine lowers the seizure threshold. Cocaine can also induce hyperpyrexia, hyperkinesis, and rhabdomyolysis. Cocaine abuse typically induces a psychological rather than physical dependence. Abusers typically have depleted dopamine stores in the pleasure centers of the brain. Hence, continued cocaine ingestion is required in order to enjoy basic functions (sexual drive, hunger, thirst).

Benzodiazepines

The use of benzodiazepines is as commonplace as the use of a scalpel in most orthopaedic practices. SAMHSA data suggest that from 1992 to 2002, drug-related ED visits involving benzodiazepine-like agents increased by 41%. For drug-related ED visits occurring in 2009, SAMHSA data reports the likelihood of polydrug, also referred to as multiple drug, involvement varied depending on the type of drug involved. The majority of visits associated with use of cocaine or marijuana involved polydrug use (68% and 73%, respectively), whereas slightly more than half of heroin-related visits involved polydrug use (52%). The majority of visits associated with the types of pharmaceuticals included in this data involved polydrug use (narcotic pain relievers: 63%, benzodiazepines: 79%). Withdrawal from benzodiazepine agents is a serious complication that often goes unrecognized. Benzodiazepine withdrawal has no associated signs and symptoms that can be considered pathognomonic. As with other substance abuse syndromes, great variability exists in its presentation. Patients at risk of developing clinically relevant withdrawal symptoms from benzodiazepines typically have been administered daily therapeutic dosages for more than 4 months or doses of more than twice the recommended level for more than 2 months. Patients who require a period of intensive care during their hospitalization, especially those who have required prolonged mechanical ventilation and continuous intravenous sedation, are at particular risk for postoperative withdrawal.

RECOGNITION—EARLY IDENTIFICATION OF SIGNS AND SYMPTOMS

How do I recognize the onset and development of withdrawal syndromes in my preoperative or postoperative patient?

The physician must remain alert for the development of early signs of withdrawal. Early intervention has the greatest chance for success. Because of the nonspecific nature of the signs and symptoms associated with withdrawal syndromes (i.e., agitation, tachycardia, tremor, and delirium), the development of withdrawal can easily go unrecognized.

Alcohol

Symptoms of AWS range from mild anxiety and tremors to seizures, delirium, and death. Early signs of AWS most often involve tremulousness and seizures, the former starting approximately 6 to 8 hours after a significant drop in serum ethanol level. The clinical picture is colored by excessive sympathetic or adrenergic stimulation resulting in tachycardia, diaphoresis, and severe hypertension (Fig. 14D-1). Associated signs include tremors, irritability, and hyperreflexia. Tremulous patients usually have a clear sensorium. Nausea, anxiety, or insomnia may be dominant complaints but are relatively nonspecific findings in the hospitalized, injured, or postoperative patient. Once a patient begins to demonstrate signs and symptoms of withdrawal, the clinical course should be documented using the Clinical Institute Withdrawal Assessment

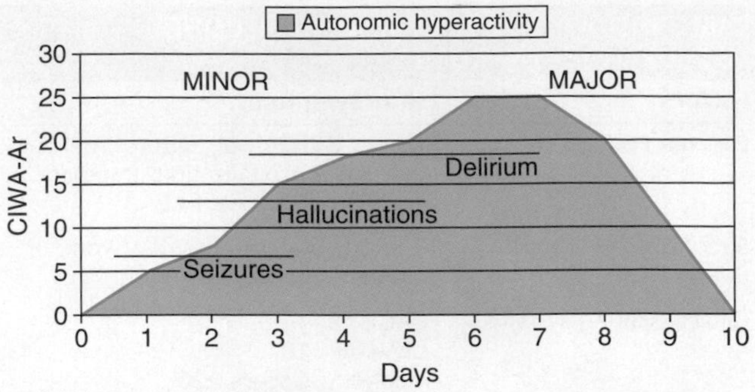

Figure 14D-1. Time course for alcohol withdrawal syndrome (AWS). Initial signs include tachycardia and tremor secondary to the autonomic hyperactivity. Seizure activity can occur very early in the time course of development of AWS, even while the Clinical Institute Withdrawal Assessment for Alcohol revised scale (CIWA-Ar scale) score is relatively low, e.g., 5 to 10. A CIWA-Ar score of ≥15 to 20 signifies major AWS and requires intensive care unit (ICU) monitoring. Most AWS will be mild and peak at 2 to 4 days. Detoxification occurs by 5 to 10 days with a 10% acute relapse rate. *(Redrawn from Lohr RH: Treatment of alcohol withdrawal in hospitalized patients, Mayo Clin Proc 70:777–782, 1995.)*

for Alcohol revised scale (CIWA-Ar scale; Fig. 14D-2).[42] This tool is widely available in most general hospitals and should be performed every 8 hours until signs and symptoms of AWS have resolved. This tool is also used to measure response to therapy (see later). AWS is generally (80%) mild, typically peaking at 24 to 36 hours and resolving by 72 hours, but it can last from days to longer than a week.[43] Without treatment, symptoms may last as long as 10 to 14 days.[44] However, 25% of patients may have an escalation in symptoms and severe manifestations including hallucinations, acute confusion, and DTs. Currently, there is no method to predict which patients with mild AWS will progress to severe disease and DTs.

Neuropsychological symptoms include anxiety, agitation, hyperalertness, insomnia, craving for rest, self-preoccupation, inattention, and mild disorientation to time, without gross confusion. The absence of significant disorientation, confusion, and autonomic instability differentiates mild AWS from the more serious DTs. Seizures occur in 10% of alcoholics and are often the precipitating event that leads to injury. Alcohol-related seizures can be the *initial* sign of AWS (see Fig. 14D-1).[2] Seizing-alcoholic patients are prone to falls and to hip, spinal, and rib fractures. Alcoholic seizures are precipitated mainly by hypoglycemia, hypomagnesemia, and respiratory alkalosis. They are usually generalized, tonic-clonic seizures. One-third of patients who have convulsions develop DTs if not treated. Non–alcohol-related causes of seizure disorder must be investigated (metabolic, posttraumatic, and idiopathic) and ruled out before the cause is attributed to AWS. Most alcohol-associated seizures occur 6 to 48 hours following drinking cessation and are typically limited to a single event (40%). These patients can demonstrate a confusing picture, since often there is no longer any measurable alcohol in their bloodstream. Once again, a high index of suspicion is required on the part of the treating clinicians.

Delirium is a common and nonspecific acute state of confusion that complicates postoperative recovery. Delirium often goes unrecognized or misdiagnosed in the surgical patient.[45] The incidence of delirium in postoperative patients is 37%. Common precipitating factors include infection, hypoxia,

	TACTILE DISTURBANCES: Ask: "Have you any itching, pins and needles sensations, any burning, any numbness, or do you feel bugs crawling on or under your skin?" Observation. 0 None 1 Very mild itching, pins and needles, burning or numbness 2 Mild itching, pins and needles, burning or numbness 3 Moderate pins and needles, burning or numbness 4 Moderately severe hallucinations 5 Severe hallucinations 6 Extremely severe hallucinations 7 Continuous hallucinations
TREMOR: Arms extended and fingers spread apart. Observation. 0 No tremor 1 Not visible, but can be felt fingertip to fingertip 2 3 4 Moderate, with patient's arms extended 5 6 7 Severe, even with arms not extended	**AUDITORY DISTURBANCES:** Ask: "Are you more aware of sounds around you? Are they harsh? Do they frighten you? Are you hearing anything that is disturbing you? Are you hearing things you know are not there?" Observation. 0 Not present 1 Very mild harshness or ability to frighten 2 Mild harshness or ability to frighten 3 Moderate harshness or ability to frighten 4 Moderately severe hallucinations 5 Severe hallucinations 6 Extremely severe hallucinations 7 Continuous hallucinations
PAROXYSMAL SWEATS 0 No sweat visible 1 Barely perceptible sweating, palms moist 2 3 4 Beads of sweat obvious on forehead 5 6 7 Drenching sweats	**VISUAL DISTURBANCES:** Ask: "Does the light appear to be too bright? Is its color different? Does it hurt your eyes? Are you seeing anything that is disturbing to you? Are you seeing things you know are not there?" Observation. 0 Not present 1 Very mild sensitivity 2 Mild sensitivity 3 Moderate sensitivity 4 Moderately severe hallucinations 5 Severe hallucinations 6 Extremely severe hallucinations 7 Continuous hallucinations
ANXIETY: Ask: "Do you feel nervous?" Observation. 0 No anxiety, at ease 1 Mildly anxious 2 3 4 Moderately anxious, or guarded, so anxiety is inferred 5 6 7 Equivalent to acute panic as seen in severe delirium or acute schizophrenic reactions	**HEADACHE, FULLNESS IN HEAD:** Ask: "Does your head feel different? Does it feel like there is a band around your head?" Do not rate for dizziness or lightheadedness. Otherwise, rate severity. 0 Not present 1 Very mild 2 Mild 3 Moderate 4 Moderately severe 5 Severe 6 Very severe 7 Extremely severe
AGITATION: Observation. 0 Normal activity 1 Somewhat more than normal activity 2 3 4 Moderately fidgety and restless 5 6 7 Paces back and forth during most of interview, or constantly thrashes about	**ORIENTATION AND CLOUDING OF SENSORIUM:** Ask: "What day is this? Where are you? Who am I?" 0 Oriented and can do serial additions 1 Cannot do serial additions or is uncertain about date 2 Disoriented for date by no more than 2 calendar days 3 Disoriented for date by more than 2 calendar days 4 Disoriented for place and/or person

Figure 14D-2. The Clinical Institute Withdrawal Assessment for Alcohol is a clinical tool that has been recently revised—CIWA-Ar—and validated in the setting of alcohol detoxification units. This tool is widely available in general medical hospitals and is administered and recorded as part of the patient's "vital signs" by the nursing staff. The scale ranges from 0 to 50, with 15 to 20 representing the transition from mild to severe withdrawal symptomatology. The therapeutic goal is set at a score of ≤10. Any patient with a score >10 or with a score that is increasing with time should have AWS prophylaxis started.

myocardial ischemia, metabolic derangement, and anticholinergic medications. Delirium is associated with increased rates of postoperative complications, delayed functional recovery, and increased length of hospital stay. Patients developing delirium during their hospital stay experience a twofold increase in mortality rate. The development of DTs is the most feared complication of AWS and is seen in less than 5% of patients experiencing AWS. DTs are marked by autonomic hyperactivity (hypertension, tachycardia, fever, tremors, diaphoresis, and dilated pupils) and disorientation. This clinical picture can be easily confused with the presentation of a postoperative infectious complication (wound, urinary tract infection, or pneumonia). Patients can become severely agitated, uncooperative, and aggressive, thus representing a potential for harm to self and others. At this extreme stage of the disease, it is often necessary to heavily sedate and control patients with neuromuscular blockade in order to establish a safe therapeutic environment. Onset of DTs occurs 3 to 5 days following abstinence but can range from 1 to 14 days. The majority of patients (83%) recover within 3 days. Relapses occur in 10% of patients and can prolong the duration of the syndrome for up to 1 month. Mortality rates range from 5% to 15% in treated patients; however, fever and seizures are associated with the poorest outcomes. The most common causes of death are cardiac arrhythmia, pneumonia, and alcohol-related end-organ dysfunction (cardiomyopathy, pancreatitis, gastrointestinal hemorrhage, infection, and liver disease). The goal of clinical management is early recognition of AWS, prompt intervention, and prevention of DTs.

The surgeon should be alert to the need for AWS prophylaxis in any patient who is considered at risk for alcohol withdrawal and develops a mild tremor.

Opiates

Although opiate withdrawal is generally considered unlikely to cause significant morbidity or mortality, the increased level of autonomic activity often associated with this withdrawal can be life threatening in the postoperative setting. The increased demand on cardiac output and myocardial contractility can exhaust a patient's cardiac reserve and thus the ability to adequately compensate during surgery. Abrupt cessation or reduction in dosage can lead to withdrawal symptoms. These symptoms typically occur after several months of daily use. Acute opiate withdrawal typically occurs in stages. Stage one usually begins at 3 to 4 hours following abstinence and is characterized by drug craving, anxiety, and fear of withdrawal. Stage two is seen approximately 8 to 14 hours following abstinence with increased restlessness, insomnia, yawning, rhinorrhea, lacrimation, diaphoresis, mydriasis, and stomach cramps. The two final stages can occur 1 to 3 days following abstinence and are characterized by tremor, muscle spasms, vomiting, diarrhea, hypertension, tachycardia, fever, chills, piloerection, and very rarely, seizures. The early signs and symptoms of opioid withdrawal syndrome (yawning, sweating, lacrimation, rhinorrhea, anxiety, hypertension, piloerection, insomnia, and tachycardia) are generally classified as elements of autonomic hyperactivity.[31] As opiate withdrawal severity worsens, patients may then exhibit increasing restlessness, seizures, myalgias, vomiting, diarrhea, dehydration, and abdominal pain. Intense drug craving also accompanies withdrawal. Although withdrawal is not considered life threatening, it certainly will complicate the clinical course of the postoperative patient.

The pharmacologic mechanism behind opiate withdrawal relates to decreased CNS concentrations in the opiate-tolerant individual. Receptors identified in the locus ceruleus of the limbic system are influenced by exogenous opiates, decreasing noradrenergic firing. Withdrawal results from increased sympathetic discharge and noradrenergic hyperactivity. Heroin withdrawal occurs 4 to 8 hours after the last dose with symptoms peaking 36 to 72 hours later. It may take up to 10 days for symptoms to finally subside. It is important to recognize the pharmacologic specificity of the opiate-receptors (μ, κ) to fully appreciate the rationale and efficacy of methadone treatment and its relationship to the non–μ-receptor opiate agonists in the management of acute pain. This point is addressed under the treatment of opioid withdrawal.

Cocaine

Early clinical signs and symptoms preceding cocaine withdrawal can begin as abruptly as 9 hours following last ingestion. Patients are often described as being in "crash" mode. Their symptoms include agitation, anorexia, sadness, and intense drug craving. They can then progress to early withdrawal, exhibiting drug craving and a normal mood devoid of anxiety. Once again, a thorough past medical and social history is vital to the successful management of this condition. Cocaine withdrawal symptoms are a result of depleted dopaminergic neurotransmitters, causing fatigue, hypersomnolence, hunger, anxiety, paranoid behavior, resting tachycardia, and depression.[46] There are early and late components to cocaine withdrawal. Early symptoms are typically characterized by a normal mood, low anxiety, and no evidence of drug craving. Late withdrawal, which can occur from 1 to 10 weeks following last ingestion, will present with fatigue, marked anxiety, and high drug craving. Heightened clinical suspicion remains central to early identification and treatment.

Benzodiazepines

Abrupt cessation of benzodiazepines should be avoided during hospitalization. Weaning protocols are widely employed and limit the rate at which the daily dose can be decreased. The weaning protocol employed in our institution is as follows: benzodiazepine infusion is decreased by increments of 0.1 mg/h to a minimum of 0.1 mg/h while the patient's sedation score is assessed. Tapering does not exceed more than 0.1 mg/h in 8 to 12 hours.

MANAGEMENT—PROPHYLAXIS/TREATMENT

The aim of therapeutic intervention in the moderate-to-high risk patient is to manage the severity of the AWS and permit detoxification to occur (7 to 10 days). Early interventions are designed to prevent the escalation of symptoms from mild and manageable to the more severe, life-threatening manifestations. Timing is critical. The time at which abstinence is initiated should be noted and patients monitored for the appearance of early signs and symptoms of AWS. Generally speaking, several hours of abstinence are required before signs and symptoms of withdrawal appear (see Fig. 14D-1). A unique caveat related to the surgical patient is the observation that general anesthetics can delay the onset of withdrawal syndromes. Thus, a patient who undergoes

BOX 14D-2 *Child-Pugh Classification of Operative Mortality Associated with Alcoholic Liver Disease*

Variable	A	B	C
Encephalopathy	None	Slight to moderate	Moderate to severe
Ascites	None	Slight	Moderate to large
Bilirubin (mg/dL)	<2	2–3	>3
Albumin (g/dL)	>3.5	3.0–3.5	<3.0
Prothrombin index	>70%	40–70%	<40%
Operative mortality (%)	2	10	50

exploratory laparotomy on admission, followed 2 days later by operative reduction and fixation of a long bone fracture and then 2 days after that by a plastic surgical procedure, may develop AWS 7 to 10 days following initiation of abstinence.

The usual approach to AWS prevention is to provide the relevant pharmacologic agent in low-dose form *prior* to the onset of signs or symptoms of withdrawal. Titration of pharmacologic therapy is based on the patient's clinical signs and symptoms. To date there continues to be a paucity of high-quality clinical trials by which to define standard of care for the subset of patients having acute surgical needs and are deemed at moderate-to-high risk for AWS. Most published studies on pharmacologic therapy address patients whose primary medical problem is alcohol addiction.[47] The patients and settings in which care is rendered are very different from the target population that is the subject of this chapter. Often the acutely injured, critically ill, or postoperative patients are purposefully excluded from these studies. Thus, a debate continues as to the most effective and safe pharmacologic agent for the prevention and/or treatment of AWS in the surgical patient. What is clear is that early recognition and timely intervention are likely more important clinical variables than is the particular pharmaceutical agent administered and that surgical disciplines consistently underrecognize the "at-risk population" under their care. Several recent meta-analyses continue to support the use of benzodiazepines as the drug of choice for both the prevention and treatment of AWS.[48,49] A small randomized controlled trial demonstrated no difference between the efficacy of benzodiazepine versus alcohol replacement in the management of trauma patients at risk for AWS admitted to a university-based level I trauma center.[50]

To standardize the objective documentation of the patient's clinical course during treatment two standardized scoring systems are widely used. The CIWA-Ar score is a measure of the patient's withdrawal symptomatology. A CIWA-Ar score ≤10, on a scale of 0 to 50, is the therapeutic goal.[42] The Observer's Assessment of Alertness/Sedation (OAA/S) score is a measure of the patient's alertness and is used to prevent overly sedating patients in an effort to control symptoms. An OAA/S score of ≥15, on a scale of 0 to 20, is the therapeutic goal.[51]

General Medical Considerations

Prior to the administration of any pharmacologic agent for the prevention or treatment of AWS, the general medical condition of the patient should be thoroughly reviewed. Type and degree of end-organ damage should be determined (Child-Pugh classification; Box 14D-2). Metabolic and electrolyte imbalances should be identified and corrected. All patients should also receive a standardized medical protocol for the metabolic management of the alcohol-dependent diagnosis that includes vitamin supplementation (folate, thiamine, vitamin B_{12}), magnesium (Mg) sulfate for magnesium deficiency (Mg <1.5 mg/dL), sodium or potassium phosphate for phosphate deficiency (phosphate <2.7 mg/dL), haloperidol for anxiety/agitation, and nicotine replacement therapy for active tobacco users. Associated psychiatric diagnoses and treatments must also be addressed. Determination and documentation of the CIWA-Ar score should be performed every 2 to 4 hours during the initial period of hospital admission. Pharmacotherapy should include the following:

1. Folate 1 mg intravenously (IV) three times daily, then 1 mg IV or orally (PO) daily thereafter
2. Thiamine 100 mg IV three times daily, then 100 mg IV or PO daily thereafter
3. Multivitamin infusion, 1 ampule IV three times daily, then 1 ampule IV or tablet PO daily thereafter
4. Nicotine replacement therapy (NicoDerm, 21 mg/patch daily)
5. Haloperidol for management of hallucinations, 2 mg IV every 4 days
6. Psychiatric consultation for evaluation and treatment as well as alcohol addiction treatment and rehabilitation

Alcohol

Benzodiazepine Administration

The benzodiazepine class of sedatives is considered the drug of choice for the treatment and prevention of AWS. Initial therapy can be administered orally or by continuous intravenous drip. A recent study in the head and neck surgical patient population found benzodiazepine prophylaxis resulted in a 13.5% and 9.4% incidence of withdrawal and DTs, respectively.[18]

Benzodiazepine Protocol

Briefly, lorazepam (Ativan, 10 mg/100 mL 5% dextrose in water [D_5W]) can be administered intravenously according to the following guidelines based on the CIWA-Ar scoring system. Trained nurses can carry out an evaluation in less than 2 minutes, and the inter-rater reliability is high ($r > 0.8$). The titration of the lorazepam drip is based on clinical symptomatology as graded by both the CIWA-Ar score and the OAA/S score (Box 14D-3; see Fig. 14D-2).

1. Loading dose: lorazepam 2 mg IV and repeat in 30 minutes if no change or an increase in CIWA-Ar scale and begin a continuous intravenous infusion, ≈0.3 mg/h. Breakthrough coverage is provided with 2 mg IV and

patients may require a higher BAL for control of their AWS. Patients requiring BALs greater than 40 mg% should have their infusions reduced once they have responded clinically (i.e., CIWA-Ar score ≤10, or decreased by 5) for 24 hours to achieve a BAL <20 mg% while maintaining the CIWA-Ar ≤10. The purpose of a daily BAL is to ensure the alcohol level remains at a low and stable level. The initiation dose of ethyl alcohol used in this algorithm, 1 mL/kg/min (0.1 g/kg/h), is just below the level at which the metabolic capacity of the average person becomes saturated. Ethanol is metabolized via a liver enzyme system (following Michaelis–Menten enzyme kinetics, with significant variation depending on the patient's recent alcohol ingestion history); thus, a large increase in the BAL may result from a relatively small increase in the infusion rate, especially at rates >1 mL/kg/h (i.e., 0.1 g/kg/h).[64,65] The goal of performing a daily BAL measurement is to prevent a rising BAL during "maintenance" infusion. Individual patient responses may vary and thus require constant clinical and laboratory monitoring throughout the duration of ethanol administration. *No patient should receive a dose in excess of 70 mL/h of 20% ethanol.* If a patient has a detectable BAL and has continued agitation, a prompt reevaluation for other causes of mental status changes must be performed.

Opiates

Opiate withdrawal syndrome is preventable. Management of opiate withdrawal depends on modifying withdrawal symptoms. Temporary substitution with a long-acting opiate reduces symptom severity. The use of short-acting opiates is appropriate for intensive care unit (ICU) and postoperative patients, where frequent monitoring and dosing assessment can be readily accomplished.[40] Long-acting opiates, such as methadone, are currently restricted under U.S. federal regulations for the treatment of opiate addiction. They can be used for maintenance therapy or detoxification when an addicted patient is admitted to the hospital for illness other than opiate abuse. It is important to note, however, that patients with non–abuse-related physical pain, who have been treated with methadone for withdrawal prevention, must have their pain needs met by a different opiate rather than by increasing their maintenance methadone dose. Patients treated with opiates for more than 1 to 2 weeks should be instructed to gradually taper their dose, by 25% every day or two, to prevent signs and symptoms of withdrawal. If needed, clonidine (0.1 to 0.2 mg, q4–6h) can be used to attenuate the autonomic hyperactivity symptoms. Clonidine has been used successfully in suppressing the signs and symptoms of withdrawal within 24 hours, thus shortening the duration of symptoms by 5 to 6 days. Clonidine, an α_2-adrenergic receptor agonist, acts by decreasing catecholamine-associated sympathetic activity and works in synergy with low doses of appropriate opiates. Common side effects of clonidine include dryness of the mouth, orthostatic hypotension, sedation, and constipation. An alternative agent for the management of the opiate-addicted individual is buprenorphine. Buprenorphine is considered a partial agonist; unlike methadone, it acts as a pure agonist. It causes fewer withdrawal symptoms and has a reduced risk for respiratory depression with an overdose. Its long half-life allows for daily dosing as well. Some detoxification protocols use buprenorphine on longer regimens ranging up to treatment every 7 weeks.[66] Reported efficacy of buprenorphine is similar to that of methadone and clonidine. Buprenorphine, with high μ-receptor affinity, has been used widely in critically ill patients with favorable results. Buprenorphine causes very little sedation, respiratory depression, or hypotension even at supratherapeutic levels. It is important to note that ongoing substance-abuse counseling, efforts to reduce needle sharing and transmission of viral disease, along with pharmacologic management contribute to patient therapeutic success.[67]

Outpatient use typically involves administration of methadone daily for a maximum of 3 days while the patient awaits acceptance into a licensed methadone treatment clinic. Methadone has also been used successfully for more than three decades and is currently the staple of outpatient management. Nalbuphine (Nubain), pentazocine and naloxone (Talwin), and butorphanol (Stadol) are three agents to be avoided by patients on methadone owing to their ability to elicit immediate withdrawal syndromes.

Cocaine

Currently, the clinical efficacy of an agent to prevent cocaine withdrawal has not been identified. The agents that have been most studied in abating cocaine withdrawal are amantadine, bromocriptine, and naltrexone. Agents such as lithium, tricyclic antidepressants, and trazodone have been used in an attempt to manage the later phases of cocaine withdrawal. Current treatment regimens are usually directed at treatment of cocaine intoxication. Benzodiazepines have played a predominant role in preventing hyperthermia, acidosis, seizures, and cardiovascular excitation of acute cocaine intoxication.[68]

Benzodiazepines

The patient who has received continuous infusion of benzodiazepines during the hospital stay should have the dose gradually tapered. Should a patient develop benzodiazepine withdrawal during hospitalization, institution of immediate therapy and subsequent weaning is recommended according to the protocol outlined earlier for alcohol withdrawal. Once the patient's condition has stabilized, the infusion is decreased by 0.1 mg/h increments to a minimum of 0.1 mg/h while the patient's sedation score is assessed. The rate of reduction should not exceed 0.1 mg/h in 8 to 12 hours.[31]

DISCHARGE PLANS

Following recovery from AWS, the patient is now considered detoxified and should be referred to a substance abuse program for follow-up care.[21] Established programs employ a combination of behavioral and pharmacologic therapies.[53]

SUMMARY

Injured and ill patients who come to a general medical hospital frequently carry a secondary substance abuse diagnosis. The physician must remain alert and determine the risk each of these patients has for the development of a medical complication related to substance abuse. Methods to identify patients at moderate-to-high risk for development of AWS have been presented and reviewed. Risk stratification is the first step. Early recognition of signs and symptoms of acute withdrawal is important. Early signs and symptoms have been reviewed with an emphasis on their time frame of development. Finally, preventive and treatment algorithms have been presented as guidelines that can be applied to the inpatient orthopaedic and preoperative and postoperative surgical patient. The need to add substance abuse to the patient's medical record along with appropriate referral to a substance abuse program cannot be overstated in the management of these challenging patient problems.

KEY REFERENCES

The level of evidence (LOE) is determined according to the criteria provided in the preface.

5. Chang PH, Steinberg MB: Alcohol withdrawal. *Med Clin North Am* 85:1191–1212, 2001. LOE II
9. The Physician's Guide to Helping Patients with Alcohol Problems: *NIH publication No. 95-3769*, Bethesda, MD, 1995, National Institute on Alcohol Abuse and Alcoholism. <http://www.niaaa.nih.gov/publications/clinical-guides-and-manuals>.

The complete References list is available online at https://expertconsult.inkling.com.

Chapter 15

Evaluation and Treatment of Vascular Injuries

DAVID V. FELICIANO • TODD E. RASMUSSEN

Recognition of a possible vascular injury is a critical skill for any orthopaedic surgeon. This is true whether the surgeon's primary area of practice is the emergency or urgent procedures associated with orthopaedic trauma or elective reconstruction. When injured patients have fractures of long bones, the pelvis, or spine; dislocations adjacent to major vessels; or severely contused or crushed extremities, loss of limb or life can occur if recognition of the associated vascular trauma is delayed.[1] In an elective practice, many orthopaedic operative procedures occur in proximity to major vessels, where an iatrogenic injury may result in loss of limb or life.[2,3]

Major changes in diagnosis and management of vascular injuries over the past 5 years have been in imaging, increased use of temporary intraluminal vascular shunts, endovascular therapies,[4] and lessons learned during Operation Iraqi Freedom and Operation Enduring Freedom (Afghanistan).

HISTORY

Although vascular repairs in the extremities were first performed nearly 250 years ago, progress in this area was limited until the early part of the 20th century. From 1904 to 1906, Alexis Carrel (1873–1944) and Charles C. Guthrie (1880–1963) at the University of Chicago and others developed standard vascular operative techniques, including repair of the lateral arterial wall, end-to-end anastomosis, and insertion of venous interposition grafts.[5-8] Early attempts at operative repair included those by V. Soubbotitch in the Balkan Wars from 1911 to 1913, by the British surgeon George H. Makins and German surgeons in World War I, and by R. Weglowski during the Polish-Russian War of 1920.[9-11] Despite the availability of these techniques, it was not until the latter part of World War II that renewed attempts were made to perform peripheral arterial repair rather than ligation.[12] Before that time, delays in medical care for casualties, lack of antibiotics, and a significant incidence of late infection in injured soft tissues of the extremities contributed to an operative approach dominated by ligation.

With the more rapid transfer of casualties to field hospitals, the availability of type-specific blood transfusion, the introduction of antibiotics, and the increased use of the autogenous saphenous vein as a vascular conduit, vascular repairs were performed frequently in the later stages of the Korean War and routinely throughout the Vietnam War.[13,14] More recently, civilian trauma surgeons have treated large numbers of patients with peripheral vascular injuries, many associated with orthopaedic trauma, and they have been able to build on the techniques for repair of traumatic vascular injuries described originally by military surgeons.[15-17] During Operation Iraqi Freedom and Operation Enduring Freedom, multiple contributions to the field have come from military vascular surgeons (to be discussed).

ETIOLOGY

In urban trauma centers, peripheral vascular injuries are most commonly caused by low-velocity missile wounds from handguns. For example, gunshot wounds cause 55% to 75% of all vascular injuries in the lower extremities in such centers. In contrast, stab wounds account for most of the civilian peripheral vascular injuries in countries where firearms are more difficult to obtain.

Vascular injuries from blunt orthopaedic trauma, such as fractures, dislocations, contusions, crush injuries, and traction (Fig. 15-1), account for only 5% to 30% of injuries being treated (Table 15-1).[1,2,3,18-24] In particular, vascular injuries associated with long bone fractures in otherwise healthy young trauma patients are rare. The reported incidence of injuries to the superficial femoral artery in association with a fracture of the femur has been less than 1% to 2% in large series.[25] Injuries to the popliteal artery, tibioperoneal trunk, or trifurcation vessels occur in only 1.5% to 2.8% of all tibial fractures. When open fractures of the tibia are reviewed separately, the incidence of arterial injuries is approximately 10%. With dislocations of the knee joint, the incidence of injuries to the popliteal artery requiring surgical repair was less than 16% in one large series.[23] These figures are significantly lower than those reported in the past for posterior dislocations of the knee and presumably reflect, in part, the current nonoperative approach to nonocclusive lesions (i.e., intimal defect, narrowing) of the popliteal artery.

As previously noted, there are also well-documented associations between certain elective and emergency orthopaedic operative procedures and arterial injuries (Table 15-2 and Fig. 15-2).[26-30]

Some of these may be noted during surgery or in the early postoperative period (e.g., occlusion of the iliac artery during total hip arthroplasty), but others may appear weeks or months later (e.g., ruptured pseudoaneurysm of a tibial artery).

LOCATIONS AND TYPES OF VASCULAR INJURIES

The brachial artery and vein in the upper extremity and the superficial femoral artery and vein in the lower extremity are

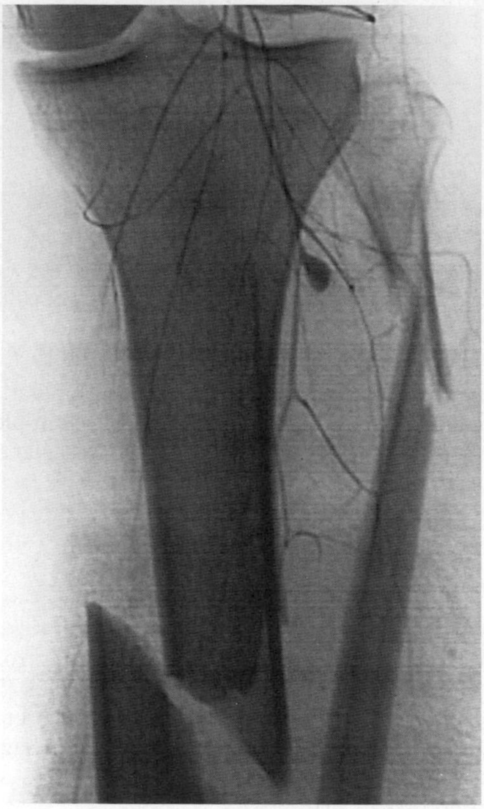

Figure 15-1. Pseudoaneurysm of left tibioperoneal trunk in patient with adjacent fracture in the fibula and midshaft fracture of the tibia.

the most commonly injured vessels in both civilian and military reports in which penetrating wounds predominate.[17] This can be explained by the length of these vessels in the extremities and by the fact that direct compression controls hemorrhage, so that few patients exsanguinate before arrival at the emergency center. Because of the low incidence of injuries to these vessels from blunt trauma, orthopaedic services most commonly encounter occlusions and occasional lacerations of the popliteal, tibioperoneal, tibial, or peroneal arteries from dislocations of the knee or severe fractures of the femur or tibia.

Intimal injuries (flaps, disruptions, or subintimal hematomas), spasm, complete wall defects with pseudoaneurysms or hemorrhage, complete transections, and arteriovenous fistulas are the five recognized types of vascular injuries. Whereas intimal defects and subintimal hematomas with possible secondary occlusion continue to be most commonly associated with blunt trauma, wall defects, complete transections, and arteriovenous fistulas are usually seen after penetrating wounds. Spasm can occur after either blunt or penetrating trauma to an extremity.

DIAGNOSIS[31-33]

History and Physical Examination

Patients sustaining peripheral arterial injuries usually have hard or soft signs of injury. Examples of hard signs of arterial injury are any of the classic signs of arterial occlusion (pulselessness, pallor, paresthesias, pain, paralysis, poikilothermy), massive bleeding, a rapidly expanding hematoma, and a palpable thrill or audible bruit over a hematoma. In patients with impending limb loss from arterial occlusion, a rapidly expanding hematoma or significant external bleeding from an extremity, immediate surgery without preliminary arteriography of the injured extremity is justified. If a hard sign is present, other than an expanding hematoma or external bleeding but localization of the defect is necessary before the incision is performed as in a patient with fractures at several levels, a rapid duplex ultrasound study or surgeon-performed arteriogram in the emergency center or operating room (OR) should be obtained.[34]

Soft signs of arterial injury include a history of arterial bleeding at the scene or in transit; proximity of a penetrating wound or blunt injury to an artery in the extremity; a small, nonpulsatile hematoma over an artery in an extremity; and a neurologic deficit originating in a nerve adjacent to a named artery. These patients still have an arterial pulse at the wrist or foot on physical examination or with use of the Doppler device. The incidence of arterial injuries in such patients

TABLE 15-1 *ARTERIAL INJURIES ASSOCIATED WITH FRACTURES AND DISLOCATIONS*

Fracture or Dislocation	Artery Injured
Upper Extremity	
Fracture of clavicle or first rib	Subclavian artery
Anterior dislocation of shoulder	Axillary artery
Fracture of neck of humerus	Axillary artery
Fracture of shaft or supracondylar area of humerus	Brachial artery
Dislocation of elbow	Brachial artery
Lower Extremity	
Fracture of shaft of femur	Superficial femoral artery
Fracture of supracondylar area of femur	Popliteal artery
Dislocation of the knee	Popliteal artery
Fracture of proximal tibia or fibula	Popliteal artery, tibioperoneal trunk, tibial artery, or peroneal artery
Fracture of distal tibia or fibula	Tibial or peroneal artery
Skull, Face, or Cervical Spine	
Basilar skull fracture involving sphenoid or petrous bone	Internal carotid artery
Le Fort II or III fracture	Internal carotid artery
Cervical spine, especially foramen transversarium	Vertebral artery
Thoracic Spine	Descending thoracic aorta
Lumbar Spine	Abdominal aorta
Pelvis	
Anterior-posterior compression	Thoracic aorta
Subtypes of pelvic fractures	Internal iliac, superior gluteal, or inferior gluteal artery
Acetabular fracture	External iliac, superior gluteal, or femoral artery

TABLE 15-2 *ACUTE OR DELAYED ARTERIAL INJURIES ASSOCIATED WITH ORTHOPAEDIC OPERATIVE PROCEDURES*

Orthopaedic Procedure	Artery Injured
Upper Extremity	
Clavicular compression plate or screw	Subclavian artery
Anterior approach to shoulder	Axillary artery
Closed reduction of humeral fracture	Brachial artery
Lower Extremity	
Total hip arthroplasty	Common or external iliac artery
Nail or nail-plate fixation of intertrochanteric or subtrochanteric hip fracture	Profunda femoris artery
Subtrochanteric osteotomy	Profunda femoris artery
Total knee arthroplasty	Popliteal artery
Anterior or posterior cruciate ligament reconstruction	Popliteal artery
External fixator pin	Superficial femoral, profunda femoris, popliteal, or tibial arteries
Spine	
Anterior spinal fusion	Abdominal aorta
Lumbar spine fixation device	Abdominal aorta
Resection of nucleus pulposus	Right common iliac artery and vein, inferior vena cava
Pelvis	
Posterior internal fixation of pelvic fracture	Superior gluteal artery
Excision of posterior iliac crest for bone graft	Superior gluteal artery

ranges from 3% to 25%, depending on which soft sign or combination of soft signs is present.[32,35,36] Most, but not all, of these arterial injuries can be managed without surgery because they are small and, by definition, allow for continuing distal perfusion. In some centers, serial physical examinations alone are used to monitor distal pulses, and no arteriogram is performed to document the magnitude of a possible arterial injury.[37] This approach has been safe and accurate in asymptomatic patients with penetrating wounds to an extremity in proximity to a major artery.[36,37] Its accuracy with the higher kinetic energy injuries associated with blunt fractures or dislocations, particularly dislocations of the knee, is similar.[23] Observation is appropriate only with complete and continuing out-of-hospital follow-up.[35,36,38] When there is concern about a distal pulse deficit, inability to properly examine for distal arterial pulses, or a combination of soft signs of an arterial injury in an extremity, either duplex ultrasonography or some type of arteriography is indicated.

Beyond the obvious hard or soft signs of vascular injury, physical examination of the injured extremity includes observation of the position in which the extremity is held, the presence of any obvious deformity of a long bone or joint, the presence or absence of an open wound or bony crepitus, the skin color of the distal extremity compared with that of the opposite side (in light-skinned persons), the time required for skin capillary refill in the distal digits, and a complete motor and sensory examination. In the lower extremity, the mobility of the knee joint should be carefully assessed as well. Increased laxity of the supporting ligaments suggests that a dislocation of the knee joint from the original trauma has spontaneously reduced (Fig. 15-3). Because of the previously noted association between posterior and other dislocations of the knee and injury to the popliteal artery, an imaging study is indicated if pedal pulses are diminished or absent after reduction.[23] Several studies suggest that routine arteriography is not indicated if normal pulses are present after spontaneous or orthopaedic reduction of a knee dislocation, although not all agree with this approach.[23,39] If the exact vascular status of the distal extremity is unclear after restoration of reasonable alignment or reduction of a dislocation, a Doppler flow detector should be applied to the area of absent pulses in the distal extremity for audible assessment of blood flow. The Doppler flow detector also can be used to compare systolic blood pressure measurements in an uninjured upper extremity with those in the injured upper or lower extremity. The arterial pressure index (API), defined as the Doppler systolic pressure in the injured extremity divided by that in the uninjured extremity, is then calculated.[40,41] In a study by Lynch and Johansen in which clinical outcome was the standard, an API lower than 0.90 had a sensitivity of 95%, specificity of 97.5%, and accuracy of 97% in predicting an arterial injury.[41] An alternative when both lower extremities are injured is to use the ankle-branchial index (ABI), which uses branchial artery pressure as the denominator. Because older patients have an increased incidence of preexisting atherosclerotic occlusive disease, the accuracy of the API or ABI is compromised.

Radiologic Studies

A noninvasive diagnosis can be made with use of duplex or color duplex ultrasonography in the emergency center, OR, or surgical intensive care unit (ICU) (Table 15-3). Duplex

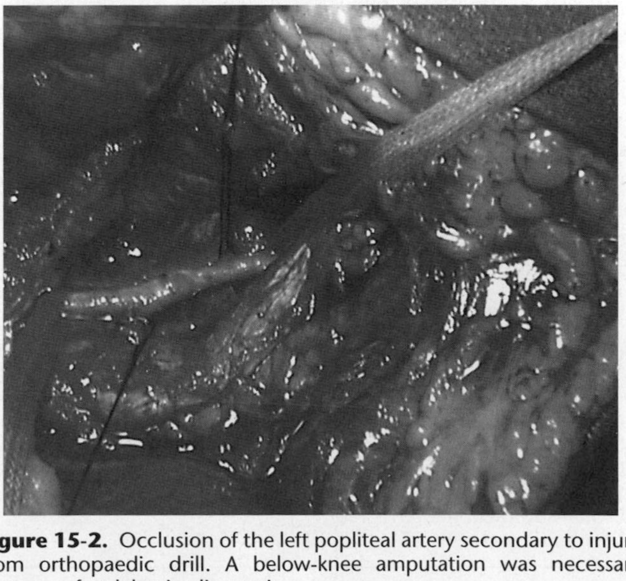

Figure 15-2. Occlusion of the left popliteal artery secondary to injury from orthopaedic drill. A below-knee amputation was necessary because of a delay in diagnosis.

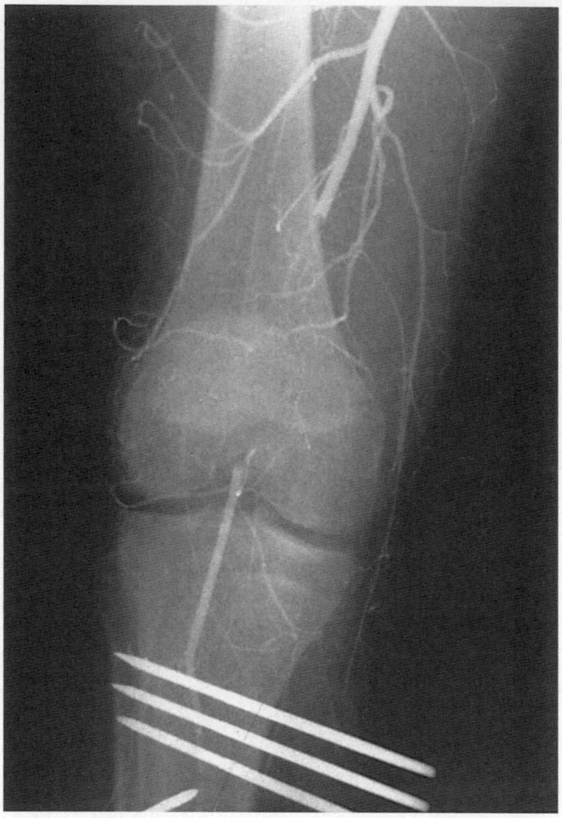

Figure 15-3. Occlusion of the right popliteal artery was missed for 48 hours because spontaneous reduction of a knee dislocation occurred before arrival in the emergency center.

ultrasonography is a combination of real-time B-mode ultrasound imaging and pulsed Doppler flow detection. Duplex or color duplex ultrasound imaging has been used to evaluate patients with possible or suspected arterial or venous injuries in the extremities for many years.[42-45] Accuracy in detection of arterial injuries, using comparison arteriography as the gold standard, has ranged from 96% to 100% in several studies.

Percutaneous arteriography performed in the emergency center or in the OR by the surgical team is infrequently used in most major trauma centers; several urban trauma centers, however, have extensive historical experience with the technique.[34,46,47] A thin-walled, 18-gauge Cournand-style disposable needle is inserted either proximal to the area of suspected injury (e.g., in the common femoral artery for evaluation of the superficial femoral artery) or distal to it (e.g., in retrograde evaluation of the axillary or subclavian arteries above a blood pressure cuff inflated to 300 mm Hg). Rapid hand injection of 35 mL of 60% diatrizoate meglumine dye is performed, and an anteroposterior radiographic view is taken. The timing for exposure of the x-ray film of the patient's extremity depends on which artery is to be evaluated. Proper evaluation of the tibial and peroneal arteries in the patient with a complex fracture of the tibia mandates that exposure not take place until 4 to 5 seconds after the injection of dye into the common femoral artery. The plane of the film is often changed before a second injection to examine the area in question more thoroughly. False-negative and false-positive results are rare when the technique is performed on a daily basis by experienced practitioners; however, this technique is rarely used in the modern era because of the availability of CT arteriography.[32] If a patient has severe combined intracranial or truncal trauma and possible peripheral arterial lesions related to orthopaedic injuries, life-threatening injuries should be treated first, followed by percutaneous *intraoperative* arteriography of the involved extremity.

Percutaneous intraarterial digital subtraction arteriography performed in a radiology suite by the interventional radiologist was the most commonly used invasive diagnostic technique in patients with suspected vascular injuries prior to the availability of computed tomography arteriography (CTA). Multiple sequential views of areas of suspected arterial injury can be obtained at differing intervals after injection of limited amounts of dye. The accuracy of this multiple-view technique has been demonstrated in many studies, although false-negative results have occurred. The disadvantages of the technique are the delays in diagnosis when on-call technicians must return to the hospital, the cost of modern equipment, and the distortion of images when metallic fragments are present (e.g., shotgun wound).

Computed tomography arteriography is replacing intraarterial digital subtraction arteriography for evaluation of cervical, truncal, and peripheral arteries in many centers.[48-51] Advantages include rapid evaluation of possible arterial injuries during CT evaluation of body parts, no need to wait for an out-of-hospital team from interventional radiology to return to the hospital, and the possibility of three-dimensional reconstructions of areas of arterial injury. One disadvantage is the presence of CT artifacts when missiles or metallic fragments are in the field of study, although one study has confirmed that this is not a significant problem.[52]

Venography is rarely performed in major trauma centers because the sequelae of missed peripheral venous injuries such as venous thromboses or pseudoaneurysms are rare. In recent years, color duplex ultrasonography has been used to evaluate veins of the extremities after penetrating trauma. Some centers choose to explore large peripheral hematomas after penetrating wounds without preliminary venography, even if arteriography results are normal, and to observe small, nonexpanding hematomas.

TABLE 15-3 *DIAGNOSTIC TECHNIQUES FOR EVALUATING POSSIBLE PERIPHERAL VASCULAR INJURIES*
Arterial pressure index
Duplex ultrasonography or color-flow ultrasonography
Emergency center or operating room arteriography by surgeon
Standard arteriography
Digital subtraction arteriography
CT multidetector or CT arteriography

CT, Computed tomography.

MANAGEMENT OF VASCULAR INJURIES[31-33,53]

The Emergency Center

The primary goal of the surgeon in the emergency center is to control hemorrhage in the patient with an extensive injury to the extremity. This has historically been accomplished by direct compression with a finger (remembering the aphorism that no vessel outside the human trunk is larger than the human thumb) or by application of a pressure dressing to the area of injury. If neither of these maneuvers controls hemorrhage, a blood pressure cuff is placed proximal to the area of injury and inflated to a pressure greater than the systolic blood pressure or a proximal tourniquet is applied as learned from the conflicts in Iraq and Afghanistan.[54-57] When hemorrhage is under temporary control, the patient is transferred to the OR for definitive vascular repair or ligation.

In a patient with pulses that are questionably palpable or audible by Doppler flow detection distal to a long bone fracture or a dislocation in an extremity, immediate reduction and splinting or application of a traction device should be performed. This relieves compression or kinking, but not spasm, in the adjacent artery. If such a maneuver restores diminished distal pulses in comparison with the uninjured contralateral extremity, the API should be measured if the bony or ligamentous injury is in the proximal extremity. If the API cannot be obtained because of a distal injury, if the API is lower than 0.90, or if distal pulses are absent after reduction, immediate arteriography is mandatory. In children, because examination of the peripheral vascular system is difficult, arteriography should be used liberally whenever fractures are present and distal arterial pulses are questionably palpable.

In an injured patient with hypotension, resuscitation is by the administration of fresh whole blood (military) or packed red blood cells—fresh-frozen plasma—platelet packs in a 1 : 1 : 1 to 3 : 1 : 1 ratio rather than the 4 : 1 ratio taught previously. This "damage control resuscitation" approach was developed by U.S. military physicians in Iraq and has changed the way injured civilian patients are resuscitated.[58,59]

Nonoperative Treatment of Arterial Injuries

If an arteriogram shows occlusion of only one major vessel below the elbow or knee when there is not a severely injured or mangled extremity, viability of the distal extremity is rarely compromised, and some centers choose to observe the patient in this situation. Because there can be retrograde flow into an area of arterial injury beyond the proximal occlusion, a repeat arteriogram should be performed within 3 to 7 days to rule out delayed formation of a traumatic false aneurysm.

As noted previously, several clinical studies have demonstrated that nonocclusive arterial injuries (e.g., spasm, intimal flap, subintimal or intramural hematoma) that often are detected in patients undergoing arteriography for soft signs of injury heal without operation in 87% to 95% of cases.[36,38] Even small, traumatic false aneurysms have been noted to heal on follow-up arteriograms in some of these patients. Arteriographic follow-up is necessary in patients who develop new symptoms while being observed.

Therapeutic Embolization

Isolated traumatic aneurysms of branches of the axillary, brachial, superficial femoral, or popliteal arteries; of the profunda femoris artery; or of one of the named arteries in the shank can be treated by therapeutic embolization instead of operation. Although such an approach has been used primarily in patients with penetrating wounds to the extremities, it is appropriate in selected patients with blunt vascular injuries as well. Patients with injuries to the arteries listed who will especially benefit from therapeutic embolization include those with multisystem injuries, closed fractures, or late diagnosis of a traumatic aneurysm after orthopaedic reconstruction. Contained aneurysms or active hemorrhage from muscular branches is treated with embolization using an absorbable gelatin sponge. When there is a need to occlude a tibial or peroneal artery proximal to a traumatic aneurysm, embolization coils are used.

Endovascular Stents and Stent Grafts

Balloon-expandable intraluminal arterial stents and stent grafts are now used routinely in patients with atherosclerotic occlusive disease. Extensive experience has been reported in patients with traumatic arterial injuries over the past 20 years as well.[4,60] For treatment of an intimal dissection or flap, an angiographic catheter is placed percutaneously across the area of injury via a transarterial sheath. This catheter is then exchanged for a separate catheter-mounted balloon inflatable endovascular stent, and the collapsed stent is expanded in place. If a traumatic aneurysm is present, an endovascular stent graft is used to occlude the orifice or trans-stent injections of microcoils are used to induce thrombosis of the aneurysmal sac.

The Operating Room

Arterial Repair

If the history, physical examination, duplex ultrasound, or arteriogram strongly suggests or documents the presence of an arterial injury that requires operative repair, the patient is given intravenous antibiotics before being moved to the OR. During the move, all open wounds are covered with sterile gauze soaked in saline or saline–antibiotic solution. In addition, all fractured or dislocated extremities are maintained in a neutral position by splinting or traction.

Skin Preparation and Draping

In the OR, an operative tourniquet can be applied in place of the blood pressure cuff for control of hemorrhage from injuries in the distal extremity. If the injuries are in the proximal extremity and exsanguinating hemorrhage resumes after removal of finger compression, a compression dressing, or a proximal blood cuff, a member of the surgical team should put on sterile operative gloves immediately. This individual then applies direct compression to a large wound with the hands or inserts fingers into an open fracture site or the entrance and exit sites of a penetrating wound to control hemorrhage as preparation of the skin and draping are performed.

Because of the possibility of an associated vascular lesion in all patients with orthopaedic injuries in an extremity, preparation of the skin and draping should encompass all potential areas of proximal and distal vascular control. Also, one or both lower extremities should be prepared and draped to allow for possible retrieval of the greater saphenous vein in case an interposition graft is required for the vascular repair. It is often helpful to have one entire uninjured lower extremity prepared and draped to the toenails, so that the greater saphenous vein may be retrieved from either the groin or the ankle. It is also helpful to drape the hand or foot of the affected extremity in a sterile plastic bag, so that color changes can be noted in light-skinned patients and distal pulses can be palpated under sterile conditions after arterial repair has been completed. The remainder of the extremity, including the area of the incision, is then covered with an orthopaedic-type stockinette.

Incisions

In patients with peripheral vascular injuries, the skin incision should be generous enough to allow for comfortable proximal and distal vascular control. To this end, it is often best for an inexperienced trauma surgeon to use the most extensive incisions.

There are a number of classic incisions for the management of peripheral vascular injuries. Those used in the upper extremity include (1) supraclavicular incision, with or without division of or resection of the clavicle, for injuries in the second or third portion of the subclavian artery; (2) infraclavicular incision for the first or second portion of the axillary artery; (3) infraclavicular incision curving onto the medial aspect of the upper arm for the third portion of the axillary artery or proximal brachial artery; (4) medial upper arm incision between the biceps and the triceps muscles for the main portion of the brachial artery; and (5) S-shaped incision from medial to lateral across the antecubital crease for the brachial artery proximal to its bifurcation. An injury to the radial or ulnar artery is usually approached by a longitudinal incision directly over the site.

In the lower extremity, the preferred incisions for arterial repair are (1) longitudinal groin incision for injury to the common femoral artery, proximal superficial femoral artery, or profunda femoris artery; (2) anteromedial thigh incision for exposure of the superficial femoral artery throughout the thigh; and (3) medial popliteal incision for exposure of the proximal, middle, or distal portions of the popliteal artery. Whereas injuries to the anterior tibial artery are approached directly over the site of injury in the anterior compartment, the posterior tibial artery is approached through a medial incision in the leg that often requires transection of the fibers of the soleus muscle. Finally, the peroneal artery is approached through a similar medial incision in the leg or through a lateral incision that requires excision of a portion of the fibula for proper exposure.

Standard Techniques of Arterial Repair

After the skin incision is made proximally and distally to the bleeding site or area of hematoma, dry skin towels are placed to cover all remaining skin edges if a plastic adherent drape has not been applied. If hemorrhage can be controlled by finger or laparotomy pad compression applied by an assistant, proximal and distal vascular control is usually obtained before the area of injury is entered. Not dissecting far enough proximally and distally from an area of injury is a common error. It is frequently necessary for an inexperienced vascular trauma surgeon to move proximal and distal vascular occlusion clamps or loops repeatedly as débridement of the injured artery is extended back to noninjured arterial intima.

In patients with an extensive hematoma overlying the arterial injury, it can be difficult to obtain proximal and distal vascular control close enough to the injury to prevent backbleeding from collateral vessels. In addition, there are patients in whom external hemorrhage cannot readily be controlled during meticulous dissection. Therefore, if dissection is proceeding extremely slowly through a very large hematoma or the assistant can no longer maintain control of exsanguinating hemorrhage by direct compression, the hematoma or site of hemorrhage should be entered directly. The site of arterial bleeding is visualized and compressed with a finger or vascular forceps, and a proximal vascular clamp or vessel loop is applied. The dissection is then completed starting from the center rather than waiting for proximal and distal control to be obtained at a distance from the hematoma or bleeding site.

After vascular control is obtained in either classic or rapid fashion, vascular occlusion can be maintained by application of small, angled vascular clamps (such as those found in an angioaccess tray), bulldog vascular clamps, Silastic vessel loops, or umbilical tapes. Occasionally, with complex arterial injuries at bifurcations, vascular control of major branches can be obtained by passage of an intraluminal Fogarty balloon catheter or a calibrated Garrett dilator.

In general, lateral arteriorrhaphy (or venorrhaphy) with 5-0 or 6-0 polypropylene sutures placed transversely is used for small lacerations or for small puncture, pellet, or missile wounds, especially in the smaller vessels of the extremities. If a transverse repair results in significant narrowing of the injured vessel, patch angioplasty is a useful alternative that is rarely used because of concerns about sizing. Any segment of injured vein that has been resected or of autogenous saphenous vein from the ankle or groin of an uninjured lower extremity can be used to create an oval patch to increase the size of the lumen of an injured vessel. The patch is usually sewn in place with 6-0 polypropylene suture.

Resection of injured peripheral vessels is often required in patients with blunt orthopaedic trauma because of the magnitude of the forces applied to cause both bony and vascular injuries. An increasing number of vascular injuries from penetrating wounds also require resection of the injured segment because of the greater wounding power of firearms now used in the United States. Resection with an end-to-end anastomosis is performed whenever a segment of a vessel has extensive destruction of the wall or a long area of disrupted intima (e.g., from blunt traction injury or through-and-through injury from a penetrating wound). Despite the elasticity of peripheral vessels in the typical young trauma patient, many collateral vessels must be ligated for an end-to-end anastomosis to be performed if more than 2 to 3 cm of the vessel is resected. An end-to-end anastomosis sewn under tension results in an hourglass appearance at the suture line and often leads to thrombosis of the repair in the postoperative period. Although an interrupted suture technique for end-to-end anastomosis is routinely used in growing children, continuous suture techniques with two-point fixation 180 degrees apart are used by experienced trauma surgeons for small vessels of the extremities (4–5 mm diameter) in adults.[61]

If exposure is difficult, as in the axillary artery near the clavicle or the popliteal artery behind the knee joint, it is often helpful to perform the first third of the posterior anastomosis with an open technique (i.e., one in which no knot is tied). This allows for precise suture bites of the posterior walls, and it prevents leaks after arterial inflow is restored. On completion of the posterior third of the anastomosis, the two ends of the suture are pulled tight, drawing the two ends of the artery together.

Both ends of the artery are then stabilized, and Fogarty embolectomy catheters are passed proximally and distally to remove any thrombotic or embolic material from the arterial tree. The amount of debris distal to an arterial injury can be extensive, especially after a prolonged period of preoperative occlusion. After both ends of the vessel have been cleared, 15 to 20 mL of regional heparin (50 units/mL) is injected into each end, and the vascular clamps are reapplied. Injection of

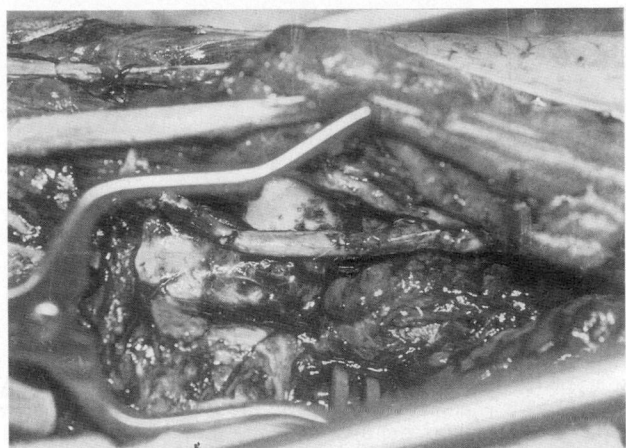

Figure 15-4. Saphenous vein graft inserted into the left anterior tibial artery in patient with Gustilo type IIIC tibial fracture.

a total of 30 to 40 mL of this solution (1500–2000 units or 15–20 mg heparin) provides significantly less anticoagulation than the 1 to 2 mg/kg of heparin used in many elective vascular procedures. More aggressive systemic heparinization is avoided in selected trauma patients because of the risk of hemorrhage from other injuries.

The end-to-end anastomosis is completed by running the two ends of the suture along the two sides of the approximated artery, leaving the last few loops of suture loose to allow for flushing before final tying. The proximal vascular occlusion clamp is first removed and reapplied after completion of flushing. The distal vascular clamp is then removed to allow for flushing from the distal end of the vessel and to clear any residual air underneath the suture line. As blood from the distal arterial tree fills the area that was between the two clamps or loops, the two suture ends are pulled up tightly and tied. The proximal arterial clamp is not released until the first knot is in place. If small suture hole leaks are present at that time, topical hemostatic agents can be applied temporarily.

If an end-to-end anastomosis cannot be performed with minimal tension, a substitute vascular conduit should be inserted into the defect between the two débrided ends of the injured vessel. An autogenous reversed saphenous vein graft from an uninjured lower extremity remains the conduit of choice for most peripheral vascular injuries (Fig. 15-4).[53] If the vessel to be replaced has a small lumen (4–5 mm), the greater saphenous vein at the medial malleolus is a good choice. If the artery or vein to be replaced has a much larger lumen, the greater saphenous vein in the proximal thigh is a better choice. Major advantages of the autogenous saphenous vein include its ready availability, the superiority of natural tissue in maintaining patency, and a long record of success in vascular and cardiac surgery. The patency of the saphenous vein graft can be improved by using gentle dissection, by avoiding overdistention during flushing, and by using only heparinized autologous blood containing papaverine for flushing before insertion.

If a saphenous vein graft is to be inserted, it is often helpful to perform the more difficult distal anastomosis first. Because of the floppy nature of a collapsed saphenous vein graft, it is useful to place two 6-0 polypropylene sutures 180 degrees apart at the two corners of the anastomosis. Another option is to use the classic trifurcation technique originally described by Guthrie and Carrel in the History section earlier. After anastomosis of the graft to the distal end of the artery has been completed, a Garrett dilator can be passed through it to ensure adequate luminal size. The proximal anastomosis is then performed. As with a simple end-to-end anastomosis, passage of a Fogarty catheter, injection of heparinized saline solution, and flushing should be performed before completion of the second anastomosis (Fig. 15-5).

If the saphenous vein is surgically absent, injured bilaterally, too small, or of an inappropriate size to fit into the injured vessel, or if the patient is critically injured and the speed of repair is important, many trauma centers use polytetrafluoroethylene (PTFE) grafts for interposition.[16] The early complication and infection rates with the use of PTFE prostheses appear to be the same as those with saphenous vein grafts, but long-term patency is less. If a PTFE graft is to be used, it is best to cut it to an appropriate length with a #11 scalpel blade rather than a pair of scissors. The rigid, open nature of PTFE allows for rapid performance of an arterial anastomosis, and no fixation sutures are needed. The passage of a Fogarty catheter and regional heparinization are performed as previously described. Laboratory and clinical studies have demonstrated that neointimal hyperplasia occurs at PTFE-artery suture lines, and patients in whom such a graft is placed are started on aspirin by rectal suppository every 12 hours while in the ICU. Two 81-mg aspirin tablets are taken orally each day for the first 3 postoperative months in the absence of a history of gastric or duodenal ulcers.

Although bypass grafting can be applied in selected circumstances of extensive vascular injuries, this technique is rarely used. For example, if ligation around an area of injury is required to prevent exsanguinating hemorrhage, a saphenous vein bypass graft can then be inserted in an end-to-side fashion proximally and distally instead of resection of the injured segment and placement of an interposition graft.

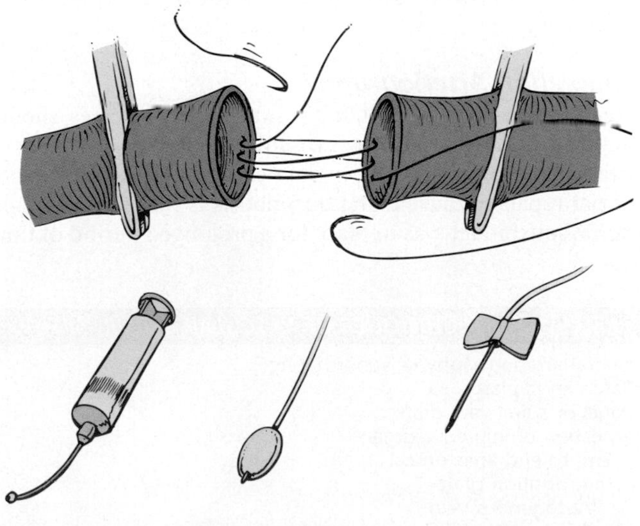

Figure 15-5. Fine points in peripheral arterial repair include use of small vascular clamps or Silastic vessel loops, open anastomosis technique, regional heparinization, passage of a Fogarty catheter proximally and distally, and arteriography on completion. *(Courtesy of Baylor College of Medicine, 1981.)*

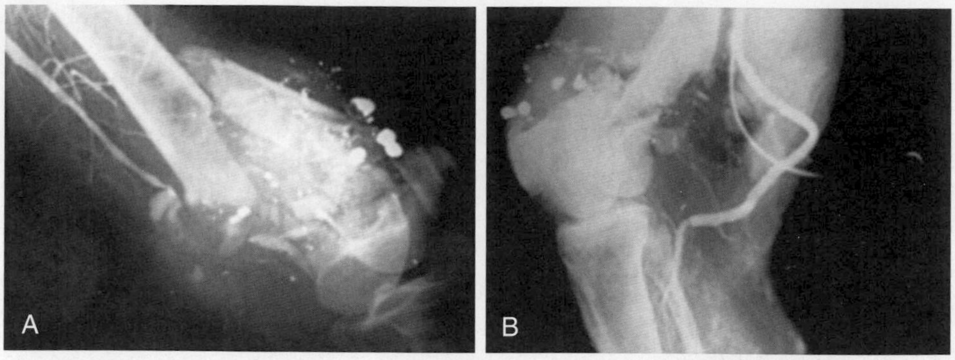

Figure 15-6. A, This shotgun wound that disrupted the distal femur also avulsed the popliteal artery, as seen on the arteriogram. **B,** An extraanatomic saphenous vein bypass graft inserted around the posterior aspect of the knee joint is shown on the completion arteriogram. *(**B**, from Feliciano DV, Accola KD, Burch MJ, et al: Extra-anatomic bypass for peripheral arterial injuries, Am J Surg 158:506, 1989.)*

Extraanatomic bypass grafting is used when extensive injury to soft tissues in the antecubital, groin, or below-knee area is accompanied by injuries to the underlying brachial, femoral, popliteal, or tibioperoneal vessels. In such instances, vigorous débridement of the wound in soft tissue is carried out at the first operation, and the extraanatomic saphenous vein conduit is inserted around the wound underneath healthy soft tissue, with both end-to-end anastomoses also covered by such tissue (Fig. 15-6).[62] The defect in soft tissue is then managed with a vacuum-assisted closure device until delayed primary closure or application of a split-thickness skin graft is performed.[62,63] Care of the wound is made easier with this approach, and the danger of graft or suture line blowout is decreased by use of the extraanatomic bypass through noninjured tissue.

Ligation is reserved for injury to the distal profunda femoris artery in the thigh or to main arteries below the elbow or knee when at least one other named vessel to the hand or foot is still patent and there is not a severely injured or mangled extremity. The technique is used in patients with a coagulopathy and in those who are so unstable that the operation must be terminated. See Table 15-4 for a list of all repair techniques.

Completion Arteriography

After arterial inflow has been restored, distal pulses should be present. In the upper extremity, palpation of normal distal pulses is usually acceptable evidence of a satisfactory arterial repair because distal thrombosis is rare unless a tight arterial tourniquet was in place for a prolonged period of time preoperatively. Most experienced trauma surgeons, however, use completion arteriography after an end-to-end anastomosis or insertion of an interposition graft of any type in an artery of the lower extremity. This is done to rule out technical mishaps at the one or two suture lines and problems such as distal embolism or in situ thrombosis in the small vessels of the shank. It is helpful to place a small metal tissue clip near any anastomosis, so that it can be localized precisely on the arteriogram. This enables the surgeon to distinguish a narrowed anastomosis from a mark produced by a vascular clamp.

Operative arteriography is easily performed after insertion of a 20-gauge Teflon-over-metal catheter into the artery. Usually, the artery is punctured proximal to the repair, and the Teflon catheter is slipped over the needle into the lumen of the artery. It is particularly useful to stabilize the artery with vascular forceps as the anterior wall of the artery is entered. This maneuver usually prevents posterior perforation of the artery, which commonly occurs when metal or larger arteriography needles or catheters are inserted into an unstable artery. The Teflon catheter is attached by a short piece of intravenous extension tubing to a 50-mL syringe filled with heparinized saline solution. This is injected through the Teflon catheter before arteriography to ensure proper catheter placement in the lumen. Free return of pulsatile blood into the plastic tubing confirms the position of the catheter. The extremity is aligned in an anterior-posterior direction over the film cassette or under the fluoroscopy unit. An excellent operative arteriogram (hard copy) can usually be obtained by exposing the film as the last several milliliters of a 35-mL bolus of 60% diatrizoate meglumine dye are injected rapidly[34] (Fig. 15-7). If the lower extremity is allowed to rotate externally during arteriography, the overlying bone may obscure the arterial repair in certain areas around and below the knee joint.

After arteriography has been completed, a syringe containing heparinized saline solution is attached to the extension tubing and the artery is flushed with the solution. The Teflon arteriography catheter is not removed until the arteriogram has been returned and is noted to be of satisfactory quality. If the completion arteriogram is satisfactory, a small U-stitch of 6-0 polypropylene suture is placed around the Teflon catheter and tied down tightly as the catheter is removed.

If a technical problem such as an intimal flap, a thrombus at the site of anastomosis, or a distal embolus is present on the completion arteriogram, vascular clamps are reapplied, the

TABLE 15-4 ***TECHNIQUES OF VASCULAR REPAIR***

- Lateral arteriorrhaphy or venorrhaphy
- Patch angioplasty
- Panel or spiral vein graft
- Resection of injured segment
  - End-to-end anastomosis
  - Interposition graft
    - Autogenous vein
    - Polytetrafluoroethylene
    - Dacron
- Bypass graft
  - In situ
  - Extraanatomic
- Ligation

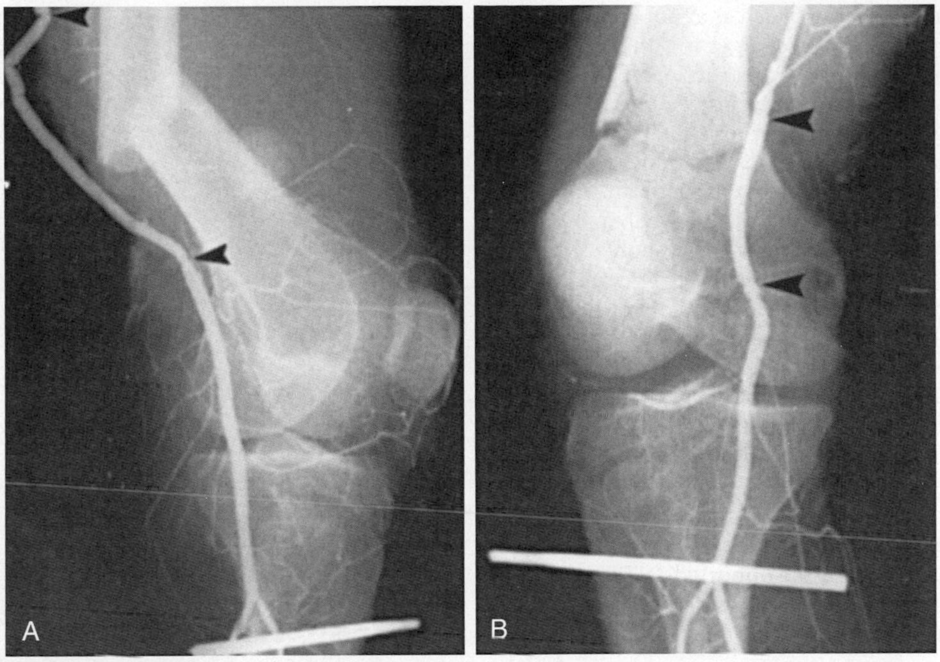

Figure 15-7. Bilateral occlusions of the superficial femoral arteries associated with fractures of the femurs were repaired with autogenous saphenous vein grafts (**A** and **B**). The graft in the left thigh appears too long but was of appropriate length after the fractured femur was realigned (**A**). *Arrowheads* indicate the proximal and distal anastomoses of saphenous vein grafts. *(From Feliciano DV: Managing peripheral vascular trauma, Infect Surg 5:659-669, 682, 1986.)*

arterial repair is opened, and the problem is corrected. If distal spasm is present but arterial flow to the foot or hand is adequate, no further therapy is required because spasm usually resolves within 4 to 6 hours. If the spasm is severe and distal flow is compromised, measurement of the below-elbow or below-knee musculofascial compartment pressures to rule out a compartment syndrome is worthwhile.

Venous Injuries

Venous occlusion or ligation in the groin has a significant adverse effect on femoral arterial inflow in the canine.[64] For this reason and because of the known adverse effect of popliteal venous ligation on viability of the leg, there is more effort to perform peripheral venous repair rather than ligation in the modern trauma center,[65] although not all agree with this approach.[66] Of interest, follow-up venography after extremity venorrhaphy has documented that more than 25% of simple venous repairs and almost 35% of interposition grafts inserted for venous repair are temporarily occluded in the postoperative period. Fortunately, many of these recanalize over time. Therefore, the consensus is that venous injuries in the groin or popliteal area should be repaired if the patient is stable and has no life-threatening intraoperative complications such as hypothermia or a coagulopathy. If the patient is unstable or has a life-threatening complication that could be aggravated by prolonging general anesthesia, venous ligation or insertion of an intraluminal plastic shunt (see later) should be performed. Although this issue is continually debated, the long-term sequelae of venous ligation in young victims of civilian trauma appear to be fewer than originally reported from the Vietnam experience.[65,66]

Venous injuries are often difficult to manage because of hemorrhage from the large lumen, the fragile nature of the wall, and the many small branches. Excessive manipulation of the injured vein often leads to further hemorrhage. It is helpful to use finger or sponge-stick compression around the area of perforation for vascular control rather than to attempt application of vascular clamps to all branches feeding the area of injury. After the area of injury has been isolated, lateral venorrhaphy in a transverse direction remains the most common technique of repair for peripheral venous injuries. Occasionally, a more complex repair such as patch venoplasty, resection with end-to-end anastomosis, or resection with insertion of some type of substitute conduit is necessary.[65] The principles of repair for major venous injuries are similar to those for arterial injuries except that Fogarty catheters are not passed, and completion venograms are not obtained.

If resection of an injured segment of a peripheral vein is required, ligation of local collateral vessels is necessary to allow for the performance of an end-to-end anastomosis with only modest tension. If a substitute vascular conduit is required to replace a segmental injury in a critical vein (e.g., popliteal, distal femoral), the surgeon must choose from a variety of less satisfactory alternatives. An autogenous saphenous vein graft from an uninjured lower extremity would appear to be an ideal conduit. The diameter of the greater saphenous vein in the groin, however, is often too small to match the size of the proximal femoral or common femoral vein in the lower extremity or the axillary or subclavian vein in the upper extremity. Such a small conduit in a much larger vein would be patent for only a short time.

Two other choices for replacement of an injured vein with autogenous tissue involve the creation of a spiral vein graft or a panel graft. The spiral vein graft is created by opening the harvested autogenous saphenous vein from an uninjured lower extremity longitudinally over its entire length, wrapping it around a rigid tubular structure such as a thoracostomy tube in a spiral fashion, and sewing the edges together to create a tube of a larger luminal diameter. Construction of a spiral vein graft is time consuming and cannot be justified for routine use in peripheral venous injuries in light of its 50% patency rate. A panel graft is created by longitudinally opening two separate segments of autogenous saphenous vein from an uninjured lower extremity, placing one on top of the other, and sewing the two side edges together to create one tubular structure of a larger luminal diameter. Again, this technique is time consuming and is rarely justified in the repair of peripheral venous injuries. If the surgeon is willing to insert a "temporary" venous conduit, an externally supported PTFE graft can be placed into large luminal veins of a proximal extremity. These grafts are available in appropriate sizes, but they remain patent for only 2 to 3 weeks if the type without external support is used.[16] If an externally supported PTFE graft is inserted, there is long-term patency for months and possibly years. To encourage dilatation of collateral veins during the period of slow occlusion of an unsupported PTFE graft, it is mandatory to keep the injured extremity elevated and to place elastic wraps around the extremity while the patient is in the hospital.

Indications for Fasciotomy

The diagnosis of a compartmental syndrome and techniques of fasciotomy are discussed in Chapter 16.

Combined Orthopaedic–Vascular Injuries

There has been much discussion about the preferred order of repair, that is, orthopaedic stabilization followed by arterial repair or the reverse.[18,67] A number of authors have emphasized the need for early arterial repair to limit distal ischemia and lessen the risk of in situ thrombosis.[68] Others have noted that early orthopaedic repair stabilizes the extremity and improves exposure of the vascular injury. This approach also lowers the risk of thrombosis in a recently completed vascular repair during subsequent manipulation to reduce a fracture (Fig. 15-8). With either approach, the ultimate amputation rate is substantial.

In a patient with neither cold ischemia (pulseless without capillary refill) nor a prolonged period of warm ischemia (capillary refill present), the choice of arterial or orthopaedic repair depends primarily on the stability of the fracture site. If the area of the fracture is reasonably stable and the trauma team is experienced in rapid vascular repair, it is appropriate to perform the arterial repair first. If the fracture is comminuted and the extremity cannot be stabilized for proper exposure of the vascular injury, the orthopaedic repair is performed first. In trauma centers with extensive experience in the management of combined injuries in the extremities, consultation among attending surgeons, fellows, or senior residents is mandatory and allows for proper sequencing of repairs.

In a patient with a cold, pulseless hand or foot and little or no capillary refill or in a patient who has undergone a prolonged period of either cold or warm ischemia, restoration of arterial inflow has the highest priority and should be accomplished first by formal repair or by the insertion of a temporary intraluminal vascular shunt. Formal arterial repair is preferred if the extremity is reasonably stable despite the presence of a fracture. If an unstable fracture that precludes appropriate

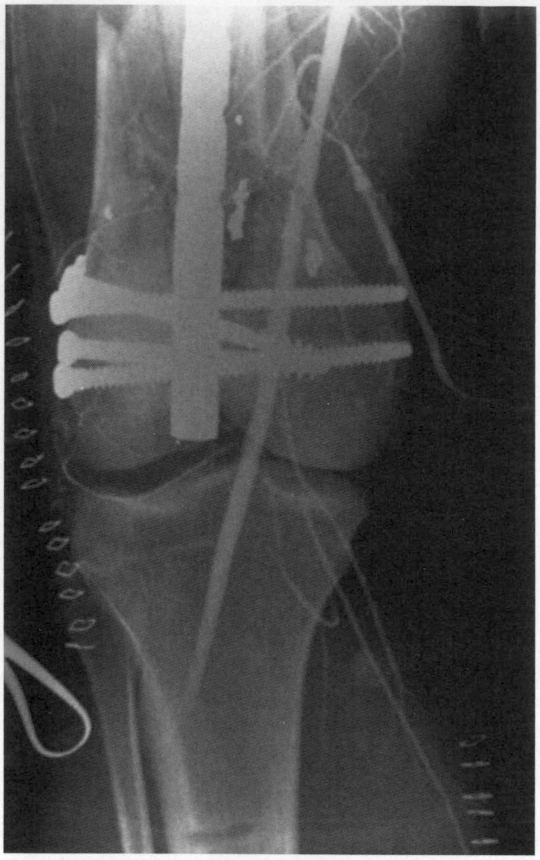

Figure 15-8. Occlusion of distal arterial bed occurred during orthopaedic manipulation after graft repair of the right popliteal artery. The patient eventually needed an above-knee amputation.

exposure of the vascular injury is present, shunts are inserted to allow for continued arterial inflow and venous outflow during the period of orthopaedic stabilization.

Temporary Intraluminal Vascular Shunts

A shunt is defined as an intraluminal plastic conduit for temporary maintenance of arterial inflow or venous outflow, or both, to or from a body part. First described for use in peripheral arterial injuries in 1919, there has been a significant increase in the use of these devices in trauma centers over the past 25 years.[69-72] At this time, suggested general indications for the use of shunts include (1) combined orthopaedic–vascular injuries, including mangled extremities; (2) preservation of an amputated upper extremity at the arm, forearm, or wrist level before replantation; or (3) rapid restoration of arterial inflow or venous outflow, or both, as part of a life-saving peripheral or truncal "damage control" operation.

As described earlier, insertion of intraluminal shunts in a patient with a combined orthopaedic–vascular injury promptly restores arterial inflow or venous outflow, or both, and allows for appropriate orthopaedic stabilization, reconstruction, or débridement. A properly fixated shunt will withstand vigorous realignment maneuvers. When the orthopaedic operative procedure is completed, the trauma vascular surgeon can then choose one of two options. In a hemodynamically stable patient without intraoperative hypothermia, metabolic acidosis, or a coagulopathy, the shunts are removed, and interposition vascular grafts are inserted under the same general anesthetic. When the injured patient is hemodynamically unstable with a body temperature lower than 35°C, a base deficit less than −10 to −15, or a coagulopathy, the original operative procedure is terminated.[73] Removal of the shunts and vascular repairs are then performed at a reoperation in 24 to 48 hours. In patients with mangled extremities, this time delay will allow for combined consultation by orthopaedic and vascular surgeons and discussions with the patient and family.

The value of temporary intraluminal shunts to maintain viability in amputated parts of the upper extremity is obvious. Identification and tagging of nerves and tendons, débridement of crushed tissue, and orthopaedic stabilization can all be completed while the shunts are in place.

With improvements in prehospital emergency medical services in urban environments, more injured patients with near-exsanguination are admitted to the emergency center than in the past. The insertion of temporary intraluminal shunts in the vessels of the arm, antecubital area, groin, thigh, or knee adjacent to a fracture or dislocation will prevent the need for ligation in the injured patient with profound shock. Indications for peripheral (or truncal) "damage control" shunts are (1) body temperature lower than 34° to 35°C (on admission or developing during operation), (2) arterial pH less than 7.2 or base deficit less than −15 in patients younger than 55 years of age or less than −6 in patients older than 55 years of age, and (3) intraoperative international normalized ratio or partial thromboplastin time greater than 50% of normal. Any trauma operative procedure is terminated whenever one of the listed abnormalities is present. Resuscitation including rewarming, hemodynamic monitoring, transfusion, use of inotropes, and correction of coagulopathy is then performed in the surgical ICU rather than the OR. The third stage of damage control is the return to the OR for definitive repairs when the patient's previous metabolic failure secondary to hypovolemic shock has been corrected.[73]

Intraluminal shunts are readily available in any OR in which elective surgery on the carotid artery is performed. They range in size from 8 to 14 Fr and are held in place with 2-0 silk ties compressing the end of the transected artery or vein onto the shunt. When a large shunt is needed for insertion into the popliteal, superficial femoral, or common femoral veins, standard thoracostomy tubes are used (Fig. 15-9).

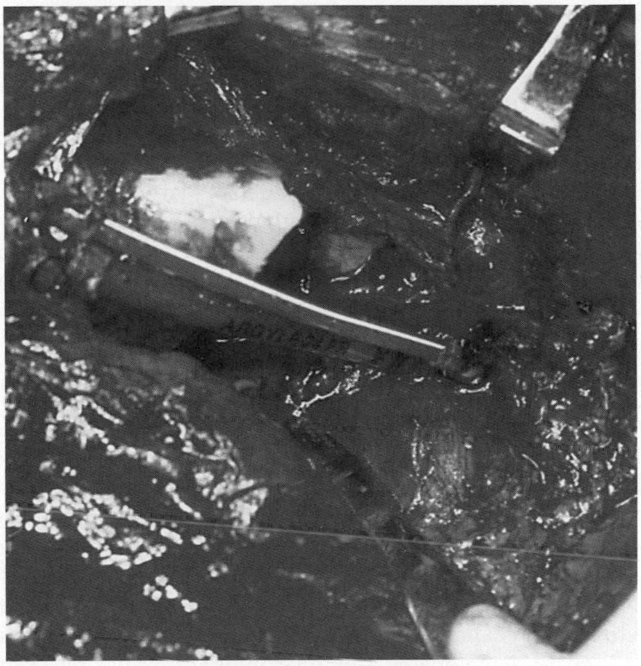

Figure 15-9. Patient with open fracture of the left femur from a crush injury who also had transection of the proximal popliteal artery and vein. A 14-Fr carotid artery shunt was placed into the popliteal artery, and a 24-Fr thoracostomy tube was placed into the popliteal vein. Because of intraoperative hypothermia, removal of shunts and insertion of interposition grafts were delayed for 18 hours.

Mangled Extremities

A mangled extremity results from high-energy transfer or crushing trauma that causes some combination of injuries to artery, bone, soft tissue, tendon, or nerve. Approximately two-thirds of such injuries are caused by motorcycle, motor vehicle, or vehicle–pedestrian accidents, reflecting the significant transfer of energy that occurs during such incidents. More than 3 decades ago, Chapman emphasized that the kinetic energy dissipated in collision with an automobile bumper at 20 mph (100,000 ft-lb) is 50 times greater than that from a high-velocity gunshot (2000 ft-lb).[74]

When a patient with a mangled extremity arrives in the emergency center, the trauma team must work its way through the following series of decisions in patient care:

1. If the patient's life is in danger, should the mangled limb be amputated?
2. If the patient is stable, should an attempt be made to salvage the mangled limb?
3. If salvage is to be attempted, what is the sequence of repairs? (See previous section.)
4. If salvage fails, when should amputation be performed?

The most difficult decision is whether to attempt salvage of the limb. Since 1985, at least five separate scoring systems that describe the magnitude of injuries in a mangled extremity have been published.[39,68,75-77] All attempt to predict the need for amputation based on a total score derived from the combination of injuries in the extremity and other factors. Only one system, the Mangled Extremity Severity Score developed by Johansen and coworkers,[40] has been studied in a prospective manner. Additionally, the applicability of any of these systems outside the institutions in which they originated has been questioned.

Two major criteria are used most frequently in clinical decisions regarding immediate amputation versus attempted salvage. If either of the following factors is present, amputation is a better choice than prolonged attempts at salvage.[78]

1. Loss of arterial inflow for longer than 6 hours, particularly in the presence of a crush injury that disrupts collateral vessels[79]
2. Disruption of the posterior tibial nerve[40,79]

Hansen[78] and Lange[79] have described *relative* indications for immediate amputation in patients with Gustilo type IIIC tibial fractures as well. These include serious associated polytrauma, severe ipsilateral foot trauma, anticipated protracted course to obtain soft tissue coverage, and need for extensive tibial reconstruction.[80] If two of these are present, immediate amputation is again recommended.

The management of mangled extremities based on outcomes has been clarified considerably by numerous publications in recent years,[81-83] especially those from the LEAP (Lower Extremity Assessment Project) Study Group.[84]

Bleeding or Edema in Soft Tissues

In patients with major peripheral vascular injuries and a coagulopathy, extensive oozing often occurs in soft tissue as the operation is completed. In such patients, placement of closed or open drains into the blast cavity or area of dissection may be required for several hours after surgery. The placement of drains prevents formation of a postoperative hematoma that could compress and possibly occlude the vascular repairs.

If a large blast cavity is present in soft tissue near the vascular repairs, some muscle or soft tissue should be sutured in a position that separates the two. A closed or open drain or open packing of the cavity exiting on the opposite side of the extremity from the skin incision and vascular repairs should then be inserted. This allows for drainage of the large blast cavity away from the vascular repairs and helps to avoid the problems of compression by hematoma and of cellulitis and late abscesses near a vascular repair.

Occasionally, primary wound closure is undesirable in patients with extensive muscle hematomas, soft tissue edema, or a severe coagulopathy after a peripheral vascular repair. In such patients, porcine xenografts (pigskin) are placed over the vascular repairs, and the wound is packed open with antibiotic-soaked gauze.[85] After 24 hours of elevation of the injured extremity, the patient is returned to the OR for delayed primary closure or closure with a myocutaneous flap performed by the plastic surgery service.

Heroic Techniques to Save a Limb

If vascular repair is satisfactory on the completion arteriogram but the distal extremity has borderline viability because of vascular spasm, extensive destruction of collateral vessels in soft tissue, or prolonged ischemia, various adjuncts for salvage should be considered after a primary or secondary compartment syndrome has been ruled out. Included among these are proximal arterial infusion with a heparin–tolazoline–saline solution (containing 1000 units of heparin and 500 mg of tolazoline in 1000 mL saline) at a rate of 30 mL/hr[86] and venous infusion with low-molecular-weight dextran at a rate of 500 mL/12 hr.

Postoperative Care

After the patient has been returned to the ward or ICU, the injured extremity should be elevated and wrapped with elastic bandages if venous ligation was performed. Care must be taken to monitor intracompartmental pressure in such a situation because the combination of venous hypertension, external compression, and elevation may create an early compartment syndrome.[87] Distal arterial pulses are monitored by palpation or with a portable Doppler unit. Intravenous antibiotics are continued for 24 hours if a primary repair or end-to-end anastomosis was performed. If a substitute vascular conduit was inserted, intravenous antibiotics are continued for 72 hours in some centers, much as in elective vascular surgery.

Complications

Early Occlusion of Arterial Repair

Intraoperative or in-hospital occlusion of an arterial repair is almost always related to delayed presentation of the patient after injury, delayed diagnosis of the injury by a physician, a technical mishap in the OR, or occlusion of venous outflow from the area of injury. In a patient with a delay in presentation or diagnosis, in situ distal arterial thrombosis may occur within 6 hours. The passage of a Fogarty embolectomy catheter may not be helpful in such a situation because it does not remove thrombi from arterial collateral vessels.

Technical mishaps during the operation that lead to postoperative thrombosis of a repair include too much tension on an end-to-end anastomosis, failure to remove any thrombi or emboli in the distal arterial tree with a Fogarty embolectomy catheter, narrowing of a circumferential suture line, and failure to flush the proximal and distal arteries before final closure of the repair. Also, ligation or occlusion of a repair in the popliteal vein can lead to occlusion of an arterial repair at the same level.

If distal pulses disappear, the patient is returned immediately to the OR for distal thrombectomy or embolectomy or revision of the repair as necessary. If there is not an obvious reason for occlusion of the arterial repair during a reoperation, standard coagulation tests are performed immediately to screen for a thrombotic disorder. Examples include heparin-associated thrombocytopenia, antithrombin III deficiency, deficiency of protein C or S, and the antiphospholipid syndrome.

Delay in Diagnosis of an Arterial Injury

Occasionally, a patient presents with a traumatic false aneurysm or an arteriovenous fistula from a previous arterial injury that was not diagnosed.[88] The insertion of an endovascular stent with or without trans-stent angiographic embolization is possible for many of these lesions, and it can be accomplished readily by an experienced interventional radiologist. If a major artery is involved, operative intervention using the principles described previously may be necessary.

Soft Tissue Infection over an Arterial Repair

A dreaded complication of combined orthopaedic–vascular injuries, particularly in the lower extremity, is infection in the soft tissue overlying the arterial repair. If débridement of the soft tissue infection results in exposure of the arterial repair, one option is to attempt coverage of the arterial repair with a porcine xenograft and hope for the gradual growth of granulation tissue over the healthy artery. If the arterial repair starts to leak or sustains a blowout, the patient is returned to the OR. The exposed portion of the artery is resected, and the aforementioned extraanatomic saphenous vein bypass graft is placed around the area of soft tissue infection, making sure that both end-to-end anastomoses are covered by healthy soft tissue outside the wound, as described previously.[62]

Another option after débridement of infected soft tissue when the underlying arterial repair is intact is for immediate coverage with a local muscle or myocutaneous rotation flap or for coverage with a free flap performed by the plastic surgery service.

Late Occlusion of Arterial Repair

Because saphenous vein grafts placed in peripheral arteries undergo the degenerative changes of atherosclerosis over time, late occlusions of some of these grafts can be expected.

Management is the same as if the patient had occlusion of a primary artery—arteriography is performed based on symptoms. Bypass grafting is chosen for occlusion of long segments if runoff is adequate to support another graft. Short-segment occlusions may be amenable to endovascular stenting.

SUMMARY

Experience with peripheral arterial injuries in the absence of an associated bony injury documents that limb salvage is possible in almost all such patients without shotgun wounds or near amputations who are treated using the principles outlined in this chapter. These principles include early diagnosis by examination, preoperative arteriography or duplex ultrasonography, frequent use of interposition grafting for arterial repair, completion arteriography, repair of venous injuries in stable patients, and liberal use of fasciotomy. If bony injuries accompany arterial injuries, limb salvage is less likely because of delays in diagnosis, a greater magnitude of arterial injury, disruption of vascular collateral vessels in soft tissue, and associated postoperative problems such as infection in adjacent soft tissue or bone. Even so, limb salvage can be accomplished in most properly selected patients in modern trauma centers using the techniques described.

KEY REFERENCES

The level of evidence (LOE) is determined according to the criteria provided in the preface.

16. Feliciano DV, Mattox KL, Graham JM, et al: Five-year experience with PTFE grafts in vascular wounds. *J Trauma* 25:71–81, 1985. LOE III
23. Miranda FE, Dennis JW, Veldenz HC, et al: Confirmation of the safety and accuracy of physical examination in the evaluation of knee dislocation for popliteal artery injury: A prospective study. *J Trauma* 52:247–252, 2002. LOE III
38. Frykberg ER, Vines FS, Alexander RH: The natural history of clinically occult arterial injuries: a prospective evaluation. *J Trauma* 29:577–583, 1989. LOE III
40. Johansen K, Daines M, Howey T, et al: Objective criteria accurately predict amputation following lower extremity trauma. *J Trauma* 30:568–573, 1990. LOE III
49. Inaba K, Branco BC, Reddy S, et al: Prospective evaluation of multidetector computed tomography for extremity vascular trauma. *J Trauma* 70:808–815, 2011. LOE III
52. White PW, Gillespie DL, Feurstein I, et al: Sixty-four slice multidetector computed tomographic angiography in the evaluation of vascular trauma. *J Trauma* 68:96–102, 2010. LOE III
53. Feliciano DV, Moore EE, West MA, et al: Western Trauma Association critical decisions in trauma: evaluation and management of peripheral vascular injury, part II. *J Trauma Acute Care Surg* 75:391–397, 2013. LOE V
56. Kragh JF, Walters TJ, Baer DG, et al: Survival with emergency tourniquet use to stop bleeding in major limb trauma. *Ann Surg* 249:1–7, 2009. LOE III
81. Doukas WC, Hayda RA, Frisch HM, et al: The military extremity trauma amputation/limb salvage (METALS) study. Outcomes of amputations versus limb salvage following major lower-extremity trauma. *J Bone Joint Surg Am* 95:138–145, 2013. LOE III
84. Castillo RC, MacKenzie EJ, Bosse MJ, et al: Orthopaedic trauma clinical research: is 2-year follow-up necessary? Results from a longitudinal study of severe lower extremity trauma. *J Trauma* 71:1726–1731, 2011. LOE III

The complete References list is available online at https://expertconsult.inkling.com.

Chapter 16

Compartment Syndromes

MICHAEL SIMMS SHULER • MELLISA ROSKOSKY • BRETT A. FREEDMAN

Additional videos related to the subject of this chapter are available from the Medizinische Hochschule Hannover collection. The following videos are included with this chapter and may be viewed at https://expertconsult.inkling.com:

16-1. Intracompartmental pressure measurements.
16-2. Stryker Stic device assembly.
16-3. Pressure measurement with Stryker.
16-4. Compartment syndrome: diagnosis and operative therapy.

INTRODUCTION

Acute compartment syndrome (ACS) can be a devastating injury if diagnosis and treatment are delayed or missed. Physicians evaluating patients with acute, long bone fractures, especially of the tibia, should keep ACS in the forefront of their mind when examining the traumatized patient. While the ability to define ACS has become clearer, still much controversy and confusion remains regarding when ACS exists and when intervention is required. As with many conditions associated with severe loss of function, ACS is a highly litigious topic.[1,2] Because fasciotomies are not benign procedures, both failing to treat ACS and unnecessary treatment when ACS is not present can lead to significant dysfunction.[3-5] The goal of this chapter is to provide a review of the pathophysiology of ACS, its diagnosis, and the methods for performing fasciotomy to various areas of the limbs.

In addition, we will provide lessons learned and a military perspective on ACS, which is a disease process that has been defined in war. Due to the sheer volume (density of exposure) of injuries, as well as the severity of injury associated with the recent conflicts throughout the world, much has been learned about the diagnosis, treatment, management, and mismanagement of ACS, but unfortunately much remains to be learned about this condition. This chapter will discuss lessons learned on the management of ACS in both the civilian and military setting, and highlight areas requiring further research and understanding.

HISTORY

In 1881, Richard von Volkmann published an article in which he attempted to relate the state of irreversible contractures of flexor muscles of the hand to an ischemic process occurring in the forearm.[6] In 1906, Hildebrand first used the term *Volkmann's ischemic contracture* to describe the end point of an untreated compartment syndrome and suggested that elevated tissue pressure may be causally related to the ischemic contracture.[7] In 1914, Murphy was the first to suggest that fasciotomy, if done before the development of the contracture, may prevent the contracture from occurring.[8] After almost 100 years of investigation, advancements have been made in the field of ACS, but still the ability to definitively and objectively diagnose and treat ACS has remained a challenge.

During and after World War II (WW II), high velocity gunshot wounds and their concomitant soft tissue injuries were identified as causes for residual muscle contractures of both the upper and lower extremities[9] (Fig. 16-1). Although the existence of arterial trauma complicating a fracture was well known, the concomitant need for fasciotomy at the time of arterial repair was not generally appreciated. During the Korean War, the advancements in vascular surgery allowed for the better restoration of blood flow to ischemic limbs, but the insight into reperfusion injuries was limited.[10] Similar observations were made in 1967 during the Vietnam War by Chandler and Knapp, who also suggested that had more fasciotomies been performed after arterial repair to the extremities, the long-term results might have been better.[11]

In 1958, Ellis brought attention to the existence of ACS in the lower extremity by describing a 2% incidence of ACS associated with tibial fractures.[12] In 1966 and 1967, two different reports described the existence of four separate compartments within the lower leg and the need for addressing each injured compartment.[13,14] After helping describe the compartments of the lower leg, Whitesides and colleagues went on to postulate a perfusion model for ACS as well as guidelines for decompression, which have been the basis for our understanding of ACS for nearly four decades.[15,16]

PATHOPHYSIOLOGY

Compartment syndrome is a condition that involves increased pressure within a confined tissue space, resulting in ischemia. This increased pressure can come through adding volume to the compartment or by decreasing the volume through external forces. There are many causes of compartment syndrome, yet ultimately, all lead to the increased pressure within a closed compartment resulting in ischemia.[16,17] The excess tissue pressure within the compartment leads to venous obstruction. If the pressure is left untreated, prolonged muscle and nerve ischemia will lead to irreversible damage to the compartment components.

Any condition increasing the content or reducing the volume of a compartment could lead to compartment syndrome, but the most prevalent cause of compartment syndrome is trauma associated with a fracture. In the cases of fracture, energy from the trauma is dissipated into the bone

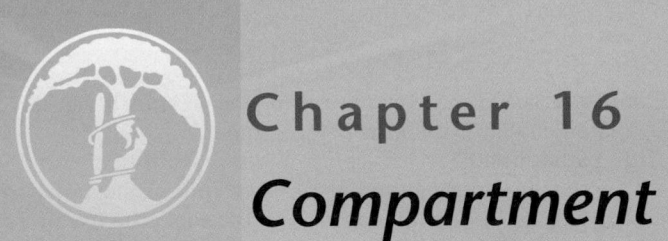

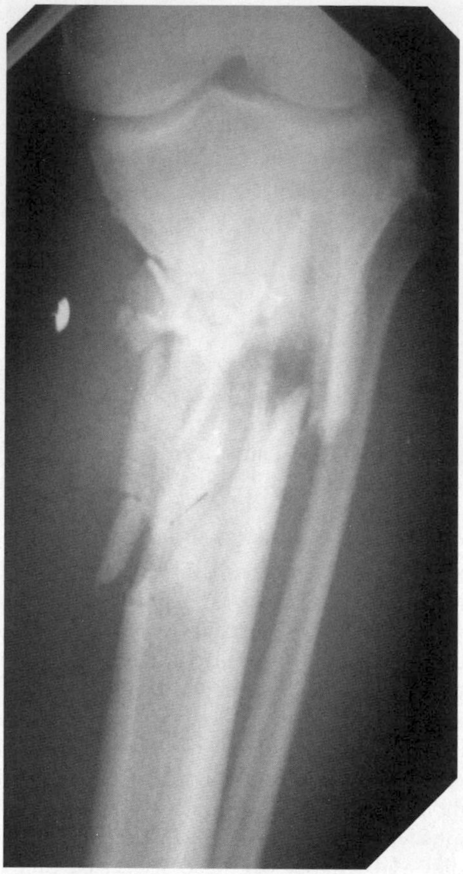

Figure 16-1. This radiograph shows a comminuted proximal tibia fracture resulting from a gunshot wound. This type of high-energy injury has a high risk of developing acute compartment syndrome (ACS). *(Courtesy of Dr. Michael S. Shuler.)*

and muscle, inducing intracellular swelling at the site of the trauma. The fracture site is also susceptible to hematoma after the injury, further amplifying the problem by increasing the volume and therefore pressure of the compartment.[18-21] High-energy tibial fractures are the most common type of injury associated with compartment syndrome, and more specifically, bicondylar plateau fractures and segmental or comminuted tibial shaft fractures (Figs. 16-2 and 16-3). ACS has been reported to complicate tibia fractures in as few as 1% to 9% of all cases and as high as 24% of polytrauma patients.[22-24] However, it is important to consider that compartment syndrome can also develop secondary to arterial injury, occlusions, reperfusion injury, crush injuries, prolonged malposition, burns, electrocutions, snake venom, stressful athletic activity, contusions, and infiltrations from intravenous (IV) sites. There is also the potential for a compartment syndrome to arise from postresuscitation systemic inflammatory response syndrome after massive blood and fluid resuscitation.[10]

Compartment syndrome may result as a complication of an arterial injury (Fig. 16-4). When it occurs, it is often observed after restoration of arterial inflow to the compartment termed *reperfusion injury*. Prior to the restoration of arterial inflow, there is a period of nerve and muscle ischemia. During hypoxia, transudation of fluid through the capillary basement membranes and the capillaries of striated muscle can occur. Once arterial inflow has been reestablished, the fluid continues to leak through the basement membrane into the interstitial space, subsequently raising the pressure because of increased content within the compartment.[25]

The pathophysiology of compartment syndrome was poorly understood during the Korean War, and misdiagnosis would often lead to poor outcomes.[10] At the time, the five or six "P's" (pain, pallor, pulselessness, paralysis, paresthesia, and poikilothermia) were most commonly used to identify compartment syndrome.[26] However, in most cases, all of the "P's" except pain are signs and symptoms associated with severe ischemia and occur too late in the process to serve as the trigger for optimal intervention and recovery. A series of tourniquet studies by Whitesides in 1971 improved our understanding of the condition.[27] By using a long cuff tourniquet and radioactive xenon imaging, the study evaluated blood reabsorption at different pressures. When the cuff pressure was at or above diastolic pressure, there was no reabsorption of xenon in the calf. However, once the cuff pressure was lowered below the diastolic pressure, xenon reabsorption was recovered. This study established the relevance of perfusion pressure (i.e., perfusion pressure = diastolic blood pressure − intracompartmental pressure) when considering compartment syndrome.[21,28]

There has been significant controversy over the pressure threshold for the diagnosis of ACS. Two theories have been proposed. One is based on an absolute value of 30 mm Hg for intracompartmental pressure,[29-31] and the other theory

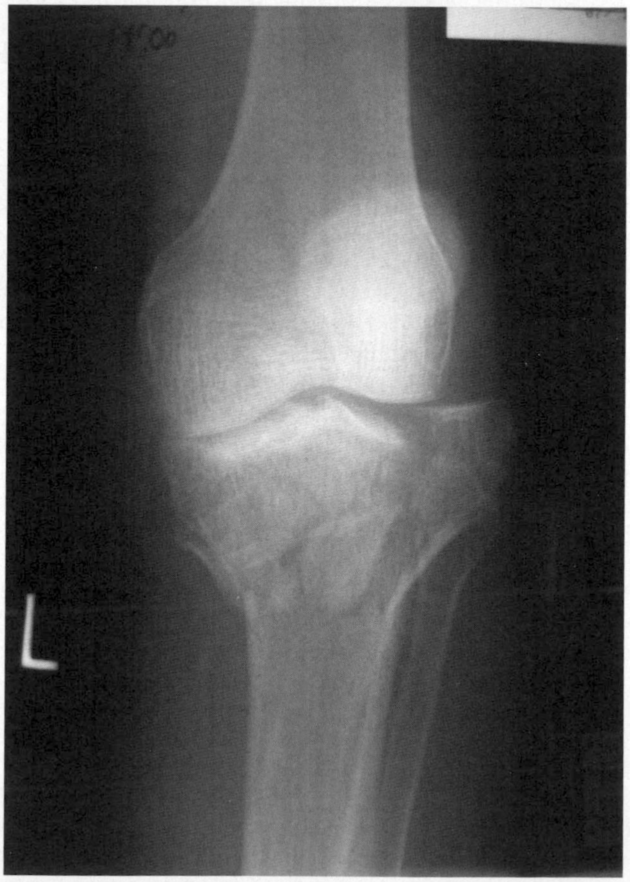

Figure 16-2. This radiograph shows a comminuted bicondylar plateau fracture. This type of high-energy injury has a high risk of developing acute compartment syndrome (ACS). *(Courtesy of Dr. Michael S. Shuler.)*

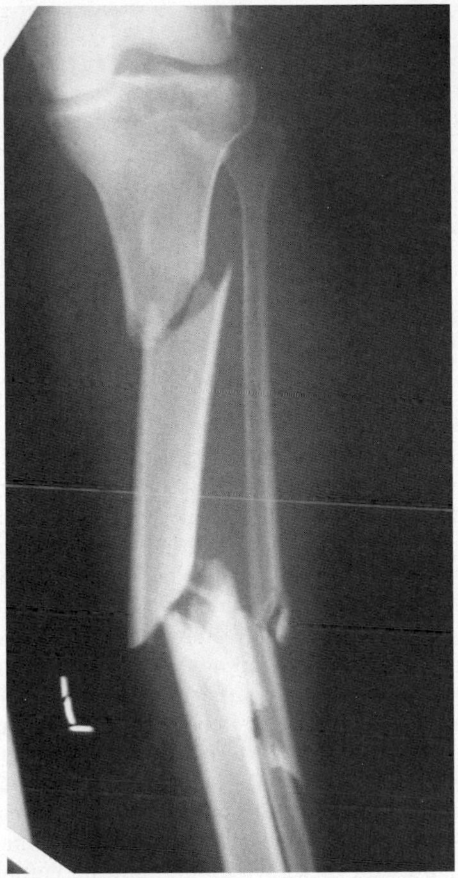

Figure 16-3. This radiograph shows a segmental tibial shaft and fibula fracture. This type of high-energy injury has a high risk of developing acute compartment syndrome (ACS). *(Courtesy of Dr. Michael S. Shuler.)*

is based on a differential value of pressure also termed *perfusion pressure* or ΔP.[16] As the body of evidence has grown, the theory of perfusion pressure has been borne out to be the more reliable and diagnostically accurate threshold for determining ACS.

Initially proposed by Whitesides and colleagues, the perfusion pressure theory was based on the fact that decreased blood flow occurs as intracompartmental pressures near the diastolic blood pressure.[16] Dahn showed that flow measured with xenon clearance stops as a cuff pressure reaches diastolic pressure.[28] Clayton and colleagues showed similar findings in a rabbit model using xenon washout.[32]

McQueen and Court-Brown reported on 116 diaphyseal tibia fractures with prospective continual monitoring of the anterior compartment.[33] Within the first 12 hours, 53 patients had absolute intracompartmental pressures higher than 30 mm Hg, 30 patients had pressures higher than 40 mm Hg, and 4 patients had pressures higher than 50 mm Hg. However, only one patient had a perfusion pressure less than 30 mm Hg, and he underwent fasciotomy without complication. Similar elevated absolute pressures were observed over the following 12 hours out to 24 hours after injury with only two patients requiring fasciotomy for perfusion pressures less than 30 mm Hg. No sequelae associated with missed ACS were reported. Previously, this group had shown that continual anterior compartment pressure monitoring leads to earlier diagnosis of ACS (diagnosed on average 16 hours from injury) and substantially less (none in their series), long-term sequelae of ACS compared to a group of patients who were not monitored and who were diagnosed much later (average, 32 hours from injury).[34] These long-term sequelae include weakness, stiffness and contracture, as well as negative effects on bone healing (delayed and increased risk of nonunion). Based on this work, McQueen and Court-Brown recommended a perfusion pressure of less than 30 mm Hg as the threshold for diagnosing ACS in the leg.[35]

White and colleagues compared two groups with continual pressure monitoring.[36] The control group consisted of 60 tibia fractures with absolute intracompartmental pressures that remained below 30 mm Hg. The study group consisted of tibial fractures with pressures greater than 30 mm Hg for at least 6 hours. No fasciotomies were performed, and there were no differences at final follow-up between groups with regard to recovery and strength. The work of these different groups provided a clinical evidence base for the superiority of perfusion pressures over absolute pressures in assessing for ACS; yet, absolute pressure thresholds remain commonly applied and commonly described in texts and articles.

Accepting perfusion pressure as the optimal means for applying information obtained from intracompartmental pressure monitoring, subsequent clinical and basic science research has been aimed at defining the most diagnostically

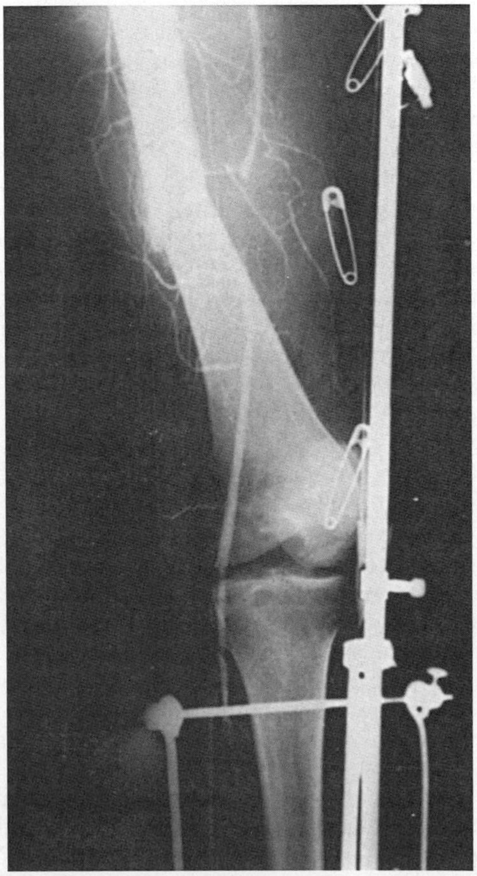

Figure 16-4. An arteriogram showing arterial disruption at the site of a fractured femur. *(From Seligson D, editor: Concepts in intramedullary nailing, Orlando, FL, 1985, Grune & Stratton, p 111.)*

accurate perfusion pressure threshold. Prayson and colleagues continually monitored 19 alert patients with tibial fractures.[37] All remained asymptomatic for ACS and showed no signs of missed ACS. Of patients, 95% had pressures of higher than 30 mm Hg; 84% had pressures that were within 30 mm Hg from diastolic pressure; and 58% had intracompartmental pressures within 20 mm Hg of diastolic. Prayson's clinical study is consistent with animal studies that suggest the threshold for ischemia and irreversible muscle damage occurs between perfusion pressures of 10 and 20 mm Hg based on diastolic blood pressure.[38,39] Despite these findings, 30 mm Hg has remained the most commonly recommended perfusion pressure threshold. This more conservative threshold increases sensitivity (i.e., maximizes chance of finding all true positives) in an attempt to ensure that a fasciotomy will be performed prior to permanent muscle and tissue damage. Because pressure measurements are typically performed as a single measurement, the goal in setting the 30 mm Hg threshold was to allow for enough time to perform an appropriate fasciotomy after a critical perfusion pressure has been recorded.[16]

The culmination of ACS research to date was a validation that perfusion pressure is the best means for using intracompartmental pressure data in the diagnosis of ACS. While perfusion pressure seemed to have been a leap forward in our understanding of how best to objectively diagnose ACS, we still have more to learn. The ambiguity in clinical and basic science research findings highlights the fact that pressure monitoring is ultimately an indirect measure or surrogate of the physiologic parameter that is at the source of ACS—perfusion.

At this point, based on the current evidence, the utility of an absolute threshold of 30 mm Hg can be considered historical. While the exact effects of moderately elevated intracompartmental pressures on muscle tissue are unknown, it seems evident that this condition does not result in significant permanent dysfunction consistent with ACS. The necessity of interpreting the intracompartmental pressure in the setting of the patient's blood pressure is vital. Understanding that blood flow is significantly decreased between 20 and 10 mm Hg perfusion will assist the surgeon in managing a potentially catastrophic disorder. By using the perfusion method in conjunction with available clinical examination, the clinician can attempt to minimize unnecessary fasciotomies while preventing missed compartment syndromes.

DIAGNOSIS: CLINICAL ASSESSMENT

The clinical diagnosis of ACS is not always obvious. Typically, the patient is polytraumatized, and ascertaining which injury is causing pain can be difficult. In many cases, the patient may be obtunded or sedated. Because of these conditions, frequent delays in ACS diagnosis can occur.[25,40-43] The subjective nature of this decision process was highlighted by O'Toole and colleagues, who examined the rate of ACS diagnosis associated with tibia fractures at a single, level I trauma center. The rate of ACS, as well as use of intracompartmental pressure measurements, varied based on the surgeon. The attending surgeons were all fellowship-trained faculty at an orthopaedic trauma fellowship program, yet the rate of ACS diagnosis in essentially the same patient population, with the same injury, varied from 2% to 24% between surgeons.[24]

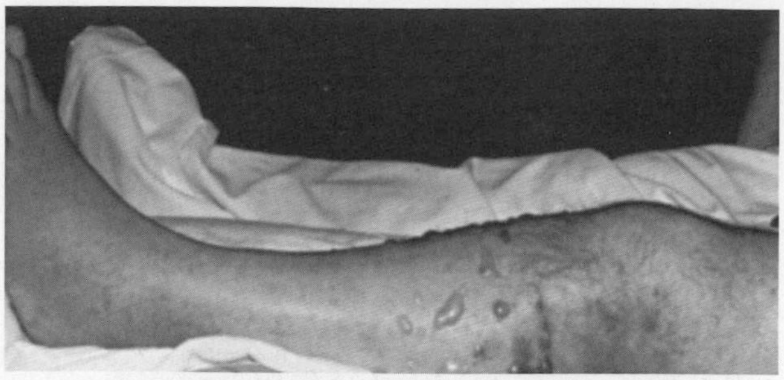

Figure 16-5. Image of a swollen leg with fracture blisters showing signs concerning for acute compartment syndrome (ACS).

The first feature of the clinical assessment is serial examination. ACS does not occur instantaneously and pressures can increase for up to 48 hours after injury or surgical procedure.[44] Identifying a change in clinical findings over time can be key to the accurate and timely diagnosis of ACS. Outcomes are directly correlated to the prompt diagnosis and treatment of ACS. If treatment is not instituted within 12 hours of symptoms, the clinical outcomes are substantially reduced.[45,46]

Clinical signs of an impending ACS include pain on palpation of the swollen, tense compartment and reproduction of pain with passive muscle stretch (Fig. 16-5). Later findings include sensory deficit in the territory of the nerves traversing the compartment and muscle weakness (Fig. 16-6). Pallor, pulselessness, paralysis, and poikilothermia (decreased temperature) are all late-stage signs that may or may not be present. If present, these symptoms indicate complete ischemia and should be considered a sign of poor prognosis.[10]

ACS is typically encountered within the first 36 to 72 hours after a traumatic injury. Peak pressures were measured between 24 and 48 hours after injury and initial pressure measurements did not correlate with maximum pressures.[44] ACS is 10 times more common in men than women and has a propensity for younger subjects, with the average age being 30 years in men and 44 years in women. High-energy injuries of the tibia followed by those of the forearm are the fractures most commonly associated with ACS. Bleeding disorders or anticoagulation are also risk factors for ACS.[47]

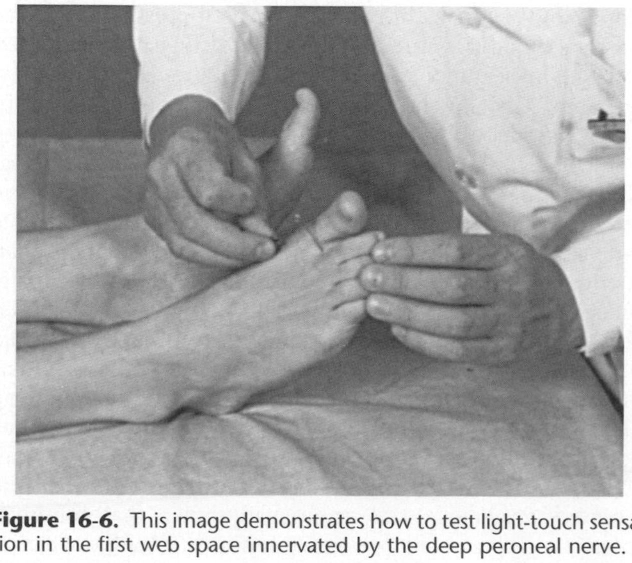

Figure 16-6. This image demonstrates how to test light-touch sensation in the first web space innervated by the deep peroneal nerve.

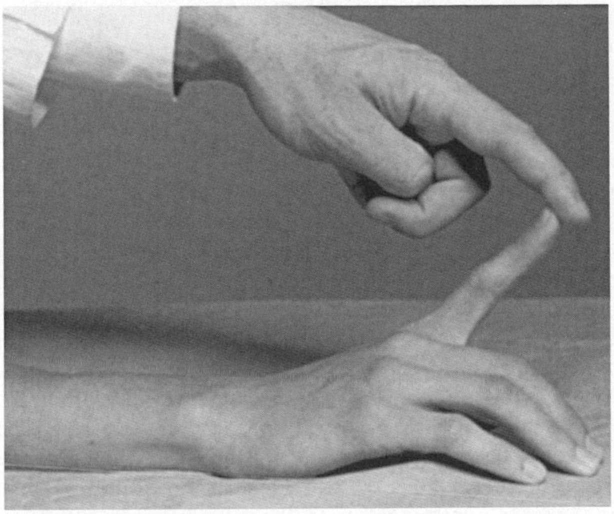

Figure 16-7. Passive stretch testing can cause pain within the associated compartment when there is decreased blood flow or ischemia.

ACS should be considered in any traumatized patient. While clinical findings are considered the gold standard, these signs cannot always be relied on. Sensitivity (13% to 19%) and positive predictive value (11% to 15%) are quite low in the traumatized patient while specificity (97%) and negative predictive values (98%) are much better.[48] In other words, if the patient has all the clinical signs, you can be fairly certain they have ACS, but the absence of signs does not necessarily imply absence of ACS. Additionally, in many instances, the patient may be obtunded or sedated leaving minimal information to gain from the clinical examination.

The earliest clinical signs associated with ACS are typically a tense compartment or extremity with increasing pain at rest and with passive stretch[18] (Fig. 16-7). The term "pain out of proportion" is commonly used to describe symptoms associated with ACS; however, in advanced ACS, this symptom may be absent.[49] Additionally, it can be difficult to assess what is "out of proportion" for any single individual. A more worrisome pain finding is progressive pain, especially when it is not well controlled by pain medications. Pulses and capillary refill are not reliable signs. They should be examined but not used to determine the existence of an ACS. Shunting can occur through vessels outside of the affected compartment(s) allowing for distal pulses and capillary refill.[50] Further, alteration in pulse, or in the extreme case, pulselessness, is an end-stage sign of ACS, and its presence may indicate a delayed diagnosis.

Any evaluation of an injured extremity, especially penetrating injuries, should include an assessment of the vascular status. Arterial injuries can be confused with or associated with ACS. Johansen and colleagues[51] demonstrated the value of measuring the Doppler-assessed ankle-brachial index (ABI) (the systolic arterial pressure in the injured extremity divided by the arterial pressure in the uninvolved arm). A value less than 0.90 necessitates further arterial investigation; 94% of patients with an index this low have positive arteriographic findings. No major arterial injuries were missed using these criteria[51] (see Fig. 16-4).

The presence of an open wound associated with the fracture should not eliminate the possibility of ACS. Between 6% and 9% of open tibial fractures are complicated by compartment syndrome, with the incidence being directly proportional to the severity of the soft tissue injury[52,53] (Fig. 16-8). Special consideration should be given to patients after fracture stabilization. In most cases, initial fracture stabilization aims to restore alignment for definitive management or for temporary management with permanent stabilization once the soft tissues are ready. It is common for ACS to develop after alignment has been restored in fractured extremities (Fig. 16-9). Intramedullary compartment pressures have been shown to increase with manipulation during intramedullary nailing of a tibia.[54] While this study showed a rapid return to lower levels of pressure, a reduction of overlapping bones will typically elongate the compartment. With elongation (i.e., distraction), a potential decrease in compartment volume can occur placing a limb at risk for ACS.[54]

Postoperative increases in pain medicine should be monitored, and patients, as well as floor staff, should be warned to monitor the injured extremity closely. The use of epidural and regional anesthetic techniques, such as pain catheters, in these patients has been a subject of debate, with case reports of delayed ACS diagnosis following each of these techniques, but systematic review of the literature calls into question the putative role of regional anesthetics in the diagnostic delays.[56] Postoperative blocks and pain pumps should be used with caution in patients for whom ACS may be concerning, specifically, upper extremity injuries such as both-bone forearm fractures. The fear is that regional or epidural anesthetics will decrease the patient's ability to detect increasing pain associated with ACS. That being said, ischemic pain tends to overcome nerve blockade, and the presence of pain (especially breakthrough pain) over a functional pain catheter should be viewed as very worrisome for ACS.[57] Over the last decade of war, the need to transport combat-injured patients great distances by land and ground transport in the initial 72 hours following injury has progressed the use of regional pain catheters in patients with injury patterns that are considered prone to ACS (like tibial shaft fractures) without an observed increase of ACS diagnosis delay related to this pain modality.[58,59] Last, a thorough postoperative evaluation or multiple

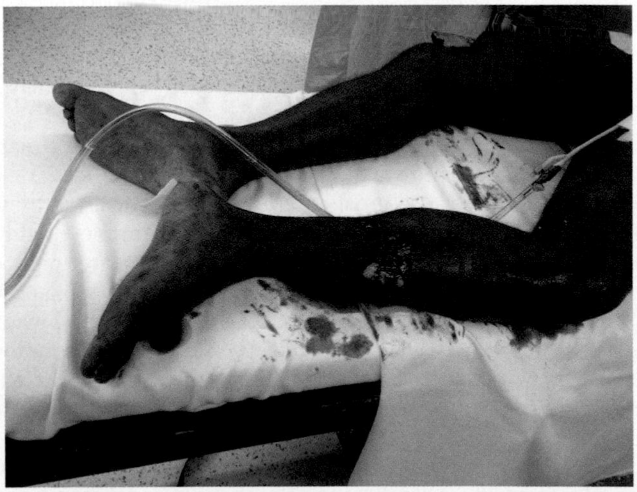

Figure 16-8. This image demonstrates an open left tibia fracture as well as an open right femur fracture. Despite the fracture being open, there is still a high risk for acute compartment syndrome (ACS). *(Courtesy of Dr. Michael S. Shuler.)*

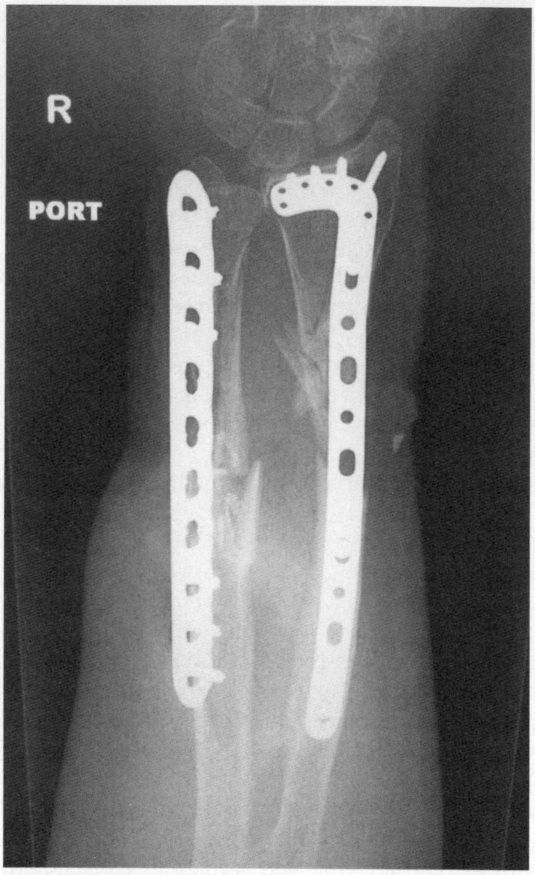

Figure 16-9. This image demonstrates a severely comminuted both-bone forearm fracture. Both-bone forearm fractures and distal radius fractures are the second most common cause of acute compartment syndrome (ACS). Care should be taken postoperatively if increasing pain occurs. Blocks should not be used postoperatively. *(Courtesy of Dr. Michael S. Shuler.)*

evaluations in the obtunded patient should be performed to detect early signs of ACS.

CRUSH SYNDROME

Crush syndrome is a medical term used specifically to describe a type of injury that can ultimately lead to devastating consequences, including death, if not managed appropriately.[60] Crush injury is typically produced by continuous and prolonged pressure and is most prevalent in the setting of mass casualties such as with earthquakes or military conflict. Crush syndrome is the second most common cause of death in these situations, behind direct injury from the catastrophe.[61] Additionally, this syndrome can occur in persons who are trapped in one position for a prolonged period or who have collapsed or fallen asleep in one position for an excessive period when under the influence of alcohol or drugs. Careful consideration should be made based on the timeline of the injury, as well as the resources available, prior to administering any medical treatments.[60]

The first step in managing the patient is to administer intravascular support. Typically, the patient experiences significant systemic hemodynamic complications such as acute renal failure and cardiac arrhythmias or collapse because of the influx of toxins and myoglobin secondary to large muscle damage.[60,62] If possible, IV catheters should be begun prior to releasing the compressive force, as once the force is released, the damaged muscle will begin to release cellular metabolites into the bloodstream.[60] It is important to remember that although elevated pressures cause muscle damage in ACS, the elevated pressures in crush syndrome are a result of already damaged muscle resulting in leaky vasculature.[63]

Appropriate management will require an understanding of both the timeline of the injury as well as the medical resources available. Surgical treatment in a crush syndrome should mirror that of an ACS with regard to timelines. Surgical release should be performed if the crush period was less than 6 to 12 hours. After 6 hours but before 12 hours of compression, the benefit of surgical release is controversial as significant muscle damage will have already occurred.[60] Surgical release after 12 hours of compression is considered contraindicated, as irreversible muscle death has already occurred and surgical release only exposes necrotic tissue to the outside environment and increases the likelihood of infection.[60] Additionally, if the compression period was less than 6 to 12 hours but elevated pressures have persisted for extended periods (greater than 6 hours), consideration for nonoperative management should be given. When in doubt and if possible, a discussion with the patient or family members regarding the potential need for revision surgery and amputation if significant necrotic muscle is encountered should take place.

In the case of a mass casualty setting, management from a surgical perspective should again center on the timeline, the time of crush and the availability of continued care and medical resources. Typical humanitarian responses can be delayed by several hours to days. In these settings and when resources are limited for continued management such as wound care and surgical closure of fasciotomies, surgical intervention should not be performed.[60,64,65] In the setting of a patient found unresponsive, an attempt at determining an accurate timeline is critical to managing the patient. If compression is alleviated within a 6-hour time frame, release of the affected compartments should be performed in an urgent manner assuming the patient is stable to undergo surgical intervention (Figs. 16-10 and 16-11). Releases after 12 hours of ischemia should be avoided because of the increased risk for infection and amputation.

The clinical examination can be very similar to ACS in crush syndrome. The patient usually suffers no pain initially and may have no physical complaints. Initially there is flaccid paralysis of the injured limb and a patchy sensory loss. Over the course of hours, swelling rapidly ensues, often far more dramatically than would be seen in compartment syndrome. The swelling is caused by rapid release of fluid because of the failure of intracellular mechanisms that allow cells to retain water. The result is clinical evidence of muscle damage with darkening of the urine related to myoglobinuria and rapid deterioration of renal function. In summary, the viability of the muscle and the ability to provide follow-up wound care and management should guide surgical intervention when managing crush syndrome.

COMPARTMENT SYNDROME IN COMBAT

While Volkmann (1881) is credited with the initial description of the aftermath of a missed compartment syndrome (the

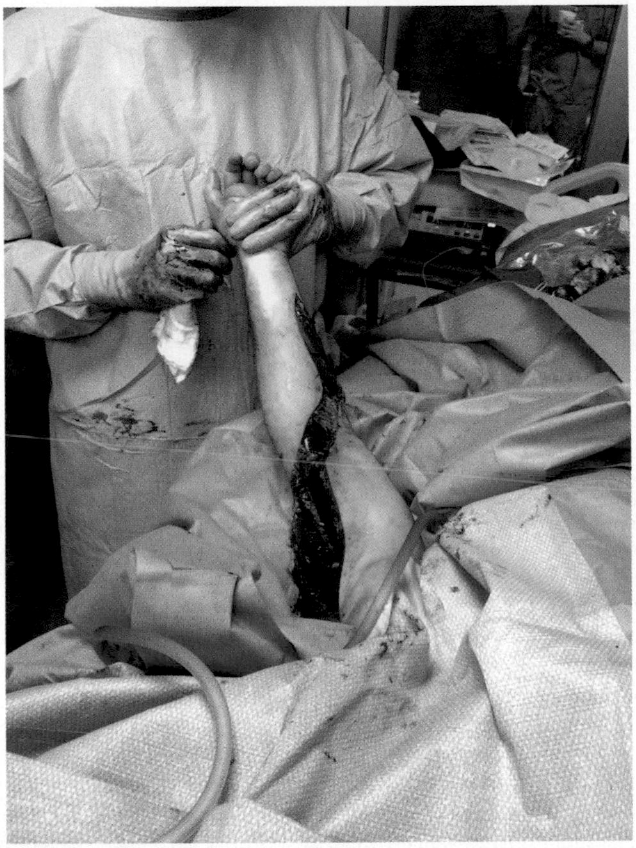

Figure 16-10. This image depicts an upper arm fasciotomy after the patient was found unconscious after intoxication. Fasciotomy was performed early and muscle necrosis was prevented. *(Courtesy of Dr. Bradley Register.)*

eponym for which is a *Volkmann contracture*), ACS has and will always remain a disease of the military surgeon. Since the Napoleonic era, when Desault and others coined the term "débridement," which described the "unbridling" of the swollen soft tissues under the nonelastic fascia following severe traumatic injury, compartment syndrome and its

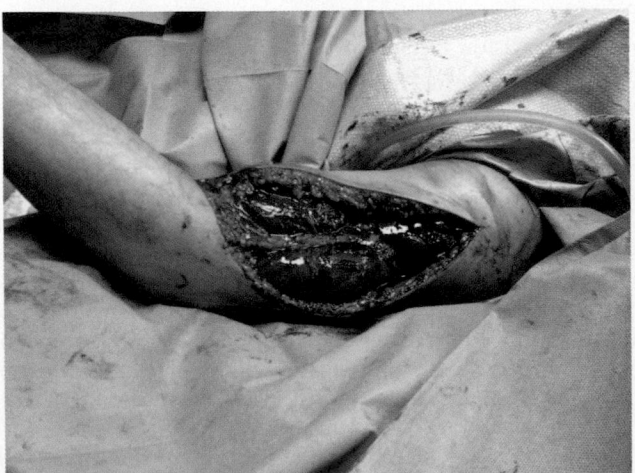

Figure 16-11. This image depicts an upper arm fasciotomy after the patient was found unconscious after intoxication. Fasciotomy was performed within the intensive care unit (ICU) because of instability secondary to myoglobinuria. *(Courtesy of Dr. Bradley Register.)*

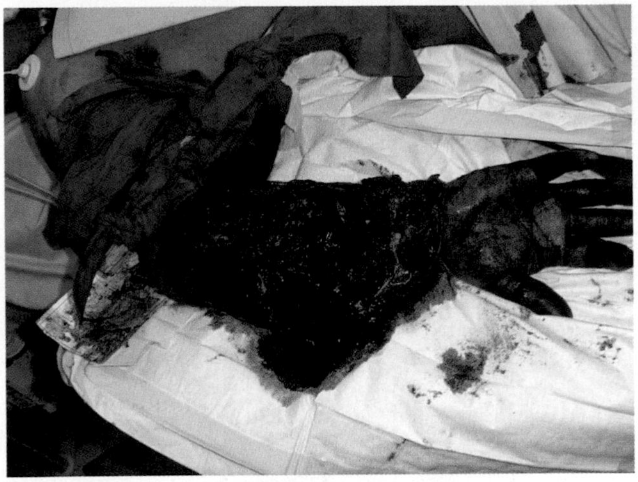

Figure 16-12. This image depicts the type of high-energy blast type injuries encountered in the combat setting.

diagnosis and management have been a constant bane of combat casualty care. Fast-forward 200 years or more to the conflicts in southwest Asia (Iraq and Afghanistan); military surgeons continue to struggle with the ideal method for diagnosing this condition.

Between September 1, 2011, and March 18, 2013, review of the Joint Theater Trauma Registry (JTTR), which is a prospectively maintained trauma registry that collects data from all echelons of care (i.e., from the battlefield support medical facilities to the major medical centers in the United States), reveals that 31% of soldiers with tibia fractures (65 out of 211) were recorded as having undergone fasciotomy. Ritenour and colleagues found that in the lead up to the "surge" in Operation Iraqi Freedom, 336 soldiers in a similar length of time (January 1, 2005, to August 21, 2006) underwent fasciotomy, with 49% being in the leg.[66] This rate of fasciotomy, a surgery whose only indication is the treatment or prophylaxis of compartment syndrome, is substantially higher than that reported in the civilian level I trauma setting. For example, O'Toole and colleagues reported a rate of 2% to 24% for tibial shaft fractures at a single major trauma center in the United States.[24] There are several explanations for this increase in fasciotomy rate in the combat setting. In some cases, the amount of energy imparted by military wounding mechanisms (i.e., improvised explosive devices [IED] blasts) is simply substantially greater than that seen in the civilian setting (Fig. 16-12). Additionally, two primary reasons for the difference in fasciotomy rates between combat and civilian casualties are the concept of a "completion" fasciotomy and the concern for transit times between echelons of care.

One of the most likely explanations for the divergence is a semantic one. The most common mechanism of injury in today's combat setting is blast related, most commonly from an IED.[66] These blast injuries produce devastating lower extremity trauma, yielding highly contaminated, grade IIIB/C fractures with large "out-to-in" open wounds (Fig. 16-13). The blast wave spontaneously rips open the fascia in many cases, at least at the injury zone. In the process of wound care, extension of the wound margins provides ready access to remaining intact fascia proximal and distal to the zone of injury. This intact fascia can act as a tourniquet, and because the wound

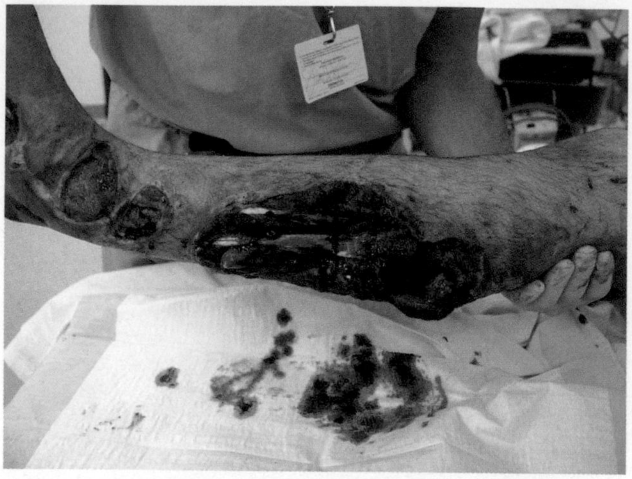

Figure 16-13. This image demonstrates the extent of soft tissue damage that is typically encountered with combat wounds.

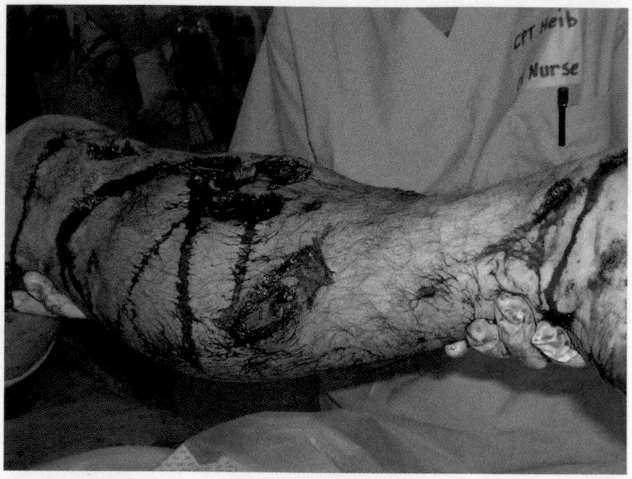

Figure 16-15. This image demonstrates the types of wounds experienced with penetrating wounds, such as shrapnel and gunshot wounds.

and wounding mechanism has introduced all of the negative aspects of fasciotomy, the benefit of completing the fascial release for the length of the compartment comes with little increased risk[3-5] (Fig. 16-14). Thus "completion" fasciotomy is one of the more common types of fasciotomies performed over the last decade of combat surgery.

While direct blast injury is the most common mechanism, there are certainly many other injuries, like gunshot wounds (Fig. 16-15), motor vehicle (land and air) accidents, and direct blows. Likewise, IED blasts that hit armored vehicles produce blunt injuries similar to civilian high-speed motor vehicle collisions. These mechanisms of injury produce long bone fractures and soft tissue responses that are similar to the civilian setting; however, these injuries also receive a higher than expected rate of fasciotomy. In this situation, one of the most cited concerns from combat surgeons is the process of aeromedical evacuation, where surgical access to the patient is lost for about 8 hours in the prime window for the development of ACS (i.e., the first 72 hours after injury). In addition,

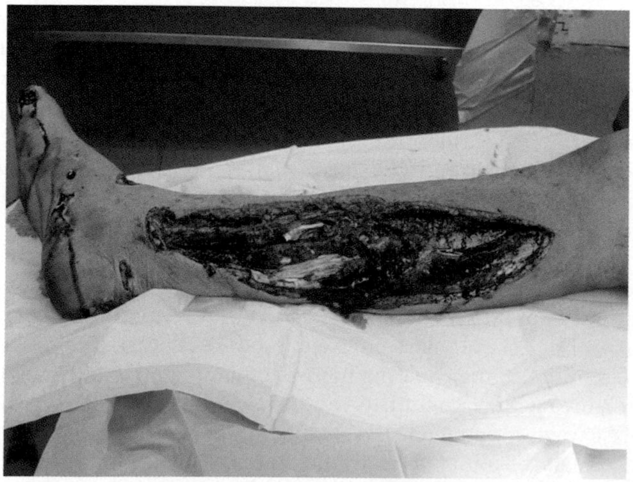

Figure 16-14. As with many combat injuries, fasciotomies are performed as a completion of fasciotomy that is partially performed during the injury.

patients are flown at altitude (cabins are typically pressurized to 8000 feet) and access to the patient to complete detailed compartment assessments is diminished. Cognizant of the theoretical potential for aero-evacuation increasing the risk of missed or delayed diagnosis of ACS and based on the results of a study conducted in the U.S. military, the U.S. Army Surgeon General issued an *All Army Activities* (ALARACT) message in May 2007 directing combat surgeons to apply "liberal use of complete fasciotomy," especially for those at highest risk. In addition, delay in evacuation of 24 hours should be considered for patients at high risk, to allow continued serial monitoring. The military retrospective study cited in this ALARACT showed that when complete fasciotomy was delayed until reaching Landstuhl Regional Medical Center, in Germany, the rate of amputation doubled (31% vs. 15%) and the rate of mortality quadrupled (19% vs. 5%), as compared to the cohort of patients who were successfully released in theater. The effect of this ALARACT was the routine and frequent use of prophylactic fasciotomy for many tibial fractures.

One of the most telling findings of the Ritenour study was that 17% of patients who underwent fasciotomy in theater, had need for revision fasciotomy to most commonly extend the fascial release (63%) or skin incision (14%). In 41% of these patients, an entire compartment was not released at the index procedure, with the anterior (40%) and deep posterior (37%) being the most commonly missed compartments. Thus, the real message was not the lack of diagnosis and fasciotomy performed on soldiers with ACS; instead, the issue was with the adequacy of surgical technique. Missing a compartment, most commonly in the leg (especially the deep posterior) and forearm, is not unique to the combat setting or surgeon, nor is the several-fold increase in amputation rate when this occurs.[67,68] The results of this study did prompt the development of a combat extremity surgery course in the U.S. Army that uses didactic and cadaver training to reinforce the proper technique for a double-incision fasciotomy of the leg, as well as fasciotomies of the other extremities, for surgeons preparing to deploy to combat medical treatment facilities.

An important lesson from this pivotal study is that simply making the incisions on the leg or other limb does not ensure that a fasciotomy has been successfully performed. This fact is most important in the setting of prophylactic fasciotomy, where the patient who receives an incomplete fascial release is exposed to all of the risk and morbidity of the procedure without the maximal potential benefit.[67] While the improved training and attention to detail that has emerged as a result of Ritenour's study has benefited combat casualties, the use of this data to reinforce an exaggerated use of fasciotomy, many of which are prophylactic, is a lasting undesirable effect of this study. Conversely, possibly the most beneficial impact of this study is that it has generated substantial commitment of Department of Defense (DoD) research dollars directed toward finally understanding ACS and developing a gold standard for diagnosis that uses reliable, readily attainable objective information to define the presence or absence of this purely physiologic disease.

MEASUREMENT TECHNIQUES

Reliable and accurate intracompartmental pressures can be difficult to obtain in the hands of an experienced clinician.[69] Practice and attention to detail during measurements can help avoid errors in measurement. Measurements taken when pressure is erroneously elevated may prompt a surgeon to act inappropriately and perform an unnecessary fasciotomy; therefore, it is critical to obtain accurate measurements.

As described by Heckman and colleagues, the measurement should be performed within 5 cm of the fracture site when evaluating fracture patients.[70] Highest pressures were obtained within 5 cm of the fracture and dissipated as pressures were recorded further away from the fracture site. Additionally, deeper values have been shown to be higher than more superficial values.[71]

At the time of measurement, the position of the foot (in the case of leg ACS) should be maintained in a neutral position without extreme dorsiflexion or plantar flexion. Dorsiflexion will increase posterior compartment pressures, whereas plantar flexion will increase the anterior and lateral compartments. The ideal position is between neutral and the resting position or between 0 and 37 degrees of plantar flexion.[72] Additionally, when measuring the posterior compartments, a rolled sheet or towel should be placed under the heel to remove any pressure associated with the weight of the leg pressing down on the bed (Fig. 16-16). The injured extremity should not be elevated to decrease edema, as this maneuver will increase the intracompartmental pressure in, and decrease perfusion to, the extremity.[73,74]

The injured extremity should have all constrictive or circumferential dressing removed. Garfin and colleagues showed in an animal model that removal of a plaster cast resulted in a 60% reduction in intracompartmental pressures. Cutting the cast, spreading the cast, cutting the cast padding, and ultimately, cast removal all resulted in sequential decreases in intracompartmental pressure.[75]

There have been several studies examining the difference between different pressure measurements. The Stryker Stic and arterial lines have been shown to provide reliable and reproducible readings.[69,76] Straight needles as well as smaller gauge needles have shown a propensity to overestimate the intracompartmental pressure.[69,77] Wick catheters and side port needles have shown a more reliable reading when compared to an 18-gauge needle.[69,77] Regardless of instrument used, once the needle is inserted into the limb, a small amount of fluid (roughly 0.1 to 0.2 mL) should be injected through the needle to clear the needle of any soft tissue that may have been trapped in the needle during insertion. If this maneuver is not performed, erroneously high measurements may be obtained.

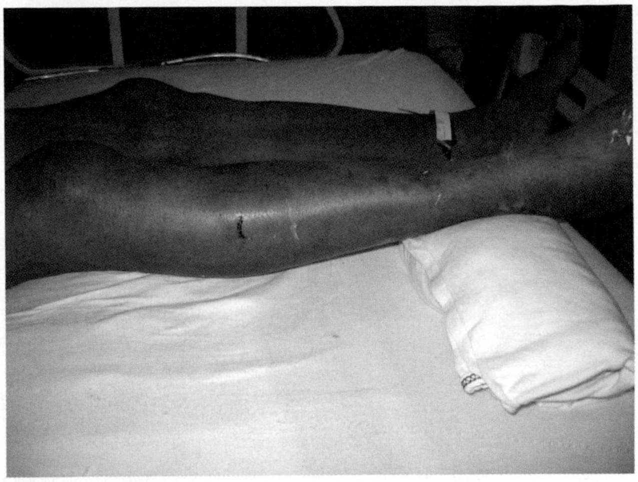

Figure 16-16. A towel or sheet can be rolled and placed under the heel to reduce the pressure in the posterior compartments when measuring the pressures. Elevation should be avoided, as this increases the pressure and reduces blood flow in the injured extremity. *(Courtesy of Dr. Michael S. Shuler.)*

Needle Manometer

The first direct attempt at measurement of interstitial compartment pressure was by Landerer in 1884.[78] Subsequently, French and Price[79] reported on the usefulness of the technique in diagnosis of chronic compartment syndrome. Whitesides and colleagues[15,16] first applied the needle manometer technique to the diagnosis of ACS. In their original description, an 18-gauge needle was connected to a 20-mL syringe by a column of saline and air, and this column was then connected to a standard mercury manometer. After the needle was injected into the compartment, the air pressure within the syringe was raised until the saline-air meniscus was seen to move. The pressure was then read off the mercury manometer (Fig. 16-17). Details of the technique have been well described.[15,16]

Arterial Line Catheter

A common means of measuring intracompartmental pressures without specialty devices is through the use of an arterial line. An arterial line is attached to any standard critical care or pressure-sensing monitor. The IV tubing is then connected to an IV bag. The tubing is attached to a stopcock valve and a 10-cc syringe full of saline is attached to the stopcock. A 16-gauge needle is attached to the stopcock needle. The system is then primed and zeroed at the level of the extremity (Fig. 16-18). Care must be taken to have the transducer at the level of the injured extremity as well. Once zeroed, the needle is inserted and a small amount of saline is injected through the needle with the stopcock opened to the syringe. The stopcock is then switched to allow free flow between the needle tip and the IV tubing and transducer (Video 16-1).

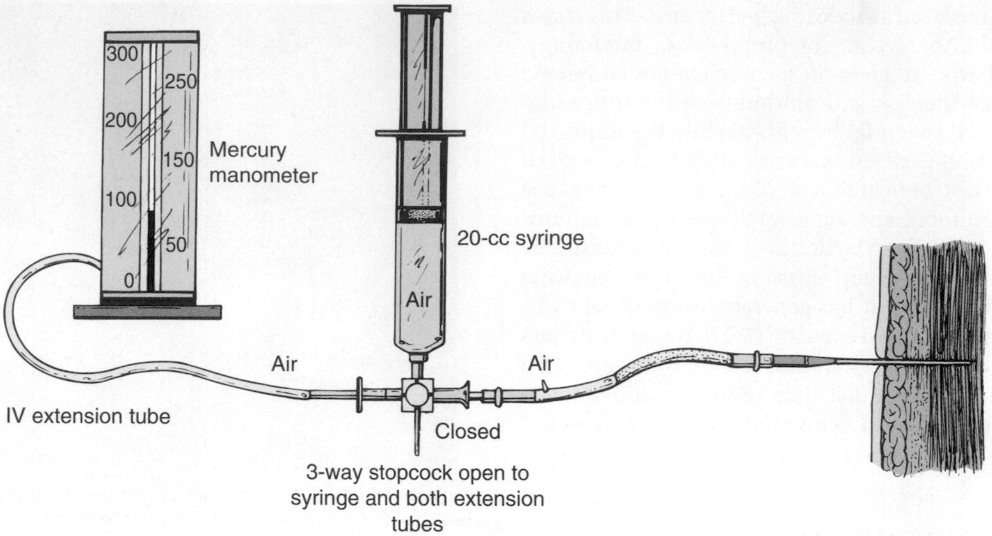

Figure 16-17. The needle injection technique measures compartment pressure by looking for movement of the air-saline meniscus. *IV,* Intravenous. *(Redrawn from Whitesides TE Jr, Haney TC, Morimoto K, Hirada H: Tissue pressure measurements as a determinant for the need of fasciotomy, Clin Orthop Relat Res 113:46, 1975.)*

Stryker Stic Catheter System

The Stryker Stic catheter system manufactured by Stryker is a handheld device that allows the surgeon to measure intracompartmental pressures quickly and simply (Fig. 16-19). The device is easy to use; it can be carried in the pocket and used in the emergency department without having to search for pieces of equipment. It has been shown to be reliable and accurate.[69,76]

The method of use is relatively simple, which has led to its increase in popularity. The device needs to be adequately "charged" for accurate use. A disposable syringe preloaded with fluid is connected to the measuring instrument, and a disposable needle-catheter that comes as part of the set is then added to the other end (Video 16-2). After the system is purged with some fluid, the monitor is zeroed at the level of the compartment to be tested and the needle is then inserted through the fascia (Fig. 16-20). The numbers on the monitor screen fall reasonably rapidly, and as the descent levels off, a reading of the compartment pressure can be made. The pressure reading on the monitor may continue to drop slowly with time and some individual variation may occur in determining the pressure at which leveling off has occurred (Video 16-3).

Microporous Catheter

The catheter system designed by Twin Star Medical has been shown to allow for continuous pressure measurements. A catheter is inserted using a needle and sheath to insert the catheter. The sheath is then peeled away to leave the soft microporous catheter to constantly record pressures (Fig. 16-21). The catheter is then attached to the skin to prevent

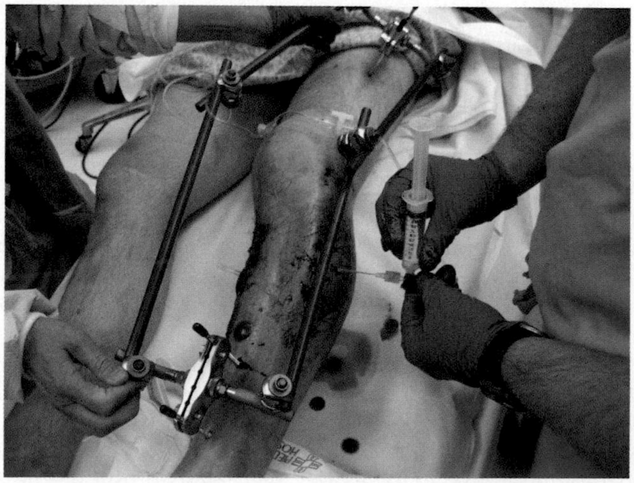

Figure 16-18. Pressure measurements can be obtained using an arterial line and a 16-gauge needle as depicted in this image (lateral compartment). The pressure transducer should be at the level of the injured extremity and the line should be flushed and zeroed with the needle ready to insert. *(Courtesy of Dr. Michael S. Shuler.)*

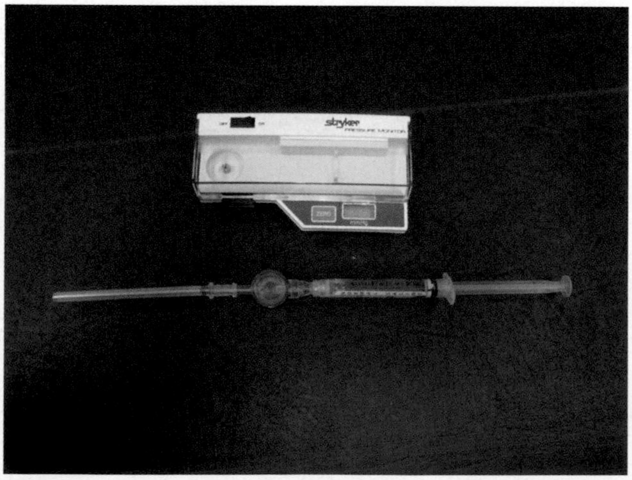

Figure 16-19. The Stryker Stic unit comes in three pieces that are assembled into a single syringe and needle unit. *(Courtesy of Dr. Michael S. Shuler.)*

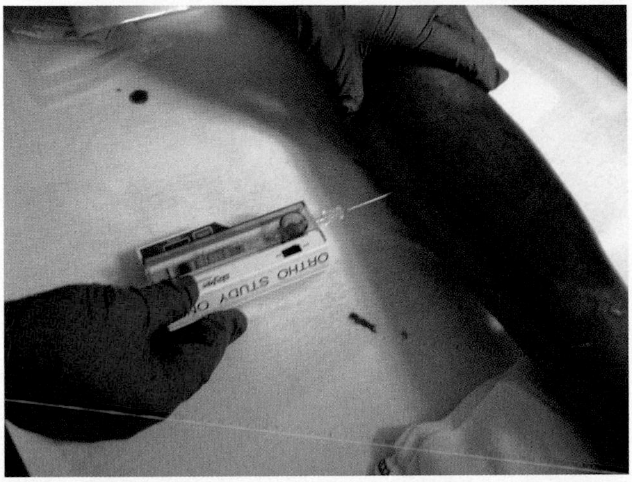

Figure 16-20. This image demonstrates the Stryker Stic device being used to measure the lateral compartment of an injured leg. *(Courtesy of Dr. Michael S. Shuler.)*

inadvertent removal.[81,82] This indwelling catheter allows for continual pressure monitoring without the necessity of continual nursing involvement. It also eliminates the risk of increasing pressures through the continual infusion of fluids required in traditional continual pressure monitoring using an IV catheter. Additionally, this technology allows for tissue ultrafiltration through the catheter. By removing some of the fluid from the compartment, tissue ultrafiltration may allow for prevention of ACS by reducing the volume within the compartment.[81,82]

NEW TECHNOLOGIES

The ideal monitoring system for ACS would allow for a reliable method for monitoring muscle and tissue perfusion in a noninvasive, continual fashion with real-time responsiveness. Many different approaches have been suggested as viable options for monitoring at-risk extremities and diagnosing

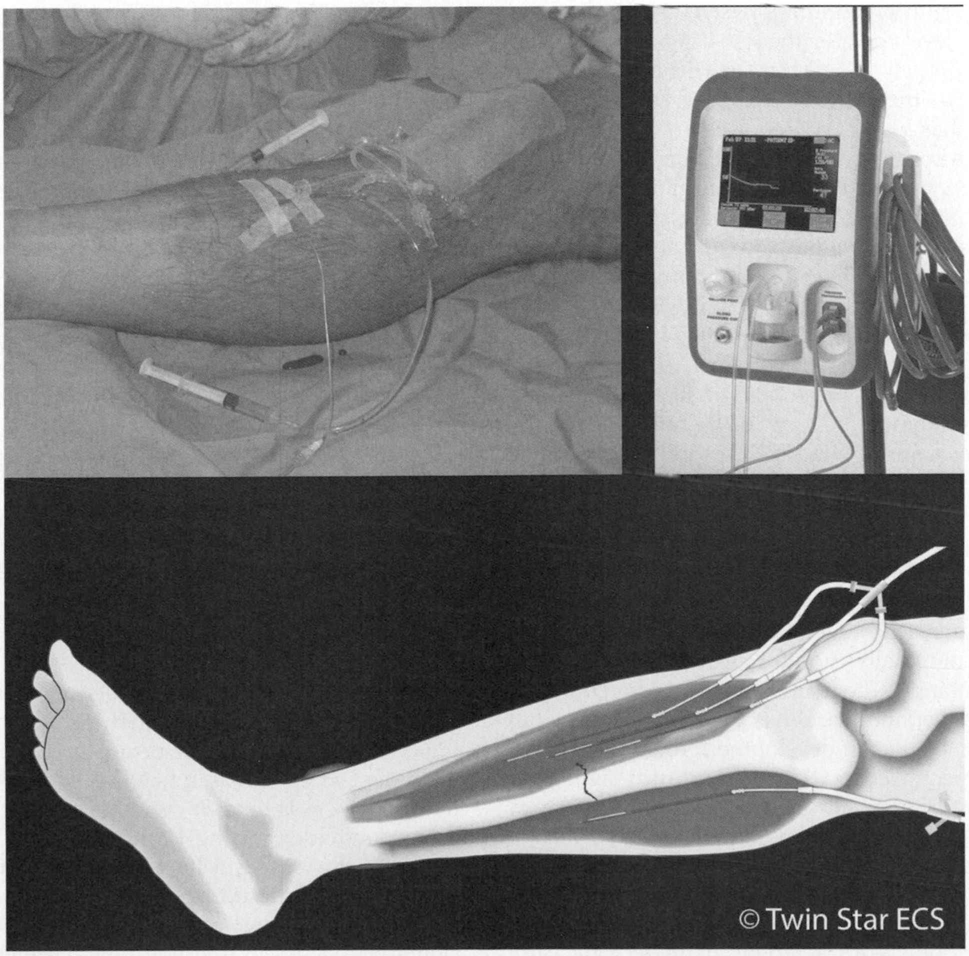

Figure 16-21. Continuous pressure monitoring using a combined solid state pressure sensor and tissue ultrafiltration (TUF) catheter. Clinical photo of a catheter in the anterior compartment of a patient's left leg *(upper left)*. The catheters are connected to a monitor that displays pressure over time *(upper right)*. A drawing depicting placement of a combined pressure and TUF catheter in both the anterior and deep posterior leg compartments, with additional small TUF-only catheters in the anterior compartment *(lower panel)*. *(Images © Twin Stat ECS, used with permission; courtesy of Dr. Andrew Schmidt.)*

ACS. This section will cover several newer technologies. At this point, no technology has been proven to provide reliable and timely information for the diagnosis of ACS.

ACS is by definition an inflammatory process that occurs in the setting of significant chemical and physiologic changes from an uninjured baseline. Recent studies have focused on the potential benefits of combating the inflammatory phase of injury to minimize or prevent muscle and tissue damage. Animal studies have shown that neutropenic rats showed significantly less muscle damage when compared to immune-competent rats when ACS was induced using an infusion technique.[83] Additionally, the use of indomethacin has shown some ability to reduce the effects of ACS in animal models. The pretreatment showed higher benefits than in a delayed fashion.[84] Other medical managements have been suggested in order to increase the perfusion pressure. Potential options are the use of mannitol, diuretics, or modalities to increase blood pressure. The risks of possible adverse effects associated with bleeding, immune suppression, or organ damage based on associated injuries must be weighed when considering any of these systemic medical managements.

Blood and serum markers have also been investigated as potential indications of impending compartment syndrome. There have been many laboratory measures that have been suggested as possible indicators for ACS. In a retrospective study, maximum serum creatinine kinase (CK) levels above 4000 U/L, chloride levels greater than 104 mg/dL, and minimum blood urea nitrogen (BUN) less than 10 mg/dL showed a high correlation to the development of ACS.[85] Ischemia-modified albumin has also been reported to correlate with limb ischemia when compared to uninjured healthy individuals.[86] Serum markers may prove to play an important role in the diagnosis of ACS; however, serum markers may be difficult to interpret in the setting of the polytrauma patient with multiple muscular skeletal injuries. Tissue ultrafiltration has been used to evaluate CK levels as well as lactate dehydrogenase. These markers have been shown to be elevated in ACS, but the details are still being worked out for how to use this new information.[81,82] Serial laboratory levels will likely be required to monitor the development of ACS in the future. The challenge will be in determining markers that indicate ischemic muscle prior to permanent muscle injury.

Radiofrequency identification (RFID) chips are a common means of transferring data or identification without the necessity of battery power. With the development of miniature sensors that allow for pressure monitoring, the coupling of RFID and miniature sensors could allow for implantable sensors that can continually monitor pressures without the need for wires or tubing.[87] The potential to allow for continual pressure monitoring without wires has substantial appeal, but this option still has significant development requirements.

Near-infrared spectroscopy (NIRS) has shown significant potential for monitoring tissue perfusion in the setting of ACS.[88-95] NIRS uses technology and physical laws that are similar to that used in pulse oximetry to solve for the percent of oxygenated and deoxygenated hemoglobin.[96-98] While pulse oximetry measures light that passes through tissue, such as a finger, toe or earlobe, NIRS regional oximeters measure reflected light that travels in arcs outward from the point it is emitted into the tissue. This method is validated, and U.S. Food and Drug Administration (FDA)-approved devices exist for measuring oxygen saturation in the brain and somatic (i.e., extremity) tissues up to 3 cm deep; however, existent technology has been validated for nontraumatized tissues, which is not the state that is relevant to monitoring for ACS. The depth of measurement can be up to 3 cm with some devices and is directly related to the distance between the light emitter from the photoreceptor, both located on the sensor pad.[96-98] The greater this distance, the greater the depth of tissue being monitored. This depth is sufficient to measure muscular tissue in all four compartments of the leg regardless of body habitus and weight.[99] NIRS has also shown the ability to isolate oxygenation levels in specific compartments in an extremity.[100] The appeal of NIRS is it provides a continual noninvasive, nonpainful means for measuring the physiologic parameter that dictates ACS, that being perfusion/tissue oxygenation[101] (Fig. 16-22). Ideal methods for NIRS monitoring of traumatized tissues, as well as guidelines and indications, still need to be elucidated before NIRS becomes a reliable instrument in the management of ACS. This vital research is ongoing.

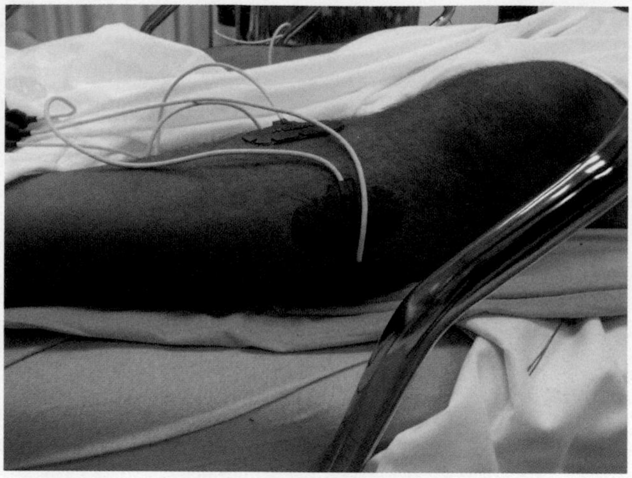

Figure 16-22. This image demonstrates the configuration used to monitor the lower extremity using near-infrared spectroscopy (NIRS) sensors. NIRS offers a noninvasive, continual real-time monitoring system. *(Courtesy of Dr. Michael S. Shuler.)*

As NIRS technology advances, there may be a role for using postfasciotomy NIRS values to assess adequacy of decompression, timeliness, and possibly need for fasciotomy. In patients whose regional muscle oxygenation values are reduced because of compromised blood supply from ACS, complete release of the compartments in a timely fashion should result in restoration (and possibly hyperemic increase) of the normal oxygenation values. Failure of NIRS values to restore to normal or to increase a significant amount from preoperative levels may indicate incomplete release or myonecrosis.[91]

In the end, ACS is akin to a "heart attack" of the leg. Using this analogy, it is hard to conceive of an acute coronary syndrome unit today using laying of hands, auscultation, and clinical history as a means of diagnosing myocardial infarction. It would be unthinkable not to use validated, objective physiologic measures, such as electrocardiogram (ECG) and laboratory values as the gold standard for diagnosing this purely physiologic disease. Unfortunately, despite centuries of medical awareness of ACS, we have yet to develop a physiomonitoring technology that has the same level of accuracy and reliability that we have for myocardial infarction. With

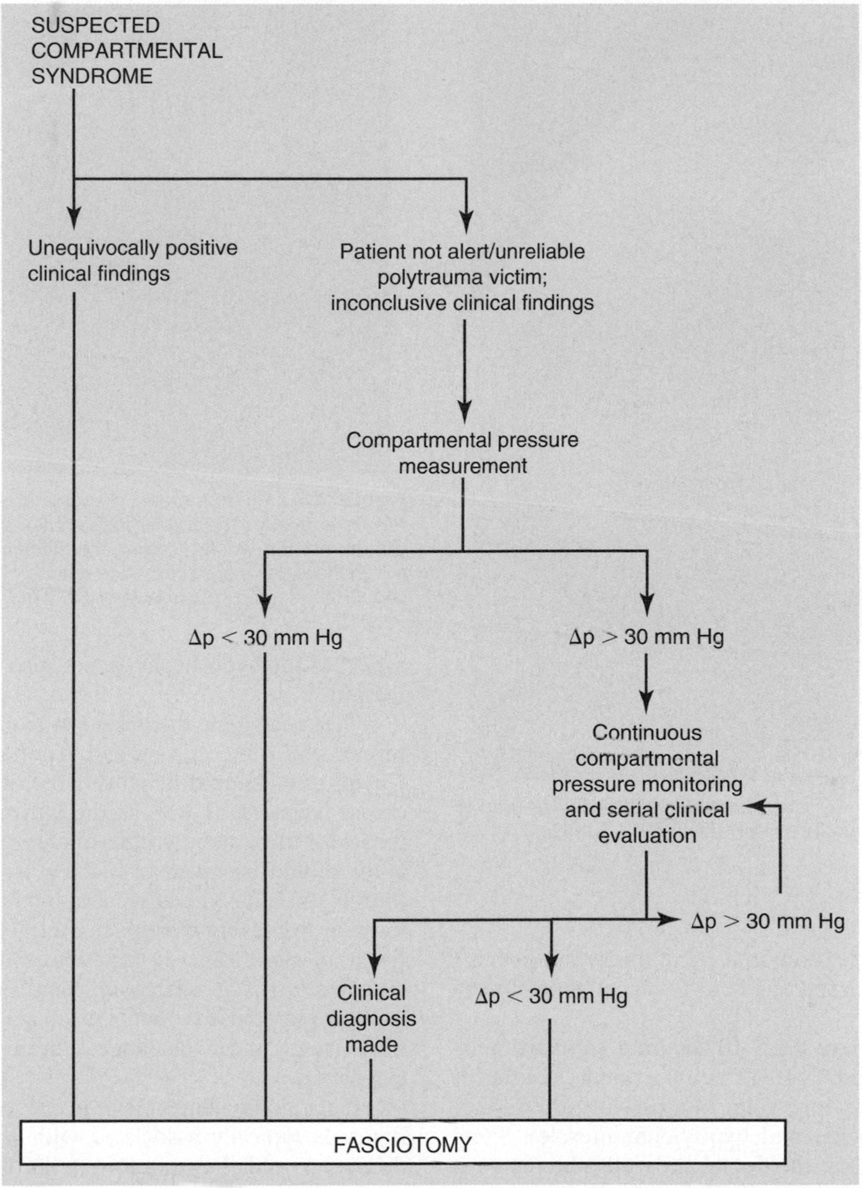

Figure 16-23. An algorithm for management of a patient with suspected compartment syndrome. Δp is defined as the difference between the diastolic pressure and the measured compartment pressure in mm Hg as documented by McQueen and Court-Brown.

continued DoD funding and the ongoing research alluded to earlier, an accurate diagnostic algorithm that uses reliable physiological measures to successfully identify those who will and just as importantly, those who will not, benefit from the morbidity of a fasciotomy procedure is nearing.[99,100]

FASCIOTOMY TECHNIQUES

A patient with an established compartment syndrome has the clinical signs and symptoms of nerve and muscle ischemia in conjunction with elevated compartment pressure. A treatment algorithm (Fig. 16-23) is a useful guide for management of such patients.

Any surgical decompression for ACS must adequately decompress all compartments that are at risk or likely to become at risk. Skin, fat, and fascial layers must all be widely decompressed and left open. Matsen and coworkers[103,104] have shown that each layer contributes to the constriction of the muscle compartment, and attempts at closure of part or all of any one of these layers at the time of fasciotomy risk endangering muscle.

Compartment Syndrome of the Hand

The first description of ACS of the hand was made by Bunnell in 1948 after WW II. While examining injured veterans, he noticed many wounded warriors had contractures of the hand associated with upper extremity injuries that were treated in a circumferential plaster cast that extended past the fingertips.[105] The diagnostic triad described by Spinner and associates is pain, paralysis, and increased pain with passive stretch of the intrinsic muscles. The hand is typically severely swollen and rests in the intrinsic minus position (metacarpal phalangeal joints extended and interphalangeal joints flexed). Hand

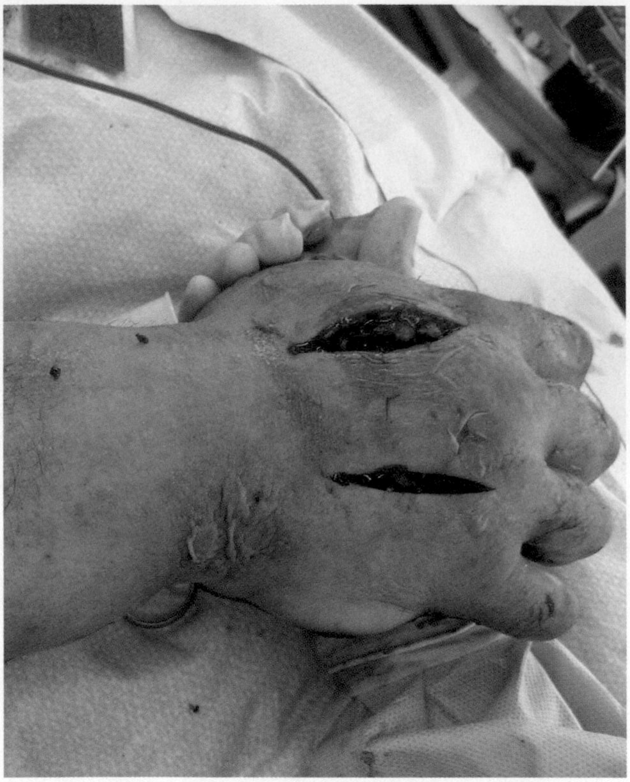

Figure 16-24. This image demonstrates the dorsal incisions used to release the interosseous muscles within the hand. *(Courtesy of Dr. Michael S. Shuler.)*

ACS normally occurs as a result of a crush injury but can also occur in association with fractures of the carpal bone or venomous bites.[106,107]

Traditionally there have been 10 separate compartments associated with the hand.[108] These compartments consist of four dorsal interosseous, three volar interosseous, the adductor pollicis, and the thenar and hypothenar muscles. Some research has suggested that the dorsal and volar interosseous muscles as well as the adductor pollicis do not contain separate fascias, reducing the number to six compartments.[109,110]

Surgical release should be made through four separate incisions when releasing compartments of the hand. Two dorsal incisions, one over the index metacarpal and one over the ring metacarpal, should be made. Through the index incision, the first and second dorsal interosseous can be released by making incisions on each side of the index metacarpal. Also, the adductor pollicis and volar interosseous compartments can be released as needed through blunt dissection volarly on the radial side of the index metacarpal. The second incision over the ring metacarpal can be used to release the third and fourth dorsal interosseous by making incisions on either side of the ring metacarpal. Additionally, the volar interosseous muscle can be released as needed through deep dissection on the radial side of the ring and small finger metacarpal[111] (Figs. 16-24 to 16-26).

Two separate longitudinal incisions for the thenar and hypothenar eminence should be made. The thenar incision should be made along the glabrous skin edge (where the hair stops at the edge of the palm) on the radial edge of the thenar muscles. The hypothenar release should be made on the ulnar

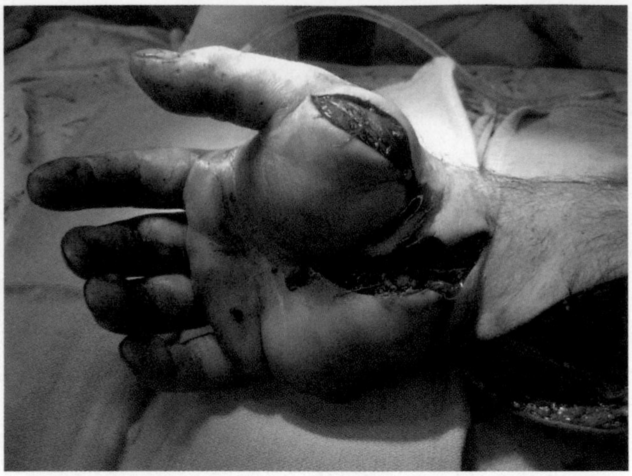

Figure 16-25. This image demonstrates the open carpal tunnel release as well as the thenar incision along the glabrous skin edge of the thumb. If possible, keeping the median nerve covered at the wrist is beneficial. However, complete release of the pressure on the nerve should be insured. *(Courtesy of Dr. Michael S. Shuler.)*

aspect of the hypothenar aspect, also along the glabrous skin margin.[111]

When managing hand injuries requiring fasciotomy, carpal tunnel syndrome as well as ulnar nerve compression at the Guyon canal should be considered. Release of the transverse carpal ligament as well as the Guyon canal should be performed if there are any signs of nerve compression. Consideration should be given to placing an external fixator on the thumb and index metacarpal to hold the first web space apart in order to prevent web space contracture. This deformity can result in significant dysfunction and proves to be difficult to correct. If left untreated, hand compartment syndrome results in interosseous contraction and an intrinsic plus deformity (metacarpal phalangeal flexion and interphalangeal extension).

Finger compartment syndrome can occur as well. This injury is typically associated with hand compartment syndrome. A midaxial incision at the end of the volar flexion crease should be performed. By placing the incision at the

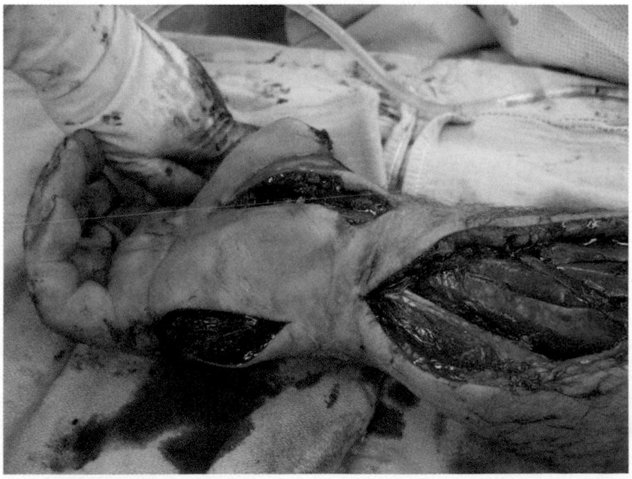

Figure 16-26. This image demonstrates the open carpal tunnel release as well as the hypothenar incision along the glabrous skin edge of the hand. *(Courtesy of Dr. Michael S. Shuler.)*

edge of the flexion crease, the neurovascular bundle should be protected volarly. Release of the Cleland ligament and the transverse retinacular ligament will assist in preventing neurovascular injury. Incisions should be placed on the radial side of the thumb and small finger and ulnarly on the index, middle, and ring fingers. Incisions in the first web space as well as the ulnar side of the small finger should be avoided.[112]

Compartment Syndrome of the Forearm

Compartment syndrome of the forearm is the second most common area to develop ACS behind the lower leg.[47,66] It is usually associated with a fracture with a direct blow or crushing component of the injury. Court-Brown and McQueen's review of their experience showed that forearm compartment syndrome tended to occur with associated fractures of the distal radius.[47] It has also been seen with inadvertent soft tissue fluid infiltration, grease-gun injuries, deep infection often associated with IV drug abuse, venomous bites, and burns resulting in inelastic eschars. Attempted closure of a tight surgical wound after internal fixation of forearm injuries may also place these compartments at risk.[112]

The forearm consists of three compartments, the volar, dorsal, and the mobile wad. The volar compartment can be subdivided into the superficial (pronator teres, the flexor carpi radialis, flexor digitorum superficialis, and the flexor carpi ulnaris) and the deep compartment (flexor digitorum profundus, flexor pollicis longus, and pronator quadratus). The mobile wad consists of the brachioradialis, as well as the extensor carpi radialis brevis and longus. The dorsal compartment consists of the rest of the extensors of the forearm.

The volar compartments can be addressed using a Henry approach or through a volar ulnar approach. In either approach, the deep flexors need to be released. Once the volar compartments are released, the dorsal and mobile wad should be reassessed. Often, the volar release reduces the pressure in the remaining two compartments. If necessary, a dorsal Thompson approach should be performed. With any forearm release, the carpal tunnel should also be released. Complete release of the median nerve as well as the ulnar nerve in the Guyon canal should be performed to prevent neurologic deficits. Surgical planning should be made preoperatively if possible to allow skin coverage of the nerves and prevent extended exposure of the nerves to the outside environment allowing for desiccation.

Volar (Henry) Approach

Decompression of the superficial and deep volar flexor compartments of the forearm can be done through a single incision (Fig. 16-27). The skin incision should begin proximal to the antecubital fossa and extend to the palm across the carpal tunnel. Compartmental pressure measurements can be taken intraoperatively to confirm decompression. No tourniquet should be used. The skin incision begins medial to the biceps tendon, crosses the elbow crease, is carried toward the radial side of the forearm, and extends distally along the medial border of the brachioradialis, continuing across the palm along the thenar crease. The fascia overlying the superficial flexor compartment is readily incised, beginning at a point 1 or 2 cm proximal to the elbow and extending distally across the carpal tunnel into the palm. Anything short of this is viewed as an inadequate decompression (Figs. 16-28 and 16-29).

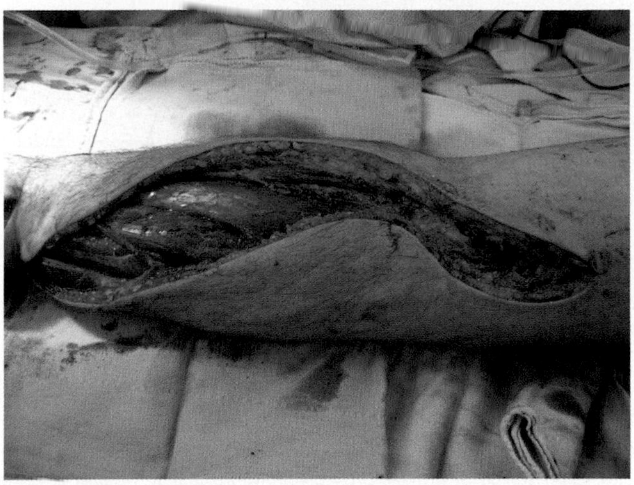

Figure 16-27. This image shows a forearm fasciotomy using the Henry approach. *(Courtesy of Dr. Michael S. Shuler.)*

The superficial radial nerve is identified under the brachioradialis, both are retracted to the radial side of the forearm, and the flexor carpi radialis is retracted to the ulnar side. The radial artery can be retracted either radially or ulnarly. This action exposes the flexor digitorum profundus and flexor pollicis longus in the depths, the pronator quadratus distally, and the pronator teres proximally. Because the effects of forearm compartment syndrome most commonly involve the deep flexor compartment in the forearm, it is imperative to decompress the fascia over each of these muscles to ensure that a thorough and complete decompression has been performed. Eaton and Green[113] recommended epimysiotomy in addition to fasciotomy, but this is not usually necessary in the acute case. Muscle viability is difficult to ascertain intraoperatively. Questionably viable muscle should be excised with caution at the time of fasciotomy. The patient should be brought back to the operating room 24 to 48 hours later for a dressing change and further débridement of muscle. The median nerve should be carefully inspected; if it appears excessively swollen, a neurolysis of the nerve should be performed.

Skin flaps can be elevated radially and the mobile wad can be released through this approach as well. The mobile wad

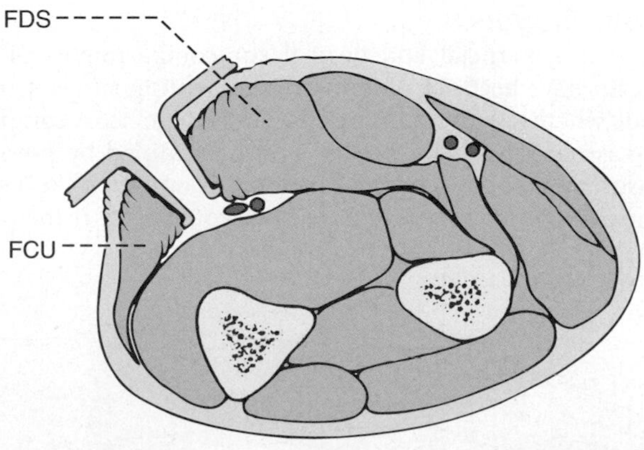

Figure 16-28. The Henry approach to the volar aspects of the forearm. *FCU,* Flexor carpi ulnaris; *FDS,* flexor digitorum superficialis. *(Modified from Whitesides TE Jr, Haney TC, Morimoto K, Hirada H: Tissue pressure measurements as a determinant for the need of fasciotomy, Clin Orthop Relat Res 113:46, 1975.)*

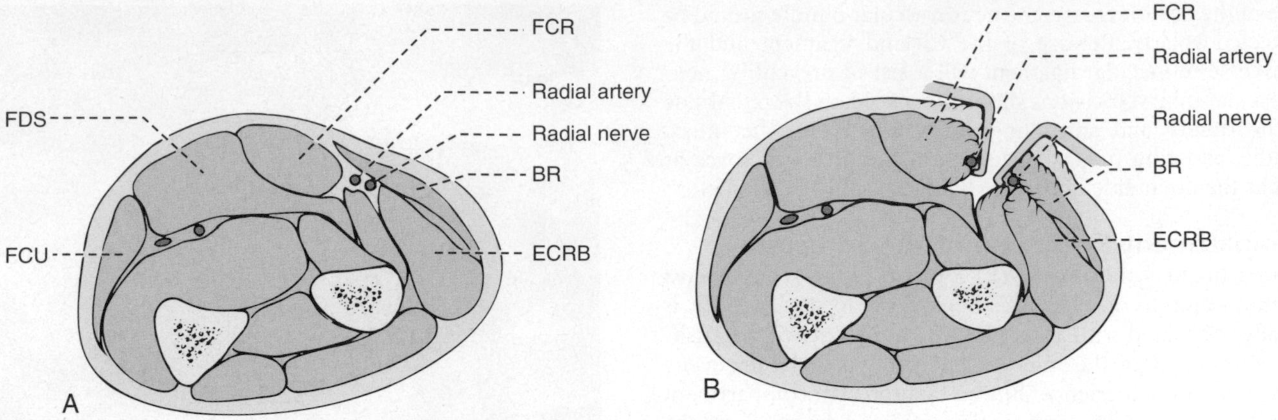

Figure 16-29. A, A transverse section through the midforearm illustrating relevant anatomy of the volar flexor compartment. *BR,* Brachioradialis; *ECRB,* extensor carpi radialis brevis; *FCR,* flexor carpi radialis; *FCU,* flexor carpi ulnaris; *FDS,* flexor digitorum sublimis. **B,** The Henry approach to superficial and deep compartments of the forearm. *(Modified with permission from American Academy of Orthopaedic Surgeons (AAOS): Instructional course lectures, vol 32, St. Louis, 1983, Mosby, p 106.)*

consists of the extensor carpi radialis longus and brevis as well as the brachioradialis.

Volar Ulnar Approach

The volar ulnar approach is performed in a similar fashion to the Henry approach. The arm is supinated and the incision is begun proximally medial to the biceps tendon, passes the elbow crease, extends distally along the ulnar border of the forearm, and proceeds across the carpal tunnel along the thenar crease (Fig. 16-30). The superficial fascia overlying the flexor carpi ulnaris is incised along with the elbow aponeurosis proximally and the carpal tunnel distally. The interval between the flexor carpi ulnaris and flexor digitorum superficialis is identified. Lying deep to the flexor digitorum superficialis and approaching from the radial to the ulnar side are the ulnar nerve and artery, which must be identified and carefully protected. The fascia overlying the deep flexor compartment is now incised. If necessary, the ulnar nerve can be decompressed distally at the level of the wrist and a neurolysis of the median nerve at the level of the carpal tunnel can be performed (Fig. 16-31). The extensor tendons can be released by creating an ulnar skin flap to expose the dorsal compartments.

Dorsal Approach

After the superficial and deep flexor compartments of the forearm have been decompressed, the treating surgeon must decide whether a fasciotomy of the dorsal (extensor) compartment is necessary. The need is best determined by pressure measurements made in the operating room after the flexor compartment fasciotomies have been completed. If the pressure continues to be elevated in the dorsal compartment, fasciotomy should be performed with the arm pronated. A straight incision from the lateral epicondyle to the Lister tubercle at the wrist is used. The interval between the extensor carpi radialis brevis and the extensor digitorum communis is identified, and fasciotomy is performed (Fig. 16-32). The mobile wad can be released by elevating skin flaps to allow for complete release of this compartment.

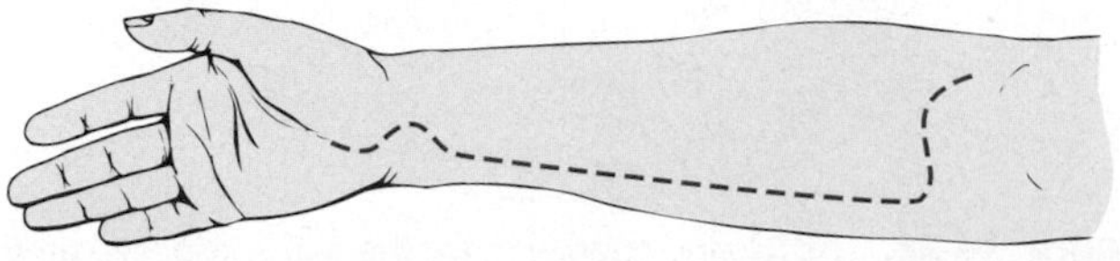

Figure 16-30. Ulnar approach to the volar flexor compartment of the forearm. *(Modified from Whitesides TE Jr, Haney TC, Morimoto K, Hirada H: Tissue pressure measurements as a determinant for the need of fasciotomy, Clin Orthop Relat Res 113:46, 1975.)*

Compartment Syndrome of the Upper Arm

ACS of the upper arm is significantly less common than the forearm and hand. There are three compartments to consider when releasing the upper arm. The anterior compartment (biceps and brachialis and the coracobrachialis) is innervated by the musculocutaneous nerve and sits anterior to the humerus. The posterior compartment (triceps) is innervated by the radial nerve and contains the ulnar nerve, the posterior antebrachial cutaneous nerve, and the nerve to the anconeus. Lastly the deltoid should be considered a separate compartment with three separate sections (the anterior, middle, and posterior). Release of the three compartments can be obtained through two separate incisions (anterior and posterior) or through a single lateral incision where both sides can be addressed. The deltoid can be released through a deltopectoral incision that can be extended to an anterior incision. Release of all the neurovascular structures in the antebrachium should be confirmed prior to completing the fasciotomy[112] (see Figs. 16-10 and 16-11).

Compartment Syndrome of the Leg

Unlike the significant and longstanding debate over the best means for diagnosing ACS of the lower extremity, there is universal consensus regarding what to do when it has been diagnosed—complete longitudinal release of all the fascial compartments in an urgent (ideally <6 to 12 hours from onset) fashion.[114-116] The seriousness of sequelae following missed and/or delayed compartment syndrome, and the universal opinion regarding the best means for treating it when diagnosed, has made this one of the most litigious orthopaedic conditions.[117] Thus, one should be familiar with the elements of diagnosing this condition and the surgical techniques for treating it. While fasciotomy should be performed in the

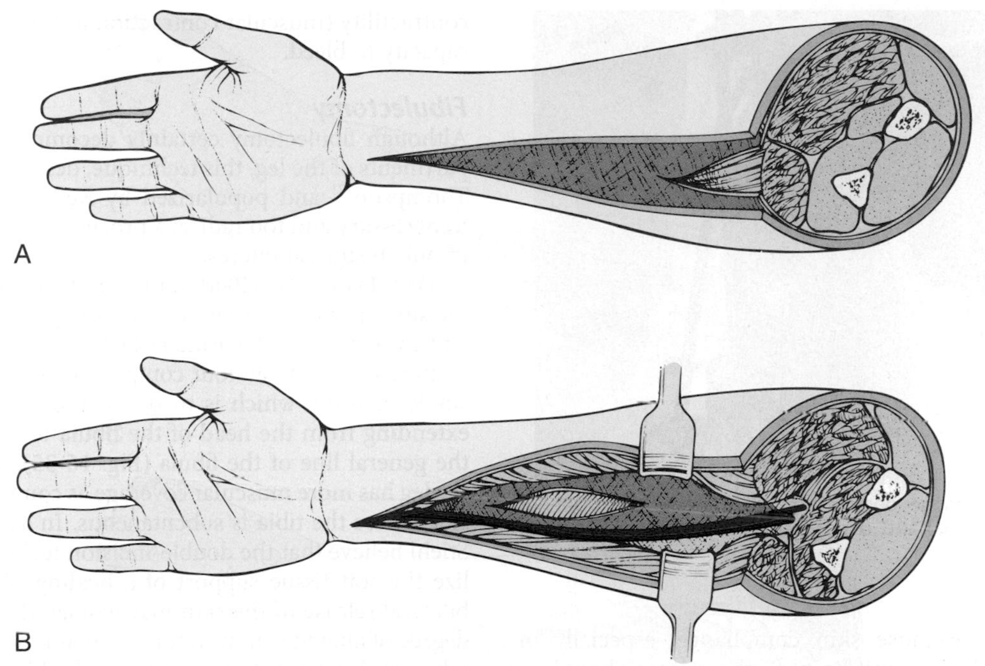

Figure 16-31. Ulnar approach to the forearm between the flexor carpi ulnaris and the flexor digitorum sublimis. *(Modified with permission from American Academy of Orthopaedic Surgeons (AAOS): Instructional course lectures, vol 32, St. Louis, 1983, Mosby, p 105.)*

operating room, Ebraheim and colleagues have reported successful performance of this at bedside under local anesthesia for patients at risk for prolonged delay for getting to the operating room.[118] In the leg, four-compartment fasciotomy can be achieved by one of two means: single-incision or double-incision four-compartment fasciotomy. While seemingly a simple procedure, it requires knowledge of the anatomy at risk:

Superficial:

Anterior compartment—deep peroneal nerve, anterior tibial artery (Fig. 16-33)

Lateral compartment—superficial peroneal nerve (see Fig. 16-18)

Superficial posterior compartment—sural nerve

Deep posterior compartment—posterior tibial and peroneal artery, tibial nerve (Fig. 16-34)

It is also important to appreciate that the most serious complication of fasciotomy is failure to completely release all compartments, which occurred in 17% of cases (anterior and deep posterior most commonly), doubling amputation rates and quadrupling mortality rate in casualties initially operated on at combat support hospitals in Iraq and Afghanistan.[66,104] For this reason, it is important to fully release all fascial compartments. Thus, surgeons should use surgical techniques that they are most familiar with, which ensures this basic goal, while minimizing the risk of iatrogenic injury and morbidity

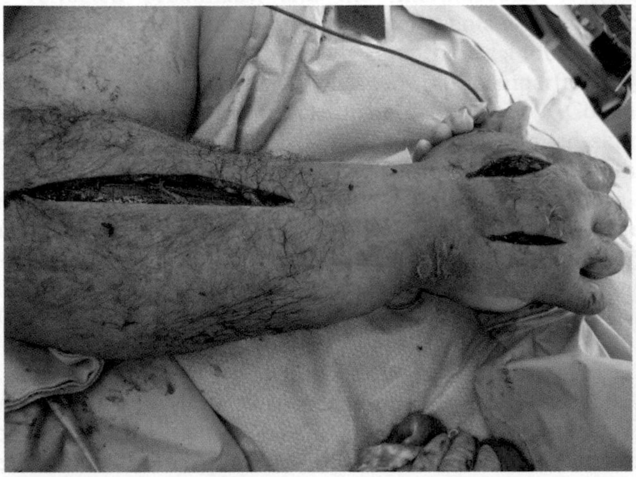

Figure 16-32. This image demonstrates a dorsal fasciotomy of the forearm. *(Courtesy of Dr. Michael S. Shuler.)*

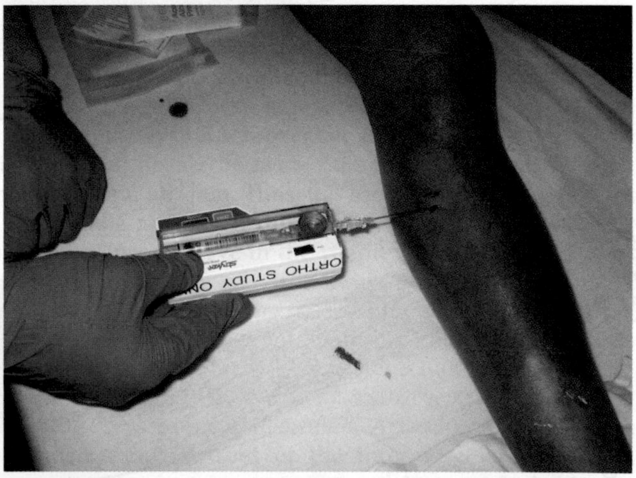

Figure 16-33. This image demonstrates the anterior compartment being measured using a Stryker device. *(Courtesy of Dr. Michael S. Shuler.)*

length of the leg. Making an initial incision through the fascia at the middle third level of the leg, where the nervous structures at risk are in their safest position is recommended. This technique allows the surgeon to enter the anterior and the lateral compartment. Closed, long Mayo scissors can then be inserted and passed subfascially in a distal and proximal direction to identify and/or create a safe plane for the fascial incision. Then the scissors can be partially opened about the fascia and pushed distally and proximal to complete the fascial release. The tips of the scissors are aimed anteriorly in the proximal direction and posteriorly in the distal direction, staying in the line of the fibula in both directions.

Next, the skin flap is developed posterior to the lateral compartment, to expose the fascia overlying the superficial posterior compartment, and a full-length fascial release is performed (Fig. 16-35, *C*). Care must be taken distally when developing the subcutaneous flap, as the sural nerve pierces the fascia in the posterior midline proximally, well away from the single lateral skin incision, but migrates laterally (toward the fibula) as it extends distally, coming to rest lateral to the Achilles tendon at the level of the ankle. To complete the deep posterior compartment release, the interval between the lateral compartment and the superficial posterior compartment is bluntly separated distally by retracting the peroneal muscles anteriorly and the gastrocsoleus complex posteriorly to expose the fibula. Develop this interval proximally by releasing some of the soleus from the fibula. The deep posterior compartment is now reached by following this interval to the posterior aspect of the fibula. The compartment is then released by subperiosteally elevating the flexor hallucis longus (FHL) and then the posterior tibialis (PT) origins from the fibula (Fig. 16-35, *D*). Care must be taken in this area, as the peroneal vessels run just medial to the fibula in the plane between the FHL and the PT muscles. Once the FHL is released, the peroneal vessels should be retracted posteriorly prior to releasing the PT from the fibula and the interosseous membrane.

Double-Incision Technique. The double-incision fasciotomy employs two vertical skin incisions separated by a bridge of skin at least 8 cm wide (Figs. 16-36 and 16-37).[13,125] The first skin incision extends from the knee to the ankle and is centered over the interval between the anterior and lateral compartments, which is the line along the anterior border of the fibula. This is the single lateral incision described in the preceding section. See the single-incision technique for greater detail about structures at risk related to this skin incision. The second incision also extends from the knee to the ankle and is centered 1 to 2 cm behind the posteromedial border of the tibia. The primary subcutaneous structures at risk with this incision are the (greater) saphenous vein and the saphenous nerve, which innervates the medial instep of the foot. This nerve, which is the distal termination of the femoral nerve, runs opposed to the posterior aspect of the vein through the leg and divides into an anterior and posterior branch 3 cm from the tip of the medial malleolus.[126] The nerve and vein should be contained in or retract with the anterior portion of the skin flap. The skin and subcutaneous tissue for both incisions are separated from the fascia overlying the

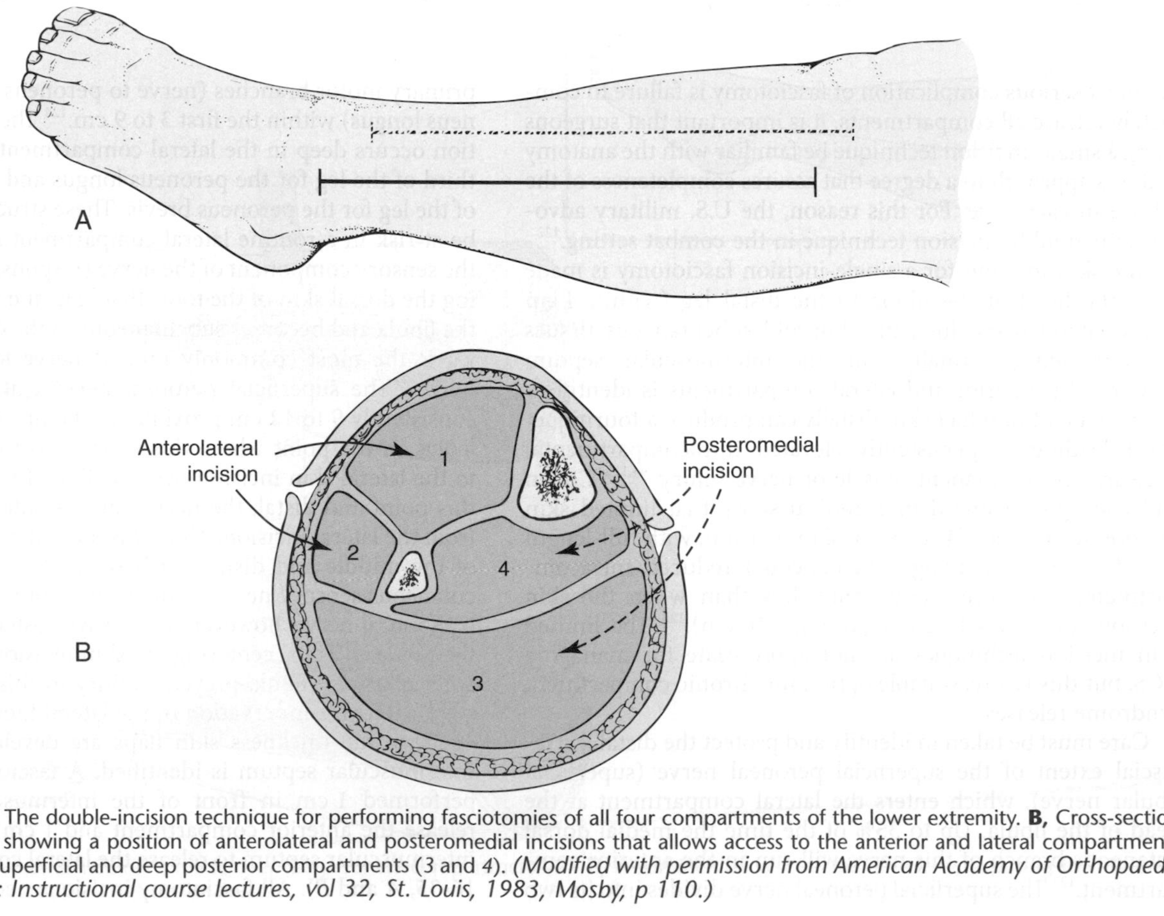

Figure 16-36. A, The double-incision technique for performing fasciotomies of all four compartments of the lower extremity. **B,** Cross-section of lower extremity showing a position of anterolateral and posteromedial incisions that allows access to the anterior and lateral compartments (*1* and *2*) and the superficial and deep posterior compartments (*3* and *4*). *(Modified with permission from American Academy of Orthopaedic Surgeons (AAOS): Instructional course lectures, vol 32, St. Louis, 1983, Mosby, p 110.)*

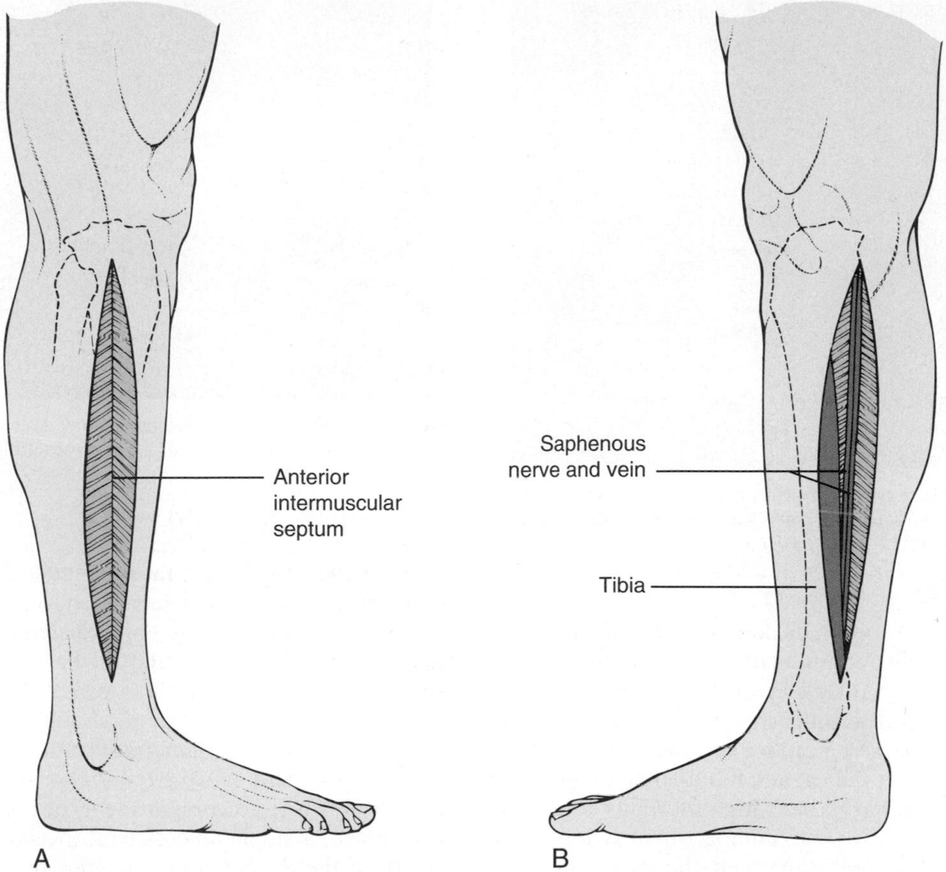

Figure 16-37. **A,** A vertical anterior incision is centered midway between the tibia and the fibula. The anterior intermuscular septum is identified, and two fasciotomy incisions are made, one anterior and one posterior to the septum. **B,** A vertical posteromedial incision is centered 2 cm to the rear of the tibia. Care is taken to avoid injury to the saphenous vein and nerve. *(Redrawn with permission from American Academy of Orthopaedic Surgeons (AAOS): Instructional course lectures, vol 32, St. Louis, 1983, Mosby, pp 519–520.)*

compartments after completion of the longitudinal skin incisions. Care must be taken to identify and protect the superficial nerves. Through the lateral incision, a fasciotomy of the anterior compartment 1 cm in front of the intermuscular septum is performed, followed by a fasciotomy of the lateral compartment 1 cm behind the intermuscular septum (Fig. 16-38). Through the medial incision, the fascia overlying the gastrocnemius-soleus complex is incised releasing the superficial posterior compartment and exposing the deep posterior compartment. It is imperative to extend the fasciotomies distally beyond the musculotendinous junction and proximally to the level of the knee joint.[119,120] To decompress the deep posterior compartment adequately in the proximal direction, it is necessary to detach part of the soleal bridge from the back of the tibia. Doing so exposes the fascia overlying the flexor digitorum longus and the deep posterior compartment, which is then incised, completing the fasciotomy of the deep posterior compartment of the leg (Fig. 16-39). The double-incision technique has the advantage of being relatively easy to perform, but the disadvantage of requiring two incisions that may (especially on the medial side) leave bone, nerve, or vessel exposed (Fig. 16-40).

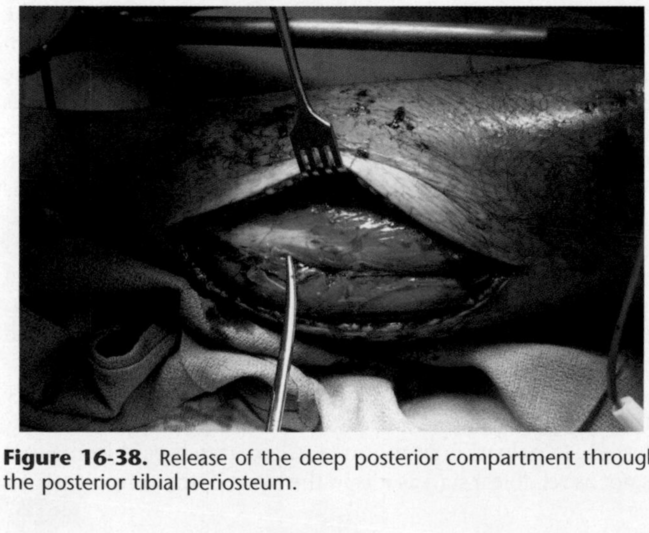

Figure 16-38. Release of the deep posterior compartment through the posterior tibial periosteum.

Compartment Syndrome of the Thigh

Compartment syndromes of the thigh, are relatively rare, but very serious conditions.[127-131] Ojike and colleagues completed a recent systematic review of the literature, which identified only nine studies with a total of 89 patients that met their inclusion criteria for quality of data (two or more patients, acute setting, all retrospective).[130] According to Schwartz and colleagues,[131] compartment syndrome can occur in patients undergoing closed intramedullary nailing of the femur; to some extent, its development depends on the Injury Severity

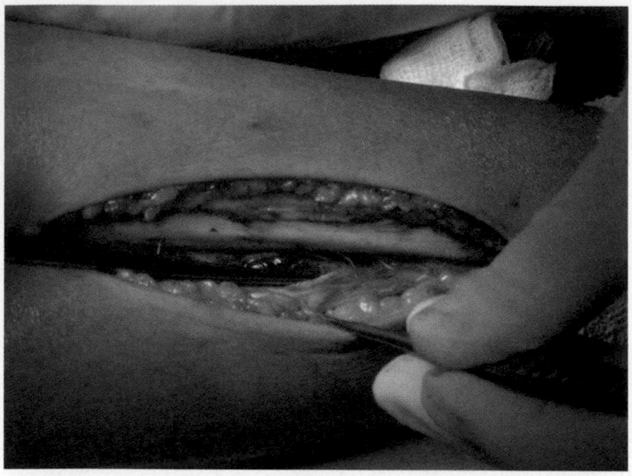

Figure 16-39. This image demonstrates how the medial incision can make a previously closed fracture an open fracture with exposed bone. *(Courtesy of Dr. Michael S. Shuler.)*

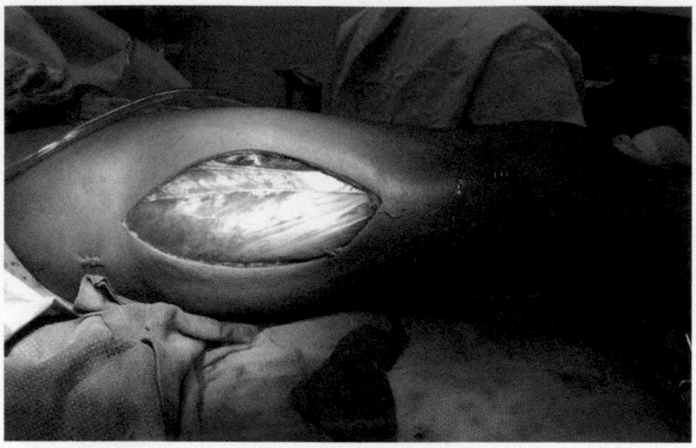

Figure 16-41. Thigh fasciotomy lateral: This image depicts a lateral release of the thigh after a femoral intramedullary nail. *(Courtesy of Dr. Michael S. Shuler.)*

Score and the amount of soft tissue damage to the thigh. There is a concern that overdistraction at the time of closed intramedullary nailing, which, in effect, decreases the compartment volume, can produce a compartment syndrome. Further, in the study with the largest number of cases from a single institution, Schwartz and colleagues found that thigh compartment syndrome can have a very high mortality rate (47% of their 17 patients).[132] Thus, thigh compartment syndrome is likely an indicator of severe injury and the large muscular volume contained within the thigh can lead to profound negative sequelae (i.e., crush syndrome) when myonecrosis occurs. While delays in diagnosis are not uncommonly reported in cases of thigh compartment syndrome, prompt diagnosis and release is important to reverse this life-threatening process.

The thigh consists of three muscle compartments—the anterior (quadriceps), posterior (hamstrings), and medial (adductors). McLaren and coworkers[128] reported an isolated case of adductor compartment syndrome of the thigh, but compartment syndromes seen as a complication of closed intramedullary nailing usually involve the anterior compartment.

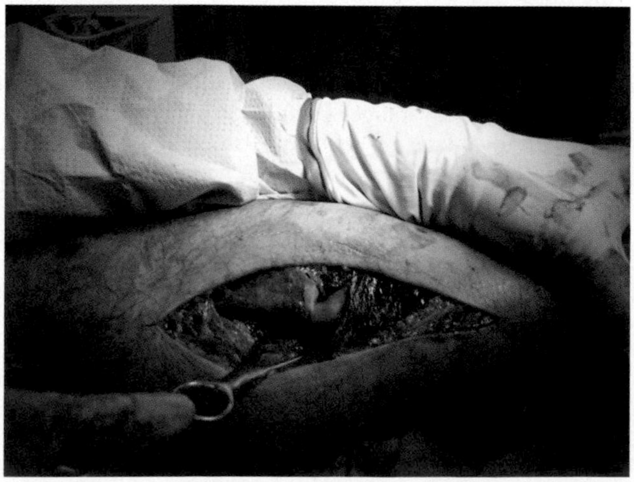

Figure 16-40. This image depicts the lateral incision with the superficial peroneal nerve highlighted. *(Courtesy of Dr. Michael S. Shuler.)*

The surgical approach recommended depends on the compartment involved, which can be determined by pressure measurements. One-incision (anterolateral) and two-incision techniques (anterolateral and medial) are reported. In Ojike and colleagues' review, unlike ACS of the leg, where it is well accepted that all compartments should be released, 86% of the cases used a single incision, most commonly opening the anterior compartment +/− the other two.[130] If the anterior (most commonly involved compartment) or posterior compartment is involved, a single anterolateral incision is made along the length of the thigh (from iliac crest or greater trochanter to the lateral epicondyle of the knee), splitting the iliotibial band in line with the incision, and the fascia overlying the vastus lateralis (anterior compartment) is divided along its length (Fig. 16-41).[133] The hamstring compartment can then be entered by retracting the vastus lateralis and dividing the lateral intermuscular septum, taking care to avoid further injury to perforating vessels. Release of the adductor compartment, if it is necessary, should be performed through a separate longitudinal incision along its length. The skin incision can be closed primarily in about three-quarters of cases, on average 5 days after fasciotomy.[130]

Compartment Syndrome of the Foot

Like those of the hand, the muscles of the foot are bound and contained within up to nine named compartments.[134,135] Failure to diagnose an ACS of the intrinsic muscles of the foot can result in myoneural necrosis with subsequent claw-toe deformity and paresthesias or hypoesthesia of the foot.[136,137] It is seen most commonly after calcaneal fractures (especially highly comminuted, intraarticular fractures), Lisfranc injuries, or significant blunt trauma or crush injury to the foot, but it can occur from more innocuous mechanisms as well, like a severe ankle sprain.[134,138-140] Rosenthal and colleagues evaluated 47 consecutive patients with calcaneus fractures and found that evidence of missed compartment syndrome of the foot (i.e., claw toes, decreased plantar sensation) were present in 10% of patients, and these patients had significantly worse functional outcomes.[139]

The clinical findings for a patient with ACS of the foot are usually equivocal. It is difficult to sort out local pain and tenderness to palpation in this area. Also, stretch pain in the foot is not as reliable a sign as it is in the hand. Intracompartmental

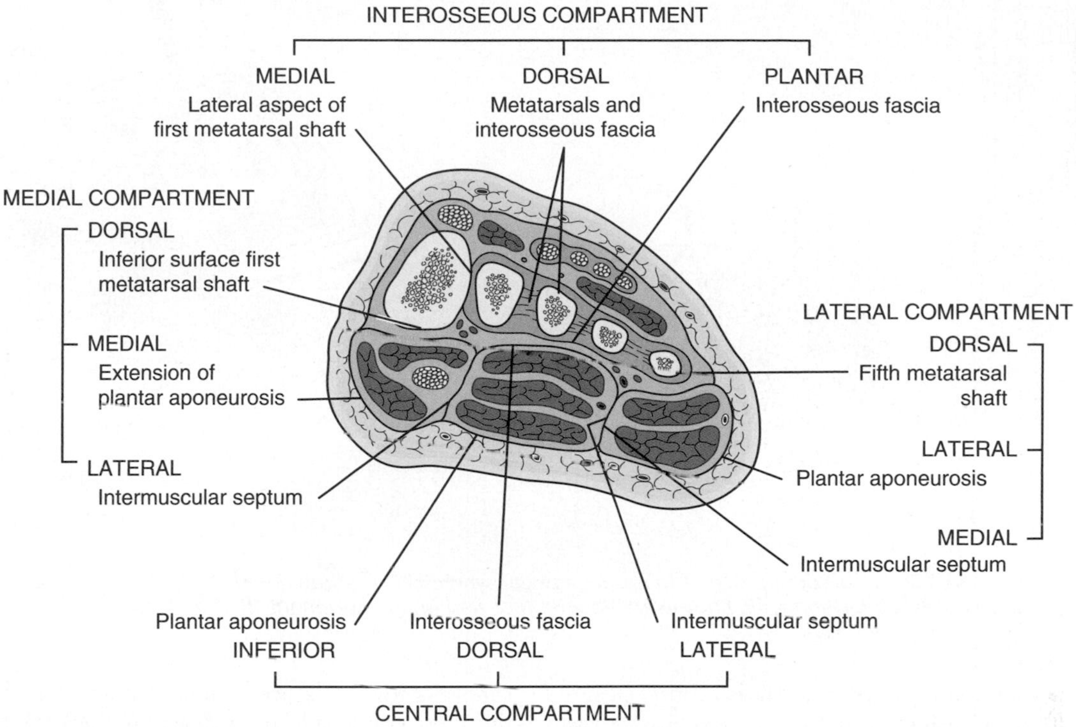

Figure 16-42. Compartments of the foot. Similar detail can be seen with magnetic resonance imaging. *(Redrawn with permission from American Academy of Orthopaedic Surgeons (AAOS): Orthopaedic knowledge update: foot and ankle, Rosemont, IL, 1994, AAOS, p 263.)*

pressures can be measured. Similar to the leg, 30 mm Hg has been advocated as an absolute pressure threshold.[141] In the end, the decision is a clinical one, based on pain out of proportion, worse with passive stretch, and a tense feel to the foot, with or without intracompartmental pressure (ICP) measurement.[138] While Myerson and colleagues have reported that the use of a pneumatic intermittent impulse compression device on the foot following calcaneus fracture significantly reduces intracompartmental pressure, this is a means of reducing swelling and the risk of compartment syndrome; it is not a treatment.[142] As with other areas of the body, the treatment of choice for ACS of the foot is fasciotomy.

The classic compartments of the foot are the medial, central, lateral, and interosseous, all of which may need to be decompressed (Fig. 16-42).[143] A calcaneal compartment that includes the quadratus plantae muscle has also been described.[134] Previously felt to be part of the central compartment, the role ischemic contracture of the quadratus plantae plays in clawtoe deformity and the presence of this contracture despite seemingly adequate release of the central compartment has demonstrated that this is a distinct fascial compartment.[143] After the diagnosis has been made, decompression of the foot can be carried out by a variety of techniques. Two dorsal incisions (centered over the second and fourth metatarsal) provide excellent access to release the four interossei compartments, and the deeper, plantar compartments can be reached with blunt dissection between and lateral to the metatarsals. Elevating the interossei off the metatarsals improves the decompression of these compartments. A medial incision, starting distal to the medial malleolus along the inferior border and extending to the neck of the first metatarsal, allows release of the medial, superficial, central, calcaneal, and lateral compartments (Fig. 16-43). In the setting of a calcaneus fracture, the medial incision alone may be sufficient. Starting at the posterior tuberosity of the calcaneus and using only the proximal half of the medial incision, one can access and release the fascia overlying the quadratus plantae by releasing the fascia about and retracting the abductor hallucis. Likewise, in the setting of ACS following metatarsal fractures or a Lisfranc injury, the two dorsal incisions may be sufficient. In crush injuries, it may be best to perform all three incisions to ensure that all compartments are released. Lastly, there is controversy regarding the best treatment for ACS of the foot that is delayed in presentation (i.e., >24 hours from onset). Some advocate not performing fasciotomy in this situation, as prolonged ischemia has already produced myonecrosis and/or permanent neural injury and the intact skin overlying the necrotized muscle below is the best defense against infection. The best treatment for this morbid condition has not been determined in clinical study.

Closure and Aftercare of Fasciotomy Wounds

In general, fasciotomy incisions are left unclosed for 3 to 5 days following fasciotomy, to allow injured muscle to dissipate edema and declare its viability.[104] During this time, the wounds have classically been packed open with damp-to-dry cotton gauze and a loose, bulky dressing and/or splint. The extremity should be maintained at heart level, and passive range of motion of the affected joints can be performed to limit stiffness and contracture.[74] That being said, some surgeons immediately close the skin over the released fascia in certain cases. This approach is not recommended, and clinical settings where it would seem appropriate call into question the necessity of "unbridling" the intracompartmental swelling by the

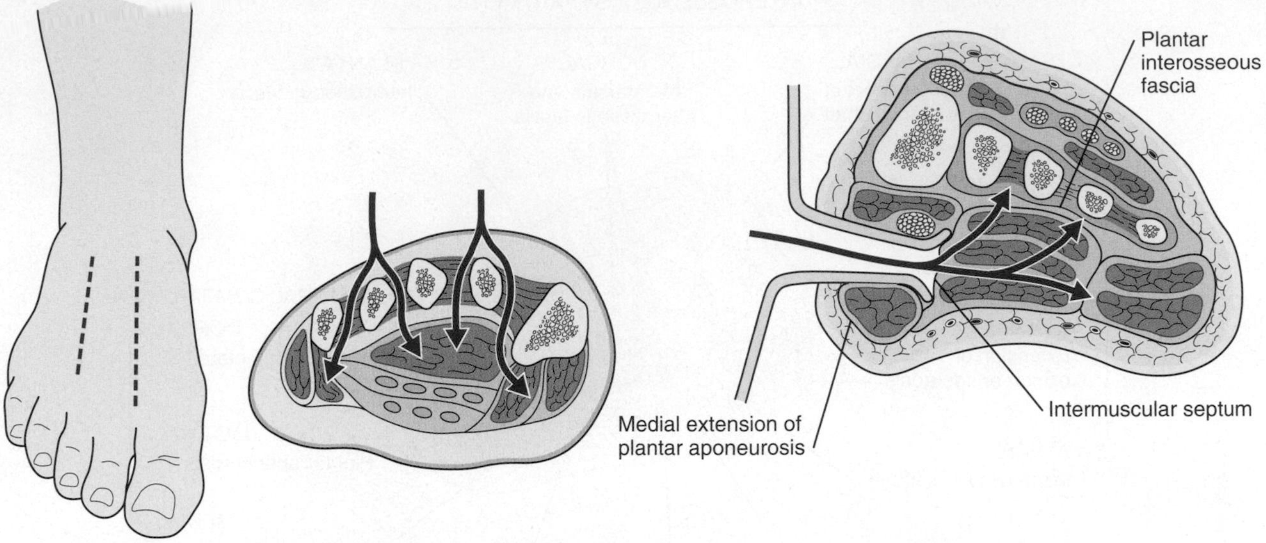

Figure 16-43. Incisions available for decompression of foot compartment syndromes. *(Redrawn with permission from American Academy of Orthopaedic Surgeons (AAOS): Orthopaedic knowledge update: foot and ankle, Rosemont, IL, 1994, AAOS, p 264.)*

morbid process of fasciotomy in the first place. Wound closure in a delayed primary fashion can be achieved in the vast majority of thigh fasciotomies, most leg fasciotomies, and only some foot fasciotomies. Where primary closure cannot be achieved, split-thickness skin grafts are used. If bone, tendon, or neurovascular structures are exposed, more advanced soft tissue coverage options may be needed, such as rotational or transpositional flaps.

Typically at 48 to 72 hours after fasciotomy, the patient is brought back to the operating room to inspect and débride the fasciotomy sites. At the time of fasciotomy, muscle that is clearly dead (absent all four "C's") should be excised. In a controlled setting (i.e., level I or II trauma center, hemodynamically stable patient), where second-look operations can be reliably performed within 48 to 72 hours, muscle at risk or of indeterminate viability can be left at the index procedure. When the swelling has reduced and the wounds appear clean and healthy with all nonviable tissue débrided, the wound is ready for closure or coverage. Internal fixation of underlying long bone fractures can safely and reliably be performed at the time of the initial fasciotomy, especially in cases in which diagnosis and fascial release occur in a timely fashion (<6 to 12 hours from onset of symptoms). The exception to this is open reduction and internal fixation (ORIF), especially at the level of the foot (i.e., calcaneal fractures) and ankle. In this situation, the customary 7- to 21-day delay to allow for soft tissue swelling to resolve should be observed following fasciotomy. In complex open long bone fractures, like those seen in combat and mangled extremities, application of a monolateral external fixator can be performed to provide relatively rigid stabilization and unhampered access to the fasciotomy wounds. This can be a successful temporizing measure, if definitive fixation can be achieved within 1 to 2 weeks.[144]

Since the mid-1990s, a new method for covering and closing wounds has been clinically available, which has revolutionized the care of acute (and chronic) large open wounds, such as those created by a fasciotomy in a patient with ACS. In fact, the standard leg fasciotomy wound is the prototypical acute wound for treatment with this novel form of wound care. Negative pressure wound therapy (NPWT), for which the most commonly used device is the KCI Wound V.A.C. (Kinetic Concepts, Inc., San Antonio, TX) device, uses simplistic medical truths intuitively known since the time of Archimedes, to significantly improve outcomes in patients with large open wounds.[145-147] All NPWT devices use a porous dressing material (in the case of KCI, this is an open-cell polyurethane sponge; other vendors use cotton gauze) that is used to fill the wound and then an airtight sealing sticker is placed over the wound. This creates, or is intended to create, a single closed chamber. Then, suction tubing is attached to the closed dressing and a metered vacuum (typically 125 mm Hg, continuous) is applied via a vacuum pump. This construct results in the removal of exudate from the wound, as well as a hyperemic and prohealing response to the continuous negative pressure environment that may be mechanical, physiologic, or both.[147] The net effect of this process is that wounds heal faster, wound area reduces more (allowing for more primary closures vs. skin grafts), and infection rates may be lower when large open wounds are treated with NPWT versus traditional damp-to-dry dressing.[145,146,148,149] This clinical superiority also comes with a substantial savings in patient pain and human resource allocation, as NPWT dressings require change every 48 to 72 hours, typically in the operating room, versus three painful daily bedside changes for damp-to-dry dressing. In fact, the safe interval for NPWT dressing change is dictated not by infection risk, but by granulation tissue ingrowth into the dressing, a process that is particularly encouraged by open-cell foam sponges. This ingrowth produces pain and can lead to gross or microscopic retention of sponge particles at dressing changes. As NPWT continues to mature and becomes the cornerstone of complex wound care, weaknesses in the current embodiments will be overcome.

The overall case for the superiority of NPWT over traditional methods of wound care was made emphatically clear over the last decade of combat in Iraq and Afghanistan, where it became the standard of care. The high volume of casualties and the high number of large open wounds per casualty that occur following blast injury, which has been responsible for more than 75% of U.S. combat casualties over the last decade, would have overwhelmed the U.S. military health system resources, if we remained reliant on the method of wound care that was popularized in the First World War—cotton gauze dressings, with or without additives, such as Dakin solution (dilute sodium hypochlorite). By necessity, combat surgeons over the last decade have done more to advance the applications and utility of NPWT in the treatment of acute complex wounds than any other group of physicians. The work of Fang and colleagues in 2010 finally filled the hole in our ability to provide seamless treatment with NPWT from the battlefield to U.S. military medical centers, when they showed that the KCI Freedom V.A.C. was safe for use on aeromedical flights.[150] Prior to this, NPWT dressings were used between medical treatment facilities in the combat zone, removed for the flight, reapplied in Germany (Landstuhl Regional Medical Center), and then this process was repeated for the flight to the United States a few days later.

The unprecedented exposure to complex wounds over the last decade of war has resulted in many lessons learned about the benefits and weaknesses of NPWT. Forsberg and colleagues prospectively followed 50 patients with combat wounds treated by NPWT that were then closed primarily.[151] Four (8%) of these went onto dehisce within the first 6 weeks after primary wound closure. They identified a set of cytokines (procalcitonin, interleukin-13 [IL-13], RANTES) in the wound vacuum-assisted closure (VAC) effluent that was predictive of this wound complication and currently are studying statistical methods to establish a predictive model of this event. This group went on to describe another significant complication of combat wounds treated with NPWT—the development of heterotopic ossification (HO). The rate of this morbid complication of severe soft tissue injury is substantially higher following military-related blast injuries (38% in this prospective study of 24 patients, but reported in up to two-thirds in other case series).[152,153] The pathophysiology of this process is not known, but Evans and colleagues showed that a wound-specific prolonged hyperinflammatory state (as marked by elevated inflammatory cytokines in serum and effluent) was a primary contributor to this phenomenon.[154,155] Bacterial colonization was a highly significant ($P < 0.001$) independent cofactor in the development of HO, and current NPWT devices have been shown to unreliably reduce bacterial colonization, especially from *Staphylococcus aureus,* which is the most common pathogen.[154,156,157] Effective modes of closed irrigation under a NPWT dressing may better reduce bacterial loads, because irrigation is the standard surgical method for diluting bacterial colonization. Oftentimes, this HO is very robust, especially in lower extremity amputees.[152,153] This phenomenon can produce large chunks of symptomatic HO that require major surgical resection. In addition, a unique plate-like superficial HO has been seen in areas underlying some wounds that have received repeated (sometimes as many as 10 or more) applications of the KCI Wound V.A.C. One possible explanation is that microscopic retention of polyurethane sponge particles encased in granulation tissue contributes to the hyperinflammatory response. While there is still a lot to learn about the pathophysiology of wounds sustained and survived in modern combat, what is clear is that blast injuries, especially to dismounted soldiers, produce a severe soft tissue injury that is unique to combat casualty and at substantial risk for wound and deep soft tissue–related complications. While current attributes of available NPWT systems may have some association with these risks, their overall benefit at the population and individual level have clearly outweighed any negative effects. That being said, it is incumbent on surgeons to continue to advance the understanding of the physiology of wound healing in a negative pressure environment, so that we can improve the device and methods for applying this concept in the most effective and economical manner.

One final consideration regarding management of the fasciotomy wound is the concept of wound approximation. Skin is an elastic tissue, which tends to retract when incised. The magnitude of this retraction is increased by swollen muscle bellies that protrude at the level of the fasciotomy incisions in patients who have ACS released. With time, wounds will contract through a cellular fibroblastic response (heal by "secondary intent"), but this is a long and slow process that rarely fully reapproximates the wound, and it leaves dystrophic reepithelized skin on the surface. This is particularly problematic in the leg, which is the area of the body most likely to undergo fasciotomy for trauma.[158] When a double-incision technique is used, the medial incision should be closed first, as it has the least amount of muscular tissue envelope (i.e., subcutaneous border of the tibia). Because both incisions tend to retract, especially if no countermeasure is employed, these incisions can reach inches in width. When the surgeon closes the medial incision, the lateral incision tends to enlarge in area. Further, the edema from the injury and the disrupted venous return tends to make the skin flaps brawnier and less supple, which also limits the ability to close both wounds by primary intention. When an incision cannot be closed, a split-thickness skin graft must be harvested and placed over the lateral incision. This coverage technique is another procedure with its own morbidity and complication profile. In the young healthy person, the significance of skin grafting on cosmesis and skin health (skin in the area of healed grafts remains thin, atrophic, anesthetic and/or paraesthetic, and dry, making it prone to ulceration) should not be diminished.[159] As a result, a multitude of techniques (from field-expedient to commercially available devices) have been introduced that allow for some degree of tension to be applied to the skin margins.

A common technique, one used regularly in the military, is known as the shoelace or Roman sandals technique (Figs. 16-44 and 16-45), in which a NPWT dressing is placed into the wound, typically cut to be smaller than the volume of the wound, and then vessel loops are stapled to the margins of the skin in a crisscross fashion, that resembles the lacing on a Roman sandal. Start at one end with both "laces," and then in an alternating sequence, pull one diagonally across and staple it to the far skin margin. Follow with the next and proceed the whole length of the wound in this fashion until you reach the other end, where you can tie the two loops together. Prior to the advent of NPWT, the ends were left free, so that providers could apply daily increase to the tension in the loops.[160] However, this method of sequential tensioning does not work well or at all under current NPWT dressings.

The propensity of NPWT dressings to reduce the volume of wounds at a rate that that is significantly faster than the healing by secondary intention, along with the vessel loop Roman sandals technique (in which the ends are tied off at each application), has been adequate to close many combat casualty fasciotomy incisions. The intent is to tension the

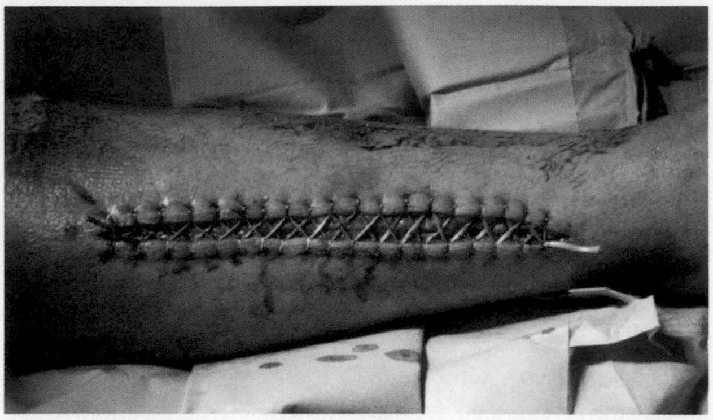

Figure 16-44. Use of the shoelace technique to assist with partial closure of a fasciotomy wound.

Roman sandals at each NPWT dressing change procedure to close down the surface area of the wound by about 50%, or as much as the surgeon feels comfortable. In advanced cases of ACS, it may be prudent to postpone this tensioning technique until the initial second-look procedure. When stapling the vessel loop, aim to pin it against the skin, not to perforate the loop, as this will cause it to break, requiring one to start over. This technique is often most effective in a serial fashion, with increased wound surface area reduction obtained at each subsequent dressing change, until the margins are close enough and the wounds are healthy enough to support primary closure. Bulstrode and colleagues reported another field-expedient method, in which they apply an OPSITE dressing over cotton gauze placed in the wound and a metal rod along the midline length of the wound.[159,161] This rod is rotated daily, applying tension through the adhesive sheet and leading to wound approximation in a controlled fashion over a course of 3 to 10 days. When tension is applied to the skin margins solely through the adhesive sheets, skin blisters can develop that complicate the healing process.[162]

CHRONIC EXERTIONAL COMPARTMENT SYNDROME

Chronic exertional compartment syndrome (CECS) has many similarities to ACS. CECS is a painful condition associated with muscle ischemia caused by tight fascial compartments. CECS does not occur due to trauma but is typically seen in high-level athletes as well as military recruits.

Clinical presentation typically involves a reproducible pain at a reproducible level of exertion. Pain resolves quickly after the inciting activity is stopped and rest begins. The pain results from an increased demand for oxygen by exercising muscles and an inability to provide blood flow to the compartment secondary to muscle swelling.[163]

The clinical history is the most useful part of the diagnosis. The lateral and anterior compartments of the leg are the most common compartments involved, but upper extremity, thigh, and gluteal CECS can occur. Intracompartmental pressures can be measured in symptomatic limbs. Pedowitz and colleagues defined elevated pressures based on three criteria: a rest preexercise pressure of greater than 15 mm Hg, a one minute postexercise pressure greater than 30 mm Hg, or a five minute postexercise pressure of greater than 20 mm Hg.[164] When the diagnosis is made for CECS, activity modification or cross-training can be attempted as a conservative measure. If conservative measures do not resolve the symptoms, a fasciotomy can be performed and typically resolves most, if not all, of the symptoms associated with the activity. In the chronic setting, endoscopic-assisted fasciotomies may allow for quicker returns to activities and less morbidity than the standard open fasciotomy.[165]

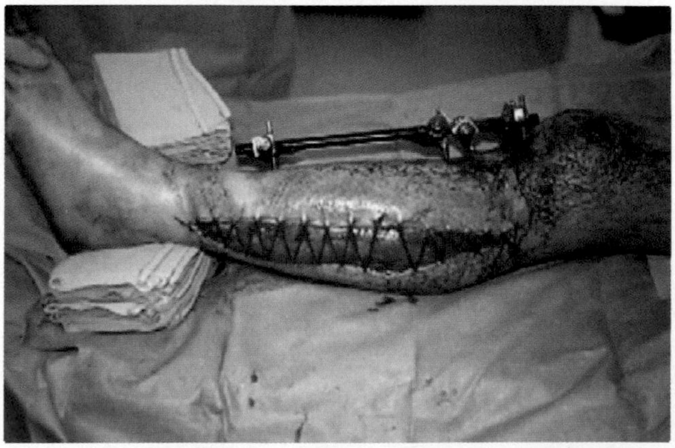

Figure 16-45. Provisional stabilization of fractures associated with compartment syndrome with an external fixator.

FUTURE DIRECTION

Much has been learned over the last century about ACS, but much is still left to do. Far too many fasciotomies are performed unnecessarily and still other cases, even in major trauma centers, are missed.[23] The first advancement that needs to be established is a reliable, accurate, and objective means for definitively diagnosing ACS. The current gold standard of "clinical diagnosis" is simply not good enough. Most published clinical research has considered ACS to be present if a fasciotomy, specifically a nonprophylactic one, is performed. This methodology has significant limitations, since O'Toole and colleagues have shown that experts in the field, looking at the same injury pattern, have a widely variant diagnostic conclusion in regard to ACS.[24]

Additionally, research should be performed on traumatized tissue. While this factor can make clinical studies difficult, uninjured tissue used to simulate ACS does not incorporate the multiple physiologic factors associated with ACS and traumatized tissue.[85,86,94] It is clear that traumatized tissue provides a completely different environment for perfusion and oxygen management. Without appreciating this physiologic state and accounting for it, any research performed will not clearly replicate the many factors involved in the development of ACS.

Finally, while intracompartmental pressure certainly plays an indirect role in the development of ACS, tissue perfusion, or the lack thereof in an extremity, is the physiologic event that produces ACS. Factors such as inflammatory mediators, hemoglobin concentration, as well as saturation, tissue oxygen consumption, vascular spasm, and cardiac output, all play a role in muscle and tissue perfusion. Pressure alone does not give a complete picture regarding the health and perfusion of an injured extremity. Future research should strive to better understand the global environment in which ACS occurs and the most accurate and reliable means to define it.

ACKNOWLEDGMENT

We would like to acknowledge the work of Bruce C. Twaddle, MD, FRACS, and Annunziato Amendola, MD, FRCS(C), in preparing the text of this chapter in the previous edition and allowing us to revise it for this edition.

KEY REFERENCES

The level of evidence (LOE) is determined according to the criteria provided in the preface.

15. Whitesides TE Jr, Haney TC, Harada H, et al: A simple method for tissue pressure determination. *Arch Surg* 110(11):1311–1313, 1975. LOE V
16. Whitesides TE, Haney TC, Morimoto K, et al: Tissue pressure measurements as a determinant for the need of fasciotomy. *Clin Orthop Relat Res* 113:43–51, 1975. LOE I
17. Matsen FA 3rd: Compartmental syndrome. A unified concept. *Clin Orthop Relat Res* 113:8–14, 1975. LOE II
24. O'Toole R, Whitney A, Merchant N, et al: Variation in diagnosis of compartment syndrome by surgeons treating tibial shaft fractures. *J Trauma* 67(4):735–741, 2009. LOE I
33. McQueen MM, Court-Brown CM: Compartment monitoring in tibial fractures. The pressure threshold for decompression. *J Bone Joint Surg Br* 78(1):99–104, 1996. LOE I
34. McQueen M, Christie J, Court-Brown C: Acute compartment syndrome in tibial diaphyseal fractures. *J Bone Joint Surg Br* 78(1):95–98, 1996. LOE II
37. Prayson MJ, Chen JL, Hampers D, et al: Baseline compartment pressure measurements in isolated lower extremity fractures without clinical compartment syndrome. *J Trauma* 60(5):1037–1040, 2006. LOE I
44. Halpern AA, Nagel DA: Anterior compartment pressures in patients with tibial fractures. *J Trauma* 20(9):786–790, 1980. LOE I

The complete References list is available online at https://expertconsult.inkling.com.

Chapter 17

Open Fractures

CLIFFORD B. JONES • JOSEPH C. WENKE

Additional videos related to the subject of this chapter are available from the Medizinische Hochschule Hannover collection. The following video is included with this chapter and may be viewed at https://expertconsult.inkling.com:

17-1. Vacuum techniques for acute traumatic wound management.

INTRODUCTION

Approximately 6 million fractures and 7.5 million open wounds occur annually in the United States.[1] Extrapolating from European studies, about 4% of all fractures are open, or about 250,000 open fractures occur annually in the United States.[2] Other studies note that open fractures occur at a rate of 11.5 per 100,000 persons per year.[3,4] Open fractures are unique, complex, and emergently presenting injuries that expose sterile bone to the contaminated environment. Because a fracture disrupts the intramedullary blood supply, the additionally stripped soft tissue envelope further devitalizes the bone.[5] The more severe the soft tissue injury or open wound, the more severe the osseous injury.[6-9] Historically, open fractures were associated with infection, delayed union, nonunion, amputation, or death.[10-17] Because of these complications, infections have an associated health care burden with a reported lifetime cost of a severe open fracture being as high as $680,000.[18] Many techniques have been established to lessen or eradicate these complications. The goals of treatment are patient assessment, injury classification, wound management, fracture stabilization, and osseous regeneration when needed.[19] With time, though, an increase in motorized vehicle collisions, especially in developing countries, and types of war injuries have increased open fractures. Motor vehicles have become safer, but collisions have produced more survivable injuries. With war and improved body armor, new ways to treat open injuries have developed. This chapter reviews the current state-of-the-art evaluation, treatment, and outcomes for open fractures.

MECHANISM

Open fractures can occur because of an extreme amount of force imparted to the bone via an axial load or bending moment. This type of fracture could be considered an "in-to-out" fracture. A crush injury or an explosion can create enough external force to cause a direct integument injury and an associated fracture. This type of fracture is termed an "out-to-in" fracture. Because the bone ends protrude through the skin from the inner sterile to the outer unsterile environment, the "in-to-out" fracture is theoretically "cleaner" than the "out-to-in" fracture.

Direct Blow

A direct blow causes a local area of injury with limited extension. The open wound can be from the direct blow site causing an "out-to-in" mechanism or the potentially contracoup injury opposite from the direct blow site with an "in-to-out" injury (Fig. 17-1). Both injuries are serious, but the direct site may be more contaminated and have a more serious associated soft tissue injury.

Crush Injury

Crush injuries create immediate and sometimes irreversible associated soft tissue injury. If prolonged or severe enough, the injury will be similar to an internal amputation with an associated open fracture of varying severity. The fracture can be a simple pattern. The circumferential crush injury creates problematic limb salvage options. Complete musculotendinous, venous, and cutaneous disruption can be present, requiring assessment, and may worsen with time (Fig. 17-2).

Explosion and Blast Injury

The pathophysiology of explosion or blast injuries depends on the force and location to the source and evolves with time. It starts with the detonation followed by the blast wave, blast wind, and anatomic stress wave. The detonation is from a high-speed chemical decomposition of an explosive gas. Space occupied by the explosive is now occupied by gas under high pressure and temperature. The blast wave is a pressure pulse a few millimeters thick that travels at supersonic speed radially from the center of the blast. The leading edge rapidly decreases in pressure and becomes an acoustic wave. The local effect is a positive destructive shock wave followed by a negative pressure wave. The pressure drops below ambient pressure, and a vacuum effect takes place. The mass movement of air causes a blast wind that can propel objects and people considerable distances. Anatomic stress wave caused by blast wave interaction with the person with local overpressure has increasing pressure up to eight times normal. The stress wave causes rapid acceleration of body surface and a stress wave. The positive pressure shock wave creates immediate muscle damage while the negative pressure shock wave takes time to allow the full destructive pattern to evolve and determine.

Three types of blast injuries are noted: primary, secondary, and tertiary.[20,21] The primary blast wave is caused by the direct effect of the blast wave on the body. The effect depends on distance. The lethal radius is three times in water.[22] It is increased at the reflecting surface. The injury is seen almost exclusively in air-filled structures. The ear is the most sensitive, but injuries to the respiratory system are the most common causes of morbidity and mortality. Injuries to gastrointestinal tract are the most common causes of delayed morbidity and mortality. Major limb amputation occurs as a result of the blast wave–induced fracture followed by the blast wind avulsing the

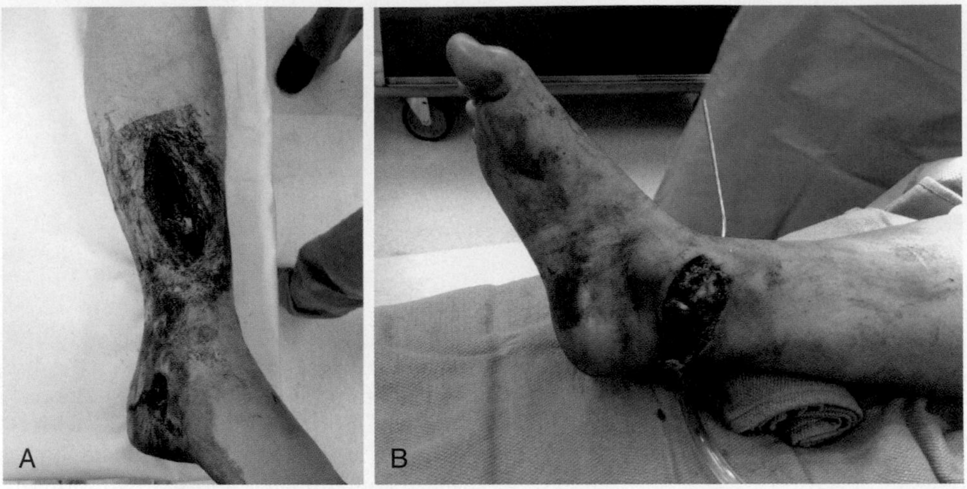

Figure 17-1. A, Clinical picture of a high energy, open tibial fracture from a high-low "out-to-in" impact. The wound edge is irregular and contaminated. The soft tissue compartment are disrupted and injured. **B,** Clinical picture of an open bimalleolar ankle fracture with "in-to-out" medial transverse laceration from low energy twisting mechanism. The wound edge is sharp and clean, without extensive contamination, and minimal deeper soft tissue damage.

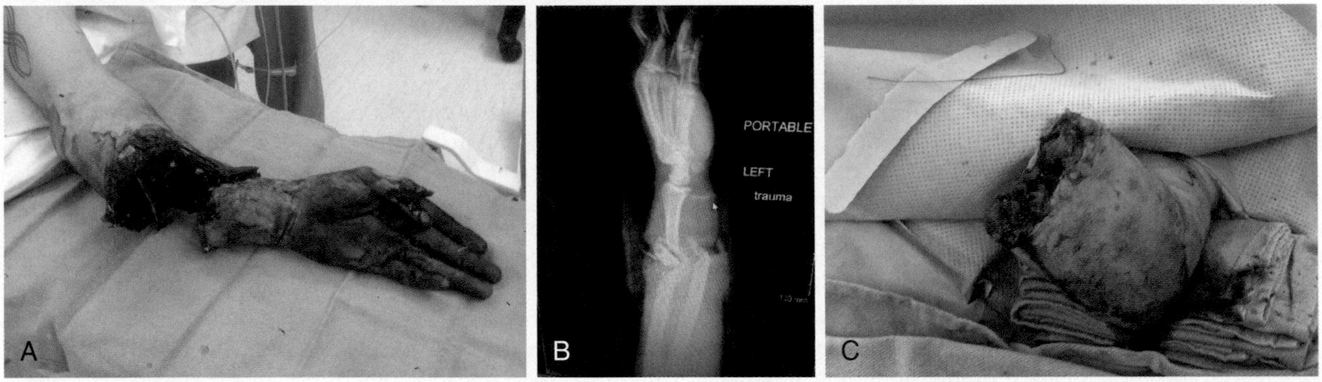

Figure 17-2. A, Forearm of a crushing conveyor belt injury to the left forearm. The volar compartment is completely destroyed and nonfunctional. The dorsal compartment is transected with only a small amount of dorsal integument remaining. **B,** Images demonstrate a complex fracture with comminution of the distal forearm. **C,** The arm was not salvageable and resulted in a below elbow amputation.

fractured limb.[23] The secondary blast injury occurs from the casualty of being struck by fragments from the explosive device or by secondary missiles being energized by the blast. This has the same principles of diagnosis and care as for bullets or open wounds. Flying casing fragments and debris are irregularly shaped and less aerodynamically stable. The drag slows the fragments' speed; therefore, they travel shorter distances. The fragments can tumble upon contact with tissue, so they are associated with potentially greater tissue damage than a bullet. A higher risk of environmental debris being dragged into the wound, causing higher contamination, is present. A large, slow-moving projectile may crush a larger amount of tissue. Missile fragmentation can increase temporary cavitation effects. The tertiary blast injury occurs when the victim is thrown against the ground or solid objects. The injuries are similar to blunt trauma or falls. Care follows blunt trauma guidelines. The tertiary blast wave causes fractures, crush injuries, amputations, and associated lacerations as people tumble and impact stationary objects (Fig. 17-3). Therefore, a patient with a blast injury can present with a spectrum of acuity (blast injury with all three components in varying degrees) and injuries (thermal, chemical, biologic, and multisystem). Patients require a multidisciplinary team

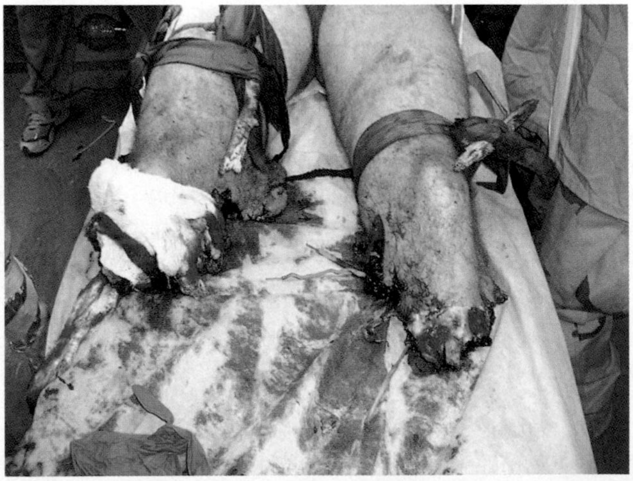

Figure 17-3. Clinical picture of a war blast injury from an improvised explosion device (IED) resulting in immediate, bilateral, below knee amputations.

secondary to the obvious and subtle injury patterns. Even though this injury is mainly associated with war injuries, terrorist (e.g., Boston City Marathon Bombing, 2013) or industrial explosions can generate forces similar to war casualties.

PATHOPHYSIOLOGY

Infection

All open fractures are contaminated. The number of bacteria initially present, the virulence of the bacteria, the severity of the wound, and the immune status of the host are important variables that contribute to the risk of infection that surgeons cannot change. Bacteria replicate quickly and can form a biofilm within 5 hours.[24] The biofilm phenotype is sessile and has a lower metabolic rate and higher resistance to antibiotics[25] and mechanical removal from irrigation.[26] To add to the difficulty of managing open wounds, bacteria that are in the biofilm phenotype do not replicate on culture plates; this may help explain why culturing of wounds has little value.[27] Colonization of bacteria or infection interferes with normal healing by heightened or prolonged inflammation or direct interference with host cells.

CLASSIFICATION

Gustilo and Anderson

Veliskakis proposed the initial open fracture classification based on three types and worsening severity.[28] Gustilo and Anderson formulated and confirmed the classification in the 1960s and 1970s.[10,29] Gustilo modified the classification further.[30] The classification was based on open tibial fractures and the size of the wound. They determined a relationship between an increasing wound size and the risk of infection or osteomyelitis. The classification did not determine outcome or treatment.

Type I fractures have a skin laceration of less than 1 cm. This is usually a poke hole through the skin from the bone poking out or a direct blow from out to in. Type II fractures have a laceration greater than 1 cm and less than 10 cm. Type III fractures fall into a large and varied category, including extensive skin damage with muscle involvement, high-energy injury, crush injury, segmental or highly comminuted fracture, segmental diaphyseal osseous defect, high-velocity weapon, extensive contamination of the wound, or farm yard injury. Type IIIA fractures have lacerations greater than 10 cm, but the integument can be closed or reapproximated. Type IIIA also includes any wound size with heavy contamination with or without segmental or comminuted fracture patterns. Type IIIB fractures have lacerations greater than 10 cm, but the wound cannot be reapproximated and requires a rotational or free tissue transfer for closure. Skin grafting closure does not make the wound a type IIIB. Modifications of this classification can be considered if using a circular frame for treatment. If the fracture is treated with an external fixator that allows for bending or shortening, the wound can then be closed. This is then considered a type IIIB converted to a type IIIA wound. The amount of bending and shortening is restricted before secondary consequences such as vascular kinking and congestion can result in a limb at risk. Type IIIC fractures are open wounds with an associated vascular injury

TABLE 17-1 *GUSTILO-ANDERSON CLASSIFICATION TYPES AND DESCRIPTIONS*

Type	Description
1	Open clean wound <1 cm length
2	Open wound >1 cm and <10 cm without extensive soft tissue damage
3A	Open wound >10 cm that is able to be reapproximated with extensive soft tissue damage, special circumstance for gun shot wounds and farm/contaminated wounds
3B	Open wound that requires rotational or free tissue transfer for osseous coverage
3C	Associated vascular injury that requires repair for viability of limb

From Gustilo RB, Anderson JT: Prevention of infection in the treatment of one thousand and twenty-five open fractures of long bones: retrospective and prospective analyses. J Bone Joint Surg Am *58(4):453–458, 1976.*

requiring repair for limb salvage (Table 17-1). Gustilo also classified an open fracture that presents longer than 8 hours after injury as a special type III open fracture.[30]

The Gustilo-Anderson classification has been able to recommend antibiotic usage based on the type of fracture.[10] The more severe wound requires broader spectrum antibiotic coverage. Type I and II wounds with mainly gram-positive bacteria require only a cephalosporin. Type III wounds require gram-negative coverage in addition. Contaminated wounds require penicillin for *Clostridium* and group A streptococcus coverage. Increasing wound size and classification severity was correlated with wound infection and amputation rates.[30] Therefore, the classification was subdivided later (1970–1980s) into three types (A, B, C) of type III injuries. The risk of wound infection was type IIIA, 4%; type IIIB, 53%; and type IIIC, 42%.[11] The risk of amputation was type IIIA, 0%; type IIIB, 16%; and type IIIC, 42%.[11] Despite the correlative increasing severity, the classification has a poor interobserver reliability at only 60%.[31,32] Even though this problem exists, the classification has generated worldwide acceptability. It is simple and logically stratifies open fractures. Despite originally determined to describe open tibial fracture patterns only, it has, rightly or wrongly, expanded to classify other fractures of the body. The system does recommend methods for closure (primary, delayed, free tissue transfer) but does not recommend overall treatment methods. Treatments do change over time and can change the classification type today. For example, vacuum-assisted closure (VAC) allows us to close many wounds today (type IIIA) that would have required free tissue transfer (type IIIB) without this method. In addition, circular external fixator frames with or without proximal corticotomy facilitate fracture manipulation to close the wound and accelerate local blood flow.

Other Open Fracture Classifications

Tscherne and colleagues developed an open and closed fracture classification.[33,34] The types were type I, puncture hole; type II, moderate contamination; type III, heavy contamination, soft tissue problems; and type IV, incomplete or complete amputation. This was combined with a closed fracture, soft tissue injury classification. The types were type 0, minimal soft tissue damage with indirect violence, simple fracture pattern (e.g., torsion fracture of the tibia in skiers); type I, superficial abrasion or contusion caused by pressure from within, mild to moderate severe fracture pattern (e.g., ankle pronation fracture-dislocation with soft tissue over medial malleolus); type II, deep contaminated abrasion associated with localized skin or muscle contusion, impending compartment syndrome (e.g., segmental "bumper" tibial fracture); and type III, extensive skin contusion or crush, underlying muscle damage may be severe, subcutaneous avulsion or degloving, associated major vascular injury, severe or comminuted fracture pattern. The injury systems are complete, but the categories contain too much variability and subjective discrimination.

The Arbeitsgemeinschaft für Osteosynthesefragen (AO) classification[35] system is a modification of the Tscherne classification[34] and uses a grading system based on skin (I), muscles and tendons (MT), and neurovascular (NV). Each grade is further divided into five degrees of severity. This is the first system to grade wounds more on severity than just size. In addition, it indirectly attempts to measure the amount of function based on the soft tissue injury to the muscle and nerves. The problem with this classification is the complexity of the multiple choices for different categories and therefore the inability to deploy or use it for daily practices or consumption.

Arbeitsgemeinschaft für Osteosynthesefragen/Orthopaedic Trauma Association Open Fracture Classification

Despite the widespread use of the Gustilo-Anderson classification, a better way to quantify the severity of open fractures is needed. For example, a Gustilo open IIIB tibial fracture with a small-sized anterior pretibial defect, no bone loss, and minimal contamination but requiring a soleus muscle rotational flap is typed the same as a Gustilo open IIIB tibial fracture with extensive degloving and contamination, more than 4 cm of segmental bone loss, and loss of the entire anterior compartment and requiring bone transport or massive autografting, free tissue transfer, and extensive split-thickness skin grafts (STSGs). To address these limitations and better define these injuries, the Orthopaedic Trauma Association (OTA), in collaboration with the AO group, created the OTA Open Fracture Study Group. With the use of the three electronic databases (PubMed, EMBASE, and Web of Science), factors used to evaluate open fractures of the upper extremity, pelvis, and lower extremity were compiled. Based on their clinical experience and the existing literature, seven fellow-trained orthopaedic trauma surgeons independently examined and prioritized factors for inclusion or exclusion for this new open fracture classification (Table 17-2). A rank-order mean for each factor was calculated and measured as to its relative importance (Table 17-3). The other factors were simplicity, pathoanatomy, the exclusion of systemic issues, and anatomic characteristics of the injury. This group recently finalized a new open fracture classification system to facilitate consistent application and communication in assessment, treatment, and research. The new OTA/AO Open Fracture Classification (OFC) includes five assessment categories: (1) skin defect, (2) muscle injury, (3) arterial injury, (4) bone loss, and an additional (5) contamination with each category subdivided into three descriptors (mild, moderate, and severe) of increasing severity (Table 17-4).[36] The classification was successfully tested for feasibility and ease of clinical data collection. The advantage of this classification is better classifying the injury severity, which is a continuous variable, into different groupings of severity instead of just three categories.

Furthermore, the OFC could also determine treatment implications instead of just infection such as the Gustilo classification. A recent study prospectively evaluated 356 patients with open fractures of different areas of the body instead of just open tibial diaphyseal fractures.[37] The use of VAC, multiple débridements, antibiotic bead placement, and early amputation was evaluated. The OFC was related to the type of treatment used to treat this cohort of open fractures. Skin injury was the strongest predictor of VAC utilization. Skin injury and muscle injury were predicted multiple débridements. Bone loss was a strong predictor of antibiotic bead placement. The combination of skin injury, contamination, and arterial injury were the strongest predictors of limb amputation. Further analysis will determine how these variations in the five subgroups will determine how an open fracture is treated.

At the 2013 annual OTA meeting, two research projects concerning the OFC were presented. Both have important and different take-home messages. The OFC was validated in a population of severe limb-threatening tibial fractures.[38] The study used the original prospective data collection from the Lower Extremity Assessment Project (LEAP) study. LEAP data included the Anderson-Gustilo open fracture classification,[29,39] the Tscherne closed and open fracture classification,[33,40,41] the AO classification of soft tissue injury of the tibia (closed and open lesions), Hannover fracture scale,[42] Limb Salvage Index,[43] Predictive Salvage Index,[44] and the Mangled Extremity Severity Score (MESS).[45,46] The cohort data retrospectively classified the fractures using the OFC scheme. From available LEAP study data, the authors identified the most appropriate classifications and response categories from the LEAP study that would correspond to each of the five arrays of the OFC. A crosswalk between the classifications used in LEAP and the OFC were performed. As expected, each of the five OFC components showed a statistically dependent relationship with the Gustilo type and revealed variation in the OFC classification within Gustilo type. The polychoric correlation between each of the OFC components was low to moderate. Examining the predictive capacity of the OFC against two important outcomes assessed criterion validity: early amputation and function at 2 years after trauma. An increased severity of each OFC component score was significantly associated with amputation. The predictive power of each OFC component with respect to amputation, as measured by predictive area under the curve (AUC), was comparable to that of the Gustilo-Anderson classification. The new OFC provides a system to classify soft tissue injuries within five clinically meaningful domains, each of which is strongly predictive of amputation, a major clinical outcome. Among salvage patients, having the highest level of the muscle, bone loss, and arterial disruption, the OFC component was associated with 2.9-, 3.8-, and 5.8-point increases, respectively, in disability at 2 years based on functional outcomes as defined by the physical and psychosocial domains of the Sickness Impact Profile (SIP).[47] A combination criterion of the highest levels of the arterial and bone loss components was developed, which occurred in 23% of this severely injured population. The data suggest that several OFC components are predictive of clinically and statistically significant differences in long-term functional outcome. Overall, the results of this analysis show that the OFC has strong content, construct, and both concurrent and predictive criterion validity.

The other OTA presentation used the same LEAP data but evaluated how soft tissue injury or loss predicts amputations in severe open tibial fractures.[48] A logistic regression model of the 19 tibial compartment soft tissue items (muscle, vein, artery, and nerve) was developed in order to examine their independent contributions to the risk of amputation. When included in a single model, all 19 items were able to predict amputation with an AUC of 0.833 (roughly equivalent to 80% sensitivity and specificity). Two components, the posterior tibial artery and the tibial nerve, were so highly correlated that it would have been impossible to include them as separate items in any model, and they were merged for the analysis. Using logistic regression a subset of six items (flexor hallucis longus, peroneal artery or vein, posterior tibial artery or vein, superficial peroneal nerve, and gastrocnemius) accounted for 98% of the predictive power of the larger model (AUC, 0.815). Injury to the flexor hallucis longus muscle or any anterior compartment muscles severe enough to render them nonfunctional as well as a nonfunctional tibial nerve were predictive of patients who ultimately underwent amputation. As a general finding, as the numbers of individual muscles injured increased, the patient was more likely to undergo an amputation. These results may allow surgeons to more accurately counsel their patients on what to expect and enable them to maximize the predicted functional outcome for a patient with a mangled lower extremity. Therefore, the OFC may be able to predict outcomes based on the severity of injury.

The OFC is a new and validated open fracture classification, which allows for improved subgrouping over the Gustilo classification. It may be able to predict operative treatment, outcomes, and potential for amputation. It will be used in parallel with, if not replacement of, the Gustilo classification for future research and publications (Figs. 17-4 and 17-5).

BASIC PRINCIPLES OF OPEN FRACTURE MANAGEMENT IN THE EMERGENT SETTING

Initial Trauma Assessment

Patients with open fractures require a full trauma assessment. One should be familiar with the Advanced Trauma Life Support (ATLS) protocols. A parallel and proactive orthopaedic assessment should be performed. The mechanism required to produce an open fracture is more than the usual twisting or fall mechanism. Therefore, looking for subtle, progressing, or serious life-threatening injuries should be performed in all patients. As an orthopaedist experienced in associated injuries, a proactive and helpful consultant is beneficial to the trauma team. Large-bore intravenous (IV) lines are required for resuscitation and antibiotic delivery. Tetanus prophylaxis is initiated as soon as possible.[49]

Prompt Diagnosis

In assessment of any fracture, the limb must be assessed circumferentially with complete removal of all clothing and splints. Do not miss an open fracture. Open fractures are surgical emergencies. Determine the time of injury and facilitate all phases of patient assessment and injury imaging. A wound oozing venous blood, especially with fat droplets, is suspicious for an open fracture. Despite varying sizes of open wounds, check to make sure no clothing or foreign body is entrapped within the wound. Open wounds can have local or distant open communicating sites. After the diagnosis is made, cover the wound with saline-soaked gauze or toppers. The saline will diminish the desiccation of the tissues. Because antibiotic, chlorhexidine, and povidone–iodine addition can affect the tissue viability,[50,51] saline is preferred to other methods of gauze preparation. After the sterile dressing is applied, do not remove it for additional provider visualization because this can be performed in the operative suite. In addition, reapplying dressings in the emergency department increases the risk of infection three- to fourfold.[34]

Imaging studies should be evaluated for any soft tissue abnormality or air consistent with an open fracture. Furthermore, imaging the entire bone along with associated joints will lessen missed fractures. After the diagnosis of an open fracture is completed, appropriate treatment options and timing can be initiated.

Control Bleeding

After initial visual assessment, apply sterile gauze or toppers to the open wound. After this, apply a mildly compressive splint to control bleeding with the compression and realignment of the limb. This will also reduce pain with immobilization of the fracture and swelling with utilization of hydrostatic forces. Remove any skin entrapped within the wound to avoid necrosis of skin edges. On rare occasions, hemostat or ligation of a bleeding vessel is required to minimize blood loss and even exsanguination. For uncontrollable hemorrhage or amputation, a temporary tourniquet can be applied and inflated proximal to the bleeding and wound (Fig. 17-6). The positive effects of tourniquet utilization need to be compared to the negative effects of worsening ischemia, muscle damage, and pain.

Injury Assessment

Integument

The extent of injury should begin with the open wound. Determine the length, width, skin loss, degloving, and counter or other wounds. Cool, mottled, or ischemic skin prompts further evaluation into the vascular integrity. Limbs lacking or having sparse hair can be associated with long-term vascular compromise or claudication. Reduce fractures to avoid compression and compromise of skin edges. Cover with sterile dressing and leave in place until the patient is in the operating room.

Contamination

Even if the wound is a low-energy twisting or small open puncture wound, contamination can be present. Note the setting of the injury such as water (e.g., lake, stream, pool, or brackish water), work (e.g., grease, paint, or dirt), or nature (e.g., farm).[52,53] Confirm the mechanism such as lawnmower, crush, or gunshot, which may have forced contamination remote or distant from the fracture or open wound. Impact injuries such as motor vehicle and cycle may have pavement, paint, or metal burnished onto a small or large area of the exposed bone end. Loose and superficial debris or contamination should be mechanically removed and washed off initially to potentially lower the bacterial count.

Vascular

Initially palpate the pulses distally to the limb and compare them with those of the contralateral extremity. Absent pulses

Text continued on p. 474

TABLE 17-2 *COMPREHENSIVE LIST OF FACTORS DESCRIBING OPEN FRACTURE TISSUE INJURY OR TREATMENT CHARACTERISTICS FROM THE LITERATURE*

Reference	AAAM	Bosse, et al.	Bosse, et al.	Byrd, et al.	Castillo, et al.	Collins, et al.	Gregory, et al.	Gustilo, et al.	Hamson, et al.	Howe, et al.
Mechanism of soft-tissue/muscle injury								X		X
Fracture pattern							X	X		X
Neurologic injury					X		X			
Arterial injury							X	X		X
Age		X	X				X			
Contamination										
Warm ischemic time										
Comorbidities							X			
Injury-to-OR interval							X			X
Seventy and duration of shock							X			
Venous injury							X			
Bone loss							X			
Injury Seventy Score (ISS)							X			
Skin injury										
Skin laceration								X		
Smoking status		X	X			X				
Amputation							X			
Energy of injury								X		
Injury location									X	
Injury status of ipsilateral foot										
Skin defect										
Occupational considerations										
Patient/family desires										
Wounding mechanism (blunt vs. penetrating)										
Loss of soft tissues of foot										
Muscle viability at operation										
Intercaiary ischemic zone after revascularization										
Transport time										
Delay of revascularization										
Bacteriologic smear										
Trauma center vs. community hospital										
Psychosocial factors			X							
AIS seventy category	X									
Open joint injury/fx				X						

From Orthopaedic Trauma Association: Open Fracture Study Group: A new classification scheme for open fractures. J Orthop Trauma *24(8):457–464, 2010, Fig. 1.*

Johansen, et al.	Johansen, et al.	Lange, et al.	McNamara, et al.	Muller, et al.	Russell, et al.	Slauterbeck, et al.	Suedkamp, et al.	Swiontkowski, et al.	Togawa, et al.	Tscherne, et al.	Tally
	X	X	X	X	X	X	X	X		X	11
		X	X		X	X	X	X			9
	X	X			X		X	X		X	8
	X	X			X					X	7
	X	X	X								6
			X			X	X	X		X	5
	X	X	X				X	X			5
X	X	X									4
	X						X				4
	X	X	X								4
	X				X			X			4
							X	X			3
	X	X									3
					X		X			X	3
				X		X					3
											3
							X				2
	X										2
									X		2
		X						X			2
							X	X			2
		X									1
		X									1
	X										1
	X										1
	X										1
		X									1
	X										1
	X										1
							X				1
	X										1
											1
											1
											1

TABLE 17-3 *OPEN FRACTURE CLASSIFICATION RANK ORDER MEAN BY COMMITTEE MEMBERS*

Item	Variable	Rank Order Mean (ROM)	7/7 in Top 10	6/7 in Top 10	5/7 in Top 10	4/7 in Top 10	3/7 in Top 10	2/7 in Top 10	1/7 in Top 10	0/7 in Top 10
1	Muscle viability at operation	5.571		X						
2	Mechanism/soft-tissue injury kinetics/muscle injury	3.286	X							
3	Energy of injury	6.571		X						
4	Arterial jnjury	8.571			X					
5	Severity and duration of shock	8.571			X					
6	Delay of revascularization	12.143				X				
7	Loss of soft tissues of distal part	15.571					X			
8	Injury status of ipsilateral part	17.429							X	
9	Intercalary ischemic zone after revascularization	16.000						X		
10	Warm ischemic time	10.571			X					
11	Venous injury	21.143								X
12	Neurologic injury	17.000							X	
13	Open joint injury/fx	16.429								X
14	Injury location	11.714						X		
15	Skin injury	18.143						X		
16	Skin defect	16.429						X		
17	Skin laceration	21.000						X		
18	Contamination	11.000			X					
19	Age	17.000							X	
20	Fracture pattern	12.714						X		
21	Bone loss	9.000			X					
22	Occupational considerations	29.429								X
23	Psychosocial factors	27.429								X
24	Injury-to-OR interval	25.714								X
25	AIS severity category	20.571								X
26	Transport time	28.714								X
27	Patient/family desires	26.714								X
28	Bacteriologic smear	28.857								X
29	ISS	17.000						X		
30	Amputation	25.000							X	
31	Trauma center vs. community hospital	27.571								X
32	Wounding mechanism (blunt vs. penetrating)	18.000						X		
33	Smoking status	20.286								X
34	Co-morbidities	20.571							X	

From Orthopaedic Trauma Association: Open Fracture Study Group: A new classification scheme for open fractures. J Orthop Trauma *24(8):457–464, 2010, Fig. 2.*

TABLE 17-4 ***PROPOSED CLASSIFICATION OF OPEN FRACTURES***

Factor	Subgroup	Description
Skin	1	Mild, <5 cm and approximates
	2	Moderate, >5 cm and approximates
	3	Severe, does not approximate
Muscle	1	Mild, no muscle injured or necrotic
	2	Moderate, localized damage requiring debridement but muscle unit functional
	3	Severe, extensive damage requiring debridement, muscle unit excised and no longer functional
Arterial	1	Mild, no major vessel disruption
	2	Moderate, vessel injury but does not require repair
	3	Severe, vessel injury requires repair for limb viability
Comtamination	1	Mild, none or minimal contamination
	2	Moderate, surface contamination easily removed and not imbedded
	3	a. Severe, imbedded in bone or soft tissues
		b. Severe, high risk environmental conditions such as farm, fecal, dirty water, etc.
Bone loss	1	None
	2	Moderate, bone missing but still some contact between proximal and distal segments
	3	Severe, segmental bone loss without any osseous contact

Overall severity: Any two above makes it a Type 2, Any three above makes it a Type 3.
Type 1 = Mild; Type 2 = Moderate; Type 3 = Severe.
From Agel J, Rockwood T, Barber R, et al: Potential predictive ability of the Orthopaedic Trauma Association Open Fracture Classification. J Orthop Trauma 28(5): 300–306, 2014, Appendix 1.

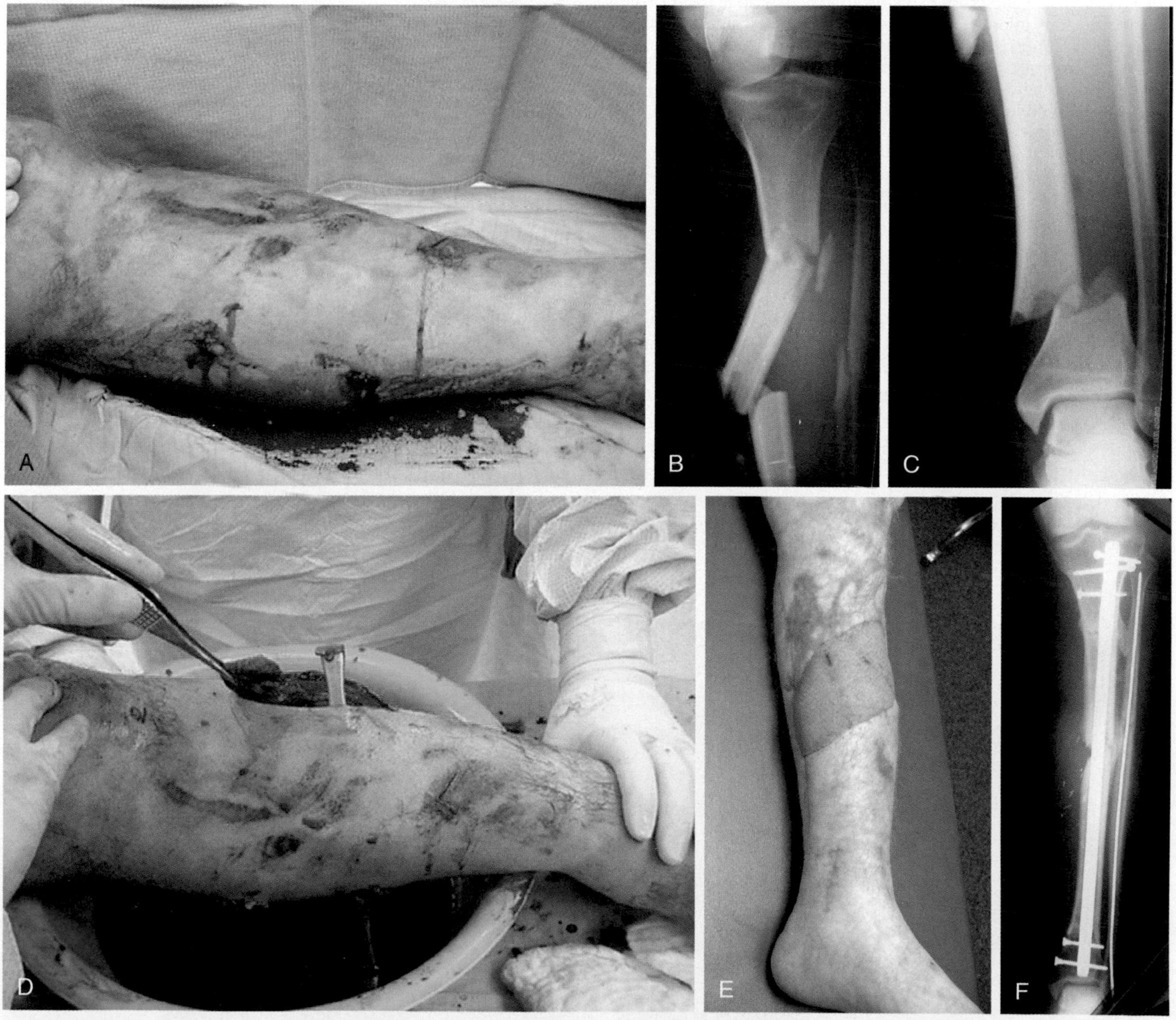

Figure 17-4. Clinical picture (**A**) and image (**B** and **C**) of a Gustilo Type IIIB tibial fracture. Initial debridement (**D**) noted a severe degloving injury that resulted in loss of the anteromedial skin over the segmental tibial fracture. After serial debridements, tibial and fibular nailing, and a rotational soleus muscle transfer, the patient healed his wounds (**E**), regained function of his tibia, and united his fractures (**F**) at the 6-month interval. Using the New OTA Open Fracture Classification, the injury would have been evaluated because skin did not reapproximate and needed a rotational muscle coverage (3), anterolateral muscle group was damaged but was still functional (2), did not have a repairable arterial injury (1), had minimal contamination (1), and had moderate bone missing at the mid-diaphyseal fracture region (2). This injury is an OTA/OFC Type 3, but the subgroupings define the injury better than the Gustilo-Anderson classification.

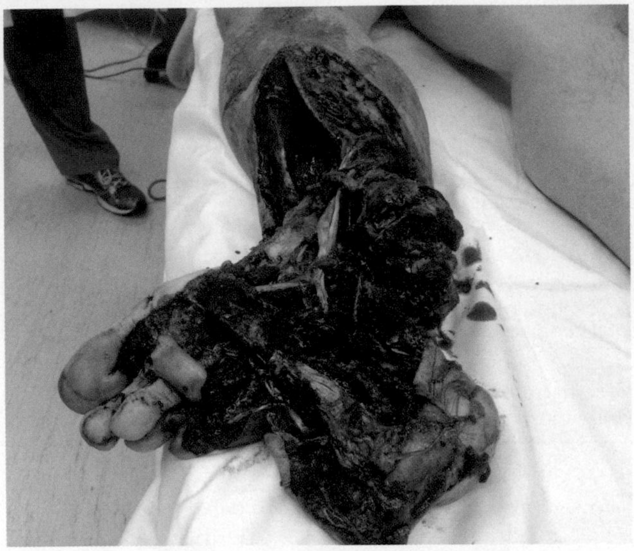

Figure 17-5. Clinical picture of a Gustilo Type IIIB tibial fracture with an associated foot injury. The foot had pulses. Using the OTA Open Fracture Classification, the injury would have been evaluated because skin did not reapproximate (3), the posterior and deep posterior muscle compartments were damaged and did not function (3), did not have a repairable arterial injury (1), had severe imbedded contamination and road debris (3), and had multiple areas of bone loss that without osseous contact possible (3). This injury is an OTA/OFC Type 3 that was deemed not salvageable and resulted in a below knee amputation after serial debridements.

or cadaveric skin confirms an avascular limb. The skin should be checked for ischemic, cyanotic, mottled, and cold characteristics (Fig. 17-7). Collateral circulation can often mask or confuse manual palpation of pulse quality. Lessened pulses, especially in patients with peripheral vascular disease or in the setting of hypotension, can be confusing. Again, a comparison with the contralateral limb for symmetry is helpful. Straighten shortened and angulated limbs to unkink or unimpinge threatened vessels. Ongoing bleeding with a severed vein or artery should be gently clamped with a hemostat to lessen further blood loss. To confirm the diagnosis or integrity, perform an ankle-brachial index (Fig. 17-8). Distal extremity injuries or wounds complicate and potentially obviate the test. When in doubt, obtain an angiogram or computed tomography angiogram to qualify and quantify the injury (Fig. 17-9).

Muscle Integrity and Function

In awake and cooperative patients, check, confirm, and document nerve function of sensation and motor. Check all dermatomes of the affected extremity for altered or absent sensation. Of course, injured limbs will have altered and potentially absent motor function secondary to inhibition or pain. Appropriate pain reduction with pain medicines and limb splinting may improve motor and functional assessment. Tendons entrapped within the fracture or dislocation will hinder the examination. An open extremity with open fascial compartments should correlate with muscle loss and muscle function (Fig. 17-10). Remember that an open fracture can have an associated compartment syndrome and elevated compartmental pressures.[30] Evaluate all muscular compartments proximally and distally from the injury.

Bone Loss

Completely devitalized bone outside the limb and wound should be discarded. Questionably devitalized bone or bone within the wound should be gently placed within the wound, under the muscle, and covered with saline-soaked gauze or toppers for complete assessment under more sterile and optimal conditions in the operative suite. Further bone loss will be assessed after the wound is cleaned and the fracture reduced operatively.

Splinting

Reduce all dislocations and fractures with long plaster splints to obtain as much length and alignment as possible. The stabilized limb will lessen the pain and facilitate transportation, vascularity, and motor examination. A straightened limb in a splint can enhance surgeon assessment of the injury with imaging and treatment options.

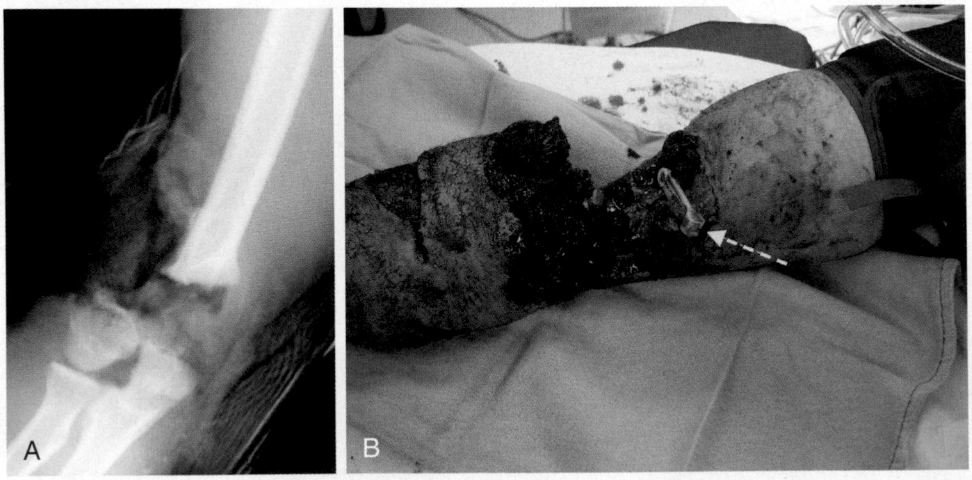

Figure 17-6. A, Open distal humeral fracture from a conveyor belt injury noting an associated humeral fracture. **B,** A tourniquet *(far right proximal portion of field)* and vessel clamp *(arrow)* are applied to control the hemorrhaging and save the patient's life. Despite saving his life, he lost his limb and ended up with an above elbow amputation.

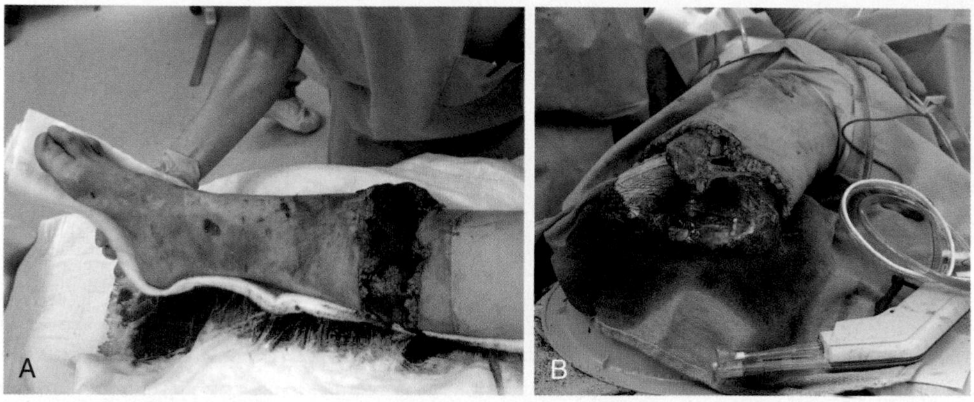

Figure 17-7. Open tibial fracture with complete disruption of the anterior and anterolateral compartments with complete vascular disruption of the tibial arterial trifurcation. **A,** Ischemia is noted distal to the site of injury with cyanosis and mottling of the skin. **B,** The injury resulted in a complex below knee amputation.

WOUND INFECTIONS AND ANTIBIOTICS

The skin and wound associated with open fractures have a contamination rate of up to 65%.[10,12,51] The risk of infection is related to the severity of the injury with rates of infection of 2% for type I, 2% to 10% for type II, and 10% to 50% for type III.[10,54] Patients with associated comorbidities are at even higher risk of infection.[55] In a study evaluating the risk factors for osteomyelitis, three classes were developed: class A, no immune compromising factors; class B, one or two immune compromising factors; and class C, three or more compromising factors. The infection rates were 4%, 15%, and 30% for class A, B, and C, respectively. The Gustilo open fracture classification, location, and tobacco abuse were all factors associated with infection (Fig. 17-11). Open fractures in the lower extremity compared with the upper extremity are three times more likely to get infected.[56] In addition, infection was related to increasing severity of Gustilo types. Infection occurred in 7% of type 1, 11% of type II, 18% of type IIIA, and 56% of types IIIB and IIIC open fractures.

Wound cultures should not be routinely obtained and are of little value. The reason for this is multifactorial based on early broad-spectrum antibiotic utilization, multiple wound débridements, and late contamination with nosocomial pathogens.[57] Despite presenting with an open wound, cultures obtained while in the emergency department are positive only 60% to 70% of the time.[54,58] Furthermore, the cultures obtained in this initial setting grow saprophytic organisms, which are clinically irrelevant organisms.[41] If the original predébridement culture becomes positive, only 40% to 73% of these

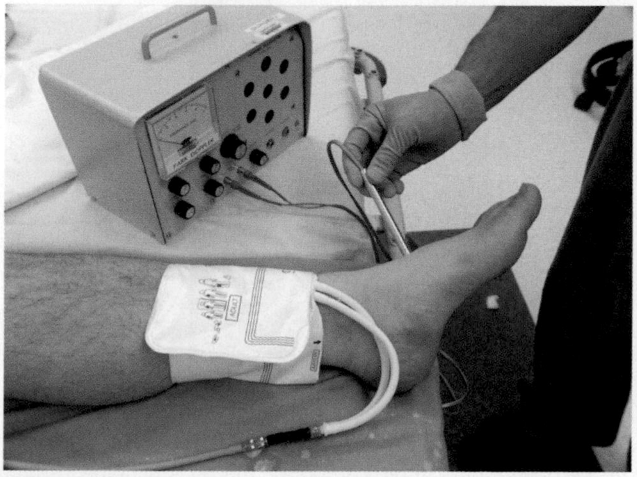

Figure 17-8. Using a manual blood pressure cuff, an ultrasound unit is utilized for the determination of the ankle brachial index (ABI).

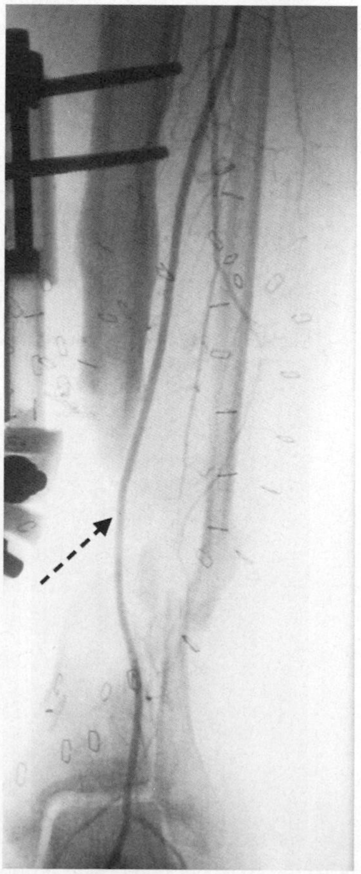

Figure 17-9. An angiogram of a severe open distal tibial fracture demonstrates a dominant, single, anterior tibial artery limb *(arrow)*. The posterior tibial artery was disrupted and not repaired initially.

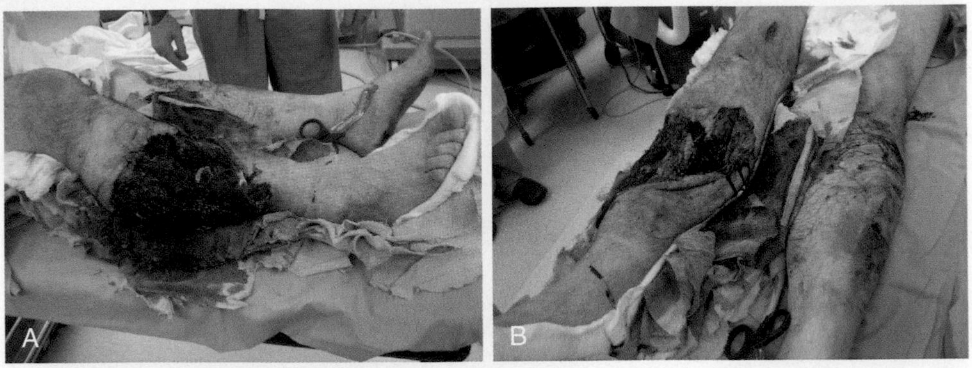

Figure 17-10. Clinical picture of an open tibial fracture that resulted from a car bumper injury crush resulting in loss of muscle compartment function of the anterior, anterolateral, and deep posterior compartments (**A**) and stripping of the tibial soft tissue attachments (**B**).

fractures become infected with one of the original pathogens.[40,57] Another study demonstrated only 8% positive predébridement cultures eventually causing infection.[57] Of the cases that become infected, only 22% of the time was the predébridement correlative with the final infecting organism. This could be because of new organisms or that conventional cultures do not identify bacteria within the biofilm.[27]

What and Type

In a randomized controlled trial, Patzakis was the first to demonstrate the importance and effectiveness of systemic antibiotics in the prevention of posttraumatic wound infections.[12,13,54] Infection rates of 14% (no antibiotics) and 9.8% (penicillin and streptomycin) were reduced to 2.4% with cephalosporin usage. The routine use of IV antibiotics for a postoperative

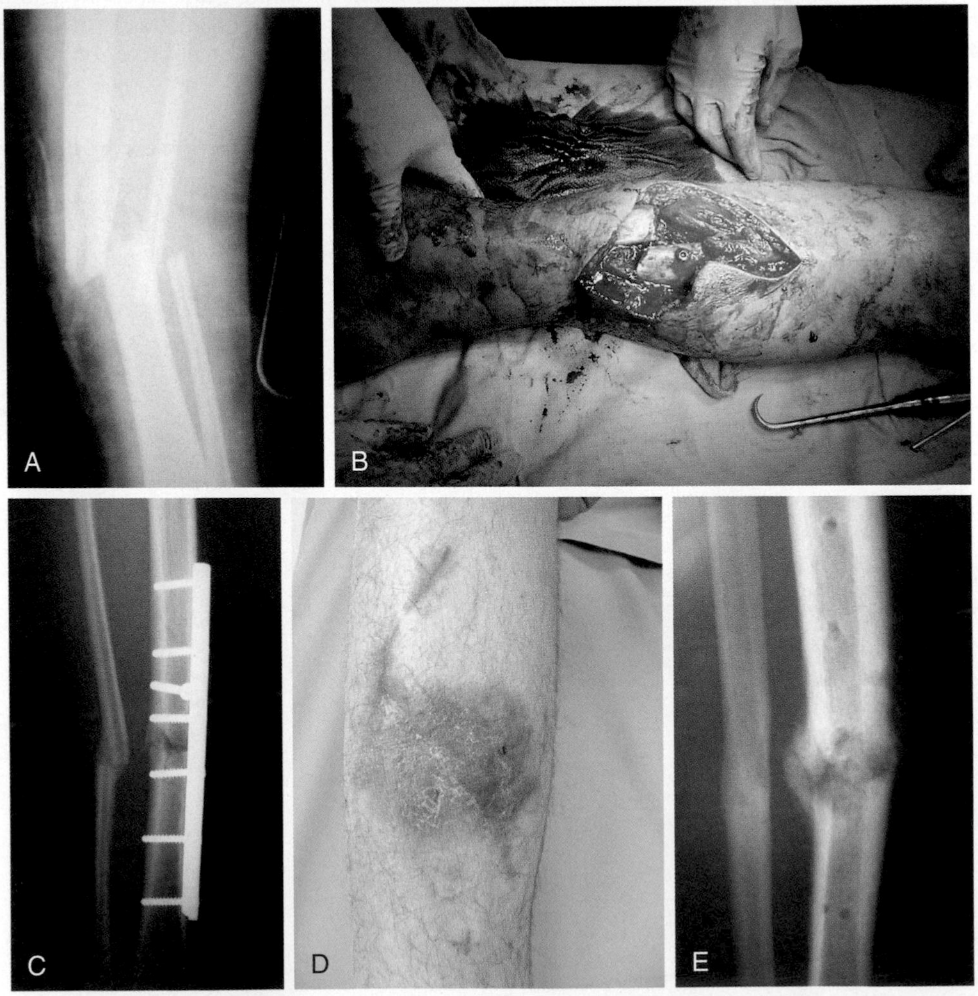

Figure 17-11. A young man presented with an open tibial fracture (**A**), which had extension of the wound (**B**), debridement, and a classic open reduction internal fixation (**C**) with a broad 4.5-mm plate. Because of the open injury, surgical stripping, medial subcutaneous broad plating, and pre-existing steroid treated reactive airway disease, a painfully red tibial developed (**D**) that required debridement, plate removal, and an infected tibial nonunion (**E**).

period of time has been replicated and confirmed.[10,54,56,59-61] Antibiotics should be initiated as soon as possible. In a recent survey, surgeons from the OTA believe that IV antibiotics should be initiated within 1 hour of injury and in the emergency department.[62] Early timing of antibiotics has been demonstrated as the single most important facture in reducing the infection rate.[54,63] Based on a retrospective study of 240 fractures, antibiotic timing was not as important as wound care.[56] If able, the emergency medical services personnel in the field or the physician at the referral hospital should begin some type of antibiotic regimen.

Optimal antibiotic determination depends on injury severity, contamination, local flora, and host factors.[64,65] Broad coverage antibiotics with bactericidal action are preferential.[66] Providing coverage against most gram-positive and many gram-negative bacteria, first- or second-generation cephalosporins are preferred alone for types I and II open fractures. Cefazolin dosing is 2 g preoperatively, every 4 hours intraoperatively, and every 8 hours postoperatively.[67] If the patient weighs more than 120 kg, the dosing regimen increases to 3 g. Cefuroxime (1.5 g), cefotaxime (1 g; 2 g if the patient weighs more than 120 kg), cefotetan (2 g), and ceftriaxone (2 g) dosing is also every 8 hours. These cephalosporins are not effective against *Pseudomonas* spp., though. An aminoglycoside (gentamicin or tobramycin), which increases gram-negative coverage, should be added for type III open fractures. Dosing for aminoglycosides is 5.1 mg/kg daily. Substitutes for aminoglycosides are quinolones, aztreonam, and third-generation cephalosporins.[19] Quinolones are potentially an important alternative because of their broad-spectrum coverage; also, they are bactericidal, tolerated clinically, and provide daily oral (not IV) administration. In a randomized control trial, ciprofloxacin alone compared with cefamandole and gentamicin combination resulted in similar infection rates (6%) for type I and II open fractures.[68] This single ciprofloxacin therapy was inferior to the combination therapy for type II open fractures at 31% versus 8%, respectively. Therefore, patients with type III open fractures should have cephalosporin and aminoglycoside therapy or ciprofloxacin with a third-generation cephalosporin (as a substitute for the aminoglycoside). Ciprofloxacin could be used as alternative therapy for low-velocity gunshot–induced fractures.[69] The inhibitory fracture healing and osteoblastic activity effects may offset the benefits of oral quinolones.[70] The OTA survey documented the need for an aminoglycoside in 2.4% of type I, 15% of type II, 59% of type IIIA, and 69% of type IIIB fractures.[62] Penicillin G (2–4 million units every 4 hours) or ampicillin should be added for open fractures with a higher potential for anaerobic infections such as *Clostridium* spp. myonecrosis from farm environment, vascular compromise (ischemia, low-oxygen tension, necrotic tissues), or associated soft tissue crush injuries (necrotic tissue, vascular compromise).[19] A recent recommendation for preventing infection in combat-related extremity injuries suggests a dose of 2 g of cefazolin.[71]

How Long?

Traditionally, routine antibiotic coverage has ranged from 3 to 5 days.[10,54,56,59-61] In an OTA survey, continuation of IV antibiotics for 48 hours was preferred in 29% of type I, 33% of type II, 39% of type IIIA, and 38.5% of type IIIB open fractures.[62] One in four surgeons recommends antibiotics for 72 hours or more. Prolonged antibiotic use has been associated with an increased risk of resistant pneumonia and other systemic bacterial infections.[72-75] Despite traditional antibiotic coverage lasting 1 to 5 days in simple, noncontaminated open fractures, a first-generation cephalosporin given for 24 hours is as effective as one given for 5 days.[59] The regimen and type of antibiotics should be reevaluated every time the patient returns to the operative suite based on the type of procedure and wound characteristics.[15,76]

BASIC PRINCIPLES OF OPEN FRACTURE MANAGEMENT IN THE OPERATING SUITE

Débridement

The timing of débridement should be performed urgently or emergently. Early and thorough débridement has been shown to lessen risk of infection and healing problems. This time zone has been established to be at a point less than 6 hours from the time of injury.[54,77,78] This originated from an open wound study of guinea pigs noting that all animals remained healthy if the wounds were débrided within the first 6 hours.[79] Furthermore, wound bacterial counts reached an open fracture infection threshold at a mean of 5.17 hours after an injury.[80] In an earlier study of 47 grade II and III fractures, 7% of the fractures débrided less than 5 hours from injury become infected compared with 38% of the fractures débrided longer than 5 hours from time of injury.[78] Timely admission to a trauma center for definitive initial treatment was deemed more important than timing of first debridement.[81] Some have demonstrated no effect of débridement timing on infection or outcome.[68,77,82-85] Delays alone did not have an effect, but delays to débridement in the setting of a polytrauma patient with increased injury severity did have increasing infection rates.[86] In a review of the National Trauma Data Bank Version 3.0, 6099 blunt trauma patients with open tibial fractures were evaluated.[87] The median time to initial débridement was 4.9 hours. Delays of more than 6 and 24 hours occurred 42% and 24% of the time, respectively. Risk factors for delays were older age, head or thoracic injury with abbreviated Injury Severity Score greater than 2, and off-hour presentation (between 6 PM and 2 AM). Interestingly, level 1 and university trauma centers had an independent risk factor of delayed time to débridement. In an OTA survey, 16% of surgeons believed débridement should be performed as soon as possible, and 41% of the surgeons recommended immediate débridement.[62] The majority of surgeons (99.7%) agree that less than 12 hours (not 6 hours) is acceptable for initial formal débridement. The quality of initial débridement was determined as one (the other was time to definitive closure) of the most important principles in preventing deep infection. Delays and inadequate débridement are deleterious to the patient and the creation of a clean wound that sets the stage for reconstruction.[88] Therefore, the timing of initial appropriate débridement with the historical "6-hour rule" should be changed to being done as early or urgently as possible without increasing risk to polytrauma patients.[89] These complex patients may benefit from an initial bedside débridement of all large particulate debris and nonviable tissue followed by limited irrigation and sterile dressing.

Débridement should be adequate with sharp débridement to remove all debris and devitalized tissue. Débridement should begin superficially and then extend deep to the bone. When débriding the skin, remove only what is nonviable

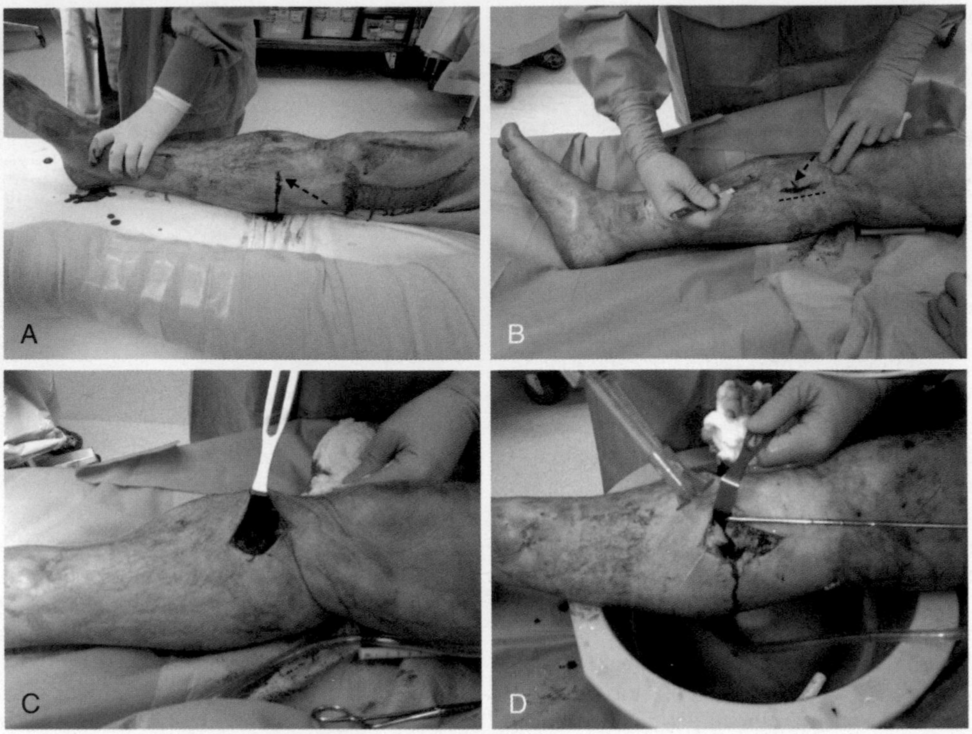

Figure 17-12. **A,** A small "in-to-out" 5-mm open proximal medial tibial wound is noted from a motorcar crash. **B,** The wound is extended both proximally and distally. **C,** The wound is then carefully retracted to explore the wound depth and extent. **D,** The bone edges are then exposed to allow for manual and saline irrigation of the canal and surface.

and keep the questionable skin until the final portion of the procedure. The incision is extended to facilitate wound assessment and delivery of bone for visualization (Fig. 17-12). Remove all degloved and damaged fat sharply. Explore for potential spaces and further areas of degloving to avoid embedded foreign bodies and contamination. Remove only contaminated, nonviable, or nonfunctional fascia. Despite being stripped from the muscle and bone, this fascia can still be functional and beneficial for muscle containment, osseous coverage, and a potential bed for future granulation tissue. Nonviable muscle is removed both sharply and bluntly. Check for muscle viability based on color, consistency, contractibility, and bleeding. Muscle usually dies from the deep to superficial. Therefore, check all damaged, contused, or stripped muscle carefully. Using an Army-Navy retractor or pointed tenaculum clamps, deliver the each bone end into the wound for visualization, débridement, and viability without further damage. Remove the fascia, muscle, and contamination from the ends and canal of the bone. Using a pick-up and knife, embedded sort tissue is removed. A small curette facilitates contamination removal from the bone ends. Make sure to remove all the dark-colored "tattooing" of the bone ends from pavement, paint, or metal impaction. Using a pituitary rongeur, remove debris within the canal. All completely stripped and nonviable bone fragments should be kept in a container of saline to assist further reconstruction concerning length and rotation of the bone. If deemed a vital part of the reduction, it can be removed after osseous stability is achieved with internal fixation. Keep all periarticular fragments, especially articular fragments. Even though nonviable, these fragments are paramount for articular reconstruction and function. During reconstruction, these metaphyseal fragments will revascularize and become functional. If deploying damage control or staged fixation of the articular surface, create a mental and written note of these fragments and place them within the joint after the débridement and before the closure or coverage. This process may take 30 to 90 minutes if not longer with more complex injuries. Do not underdébride or overdébride. This process requires years of experience or oversight from an experienced surgeon.

Irrigation

Irrigation should be performed after all devitalized soft tissue, debris, and loose contamination is removed. Wound irrigation is an essential and universally accepted part of open fracture care.[26] Because little is known concerning options for irrigation, type, additives, pressure, and volume are debatable. Despite this, some accepted guidelines exist.

The standard irrigation type is normal saline (NS). A recent survey of nearly 1000 international surgeons revealed that 71% use NS.[90] Other types of fluid have consisted of chelating agents, antiseptics, antibiotics, and surfactant (soap) solutions. Chelating agents have been demonstrated to be of no or detrimental value.[91] The goals of antiseptics are to kill bacteria, lessen the bacterial load, and therefore lessen the rate of clinical infection. Antiseptics are povidone–iodine (Betadine) solution, povidone–iodine scrub, hexachlorodine gluconate (Hibitane), hexachlorophene (pHisoHex), sodium hypochlorite (Dakin's solution), benzalkonium chloride (Zephiran), and alcohol-containing solutions.[92] By damaging the cell wall or cell membrane of the pathogen, antiseptics change the permeability of the cell and kill the pathogens in the wound. They provide a broad spectrum of activity against bacteria, fungi, and viruses but are also toxic to host cells such as leukocytes, erythrocytes, fibroblasts, keratinocytes, and osteocytes. The effects are concentration dependent, and some lose the bactericidal activity before losing the tissue toxicity function.[93,94] Antiseptics detrimentally affect microvascular flow, endothelial integrity, wound healing, and efficacy in preventing infection.[95] Antiseptics have been demonstrated to have varying effects on wound infection but have substantial deleterious effects on host tissue; therefore, antiseptics should not be used in open wound irrigation. Antibiotics (bacitracin, polymyxin, and neomycin) are bactericidal or bacteriostatic based on concentration and duration in the wound. Bacitracin interferes with bacterial cell wall synthesis. Polymyxin alters cell membrane permeability. Neomycin acts topically through an unknown mechanism. Most studies note lower infection rates with antibiotics in in vitro studies and general surgery studies.[96] A paucity of data exists in the orthopaedic literature.[97] Antibiotic irrigation has three negative aspects: patient safety (anaphylaxis), cost containment, and potential development of surfactants (castile soap, green soap, benzalkonium chloride) interfere with bacterial adhesion to the wound surface and assist irrigation to emulsify and remove debris. Surfactants directly disrupt the hydrophobic forces that propel the initial stages of adhesion and clumping of bacteria to surfaces. Therefore, surfactants do not kill bacteria, but they potentially reduce the bacterial load remaining in the wound after débridement. Since the era of antibiotics, the frequent use of soaps to clean wounds has diminished.[98] Castile soap has proven to be more effective than jet lavage alone at removal of various bacterial species and from different surfaces.[99,100] It also was effective at removing glycocalyx-producing adherent bacteria from stainless steel screws. Surfactants are more effective at removing bacteria than NS alone and should be considered for heavily contaminated wounds with little negative effect on host tissue. Although castile soap helps remove bacteria from the wound, this benefit does not reduce later deep infection rates.[101]

The pressure can be gravity flow, low, or high pressure (Fig. 17-13). Sixty-three percent of surveyed surgeons prefer to not use high pressure. Increased pressure removes more debris and bacteria but at the cost of damaging bone and delaying fracture healing and may increase infection from soft tissue injury.[92,102] Pulsatile flow has not been shown to be more effective than continuous flow delivery.[91] High-pressure (jet lavage) is more effective than low pressure (bulb syringe) at removing debris and bacteria.[91,103-108] This is especially true when delays in initial wound irrigation are present. This comes at a price because high-pressure flow can impair the infection-fighting ability of the soft tissue and can propel fluid (not bacteria) into the damaged soft tissues.[102,109] High-pressure irrigation damages cortical bone based on osteocyte death and microscopic fissures.[105] Based on an osteotomy model, new bone formation is delayed with high-pressure compared to bulb syringe irrigation.[110] In contradistinction, the same study group noted that high-pressure irrigation did not affect new bone healing based on an intraarticular fracture model.[111] A large animal study suggests that although higher pressures remove more bacteria from the wound initially, there is a rebound effect in the bioburden. Two days after irrigation, the wounds that were irrigated with higher pressure had more bacteria than those that received lower pressure irrigation. It is believed that the higher pressure damaged the tissue within the wound, which provided a good environment for the

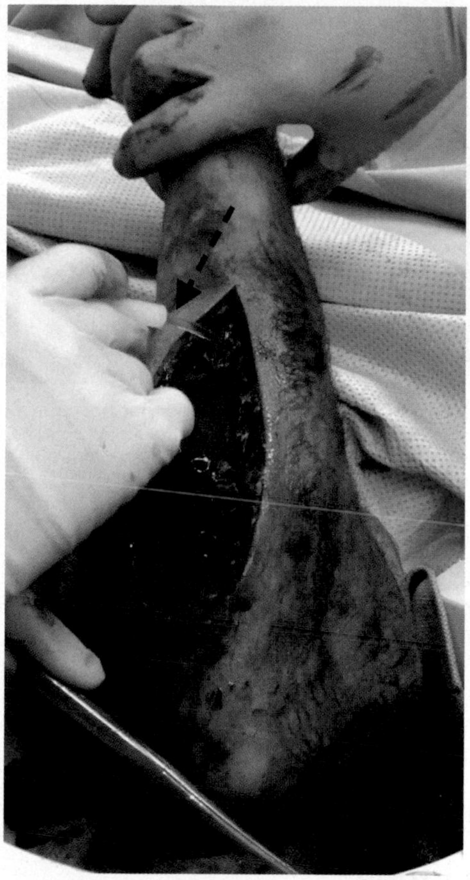

Figure 17-13. A gravity driven normal saline irrigation of an open forearm fracture is noted without pulsatile damage to soft tissues.

bacteria to grow.[101] A pilot study investigating irrigants and irrigation pressures suggests that the high pressure causes more adverse events.[112] The fully powered Fluid Lavage of Open Wounds (FLOW) trial has enrolled all of the 2500 patients and will provide greater evidence to the most effective irrigation solution and pressure to use on open fractures.[113]

The amount to be delivered has been described as "adequate," "copious," or "ample" without further finite descriptors. Although some studies have recommended 6 to 15 L per wound, others have described the amount as being "arbitrary."[114] Although only animal and not human studies have been performed, increases in irrigation volume do remove more debris and bacteria in a corresponding manner up to a point and then plateaus at a certain point depending on the system.[99,115] Truly, volume amount is variable and related to the amount needed for the job and wound involved. A small wound with an associated phalanx fracture would not require nor receive the same amount of fluid required for a contaminated wound with extensive soft tissue injury. As a general rule and based on delivery in 3-L NS bags, use 3 L for type 1, 6 L for type 2 wounds, and 9 L or more for type III injuries.[92] Avoid removal of precariously attached periarticular osseous fragments. Avoid generation of an irrigation-induced muscle injury or compartment syndrome from surgeon-directed high-flow irrigation. Make sure an effluent and influent flow is functional. Use a large basin or modified basin to collect the fluid and avoid further contamination of the room and team.

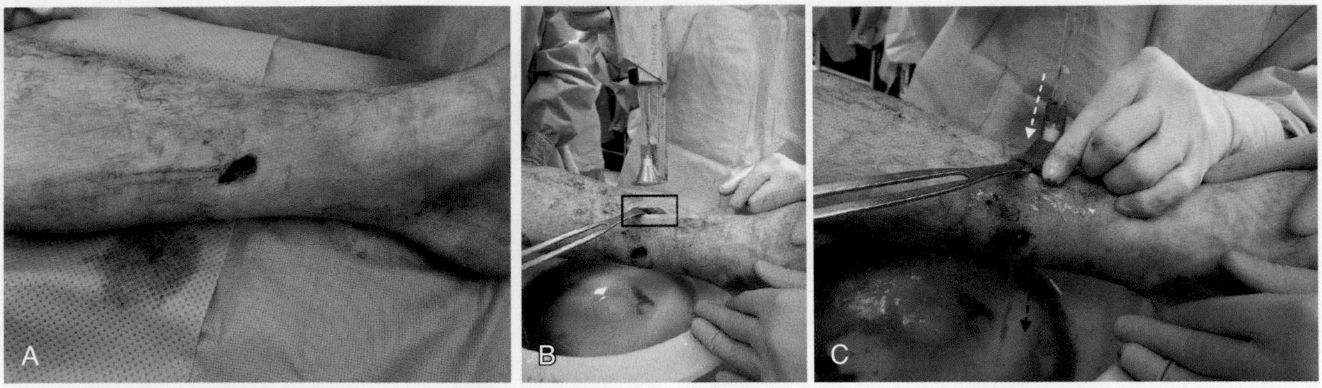

Figure 17-14. A, Open tibial fracture with a posterior open wound. **B,** A counter incision (rectangle) was created to avoid opening the posterior incision or creating further stripping along the medial subcutaneous border. **C,** Irrigation *(white arrow)* is then performed to the open fracture anteriorly to facilitate mechanical debridement and outflow *(black arrow)* through the posterior open wound.

In conclusion, animal studies have demonstrated that high-volume, high-pressure irrigation is more effective at removing debris and bacteria than low-volume, low-pressure irrigation. The high pressure damages host tissue and results in a greater amount of bacteria within the wound at later time points. The irrigation should be done effectively with attention to avoiding further damage to the bone and soft tissues. At this time, low-pressure irrigation with saline is recommended until the results of the FLOW study are published.

Tips and Tricks

The combination of a thorough surgical débridement and irrigation is required to remove debris and lower the bacterial burden in the wound. The wound location and size determine the method of incisional enlargement, wound inspection, bone delivery, and irrigation. Small type I wounds require opening larger for complete wound inspection and débridement. Avoid a small opening with insertion of the irrigation system tip without proper efflux of the fluid. If the wound is along the subcutaneous border as a small open tibial fracture with a puncture wound with or without degloving, a counter-incision laterally either proximally or distally may create less disruption of the precarious blood supply medially with wound extension, avoid a small soft tissue bridge, and facilitate irrigation affluent and effluent (Fig. 17-14). If the open fracture extends intraarticularly with air in the joint or perichondral fracture fragments based on imaging studies such as an open tibial pilon fracture, determine and mark future incisions required for joint reconstruction. If feasible, use one or more of these incisions to facilitate débridement and irrigation of the joint again with an influent and effluent. Not débriding or irrigating the joint underestimates wound and contamination extension.

With larger wounds or degloving, the problem is removing the contaminated and devitalized tissue without removing too much tissue beneficial for coverage and limb salvage. Débride over a bucket or grate to salvage important fragments and contain the irrigation debris. Initially, débride dead muscle and completely devitalized bone. Salvage periarticular bone with chondral fragments for articular reconstruction. Salvage large diaphyseal fragments for assistance in length and rotational reconstruction. The diaphyseal fragments can then be discarded after plate or nail stabilization. If a complete segmental diaphyseal fragment is noted, it can be cleaned, irrigated, and reinserted for medullary nail stabilization. After interlocking screws are inserted, the fragment can be removed using an osteotome or saw. Be careful not to notch or damage the nail on removal to avoid early fatigue failure. The osseous void can then be filled with antibiotic beads. Degloving wounds with degloved fat, partially vital muscle, embedded debris, and contamination may benefit from a surface débriding, hydrosurgery device such as a Versajet (Richards Smith Nephew, Memphis, TN). Viable but defatted skin may be used for further coverage and reconstructive procedures.

Future Studies

Currently, the FLOW study, a large (>2500 patients) multicenter, multinational, blinded, randomized, and factorial trial comparing alternative irrigation solutions and pressures in patients with open fractures, is being conducted.[90,112] Randomization of pressure types (high pressure, low pressure, and gravity flow) and NS additives (soap vs. NS) to the irrigant is being evaluated. The functional outcomes and health-related quality of life will be evaluated. Results of this study will be available in 2014 or 2015.

Open Fractures with Compartment Syndrome

Just because an open fracture disrupts the soft tissue envelope, increased compartmental pressures and compartment syndromes can simultaneously exist.[116] Open tibial fractures have an associated compartment syndrome ranging from 2% to 16% of the time.[117-120] Increasing risk of elevated compartmental pressures correspondingly occurs with increasing severity of injury.[121] In polytrauma settings, higher energy injuries such as open type III, automobile versus pedestrian, crush injuries, segmental, or highly comminuted fractures, these combined injuries can exist. Delayed diagnoses occur in the polytrauma, altered mental status, traumatic brain injury, prolonged procedures, and prolonged resuscitation settings. The leg should be maintained at the level of the heart to lessen the risk of elevated limbs altering the inflow and the dependent limbs altering the outflow. If in doubt, compartmental pressures should be obtained at the time of injury and sequentially to avoid a missed compartment syndrome.[122] If in doubt, multiple measurements should be obtained to improve accuracy.[123]

Continuous monitoring is favored but requires experience and staffing to facilitate the care.[124] Measurements should be obtained at the appropriate depth and location to the fracture.[125] Because the reduction maneuver and nailing can transiently increase compartmental pressures, compartmental pressures should be checked at the end of the initial and subsequent procedures.[126] Patients undergoing anesthesia or intubated patients in the intensive care unit can have transient blood pressure decreases that can initiate increased compartmental pressures in compromised patients with preexisting increased compartmental pressures.[127] After a compartment syndrome is diagnosed, all compartments of the limb should be released and decompressed.[128]

Osseous Stabilization

Stabilization of the bone will allow for stabilization and healing of the soft tissue injury. The osseous stabilization should occur without further insult or damage to the patient, soft tissues, or bone. Osseous stabilization also reduces pain and facilitates mobilization and return to function. Traction allows for osseous alignment and stabilization but usually for limited, short time periods. Traction impedes mobilization of the patient and therefore increases morbidity of recumbency. The method of osseous stabilization should allow for limb alignment, length, and rotation without further soft tissue injury or damage to the periosteal blood supply. Temporary initial casting and splinting can be used until operative intervention but should be avoided for longer periods or permanent treatment because monitoring of soft tissue swelling, increasing compartmental pressures, and vascular impairment is difficult. Splinting can be used after internal fixation to avoid soft tissue contractures.

Internal Fixation

Internal fixation with plates is best suited for upper extremity diaphyseal, periarticular, or articular fractures.[17,129,130] Lower extremity articular fractures demand rigid internal fixation with screws, plates, or both.[131,132] Intramedullary nails (IMNs) fare better clinically than plates for diaphyseal fractures, especially with bone loss.[133] For open fractures requiring delayed soft tissue coverage (type IIIB) or precarious vascularity (type IIIC), plating should be avoided or delayed until a stable and covered wound develops. Temporary staged external fixation is preferable in these situations. Plate application should occur without further periosteal stripping or damage (Fig. 17-15).[134] The incision used for plate application should be closable and preferably using a muscular coverage (not subcutaneous).[135,136] If plate application is required for stabilization, definitive soft tissue coverage should be performed before secondary colonization occurs.[137]

Intramedullary Nailing

Intramedullary nails are the treatment of choice for long bone or diaphyseal fracture locations (Fig. 17-16).[138-142] Because the normal centripetal blood flow from inner endosteal and medullary portions to the outer cortical and periosteal portions is disrupted with a fracture,[5] IMNs should be used cautiously because of potential further damage to the intramedullary blood flow return, especially in the setting of periosteal stripping of the fracture ends. Therefore, a temporary nonreamed nail (NRN) was developed of a solid core (noncannulated) and inserted without reaming of the canal. The nail sizes and corresponding interlocking screw sizes were smaller to accommodate insertion. Compared with external fixation, IMN provides excellent healing rates and improved reduction

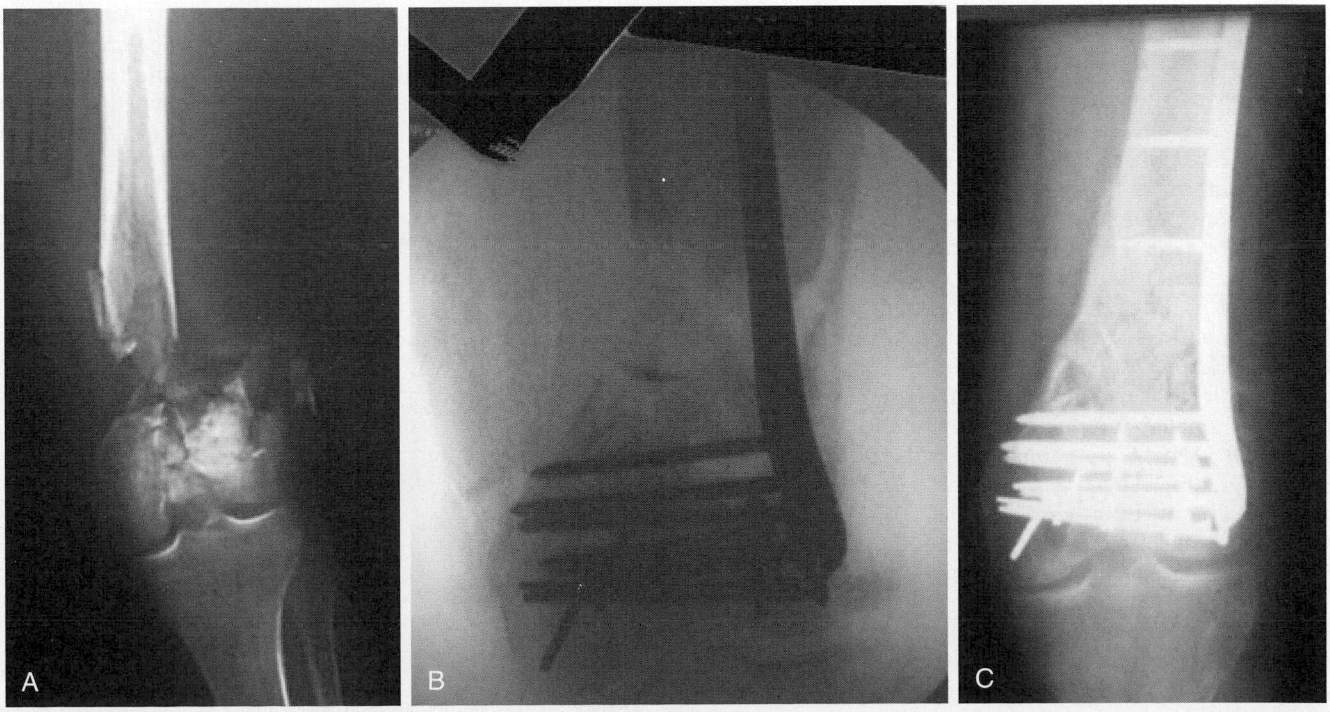

Figure 17-15. A, Open distal femoral fracture with bone loss after a motorcar crash. **B,** Initial debridement, spanning external fixation, staged open reduction internal fixation of the articular surface, and submuscular plating of the meta-diaphysis. **C,** Initial antibiotic beads were replaced with bone grafting at 6 weeks followed by uneventful osseous union and healing.

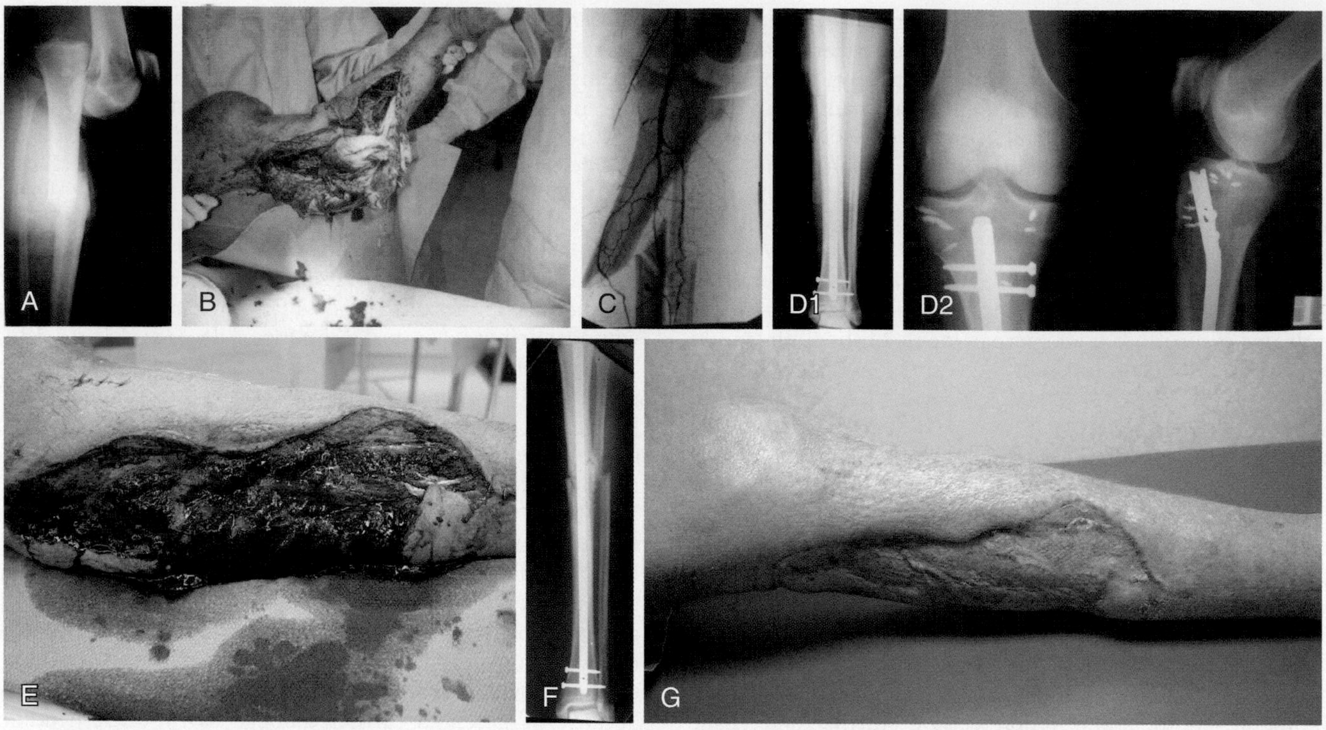

Figure 17-16. **A,** A middle-age man presented after a motor cycle accident resulting in an ipsilateral knee dislocation and open mid-diaphyseal tibial fracture. **B,** A large open posteromedial wound with degloving and partial disruption of the posterior compartment. **C,** Despite having thready pulses and an abnormal ankle brachial index, a normal angiogram was noted. After initial debridement, a tibial nail was inserted (**D1**), knee ligaments were repaired (**D2**), and an initial vacuum assisted closure was applied (**E**). Final images of tibia (**F**) and leg (**G**) demonstrate osseous union and soft tissue healing. He returned to pain-free ambulation without assistive devices but was unable to return to active sports.

quality.[17,143] Cortical temperature increases with reaming.[144] Although tibial thermal necrosis is anecdotal with reaming and tourniquet use,[145] tourniquet usage for reamed open fracture tibial nailing is common and should be discouraged.[146] In canine studies, cortical porosity, which is related to damage, is increased with reamed compared with nonreamed tibial IMN.[147] At 11 weeks after IMN, equal healing rates and similar biomechanical stiffness are noted.[148] For clinical studies of open tibial fractures, a stepwise progression is noted. For type I and II open fractures, the NRN was found to be better than external fixation.[17,143] For type II and III open fractures, the NRN demonstrated better outcomes than external fixation.[149,150] For type II and III open fractures, a reamed IMN was deemed better than external fixation.[118,151] In a randomized control trial of tibial fractures (excluding type IIIB and IIIC open fractures), NRN compared with reamed tibial nails had no difference to union or complications. NRNs are inserted with smaller diameters (9 mm vs. 11.5 mm), correspondingly smaller interlocking screws, and higher fixation failure rates (29% vs. 9%) compared with reamed IMN.[152] In a study including type IIIB open fractures, NRN had a 96% union rate, 8% infection rate (all type III), 10% screw failure rate, and 6% nail failure rate.[153] In a more recent study, an increased risk of negative events was noted in patients with high-energy mechanisms of injury.[154] Reamed IMN had an increased risk of adverse events compared with NRN. In conclusion, NRN and reamed IMN are safe procedures for type I, II, and IIIA open tibial fractures. Because type IIIB and IIIC are complex fractures with increased complications and adverse events, temporary external fixation may be prudent until a medically stable patient and wound develops.[77,155]

External Fixation

External fixation allows for immobilizing and straightening of open fractures without placing foreign objects within the injury zone (Fig. 17-17). These devices have been used for fractures with associated soft tissue injuries.[156] Advancements with modularity and techniques have lessened complications (malunion, nonunion, joint stiffness) and improved healing rates.[157-159] The best indication is for Gustilo type IIIB and IIIC fractures with contamination.[156] The fracture can be stabilized,

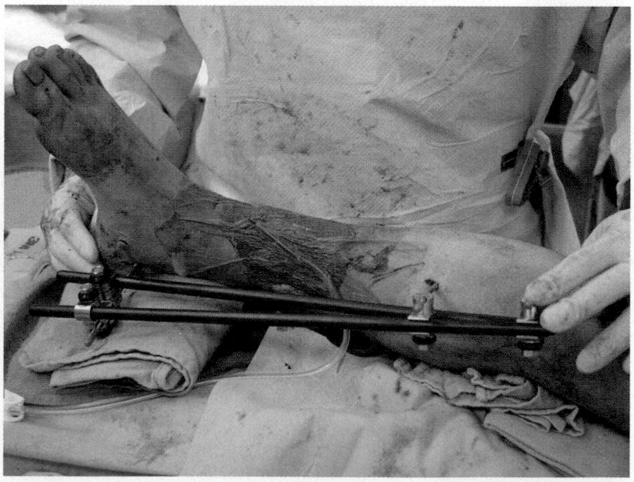

Figure 17-17. A medial-based uniplanar external fixator is applied to a severe Gustilo IIIB or OTA OFC Type 3 open tibial pilon fracture. The pins are out of the zone of injury and allow for soft tissue management, here being a temporary vacuum-assisted closure device.

realigned, and brought out to length quickly and efficiently to facilitate débridement, vascular repair, and wound coverage. Minimal soft tissue dissection is required for pin insertion. Predrilling the pin sites can lessen thermal necrosis, infection, and pin loosening. The frame can be removed to facilitate additional débridements. Staged fixation of open periarticular, metaphyseal, and joint injuries is beneficial.[160-163] Furthermore, no further vascular disturbance is noted with intramedullary (IMN) or extramedullary (plate) fixation of the fracture. The fixators can be removed when short-term tissue stability has plateaued and be converted to an IMN or plate fixation. Conversion to an IMN can be complicated by intramedullary infection with rates as high as 70%.[164-168] Conversion timing of less than 2 weeks is best but can be delayed as long as 8 weeks if no fracture site or pin tract infections are noted.[167] Experimentally, the earlier (<2 weeks) conversion cases have higher healing rates with higher mineralization and improved biomechanics.[169] Femoral shaft fracture conversion results in high healing rates with minimal infection rates but substantial knee stiffness caused by knee manipulation.[170] Do not convert too early when the soft tissues are still in transition or when polytrauma multisystem issues are present.[171] In addition, the fixator can be converted to a modular fixator (Ilizarov or Taylor Spatial Frame) to improve stiffness, longevity, and alignment. Early bone grafting and cyclic loading can enhance healing and lessen fixator failure.

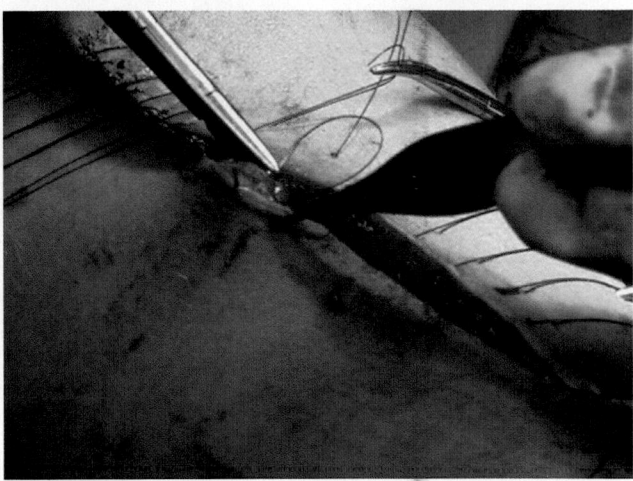

Figure 17-18. Closure of a proximal tibial wound with Allgöwer-Donati sutures of 3.0 nylon. The knot portion of the suture goes on the least damaged or compromised side of the wound.

WOUND MANAGEMENT

Primary Closure

Historically, all open fractures were kept open and returned to the operative suite 2 to 3 days later for second look, redébridement, and possible closure. Wounds with delayed primary closure had lower infection and complication rates. Returning to the operative suite for redébridement translates into incomplete débridement initially. The initial débridement is the most important and requires an experienced surgeon. Of course, crush injuries, blast injuries, and temporary external fixation require repeat débridements and staged surgeries. Returning on postoperative day 2 or 3 corresponds to peak inflammation. Trying to close on these days is difficult and may require a third operative procedure for closure later after the swelling is decreased. Closure should be performed with techniques to preserve the soft tissue integrity and viability. A drain should be inserted deep to reduce swelling and hematoma and seroma accumulation. Allgöwer-Donati sutures are preferred without any dissolvable subcutaneous sutures (Fig. 17-18). Compared with simple, vertical mattress, and horizontal mattress sutures, the Donati sutures had the least effect on cutaneous blood flow. Place the knot on the safest side (e.g., away from the subcutaneous border, apex of a flap, or opposite another incision) of the wound. If able, apply stretchy Steri-Strips to facilitate wound closure and dissipate closure forces.

Using these techniques, immediate wound closure has been noted in small series of open fractures with similar complications. In a study of 119 open fractures, the wound was closed at the initial setting based on surgeon discretion in 22 of 25 grade I open fractures (88%), 37 of 43 grade II fractures (86%), 24 of 32 grade IIIA fractures (75%), 4 of 12 grade IIIB fractures (33%), and 0 of 7 grade IIIC fractures (0%).[172] Eight fractures (7%) developed a wound infection, and 19 fractures (16%) developed a delayed or nonunion. These numbers were similar to those for wounds treated with delayed closure. In a larger prospective randomized multicenter trial, 451 open grade II and IIIA tibial diaphyseal fractures were treated with standardized débridement, nailing, and wound closure.[173] Infection developed in 17 (9%) and 18 (10%) of the immediate compared with the delayed closure groups, respectively. Delayed union or nonunion developed in 61 (31%) versus 52 (27%) of the immediate and delayed closure groups, respectively. Wound complications were more common in the delayed (nine STSGs, two flaps) compared with the immediate (two STSGs, two flaps) closure group. The immediate closure group had similar infection and union rates but fewer wound complications. In a large evaluation of tibial fractures treated with IMN, primary closure without additional soft tissue procedures had a decreased risk of adverse events compared with more complex soft tissue reconstructions.[154] In an OTA survey, 35% of the surgeons believed that the most effective time to closure was within the first 3 days, and time to definitive closure was one of the most important principles in preventing deep infection.[62] The delayed primary closure protocol should be reconsidered. The results of the FLOW study will help determine which doctrine is better.

Tips and Tricks

Ankle Fractures

Transverse medial wounds, especially over the medial tibia, should be closed immediately after débridement and irrigation (Fig. 17-19). Keeping the wound open potentiates skin and wound contracture. If not closed during the first operative setting, many of these wounds will never be able to be closed and will require a skin graft or soft tissue transfer procedure. In elderly patients or vasculopaths who cannot undergo free tissue transfer and have limited peripheral vascularity, the inability to close the wound may lead to an amputation.

Delayed Primary Closure

Vacuum-Assisted Closure and Negative-Pressure Wound Management

Negative-pressure wound therapy (NPWT) has been used for treatment of wounds for 2 decades. Since that time, it has

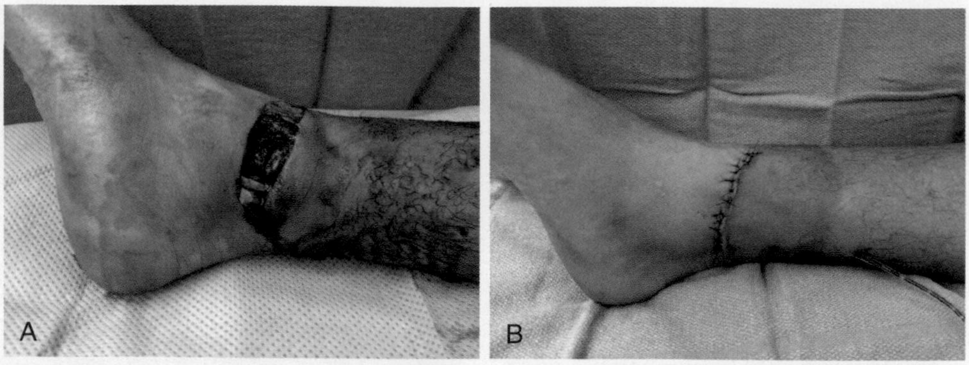

Figure 17-19. **A,** An open bimalleolar ankle fracture was debrided and stabilized with internal fixation. **B,** Since the wound edges and vascularity were minimally compromised, the skin edges were closed with Allgöwer-Donati sutures over a drain and without tension to avoid the potential need for secondary soft tissue coverage.

become widely accepted in the treatment of large, musculoskeletal wounds such as open fractures (Fig. 17-20). Until recently, only preclinical animal studies supported its use on wounds, and some of the possible benefits of NPWT include increased blood flow to damaged tissue, decreased interstitial edema, increased granulation of wound beds, increased flap survival, and increased bacterial clearance.[174-180] A recent prospective randomized clinical study in 70 patients demonstrated that NPWT reduced the infection rate of open fractures.[181] The control group underwent initial irrigation and débridement followed by standard fine mesh gauze dressing, with repeat irrigation and débridement every 48 to 72 hours until wound closure. Patients randomized to the NPWT group had identical treatment except that negative pressure was applied to the wounds between irrigation and débridement procedures until closure. The control and NPWT had infection rates of 28% and 5%, respectively ($P = 0.02$). Intermittent pressure has been shown to improve granulation of the wounds in animal models but often causes pain in patients. Continuous pressure at 125 mm Hg is commonly used. Care should be taken to ensure proper seal of the wounds because loss of suction can increase wound complications such as infection.[182] Loss of suction can occur with intermittent pressure, angular areas of body contour (e.g., toes, ankle, groin, and axilla), proximity to external fixator pins, and large areas of high-volume output (especially hematoma) and limited effluent drains (e.g., large degloving area of the leg using only one NPWT sponge and drain tube). Angular areas of the body require hair removal, sealing noncontoured edges, and extending the area of suctioning. Suturing the pin site incision or sealing the external fixator pin within the system can lessen a leak. Large high-volume areas benefit with use of more drain connectors to a single pump via a 2 : 1 connector or utilization of an additional pump.

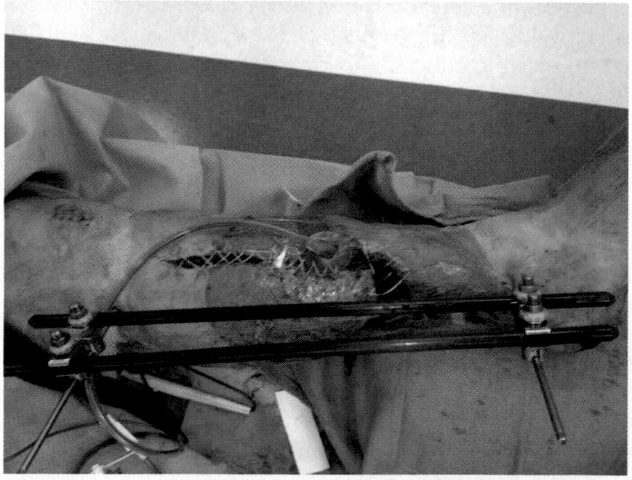

Figure 17-20. A severe open tibial fracture with tibial osseous and medial soft tissue defect is temporarily spanned with an external fixator and a vacuum-assisted closure dressing. Rubber bands are applied over the sponge to keep tension on the soft tissues to aid in reduction of swelling and wound edge retraction.

Local Antibiotics

Antibiotic administration to the wound can be via powder or antibiotic-laden (AL) polymethylmethacrylate (PMMA). Local application of vancomycin has been demonstrated to lower postoperative wound infection rates without deleterious effects on bone healing.[183-186] The addition of 1 g of vancomycin powder to the wound edges before closure was associated with a very low postoperative infection rate without any deleterious effect on the thoracolumbar instrumented fusions.[186] This study was repeated in an elective, posterior cervical, instrumented spinal fusion study; 1 g of vancomycin powder was added to the incision on closure, resulting in lowering infection rates from 10.9% to 2.5% in the control versus treated incision groups, respectively.[184] Nonunion rates were similar at about 5%.

Mixing a heat-stable, water-soluble antibiotic powder (vancomycin and tobramycin) with PMMA can generate a long eluting of antibiotic up to 4 to 6 weeks.[187,188] Because the Food and Drug Administration (FDA) has not approved AL-PMMA, the surgeon must create a preferred combination, dosage, and size. Combining 40 g of PMMA with 1 to 4 g vancomycin and/or 1.2 to 4.8 g tobramycin in a mixing bowl is sufficient to create a stable AL-PMMA compound. The doughy compound is then applied to a 24-gauge wire or #1 suture in beads or via a bead mold. After it has hardened, the beads can then be placed into the wound and sealed with film dressing or semipermeable barrier creating a "bead pouch" (Fig. 17-21). Ioban (3M, St. Paul, MN), which comes in varying sizes and shapes, is a great covering agent to avoid leakage and improve sealing the wound. The "bead pouch" technique has advantages.[19] It provides high concentration (10–20 times) of local antibiotic

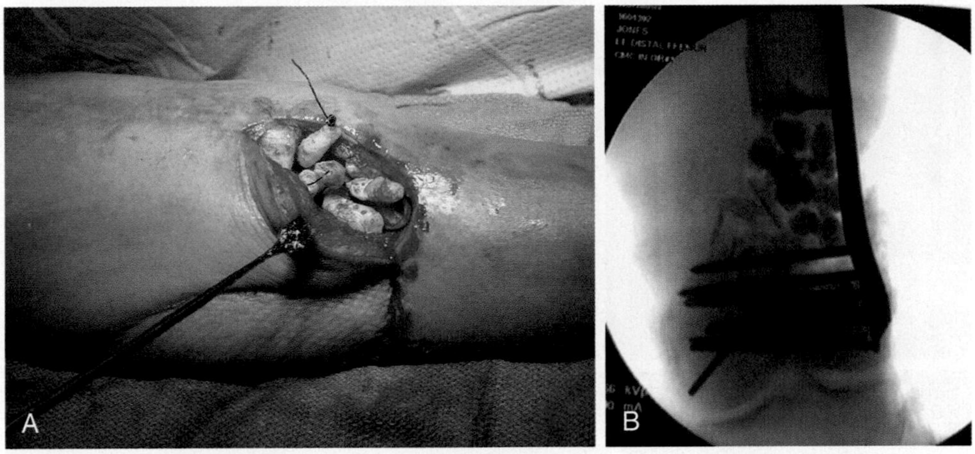

Figure 17-21. A, Antibiotic beads are inserted into a tibial defect in preparation of staged bone grafting and after soleus muscle transfer. **B,** Antibiotic beads are inserted into a large osseous defect in the metaphyseal area of an open supracondylar femoral fracture after submuscular plating and in preparation of a staged bone grafting.

compared with systemic IV antibiotics. The low systemic levels of antibiotic lessen the potential systemic side effects, especially with aminoglycosides. Usage also lessens the amount and duration of systemic antibiotics that could lessen the length of hospital stay and overall cost. The wound is sealed from the environment, lessening contamination and nursing care. Lessening the relative amount of liquid monomer and delaying the addition of the antibiotic powder 30 seconds after polymerization can increase the cumulative elution of antibiotic over 6 weeks.[189] In a large study of open fractures, IV antibiotics alone were compared with IV antibiotics and local aminoglycoside-impregnated PMMA.[190] The overall infection rate dropped from 12% to 3.7% with the use of PMMA in the wound. Both acute infection and local osteomyelitis were decreased in type IIIB and IIIC open fractures. Chronic osteomyelitis was decreased in type II and IIIB open fractures. Therefore, the authors recommend additional antibiotic-laden PMMA beads locally in the wound for the more severe open fractures. In that study, the patients with impregnated beads had their wounds closed earlier, which introduced a potential bias into the study conclusions, and other clinical studies have not demonstrated an added benefit of adding antibiotic beads to the wound.

The AL-PMMA compound can be used for local antibiotic beads, temporary antibiotic IMN, or antibiotic spacer (Fig. 17-22).

Comparison of Different Options for Initial Wound Management

Although it is favorable to close wounds after initial débridement, it is not always possible with severe or highly contaminated injuries. Many different options to manage the soft tissue injury or attempt to reduce bacterial contamination are available. A series of studies evaluated some of the most common therapies using the same animal model and assessment tools.[180,191,192] Briefly, a large musculoskeletal wound was created on the proximal leg of goats and inoculated with a bioluminescent strain of *Staphylococcus aureus*. Six hours after injury and contamination, the wound was débrided and irrigated with saline and assigned to treatment group. Two days later, the bacteria within the wounds were quantified using a photon-capturing camera; this technique has high correlation to quantitative cultures and assesses the entire wound surface. Wet-to-dry dressings were the least effective against the bacteria, and the standard bead pouch described earlier reduced the most bacteria (Fig. 17-23).

Immediate Shortening

Immediate shortening can lessen the relative soft tissue void and facilitate soft tissue closure and osseous healing. Shortening of up to 2.5 cm in the humerus is tolerated well. Shortening in the forearm requires equal shortening to avoid proximal or distal radial ulnar disruption or tendinous imbalance or weakness to the digits. Lower extremity shortening creates leg length discrepancy, which would benefit from future reconstructive procedures to lengthen the involved limb or shorten the contralateral limb.[193] Aggressive limb shortening can result in vascular congestion from vessel redundancy and potential ischemia. Plates and nails can immediately shorten a limb. Modular external fixators can shorten, angulate, straighten, and then lengthen a limb. These frames can change a Gustilo type IIIB fracture into a type IIIA fracture based on modulation of the limb length and alignment. Therefore, the patient may have a greater chance of limb salvage without free tissue transfer.

FUTURE DEVELOPMENTS

Bacteria Identification Using Molecular Platform

Culturing of wounds currently has little value because it is a poor predictor of infection and the ultimate infecting organism. Bacteria that are within the biofilm phenotype are in a quiescent state and grow poorly, if at all, when cultured on agar plates. Molecular techniques that amplify the nucleic acids, which allows for identification of small amounts of bacteria, can identify various ways such as primers or mass spectrometry and can identify bacteria within a biofilm.[194] A large clinical trials consortium, the Major Extremity Research Consortium (METRC), has an ongoing study that will prospectively assess the value of molecular diagnostics and traditional cultures in 600 lower extremity wounds and should determine the value of this approach.

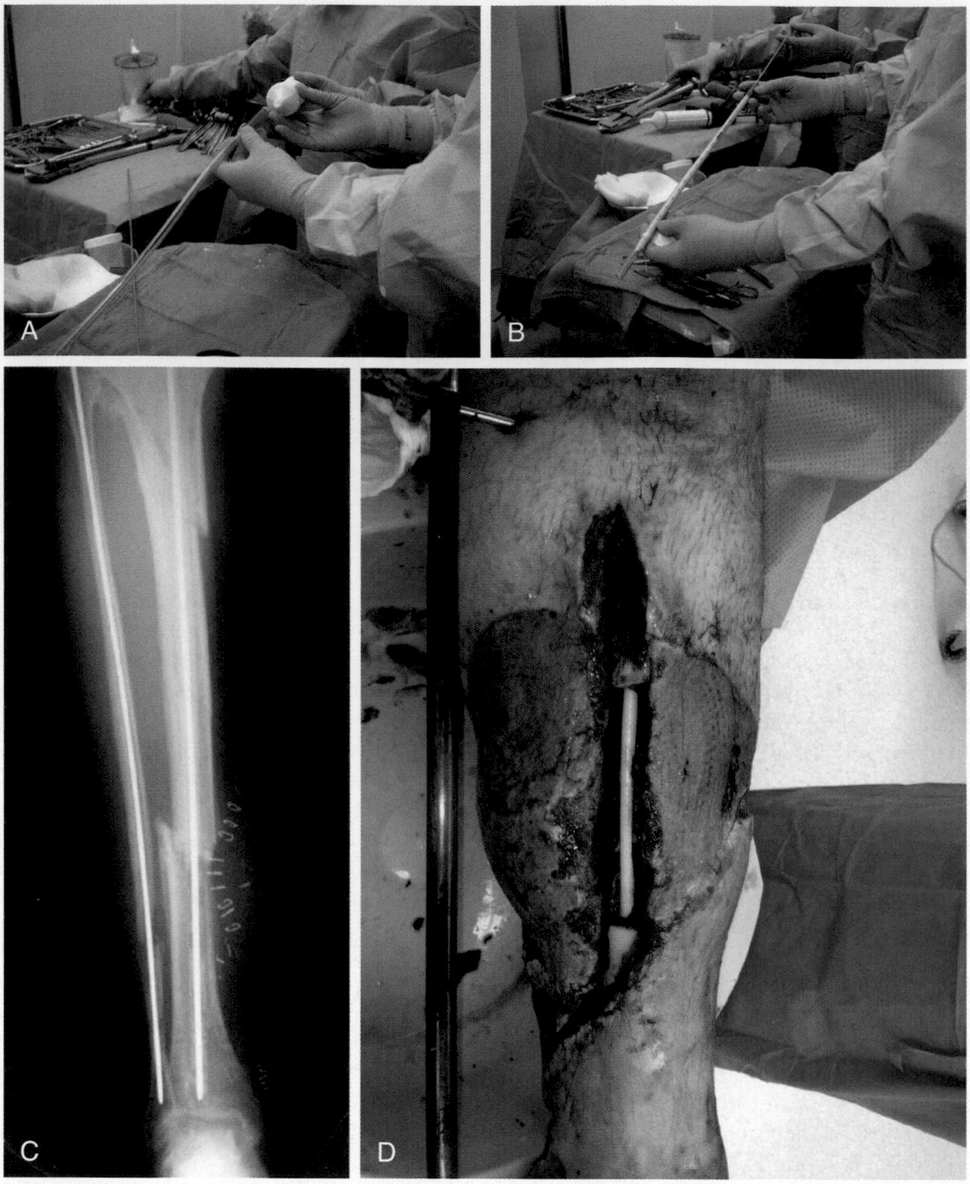

Figure 17-22. An antibiotic nail is generated with initial mixture of 2 bags of PMMA, 2.0 grams of vancomycin powder, and 2.4 grams of tobramycin powder. This mixture is then inserted into cement gun while still "runny" or liquidly (**A**) and injected into a 32-French chest tube. **B,** A 3.2-mm guide pin is then inserted down the middle of the chest tube to provide stability for insertion, temporary fixation, and removal. **C,** Segmental tibial fracture stabilized with an antibiotic nail secondary to initial contamination and serial debridements. **D,** Complex open tibial fracture stabilized with both a medial external fixator, an intramedullary antibiotic IMN. Prior split thickness skin grafting has been applied in preparation of the soft tissues for closure and bone grafting the tibial defect.

Antimicrobial Implants

There is concern that IMN fixation increases the risk for infections in severe open fractures, and ring fixation is extremely expensive and can be difficult for the patient. Various strategies to protect the hardware from colonization of bacteria are being explored. An antibiotic plate sleeve, hardware coating doped with an antimicrobial, and strategies that do not allow bacterial adhesion are being explored.[195,196]

Local Antibiotic Delivery Devices

An FDA-approved local antibiotic delivery device in the United States is currently not available. Surgeons have to individually make these devices on the back operative table and generally add antibiotic to the PMMA (AL-PMMA) or calcium sulfate. Antibiotic gels and sponges have been shown to reduce more of the amount of bacteria within a wound compared with PMMA beads.[197,198] The bead depot relies on diffusion of the antibiotic throughout the wound and does not work well with simultaneous NPWT utilization.

Antibiofilm Agents

The development of a biofilm may allow the cells within the colony to be increasingly resistant to antibiotics and the host immune system. The development and dispersal of the biofilm is a coordinated effort through quorum sensing using various products. Great strides have been made toward identifying these dispersal agents.[199] These agents can be effective at low doses, and several appear to have a fairly broad activity.[200]

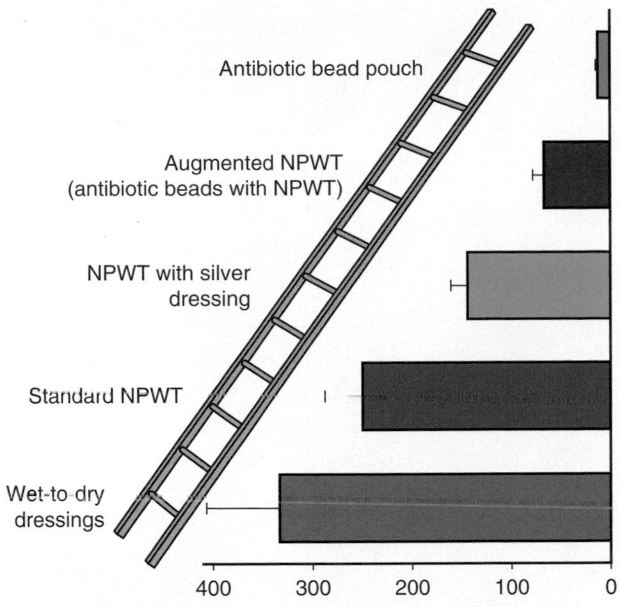

Figure 17-23. Ladder of effectiveness. There are many different options for managing open wounds. A large animal open fracture model was used to determine the effect of different approaches on amount of *Staphylococcus aureus* within the wound. With wet-to-dry dressings, dressings were changed twice a day. In standard negative-pressure wound therapy (NPWT), continuous negative pressure was applied to the wound. With NPWT with silver dressing, a silver dressing was placed in contact with the wound. Augmented NPWT consisted of vancomycin-loaded PMMA beads being placed within the wound and negative pressure being applied to the wound. For the antibiotic bead pouch, vancomycin-loaded PMMA beads were placed within the wound, and the wound was closed with a semipermable membrane. *(Data from Laliss SJ, Stinner DJ, Waterman SM, et al: J Orthop Trauma 24(9):598–602, 2010; Stinner DJ, Waterman SM, Masini BD, et al: J Trauma 71(1 Suppl):S147–150, 2011; and Stinner DJ, Hsu JR, Wenke JC: J Orthop Trauma 26(9):512–518, 2012.)*

Potent biomimetic biofilm disruptors have been developed that work at much lower levels than the naturally occurring dispersal agents.[201]

Dual-Purpose Bone Grafts

Grafting large bone defects is often required for union. On implantation of an avascular graft, a race to the surface commences between bacterial and host tissue cells. If bacteria colonize the surface of the implant before tissue cells, an infection can result. Thus, an unintended consequence of implantation of a bone graft is its potential to function as the nidus for biofilm formation and infection.[202] Dual-purpose bone grafts are devices that both promote bone growth and prevent bacteria from colonizing the graft. Antimicrobials,[203] antibiotics,[204] or biofilm dispersal agents[205] can be released from the graft for up to several months, which will prevent bacteria from colonizing the graft before it becomes vascularized.

Tissue Engineering and Regenerative Medicine Approaches

Tissue engineering and regenerative medicine are two of the most active fields of research. The approaches generally use a scaffold, stem cells, growth factors, or a combination of these. More effective release kinetics of recombinant human bone morphogenetic protein, which is thought to be a burst and sustained release, has shown to improve bone formation compared with the collagen sponge. Developing injectable, settable, weight-bearing scaffolds is another effort that may help with open fractures that involve the joint. To date, the vast majority of regenerative approaches that are pertinent to open fractures have focused on bone. Recently, efforts have been made to regenerate skeletal muscle. Implanting scaffolds is a common approach and is clinically available.[206] Although this approach probably does not form new muscle, it appears to help the muscle mass remaining to produce force by acting as a functional scar in large volumetric muscle defects.[207] Mincing autologous muscle into 1-mm defects and implanting them within the muscle defect has shown to improve the strength of the affected limb and to regenerate skeletal muscle.[208] This approach may be able to be transitioned to practice quickly because the FDA regulates products, not practice.

CONCLUSION

Open fractures are complex, complicated, and costly. Avoiding complications during the process of wound coverage, osseous healing, and functional rehabilitation is important. Sacrosanct principles of time to surgery and to wound closure are being debated. The FLOW study results should shine a light on many areas of open fracture care and outcomes. METRC studies will help determine salvage and reconstruction of traumatic lower extremity wounds and fractures.

KEY REFERENCES

The level of evidence (LOE) is determined according to the criteria provided in the preface.

10. Gustilo RB, Anderson JT: Prevention of infection in the treatment of one thousand and twenty-five open fractures of long bones: retrospective and prospective analyses. *J Bone Joint Surg Am* 58(4):453–458, 1976.
17. Chapman MW, Mahoney M: The role of early internal fixation in the management of open fractures. *Clin Orthop Relat Res* 138:120–131, 1979.
19. Zalavras CG, Patzakis MJ: Open fractures: evaluation and management. *J Am Acad Orthop Surg* 11(3):212–219, 2003.
54. Patzakis MJ, Wilkins J: Factors influencing infection rate in open fracture wounds. *Clin Orthop Relat Res* 243:36–40, 1989.
56. Dellinger EP, Miller SD, Wertz MJ, et al: Risk of infection after open fracture of the arm or leg. *Arch Surg* 123(11):1320–1327, 1988.
62. Obremskey WT, Molina CS, Collinge C, et al: Current practice in the initial management of open fractures among orthopaedic trauma surgeons. *J Orthop Trauma* Nov 13, 2013 [Epub ahead of print].
77. Bednar DA, Parikh J: Effect of time delay from injury to primary management on the incidence of deep infection after open fractures of the lower extremities caused by blunt trauma in adults. *J Orthop Trauma* 7(6):532–535, 1993.
91. Rodeheaver GT, Pettry D, Thacker JG, et al: Wound cleansing by high pressure irrigation. *Surg Gynecol Obstet* 141(3):357–362, 1975.
92. Anglen JO: Wound irrigation in musculoskeletal injury. *J Am Acad Orthop Surg* 9(4):219–226, 2001.

The complete References list is available online at https://expertconsult.inkling.com.

Chapter 18

Soft Tissue Reconstruction

RAJIV CHANDAWARKAR • GEORGE P. NANOS III

Additional videos related to the subject of this chapter are available from the Medizinische Hochschule Hannover collection. The following video is included with this chapter and may be viewed at https://expertconsult.inkling.com:
18-1. Soleus flap.

INTRODUCTION AND GENERAL PRINCIPLES

Introduction

The optimal soft tissue characteristics required for coverage of defects involving the upper and lower extremity vary according to the site and location of the defect. Characteristics of interest include pliability, durability to withstand the wear and tear of movement and friction (from work as well as clothing), the ability to cover large surface areas with minimal thickness, and cosmetic appearance. These features allow the best functional outcome, maximally protect the vital structures of the extremity, and optimize the aesthetic result. In addition, the general requirements of any soft tissue reconstruction, including minimal donor site morbidity and minimal disruption of local vasculature, become more critical when considering the functional restoration of the extremity.[1-4] Although soft tissue defects can occur from a variety of conditions (trauma, tumor, or infection), soft tissue coverage remains a vital operative intervention that protects underlying vital structures, such as nerves, tendons, blood vessels, and bone, preserves the integrity and continuity of musculoskeletal elements, prevents functional disability, and promotes an acceptable aesthetic result. Techniques include primary wound closure, delayed primary wound closure, skin grafting, local random flaps, axial pattern flaps, island adipofascial and fasciocutaneous flaps, muscle or myocutaneous pedicled flaps, and microvascular free-tissue transfer, or free flaps. Optimal choices depend on the extent of the defect and available soft tissue donor sites.

The concept of the "reconstructive ladder," or choosing the simplest closure or coverage option available, has been at the forefront of soft tissue reconstruction since its description by Mathes and Nahai in 1982, and assists the surgeon in choosing the best coverage option.[5] However, this approach assumes the coverage technique as the important outcome of interest, and may not optimize the reconstruction plan or optimize the functional result in more complex cases. When this is the case, it may be prudent to choose the more complex option to facilitate the reconstruction plan and functional outcome. This paradigm has been described as the "reconstructive elevator"[6] (Table 18-1).

Initial Evaluation

The detailed patient assessment is critical to the success of any soft tissue repair or reconstruction. The general condition of the patient and the ability to withstand reconstruction must be carefully determined. Included in this analysis is the causative aspect of the defect. In cases of trauma, the antecedent injuries need to be factored; mechanism of injury, degree of energy imparted to the soft tissues, and presence of contamination will significantly impact the surgical plan. A quick analysis of the clinical problem with a template of reconstructive choices is an important and essential step at this point. Ensuring treatment will occur in the correct facility, with the appropriate resources and expertise emphasizing a multidisciplinary approach to care, will ensure the optimum outcomes.

The typical approach used by plastic and reconstructive surgeons is to devise a patient-specific surgical plan that includes contingencies for every possible extent or type of defect. This is particularly important in extensive trauma, wherein the final defect after required tissue débridement may be quite different than anticipated. An algorithm, or list of options, for soft tissue reconstruction is often useful and will help the surgeon organize the surgical plan, but in the end, all plans must take a customized approach to the patient. A reconstructive management strategy is based on the evaluation of the defect and the patient's specific functional needs. The mechanism of injury, the location and extent of the wound, tissue viability, contamination, and exposure of vital structures are all critical considerations. A plan for concurrent acute and definitive fracture care must be coordinated with the trauma team, and within the scope of wound care.

Most reconstructive surgeons favor immediate reconstruction, except when the defect demands a delay. In high-energy injury patterns, in cases of infection, or in heavily contaminated wounds, it may be necessary to delay definitive wound closure or coverage until an adequate, multistaged evaluation and débridement may be performed. Vacuum-assisted closure (VAC) dressings have improved treatment of open wounds, and may allow some additional delay in flap reconstruction without expectation of further morbidity. However, the general trend supported by the literature remains to cover tissue as soon as the injured patient and limb are optimized, even if this extends past the 72-hour window proposed by Godina.[7-9]

WOUND PREPARATION

A healthy wound bed begins with the meticulous and complete surgical removal of foreign material, infection, and devitalized tissue.[10] Chronic wounds should be converted to acute wounds to promote healing. In acute injury, wounds must be extended past the zone of injury to ensure complete treatment as well as effective débridement is accomplished. Judicious use of lavage may help remove foreign matter, but care must be taken not to extend the zone of contamination by forcing debris into the surrounding tissue. Use of a tourniquet early

TABLE 18-1 *THE RECONSTRUCTIVE ELEVATOR*
Free flap
Pedicled flap
Local fasciocutaneous flap
Skin graft
Primary closure
Wound care
Reconstructive elevator

in the case in important to best visualize all contaminants and devitalized tissue and avoid injury to vital structures such as nerves and blood vessels. The tourniquet should be released prior to closure or dressing application to confirm removal of all devascularized tissue and to ensure adequate hemostasis.

A systematic approach to wound débridement achieves the best results, and sharp débridement is the cornerstone of this surgical technique. Excision of all devitalized tissue to a healthy tissue margin, instead of a "wait and see" approach to suspect tissue, will limit persistent contamination and infection. All nonviable or suspect tissue is sharply débrided from the wound until a healthy margin of viable tissue is achieved. Every effort to preserve nerves and blood vessels crossing the zone of injury is made, and if they are transected, these structures are carefully tagged with dyed monofilament suture and documented in the operative records so that they may be more easily visualized during later wound débridement or reconstructive efforts.[11]

Identification of nonviable tissue remains a challenge, and there is no substitute for experience. Knowledge of anatomy and local blood supply is paramount in this endeavor as overly aggressive débridement within muscle compartments may devascularize previously viable tissue. Tendon débridement must be carefully considered due to potential loss of function. Tendons are also easily desiccated, especially if overlying paratenon or sheath is missing. Injured blood vessels or nerves must be carefully assessed for primary or delayed repair or grafting. Smaller sensory nerve branches may not be amenable to salvage, and if so, we like to pull traction on the proximal end, cut sharply, and allow retraction into the soft tissues. If the stump cannot be retracted, we make every effort to bury it in muscle. Local soft tissues should be used to cover exposed tendons, nerves, and vessels to prevent further injury.

Devascularized bone fragments must be removed from the wound bed, with the exception of substantial articular fragments, which should be retained in an attempt to preserve the articular surface. Curettes, rongeurs, and burs are useful to check for punctate bleeding indicative of healthy bone that should be preserved. Culture of any contaminated or osteolytic bone will help guide antibiotic selection.

Strict hemostasis is critical to prevent hematoma and limit further infection and morbidity caused by blood loss. Suture ligatures and surgical clips should be used for larger vessels, Bovie or bipolar cautery for smaller vessels. Braided suture is typically avoided when possible to avoid harboring bacteria. Judicious use of a tourniquet is helpful to identify and control large bleeding vessels and includes release to assess hemostasis prior to closure, grafting, or dressing application. Adjunctive topical hemostatic agents are available and have been used successfully in some of our most severely war injured patients. Lavage is important for removal of foreign debris and lowering bacterial counts. Gravity or bulb irrigation is considered the standard, whereas pulsatile lavage can further damage delicate tissues exacerbating the potential for adhesions and functional loss.[12]

Negative-pressure wound therapy dressings are a great advance in the treatment of wounds not amenable to primary closure. V.A.C. Therapy dressing is commonly used to manage large wounds from high-energy injuries. It continues to débride wounds, reducing edema and local bacterial counts, while promoting growth of healthy granulation tissue.[13,14] It also eliminates the need for multiple daily dressing changes, thereby reducing the patient's discomfort and nursing staff workload. It is prudent to limit exposure of blood vessels, nerves, or tendons to the wound VAC and try to rotate available local tissue to provide coverage prior to placement of the wound VAC.

Eliminating contamination and infection is essential to successful wound treatment. In addition to appropriate broad-spectrum antibiotic use, there are many different options available that can be tailored to the clinical or surgical situation to provide local infection control. Antibiotic bead pouches or fracture spacers have been used effectively to provide local infection control in cases of wounds with associated high-energy fracture patterns. With comminution and bone loss, soft tissue space can be maintained for future reconstruction and enhanced mechanical stability provided. In highly resistant bacterial infection silver-impregnated films, colloidal materials, wound VAC sponges, and distillation solutions are additional options for the surgeon and have been used with great frequency at our institution. For extremely large wounds with highly resistant bacterial colonization or infection that are not amenable to wound VAC treatment, mafenide acetate (Sulfamylon) or Dakin's soaked wet-to-dry dressings have proven effective and resulted in successful wound closure. Infectious disease specialty assistance is recommended in such cases.

When wounds are associated with fractures in the acute setting, provisional stabilization should be attempted to maintain soft tissue space, prevent mechanical agitation of the surrounding tissues, and optimize pain control when definitive fixation is not advisable. In general, external fixators and Kirschner wires are preferred acutely with conversion to definitive fixation as indicated by the injury, especially in the setting of high-energy injuries, such as blast injuries, when large amounts of debris are forced into the wounds with tremendous energy and the level of contamination is typically higher than that seen in most blunt open trauma.

For highly contaminated wounds, or when there is concern for viability in critical areas or structures, repeat operative débridement should be planned every 24 to 36 hours until a healthy, vascularized soft tissue bed is achieved (Table 18-2).

WOUND COVERAGE TYPES

Skin Grafts

Split-thickness skin grafts are a good coverage option for simple wounds that cannot be closed primarily and have a

TABLE 18-2 *WOUND COVERAGE TREATMENT PITFALLS*
1. Inadequate clinical and surgical resources for proper treatment
2. Failure to recognize and optimize host factors
3. Failure to recognize and treat vascular compromise
4. Inadequate débridement
5. Failure to recognize and treat infection
6. Wound closure with excessive tension
7. Inadequate soft tissue rest
8. Prominent bone or hardware

healthy wound bed. By definition, split-thickness skin grafts remove the epidermis, but only partially harvest the dermis, allowing for regeneration of epidermis at the harvest site. The thickness of the graft will determine the potential of graft contraction, with thinner grafts contracting more and thicker grafts contracting less. This thinner graft may be advantageous when the wound condition dictates contracture to a smaller wound; conversely, a thicker graft may be preferred when wound contracture is not desired, such as crossing a joint. In a healthy wound bed, split-thickness skin grafts are reliable, and can be meshed to cover a larger area than harvested from the donor site. Graft harvest requires specialized equipment, and cosmetic donor site morbidity can be expected when a large volume of skin graft is required.

Full-thickness skin grafts, by definition, remove the entire epidermis and dermis of the affected area, requiring primary closure. Advantages of full-thickness skin grafts are reduced graft contracture and enhanced durability. For this reason, they are typically employed in the hand. Disadvantages include limitation in recipient site coverage.

Dermal Substitutes

The past several decades have seen significant research and interest in dermal substitutes for a variety of applications, including burns and complex wounds. Perhaps the most commonly reported dermal substitute for wound coverage is Integra (Integra Life Sciences, Plainsboro, NJ), an acellular bilaminate membrane composed of cross-linked bovine tendon collagen and chondroitin-6-sulfate. Integra is most commonly used in a meshed bilayer construct with the addition of a silicone layer to prevent desiccation. Dermal substitutes such as Integra are easy to use or apply, limit donor site morbidity, are readily available, and have a proven track record in burn patients and complex extremity wounds.[15,16] In many cases, use of Integra has eliminated the need for complex flap reconstruction and its associated morbidity.[17] Coupled with a split-thickness or full-thickness skin graft, usually performed 14 to 21 days after initial application, Integra has provided reliable coverage of complex wounds with exposed muscle, tendon, and even bone. However, successful coverage has not been proven with application directly over fracture. The disadvantages of dermal substitutes are the financial cost of implant, and the inherent lack of antimicrobial properties prompting the use of additional antimicrobial dressings that may increase cost.[18] Negative-pressure wound therapy is now commonly used with Integra application, and may accelerate healing and time to skin graft placement.[19] In addition to primary coverage of complex wounds, Integra has been used to decrease donor site morbidity in flap surgery by providing a more supple, durable coverage.[20] Integra has also been used effectively to provide durable coverage of amputation stumps that allow functional prosthetic usage.[21]

Random Pattern Flaps

By definition, random skin flaps have no named blood vessels, and rely on the subdermal vascular plexus for perfusion. This limits the geometry of the flap, requiring that the length of the flap be no more than twice the base of the flap to ensure flap blood flow. Longer flap geometries have been described, but flap viability may be compromised, and when this occurs, it will be at the distal extent of the flap. This type of flap requires mobile skin, and the donor defect can usually be closed, although the addition of a Z-plasty may be required.

Axial Pattern Flaps

Axial pattern flaps are fasciocutaneous flaps designed around a named artery and vein. The groin flap is a classic example of this flap, designed around the circumflex scapular artery and vein. Axial pattern flaps have the advantage of supplying a much larger flap than random pattern flaps, and due to a larger, more robust vascular system, can be converted to free flaps if required.

Island Pattern Flaps

Island pattern flaps are similar to axial pattern flaps, in that the flap is supplied by a named artery and venous outflow. However, as the name would imply, island flaps can be separated completely from the harvest site, and transposed somewhat distantly on its named arteriovenous pedicle. The advantage is usually ease of flap harvest and inset. The disadvantage is the potential loss of a named artery supplying distant structures. Common examples include the radial forearm flap in the upper extremity, and the reverse sural artery flap in the lower extremity. Island pattern flaps may be fasciocutaneous, involving the skin and fascia, or adipofascial flaps, preserving the skin at the donor site.

Perforator Flap

Perforator flaps are fasciocutaneous flaps that derive their blood supply from intramuscular and intermuscular septal perforators from the deep vascular arterial system. The most common example of this type of flap is the anterolateral thigh flap. Perforator flaps can be pedicled or used as free flaps. Propeller flaps are a subgroup of perforator flaps, defined as perforator flaps that are islanded and rotated into a defect. These flaps have seen increased popularity for reconstruction of small soft tissue defects in the upper and lower extremity.

Free Flap

By definition, a free flap is harvested, its blood supply divided, and then reanastomosed to an arteriovenous supply at the flap recipient site, usually requiring microsurgical techniques. Free flaps, or free tissue, is usually classified by its blood supply. Free flaps can include skin, fascial and subcutaneous fat, muscle, bone, or combinations of any tissue type based on its blood supply. Muscle flaps, such as the latissimus dorsi muscle flap, continue to be commonly employed in reconstructive surgery. Muscle flaps have the advantage of covering large defects, and filling three-dimensional volume defects, but may not be the best coverage option when staged reconstructive procedures, such as tendon or nerve reconstruction procedures are anticipated. Because of these limitations, fasciocutaneous and adipofascial flaps based on large named arteriovenous pedicles, or even smaller flaps based on smaller perforator vessels, have recently gained popularity among reconstructive surgeons.

SOFT TISSUE RECONSTRUCTION OF THE UPPER EXTREMITY

Surgical Planning

Selecting the optimal reconstructive option depends heavily on the location of the defect. For simplification, the following algorithmic approach divides the upper extremity into five anatomic zones: shoulder, arm (within 6 to 8 cm from elbow),

TABLE 18-3 *OPTIONS FOR SOFT TISSUE RECONSTRUCTION OF THE UPPER EXTREMITY BY LOCATION*

Simple Wound (No Exposed Bone, Tendons, or Neurovascular Structures)	-Use split-thickness skin grafting in the arm and forearm -Use full-thickness skin graft for the palmar hand and digits -Can use dermal substitutes to increase thickness and durability of graft
Complex Wounds (Exposed Bone, Tendons, or Neurovascular Structures)	**Shoulder** -Scapular/parascapular flap -Latissimus dorsi muscle flap -Free flap **Brachium/Arm** -Latissimus dorsi muscle flap -Pectoralis muscle flap -Free flap **Elbow** -Radial forearm flap -Lateral arm flap -Latissimus dorsi muscle flap -Anconeus muscle flap -Free flap **Forearm** -Groin flap -Free flap **Wrist and Hand** -Reverse radial forearm flap -Posterior interosseous artery flap -Dorsal metacarpal artery flap -Groin flap -Fillet flap -Free flap

elbow (including lower 6 to 8 cm of arm), forearm, and hand. Specific flaps as shown in Table 18-3 can effectively reconstruct each anatomic region.

A defect that involves bone, blood vessels, and/or nerves will need a careful assessment and stepwise treatment plan. Reconstruction typically involves skeletal fixation as the starting point. All vascular repairs typically require autologous grafts. Determination for acute repair versus delayed reconstruction of any nerve or tendon injuries must be determined prior to definitive wound closure or coverage.

Intuitively, the lack of local available soft tissue generally precludes a simple reconstruction method. However, certain anatomic areas are easier to reconstruct with fasciocutaneous flaps, which provide durable coverage. These areas include shoulder, limited defects on dorsal elbow, or even in the cubital fossa. In certain situations wherein there is a healthy well-vascularized soft tissue bed comprising healthy muscle or even paratenon, a simple skin graft may be an easy reconstructive strategy. Of course, the long-term problems with graft contractures and lack of durability, usually due to thin, insensate coverage, adversely impacts the outcome.

In two critical ways, understanding the vascular roadmap becomes essential to upper extremity reconstruction: (1) identification of donor vessels and (2) understanding the impact of sacrificing a vessel for flap anastomoses. Methods of assessing vascular integrity include a simple physical examination of the pulses, an Allen test (using Doppler ultrasound confirmation both preoperative and intraoperatively), and when needed an angiogram or a magnetic resonance angiogram (MRA) is available.[22] More recently, indocyanine green fluorescence angiography used in the SPY imaging system has gained increasing interest and use for flap design and intraoperative and postoperative flap assessment.[23] Further work is ongoing to define its role as a reliable tool for the surgeon.[24]

The Shoulder

In many cases, soft tissue defects about the shoulder can be effectively addressed with local fasciocutaneous flaps. The donor site is usually amenable to primary closure (for defects <6 cm in diameter) and may need skin grafting for those that are larger than 6 cm.

Scapular and Parascapular Flap

The scapular or parascapular flap is an excellent choice for larger defects on the shoulder. It can be used as a pedicle flap or free flap, and may include bone. The pedicled parascapular flap is more commonly used for reconstruction of defects of the shoulder and axillae. Either flap easily provides a fasciocutaneous flap 15 cm in length, and has been harvested as long as 25 cm.[25,26] The anatomy of the parascapular flap allows it to be harvested as a chimeric flap, soft tissue or bone harvested on a single pedicle, allowing for reconstruction of large composite tissue defects in the shoulder region. The superior aspect of the flap is centered over the triangular space, where the circumflex scapular artery nourishes the parascapular flap after it travels through the triangular space. The borders of the triangular space are made up of the teres minor, teres major, and long head of triceps. The parascapular flap may be combined with the following tissues as a chimeric flap on the subscapular vessel axis: scapular flap, scapular bone, latissimus muscle, serratus muscle, and serratus muscle with rib.

The latissimus and teres major muscles are important landmarks because flap dissection proceeds from inferior to superior and these are identified early in the dissection. The elevation of the flap is performed in the areolar fascial layer just above the thick muscular fascia of the back. The infraspinatus fascia overlying the infraspinatus muscle and the teres minor fascia overlying the teres minor are particularly thick. If the flap is elevated deep to the muscular fascia, the dissection can become confusing and especially difficult around the pedicle where the fascia surrounds the triangular space.

The circumflex scapular artery is a branch of the subscapular artery, which originates from the axillary artery. The circumflex scapular arises about 1 to 4 cm from the origin of the subscapular artery, but can on occasion arise directly from the axillary artery. After the circumflex scapular artery pierces the triangular space, it sprouts a transverse cutaneous scapular branch and a vertical parascapular branch. The parascapular branch forms the basis of the parascapular flap.

The subscapular artery pedicle can be from 3 to 7 cm in length with vessel circumference at this level up to 4 mm in size. Although the circumflex scapular artery is usually accompanied by two venae comitantes, the subscapular artery is typically accompanied by one vein. This flap can be rotated into the shoulder area easily and provide durable coverage with low morbidity.

The Brachium and Arm

Pedicled Latissimus Dorsi Muscle Flap

The brachium, or arm, is defined as distal to the shoulder and at least 6 cm proximal to the elbow. Defects in this region are best reconstructed with a pedicled latissimus dorsi muscle

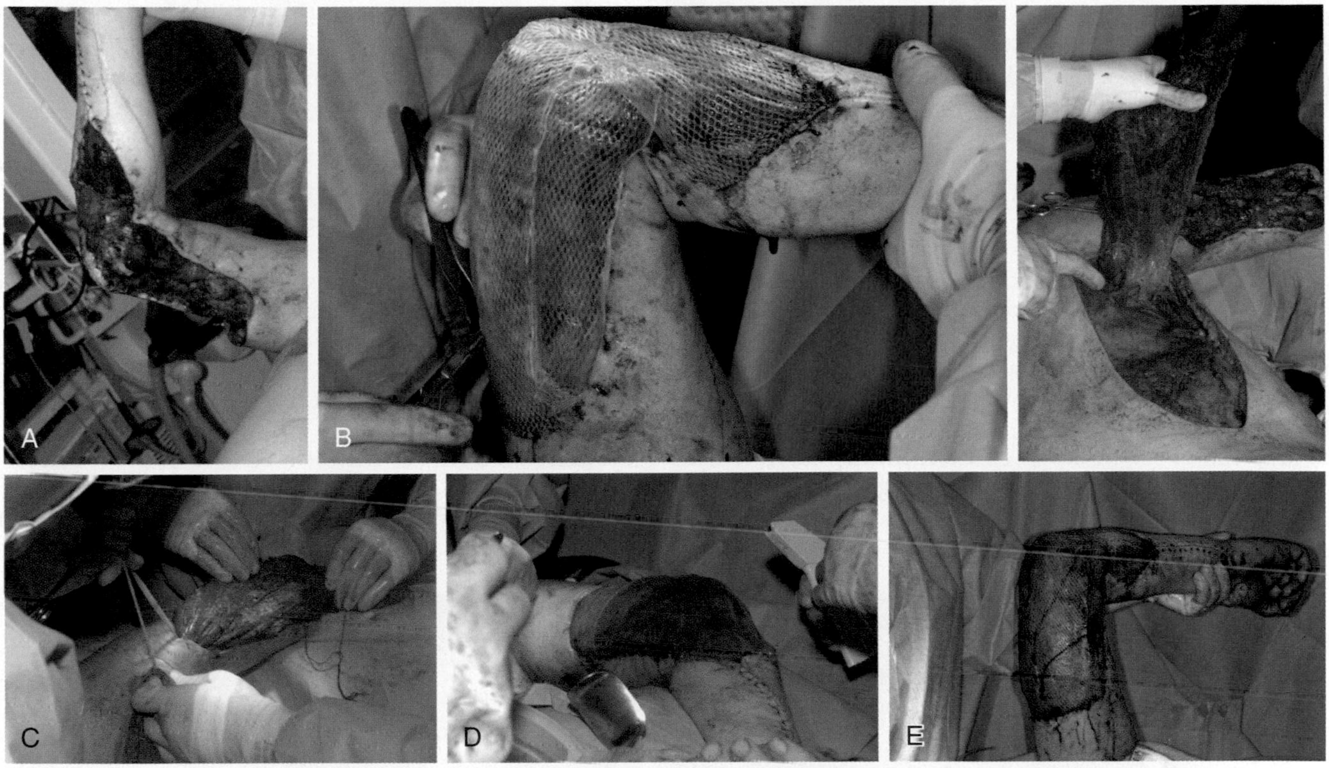

Figure 18-1. Pedicled latissimus dorsi muscle flap. **A,** A large defect of the medial arm and elbow. **B,** Latissimus dorsi muscle pedicle flap harvest. **C,** Flap inset. **D,** Dermal substitute applied to flap at time of inset. **E,** Split-thickness skin grafting performed 2 weeks later.

flap. It provides excellent coverage with generous amounts of soft tissue that can envelope the entire circumference of the upper arm if needed.[27,28] A skin paddle can be added to monitor the flap postoperatively, and to add additional fasciocutaneous coverage. The donor site on the flank is amenable to primary closure with minimal morbidity.

The blood supply is derived from a single constant vascular pedicle (thoracodorsal artery) and the flap can be rotated into the upper arm with ease because of its long neurovascular pedicle, large size, ease of mobilization, and expendability. In some cases, it can cover soft tissue defects involving the shoulder, arm, and even sometimes the elbow. As an innervated functional muscle flap, it can improve shoulder abduction, or when rotated to the elbow, it can restore elbow flexion or extension. Detaching the humeral attachment can extend the reach of the muscle (Fig. 18-1).

Pedicled Pectoralis Muscle Flap

Other options include a pedicled pectoralis muscle flap (or sometimes along with a skin paddle, which may or may not be a reliable option). Based upon the thoracoacromial trunk, this muscle extends into upper arm defects easily. Its availability is limited by the anchor point on the clavicle from, at which point the blood supply enters the muscle.

The Elbow

Common flap options for coverage include the reverse radial artery flap, reverse lateral arm flap, and the pedicle latissimus dorsi muscle flap. Drawbacks of these flaps include sacrifice of the radial artery, donor site morbidity, bulky flaps requiring secondary thinning, nonaesthetic donor sites, and the inability to provide sensate coverage in most cases.

Radial Forearm Flap

The traditional radial forearm flap is a common flap for coverage of large defects about the elbow. It sacrifices the radial artery and cannot be performed if the ulnar artery is insufficient to perfuse the hand. The flap is designed over the radial distal forearm and is designed to include a branch of the cephalic vein. Care is taken to preserve the paratenon during dissection over the flexor carpi radialis and brachioradialis to facilitate skin graft take over the donor site. The cephalic vein and lateral antebrachial cutaneous nerve are included in flap dissection to improve venous outflow and provide sensation to the flap. The flap is pedicled and inset into the donor site after subcutaneous transposition of the ulnar nerve. The donor site is covered with a split-thickness skin graft. Use of a dermal substitute may improve the cosmetic donor site result.

Anconeus Muscle Flap

The anconeus muscle flap may be used for the coverage of small traumatic defects around the elbow.[29] The anconeus muscle is approximately 4 by 10 cm, and can reliably cover up to 7-cm defects.[30] Both the medial collateral artery and the recurrent posterior interosseous artery perfuse the anconeus muscle, which anastomose within the muscle, allowing surgeon flexibility to rotate the flap on either pedicle. Common uses are to cover the radiocapitellar joint, the olecranon, and the distal triceps tendon. Primary closure is performed when possible, or in some cases, skin grafting may be required.

Pedicled Latissimus Dorsi Muscle Flap

As previously mentioned, the pedicled latissimus dorsi muscle flap may not easily reach the elbow. Detaching the humeral insertion can extend the reach. Flap elevation is performed through a posterior lateral incision. Transposition through an axillary skin tunnel and insetting over the elbow is followed by a split-thickness skin graft applied directly over the muscle. Alternatively, a skin paddle may be taken with the latissimus dorsi muscle, but the more distal it is placed (to reach the elbow), the more tenuous is the blood supply to the distal tip (which at inset covers the most important area of the defect).

Forearm

Soft tissue defects in this zone with exposed vital structures (bone, blood vessels, nerves, or hardware) require free flap reconstruction. There are numerous options available depending on available soft tissue donor sites.

Anterolateral Thigh Flap

The anterolateral thigh flap is an excellent flap for coverage of forearm soft tissue defects because of its generous size, large donor vessel, and low morbidity to the patient. The perforator for the flap is located at the midpoint between the upper lateral margin of the patella and the anterior superior iliac spine (ASIS). The lateral femoral circumflex artery is easily identified by retracting the rectus femoris muscle medially. The flap can be harvested with a cuff of vastus lateralis muscle in two situations: to provide additional muscular tissue for dead space obliteration or when the perforator actually travels through the muscle itself. Harvested flap width up to an 8-cm width can usually be closed primarily. Occasionally the lateral femoral cutaneous nerve can be harvested for sensory neurotization. The flap is then inset into the defect while the vessels are anastomosed end-to-side into the brachial system[31-34] (Fig. 18-2).

Lateral Arm Flap

The lateral forearm flap may be used to reconstruct defects of the forearm, hand, and wrist. Substantially large defects ranging from a minimum of 5 cm to a maximum of 15 cm can

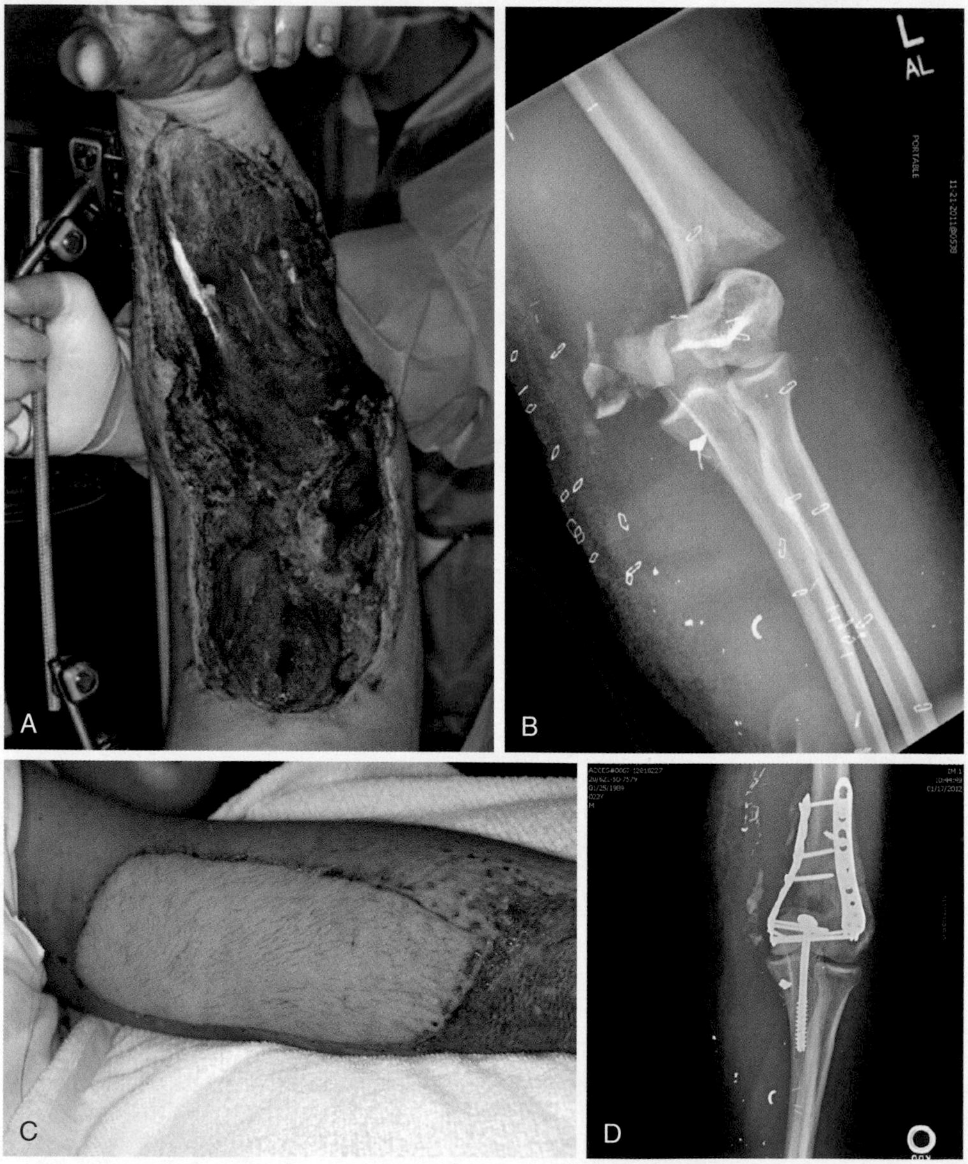

Figure 18-2. Anterolateral thigh flap. **A,** Large soft tissue defect of the anterior elbow and forearm. **B,** Distal humerus fracture. **C,** Soft tissue coverage with a combined anterolateral thigh fasciocutaneous flap and dermal substitute with overlying split-thickness skin graft. **D,** Fracture fixation.

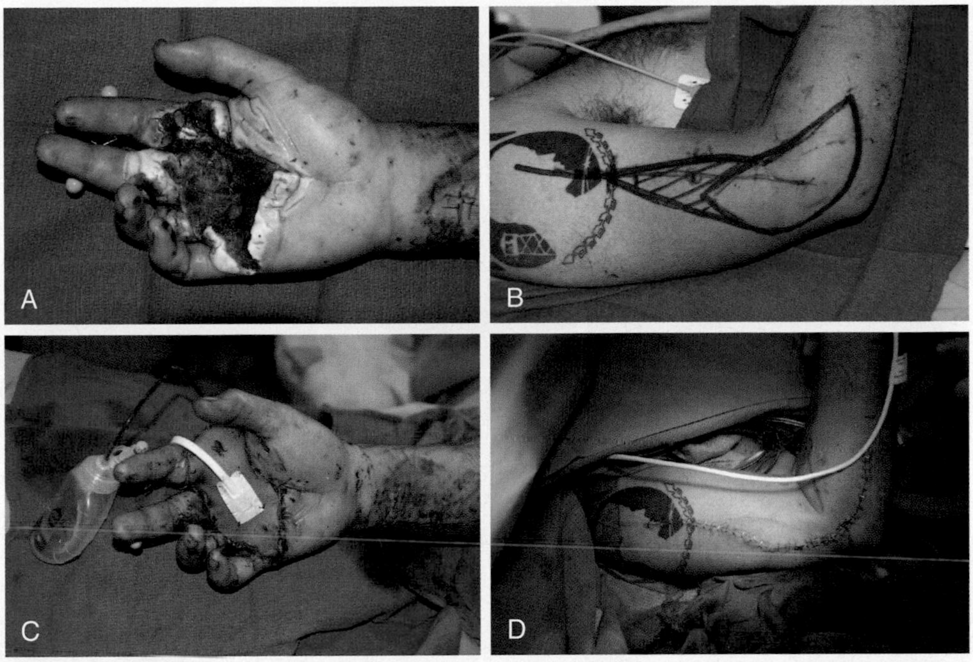

Figure 18-3. Lateral arm flap. **A,** Complex soft tissue defect in the palm. **B,** Lateral arm flap donor site. **C,** Lateral arm flap inset. **D,** Primary closure of donor site.

be covered.[35,36] The radial collateral artery, a branch of the brachial artery, supplies the flap. It wraps posteriorly around the humerus, descends on its lateral aspect and divides into anterior and posterior branches. The posterior branch supplies the lateral arm and lateral forearm flaps. The skin incision is based on the long axis of the humerus in line with the deltoid muscle insertion along the lateral intermuscular septum. Dissection identifies the biceps, brachialis, and brachioradialis muscles along the anterior plane and the triceps muscle posteriorly. The radial nerve courses posterior to the humerus from its origin at the brachial plexus and runs over the lateral aspect of the humerus. The lateral arm flap can also be harvested as an osteocutaneous flap. The wedge of bone with periosteal cuff is harvested under the septum and septal pedicle. A narrow portion of bone approximately 1- to 1.5-cm wide can be harvested (Fig. 18-3).

Scapular and Parascapular Flap

The scapular or parascapular flap is indicated for reconstruction of complex soft tissue and bone defects of the forearm. As described earlier, both flaps are based on the circumflex scapular artery, a branch of the scapular artery, and may be combined with bone harvest from the lateral scapular via osseous branches of the circumflex scapular artery. As an osteocutaneous flap, up to 10-cm length of bone, and up to 3- to 4-cm in width may be harvested without significant morbidity to the patient.[37] Additional flaps, such as the parascapular flap, latissimus dorsi muscle, or serratus anterior and ribs may be combined as a chimeric flap based on the scapular artery. This flap has proven versatile in the treatment of high-energy blast injuries seen in recent conflicts[38] (Fig. 18-4).

Omental Flap

The omental flap is a choice available when all other tissues are unavailable. The omentum does offer unique advantages, which are a long vascular pedicle; abundant pliable tissue that can contour complex defects; laparoscopic-assisted harvest (reducing donor site morbidity); and finally, physiologically creating a barrier to infection that facilitates healing, reduces edema, and fights infection.[39] Because of its vascularity, it may be used to reconstruct segmental radial or ulnar artery defects in the forearm, in addition to providing a large area of coverage. Split-thickness skin grafting is required, and use of a dermal substitute with skin grafting provides a more aesthetically uniform and durable result (Fig. 18-5).

Wrist and Hand

Soft tissue reconstruction seeks to restore both the aesthetic appearance and the function of the hand. Skin grafts and skin substitutes both are useful reconstructive options for certain defects. The radial forearm flap and posterior interosseous artery island flap are commonly used local flaps for coverage of large defects of the wrist and hand. The groin flap remains a mainstay of reconstruction in the wrist and hand.[40] The lateral arm flap is the most commonly used free flap in the wrist and hand because of its size and thin tissue characteristic (Fig. 18-6).

Reverse Radial Forearm Flap

Previously described in this chapter, the radial forearm flap provides robust fasciocutaneous coverage, most commonly for the dorsum of the hand. The flap is similar to that described for coverage of the elbow, with the exception of harvesting the flap from the proximal forearm, and dividing the radial artery and cephalic vein proximally to rotate the flap into the wrist and hand. Recently more popular, the radial forearm flap can be harvested as an adipofascial flap, allowing the donor site to be closed primarily, and preventing the "shark bite" appearance of the forearm.[41] However, a skin graft will be required at the recipient site. The surgeon must weigh the benefits of flap

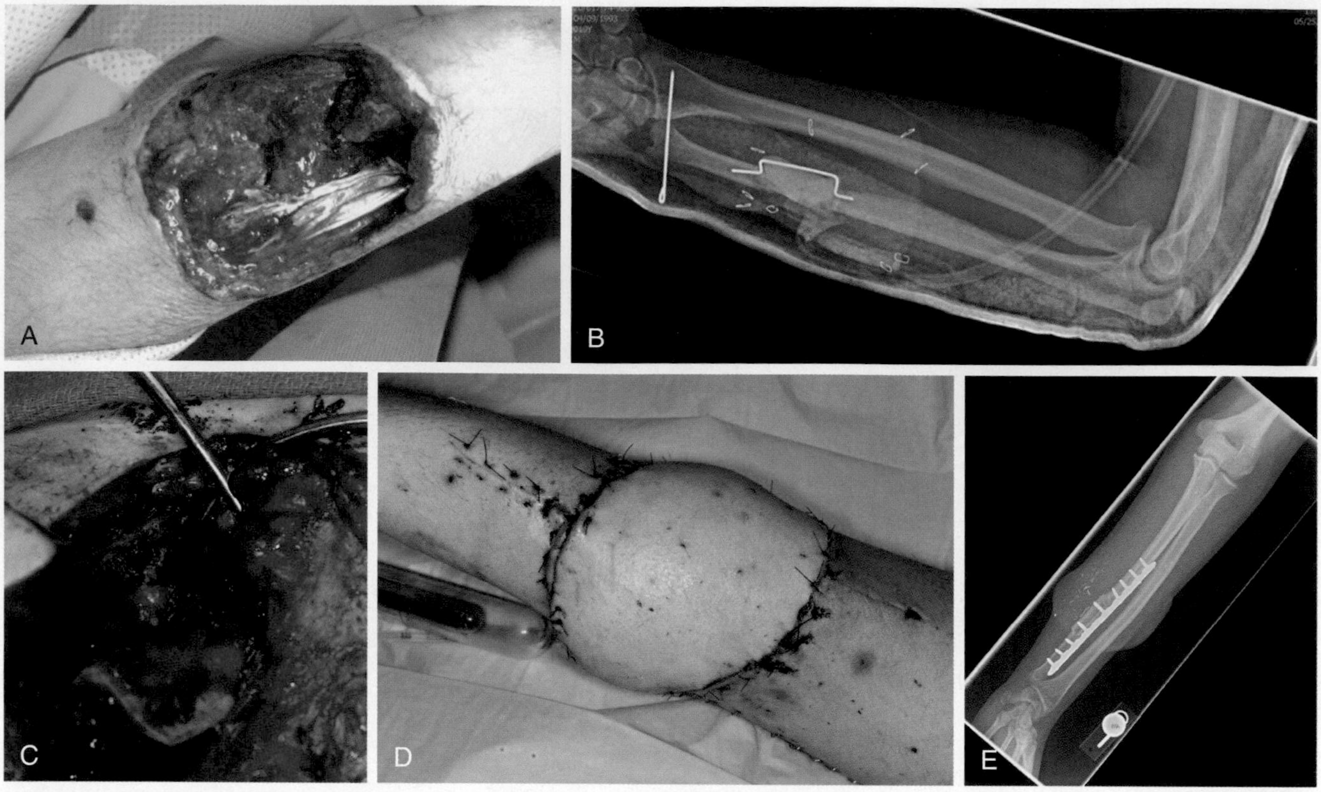

Figure 18-4. Osteocutaneous scapular flap. A and **B,** A large soft tissue defect of the arm with ulnar bone loss secondary to blast injury. **C,** An osteocutaneous scapular flap is used to reconstruct the soft tissue and bone defects. **D,** Flap inset. **E,** Radiograph demonstrating incorporation of the bone graft.

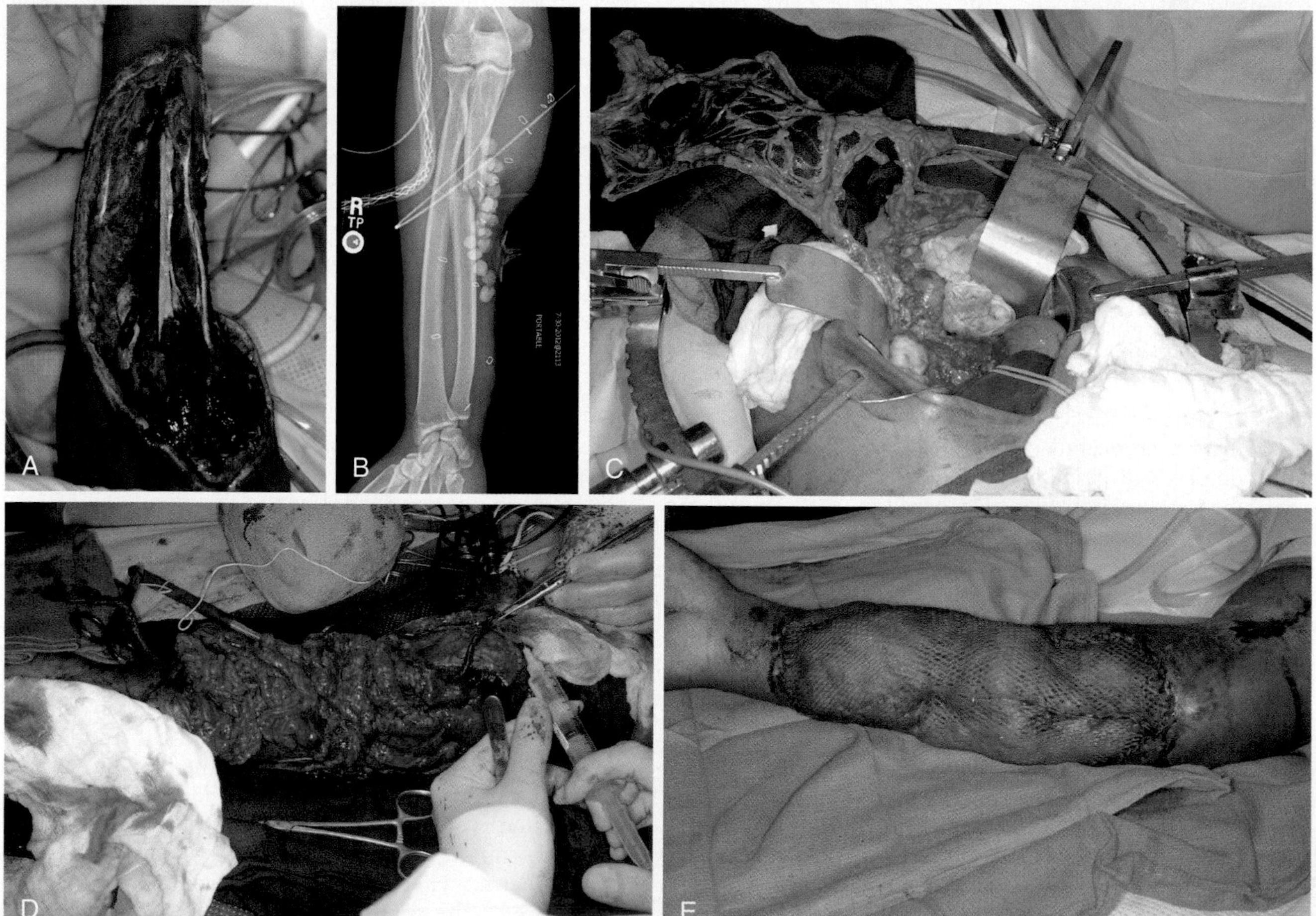

Figure 18-5. Omental flap. A and **B,** A large soft tissue defect of the forearm with large segmental ulnar artery loss, ulnar nerve segmental defect, and ulna fracture. **C,** Omental flap harvest. **D,** Omental flap inset. **E,** Dermal substitute with split-thickness skin graft.

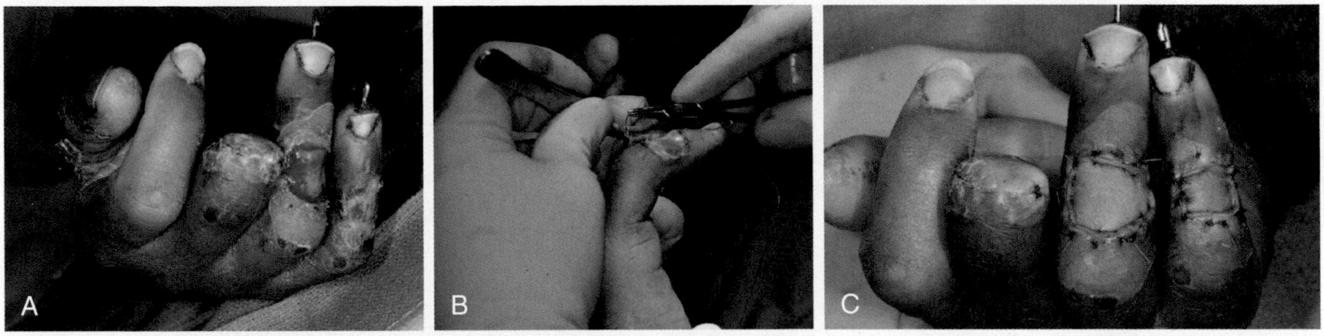

Figure 18-6. A, Soft tissue defect on dorsum of the small finger in a mangling hand injury precluding use of local flaps. **B,** Placement of a skin substitute. **C,** Full-thickness skin graft over dermal substitute.

durability and cosmesis with donor site morbidity when deciding on the type of radial forearm flap to employ (Fig. 18-7).

Posterior Interosseous Artery Flap

The reversed-flow posterior interosseous artery island flap, sometimes termed the *posterior forearm flap,* is commonly deployed to cover large soft tissue defects of the wrist and hand, and to reconstruct the thumb web space.[42-44] The distal extent of the flap is considered to the level of the metacarpophalangeal joint of the hand, although more distal reach has been described. It is based on the posterior interosseous artery, located in a line extending from the lateral epicondyle to the distal radioulnar joint, with the medial posterior interosseous perforator commonly identified 1 cm distal to the midpoint of this axis. Flap width can be up to 5 to 7 cm, but beyond 4 cm, the donor site is difficult to close. The pivot point for the pedicle is 2 cm proximal to the distal radioulnar joint. Flap harvest generally proceeds from radial to ulnar, with great care expended to ensure the septocutaneous perforators, located in the intermuscular septum between the extensor carpi ulnaris and the extensor indicis proprius, are not disturbed. Because the flap vascular pedicle is rotated 180 degrees, venous congestion may be encountered. In such cases, a flap delay prior to transfer may be indicated.[45]

Groin Flap

Described by McGregor in 1972, the groin flap is the first-described axial pattern flap, and still remains a mainstay of reconstructive surgery of the upper extremity, including the distal forearm, wrist, and hand. Reliability and ease of flap

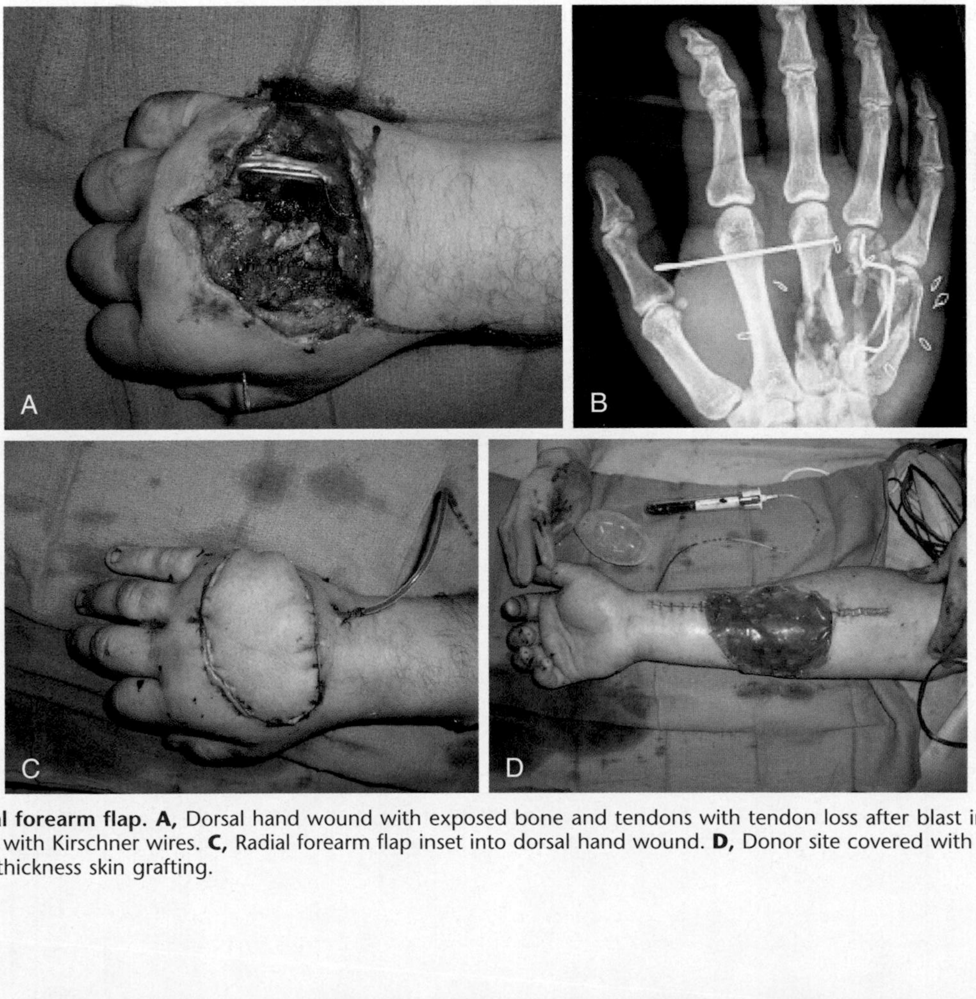

Figure 18-7. Radial forearm flap. A, Dorsal hand wound with exposed bone and tendons with tendon loss after blast injury. **B,** Right hand fracture stabilization with Kirschner wires. **C,** Radial forearm flap inset into dorsal hand wound. **D,** Donor site covered with dermal substitute in anticipation of split-thickness skin grafting.

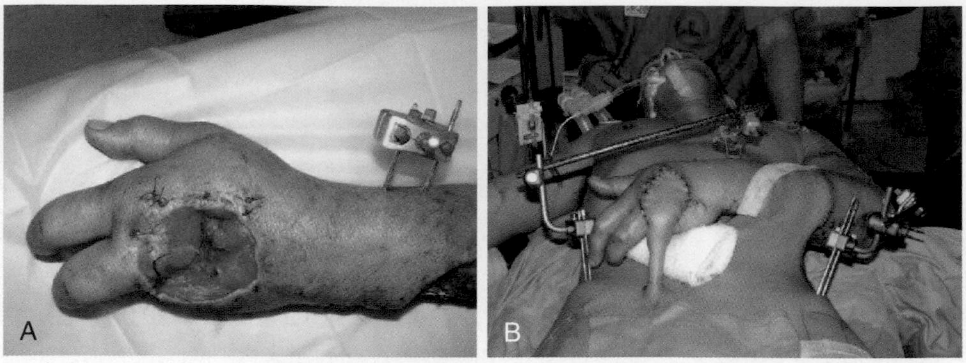

Figure 18-8. **A,** Dorsal hand and forearm wounds requiring coverage in a critically injured polytrauma patient. **B,** Groin flap coverage with concurrent thoracoepigastric random pattern flap coverage. Note adjunct use of external fixation to protect flap in the obtunded patient.

harvest without need for microsurgical techniques are its main advantages. The main disadvantages are considerable flap bulk in some cases, and patients unwilling to have their upper limb joined to the flap for 2 to 3 weeks before the flap is divided and finally inset. The groin flap is based on the superficial circumflex iliac artery, a branch of the femoral artery located approximately two fingerbreadths below the inguinal ligament.[46]

Based on this vascular distribution, flap sizes can be quite wide and extend well lateral to the ASIS. However, flap width greater than 10 cm can be difficult to close primarily and may require a skin graft. Hip flexion assists in primary closure. The flap is generally tubed in its midsection to minimize flap leakage during the phase prior to flap division, and the flap is inset into the defect. Care must be taken with postoperative dressings and positioning to avoid flap complications. The flap is usually separated from the groin at 2 to 3 weeks, followed by flap inset, and the donor site finally closed. Mild shoulder and elbow stiffness is to be expected, but usually resolves in most cases[47] (Fig. 18-8).

First Dorsal Metacarpal Artery Flap

A network of arteries arising from the radial, ulnar, and posterior interosseous arteries supplies the dorsum of the hand. The first dorsal interosseous artery consistently arises from the radial artery or the princeps pollicis artery, and courses radial to the index finger metacarpal over the interosseous muscle fascia, before it arborizes distal to the metacarpophalangeal joint on the dorsum of the finger. Sometimes called the "kite flap," this reliable flap can be designed and harvested from the dorsum of the index finger and transposed locally or used as a free flap. This flap is typically indicated for reconstruction of defects of the thumb or thumb web space. In a one-stage procedure, the donor site is typically covered with full-thickness skin graft[48-51] (Fig. 18-9).

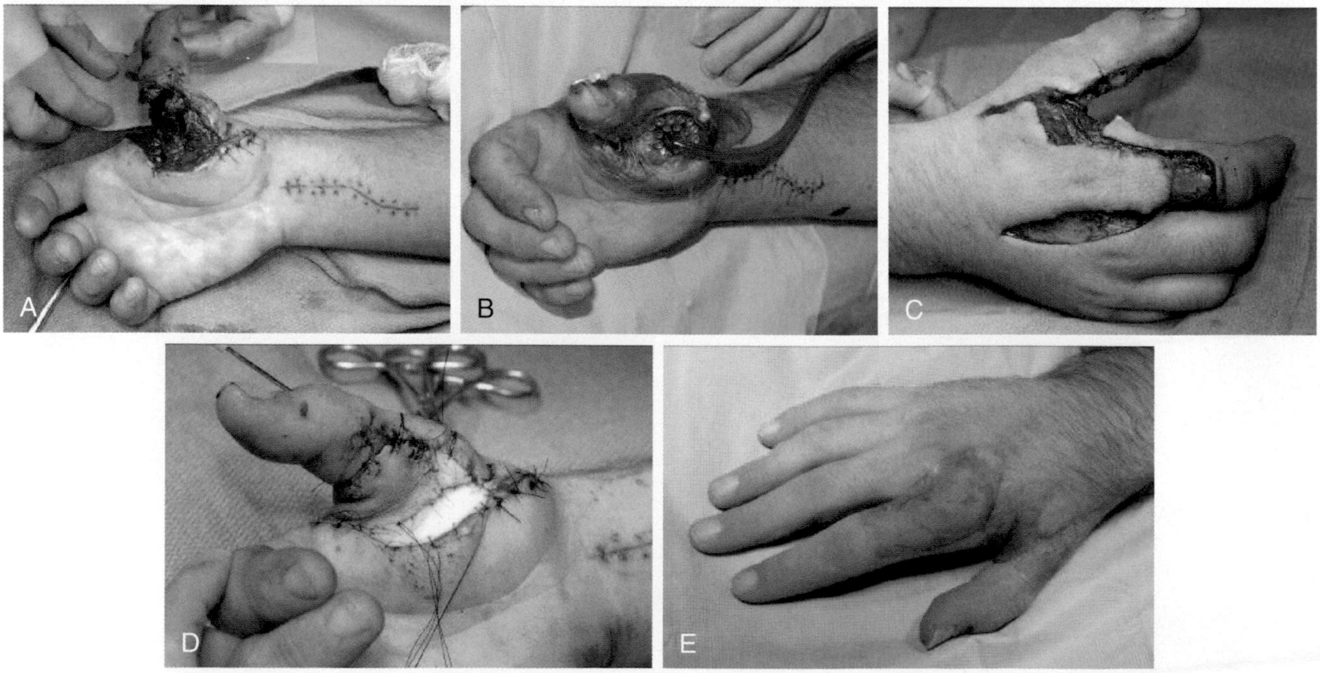

Figure 18-9. First dorsal metacarpal artery flap. **A,** Complex wound of the thumb and web space due to gunshot wound. **B,** Vacuum-assisted closure dressing of thumb. **C,** First dorsal metacarpal artery flap harvest. **D,** Flap inset. **E,** Result. *(Courtesy of Dr. Patricia McKay, MD, CDR, MC, USN.)*

LOWER EXTREMITY SOFT TISSUE RECONSTRUCTION

Introduction

A clinically applicable situation wherein soft tissue reconstruction of the lower extremity is needed arises from trauma, tumor, infection, diabetes, or rarely, defects resulting from joint replacement surgery.[52-54] Although each of the clinical entities is vastly different, the defects that are produced that need complex reconstruction (as opposed to simple primary closure) share certain common characteristics. These characteristics are all not essential but, in and of themselves, sufficient to warrant reconstructive attention. They include missing tissue elements leading to exposure of vital structures in the extremity (bone, blood vessels, nerves, tendons, joint, and hardware); their location would guarantee limitation of mobility if left to heal via secondary intention; considerations of durability to withstand the wear and tear of weight-bearing and friction (from work as well as clothing) demand that the tissues must retain optimal thickness; finally, if possible, the use of neurotized tissue instead of insensate skin cover assumes a great role in creating a reconstructed defect that is fully functional as opposed to one that is prone to constant breakdown. As noted in the reconstructive requirements in the upper extremity, the site and location of the defect plays a vital role in the selection of the reconstructive tissues. Techniques include primary closure, skin grafting, local cutaneous flaps, fasciocutaneous transposition flaps, island fascial or fasciocutaneous flaps, muscle or myocutaneous pedicled flaps, and microvascular free-tissue transfer. Optimal choices depend on available tissue as well as the location and extent of the defect. Timing of reconstruction is an important consideration and one-stage reconstruction has distinct advantages and must be preferred whenever feasible.[55]

Surgical Planning

Selecting the right reconstructive option depends heavily on the location of the defect on the lower extremity. Thigh defects are largely divided into upper two-thirds thigh defects and those that involve the lower one-third thigh, which are reconstructed with techniques similar to defects around the knee joint. The leg below the level of the knee itself is divided into thirds again, upper, mid, and lower third defects that conjure up distinct reconstructive options. Foot and ankle defects mark a separate zone, and reconstruction of these defects usually involves free flap microvascular reconstruction, or an array of local skin and fascial flaps when available. Refer to Table 18-4 for the list of coverage options for the lower extremity based on anatomic location.

As delineated in the section on upper extremity reconstruction defects, the lower extremity defects that involve bone, vessels, and nerves need careful assessment and as emphasized earlier, the reconstruction involves skeletal fixation as the starting point. All vascular repairs typically require autologous grafts. Nerve repairs again need to be addressed along with soft tissue reconstruction and may involve direct repair or the interposition of nerve grafts using sural nerves as common donor sites. Tendons that have to be sacrificed as part of the resection or débridement should be tagged distally as well as proximally if a delayed tendon repair is anticipated.

TABLE 18-4 *OPTIONS FOR SOFT TISSUE RECONSTRUCTION OF THE LOWER EXTREMITY BY LOCATION*

Simple Wound (No Exposed Bone, Tendons, or Neurovascular Structures)	-Split-thickness skin graft except in weight-bearing areas -Use dermal substitute to increase thickness and durability of graft
Complex Wounds (Exposed Bone, Tendons, or Neurovascular Structures)	**Thigh (Lower Third) and Knee** -Gastrocnemius muscle flap -Vastus lateralis muscle flap -Fasciocutaneous flap -Free flap **Leg** ***Upper Third*** -Gastrocnemius muscle flap ***Middle Third*** -Soleus muscle flap -Cross leg flap (rarely indicated in modern times) -Free flap ***Lower Third*** -Reverse sural artery flap -Free flap **Foot** ***Dorsum, Sole, and Heel*** -Medial plantar flap for the heel -Distally based sural artery flap for the heel -Local random fasciocutaneous flaps for small defects of the sole -Free flap **Ankle and Malleolus** -Reverse sural artery flap -Dorsalis pedis flap -Median plantar flap -Free flap

Intuitively, the lack of local available soft tissue precludes any easy reconstruction; that said, certain anatomic areas are easier to reconstruct with fasciocutaneous flaps, which provide durable coverage, or muscle flaps that cover very large areas or reconstruct defects to fill volume, but associated donor site morbidity must be considered in each patient.[56] If there is a healthy, well-vascularized soft tissue bed comprising healthy muscle or paratenon, a simple skin graft may be an easy reconstructive strategy. Of course, the long-term problems with graft contractures and lack of durability (due to thin, insensate coverage) adversely impact the outcome. As in upper extremity reconstruction, understanding the vascular roadmap becomes essential to lower extremity reconstruction.

Hip and Thigh

Soft tissue defects requiring flap coverage are uncommon about the hip and upper thigh. When tissue is required, most defects in this region can be effectively addressed with local fasciocutaneous flaps. The donor site is usually amenable to primary closure for defects less than 8 cm in diameter and may need skin grafting for those that are larger than 8 cm. An array of muscles, including the vastus lateralis, gracilis, sartorius, tensor fascia lata, and even the rectus femoris can be raised and rotated to cover exposed vital structures, followed by a split-thickness skin graft. Irradiated tissue is a notable contraindication because of compromised tissue health and poor vascular perfusion. Free tissue transfer may be more appropriate in these cases.

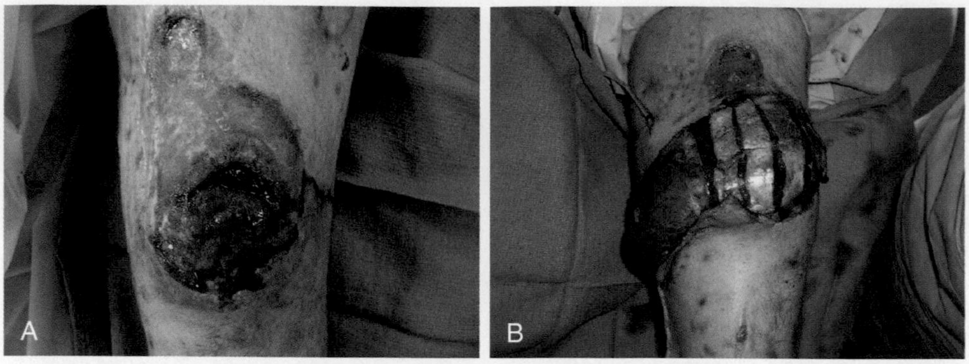

Figure 18-10. Pedicled gastrocnemius muscle flap. **A,** Soft tissue defect of the anterior knee with exposed open knee joint and patella fracture secondary to blast injury. **B,** Medial gastrocnemius muscle flap rotation with fascial lengthening.

Lower Thigh, Knee, and Proximal Third of the Leg

Gastrocnemius Muscle Flap

The gastrocnemius muscle flap is the workhorse of all muscle flaps for soft tissue coverage around the knee.[57] The medial gastrocnemius flap is most effective for coverage of distal defects over the tibial tubercle or patellar tendon. Defects that extend more proximally over the patella or quadriceps tendon usually require an extension of the gastrocnemius muscle by detaching the tendinous attachment to the condyles to achieve adequate soft tissue coverage. In situations that result in an open wound with exposed hardware and sometimes even a fracture (e.g., revision or infected total knee arthroplasty surgery, or double-plate fixation via a two-incision approach in the treatment of complex tibial plateau fractures), higher success rates of wound healing with solid bony union are seen when a gastrocnemius muscle flap is performed.[58,59] The sural arteries supply this flap, arising from the popliteal artery above the level of the knee joint. Each vessel courses a few centimeters with its venae comitantes before entering the proximal muscle belly with the innervating branches of the tibial nerve.[60] Transfer does not adversely impair function of the limb, making it an ideal flap to cover a large wound in this region. For the medial gastrocnemius muscle flap, incision is made 2 to 3 cm behind the medial border of tibia from the popliteal fossa and carried downward to below mid-calf level. Deep fascia and medial head of gastrocnemius are identified and separated from under soleus muscle. The distal end of muscle is sharply divided from the Achilles tendon leaving a cuff of 1 to 2 cm of tendon at the flap edge for improved suture fixation on inset. It is then divided and separated from the lateral gastrocnemius at the midline raphe, taking care to avoid injury to the sural nerve and short saphenous vein. The inset of the muscle is completed and the muscle is covered by a meshed skin graft.

Harvest of the lateral gastrocnemius muscle flap requires that the common peroneal nerve to be positively identified and retracted gently to avoid injury. The remainder of the procedure is similar to flap harvest on the medial side. Suction drains are typically used, and then the limb is usually immobilized for 1 week. Typically, the first flap check is made at the third postoperative day. This is a hardy flap, and can be extended either by scoring the overlying fascia transversely, or fascial lengthening, or for greater length, by incising the proximal insertion to the condyle. In the extended form, it can reach lower thigh defects easily and can be used for more extensive defects (Fig. 18-10).

Vastus Lateralis Muscle Flap

This flap is an excellent choice for knee defects when the gastrocnemius flap is not available or sufficient for coverage. It can be combined with the gastrocnemius flap for larger defects when necessary.[61] In addition, it can be used with other flaps harvested from the thigh for greater coverage.[62] When the gastrocnemius muscle is unavailable for transfer (vascular injury to popliteal, previous surgery, amputation), the vastus lateralis can provide muscular tissue for soft tissue coverage. Donor site morbidity is limited as this muscle is one of at least four extensors of the knee. In addition, it has adequate mass and can be extended to reach the desired length for coverage of the defect.[63]

The muscle is located between the vastus intermedius and the biceps femoris muscles and beneath the tensor fascia lata originating from the greater trochanter, intertrochanteric line, gluteal tuberosity, and lateral intermuscular septum, and inserts into the patella. The dominant pedicle is the descending branch of the lateral circumflex femoral artery and venae comitantes. It is located in the superior one-third of the muscle extending inferiorly along the medial border of the muscle belly. The pedicle enters the medial deep aspect of the muscle approximately 10 to 15 cm below the ASIS. The vastus lateralis is a type II flap and can also be based on a distally located minor pedicle. There are three named minor pedicles. The first, the transverse branch of the lateral circumflex femoral artery, enters the muscle in its superior one-fourth on the deep surface. The second, the posterior branch from the profunda femoris artery, is located at the inferior half of the posterior muscle at the lateral intermuscular septum. And the third, the superficial branch of the lateral superior genicular artery, courses around and superior to the lateral condyle of the knee deep to the biceps femoris and provides a superficial branch to the distal muscle, entering the lateral posterior aspect of the vastus lateralis muscle. Unlike the medial thigh, which has a segmental blood supply from branches of the superficial femoral artery (SFA), the vastus lateralis is devoid of significant vascular contributions in its midportion. Based upon the minor pedicles, it can reach the knee and a few centimeters beyond quite easily with a radius of rotation of approximately 15 cm. Typically, the flap sacrifices only the mid muscle belly. In very large defects, microvascular anastomosis of the dominant pedicle to suitable receptor vessels at the defect site can allow the use of the entire muscle.

The flap is ideally suited for use in the popliteal fossa posteriorly and in the inferior portion of the knee anteriorly. Approach to the muscle is through a thigh incision from a point 10 cm below the ASIS at the level of the greater trochanter to the lateral condyle of the femur. The incision is carried through the deep fascia at the medial edge of the tensor fascia lata muscle in the proximal one-fourth of the leg and the iliotibial tract distally. The border between the vastus lateralis and medialis is identified and separated. The anterior portion of the tensor fascia lata is divided through a midlateral thigh incision, exposing the vastus lateralis muscle. In the distally based flap based on the minor pedicle, isolating and preserving a segment of the descending branch of the lateral circumflex femoral artery associated venae comitantes is performed. The donor site can usually be closed primarily.

Saphenous Artery Fasciocutaneous Flap

The saphenous flap is based on the saphenous artery originating from the descending genicular artery. It covers defects on both the anterior and posterior surfaces of the leg, including the popliteal fossa and knee joint. First described in the 1980s, the saphenous flap is a reliable local flap for soft tissue coverage of the knee with a versatile range.[64,65] It is a simple one-stage operation. Retrograde flow through the saphenous artery is supplied by anastomoses with the medial inferior genicular artery in a distally based, reversed-flow saphenous island flap based on the medial inferior genicular artery, and rarely, a venous saphenous flap based solely on the saphenous vein. The saphenous artery flap is located on the medial aspect of the knee and upper leg. The typical size of the flap is approximately 7 by 20 cm, but flaps up to 29 by 8 cm and 15 by 11 cm have been reported.

The dominant pedicle, measuring 5 to 15 cm, is the saphenous artery branch of the descending genicular artery, a branch of the SFA, and venae comitantes. The saphenous artery pierces the sheath of the adductor canal and then joins the saphenous nerve and passes deep to the sartorius muscle between the sartorius and gracilis muscles to supply the inferior medial aspect of the leg. At the level of the joint line, the sartorius muscle becomes tendinous, and the saphenous artery runs out from beneath the tendon. The descending genicular artery originates from the SFA 14 to 15 cm above the medial joint line of the knee. It then runs distally for 0.5 to 2 cm, dividing into two to three branches that include the saphenous artery, osteoarticular branch, and muscular branch. The subcutaneous perforators are identified by Doppler (preferred over invasive angiogram) since the vessels are superficial with little subcutaneous fat between them and the overlying skin.

The saphenous artery flap has less subcutaneous fat than other flaps, facilitating easy detection of the perforators with Doppler imaging. Angiography is more necessary in patients with a history of trauma, surgery, or arteriosclerosis. In designing the flap, a line is first drawn from the ASIS to the medial condyle of the tibia, outlining the course of the sartorius muscle. The skin island is centered over the distal portion of the sartorius, with the upper border as much as 10 to 15 cm above the knee joint. The incision is made in the medial thigh over the sartorius muscle along the line from the ASIS to the medial tibial condyle and continues down to the deep fascia of the sartorius. Blunt dissection of the anterior border of the sartorius muscle exposes the septocutaneous branches of the saphenous artery. The deep fascia is divided anterior to the sartorius muscle, and the saphenous artery is visualized between the sartorius and vastus medialis. The pedicle courses deep to the sartorius muscle several centimeters superior to the skin island, with perforating vessels coursing on either side of the muscle supplying the skin. The medial femoral cutaneous nerve and saphenous vein run along the posterior border of the sartorius muscle. The distal saphenous artery is identified next. The skin and deep fascia are then divided cautiously up to within 6 cm of the knee joint while searching carefully for the arterial branching pattern. Next, identify which cutaneous vessels predominate. If the perforators emerging anterior to the sartorius are predominant, the skin island is placed anterior to the muscle. If the perforators emerging posterior to the sartorius are predominant, the skin island is placed posterior to the sartorius. If the anterior and posterior vessels are equal in size, the skin island is centered on the sartorius and a portion of muscle is included within the flap. Dividing or including portions of the sartorius with the flap may be necessary to preserve the cutaneous branches. Distally, the saphenous vein is divided at the distal flap margin for inclusion proximally to enhance venous outflow. The flap is dissected from below upward. The arc of rotation can be based on its dominant pedicle and transposed to the knee. The saphenous flap can also be based on a reverse flow based on collateral vessels around the knee that can communicate with the terminal branches of the saphenous artery. The skin island for the reverse flap is usually located higher than for the standard flap. The saphenous vein and artery are identified and divided at the proximal flap border. This modification covers upper portions of the leg and is useful for amputation stump coverage. Although the saphenous vein flap can be used for more proximal coverage, it should not be the first choice, as a relatively high complication rate can be expected.

Early reports of the unipedicled venous flaps postulated a to-and-fro flow pattern in the vein, seemingly supported by experimental and mathematical models. The survival of unipedicled type I venous flaps has now been attributed to either a perivenous or perineural capillary network. The large venous flap is a modification of the saphenous artery flap in which the entire skin island is elevated to include the saphenous vein. The skin island is centered over the course of the saphenous vein in the inferior medial thigh. The saphenous vein is identified at the distal flap border and divided. The flap is then elevated and transposed, including the saphenous vein. The distal vein may be anastomosed to a suitable receptor artery if an arterialized venous flap is planned. The donor site has been reported to cause problems occasionally, including sensory disturbance of the medial leg and the stretched donor scar around the joint. Sacrifice of the saphenous nerve leads to a bothersome area of anesthesia at the anteromedial leg. Therefore, when not required, attempt to safely dissect the nerve from the saphenous artery. Otherwise, the saphenous flap is very useful because it has a dependable vascular supply, is a one-step procedure, and can be performed with the patient in the supine position.

Sural Artery Fasciocutaneous Flap

The sural artery fasciocutaneous flap offers several distinct advantages over the gastrocnemius muscle flap. It has a longer arc of rotation than the gastrocnemius and is capable of resurfacing defects proximal to the patella. This flap is located between the popliteal fossa and the midportion of the leg, centered over the midline raphe between the medial and lateral heads of the gastrocnemius muscle. The sural artery fasciocutaneous flap can be used as a pedicled island or free flap. Dissection of this flap is simple, takes minutes, the flap is pliable, and it can be innervated. The flap covers large defects and reaches defects in the popliteal fossa and upper one-third of the leg. Tissue expansion has been described to further increase the flap dimension prior to flap elevation, but the authors do not recommend this.

The vascular pedicle is based upon the descending cutaneous branches of the popliteal artery. The dominant pedicle, either the medial or a lateral superficial sural artery with its venae comitantes, is located in the popliteal fossa entering the deep fascia between the medial and lateral heads of the gastrocnemius muscle. The pedicle generally courses slightly lateral to the posterior midline over the lateral gastrocnemius muscle. The venous drainage typically consists of paired venae comitantes emptying into the popliteal or sural veins. The flap is innervated in the superior calf by the posterior cutaneous nerve of the thigh and in the middle and inferior calf by the posterior branch of the medial cutaneous nerve of the thigh and the lateral sural cutaneous branch of the common peroneal nerve. Preoperatively, the superficial sural artery is first detected with a Doppler. The flap is designed in the calf and includes a line representing the course of the superficial sural artery either in the center or in the lateral part of the calf. Medially and laterally, the midaxial lines serve as the anterior limits. After marking the flap boundaries according to the above guidelines, elevate the flap distally with an incision through the skin, subcutaneous tissues, and deep fascia. The flap is elevated in the subfascial plane to avoid damaging the vessels. When incising both sides and exposing the pedicle, take care to prevent injury to the common peroneal nerve and the pedicle of the flap, preserving both medial and lateral superficial sural arteries until both are observed. Furthermore, both fasciocutaneous vessels may unite before their junction with the popliteal artery and vein. Once clearly defined, the larger vessel is included in the midaxis of the flap. Proximal superficial draining veins are also preserved to enhance venous drainage. Deep to the fascia, the distal lesser saphenous vein is identified, divided, and included with the flap. The sural nerve, which runs in close proximity to the arterial supply, is also transected distally and included. Myocutaneous perforators are carefully ligated only as needed as ligating all of them could potentially harm venous occlusion. If venous congestion, which is uniformly noted after initial flap elevation, is irreversible or the venae comitantes prove to be exceedingly small, then a subcutaneous vein should be included with the flap proximally to serve as an additional source of venous outflow. Typically the flap can be transposed as an island flap, pivoted on the pedicle point located at the popliteal fossa. Primary closure of the donor site is possible with a flap having a width of 6 cm or less, but larger flaps usually require skin grafting.

Popliteal-Based Posterior Thigh Fasciocutaneous Flap

Several fasciocutaneous flaps have been described involving the lower posterior and lateral thigh and deriving inflow from branches arising from the knee region. The popliteal–posterior thigh fasciocutaneous island flap covers the knee and reaches to the upper and middle thirds of the calf. A direct ascending branch of the popliteal artery arising 7 to 11 cm above the knee supplies the popliteal–posterior thigh fasciocutaneous flap. The vessel emerges between the semimembranosus muscle and biceps femoris muscles at the level of the popliteal fossa. The posterior femoral nerve can potentially provide sensation to the flap. The flap is designed using Doppler ultrasound and may include the vessel origin inferiorly and can extend superiorly to the gluteal crease. Laterally, it lies over the hamstring musculature. The incision is carried down through the subcutaneous tissue and deep fascia of the thigh. The distal incision is made, and the distal end of the flap is gently turned upward. The intermuscular septum between the hamstring muscles is divided between the muscles. The fascial septum is included to augment the circulation, but do not rely on the fasciocutaneous branches along the fascial septum. Local rotation on its vascular pedicle has allowed coverage about the knee. A defect up to 10 cm can be closed primarily.

Superior Lateral Genicular Artery Fasciocutaneous Flap

The superior lateral genicular artery (SLGA) fasciocutaneous flap is an excellent choice for flap reconstruction of defects around the knee.[66] It provides excellent contour of the recipient site. The SLGA flap is supplied by the SLGA, a branch of the popliteal artery or the sural artery located approximately 4 cm above the knee. The point at which the cutaneous perforator of the SLGA penetrates the deep fascia ranges from 3 to 8 cm from the knee joint. The cutaneous perforator is typically located in the triangle framed by the superior margin of the lateral femoral condyle, the posterior margin of the vastus lateralis, and the anterior margin of the short head of the biceps femoris. The cutaneous perforators of the SLGA anastomose with multiple local vessels: the rete patellae, the lateral perforator of the profunda femoris artery, the musculocutaneous perforators from the popliteal artery, and the musculocutaneous or septocutaneous perforators from the descending branch of the lateral circumflex femoral artery. The flap is designed on the lateral aspect of the lower thigh and includes the triangle containing the vascular pedicle formed by the vastus lateralis anteriorly, the biceps femoris posteriorly, and the lateral femoral condyle inferiorly. The proximal end of the flap can be extended safely to the midpoint between the greater trochanter and the lateral condyle of the femur. The incision extends from the proximal apex of the flap, in the loose areolar layer over the deep fascia distal to the point 10 cm above the knee joint, and the dissection should be carried down to the iliotibial tract for the safe dissection of the intermuscular septum between the vastus lateralis and the short head of the biceps femoris. Dividing the vastus lateralis and the short head of the biceps femoris, the vascular pedicle can be identified just above the lateral condyle of the femur. The islanded lateral genicular artery flap is then elevated and transferred to the defect. The rotation arc of the flap reaches the distal one-third of the thigh, the knee, and the popliteal fossa and the proximal one-third of the lower leg, with the exception of the medial aspects of these regions. A 10-cm-wide donor defect can be closed primarily. Otherwise, a skin graft is applied to the donor site.

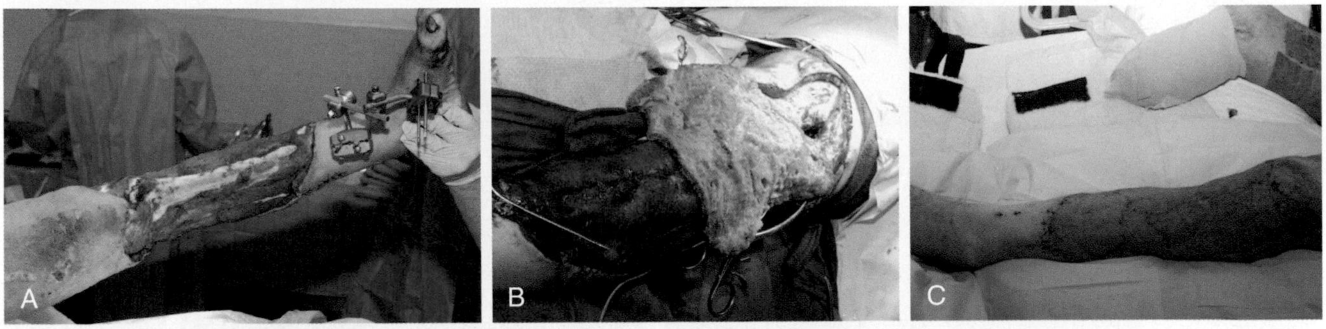

Figure 18-11. Latissimus dorsi muscle free flap. **A,** Large soft tissue defect over exposed tibia. **B,** Latissimus dorsi muscle free flap coverage. **C,** Defect after split-thickness skin grafting.

Middle Third of the Leg

Soleus Flap

Typically, the medial or lateral head of the gastrocnemius are inadequate options for reconstruction of these defects. The best choice remains the proximally based soleus flap. It is a type II muscle flap; the posterior tibial artery, the dominant pedicle, enters the muscle proximally, with multiple additional segmental perforators from the posterior tibial and peroneal artery. Either half of the muscle can be transferred individually. Potential donor site morbidity should be considered, as the soleus muscle is an important participant in the venous pump, posture stabilization, and gait, with potential impact on these functions. Although distally based soleus flaps are described, success rates are variable. Free flap reconstruction is usually recommended in these cases. In situations wherein the soleus flap is not available, or the defect is large and extends onto the lower third of the leg, free flap transfer using a variety of options including radial forearm, lateral arm, rectus abdominis, and parascapular flaps are robust choices (Fig. 18-11).

Lower Third of the Leg and Ankle

Defects in this region are challenging because of several factors: nonavailability of local tissue, presence of vital structures in close proximity, and an inherent lack of thick muscular soft tissue cover. Lower third defects on the leg wounds are best reconstructed with microvascular free-tissue transfer. Distally based pedicled muscle flaps are largely ineffective.

The choice of which free flap to use depends on the requirement of the defect. Small defects can be reconstructed using a variety of options including radial forearm and lateral arm flaps. Larger defects requiring a deeper volume restoration caused by missing bone cortex or large cavities caused by resected soft tissue may need a bulky muscle flap, such as a rectus abdominis flap. Defects that are larger in the surface area but not deep are best reconstructed using a latissimus dorsi muscle flap, anterolateral thigh flaps, or parascapular flaps, all providing well-vascularized coverage.

Propeller Flaps

Propeller flaps allow the coverage of wide defects for a large number of indications including trauma, diabetes, and even patients with vascular disease, and can be raised with a relatively simple surgical technique, have a high success rate, and good cosmetic results without functional impairment.[67-70] There is a significant shift toward the use of these flaps in terms of the strategy for lower extremity reconstruction.[71,72] In the light of this, they can be considered among the first surgical choices to resurface complex soft tissue defects of the leg.[73] After the introduction of the perforator-based flap concept, new flaps have also been described for the leg. An evolution and simplification of the perforator flap concept, together with the "freestyle" flap harvesting method, are the propeller flaps, that is, local flaps, based on a perforator vessel, which becomes the pivot point for the skin island that can, therefore, be rotated up to 180 degrees.[74] The blood supply of the distal lower leg and foot is ensured by the contribution of the peroneal artery (PA), anterior tibial artery (ATA), and posterior tibial artery (PTA) through their musculocutaneous (MC) and septocutaneous (SC) perforators. This vascular supply occupies three vascular territories organized as a series of longitudinal rows within the intermuscular septa of the lower leg. The most distally located perforators and especially those emerging from the PA approximately 5 cm above the lateral malleolus and from the PTA approximately 5 cm above the medial malleolus represent a very good vascular source for perforator flaps.[75] Critics argue that the freestyle dissection has its price in terms of a larger proportion of flap loss unless the perforating vessels are well defined.[76] However, when used appropriately, propeller flaps present an ever-expanding array of reconstructive choices in difficult cases.

Reverse Sural Artery Flap

The distally based sural artery fasciocutaneous flap has been effectively used to resurface distal leg and ankle defects, and is useful for the treatment of severe and complex injuries and their complications in diabetic and nondiabetic lower limbs.[77,78] The technique is based on the use of a reverse-flow sural artery, creating an island fasciocutaneous flap used alone or combined with other flaps, such as the cross-leg flap, the peroneal fasciocutaneous flap, or the gastrocnemius muscle flap. The fasciocutaneous flap constitutes the sural artery pedicle, the superficial and deep fascia, the sural nerve, the lesser saphenous vein and skin.

Operative details include the following essential steps:

1. Identify perforators in a line that runs along the vertical axis and is in the midspace between the lateral border of the Achilles tendon and the lateral malleolus. Typically, they are between 5 and 8 cm above the malleolus. These perforators are then incorporated in a subcutaneous fascial pedicle with a width of 2 to 3 cm and must include the sural vessels.

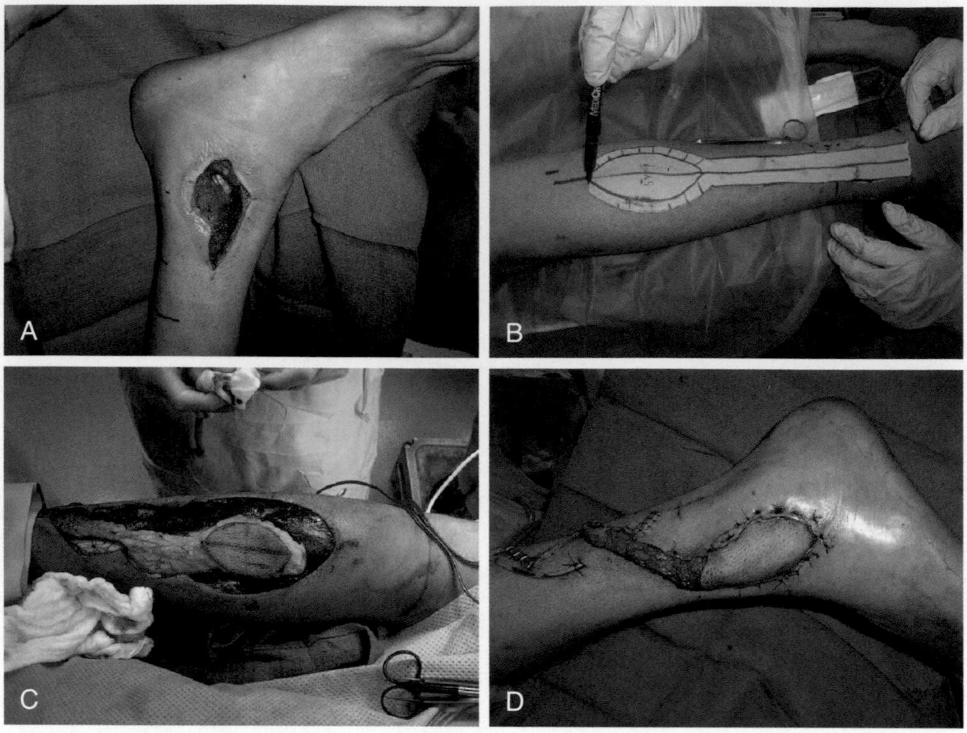

Figure 18-12. Reverse sural artery flap. **A,** Soft tissue defect over the lateral ankle. **B,** Template for design of reverse sural artery flap. **C,** Reverse sural artery flap harvest. **D,** Flap inset.

2. The skin paddle is outlined at the junction of two heads of gastrocnemius and includes the sural nerve and lesser saphenous vein.
3. The pivotal point of the pedicle is 5 to 8 cm proximal to the tip of lateral malleolus.
4. The fascial layer overlying the muscle is included in the pedicle, and after careful dissection, the flap is ready for inset.
5. The inset requires that the flap be rotated without compromise of the pedicle. Most often, this requires an incision over the interposing skin between the donor site and recipient rather than tunneling through, which may kink or compress the pedicle.[79]

The donor site can be closed primarily if it is less than 4 cm in width, but typically wider defects need a skin graft.

The reverse sural artery flap has several technical advantages. The dissection is easy, while preserving important vascular structures in the limb, and complete coverage of the soft tissue defect can be made in just one operation without the need for microsurgical anastomosis.[80] It is not uncommon to encounter venous congestion with this flap. "Supercharging" the venous outflow of the flap by preserving the lesser saphenous vein may prevent venous congestion, as can consideration for delaying transposition of the flap if this is encountered. In many instances, it has obviated the need for free tissue transfer. The distally based superficial sural artery flap is a versatile, reliable procedure, useful in reconstruction of lower third of the leg, heel, malleoli, and hind-foot defects (Fig. 18-12).

The Foot

Distally Based Sural Artery Flap

As discussed in the preceding section, this fasciocutaneous flap provides excellent coverage for heel and proximal plantar foot defects. Its reach is somewhat limited by the location of the pedicle, which is a pivot point beyond which this flap cannot be dissected[81] (Table 18-5).

Dorsalis Pedis Flap

The dorsalis pedis flap has been used successfully for many years as both a pedicled transfer for local foot reconstruction and as a free microvascular transfer.[82] Proponents cite the reliable vascular pedicle, flap versatility, and ease of harvest, and it is a thin flap.[83] Flap length may reach 8 to 10 cm in an

TABLE 18-5 *SOFT TISSUE COVERAGE OF THE FOOT: A CLASSIFICATION BASED ON DEFECT SITE, SIZE, AND EXTENT*

Size	Extension	Site	Type of Flap
<3 cm^2	Soft tissue	Weight-bearing areas	Local flap
<3 cm^2	Soft tissue	Non–weight-bearing areas	Skin grafts
>3 cm^2	Soft tissue	Weight-bearing areas	Free flap (free fasciocutaneous, musculocutaneous flaps, muscle free flap plus skin graft)
>3 cm^2	Soft tissue and bone loss	Weight-bearing areas	Free osteocutaneous flap

average-size individual, and including the first web provides additional length. Although significant donor site morbidities (including graft loss, exposure of tendons and vessels, and an overall long-term failure of the graft caused by two main reasons: friction breakdown of the thin graft with footwear and lack of sensation on the graft that further exacerbates the breakdown) have been recognized, it is a useful flap when no other choices are available.

The dorsalis pedis artery courses plantar at the level of the base of the first and second metatarsals. The first dorsal metatarsal artery originates from the dorsalis pedis at this level. Using the skin over the first and second metatarsals requires the presence of a first dorsal-metatarsal artery, which can be confirmed by Doppler ultrasound or arteriogram. The donor site skin on the foot requires a skin graft and postoperative elevation of the foot. Use of a dermal substitute can make the area of skin grafting more durable for shoe wear. The dissection, although quite simple, has two risks. First, if the surgeon is not careful, the fasciocutaneous skin paddle can be separated from the vascular pedicle. Second, the connective tissue overlying the extensor tendons can be quite flimsy, leading to exposure of the bare tendons on the dorsum of the foot affecting subsequent skin graft take and contributing to concerns for donor site morbidity.[84] A dermal substitute may be required in these cases prior to skin grafting.

Medial Plantar Flap

Full-thickness defects on the plantar surface of the foot present a challenge for the reconstructive surgeon. Skin grafts and a variety of flap procedures have been described to resurface this site, but not all achieve a return to normal foot function. The skin and fascia over the medial aspect of the foot is thin, providing glabrous tissue for reconstruction of a variety of small soft tissue defects. This skin can be raised as a V-Y flap as well.[85] Perforators from the medial plantar branch of the PTA supply the skin. The venous system is quite thin and small, and the subcutaneous system is easily incorporated into the flap and used for venous drainage. The flap length varies by defect size, with the width allowing primary closure at most at 2 cm. If a wider flap is necessary, the defect must be skin grafted. The medial plantar flap is capable of providing durable, sensate coverage of plantar hind-foot defects with minimal donor-site morbidity.[86] The flap is raised starting at the plantar aspect first, dissecting toward the dorsal aspect of the foot while deep to the muscular fascia over the flexor hallucis brevis muscle. Dissection proceeds distally to reach the dorsum of the foot wherein the perforator emerges between the heads of the flexor hallucis brevis and abductor hallucis muscles. A cutaneous nerve branch from the posterior tibial system can be incorporated. Furthermore, that sensation remains identical to that of the instep donor site and superior to that of the normal heel pad.

Free Flap

Again, the selection of the type of free flap is dictated by the needs of the defect. In the foot, it is important to take into consideration that the microanastomosis needs to be performed well beyond the "zone of injury." Specifically, this means that the recipient vessels must be in a relatively unaffected portion of the leg. Sometimes, depending on the current injury, or preexisting trauma or comorbidities, it may be necessary to dissect out the vessels proximally and hence mandate the free flap to have a longer vascular pedicle rather than a short leash. This may require a vein graft to extend the pedicle, or use of vascular loop.[87,88]

Many of the flaps described previously may be used for coverage defects of the foot.

Finally, performing a duplex ultrasound examination is needed in situations wherein a deep venous thrombosis is suspected. High venous pressures in the recipient veins can seriously impact free flap viability and may hasten its failure by venous compromise.[89]

REHABILITATION AND OUTCOMES

The ultimate goal of soft tissue reconstruction is to facilitate a near-complete functional recovery while optimizing the aesthetic result. Early rehabilitation with a multidisciplinary approach achieves the best outcome. It is important to be cognizant of this goal at all times, from the beginning of the strategic planning to the postoperative recovery phase wherein delay could significantly hamper the long-term results. As important is consideration of cases that may require further reconstructive procedures. In this regard, soft tissue coverage options with durable fasciocutaneous or adipofascial flaps with durable skin grafts are more amenable to flap revisions and gaining access for additional limb reconstruction. In this situation, a team approach with an agreed-on reconstructive plan will facilitate the best outcomes.

Outcome Studies

Evidence-based outcome studies of soft tissue reconstruction of upper extremity defects are scarce, partly because of the heterogeneity of the defects and a lack of comprehensive approaches to this problem. Future directions must include a strategy that can objectively assess outcomes in a multi-institutional setting to understand more fully the scope and range of options that will allow a full functional recovery following what remains a tough clinical challenge.

KEY REFERENCES

The level of evidence (LOE) is determined according to the criteria provided in the preface.

1. Wolf JM, Athwal GS, Shin AY, et al: Acute trauma to the upper extremity: what to do and when to do it. *Instr Course Lect* 59:525–538, 2010. LOE V
4. Bumbasirevic M, Stevanovic M, Lesic A, et al: Current management of the mangled upper extremity. *Int Orthop* 36(11):2189–2195, 2012. LOE V
7. Godina M: Early microsurgical reconstruction of complex trauma of the extremities. *Plast Reconstr Surg* 78(3):285–292, 1986. LOE IV
8. Liu DS, Sofiadellis F, Ashton M, et al: Early soft tissue coverage and negative pressure wound therapy optimizes patient outcomes in lower limb trauma. *Injury* 43:772–778, 2012. LOE V
10. Attinger CE, Janis JE, Steinberg J, et al; Clinical Approach to Wounds: Debridement and Wound Bed Preparation Including the Use of Dressings and Wound-Healing Adjuvants. *Plast Reconstr Surg* 117(Suppl):72S–109S, 2006. LOE V
22. Bogdan MA, Klein MB, Rubin GD, et al: CT angiography in complex upper extremity reconstruction. *J Hand Surg [Br]* 29(5):465–469, 2004. LOE V
26. Cerkes N, Erer M, Sirin F: The combined scapular/parascapular flap for the treatment of extensive electrical burns of the upper extremity. *Br J Plast Surg* 50(7):501–506, 1997. LOE V
29. Elhassan B, Karabekmez F, Hsu CC, et al: Outcome of local anconeus flap transfer to cover soft tissue defects over the posterior aspect of the elbow. *J Shoulder Elbow Surg* 20(5):807–812, 2011. LOE V

31. Yildirim S, Taylan G, Eker G, et al: Free flap choice for soft tissue reconstruction of the severely damaged upper extremity. *J Reconstr Microsurg* 22(8):599–609, 2006. LOE V
32. Gideroglu K, Cakici H, Yildirim S, et al: Functional reconstruction in large and complex soft tissue defects of forearm and hand with multifunctional anterolateral thigh flap. *Eklem Hastalik Cerrahisi* 20(3):149–155, 2009. LOE V
34. Yokota K, Sunagawa T, Suzuki O, et al: Short interposed pedicle of flow-through anterolateral thigh flap for reliable reconstruction of damaged upper extremity. *J Reconstr Microsurg* 27(2):109–114, 2011. LOE V
43. Dap F, Dantel G, Voche P, et al: The posterior interosseous flap in primary repair of hand injuries. *J Hand Surg* 18(4):437–445, 1993. LOE V
48. Foucher G, Braun JB: A new island flap transfer from the dorsum of the index to the thumb. *Plast Reconstr Surg* 63:344–349, 1979. LOE V
49. Germann G, Levin LS: Intrinsic flaps in the hand: new concepts of skin coverage. *Tech Hand Up Extrem Surg* 1(1):48–61, 1997. LOE V
50. Sherif MM: First dorsal metacarpal artery flap in hand reconstruction. I. Anatomical study. *J Hand Surg* 19A:26–38, 1994. LOE V
51. Sherif MM: First dorsal metacarpal artery flap in hand reconstruction. II. Clinical application. *J Hand Surg* 19(1):32–38, 1994. LOE V

The complete References list is available online at https://expertconsult.inkling.com.

Chapter 19

Gunshot Wounds and Blast Injuries

GREGORY A. ZYCH • STEVEN P. KALANDIAK • PATRICK W. OWENS • ROBERT BLEASE

INTRODUCTION

Although violent crime continues to decline, approximately 74,000 nonfatal gunshot injuries were reported to the Centers for Disease Control (CDC) in the United States in 2011, an increase of 10,000 compared to 2004. Estimates of total cost of injury indicate that firearm and gunshot injuries account for 9% or 41.4 billion dollars per year.[1] An unknown but substantial number involved the musculoskeletal system. Gunshot fractures are most common in urban areas and theaters of war but may be encountered in almost any region. In one retrospective study by Bartkiw and colleagues, 44% of all gunshot injuries treated at their urban trauma center involved fractures.[2] The orthopaedic surgeon should therefore have a working knowledge of the various types of gunshot injuries and their treatment.

BALLISTICS

The purpose of a firearm projectile is to crush tissue. Secondary effects are laceration of structures and tissue stretching. When a projectile strikes the body, a permanent cavity, which is variable in size, is created in the tissues. This cavity is particular to the projectile type and represents the amount of crushed tissue. Some tissue, peripheral to the permanent cavity, will undergo elastic deformation (stretching) and is termed the *temporary cavity*. The amount of tissue damage is mainly related to the projectile velocity, projectile mass, tissue density, and projectile design.

The kinetic energy (KE) of a projectile is defined by $KE = 1/2mv^2$. This equation shows that, in general, the velocity is more important than the mass since doubling the velocity quadruples the kinetic energy while doubling the mass only yields twice the kinetic energy. Bullets have been classified, based on muzzle velocity, into low velocity (<2000 fps) and high velocity (>2000 fps). Much of the previous literature focused on the velocity of the bullet as the most important determinant of tissue damage, but this factor is only one of several that must be considered. What appears to be more important is the degree of kinetic energy transmitted to the body tissues.[3] The human body has many differing tissue densities. Low-density tissues include lung, fat, and muscle and are not so easily damaged by a projectile as the denser tissues of bone and solid organs.

High-velocity bullets may pass through certain low-density tissues such as lung or muscle with minimal damage owing to minimal transfer of the kinetic energy. A low-velocity bullet can produce considerable tissue injury if the majority of the kinetic energy is transmitted to the tissues.

The mass of the projectile also bears importance. An average 9-mm handgun may have a bullet weighing 150 grains; a 0.44 Magnum revolver, 230 grains; and a shotgun load as much as 650 grains. A large increase in mass yields substantially greater kinetic energy and the probability of greater tissue crush.

Design of projectiles has a profound effect on wounding potential. Bullets that deform on impact present a greater cross-sectional area capable of crushing more tissues. This is also true of bullets that fragment, resulting in many secondary "bullets" that scatter throughout the tissues, each creating its own path of destruction. Some bullets will oscillate or yaw before or after encountering the body, increasing the cross-sectional area of tissue contact and leading to more tissue crushing.

Low-velocity handguns cause most civilian gunshot wounds, with minimal soft tissue damage, and these are the most common that the orthopaedic surgeon will encounter. Direct hits onto bone may cause impressive comminution owing to the relatively high density of bone and its physical property of brittleness. The diaphysis is more prone to comminution than the metaphysis. Some types of higher power handguns, such as the 0.357 and 0.44 Magnum revolvers, have more destructive potential from larger bullet size and more propellant load.

Assault and hunting rifles with higher muzzle velocities and expanding or fragmenting bullets are designed to produce severe internal tissue damage with nearly complete retention of all bullet fragments, a measure of killing potential.

Shotguns can fire loads of either multiple small pellets or single large slugs. The muzzle velocity is classified as low (1200 fps), but the destructive power arises from the multiple or large and heavy projectiles that are used. Shotgun loads vary tremendously, but in general, the most tissue destruction occurs within a short barrel-to-target distance. At greater distances, the pellets spread out, and tissue damage will be minimized.

Close-range shotgun injuries have extensive wounds. The design of most shot shells incorporates some type of wadding between the lead load and the propellant. This wadding can be either plastic or fiber and will follow the pellets into the tissues. As part of the débridement process, the surgeon should explore for the retained wadding, since this material can become a focus of infection.

DIAGNOSIS

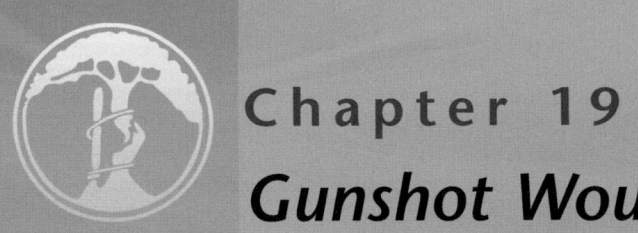

The history of a gunshot injury may yield important clues that will assist in diagnosis and treatment. If possible, the type of weapon, number of rounds, and distance from the weapon to the victim should be elicited from the patient, first responders, or law enforcement officers. High- or intermediate-velocity or shotgun weapons may lead to more tissue injury, but this is not absolutely certain. Most handgun injuries occur within a few feet so the wounding potential of even small-caliber handguns can be significant.

Standard Advanced Trauma Life Support (ATLS) protocol should be followed for the initial physical examination and the treatment. Some special aspects of the physical examination in patients with gunshot wounds should be amplified. The skin should be searched for wounds of entrance and exit, and their location, size, and appearance documented. More than two wounds suggest multiple gunshots. An attempt should be made to match each entrance wound with its corresponding exit wound. Occasionally, bone fragments may be seen within the wound if the gunshot caused a comminuted fracture in a subcutaneous location. Pulsatile bleeding may be an early indication of a major vascular injury.

The gunshot pathway through the patient's body should be determined. All structures that could be violated require close evaluation. Detailed neurologic and vascular examination will detect any deficits. In the absence of obvious fracture, the extremities should be put through a full range of motion. Extremity joints that have been penetrated by the gunshot will typically be painful with an effusion.

After the initial physical examination is completed, the skin wounds should be sterilely dressed. The time-honored technique of securely placing a metallic marker (paper clip, coin) on the dressing surface can be helpful in determining the relationship of the skin wounds to the underlying anatomic structures on subsequent imaging studies (Fig. 19-1).

Immobilization via splinting or skeletal traction of all fractures is the next priority.

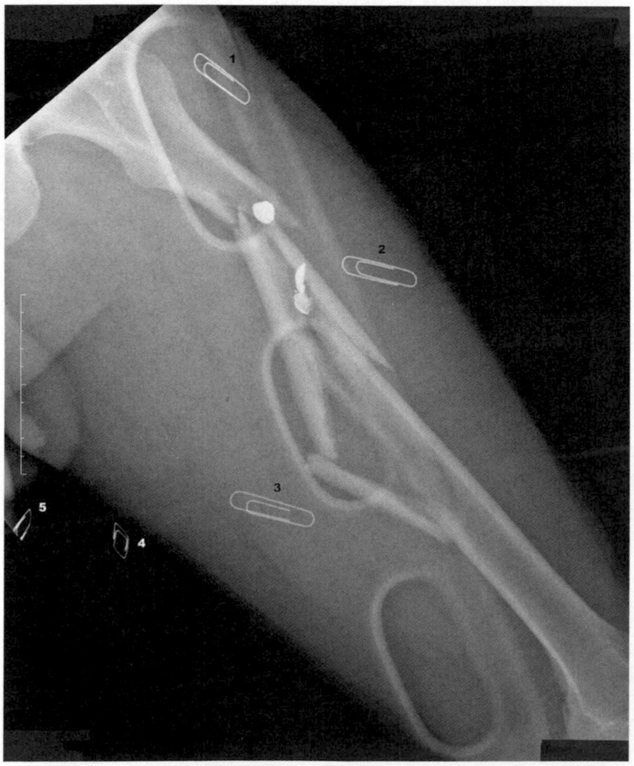

Figure 19-1. Anteroposterior femoral radiograph in a patient with multiple gunshots to the thigh. Each paper clip, five in total, denotes an entrance or exit wound.

Plain extremity radiographs, two views at right angles, including the joints above and below, are obtained for all possible involved regions or extremities. Special radiographic views can be taken as needed to assess the pelvis or spine. The imaging studies are scrutinized for the location and number of all metallic gunshot fragments. Certain gunshots will leave an obvious trail of lead particles as they pass through the body tissues. In cases with only an entrance wound, there must be a retained gunshot fragment somewhere in the body. A gunshot fragment that is within the anatomic confines of a joint capsule on the two plain radiographs (perpendicular to each other) must be assumed to be intraarticular. In trauma situations, whole-body multidetector computed tomography (CT) scans will often be done and have been shown to be quite reliable in locating metallic fragments, although less effective at visualizing the path of the gunshot wound.[4] Arthrocentesis and aspiration may reveal occult joint violation in suspicious cases. Standard musculoskeletal imaging studies should be done on the basis of the joint injury or fracture, regardless of the gunshot mechanism.

GENERAL TREATMENT PRINCIPLES

Antibiotic Usage

As early as 1892, Lagarde[5] demonstrated that bullets were not sterile, neither before nor after being fired from a gun. Recently, Vennemann, Grosse Perdekamp, and Kneubuehl[6] have shown that skin particles and the subsequent bacteria adhering to them from the entrance and exit wounds can be found in the bullet tracks within the body. Therefore, it is reasonable to believe that gunshot wounds are contaminated with bacteria and if associated with a fracture, then the fracture should be classified as open. However, the majority of civilian gunshot wounds are small in size with limited tissue damage and would fit the criteria for a type I open fracture according to the classification of Gustilo and Anderson.

Howland and Ritchey[7] studied nonsurgical management and antibiotic prophylaxis in patients with stable low-velocity gunshot fractures, and they concluded that it was not necessary to surgically débride the wounds or administer antibiotics. However, they did stress the importance of distinguishing between civilian and military gunshot fractures.

Dickey and associates[8] treated 73 patients with gunshot fractures that did not require surgical repair and were randomized prospectively into two groups: intravenous antibiotics and no antibiotics. Two infections occurred, one in each group. They concluded that intravenous antibiotic prophylaxis was of no significant benefit.

Knapp[9] reported a series of 190 patients with 222 extraarticular long bone gunshot fractures that did not require operative fixation. They were randomized to both intravenous cephapirin and gentamicin for 72 hours or oral ciprofloxacin for 72 hours. Each group had two infections (2% for each), and it was concluded that these injuries could be treated with oral antibiotics.

Therefore, it appears that the evidence for antibiotic prophylaxis of low-caliber (velocity) gunshot fractures not requiring surgical fixation is weak. Nevertheless, in the urban penetrating trauma population, a brief period, 24 to 48 hours, of antibiotics is often used. This protocol has been thought to

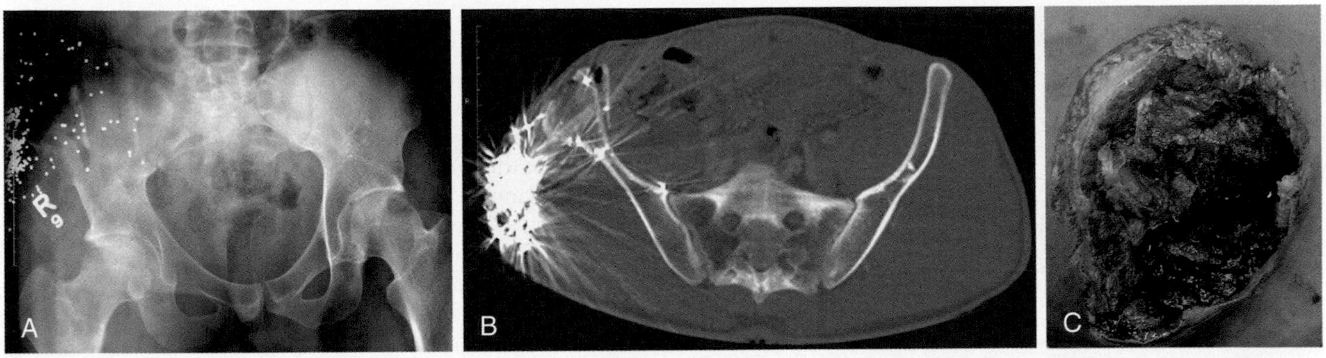

Figure 19-2. Close-range shotgun injury to iliac region **A,** Radiograph shows large amount of metallic pellets around the right ilium. **B,** Computed tomography (CT) scan demonstrates a comminuted iliac fracture and shotgun pellets. **C,** Clinical photograph of the extensive wound with massive soft tissue loss.

be efficacious to treat the wound contamination characteristic of these injuries in these often nutritionally and medically compromised patients. Patients who require surgical fracture fixation should receive standard perioperative antibiotic prophylaxis according to the surgeon's discretion. Shotgun and high-velocity gunshot fractures benefit from intravenous antibiotic treatment for 24 to 48 hours and, in most situations, surgical débridement.

Wound Assessment

One problem facing the surgeon is the assessment of the character of the gunshot injury. The presence of a large wound is an obvious indicator of tissue damage. However, the skin wounds can be deceptive, with many significant injuries presenting with small entrance and exit wounds. In these cases, it is the intercalary tissue appearance and integrity that needs close scrutiny.

Extensive ecchymosis and severe local swelling are potential indications of the need to surgically explore a gunshot wound. Recent authors have stressed the importance of "treating the wound" and not treating the history of the wound mechanism. That is to say, gunshot velocity is only one factor in the decision for surgical exploration.

Some "low-velocity" gunshot tibial fractures can have extensive bone comminution with fracture fragments having been rendered avascular since most of the energy was transmitted to the bone. These fractures do require débridement and excision of nonviable fragments. Reconstruction of the skeleton may become necessary due to residual segmental defects.

Close-range shotgun injuries require thorough débridement and exploration for the retained wadding, which must be removed. Generally, it is futile to attempt removal of all retained pellets, since normal tissue will be violated in the process. Devitalized bone fragments are best excised unless they are intraarticular and possibly suitable for internal fixation (Fig. 19-2). Longer distance shotgun wounds have multiple pellet entrance wounds without exit wounds. Pellet removal is indicated only if proven to be intraarticular.

High-power handguns, machine pistols, and assault rifles constitute the other end of the spectrum seen in civilian trauma. Some of the wounds associated with these weapons have a completely benign appearance. Large exit wounds are pathognomonic of severe soft tissue crush and laceration and are generally good indications for wound exploration and débridement (Fig. 19-3).

Krebsbach and colleagues demonstrated in a gelatin extremity surrogate model that higher velocity projectiles tend to have greater bacterial contamination deeper into the projectile track and closer to the exit wound.[10] This lends support for thorough exploration and débridement of the entire ballistic wound. Diaphyseal comminution is not uncommon, and judgment must be used if this is the only apparent criterion for exploration.

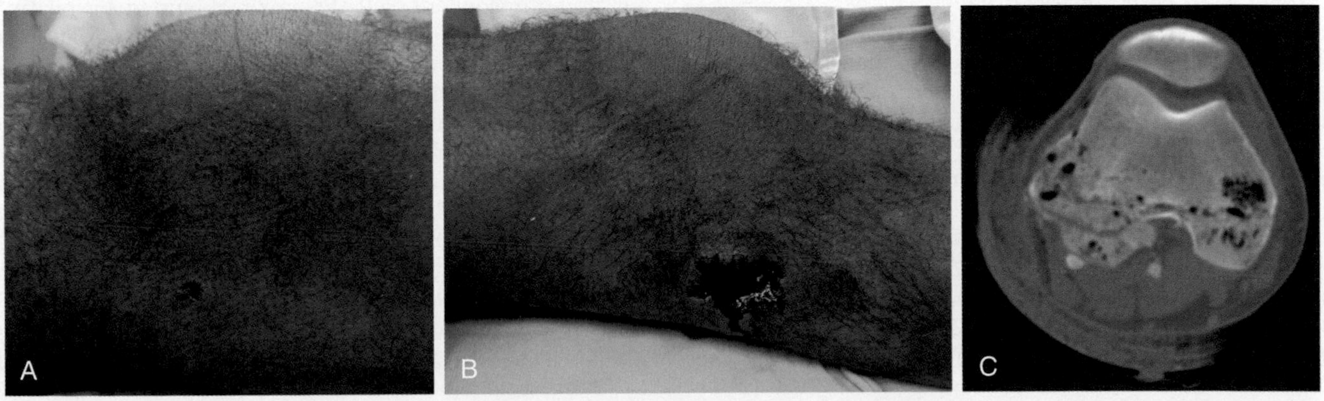

Figure 19-3. Gunshot injury to knee. **A,** Entrance wound laterally less than 1 cm in diameter. **B,** Medial exit wound much larger suggestive of higher energy injury. **C,** Computed tomography (CT) scan demonstrates the bullet pathway, fracture comminution, and soft tissue injury.

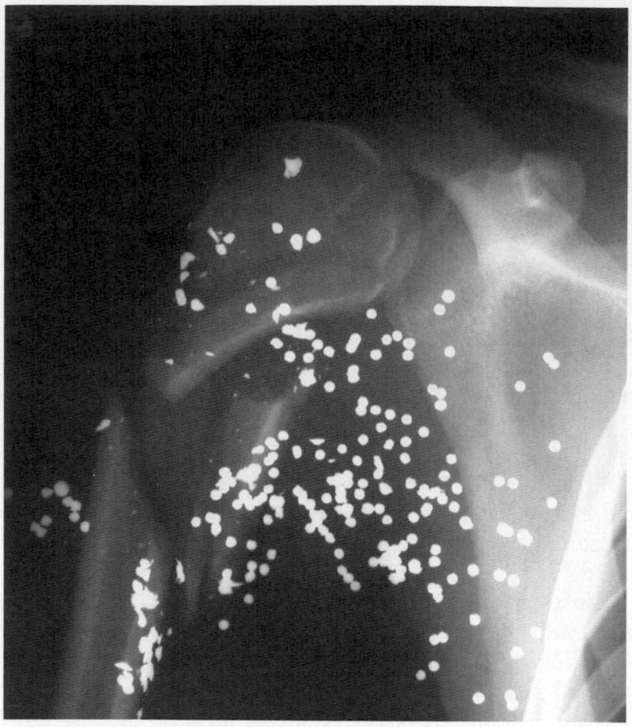

Figure 19-4. Shotgun blast to shoulder.

UPPER EXTREMITY

Proximal Humerus and Shoulder Joint

Vessel and Nerve Injury

When vascular injury near the shoulder is present, it is often accompanied by nerve injury. Hardin and associates[11] reviewed 99 low-velocity, upper extremity vascular injuries. Eleven (52%) of the 21 patients with axillary artery lesions and 27 (63%) of the 43 limbs with brachial arterial injuries had concomitant nerve injury. At final follow-up, only one patient (9%) had complete return of function. Shotgun injuries produced the most extensive tissue destruction (Fig. 19-4), almost always resulting in permanent functional impairment and often resulting in amputation of all or part of a limb. Borman and coworkers[12] reported numerous successful arterial reconstructions but permanent and severe limitation of function when accompanying nerve or plexus injury was present.

There is no clear consensus about whether and when to explore brachial plexus injuries after a gunshot. Armine and Sugar[13] recommended primary repair of the brachial plexus when there is an associated vascular injury requiring exploration and repair. However, if no vascular or pulmonary injury is present, Leffert[14] recommended that initial management be conservative, with wound and fracture care and physical therapy as needed.

In a study of patients with brachial plexus injury during World War II, Brooks[15] found only 4 of 25 who underwent surgical exploration for plexus lesions to have divided nerves. In an effort to relate the prognosis to the location of the nerve lesion, Brooks suggested three groups: (1) lesions of the roots and trunk of C5 and C6, (2) lesions of the posterior cord, and (3) lesions of C8 to T1 of the medial cord. The recovery in the first group was good; in the second, fair; and in the third, poor. Recovery in the small muscles of the hand did not occur if severance of the nerves occurred. Brooks, therefore, concluded that routine exploration of open wounds of the plexus was rarely indicated.

When managing nerve injuries nonoperatively, we have found that the most useful clinical indication of axonal regeneration in nerve injuries is evidence of an advancing Tinel sign. Percussion over the site of the nerve injury produces the sensation of radiating "electrical shocks" because of stimulation of the free nerve endings. If there is no recovery by 3 months, if the lesion is incomplete with a major area of neurologic deficit, or if a Tinel sign fails to advance for three consecutive monthly examinations, the nerve should be considered for exploration.

When exploration is performed, nerves found transected may be either repaired primarily or grafted. If a neuroma in continuity is found, either it may be resected and repaired or neurolysis may be performed. Whatever the finding at exploration, the outlook for a high nerve injury that fails to recover spontaneously is often poor, and tendon transfers may be an appropriate treatment.

Fracture

Low-energy gunshot injuries are treated with local wound care and intravenous or oral antibiotics. Formal irrigation and débridement are unnecessary; the surgeon should choose nonoperative or operative treatment as if the injury were closed. If surgery is selected, the bullet track remains unexplored unless it lies in the path of the surgical approach. In contrast, high-energy gunshot wounds are treated as grade III open fractures, with prompt irrigation and surgical débridement, frequent use of temporizing external fixation, and definitive fixation only if and when the condition of the soft tissues permits.

With low-energy gunshots, nondisplaced and minimally displaced proximal humeral fractures are treated nonoperatively. The indications for surgery of displaced fractures of the humeral head and neck are the same as those used for closed fractures–displacement of more than 1 cm of a "part" of the proximal humerus and angulation greater than 45 degrees are generally considered indications for operative treatment. Plate and screw fixation, closed or open intramedullary nailing, or closed reduction and percutaneous pinning may all be appropriate, according to the experience and preference of the surgeon. Comminution of the surgical neck without bone loss may be bridged with either a locked plate or an intramedullary nail. The proximal humerus is relatively tolerant of shortening, and when bone loss at the surgical neck is present, it may often be treated by simply shortening the humerus by a centimeter or two (Figs. 19-4 and 19-5).

Although most low-velocity gunshot injuries to the shoulder girdle can be treated conservatively, if the gunshot wound involves the glenohumeral joint itself, the joint should be explored either arthroscopically[16] or through a formal arthrotomy. The path of the bullet itself can sometimes be a useful portal into the joint.[17] Intraarticular bullets should be removed, because lead may leach out into the joint and deposit within the synovial tissues, causing either periarticular fibrosis or toxic effects to the articular cartilage.[18] Osteochondral fragments that are small and irreparable should be excised, but larger, more significant pieces of the joint surface should be repaired. Countersunk or headless screws are often useful in

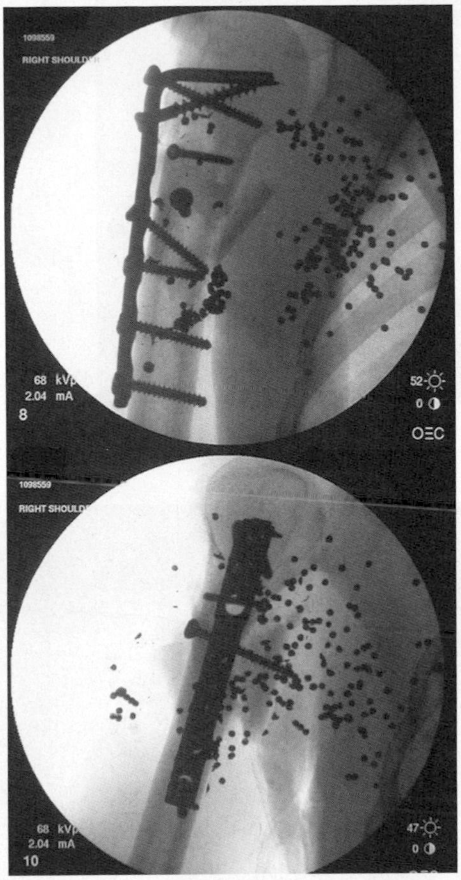

Figure 19-5. Treatment with primary shortening and blade plate fixation.

these unusual circumstances (Figs. 19-6 and 19-7). In cases of extreme comminution of the articular surfaces, prosthetic replacement or resection arthroplasty may be the only options. Placing either vancomycin or tobramycin in cement used for the prosthesis may decrease the risk of infection.

External fixation is an option for both temporary and definitive treatment of proximal humerus fractures, especially when soft tissue injury or bony comminution is severe (Fig. 19-8). Although we have little experience with it at most U.S. centers, recent war experiences in the Balkans and Middle East have given us a significant literature on the use of external fixation in high-energy gunshot injuries of the upper extremity[19] reported as external fixation of severe gunshot and blast injuries. Surgeons were able to use the proximal humerus for pin placement in half of their patients but needed to use the scapula and/or clavicle for the most severe injuries. Large soft tissue defects around the shoulder can be covered by rotation of a latissimus dorsi myocutaneous flap on its vascular pedicle. Once a favorable soft tissue environment has been established, the temporizing fixator can be converted to a more elaborate, definitive frame or to internal fixation if desired. Because long-term use of pins or wires in the humeral head can cause soft tissue irritation or infection, if external fixation is to be used until fracture healing has occurred, pin care must be meticulous.

Humeral Shaft and Arm

Vessel and Nerve Injury

As in the shoulder, gunshot wounds in the upper arm frequently injure arteries and nerves in addition to the bone itself. If vascular injuries are treated promptly, critical limb ischemia is rare.[20] Although some[21] have advocated that a fracture be stabilized first if there is an associated vascular injury in order to protect the repair, others have found different results. McHenry and colleagues[22] reviewed their upper and lower extremity fractures with associated vascular injuries. They definitively repaired five fractures first, shunted 13 of the 22 vascular injuries that were addressed before fracture repair, and repaired 9 of 22 vascular injuries definitively first. The need for fasciotomy and the length of hospitalization were both reduced when revascularization preceded care of the orthopaedic injury. Definitive fracture treatment, performed after the revascularization, did not disrupt the shunt or the definitive vascular repair in any case. Despite this, to maximize the safety of the vascular repair, our institution favors shunting of the vascular injury first, followed by either definitive fracture repair if the soft tissues allow or external

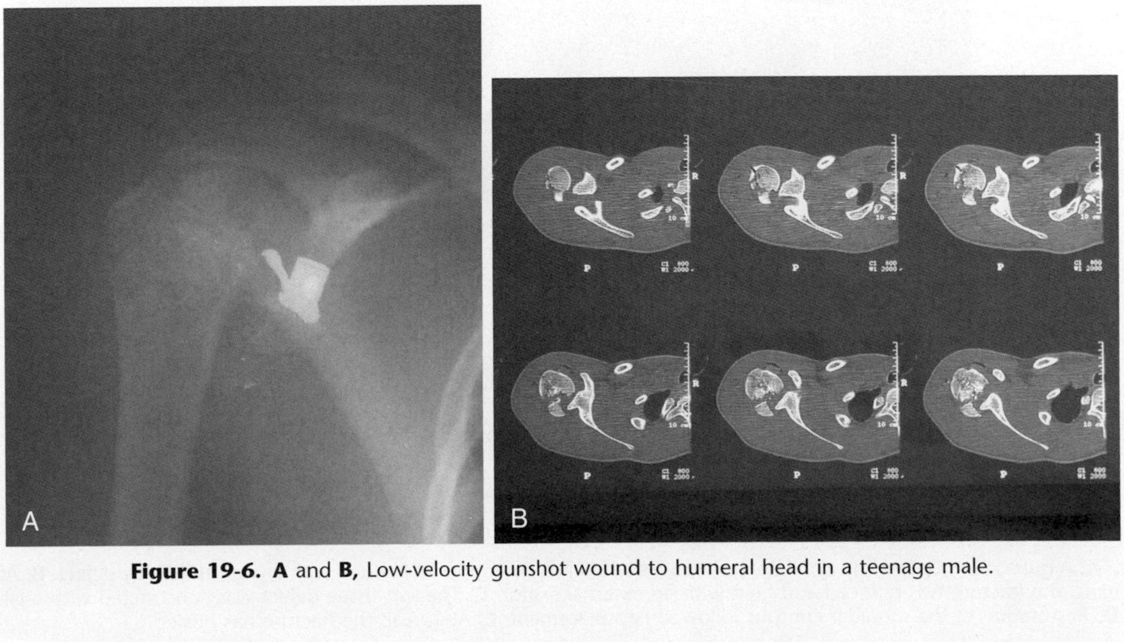

Figure 19-6. A and **B,** Low-velocity gunshot wound to humeral head in a teenage male.

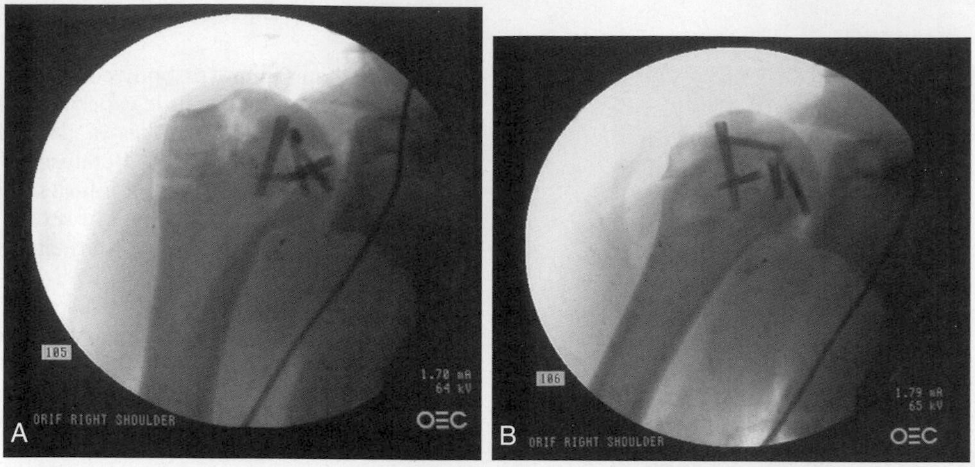

Figure 19-7. **A** and **B,** Treatment with open reduction and internally fixed with headless screws.

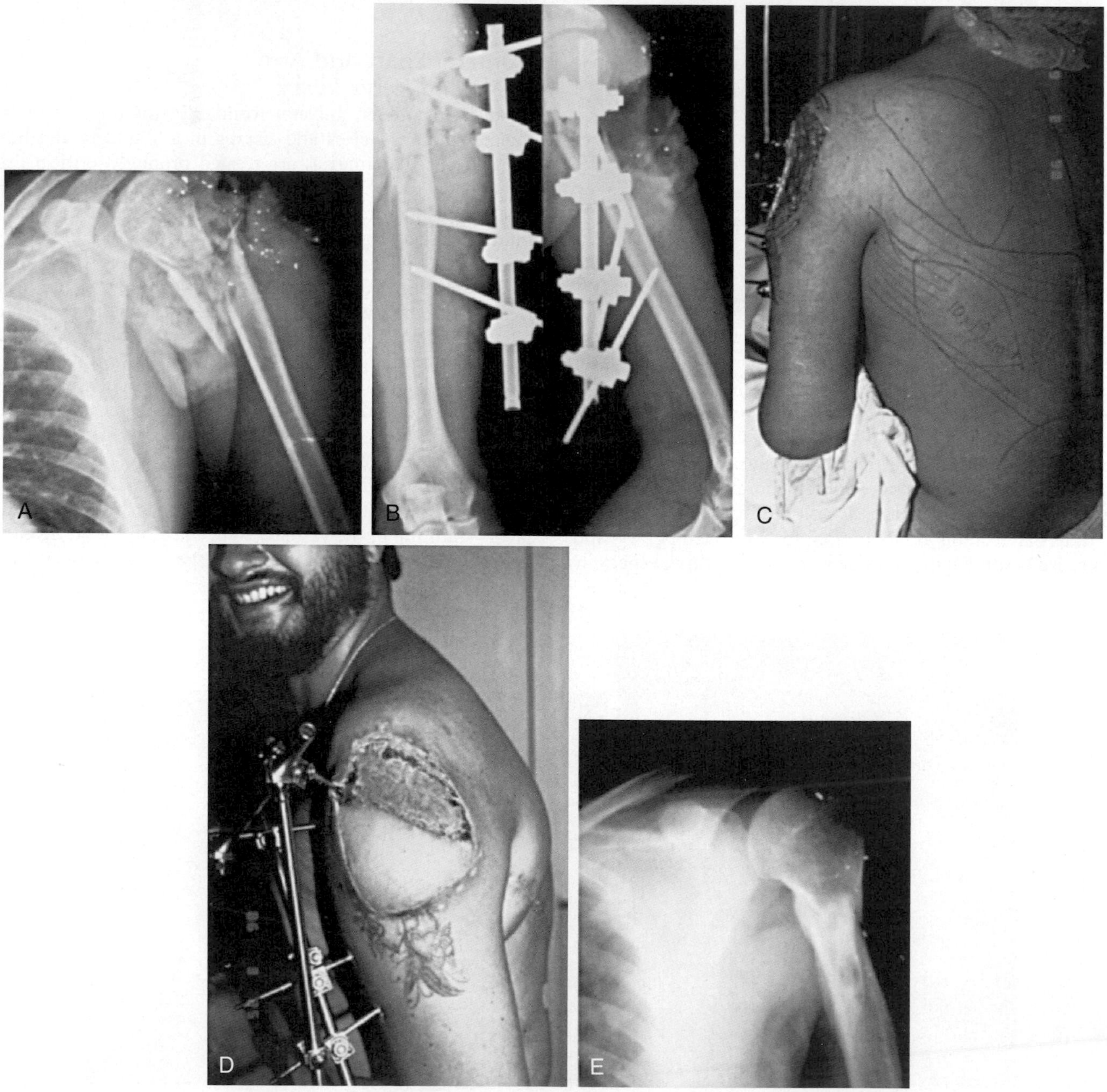

Figure 19-8. **A,** A gunshot wound to the proximal humerus resulted in a comminuted fracture with a large soft tissue defect. **B,** After irrigation and débridement, the fracture was reduced and held with an external fixator. **C,** The soft tissue defect was constructed with a latissimus dorsi pedicle flap. **D,** Restoration of the shoulder contour followed flap placement. **E,** At 1 year, the fracture has healed.

fixation if not, and then definitive vascular repair. More recent reviews of the use of temporary vascular shunting in both the global war on terror[23] and in a civilian level I trauma center[24] have suggested benefit from the use of temporary shunts, particularly in cases requiring stabilization of high-grade open fractures.

When fracture and vascular injury are both present, complication rates for the vascular injury may increase. McNamara and coworkers[25] found no amputations in 64 patients without humeral fracture who underwent brachial artery repair, but 10% of the 20 patients with humeral fractures had amputations. There was one failure of repair (2.3%) among the 44 patients without fracture, and there were two failures (10%) among those with fracture.

Humeral shaft fractures combined with ipsilateral brachial plexus injuries pose special problems. Of 19 patients with brachial plexus injuries and ipsilateral humeral shaft fractures treated at the Los Angeles County–University of Southern California Medical Center and Rancho Los Amigos Hospital, 3 were treated by compression plate, 4 by intramedullary nail, 2 with external fixation, and 10 with a cast or brace. All fractures treated by compression plating healed, but 4 of the 6 treated with intramedullary rods or external fixation and 4 of the 10 treated with a cast brace failed to unite.[26] All of the nonunions required open repair with compression plating to achieve union.

The question of whether or not the presence of a nerve injury associated with a gunshot wound and fracture merits exploration has been controversial. A 4-year review of all gunshot fractures of the humerus at an urban trauma center identified three isolated single nerve palsies, which all resolved with observation. Three nerve injuries were associated with brachial artery lacerations, and all required secondary nerve procedures. Based on this, the authors recommended observation for nerve injury alone, with early exploration for nerve injury associated with vascular injury.[27]

If the peripheral nerves traversing a high-energy gunshot wound in the upper arm are not functioning, and the wound is to be débrided because of the severity of the soft tissue injury, the nerves may be explored at the time of débridement. While repair can sometimes be carried out primarily, the extent of injury to the nerve is typically unclear, so the nerve ends are usually tagged for later repair. When fractures result from lower energy missiles, they can often be treated nonoperatively. In this case, peripheral nerve injuries are usually managed expectantly. Although some have found little benefit to exploration and repair of nerve injury in the upper arm, others have reported large series with better prognosis if the nerve injury is in the arm or more distal.[28,29]

Fracture

Fractures of the humeral shaft, when not complicated by vascular injury, are often best treated with local wound care and plaster or cast-brace immobilization. Humeral fracture bracing may be started as soon as the wound permits. There is no significant difference in the rate of union between closed humeral fractures and uncomplicated humeral fractures caused by a low-velocity gunshot, even if appreciable comminution or displacement is present.[30] When low- or even moderate-energy soft tissue injury is present, operative stabilization with either a nail or plate may be carried out both promptly and safely if the pattern of fracture merits. In cases of severe soft tissue injury, débridement and external fixation is almost always the initial treatment of choice for the fracture, facilitates subsequent wound and soft tissue care, and may provide definitive fixation. Half-pin frames in the arm often have pin track problems as the patient begins to mobilize the shoulder and elbow, and our preference is to convert to a plate when possible, or to an intramedullary nail, because time required for healing is often prolonged, and the pins may be difficult to maintain for these long periods. However, with careful attention to the frame and appropriate treatment of the anticipated pin track problems, external fixation can certainly be used as definitive treatment.

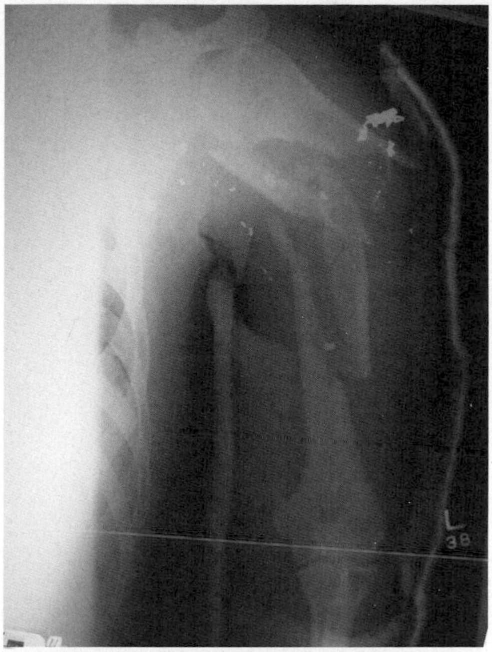

Figure 19-9. Comminuted proximal humeral shaft fracture without significant neurovascular or soft tissue injury.

In centers experienced with their use, Ilizarov type frames can also be used with good results.[31] The care of these complex injuries is difficult, and decisions regarding care must be individualized to the patient, the fracture, and the injury (Figs. 19-9 through 19-12).

In addition to neurovascular injury and soft tissue loss, high-energy gunshot wounds can also cause significant loss of diaphyseal bone. Although there are reports of spontaneous reconstitution of humeral bone loss, some type of surgical intervention is generally required to restore bony continuity. Numerous techniques have been proposed to deal with this challenging situation, including wave plating with cancellous grafting,[32] interposition of a titanium mesh cage with bone graft,[33] transposition of composite flap including the lateral border of the scapula,[34] transfer of a segment of vascularized fibula,[35] and bone transport using an Ilizarov type external fixator.[36]

At present, there is no large series or body of evidence to suggest the superiority of any one method of reconstituting humeral bone loss.

Elbow

Because of its complex bony anatomy and propensity for stiffness following injury, gunshot wounds about the elbow are

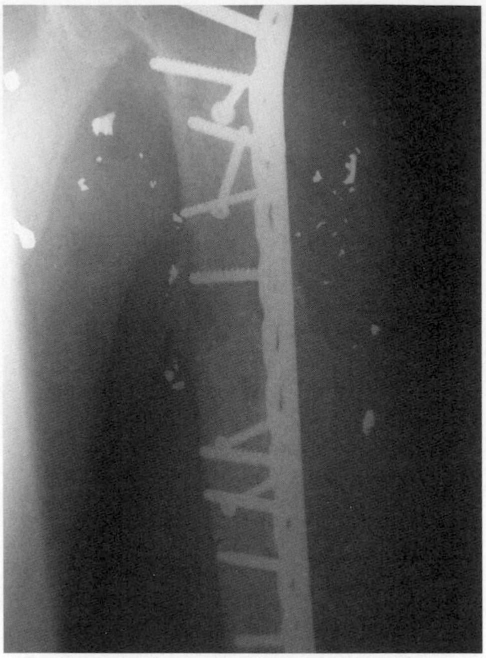

Figure 19-10. Treatment with a plate.

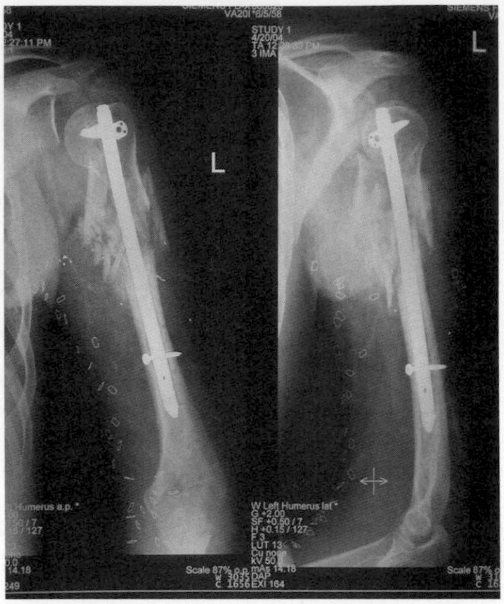

Figure 19-12. After serial débridement to resolve the infection, the patient in Figure 19-10 underwent pedicled latissimus coverage and conversion to an intramedullary nail.

particularly difficult. Following severe elbow injuries, the goal of achieving the flexion and extension and forearm rotation required for most activities of daily living is often not realized. Although secondary procedures, such as capsular release and resection of heterotopic bone, can sometimes help regain lost motion, articular injuries are sometimes so severe that achieving a stable and pain-free elbow with any motion at all may be a victory.

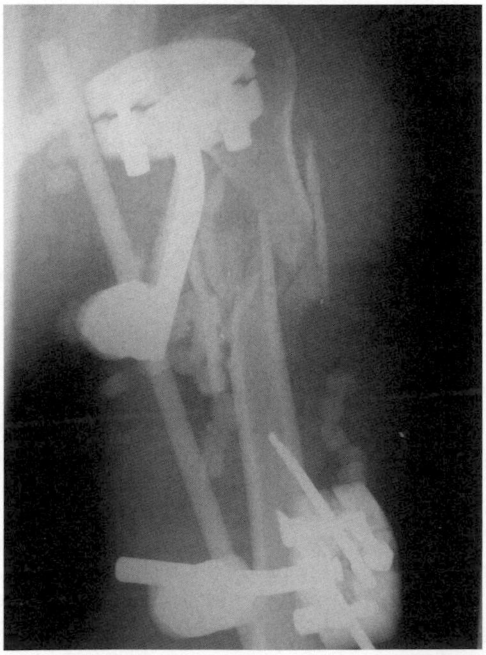

Figure 19-11. Comminuted proximal humeral shaft with vascular injury and delayed revascularization and external fixation. Patient developed infection and compartment syndrome and lost most of the muscle below the deltoid.

The brachial artery at the elbow is particularly vulnerable because of its location. In addition to trauma from the missile itself, displacement of fracture fragments about the elbow can lacerate or completely tear the artery as well. Compression or occlusion of the brachial artery can also result from entrapment between fracture fragments and from the edema that may follow restoration of arterial flow after prolonged ischemia, leading to forearm compartment syndrome.[37] Six compartment syndromes that developed in association with isolated proximal ulna fractures have been reported. Five of the six developed in a delayed fashion; all five were associated with low-velocity gunshots. If a nerve injury is also present at the elbow, pain and paresthesias from forearm compartment syndrome may be absent, and the only reliable way to detect it is with a high degree of suspicion and direct compartment monitoring. In a review of vascular injuries about the elbow, Ashbell and colleagues[38] reported that 86% of those who sustained arterial injury also had injury to muscle, nerve, or bone in the same area. Concomitant injuries to one or more major nerves in the arm occurred in 69% of patients, with muscle injuries next in frequency (66%). Combined injury to both nerve and muscle was seen in 45% of patients.

When there is severe soft tissue and muscle damage, we recommend initial external fixation across the elbow joint. This approach protects arterial repair and allows soft tissue management and recovery. If there is soft tissue loss, an intact soft tissue envelope must be reestablished before further reconstruction can occur. For smaller defects in the surrounding soft tissue, local flaps may be an option. For larger areas of bone and soft tissue loss around the elbow, a composite latissimus flap, such as that described by Evans and Luethke,[39] offers an option for coverage and for osseous reconstruction as well. When soft tissues recover sufficiently to allow it, the surgeon may undertake fixation of the articular injury and reconstruction of any juxtaarticular bone loss. Although a significant loss of elbow motion often results if the fixator is left on for more than 4 to 6 weeks, there are times when the severity of the injury allows no other treatment.

Distal Humerus

Although earlier texts adopted a fairly nihilistic approach toward the reconstruction of these complex articular injuries, techniques and implants have improved to a point where many extremely complex articular injuries can be reconstructed.

For comminuted juxtaarticular fractures, external fixation has been described as a means of restoring limb alignment and permitting immediate motion while minimizing dissection in the zone of injury.[40] When the articular surface is comminuted, open reduction of even the most comminuted joint is often possible once the soft tissues have recovered to a point that permits a safe operation. In cases where the soft tissue injury is too severe to permit the safe placement of plates and screws, the use of Ilizarov fine-wire fixation has been reported in areas such as the Middle East, where blast and high-energy gunshot wounds are more common.[41,42]

Triceps splitting or olecranon osteotomy can be used at the surgeon's discretion. Multiple fine, threaded Kirschner wires, buried screws, and absorbable pins can be used to build small osteochondral fragments onto the epicondyles until the medial and lateral halves of the articular spool can be mated. The repaired articular segment can then be fixed to the humeral shaft, typically with a 3.5 plate on each column. Fixation of a comminuted medial or lateral column may be aided with use of an additional minifragment or modular hand plate on the column. Moderate supracondylar bone loss can be addressed with a shortening osteotomy of the supracondylar humerus, with a burr used to recreate the olecranon and coronoid fossae. Columnar bone loss can be grafted with a structural piece of tricortical iliac crest or bridged with a plate and the column grafted with cancellous bone. The goal is to obtain fixation that is sufficiently stable to allow immediate range of motion. When this quality of fixation cannot be obtained, the elbow can be immobilized, although this tends to cause stiffness rapidly and may require secondary release.

Despite improvements in both techniques and implants, some distal humeral injuries remain unreconstructable because of articular loss or comminution or severe soft tissue injury. In these cases, the older technique of skeletal traction applied through a proximal ulnar pin, which allows some early motion and can maintain reasonable alignment of the fracture fragments, can be used.[42]

Ulna

Gunshot wounds of the olecranon and proximal ulna present difficulties for the orthopaedist as well. In simple, low-energy injuries with minimal comminution, standard open reduction and internal fixation can be carried out with either a modified tension band or with plate and screw fixation. When olecranon comminution is extensive (75% to 80% of the articular surface), it can be managed by excision and the triceps advanced to the remaining bone.[43,44] If the articular surfaces of the olecranon and coronoid can be reconstructed, plates may be used to bridge areas of periarticular comminution. The coronoid is of primary importance in this area, and every effort should be made to preserve it if possible. Figures 19-13 and 19-14 illustrate this point, with use of mini screws, fine-wire fixation, and an intramedullary miniplate on the comminuted coronoid to reconstruct the joint surface and plate fixation to bridge the periarticular comminution. Fixation was adequate to begin early motion, and the patient illustrated recovered nearly full range of motion.

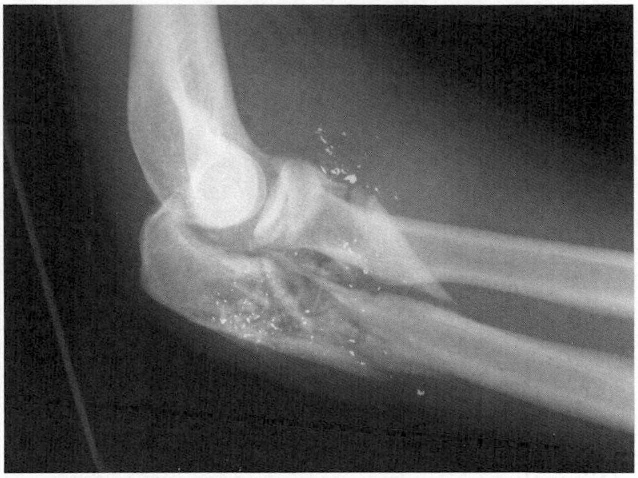

Figure 19-13. Gunshot wound through proximal ulna.

Additional techniques are available for salvage of the severely injured elbow. None present ideal solutions for these difficult injuries, and the choice of treatment must be individualized according to the injury and the experience of the surgeon. Arthrodesis can relieve pain and provide strength and stability, but the loss of elbow motion is extremely limiting. Techniques of elbow fusion are described using internal,[45] external,[46] and combined[47] methods of fixation, as well as using vascularized free fibulae to make up bony defects.[48]

Hinge distraction can be used to help regain motion after release of contractures or repair of instability or in conjunction with excisional or fascial interposition arthroplasty to obtain motion in stiff elbows with loss of the articular surface of the distal humerus. This technique is particularly helpful in patients who are thought to be too young or too unreliable for total elbow arthroplasty and in those who refuse arthrodesis.

Cadaveric elbow allografts have been used as an alternative to arthrodesis as a final salvage attempt when there is significant bone loss. Dean and colleagues[49] have reported a 20-year

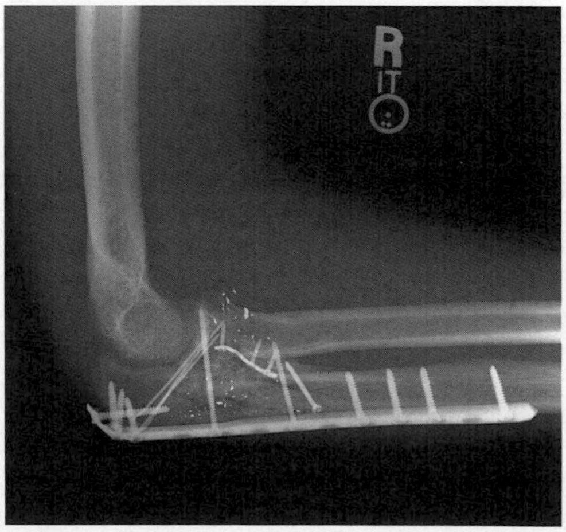

Figure 19-14. Treatment with open reduction and internal fixation.

experience with 23 whole elbow allograft reconstructions. Complications were observed in 16 and removal of the allograft was required in 6. Ten of 14 patients followed an average of 7.5 years had satisfactory results. They viewed the operation as salvage only and noted that it reestablishes bone stock for future arthrodesis or arthroplasty. Finally, although the indication is rare, total elbow arthroplasty can be done in the older patient who will not place great physical demands on the elbow if adequate bone and soft tissue coverage are present. Reports of using total elbow replacement in younger, more active patients have yielded good results in the very short term, but in these higher demand patients, midterm failure, with need for revision surgery, was almost inevitable.[50]

Forearm

Forearm fractures after gunshots have a high incidence of concomitant peripheral nerve injury and resultant loss of hand function. Initial evaluation should include a careful neurologic examination as well as an accurate assessment of swelling in the forearm. Compartment syndromes are common, and a high index of suspicion is essential, especially for fractures in the proximal third of the forearm. Moed and Fakhouri[51] found a 10% incidence of compartment syndrome in a series of 131 low-velocity gunshot wounds to the forearm (60 with fractures, 71 without bone injury). Location was the only significant fracture-associated risk factor predicting the development of compartment syndrome; displacement, comminution, and metallic foreign bodies in the wound had no effect. If any doubt exists, intracompartmental pressure measurements are indicated. If there is a possibility of vascular injury, an angiogram should be obtained.

Elstrom and coworkers[52] reviewed 29 extraarticular gunshot fractures of the forearm. Eighty-eight percent of the nondisplaced fractures did well and healed after approximately 7 weeks. Displaced fractures did not do so well, with 77% unsatisfactory results. The results in the patients with displaced fractures treated by delayed primary open reduction and internal fixation were superior to those of patients treated by closed methods. Twenty-seven percent had long-term disability secondary to the sequela of nerve injury or difficulty in obtaining fracture union. Lenihan and associates[53] reviewed 32 patients with gunshot fractures of the forearm. They also found nonoperative treatment to be satisfactory for almost all nondisplaced fractures and unsatisfactory for those displaced. Of nine nerve injuries, 55% resolved spontaneously. Two patients (7%) underwent fasciotomy for compartment syndrome in the forearm.

Our recommendation for the treatment of uncomplicated, nondisplaced gunshot fractures of the forearm without vascular injury includes local wound care, antibiotics, and cast immobilization. However, displaced fractures of the radius or ulna and injuries involving both bones are best treated by immediate splinting and early open reduction and internal fixation. The patient should be observed for at least 24 hours for signs of ischemia or impending compartment syndrome.

When soft tissue injury is severe, external fixation confers quick and efficient stabilization, facilitates nursing, and aids recovery of both the patient and the injured limb.[54] The fixator may be definitive or may be changed later to plate fixation once soft tissues recover.

Because the majority of nerve injuries recover, they are generally treated expectantly. If open treatment of the fracture is undertaken, the nerve may be explored, but in the acute setting, it can be difficult or impossible to determine the extent of damage. While awaiting recovery from nerve injury, paralyzed joints should be splinted appropriately, and passive range-of-motion exercise should be performed regularly to prevent contracture. The most useful splints are the lumbrical bar splint for ulnar nerve palsy (to prevent flexion contracture of the proximal interphalangeal joints of the fourth and fifth fingers) and the thumb opposition splint for median nerve injury (to prevent thumb web contracture). Patients with radial nerve palsy often do not need splinting, as contracture can usually be prevented by passive range-of-motion exercise.

When bone loss is present in the forearm, a number of strategies may be used to gain union across these gaps. If the soft tissue envelope is compliant, has limited scar, and consists largely of healthy muscle with a good vascular supply, autogenous cancellous bone grafting and stable internal plate fixation results in a high rate of union and improved upper limb function in patients with diaphyseal defects of the radius and/or ulna.[55] For contaminated segmental forearm fractures of up to 6 cm, the use of an antibiotic-impregnated cement spacer followed by delayed cancellous bone grafting has been reported by Georgiadis and DeSilva.[56] To improve stability and decrease the time to fracture union and the possibility of mechanical failure or loosening of the implants, a structural tricortical autogenous iliac crest graft may also be used.[57]

Finally, both Jupiter and colleagues[58] and Adani and colleagues[59] have reported on the use of vascularized fibular autograft for forearm defects ranging from 6 to 13 cm.

GUNSHOT FRACTURES OF THE HAND AND WRIST

Introduction

Gunshot wounds of the hand have been more common in recent years as a result of the growing number of civilian injuries in inner city trauma centers. An estimated 20% of missile injuries involve the hand. Although these are typically low-velocity injuries, high-velocity injuries do account for a number of civilian injuries. The economic impact of these injuries can be substantial, with one study calculating the average direct hospital costs for hospitalization and operative care at $14,000 per gunshot hand fracture.[60] Treatment of these patients is also challenging because of poor patient compliance. In one study of urban civilian hand gunshot injuries, 85% of patients were lost to follow-up before documented fracture healing, and 26% were lost to follow-up with removable fixation devices in place.[61] There is also an increase in battlefield survival, making it more likely that these patients will have ballistic injuries to the hand that need to be addressed. Fragmentation type injury is also an increasing percentage of combat wounds, and may be seen outside of the battlefield in the case of terrorist bombings.

Gunshot wounds to the wrist and hand can be complicated owing to the multitude of important structures contained within a small area. Frequent involvement of bone, tendons, nerves, and arteries is found with both high- and low-velocity injuries. On presentation to the emergency department, a

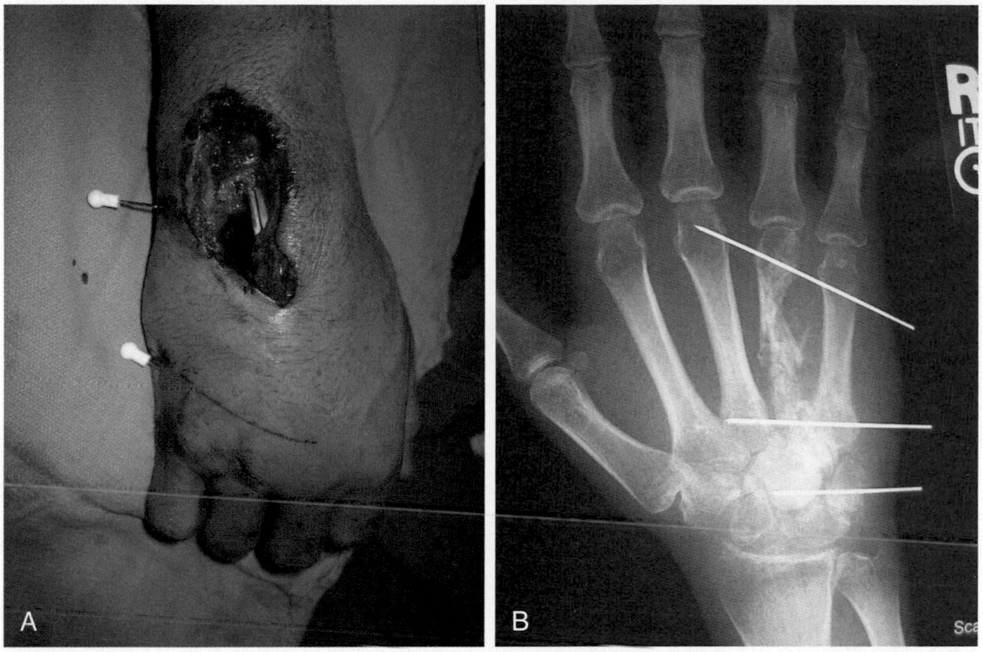

Figure 19-15. A, This patient sustained a high-energy gunshot to the hand that resulted in a large soft tissue defect, extensor tendon injury, and highly comminuted fractures of the metacarpal, capitate, and hamate. **B,** One week after initial débridement, the patient underwent bone grafting, tendon repairs, and wound closure.

thorough examination of the patient is crucial. The patient's account of the injury should also be documented for medicolegal reasons. Assessment of the soft tissue envelope, motor, sensory, and circulation is necessary for treatment planning. Adequate radiographs should be obtained to evaluate the presence and severity of the skeletal injury. For more extensive injuries, CT scanning is helpful in planning skeletal reconstruction.

Initial Treatment

After assessment of the patient and the injury, the wound should be treated with local superficial wound cleansing and local wound care. Simple wounds should be allowed to heal by secondary intention. Prophylactic antibiotics, frequently used because the degree of contamination may not be obvious, may not be necessary.[62] Fracture of the hand may have a higher rate of infection than in other areas of the body. Fracture stability and associated injuries guide further treatment. Stable fractures of the hand can be treated nonoperatively in appropriate casts or splints. A bulky dressing is applied with a dorsal splint maintaining the metacarpophalangeal joints in 70 to 90 degrees of flexion, the interphalangeal joints in extension, and the wrist in 20 degrees of extension.

Low-velocity firearms, such as handguns, cause the majority of civilian gunshot wounds. Injuries caused by handguns cause much less damage to the soft tissues and less bony comminution. Thus, many of these fractures can be treated nonoperatively.[60,61]

Surgical Treatment

Gonzalez and colleagues[63] defined operative indications for gunshot metacarpal fractures as follows: 50% or more comminution, angulation greater than 15 degrees, less than 50% bony apposition, shortening greater than 5 mm, and multiple fractures. Similar guidelines can be applied to proximal phalangeal fractures[63,64] (Fig. 19-15).

For injuries that require surgical treatment, care should be taken to remove only clearly devitalized tissue. Consideration of the function of structures in the zone of injury is important so that questionable tissue is left because the hand has an amazing capacity to heal. In the hand and wrist, removal of bullet fragments from synovial compartments should be considered (Fig. 19-16). Lead arthropathy and toxicity have been reported with intraarticular bullets and may also occur with retained fragments in tenosynovium.[65]

Tendon injuries are present in 20% to 30% of gunshot wounds.[66] Most injuries can be treated with primary repair, but some injuries require single- or two-stage grafting or even late tendon transfers. Tendon repair should be performed if possible at the time of bone reconstruction. In the dorsal aspect of the hand and in the fingers, the tendons are in close proximity to the bone. Even in the absence of direct tendon injury, the tendons can be secondarily affected by entrapment in scar or bony callus. Thus, it is imperative to promptly initiate digital motion to lower the likelihood of tendon adhesion. Bone fixation should be rigid enough to allow for rehabilitation of the tendon injury. Functional results will suffer if appropriate postoperative therapy cannot be instituted in a timely fashion. If there is significant tendon loss, grafting or tendon transfer should be performed.

For the flexor tendons, the A2 and A4 pulleys are crucial for efficient digital flexion, and the tendons should be repaired or reconstructed with local mobilization of tissues.[67] For flexor tendon injuries that cannot be repaired primarily without undue tension, a tendon graft should be employed. For injuries in the pulley region, the graft should extend from the palm to the insertion of the flexor digitorum profundus (FDP) on the distal phalanx. For injuries in the palm or wrist, segmental

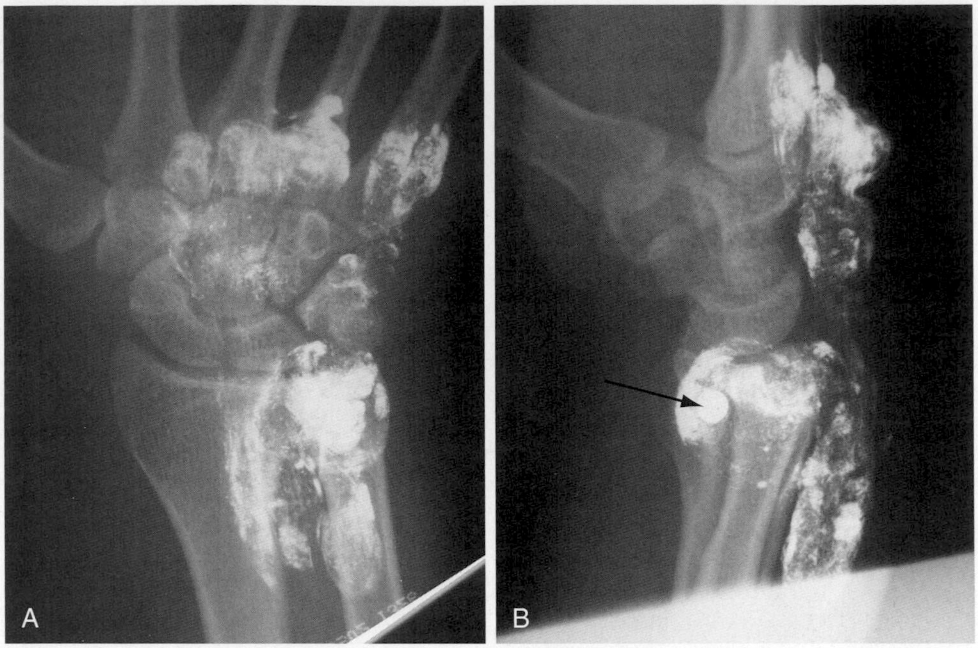

Figure 19-16. A and **B,** This patient had a 1-year history of dorsal wrist swelling. Ten years earlier, the patient had sustained a shotgun wound to the wrist. The extensor tenosynovium of the fourth and fifth compartments as well as the distal radioulnar joint are well outlined by the lead from the degraded shot, with one pellet still visible *(arrow)*.

grafting should be performed to avoid tendon anastomosis within the carpal tunnel. Extensor tendon injuries of the fingers associated with fractures often have poor motion at the proximal interphalangeal (PIP) joint. For extensor damage on the dorsum of the hand or wrist, tendon loss can be treated with segmental grafts, transfer of the extensor indicis proprius (EIP) or extensor digiti quinti (EDQ), or side-to-side repair with the adjacent digital extensor.

Muscle involvement in the hand is not uncommon, mainly injuries to the interosseus muscles. Damage to these muscles can result in loss of grip strength and usually does not require further treatment. Damage to the thenar and hypothenar muscles may result in loss of abduction and opposition of the thumb and small finger and, if severe, may require tendon transfers to restore function.

Compartment syndrome of the hand can occur following gunshot wounds. This may be difficult to diagnose owing to the lack of distal sensory and vascular changes or pain due to the injury itself or in the obtunded patient. The clinician should measure interosseus muscle pressures when the diagnosis is in question. Release of the interosseus muscle fascia is satisfactory to allow room for muscle swelling.

Nerve injuries are commonly found in association with hand gunshot fractures with a frequency of around 30% to 40%. Seventy to ninety percent will resolve spontaneously.[68] If a complete nerve transection is encountered during surgical exploration, the nerve should be repaired with minimal tension. For high-energy injuries, immediate vein grafting or another nerve conduit can be used with a high rate of satisfactory results.[69]

Soft Tissue Management

Damage to the skin and subcutaneous tissues can vary greatly from small, uncomplicated wounds to large areas of soft tissue loss. Treatment for uncomplicated wounds should proceed as described earlier. For areas of larger soft tissue loss, there are a number of options.[66] Closure by secondary intention, which has a low rate of complications and satisfactory motion for wounds of the hand and fingers, is recommended.[66] Early and intensive hand therapy as well as patient cooperation are necessary for good results. Other options include split-thickness skin grafts, staged coverage with dermal templates with delayed skin grafting, vacuum-assisted closure, and flap coverage. Flaps are preferred in many cases to provide immediate coverage of tendons, nerves, and bone reconstruction, which may facilitate early motion. The groin flap was the workhorse in the past, but pedicled radial forearm, perforator flaps, or posterior interosseus flaps can provide excellent coverage while allowing for elevation of the hand and more effective postoperative therapy.[70] Delayed reconstruction with distant tissue transfer, either free or pedicled, has been shown to be effective in injuries sustained on the battlefield.

Fracture Treatment

Fractures of the wrist and hand should be treated with the goal of early rehabilitation. For stable nondisplaced or minimally displaced fractures of the wrist, a short arm cast or splint is satisfactory. For stable fractures of the metacarpals or proximal phalanges, immobilization should be placed dorsally with the metacarpophalangeal (MCP) joints in 70 to 90 degrees and the PIP joints in extension. Flexion exercises can be started in the cast to maintain joint mobility. Stable fractures of the middle and distal phalanges should be splinted with the next proximal joint free.

Many fractures of the metacarpals and phalanges are unstable owing to comminution or bone loss. Rigid internal fixation with plates, screws, intramedullary rods, or a combination should be attained whenever possible. Grafting with cancellous or corticocancellous bone should treat bone loss. Studies of the use of bone graft substitutes in these types of fractures have not been reported. Early bone grafting has a low complication rate and high union rate.[63,64] In cases treated late, bony union and satisfactory motion can still be achieved. Some fractures are not amenable to rigid internal fixation and may require temporary Kirschner wire spacers, pinning to an adjacent metacarpal, or the use of external fixation. External fixation is especially helpful in patients with complex soft tissue injuries.[71]

Articular fractures in the wrist and hand can be challenging. Essentially all gunshot carpal fractures are articular fractures and may require limited or total wrist arthrodesis. For many injuries, distraction through the use of external fixation can restore articular congruity.[67] If joint congruity can be obtained with traction, PIP joint injuries can potentially be treated with dynamic external fixation that allows for early motion. For nonreconstructable articular injuries of the thumb MCP or interphalangeal (IP) joint, and for distal interphalangeal (DIP) joints, arthrodesis is preferred. For similar injuries to the MCP or PIP joints of the fingers, external fixation can be used to maintain length and alignment prior to arthrodesis. Arthroplasty may be useful in some select cases to maintain MCP or PIP motion in select cases.

LOWER EXTREMITY

Pelvis

Gunshot wounds of the pelvis are rarely encountered in civilian settings. Many different anatomic structures are present within and surrounding the pelvic ring. Thorough assessment of all potentially violated organ systems is indicated. This includes the genitourinary, neurologic, vascular, and gastrointestinal systems. The greatest danger zones for injury are central within the true pelvic cavity, in the area bounded by the sacroiliac joints posteriorly and anteriorly, and lateral to the pectineal tubercle/prominence. Fragments can penetrate four joints: two sacroiliac and two hip. Typically, because of the direct nature of the trauma, there is disruption of either the anterior or posterior pelvic ring but rarely both. More central bullet pathways tend to produce more important tissue disruption. The surgeon needs to evaluate all the potential structures within the bullet pathway. Abdominal or peritoneal cavity penetration is possible. Controversy exists over whether patients with gunshots to the abdominopelvic region require acute laparotomy or can be managed expectantly.

All patients with gunshot injuries to the pelvis require consultation by a general trauma surgeon to evaluate for significant abdominal or vascular damage.[72] Patients with hemodynamic instability require appropriate and complete resuscitation, according to ATLS guidelines, a trauma team approach, and often, emergent laparotomy. Intravenous broad-spectrum antibiotics are administered immediately after the diagnosis is made. Stable patients can be evaluated carefully to determine the extent of injury and the necessary imaging studies.

Imaging Studies

Initially a high-quality anteroposterior (AP) pelvis radiograph is obtained to survey the pelvic region and to direct subsequent imaging studies. Bullet location, number of fragments, and obvious fractures are noted. Detailed CT scans with contrast are essential in the determination of (1) bullet trajectory

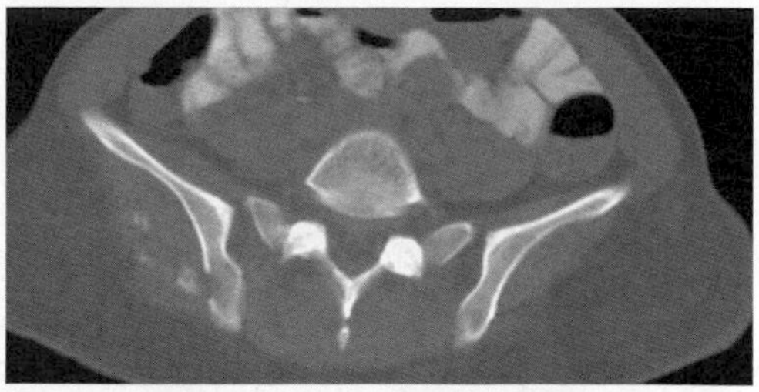

Figure 19-17. Computed tomography (CT) scan axial image of extraarticular gunshot fracture to posterior ilium.

through the pelvis, (2) bone or joint violation, (3) solid or hollow viscus injury, and (4) significant arterial bleeding (Figs. 19-17 and 19-18). Metallic artifacts may preclude precise localization of the fragments. CT reconstructions in the sagittal and coronal planes will reduce some of the metallic artifact effect, especially important in diagnosis of intraarticular fragments. Additional imaging studies should be done as appropriate. Magnetic resonance imaging (MRI) of the pelvic area is probably not indicated owing to the possible deleterious effect on ferromagnetic fragments from the bullet.

Intraarticular Bullets

Most bullets that penetrate the pelvic joints will be "stopped" by the relatively dense bones. There may be associated fractures or simply intraarticular penetration by the bullets. The adverse effects of lead in contact with synovial fluid and the direct mechanical effect of the bullet fragments on the articular cartilage mandate bullet fragment removal. This has been accomplished in several reports using arthrotomy, minimal surgery, or arthroscopy.[73-75] Regardless of the method, removal of all bullet fragments and, if possible, joint débridement and thorough joint irrigation are the goals (Fig. 19-19). A brief period (24 to 48 hours) of antibiotics is indicated. Displaced intraarticular acetabular fractures should be anatomically reduced and stabilized. The surgeon must be aware of the possibility of unrecognized comminution and bone loss and be prepared to handle this intraoperatively.

Intestinal Contamination

Bullets may penetrate the intestinal tract before lodging in the pelvic bones. This information will be known only after a laparotomy has been performed. The question arises as to the proper method of treating a pelvic fracture that is caused by one of these contaminated bullets. It is logical to assume that if a contaminated bullet does violate a pelvic joint, especially the hip, the fracture should be débrided, all accessible bullet fragments removed, and the joint irrigated. However, a bullet or fragments that penetrate the extraarticular pelvic bones may not pose a serious risk of infection after treatment with a course of prophylactic antibiotics. The bone structures of the pelvis are principally cancellous bone, which has an abundant vascular supply. Antibiotic concentration in this type of bone should be optimal and the relative therapeutic effect maximized.

One study by Watters and colleagues found no increased incidence in infection in patients with pelvic gunshots and fractures whether or not they were surgically débrided. However there was a trend for patients with abdominal perforations to have more infectious complications than those without abdominal perforations.[76] Another study by Rehman

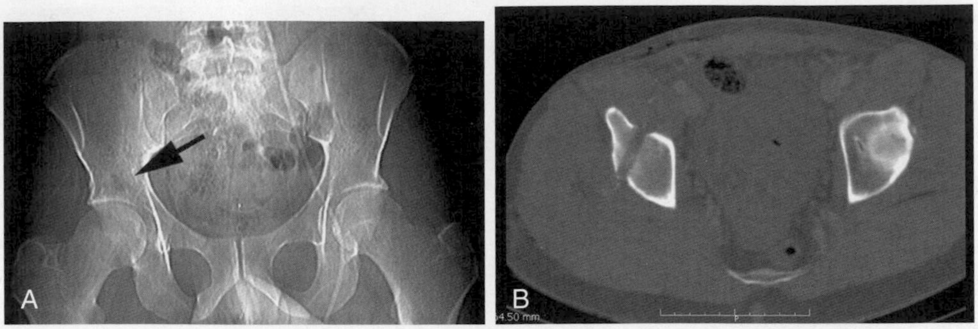

Figure 19-18. **A,** Gunshot to supraacetabular hip region without joint involvement. The plain anteroposterior pelvic radiograph does show radiolucent defect *(black arrow)* but does not clearly delineate the bullet pathway. **B,** Corresponding computed tomography (CT) axial image does show the bullet track through the supraacetabular bone without extension into the hip joint.

and colleagues concluded that surgical débridement was not necessary in pelvic fractures caused by gunshots even with associated abdominal viscus injuries.[77]

However, with the higher energy (velocity) gunshots, there may be stronger indications for débridement. The surgeon must analyze the risk-benefit ratio to determine the most appropriate treatment strategy for the particular clinical situation.

Fracture Management

Pelvic fractures that are secondary to gunshots should for the most part be managed on the basis of the specific fracture pattern and not the gunshot mechanism. Nondisplaced fractures are treated with protected weight bearing for several weeks. Disruptions of the pelvic ring are rarely caused by civilian gunshots and, if present, either indicate severe high-velocity and/or high-energy projectile injury (e.g., from a shotgun or assault rifle) or are secondary to nongunshot trauma, which may occur subsequently to the gunshot. A skeletally unstable pelvic ring should be stabilized by one of three methods: skeletal traction, external fixation, or internal fixation. The method chosen depends on the surgeon's expertise and preference and evaluation of the degree of soft tissue and bone damage. Most cases of this magnitude should be referred to a trauma center with orthopaedic traumatologists who specialize in pelvic trauma.

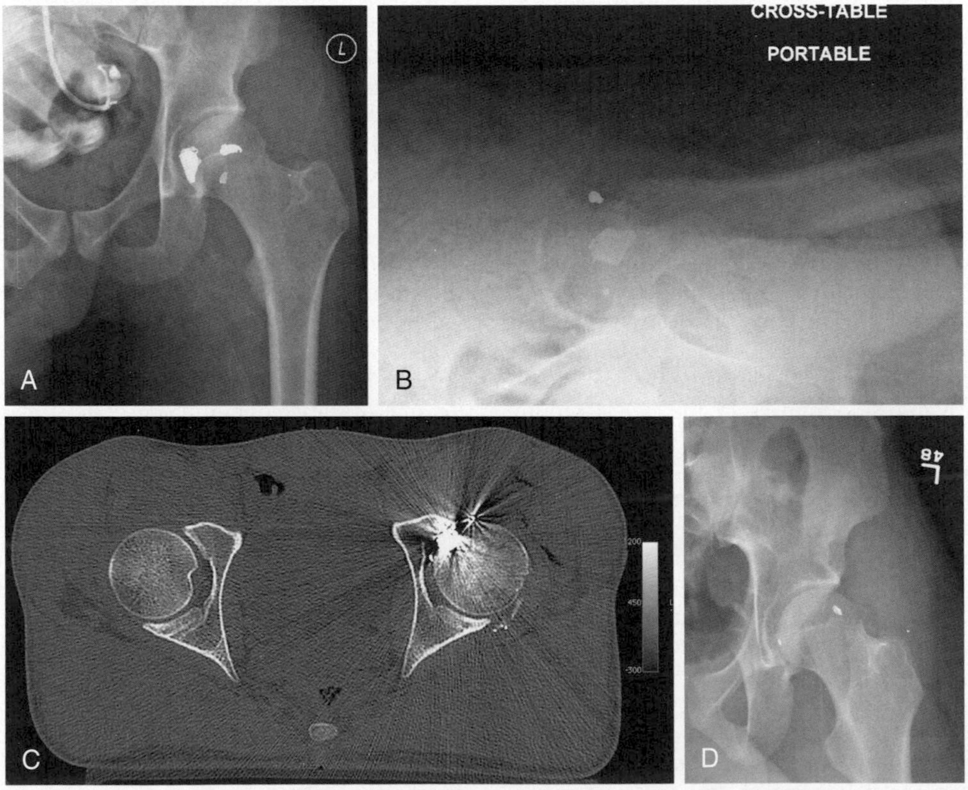

Figure 19-19. Gunshot injury to hip. **A,** Multiple bullet fragments seen on anteroposterior plain radiograph. **B,** Cross-table lateral plain radiograph suggests that fragments may be intraarticular. **C,** Computed tomography (CT) scan shows definite intraarticular fragments located in the anterior hip region. **D,** An anterior hip approach was performed and the postoperative anteroposterior radiograph indicates removal of the intraarticular hip fragments.

Femur

The femur is one of the long bones more frequently affected by gunshots. The thigh is a relatively easy target because of its large size. Inexperienced shooters will attempt to aim for the "kill zone" (the area of the chest and abdomen) and instead will hit the lower extremities, often the thigh. Typical civilian handgun bullets will strike the femur and often fragment on impact in the diaphysis and pass through the metaphyseal areas. The stress riser created in the bone cortex leads to a secondary extension to a complete fracture from the combination of weight-bearing forces and muscle contraction, especially during an attempt to "flee" from the firearm. Another mechanism occurs when the bullet imparts all the energy to the bone and leads to a fracture with significant comminution.

Long and colleagues[78] proposed a classification system for gunshot injuries to the femoral diaphysis based on wound size and radiographic appearance. Grade I injuries had entrance and exit wounds that were less than 2 cm with minimal radiographic changes. Grade II injuries were entrance and exit wounds less than 5 cm with greater radiographic changes. Grade III injuries had necrotic muscle by physical examination and extensive soft tissue disruption and segmental bone destruction on radiographs. This classification was used to guide the treatment of 100 femoral diaphyseal gunshot fractures. Although the grade III fractures were treated with repeated surgical débridement and skeletal stabilization, 50% developed deep infection, underscoring the severity of these injuries. This classification has not been validated or reported in any other series.

History and Physical Examination

An attempt should be made to obtain as much information as possible from the history and physical examination. The patient will frequently know the type of weapon and the shooting distance. This information may also be available from law enforcement. Usually the patient will be unable to stand or walk although some may actually run a short distance before they fall to the ground.

Emphasis during the physical examination should be placed on neurologic function and vascular status. Soft tissue swelling needs to be evaluated, and the opposite thigh can be used for comparison. The wounds of entrance and exit require inspection for size and character of the wound edges. Large exit wounds greater than the diameter of the suspected bullet strongly suggest higher energy transfer to the bone and soft tissues.

Imaging

Standard radiographs include anteroposterior and lateral views of the entire femur. Additional views of the hip and knee may be necessary if the fracture is in proximity to these joints. The number of bullets or fragments, location, and distance from the femur should be noted. Fracture comminution per se is not a positive indicator of either the type of bullet or the amount of soft tissue injury. Multiple bone fragments that are displaced away from the femur can be considered a more reliable sign of energy transfer known as "secondary missiles." Bone and bullet fragments that follow the presumed path of the projectile are due to the suction created by the cavity formation and subsequent collapse that accompanies higher velocity or more destructive bullets. A full-length anteroposterior view of the opposite femur will be helpful in estimation of femoral length prior to stabilization of comminuted diaphyseal fractures.

Initial Treatment

An intravenous antibiotic appropriate for open fractures should be administered as soon as the diagnosis of gunshot fracture is made. A first- or second-generation cephalosporin would be a good choice. Displaced fractures are only satisfactorily stabilized by application of skeletal traction via proximal tibial (preferred) or distal femoral pin. An average adult requires a minimum of 15% of body weight, approximately 9 kg (20 lb) for a 70-kg (154 lb) individual. Delayed application of skeletal traction will permit more bleeding within the soft tissue thigh envelope and possibly be a causative agent in development of compartment syndrome of the thigh. Nondisplaced or incomplete fractures are immobilized with splints, or if the fracture is distal, knee orthoses. The entrance and exit wounds should be sterilely dressed. Skin débridement is not indicated for small typical wounds. Hemograms should be followed serially, since it is not uncommon to see substantial drops in blood volume from internal thigh bleeding.

Definitive Treatment

Definitive treatment of the gunshot femoral fracture generally follows the established principles of open fracture management with a few exceptions. Low-energy (velocity) gunshots are treated similarly to closed femoral shaft fractures. High-energy (velocity) gunshots mandate surgical débridement of the soft tissues and bone. Fracture stabilization can be accomplished by the surgeon's choice of either external or internal fixation. Antibiotic coverage should be given as for any open fracture. Soft tissue coverage may be necessary in more severe cases involving tissue loss.

Diaphyseal and Subtrochanteric Fractures

Closed intramedullary nailing has become the treatment of choice for most closed and many open femoral fractures. Functional and clinical outcomes have been highly satisfactory, even in high-energy fractures (Fig. 19-20). Formerly, there was concern that gunshot fractures were a unique kind of open fracture and should be treated with a short course of antibiotics and delayed intramedullary nailing. It has been established through several studies that acute intramedullary nailing of low- to mid-velocity (energy) gunshot femoral fractures produces results that are essentially equivalent to intramedullary nailing of closed fractures.[79] Practical experience in major urban trauma centers has borne out the fact there is no advantage to delayed nailing.[80] The timing of intramedullary nailing of low- to mid-velocity (energy) gunshot femoral fractures is therefore at the discretion of the surgeon and the available resources.

High-velocity (energy) fractures whether caused by handguns, shotguns, or rifles should be considered as serious, or grade III, open fractures because of the significant bone and soft tissue damage that typically occurs. Cavitation and crushing from the projectile produce large amounts of necrotic muscle and devitalized bone fragments that must be débrided. Large entrance or exit wounds are débrided and can be extended in an anatomic manner, as necessary. Thorough pulsatile lavage irrigation assists in removal of loose tissue

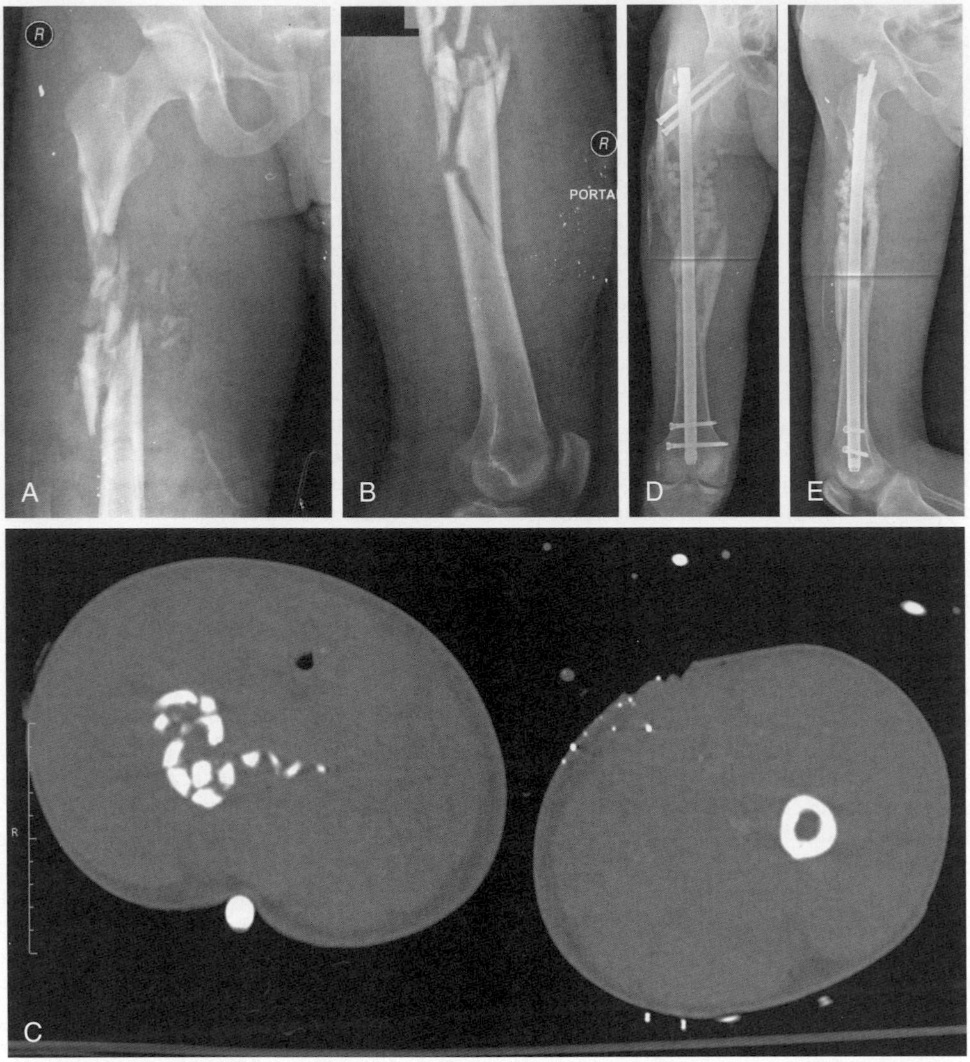

Figure 19-20. Documented assault rifle injury to right thigh. **A** and **B,** Radiographs demonstrating severe comminution and bone loss to the femoral diaphysis. **C,** Computed tomography (CT) scan done for evaluation of possible vascular injury indicates the extent of comminution. **D** and **E,** After initial half-pin external fixation and multiple serial débridements, definitive fracture stabilization was performed with a cephalomedullary nail technique as seen in the radiographs.

fragments. The authors prefer to leave the original entrance and exit wounds open for delayed closure and primarily close the surgical extensions only if wound tension permits.

Numerous options exist for fracture stabilization after surgical débridement. Skeletal traction, a time-honored method of femoral immobilization, is useful when the definitive method of fracture fixation has not been determined or there is concern about the status of the soft tissues. Wound care may be difficult in skeletal traction. It will "buy time" but rarely is used for definitive treatment.

External fixation has emerged as an excellent alternative method of fracture stabilization mainly for temporary (and occasionally definitive) purposes. "Damage control" is widely practiced in the management of multiple trauma patients, including those with gunshot injuries. Acute external fixation permits rapid bone fixation, facilitates access to the soft tissues, and eases patient mobilization. Miric and Nikolic[81,82] have reported experience in the use of external fixation with massive war wounds of subtrochanteric and supracondylar femoral fractures. They noted that the final outcome was mainly due not to the skeletal injury but to the soft tissue damage. These studies indicate, at least for severe gunshot wounds, that external fixation generally achieved fracture healing but limitation of joint motion, contractures, and persistent nerve deficits were a common outcome.

There are some physiologic advantages of external fixation and several options for further fracture care. Occasionally, the initial external fixator can be maintained until complete fracture healing in patients in whom internal fixation is not suitable or possible. A half-pin external frame can be converted to a circular ring system, which will permit distraction osteogenesis in those fractures with large bone defects. However, most common and most appropriate for diaphyseal fractures is conversion to intramedullary nailing, if performed within 2 weeks of the acute injury. Plate fixation can also be performed after external fixation in suitable fracture patterns.

The only series of plate fixation reported for gunshot femoral fractures is the study by Necmioglu and colleagues.[83] They had 17 patients with high-velocity gunshot fractures distributed as subtrochanteric (7), supracondylar (7), and diaphyseal (3). All patients initially had surgical débridement. Seven of the patients underwent minimally invasive percutaneous plate fixation at a mean of 1.3 days, and the remaining 10 patients at a mean of 11.5 days. Follow-up averaged 25 months. Fracture union was noted at a mean of 4.4 months in 16 patients. One patient had autogenous bone grafting for a delayed union in the early group, and four in the later group required grafting at the time of plate fixation for bone loss. Eight patients had angulatory malunions (mean, 5 degrees; range, 3 to 8 degrees). There were two infections: one superficial and one deep. The authors concluded that plate fixation was an alternative method of fracture treatment in high-velocity femoral fractures.

Patients who have femoral fractures with associated vascular injury that require repair pose special problems. Rehman and colleagues[84] studied 24 patients retrospectively with such injuries. Patients who had vascular repair first prior to fracture stabilization had more complications with two vascular repairs being disrupted after femoral fixation. Our policy is to rapidly apply a half pin external fixator to establish femoral length and alignment. This facilitates the vascular repair at the correct length and in a stable surgical field. If the decision is to proceed with vascular repair first, then at the minimum, the femoral fracture should be brought to length grossly and temporarily stabilized with towel bundles. Subsequently careful application of external fixation is performed. In rare cases, the patient may be hemodynamically unstable precluding any further surgery after vascular repair and skeletal traction can be applied via a proximal tibial pin. The traction weight must be minimized to only that sufficient to maintain femoral length. It must be emphasized that this is a suboptimal technique.

Distal Femoral Fractures

Gunshots to the lower thigh may produce either extraarticular or intraarticular fractures. A series by Tornetta and colleagues[79] used anterograde intramedullary nails for distal shaft and metaphyseal fractures. The distance from the fracture to the distal locking screws was less than 5 cm in all cases, emphasizing the distal fracture location. All 38 patients healed in an average of 8.6 weeks. Many of these fractures would now be treated with a retrograde nail or newer generation distal femoral plate.

Supracondylar fractures with intraarticular extension secondary to gunshots are often deceptive (Fig. 19-21). Fracture comminution may not be appreciated on preoperative radiographs, and limited CT axial, coronal, and sagittal reconstructions are recommended to evaluate all aspects of the fractures. Both retrograde intramedullary nails and precontoured distal femoral plates with some locking capability are effective in achieving stable fixation in these fractures. The method chosen relates to the surgeon's preference and the integrity of the femoral notch region.

Tibia

The tibia is commonly injured by gunshots. The anteromedial aspect of the leg is quite vulnerable to bullets with dissipation of kinetic energy directly into the tibia not dampened by surrounding muscles. Many gunshot victims are in an upright position at the time of wounding, and the force of body weight acts on the tibia to create more fracture displacement. The diameter of the leg is considerably less than that of the thigh, and the probability of neurologic deficits is greater. Nondisplaced and minimally displaced fractures are clear indications for nonoperative treatment with casting or fracture bracing. Displaced fractures are treated as the surgeon would treat other open tibial fractures. Assessment of the associated soft tissue injury in gunshot tibial fractures can be challenging. Comminuted fracture patterns are frequent and may be indicative of significant soft tissue injury. As with all other gunshots, a large exit wound is highly suggestive of deep soft tissue disruption. The safest course of action, if there is doubt, is to surgically explore the soft tissue and bone and débride as indicated.

Leffers and Chandler[85] did a retrospective review of 41 tibial gunshot fractures at an urban trauma center. They divided the patients into three groups on the basis of the projectile velocity: low, intermediate, and high. They found that low-velocity gunshots had a characteristic fracture pattern with minimal comminution and that all other gunshots created highly comminuted fractures. Fracture treatment was usually casting, with external fixation used in a minority of patients. Increased length of hospital stay, time to union, and morbidity were associated with the intermediate- and high-velocity groups. Both nonunions in this series occurred in patients with low-velocity fractures.

In a study by Meskey and colleagues, retrospective review of all gunshot fractures over a 6-year period yielded a 2.8% incidence of compartment syndrome.[86] The most likely fractures to develop a compartment syndrome were fractures of the proximal fibula and proximal tibia. Therefore, the orthopaedic surgeon should maintain a high suspicion for possible compartment syndromes in these fractures.

Displaced gunshot fractures of the tibial diaphysis have been treated with various forms of fixation. There are no specific prospective or retrospective studies of the treatment of gunshot fractures of the tibia with intramedullary fixation. Most major series of tibial intramedullary nailing have included a few cases of gunshots (of low velocity), with no apparent difference in outcome when compared with other open fractures in the series.

Direct evidence in the literature is lacking for the specific results of internal fixation of gunshot tibial fractures. The reported clinical experience with the other mechanisms of injury for open tibial fractures should be a reasonable approximation of the anticipated results with gunshot fractures.

External fixation has been reported recently to be clinically effective in the more severe tibial fractures, especially with bone loss. Circular external fixation, flap coverage, and distraction osteogenesis have been used to reestablish bone length and continuity with minimal morbidity. Circular external fixation generally permits early weight bearing with its attendant advantages (Fig. 19-22).

Atesalp and colleagues[87] reported on seven patients with comminuted gunshot tibial fractures managed with circular external fixation and compression-distraction technique. All fractures united at an average of 3.5 months without infection. These were low-velocity injuries and would be anticipated to unite in this time frame. The major problems associated with circular external fixation are pin track infection and the requirement for additional surgery at the docking site in fractures that required distraction osteogenesis. It remains a suitable alternative in any displaced fracture.

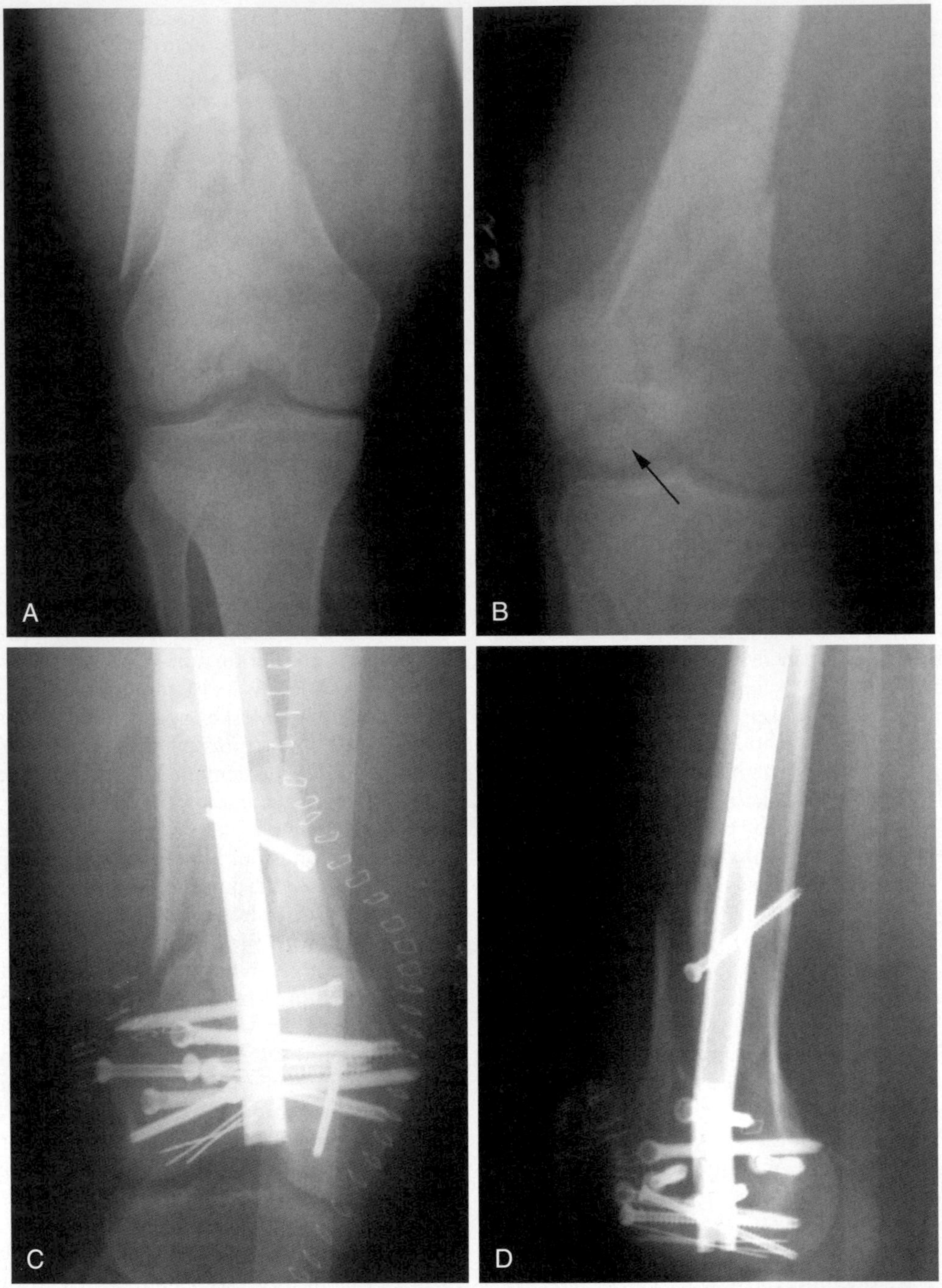

Figure 19-21. **A,** Single through-and-through gunshot to the distal femur in an obese patient. Initial radiographs (**A** and **B**) show what appears to be a mildly comminuted supracondylar fracture with intercondylar extension *(arrows)*. A computed tomography (CT) scan could not be obtained owing to the patient's body weight. At the time of arthrotomy, severe comminution was present with multiple osteochondral fractures. Fracture fixation was performed with a retrograde intramedullary nail supplemented by multiple lag screws and free wires. **C,** Anteroposterior view. **D,** Lateral view.

Intraarticular Fractures

Gunshot fractures of the proximal and distal tibia with intraarticular involvement are unusual. Unfortunately, in the author's experience, there can be a great deal of loss of articular surface and metaphyseal bone. Acute arthrotomy or arthroscopy is indicated for débridement of bone fragments and any lead pieces that are loose or in contact with the joint fluid. However, any fracture fragments with articular cartilage should be retained for definitive joint fixation. Temporary bridging external fixation will maintain fracture length and position. When the soft tissues permit, anatomic restoration of the articular surface is the goal but may not be possible. Bone defects should be filled with either autogenous bone or bone substitutes. Stable internal fixation alone or the combination of limited internal fixation and circular external fixation is recommended. Some degree of early joint motion is preferable for surface lubrication and nutrition. Fracture healing is achieved in the majority of patients, but there is a high

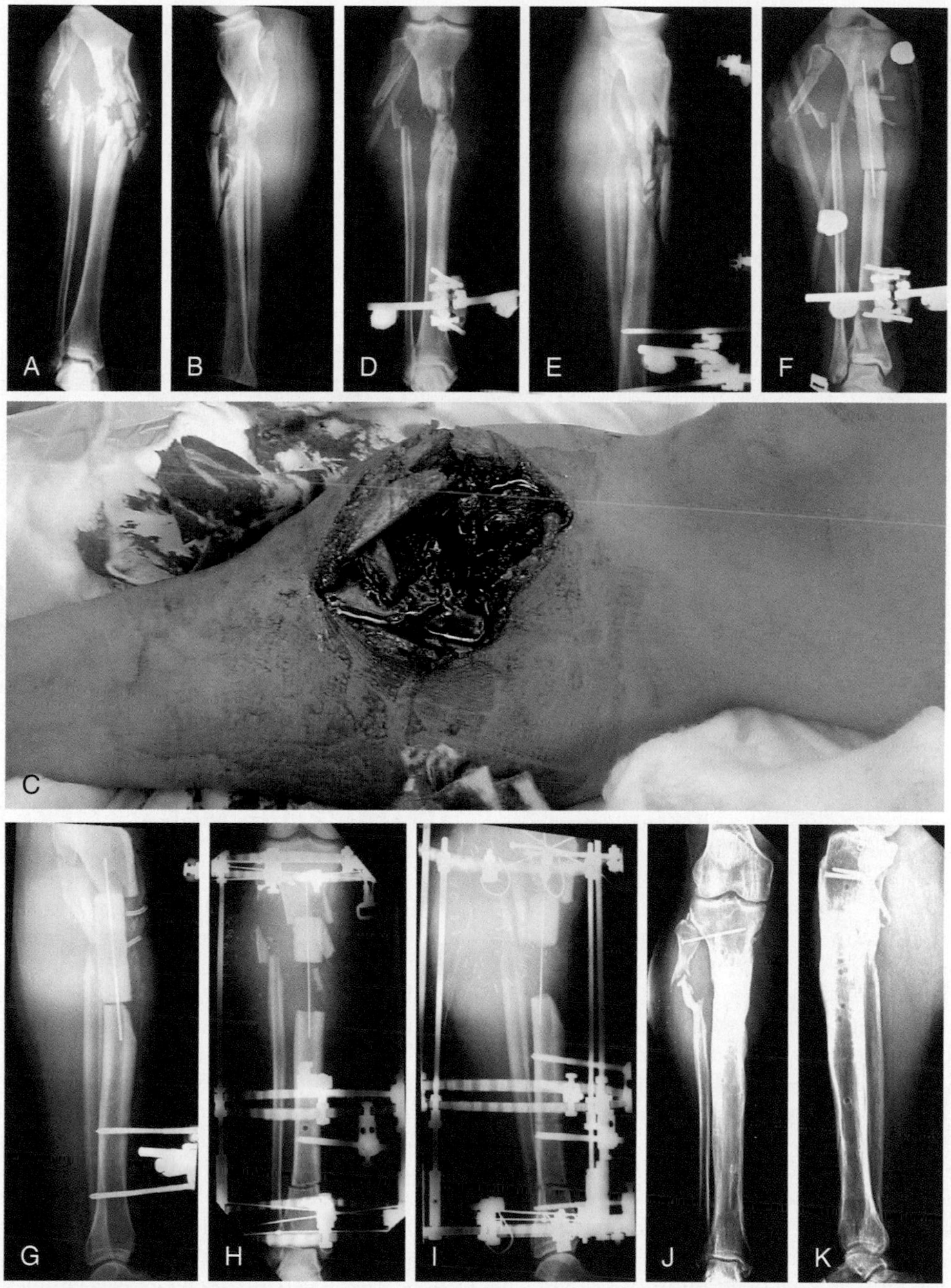

Figure 19-22. Documented assault rifle injury to the tibia. **A** and **B,** Radiographs shows severely comminuted fractures of the proximal tibia and fibula with minimal metallic fragments. **C,** Exit wound with massive soft tissue damage and protruding bone fragments. **D** and **E,** Initial débridement and half-pin external fixation were followed by serial débridements until only viable tissues remained. **F** and **G,** An antibiotic cement spacer maintained length of the 11-cm bone defect. **H** and **I,** Reconstruction of the extremity proceeded with revision to circular external fixation with a distal to proximal bone transport distraction osteogenesis. **J** and **K,** Radiographs at 3-year follow-up examination with complete reconstruction of the extremity with normal length and alignment, no infection, and function restored.

incidence of traumatic arthrosis due to irreparable articular cartilage damage and poor functional outcome in the more severe injuries.

Yildiz and colleagues[88] reported their retrospective results in 13 patients with high-velocity gunshot fractures of the tibial plafond. There were 11 grade IIIA and 2 grade IIIB open fractures. Treatment consisted of débridement, primary wound closure, and Ilizarov fixation. Intraarticular fractures were manipulated indirectly by frame distraction or directly by Kirschner wires; however, no screw or plate fixation was used. Three patients required distraction osteogenesis for bone loss. All fractures healed with an average tibiotalar motion of 30 degrees. Four patients had radiographic arthritis at a mean follow-up of 38.4 months. Pin track infection was seen in the majority of patients. Superficial wound infection occurred in two patients. This group of fractures was probably incorrectly classified in terms of the degree of joint involvement, as it is quite uncommon, in the author's experience, for intraarticular

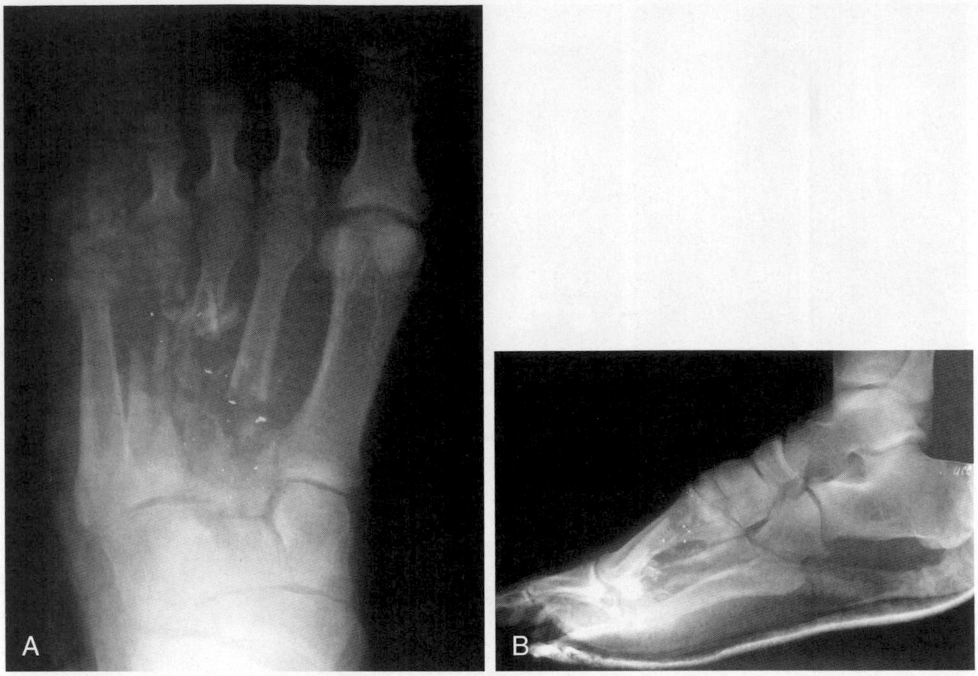

Figure 19-23. Low-velocity tangential gunshot to the dorsal foot with severe comminution and bone loss of multiple metatarsals. **A,** Anteroposterior view. **B,** Lateral view.

distal tibial fractures to not require some limited internal fixation to restore joint congruity.

Foot

Low-velocity gunshot wounds to the foot are often self-inflicted, accidentally or intentionally. Fractures are usually comminuted with minimal displacement. There are many joints within the foot and they are often violated by the gunshot. In most cases, the soft tissues do not sustain significant damage. Some gunshots, however, have such a trajectory through the foot that there can be bone loss and severe comminution (Fig. 19-23).

Bullet fragments are not well tolerated in the foot and interfere with weight-bearing and shoe wear. This is one of the few surgical indications to "take the bullet out" especially if the fragment(s) are in a superficial location.

The treatment for most low-velocity gunshot fractures to the foot should follow the principles for closed foot fractures. A variable period of immobilization in a cast, weight bearing if possible, will achieve fracture healing in a relatively short period of time. Stiffness of the articulations that were violated by the gunshot is fairly common but rarely disabling. Higher-grade injuries with bone loss and skeletal deformity require appropriate surgical reconstruction and possibly soft tissue coverage.[89]

Boucree and colleagues[90] reviewed 101 patients with gunshot wounds of the foot, with 81 fractures. Infection was encountered in approximately 12%, equally divided between low-velocity and high-velocity or shotgun injuries. From this experience, they recommended a course of intravenous antibiotic for 72 hours for low-velocity gunshot and shotgun injuries. They suggested that high-velocity gunshot and shotgun injuries receive surgical débridement and intravenous antibiotics.

ORTHOPAEDIC MANAGEMENT IN THE BLAST TRAUMA PATIENT

In the wake of the 9/11 attacks against the United States and the subsequent War on Terrorism, blast trauma has become the most common mechanism of wounding among U.S. and coalition troops, contractors, and civilians.[91] The magnitude, frequency, and sophistication of these devices has increased as well throughout the course of the conflict as enemy combatants have improved their techniques in the attempt to maximize the effects of their attacks and have also been forced to attempt to counter coalition antiexplosives countermeasures. By far, the most commonly deployed explosive device used by enemy combatants has been, and continues to be, the improvised explosive device (IED). This constitutes a broad range of devices, deployment methods, size, and sophistication. The spectrum includes everything from bombs using everyday household items, to buried and repurposed artillery shells with remote triggering devices, to suicide and homicide bombers (with increasingly frequent use of women and children in this capacity), to the more massive and lethal vehicle-borne IEDs, and to even more sophisticated, armor-piercing explosively formed projectiles. The reasons for the incremental increase in the deployment of these destructive devices is multifactorial, but can be attributed to the ready availability of materials, the devastation that they are capable of providing, and the relatively low risk to the attackers versus engaging in force-on-force combat with coalition forces (Fig. 19-24, *A*).

The net effect of these attacks on both the intended and unintended victims has been to impart a devastating amount of trauma, resulting in massive soft tissue injury, multiple fractures and/or amputations, heavily contaminated wounds, as well as injuries to multiple other organ systems to include

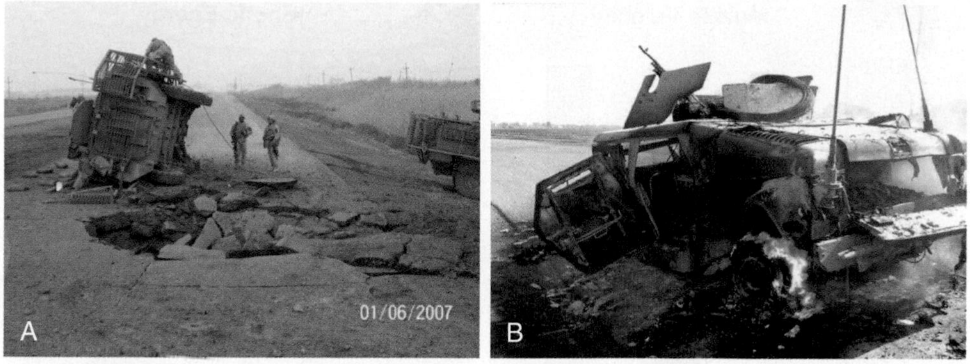

Figure 19-24. Mechanisms of blast trauma include the initial blast wave, primary and secondary debris, and victim collision with fixed objects as a result of being tossed by the blast wave, burns, and other late effects. **A,** This military Stryker vehicle, weighing 16 to 20 tons, was flipped and destroyed by an improvised explosive device (IED) blast. **B,** The armored military high mobility multipurpose wheeled vehicle (HMMWV) pictured was destroyed by an IED blast.

the bowel, the middle ear, and the lungs. As our experience with, and understanding of, these injuries has increased, there has been a concurrent improvement in both our treatment stratagems and techniques. Significant advances have been made in the areas of soft tissue management techniques, staged multidisciplinary management of these complexly injured patients, and specifically within the area of nontraditional amputation and débridement strategies, rehabilitation, and prosthetics (Fig. 19-24, *B*).

Perhaps one of the most important questions is, how does this affect the civilian orthopaedic surgeon? In addition to the translation of specific technical advances, the incidence of terrorism and blast trauma within the civilian sector is also increasing and may be experienced by any surgeon both domestically and abroad. Having a working understanding of the injury mechanisms and treatment stratagems developed on the battlefield and within the military evacuation and echelons of care system may help the civilian orthopaedic surgeon in the management of multiple, severely injured patients in a mass casualty situation. This can be focally highlighted by the recent terrorist attack at the finish line of the 2013 Boston Marathon. This particular attack may, sadly, provide a template that is likely to be seen with increasing frequency within the civilian sector. A large and difficult to monitor crowd, which is spread out over a geographically challenging area to control, provides a tactically enticing target wherein placement of an IED can wreak great devastation, yet provide easy cover for the attacker's egress from the scene. As was seen in Boston, well-placed relatively small devices resulted in a large number of casualties from a combination of the various blast mechanisms that will be subsequently discussed.

Blast Trauma Mechanisms of Injury

Blast devices can be broken down into two broad categories based on the speed and magnitude of their energy dispersion. These two categories can be defined as either low-energy (LE), or high-energy (HE) devices. The principal differentiation between the two categories is determined by the speed at which they burn. A LE explosive burns, or deflagrates at a speed of 1000 m/s (meters per second) or less. Common examples include black gunpowder, smokeless gunpowder, and gasoline. They tend to produce large amounts of gas that explode only when confined such as that which occurs in a common pipe bomb. Conversely, HE explosive burns at a speed in excess of 4500 m/s. This creates a hypersonic blast wave (shock wave) even if the ignited explosive is unconfined. Typical examples include TNT, dynamite, ammonium nitrate, fuel oil, and plastic explosives such as C4 and Semtex. These explosions impart an enormous amount of injury to the soft tissues and skeletal system incorporating sufficient energy to create a shattering effect termed *brisance*.[3] The most devastating and common terrorism-based injury patterns are secondary to HE explosives and will be the primary focus of the continuing discussion.

There are four relatively distinct phases of injury that occur secondary to a HE explosion.

1. Primary Blast Injury: The initiation of HE explosions creates an almost instantaneous, hypersonic, circumferential shock wave of blast overpressure that, in an open environment, dissipates at a predictable rate as it expands over time and distance. This is known as a Friedlander curve or wave. At the point of detonation, pounds per square inch (psi) may exceed 14 million psi, with as little as 60 to 80 psi being frequently fatal. Thus, those in closest proximity to the detonation have little chance of survival. Much of the devastating soft tissue trauma that occurs during a blast is due to the effects of this pressure wave as it passes through soft tissue. Several mechanisms have been postulated as causing injury during this phase. Covey and Born[92] describe the mechanism of injury as the pressure wave passes through tissues of different densities, notably at air/fluid interfaces as a combination of spalling (forced, explosive movement of fluids from more dense to less dense tissues, i.e., lung tissue), and implosion (sudden and forcible collapse of hollow organs, followed by rapid re-expansion and tissue injury after the pressure wave passes). Further, the mechanism of brisance, or shattering as the pressure wave passes has been well described. This can result in fracturing throughout the appendicular skeleton (most notably in the subpatellar tendon/proximal tibia region). When combined with the shearing and stretching forces applied to the soft tissue envelope, this combination of forces can result in partial and/or complete traumatic amputations. Because of the high amount of energy required to impart this amount of

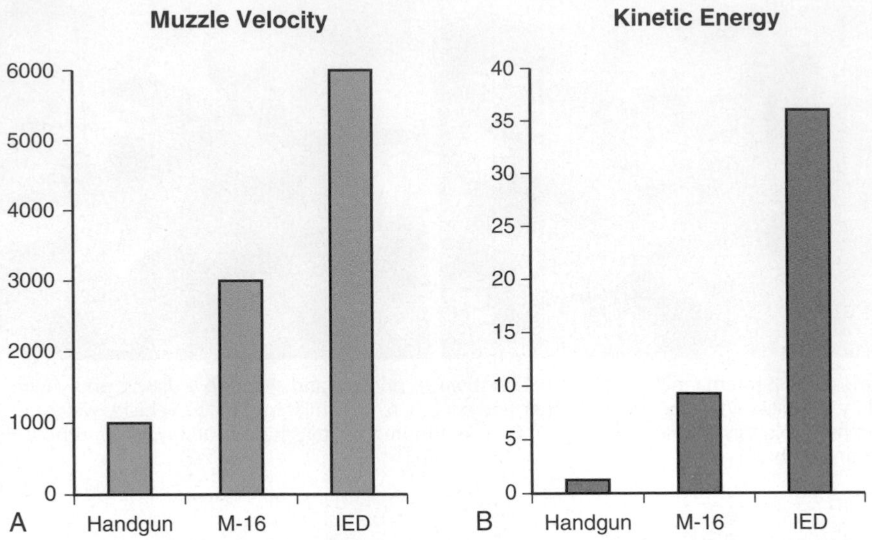

Figure 19-25. Generalized initial velocities of common wounding mechanisms, with their imparted kinetic energy *(KE)* based on $KE = \text{Mass} \times \text{Velocity}^2$. *IED,* Improvised explosive device.

energy as well as to the concomitant injury to the lungs and other hollow organs, survival of a victim who has sustained a blast injury amputation is tenuous at best (Fig. 19-25).

Several notable facts to understand about blast waves are that they do in fact act much like waves. They can be deflected by large, fixed structures. They will flow around obstacles, resulting in a concentration of forces. They will deflect off of fixed structures, likewise causing a multifold increase in the concentration of force at the areas of deflection. Persons who are protected by a fixed object that is capable of deflecting the force of a blast wave are subjected to an order of magnitude less energy. Blast waves set off within closed spaces do not exhibit a typical Friedlander wave pattern and will continue to bounce off of opposing walls causing retention of energy, higher peak pressures, and a blast wave of longer duration of within that confined space, resulting in much poorer chances of survivability. A blast wave set off in a liquid medium, such as a body of water, tends to travel much more quickly, and to dissipate energy much more slowly, again resulting in poorer chances of survival for the victims of such incidences.

2. Secondary Blast Injury: For the person who survives the primary blast injury, secondary blast injury may be of even more significant concern. Secondary blast injury is caused by both primary fragmentation (flying debris from the explosive device itself) and secondary fragmentation (those objects that are picked up by the blast wave and propelled in its wake). In the case of the IED, this may include random household or industrial objects such as bolts, nuts, finishing nails, ball bearings, marbles, and jacks. Secondary fragmentation may consist of both organic and nonorganic substances, and in the case of the suicide or homicide bomber, may include tissues from the bomber himself. Both primary and secondary projectiles will act somewhat in accordance with well-recognized ballistic characteristics as they penetrate soft tissues based on both their mass and velocity at time of impact. However, as opposed to regularly formed, aerodynamic rifle or handgun projectiles, these fragments will be more irregularly shaped, often are larger, and may be flying in irregular patterns. This can result in a host of bizarrely implanted projectiles, greater cavitation effect, amputations from flying debris, and in combination with primary blast injury, highly contaminated and extensive soft tissue injuries in addition to highly comminuted fractures (Figs. 19-26 and 19-27).
3. Tertiary Blast Injury: This third phase of blast injury can be most succinctly described as those injuries which are sustained by the victim as he or she is thrown outward by the blast wave and strikes hard structures such as walls, fixed objects, and/or the ground. This can result in a large number of orthopaedic injuries in and of its own right.
4. Quaternary Blast Injury: The final phase of blast injury has perhaps the widest diversity of definition. In general,

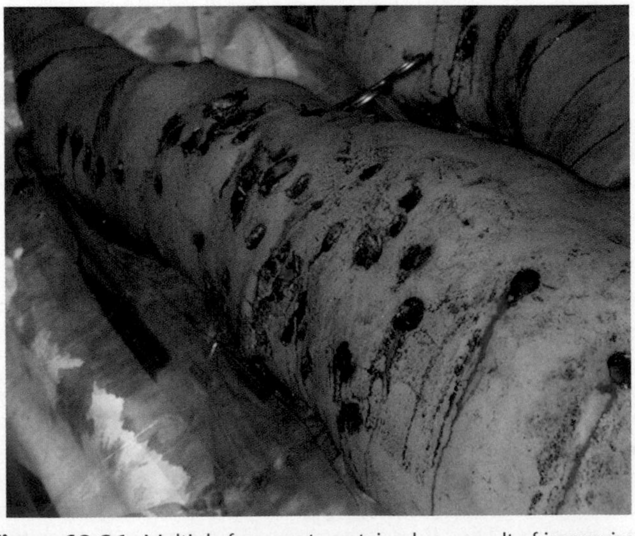

Figure 19-26. Multiple fragments sustained as a result of improvised ball bearings placed within an improvised explosive device (IED).

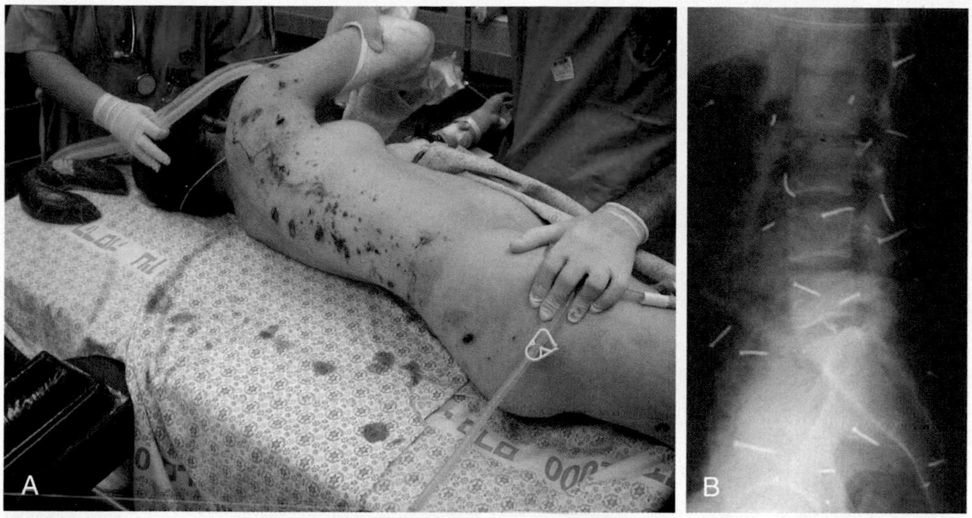

Figure 19-27. A, Blast trauma victim shows little external damage during her initial emergency department presentation. **B,** The same patient shows multiple penetration of finishing nails throughout her body secondary to improvised shrapnel placed within the improvised explosive device (IED).

it is the late effects of the first three phases and their resultant injuries. In the realm of orthopaedics, this could be compartment syndromes, myonecrosis, or burns.

Modern, deployed coalition militaries have several unique advantages when coping with a terrorist bombing versus civilian medical infrastructure. Primarily they are expecting mass blast trauma as a normal course of their activities and are medically prepared and deployed for this eventuality. They have forward-placed surgical assets within minutes of the point of injury with blood transfusion capabilities. Medevac capability is readily available in most instances and within close proximity to the point of injury. Patrolling service members routinely wear advanced body armor and antiballistic helmets with resultant protection to the chest, abdomen, and head.

Body armor and helmets have played a significant role in protecting soldiers in combat situations from multiple mechanisms of injury, potentially resulting in an increased incidence of survivable extremity trauma.

Additionally, medics are ubiquitous within the maneuver units themselves. The rapid application of tourniquets by these medics, as well as by the trained service members themselves has saved many lives, and nearly all deployed U.S. service members are supplied with these and are instructed on their use. One final advantage that the military has is that they have a relatively young, motivated, and underlying disease-free population, which is not necessarily reflective of the typical patient who will be seen in a civilian hospital facing similar circumstances.

These described advantages have resulted in a paradoxically high survival rate among some of those service members who have been the most highly injured secondary to HE explosions. This has led to increased recognition of several injury patterns that may not have been significantly recognized during previous conflicts, due to significantly poorer survival rates. As resources were shifted from the Iraqi Theater of Operations (ITO) to the Afghanistan Theater of Operations (ATO) in 2009-2010, there was a sharp increase noted in the severity of injury seen in patrolling service members who were subjected to blast trauma versus their counterparts in the ITO. Theory points to the likely culprit of this phenomenon as the shift from vehicle-mounted patrols, which were in primary use in the ITO toward primarily dismounted patrols that were forced by the terrain of the ATO. As the insurgents in Afghanistan became more sophisticated and well supplied, they quickly began deploying IEDs against the dismounted troops in Afghanistan that were of similar size and sophistication as those that were faced by the mounted troops in Iraq. The result of this relatively increased level of blast energy to patrolling service members has been the recognition of a category of blast trauma patients that fit what is now recognized as dismounted complex blast injury (DCBI)[93-95] (Fig. 19-28).

Specifically, two patterns of injury have been described. The first has been well described by Mamczak and colleagues and consists of bilateral (generally high above knee) lower extremity amputations in combination with open pelvic fractures, genitourinary injuries, and massive exsanguination.[95] During the 2009-2011 surge of troops into the ATO, a relatively large number of these patients presented to both level II+ (austere forward surgical teams) as well as more capable level III

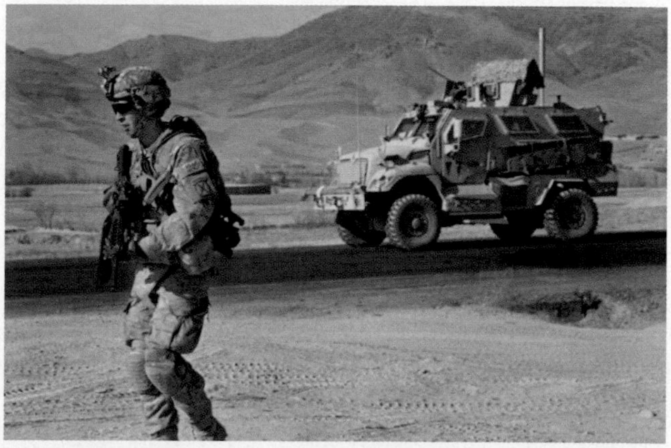

Figure 19-28. Stark contrasts exist in the amount of energy imparted to the soldiers protected by armored, blast-resistant vehicles, and that which is imparted to the dismounted soldier.

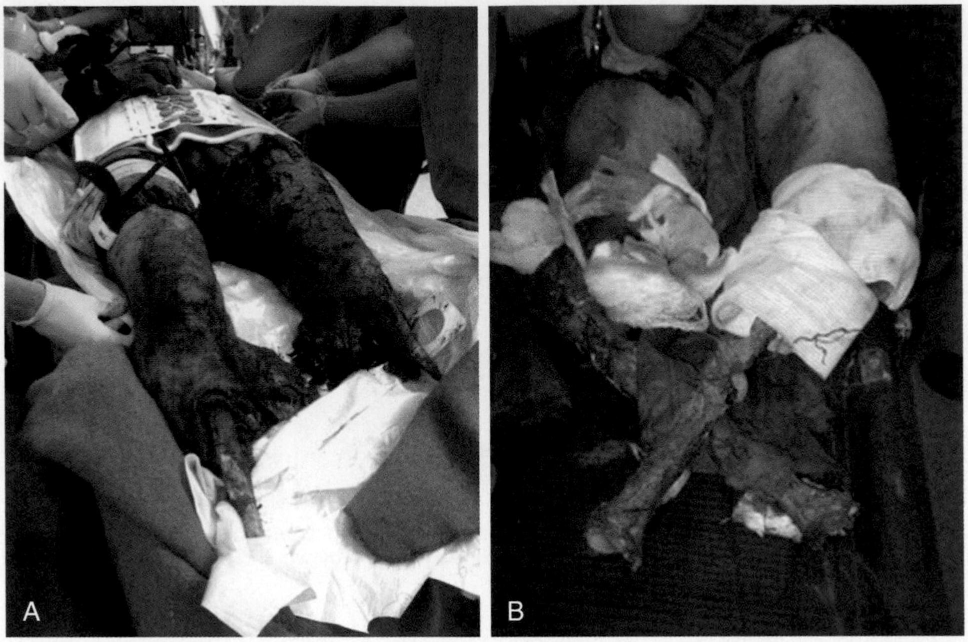

Figure 19-29. Dismounted complex blast injury (DCBI) victims with multiple amputations, severe extremity trauma, open pelvic fractures, and potentially urogenital injuries are an increasing percentage of patients being treated on the battlefield.

(combat support hospitals) facilities. These patients presented in extremis and required intensive, staged treatment efforts, both surgical and resuscitative, to offer even a chance of survival. Control of hemorrhage, up to and including cross-clamping of the descending aorta and/or the iliac arteries, and pelvic packing, in combination with pelvic ring external fixation and massive transfusion was required during the initial resuscitation phase of care. This initial treatment was followed by staged washouts of extremity and soft tissue wounds, further resuscitation, frequent revision of amputations as tissue necrosis and the soft tissue wounds evolved. Those who survived the initial insult and resuscitation still sustained a high incidence of mortality secondary to multisystem organ failure and/or sepsis. Of note, *Mucor* species fungal infections were noted to occur frequently, with a resultant need for aggressive débridement and often revisions of amputations to higher levels up to and including full or partial hemipelvectomy. The second major category of DCBI patient noted and described by Andersen and others has been the multiple major amputation patient.[93] Concurrent with the increase in relative blast energy and imparted blast trauma noted earlier, a statistically significant increase in double, triple, and quadruple amputees has been noted. These patients likewise have presented in extremis, required a robust team approach to their management, and present significant treatment, rehabilitation, and prosthetic challenges (Fig. 19-29).

Lessons Learned

Several key factors have been identified during the course of the War on Terrorism as being key to the improved survival and posttrauma function of blast injury patients. Included on this list are:

1. Tourniquets applied liberally and effectively have resulted in the saving of lives and the loss of relatively few limbs.[96] With nearly every service member supplied with and trained in their use, as well as with other hemostatic agents such as combat gauze, the loss of life from compressible exsanguination has dropped significantly (Fig. 19-30).
2. Junctional bleeding (groin and axilla) is still a source of concern and is poorly managed outside of the operating room. Significant further work remains in this realm.
3. Blood transfusion is critical.[3] Both the specific ratio of transfused components (a 1 : 1 : 1 ratio of packed red blood cells/plasma/platelets) as well as the amount and rapidity of transfusion have been described in the literature as saving lives. Whole blood transfusion from a predesignated donor pool has also been noted to be significantly beneficial to the patient in extremis, but is fraught with many potential complications, and should only be used in those circumstances when other supplies have been, or are likely to be, exhausted. A

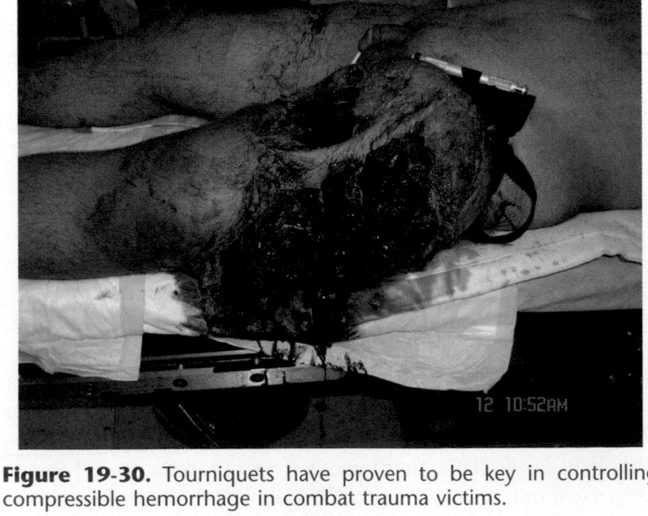

Figure 19-30. Tourniquets have proven to be key in controlling compressible hemorrhage in combat trauma victims.

well-designed and practiced whole blood drive program, like any successful disaster contingency program, is essential for proper functioning of the system during instances of actual need.

4. Surgical care and resuscitation prepositioned as close as possible to the point of injury has likewise resulted in the saving of lives.
5. The blast trauma patient in extremis cannot tolerate extended time in the operating room. The patient is likely in or bordering the "triad of death"—hypovolemia, hypothermia, and hypocoagulability. Despite the ongoing and aggressive resuscitation that will be carried out in the operating room, a patient's physiologic reserve will not tolerate much further insult. As opposed to a typical civilian trauma where each surgical service (general, vascular, orthopaedic, urology, etc.) tends to operate in turn in a priority-based serial approach, the blast trauma patient needs a prioritized, yet parallel effort in order to maximize the use of limited surgical time. Once the trauma team conducts the initial evaluation, the principal surgical services must agree and execute a planned and coordinated resuscitation and surgical stabilization of the patient. Often, all that must be done cannot occur in the initial surgical setting because of the patient's tenuous physiologic condition, and further resuscitation must be carried out in the intensive care unit prior to a second or third round of surgery. This need not take days, but hours, dependent on the patient's condition (Fig. 19-31).

The hallmark of the extremity blast injury is massive soft tissue injury and loss. Frequently, the management of a relatively simple fracture is made significantly more complex due to the loss of skin, subcutaneous tissue, and/or muscle that can frequently be measured in square feet as opposed to square inches. These injuries are highly contaminated and continue to evolve for days to weeks. Early definitive fixation results in a high rate of infection, failure, and potential amputation. Thus, multiple staged washouts, antibiotic management, antibiotic bead pouch placement, and/or wound vacuum-assisted closure therapy are required until the wounds appear healthy and viable. At this point, coordinated care between plastic surgery and the orthopaedic surgeon is required prior to definitive internal or thin-wire external fixation and soft tissue coverage either via free or local flap coverage (Fig. 19-32).

6. Completion of partial amputations versus limb salvage continues to be a controversial issue both in military and civilian trauma settings.[97] In the blast trauma patient, amputation should be considered at the far end of the débridement spectrum and not separate from it. The basic rule of thumb taught to deploying military providers is to retain what appears viable and to discard anything that does not. Completion of a partial amputation can occur anywhere along the echelons of care (or at subsequent surgical settings in the civilian sector) and need not occur at the patient's initial interface with surgical care. Often an extremity headed for eventual amputation may retain viable tissues, particularly skin, muscle, subcutaneous tissues, and bone that may be used in the coverage or reconstruction of other wounds or amputations and thus should be spared until that definitive procedure if at all practical. Similarly, with advances in modern prosthetics, traumatic amputations should not be converted to standard below knee, or above knee amputations. These traumatic amputations should be débrided according to standard principles as discussed, retaining any viable muscle, tendon, and skin tissue in order to preserve residual limb length and thus function. Similarly, completion of amputations should not necessarily occur through the sight of a more proximal fracture. Hsu and colleagues demonstrated a high rate of curable infection secondary to definitive fixation in these circumstances, but with demonstrably improved

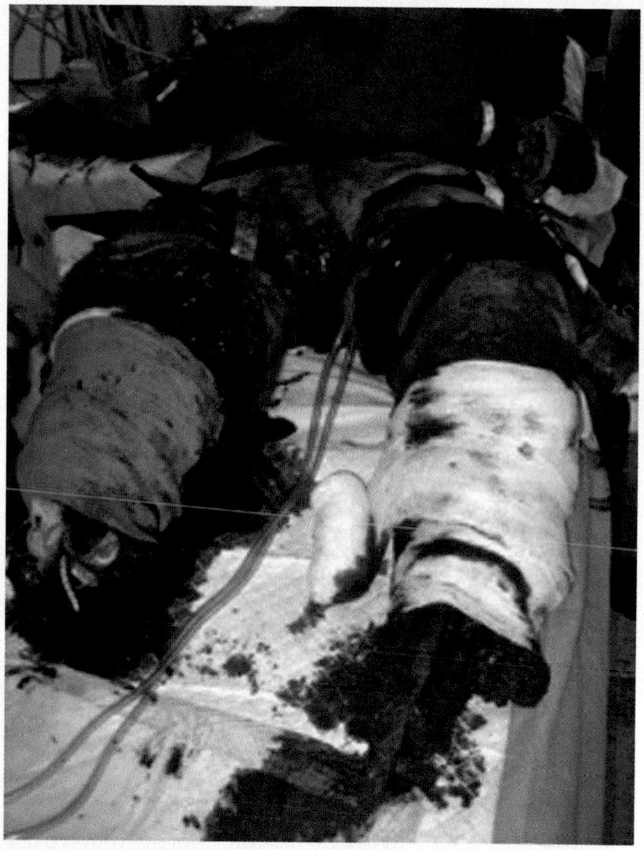

Figure 19-31. Multiply injured blast trauma patients are in extremis and cannot tolerate extended surgical procedures. A coordinated team approach is required to minimize surgically related physiological insult.

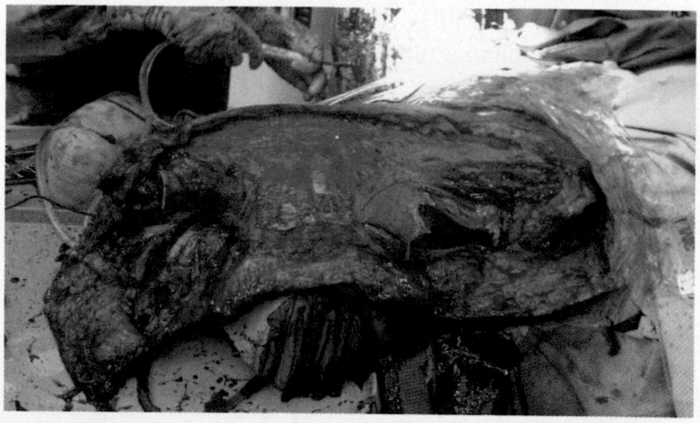

Figure 19-32. Complex, severe soft tissue injury and traumatic amputations are the major hallmarks of combat blast trauma.

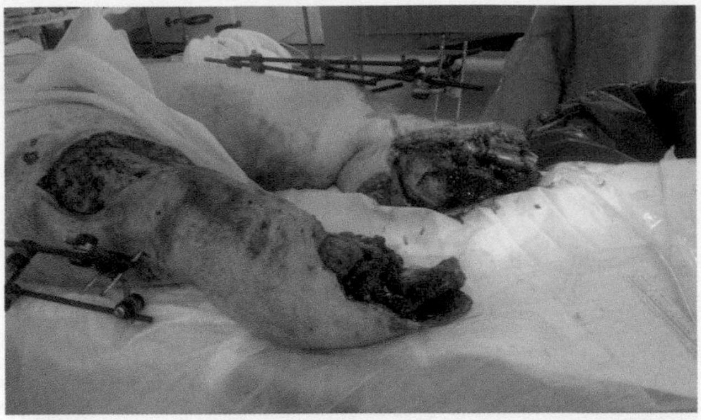

Figure 19-33. Combat blast trauma patient following multiple washouts and débridements, in preparation for further soft tissue closure and management of more proximal skeletal injuries.

function secondary to preservation of length one to two amputation levels above what may otherwise have been performed. One significant outcome of the Lower Extremity Impairment (LEAP) study was the poor long-term outcome of those patients who had sustained a complex, open tibia fracture above a mangled foot, and who underwent limb salvage. Patzowski and colleagues have developed and studied a unique prosthetic for this subcategory of trauma patient that is termed the *Intrepid Dynamic Exoskeletal Orthosis* that has resulted in instances of remarkable preservation or return of function versus that which would normally have been expected.[98] Although this device continues to be studied and made more widely available, it may present a viable alternative to amputation in the relatively young, fit, and compliant patient (Fig. 19-33).

The energy imparted by blast trauma has a high propensity to stimulate heterotopic bone formation.[99] This occurs in both the limb salvage and the limb preservation patient and often causes extreme discomfort and complications to the patient's rehabilitation course. This may frequently result in the need for later surgical excision of the affected tissues and, on occasion, result in the need for a higher level of amputation. Although prophylactic irradiation is not available on the battlefield, this may be a consideration for civilian victims of blast trauma, where available.

7. Long-term outcome for the military blast trauma patient population from the recent conflicts remains to be determined. They have frequently sustained significant injuries to other organ systems to include traumatic brain injury (TBI), loss of hearing, and pulmonary insult, which may affect their rehabilitation. The amputee population will continue to require advanced and intensive prosthetic care and the limb salvage population will continue to require care for some degree of long-term disability. Their eventual transfer from the active duty care system to the Veterans Affairs (VA) or civilian systems may play a significant role in long-term functionality and outcomes.

CONCLUSIONS

Blast trauma is becoming increasingly more ubiquitous in both military and civilian settings. The force and devastation that is wreaked upon the victims of an HE blast by the blast wave mechanism cannot be understated. The amount of force imparted can be massive, is frequently fatal, and is responsible for a large percentage of the overwhelming injuries that are sustained during either a terrorist IED attack or a large-scale industrial explosive accident. A thorough understanding of the mechanics of blast waves and their effects on physiology and soft tissues will help providers in both settings appreciate and properly manage these complexly injured patients. Further understanding of the secondary, tertiary, and quaternary mechanisms of blast injury trauma likewise will aid in the evaluation and management of these patients throughout the spectrum of their initial care and through their often long and complex rehabilitations.

KEY REFERENCES

The level of evidence (LOE) is determined according to the criteria provided in the preface.

7. Howland WS Jr, Ritchey SJ: Gunshot fractures in civilian practice: an evaluation of the results of limited surgical treatment. *J Bone Joint Surg Am* 53:47–55, 1971. LOE IV
8. Dickey RL, Barnes BC, Kearns RJ, et al: Efficacy of antibiotics in low-velocity gunshot fractures. *J Orthop Trauma* 3:6–10, 1989. LOE IV
9. Knapp TP, Patzakis MJ, Lee J, et al: Comparison of intravenous and oral antibiotic therapy in the treatment of fractures caused by low-velocity gunshots: a prospective, randomized study of infection rates. *J Bone Joint Surg Am* 79:1590, 1997. LOE II
24. Subramanian A, Vercruysse G, Dente C, et al: A decade's experience with temporary intravascular shunts at a civilian level I trauma center. *J Trauma* 65(2):316–324, 2008. LOE IV
92. Covey DC, Born CT: Blast injuries: mechanics and wounding patterns. *J Surg Orthop Adv* 19(1):8–12, 2010. LOE III
95. Mamczak CN, Elster EA: Complex dismounted IED blast injuries: the initial management of bilateral lower extremity amputations with and without pelvic and perineal involvement. *J Surg Orthop Adv* 21(1):8–14, 2012. LOE III

The complete References list is available online at https://expertconsult.inkling.com.

Chapter 20

Pathologic Fractures

ROBERT J. STEFFNER • ANDRE R. SPIGUEL • TESSA BALACH

INTRODUCTION

Pathologic fractures can be a source of diagnostic and therapeutic challenge to the practicing orthopaedic surgeon. These often unexpected fractures can be a significant cause of anxiety for patients, who are told they have a tumor, as well as for surgeons. Pathologic fractures, by nature, occur through bone that is biologically abnormal and where the response to and potential for healing can be dramatically different from normal bone for a variety of reasons, including neoplastic and nonneoplastic processes. As a result of this inherent biologic difference, the treatment of pathologic fractures needs to be considered from a different perspective with a different evaluation and treatment algorithm compared to typical fractures.

In these cases, the bone is abnormal for any number of reasons, including metabolic processes that affect the mineralization of bone such as osteoporosis or osteomalacia; medications such as bisphosphonates that suppress bone turnover and affect bone remodeling; treatments such as external beam radiation therapy for treatment of a malignancy; and bone replacement by a neoplasm, which can be either benign or malignant. Benign bone diseases that can predispose a patient to fracture are fibrous dysplasia, unicameral bone cysts, giant cell tumors of bone, and many others. The malignant neoplastic processes encompass diagnoses such as primary bone sarcomas, metastatic bone disease, multiple myeloma, and lymphoma.

Effective and successful treatment of pathologic fractures depends greatly on the reason for which the underlying bone is pathologic, as this has a significant effect on quality of bone stock, potential for healing, and, in the case of malignancy, life expectancy and prognosis.

In the setting of fracture through a benign lesion, an understanding of the natural history of the specific lesion can help to guide treatment. The Enneking staging system for benign tumors can help to provide an understanding for this history as well as guide its treatment.[1,2] Latent benign lesions (stage I), such as a nonossifying fibroma, can be treated nonsurgically if the fracture pattern allows, as these lesions will heal and regress spontaneously. If the fracture requires surgical stabilization, it can be applied as the fracture pattern dictates, occasionally with concomitant curettage and bone grafting. More biologically active lesions (stage II and III), such as giant cell tumors of bone or aneurysmal bone cysts, require that the surgeon treat both the fracture and the tumor itself. This can be accomplished with immediate treatment of the tumor, often with curettage and stabilization of the fracture; alternatively, the fracture can be allowed to heal nonsurgically and the tumor treated once healing has occurred. Because the bone surrounding these lesions is often normal, healing can occur reliably.

Within the spectrum of fractures through malignant neoplasms, the vast majority are encountered within the setting of metastatic cancers. According to recent data from the Surveillance, Epidemiology, and End Results (SEER) National Cancer Institute database, more than 675,000 cases of lung, breast, and prostate cancer are estimated to be diagnosed in 2013.[3] The rate of metastatic bone disease in these cancers ranges from 30% to 80%.[4] The disease burden, therefore, is significant, and the practicing orthopaedic surgeon will encounter these lesions more commonly than any other.

A fracture through a malignant neoplasm must be treated aggressively. The differentiation between a fracture through a metastatic bone lesion, multiple myeloma, or lymphoma versus one through a primary bone sarcoma must be made before treatment is initiated. In the setting of a primary bone sarcoma, an accurate diagnosis must be established through careful staging and biopsy. These fractures should be stabilized with a cast or minimal internal fixation that can be resected at the time of definitive surgical treatment of the bone sarcoma.

Fracture through bone metastases, multiple myeloma, or a lymphoma of bone are treated with a variety of methods. It is critical to identify the underlying biologic etiology of the fracture because healing rates and treatment options vary widely depending on the type of pathologic bone through which the fracture has occurred. Goals of treatment for impending or actualized pathologic fractures in metastatic disease revolve around palliation and providing the patient sufficient stability of the fracture to allow for immediate, full weight bearing and restoration of function. In these cases, the treating physician cannot rely on the bone to heal, should work under the assumption that local disease progression will occur, and that a construct must be durable enough to last the patient's lifetime without a need for reoperation. It is important to recognize these fractures and impending fractures and have a treatment strategy for these patients. This chapter will focus on providing a strategy for the evaluation and management of pathologic fractures from metastatic cancers and multiple myeloma.

METASTATIC BONE LESIONS

Cancer is a major public health problem, causing one in four deaths in the United States today. Breast and prostate cancers continue to be the most commonly diagnosed, although lung cancer continues to be the number one killer in both men and women.[5] Prostate, breast, lung, kidney, and thyroid cancers account for 80% of all skeletal metastasis; and after lungs and liver, the skeleton is the most common site of metastatic disease. The most commonly affected sites are the femur, spine, humerus, pelvis, ribs, and skull, in that order.[6] In regard to breast and prostate cancers, bone is the most common site of metastasis; postmortem examinations show 70% of patients with metastatic bone disease. Carcinomas of the thyroid, kidney, and bronchus have an incidence of 30% to 40% skeletal metastasis at postmortem examination. Furthermore, once tumors metastasize to bone, they usually are incurable. Only 20% of patients with breast cancer are alive at 5 years after the diagnosis of skeletal metastasis.[7]

The exact incidence of bone metastasis is unknown, although it is estimated that 350,000 people with bone metastases die annually in the United States.[8] With the improvement of medical therapies of many cancers, the life expectancy of these patients has increased, which has led to an increasing number of cancer patients surviving with metastatic bone disease. As a result, metastatic bone disease is estimated to cost as much as 17% of the total direct medical costs of cancer treatment in the United States.[9] The consequences of skeletal metastasis are often devastating and can be a major contributor to the deterioration of the quality of life of patients with cancer. Patients can develop severe pain, pathologic fractures, life-threatening hypercalcemia, spinal cord compression, as well as other nerve compression syndromes. Impending and actual pathologic fractures can initiate the period of dependent care for many cancer patients. For all of these reasons, bone metastases are a serious and costly consequence of cancer.[10]

Prognosis

Patient survival after metastasis to bone varies greatly depending on the tumor type and sites of involvement. Mean survival ranges from 6 months, for those with lung carcinoma, to several years, for those with bone metastasis from prostate, thyroid, or breast carcinoma. Also, in breast cancer, prognosis after the development of bone metastasis is considerably better than that after recurrence in visceral sites. Coleman and colleagues found that the median survival of patients with first recurrence of breast cancer in the skeleton to be 24 months, compared to 3 months after relapse in the liver. They also found the probability of survival to be influenced by the development of metastasis at extraosseous sites. Patients with metastatic disease confined to the skeleton had a median survival of 2.1 years, compared to those who later developed extraosseous disease and had a median survival of 1.6 years.[7,11,12] When examining lung cancer and skeletal metastasis, Sugiura and colleagues found a mean survival of 9.7 months, with a median survival of 7.2 months. Approximately 70% of patients died within 1 year after skeletal metastasis, and only 6% survived at least 2 years. The mean length of survival was substantially longer in patients with solitary site of metastasis versus patients with multiple sites of disease.[13] The importance of the extent of bone metastasis can also be seen with renal cell metastasis where patients with solitary sites of bone disease treated with wide excision can survive for many years, whereas patients with multiple sites of disease or pathologic fracture have a much shorter survival.[14]

The importance of prognosis for guiding treatment decisions involving these patients cannot be underestimated and many have tried, with little success, to develop models to assist in the decision making for end-of-life orthopaedic care. This information is sought after to help set appropriate expectations for the patient, family, and medical staff. The goal is to maximize function and quality of life for the greatest amount of time. The data about cost, risk, and quality of life are often conflicting, but properly weighed, could help define the most appropriate treatment for an individual with metastatic bone disease.[15]

The decision to pursue surgery, as well as the type of surgery, is strongly influenced by the expected survival of the patient and the need for surgical stabilization. Falsely optimistic survival estimates may influence patients and clinicians to pursue more aggressive therapies, rather than more conservative ones and could result in a higher proportion of both major perioperative complications and death. Conversely, falsely pessimistic survival prognoses could persuade a surgeon to choose a less invasive, less durable fixation technique that lacks sufficient biomechanical durability to outlast the patient.

Nathan and colleagues evaluated patients who had been operated on for pathologic fractures to determine if well-recognized prognostic parameters had any value in determining the survival in this patient population. Median survival in their cohort was 8 months and 60% of the fracture-related consultations to the service underwent operative intervention of both fractures and impending fractures. Independent predictors for survival were diagnosis (or primary site of disease), Eastern Cooperative Oncology Group (ECOG) performance status, number of bone metastases, presence of visceral metastases, and hemoglobin level. Patients with lung cancer fared the worst, and patients with renal cancer fared the best. They concluded, at the end of their study that justification for surgery on the basis of survival prognostication can be dangerously inaccurate and that more accurate prognostic indices are needed for patients undergoing surgery for bone metastases.[15] Forsberg and colleagues attempted to tackle this issue by evaluating three different prognostic models to assist in the decision to offer surgery and also whether a more durable implant was appropriate based on the prediction of 3- and 12-month survival.[16] Ultimately, the treating orthopaedic surgeon makes this difficult decision with input from the rest of the oncology team and careful consideration for the family's wishes and best interest of the patient.

Biology of Bone Metastases

Metastases can be characterized as either osteolytic or osteoblastic, which represent two extremes within a continuum where the dysregulation of normal bone remodeling occurs. Tumor cells can unbalance coupling in the bone microenvironment leading to bone formation or bone loss. Patients with skeletal metastasis can have either type of lesion or can have mixed blastic/lytic lesions. Specific cancers also have a predilection toward one type or the other. Breast cancer presents with predominately osteolytic lesions, although 15% to 20% can be osteoblastic. In contrast, the lesions in prostate cancer are predominately osteoblastic. Only in multiple myeloma do purely lytic bone lesions develop.

With osteolytic metastasis, the destruction of bone is mediated by osteoclasts rather than tumor cells. Several osteoclastogenic factors have been implicated including interleukin-1, interleukin-6, receptor activator of nuclear factor κB (NF-κB) ligand (RANKL), and macrophage inflammatory protein-1α. Parathyroid hormone-related peptide is also produced by most solid tumors and breast cancer cells and is most likely the factor that stimulates the formation of osteoclasts. The mechanism of formation of osteoblastic metastasis remains unknown, but factors such as endothelin-1, platelet-derived growth factor (PDGF), transforming growth factor-β

(TGF-β), urokinase, and prostate-specific antigen (PSA) are thought to be involved.[8,10]

More than 100 years ago, Paget first noted that the spread of different cancers to distinct organs within the body was not random. He proposed an explanation for this and called it "the seed and soil hypothesis." The "seed," the cancer cell, which circulates in the bloodstream, can only "grow," and metastasize, in particular compatible areas of the body, the "soil." Not all cancers can grow on all "soil," which leads to site-selected metastasis.[17]

There are a series of inefficient steps that need to occur for a cancer cell to metastasize. The cell must detach and extravasate from the primary tumor; invade through the extracellular matrix and endothelium to enter the bloodstream; survive within the bloodstream; arrest at a distant site by adhesion to the endothelium; intravasate again through the endothelium and additional extracellular matrix; and finally grow at a distant site. The primary tumor is a heterogeneous population of tumor cells with varying ability to metastasize; some of these cells express prometastatic genes that enable the cells to survive this process and metastasize to bone.[18]

Hematogenous dissemination of cancer to bone is influenced by several factors. Batson described a high-flow, low-pressure, valveless plexus of veins that connects the visceral organs to the spine and pelvis. This vertebral venous system, referred to as "Batson's plexus," runs parallel to the vertebral column and forms extensive anastomoses with the venous system of the vertebrae, pelvis, thorax, and brain.[19] However, circulatory anatomy alone does not predict metastasis to bone. Bone receives 5% to 10% of the cardiac output, and as a consequence, most tumor cells that enter the circulation will pass through the bone marrow. Studies comparing perfusion criteria of various organs with metastatic frequency showed no correlation, as there are also other highly vascularized organs to which tumor cells rarely metastasize. Therefore, it is probable that bone provides a particularly fertile microenvironment "soil" for the growth and aggressive behavior of the tumor cells that survive the metastatic process and are able to reach it.[8,17]

EVALUATION

Examination

Clinical Features and Presentation

Pain is the most common presenting symptom of metastatic disease to bone. The pathophysiologic mechanism for this pain is poorly understood but includes tumor-induced osteolysis, cytokine and growth factor production, direct infiltration and irritation of endosteal nerve endings, mass effect causing periosteal stretch and elevated intraosseous pressures, stimulation of ion channels, and production of local tissue factors such as endothelin.[7,20,21] The pain is usually well localized but can also be a diffuse ache, typically worse at night and not relieved by rest. Eventually the pain worsens with any weight-bearing activity and becomes functional pain. Functional pain is caused by the mechanical weakness of bone that can no longer support the normal stresses of daily activities. Functional pain is typically considered to be an indicator of bone at risk for pathologic fracture.[12]

As a direct result of bone destruction and osteolysis seen with metastatic bone disease, hypercalcemia is a common metabolic complication. One breast cancer study found hypercalcemia in 17% of breast cancer patients with first-time recurrence in bone. Unrecognized, it can be a significant source of morbidity. The signs and symptoms are nonspecific and clinicians should always maintain a high index of suspicion. Mild hypercalcemia may cause unpleasant side effects related to dysfunction of the gastrointestinal tract, kidneys, and central nervous system. As the calcium levels increase, this can lead to renal insufficiency and calcification in the kidneys, skin, blood vessels, lungs, heart, and stomach. Severe hypercalcemia is a medical emergency, and death may ensue as a result of cardiac arrhythmias and renal failure.[7,20,22]

Finally, a patient may present with a pathologic fracture; this may be the first sign of metastatic bone disease. Breast, lung, renal, and thyroid cancers are the most common cancers that lead to pathologic fractures. Thirty-five percent of breast cancer patients with metastatic bone disease will sustain a fracture. Patients with bone metastases from prostate cancer usually do not sustain pathologic fractures because of the osteoblastic nature of the disease. However, those with castrate-resistant prostate cancer, where osteoblastic metastasis is typical, annual fracture rates in excess of 20% may be seen.[7,12]

DIAGNOSIS

Diagnostic Evaluation

It is important to understand the differential diagnosis for an adult patient who presents with radiographic findings consistent with an aggressive-appearing skeletal lesion. These include metastatic bone disease, multiple myeloma, lymphoma, primary malignant bone tumor, destructive benign bone lesions, and nonneoplastic conditions (e.g., infection, stress fracture, myositis ossificans, metabolic bone disease, and osteonecrosis). In 2012, there were an estimated 1.64 million new patients with a diagnosis of cancer; of these, it is estimated that greater than 50% are likely to develop bone metastasis. In contrast, only 2890 of these new cases were of patients who presented with primary bone and joint malignancies. Therefore, the chance that a solitary bone lesion is a metastatic carcinoma, especially in an individual older than 40 years of age, is approximately 500 times greater than the chance that it is a primary bone sarcoma.[5] Knowledge of this differential diagnosis helps to guide the diagnostic evaluation of an adult with an aggressive-appearing bone lesion.

Usually, there are three types of patients who are ultimately diagnosed with skeletal metastasis. First is the patient with a remote history of cancer who seeks an opinion regarding an occult or painful osseous lesion. The second has a known cancer history and presents with an asymptomatic skeletal lesion found on routine staging studies. The third type of patient is found to have a skeletal lesion without a prior history of cancer and likely an undiagnosed carcinoma.[23] Regardless of how the patient presents, a thorough history and physical examination is essential to initiate the diagnostic workup. It is important to collect information about current symptoms, cancer history, constitutional symptoms, changes in bowel or bladder function, smoking history, and exposure to chemicals, such as asbestos.

Laboratory studies are part of the diagnostic workup for a patient with a new bone lesion, and although usually not definitively diagnostic, may be helpful and offer clues that will help facilitate staging. Important laboratory values to evaluate include a complete blood count, urinalysis, and chemistry panel. Determination of the erythrocyte sedimentation rate and C-reactive protein are helpful; they are often elevated in individuals with infection, immunologic disorders, or marrow cell neoplasms such as lymphoma or Ewing sarcoma. Metabolic bone diseases such as osteomalacia, hyperparathyroidism, and rickets may be identified with abnormal serum or urine calcium and phosphorus levels. If multiple myeloma is suspected, serum and/or urine protein electrophoresis with immunofixation may confirm this diagnosis. These patients may also have impaired renal function secondary to the presence of Bence Jones proteins. There are also specific blood and tumor markers that can evaluate specific primary sites of disease including thyroid function tests, PSA, carcinoembryonic antigen, α-fetoprotein, β-human chorionic gonadotropin, and cancer antigen–125. These known tumor markers lack specificity and their value usually lies in the assessment of response to therapy more so than in the identification of a primary site of disease.[20,24,25]

Imaging

The clinical imaging evaluation of skeletal metastasis is usually accomplished in one of four ways: plain film radiography, radioisotope scanning, computed tomography, and magnetic resonance imaging. More recently, positron emission tomography (PET) scans have been introduced as another imaging modality to assist in the staging of patients with diagnosed malignant tumors and to evaluate infections and other physiologic processes in the skeleton and soft tissues.

The most important initial imaging modality for evaluation of a bone lesion is a plain radiograph in two planes for any painful lesion. It is important to image the entire bone involved, so as not to miss any discontinuous sites of disease. Plain radiographs can yield more information about a bone tumor than any other diagnostic modality, allowing the clinician to evaluate the anatomic site, the zone of transition between the tumor and the host bone, the internal characteristics of the tumor, and the nature of the matrix that it produces. One can look for aggressive features that include size of the tumor, cortical destruction, periosteal reaction, and pathologic fracture.

Additional three-dimensional imaging of a metastatic bone lesion is typically not needed, unless more precise definition of the soft tissue component is helpful in preparation for surgical or radiation treatment. In these cases, computed tomography (CT) scan or magnetic resonance imaging (MRI) can then be obtained. Once a skeletal metastasis is identified, a bone scan is also typically warranted to evaluate the patient for other bony sites of disease. It should be noted that bone scans identify osteoblastic activity, and disease processes, such as multiple myeloma, with minimal osteoblastic activity, require a skeletal survey for evaluation to prevent falsely negative findings.

PET is an emerging technology that has a high sensitivity for identifying tumors; however, its specificity is quite low. It has been found to be superior to bone scan in detecting bone involvement in various malignancies, and because tracer uptake is not restricted to the skeleton, it has become the mainstay of staging in several malignancies.[26] It can detect lytic, blastic, and mixed lesions because it identifies the presence of tumor directly by measuring its metabolic activity. This method allows for earlier detection of metastatic foci than other studies that indirectly identify tumor by highlighting bone loss as a result of the presence of tumor.[27] It is also much more sensitive than bone scintigraphy, especially in the detection of myeloma or renal cell carcinoma, which are predominately osteolytic. Recent studies have compared PET scans to bone scans and found that PET scans have increased specificity and sensitivity and overall better metastatic lesion detection. However, skeletal scintigraphy, or bone scan, still remains the most commonly used diagnostic imaging modality for the evaluation of the entire skeleton for bony metastases, which is likely due to familiarity with its use compared to the more limited availability and relatively high cost of PET scans. However, with the recent surge in interest, gradually increasing availability, and increasing spectrum of applications for PET scans, this is rapidly changing and newer imaging and treatment modalities are constantly evolving.[26]

Understanding that many patients with skeletal metastasis are older than 40 years of age, present with a destructive painful bone lesion, and have an unknown primary, Rougraff and colleagues developed a diagnostic protocol to assist the orthopaedic surgeon who will have the task of determining the primary site of malignancy. By obtaining an adequate history and physical, routine laboratory analysis, plain radiographs of the involved bone and chest, whole body bone scan, and CT scan of the chest, abdomen, and pelvis with oral and intravenous (IV) contrast, they were able to identify the primary tumor site in 85% of patients.[28]

Biopsy

A biopsy is performed only once all of the workup has been done and the data necessary to assist in the diagnosis has been collected. There are several reasons why it is critical to conduct a staging workup prior to the biopsy. First, the tumor may be a primary sarcoma of bone and an ill-planned biopsy could compromise the ability to perform a limb-sparing procedure and to obtain high-quality imaging studies. Second, there may be another site of disease that is easier to biopsy and associated with less morbidity. Third, preoperative embolization may be helpful to prevent bleeding during biopsy or treatment, such as in the case of presumed renal cell metastases. Fourth, an unnecessary biopsy can be avoided if the diagnosis can be made based on laboratory analysis alone, such as with multiple myeloma. Fifth, histologic analysis alone identified the primary site of disease in only 3% of patients. Sixth, the increased information, as a result of combining laboratory studies with imaging results and histopathology, make it more likely that an accurate diagnosis is obtained.[25,28]

There are multiple ways to perform a biopsy and specific guidelines that must be adhered to. Biopsy techniques include fine-needle aspiration, image-guided core-needle biopsy, or open incisional biopsy. Proper oncologic principles should always be followed. The advantage of fine-needle aspirations or core-needle biopsies is that general anesthesia is not required, they are less morbid procedures, and they reduce the potential for contamination of the tumor site. The main disadvantage is a potential for sampling error due to the smaller tissue sample resulting in lower rates of accurate diagnosis compared with open biopsy. When performing an open incisional biopsy, the incision should be as small as possible, should be oriented in a longitudinal fashion with minimal disruption of the surrounding tissues, and should avoid major neurovascular structures. The location of the biopsy must be chosen cautiously, so it can be excised en bloc with the tumor, if necessary. It is important to maintain hemostasis throughout the procedure using electrocautery and bone wax to minimize contamination and tumor cell spillage.[24,29]

MANAGEMENT

Impending Fractures

The majority of metastatic bone lesions are treated effectively with nonsurgical modalities such as radiation therapy, chemotherapy, immunotherapy, hormonal therapy, and bisphosphonates. Operative treatments are palliative procedures with the goals of achieving local tumor control and structural stability, allowing the patient immediate function and weight bearing with the least possible morbidity and need for rehabilitation.[6] The question is always, when to operate? To help with this decision, many physicians rely on Harrington's classic definitions of impending pathologic fractures of the long bones or the Mirels classification system. Harrington's criteria for impending pathologic fracture includes a bone lesion that measure 2.5 cm or greater in the proximal femur, occupies 50% or more of the bone diameter, is accompanied by an adjacent lesser trochanter fracture, and has not responded to treatment with radiotherapy. However, subsequent studies have failed to prove a strong relationship between these factors and risk of fracture.[30,31]

The Mirels scoring system is based on four parameters: site, radiographic appearance, size, and related pain. Mirels reviewed 78 patients with radiated lesions of the long bone and devised a scoring system to predict the risk of pathologic fracture. This numerical scoring system has a maximum of 12 points. For scores greater than 8, prophylactic stabilization of impending pathologic fracture was recommended, while for scores of 7 or less, nonsurgical treatment was recommended due to the low fracture risk. For a score of 8, the decision must be individualized. Mirels' scoring system has the advantage of being simple, reproducible, and valid across experience levels. The disadvantages are that it has never been evaluated prospectively and, although highly sensitive as a screening tool, it has relatively poor specificity in predicting actual fracture.[31,32]

Unfortunately, impending and actual pathologic fractures often initiate the period of dependent care for many cancer patients, which is why this decision is of the utmost importance. Identifying an impending fracture and recommending prophylactic fixation is an important issue. Elective fixation prevents the pain and suffering associated with a pathologic fracture, and prophylactic fixation is often easier to perform. Ward and colleagues noted in a retrospective, nonrandomized study, that treatment of impending pathologic fractures yielded better results than treatment of complete fractures. There was less average blood loss, shorter postoperative hospital stay, greater likelihood of discharge to home as opposed to an extended care facility, and a greater likelihood of resuming support-free ambulation. Patients with impending fractures also fared better in terms of survival at 1 and 2 years.[33]

Pathologic Fractures

Goals

The treatment of bone lesions before or after fracture depends on the underlying lesion and its location. If the suspicion is high for a primary bone tumor, whether benign or malignant, it is best to refer to an orthopaedic oncologist. Common benign lesions include nonossifying fibromas, bone infarcts, unicameral bone cysts, fibrous dysplasia, aneurysmal bone cysts, and giant cell tumors of bone. The decision to observe, curettage and graft, and/or internally fix should be determined by someone familiar with these uncommon entities. Malignant primary bone tumors, such as osteosarcomas or chondrosarcomas, benefit from multidiscipline care, which may include chemotherapy, radiation, surgical resection, and soft tissue coverage procedures. The modern orthopaedic oncologist is able to pursue curative intent with limb salvage in 95% of cases.[12] Pathologic fractures sustained in the setting of a primary bone sarcoma are no longer an immediate indication for amputation because of the effectiveness of modern-day systemic therapies. Consequently, many orthopaedic oncologists will splint or perform limited internal fixation of these pathologic fractures and wait to see how patients respond to neoadjuvant treatment before deciding on definitive surgical management. Secondary bone lesions from metastatic carcinoma and the primary bone marrow malignancies are the most common cause of pathologic fractures. While specialized care for these lesions is also appropriate, they can also be appropriately treated at nonspecialty centers, if basic principles are acknowledged.

The most important first step is establishing the underlying cause of a pathologic fracture. There can be many reasons for bone to be weak such as osteoporosis, prior radiation, medication use, metabolic derangements, infection, and malignancy from, or traveling to, bone. If there is any uncertainty, an open biopsy must be performed first. Principles of biopsy were discussed earlier. It is not acceptable to send intramedullary reamings to establish diagnosis because the whole bone has already been violated if the lesion turns out to be a primary sarcoma (Fig. 20-1). In the setting of a known metastatic tumor, it may be appropriate to send reamings in order to assess tumor response to treatment. Treatment varies depending on the diagnosis of the primary tumor. Primary bone lesions and solitary metastatic tumors from thyroid and renal cell carcinoma metastatic lesions to bone are sometimes treated with local surgical resection and curative intent.[14,34] Other secondary bone lesions from carcinoma and widespread bone marrow malignancies are treated with palliative intent. The surgical goals are unique for these patients and the principles of fracture management differ from conventional management of long bone fractures.

The vast majority of patients with metastatic disease to bone, with the uncommon exception of isolated lesions from thyroid or renal cell primaries, are not going to be cured through surgery. The orthopaedic surgeon needs to view these patients and goals of surgery differently. First, quality of life and the maintenance of function are the primary goals, not the prolongation of life. Surgical strategies to allow immediate, full weight bearing, minimize pain, facilitate mobility, and minimize time in the hospital are the priority. Second, the benefit of surgery and time to recover should be weighed against the expected patient survival. If the latter is less than the recovery time, a less invasive strategy to address pain

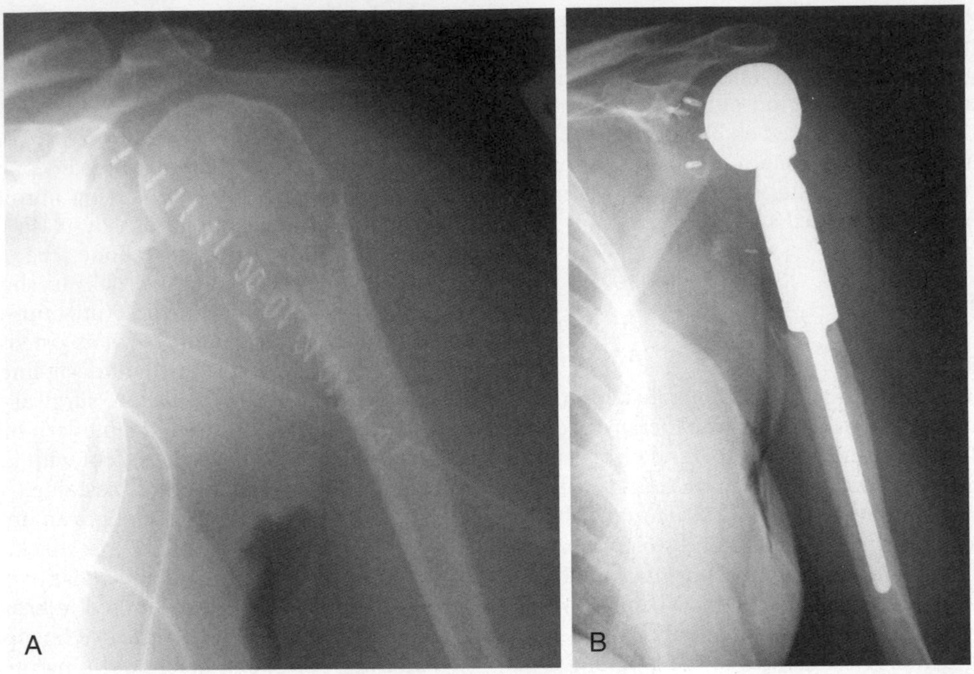

Figure 20-1. A, A 62-year-old female with a pathologic fracture of the proximal humerus. Suspicion was high for a metastatic carcinoma, however, open biopsy demonstrated a leiomyosarcoma. **B,** She was treated with wide resection and endoprosthetic reconstruction.

should be planned. Third, pathologic bone is weak, of poor quality, and cannot be relied upon to heal. Further, additional measures in the form of chemoradiation can worsen the healing potential. At best, healing is significantly delayed, often taking longer than 6 months.[35] Fixation needs to be durable, tolerate a greater load for a longer period of time, allow immediate full weight bearing, outlive the patient, and avoid reoperation. Fourth, endoprosthetic reconstruction is a consideration for initial management[36,37] (Fig. 20-2). Extensive pathologic bone, likely disease progression in treatment-resistant tumors, and limited alternatives that could allow immediate weight bearing are all instances in which to consider an endoprosthesis as first-line treatment. Fifth, there must always be an attempt at local control of the tumor. This can be from complete wide resection, curettage, systemic therapies, or with external beam radiation therapy (EBRT). Radiation is most commonly used after surgery and the field frequently encompasses the entire length of the surgical implant. Sixth, these patients need careful soft tissue management. Providing a setting for uncomplicated healing after surgery facilitates early adjuvant treatment, prevents wound breakdown from radiation, and protects against infection when patients are immunosuppressed. Consideration of these factors goes a long way in keeping patients out of the hospital and improving quality of life.

Determining the best treatment for metastatic disease requires knowledge of both the tumor biology and the surgical technique. Life expectancy is more favorable in those with solitary bone lesions, without visceral metastases, and in those with treatment-responsive subtypes, such as prostate, breast, and multiple myeloma.[38] The capacity to heal should be considered in these patients. Gainor and colleagues showed that 60% to 70% of pathologic fractures from these histologic subtypes will heal in longer than 6 months. Internal fixation enhanced healing, whereas adjuvant radiation did not appear to have an influence.[35] On the contrary, lung cancers and melanoma have poor prognoses and are notoriously resistant to systemic treatments and radiation.[39] These patients have shorter life expectancies and disease that is likely to progress. Early aggressive surgery is favored in those medically fit for such intervention, as healing cannot be relied upon. Renal cell carcinoma has traditionally been associated with a poor prognosis. However, new targeted therapies that inhibit angiogenesis have improved disease control and patient longevity.[40] Local management of renal cancer metastatic to bone remains a challenge and will be discussed later in additional detail.

In all these patients, a few simple surgical techniques should be considered. As noted earlier, implants should be expected to bear a greater load for a longer period of time and should provide immediate axial and rotational stability. Therefore, long, load-sharing implants are preferred when possible. They are durable and can prophylactically protect long segments of bone to avoid future fractures in the event of disease progression (Fig. 20-3). These devices are strongest when made from stainless steel but this strength must be weighed against the need for future imaging with MRI, where a titanium implant may be more appropriate. Significant tumor load may benefit from open debulking to decrease the local disease burden and enhance the effectiveness of adjuvant radiation for local tumor control. The remaining defect(s) can be supplemented with polymethylmethacrylate (PMMA) to improve the rigidity of the construct and facilitate early weight bearing. PMMA is not weakened by radiation and, when used to fill cavities, does not prevent bone healing.[41,42]

Amputation is rarely done for pathologic fractures from metastatic disease. It is primarily considered in tumors that progress and ulcerate through the skin despite treatment, painful nonunions after failed fixation without other reconstruction options, extensive bone loss or neurovascular

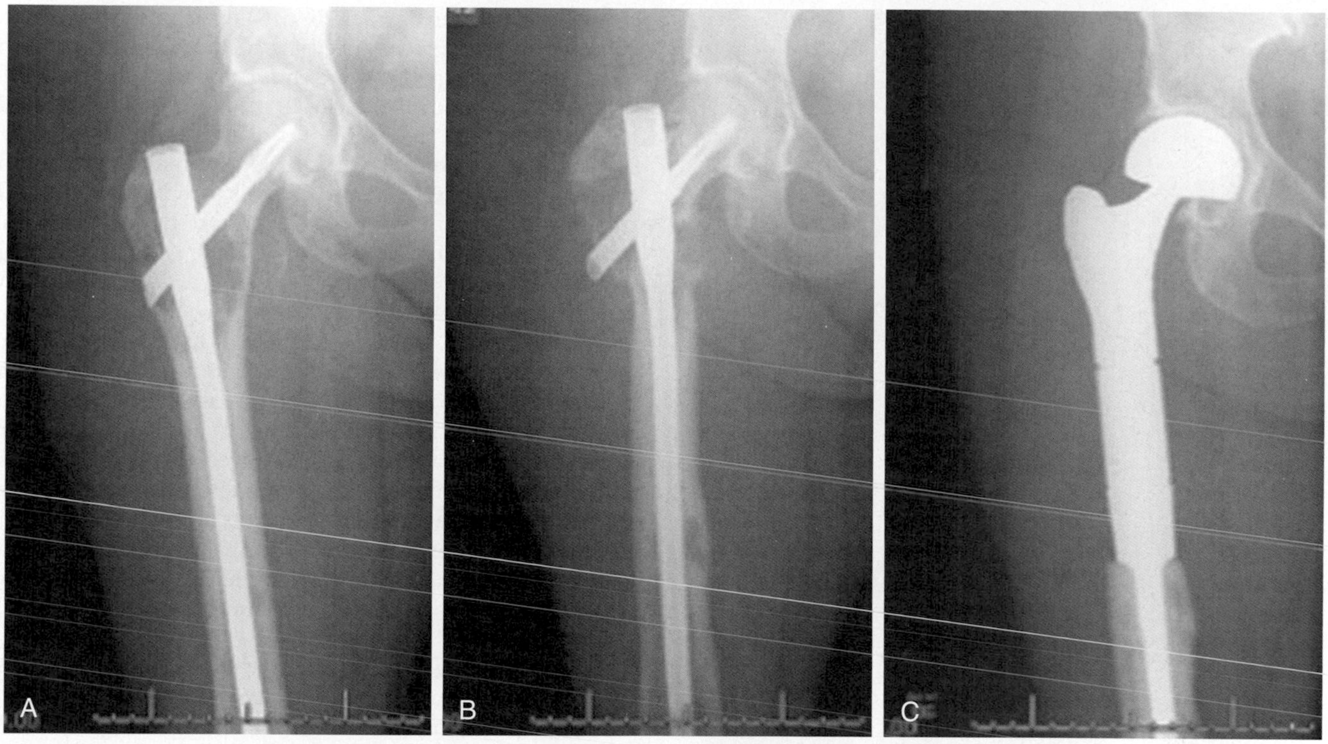

Figure 20-2. A 62-year-old female with treatment-resistant clear cell renal cell carcinoma. **A,** Initial treatment of an impending fracture of the proximal femur with a cephalomedullary nail followed by radiation. **B,** With disease progression, the implant is under tremendous stress and the patient developed intractable pain. **C,** She subsequently underwent reoperation for a proximal femur endoprosthesis. An additional surgery could have been avoided with an initial endoprosthesis.

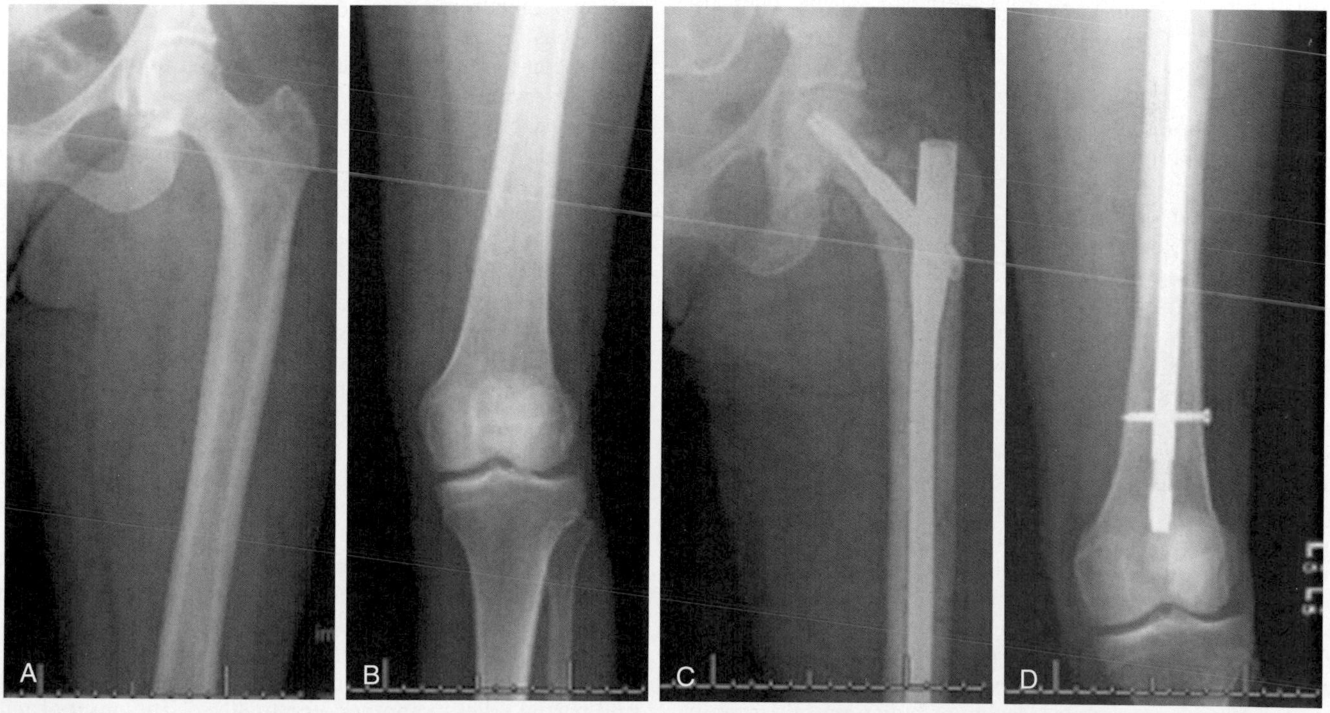

Figure 20-3. A 46-year-old female with metastatic breast cancer. **A** and **B,** Diffuse poorly defined radiolucent metastatic lesions throughout the left femur. **C** and **D,** Treatment with a long wide-diameter cephalomedullary nail to protect the entire bone and facilitate immediate weight bearing.

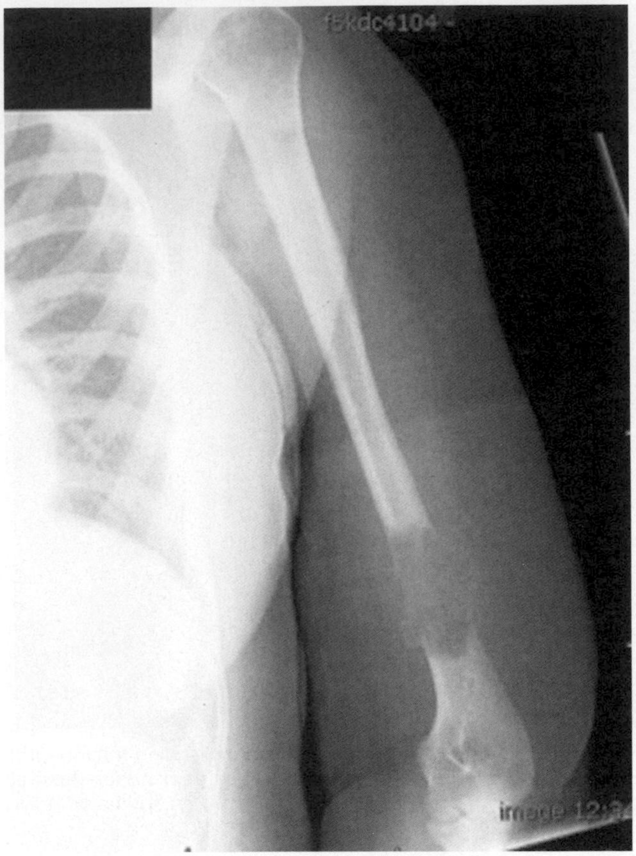

Figure 20-4. A 42-year-old female with metastatic breast cancer to the distal humeral metadiaphysis of her nondominant extremity. With well-maintained alignment and minimal discomfort in a functional brace, she was treated with radiation, systemic hormonal therapy, and bracing.

involvement, and for postradiation changes that result in a painful, nonfunctioning extremity.

Nonoperative Treatment

Although pathologic fractures are nearly all indicated for operative intervention, certain fractures in treatment-sensitive malignancies can be treated without surgery. Fractures of the upper extremity, ribs, and clavicle are nonweight bearing areas that can be well managed with casting, bracing, or pain-control measures. Patients can remain quite functional and have a favorable quality of life during treatment. Humeral shaft fractures are particularly well tolerated despite the long course of treatment with functional bracing (Fig. 20-4), and many pathologic vertebral compression fractures can be treated nonsurgically with good results. Small, nondisplaced fractures in low stress areas of the lower extremities or hard-to-reach areas of the pelvis, such as the ischium, pubis, and sacroiliac joint, can be considered in patients with favorable life expectancies as long as their pain is mild, cortical destruction is minimal, and they are willing to adhere to weight-bearing restrictions while receiving radiation or systemic therapies (Fig. 20-5). Close follow-up is necessary to monitor the response to treatment and assure patient function and quality of life is not being compromised.

There are times where surgery is indicated but the poor health status of patients renders them medically unfit for an operative procedure, which is usually because of extensive comorbidities and/or advanced state of the malignancy leading to a poor life expectancy. Comfort measures become the priority with a focus on local disease control and pain management.

Local tumor control without surgery puts the focus on adjuvant treatments. Chemotherapy is an option for all metastatic cancers and is specific to each tumor type. The systemic action leads to diminished tumor load and a decrease in musculoskeletal pain. Lymphoma is particularly sensitive to chemotherapy and often does not require any additional treatments even when bone is involved. Use of chemotherapy is limited by the severity of toxicity. As a result, elderly and medically complicated patients are often not candidates. Hormone therapy is an option in breast and prostate cancers. Agents for breast cancer include estrogen-receptor antagonists and aromatase inhibitors, which are effective in around 50% of patients.[39] Prostate cancer treatments include gonadotropin-releasing hormone (GnRH) analogs, cytochrome P450 inhibitors, androgen antagonists, and 5α-reductase inhibitors. They decrease bone pain from prostate cancer metastases in 70% to 80% of patients.[39]

Another strategy is to target the tumor activation of host osteoclasts that leads to bony destruction. Bisphosphonates and RANKL inhibitors are used to combat this process and have been shown to decrease bone destruction and the incidence of pathologic fracture.[43-45] Bisphosphonates work by binding bone mineral and being internalized by osteoclasts and ultimately induce apoptosis. They are effective in preventing progression in both osteolytic and osteoblastic bone lesions.[46] Although best studied in breast cancer and multiple myeloma, they have proven effective across a wide range of cancers. Zoledronic acid (Zometa, Novartis, Basel, Switzerland) has proven to be effective in achieving pain relief, decreasing the need for radiation, preventing hypercalcemia, and preserving function.[47] Administered as a 4-mg IV infusion every 3 weeks, skeletal-related events (SREs), defined as pathologic fracture, surgery for bone complication, use of radiation, or hypercalcemia, can be diminished by 35% and the time to the first SRE is delayed by 70 days.[48] There may be some direct antitumor effect from bisphosphonates as well, but this has been debated.[49-52] Denosumab (Xgeva, Amgen, Thousand Oaks, CA) is another medication able to interfere with tumor activation of host osteoclasts. It is a human immunoglobulin G (IgG) monoclonal antibody to RANKL and prevents the activation of RANK receptors on osteoclasts. Given as a 120-mg subcutaneous injection once a month, it has proven more effective than bisphosphonates in the reduction of SREs and time to first SRE. There is no difference between the two medications in regard to disease progression or overall patient survival.[53]

Direct local control in impending and pathologic fractures not treated with surgery either due to location, minimal symptoms, or patient comorbidities is most commonly treated with EBRT. Radiation, administered in single or multiple fractionated doses, achieves complete pain relief in around 30% and partial relief in another 30% to 40%.[39] The onset of relief takes 2 to 4 weeks and the average duration is 6 months.[54,55] A single fraction of 8 Gy is as effective as multifraction radiation for pain relief but has a higher incidence of retreatment.[56,57] Multifractional treatment is generally preferred for neuropathic pain and in patients with longer life expectancies.[58]

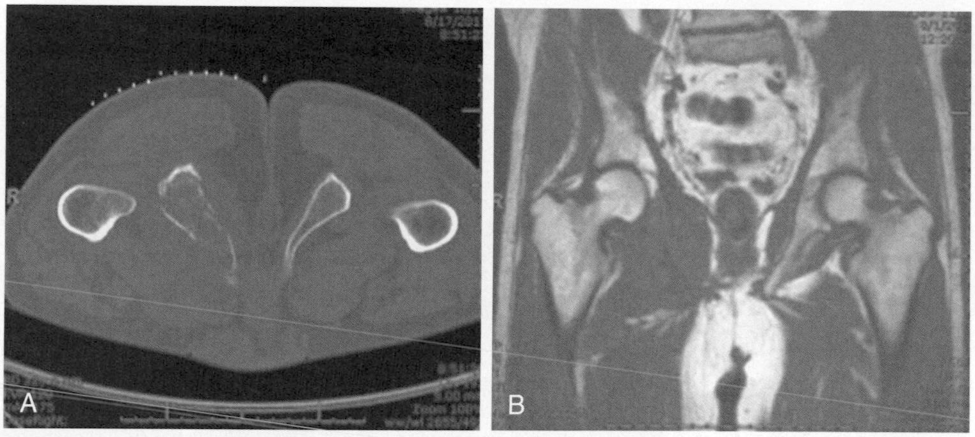

Figure 20-5. A 60-year-old male with metastatic head and neck squamous cell carcinoma to the right ischium. (**A**) Axial computed tomography (CT) scan and (**B**) T1-weighted coronal magnetic resonance imaging (MRI) demonstrating the lesion and associated pathologic fracture. Because of the location away from the weight-transfer axis and hip joint, this was treated with radiation alone and the patient was weight bearing as tolerated.

EBRT for palliation has the additional benefit of assisting bone repair by interfering with osteoclasts and ossifying collagen strands from the proliferative fibrous tissue that replaces metastatic cells.[59] Use can decrease the risk of reoperation from 15% to 20%.[60] Stereotactic radiation utilizing steep dose gradients to protect vital structures has been adopted from the treatment of brain malignancies to palliate disease to the spine (Fig. 20-6).

Various techniques exist to address metastatic lesions through percutaneous or endovascular techniques. Each has specific indications and is useful in isolation or as an adjunct to surgery. Radiofrequency ablation (RFA) is considered in small (≤5 cm), contained lesions that are painful. In management of pathologic fractures, this technique is primarily used in pelvic lesions with associated insufficiency fractures (Fig. 20-7). Performed percutaneously with CT, ultrasound, or fluoroscopic image-guidance, heat is generated within the lesion to directly ablate tumor as well destroy local sensory nerves. This ablation is often followed by injection of PMMA to provide increased structural stability at the tumor site. RFA can spare exposure to EBRT and is effective, with 95% achieving pain relief lasting for 6 months.[61]

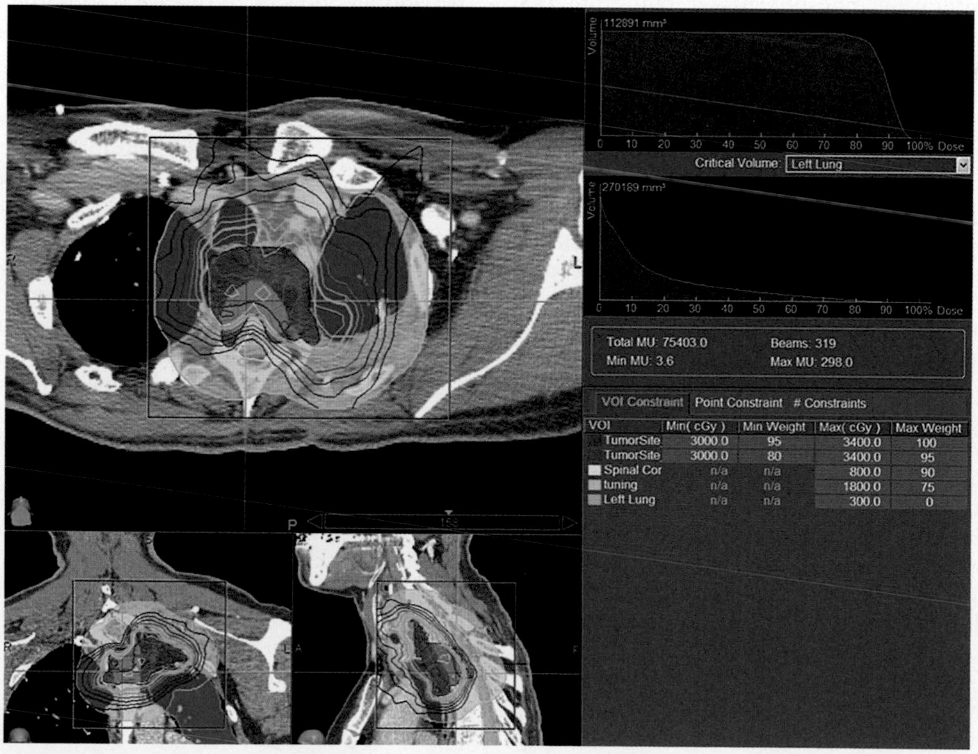

Figure 20-6. Stereotactic body radiotherapy being given to the upper thoracic spine for a recurrent tumor. The isodose lines bend around the dural sac to spare sensitive structures from high-dose radiation.

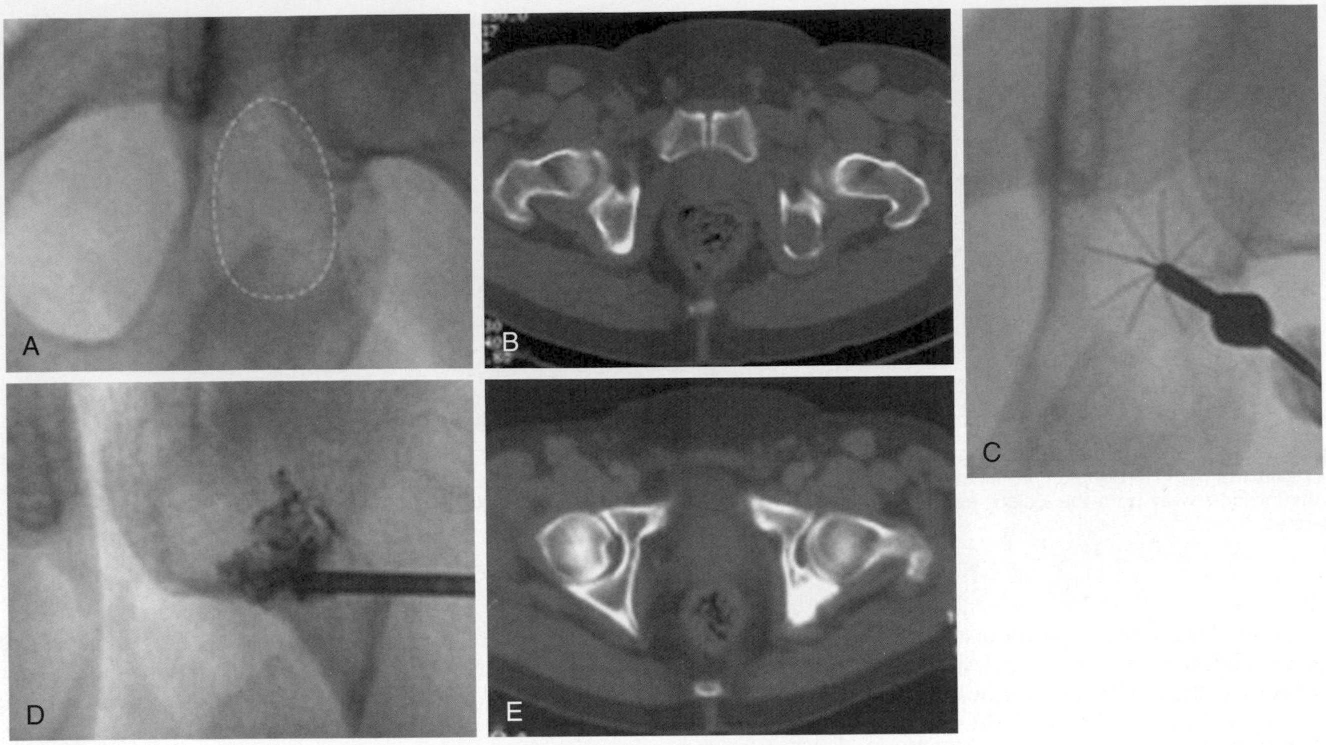

Figure 20-7. Patient with metastatic renal cell carcinoma. **A,** Painful radiolucent lesion in the left ischium on radiography and (**B**) axial computed tomography (CT) scan. **C,** Treated with radiofrequency ablation (RFA) and (**D**) injected with cement at the end of the procedure. **E,** Five years after RFA there has been no recurrence of the lesion and the patient remains pain free.

Administration of radioisotopes is another technique used to address symptoms from multifocal metastatic lesions too numerous for EBRT and resistant to other systemic medical therapies. The radioisotopes, given as a single outpatient injection, include strontium-89, phosphorus-32, samarium-153, and radium-223, and are most effective in prostate and breast carcinomas.[39] The isotopes have an affinity for bone and emit radioactive particles in a range of 0.2 to 3 mm, which helps localize the radiation and minimize side effects, which are primarily myelosuppression and thrombocytopenia.[12] Treatment is contraindicated in those with a poor performance status, less than 2-month survival, extensive soft tissue metastases, a platelet count below $60 \times 10^3/\mu L$, recent disseminated intravascular coagulation, impending fractures, and cord compression.[12] Most patients respond in 2 to 4 weeks and 60% to 80% achieve modest pain relief that lasts longer than 6 months.[39,62] Radioisotopes have been associated with decreased use of pain medications, less need for EBRT, and the development of fewer new bone metastases.[63,64] Retreatment can occur every 10 weeks. Bone marrow recovery must occur after administration, which limits use of this modality in conjunction with EBRT and chemotherapy.

Embolization is another modality that can be utilized on its own to address difficult-to-reach anatomic areas or in preparation for surgery to decrease blood loss. Using percutaneous endovascular techniques, interventional radiologists use polyvinyl alcohol, coils, or gel foam to occlude large feeding vessels to the tumor. Pathologic fractures secondary to thyroid, renal, lung, and myeloma malignancies should receive preoperative embolization to reduce blood loss (Fig. 20-8). Surgery should take place within 48 to 96 hours, before revascularization occurs.[65]

Surgical Treatment

Orthopaedic intervention for impending and pathologic fractures decreases pain and improves mobility in 90% of patients.[66] As a result, surgical stabilization is recommended unless patients are too sick or disease is too progressive with a poor life expectancy. Surgical approach and recommended fixation varies by location and therefore, our discussion will consider specific anatomic areas. It is important to note that most surgically treated impending and pathologic fractures are treated postoperatively with EBRT within 2 to 3 weeks of surgery, once wounds have healed. Further, almost all patients are made weight bearing as tolerated immediately after surgery.

Upper Extremity. Twenty percent of metastatic lesions to bone occur in the upper extremities. Impending and pathologic fractures occur most commonly in the proximal humerus and humeral shaft. Distal lesions can occur and often result from lung and renal primaries. While less devastating than fractures in the lower extremity due to lower stress and limited need for weight bearing, patients have improved pain control and maintained function after operative stabilization of pathologic fractures.[67-70] The mode of fixation is dependent on the location of fracture and extent of destruction.[68,71-73]

Fractures in the humeral head and anatomic neck are indicated for a cemented hemiarthroplasty[65,68-70] (Fig. 20-9). The length of the stem should bypass all lesions in the humerus, ideally by two cortical diameters. It is imperative to obtain radiographs of the entire long bone before determining the length of the stem. Lesions on the glenoid side can be treated with curettage and cementation with or without resurfacing. An active patient with a rotator cuff deficient shoulder with an intact deltoid warrants consideration for a cemented reverse total shoulder to maximize abduction and forward flexion.

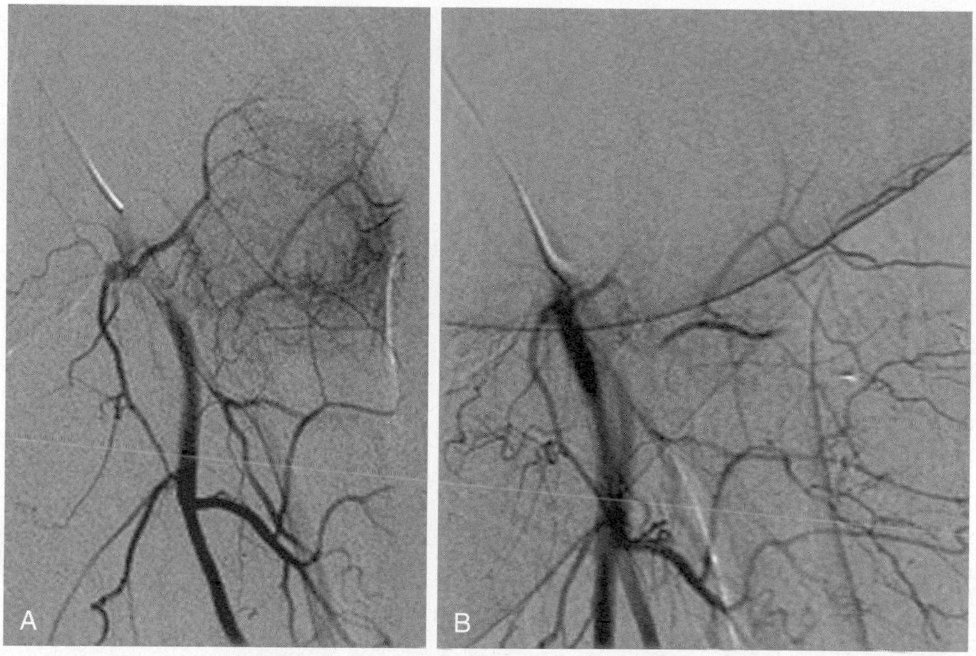

Figure 20-8. A 69-year-old male with metastatic renal cell carcinoma with an impending fracture of his left proximal femur. He was sent for preoperative embolization. **A,** A significant blush seen on his initial angiogram. **B,** Absence of blush after embolization.

Historically, hemiarthroplasty has been favored over total and reverse shoulder arthroplasty due to reliable pain relief and stability. Function, however, was rather poor. A growing focus on patient-derived outcomes has pushed thinking toward techniques with better functional outcomes. Because resections for metastatic lesions are intralesional, surgeons are able to maintain more structures to aid stability, such as the joint capsule and rotator cuff tendons, improving stability in total and reverse shoulder arthroplasties. When used for proximal humerus malignancies and at a mean follow-up of 7.7 years, the reverse total shoulder provided a mean abduction of 157 degrees and significantly improved activities of daily living.[74] Advanced disease in the proximal humerus with a large soft tissue mass and extensive bone loss is a reason to consider an endoprosthesis (Fig. 20-10). If remaining diaphyseal segment is very short, options include a compliant prestress fixation-type endoprosthesis, shortening the stem with a high-speed cutting burr on a conventional endoprosthesis, or a total humeral replacement.

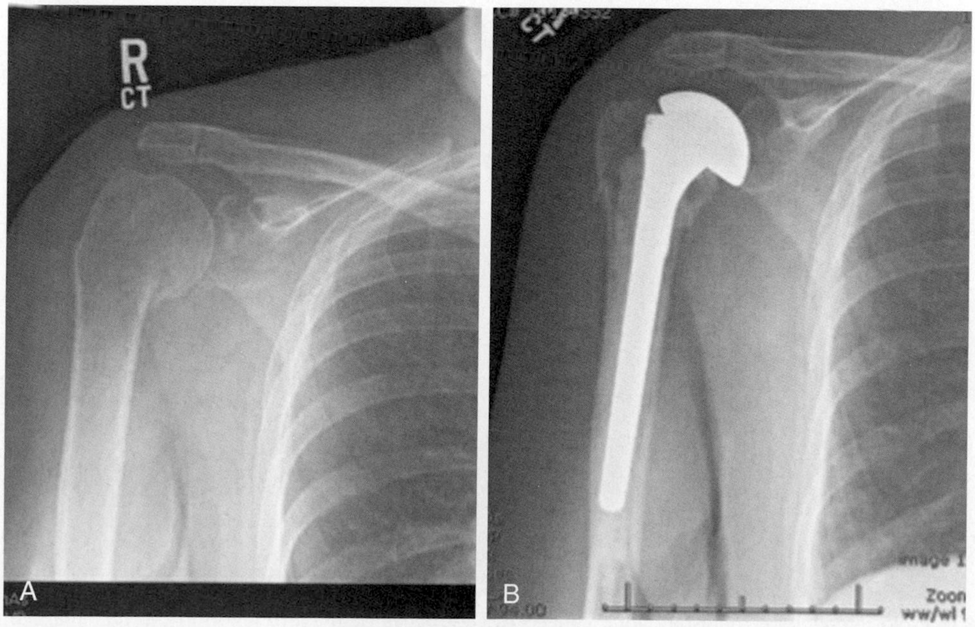

Figure 20-9. A 61-year-old female with metastatic lung cancer. **A,** Pathologic fracture of her right humeral surgical neck with disease extension into the greater tuberosity and humeral head. **B,** She was treated with a cemented hemiarthroplasty.

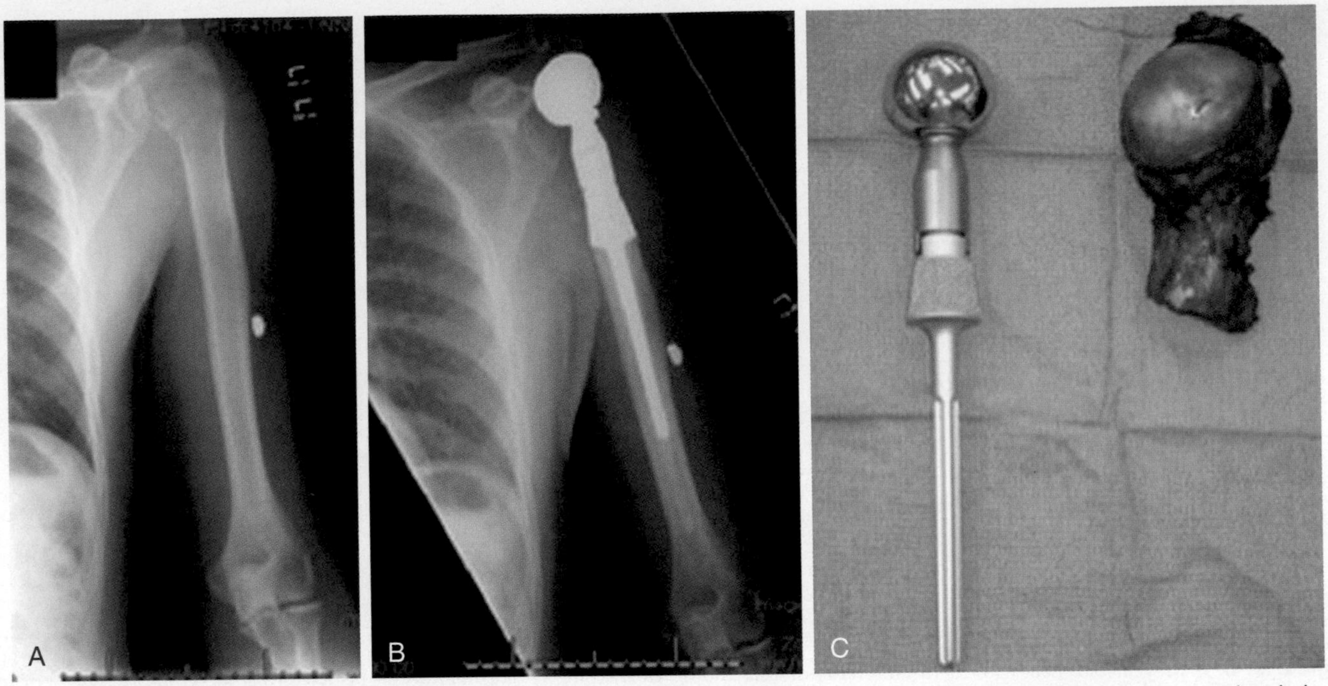

Figure 20-10. A 45-year-old male with metastatic acinic carcinoma. **A,** Permeative lesion of the proximal humerus with associated pathologic fracture of the surgical neck. Patient had a previous gunshot wound with retained shrapnel to his left arm. **B,** Postoperative radiographs after resection of proximal humerus with cemented endoprosthetic reconstruction. **C,** Pathologic specimen next to prosthesis.

Fractures in the proximal humerus encompassing the surgical neck to the proximal-third shaft of the diaphysis that are minimally displaced with maintained bone stock can be debulked with curettage and then stabilized with anatomically contoured proximal humerus plates with fixed-angle locking screws into the humeral head and hybrid compression screws in the shaft augmented by locking screws to improve torsional strength (Fig. 20-11). Longer plates are preferred because load is shared over a greater surface area and more distance is created between the first and last screws increasing the strength of the construct. Defects should be filled with fixed-angle screws through the plate, which then function as a rebar when the space is filled with PMMA cement. Alternatively, a calcium phosphate cement that converts to hydroxyapatite can be used and then drilled for screws after hardening.

Diaphyseal lesions are treated with locked antegrade intramedullary nails (Fig. 20-12). These are load sharing and associated with immediate stability, good pain relief, and early

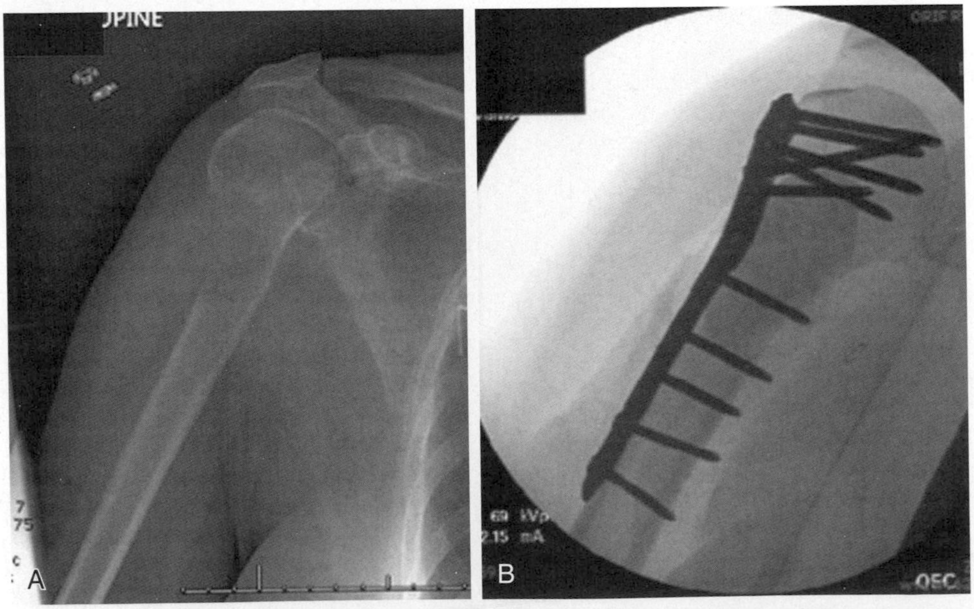

Figure 20-11. A 58-year-old female with metastatic lung cancer. **A,** Destructive permeative lesion in the proximal humerus with associated pathologic fracture in the proximal humeral shaft. **B,** Fluoroscopic images after repair with hybrid plating; cement was placed around locking screws into the area of defect to provide compressive strength.

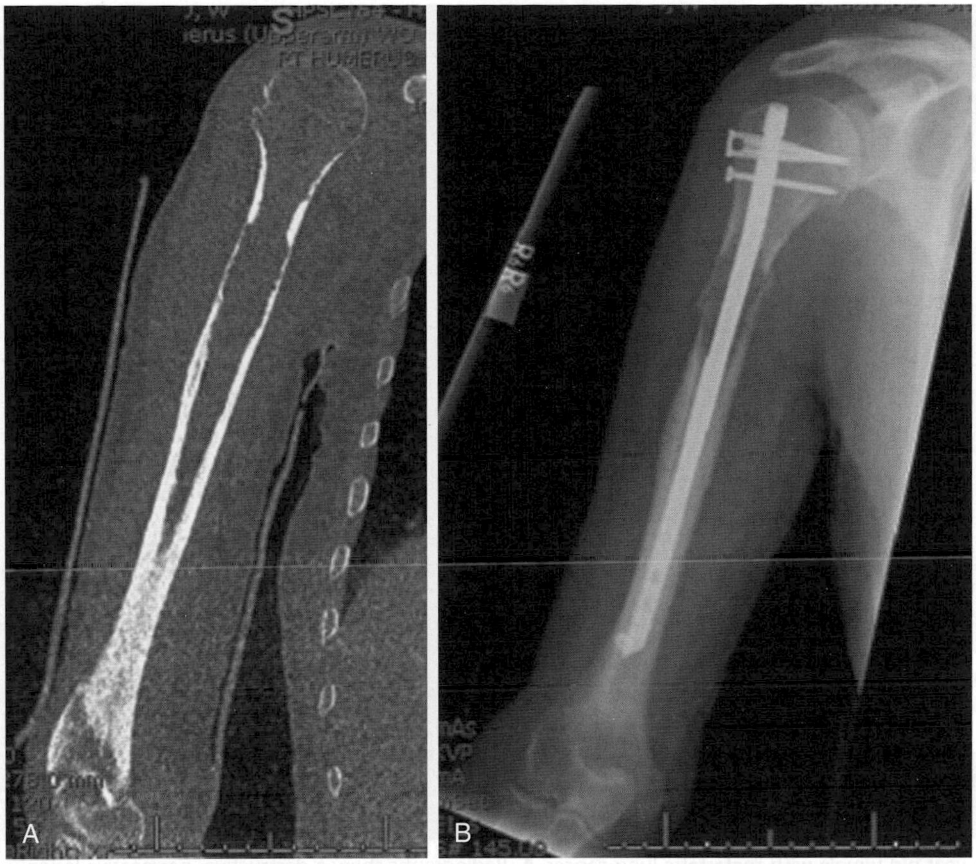

Figure 20-12. An 85-year-old male with multiple myeloma. **A,** Coronal computed tomography (CT) shows an impending fracture of the right proximal humerus diaphysis. **B,** Anterior-posterior (AP) radiograph after intramedullary nail placement.

return to function.[75] Success in maintaining function and minimizing rotator cuff morbidity is completely dependent on technique. Using an approach extending from the anterolateral acromion between the anterior and medial deltoid raphe makes it easier to identify the rotator interval. Once identified, the rotator cuff should be carefully split, tagged, and retracted to avoid damage from entry reaming. Use of a soft tissue protector and maintaining tendon retraction with K-wires into the humeral head can assist in this task. Reaming should be minimized or avoided altogether to avoid iatrogenic bone loss. Once placed, the nail should be adequately buried to avoid prominence and prevent rotator cuff irritation. This also facilitates placement of bicortical interlocking screws in the calcar, which helps increase torsional strength of the construct. The tumor at the fracture site can be debulked and supported with PMMA, but this is only done if the local disease load is significant. It is preferred to minimize the number and length of incisions to expedite healing and time to adjuvant EBRT. Contemporary nails are better suited for pathologic fractures as they are more rigid and allow multiple areas of fixed-angle interlocking both proximally and distally. Further, improved anatomic design of the nails allows use of an entry site that is easier to access and provides better alignment at fracture sites, most notably at the medial calcar where varus deformity can commonly occur. If necessary, compression can also be obtained through the nail either by placing distal interlocks and backslapping in a controlled manner over the nail itself. Shortening is well tolerated in the upper extremity and can reduce the size of a bony defect from tumor in order to improve bony apposition and the prospect of healing. Retrograde nailing is rarely performed and not recommended as it requires removal of significant bone distally to create a proper entry site above the olecranon fossa. This bone loss puts the patient at significant risk of a supracondylar humerus fracture, which is a difficult problem to treat and would subject a patient with an already limited life span to additional surgery.[76] Failure of an antegrade nail can be salvaged with a proximal humeral endoprosthesis, which is more functional than a distal humerus endoprosthesis with a total elbow replacement.

Distal humeral lesions are challenging and often surgically treated with curettage and parallel bridge plating with anatomically contoured hybrid 3.5-mm column plates that are long, stainless steel, and allow rebar-type locking screws into fracture defects that can support cement. This construct has been shown to have better torsional strength than plates placed in a ninety-ninety configuration.[77] Significant bone loss warrants consideration for distal humeral replacement with total elbow arthroplasty. This scenario is extremely uncommon and likely to only occur in neglected metastatic lesions that do not receive standard systemic treatments.

Pathologic fractures of the radius and ulna are rare and are treated with plating using the same principles for the proximal and distal humerus (Fig. 20-13). Long plates are preferred, and ninety-ninety plating should be considered for areas of significant bone loss. Pathologic fractures of the wrist and hand are even more uncommon and can be treated nonsurgically with

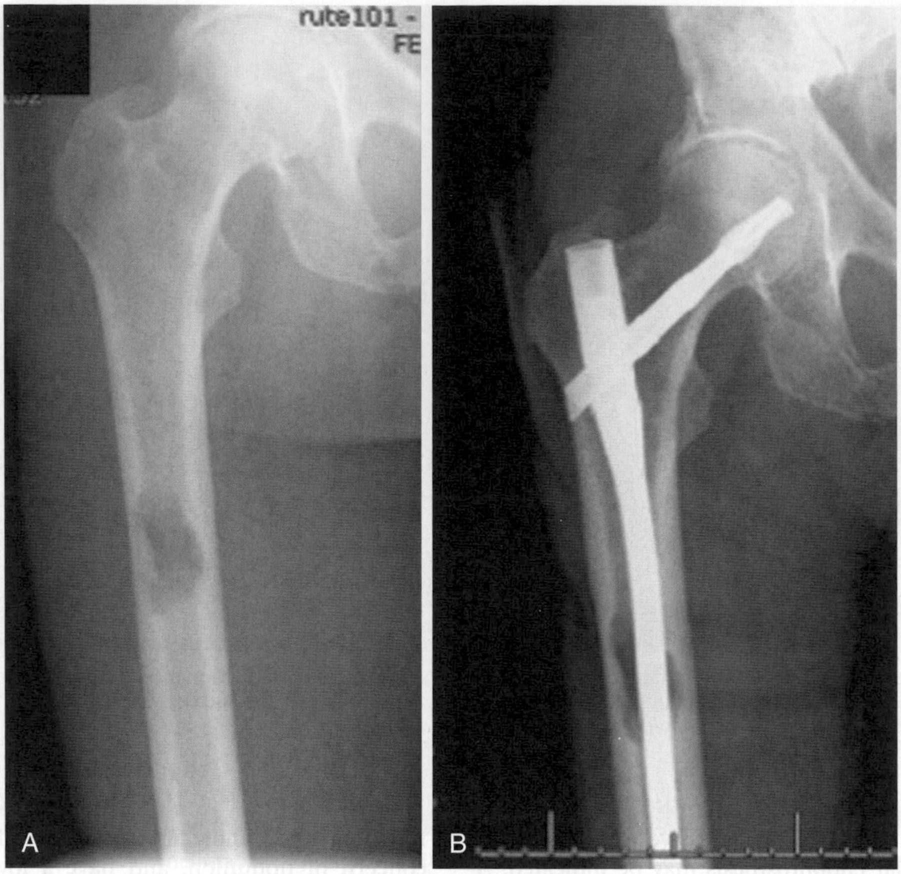

Figure 20-16. An 83-year-old male with multiple myeloma. **A,** Impending fracture from a radiolucent lesion in the proximal femoral diaphysis. **B,** Radiograph after prophylactic fixation with a long cephalomedullary nail.

of elasticity than titanium. Larger diameter and longer length increase bending rigidity. A low neck-shaft fixed-angle screw into the femoral head makes it easier to achieve a low tip-to-apex distance. It is also important to appreciate that different nail systems have varying proximal diameters, often from 15.5 to 17 mm. The larger proximal diameter will provide the greatest strength and will help avoid fatigue failure from repetitive loading. Start site is also crucial. Moving the start site slightly more posterior will better accommodate the nail's radius of curvature and decrease hoop stresses on the proximal femur thus reducing stresses on the implant. Many of these concepts are counter to nail use in trauma where preservation of bone with smaller diameter nails and titanium implants with elasticity closer to cortical bone are preferred.

Intramedullary nails are advantageous because they can protect the entire femur and require few incisions, which minimizes the risk of wound complications. Their use is preferred but not always possible. Osteoblastic bone lesions may result in an obliterated canal. When the areas are focal, use of small cutting reamers or employing a separate lateral incision and burring the canal open will allow use of a nail. Extensive canal sclerosis, morbidly obese patients where a start site cannot be obtained, or patients with implants about the knee are instances where a nail cannot be utilized. In these cases, a sliding hip screw with a trochanteric side plate or a proximal femoral locking plate, both of adequate length to bypass the most distal area of disease, are reasonable alternatives. When an implant already exists about the distal femur, it is important to overlap with that implant to avoid a stress riser. If overlap cannot be achieved, a separate plate at 90 degrees should be placed to span the proximal and distal femoral implants. Augmenting defects with cement has greater value when load-sharing implants are used. Such implants are also to be considered if there is any uncertainty over the diagnosis. Use of a plate or sliding hip screw of short length until definitive pathology is known provides pain relief for the patient and preserves surgical treatment with resection and reconstruction in the event the pathologic fracture is from a primary bone tumor (Fig. 20-17).

Impending fractures treated with CMNs are at risk for embolization of marrow contents to the lung due to increased intramedullary pressures during instrumentation. This can lead to cardiopulmonary dysfunction.[86] Informing the anesthetic service of this possibility, reaming at small 0.5-mm intervals, advancing the reamer slowly, and using fluted nails helps to reduce the risk.[87] Risk can be additionally mitigated with placement of a vent hole above the distal femoral metadiaphysis with a 5-mm drill bit and connecting it to a top hat–type drill guide.[88] Patients with bilateral impending or pathologic femur fractures will require a CMN on each site. It is best to stage the procedures by at least a few days in order to reduce the risk of cardiac and pulmonary complications and the risk of death.[89]

Impending and pathologic fractures in the distal third of the femoral shaft can be treated with retrograde nails.[90] The

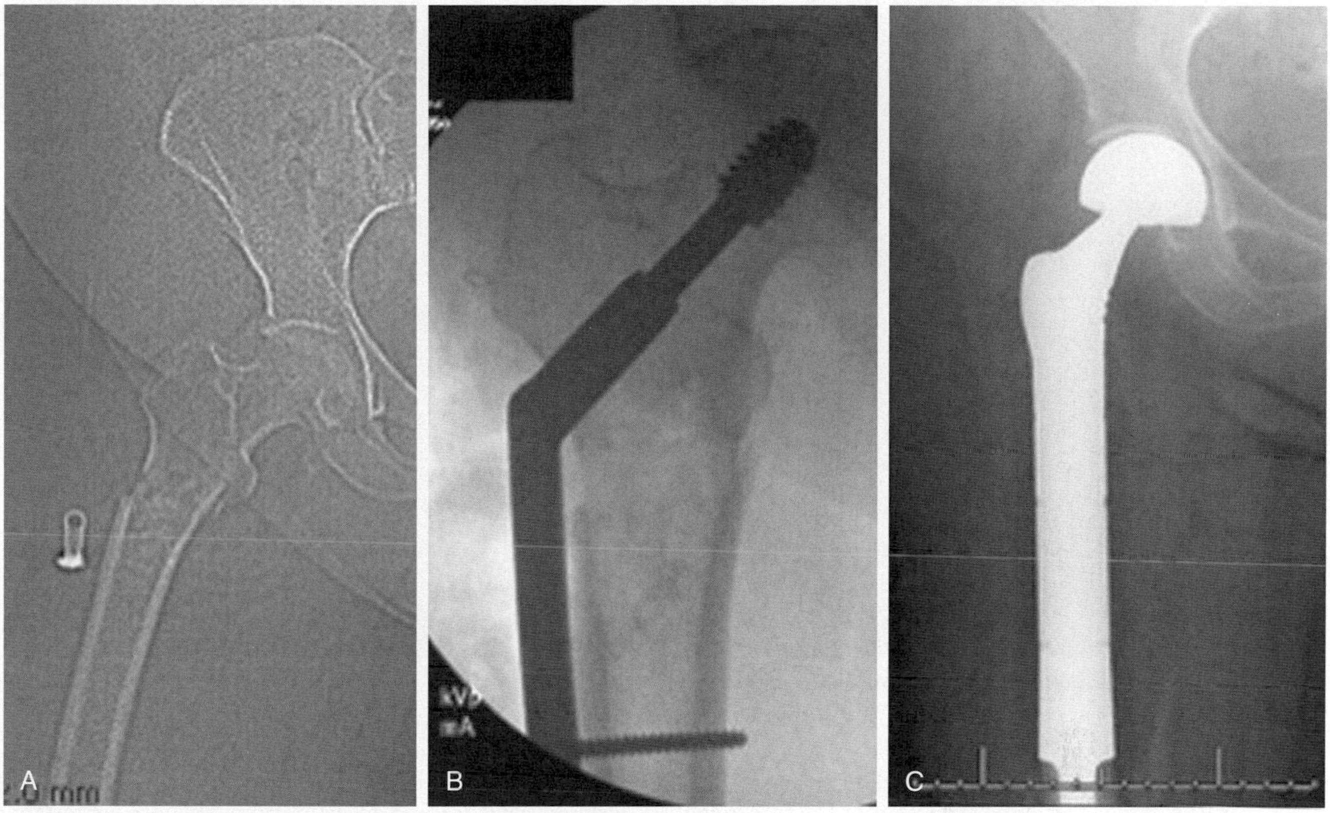

Figure 20-17. A 63-year-old female (**A**) sustained a pathologic fracture of her right subtrochanteric femur. **B,** The diagnosis was unclear on frozen section so a sliding hip screw was used for fixation. The final pathology report diagnosed the lesion as a chondrosarcoma. **C,** The patient underwent wide resection with an endoprosthetic reconstruction. If an intramedullary device had been used at the initial fracture fixation, an amputation would have been necessary.

same principles discussed earlier apply to implant selection. Newer designs now allow multiple points of fixation to be obtained in very short segments of the distal femur. One drawback of this implant is that it does not protect the femoral neck. Separate screws can be placed under the same anesthetic across the neck straddling the nail to provide this protection. Fractures in the supracondylar region of the femur are best treated with curettage of gross tumor and hybrid plating with long, stainless steel, distal femur periarticular plates (Fig. 20-18). Use of new plates that allow placement of variable-angle fixed-angle screws makes it easier to reinforce bone defects and achieve more points of fixation distally. Typically, bicortical compression screws are used to bring the plate down to bone and then bicortical locking screws are placed with a short working length in order to create a rigid construct with good torsional strength to allow immediate weight bearing. Cement is used to provide compressive strength to bone defects.[71,91-93] Similar scenarios to those discussed in the proximal femur point to consideration of a cemented endoprosthesis in the distal femur (Fig. 20-19). Although rare, extremely extensive bone loss in the femur can be addressed with a total femur replacement or amputation.

Pathologic fractures of the tibia are uncommon and are typically due to melanoma, lung, or thyroid cancers. Proximal and distal periarticular tumors are treated with curettage and internal fixation with long hybrid stainless steel locking plates. Diaphyseal defects are treated with a full-length intramedullary nail placed with the same implant characteristics and surgical goals noted for femoral CMNs (Fig. 20-20). Newer tibial nails have multiple interlocking options that have broadened their application to include fractures with short proximal and distal segments. Cement is used to fill and augment defects in the bone given the weight-bearing nature of the tibia. An endoprosthesis can be used if disease is extensive in the proximal tibia, but this requires reconstruction of the extensor mechanism and a prolonged course of rehabilitation. Because of a lack of endoprosthetic options for the distal tibia, destructive lesions that cannot be adequately managed with curettage and internal fixation may need to be considered for amputation. Pathologic fractures of the foot are exceedingly uncommon. Minimally displaced fractures can be treated with a walking cast and systemic therapy. The weight-bearing nature of the foot makes the treatment of fractures in this location different than the hand. As a result, a lower threshold for curettage and internal fixation with cement augmentation exists. Radiation alone or postoperatively can also produce scarring, edema, and arthrofibrosis, and should be used judiciously in the foot. If a lesion is very destructive and resistant to treatment, amputation may be considered.

Pelvis and Acetabulum. Impending or pathologic fractures should be aggressively addressed as neglect can result in difficult problems in the way of bone loss, acetabular protrusio, and pelvic discontinuity. Further, inadequate pain control risks secondary problems from prolonged immobilization, such as pneumonia, decubitus ulcers, and pulmonary emboli. As noted earlier, small metastatic bone lesions to the ischium,

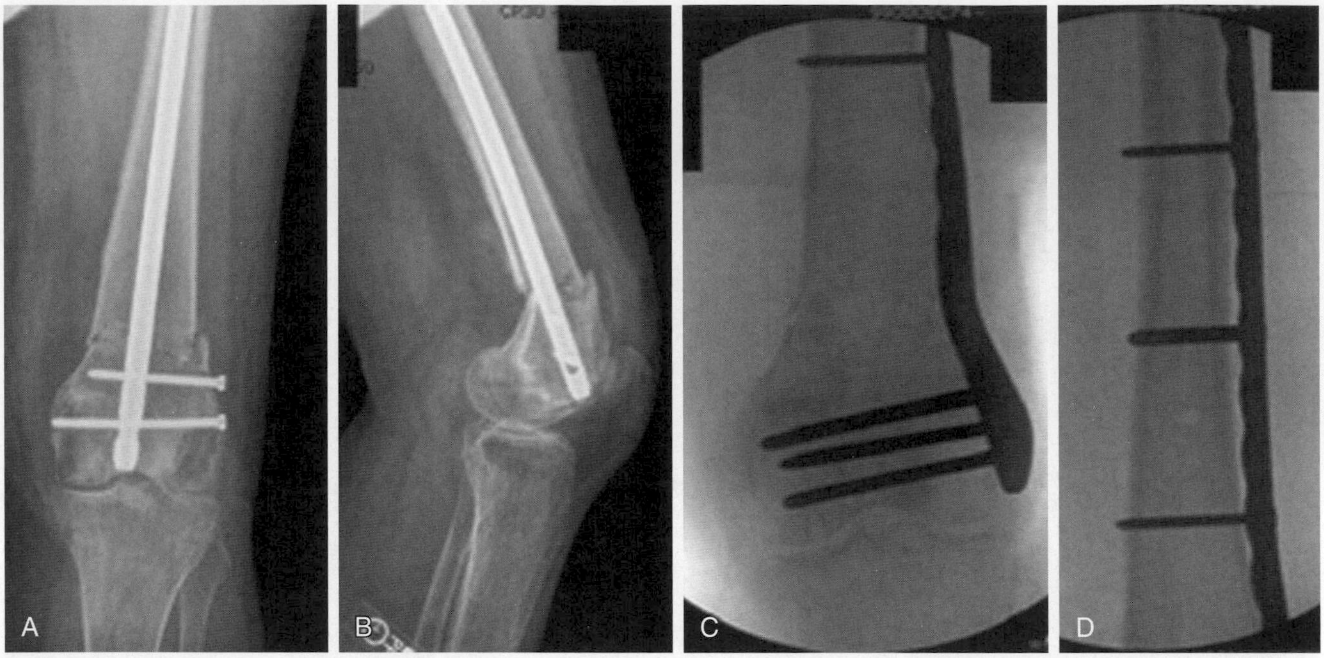

Figure 20-18. A 56-year-old female with lymphoma. **A** and **B,** Pathologic fracture with failed intramedullary nail of the right supracondylar femur. **C** and **D,** Fluoroscopic images after hardware removal and hybrid distal femoral plating.

pubis, and sacroiliac region causing pain can be treated with radiation or RFA. Radiation alone for lesions or fracture in the region of weight-bearing transfer in the pelvis often proves inadequate with short periods of pain relief and ultimately leads to the accumulation of microfractures and catastrophic failure with joint collapse.[94] This treatment makes subsequent surgery more difficult due to scarring and increases the risk of infection. Generally, any patient who is medically stable with a reasonable life expectancy should be considered a candidate for stabilization. The goal is to create a construct that supports a weak area of bone, transfers stress to stronger bone toward the spine, and avoids loosening. Early surgery is associated with faster pain relief, immediate weight bearing, and decreased wound healing complications.

The anatomy of the pelvis is complex, and achieving a good understanding of bone loss and fracture lines is important. Judet radiographs and a fine-cut CT are most helpful at characterizing the deficiencies. Lesions and fractures of the posterior ring leading to pain from pelvic ring instability should be addressed. Sacral ala fractures should receive transsacral screws with cement injected into the deficient areas. Lesions of the posterior ilium can be supported with fully threaded column screws from the posterior superior iliac spine (PSIS) over the sciatic buttress toward the anterior inferior iliac spine (AIIS), and defects are supported with cement. Extensive damage in the posterior ring warrants a discussion of spinopelvic fixation. Anterior ring lesions and fractures can often be treated without surgery but sometimes require treatment if pain persists despite conservative measures. An anterior column screw above the acetabulum into the superior ramus can provide reinforcement.

The periacetabular pelvis is the most common location for pelvic metastases and they are certainly among the more difficult to treat. The main concern from the surgeon's

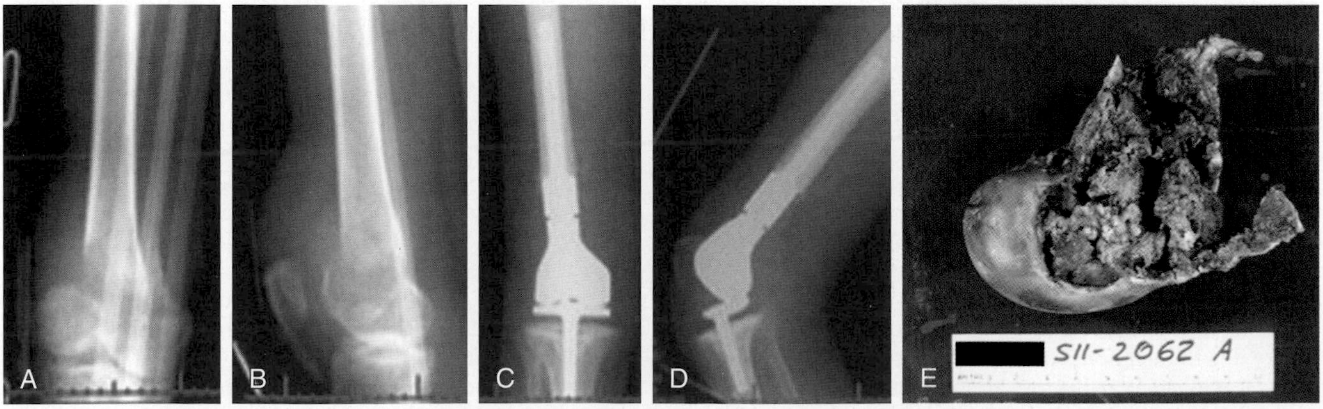

Figure 20-19. A 72-year-old male with metastatic renal cell carcinoma. **A** and **B,** Destructive lesion of the right distal femur with pathologic fracture and severe bone loss of the lateral femoral condyle. **C** and **D,** Radiographs after resection and distal femoral endoprosthesis. **E,** Gross pathologic specimen.

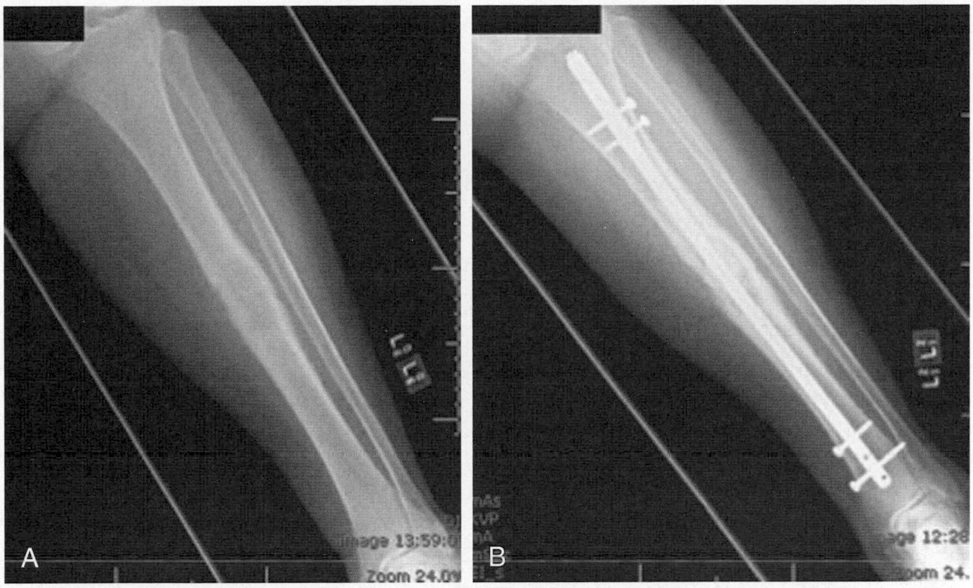

Figure 20-20. A 66-year-old female with metastatic lung cancer. **A,** She sustained a pathologic fracture of her left midshaft tibia. **B,** Postoperative radiographs demonstrate an intramedullary nail with cement packed into the midshaft bone defect.

standpoint is disruption of the weight-bearing transfer from the hip joint to the superior acetabular dome to the sciatic buttress to the sacroiliac joint up into the lumbar spine. Loss of this weight transfer leads to pain and immobility. Assessment starts by examining the integrity of the medial wall of the acetabulum, superior weight-bearing dome (Fig. 20-21), and acetabular rim. Presence or absence of these structures dictates treatment.

An intact dome, rim, and medial wall with a painful focal lesion in the periacetabular pelvis can undergo curettage and cementation if the subchondral surface is intact. This is effective in pain relief.[41,95] With disruption of the subchondral surface, a cemented THA is more reliable for pain relief and function.[96] After the femoral neck cut and reaming of the acetabulum, tumor defects are curetted and filled with cement. Both the femoral and acetabular components are generally cemented in place, as bony ingrowth is less reliable in the face of chemotherapy and radiation treatment. When there is good bone stock, favorable patient prognosis, and treatment options that allow chemotherapy or radiation to be withheld, press-fit implants with ingrowth potential may be considered.[97]

Medial wall deficiency is common. It is frequently observed leading to fracture and progressive migration of the femoral head proximally and medially. Reconstruction depends on the status of the rim and superior dome, tumor response to systemic treatment, and life expectancy of the patient. If the superior weight-bearing acetabulum and rim are intact, there is still an area in which to affix an acetabular component. Further, a patient with a favorable life expectancy and tumor responsive to systemic treatment may be viewed more as a patient with acetabular deficiency and less as a pathologic entity. In these cases, trabecular metal revision cups with augments or jumbo cups that can achieve a pinch fixation between the ilium and ischium and be supported with multiple long-column screws can be considered as biologic ingrowth is a reasonable expectation. There is evidence that such reconstructions can provide durable reconstruction in pathologic fields.[97,98] An intact rim in a patient with a poor expected

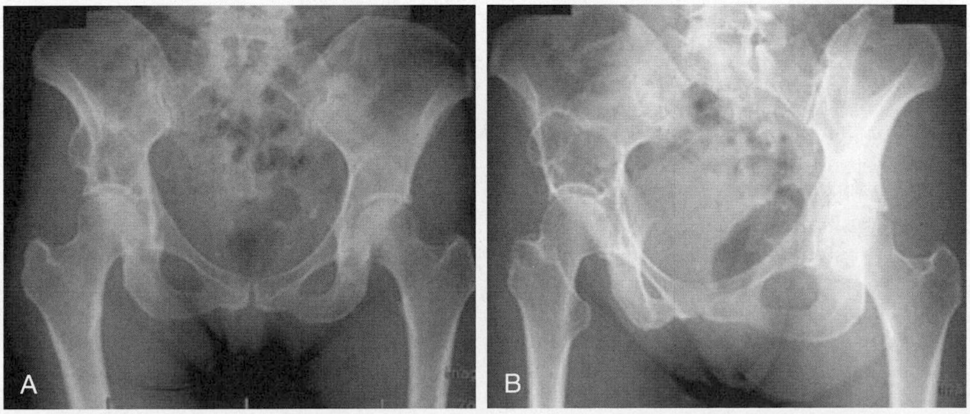

Figure 20-21. A 55-year-old female with metastatic breast cancer. **A** and **B,** Anterior-posterior (AP) and iliac oblique radiographs demonstrating a radiolucent expansile lesion in the superior dome of the acetabulum.

survival or with a tumor unresponsive to treatment warrants a flanged cage that is cemented and supported with screw fixation into areas of stronger bone around the acetabulum. These cages are often referred to as *protrusio rings*, *antiprotrusio cages*, or *reconstruction cages*. A polyethylene liner is then cemented into place. Positioning the cup in slightly more abduction than normal is recommended as it maximizes the compressive strength of cement. Use of a constrained liner can be effective in these lower demand patients and alleviates dislocation concerns. This strategy allows most patients to return to walking.[99] Loss of either the superior dome and/or acetabular rim creates a break in the weight transfer from the lower extremities to the spine and also provides no reliable bone to buttress a cup. A new bridge must be created and then used to support the acetabular reconstruction. Most commonly, this is done by placing partially threaded 5-mm Steinmann pins or fully threaded screws from the iliac crest into the area of acetabular defect. A pin is also frequently placed from the defect over the sciatic buttress and into the PSIS (Fig. 20-22). Additional column screws can be placed to further reestablish the weight transfer; these include inner ilium down the posterior column, AIIS to PSIS, upper retro-acetabulum to the superior pubic ramus, and greater sciatic notch toward the pelvic brim. The remaining defect is filled with cement. Depending on the degree of deficiency, a liner can be cemented in place or a flanged cage can be placed for additional medial support and then the liner cemented (Fig. 20-23). Orientation of the cup can be difficult, and it is best to use any remaining rim to get a sense of location. Use of trial implants and fluoroscopy takes away any guesswork when setting offset and cup position. In the circumstance of rim, dome, and medial wall loss in a patient with favorable longevity who can receive minimal or no radiation due to a good response to systemic treatments, a trabecular metal cup and cage or triflange reconstruction can be discussed.[100] Cementing the liner into these implants converts the screws through the cup into fixed-angle implants improving construct strength and making them a viable option.[101] Patients on the opposite side of the spectrum with short life expectancies and treatment-resistant malignancies with loss of the dome, rim, and medial wall could be considered for a saddle prosthesis. These do well with respect to pain control and preserving ambulation[102,103]; however, ambulation is not normal and over time, function worsens and there is a high rate of complications.[104] Patients unfit for such a large surgery may receive pain relief with a Girdlestone resection arthroplasty.

Management of the femoral side is influenced by many of the factors discussed earlier. Those with disease in the proximal femur or with poor estimated survival are treated with a cemented femoral stem, which provides immediate stability and withstands radiation reliably. The length is determined by the most distal site of disease in the femur. If there is no disease on the femoral side, a favorable patient life expectancy, and tumor responsive to systemic treatment obviating the need for radiation, a press-fit stem can be used.[97]

The surgical approach for periacetabular work is most often posterolateral or straight lateral. A trochanteric osteotomy can improve exposure and allow access to the retro-acetabulum and superior rim. The Levine anterior approach, which is a modified Smith-Peterson approach with extension to the ASIS and up along the ilium, is an alternative that is particularly useful with rim and superior dome deficiencies requiring Steinman pins or long screws with cement to reestablish the weight-bearing transfer of the pelvis.[105] Further, being an anterior approach, the Levine approach provides greater postoperative stability to the hip and earlier functional returns.

Complications such as periprosthetic infection, dislocation, and construct failure in the setting of these surgeries can be devastating. They delay adjuvant treatment with radiation and/or chemotherapy and prolong time in the hospital taking patients away from family and quality of life activities. Several measures can be useful to minimize risk. Antibiotics can be placed in the cement to provide prophylaxis from infection. A large prosthetic femoral head and increased offset can aid hip stability and prevent dislocation. Careful soft tissue repair of the capsule, short external rotators, and imbrication of the iliotibial band can enhance hip stability.

Reconstructions for periacetabular bone loss or fracture from metastatic disease can help maintain ambulation and provide pain relief in the majority of patients at 6 months. Healey and colleagues reviewed 55 patients with acetabular reconstructions for metastatic disease and found 83% had significant pain relief at 3 months. Of those alive at 2 years, 86% continued to have pain relief.[106]

Spine. The most common site of metastatic spread to bone is the spinal column, which predominately occurs in the thoracic and lumbar spines. Most lesions are occult with 10% to 20% becoming symptomatic and 5% to 10% causing symptoms from epidural compression.[107] Prostate is the most common primary malignancy, metastasizing to the spine 90% of the time.[108] Across all tumor subtypes, treatment of symptomatic lesions has proven beneficial and durable in maintaining patient function and pain relief.[109]

Patients with spine metastases often have more advanced disease and a poorer prognosis. The overall 3-month mortality with spine metastases is 29% and the mean survival for patients with spine metastases is 15.9 months.[110] Therefore, it is very important to identify the appropriate level of intervention for each individual patient. The expected life span, general medical condition, age, tumor subtype, status of radiation, preoperative examination, and number of levels involved are key factors in decision making. Metastases from melanoma, lung, and the upper gastrointestinal track cancers have a poor prognosis whereas those from breast, prostate, myeloma, and lymphoma are more favorable.[111] One-year survival with a primary lung cancer is 22% versus 78% and 83% for breast and prostate primaries.[112] Other indicators of a poor outcome include metastatic spread to visceral organs, immunosuppressed patients with poor nutrition and multiple comorbidities, and advanced age. These are associated with a higher risk of death within 30 days of surgery.[111] Those treated with radiation before surgery have a greater risk of infection postoperatively and patients with a neurologic deficit before surgery have a lower mean survival at 1 and 3 years after surgery.[110,111,113,114] Multiple levels of spine involvement, most notably cord compression at two noncontiguous levels, is an indicator of poor functional prognosis that needs to be factored into surgical decision making.[115] Palliative treatment with pain medication, radiation, and bracing are preferred for patients with several of these risk factors. Tokuhashi and colleagues developed an algorithm to predict the survivability of patients after surgery (Table 20-1). They identified general medical condition; number of extraspinal bone, vertebral, and visceral metastases; primary site of malignancy; and severity of spinal cord compression as

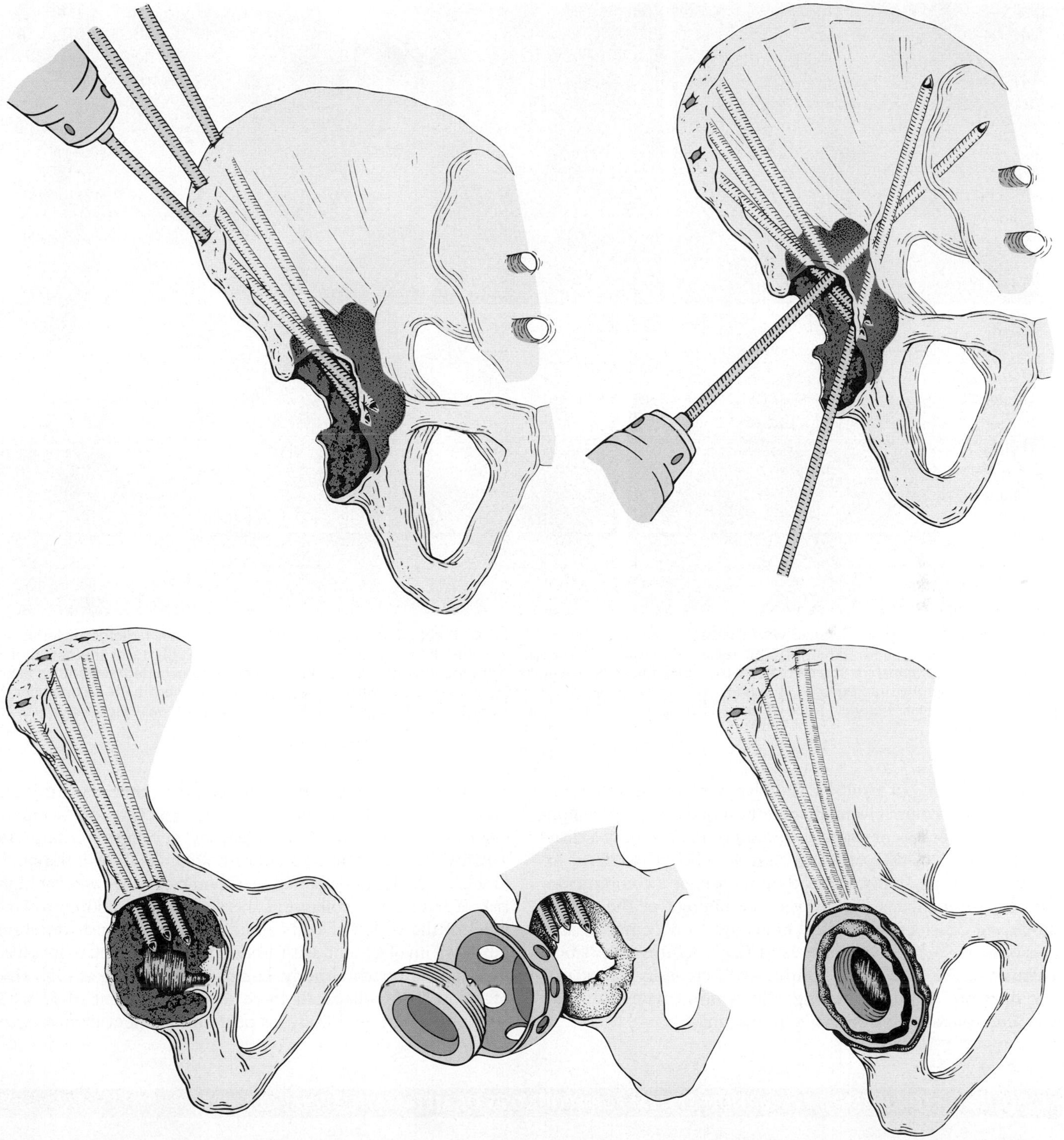

Figure 20-22. Placement of Steinmann pins to reconstruct the medial wall and superior dome of the acetabulum. A protrusion cage with a cemented liner is placed into the remaining defect.

important factors. A scoring system was established and a score less than or equal to 5 estimated an average survival of 3 months or less. A score of 9 or greater predicted a survival of 12 months or longer.[116]

Patients with a life expectancy longer than 3 months and general health capable of tolerating surgery with a progressive neurologic deficit, spinal instability with mechanical pain, fracture-dislocation, enlarging radioresistant tumor, or intractable pain despite nonsurgical measures are candidates for surgery. Evaluation begins by assessing for radiculopathy or myelopathy, which suggest epidural compression. Standing and/or flexion and extension radiographs can show fractures and subtle signs of instability. Advanced imaging should be performed with a CT scan to evaluate structural bone integrity and an MRI with contrast to evaulate soft tissue involvement and neural compression. These images help the surgeon gain

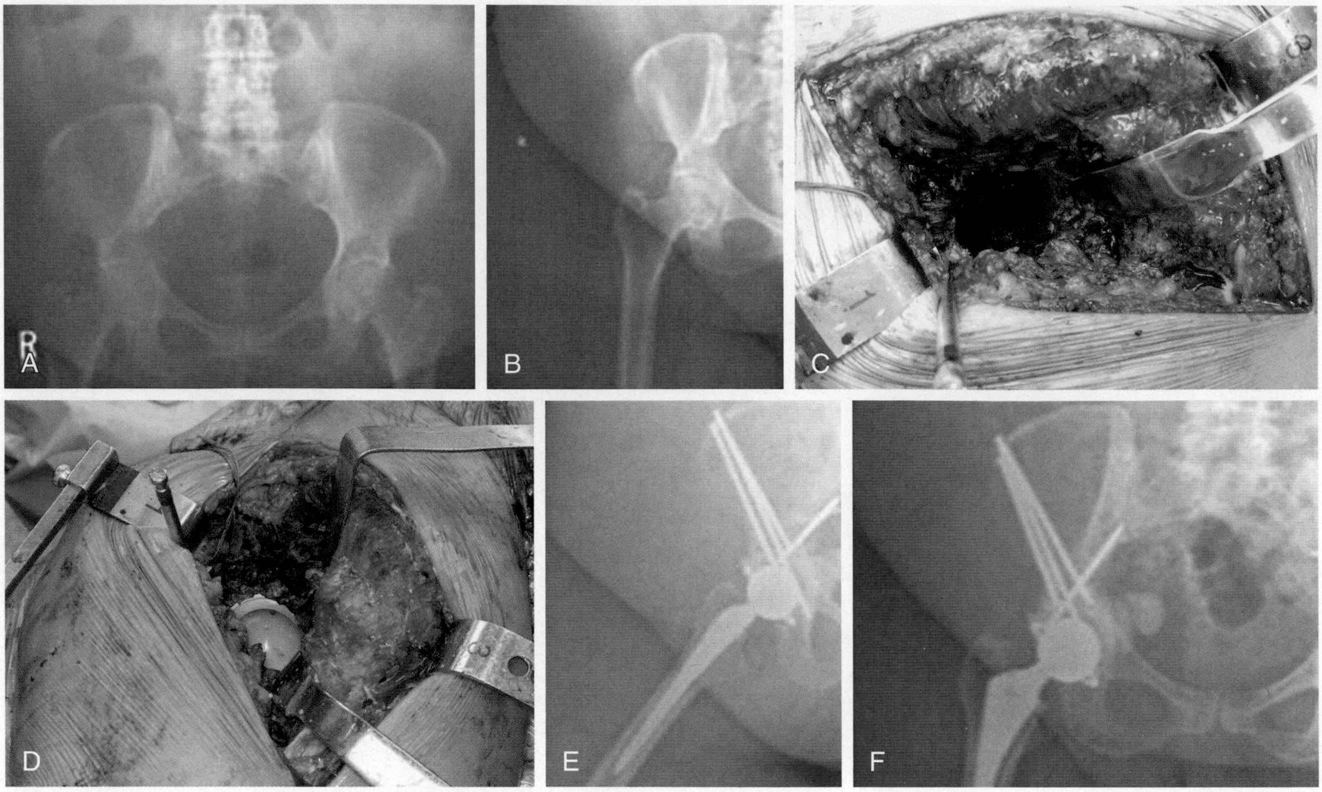

Figure 20-23. A 54-year-old male with metastatic prostate cancer. **A** and **B,** Preoperative radiographs show a subtle radiolucent lesion in the supra-acetabulum with extension into the medial wall with disruption of the iliopectineal line. **C,** Intraoperative photo of the acetabular defect with Steinmann pins directed from the ilium into the defect. **D,** Intraoperative photo of the cemented constrained acetabular liner. **E** and **F,** Postoperative radiographs showing the reconstructed supra-acetabulum and medial wall with pins and cement with a constrained, cemented acetabular liner with press-fit femoral component. There was no disease on the femoral side and the patient was responding well to systemic therapy.

an understanding of level(s) of involvement, extent of tumor, posterior element involvement, direction of cord compression, and presence or risk of fracture. The surgeon must have a clear understanding of the pathology and whether it is related to compression, instability, impending failure, or a combination of these mechanisms. As always, the biology of the tumor should be considered. Surgical goals are to decompress any sites of neurologic compression, stabilize fractures or instability, and achieve local tumor control while creating a construct that does not rely upon healing, allows immediate mobilization, and tolerates postoperative radiation.

Impending failure of the spinal column can lead to an acute event often in the form of a burst fracture or fracture-dislocation. Taneichi and colleagues developed criteria to identify patients at high risk of pathologic fracture of the spine (Table 20-2). He determined that thoracic lesions were at high risk of failure and collapse if there was 50% to 60% involvement of the vertebral body alone or there was costovertebral junction involvement with associated 25% to 30% involvement of the vertebral body. Lumbar lesions were at high risk of failure and collapse if there was involvement of 35% to 40% of the vertebral body, or posterior element involvement

TABLE 20-1 *TOKUHASHI'S EVALUATION SYSTEM FOR PROGNOSIS OF METASTATIC SPINAL TUMORS*

	Score		
Symptoms	*0*	*1*	*2*
General condition (performance status)	Poor (10–40%)	Moderate (50–70%)	Good (80–100%)
Number of extraspinal skeletal metastases	>3	1–2	0
Metastases to internal organs	Unremovable	Removable	No metastases
Primary site of tumor	Lung, stomach	Kidney, liver, uterus, unknown	Thyroid, prostate, breast, rectum
Number of metastases to spine	>3	2	1
Spinal cord palsy	Complete	Incomplete	None

9 to 12 points: >12 months' survival; 0 to 5 points: <3 months' survival.

From Tokuhashi Y, Matsuzaki H, Tonyama S, et al: Scoring system for the preoperative evaluation of metastatic spine tumor prognosis, Spine (Phila Pa 1976) 15:1110–1113, 1999.

TABLE 20-2 *RISK FACTORS FOR COLLAPSE WITH METASTATIC DISEASE OF THE THORACIC AND LUMBAR SPINE*

Thoracic Spine
Risk Factors
Costovertebral joining destruction
Percent of body involvement
Criteria for impending collapse
50% to 60% body involvement alone
25% to 30% of body with costovertebral involvement
Lumbar Spine
Risk Factors
Pedicle destruction
Percent of body involvement
Criteria for impending collapse
35% to 40% body involvement alone
25% with pedicle and/or posterior element destruction

From Taneichi H, Kaneda K, Takeda N, et al: Risk factors and probability of vertebral body collapse in metastases of the thoracic and lumbar spine, Spine (Phila Pa 1976) 22(3):239–245, 1997.

with an associated lesion involving 20% to 25% of vertebral body. This risk is amplified if the tumor is between L1 and L3, of poorly differentiated histology, or involves both sides of the vertebrae.[117]

Patients with an asymptomatic lesion identified on staging or surveillance imaging should be evaluated for risk of impending fracture. If risk is low and there is no sign of posterior element compromise, minimal vertebral body involvement, and no evidence of instability, the patient may be observed and receive systemic treatment only. If there is vertebral body involvement greater than 50%, even if asymptomatic, radiation should be discussed because of concern for impending failure. Tumors resistant to conventional radiation are at greater risk of local recurrence and should be evaluated for embolization, brachytherapy, or stereotactic body radiation therapy (SBRT).[118,119] SBRT involves multiple beams that can be concentrated under image guidance on a single target tissue to provide high doses while minimizing toxicity to the surrounding spinal cord and normal tissues. Doses are usually greater than 5 Gy per fraction and administered in multiple fractions to achieve a total dose of 15 to 35 Gy. This allows the delivery of up to six times the dose of conventional EBRT.[61] Use of SBRT is becoming more common and is now being considered for preoperative use as it has a lower incidence of wound complications. However, its use is still limited by cost and technical skill involved. The higher doses create a greater potential for toxicity, which include radiation myelopathy, esophageal necrosis, bronchial stenosis, and vertebral compression fractures and this requires a radiation oncologist comfortable with this technology.[120-122] While there is much enthusiasm about the potential of SBRT to palliate metastatic disease to the spine, there is currently sparse evidence demonstrating improved outcomes over EBRT.

A symptomatic patient should raise concern of neural compression, fracture, and/or bony instability. If the patient has pain without neurologic compromise, the assessment centers on the stability of the spinal column, which can be compromised by tumor invasion. A stable column without cord compression with vertebral body destruction less than 50% can be treated with radiation alone. A regimen of 2 Gy in five fractions is frequently used.[109] Vertebral body involvement greater than 50% with pain is at risk of impending fracture and is likely to have instability.[117] Instability, defined as insufficient structures to support physiologic loading, warrants a discussion about surgical intervention. When there is pain from fracture or instability but no neurologic deficit, outcomes after surgical intervention are more favorable and lead to more predictable outcomes. In these cases, posterior fixation only with pedicle screws followed by radiation provides good tumor control and pain relief. This approach is associated with a reduction in patient morbidity, decreased hospital time, and quick returns to chemotherapy. Neurologic compromise in the way of radiculopathy or myelopathy should alert the physician to look for epidural compression, burst fracture, and instability leading to symptomatic compression from kyphosis (Fig. 20-24). A whole spine MRI is necessary and is often able to localize the level and direction of compression. Patients with single levels of compression, a recent neurologic deficit, and with satisfactory bone quality above and below the level involved to support fixation in an individual with a life expectancy longer than 3 months do better with surgery compared to treatment with radiation alone. A neurologic deficit makes recovery less predictable, but a favorable recovery is associated with incomplete paraplegia, intact sphincter control, and gradual onset of deficit. Poor neurologic recovery is associated with complete paraplegia, loss of sphincter control, and rapid onset of deficit.[123] Radiation only improves about 50% of neurologic impairment from compression, while surgery is associated with restored ability to walk and improved quality of life.[124-129] Ambulatory status after surgery is best predicted by preoperative neurologic status.[130] High-dose dexamethasone can be used in patients with acute neurologic deficits from spinal cord compression and is associated with improved postoperative ambulation. Use should be restricted to acute deficits as patients are at risk of medication side effects such as peptic ulcer and bleeding.

Surgery should use the most appropriate approach to achieve direct decompression of tumor. The direction of compression on the dural sac is most often anterior followed by posterolateral and posterior.[131] Vertebral body metastases necessitate an anterior approach with corpectomy and an anterior column reconstruction with structural support in the form of cortical allograft, cage with bone graft, cement, or prosthesis; a plate is often placed for rotational control (Fig. 20-25). Cement or prosthesis is often preferred in this setting as they provide immediate structural stability and are not affected by radiation. Bone graft should only be used in patients with a long life expectancy and in tumors with a good response to systemic therapy because radiation will have to be either withheld or delayed to allow incorporation.[132] Anterior decompression with reconstruction of the anterior spinal column can also be supported with posterior instrumentation when instability or tumor progression remains a concern. This technique does require a second approach and results in a greater surgical burden on the patient.

Posterior or posterolateral compression requires removal of posterior elements for adequate decompression followed by stabilization with pedicle screws.[133] Laminectomy alone for these cases, even with radiation, is not effective because patients may develop instability.[124,134-137] Patients with a large tumor load may need anterior and posterior approaches to

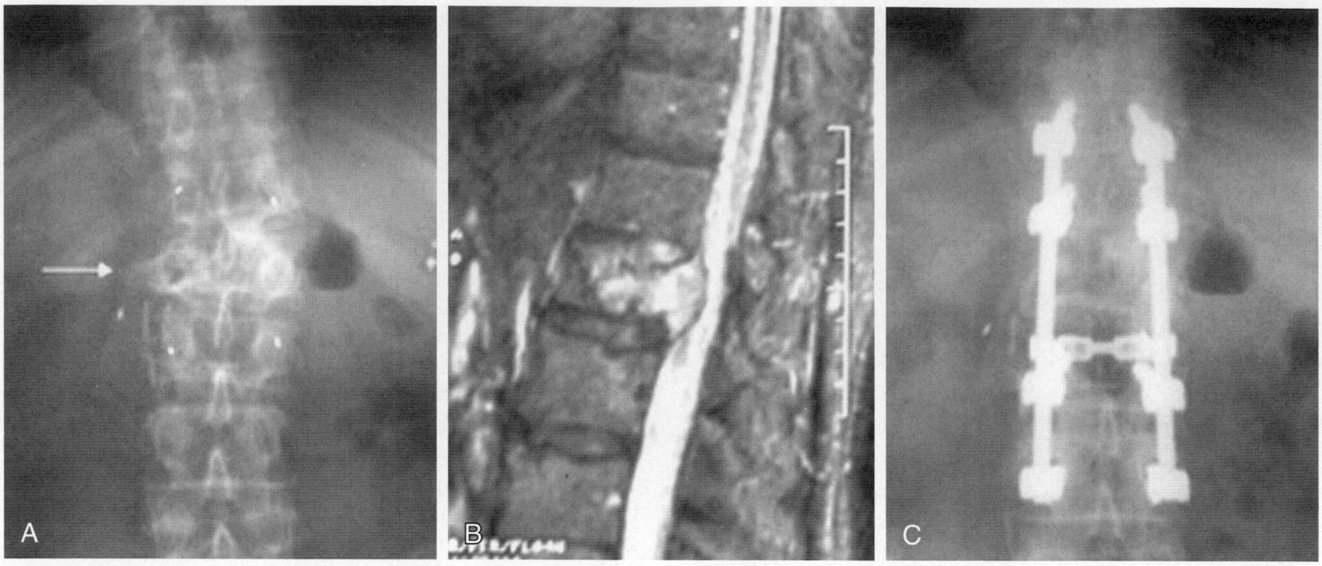

Figure 20-24. Patient with renal cell carcinoma presented with pain and myelopathy. **A,** Standing radiographs demonstrated lateral subluxation and scoliosis. **B,** Sagittal T2 magnetic resonance imaging (MRI) showed a destructive vertebral body lesion with epidural extension and dural compression. **C,** Postoperative radiographs after anterior decompression and posterior fixation.

achieve adequate decompression as well as fixation stable enough to allow immediate mobilization. When symptomatic spine involvement extends into the lower lumbar spine and upper sacrum, spinopelvic fixation must be considered (Fig. 20-26). Radiation is administered postoperatively to facilitate local tumor control and minimize wound complications. Surgery with radiation leads to improvement in 80% of patients, most notably in walking, continence, strength, function, and reduced use of pain medications.[138-140] Pain relief is the major benefit of surgery and it is often maintained for at least 6 months.[141] As always, the magnitude of the surgery must be weighed against the patient's prognosis, overall health, and potential for recovery.[142] Patients with multiple nonadjacent levels of compression, poor bone stock, extensive disease, short life expectancy, or a complete neurologic deficit have a poor prognosis for recovery and are a relative contraindication for surgery[115] (Fig. 20-27). Operative efforts often prove futile in these cases with failed fixation leading to problems with skin breakdown, infection, and pain; here, radiation therapy and bracing is often the best treatment.

An alternative for those with pain and destructive bone lesions of the vertebrae or sacrum is vertebroplasty or kyphoplasty. These procedures are primarily indicated for poor surgical candidates, multilevel disease, and profound neurologic deficits. These patients must have an intact posterior vertebral

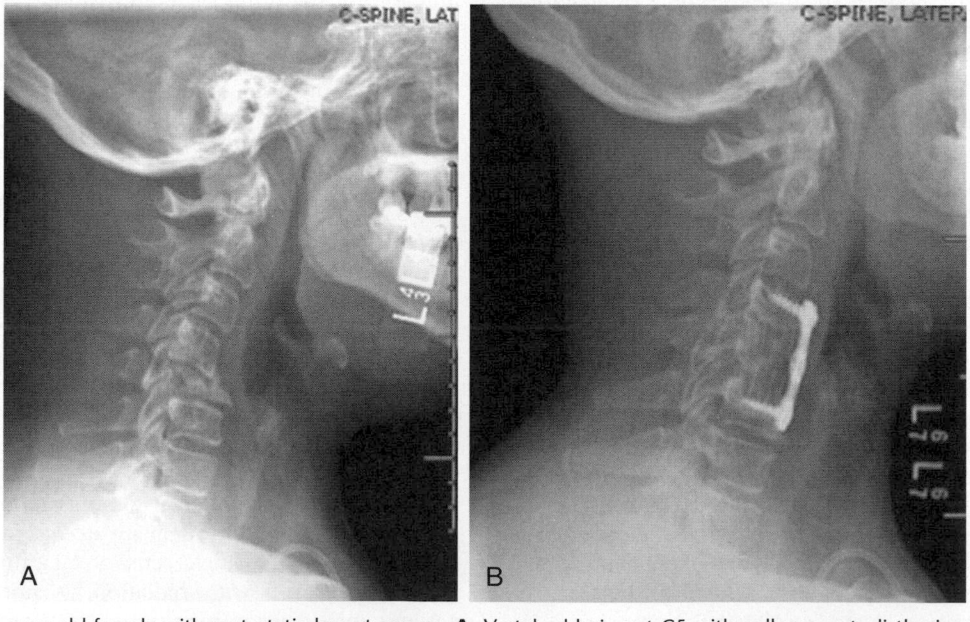

Figure 20-25. A 51-year-old female with metastatic breast cancer. **A,** Vertebral lesion at C5 with collapse, retrolisthesis and kyphosis. **B,** Postoperative radiograph after anterior corpectomy and fusion.

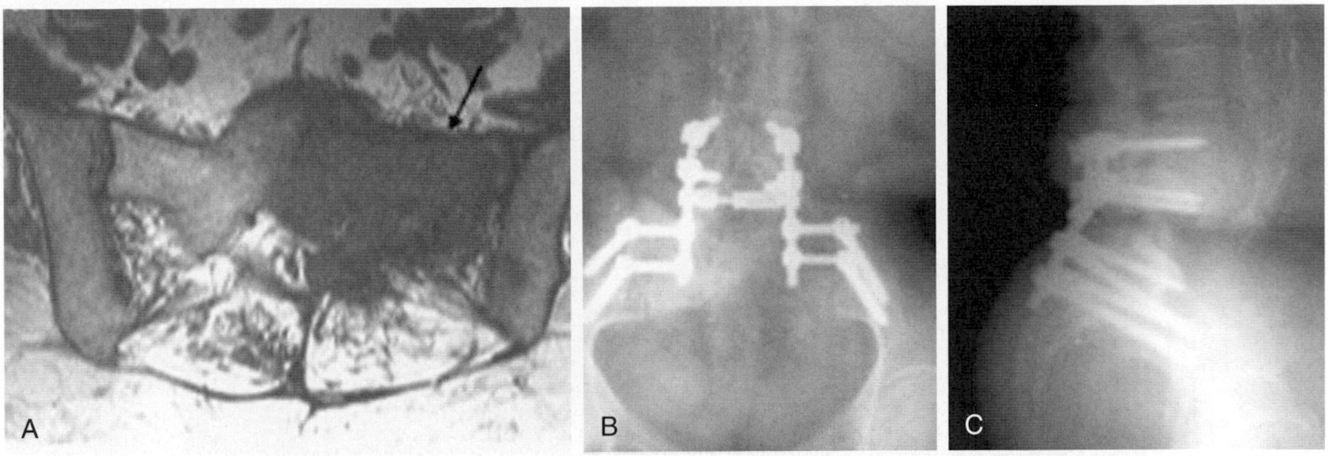

Figure 20-26. Patient with metastatic breast cancer. **A,** Complete infiltration of left sacral ala by tumor with associated destruction of the left L5-S1 facet joint. As a result, the patient had instability and intractable pain. **B** and **C,** Radiographs after spinopelvic posterior fusion bypassing the area of tumor and restoring stability and the weight transfer axis. The patient was treated a few weeks later with adjunctive stereotactic body radiotherapy (SBRT).

wall and have intractable pain from vertebral collapse without cord compression or gross instability. Vertebroplasty is the percutaneous injection of acrylic cement into the vertebral body (Fig. 20-28). Kyphoplasty uses a balloon to restore height to a collapsed vertebra and then fills the balloon with cement for support. Less pressure is generally needed for the latter.

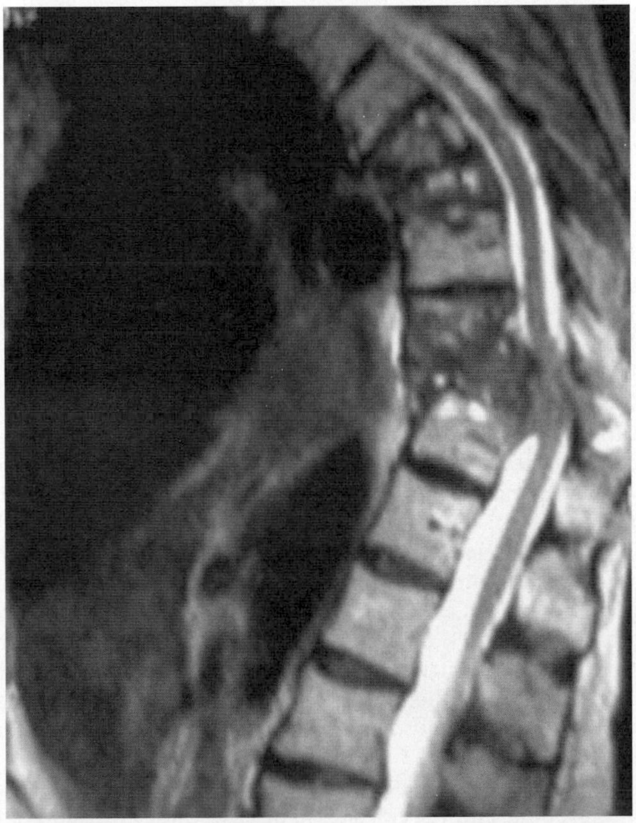

Figure 20-27. Elderly female with many comorbidities and extensive metastatic breast cancer including a destructive vertebral lesion with dislocation and dural compression at the thoracolumbar junction. Given the multiple areas of vertebral involvement, poor bone stock, complete neurologic deficit, and poor life expectancy, the patient was treated with palliative external beam radiotherapy (EBRT) and bracing.

Injection of cement restores mechanical integrity to the vertebral body and helps prevent further collapse. These procedures can be performed in a radiology suite or operating room with IV sedation under fluoroscopic guidance via a parapedicular or transpedicular approach. There is an approximately 10% risk of cement extravasation into neural foramina or the spinal column as well as a risk of respiratory compromise from particle embolization with cement pressurization.[143] These complications are best prevented with use of barium to visualize cement injection, use of live fluoroscopy, slow cement injection, use of viscous cement, limiting cement volume, and use of intraosseous venograms.[144] Pain control is effective with approximately 70% of patients achieving sustained relief for 6 months or longer.[145-148] The success of these techniques has led some surgeons to consider a new approach in poor surgical candidates with multilevel metastatic spine disease with focal cord compression; using a posterolateral approach, an open decompression is performed followed by a vertebroplasty for anterior column support. This procedure avoids posterior multilevel instrumentation and appears to provide relief.[109] There are no studies yet comparing this treatment to radiation alone.

COMPLICATIONS

As has been discussed, pathologic fractures through malignant bone lesions present unique medical and biologic challenges to the treating physician. Many of the potential complications associated with specific treatments have been discussed. One of the most clinically important complications is failure of fixation or reconstruction because of unreliable healing and local disease progression. Both of these can jeopardize fixation and stabilization and subject these already unwell patients to another, more complicated surgical procedure. In an effort to minimize this complication, surgeons should work with the assumption that disease progression will occur and aim to provide a reconstruction that is durable and long lasting.

In addition, from a general health perspective, these patients often have multiple medical problems, many

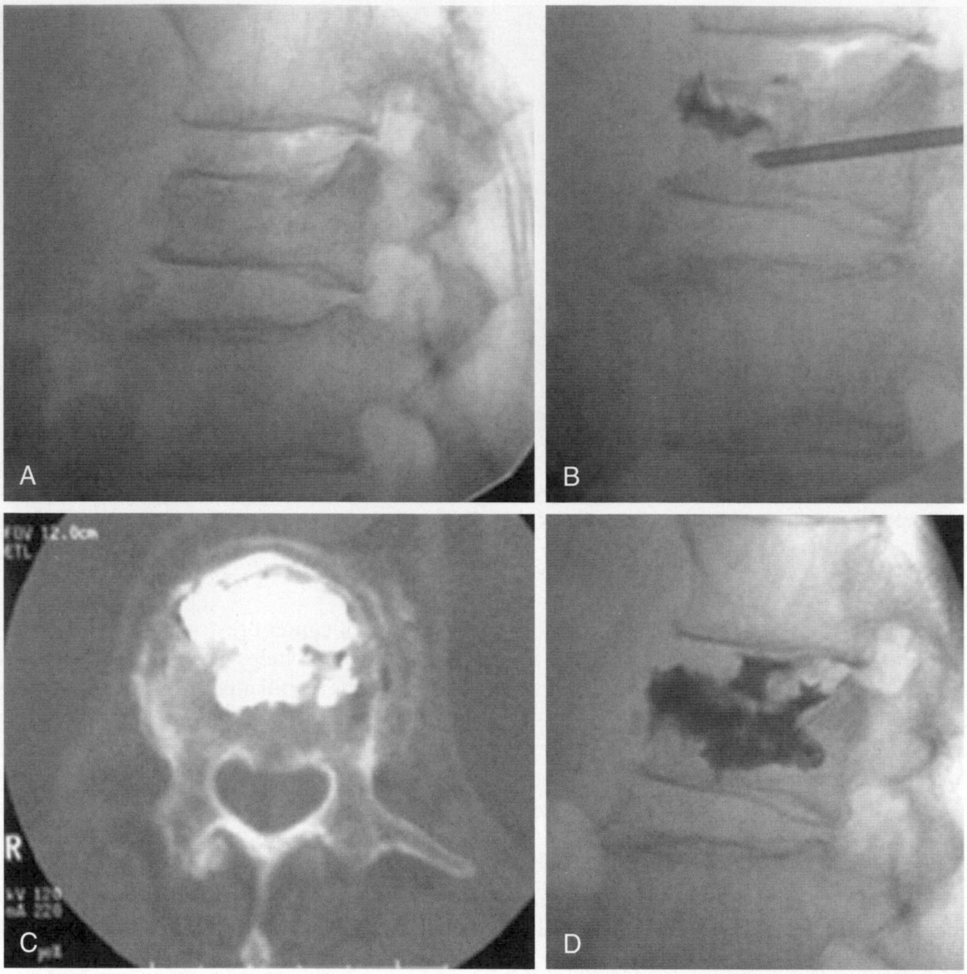

Figure 20-28. Elderly patient with multiple myeloma and significant back pain. **A,** Radiograph demonstrating vertebral body collapse without evidence of instability and an intact posterior wall. The patient had no epidural compression from tumor. **B–D,** Percutaneous vertebroplasty was performed with cement injection into the vertebral body. The patient's pain improved afterward.

specifically related to their malignancies. Generalized decompensation as a result of widespread cancer puts these patients at a high risk for perioperative medical and surgical complications. Often, because the planned procedures are urgent, there is little time to optimize modifiable risk factors, making surgical intervention more dangerous. Additionally, compared to the general population, they are at increased risk of wound healing problems, infection, and venous thromboembolism. This risk should be assessed preoperatively and an appropriate prophylactic strategy employed. Prophylaxis against thromboembolic events can range from chemoprophylaxis (e.g., aspirin, warfarin, or enoxaparin), to mechanical prophylaxis with sequential compression devices, or to the placement of an inferior vena cava filter.[149,150] There are no clear evidence-based guidelines for the best or most appropriate prophylactic regimen in these medically complicated patients.

SPECIAL CONSIDERATIONS

There are a few subtypes of pathologic fractures that require special consideration. Renal cell carcinomas, radiation-induced fractures, and bisphosphonate-related fractures fall into this category. Fractures in the setting of these diseases are treated with a slightly different approach and can have different outcomes compared to those discussed earlier in this chapter.

Renal Cell Carcinomas

Although within the category of metastatic carcinoma, solitary bone metastases from renal cell carcinomas are approached with a treatment strategy different to that for other metastatic carcinomas. In the setting of a solitary bony metastasis with no visceral disease, there is data to suggest that complete surgical resection of the tumor may improve survival.[151-153] Data from the Mayo Clinic demonstrated the risk of death from disease to be <20% after complete metastasectomy at 5 years compared to 49% in those who did not have all disease surgically resected.[153] Therefore, within this subset of patients, aggressive, potentially curative or life-prolonging resection should be considered.

When there is widely metastatic disease as indicated by multiple bone and visceral sites of disease, these are lesions are treated with palliative intent. The challenge that a surgeon may encounter is that these cancers are not traditionally responsive to systemic therapies or radiation therapy and can have a higher risk of local disease progression. Therefore, it is often recommended that more aggressive reconstruction techniques be considered to decrease the rate of local recurrence and failure of the reconstruction.[151,154-156] For example, in the setting of a lesion in the intertrochanteric femur, a proximal femoral replacement with endoprosthetic reconstruction could be considered as opposed to an intramedullary nail. This option may offer a more durable reconstruction without the risk of local disease progression and additional bony destruction. If intralesional work is to be done, preoperative embolization should be performed to prevent massive intraoperative hemorrhage from these very vascular tumors.

Radiation-Induced Fractures

Radiation-induced fractures can, at times, be more challenging to treat than fractures through malignant lesions. Although these are a rare subtype of pathologic fractures, they are most commonly encountered after a patient has received very high doses of radiation as part of the treatment of a soft tissue sarcoma.[157] In addition to the insult of radiation to the bone, the surgical resection of the sarcoma may necessitate removal of a significant portion of the periosteum or even a partial bony resection.[158] This combination of biologic offenses creates a situation where pathologic stress fractures and complete fractures can occur and also creates an environment in which bone healing is extremely unreliable. Failure rates after surgical stabilization of these fractures with traditional internal fixation techniques range from 45% to 63%.[159-161] Therefore, consideration of more aggressive techniques to manage these fractures, such as resection of the affected bone and endoprosthetic reconstruction may need to be considered. Alternatively, some have suggested prophylactic stabilization of these impending fractures to avoid the complications of nonunion and construct failure discussed previously.[161-163]

Bisphosphonate-Associated Fractures

Bisphosphonate-associated fractures or atypical femoral fractures have been seen in increasing numbers over the last few years. These subtrochanteric femur fractures present either as an incomplete stress fracture or complete fracture through an area of stress reaction in the femur. It is believed that the suppression of bone remodeling that occurs as a result of prolonged bisphosphonate use prevents the normal response to stresses within the bone of the subtrochanteric femur resulting in a stress fracture.[164] The fractures have a characteristic appearance described as a transverse fracture in the subtrochanteric femur with associated lateral cortical thickening (Fig. 20-29).[165] Treatment of acute fractures does not differ from that of any other subtrochanteric femur fracture and long cephalomedullary or reconstruction nails are often used as the first-line method for fracture stabilization. Some series have demonstrated decreased rate of union compared to more typical subtrochanteric femur fractures (approximately 50% vs. nearly 99%).[166,167] This difference in union rate is believed to be the result of the altered biology of bone turnover because of bisphosphonate use.

The controversy in treatment of these fractures lies in those that are at the stage of stress reaction or stress fracture with impending pathologic fracture. The role of surgical versus nonsurgical treatment medical therapies has not been conclusively borne out in the literature. It has been recommended that when these fractures are encountered, bisphosphonate use should be discontinued.[168,169] There are, otherwise, no evidence-based recommendations for the surveillance or treatment of these lesions. There are a few case reports of use of anabolic agents (i.e., parathyroid hormone analogs) and small case series about prophylactic stabilization, but it is difficult to determine which is the most appropriate method of treatment for these patients.[170,171] More work needs to be done to quantify risk of these fractures, more clearly document their outcomes, and provide more evidence-based treatment recommendations for the treatment of these pathologic fractures.

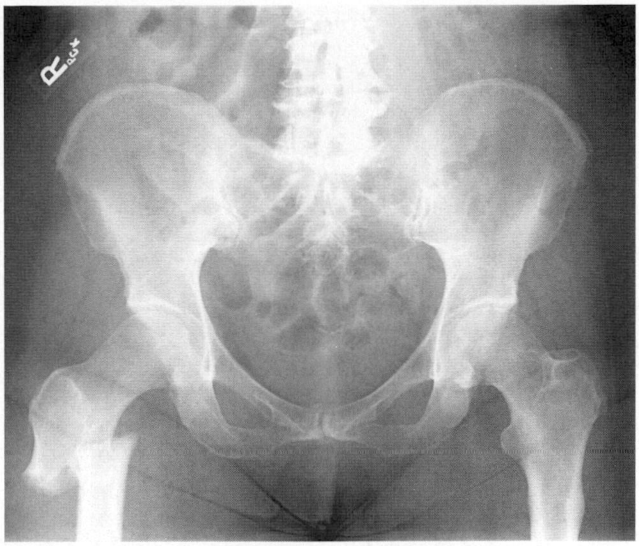

Figure 20-29. Anterior-posterior (AP) pelvic image of a woman who sustained a pathologic fracture of the right subtrochanteric femur. She had a history of prolonged bisphosphonate use and was found to have had a bisphosphonate-related pathologic fracture on the right characterized by its transverse nature through an area of lateral cortical thickening. Additionally, she had a stress fracture on the left as evidenced by the lateral cortical thickening within the subtrochanteric femur.

CONCLUSION

Pathologic fractures arise in the setting of bone that is abnormal for a large variety of reasons. It is essential for the treating surgeon to identify the underlying etiology of the pathologic bone as this has a significant influence on treatment, outcome, and eventual prognosis. An aggressive solitary bone lesion in an adult older than 40 years of age should be evaluated with a routine protocol that includes laboratory tests, CT chest, abdomen and pelvis, and a whole body bone scan followed by a biopsy to establish an accurate diagnosis prior to any surgical intervention. For impending or actualized pathologic fractures, the main treatment goals include pain relief and return of function with a reconstruction that will minimize complications, potential for return to the operating room, and one that will last the patient's lifetime.

KEY REFERENCES

The level of evidence (LOE) is determined according to the criteria provided in the preface.

48. Rosen LS, Gordon D, Tchekmedyian S, et al: Zoledronic acid versus placebo in the treatment of skeletal metastases in patients with lung cancer and other solid tumors: a phase III, double-blind, randomized

trial–the Zoledronic Acid Lung Cancer and Other Solid Tumors Study Group. *J Clin Oncol* 21(16):3150–3157, 2003. LOE I

53. Fizazi K, Carducci M, Smith M, et al: Denosumab versus zoledronic acid for treatment of bone metastases in men with castration-resistant prostate cancer: a randomised, double-blind study. *Lancet* 377(9768):813–822, 2011. LOE I
56. Sze WM, Shelley MD, Held I, et al: Palliation of metastatic bone pain: single fraction versus multifraction radiotherapy—a systematic review of randomised trials. *Clin Oncol (R Coll Radiol)* 15(6):345–352, 2003. LOE I
98. Joglekar SB, Rose PS, Lewallen DG, et al: Tantalum acetabular cups provide secure fixation in THA after pelvic irradiation at minimum 5-year followup. *Clin Orthop Relat Res* 470(11):3041–3047, 2012. LOE IV
116. Tokuhashi Y, Matsuzaki H, Toriyama S, et al: Scoring system for the preoperative evaluation of metastatic spine tumor prognosis. *Spine (Phila Pa 1976)* 15(11):1110–1113, 1990. LOE IV
117. Taneichi H, Kaneda K, Takeda N, et al: Risk factors and probability of vertebral body collapse in metastases of the thoracic and lumbar spine. *Spine (Phila Pa 1976)* 22(3):239–245, 1997. LOE IV
126. Patchell RA, Tibbs PA, Regine WF, et al: Direct decompressive surgical resection in the treatment of spinal cord compression caused by metastatic cancer: a randomised trial. *Lancet* 366(9486):643–648, 2005. LOE II
141. Wai EK, Finkelstein JA, Tangente RP, et al: Quality of life in surgical treatment of metastatic spine disease. *Spine (Phila Pa 1976)* 28(5):508–512, 2003. LOE IV
150. Ramo BA, Griffin AM, Gill CS, et al: Incidence of symptomatic venous thromboembolism in oncologic patients undergoing lower-extremity endoprosthetic arthroplasty. *J Bone Joint Surg Am* 93(9):847–854, 2011. LOE III
164. Shane E, Burr D, Abrahamsen B, et al: Review. Atypical subtrochanteric and diaphyseal femoral fractures: second report of a task force of the American Society for Bone and Mineral Research. *J Bone Mineral Res* 2013.

The complete References list is available online at https://expertconsult.inkling.com.

Chapter 21

Osteoporotic Fragility Fractures

KENNETH J. KOVAL • JOHN T. RIEHL • PAUL C. BALDWIN III • STEPHEN L. KATES

DEMOGRAPHICS OF OSTEOPOROTIC FRAGILITY FRACTURES

Fragility fracture refers to those fractures that result from a fall from standing height or less and frequently occur in the hip, wrist, and spine. Osteoporosis is characterized by a combination of both a decrease in bone density as well as qualitative defects in bone. Fractures secondary to osteoporosis are, by strict definition, pathologic fractures. They occur in bones whose structural integrity and strength have been diminished by an underlying disease process. Osteoporotic fragility fractures have become a major health and economic concern in the United States that has reached epidemic proportions. Currently, osteoporotic fragility fractures occur more frequently than heart attacks, strokes, and breast cancer combined.[1] Strategies are continually being developed and refined to both prevent these fractures, as well as to manage them when they occur.

The impact of osteoporotic fragility fractures in the United States will likely be felt more in the decades to come than ever before. Following World War II and in the ensuing 18 years, the United States saw a dramatic increase in childbirth rates. In 2011, the first of these "baby boomers" turned 65 years of age; at that time, approximately 13% of the U.S. population was age 65 or older.[2] In contrast, as more of the baby-boomer population reaches this milestone, it is estimated that by 2030, roughly 18% of the U.S. population will be age 65 or older. During the period from 2011 to 2026, 78 million baby boomers will reach the age of 65 years in the United States alone. During the 20-year period from 2010 to 2030, it is expected that the United States will see a rise in the elderly population significantly higher than that of the prior 20 years or of the following 20 years (Fig. 21-1). The health concerns associated with an aging population, including fragility fractures, are not isolated to the United States. Osteoporotic fragility fractures are or will become a major health issue in all regions. In particular, nearly half of the world's hip fractures will occur in Asia by 2050,[3] as that region is expected to see a dramatic increase in its total number of hip fractures. The aging of the population, along with the economic burden of providing healthcare that goes with it, will make prevention and management of osteoporotic fragility fractures an important health issue for many years to come.

Concurrently with the aging of the baby boomers, life expectancy in the United States is at an all-time high. In 1980, the life expectancy of a female living in the United States was 77.4 years of age. In 2009, that number had risen to 80.9. Furthermore, life expectancy increases as an individual ages. Therefore, for a woman in the United States who has already made it to 65 years old, life expectancy increases to 85.3 years.[4]

Along with the increasing age of the population, one can find an increase in the activity level and health expectations of seniors in the United States. Advancing age is no longer synonymous with physical and functional decline. The health benefits of physical activity late in life are well described.[5] Aging seniors expect to be active following retirement. Many delay retirement or take on new employment following departure from their lifelong careers. Recreational options for seniors today often include nearly everything that was possible at a younger age. These increased expectations of overall health and quality of life continue for many following a fragility fracture, with expectations to return to a level of functioning equal to that before their fracture. The reality of the situation currently, however, does not always live up to these expectations (Fig. 21-2). With hip fractures, many do not regain their preoperative physical function, are at increased risk of sustaining an additional osteoporotic fracture, and approximately 20% of seniors who sustain a hip fracture die within 1 year.[6] In addition to the physical morbidity associated with hip fractures in the elderly, psychosocial consequences and loss of independence are common issues.

TRENDS OF FRAGILITY FRACTURES

Recent evidence has suggested there may be a decreasing incidence of hip fracture and subsequent mortality over the past 10 years.[7-10] The reasons for this are not entirely known, but are likely to be multifactorial. While bisphosphonates have been shown to reduce the risk of hip fracture,[11] it is unlikely that the reduction in hip fracture incidence is entirely due to bisphosphonate use alone.[2] Supplementation and lifestyle changes, such as fall prevention, smoking cessation, healthy diet and exercise, and calcium and vitamin D supplementation, all contribute to better bone health[6] and probably play some role in this decreased incidence. Temporal and geographic variations have been shown to affect rates of hip fracture as well.[12]

Despite the recent reports showing a decreased incidence of hip fractures, it is unclear if this reduced incidence will continue with time. Regardless, the population in the United States and much of the world continues to age. As it does, it is projected that the number of osteoporotic fragility fractures will markedly increase over the next 30 to 40 years.

Although the use of bisphosphonates has contributed largely to a decreased incidence of hip fractures, it has also resulted in the emergence of atypical patterns related to their use.[13,14] A characteristic fracture pattern, first reported on in 2005, has been observed and linked to the chronic use of this class of medications. By 2009, the American Society for Bone and Mineral Research (ASBMR) created a task force to study this issue and their report was published in 2010 delineating criteria for diagnosis of atypical femoral fractures.[15] This distinct fracture type has been described by the following:

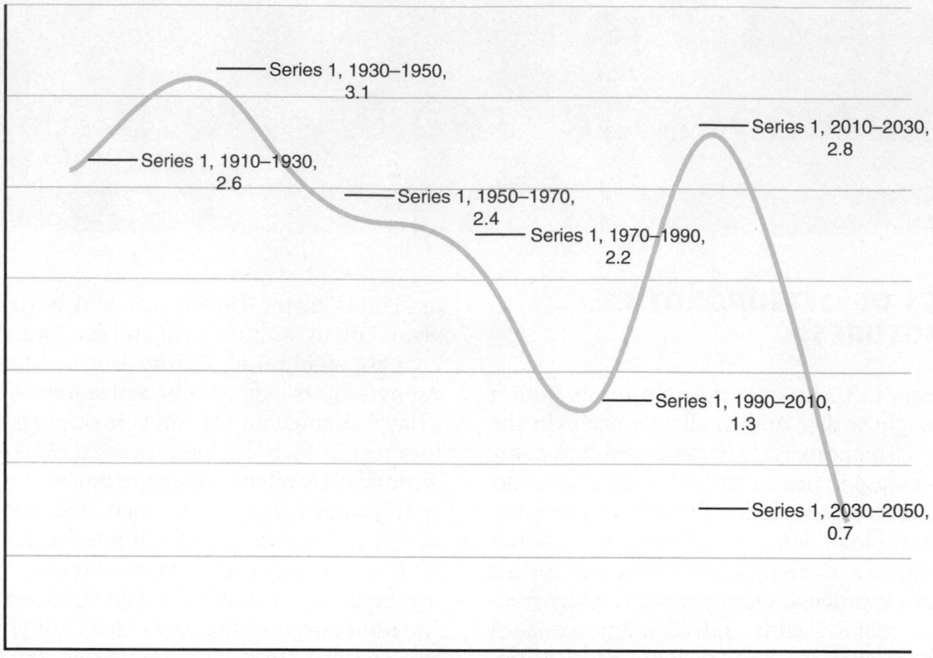

Figure 21-1. The average annual growth rate, in percent, of the elderly population in the United States. *(**Source:** Adapted from U.S. Census Bureau, Statistical brief: Sixty-five plus in the United States. Available at:* www.census.gov/population/socdemo/statbriefs/agebrief.html. *Accessed February 22, 2014.)*

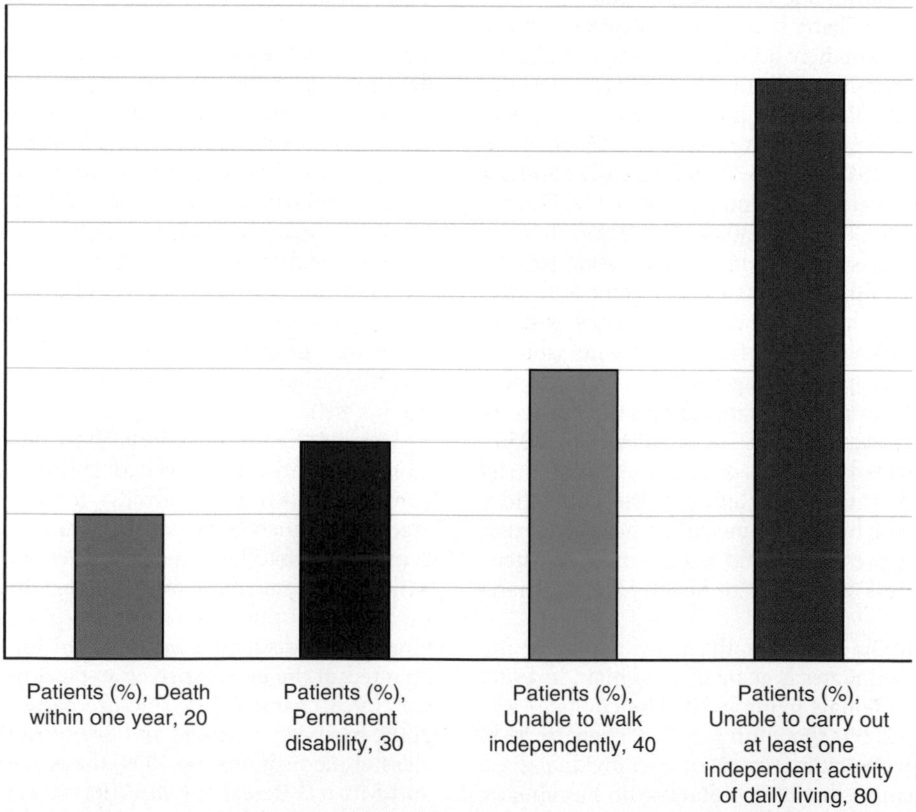

Figure 21-2. Morbidity and mortality as a percentage of patients 1 year after sustaining a hip fracture. *(**Source:** Shane E, Burr D, Ebeling PR, et al: Atypical subtrochanteric and diaphyseal femoral fractures: report of a task force of the American Society for Bone and Mineral Research, J Bone Miner Res 25(11):2267–2294, 2010.)*

a transverse or short oblique fracture line, focal callus reaction, medial spike, and a lack of comminution.[16,17] The prevalence of atypical fracture is not truly known at this time. It is suspected to occur in less than 1% of patients with chronic bisphosphonate use.[18] Widespread publicity about this problem has caused many patients and physicians to become reluctant to employ bisphosphonates as an antiresorptive therapy, and has led some experts to recommend a bisphosphonate drug holiday in select patients with a history of chronic bisphosphonate use.[19]

RESULTS OF FRAGILITY FRACTURES

Most of the literature reporting results after fragility fracture has looked at the effect of hip fracture on morbidity, mortality, and functional outcome in older individuals. The lifestyle and quality of life of a patient following hip fracture is drastically altered.[20] Postfracture independence is often reduced. Patients require increased levels of care and attention secondary to loss of mobility and ability to perform independent activities of daily living (ADLs). Often, the extent of these functional losses dictates whether or not discharge to a short-term rehabilitation facility or skilled nursing facility is necessary.

Mobility and ambulatory status following surgical stabilization of a hip fracture have significant importance for a patient's functional recovery. Ability to ambulate is fundamental to a patient being able to perform ADLs. In a prospective study of 336 patients, who were prefracture community ambulators, only 41% regained their preinjury ambulatory status following surgery, while the remaining 59% of patients all lost varying degrees of their preinjury ambulatory functional status.[21,22] Some reports state up to 22% of patients become nonambulators 1 year after suffering a hip fracture.[23] Several risk factors have been identified as independent predictors of a patient regaining their preinjury ambulatory status at 1-year follow-up. These included patient age, American Society of Anesthesiologists (ASA) physical status classification level, type of fracture, timing of surgery, and preoperative ambulatory status.[21,24,25] Patients 85 years or older, those with an ASA level of III or IV, those sustaining a femoral neck fracture, and patients with a delay in surgical treatment are less likely to obtain their prefracture ambulatory capacity at 1-year follow-up than patients aged younger than 85 years, those with an ASA level of I or II, an intertrochanteric fracture pattern, and those receiving prompt surgical treatment.[21,25] In addition, female gender, cognitive limitations, including a history of dementia and postoperative delirium, as well as a readmission to the hospital negatively affect a patient regaining their prefracture ambulatory status.[26] A history of cerebrovascular accident with associated physical or cognitive limitations has also been shown to limit a patient's ability to regain ambulatory function following a hip fracture.[27] Other factors, such as the surgical implant utilized and the type of anesthesia administered have not been shown to influence the recovery of ambulatory function in patients 1 year following surgical treatment of a hip fracture.

Disposition of a patient following treatment of a hip fracture is largely dictated by the patient's functional status at the time of discharge. The abilities to ambulate and independently perform ADLs are two of numerous factors that help determine the discharge disposition of a patient. The ADLs required for functional independence include two groups: basic ADLs (BADLs) and instrumental ADLs (IADLs). BADLs include feeding, bathing, dressing, and toileting, while IADLs incorporate more advanced activities such as shopping for food, cooking, banking, use of public transportation, and doing laundry. Multiple studies have shown that most patients who suffer a hip fracture lose functional independence, with 33% to 73% of patients regaining their preinjury function in BADLs and 21% to 48% of patients regaining their baseline capacity in IADLs.[28,29] Poor prognostic indicators for return to prefracture function in both BADLs and IADLs after a hip fracture have been identified. These factors include patient age older than 85 years, low preinjury physical function, history of postoperative complication, one or more preexisting medical comorbidities, institutionalization on discharge, and living alone prior to injury.[28,29]

Following surgical treatment, 24% to 72% of patients are discharged to home.[30-32] Of patients who lived in the community prior to sustaining a hip fracture, poor baseline cognitive function most strongly predicted being discharged to an institution for at least 6 months.[33] A lack of baseline social supports prior to injury, such as family involvement or a caretaker, was also predictive of a patient being institutionalized at discharge for at least 6 months.[34-37] Permanent institutionalization following a hip fracture has been associated with patient age older than 80 years, poor cognitive function, requiring assistance with ADLs, inadequate physical therapy, and lack of family support.[34] A strong social support network, being married, and normal preinjury cognitive function are factors that have been found to be protective against institutionalization at discharge following treatment of a hip fracture.[33] In addition, patients younger than 85 years of age, those independently ambulating at the time of hospital discharge, and those with three or less medical comorbidities are more likely to resume living independently after discharge.[31]

Despite advances in medical care and surgical treatments of major fragility fractures, such as hip fractures, overall patient outcomes have not drastically improved over the past 40 years. The 1-year mortality rates after a hip fracture remain nearly 24%, and 30-day mortality rates approach 10%. As with other diagnoses, length of stay during the acute hospitalization for hip fractures has decreased over the past two decades, but patient outcomes have not improved. Readmission following discharge for hip fracture occurs more than with any other associated orthopaedic diagnosis, with rates estimated as high as 14.5% in 2011.[38] Even with the development of new surgical implants and implant design improvements, implant failure is a common occurrence with hip fracture treatments and complication rates remain high. Following the index surgery, 3% to 10% of patients will require a revision surgery due to implant or fixation failure.[39] Similarly, mortality rates have not improved with the development of more novel surgical implants and techniques.[40] When comparing cemented to noncemented hip hemiarthroplasty implants in the treatment of patients with femoral neck fractures, the mortality rates for patients undergoing noncemented hip hemiarthroplasty was lower only during the first 2 postoperative days when compared to patients treated with cemented implants. Longer follow-up at 6 years showed no difference in the mortality rates between the two implant designs.[41] Other studies comparing cemented to noncemented implants have shown no difference in mortality rates, pain scores, and functional outcomes such as independence levels at any point in time during a 2-year follow-up period. In addition, the more modern, noncemented, implants were found to have higher rate of complications, such as subsidence related to fracture, than the cemented implant group.[42] While there is a better understanding of why hip fracture surgical fixations fail, the more novel implant designs and techniques have yet to improve patient outcomes.

Patients who present with a single fragility fracture, such as a hip fracture, will often sustain additional fragility fractures in the future.[43] The risk factors that placed the patient at risk for the initial hip fracture remain present after treatment of the original injury, increasing the risk for future fractures. Patient factors such as history of a previous fracture, diminished bone mineral density, cognitive impairment, functional disability, decreased visual acuity, and the presence of sedating medicines create the perfect milieu for mechanical falls, resulting in subsequent fractures.[44] The rate of secondary fractures in some populations has been estimated at 3% within 3 months, and 9.2% within 2 years of the index hip fracture. These secondary injuries often include fractures of the wrist, hip, and vertebral column.[45,46] Many of the factors placing a patient at increased risk for secondary injuries are difficult to modify. Even in the best-case scenario, where the orthopaedic surgeon can refer the patient to an orthopaedic osteoporosis clinic after a hip fracture, only 58% of patients were found to be on pharmacologic therapy for osteoporosis 6 months after discharge. When patients were referred to their primary care physician for osteoporosis therapy, the rate dropped to 29% at 6 months.[47] Initiating evaluation of a patient following a fragility fracture by ordering a bone mineral density study in the orthopaedic clinic has been shown to improve osteoporosis evaluation and treatment rates.[48] The failure to modify these risk factors places patients at continued risk for secondary fractures.

SOCIOECONOMIC IMPLICATIONS OF FRAGILITY FRACTURES

Fragility fractures represent an extraordinarily expensive diagnosis to care for both in terms of direct costs of care and also in terms of lost wages for those who are still employed. The high prevalence of these fractures and the prolonged healing time combined with the high costs of care, make treatment of fragility fractures extraordinarily expensive. In the United States, it has been estimated that 2 million osteoporotic fractures occur annually, with an estimated annual cost of $17 to $18 billion.[1,49] By 2025, the direct costs from osteoporosis are expected to reach $25.3 billion in the United States.[50] Hip fracture is the most costly of the osteoporotic fractures.[51] In the United States, there are approximately 330,000 hip fractures per year.[52] The average length of stay is 6.4 days,[52] which means that 2.1 million bed-days are occupied by hip fracture patients per year. The readmission rate for hip fracture is 14.5%; the highest readmission rate for any orthopaedic diagnosis according to recent data.[38] There is considerable variation in both the length of stay and readmission rates following hip fracture. Interestingly, this variation occurs in both academic medical centers and community hospitals and likely represents a significant cost to the healthcare system. These findings have resulted in hip fracture being the third most costly diagnosis in American medicine in 2012.[53]

Hip fracture is expensive in many other ways. Hip fracture is frequently the sentinel event for an older individual's decline or death. Although the death may not be directly attributed to the hip fracture, the fracture nonetheless is associated with a 20% to 24% 1-year mortality rate in many studies.[7,54,55] The specific causes of death are often very costly to care as well. Pneumonia represents a very common cause of readmission and death following hip fracture. Congestive heart failure and renal and urinary complications are also common.[56] It is known these are very costly diagnoses as well. Following a fragility fracture, most patients are unable to return directly back to their prior living situation. This necessitates a stay in a subacute nursing care facility or occasionally an acute rehabilitation unit. These costs are typically somewhat less than the acute hospital stay but can account for the second most expensive aspect of care following a fragility fracture. Rehabilitation costs after discharge from a nursing facility and additional medical care add to the cost burden. If an individual is still employed, they nearly always lose significant time from their employment which is quite costly to society as well.

For 20% or more of patients who have sustained a hip fracture or other major lower extremity fracture, loss of independence is an ongoing problem.[31,57,58] This creates a significant cost burden on society and the family as well as the patient themselves. The costs of nursing home care are $66,000 to $140,000 per year.[58] Assisted living care costs approximately half of that.[58]

IS THE MEDICAL SYSTEM PREPARED FOR THIS CHANGE?

There are several traditional models of inpatient fracture care that are prevalent in the United States and other countries.[59] These include a multidisciplinary approach to the patient with a hip fracture. In the first traditional model, the patient with a hip fracture is admitted through the emergency department to an orthopaedic surgeon for care. Once admitted to the surgeon, a medicine specialist is requested to consult on the patient's fitness for surgery.[59] The medicine specialist may be a family medicine physician, an internist, or a hospitalist physician. Rarely, a geriatrician is involved in the patient's care. Often the physician consulted is the patient's own primary care doctor who will need to see the patient before or after office hours. It is not uncommon that a cardiology consultation is requested if there is any cardiac history. This may result in a request for an echocardiogram as well. Once the patient has been medically cleared for surgery by the medicine physician, surgery is scheduled and performed on an urgent basis. Postoperatively, the hip fracture patient is typically managed by the surgeon with or without ongoing medicine consultation. Typically, the cardiologist will not follow the patient postoperatively unless there is an active cardiac condition. The patient is discharged from the hospital after discharge planning arrangements have been accomplished. The reported length of stay is 6.4 days with usual care in the United States.[60]

Similarly, some patients with a hip fracture may be admitted to the medicine service preoperatively. This is particularly true of cases in which the patient is medically complex (many

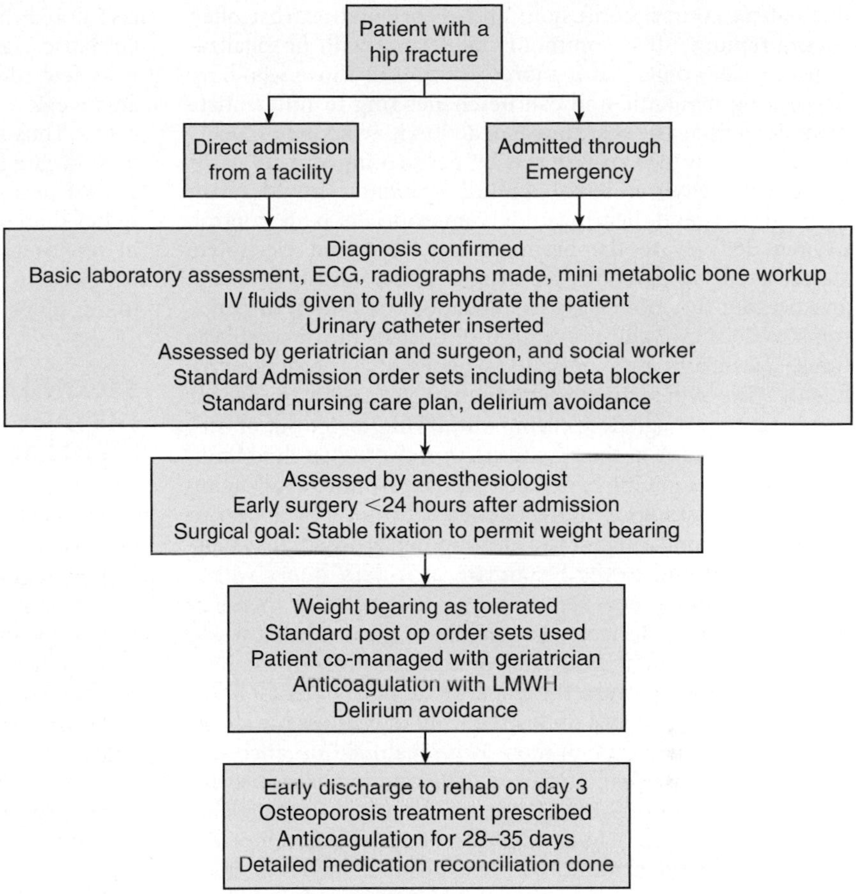

Figure 21-3. Geriatric Fracture Center or Rochester model of care. *ECG,* Electrocardiogram; *IV,* intravenous; *LMWH,* low molecular weight heparin.

comorbidities) or medically unstable. The surgeon then becomes a consultant and performs the surgery when the patient has been medically optimized for surgery. In some cases the patient will return postoperatively to the medicine service for postoperative management and discharge planning. The above two models of care are commonplace in the United States and have been in use for the past 50 years.[59] While multiple different disciplines or services may see the patient and treat them, the care is termed *multidisciplinary* as they tend to work "in silos" rather than in a concerted manner.

A newer model of care is termed the *Geriatric Fracture Center or Rochester* model of care.[61] In this model, patients are co-managed throughout the hospital stay by a team of healthcare providers including the orthopaedic surgeon, a geriatrician, nurses, therapists, and an anesthesiologist to provide interdisciplinary care[62] (Fig. 21-3). Interdisciplinary care involves healthcare providers working together seamlessly as a team with a focus on the patient and their needs.[63] During the hospital stay, standardized order sets are utilized at each phase of care to reduce the likelihood of errors and adverse events.[62] Such standard order sets include emergency department orders, admission orders, and postoperative orders. The nursing care plan is mapped out as a team so that the nursing care mirrors the standard order sets. All members of the team have identical expectations for the patient's hospital course. Discharge planning is done when the patient is admitted and expectations for a short length of stay are expressed by all members of the team to the patient and their family. A focus on early surgical intervention is made in this model. It has been definitively shown that early surgery (<24 hours) reduces the risk of adverse events experienced by the hip fracture patient.[62,64]

Additional important principles of this model are as follows: most hip fractures require surgical stabilization, patients should be made weight bearing as tolerated postoperatively, co-managed care results in reduced iatrogenic problems, and total quality management should be performed for each stage of care.[62,65] Following surgery, it is important that patients be permitted to weight bear as tolerated on their surgical repair or replacement. Fortunately, hip fracture surgery has many options dependent on fracture pattern and location. In general, it is best that choice of procedure be the one that permits immediate weight-bearing by the patient.[66] Sometimes this may necessitate an alteration of the surgical plan. Additionally, with older adults, "single shot" surgery is important. When older adults need revision procedures, they often experience tremendous loss of function and often will experience a complication. Therefore performing the surgery as a single procedure rather than a staged procedure is highly desirable and should be a goal of care for fragility fracture surgery. It has been shown that immediate weight bearing improves patient outcomes after hip fracture.[67,68]

Another important consideration with the Geriatric Fracture Center care model is avoidance of delirium.[69] Delirium frequently occurs following a hip fracture and has been reported in up to 61% of cases. There is no specific treatment for delirium, so it must be avoided if possible. Delirium is an acute confusional state characterized by inattention, fluctuating course, confusion, and disorientation that often occurs rapidly.[70] It is commonly associated with hospitalization in older adults.[70] It is more common in those who have preexisting dementia and can be challenging to differentiate from dementia. The best course of action is avoidance.[70] Delirium can be avoided or reduced by performing surgery early, appropriate environmental stimuli (patients should retain their glasses and hearing aids), appropriate pain control, oxygen delivery to the brain, proper fluid and electrolyte status, avoiding psychotropic drugs, proper nutrition, bowel and bladder function, early mobilization, treatment of symptoms of delirium, and prevention of postoperative complications.[71] Delirium may present as hyperactive or hypoactive forms.[70] The hyperactive variant is characterized by the patient being extremely agitated, crying out, trying to get out of bed, picking or pulling at their bedding or intravenous fluid lines, and hallucination. The hypoactive variant is more challenging to diagnose. Patients with hypoactive delirium may appear to be somnolent and difficult to arouse. When aroused, they typically will respond to the healthcare providers' query with a short and sometimes appropriate response and then fall immediately back to sleep. Hypoactive delirium has a worse prognosis. It is often associated with aspiration pneumonia and therefore may cause the patient's demise. Overall, delirium increases the length of hospitalization, reduces the ability of patients to participate in their own rehabilitation, increases the risk of readmission, increases costs, and increases the risk of complications or death.[70] There is a chronic variant of delirium that may persist long after the hospital stay. Once the patient has had delirium on a prior hospital stay, it is much more likely they will have delirium on subsequent hospitalizations. Delirium avoidance includes avoiding harmful medications such as diphenhydramine, meperidine, benzodiazepines, and histamine type 2 (H2) blockers.

Published outcomes of this care model have shown a lower than expected length of hospital stay, reduced complications, reduced readmissions, and reduced costs compared to usual care models.[61,62,69,72] In the era of healthcare reform, this combination of improved quality and safety with reduced costs make this care model attractive to many hospitals to adopt.

Changes in the care model and payment model have been associated with improved patient outcomes coupled with reduced costs in the National Health Service in the United Kingdom.[73] The Best Practice Tariff has been implemented for fragility hip fractures. Suggested actions for healthcare professionals in this program include[73]:

- Time to surgery within 36 hours from arrival in emergency department
- Admitted under the joint care of a consultant geriatrician and a consultant orthopaedic surgeon
- Admitted using an assessment protocol agreed on by geriatric medicine, orthopaedic surgery, and anesthesia
- Assessed by a geriatrician in the preoperative period within 72 hours of admission
- Postoperative geriatrician-directed multiprofessional rehabilitation team
- Fracture prevention assessments—falls and bone health

To achieve the full hospital reimbursement, all of the above assessments must be performed on each patient.[73] This approach to system management has resulted in a reduced mortality at 30 days from 12% in 2008 to 9% in 2012. It is also noted that this approach is very similar in content to the Geriatric Fracture Center model of care.

A few additional comments are appropriate here. There is an inverse relationship between quality of care and cost of care.[72] Thus it is less costly to care for a fragility fracture well than to care for it poorly.[74] Additionally, orthopaedic surgeons should be focusing on improvements in the system of care rather than on the traditional focus on specific implants used in care as a means of improving our patient outcomes. Only with system changes will we be able to improve quality of care to our older adults with a fragility fracture.

SECONDARY FRACTURE PREVENTION: DIETARY SUPPLEMENTATIONS AND MEDICAL THERAPIES

Patients who sustained a fragility fracture are at markedly increased risk of developing a subsequent fracture.[75] Patients with a fragility fracture should be advised of their diagnosis of osteoporosis.[47] Although simple to carry out, this is not often done in practice. Orthopaedic surgeons are typically the first medical care providers to treat patients with a fragility fracture and should discuss the diagnosis of osteoporosis.[47]

Secondary prevention of fracture involves a two-pronged approach to the patient. The first should be postfracture osteoporosis management and the second is fall prevention. These two approaches will be covered in some detail in the following sections.

Vitamin D and Calcium

Following a fragility fracture, common causes of secondary osteoporosis should be sought. The most common cause of secondary osteoporosis is vitamin D deficiency or insufficiency.[76] Testing for vitamin D insufficiency or deficiency can easily be accomplished by ordering a small number of laboratory tests when the patient is initially hospitalized.[76] These include a calcium level, parathyroid hormone (PTH) level, and a 25-OH vitamin D level. A low 25-OH vitamin D level combined with a lower value of serum calcium will establish the diagnosis of vitamin D deficiency or insufficiency. There is some dispute as to what level constitutes deficiency and what level constitutes insufficiency in the published literature. A deficient state implies that the patient is experiencing some symptoms of the condition, whereas the insufficient state may be asymptomatic.[77] Frequently, the PTH level will also be elevated as a marker of vitamin D deficiency. With this same set of laboratory tests, a diagnosis of primary hyperparathyroidism can be established. This would include an elevated calcium and elevated PTH level. A thyroid-stimulating hormone (TSH) level is another reasonable laboratory test to evaluate for hyperthyroidism. Other common causes of secondary osteoporosis include prolonged anticonvulsant usage, glucocorticoid use for more than 6 months, renal failure, Parkinson disease, and use of antiretroviral medications in the treatment of human immunodeficiency virus (HIV).[66] The more complex the cause of the secondary osteoporosis, the more the patient would benefit from assessment and treatment in a metabolic bone clinic.[66] Most hip fracture patients will require supplementation with vitamin D to help them heal their new fracture. Table 21-1 offers guidance on management of vitamin D deficiency and insufficiency.[66]

TABLE 21-1 *RECOMMENDATIONS FOR VITAMIN D SUPPLEMENTATION*

25-OH Vitamin D Level	Dose (IU)	Type	Frequency
0–10 ng/dL	50,000	Vitamin D_2	Three times per week
11–20 ng/dL	50,000	Vitamin D_2	Twice per week
21–32 ng/dL	50,000	Vitamin D_2	Once a week
Maintenance	2000	Vitamin D_3	Daily

It is recommended to recheck the level of 25-OH vitamin D after 6 to 8 weeks of the described treatment to ensure that you are adequately repleting the patient's level.[66] It should be remembered that vitamin D is a fat-soluble vitamin that is widely distributed and metabolized in the human body.[66] Therefore it can take a prolonged treatment period to correct a deficient or insufficient state.[66] There is much controversy about the correct maintenance level to use. However, when treating patients who have already experienced a fragility fracture, correction of this abnormal state will benefit their healing and help prevent secondary fractures.[66]

Inadequate dietary consumption of calcium is common. The appropriate total consumption of calcium should be 1000 to 1500 mg per day. This includes the dietary source plus supplemental calcium. Calcium alone is not protective for fracture.

Bisphosphonate Therapy

Bisphosphonates are a commonly used first-line therapy for treatment of postfracture osteoporosis.[78] Bisphosphonates are analogs of hydroxyapatite and bind to bone permanently. They typically have very long half-lives of 3 to 11 years. They inhibit osteoclast-mediated resorption of bone. They also increase osteoclast apoptosis. Bisphosphonates inhibit bone remodeling but not bone healing.[79] It is safe to start the oral bisphosphonate therapy immediately after fracture on a patient who is bisphosphonate naïve. It will take approximately 6 months after oral dosing for the patient to develop adequate levels of bisphosphonate in their bones to prevent secondary fractures. Bisphosphonates have been shown to be extremely effective at preventing hip fracture, vertebral fracture, and other types of fracture. However, oral dosing of bisphosphonates can be problematic.[79] Poor compliance to bisphosphonate therapy has been reported, with upward of 50% of patients stopping the medicine within the first 6 months. Proper dosing of bisphosphonate medication involves drinking the tablet with a full glass of water while sitting in an upright position for 1 hour. The medication is only appropriate in patients who have fairly normal renal function. Patients with advanced renal disease or who cannot sit upright for an hour after taking the medication should be considered for alternative therapy. Bisphosphonates can be administered intravenously on a yearly basis and this route of administration is not associated with negative upper gastrointestinal side effects. It is not recommended for patients with advanced renal disease. Intravenous administration of bisphosphonates can be associated with a short duration of a flulike illness.[79]

Bisphosphonates are the preferred treatment to prevent glucocorticoid-induced osteoporosis and are the first-line treatment for postfracture osteoporosis management.[66] Some patients, as mentioned earlier, may benefit from other types of treatment.

Side effects of bisphosphonates are concerning. A small percentage of patients treated with bisphosphonates for a prolonged period (>5 years) may develop an atypical fracture of the femur.[15] The atypical fracture is seen between the lesser trochanter and the supracondylar region of the femur. It typically has a simple fracture pattern such as transverse or short oblique and may have a "medial spike."[15] There may be prodromal symptoms, such as aching in the thigh, which precede the fracture.[15] The fracture always initiates from the tensile, lateral, side of the femur and propagates medially. There may be a lateral periosteal reaction.[16] In some cases, a black line appears through the lateral cortex, and this has been termed the "dreaded black line."[16] A full list of criteria for the atypical fracture has been nicely described by the ASBMR task force in 2010.[15] Treatment of the atypical fracture includes stopping the bisphosphonate therapy immediately, reduction and intramedullary nailing of the fracture, and managing delayed healing in some cases with anabolic therapy such as the PTH analog teriparatide. The contralateral femur should be closely followed as it may also fracture. Prophylactic nailing of the contralateral femur is controversial and should only be undertaken if there is a high probability of fracture.

Selective Estrogen Receptor Modulators

Selective estrogen receptor modulators (SERMs) are serum estrogen receptor modulators. They are a second-line, hormonally based therapy used in postmenopausal women with osteoporosis in whom bisphosphonate therapy is contraindicated. These medications stimulate the estrogen receptor and bone but are associated with antiestrogen affects in the breast.[80] It is considered an antiresorptive therapy. SERMs are associated with an increased incidence of venous thromboembolism (VTE) for the first 4 months of therapy. Raloxifene is the most commonly used medication in this class.

Calcitonin

Calcitonin is a hormone that stimulates bone formation. Based on recent recommendations, it has no place in osteoporosis management at this time.

Antiresorptive Monoclonal Antibodies

Denosumab

Denosumab is a monoclonal antibody that inhibits bone resorption by binding to receptor activator of nuclear factor κB (RANK) ligand.[81] It is administered as a subcutaneous injection every 6 months. It has profound antiresorptive effects on bone and will likely be associated with a similar side effect profile to bisphosphonates in this regard. Already, there have been a few reports of atypical fractures.[82] Denosumab can be used in patients with renal impairment. When the medication is stopped, the effects will be gone after 6 months. It is considered a second-line therapy at this time and should be used with the guidance of a metabolic bone expert.

Anabolic Agents

Teriparatide

Teriparatide is an analog of PTH containing amino acids 1 through 34 of PTH. Teriparatide is administered as a daily subcutaneous injection of 20 μg with a premetered injection

TABLE 21-2 *PATIENT RISK FACTORS FOR FALLS*

Risk Factor for Falls	Potentially Modifiable?
Advanced age	No
Female gender	No
Low body mass index (BMI)	Possibly
Medical comorbidities	Possibly
Musculoskeletal diseases	Yes
Cognitive impairment	No
Gait/balance disorder	No
Sensory impairment	No
Hypotensive episodes	Yes
Psychotropic drugs	Yes
Vitamin D deficiency	Yes
Deconditioning	Yes
Cataracts	Yes

*(**Source:** Karlsson MK, Magnusson H, von Schewelov T, Rosengren BE: Prevention of falls in the elderly—a review, Osteoporos Int 243:747–762, 2013.)*

TABLE 21-3 *ENVIRONMENTAL RISK FACTORS FOR FALLS*

Environmental Risk Factor	Modifiable?
Throw rugs	Yes
Irregular/slippery floor	Yes
Inadequate lighting	Yes
Electrical cords	Yes
Troublesome chairs	Yes
Objects on floors	Yes
Stairs with loose carpeting	Yes
Stairs without handrail	Sometimes
Pets	Potentially

*(**Source:** Karlsson MK, Magnusson H, von Schewelov T, Rosengren BE: Prevention of falls in the elderly—a review, Osteoporos Int 243:747–762, 2013.)*

pen. The treatment is costly and can be associated with side effects of hypercalcemia, nausea, or pruritus. Teriparatide is anabolic to bone and stimulates the formation of new bone, particularly on the periosteal side of the bone. It is only approved for 24 months of use in the United States. It is contraindicated in patients with open growth plates, history of radiation therapy, or patients with Paget disease of bone.

PREVENTION OF FALLS

The other arm of secondary fracture prevention is the prevention of falls. Nearly all major osteoporotic fractures occur with a fall.[83] Prevention of falls therefore should assume a significant role in secondary fracture prevention. See Table 21-2 for fall risk factors.

Comprehensive Falls Assessment

A comprehensive falls assessment requires a detailed assessment of the patient's overall health as well as the patient's environment at home. This often will involve assessment of vision, gait, balance, medical comorbidities, and medications. As listed in Table 21-2, some of these factors can be intentionally modified to reduce the risk of falls. Some problems are not modifiable and must be accepted as risk factors for future falls. Experts suggest that intervention in multiple areas represents the best strategy to prevent falls in community-dwelling older adults.[84]

Modification of the Home

The patient's residence is a frequent source of fall risk. As listed in Table 21-3, many of the environmental risk factors can be mitigated based on a home risk assessment. Unfortunately, seniors often are unwilling to permit some of these modifications to their residence. On meta-analysis, environmental interventions for community-dwelling elderly individuals favor such home safety interventions strongly.[83]

Exercise Programs

Exercise programs that include balance training and strength training have been shown in many randomized control trials to reduce the risk of falls. Tai chi in particular seems to be extremely effective in fall prevention in community-dwelling elderly individuals.[83] Walking alone does not seem to reduce the risk of falls. An excellent review of these exercise programs was recently conducted by Karlsson and colleagues.[83] Individuals who report frequent falls should be encouraged to participate in balance and strength training to reduce their falls risk.[84]

MEDICAL AND SURGICAL INTERVENTIONS

There are several surgical procedures that are associated with falls risk reduction. These include cataract extraction for at least one eye,[85] cardiac pacemaker insertion for appropriate causes of cardiac syncope, and appropriate foot and ankle intervention for painful foot conditions.[83]

Unsuccessful Interventions

Use of assistive devices such as canes and walkers have not been shown to reduce fall risks.[83] However, such devices should be prescribed when needed for safety. Nutritional supplementation has also not been shown to reduce the risk of falling. Finally, educational interventions about falls have not been shown to reduce fall risks.[83]

Implementing Secondary Fracture Prevention as a System: The Fracture Nurse Liaison Model

Numerous articles have shown that orthopaedic surgeons have intervened infrequently in the prevention of secondary fractures.[47] Rates of intervention have consistently been reported in the 15% to 20% range. This begs the question as to how to improve such a serious deficit in care. The most successful model of care reported for secondary prevention is the Fracture Nurse Liaison Model.[86,87] This has been in use for more than 20 years in Glasgow, Scotland, and is now gaining attention as the appropriate system of care for secondary fracture prevention in many parts of the world.[86,87]

This model is delivered by a specially trained nurse and supported by a physician trained in osteoporosis management.[87] The nurse identifies patients who have been admitted or treated for a new fragility fracture. The nurse then arranges for follow-up in clinic where a bone mineral density scan can be obtained and fracture risk is assessed. The patient's history and lifestyle are assessed and osteoporosis treatment is arranged. Patients are also referred to a falls prevention service to implement appropriate interventions to reduce the risk of falls.[87] In the United Kingdom, this model is becoming commonplace and pays for itself by fracture risk reduction. In the United States, a similar program has successfully been implemented at Kaiser Permanente by Dr. Richard Dell. This program has been shown to tremendously reduce the number of hip fractures experienced by patients within the Kaiser Permanente health system.[88] The program is termed "Healthy Bones" and uses Kaiser's robust electronic medical record system to perform the fracture case finding on a daily basis.[88]

Obtaining Dual-Energy X-Ray Absorptiometry Scans

Dual-energy x-ray absorptiometry (DXA) scan remains the gold standard for measuring and following progress of osteoporosis treatment.[66] It should be considered for all patients with a fragility fracture who are older than age 50 years and for all women older than age 65. When reordering a DXA scan, it is beneficial to have the scan performed on the same machine as the prior study to standardize the result.

Intradisciplinary Team Communication

When a patient experiences a fragility fracture, it is the treating surgeon's responsibility to inform patients that they have a diagnosis of osteoporosis. This diagnosis should be entered into the electronic medical record and should be shared in writing with the primary care physician.

Initiation of Medical Management

Medical management may be safely initiated immediately after the fracture. In nearly all cases, vitamin D and calcium should be ordered and oral bisphosphonates should be considered if the patient is bisphosphonate naïve.

Medical Therapy Compliance

It is common for patients to stop oral bisphosphonate therapy due to side effects. It should be remembered that osteoporosis is a silent disease unless the patient experiences a fracture.[89] A common reason for stopping therapy is that another physician tells the patient that it is not necessary. Oftentimes this is based erroneously on a DXA scan showing osteopenia ($-1 > T > 2.5$) rather than osteoporosis ($T < 2.5$). Rather, the bone mineral density (BMD) results from the DXA scan may be used as a target to improve adherence.[89]

The Role of a Metabolic Bone Clinic

In some cases, it will be necessary for the orthopaedic surgeon or primary care physician to refer their patient to a metabolic bone clinic for management. Below are listed three such scenarios. Also, there may be challenging patients who would benefit from assessment at a metabolic bone clinic.[66]

1. When to do a drug holiday from bisphosphonates or what to do after a drug holiday
2. *Special problematic cases*
3. *Failure of treatment on standard therapies*

SUMMARY

Osteoporosis and fragility fractures present a widespread problem throughout the world that is expected to become more prevalent as the world's population continues to age. Strategies continue to be developed in an effort to decrease the occurrence of these fractures, as well as to better treat these fractures when they occur. A multidisciplinary approach with an active role by the orthopaedic surgeon in treatment initiation has been shown to be highly beneficial for patients sustaining fragility fractures.

KEY REFERENCES

The level of evidence (LOE) is determined according to the criteria provided in the preface.

11. McClung MR, Geusens P, Miller PD, et al: Hip Intervention Program Study Group. Effect of risedronate on the risk of hip fracture in elderly women. *N Engl J Med* 344(5):333–340, 2001. LOE I
17. Schilcher J, Michaelsson K, Aspenberg P: Bisphosphonate use and atypical fractures of the femoral shaft. *N Engl J Med* 364(18):1728–1737, 2011. LOE III
21. Egol KA, Koval KJ, Zuckerman JD: Functional recovery following hip fracture in the elderly. *J Orthop Trauma* 11(8):594–599, 1997. LOE III
29. Koval KJ, Skovron ML, Aharonoff GB, et al: Predictors of functional recovery after hip fracture in the elderly. *Clin Orthop Relat Res* 348:22–28, 1998. LOE IV
47. Miki RA, Oetgen ME, Kirk J, et al: Orthopaedic management improves the rate of early osteoporosis treatment after hip fracture. A randomized clinical trial. *J Bone Joint Surg Am* 90(11):2346–2353, 2008. LOE I
56. Boockvar KS, Halm EA, Litke A, et al: Hospital readmissions after hospital discharge for hip fracture: surgical and nonsurgical causes and effect on outcomes. *J Am Geriatr Soc* 51(3):399–403, 2003. LOE IV
59. Giusti A, Barone A, Razzano M, et al: Optimal setting and care organization in the management of older adults with hip fracture. *Eur J Phys Rehabil Med* 47(2):281–296, 2011. LOE V
62. Friedman SM, Mendelson DA, Bingham KW, et al: Impact of a comanaged Geriatric Fracture Center on short-term hip fracture outcomes. *Arch Intern Med* 169(18):1712–1717, 2009. LOE IV
66. Bukata SV, Kates SL, O'Keefe RJ: Short-term and long-term orthopaedic issues in patients with fragility fractures. *Clin Orthop Relat Res* 469(8): 2225–2236, 2011. LOE IV
86. McLellan AR, Gallacher SJ, Fraser M, et al: The fracture liaison service: success of a program for the evaluation and management of patients with osteoporotic fracture. *Osteoporos Int* 14(12):1028–1034, 2003. LOE IV

The complete References list is available online at https://expertconsult.inkling.com.

Chapter 22

Surgical Site Infection Prevention

CALIN S. MOUCHA

Surgical site infection (SSI) is one of the most common and devastating complications of orthopaedic surgical procedures. The Centers for Disease Control and Prevention (CDC) estimates that 22% of all healthcare-associated infections are SSIs. More than 290,000 SSIs occur annually in the United States, resulting in $1 billion to $10 billion in direct and indirect medical costs.[1] In 2002, there were more than 43 million procedures in the United States, of which more than 600,000 included open reduction and internal fixation.[2]

Although advances in infection prevention have occurred over recent years, SSIs remain a substantial cause of morbidity and mortality. Patients with SSIs are 60% more likely to spend time in an intensive care unit, twice as likely to die, and five times more likely to be readmitted compared with patients without an SSI.[3] In surgical patients with an SSI who died, 89% of the deaths were attributable to the infection.[4] These statistics translate not only into significant losses for the individual patient but also a dramatic burden on societal healthcare costs as a whole.

The pathogens involved in SSIs did not change much between 1986 and 1996.[5] Staphylococcus species, including *Staphylococcus aureus,* are the leading nosocomial pathogens in hospitals worldwide. Coagulase-negative staphylococci, *Enterococcus* species, and *Escherichia coli* are also commonly isolated pathogens. Gram-negative organisms are reported to account for approximately 30% of SSIs in cardiac surgery and total joint arthroplasty.[6] More recently there has also been an increase in infections related to antimicrobial-resistant pathogens such as methicillin-resistant *S. aureus* (MRSA) and vancomycin-resistant enterococci, both of which colonize the skin and are spread by direct contact.[7] In the United States, it has been estimated that 94,360 invasive MRSA infections occurred in 2005 and that 86% of these were healthcare associated.[8] The death rate from MRSA is 2.5 times greater than from nonresistant *S. aureus,* and more than 18,000 MRSA deaths were documented in 2005.[1,8]

In the United States, prevention and treatment of these infections has become a national priority. The Healthcare Infection Control Practices Advisory Committee (HICPAC) is a federal advisory committee that consists of 14 external infection control experts. The HICPAC works together with the CDC and the Secretary of the Department of Health and Human Services to formulate best practices for health care–associated infection prevention, control, and surveillance. The CDC's National Nosocomial Infections Surveillance System (NNIS), established in 1970, monitors nosocomial infection trends.

In an effort to make evidence-based recommendations on infection prevention, the CDC published the "Guideline for Prevention of Surgical Site Infection, 1999."[7,9] In 2002, the CDC collaborated with the Centers for Medicare and Medicaid Services (CMS) to implement the Surgical Site Infection Project. The goal of the project was to decrease mortality and morbidity associated with SSIs by promoting appropriate prophylactic antibiotic choice and timing. Effective July 1, 2006, The Joint Commission expanded the Surgical Site Infection Project to the Surgical Care Improvement Project (SCIP). SCIP is a partnership of many organizations dedicated to improving surgical care. The American Academy of Orthopaedic Surgeons (AAOS) is one of more than 30 organizations represented. The goal of SCIP was to reduce the incidence of surgical complications nationally by 25% by the year 2010. Some of the SCIP target areas pertinent to orthopaedic surgery are shown in Table 22-1.[10]

DEFINING SURGICAL SITE INFECTIONS

The National Nosocomial Infections Surveillance System (NNIS) has provided standardized surveillance criteria for defining SSIs (Fig. 22-1 and Table 22-2). These definitions, applied consistently by surveillance personnel, have become a national standard. SSIs are classified as superficial if they involve only the skin and subcutaneous tissue and deep if the infection is within the fascia or muscle. Organ/space SSIs involve any part of the anatomy other than incised body wall layers that were manipulated during surgery. Septic arthritis, septic bursitis, diskitis, epidural abscess, and osteomyelitis are considered organ/space SSIs. Infection occurs within 30 days after the procedure if no implant is left in place or within 1 year if an implant is in place and the infection appears to be related to the operation.

It is important to note that other organizations have also formulated evidence-based definitions of orthopaedic infections. The AAOS[11] and the Musculoskeletal Infection Society[12] have specific recommendations and definitions for diagnosing periprosthetic joint infections (PJIs) (Table 22-3). Although these definitions are not currently used by government agencies, it is anticipated that they will be used in the future during data collection for the American Joint Replacement Registry (AJRR).

PREOPERATIVE INTERVENTIONS

Infection control is best integrated into a clinical practice using an outside-to-inside methodology.[13] The AAOS Patient Safety Committee has identified a variety of modifiable risk factors for SSI (Fig. 22-2).[14,15] Certainly, not all of these risk factors can be applied to the acute trauma setting. Many orthopaedic patients, however, are unhealthy hosts, and optimizing these patients as best possible before surgery may be the most important and tangible aspect of SSI prevention. Although direct scientific evidence showing that risk

TABLE 22-1 *SURGICAL CARE IMPROVEMENT PROJECT (SCIP) MILESTONES: SCIP IDENTIFIER PROCESS OR OUTCOME MEASURES*

Infection	
SCIP INF 1	Prophylactic antibiotic received within 1 h before surgical incision
SCIP INF 2	Prophylactic antibiotic selection for surgical patients
SCIP INF 3	Prophylactic antibiotics discontinued within 24 h after surgery end time (48 h for cardiac patients)
SCIP INF 4	Cardiac surgery patients with controlled 6 AM postoperative serum glucose measurement
SCIP INF 5a	Postoperative surgical site infection diagnosed during index hospitalization
SCIP INF 6	Surgery patients with appropriate hair removal
Venous Thromboembolism	
SCIP VTE 1	Surgery patients with recommended venous thromboembolism prophylaxis ordered
SCIP VTE 2	Surgery patients who received appropriate VTE prophylaxis within 24 h before surgery to 24 h after surgery
SCIP VTE 3a	Intraoperative or postoperative PE diagnosed during index hospitalization or within 30 days of surgery
SCIP VTE 4a	Intraoperative or postoperative DVT diagnosed during index hospitalization or within 30 days of surgery
Global	
SCIP Global 1	Death within 30 days of surgery
SCIP Global 2	Readmission within 30 days of surgery

DVT, Deep vein thrombosis; *PE,* pulmonary embolism; *VTE,* venous thromboembolism.

From Fry DE: Surgical site infections and the Surgical Care Improvement Project (SCIP): evolution of National Quality Measures, Surg Infect 9(6):579–584, 2008.

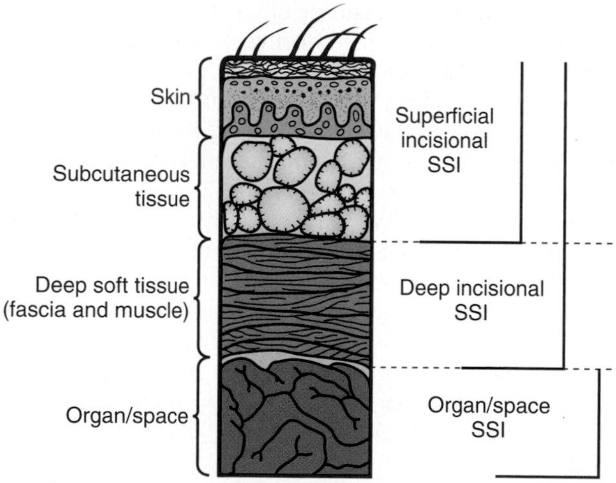

Figure 22-1. Cross-section of the abdominal wall. Wounds are classified as superficial incisional, deep incisional, and organ/space infections. *SSI,* Surgical site infection. *(From Mangram AJ, Horan TC, Pearson ML, et al: Guideline for Prevention of Surgical Site Infection, 1999. Centers for Disease Control and Prevention (CDC) Hospital Infection Control Practices Advisory Committee, Am J Infect Control 27(2):97–132, 1999.)*

TABLE 22-2 *CRITERIA FOR DEFINING A SURGICAL SITE INFECTION (SSI)*

Superficial Incisional SSI

Infection occurs within 30 days after the operation *and* infection involves only skin or subcutaneous tissue of the incision *and* at least *one* of the following:

1. Purulent drainage, with or without laboratory confirmation, from the superficial incision
2. Organisms isolated from an aseptically obtained culture of fluid or tissue from the superficial incision
3. At least one of the following signs or symptoms of infection: pain or tenderness, localized swelling, redness, or heat *and* superficial incision is deliberately opened by surgeon *unless* the incision is culture negative
4. Diagnosis of superficial incisional SSI by the surgeon or attending physician

Do *not* report the following conditions as SSI:

1. Stitch abscess (minimal inflammation and discharge confined to the points of suture penetration)
2. Infection of an episiotomy or newborn circumcision site
3. Infected burn wound
4. Incisional SSI that extends into the fascial and muscle layers (see deep incisional SSI)

Note: Specific criteria are used for identifying infected episiotomy and circumcision sites and burn wounds.

Deep Incisional SSI

Infection occurs within 30 days after the operation if no implant* is left in place or within 1 year if the implant is in place and the infection appears to be related to the operation *and* infection involves deep soft tissues (e.g., fascial and muscle layers) of the incision *and* at least *one* of the following:

1. Purulent drainage from the deep incision but not from the organ/space component of the surgical site
2. A deep incision spontaneously dehisces or is deliberately opened by a surgeon when the patient has at least one of the following signs or symptoms: fever (>38°C), localized pain, or tenderness unless the site is culture negative
3. An abscess or other evidence of infection involving the deep incision is found on direct examination, during reoperation, or by histopathologic or radiologic examination
4. Diagnosis of a deep incisional SSI by a surgeon or attending physician

Notes

1. Report infection that involves both superficial and deep incision sites as deep incisional SSI.
2. Report an organ/space SSI that drains through the incision as a deep incisional SSI.

Organ/Space SSI

Infection occurs within 30 days after the operation if no implant* is left in place or within 1 year if the implant is in place and the infection appears to be related to the operation *and* infection involves any part of the anatomy (e.g., organs or spaces) other than the incision, which was opened or manipulated during an operation *and* at least *one* of the following:

1. Purulent drainage from a drain that is placed through a stab wound† into the organ/space
2. Organisms isolated from an aseptically obtained culture of fluid or tissue in the organ/space
3. An abscess or other evidence of infection involving the organ/space that is found on direct examination, during reoperation, or by histopathologic or radiologic examination
4. Diagnosis of an organ/space SSI by a surgeon or attending physician

*National Nosocomial Infection Surveillance definition: a nonhuman-derived implantable foreign body (e.g., prosthetic heart valve, nonhuman vascular graft, mechanical heart, or hip prosthesis) that is permanently placed in a patient during surgery.

†If the area around a stab wound becomes infected, it is not an SSI. It is considered a skin or soft tissue infection, depending on its depth.

TABLE 22-3 *MUSCULOSKELETAL INFECTION SOCIETY DEFINITION OF PERIPROSTHETIC JOINT INFECTION*
Based on the proposed criteria, definite Periprosthetic Joint Infection exists when: 1. There is a sinus tract communicating with the prosthesis; or 2. A pathogen is isolated by culture from at least two separate tissue or fluid samples obtained from the affected prosthetic joint; or 3. Four* of the following six criteria exist: a. Elevated serum ESR AND serum CRP concentration b. Elevated synovial leukocyte count c. Elevated synovial neutrophil percentage (PMN%) d. Presence of purulence in the affected joint e. Isolation of a microorganism in one culture of periprosthetic tissue or fluid f. Greater than five neutrophils per high-power field in five high-power fields observed from histologic analysis of periprosthetic tissue at >400× magnification.

*A periprosthetic joint infection may be present if fewer than four of these criteria are met.
CRP, C-reactive protein; *ESR,* erythrocyte sedimentation rate; *PMN,* polymorphonuclear neutrophils.
Adapted from Parvizi J, Zmistowski B, Berbari EF, et al: New definition for periprosthetic joint infection: from the Workgroup of the Musculoskeletal Infection Society, Clin Orthop Rel Res 469(11):2992–2994, 2011.

factor modification will lead to a lower SSI rate is lacking in some instances, extrapolating data from other fields such as cardiac surgery has been helpful in raising awareness among orthopaedists and mobilizing future orthopaedic research on this topic.

Smoking is a well-known risk factor for multiple surgical complications, including infection.[16] A recent large prospective report has confirmed the significant association between smoking and organ/space SSI in orthopaedic surgery with implants.[17] Tobacco products cause microvascular vasoconstriction via the effects of nicotine on the sympathetic nervous system. Tissue hypoxia is caused by carbon monoxide binding to hemoglobin and creating carboxyhemoglobin.[18-20] Smoking intervention programs, even when instituted as briefly as 4 weeks before surgery, can diminish the risk of complications.[21-24] A patient in an external fixator who is awaiting definitive fixation of a pilon fracture, for example, would be an ideal patient to enroll in a smoking cessation program.

Obesity, defined as a body mass index of 30 kg/m^2 or greater, is a known risk factor for orthopaedic postoperative infections.[25-27] The pathogenesis by which many obese patients go on to have a postoperative infection is multifactorial. The diet many of these patients follow is devoid of essential nutrients. Surgical time is often longer for these patients,[26] and hematoma or seroma formation leading to prolonged drainage is more common.[28] The subcutaneous layer in these patients is often poorly vascularized, and they require a significantly greater fraction of inspired oxygen (FiO_2) to reach an arterial oxygen tension of 150 mm Hg.[29] Meticulous treatment of soft tissues and expedited surgeries by experienced surgeons should be considered whenever possible. Obese patients should have properly dosed prophylactic antibiotics[30] and nutritional counseling perioperatively. Last, these patients need to be counseled never to try to lose weight while healing their surgical wounds because this may lead to a catabolic state.

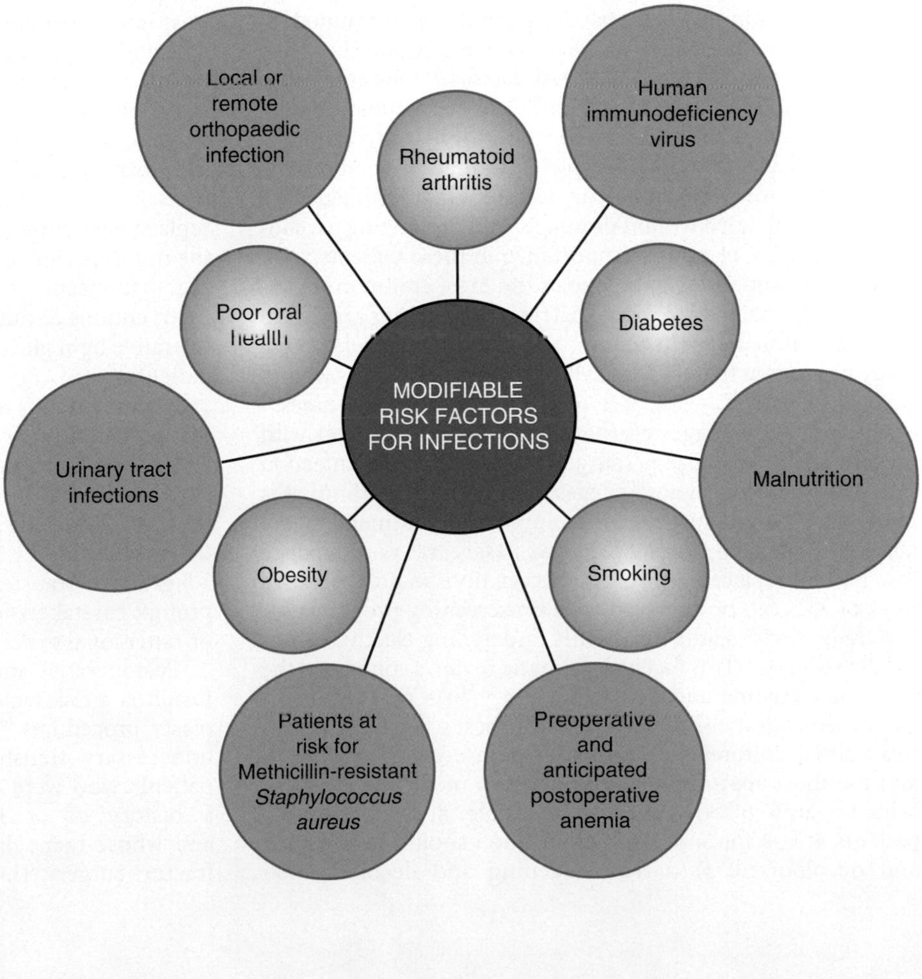

Figure 22-2. Modifiable risk factors for surgical site infection. *(Redrawn from Moucha CS, Clyburn T, Evans RP, Prokuski L: Modifiable risk factors for surgical site infection, J Bone Joint Surg Am 93(4):398–404, 2011.)*

Patients with rheumatoid arthritis have an increased risk of infection after orthopaedic procedures such as joint replacement. Many of these patients are treated with complex drug regimens that have an effect on wound healing. Antiinflammatory medications should be held perioperatively both because of wound healing complications that can lead to infection as well as their potential effects on wound healing.[31] Although corticosteroids have been shown to increase infection rates and affect wound healing,[32] these medications should be continued. Although the use of steroid stress doses remains controversial, they should probably not be routinely administered. Rather, each patient should be dealt with individually, keeping in mind the chronicity and dose of steroid usage, anticipated stress level of the surgery, and the presence of other risk factors for infection.[31,33] Methotrexate should not be discontinued perioperatively except in patients with renal insufficiency, poorly controlled diabetes, lung or liver disease, or a history of alcohol abuse.[31,33] One study has described serious postoperative orthopaedic infections in patients taking tumor necrosis factor (TNF).[34] Another study, however, did not show an increased risk of infection in patients undergoing foot and ankle surgery while taking TNF inhibition therapy.[35] Perioperative consultation with a rheumatologist who has experience with these medications is recommended.

The number of patients infected with human immunodeficiency virus (HIV) who are undergoing orthopaedic procedures is on the rise.[36] Some studies, many in arthroplasty patients, done on these patients have shown a higher SSI risk, and others have not.[37-42] A recent study of orthopaedic trauma patients who were HIV positive revealed that CD4 counts less than 300 cells/μL were associated with development of postoperative infection at a higher risk than those without HIV.[43] Routine screening of orthopaedic patients for immunodeficiencies has not been shown to be cost effective and should be reserved for patients with other risk factors.[44] One study suggested that to diminish the risk of SSI in this patient population, we should administer prolonged prophylactic antibiotic therapy and antiretroviral therapy.[45] Eliminating or modifying other risk factors (injection drug use, smoking, serum glucose level, and prolonged wound drainage) and optimizing psychosocial issues are of utmost importance in these patients.[40]

S. aureus continues to be one of the most common organisms in orthopaedic SSI. Nasal carriers of *S. aureus* are two to nine time more likely to acquire SSIs than noncarriers.[46] One study has shown that 80% to 85% of the time, *S. aureus* wound isolates in patients with SSIs match those from the nares.[47] One early study suggested that prophylactic treatment with mupirocin in orthopaedic surgery can reduce the infection rate.[48] Rao and colleagues[49] suggested that chlorhexidine baths for 5 days before surgery with mupirocin ointment to the nares twice daily in positive *S. aureus* nasal carriers will reduce SSIs in joint replacement surgery. Reductions in postoperative rates of SSIs can be achieved with prescreening programs for *S. aureus* carrier status in patients undergoing elective orthopaedic surgery.[50] Two recent systematic reviews confirmed the value of screening and decolonization.[51,52] As new technologies evolve, questions remain about the best screening method (traditional cultures vs. rapid polymerase chain reaction)[53] and the most appropriate decolonization medication (antibiotics vs. antiseptics). Whenever possible, at the very least, patients at risk for *S. aureus* colonization should be screened and decolonized. *S. aureus* screening and decolonization protocols must be repeated before any readmission, regardless of prior colonization status.[54] Risk factors include previous MRSA infection; being a healthcare worker, nursing home patient, or prisoner; and being in contact with a patient who has MRSA colonization. Patients found to be carriers of MRSA, in addition to either mupirocin or povidone–iodine nasal decolonization, should be considered candidates for vancomycin prophylactic antibiotics in place of (or possibly in addition to) a cephalosporin, although strict guidelines cannot currently be established. Hospitals with antibiograms showing a high percentage of resistant bacteria should also consider altering their prophylactic prophylaxis regimen appropriately.[55]

Diabetes and hyperglycemia have been known risk factors for orthopaedic SSI for some time. Although the pathologic effects of diabetes on surgical hosts are clearly detrimental, the acute effects of perioperative hyperglycemia are both more detrimental and more readily addressed.[56] In fact, a recent registry study examining the effects of diabetes (as coded in the registry) on total knee replacements did *not* show a higher risk of revision arthroplasty or deep infection.[57] Hyperglycemia is probably more important and more prevalent than the diagnosis of diabetes itself. It has been defined in many studies as blood glucose levels above 200 mg/dL. In the trauma setting, elevated blood glucose level occurs in up to 50% of patients in the intensive care ward,[58] and the etiology of this stress-induced hyperglycemia is multifactorial.[59,60]

The pathogenesis of hyperglycemia leading to infection has been well described. Chemotaxis, phagocytosis, and oxidative bacterial killing are all diminished by high serum glucose levels.[61-63] Hyperglycemia leading to glycosylation of complement proteins and immunoglobulin results in overall host immunosuppression.[64] Multiple studies have shown the advantage of tight glycemic control in critically ill patients.[65,66] Cardiac surgery studies have confirmed that sternal wound infections are more likely to occur in hyperglycemic patients.[67] In these patients, implementation of continuous insulin infusion protocols reduce the rates of deep sternal wound infections.[68] Several recent studies in orthopaedic spine,[25] joint replacement surgery,[69,70] and ankle fracture surgery[71] support the role of perioperative glycemic control in patients undergoing orthopaedic surgery. Even though studies supporting interventions at multiple points of care are still needed, perioperative tight glucose control is clearly critical in orthopaedic patients.[72]

Malnutrition is a known risk factor as well after orthopaedic procedures. Screening should be done in patients at risk of malnutrition, such as elderly adults and those with gastrointestinal diseases, renal failure, alcoholism, cancer, or any chronic disease.[73-75] Total lymphocyte count of less than 1500/mm^3 (1.5×10^9/L), serum albumin level less than 3.5 g/dL, or transferrin level of less than 226 mg/dL should prompt caretakers to initiate consultations with an endocrine or nutritional expert.

Postoperative anemia treated with allogeneic blood transfusion is a risk factor for SSI in patients undergoing arthroplasty procedures.[76,77] It is likely that many patients receive unnecessary transfusions. A recent study[78] enrolled 2016 patients who were 50 years of age or older who had either a history of or risk factors for cardiovascular disease and whose hemoglobin levels were below 10 g/dL after hip fracture surgery. The investigators randomly assigned patients to a liberal transfusion strategy (a hemoglobin threshold of 10 g/dL) or a restrictive transfusion strategy (symptoms of anemia or at physician discretion for a hemoglobin level of <8 g/dL). A liberal transfusion strategy, as compared with a restrictive strategy, did not reduce rates of death or inability to walk independently on 60-day follow-up or reduce in-hospital morbidity. Postoperative risk of transfusion can be diminished with perioperative interventions. Epoetin alfa directly increases preoperative red blood cell mass, hemoglobin concentration, and hematocrit levels. It has been shown to be useful for lowering transfusion requirements in total joint replacement procedures[79] but not in pediatric neuromuscular scoliosis patients.[80] A recent pooled observational analysis of very-short-term perioperative administration of intravenous (IV) iron in patients undergoing major orthopaedic surgery has renewed interest in this important modality.[81] Tranexamic acid, an antifibrinolytic included on the World Health Organization's list of essential medicines, has been shown to be a useful adjuvant in the prevention of postoperative allogeneic blood transfusions in spinal[82] and joint replacement[83] surgeries.

Poor oral health, urinary tract infections, and local or remote orthopaedic infections have also been identified by the AAOS as being modifiable risk factors for SSI. Whenever possible, decayed teeth, untreated dental abscesses, advanced gingivitis, and periodontitis should be taken care of before surgical intervention; this practice is commonly advocated in cardiac surgery.[84,85] Urinary tract infections and a subsequent delay in surgical intervention should be handled based on the type of symptoms (obstructive vs. irritative) and bacterial colony count.[86,87] Although it is not the topic of this chapter to discuss the diagnosis of infection for all types of orthopaedic procedures, one should consider at the very least obtaining a C-reactive protein level and an erythrocyte sedimentation rate in all patients undergoing conversion of previous surgery to total joint replacement and in all patients undergoing nonunion surgery.

It may not always be possible to optimize patients completely in the trauma setting. There is almost always something that can be addressed, however, to improve the surgical host and diminish the risk of SSI.

PROPHYLACTIC ANTIBIOTICS

All surgical wounds are at risk of bacterial contamination. Normal skin transmits aerobic gram-positive cocci, and body orifices contaminate wounds with enteric bacteria.

Prophylactic antibiotics do not sterilize the wound; rather, their administration allows the host to fight off inevitable bacterial contamination more effectively.[88] The ideal antibiotic should be active against the most common pathogens in wounds, have minimal side effects, achieve adequate concentrations in the tissue during the entire time that the wound is open, and carry the smallest impact possible on the patient's normal bacterial flora. Poor antibiotic selection and timing will lead to ineffective prophylaxis.[89]

Studies on the topic of antibiotic prophylaxis are mostly seen in the field of joint replacement surgery[90-93] and closed fracture fixation.[94-97] The Dutch Trauma Trial,[98] a prospective, randomized, double-blind, placebo-controlled study, looked at 2195 closed fractures. Patients received either preoperative ceftriaxone or placebo. The infection rate was 3.6% in the antibiotic group and 8.3% in the placebo group. A more recent meta-analysis[99] supports these findings. In lower extremity arthroplasty cases and in closed fracture procedures, administration of prophylactic antibiotics is the standard of care in the majority of cases. Routine use of prophylactic antibiotics in spine surgery has also been supported by multiple studies.[90,100-103]

Fields such as foot and ankle surgery[104,105] and nontraumatic upper extremity surgery[106-108] tend not to advocate *routine* use of prophylactic antibiotics, although studies are limited. It has been the author's observation that most surgeons appear to give prophylactic antibiotics for ankle and hand arthroplasty procedures as well as for extensive reconstructive procedures in any field.

Timing of Administration

Burke,[109] building on work of Lister,[110] investigated the effects of parenteral antibiotics on surgical incisions contaminated with *S. aureus*. This seminal study discovered the importance of adequate tissue levels of antibiotics *before* incision. Several years later, Stone and colleagues critically evaluated 400 nonorthopaedic patients and clearly showed a reduction of infection rates with preoperative antibiotics.[111] The lowest rate of SSI has been observed with antibiotics given briefly before incision. Classen and colleagues prospectively studied the timing of antibiotic prophylaxis in 2847 patients and found that those receiving antibiotics during the 2 hours before the incision had the lowest risk of wound infection.[112] Cephalosporin and clindamycin infusions should begin within 60 minutes of incision and be completed just before the incision. Vancomycin infusion should begin 1 to 2 hours before the incision because fast administration may result in "red man" syndrome, a condition characterized by hypotension and a rash. Last, tourniquet usage affects tissue concentrations of antibiotics. Johnson[113] studied cefuroxime concentration in bone and subcutaneous fat during knee arthroplasty. Patients were randomized to receive the antibiotics 5, 10, 15, and 20 minutes before tourniquet inflation. Bone concentrations were above the minimum inhibitory concentration (MIC) for *S. aureus* in all groups. Subcutaneous fat levels were lower than MIC for *S. aureus* in 86% of patients who received antibiotics at 5 minutes before tourniquet inflation. The authors concluded that at least 10 minutes is needed between administration of antibiotics and tourniquet inflation to achieve adequate tissue levels of cefuroxime. Two other studies support these findings[114,115]; investigations in the foot and ankle literature[116,117] suggest that administration of antibiotics after tourniquet inflation may not be detrimental.

Even though there is enough evidence showing that preoperative antibiotics should be administered before incision, reports show that this still does not happen routinely.[118,119] Although educating team members, instituting organized perioperative checklists, and providing feedback to surgeons has raised compliance in some countries,[120] more work remains to be done.

Antimicrobial Choices

Cephalosporins are the most commonly used antibiotics in orthopaedic surgery. First-generation cephalosporins provide excellent bactericidal activity against aerobic gram-positive cocci that usually contaminate these wounds. Second- and third-generation cephalosporins have a broader spectrum but are not as effective against gram-positive bacteria. Cunha and colleagues investigated several antibiotics during total hip replacement and showed that 25 to 40 minutes after injection of cefazolin, a first-generation cephalosporin, the peak bone level was 60 times the MIC of penicillin-resistant staphylococci.[121] The half-lives of cephalosporins are sufficiently long enough that adequate tissue levels remain throughout most orthopaedic procedures. The cost of these agents is relatively low as is the risk of adverse effects. As such, they continue to be widely used and recommended for prophylaxis in orthopaedic surgery.[122] Although patients sometimes have concerns about allergic reactions, it is important to delineate whether these are true allergic reactions or not. The incidence of adverse reactions to cephalosporins in patients with reported penicillin allergy is rare. If skin testing or history points to a true allergy (e.g., hypotension, bronchospasm, pruritus, urticaria), then other agents, such as vancomycin, should be considered. Penicillin allergy testing can decrease prophylactic vancomycin use in patients treated with elective orthopaedic surgery.[123]

Clindamycin and vancomycin are alternative agents that can be used as prophylaxis when cephalosporins are contraindicated. Compared with cephalosporins, bone penetration of vancomycin appears to be inferior, but that of clindamycin is comparable. Clindamycin[124,125] and vancomycin[126] both exceed the MIC of gram-positive organisms that cause orthopaedic infections. However, increased use of vancomycin leads to increased resistance and emergence of vancomycin-resistant enterococcus infections.[127] Vancomycin should be reserved for patients with known MRSA colonization, those in facilities with recent MRSA *outbreaks,* and those with known risk factors for MRSA. Risk factors for community- and hospital-acquired MRSA include athletes in contact sports, children at day care centers, homeless patients, IV drug users, men who have sex with men, military personnel, prison inmates, antibiotic use within the preceding year, crowded living conditions, chronic wounds, those who have been recently hospitalized or dialyzed, and those with indwelling catheters or percutaneous medical devices.[128-130] A cardiac surgery study showed that the choice of antimicrobial used (cefazolin vs. vancomycin) changed the infecting organism and not the rate of SSI.[131] To date, there is insufficient evidence that changing the antibiotic prophylaxis from cephalosporins to vancomycin in institutions with perceived high rates of MRSA will result in fewer SSIs.[132]

Dosing

Because of the historic "one size fits all" strategy, many patients are routinely underdosed with prophylactic antibiotics. Many patients are obese, and this group in particular is at risk for antibiotic treatment failure. Appropriate dosing is most likely one of the contributing factors.[133] Clinicians need to consider the relative risks of overdosing and underdosing. Obesity causes a number of changes, including an increase in volume of distribution and changes in hepatic metabolism and renal excretion.[134] Cefazolin should be dosed at 1 g for patients weighing less than 80 kg and 2 g for patients over that limit.[7,122] Clindamycin and vancomycin dosing is based on the patient's body mass, as is pediatric dosing. Consultation with infectious disease and pharmacy experts at the surgeon's institution is advised. Redosing of antibiotics can lead to suboptimal tissue levels[135] and should be done whenever the procedure exceeds one to two times the half-life of the antibiotic[131,136] or if there is significant blood loss.[137]

Duration

For a while there has been a trend to administer prophylactic antibiotics for longer periods than necessary. In the recent past, for example, patients undergoing arthroplasty procedures would be given antibiotics until either the drains were removed or the wounds were dry. This has been shown to be unnecessary.[122,138] In nonorthopaedic procedures,[139] joint replacement surgery,[140-143] and hip fracture surgery,[95,144] prolonged prophylaxis has not been shown to be important in reducing SSI rates. Although we do not know the shortest course of antibiotics for prevention of SSI,[122,145] we do know that prolonged antibiotic usage leads to increased microbial resistance. The current recommendation by the AAOS and SCIP is to discontinue antimicrobial agents within 24 hours postoperatively after elective primary joint replacement.

INTRAOPERATIVE MEANS OF REDUCING INFECTION

Surgeons, nurses, anesthesiologists, and other members of the operating room (OR) team are *all* responsible for preventing SSIs. There is not one single aspect of the OR experience that can be singled out to make the most difference in SSI prevention and control. Attention to small details before, during, and after a surgical incision is critical because there is much room for errors to occur.

The Operating Room Environment

Sir John Charnley was one of the first to study airflow in an OR; his experience favored laminar ultra-clean air systems in joint replacement surgery.[146] Several studies have shown a correlation between airborne bacterial contamination and postoperative PJI.[147-150] Although laminar airflow (LAF) results in a statistically significant reduction in airborne bacterial colony-forming units (CFUs), a statistically significant decrease in SSI has not been shown.[151] The absence of a high level of evidence from randomized trials is not proof of ineffectiveness.[152] Many of the studies on laminar flow included personnel dressed in body exhaust suits. Body exhaust suits provide the patient with protection against bacterial shedding, hair, exposed skin, and mucous membranes of OR staff.[153,154] Although most would agree that these suits appear to reduce bacterial counts in the air, SSI reduction has not been observed.[155] To note, one recent study suggests that modern body exhaust suits that use a fan may in fact increase contamination.[156] People in the OR are the primary source of particulate matter.[157] CFUs in the OR directly correlate to the number of people in the OR.[88,158-160] Although all people shed particulate matter from their bodies, some, known as "shedders," produce more than others. The presence of a "shedder" in the OR is associated with an increased risk of SSI.[161,162] OR traffic has been shown to be a major concern during arthroplasty procedures, especially during revision cases.[163] Limiting the number of people in the OR is critical in preventing SSIs[159,164] and is likely more important than LAF.[165,166] Last, although ultraviolet light (UVL) has been shown to be effective in creating a clean-air environment in some studies, others have not supported this argument.[167-169] A study surveying almost 300 hospitals across four states showed that during total knee replacement surgery, 30% reported regular use of LAF, 42% reported regular use of body exhaust, and 5% reported regular use of ultraviolet lights.[170] The CDC recommends further study of LAF but recommends UVL not be used secondary to documented potential health risks to personnel.[152]

The role of facemasks has been surprisingly controversial. Several studies have not definitively shown that CFUs are reduced with surgical masks.[171-173] One study, quoted by the CDC, showed that a fresh facemask almost completely abolished bacterial contamination of agar plates 30 cm from the mouth.[174] Interestingly, a recent study looking at more than 800 surgical cases in an Australian tertiary care center found no difference in infection rates when nonscrubbed staff wore masks and when they did not.[175] Another study favored wearing a *hood* over a mask to reduce contamination.[176] Because available data are sparse in this field, this chapter's author routinely uses a facemask while entering an arthroplasty room and has it removed after the body exhaust suit is wrapped up. He also mandates that all OR personnel wear a facemask throughout the extent of the procedure.

The Surgical Team

Surgeons have advocated the surgical hand scrub since Lister used carbonic acid to clean his hands.[177] Considering that glove perforation continues to be an issue,[178] reducing resident and transient flora on the skin before the incision and achieving persistent antimicrobial activity throughout the length of the procedure are critical. Data on the clinical effects of a variety of surgical hand scrub protocols are lacking, and most studies have looked at bacterial counts on the skin. Because of the high variability of available products, there is no standard recommended scrub. Several studies have demonstrated that scrubbing for 5 minutes with an antimicrobial soap without a brush reduces bacterial counts as effectively as a 10-minute scrub.[179,180] Chlorhexidine-containing soap has shown excellent results in bacterial load reduction and continues to work throughout the procedure.[181] Alcohol-based hand rubs that require less time than washing hands have shown greater effectiveness, less irritation to the hands, and no risk of recontamination by rinsing hands with water that may not be of the best quality.[182] If one chooses to use an alcohol-based rub, it is important to prewash the hands and allow them to dry completely before application. Whichever surgical scrub or rub is used, it is critical that all staff is well educated about the manufacturer's recommended application technique.

Double gloving has been shown to reduce blood contact to the hands of the operating team members by nearly 90%.[183] The risk of contamination from blood can be 13 times higher when using single compared with double gloves, and double indicator gloves appear to be better than two regular gloves.[184] Double gloving, however, has shown a *similar* incidence of *wound* contamination compared with single gloving.[185] Cloth gloves placed *over* latex gloves appear to result in fewer punctures of the inner glove.[186] The puncture rate of gloves increases in longer procedures,[186] and systematic glove changes at key phases of certain procedures such as hip arthroplasty do reduce the frequency of occult perforations and bacterial loading of glove surfaces.[187] Considering that double gloving does not significantly impact manual dexterity or tactile sensitivity compared with single-gloving,[188] given the available data, it appears reasonable to recommend double gloving for the majority of orthopaedic cases in which glove perforation is likely to occur. Scrub staff–assisted donning of gloves should be done whenever possible because it appears to lead to less gown contamination.[189] It appears best that gowns should be occlusive, water repellent or impervious, and nonwoven.[190,191] More data are needed to determine the benefits of single-use versus reusable gowns.[192,193]

The Surgical Site

For elective cases, surgical site preparation should start at home before admission. Cleaning the surgical site with an antiseptic the night before surgery has been shown to significantly decrease skin bacterial counts of staphylococci and yeast.[194] Repeated applications increase the efficacy.[195] For trauma cases, it should start as soon as possible before the incision. Hair removal should only be done when there is excessive hair. Use of a safety razor more than 24 hours before surgery carries a 20% infection risk,[196] and shaving immediately before surgery carries a 3.1% risk. The lowest SSI rate is associated with no hair removal at all or with use of a depilatory method within a few hours of surgery.[197]

Four surgical preparation solutions are commonly being used: 4% chlorhexidine gluconate, povidone–iodine (Betadine), 2% chlorhexidine gluconate mixed with 70% alcohol (Chloraprep), and iodine povacrylex mixed with isopropyl alcohol (DuraPrep).[198-202] The 4% chlorhexidine gluconate solution appears to be superior to Betadine at reducing intrasurgical wound contamination. Betadine is as effective as 4% chlorhexidine gluconate in decreasing initial bacterial contamination, although the latter is less toxic and has a more cumulative effect than the former. Chloraprep appears to have better immediate and residual antimicrobial activity than 4% chlorhexidine gluconate. In a study of general surgery cases, DuraPrep was shown to have the lowest SSI rate compared with Chloraprep and Betadine.[202] Interestingly, the chlorhexidine-based solutions may lead to more erasure of surgical site markings used during time-out patient safety procedures than the iodine-based products.[203]

The use of adhesive drapes in joint replacement surgery is common, although it is not universally used in other orthopaedic subspecialties. It has been proposed that these drapes function by preventing bacterial penetration, multiplication, and lateral movement.[204] One study found a wound contamination reduction from 15% to 1.6% with use of an iodophore-impregnated drape.[205] A study out of Germany looking at 123 cases with and without a drape found no significant difference in infection rates.[206] If one chooses to use an adhesive drape, attention must be given to prevention of drape "lift-off." DuraPrep appears to be superior to both Betadine[207] and Chloraprep in terms of drape adhesion.

Although many surgeons have spread the belief that "the solution to pollution is dilution," there is disagreement about the most effective type of irrigation solution and the best method of delivery. A recent study in hip and knee arthroplasty patients suggested the benefits of dilute Betadine lavage for 3 minutes before wound closure.[208] Similar findings have been shown using the same method in spine surgery cases.[209] Although antibiotic irrigation does not appear to be effective in reducing SSI rates,[210] an in vitro animal wound model showed that surfactant irrigation was superior to saline or antibiotic solution in removing bacteria from metallic surfaces, bone, and bovine muscle. Interestingly, not much work has been done on the ideal amount of irrigation fluid. One study on removal of cement debris in knee arthroplasty procedures suggested that 4 L of irrigation solution is needed.[211] Pulsatile lavage appears to be superior to bulb-syringe irrigation[212]; however, attention should be given to maintain a relatively low pressure; high-pressure lavage can lead to deep tissue bacterial penetration and retention compared with low-pressure pulsatile lavage.[213]

Suction tips[214,215] and irrigation splash basins[216] are also sources of potential bacterial contamination. Suction tips should probably be changed during lengthy procedures, although data specifically supporting this suggestion are lacking. Culture positivity correlates directly with the duration of open exposure of uncovered OR trays.[217] Instrument tray coverage should be considered when lengthy anesthesia preparation is anticipated or when multiple procedures by different teams may prolong the time that unused instruments stay uncovered.

CONCLUSION

Surgical site infections continue to be serious, potentially life-threatening complications of surgery. The social burden of these infections is immense.[218,219] SSIs will always be present and cannot be completely eliminated. New technologies that tether prophylactic antimicrobials to implants have shown promising results,[220,221] as have simpler methods such as antibiotic-loaded bone cement in arthroplasty cases[222] and direct placement of antibiotics into the wound itself.[223,224] The emerging paradigm of infection prevention and control discussed in this chapter should serve as a foundation for minimizing this devastating complication.

KEY REFERENCES

The level of evidence (LOE) is determined according to the criteria provided in the preface.

10. Fry DE: Surgical site infections and the surgical care improvement project (SCIP): Evolution of national quality measures. *Surg Infect (Larchmt)* 9(6):579–584, 2008. LOE V
11. Parvizi J, Della Valle CJ: AAOS clinical practice guideline: diagnosis and treatment of periprosthetic joint infections of the hip and knee. *J Am Acad Orthop Surg* 18(12):771–772, 2010. LOE V
12. Parvizi J, Zmistowski B, Berbari EF, et al: New definition for periprosthetic joint infection: From the workgroup of the Musculoskeletal Infection Society. *Clin Orthop Relat Res* 469(11):2992–2994, 2011. LOE V
13. Evans RP, Clyburn TA, Moucha CS, et al: Surgical site infection prevention and control: an emerging paradigm. *Instr Course Lect* 60:539–543, 2011. LOE V
15. Moucha CS, Clyburn T, Evans RP, et al: Modifiable risk factors for surgical site infection. *J Bone Joint Surg Am* 93(4):398–404, 2011. LOE V
72. Rizvi AA, Chillag SA, Chillag KJ: Perioperative management of diabetes and hyperglycemia in patients undergoing orthopaedic surgery. *J Am Acad Orthop Surg* 18(7):426–435, 2010. LOE V
89. Polk HC Jr, Trachtenberg L, Finn MP: Antibiotic activity in surgical incisions. The basis of prophylaxis in selected operations. *JAMA* 244(12): 1353–1354, 1980. LOE V
122. Bratzler DW, Houck PM, Surg G: Infection prevention, antimicrobial prophylaxis for surgery: an advisory statement from the National Surgical Infection Prevention project. *Clin Infect Dis* 38(12):1706–1715, 2004. LOE V
202. Swenson BR, et al: Effects of preoperative skin preparation on postoperative wound infection rates: a prospective study of 3 skin preparation protocols. *Infect Control Hosp Epidemiol* 30(10):964–971, 2009. LOE II
223. Cavanaugh DL, et al: Better prophylaxis against surgical site infection with local as well as systemic antibiotics. An in vivo study. *J Bone Joint Surg Am* 91(8):1907–1912, 2009. LOE V

The complete References list is available online at https://expertconsult.inkling.com.

Chapter 23

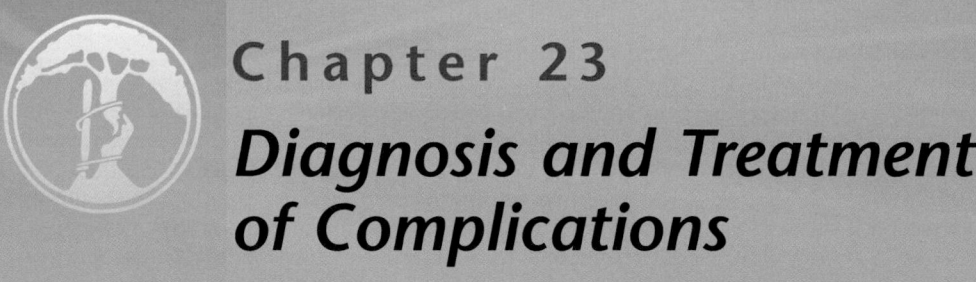

Diagnosis and Treatment of Complications

CRAIG S. ROBERTS • DAVID SELIGSON • BRANDI HARTLEY

We define a *complication* as a disease process that occurs in addition to a principal illness. In the lexicon of diagnosis-related groupings, *complications* are comorbidities. However, a broken implant complicating the healing of a radius shaft fracture hardly seems to fit either of these definitions. In orthopaedic trauma terminology, the term *complication* has come to mean an undesired turn of events specific to the care of a particular injury.

Complications can be *local* or *systemic* and are caused by, among other things, physiologic processes, errors in judgment, or fate. Codivilla described complications as "inconveniences."[1] A colleague once described a pin tract infection with external fixation as a *problem,* not a complication. Preventing pin tract drainage is indeed a problem that needs a solution, but when it occurs in a patient, it becomes a complication. Since 1995, The Joint Commission (formerly the Joint Commission on the Accreditation of Healthcare Organizations) has required the mandatory reporting of "sentinel events," a type of major complication that involves unexpected occurrences such as limb loss, surgery on the wrong body part, and hemolytic transfusion reaction. Another term, "never events," was introduced in 2001 by Dr. Ken Kizer and includes medical errors that should never occur (e.g., wrong site surgery, a retained foreign object after surgery, intraoperative or postoperative death in an American Association of Anesthesiologists class I patient, any stage 3 or 4 pressure ulcer acquired after admission).[2] These definitions beg the question, is death from any arrhythmia caused by a congenital irritable cardiac focus any more preventable on an operating table than it is on a basketball court?

Fracture care today expects perfection. These unrealistic expectations have led in part to the current adverse medicolegal situation surrounding the care of broken bones. There are many scales for judging the quality of results but none for complications. As a starter, operative misadventures can be classified as follows: (1) unexpected events that just slow things down—such as contaminating a reamer; (2) events that change the operation but have no long-term consequences—such as breaking a drill bit; and (3) events that cause long-term harm—such as cutting a nerve.

This chapter presents current knowledge about three *systemic* complications (fat embolism syndrome [FES], thromboembolic disorders, and multiple organ system dysfunction and failure) and five *local* complications (soft tissue damage, vascular problems, posttraumatic arthrosis, peripheral nerve injury, and complex regional pain syndrome [CRPS] or reflex sympathetic dystrophy [RSD]).

SYSTEMIC COMPLICATIONS

Fat Embolism Syndrome

Fat embolism syndrome is the occurrence of hypoxia, confusion, and petechiae a few days or even hours after a long bone fracture. FES is distinct from posttraumatic pulmonary insufficiency, shock lung, and acute respiratory distress syndrome (ARDS). When known etiologic factors of posttraumatic pulmonary insufficiency such as pulmonary contusion, inhalation pneumonitis, oxygen toxicity, and transfusion lung are excluded, there remains a group of patients who have FES with unanticipated respiratory compromise several days after a diaphyseal fracture.

Fat embolism was first described by Zenker in 1861 in a railroad worker who sustained a thoracoabdominal crush injury.[3] It was initially hypothesized that the fat from the marrow space embolized to the lungs and caused the pulmonary damage.[4] Fenger and Salisbury believed that fat embolized from fractures to the brain, resulting in death.[5] Von Bergmann first clinically diagnosed fat embolism in a patient with a fractured femur in 1873.[6] The incidence of this now recognized complication of long bone fracture was extensively documented by Talucci and coworkers in 1913 and subsequently studied during World Wars I and II and the Korean conflict.[7] Mullins described the findings in patients who died as "lungs that looked like liver."[8] Wong and colleagues reported on the use of continuous pulse oximeter monitoring and daily intermittent arterial blood gas to define the incidence pattern and severity of long bone fractures compared with control participants; they found that long bone fracture patients had more desaturation episodes, longer duration of total desaturation, and larger total area under desaturation curves in both the prefracture repair and the postfracture periods.[9]

Although the fat in the lungs comes from bone, other processes are required to produce the physiologic damage to lung, brain, and other tissues. Although the term *fat embolism syndrome* does not describe the pathomechanics of this condition as was originally hypothesized, embolization of active substances and fat from the injured marrow space has traditionally been thought to be the source of embolic fat. Recent studies suggest otherwise. Mudd and associates did not observe any myeloid tissue in any of the lung fields at autopsy in patients with FES and suggested that the soft tissue injury, rather than fractures, was the primary cause of FES.[10] Husebye and colleagues also noted that FES might also result from "an abnormal patient reaction to the fat intravasation."[11] ten Duis in a review of the literature stated that "future attempts to unravel this syndrome . . . should pay full attention to differences in the extent of accompanying soft tissue injuries that surround a long bone fracture."[12] In a laboratory rabbit model, Aydin and colleagues found that pulmonary contusion had more deleterious effects than fractures in the formation of cerebral fat embolism.[13]

Although there are many unanswered questions about FES, several issues are apparent. It strikes the young patients; older patients with significant upper femoral fractures do not seem at risk. It usually occurs after lower, not upper, limb fractures and is more frequent with closed fractures.[14] Russell and associates reported a case of fat embolism in an isolated humerus fracture.[15] McDermott and colleagues reported three cases of patients with tibial fractures from football injuries who also had dehydration and developed FES, and they concluded that adequate preoperative hydration, especially if injuries were sustained during heavy exercise, may reduce the risk of developing FES.[16] In a prospective study, Chan and associates found an incidence of 8.75% of overt FES in all fracture patients, with a mortality rate of 2.5%.[17] The incidence rose to 35% in patients with multiple fractures. Other investigators reported the incidence of FES between 0.9% and 3.5% in patients with long bone fractures.[18-20]

Early recognition of the syndrome is crucial to preventing a complex and potentially lethal course.[21] Clinically, FES consists of a triad of hypoxia, confusion, and petechiae appearing in a patient with fractures.[22] The disease characteristically begins 1 to 2 days after fracture after what has been called the *latent* or *lucid* period.[4] Sixty percent of all cases of FES are seen in the first 24 hours after trauma, and 90% of all cases appear within 72 hours.[23] Gurd and Wilson's criteria for FES are commonly used, with the clinical manifestations grouped into either major or minor signs of FES.[24] The major signs are respiratory insufficiency, cerebral involvement, and petechial rash. The minor signs are fever, tachycardia, retinal changes, jaundice, and renal changes. Petechiae are caused by embolic fat. They are transient and are distributed on the cheek, neck, axillae, palate, and conjunctivae. The fat itself can be visualized on the retina.[25] A fall in hematocrit levels[26] and alterations in blood clotting profile, including a prolongation of the prothrombin time, can be observed. The diagnosis of FES is made when one major and four minor signs are present (Table 23-1) along with the finding of macroglobulinemia.[27] The most productive laboratory test is measurement of arterial oxygenation on room air. When the Po_2 is less than 60 mm Hg, the patient may be in the early stages of FES.

TABLE 23-1 ***MAJOR AND MINOR CRITERIA FOR THE DIAGNOSIS OF FAT EMBOLISM SYNDROME****

Major Criteria	Minor Criteria
Hypoxemia (Pao_2 <60 mm Hg)	Tachycardia >110 beats/min
Central nervous system depression	Pyrexia >38.3°C
Petechial rash	Retinal emboli on funduscopy
Pulmonary edema	Fat in urine Fat in sputum Thrombocytopenia Decreased hematocrit

*A positive diagnosis requires at least one major and four minor signs.
Source: *Gurd AR, Wilson RI: The fat embolism syndrome, J Bone Joint Surg Br 56:408–416, 1974.*

Lindeque and colleagues[28] believe that Gurd and Wilson's criteria are too restrictive and should also include the following: (1) Pco_2 of more than 55 mg Hg or pH of less than 7.3; (2) sustained respiratory rate of more than 35 breaths/min; and (3) dyspnea, tachycardia, and anxiety. If any one of these is present, then the diagnosis of FES is made. Other supportive findings include ST segment changes on electrocardiography and pulmonary infiltrates on chest radiography.[29]

Neurologic changes have been noted in up to 80% of patients.[30] It is important to assess the neurologic status of the patient to differentiate among fat embolization, frontal concussion or contusion, and intracranial mass lesions. Although hypoxia alone can cause confusion, in FES, petechial hemorrhages, particularly in the reticular system, may alter consciousness. These changes persist despite adequate oxygen therapy.[23,31,32] Focal neurologic findings should be investigated to rule out lesions caused by associated head trauma. Persistent alterations of consciousness or seizures are a bad prognostic sign.

Clinically, fat embolism is a diagnosis of exclusion. In the first few days, sudden pulmonary compromise can also result from pulmonary embolism (PE), heart failure, aspiration, and medication reaction. When these possible causes have been excluded along with many other less likely conditions, fat embolism becomes the leading cause of morbidity in the injured patient with a long bone lower limb fracture.

Fat globules are found in blood,[33] sputum, urine, and cerebrospinal fluid. The urine or sputum can be stained for fat using a saturated alcoholic solution of Sudan III. Sudan III stains neutral fat globules yellow or orange. The Gurd test, in which serum is treated with Sudan III and filtered, is also diagnostic. These tests are of historical interest when house staff actually handled specimens.

The specificity of these tests is in question. Fat droplets are normally found in sputum.[34] In addition, Peltier believes that detection of fat droplets in circulating blood and urine is too sensitive a test for the clinical diagnosis of FES.[35] Furthermore, because the embolic phenomena associated with FES are transient and may not be detected on spot testing, these laboratory investigations are of research interest only and are not part of the usual clinical workup.

The experimental study of FES is linked historically to the study of the circulation of blood, the development of intravenous (IV) therapy, and transfusion. As early as 1866, Busch experimented with marrow injury in the rabbit tibia and showed that fat in the marrow cavity would embolize to the lungs.[36] Pulmonary symptoms have been produced in the absence of fracture by the IV injection of fat from the tibia of one group of rabbits to another.[37]

There are several reasons for uncertainty about the role of bone fat in producing FES. First, researchers have failed to develop an animal model that reproduces the human syndrome. Moreover, injection of human bone marrow fat into the veins of experimental animals has shown that neutral fat is a relatively benign substance, and it is not certain that the bones contain enough fat to cause FES. One hypothesis is that the fat that appears in the lungs originated in soft tissue stores and aggregated in the blood stream during posttraumatic shock.[38] However, chromatographic analysis of pulmonary vasculature fat in dogs after femoral fracture has shown that the fat most closely resembles marrow fat.[39] In contrast, Mudd and colleagues reported that there was no evidence of myeloid elements on postmortem studies of lung tissue in patients with FES.[10] Furthermore, extraction of marrow fat from human long bones has shown that sufficient fat is present to account for the observed quantities in the lungs and other tissues.[40] The relative lack of triolein in children's bones may explain why they have a significantly reduced incidence of FES compared with adults.[32,41,42]

Etiology

Although the precise pathomechanics of FES are unclear, Levy found many nontraumatic and traumatic conditions associated with FES.[43] The simplest hypothesis is that broken bones liberate marrow fat that embolizes to the lungs. These fat globules produce mechanical and metabolic effects culminating in FES. The mechanical theory postulates that fat droplets from the marrow enter the venous circulation via torn veins adjacent to the fracture site.

Peltier[44] coined the term *intravasation* to describe the process whereby fat gains access to the circulation. The conditions in the vascular bed that allow intravasation to take place also permit marrow embolization.[45] Indeed, marrow particles are found when fat is found in the lungs (Fig. 23-1).[46]

Mechanical obstruction of the pulmonary vasculature occurs because of the absolute size of the embolized particles. In a dog model, Teng and coworkers[46] found 80% of fat droplets to be between 20 and 40 μm. Consequently, vessels in the lung smaller than 20 μm in diameter become obstructed. Fat globules of 10 to 40 μm have been found after human trauma.[43] Systemic embolization occurs either through precapillary shunts into pulmonary veins or through a patent foramen ovale.[47]

The biochemical theory suggests that mediators from the fracture site alter lipid solubility, causing coalescence, because normal chylomicrons are smaller than 1 μm in diameter. Many of the emboli have a histologic composition consisting of a fatty center with platelets and fibrin adhered.[48] Large amounts of thromboplastin are liberated with the release of bone marrow, leading to activation of the coagulation cascade.

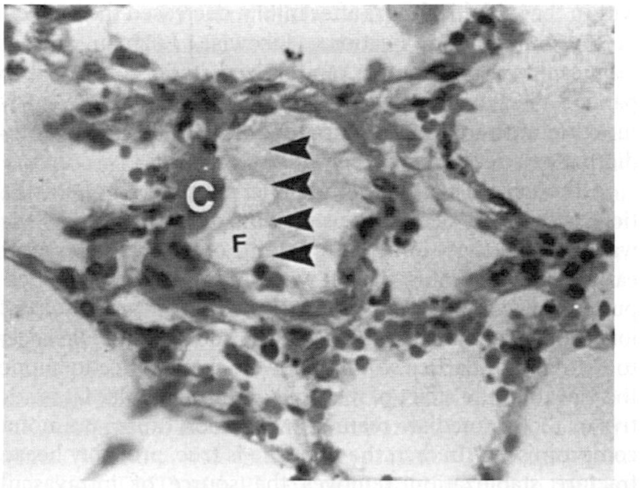

Figure 23-1. Histologic appearance of fat from a pulmonary fat embolism in a vessel of the pulmonary alveoli. *C*, Capillary; *F*, fat globules *(arrowheads)*. *(From Teng QS, Li G, Zhang BX: Experimental study of early diagnosis and treatment of fat embolism syndrome, J Orthop Trauma 9:183–189, 1995.)*

Studies of the physiologic response to the circulatory injection of fats have shown that the unsaponified free fatty acids are much more toxic than the corresponding neutral fats. Peltier hypothesized that elevated serum lipase levels present after the embolization of neutral fat hydrolyzes this neutral fat to free fatty acids and causes local endothelial damage in the lungs and other tissues, resulting in FES.[40] This chemical phase might in part explain the latency period seen between the arrival of embolic fat and more severe lung dysfunction. Elevated serum lipase levels have been reported in association with clinically fatal FES.[49,50] Alternative explanations are also possible for the toxic effect of fat on the pulmonary capillary bed. The combination of fat, fibrin, and (possibly) marrow may be sufficient to begin a biochemical cascade that damages the lungs without postulating enzymatic hydrolysis of neutral fat.[32,38,51] Bleeding into the lungs is associated with a decrease in the hematocrit level.[52] The resulting hypoxemia from the mechanical and biochemical changes in the lungs can be severe—even to the point of death of the patient.

Pape and associates[53] demonstrated an increase in neutrophil proteases from central venous blood in a group of patients undergoing reamed femoral nailing. In another study, Pape and colleagues[54] demonstrated the release of platelet-derived thromboxane (a potent vasoconstrictor of pulmonary microvasculature) from the marrow cavity. Peltier[55] demonstrated the release of vasoactive platelet amines. These humeral factors can lead to pulmonary vasospasm and bronchospasm, resulting in vascular endothelial injury and increased pulmonary permeability. Indeed, thrombocytopenia is such a consistent finding that it is used as one of the diagnostic criteria of FES. Barie and coworkers[56] associated pulmonary dysfunction with an alteration in the coagulation cascade and an increase in fibrinolytic activity.

Autopsy findings in patients who died of FES do not, however, show a consistent picture.[4] This may be caused by a lack of clear-cut criteria that define patients included in a given series but may also be because manifestations of FES depend on a wide number of patient, accident, and treatment variables.[44]

In light of the incidence of fat emboli and FES in trauma patients, it is likely that other precipitating or predisposing factors such as shock, sepsis, or disseminated intravascular coagulation are needed for the phenomenon of embolized fat to cause FES.[57] Müller and associates[58] summarized that "fat embolism syndrome is likely the pathogenetic reaction of lung tissue to shock, hypercoagulability, and lipid mobilization."

Two clinically related treatment questions arise: (1) Is there an association between intramedullary (IM) nailing, FES, and other injuries? (2) Is there an effect from different nailing methods on the incidence of FES? In 1950, Küntscher described FES as a complication of IM nailing.[59] Pape and associates[60,61] found that early operative fracture fixation by nailing was associated with an increased risk of ARDS in patients with thoracic injury. These results are in contrast with those of the group without thoracic injury. Thoracic trauma is associated with direct pulmonary injury. The pathogenic mechanisms were examined by Lozman and colleagues.[62] Thus, the timing and the associated injuries are crucial in deciding when and how to use a nail.

in total hip and knee arthroplasty patients. Recommendations from the 9th edition *Chest* supplement are for the use of one of the following antithrombotic approaches (rather than no antithrombotic prophylaxis) for a minimum of 10 to 14 days: LMWH, fondaparinux, low-dose UFH, adjusted-dose vitamin-K antagonist, aspirin, or an intermittent pneumatic compression device.[157] Interestingly, the Supplement noted a preference for LMWH compared with the other agents that they recommended.[157] In addition, they recommended that if hip fracture surgery would be delayed that LMWH would be started.[157] From an ethical standpoint, one might question if overvigorous anticoagulation is appropriate in every case. Consider, for example, an elderly, demented nursing home patient who falls and has a hip fracture. Indeed, there is potentially a wide range of mischief from the use of anticoagulation in elderly patients, who may experience bleeding, stroke, and diagnostic misadventures as a result of overzealous prophylaxis!

Isolated Lower Leg Injury Patient Distal to the Knee. Isolated extremity injuries are probably the most common injuries seen by orthopaedic physicians. The recommendation was for "no prophylaxis rather than pharmacologic thromboprophylaxis in patients with isolated lower leg injuries requiring leg immobilization."[157] On the other hand, surveillance of patients for VTE and protection or prophylaxis seems prudent, particularly for patients with risk factors such as underconditioning middle age or old, multiparity, and so on. At a minimum, one could consider simple measures (early mobilization, ankle pump exercises, graduated compression stockings, intermittent pneumatic compression (IPC) with or without graduated compression stockings) or more intensive measures (preoperative and immediate postoperative graduated compression stockings followed by a short course of LMWH, synthetic pentasaccharides, or adjusted vitamin K antagonists). Patient and office staff education are wise steps.

Spinal Cord Injury Patient. Acute spinal cord injury was the risk factor most strongly associated with the development of DVT in major trauma.[94] Rogers and colleagues[158] in their meta-analysis noted that spinal cord injuries or spinal fractures are high risk for VTE. It is recommended that "thromboprophylaxis be provided for all patients with acute spinal cord injuries."[156] The recommendations for patients with acute spinal cord injury were for pharmacologic prophylaxis (low-dose UFH or LMWH) together with mechanical prophylaxis (e.g., intermittent pneumatic compression).[157]

Treatment of Existing Deep Venous Thrombosis and Pulmonary Embolism. After DVT or PE is suspected, the clinical impression should be confirmed by diagnostic testing. Parenteral anticoagulants can be started unless contraindicated while the diagnostic testing is pending; this is the current recommendation for patients in whom there is a high clinical suspicion of acute VTE.[157] If there is an "intermediate" or "low" clinical suspicion of DVT, the recommendation is not to start parenteral anticoagulants.[157] The options for anticoagulation are parenteral anticoagulation with LMWH, fondaparinux, IV UFH, or subcutaneous UFH.[157] Furthermore, there is more focus on the specific location of the DVT (i.e., proximal or distal in the lower extremities). When there are no severe symptoms or risk factors for extension, the recommendation is for serial imagery of the deep veins for 2 weeks over initial anticoagulation.[157] If there are severe symptoms or risk factors for extension, the recommendation is for anticoagulation.[157] For patients with an acute proximal DVT, the recommendation is for LMWH or fondaparinux over IV UFH and over subcutaneous heparin.[157]

There are also now changes in the recommendation for how, when, and where the anticoagulation is administered. When patients with an acute DVT of the leg are treated with LMWH, the suggestion is for once-a-day over twice-a-day administration with the caveat that the once-a-day administration is twice the dosage of the once-a-day dose.[157] In terms of where treatment is given, the recommendation is for initial treatment at home in patients with acute DVT provided "home circumstances are adequate."[157] It has been suggested that the optimal duration of thromboprophylaxis after multiple trauma be "largely based on rational, clinical decision-making on a case-by-case basis."[159]

Although options such as thrombolytic therapy for the treatment of acute DVT may be considered, the latest recommendations are for anticoagulant therapy alone for catheter-directed thrombolysis.[157] Even if catheter-directed thrombolysis is not available, the latest recommendations are for anticoagulant therapy alone over systemic thrombolysis.[157] Operative venous thrombectomy is also deemphasized because anticoagulant therapy alone is suggested over operative venous thrombectomy.[157] Furthermore, the recommendations are for anticoagulation of the same intensity and duration in patients who undergo thrombosis removal as in patients who are comparable who did not undergo thrombosis removal.[157]

Inferior vena cava filters are used less frequently and are no longer recommended as primary prophylaxis against VTE.[156] IVC filters have associated complications such as venous stasis leading to edema, pain, varicose veins, and skin ulcers in a condition known as the *postphlebitic syndrome*.[160] Other complications include bleeding or thrombus formation at the site of insertion, migration of the filter, and perforation of the vena cava.[161,162] Martin and coworkers[141] described a case report of phlegmasia cerulea dolens as a complication of an IVC filter for prophylaxis against PE in a man with a fracture of the acetabulum. In addition, filters are not 100% effective.[163]

Vena cava interruption is performed when heparinization is contraindicated, as in patients with a preexisting bleeding disorder; severe hypertension; neurologic injury; or bleeding problems of pulmonary, gastrointestinal (GI), neurologic, or urologic etiology. If anticoagulation fails to stop pulmonary emboli, vena cava interruption is indicated.[164] Also, if patients develop complications with anticoagulation, they can be switched to vena cava interruption. An additional approach is the preoperative use of vena cava interruption in patients who are at extremely high risk for PE.

Summary

The current literature clearly indicates that certain trauma patients benefit from some form of surveillance or prophylaxis. DVT and PE are common causes of morbidity, mortality,[155,165,166] and litigation associated with the care of orthopaedic trauma patients. The complete prevention of thromboembolism in orthopaedic trauma is impossible because trauma cannot be anticipated. One or more components of Virchow's triad are usually present from the time of injury, so the concept of "DVT prophylaxis" is a misnomer for trauma patients.

Questions remain such as, "Is there a genetic predisposition to VTE?" Risk stratification is being used in other areas of medicine and is only beginning to be understood in

TABLE 23-2 *CRITERIA FOR ORGAN DYSFUNCTION AND FAILURE*

Organ or System	Dysfunction	Advanced Failure
Pulmonary	Hypoxia requiring intubation for 3–5 days	ARDS requiring PEEP >10 cm H_2O and Fio_2>0.5
Hepatic	Serum total bilirubin ≥2–3 mg/dL or liver function tests ≥ twice normal	Clinical jaundice with total bilirubin ≥8–10 mg/dL
Renal	Oliguria ≤479 mL/day or creatinine ≥2–3 mg/dL	Dialysis
Gastrointestinal	Ileus with intolerance of enteral feeds >5 days	Stress ulcers, acalculous cholecystitis
Hematologic	PT/PTT >125% normal, platelets <50,000–80,000	DIC
Central nervous system	Confusion, mild disorientation	Progressive coma
Cardiovascular	Decreased ejection fraction or capillary leak syndrome	Refractory cardiogenic shock

ARDS, Adult respiratory distress syndrome; *DIC,* disseminated intravascular coagulation; *Fio₂,* fraction of inspired air in oxygen; *PEEP,* positive end-expiratory pressure; *PT,* prothrombin time; *PTT,* partial thromboplastin time.
Source: *Deitch EA: Pathophysiology and potential future therapy, Ann Surg 216:117–134, 1992, with permission.*

orthopaedic trauma. In addition, combinations of injuries, multiple lower extremity fractures with a spinal cord injury, or a pelvic fracture together with a femur fracture likely exponentially increases the risk of VTE. Although current prophylactic regimens in trauma patients significantly reduce the relative risk for DVT and PE, no method provides 100% protection. Further randomized controlled trials of DVT prophylaxis in trauma patients are needed. Nonetheless, our ability to diagnose VTE and protect patients from it is constrained by acute hemorrhage and an inability to tolerate anticoagulation, soft tissue contusion, and extremity injuries that prevent the placement of IPC and GCS. Prophylaxis is also impossible, and the best we can do is to try for VTE protection. Nonetheless, there are many methods of DVT surveillance and protection at our disposal, and they should be considered. Although the ideal method of documentation for hospital or outpatient examinations is unknown, we have found that a note such as "no signs or symptoms of PE/DVT" along with the documentation of VTE protection or prophylaxis to be prudent and reasonable. Clinicians are also advised to stay informed of the consensus recommendations that are published every 2 to 3 years in the *Chest* supplement.

Multiple Organ System Dysfunction and Failure

Multiple organ failure (MOF) is defined as the sequential failure of two or more organ systems remote from the site of the original insult after injury, operation, or sepsis. The organ failure can be pulmonary, renal, hepatic, GI, central nervous, or hematologic.[167,168] These systems can be monitored for objective criteria for failure, but criteria vary from series to series (Tables 23-2 and 23-3).[169,170] The risk of developing MOF and the severity of the MOF can also be graded by measuring the effects on specific organ systems.[171]

Multiple organ failure is the end result of a transition from the normal metabolic response to injury to persistent hypermetabolism and eventual failure of organs to maintain their physiologic function. A 1991 consensus conference used the term *multiple organ dysfunction syndrome* (MODS) to describe this spectrum of changes.[172] Organ dysfunction is the result of either a direct insult or a systemic inflammatory response, known clinically as the *systemic inflammatory response syndrome* (SIRS),[173] which can be reversible or progress to MODS or MOF. SIRS can be caused by a variety of infectious and noninfectious stimuli[172] (Fig. 23-5). Treatment of the offending source must be undertaken early because when organ failure has begun, treatment modalities become progressively ineffective.[174] Fry identified the mortality rate for failure of two or more organ systems as about 75%. If two organ systems fail and renal failure occurs, then the mortality rate is 98%.[169] MOF has been described as the number one cause of death in surgical intensive care units (ICUs).[175]

The basic theory behind the development of MOF and the closely related ARDS has undergone modification since the 1970s and mid 1980s. Moore and Moore[176] described the earlier models, which promoted an infectious basis for ARDS and MOF, with two possible scenarios: (1) insult → ARDS → pulmonary sepsis → MOF or (2) insult → sepsis → ARDS and MOF. Current thinking promotes an inflammatory model of MOF with an inflammatory response from a number of infectious and noninfectious stimuli. Two patterns exist: the

TABLE 23-3 *DEFINITION OF ORGAN FAILURE BASED ON FRY CRITERIA*

Pulmonary	Need of ventilator support at Fio_2 ≥0.4 for 5 consecutive days
Hepatic	Hyperbilirubinemia >2.0 g/dL and an increase of serum glutamic-oxaloacetic transaminase
Gastrointestinal	Hemorrhage from documented or presumed stress-induced acute gastric ulceration. This can be documented by endoscopy; if endoscopy is not performed, then the hemorrhage must be sufficient to require 2 units of blood transfusion.
Renal	Serum creatinine level >2.0 mg/dL. If a patient has preexisting renal disease with elevated serum creatinine level, then doubling of the admission level is defined as failure.

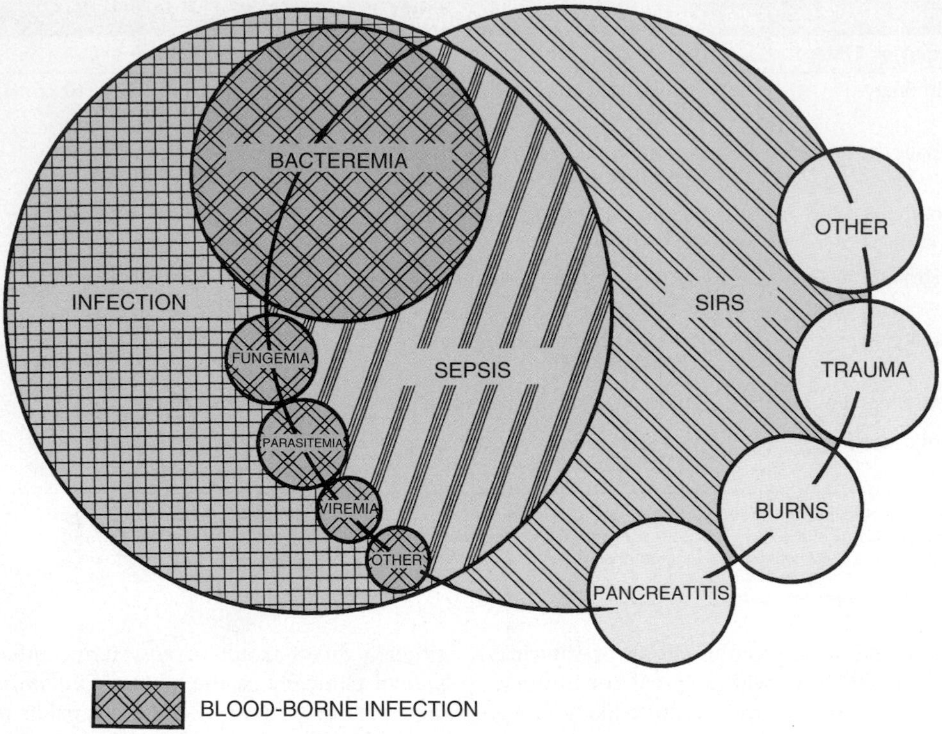

Figure 23-5. The interrelationship among systemic inflammatory response syndrome (SIRS), sepsis, and infection. *(From Bone RC, Balk RA, Cerra FC, et al: Definitions for sepsis and organ failure and guidelines for the use of innovative therapies in sepsis, Chest 101:1644–1655, 1992.)*

one-hit model (massive insult → severe SIRS → early MOF) and the more common two-hit model (moderate insult → moderate SIRS → second insult → late MOF). Research into the pathogenesis of MOF has focused on how the inflammatory response is propagated independent of infection. Moore and Moore have the global hypothesis that postinjury MOF occurs as the result of a dysfunctional inflammatory response.[176] Deitch created an integrated paradigm of the mechanisms of MOF.[175] In general, three broad overlapping hypotheses have been proposed in the pathogenesis of MOF: (1) macrophage cytokine hypothesis, (2) microcirculatory hypothesis, and (3) gut hypothesis. Further understanding of MOF must extend to the cellular and molecular levels.

Organ injury in MOF is largely caused by the host's own endogenously produced mediators and less caused by exogenous factors such as bacteria or endotoxins (Table 23-4).[175] There is increasing evidence that biologic markers for the risk of development of MOF may be more useful than anatomic descriptions of injuries. Nast-Kolb and associates[75] measured various inflammatory markers in a prospective study of 66 patients with multiple injuries (injury severity score [ISS] >18) and found that the degree of inflammatory response corresponded with the development of posttraumatic organ failure.[75] Specifically, lactate, neutrophil elastase, interleukin-6 (IL-6), and IL-8 were found to correlate with organ dysfunction. Strecker and coworkers[177] studied 107 patients prospectively and found that the amount of fracture and soft tissue damage can be estimated early by analysis of serum IL-6 and creatine kinase and is of great importance with regard to long-term outcome after trauma. These investigators found significant correlations between fracture and soft tissue trauma

TABLE 23-4 *POTENTIAL MEDIATORS INVOLVED IN THE PATHOGENESIS OF MULTIPLE ORGAN FAILURE*

Humoral Mediators
Complement
Products of arachidonic acid metabolism: lipoxygenase products, cyclooxygenase products
Tumor necrosis factor
Interleukins (1–13)
Growth factors
Adhesion molecules
Platelet activating factor
Procalcitonin
Procoagulants
Fibronectin and opsonins
Toxic oxygen free radicals
Endogenous opioids-endorphins
Vasoactive polypeptides and amines
Bradykinin and other kinins
Neuroendocrine factors
Myocardial depressant factor
Coagulation factors and their degradation products
Cellular Inflammatory Mediators
Polymorphonuclear leukocytes
Monocytes and macrophages
Platelets
Endothelial cells
Exogenous Mediators
Endotoxin
Exotoxin and other toxins

Source: *Adapted with permission from Balk RA: Pathogenesis and management of multiple organ dysfunction or failure in severe sepsis and septic shock, Crit Care Clin 16(2):337–352, 2000.*

and ICU stay; hospital stay; infections; SIRS; MOF score; and serum concentrations or activities of serum IL-6, IL-8, and creatine kinase during the first 24 hours after trauma.

Blood transfusions are a frequent part of polytrauma treatment and an independent risk factor for MOF. Zallen and associates have identified the age of packed red blood cells (PRBCs) to be a risk factor, with the number of units over 14 days and 21 days as independent risk factors for MOF.[178] Old but not outdated PRBCs prime the neutrophils for superoxide production and activate the endothelial cells, which are pathogenic mediators for MOF.

Multiple organ failure is a syndrome distinct from respiratory failure that can complicate airway injury, resuscitation, or anesthesia after an accident. With the development of improved patient categorization, transport, and emergency care, it has become recognized that there is a threshold beyond which the survival from injury is problematic. With simple injuries (e.g., an ankle fracture and laceration from a fall), the physiologic effects are not additive. However, in high-energy blunt trauma, the systemic effects—for example, of a pulmonary contusion, ruptured spleen, and fractured pelvis—become more than additive.

The ISS, used to quantify the extent of trauma,[179] was derived from the abbreviated injury score (AIS) of the American Medical Association Committee on Medical Aspects of Automotive Safety,[180] which was updated in 1985 as AIS-85. Injuries to six body regions (head and neck, face, chest, abdomen and pelvic viscera, extremities and bony pelvis, and integument) are graded as (1) mild, (2) moderate, (3) severe, (4) critical—outcome usually favorable, and (5) critical—outcome usually lethal. The ISS equals the sum of the squares of the three highest AIS grades. The ISS score has a maximal value of 75.

When the ISS is 25 or greater, the patient is at risk for MOF and will benefit from specialized trauma center care. The median lethal ISS scores have been determined by age group (in years): ages 15 to 44 years, an ISS of 40; ages 45 to 64 years, an ISS of 29; and ages 65 years and older, an ISS of 20.[181] Moore and Moore[176] identified the following variables to be predictive of MOF: age older than 55 years, ISS of 25 or greater, more than 6 units of blood in the first 24 hours after admission, high base deficit, and high lactate level. These investigators stratified patients at risk for MOF (Table 23-5).

TABLE 23-5 ***RISK STRATIFICATION FOR POSTINJURY MULTIPLE SYSTEM ORGAN FAILURE***

Category	Risk Factors	MSOF Probability (%)
I	ISS 15–24	4
II	ISS ≥25	14
III	ISS ≥25 plus >6 U RBCs/first 12 hr	54
IV	ISS ≥25 plus >6 U RBCs/first 12 hr plus lactate ≥2.5 mmol at 12–24 hr	75

ISS, injury severity score; *MSOF*, multiple system organ failure; *RBC*, red blood cell.
Source: *Moore FA, Moore EE: Evolving concepts in the pathogenesis of postinjury multiple organ failure, Surg Clin North Am 75:257–277, 1995.*

One of the consequences of MOF is the depletion of body protein reserves. Amino acids are essential components of the energy systems that maintain the body's homeostasis; this deficit cannot be replenished by IV glucose or lipids.[182] As MOF progresses, the peripheral metabolic energy source switches from the conventional energy fuels of glucose, fatty acids, and triglycerides to the catabolism of essential branched-chain amino acids. The multiple-injury patient is like a diesel submarine on the bottom of the ocean with a limited air supply. When the air supply is exhausted, damage control systems can no longer be maintained. Amino acids are lost as muscles are oxidized for energy, and the supply is not replenished.[45,183]

Tscherne emphasized the role of necrotic tissue in the pathogenesis of MOF. It is well known that a gangrenous limb, for example, can provoke a systemic catabolic response with the dramatic reversal of alarming symptoms when an urgent amputation is undertaken for gangrene. Pape and colleagues noted the importance of soft tissue injuries (extremities, lung, abdomen, and pelvis), which create a pathophysiologic cascade after blunt trauma.[184]

Dead tissue (e.g., muscle, bone marrow, and skin) provokes an inflammatory autophagocytic response.[185,186] In this setting, consumption of complement and plasma opsonins has been measured.[187-189] The complement system is activated with depletion of factors C3 and C5 with elevated levels of C3a and increased metabolism of C5a. C3a and C5a are anaphylatoxins and may cause the pulmonary edema in ARDS by affecting the smooth muscle contraction and vascular permeability.[188] Plasma opsonin activity is decreased with the consumption of the complement system. The opsonins are critical for antibacterial defense, and their consumption may lead to an increased susceptibility to infection.[187] Several investigators identified serum factors that stimulate muscle destruction.[190,191] Multiple mediators and effectors have been implicated in the pathogenesis of MOF, but exactly which mediator or combination of mediators is responsible for the hypermetabolic response is not known.[192] This response consumes the individual's energy reserve and leads to MOF. When MOF is established, the sequence of organ failure apparently follows a consistent pattern, with involvement first of the lung and then the liver, gastric mucosa, and kidney.[193]

Positive blood culture results have been documented in 75% of patients with MOF, but it is not clear whether infection is the cause or simply accompanies MOF.[193,194] Goris and associates[185] were able to induce MOF in rats by injecting a material that causes an inflammatory response. Sepsis causes tissue destruction and, therefore, similar to broken bones, releases activators of autophagic systems into the blood stream.

The immune system's response in polytrauma can be measured. Polk and colleagues[170] defined a scoring system for predicting outcome by combining points for ISS and contamination with a measurement of monocyte function (the surface expression of D-related antigen). This method appears promising in predicting survival.[195]

Because patients with identical injuries can have vastly different inflammatory responses after severe trauma, there may be a genetic predisposition for a compromised immune system after trauma. Hildebrand and colleagues[196] performed a prospective cohort study of patients with an ISS greater than 16 and noted that the IL-6-174G/C polymorphism was associated with the severity of the posttraumatic systemic inflammatory response. These authors concluded that there may be

TABLE 23-6 *PREVENTION OF MULTIPLE ORGAN FAILURE*

Resuscitative Phase
Aggressive volume resuscitation in early stages of treatment Appropriate monitoring of volume resuscitation with measurement of arterial base deficit and serum lactate level, use of pulmonary artery catheters, calculation of oxygen delivery and consumption, use of gastric tonometry
Operative Phase
Timely operative management of soft tissue injuries with débridement of nonviable and infected tissue Early fixation of all possible long bone and pelvic fractures Vigilance in preventing the missed injury
Intensive Care Unit Phase
Early nutritional support Appropriate use of antibiotics Specific organ support Timely reoperative surgery for missed injuries and complications of trauma

a genetic predisposition to an enhanced inflammatory response after polytrauma that may be associated with an adverse outcome.

A multiple system approach to the multiple-injury patient has proved valuable in preventing the development of MOF (Table 23-6). Avoidance of pulmonary failure, prevention of sepsis, and nutritional support are the keys.[197] Mechanical ventilation is regulated in a special care unit under the supervision of anesthesiologists or traumatologists with experience and training in this area of intensive care. Immediate wound débridement and constant attention to the details of wound management, pulmonary toilet, cleanliness of access lines, and urinary tract sterility are required to prevent sepsis. With open fractures, parenteral or local wound antibiotics are therapeutic. An assessment of nutritional reserve, including measurement of triceps skin fold, total lymphocytes, and serum transferrin, is helpful in determining the need for nutritional support. If possible, the GI tract should be used, but in patients with extensive intraabdominal injury and poor nutritional reserves, early total parenteral nutrition with amino acid supplementation is essential. Nutrition has an important role in preventing the translocation of bacteria and toxins from the gut into the splanchnic circulation.[72,198]

Orthopaedic Management

Early total care of significant pelvic, spinal, and femoral fractures can have a powerful role in avoiding the cascade of events leading to pulmonary failure, sepsis, and death.[199-201] Increased understanding of the metabolic consequences of fracture surgery further clarifies the timing of orthopaedic surgery in polytrauma patients; specifically, when is early total care of fractures safe, and when is DCO useful? There is optimism that the DCO approach to polytrauma patients will decrease the incidence of multisystem organic dysfunction and failure.[53,202] IM nailing of the femur has been shown to be a "second hit" to the patient.[203] Harwood and colleagues reported that DCO was associated with a lesser systemic inflammatory response.[204] Even though DCO is used in many centers for patients with the lethal triad of acidosis, hypercoagulability, and hyperthermia, there is limited scientific evidence (e.g., randomized, prospective studies) that it is effective. There are many studies that support the early fixation of fractures. Demling[205] stressed control of the inflammatory process to prevent further stimulus to MOF by early rapid removal of injured tissue and prevention of further tissue damage by early fracture fixation.

Overall, early fixation has been shown to decrease rates of respiratory, renal, and liver failure.[206] Seibel and associates showed that in the blunt multiple-trauma patient with an ISS ranging from 22 to 57, immediate internal fixation followed by ventilatory respiratory support greatly reduces the incidence of respiratory failure, positive blood culture results, complications of fracture treatment, and MOF.[207] When patients were treated with the same ventilatory support but with 10 days of traction before fracture fixation, pulmonary failure lasted twice as long, positive blood culture results increased 10-fold, and fracture complications increased by a factor of 3.5. If no ventilatory support was used and traction was used for 30 days, pulmonary failure lasted three to five times as long, positive blood culture results increased by a factor of 74, and fracture complications increased by a factor of 17. Carlson and coworkers demonstrated that fixation in less than 24 hours after injury versus nonoperative fracture management decreased the late septic mortality from 13.5% to less than 1%.[206] In a series of 56 multiple-injury patients, Goris and colleagues[208] showed that the advantage of controlled ventilation combined with early fracture fixation was greater than that of either ventilation or fracture fixation alone. The greatest advantage was observed in patients with an ISS of more than 50.[208]

Meek and coworkers[209] retrospectively studied 71 multiple-trauma patients with similar age and ISS with respect to timing of fracture stabilization. The group with long bone fractures stabilized within 24 hours had a markedly lower mortality rate than the group treated with traction and cast methods. In a prospective study, Bone and associates[172] compared the incidence of pulmonary dysfunction in 178 patients with acute femoral fractures who underwent either early (in the first 24 hours after injury) or late (>48 hours after injury) stabilization. The patients were further divided into those who had multiple injuries and those with isolated fracture of the femur. In none of the patients with isolated femoral fractures, whether treated with early or late stabilization, did respiratory insufficiency, required intubation, or needed placement in the ICU occur. In the patients with multiple injuries, those who had delayed stabilization of fractures had a significantly higher incidence of pulmonary dysfunction.

Early femoral fixation may not play as critical a role in the outcome, however, in an aggressively managed surgical ICU. Reynolds and associates studied 424 consecutive patients with femur fractures treated with IM rods, and half of these were done in the first 24 hours.[210] Of these 424 patients, 105 had an ISS of 18 or greater; these patients were studied for the relationship of fracture, fixation, timing, and outcomes. IM fixation was done in the first 24 hours in 35 of 105, between 24 and 48 hours in 12 of 105, and after more than 48 hours in 58 of 105. A few days' delay in fracture fixation did not adversely affect outcome, and pulmonary complications were related to the severity of injury rather than to timing of fracture fixation. Indeed, "fracture fixation" is a generic term for everything from open surgical intervention with extensive blood loss on a subtrochanteric fracture to the placement of a few screws through percutaneous incisions or the rapid assembly of a fixator. Only prospective research can identify which variables are truly important—anesthesia, blood loss, necrosis, ventilation, and micromotion, to name a few. The physiologic consequences of medullary nailing of the femur are the best known. Large trials in injured patients are needed to compare femoral nailing with other fixation methods.

The type of femoral fixation may play a role in risk consideration. With IM nailing, there is the risk of additional bone marrow emboli and potential associated lung dysfunction. Pape and associates found ARDS in a higher percentage of patients treated with a reamed IM femoral nail acutely performed (eight of 24, 33%) versus delayed nailing (two of 26, 8%) in patients with femur fractures and severe thoracic injuries.[53] Charash and coworkers repeated the Pape study design and reported contradictory findings with favorable results in acute reamed IM nailing versus delayed nailing: pneumonia (14% vs. 48%) and pulmonary complications (16% vs. 56%).[211] Bosse and coworkers studied severe chest-injured patients with femur fracture treated within 24 hours with reamed IM nail or plating.[212] The retrospective study was controlled for group A, femur fracture with thoracic injury; group B, femur fracture with no thoracic injury; and group C, thoracic injury with no femur fracture. The overall ARDS rate in patients with femur fractures was 10 of 453 (2%). There was no significant difference in ARDS or pulmonary complications or MOF whether the femur fracture was treated with rodding or plating. Bosse and associates found no contraindication for reamed femoral nailing in the first 24 hours even if a thoracic injury was present. Pape and associates assessed lung function in two groups of patients undergoing early (≤24 hours) IM femoral nailing.[60] One group had femoral nailing after reaming of the medullary canal (RFN), and the other group had a small-diameter solid nail inserted without reaming (UFN). These investigators found that lung function was stable in UFN patients but deteriorated in RFN patients. They concluded that IM nailing after reaming might potentiate lung dysfunction, particularly in patients with preexisting pulmonary damage such as lung contusion. In contrast, Heim and associates, in a rabbit model, compared reamed versus unreamed nailing of femoral shaft fractures and showed that both techniques resulted in bone marrow intravasation and resulting pulmonary dysfunction.[63] In sum, the pathomechanics of FES with respect to what causes the lung injury, what mode of femur fixation is best, and when to do the fracture repair has yet to be precisely unraveled. Really good evidence-based investigation in humans is required to solve this problem. Recent research regarding central mechanisms of bone regulation suggests that fracture repair depends not only on local but also on central mediators. The response of the organism as a whole to the noxious effects of injury may be needed to optimize repair systems.

When treating the patient with overt MOF, recognize that a potentially lethal condition is present and that the usual methods to control specific complications (e.g., pneumonia, renal failure, GI bleeding) will be ineffective. The patient must be assessed as a whole. Focused intervention is required to turn the situation around. In such conditions, a delay in performing operative procedures may be unwise. Significant unstable long bone, pelvic, and spinal fractures can be stabilized. However, long bone stabilization may need to be performed by means of DCO (temporary spanning external fixator) to avoid creating a "second hit" to the patient that would worsen recovery from MOF. There is a role for the use of DCO with patients who already have MODS or who are thought to be at risk for its development. With patients with diagnosed MSOS, DCO allows the possibility of skeletal stabilization of femoral shaft and tibial shaft fractures and unstable knee and ankle joints without contributing an additional fatal insult or "hit" to the patient's physiology from an invasive orthopaedic procedure. Just simply placing a fixator does not solve the physiologic problem. External fixation that provides adequate stability at the fracture site is important. Until we control for quality, we may not be able to assess the value of external fixation for immediate fracture care. In patients who are at risk of developing MOD, DCO provides a way to provide skeletal stabilization of the above injuries without causing an additional physiologic "insult" or "hit" that might cause the patient to develop MODS. DCO treatment has been reported to be associated with lesser systemic inflammatory response than early total care for femur fractures.[213,214] Patients often require blood, calories (preferably enteral when feasible), effective antibiotics, controlled ventilation, and dialysis. All of these must be continuously monitored. Keel and Trentz stated that the development of immunomonitoring will help in the selection of the most appropriate treatment for polytrauma patients.[215] Treatment measures for MOF often require careful balancing of risks and benefits. If anticoagulation prevents the propagation of thrombi, it can also be a cause of bleeding.

The orthopaedist's role is to assess fractures that are causing continued recumbency and to locate sources of devitalized tissue and sepsis in the musculoskeletal system. Sacrifice of a crushed but viable limb, loss of fracture reduction, or performance of a quick but not optimal limb stabilization are examples of the difficult choices or procedures that have to be made to save a life. The use of spanning external fixation (traveling traction),[216] so-called DCO,[51,202,216,217] is a good option because of its minimal additional tissue trauma, provisional bony stability, and improved ability to mobilize the patient.

In summary, in the presence of major thoracic and head injuries, there are potential risks of worsening a brain injury or precipitating ARDS from early orthopaedic procedures. Carlson[206] and Velmahos and associates[218] have shown no added morbidity for early fixation when chest or head injuries are present. However, Townsend and colleagues[218a] and Pape report increased risk for secondary brain injury and ARDS associated with early fixation.[60] Reynolds and associates showed that a modest delay did not affect the outcome.[210] Dunham and colleagues[219] noted no difference between early and late fracture fixation. Bhandari and colleagues[220] stated that head injury does not seem to be a contraindication to reamed IM nailing. Giannoudis and colleagues noted that the literature does not provide clear-cut guidelines for the management of orthopaedic injuries in head-injured patients. These authors stated that it was best to individualize treatment.[221] Finally, as Deitch and Goodman have noted, the best way to treat MOF is the prevention of MOF in the first place.[222]

LOCAL COMPLICATIONS OF FRACTURES

Local complications or unwanted therapeutic outcomes are simply part of taking care of fractures. Local failures of fracture treatment can manifest as immediate, delayed, or long-term adverse outcomes. Delayed complications include CRPS and disuse atrophy—the "fracture disease." Arthrosis and malunion are examples of the long-term adverse results with permanent impairment and economic importance. Any treatment program, no matter how thoughtfully conceived and carefully performed, has a failure rate that cannot be entirely eliminated. The patient, physician, and system variables inherent in each given clinical situation mean that, in practice, complication rates are usually in excess of those rates published in the literature. With multiple injuries, the rates become more than additive. This is expressed in the ISS by adding the squares of injury components.[179] The purpose of this section is to provide a framework for understanding local complications of fractures.

Soft Tissue and Vascular Problems

An accident, unlike an elective operation, causes the transmission of force of an undetermined magnitude to human tissue. However, through accident reconstruction, it is possible to estimate the magnitude of energy transfer. For example, a fall from 30 ft is equivalent to being struck by a car going 30 mph. In the immediate hours, days, and weeks after an injury, it should not be surprising that areas of skin demarcation, skin sloughing, ecchymosis, or thrombosed vessels appear. These areas, if operative interventions are appropriate, are the consequences of injury and not of its treatment. In addition, after an osteosynthesis, there is additional opportunity for the slow accumulation of hematoma from bleeding from bone surfaces. Today's shortened hospitalizations with early mobilization and less control over the postoperative activity have contributed to an increased incidence of postoperative hematoma. Postoperative hematoma manifests as swelling, pain; loss of function; and frequently, serous drainage either from a wound or from the drain tract. Hematomas may not resorb but instead continue to increase in size and cause wound separation, skin sloughing, and infection. Collections of blood or fluid can be detected with ultrasonography. It is usually best to reexplore the wound under adequate anesthesia, evacuate the hematoma, irrigate the fracture site, drain the field, and apply a compression dressing.

Arterial injuries may manifest acutely with signs of hemorrhage and ischemia, or the presentation may be delayed, as in an arteriovenous fistula or a pseudoaneurysm. In civilian injuries with associated fractures or dislocations, the arterial injury rate is from 2% to 6%. For isolated fractures or dislocations, the arterial injury rate is less than 1%. War-related extremity injuries, a high proportion of which result from high-velocity gunshot wounds, consist of a long bone fracture with associated vascular injury in about one third of cases.[223] Certain injury patterns such as a knee dislocation, especially in a posterior direction, have a 30% incidence of associated popliteal artery damage. Although standard angiography was the preferred diagnostic test for vascular injury, computed tomography angiography (CTA) is rapidly supplanting angiography. CTA avoids the hazards of arterial puncture contrast reactions and provides excellent visualization of the vascular tree. Traditional angiography at most centers has been replaced by CTA.

Rieger and colleagues retrospectively assessed the accuracy of multidetector computed tomography angiography (MDCT) as the initial diagnostic technique to depict arterial injury in patients with extremity trauma.[224] Prospective sensitivity and specificity were 95% and 87%, respectively, and retrospective sensitivity and specificity were 99% and 98%, respectively. Inaba and colleagues also studied the ability of multislice helical computed tomography angiography (MCTA) to detect arterial injury in the traumatized.[225] MCTA achieved 100% sensitivity and 100% specificity in detecting clinically significant arterial injury. No missed injuries were identified during the follow-up period, which was a mean of 48.2 days.[225] Despite these reported accuracies, there are reported concerns about the limitations of MDCT such as that reported by Portugaller and colleagues, who noted lower sensitivity in the infrapopliteal area caused by small vessel diameter.[226]

Computed tomography angiography is clearly the wave of the future for imaging the vascular system. Improvements in technique and accuracy of interpretation are likely to strengthen the available evidence to support its widespread application.

When femur fractures are associated with femoral artery injury, the results of vascular repair and limb function are characteristically good, although delayed diagnosis of pseudoaneurysm and claudication can be a problem.[227] Cases requiring amputation because of a delay in diagnosis can occur. Popliteal artery injury, even when diagnosed early, may not be amenable to vascular reconstruction. Vascular injuries distal to the popliteal trifurcation are basically not fixable and carry a much worse prognosis. Revascularization is usually not needed if one vessel is patent on angiography and the distal pressure is 50% of the brachial artery pressure. When revascularization is required, a good functional result can be expected in only about 25% of cases. In Flint and Richardson's experience, six of 16 patients undergoing revascularization distal to the trifurcation required early amputation, and six more required late amputation (total, 12 of 16) for osteomyelitis, nonunion, and persistent neuropathy and its associated complications.[227] Early amputation without revascularization is often appropriate in patients with loss of vascular inflow, long bone fracture, neurotmesis, or extensive soft tissue damage. The high rate of infection and complications can result in a delayed amputation when revascularization is performed.[228] In general, amputation after the onset of infection is at a higher anatomic level than would have been selected had the amputation been performed initially.

Posttraumatic Arthrosis

Posttraumatic arthrosis is considered a complication of fractures (Fig. 23-6). Wright, a retired judge, used a questionnaire to determine a consensus view of the factors related to the development of posttraumatic arthrosis after fracture.[229] He found the following: that lower limb joints are more likely to develop arthritis than upper extremity joints, that older patients are at higher risk for the development of posttraumatic arthrosis (although younger patients have a longer time frame to develop posttraumatic arthrosis), and that occupation is a risk factor. Kern and associates also reported the association of osteoarthritis and certain occupations.[230] Specific components of the pathomechanics of posttraumatic arthrosis include (1) incongruity of the articular surface, (2) cartilage damage from the load transfer, (3) malalignment, (4) malorientation of the joint, and (5) repetitive loading injury.

Barei and colleagues reported that residual dysfunction is common after severe bicondylar tibial plateau fractures.[231]

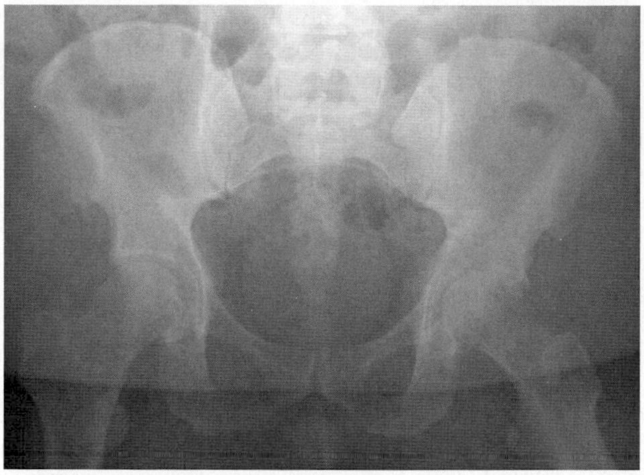

Figure 23-6. Radiograph of a 33-year-old man 3 years after nonoperative treatment of a left transverse acetabulum fracture.

They noted that accurate reduction was possible in only half of the patients and was associated with better outcomes.[231]

Weigel and Marsh reported on knee function after high-energy tibial plateau fractures in patients treated with a monolateral external fixator and limited internal fixation of the articular surface.[232] They noted that these patients had a good prognosis for satisfactory knee function in the second 5 years after injury.[232] Rademaker and colleagues reported on a series of 202 consecutive tibial plateau fractures treated with operative treatment and reported excellent long-term results independent of the patient's age.[233]

Joint Incongruity

The emphasis on anatomic reduction in fracture surgery focuses on the reestablishment of joint congruity often at the expense of the soft tissue attachments to bone. Extensive bony comminution of the articular surface, particularly of the knee and the distal tibia, can make a repair of joint congruity a formidable or even an impossible task. Acetabular fractures are a good example of articular fractures that are associated with the development of posttraumatic arthrosis[234] largely because of failure to reestablish joint congruity and the articular cartilage injury itself.[235]

Articular Cartilage Damage

Although impact to the articular cartilage at the time of injury in high-energy trauma is a likely contributor to the articular cartilage damage and the subsequent development of posttraumatic arthrosis (Figs. 23-7 and 23-8), the clinical data are not well-defined. Volpin and coworkers reported at an average follow-up of 14 years of intraarticular fractures of the knee joint that there were 77% good-to-excellent results.[236] Repo and associates stated that the impact loads sufficient to fracture a femoral shaft of an automobile occupant are nearly sufficient to cause significant articular cartilage injury (chondrocyte death and fissuring).[237]

There is an increasing appreciation of cartilage injury from impact. The advent of MRI of knee injuries has enhanced our appreciation of damage to the articular surfaces (bone bruising) (Fig. 23-9). Spindler and associates studied 54 patients with anterior cruciate ligament tears and found a bone bruise present in 80% of cases, of which 68% were in the

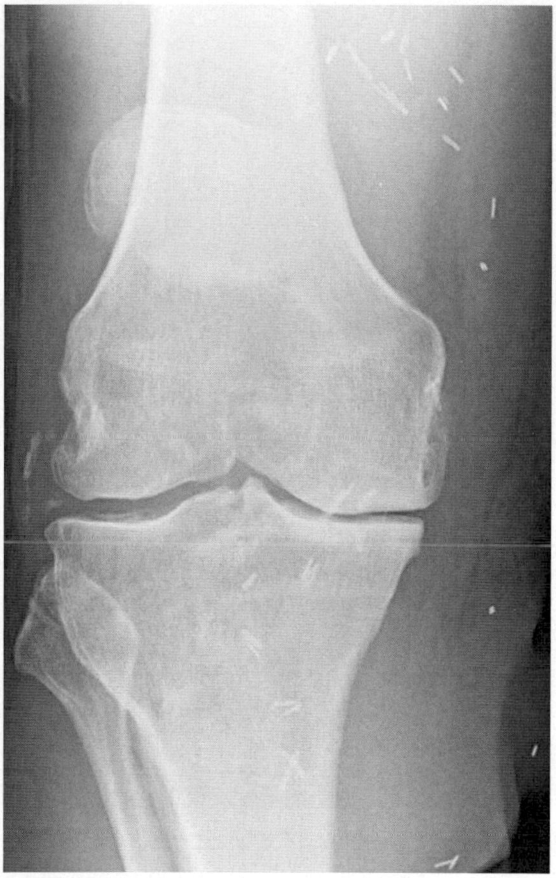

Figure 23-7. Radiograph of a 37-year-old man 6 years after a knee dislocation with vascular injury; note the varus alignment and joint space.

lateral femoral condyle.[238] Bone bruises in combination with anterior cruciate ligament tears may be harbingers of future arthritis. Miller and coworkers studied 65 patients who had MRI-detected trabecular microfractures associated with isolated medial collateral ligament injuries.[239] Although these bone bruises were approximately half as common as bone

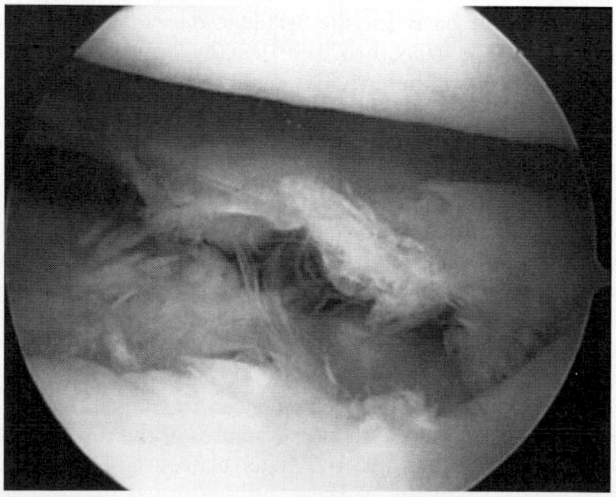

Figure 23-8. Correlative arthroscopic view of the lateral compartment of the knee in Figure 23-7, which demonstrates posttraumatic arthrosis secondary to joint incongruity, articular cartilage degradation, and meniscal degeneration 5 years after a high-energy tibial plateau fracture.

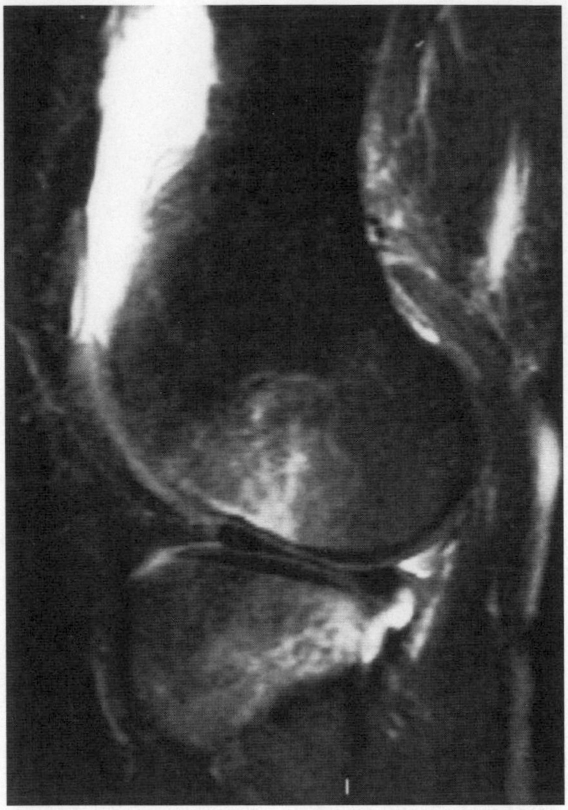

Figure 23-9. Sagittal magnetic resonance image of the lateral compartment of a knee that demonstrates a bone contusion involving the lateral femoral condyle and the lateral tibial plateau in association with a recent anterior cruciate ligament tear. *(Courtesy of Theresa M. Corrigan, MD.)*

bruises associated with anterior cruciate ligament tears, these investigators stated that medial collateral ligament–associated trabecular microfractures may be a better natural history model.[239] Wright and associates noted that isolated bone bruises not associated with ligamentous or meniscal injury may have a better prognosis than bone bruises noted in conjunction with ligamentous and meniscal injury.[240]

The biologic basis for the cartilage degradation is being studied.[241] It has been theorized that the impact at the time of injury damages the articular cartilage or its blood supply irreversibly and initiates a biologic cascade of mediators resulting in posttraumatic arthritis.[237] This etiology of impact arthritis has not been well studied.[237,242,243] Attempts to develop a model have been made. Vrahas and coworkers developed a method of quantifying blows to articular cartilage in a rabbit model.[243] Nonetheless, cartilage damage, particularly when it is unassociated with bone changes, may not necessarily progress to arthritis.[244] Radin noted that full-thickness cartilage lesions that are smaller than 1 cm usually will not progress to arthritis.[244]

Giannoudis and colleagues reviewed the current evidence regarding articular step-off after fractures of the distal radius, acetabulum, distal femur, and tibial plateau and the risk of posttraumatic arthritis.[245] These authors noted that different joints and even different areas of the same joint appear to have different tolerances for posttraumatic articular step-offs. For the distal radius, step-offs and gaps detected with precise measurement techniques in the first 5 years after injury have been correlated with higher incidence of posttraumatic arthrosis. After acetabular fractures, restoring the superior weight-bearing dome decreases posttraumatic arthrosis. For tibial plateau fractures, articular incongruities are well tolerated. Other factors only partially related to the articular reduction are more important in determining outcomes than articular step-off alone such as joint stability, retention of the meniscus, and coronal alignment.

Thomas and colleagues used novel CT-based image analysis techniques to quantify injury characterization in a prospective study of 20 patients with tibial plafond fractures.[246] These investigators reported that CT-based metrics of acute injury severity can reliably predict posttraumatic arthritis at 2 years after tibial plafond fracture.

There is a resurgence of interest in using an integrated orthotic and rehabilitation initiative in the management of end-stage posttraumatic arthritis of the ankle and subtalar joints after combat trauma.[247] The authors suggested that this clinical pathway might serve as an adjunct to arthrodesis and arthroplasty for young patients with severe posttraumatic osteoarthritis of the ankle and subtalar joints.[247]

Malalignment

Tetsworth and Paley have focused on the relationship between malalignment and degenerative arthropathy.[248] Focusing on degenerative arthritis and changes in the weight-bearing line or mechanical axis (malalignment), changes in the position of each articular surface relative to the axis of the individual segments (malorientation), and changes in joint incongruity, they noted that the joints of the lower extremity are nearly co-linear and that any disturbance in this relationship (malalignment) affects the transmission of load across the joint surfaces.[248]

The hip and shoulder joints, because of their sphericity, tolerate malalignment. The ankle joint is also fairly tolerant of deformity because of compensation through the subtalar joint. However, the knee is most vulnerable to changes in the normal coronal plane relationship of the lower extremity.[248] Malalignment of the knee, which changes the mechanical axis, creates a moment arm, which increases force transmission across either the medial or lateral compartments of the knee joint.[249,250]

Nonetheless, there are conflicting clinical data regarding whether these factors lead to posttraumatic arthrosis. Kettlekamp and associates stated that there are no data to support the position that malalignment always leads to degenerative arthritis.[251] Kristensen and coworkers reported no arthrosis of the ankle 20 years after malaligned tibial fractures.[252] In contrast, Puno and coworkers studied 27 patients with 28 tibial fractures and found that greater degrees of ankle malalignment produced poorer clinical results.[253] Merchant and Dietz stated that they did not find any support in their study for the hypotheses that angulation results in shear rather than compressive forces on articular cartilage and that these forces lead to early arthrosis.[254]

Malorientation

Another postfracture residual deformity that can contribute to posttraumatic arthrosis is malorientation (a change in the orientation of a joint to the mechanical axis). The association of malorientation of the knee and osteoarthritis has been demonstrated.[255,256] Malorientation can result from translation or rotation. When the orientation of the joint is substantially changed in relation to the mechanical axis, the theory is that abnormal loading of the articular cartilage and subchondral plate will occur, which will accelerate joint deterioration and ultimately lead to osteoarthritis. Malorientation is probably more of a problem with weight-bearing joints such as the knee, which are subject to high and frequent loading.

Repetitive Loading Injury

Articular cartilage damage can occur either by sudden impact loading or by repetitive impulsive loading.[257-260] As a result, portions of the matrix can be fractured, cause cartilage necrosis, and produce subclinical microfractures in the calcified cartilage layer.[261] The effect on cartilage homeostasis appears to lead to changes that are seen in association with osteoarthritis.[257,260,262] Fairbanks changes,[263] radiographic evidence of knee arthritis after meniscectomy, most likely result from repetitive loading to the articular cartilage after changes in load distribution of the knee joint. Deterioration of damaged articular cartilage by repetitive loading may be asymptomatic because cartilage is relatively aneural.[261]

Adult canine articular cartilage after indirect blunt trauma demonstrates significant alterations in its histologic, biomechanical, and ultrastructural characteristics without disruption of the articular surface.[258] Thompson and associates found arthritic-like degeneration of the articular cartilage in an animal model within 6 months after transarticular loads.[242] These investigators also noted that degenerative changes that occur in patients who sustained traumatic insult to the joint may represent a phenomenon similar to their animal model.[263]

Damage to articular cartilage often can occur without perceptible alteration in the macroscopic appearance of the tissue.[264] Although the traditional understanding has been that cartilage has limited capacity for self-repair, there is hope that some cartilage repair is possible, which has led to the proliferation of procedures such as autologous cartilage transplantation[265] and microfracture.[266]

Summary

We have summarized the incidence of posttraumatic arthrosis[267] associated with some common fractures and dislocations (Table 23-7). In addition, posttraumatic arthrosis is discussed elsewhere in the text.

Arthrosis is not necessarily progressive. Letournel studied a small cohort of patients with tibial pilon fractures 5 and 10 years after injury. Results trended toward improvement in time rather than progression. Posttraumatic arthrosis may be an inevitable consequence of musculoskeletal injury. It appears to be related to the magnitude of the original injury. At the present time, fracture surgery techniques cannot fully reverse the articular cartilage injury. Gelber and associates reported that an injury to the knee joint in young adulthood was related to a substantial increased risk for future knee osteoarthritis.[268] Other confounding factors in determining the relationship between fractures and the development of posttraumatic arthrosis are normal age-related changes.

Specific components of the pathomechanics of posttraumatic arthrosis include malalignment, malorientation, joint incongruity, articular cartilage destruction, ligamentous or fibrocartilaginous injury, and repetitive loading injury. Salvage procedures such as joint replacement or osteotomy are less successful for posttraumatic arthrosis than for osteoarthritis.[269] Postinjury counseling and patient education are necessary to convey realistic expectations after fracture surgery. Prospective, multicenter, long-term studies are needed to better understand the natural history of posttraumatic arthrosis and to be able to discern it from normal age-related osteoarthrosis.

Peripheral Nerve Injuries

Few entities can overshadow the outcome of the treatment of a fracture as much as a peripheral nerve injury. Whether the nerve palsy is diagnosed before or after surgery, it is certain that the patient and other healthcare providers will be inordinately focused on the nerve palsy itself. Peripheral nerve injuries in orthopaedic trauma are probably underreported because clinical assessment of peripheral lesions is often impossible or impractical. Electrodiagnostic testing is more sensitive than clinical examination alone and can facilitate the diagnosis of traumatic peripheral nerve injuries. A scientific approach to peripheral nerve injury is imperative. Electromyography (EMG) is most useful for localizing entrapment when there are multiple sites that are hard to differentiate clinically.

History of the Treatment of Nerve Injury

George Omer traces the history of the treatment of peripheral nerve injuries to William A. Hammond, Surgeon General of the U.S. Army during the American Civil War.[270] Omer traces the evolution of understanding and treatment of peripheral nerve injuries from the Civil War through the two World Wars, the Vietnam and Korean conflicts, and the development of "The Sunderland Society."[270]

Classification of Nerve Injury

Seddon is credited with the scientific classification of peripheral nerve injury into three categories: neurotmesis, axonotmesis, and neurapraxia (Table 23-8).[271] Seddon, however, noted that these three terms were coined by Professor Henry Cohen in 1941.[271] Understanding peripheral nerve injury is based on understanding the anatomy of myelinated nerves (Fig. 23-10).

Neurotmesis implies a cutting or separation of related parts in which all essential structures have been "sundered."[271] Seddon noted that although there is not necessarily an obvious anatomic gap in the nerve and the epineural sheath may appear to be in continuity, the effect is as if anatomic continuity has been lost.[271]

Axonotmesis involves a lesion to the peripheral nerve of such severity that wallerian degeneration occurs but the epineurium and supporting structures of the nerve have been "so little disturbed that the internal architecture is fairly well preserved."[271]

Neurapraxia is described as a lesion in which paralysis occurs in the absence of peripheral degeneration. Seddon noted that "neurapraxia" is preferred to "transient block" because the recovery time can be lengthy and is "invariably complete."[271]

Seddon notes that of the three terms for describing nerve injury, neurotmesis is probably the best understood, and in clinical practice, the existence of axonotmesis or neurapraxia could only be surmised.[271] The advent of electrodiagnostic testing has made the distinction between axonotmesis and

TABLE 23-7 *INCIDENCE OF POSTTRAUMATIC ARTHRITIS*

	Upper Extremity		
Shoulder	Acromioclavicular joint dislocations	25%–43%	
	Scapula fractures	Superior lateral angle	61%
	Anterior shoulder dislocation		7%
Elbow	Elbow dislocations—simple	24-yr follow-up	38%
	Elbow dislocations with a radial head fracture		63%
	Wrist		
	Colles fractures		3%–18%
	Colles fractures	Young adults	57%–65%
	Scapholunate dislocations		58%
	Transscaphoid perilunate dislocations; fracture	4.3-yr follow-up	50%
	Lower Extremity		
Acetabular fractures	6.5%–56%		
Hip dislocations	Anterior	17%	
	Posterior	<6 hr time to reduction	30%
	Posterior	≥6 hr time to reduction	76%
Supracondylar or intercondylar femur fractures			22% (patellofemoral joint) 5% (tibiofemoral joint)
Patella fractures			18%
Tibial plateau fractures	Fracture patterns	Bicondylar fractures	42%
		Medial plateau fractures	21%
		Lateral plateau fractures	16%
	Association with alignment after plateau fractures	Normal	13%
Ankle fractures	20%–40%		
Talar neck	Ankle joint	Subtalar joint	
Fractures			
Hawkins I	15%	24%	
Hawkins II	36%	66%	
Hawkins III	69%	63%	
Subtalar joint dislocations			56%
Tarsometatarsal fracture-dislocation (Lisfranc joint injuries)			78% (15-yr follow-up)

Source: *Foy MA, Fagg PS: Medicolegal reporting in orthopaedic trauma, New York, 1996, Churchill Livingstone, pp 2.1-01–4.1-16.*

neurotmesis much easier. Seddon noted that the most common variety of neurotmesis was from anatomic division. Wallerian nerve degeneration occurs peripherally, and the clinical picture is that of complete interruption of the nerve.

Axonotmesis is characterized by complete interruption of axons but with preservation of the supporting structures of the nerve (Schwann tubes, endoneurium, and perineurium). On a histologic level, there is complete interruption of the axons, preservation of the Schwann tubes and endoneurium, and wallerian degeneration peripherally. Seddon noted that clinically axonotmesis was indistinguishable from neurotmesis until recovery occurs, which in axonotmesis was spontaneous.[271] When exploration is performed, the finding of an intact nerve suggests that the lesion is an axonotmesis.[271] A fusiform neuroma finding suggests that the injury was a mixed lesion of axonotmesis and neurotmesis with the former predominating.[238] A finding of intraneural fibrosis is evidence that the lesion was a neurotmesis.

Seddon noted that with neurapraxia, there is no axonal degeneration. There is localized degeneration of the myelin sheaths. Blunt injuries and compression were the most common cause of neurapraxias.[271] He noted that the clinical picture is one of complete motor paralysis and incomplete sensory paralysis.[271] Also, he noted that there was no anatomic "march" to recovery as seen after nerve suture or axonotmesis.[271] Finally, Seddon noted that many nerve injuries were, in fact, combinations of the three different nerve injury patterns he described.[271] Of a series of 537 nerve injuries, he noted that there were 96 cases in which a neurotmesis and an axonotmesis were combined.[271]

Sunderland added to the work of Seddon by subdividing peripheral nerve injury into five degrees by basically subdividing the neurotmesis into three types (third-, fourth-, and fifth-degree injuries) while maintaining the concepts of neurapraxia (first-degree injury) and axonotmesis (second-degree injury).[272] He defined five degrees of nerve injury based on

TABLE 23-8 *TYPES OF PERIPHERAL NERVE INJURIES*

Injury	Pathophysiology	Prognosis
Neurapraxia	Reversible conduction block characterized by local ischemia and selective demyelination of the axon sheath	Good
Axonotmesis	More severe injury with disruption of the axon and myelin sheath but with an intact epineurium	Fair
Neurotmesis	Complete nerve division with disruption of the endoneurium	Poor

Source: *Brinker MR, Lou EC: General principles of trauma. In Brinker MR, editor: Review of orthopaedic trauma, Philadelphia, 2001, WB Saunders, p 8, with permission.*

TABLE 23-9 *COMMON ORTHOPAEDIC ENTITIES ASSOCIATED WITH PERIPHERAL NERVE INJURIES*

Anatomic Location	Type of Injury	Incidence of Nerve Injury
Humerus	Midshaft fracture	12%–19% incidence of radial nerve palsy
Pelvis	Double vertical pelvic fracture	46% incidence of neurologic injury
Tibia	Tibia fracture	19%–30% incidence of neurologic findings after intramedullary nailing
Ankle	Ankle eversion	86% incidence of neurologic findings

changes induced in the normal nerve. Seddon described these injuries in ascending order, which affected successively (1) conduction in the axon, (2) continuity of the axon, (3) the endoneurial tube and its axon, (4) the funiculus and its contents, (5) the entire nerve trunk.[272] The most important part of Sunderland's work is his clarification that nerve injuries previously classified by Seddon as neurotmesis were not all equal.

Sunderland also added to the knowledge of partial and mixed nerve injuries. He noted that some fibers in a nerve may escape injury while others sustain a variable degree of damage.[272] He observed that in partial severance injuries and fourth-degree injuries, it was unlikely that the remaining fibers would escape some injury. This type of injury should be described as a "mixed lesion."[272] However, fourth- and fifth-degree lesions could not coexist either together or in combination with any of the minor types of injuries.[272]

There are difficulties with the classification of peripheral nerve injury. Many nerve injuries are mixed injuries in which various nerve fibers are affected to varying degrees.[273] In addition, the subtypes of Seddon's classification are usually discernible only on histologic examination of the nerve and are seldom possible on the basis of clinical or EMG data.

Incidence of Nerve Injuries Associated with Fractures

There is a fairly high incidence of nerve injury with some common orthopaedic entities (Table 23-9). Conway and Hubbell reported EMG abnormalities associated with pelvic fracture and noted that patients with double vertical pelvic fractures (combined injury to the anterior third of the pelvic ring and the sacroiliac area) were most at risk, with a 46% incidence of neurologic injury.[274] Goodall noted that 95% of fractures with an associated nerve injury occur in the upper extremity.[275] Of all fracture types, a humerus fracture is the most likely fracture to have an associated nerve injury.[276] Omer reported, based on a collected series,[277] the following distribution of nerve injuries associated with fractures and fracture-dislocations: radial nerve (60%), ulnar nerve (18%), common peroneal nerve (15%), and median nerve (6%).[275,278,279]

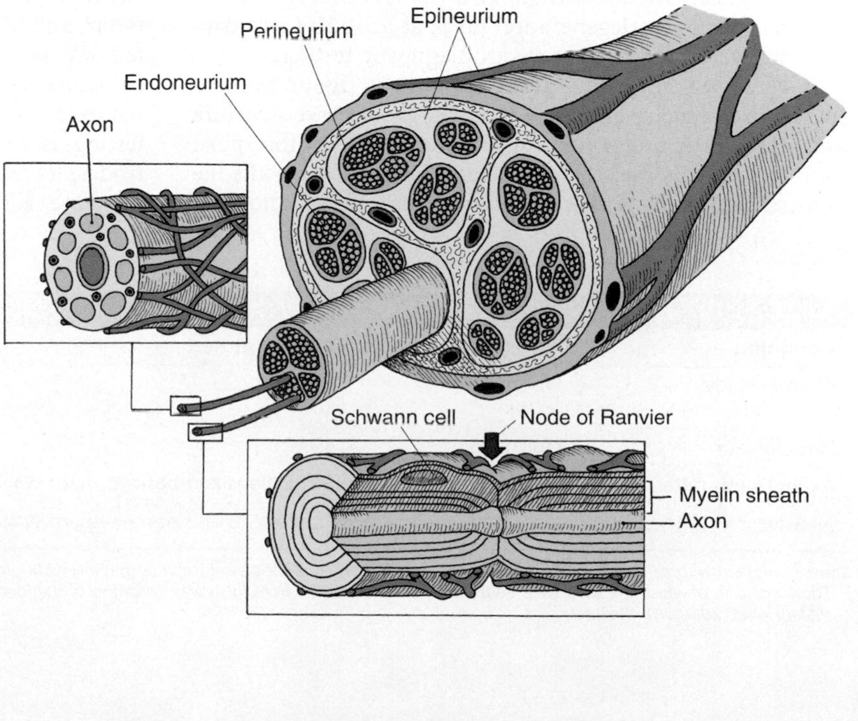

Figure 23-10. Cross-sectional anatomy of peripheral nerve. The *inset* at *left* shows an unmyelinated fiber. The *inset* at the *bottom* shows a myelinated fiber. *(From Lee SK, Wolfe SW: Peripheral nerve injury and repair, J Am Acad Orthop Surg 8:243–252, 2000.)*

Evaluation of Peripheral Nerve Injuries

In polytrauma patients, the neurologic assessment is incorporated in the initial assessment, which uses the alphabet—ABCD—where D is for disability and neurologic assessment.[280] The Glasgow Coma Scale, developed by Teasdale and Jennet, specifically assesses eye opening, motor response, and verbal response on a maximum 15-point rating scale.

The assessment of peripheral nerve injury during orthopaedic surgery rounds and emergency department assessments often is reduced to the terms *neurovascularly intact* or *N/V intact.* In our opinion, such terms, although convenient, should not be used unless a complete neurologic examination (cutaneous sensation, including light touch, pain, and temperature; vibratory sensation; motor strength in all muscles with grading; deep tendon reflexes; and special tests for clonus and so on) and a complete vascular examination (pulses, capillary refill, venous examination, tests for thrombosis, auscultation for bruits, and so on) are performed. Formal assessment of peripheral nerve injury is usually performed using electrodiagnostic testing with EMG) and nerve conduction velocities (NCVs).

Electromyography and Electrodiagnostics. In a broad sense, EMG refers to a set of diagnostic tests using neurophysiologic techniques that are performed on muscles and nerves.[281] Strictly speaking, EMG refers to one of these tests, in which a small needle is used to probe selected muscles, recording electrical potentials from the muscle fibers.[281]

Although electrodiagnostic testing has historically been of little interest to orthopaedic surgeons, there is heightened interest in electrodiagnostics as a result of intraoperative use of sensory-evoked potentials and motor-evoked potentials in spine surgery, brachial plexus surgery, and acetabular surgery.

It has been said that the best times for electrodiagnostic studies are the day before injury and then about 10 to 14 days after injury. The former is, of course, impossible but nonetheless underscores the importance of baseline studies and changes over time, particularly when one is looking for evidence of reinnervation (which would be consistent with an axonotmesis) or denervation (which would be consistent with a neurotmesis). The latter highlights the fact that reinnervation after wallerian degeneration takes at least 10 to 14 days to be able to be detected on electrodiagnostic testing.

Basic Science of Electrodiagnostics. To understand EMG, it is necessary to review some basics of nerve structure and function. A motor neuron has a cell body in the spinal cord and extends into the nerve root, an axon that exits the spine, traverses the plexus, travels within a nerve, and then forms many distinct branches.[281] A motor unit consists of one such cell and the several muscle fibers that it innervates.[281] Muscles contain many motor units that are analogous to colored pencils in a bundle.[281] Muscle forces are created by activation of an increasing number of motor units under the command of the brain.[281] When a motor unit fires, a small electrical signal is generated and can be recorded by placing a small needle through the skin and into the muscle near the motor unit fibers acting electronically like an antenna.[281] This signal is amplified, filtered, digitized, and displayed on a computer screen.[281] Single motor unit potentials are sampled first on the oscilloscope. As greater force is generated, there is recruitment of more motor units and an increase in the firing rate.[281] When full muscle force is generated, the oscilloscope screen fills with signals, which has an appearance called the *full interference pattern.*[281] Another important component of EMG interpretation is the sound of the motor potentials, which are amplified and broadcast through a speaker.[281] Experienced electromyographers can recognize characteristic sounds and audible patterns.[281]

The usefulness of EMG for trauma patients is the ability to localize neurologic lesions anatomically based on a pattern of denervated muscle. EMG is also useful for following nerve recovery over time.

Characteristic Electromyography Patterns. If there is an injury to the axon, as with axonotmesis or neurotmesis, distal degeneration of the nerve (wallerian degeneration) causes it to be electrically irritable.[281] Needle movement generates denervation potentials called fibrillations and positive waves, which have both characteristic appearances on the oscilloscope and sounds on the loudspeaker.[281] These findings are delayed, occurring at least 10 days afterward even after complete transection.[281] Sprouting and reinnervation that would occur with a recovering axonotmesis create a high-amplitude polyphasic motor unit potential (Table 23-10).[281]

Nerve Conduction Studies. Nerve conduction studies are different from EMGs. Nerve conduction studies can be used to test both sensory and motor nerves in skeletal muscle. These studies test only large myelinated nerve fiber function. Nerve fibers commonly evaluated include the ulnar, median, radial, and tibial nerves (motor and sensory fibers); the sciatic, femoral, and peroneal fibers (motor fibers only); and the musculocutaneous, superficial peroneal, sural, and saphenous nerves (sensory only). The procedure of nerve conduction testing uses surface electrodes, often silver discs or ring electrodes, to record extracellular electrical activity from muscle or nerve. EMG machines have a nerve stimulator that can

TABLE 23-10 *ELECTROMYOGRAPHIC FINDINGS RELATED TO TRAUMA*

Condition	Insertional Activity	Activity at Rest	Minimal Contraction	Interference
Normal study	Normal	Silence	Biphasic and triphasic potential	Complete
Neurapraxia	Normal	Silence	Reduced number of potentials	Reduced
Axonotmesis (after 2 wk)	Increased	Fibrillations and positive sharp waves	None	None
Neurotmesis (after 2 wk)	Increased	Fibrillations and positive sharp waves	None	None

Source: *Adapted with permission from Brinker MR, Lou EC: General principles of trauma. In Brinker MR, editor: Review of orthopaedic trauma, Philadelphia, 2001, WB Saunders, p 9, of which the data were adapted with modifications from Jahss MH: Disorders of the foot. In Miller MD, editor: Review of orthopaedics, ed 3, Philadelphia, 2000, WB Saunders.*

TABLE 23-11 *NERVE CONDUCTION STUDY RESULTS RELATED TO TRAUMA*

Condition	Latency	Conduction Velocity	Evoked Response
Normal study	Normal	Upper extremities: >48 m/sec	Biphasic
Lower extremities: >40 m/sec			
Neurapraxia			
Proximal to lesion	Absent or low voltage (if partial)	Absent or low voltage (if partial)	Absent
Distal to lesion	Normal	Normal	Normal
Axonotmesis			
Proximal to lesion	Absent	Absent	Absent
Distal to lesion (immediate)	Normal	Normal	Normal
Distal to lesion (>7 days)	Absent	Absent	Absent
Neurotmesis			
Proximal to lesion	Absent	Absent	Absent
Distal to lesion (immediate)	Normal	Normal	Normal
Distal to lesion (>7 days)	Absent	Absent	Absent

Source: *Adapted with permission from Brinker MR, Lou EC: General principles of trauma. In Brinker MR, editor: Review of orthopaedic trauma, Philadelphia, 2001, WB Saunders, p 8, of which the data were from Jahss MH: Disorders of the foot. In Miller MD, editor: Review of orthopaedics, ed 3, Philadelphia, 2000, WB Saunders.*

apply an electrical shock to the skin surface at accessible points on the nerve.[281] This stimulus depolarizes a segment of the nerve and generates an action potential, which travels in both directions from the point at which it was stimulated.[272] When a sensory nerve is tested, the action potential can be recorded from a distal point (surface electrodes or finger electrodes).[281] By measuring the distance from the stimulus point to the recording site and using the oscilloscope values of the time of latency and action potential amplitude, the examiner can determine the sensory conduction velocity.[281]

Motor NCVs are recorded from surface electrodes taped over muscles distally in the limb.[281] Normative control values for motor NCVs at different ages are used for comparison. This difference is attributable to the degree of myelination, which increases with age over the early developmental years. Although NCVs are fairly uniform from age 3 years through adulthood,[281] NCVs can vary based on several conditions. Nerve conduction values at birth are about 50% of adult values. As surface temperature decreases below 34° C, there is a progressive increase in latency and a decrease in conduction velocity.[282] Upper extremity conduction velocities are generally about 10% to 15% faster than those of the lower extremity. Conduction velocities in the proximal segments are usually 5% to 10% faster than in the distal segments,[282] which is a function of nerve root diameter.

To study motor conduction, the nerve is supramaximally stimulated at two or more points along its course where it is most superficial. At a distal muscle that is innervated by the nerve, a motor response is recorded.[177] Various parameters measured include latency, conduction velocity, amplitude, and duration. Characteristic nerve conduction study findings for various nerve injuries are shown in Table 23-11.

Sensory nerve conductions are generally unaffected by lesions proximal to the dorsal root ganglion even though there is sensory loss.[282] Sensory testing is good for localizing a lesion relative to the dorsal root ganglia: either proximal (root or spinal cord), in which case the NCV is normal, or distal (plexus or peripheral nerve), abnormal NCV. In addition, sensory nerve potential is lower in amplitude than compound motor action potentials and can be obscured by electrical activity or artifacts. Sensory axons are evaluated in four ways: (1) stimulating and recording from a cutaneous nerve, (2) recording from a cutaneous nerve while stimulating a mixed nerve, (3) recording from a mixed nerve while stimulating a cutaneous nerve, and (4) recording from the spinal column while a cutaneous nerve or mixed nerve is stimulated.[282] Variables measured include onset latency, peak latency, and peak-to-peak amplitude.

Two other parameters that are measured are the F-wave and the H-reflex. The F-wave is a late motor response attributed to a small percentage of fibers firing after the original stimulus impulse reaches the cell body. These F-waves are useful for the evaluation of the proximal segments of peripheral nerves[282] but only in the assessment of proximal nerve injuries in the absence of more distal pathology. There is also variability in the F-wave response because different fibers fire each time, making it less quantitative. The H-reflex is an electrically evoked spinal monosynaptic reflex that activates the Ia afferent fibers (large myelinated fibers with the lowest threshold for activation). The Achilles tendon reflex (S1) is the easiest to record and can differentiate between an S1 and an L5 radiculopathy.[282] Again, distal pathology must be ruled out if the latency is prolonged and being used to assess for proximal pathology.

Somatosensory-Evoked Potentials. The method of performing somatosensory-evoked potentials (SSEPs) involves an afferent pulse of large nerve fiber sensory activity that travels proximally and enters the spinal cord and then ascends to the brain via the posterior columns in the brainstem after the nerve is stimulated.[281] This postsynaptic activity ultimately reaches the thalamus and the parietal cortex of the brain.[281] A small brain wave occurs following nerve stimulation at a fixed time following nerve stimulation and is recordable from surface electrodes in the scalp.[281] These SSEPs can be recorded simultaneously from various points such as the Erb point, which overlies the brachial plexus, over the cervical spine, and from the scalp overlying the cortex.[281] SSEPs are useful for monitoring the lower extremity in spinal surgery. Upper extremity SSEPs are useful in brachial plexus surgery.

Although the use of SSEPs was popular[283] for acetabular surgery, SSEPs have been supplanted by spontaneous EMG[284] when monitoring is desired. However, the general use of SSEPs or EMG modalities does not seem to be justified.[285]

Association of Peripheral Nerve Injury with Causalgia

There is a potential after peripheral nerve injury for development of causalgia (type II CRPS). There is a 1% to 5% incidence of causalgia in association with peripheral nerve injuries.[286] Data from the Vietnam War indicate a lower incidence of causalgia than the data from World War II (1.5% vs. 1.8%–13.8%). Rothberg and associates and Bonica[286] suggest that this lower incidence was due to the more rapid transport of the wounded and the higher quality of care.

Prognosis

Nerve Injuries Associated with Open and Closed Fractures and Dislocations. Omer noted a spontaneous return of nerve function in 83% of nerve injuries associated with fractures.[287] Radial nerve palsy associated with humerus fractures is perhaps a good example in which nerve recovery can be expected in roughly 90% of cases.[168,251,288,289] There are further distinctions in prognosis, including lower recovery rates of nerve function with open fractures than with closed fractures (17% vs. 83.5% in one series).[290] Omer also reported that nerve injuries associated with a dislocation were less likely to show spontaneous recovery than nerve injuries associated with a fracture.[291] Omer noted that peripheral neuropathies associated with closed fractures are usually neurapraxias, which have an excellent prognosis.[291] Peripheral neuropathy associated with open fractures had a prognosis related to the etiology: lacerations are usually neurotmesis lesions and should be closely examined, explored, and sutured.[291]

Nerve Injuries Associated With Projectile Injuries. Data from Vietnam on 595 gunshot wounds studied by Omer had a similar (69%) spontaneous recovery rate for both low- and high-velocity gunshot wounds.[292] Proximal nerve injuries in the extremities take longer to show clinical recovery than more distal extremity injuries because cellular repair occurs from the intact viable cell body distally to the receptor.[292] Civilian peripheral nerve injuries from projectiles with associated vascular injury have a poor prognosis. In one series, only 10% of these nerve injuries resolved.[293] Shotgun injuries have a higher incidence of nerve injuries than other types of gunshot injuries, have a worse prognosis (spontaneous recovery rate of about 45%),[294] and have a higher percentage of complete nerve transection (neurotmesis) than even high-velocity missile wounds. High-velocity missiles often create axonotmesis lesions and have a better prognosis than low-velocity missile wounds.[292]

Summary

Peripheral nerve injuries associated with fractures and dislocations are probably underappreciated in the acute trauma setting. Orthopaedic surgeons should refrain from using the term *neurovascularly intact* unless a complete neurologic and vascular examination has been performed. Instead, documentation should be limited to what was observed and performed (e.g., "can dorsiflex great toe," "1+ dorsalis pedis pulse"). Heightened surveillance for neurologic injury is protective for clinicians because failure to diagnose nerve injuries may result in patient dissatisfaction, disability, and litigation. Orthopaedic surgeons need to be familiar with the lexicon of nerve injury (neurapraxia, axonotmesis, and neurotmesis) to communicate with colleagues. From a practical standpoint, evaluation of recovery after a peripheral nerve injury is best performed by serial physical examinations. However, there is a role for electrodiagnostic testing, particularly when there is no sign of recovery of nerve function. Electrodiagnostic studies should be delayed for at least 3 weeks and often need to be repeated serially. Research in nerve regeneration techniques may ultimately hold the key to the treatment of peripheral nerve injuries in the future.

Complex Regional Pain Syndrome

Pain after musculoskeletal injury usually subsides. When patients have peculiar, disagreeable, and persistent painful symptoms several weeks after injury, they may have CRPS. CRPS is increasingly recognized as a cause of disability after injury.[295] The index of suspicion in general is not high enough, and many patients are not diagnosed until the later stages when the prognosis is less favorable.[295] Advances have been made in the understanding and treatment of CRPS. Nevertheless, many treatment methods are empirical, and there is a need for research in this area.[295]

Modern Terminology

More than six dozen different terms have been used in the English, French, and German literature over the past two decades to describe CRPS type I, which used to be called RSD.[240] A complicated lexicon of RSD has evolved from the more general category of "pain dysfunction syndromes,"[296] to the terminology adopted in 1994 by the International Association for the Study of Pain into "complex regional pain syndromes."[297] CRPS is subdivided into CRPS type I (RSD) and CRPS type II (causalgia).[297] The distinction is based on the absence of a documented nerve injury for type I and a documented nerve injury for type II causalgia (Table 23-12). An additional variant of CRPS, termed complex regional painless syndrome, has been reported.[298] This variant has all the clinical findings of CRPS type I except that pain is not the presenting symptom and is minimal. How common this variant of CRPS type I will prove to be remains to be seen. The focus here is on painful CRPS type I associated with traumatic orthopaedic injuries.

Etiology and Epidemiology

Trauma secondary to accidental injury has been described as the most common cause of CRPS type I.[286] These injuries include sprains; dislocations; fractures, usually of the hands, feet, or wrists; traumatic finger amputations; crush injuries of the hands, fingers, or wrists; contusions; and lacerations or punctures of the fingers, hands, toes, or feet.[286] It has been reported that CRPS develops in 1% to 5% of patients with peripheral nerve injury, 28% of patients with Colles fractures,[299] and 30% of patients with tibial fractures, although these percentages are higher than our experience for Colles

TABLE 23-12 *INTERNATIONAL ASSOCIATION FOR THE STUDY OF PAIN: DIAGNOSTIC CRITERIA FOR COMPLEX REGIONAL PAIN SYNDROME*

Complex Regional Pain Syndrome Type I (Reflex Sympathetic Dystrophy)*
1. The presence of an initiating noxious event or a cause of immobilization
2. Continuing pain, allodynia, or hyperalgesia with which the pain is disproportionate to the inciting event
3. Evidence at some time of edema, changes in skin blood flow, or abnormal sudomotor activity in the painful region
4. The diagnosis is excluded by the existence of conditions that would otherwise account for the degree of pain and dysfunction
Complex Regional Pain Syndrome Type II (Causalgia)†
1. The presence of continuing pain, allodynia, or hyperalgesia after a nerve injury, not necessarily limited to the distribution of the injured nerve
2. Evidence at some time of edema, changes in skin blood flow or abnormal sudomotor activity in the region of the pain
3. The diagnosis is excluded by the existence of conditions that would otherwise account for the degree of pain and dysfunction

*Criteria 2, 3, and 4 are necessary for a diagnosis of complex regional pain syndrome.

†All three criteria must be satisfied.

***Source:** Adapted with permission from Pittman DM, Belgrade MJ: Complex regional pain syndrome, Am Fam Phys 56:2265–2270, 1997; which was adapted with permission from Merskey H, Bodguk N, editors: Classification of chronic pain, descriptions of chronic pain syndromes and definitions of pain terms, ed 2, Seattle, 1994, IASP Press, pp 40–43.*

TABLE 23-13 *SELECTED DIFFERENTIAL DIAGNOSIS OF COMPLEX REGIONAL PAIN SYNDROME TYPE I*

Musculoskeletal
Bursitis
Myofascial pain syndrome
Rotator cuff tear (Buerger disease)
Undiagnosed local pathology (e.g., fracture or sprain)
Neurologic
Poststroke pain syndrome
Peripheral neuropathy
Postherpetic neuralgia
Radiculopathy
Infectious
Cellulitis
Infectious arthritis
Pain of unexplained etiology
Vascular
Raynaud disease
Thromboangiitis obliterans
Thrombosis
Traumatic vasospasm
Rheumatic
Rheumatoid arthritis
Systemic lupus erythematosus
Psychiatric
Factitious disorder
Hysterical conversion reaction

***Source:** Adapted with permission from Pittman DM, Belgrade MJ: Complex regional pain syndrome, Am Fam Phys 56:2265–2270, 1997.*

and tibia fractures.[300] In a recent series, the three most common inciting events were a sprain or strain in 29%, surgery in 24%, and a fracture in 16%.[210] Interestingly, in this same series, 6% of patients could not remember an inciting event.[301] Saphenous neuralgia has been called a *forme fruste* of sympathetically mediated pain around the knee.[302] External fixators appear to be associated with CRPS in the upper extremity, although whether it is a result of the fracture immobilization, possible traction injury to the nerves, or direct neural trauma from the pins is unclear. CRPS can also be associated with arthroscopic surgical procedures[303] and prolonged usage of extremity tourniquets.

Allen and associates[301] reported on the epidemiologic variables of patients with CRPS. They noted in a series of 134 patients evaluated at a tertiary chronic pain clinic that patients had a history of having seen on average 4.8 different physicians before referral.[301] The average duration of symptoms of CRPS before presentation to the tertiary chronic pain clinic was 30 months.[301] In addition, 54% of patients had a worker's compensation claim, and 17% of patients had a lawsuit related to the CRPS.[260] Of the 51 of 135 patients who underwent a bone scan, only 53% of the studies were interpreted as consistent with the diagnosis of CRPS.[301]

Pathophysiology

Breivik noted that, as described by the International Association for the Study of Pain, CRPS is a complex neurologic disease involving the somatosensory, somatomotor, and autonomic nervous systems in various combinations, with distorted information processing of afferent sensory signals to the spinal cord.[304,305] Autonomic nervous system dysregulation occurs in only 25% to 50% of patients with CRPS.[263,305,306] The role of the sympathetic system was further clarified by Ide and associates, who used a noninvasive laser Doppler to assess fingertip blood flow and vasoconstrictor response and found that skin blood flow and vasoconstrictor response returned to normal after successful treatment of the condition.[307] These investigators suggested that the sympathetic nervous system function is altered and is different in the various stages of CRPS type I.

Many CRPS type I patients have a combination of sympathetically maintained pain (SMP) and sympathetically independent pain. SMP is defined as pain that is maintained by sympathetic efferent nerve activity or by circulating catecholamines.[263,305,306] SMP is relieved by sympatholytic procedures.[304] SMP follows a nonanatomic distribution.[308] Nonetheless, SMP is not essential in the development of CRPS, and that is why the term RSD is no longer in favor.[304] In some patients, sympatholytic procedures will not relieve their pain.[304] Breivik notes that more than half of all patients with CRPS have sympathetically independent pain. In one series, whereas symptoms of increased sympathetic activity occurred in 57% of patients, signs of inflammation and muscle dysfunction occurred in 90% of patients.[309]

Clinical Presentation

Although the differential diagnosis of CRPS type I is extensive (Table 23-13), the diagnosis of florid CRPS type I is usually not difficult.[310] However, recognizing milder cases can be challenging because of the changing clinical features of this syndrome over time (i.e., vasodilatation first, then vasoconstriction, and finally dystrophic changes); dynamic alterations, including diurnal fluctuations; and the subjectivity of some complaints.[310] Nonetheless, the importance of early diagnosis is highlighted by the fact that results of treatment are better when treatment is initiated earlier.

Sandroni and colleagues have prospectively studied whether certain clinical characteristics and laboratory indices correlate with the diagnosis of CRPS type I.[310] They found that both the clinically based CRPS I scoring system, which graded allodynia, vasomotor symptoms, and swelling, and the laboratory-based CRPS I grading system, which incorporated a sudomotor index, vasomotor index, and a resting sweat index, were sensitive and reliable tools and could be combined to provide an improved set of diagnostic criteria for CRPS I. Oerlemans and colleagues found that bedside evaluation of CRPS type I with Veldman's criteria was in good accord with psychometric or laboratory testing of these criteria.[311] Veldman's criteria are defined as follows: (1) the presence of four or five of the following signs and symptoms: unexplained diffuse pain, difference in skin color relative to the other limb, diffuse edema, difference in skin temperature relative to the other limb, and limited active range of motion; (2) the occurrence or increase of the above signs and symptoms after use; and (3) the presence of the above signs and symptoms in an area larger than the area of primary injury or operation and including the area distal to the primary injury.[309] Schurmann and coworkers studied the incidence of specific clinical features in CRPS type I patients and unaffected control patients and assessed the diagnostic value of a bedside test that measures sympathetic nerve function.[312] Sympathetic reactivity was obliterated or diminished in the affected hands of patients with CRPS type I in contrast to age-matched control participants with similar fracture patterns.[312]

Staging

CRPS type I has been separated into three stages: acute, dystrophic (ischemic), and atrophic.[313-315] These stages are generally based on chronology, with stage I lasting about 3 months, stage II from 3 to 6 months after the onset of symptoms, and stage III beginning 6 to 9 months after the injury.[316] Stages are also determined based on their symptom complexes. Stage I is characterized by swelling, edema, increased temperature in the extremity, and pain aggravated by movement. Stage I is associated with hyperpathia (delayed overreaction and aftersensation to a painful stimulus, particularly a repetitive one), exaggerated pain response, hyperhidrosis, and allodynia (pain elicited by a normally non-noxious stimulus, particularly if repetitive or prolonged).[316,317] Sympathetic blocks may be curative during this acute stage of CRPS. Stage II occurs typically after about 3 months when the initial edema becomes brawny, trophic changes of the skin appear, the joint may become cyanotic, and joint motion decreases. In the third stage, the pain may begin to decrease, trophic changes are more pronounced, edema is less prominent, the skin becomes cooler and drier with a thinning and glossy appearance, and joint stiffness occurs.[316]

Diagnostic Testing

The diagnosis of CRPS type I is usually based on clinical findings. The new criteria for diagnosing CRPS do not include the results of diagnostic testing with sympathetic blocks, and a discerning clinician may disagree on the true presence of CRPS type. Selected diagnostic tests are discussed.

Radiography. The early findings of CRPS are patchy demineralization of the epiphyses and short bones of the hands and feet.[317] Genant and associates[264] defined five types of bone resorption that may occur in CRPS type I. These are irregular resorption of trabecular bone in the metaphysis creating the patchy or spotty osteoporosis, subperiosteal bone resorption, intracortical bone resorption, endosteal bone resorption, and surface erosions of subchondral and juxtaarticular bone.[264] Radiographic findings such as subperiosteal resorption, striation, and tunneling of the cortex are not diagnostic of CRPS type 1 and may occur with any condition causing disuse.[317] When patchy osteopenia is present, the patient is usually already in stage II CRPS.[318,319] Osteopenia of the patella is the most common finding of CRPS of the knee.[316]

Bone Scanning. Three-phase bone scanning with technetium has long been used as a diagnostic study for CRPS type I, with the pervasive notion that scans will be hot in all three phases. Although this may often be the case in the acute phase, the bone scan findings in stages II and III are more subtle. There are many false-negative bone scan results in stages II and III.[320] Raj and associates noted that in stage II, the first two phases of the bone scan are normal, and the delayed images (static phase) of the bone scan demonstrate increased activity.[320] Stage III has decreased activity in phases one and two and normal activity in the third phase (delayed or static phase).[320] In contrast, a study of quantitative analysis of three-phase scintigraphy concluded that scintigraphy should not be considered as the definitive technique for the diagnosis of CRPS type I.[321]

Bone scans have been used to assess the response to treatment and have been found to have no value in monitoring treatment.[322] However, these investigators found that the bone scan had prognostic value: marked hyperfixation of the tracer indicates better final outcome.

Thermography. Thermography images temperature distribution of the body surface.[317] Gulevich and associates reported on the use of stress infrared telethermography for the diagnosis of CRPS type I and reported that as a diagnostic technique it was both sensitive and specific.[323] Further study of thermography is needed before global usage can be recommended.

Psychologic or Psychiatric Assessment

Psychologic assessment of patients with CRPS has included structured clinical interviews and personality measures such as the Minnesota Multiphasic Personality Inventory (MMPI) and Hopelessness Index.[317] The MMPI profiles of patients with CRPS resemble those of patients with chronic pain (increasing elevations on the hypochondriasis, depression, and hysteria scales).[317] Patients in stage I have more pessimism than patients in the second and third stages. More pessimism and depression are seen in younger patients than in older patients.[320]

Bruehl and Carlson examined the literature for evidence that psychologic factors predispose certain individuals to development of CRPS.[324] They did find that 15 of 20 studies reported the presence of depression, anxiety, or life stress in patients with CRPS[324] and hypothesized a theoretical model in which these factors influenced the development of CRPS through their effects on α-adrenergic activity. They could not determine whether depression, anxiety, and life stress preceded the CRPS and were etiologically related to it.

Current Concepts in Treatment

Overview. The use of daily vitamin C has been reported to be effective in preventing the development of CRPS type I in patients after foot and ankle surgery.[325-327] The first line of treatment of CRPS type I includes nonsteroidal antiinflammatory drugs (NSAIDs), topical capsaicin cream, a low-dose antidepressant, and physical therapy (contrast baths, transcutaneous electrical nerve stimulation [TENS] unit treatments, gentle range of motion to prevent joint contractures, and isometric strengthening exercises to prevent atrophy). Treatment at this time can usually be initiated by the orthopaedic surgeon. However, if the patient fails to respond, then referral to a pain specialist, generally an anesthesiologist with a special interest in pain management, should also be considered. The second line of treatment includes possible sympathetic blocks, anticonvulsants (gabapentin), calcium channel blockers (nifedipine), adrenergic blocking agents (phenoxybenzamine), and antidepressants in higher doses. The third line of treatment includes possible sympathectomy (surgical or chemical), implantable spinal cord stimulators, and corticosteroids. Table 23-14 shows the medications commonly used for CRPS type I.

TABLE 23-14 *MEDICATIONS COMMONLY USED TO TREAT REFLEX SYMPATHETIC DYSTROPHY*

Medication	Initial Dosage*
Adrenergic Agents	
β-Blocker: propranolol (Inderal)	40 mg twice a day
α-Blocker: Phenoxybenzamine (Dibenzyline)	10 mg twice a day
α- and β-blocker: guanethidine (Ismelin)	10 mg/day
α-Agonist: clonidine (Catapres-TTS)	One 0.1 mg patch/wk
Calcium Channel Blocking Agent	
Nifedipine (Adalat, Procardia)	30 mg/day
Drugs for Neuropathic Pain	
Tricyclic Antidepressants	
Amitriptyline (Elavil)	10–25 mg/day
Doxepin (Sinequan)	25 mg/day
Serotonin Reuptake Inhibitors	
Fluoxetine (Prozac)	20 mg/day
Anticonvulsant: gabapentin (Neurontin)	300 mg on the first day, 300 mg twice a day on the second day, and 300 mg three times a day thereafter
Corticosteroid: prednisone	60 mg/day; then rapidly taper over 2–3 wk

*The initial dosage may need to be adjusted based on individual circumstances. Consult a drug therapy manual for further information about specific medications.

Source: *Adapted with modifications with permission from Pittman DM, Belgrade MJ: Complex regional pain syndrome, Am Fam Phys 56:2265–2270, 1997.*

Nonsteroidal Antiinflammatory Drugs. The possibility that the inflammatory response is important in the pathophysiology of CRPS[319] highlights the role of NSAIDs in treatment. Veldman and associates[309] suggested that the early symptoms of CRPS are more suggestive of an exaggerated inflammatory response to injury or surgery than a disturbance of the sympathetic nervous system.[309] Nonetheless, Sieweke and associates found no effect of an antiinflammatory response and hypothesized a noninflammatory pathogenesis in CRPS that is presumably central in origin.[328]

Antidepressants. Antidepressants are useful in treating CRPS primarily by causing sedation, analgesia, and mood elevation. Analgesic action has been attributed to inhibition of serotonin reuptake at nerve terminals of neurons that act to suppress pain transmission, with resulting prolongation of serotonin activity at the receptor.[329]

Narcotic Analgesics. There is a potential for abuse of narcotics in CRPS because of the associated chronic pain. These agents do little to relieve sympathetically mediated pain. However, when narcotics are given epidurally in combination with local anesthetic agents, they are effective. Epidural administration of fentanyl (0.03–0.05 mg/hr) allows maximum effect on the dorsal horn with minimal plasma concentration and minimal side effects.

Anticonvulsants. Mellick reported the results of using gabapentin (Neurontin) in patients with severe and refractory CRPS pain.[330] He noted satisfactory pain relief, early evidence of disease reversal, and even one case of a successful treatment of CRPS with gabapentin alone. The specific effects noted included reduced hyperpathia, allodynia, hyperalgesia, and early reversal of skin and soft tissue manifestations. Vas and Renuka[331] reported the successful reversal of type I CRPS of both upper extremities in five patients using Lyrica.

Calcium Channel Blockers (Nifedipine) and Adrenergic Blocking Agents (Phenoxybenzamine). Nifedipine, a calcium channel blocker, has been used orally to treat patients with CRPS. At a dosage of 10 to 30 mg three times a day, it induces peripheral vasodilatation. Gellman and colleagues[332] stated that this effect of nifedipine was most likely from its effect on smooth muscles. Initial treatment is usually at a dosage of 10 mg three times a day for 1 week, which is increased if there is no effect to 20 mg three times a day for 1 week, which is increased to 30 mg three times a day the following week if there is no effect. If partial improvement or relief occurs at any of these doses, then the dosage is continued for 2 weeks and then tapered and discontinued over several days.[253] The most common side effect of nifedipine is headache, which is most likely caused by increased cerebral blood flow. Muizelaar and coworkers[333] assessed treatment of both CRPS types I and II with nifedipine or phenoxybenzamine, or both, in 59 patients. They found a higher success rate using phenoxybenzamine in 11 of 12 patients. A lower success rate of 40% was found in treating chronic CRPS. Although long-term oral use of phenoxybenzamine has been reported for the treatment of CRPS, there has been a high incidence of orthostatic hypotension (43%).[334] In an attempt to avoid these side effects, IV regional phenoxybenzamine has been used to treat patients with CRPS with good results in a small series of patients.[335]

Corticosteroids. Although the use of corticosteroids in the treatment of patients with CRPS is much less common, Raj and associates note that a trial of steroids might be a reasonable treatment for patients with long-standing pain who have not responded to blocks.[317] It has been reported that the patients who respond to corticosteroids had chronic pain of a mean duration of 25 weeks.[336]

Physical Therapy. Physical therapy has long been an integral part of treatment of patients with CRPS type I. Oerlemans and associates prospectively studied whether physical therapy or occupational therapy could reduce the ultimate impairment rating in patients with CRPS and found that physical therapy and occupational therapy did not reduce impairment percentages in patients with CRPS.[337] Nonetheless, these same investigators have also reported that adjuvant physical therapy in patients with CRPS results in a more rapid improvement in an impairment level sum score.[338] Smith[339] did a review of the literature and reported that exercise, motor feedback exercises, relaxation techniques, acupuncture, electroacupuncture, transcutaneous nerve stimulation, and combined treatment programs may help in the treatment of CRPS type I.

Electroacupuncture. There has been a resurgence of interest in electroacupuncture.[340,341]

Chan and Chow reported their results with acupuncture with electrical stimulation in 20 patients with features of CRPS.[342] They found that 70% had marked improvement in pain relief, and an additional 20% had further improvement. In addition, later follow-up reassessment of these patients showed maintenance or continued improvement of their pain relief 3 to 22 months after their course of electroacupuncture.[342]

Regional Intravenous and Arterial Blockade. The use of IV or intraarterial infusions of ganglionic blocking agents is becoming increasingly popular in the treatment of patients with CRPS.[317] Guanethidine, bretylium, and reserpine have been used with promising results.[312] Guanethidine has been substituted for reserpine in the IV regional block format to lessen side effects.[317]

Sympathetic Blocks. Sympathetic blockade has historically been useful both as a diagnostic test (placebo injections are included and documented temperature elevation after blockade) and as a basic treatment. Increasing recognition of the presence of nonsympathetically mediated pain in CRPS has contributed to the decreased use of diagnostic sympathetic blockade.

A series of injections are generally performed on an outpatient basis. Alternatively, continuous epidural infusions can be performed on an inpatient basis if the patient is unable or unwilling to have a series of outpatient nerve blocks.[303]

For upper extremity CRPS, the site of blockade is either the stellate ganglion or the brachial plexus. For lower extremity CRPS, the lumbar sympathetic chain or epidural space is the preferred site for sympathetic blockade.

Transcutaneous Electrical Stimulation. Transcutaneous electrical nerve stimulation has been useful in the treatment of CRPS. It most likely works via the gate theory of pain introduced by Melzack and Wall in 1965 in which stimulation of the larger nerve fibers transcutaneously closes the "gate" and may inhibit the transmission of pain.[343]

Topical Capsaicin. Topical capsaicin cream in concentrations of 0.025% to 0.075%, used previously for postherpetic neuralgia and painful diabetic neuropathy, has been noted to be worth considering for treating localized areas of hyperalgesia.[344,345] The effectiveness of topical capsaicin cream decreases after several weeks of daily usage. There is limited evidence (mostly case reports) to support its use with CRPS.

Chemical Sympathectomy. Neurolytic sympathetic block is an alternative for the lower extremity but usually not the upper extremity. The proximity of the cervical sympathetic chain to the brachial plexus makes a cervical neurolytic sympathectomy too hazardous unless placed under fluoroscopic or CT guidance. Neurolytic lumbar sympathetic blockade is considered to be a viable alternative to surgical sympathectomy for lower extremity CRPS.[317] However, there are potential complications with such procedures, including dermatologic problems and "sympathalgia" in the second or third postoperative weeks, which is characterized by muscle fatigue, deep pain, and tenderness.[346]

Surgical Sympathectomy. Surgical sympathectomy has been advocated for patients who do not get permanent pain relief from regional blockade as a last resort or end-of-the-road treatment. The criteria suggested before the selection of surgical sympathectomy are as follows: patients should have had pain relief from sympathetic blocks on several occasions, pain relief should last as long as the vascular effects of the blocks, placebo injections should produce no pain relief, and secondary gain and psychopathology should be ruled out.[317] Failure of surgical sympathectomy has been attributed to reinnervation from the contralateral sympathetic chain.[347,348] Recently, a new variation of surgical sympathectomy, "regional subcutaneous venous sympathectomy," has been reported in the treatment of CRPS type II.[349] Surgical sympathectomy in our opinion is less effective than chemical sympathectomy.

Electrical Spinal Cord and Motor Cortex Stimulation. Electrical spinal cord stimulation is generally reserved for patients who have severe pain that is unresponsive to conventional treatments. Kemler and associates retrospectively studied the clinical efficacy and possible adverse effects of electrical spinal cord stimulation for the treatment of patients with CRPS.[350] About 78% of patients (18 of 23) reported subjective improvement during the test period, and 50% had complications related to the device. Prospective studies are needed to assess the efficacy of spinal cord stimulation. Velasco and colleagues[351] reported on motor cortex electrical stimulation applied to patients with CRPS and noted its effectiveness with pain and sympathetic changes.

Nontraditional Therapies and Treatments. Certain patients are responsive to nontraditional treatment such as art and music therapy, herbal medicines, and massage therapy. These approaches should be viewed with an open mind because the traditional, evidence-based therapies may not be successful in relieving pain associated with CRPS.

Krans-Schreuder and colleagues[352] reported the results of amputation for long-standing therapy-resistant type I CRPS in 22 patients. They reported that amputation may positively contribute to the lives of patients with long-standing therapy-resistant type I CRPS in carefully selected patients with a 24% risk of recurrence.[352]

Prevention

It has been suggested that optimal pain relief after surgery can reduce the incidence of chronic postoperative pain syndromes, such as those that occur in almost 50% of thoracotomies.[353] This hypothesis is based on the concept that an abnormally exaggerated and prolonged hyperalgesia reaction is involved in the development of complex posttraumatic syndromes.[304] Although the potential for dose escalation and dependency has to be considered, perioperative management of pain with appropriate analgesics appears to help prevent CRPS.

Prognosis

The prognosis of CRPS has historically been grim. The prognosis has also been linked to the time of diagnosis, with early diagnosis yielding a better prognosis. The assumption has generally been that stage I CRPS will progress in most cases to stage II and then to stage III. Zyluk studied the natural history of posttraumatic CRPS without treatment and found that the signs and symptoms were largely gone in 26 of 27 patients who completed the study at 13 months after diagnosis.[354] Nonetheless, the hands were still functionally impaired, and three patients who withdrew from the study had worsening of the signs and symptoms of CRPS.[354] Geertzen and associates studied 65 patients with CRPS to analyze the relationship between impairment and disability.[355] They found that CRPS patients had impairments and perceived disabilities after a mean interval of 5 years.[355] Furthermore, these investigators found no differences in impairments in patients who were diagnosed within 2 months of the causative event and those diagnosed 2 to 5 months after it. Nonetheless, evidence suggests that the effect of treatment for sympathetically mediated pain is better during the first few months after onset.[304] Cooper and DeLee noted that the most favorable prognostic indicator in the management of CRPS of the knee was early diagnosis and early institution of treatment (within 6 months of onset).[316] de Mos and colleagues[356] reported the outcome of CRPS from a Dutch general practitioner's database of 102 patient at an average follow-up of 5.8 years. Sixteen percent of patients reported the CRPS as still progressive and 31% were incapable of working.[356]

Summary

Key for the orthopaedic surgeon is to recognize that a fracture patient may develop CRPS, distinct from another condition. Roberts and Heintzman noted that providers of musculoskeletal care "are probably in the best position to determine what is and what is not appropriate pain after musculoskeletal injury."[357] CRPS patients may take several visits to diagnose. It is important to have heightened awareness to differentiate it from an undetected additional injury; especially in polytrauma patients, making an early presumptive diagnosis of CRPS helps initiate timely, appropriate treatment. The International Association for the Study of Pain criteria for CRPS type I make the diagnosis easier but less specific. Although treatment may be in the hands of pain specialists, prevention strategies and risk reduction "are best administered by those who see the patient first."[358]

MANAGEMENT OF COMPLICATIONS

In this chapter, a complication of fracture treatment has been defined as an *undesired turn of events* in the treatment of a fracture. But because the patient, doctor, and insurer each bring a different set of values into the assessment of medical outcomes, the question might be asked, "Undesired by whom?" The patient and doctor, for example, may agree to attempt limb salvage for a difficult compound tibial fracture with contamination and arterial injury. The insurer, facing charges in excess of half a million dollars for vascular repair, free flap coverage, fracture fixation, bone grafting, and multiple reoperations if infection develops, combined with a prolonged time of total disability before the patient is able to return to work, may regard the outcome as an undesired event when compared with below-the-knee amputation, prosthesis fitting, and an early return to work.

An explicit understanding of the *desired* course of events is therefore crucial to recognizing complications. In this respect, fracture treatment is different from many other areas of orthopaedics and, indeed, medicine in general for two reasons. First, the goal of treatment is generally obvious: secure complete functional healing of a broken bone with return to full activity. Second, the patient did not anticipate the injury; therefore, patient education begins at the perioperative visit. The choice of physician is largely determined by institutional lines of case referral. Also, the patient must adjust to pain, inconvenience, and an unexpected loss of productivity. To make matters more difficult, some accident victims have associated psychopathology that makes communication difficult.[359] These patients may be stigmatized as "mentally ill," thereby setting the stage for withholding appropriate care.

Many fractures with good results of treatment yield permanent impairment. A difficult supracondylar fracture of the humerus repaired with an open reduction often has a residual loss of at least 15 degrees of elbow extension. The clinical and radiographic results are excellent in terms of present state-of-the-art treatment despite the presence of measurable permanent impairment. The chain of causation that led to this impairment began when the patient fell and landed on the elbow. It is crucial to maintain this link. When the physician does not acknowledge the presence of impairment and, even worse, fails to recognize that the patient is bothered, for example, by a prominent screw that has backed out of an olecranon osteotomy, there is a risk that the patient, or the patient's lawyer, will attempt to shorten the chain of causation to the operative event. For many patients, an understanding of the loss sustained in injury and the recognition of complications by the treating physician are crucial steps. These steps are the only chance of defusing a potentially explosive situation and allowing the process of controlling and treating complications in the most effective manner possible.

Local complications occurring late in the course of treatment are most often related to disturbances in fracture healing. These may develop insidiously over weeks or months. Often in such cases, the patient is anticipating recovery, and the orthopaedist overlooks a trend toward deformity that, on retrospective viewing of radiographs arranged in sequence, is all too evident.

Each fracture has two complementary problems that must be solved: a biologic one and a mechanical one. The biologic problem consists of providing the setting for fracture healing. In most simple closed fractures, adequate biologic factors are present so that healing will occur. In high-grade compound fractures, the biologic issue is an important one. Only a few strategies are available to improve biology; these include autogenous bone grafting, electrical stimulation, free tissue transfer, and bone morphogenetic proteins. New techniques that harness the power of gene therapy and accelerate future healing will soon be available. Their safety and cost effectiveness require incisive evidence-based research. The mechanical problem includes the selection of an operative or nonoperative treatment strategy that anticipates the mechanical behavior of a fractured bone and provides an environment that allows biologic processes to heal the fracture. Work by Goodship and associates[360] and by Rubin and Lanyon[361] has begun to define the mechanical circumstances favorable to fracture healing. Although it destroys marrow content, closed reamed IM nailing works well because it does not disturb the soft tissue envelope, and the biomechanics of fracture site loading are favorable. When the vitality of the tissues surrounding a fracture site is compromised, the margin of safety is smaller, and adverse outcomes become more prevalent. In this situation, modification of the method (e.g., eliminating reaming and using a mechanically stronger but thinner improved implant) may reduce the incidence of complications to an acceptable level.

New therapies such as absorbable antibiotic implants, biologic bone "glues," implantable proteins that stimulate fracture healing, antibiotic-coated implants, absorbable fracture fixation devices, and gene therapy hold promise for improved results.

Database management is at the heart of analyzing complications. Today's information technology advances provide a tremendous opportunity to improve fracture care information. The data collected must, however, be meaningful. What is put into a database determines what comes out. The fracture nomenclature and the proposed open fracture classification adopted by the Orthopaedic Trauma Association is an attempt to create groupings of similar cases for long-term study.

Because the risk-to-benefit ratio is at the heart of decision making in fracture treatment and in an era of results analysis, new factors will emerge that will influence the expenditure of healthcare resources for fracture care. The categorization of complications will assume great importance.[362] An approach for fracture treatment must be shaped to ensure that equal weight is given to the long-term outcome of a particular treatment pattern. The focus should be shifted away from short-term economic monitors (e.g., days in the hospital, readmission within 2 weeks, implant costs) because these factors do not disclose the true socioeconomic morbidity of this disease and the potential lasting impact of local complications of fracture treatment. The medical-industrial complex has a desire to set practice pattern algorithms to predict and control costs. The problem in trying to standardize treatment routines is that algorithms for care of human conditions are based on faulty assumptions.[363] Despite the appearance of systematization in today's microprocessor-produced output, practice patterns are dependent on human variables, and the treatment of broken limbs remains an art as well as a science.

Risk Management

No discussion about complications would be complete without reviewing the risks and medicolegal implications of complications. Many complications result in a degree of permanence (e.g., pain, decreased range of motion, muscle weakness). The mere existence of a complication potentially fulfills the criterion that there were damages, one of the triad of criteria for medical malpractice. Malpractice is simply defined as an event in violation of the "standard of care" that causes damages. Rogal noted that a theory of fault can be created for any adverse outcome that occurs while a person is under a physician's care.[364] A bad outcome after surgery itself is associated with the risk of a lawsuit.[229]

There are several reasons why orthopaedic surgeons are near the top of the list in the number of malpractice claims.[364] The work of orthopaedists is often visible on radiographs.[364] Because of the emphasis on radiographic cosmesis, fracture surgery is particularly susceptible to scrutiny by anyone. These factors, coupled with the fact that fracture surgery can rarely be performed perfectly, makes fracture surgery a target for malpractice allegations. Rogal also notes that many orthopaedic injuries are "irreconcilable" and cites the example of a decimated articular surface, which is juxtaposed with the public perception that modern technology can return any injury back to normal.[364] He also noted that in many situations, time is of the essence (e.g., neurovascular compromise, compartment syndrome), and he noted that lawsuits are often spawned when care is delayed and the outcome is minimally adverse. Related to this last scenario is the unique entity in orthopaedic traumatology of the missed injury.

Missed Injuries

Missed injuries or the delayed diagnosis of injuries has been called the "nemesis" of the trauma surgeon.[365,366] Missed injuries are reported in 2% to 9% of patients with multiple injuries.[359,365,367,368] The majority of these injuries are musculoskeletal injuries. In one series, Buduhan and McRitchie reported that 54% of the injuries were musculoskeletal and 14.3% affected the peripheral nerves (14.3%) (Fig. 23-11).[368] They noted that patients with missed injuries tend to be more severely injured and to have initial neurologic compromise. Buduhan and McRitchie reported that in 46 of 567 (8.1%) missed injuries, 43.8% were unavoidable.[368] Born and associates in 1989 reported a delay in diagnosis of musculoskeletal injuries in 26 of 1006 consecutive blunt trauma patients and a total of 39 fractures with a delay in diagnosis.[367] The most common reason for the delay in diagnosis was the lack of radiographs at admission. Enderson and associates in 1990[365] reported that a tertiary survey was able to find additional injuries in patients who had already undergone primary and secondary trauma surveys and that the use of the tertiary survey found a higher percentage of injuries (9%) than the 2% incidence in their trauma registry. These investigators noted that the most common reason injuries were missed was altered level of consciousness caused by head injury or alcohol. Ward and Nunley in 1991 reported that 6% of orthopaedic injuries were not initially diagnosed in 111 multitrauma patients.[295] Seventy percent of occult bony injuries were ultimately diagnosed by physical examination and plain radiographs alone. Risk factors for occult orthopaedic injuries were (1) significant multisystem trauma with another more apparent orthopaedic injury within the same extremity, (2) trauma victim too unstable for full initial orthopaedic evaluation, (3) altered sensorium, (4) hastily applied splint obscuring a less apparent injury, (5) poor quality or inadequate initial radiographs, and (6) inadequate significance assigned to minor signs or symptoms in a major trauma victim. These investigators noted that all orthopaedic injuries cannot be diagnosed on initial patient evaluation.

Spine injuries are a subgroup of injuries that are frequently diagnosed late. In 1996, Anderson and coworkers noted that in 43 of 181 patients with major thoracolumbar spine fractures, there was a delay in diagnosis.[369] This delay in diagnosis was associated with an unstable patient condition

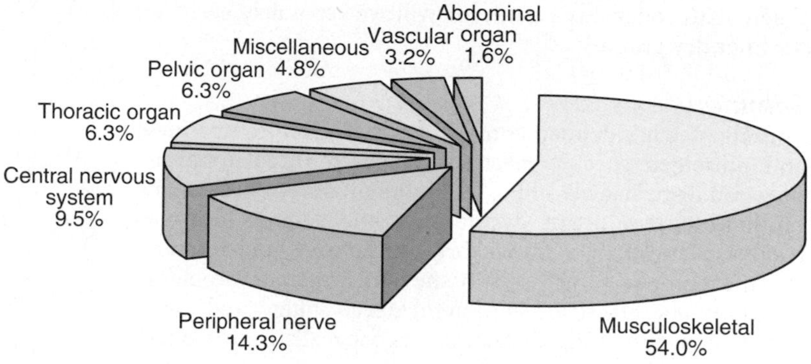

Figure 23-11. Pie diagram of the types of missed injuries in patients with multiple trauma, demonstrating that the majority of missed injuries are musculoskeletal. *(From Buduhan G, McRitchie DI: Missed injuries in patients with multiple trauma, J Trauma 49:600–605, 2000, with permission.)*

necessitating higher priority procedures than emergency department thoracolumbar spine radiographs. Lumbar transverse process fractures have also been reported to be associated with significant lumbar spine fractures in 11% of cases and can be easily missed if CT scanning is not used in addition to plain radiographs.[370]

Because many of these patients have life-threatening conditions, the initial evaluations may overlook additional bony injuries that may contribute to the development of MOF. Early missed injuries are frequent even in regional trauma centers. In a series of 206 patients, Janjua and coworkers reported a 39% incidence of missed injuries, which included 12 missed thoracoabdominal injuries, seven missed hemopneumothoraces, and two deaths from missed injury complications.[371]

A tertiary survey of the patient at 24 to 48 hours and subsequent serial examinations are needed to find these injuries. Huynh and colleagues[372] reported on the use of mid-level to contract tertiary surveys at a level 1 trauma center. Lawson and colleagues[366] reported that a "trauma scan" (high-resolution CT studies of the cervical spin, head, chest, abdomen, and pelvis) reduced (but did not eliminate) the number of missed injuries. They noted that the most common missed injury remains the bowel and noted the continued importance of tertiary trauma surveys.[366]

Documentation of Complications

In the age of the electronic medical record, several factors should be considered in documentation. One key point is documenting the precise date that the complication was discussed with the patient. Common sense and tact are critical in these discussions. It may be more difficult to have these discussions in major teaching hospitals, where the patient and family are seeing the resident physicians daily and the attending physician less frequently. Axiomatic in discussing complications with patients and their families is avoidance of self-blame. In a legal context, statements such as "I wish we had done it differently" have the force of a confession and are known as admissions. The complication needs to be disclosed but not adopted. How the recent trend for full disclosure of medical errors will affect the disclosure and discussion of complications remains to be seen. The mere presence of a complication may place the physician at risk for litigation because the more disabling the outcome of the injury, the more it costs, which enhances the chance of an accusation of medical malpractice.[229]

When multiple services are caring for a trauma patient, delineation of responsibility in the medical record is important. It may not be clear to the patient or to the family which service is responsible for which aspect of the patient's care. For example, the patient might assume that the orthopaedic trauma service is responsible for metacarpal fractures when, in fact, there is a separate hand surgery service. Nevertheless, a team approach that presents a "united front" is important when there are multiple services caring for a patient.

Another significant development is the need to satisfy federal compliance issues in the medical record for surgical billing. These rules require the documentation of the presence of the attending physician during surgery for the key and critical parts of the operation. The patient, who subsequently acquires a copy of the medical record, will then know for which part of the surgery the attending physician was present. If any complications arose intraoperatively, particularly if the attending physician was not present for that part of the operation, the situation may become a medicolegal nightmare. A clarifying discussion with the patient and family should include the fact that a team of many hands is needed to treat broken bones.

Documenting systems problems is another potential challenge for orthopaedic traumatologists. Defining such issues in the medical record, for example, that "the surgery was delayed an additional 2 days because no operating room time was available," can be risky for the physician. Often, from the patient's and the patient's attorney's perspective, the physician and the institution are inextricably linked even when the physician is an independent contractor. Furthermore, there is tremendous pressure for physicians to support and not to criticize the institution in which they work. The survival of orthopaedic trauma as a field depends on our skill in negotiating a good environment for musculoskeletal care outside of the patient record.

Doubtless the electronic medical record will create new opportunities for litigation. Healthcare providers use passwords to access the record. The time and sequence of entry into the record is documented. There is currently no assurance that the chart is being created by the designated user. Furthermore, many record systems contain narrative elements that are not actually written by the provider. Does "signing" such a record attach responsibility for the contents? Today the contemporaneous handwritten record is authoritative. Tomorrow, it is not clear what the stylized, preformatted electronic record will bring. In reality, we are not teams but competitive groups of specialists with competing interests. Some of us are independent agents, others employees of large and small companies. When complications arise, are we best served by banding together to conceal the truth, or will we separately each run for high dry ground?

Summary

This chapter has defined complications of fracture treatment and presented specific information about three important systemic disturbances—FES, thromboembolic disorders, and multiple system organ dysfunction and failure—that can result. In addition, a framework for approaching fracture-specific complications—soft tissue and vascular problems, posttraumatic arthrosis, peripheral nerve injury, and CRPS type I—was presented. Last, strategies for realistically managing complications and optimizing outcomes were suggested.

Complications, such as missed injuries, are intrinsic to fracture care and are a part of the natural history of fractures rather than markers that something went wrong. In the final analysis, the management of complications begins with understanding the scientific basis of the treatment, listening to what the patient is telling us, and accepting the fact that we as fracture surgeons cannot avoid adverse circumstances.

KEY REFERENCES

The level of evidence (LOE) is determined according to the criteria provided in the preface.

154. Bettman MA, Baginski SG, White RD, et al: ACR Appropriateness Criteria acute chest pain—suspected pulmonary embolism. *J Thoracic Imaging* 27:W28–W31, 2012. LOE V
157. Guyatt GH, Akl EA, Crowther M, et al: Antithrombotic therapy and prevention of thrombosis, 9th Ed: American College of Chest Physicians Evidence-Based Clinical Practice Guidelines. *Chest* 141:7S–47S, 2012. LOE V
214. Harwood PJ, Giannoudis PV, van Griensven M, et al: Alterations in the systemic inflammatory response after early total care and damage control procedures for femoral shaft fracture in severely injured patients. *J Trauma* 58(3):452–454, 2005. LOE III
231. Barei DP, Nork SE, Mills WJ, et al: Functional outcomes of severe bicondylar tibial plateau fractures treated with dual incisions and medial and lateral plates. *J Bone Joint Surg* 88:1713–1721, 2006. LOE III
233. Rademakers MV, Kerkhoffs GMMJ, Sierevelt IN, et al: Operative treatment of 109 tibial plateau fractures: five- to 27-year follow-up results. *J Orthop Trauma* 21:5–10, 2007. LOE IV
246. Thomas TP, Anderson DD, Mosqueda TV, et al: Objective CT-based metrics of articular fracture severity to assess risk for post-traumatic osteoarthritis. *J Orthop Trauma* 24:764–769, 2010. LOE V
327. Zollinger PE, Tuinebreijer WE, Breederveld RS, et al: Can vitamin C prevent complex regional pain syndrome in patients with wrist fractures? *J Bone Joint Surg* 89:1424–1431, 2007. LOE I
349. Happak W, Sator-Katzenschlagr W, Kriechbaumer LK: Surgical treatment of complex regional pain syndrome type II with regional subcutaneous venous sympathectomy. *J Trauma Acute Care Surg* 72(6): 1647–1653, 2012. LOE III
357. Roberts CS, Heintzman SE: Editorial. Complex regional pain syndrome after musculoskeletal trauma: Who owns the monkey? *Injury* 41:669–670, 2010. LOE V
372. Huynh TT, Blackburn AH, McMiddleton-Nyatui D, et al: An initiative by midlevel providers to conduct tertiary surveys at level 1 trauma centers. *J Trauma* 68:1052–1058, 2010. LOE III

The complete References list is available online at https://expertconsult.inkling.com.

Chapter 24

Chronic Osteomyelitis

J. KRISTOPHER WARE • BRUCE D. BROWNER • EDWARD L. PESANTI • HARLAN STOCK • CLINTON K. MURRAY

BACKGROUND

Bone infections have long been a source of challenge, and too often frustration, for patients and physicians alike. Despite significant advances over the past century in the diagnosis and treatment of osteomyelitis, multiple surgeries are often necessary and recurrence is not uncommon. The purpose of this chapter is to review our current knowledge of osteomyelitis along with methods of examination, diagnosis, and treatment of the disease. To appreciate the present understanding of osteomyelitis, a brief review of the history of bone infections is helpful.

The Edwin Smith Papyrus (3000–2500 BC) is often cited as the earliest written evidence of bone infection.[1,2] Review of the translated hieroglyphic text reveals recognition by its author of the challenges and uncertain outcomes associated with wounds extending to bone with accompanying inflammation. The unknown author describes clearly outlined management of closed fractures but in the case of an open humerus fracture instructs, this is an "ailment not to be treated."[1] Although the severity of the sequelae of open fractures appears to be recognized, limited treatment options seem to have been available.

Hippocrates (460–370 BC) is credited as the first author to describe necrosis of the bone occurring after open fractures.[3,4] His treatment involved cleaning the wound and reducing the fracture, or sawing off the protruding segment, followed by splinting. At the time, dead bone was allowed to "exfoliate" from the wound.[4] Historical texts reveal that removal of the necrotic bone was advocated as early as the third century AD.[5] Around the turn of the eleventh century, Avicenna wrote of the importance of "curetting … cutting … or sawing" bone to completely remove "corruption of the bones."[5]

Several centuries later, eighteenth-century physicians provided more complete descriptions of the characteristics and management of bone infection. Various terms were used for bone infections including "caries of the bone," "abscessus in medulla," and "boil of the bone marrow."[3,6] In 1844, Auguste Nélaton is believed to have introduced the term "osteomyelitis."[5] Additionally, following this period, the terms *sequestrum* and *involucrum* came into usage describing the fragment of necrotic bone and surrounding sheath of reactive bone formation, respectively.

In 1867, following Louis Pasteur's identification of a microbial basis of infection, Joseph Lister described his aseptic technique for surgery using carbolic and phenic acid.[7] He also discussed applying these agents to open fractures. In a case series, several cases of osteomyelitis were successfully treated with excision of the infected bone combined with application of antiseptic agents.[8] This was a significant advancement in reducing gangrene and septicemia that were exceedingly common following open fractures.[7]

Much of the early twentieth-century literature describes treatment of osteomyelitis based on the Orr method.[3,6, 9-11] H. Winnett Orr provided detailed descriptions of his surgical protocol, postoperative management, and outcomes.[6,9] His treatment approach included "saucerizing" the infected area, removing foreign and dead tissue, cleaning with iodine and alcohol, filling the defect with Vaseline gauze packs, and applying a splint. Although he was not the first to describe the surgical procedure, unique to Orr's treatment was that no dressing changes were performed for several weeks in order to avoid manipulating the fracture by opening the splint. In 76 cases of chronic osteomyelitis due to open fractures, Orr reported 62% healed, 9 did not heal, 3 required amputation, and 2 deaths occurred. [6] Other authors using the Orr method reported similar results.[10,11] However, examining photos of successfully treated patients reveals a level of persistent deformity that would not likely be tolerated by today's standards.[6]

Attempts to better characterize the differing presentations of osteomyelitis are evident from early twentieth-century literature. Chappel differentiated between primary and secondary osteomyelitis.[12] According to Chappel, primary osteomyelitis was due to direct inoculation of bone from an exogenous source. Secondary osteomyelitis occurred from hematogenous bacterial seeding. He theorized that microtrauma to bony trabeculae resulting in microvascular compromise predisposed patients to this infection. He also differentiated between acute, subacute, and chronic osteomyelitis, as well as specific forms including Brodie abscess and nonsuppurative hemorrhagic osteomyelitis. Orr also cited early classification of osteomyelitis including acute, chronic, idiopathic, fulminating, and postoperative.[6] Although these early physicians recognized that various presentations of the disease were possible, in the period prior to the introduction of antibiotics, the type of bone infection had no relevance as surgical excision was the only treatment option.[10,12]

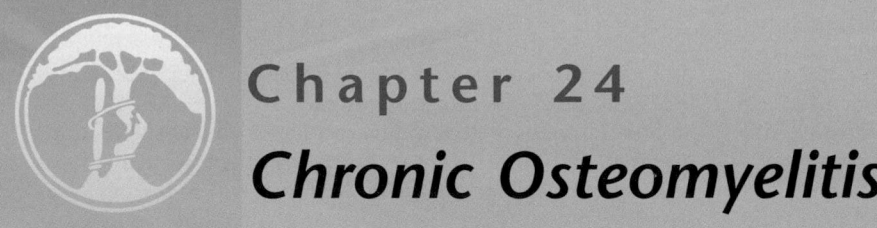

The discovery of penicillin was a pivotal point in the evolution of osteomyelitis treatment. In the 1930s, as is the case today, *Staphylococcus aureus* was recognized as the primary pathogen responsible for most cases of osteomyelitis.[11] Despite having a better understanding of the disease than their predecessors, physicians of the early twentieth century remained limited in their treatment options and control of the infection, following débridement, was purely dependent on host immune function. In 1940, Chain and colleagues[13] proved the effectiveness of penicillin in eradicating systemic staphylococcal infections in animal models. Over the course of the next decade, penicillin became widely available and was used for prevention and treatment of osteomyelitis. Suddenly, the pathophysiologic differences of acute and chronic osteomyelitis became significant.

Historically, the distinction between acute and chronic osteomyelitis was based on an ill-defined chronicity of infection. Acute osteomyelitis has been described as bone infection present for a few days to weeks.[14] Chronic osteomyelitis has in some cases been arbitrarily defined as infection lasting months to years.[2,14,15] However, the time frame is not as helpful as the character of the infection in determining treatment.[16] Acute osteomyelitis is most often due to bacterial seeding of bone from a hematogenous source. It predominantly affects adolescents with open physes.[14,17] Conservative treatment with appropriate antibiotics is the mainstay of treatment. In the majority of cases, acute hematogenous osteomyelitis can be arrested with antibiotics and without the need for surgical intervention.[2,14] In contrast, chronic osteomyelitis is marked by sequestrum formation that may be infected by an endogenous or exogenous source. It is the presence of this necrotic tissue that defines the disease rather than chronicity. This necrotic tissue allows the formation of a bacterial environment resistant to antibiotics and is the reason surgical intervention remains necessary.[14]

Where the early part of the twentieth century was marked by tremendous progress in understanding the etiology of osteomyelitis and developing different methods of débridement and postoperative care, the second half of the century was marked by improvement in diagnosis and fine-tuning of the surgical approach to create more options for limb salvage. The development and improvement of advanced imaging techniques, including magnetic resonance and nuclear medicine imaging techniques, has facilitated diagnosis and allowed precise localization of infection.[18] The use of external fixators allowed stabilization of open fractures while maintaining exposure of wounds for better soft tissue management.[19] The development of antibiotic-impregnated cement beads has allowed local delivery of antibiotics with control of dead space. In addition, advances in soft tissue closure techniques, including myocutaneous and free flap procedures, have allowed improved vascularity for systemic antibiotic delivery as well as a better opportunity for wound healing with the potential for immediate closure of wounds.[19] The introduction, and now wide usage, of negative pressure wound therapy devices has allowed temporary coverage of open wounds and facilitated multistage intervention.[20] The combined effects of these advances in the treatment of chronic osteomyelitis has allowed successful treatment of infection in 90% of patients.[19] However, even with current advances in treatment, remission rather than cure is often regarded as a successful outcome and recurrence following several years without signs or symptoms of infection is not unusual.

EPIDEMIOLOGY

Although the true incidence and prevalence of osteomyelitis is unknown, it has been reported that 50,000 hospital admissions occur annually due to the disease.[21] Additionally, bone and joint infections have been reported to be present in 1% of hospitalized patients.[15] The vast majority of cases of chronic osteomyelitis occur from an exogenous source, open fractures being the most commonly reported.[17]

Posttraumatic osteomyelitis is one of the few infectious diseases that have become more prevalent over the past century, probably due to improved survival following catastrophic injury. There are two reasons infection is so closely linked with such injuries. First, they provide ubiquitous microbes with an opportunity for breaching host defenses by exposing bone to the contamination of an accident scene. Second, once the microbes have bypassed external defenses, the trauma setting offers an ideal environment for adherence and colonization, namely, devitalized hard and soft tissues. When presented with these conditions, bacteria are able to form a biofilm layer making eradication of infection challenging.

A review by Gustilo[22] showed the deep infection rate in the setting of open fractures to be anywhere from 2% to 50%. The infection rate is influenced, to a large extent, by the severity of the injury.[23,24] Grade I and II open fractures are associated with around a 2% risk of infection as compared with 10% to 50% in grade III injuries.[22-24] In addition, type IIIC fractures have a significantly greater risk of infection compared to type IIIa and IIIb.[25,26] It intuitively seems reasonable that lack of bone coverage, massive contamination of the wound, compromised perfusion, and instability of the fracture would lead to an increased risk of infection in more severe injuries.

Because of the limited anterior soft tissues, the tibia is the most frequent location of open fractures (Fig. 24-1). Accordingly, the tibia is the most frequent site of osteomyelitis.[24] One retrospective study of 948 high-energy open tibial fractures reported a 56% posttraumatic infection rate.[27] Although not involved so often as the lower extremity, the upper extremity also is vulnerable to accidental trauma and subsequent infection.[24,28]

In addition to accidental trauma, surgery itself poses a risk for the development of bone infection. Even when attempting to provide the most sterile conditions, there is an estimated 1% to 3% risk of surgical site infection.[29] In addition to the risk posed by violating the integrity of the skin, soft tissues and potentially bone, orthopaedic implants may allow bacteria to colonize and form an environment secure from immune

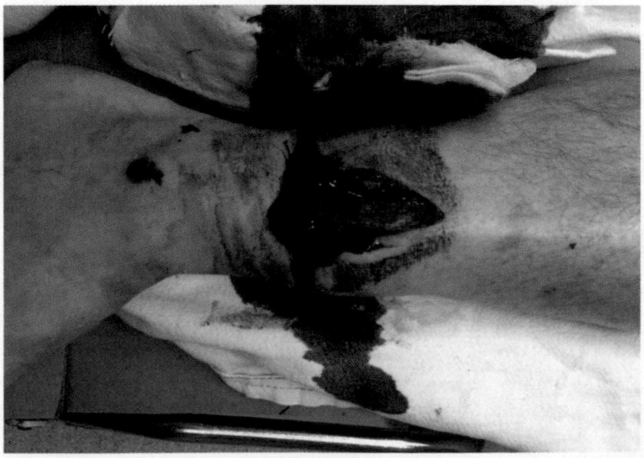

Figure 24-1. Open tibia fracture. The limited soft tissue coverage of the anteromedial tibia makes this area particularly susceptible to osteomyelitis.

surveillance.[30] Joint replacement and spine surgery was shown in one study to have the highest association with nosocomial infection.[29] Although the risk of prosthetic joint infection is greatest within 2 years of implantation, the potential for colonization from hematogenous invasion remains elevated throughout the life of the prosthesis.

Pressure ulcers, a common occurrence in the bedridden multitrauma patient, are another frequent source of osteomyelitis.[31] Despite the limited literature on decubitus ulcers and the development of osteomyelitis, this population (with limited mobility and often multiple comorbidities) comprises a significant portion of the patients with pelvic and calcaneal osteomyelitis.[32,33] Typically, the pressure ulcer is contaminated with various organisms from the external environment. In the case of pelvic osteomyelitis, this includes enteric bacteria. The infected soft tissue, combined with an often compromised vascular and immune system, allows for bone involvement through contiguous spread.

In addition to multiple potential sources of infection, a number of host factors are associated with the development of osteomyelitis. Although quality evidence is often lacking, malnutrition, obesity, drug abuse, smoking, diabetes, malignancy, and immune system compromise and/or suppression are believed to be predisposing conditions for the development of osteomyelitis.[34-38] Diabetic patients are particularly susceptible to soft tissue and bone infections. In fact, roughly 25% of diabetic patients will develop a foot ulcer in their lifetime.[35] The combination of peripheral neuropathy, which leads to loss of protective sensation, combined with microvascular disease, which impairs the ability to heal and fight infection, sets the stage for nonhealing soft tissue lesions that may quickly spread to bone.[35,39] Furthermore, hyperglycemia leads to altered cellular and humeral response to infection, thus weakening the host defenses.[39]

Patients with peripheral vascular disease from causes other than diabetes are also at increased risk of osteomyelitis.[36] Impaired bone perfusion in these patients not only functions as a barrier to immune surveillance but also impairs access to the infected tissue by systemic antibiotics. Additionally, vaso-occlusive disorders such as sickle cell anemia may lead to bone ischemia and necrosis predisposing these patients to opportunistic infection.[40,41]

As one would anticipate, immunocompromised individuals are at high risk for developing osteomyelitis. Whether immune system impairment is due to disease or medications, the host becomes susceptible to microbial invasion and spread.[37] Patients suffering from a disorder of polymorphonuclear leukocytes, for example, have been shown to be at significantly elevated risk for the development and progression of osteomyelitis.[42] Other immunocompromised individuals, such as organ transplant recipients,[43,44] patients with end-stage renal disease on hemodialysis,[21] and those receiving chemotherapy,[45] also are at an increased risk. With the development and widespread use of immune-modulating medications, such as tumor necrosis factor (TNF)-α inhibitors, patients undergoing treatment for various autoimmune diseases may be predisposed.[46] Although human immunodeficiency virus infection has not been identified as an independent risk factor in developing osteomyelitis,[47] skeletal infection in this population is clearly associated with a more severe clinical course with elevated morbidity and mortality.[38,48] Furthermore, behaviors that may be associated with human immunodeficiency virus (HIV) infection, particularly intravenous (IV) drug abuse, has been shown to increase a patient's risk of osteomyelitis.[38]

In addition to risk factors for the development of osteomyelitis, the disease itself may pose a risk for the development of certain malignancies. Patients with chronic draining sinuses often present with metaplastic changes of the sinus tract epithelium. These lesions have been reported to undergo malignant transformation in 0.2% to 1.6% of cases.[49] Squamous cell carcinoma is the most frequently reported and should be suspected in patients with the triad of elevated symptoms, foul discharge, and hemorrhage.[49,50]

PATHOGENESIS

The initial step in the pathogenesis of osteomyelitis involves bacterial penetration of the host's external barriers. An open fracture and deep wound provide guaranteed access, but bacteria may also enter through an infection at a remote site. The bacteria must then find their way to the bone. In the case of an open fracture, this typically involves direct inoculation, and with an open wound, it is from spread of the adjacent soft tissue infection. In the case of a remote infection, the bacteria infiltrate the adjacent blood vessels and are carried with the blood to the osseous microvasculature.

Next, bacteria must be presented with an environment conducive to proliferation. This is not easily found in a healthy host as a functioning immune system renders bone quite resistant to bacterial colonization.[17] It is only under certain conditions, such as a very large inoculum (>10^5 organisms),[51-53] ischemic bone and soft tissue, or the presence of a foreign body that infectious pathogens may have an opportunity to take a stand.[53-55] The accumulation of bacteria results in local edema, changes in pH, and the release of inflammatory mediators and catabolic enzymes causing destruction of bony trabeculae.[44] Although the steps involved differ slightly between the different routes of infection, the common feature in chronic osteomyelitis is the creation of devitalized bone, the sequestrum (Fig. 24-2). Around the necrotic bone forms a sheath of reactive bone, the involucrum, which effectively shields the area from the bloodstream much like a walled-off abscess.

When microorganisms are transmitted to bone via a hematogenous route, the pathogens have a predilection for infiltration of metaphyseal end arteries, especially in the skeletally immature, and the highly vascular vertebral bodies. This instigates a robust inflammatory response with an influx of inflammatory cells. This increased volume within the inelastic walls of the haversian system results in increased intraosseous pressure and an occlusion of normal blood flow.[56] The resulting ischemic condition sets the stage for the development of chronic osteomyelitis. However, in this instance, it is possible to interrupt the progression with early administration of antibiotics. As a result, in regions where modern medical care is readily available, acute hematogenous infection can be arrested before it evolves into chronic osteomyelitis.[14]

In contrast, the patient with an open fracture often presents with a high level of bacterial contamination, foreign debris, and ischemic bone due to the trauma. Surprisingly, not all of these situations actually progress to osteomyelitis.[57] For osteomyelitis to develop, the microbe must not only penetrate the

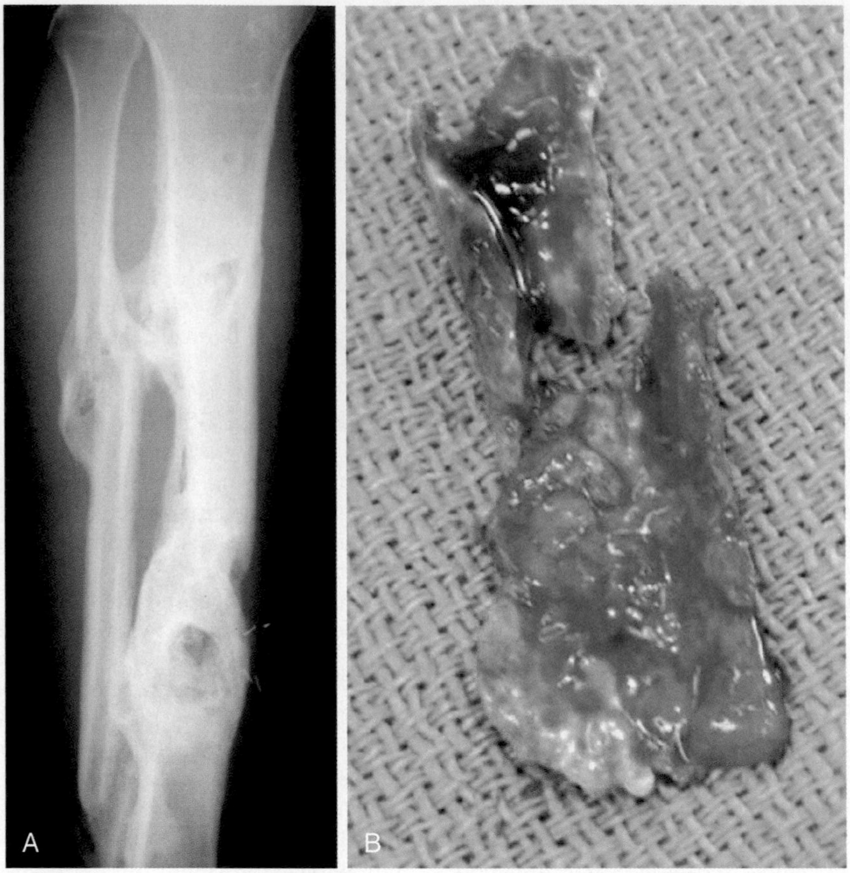

Figure 24-2. A, Radiograph of tibia and fibula chronic osteomyelitis showing sclerotic dead bone and (**B**) sequestrum removed at time of débridement.

host's external defenses but actually become adherent to the underlying bone. This involves a complex interplay of intermolecular forces that allows binding of bacterial glycoproteinaceous structures (adhesins) to cell surface receptors and the extracellular matrix of the host tissue. The bacteria-host interaction is strain specific with bacteria showing varied expression of adhesins for multiple host proteins and glycoproteins, including collagen, bone sialoprotein, elastin, fibronectin, laminin, albumin, and fibrinogen, among others.[14,53,58] These molecules are exposed to a greater degree with bone injury facilitating bacterial colonization.

Furthermore, necrotic bone fragments act as avascular foci for further bacterial adherence. Thus, as the osteonecrotic area expands, the disease is perpetuated by exposure of an increasing number of sites to which opportunistic bacteria can bind. In cases of chronic osteomyelitis secondary to internal fixation, the hardware itself serves as a surface for adhesion.[53,58-61]

Once anchored to the substratum, bacteria aggregate and proliferate within an extracellular polysaccharide matrix, known as a biofilm or "slime" layer.[62] The microbial inhabitants of this biofilm-protected environment undergo complex changes in behavior regulated through intercellular signaling. This cell-to-cell communication occurs through the release of simple hormone-like molecules and is known as *quorum sensing*.[14] The effects include altered gene expression, regulated cell growth and division, as well as lowered metabolic rate. This interaction is likely an adaptation that allows bacterial colonies the ability to manage their nutritional resources. The biofilm also provides resistance to antimicrobials resulting in a significantly elevated minimum inhibitory concentration (MIC) of antibiotics necessary for controlling the infection, usually exceeding the capabilities of systemic antibiotics. In addition, the biofilm has a direct impact on immune function by inhibiting the activity of B and T lymphocytes and resisting phagocytosis of bacterial cells.[14,16,53]

After bacteria successfully adhere to bone, they are able to aggregate and replicate in the devitalized tissue. Effectively sealed off from the host immune system, as well as from antibiotics, the organisms at the avascular focus of infection proliferate undeterred in a medium of dead bone, clotted blood, and dead space. Eventually, the bacteria disperse to adjacent areas of bone and soft tissue and the infection expands. The rapid growth of bacteria can lead to abscess and sinus tract formation. As pus accumulates and abscesses form within the soft tissues adjacent to the necrotic tissue, the patient experiences cyclic episodes of pain followed by drainage. A chronic course ensues without aggressive surgical débridement of all avascular tissue.

MICROBIOLOGY

Although cases of fungal and parasitic bone infections have been reported,[63-65] the vast majority of osteomyelitis is due to bacterial infection.[16] In contrast to acute hematogenous osteomyelitis, which is typically monomicrobial, chronic osteomyelitis involves a polymicrobial infection in a substantial proportion of patients.[66] Given that trauma is the most common cause of adult osteomyelitis, it is no surprise that a combination of bacteria from exposure to water, soil, foreign bodies, and skin flora result in most adult musculoskeletal infections. Despite this, it is important to recognize that certain bacteria may predominate in the pathogenesis of osteomyelitis for a given patient under certain conditions.

Staphylococcus aureus is the most common isolate in all types of bone infection and is implicated in 38% to 67% of chronic osteomyelitis cases.[19,23,67,68] Although coagulase-positive staphylococci *(S. aureus)* are often cultured from the wound at the time of initial inspection, superinfection with multiple other organisms, such as coagulase-negative staphylococci *(Staphylococcus epidermidis)* and aerobic gram-negatives (*Escherichia coli* and *Pseudomonas* species), also occurs.[23] In bone cultures obtained from 100 patients with osteomyelitis, Zuluaga and colleagues[68] found gram-positive aerobes in 89%, gram-negative aerobes in 45%, and anaerobes in 16% of cultures. *Staphylococcus aureus* was found in 43% followed by *Enterococcus faecalis* in 19% and *Pseudomonas* in 14%. Similarly, Cierny and coworkers[19] found staphylococci to be the most common microbiologic finding in cultures from patients with infected tibia nonunions. This was followed by gram-negative rods and anaerobes. In their review, the distribution of bacteria found remained relatively constant from 1981 to 1995, but an increased incidence of methicillin-resistant *S. aureus* (MRSA) was seen in more recent years. Patzakis and colleagues[69] grew 20 different organisms from 36 patients with posttraumatic osteomyelitis. The most frequently occurring isolates in decreasing order of frequency were *S. aureus, Pseudomonas aeruginosa, Bacteriodes* spp., and *S. epidermidis*. Interestingly, data from the University of Connecticut Multidisciplinary Bone Infection Clinic collected over the past 20 years has shown differences in the prevalence of certain organisms depending on the location of chronic osteomyelitis (unpublished data). Although *S. aureus* was the most frequently cultured organism, *Corynebacterium* and *P. aeruginosa* were found more frequently in the pelvis and proximal femur. In contrast, patients with osteomyelitis of the tibia were more likely to be infected with coagulase-negative staph ylococci and enterococci.

Staphylococci are so frequently cultured in bone infection partly because they are ubiquitous organisms and are elements of normal skin flora. Any traumatic event gives these bacteria a conduit to internal tissues. In addition, staphylococci have adapted through natural selection to be particularly virulent in regard to bone and soft tissue infection. For one, *S. aureus* has been shown to express multiple adhesins, including fibronectin-binding proteins and collagen-binding proteins, facilitating attachment to wounded tissue.[14,67] Both *S. aureus* and *S. epidermidis* also produce biofilm-associated protein and polysaccharide intercellular adhesins that facilitate aggregation and the production of a biofilm layer.[62,70] As discussed, the cells protected in this glycocalyx layer are resistant to humoral and cell-mediated immunity, as well as antimicrobial agents, allowing for chronic and recurrent infection.

Another important virulence factor designed to protect *S. aureus* is the ability to gain intracellular access to host cells. Both *S. aureus* and *S. epidermidis* have been shown to invade osteoblasts.[67] Surface proteins, specifically fibronectin-binding protein, allow staphylococci to complex with osteoblast integrins. This results in a series of enzymatic reactions resulting in internalization of the bacterium. Once intracellular, the pathogens can survive and replicate free from the danger of host immunity and antibiotics.[14,67]

Furthermore, staphylococci are highly invasive and destructive when attached to bone. *Staphylococcus* surface-associated material (SAM) has been shown to stimulate osteoclast activity, likely through interaction with host cell receptors and provoking a release of interleukin-1 (IL-1), interleukin-6 (IL-6), and TNF-α.[67] One surface protein, *S. aureus* protein A (SpA), has recently been shown to have an important role in mediating bone destruction. Widaa and colleagues[71] showed that binding of SpA to receptors on osteoblasts interferes with normal metabolic activity and proliferation. Furthermore, the interaction was shown to induce expression of receptor activator of nuclear factor kappa B ligand (RANKL) and secretion of proinflammatory cytokines leading to stimulation of osteoclastogenesis and bone resorption.[71,72]

Although staphylococci are most commonly involved in musculoskeletal infections, and as a result happen to be the most extensively studied, it is important to recognize that many other organisms are frequently involved. As can be seen in Table 24-1, both the mechanism of inoculation and the status of the host influence the microbiologic makeup of the infection. This is important to recognize when choosing empiric antibiotics for a given patient.

Like staphylococci, *P. aeruginosa* is a ubiquitous organism, with soil and fresh water serving as its primary reservoirs.

TABLE 24-1 *MICROORGANISMS AND CLINICAL ASSOCIATION*

Clinical Scenario	Microorganism
Most common in any type of osteomyelitis	*Staphylococcus aureus* (methicillin sensitive or resistant)
Foreign body associated	Coagulase-negative staphylococci or *Propionibacterium* spp.
Soil contamination	*Pseudomonas aeruginosa, Clostridium* spp., *Bacillus* spp., *Nocardia* spp.
Fresh water	*Pseudomonas* spp., *Aeromonas* spp., *Plesiomonas* spp.
Bite wounds	*Pasteurella multocida, Eikenella corrodens*
Diabetic foot lesions	Streptococci, enterococci, *Corynebacterium,* and/or other anaerobic bacteria
Sickle cell disease	*Salmonella* spp., *Streptococcus pneumoniae, Proteus mirabilis, Haemophilus influenzae, Mycobacterium tuberculosis*
HIV infection and immunocompromised patients	*Bartonella henselae, Bartonella quintana, Mycobacteria* spp., *Aspergillus* spp., *Candida albicans*
Vertebral osteomyelitis	Group B and G streptococci, gram-negative bacilli, *M. tuberculosis*

HIV, Human immunodeficiency virus.
Source: *Adapted with permission from Lew DP, Waldvogel FA: Osteomyelitis, Lancet 364:369–379, 2004.*

Puncture wounds of the foot involve *P. aeruginosa* in about 95% of cases,[73] probably because of its prevalence in soil and moist areas of skin. In addition, a soiled, sweaty shoe can serve as a repository of bacteria that are carried on a penetrating object into the patient's foot. *Clostridium, Bacillus,* and *Nocardia* species are also present in soil and have been implicated in certain cases of osteomyelitis following open fracture.[74] Conversely, *Aeromonas* and *Plesiomonas* species are more likely to be present in fresh-water infections.[74] In the event of inoculation through bite wounds, multiple organisms are often found but *Pasteurella multocida* and *Eikenella corrodens* infections may be uniquely involved.[14,74]

Intravenous drug use has long been associated with osteomyelitis likely due to the high frequency of skin puncture, lack of sterile conditions, and the presence of comorbidities commonly found in this population. Allison and coworkers[75] found bone and joint infections of injection drug abusers, as with other causes of osteomyelitis, to be primarily because of *S. aureus*. However, the frequency of infection with *S. epidermidis, P. aeruginosa, Streptococcus,* and anaerobic infections are higher than in studies of nondrug abusers.[68,69,75] Surprisingly, despite the expected hematogenous route of infection in these patients, 46% with osteomyelitis were found to have a polymicrobial infection.[75]

Although HIV has not been clearly linked to an increased incidence of osteomyelitis,[48] the microbiologic profile of the infection in those with HIV appears to be slightly different compared to those without HIV. In a sample of 23 HIV infected patients with osteoarticular infections, Busch and colleagues[38] found an increased incidence of mycobacterial and streptococcus species, although *S. aureus* remained the most frequently identified organism. Other organisms reported in patients with HIV are *Bartonella henselae* and *Bartonella quintana*. Both HIV-infected and immunosuppressed patients are also more susceptible to fungal infections including *Aspergillus* and *Candida*.[74]

Diabetic foot infections often involve a broad range of bacteria. *Staphylococcus, Streptococcus, Pseudomonas, Enterococcus,* and *Corynebacterium* have been found in a high percentage of patients.[32] However, this is not consistent across all studies. Parvez and coworkers[35] took bone cultures from 35 subjects with diabetic foot lesions. The most common organism identified was *E. coli* occurring in 22.7% followed by *Proteus* species in 18.2%. Other bacteria identified in a high number of patients included *Klebsiella pneumoniae, P. aeruginosa, Peptostreptococcus,* and *Clostridium* species. The difference in bacterial makeup found in various studies of diabetic foot infections may be in part due to regional differences, but what is important to recognize is that these infections can involve a wide range of pathogens necessitating broad empiric antibiotic coverage.

Patients with sickle cell disease represent another population at elevated risk for osteomyelitis.[41] There appears to be a predisposition to *Salmonella* infection in these patients.[40,41] Other frequently found organisms include *S. aureus, Proteus mirabilis, Haemophilus influenzae, E. coli,* and *Mycobacterium tuberculosis*.[40,41]

Surgical site infections most commonly involve skin flora. Coagulase-positive and coagulase-negative staphylococci tend to predominate,[29,74] but other organisms, including fungi, may be involved. Similarly, prosthetic-related infections most commonly involve staphylococci.[30,74] In a review of 81 total knee arthroplasty infections, gram-positive cocci including *Staphylococcus, Streptococcus,* and *Enterococcus* predominated.[30] In contrast, *Propionibacterium acnes* is a commonly recognized cause of infection after shoulder arthroplasty.[76,77] This organism may be easily missed as clinical signs are often subtle and growth on culture takes longer than many other organisms.[78,79]

Vertebral osteomyelitis is most commonly caused by hematogenous seeding. As in other infections of hematogenous route, *S. aureus* is the most common pathogen. Other bacteria include group B and G streptococci and various gram-negative bacilli.[14,74] In addition, *M. tuberculosis* involves the spine in approximately 50% of musculoskeletal tuberculosis.[74]

Other atypical causes of osteomyelitis have been reported in the literature. Cryptococcal osteomyelitis has been reported in both long bone and spine infections.[80,81] These infections have been shown to produce lytic bone lesions similar to bacterial infections. In addition, musculoskeletal brucellosis because of *Brucella* infection is a rare cause of osteomyelitis that produces an inflammatory response and subsequent osteolysis.[82] This most commonly involves the sacroiliac joint.[83] Q fever is caused by an infection by *Coxiella burnetii* and has been reported to be a potential cause of osteomyelitis.[84,85]

Widespread use of antibiotics leading to the development of multidrug-resistant organisms is creating ongoing challenges in the treatment of osteomyelitis. A dramatic rise in the frequency of MRSA infections has occurred in the past 20 years.[21,75] The presence of MRSA in patients with osteomyelitis ranges from 33% to 55%.[74] Vancomycin-resistant enterococci have also been on the rise over the past 15 years.[74] This is especially evident in military data of wartime injuries. In a study of 137 Iraqi civilians with combat-related injuries, 55% were found to be infected with multidrug-resistant organisms.[86] Resistant organisms found in this study included Enterobacteriaceae, MRSA, and *Acinetobacter baumannii*.

CLASSIFICATION

Several systems exist for classifying osteomyelitis.[14,87-90] First, a distinction is often made between acute and chronic osteomyelitis. A precise definition is lacking for what constitutes acute osteomyelitis,[16,34] but this is typically used to represent infection occurring within days to weeks of inoculation and presenting with systemic signs and symptoms of infection.[14,91] In contrast, as was previously discussed, chronic osteomyelitis describes a bone infection in the presence of necrotic bone.[14] It has been reported that chronic osteomyelitis is the consequence of untreated acute osteomyelitis. However, although this may occur in some cases, most cases of adult osteomyelitis occur because of inoculation of injured bone at the time of a traumatic event. In this case, the initial injury is likely to lead to bone ischemia and subsequent necrosis prior to the development of signs and symptoms of osteomyelitis. As a result, osteomyelitis following trauma is usually considered "chronic" from the start.

Another method of distinguishing between forms of osteomyelitis is by the route of inoculation. Pathogens may be delivered to bone by hematogenous seeding, direct inoculation, or spread from a contiguous focus.[17,44,91] Contiguous-focus osteomyelitis can be further divided into that occurring with and without vascular insufficiency.[36,44] Hematogenous osteomyelitis occurs most commonly in the pediatric population, but has been reported to account for up to 20% of adult bone infections.[91] Direct inoculation occurs when an open fracture exposes bone to the external environment. Contiguous-focus osteomyelitis is the result of direct spread from local soft tissue infection or due to a nosocomial infection occurring from a postoperative wound infection.[92] When vascular insufficiency is present, as is often the result in diabetics and those with peripheral vascular disease, the patient's ability to fight soft tissue infection is compromised resulting in a predisposition to chronic osteomyelitis.

Although differentiating between routes of infection can be helpful for communication and helping to predict the microbiologic profile, it provides little help with determining the most appropriate treatment. It is well accepted that chronic osteomyelitis will almost invariably persist without surgical intervention. However, deciding the best treatment for the patient is based on multiple factors including the status of the host, the location of infection, and the effect of the disease on patient function. For this reason, the Cierny-Mader[89] classification is helpful for guiding treatment.

The Cierny-Mader staging system classifies bone infection on the basis of two independent factors: (1) the anatomic area of bone involved and (2) the physiologic status of the host. By combining one of the four anatomic types of osteomyelitis (I, medullary; II, superficial; III, localized; or IV, diffuse) (Fig. 24-3) with one of the three classes of host immunocompetence (A, B, or C), this system arrives at 12 clinical stages.[89] As described by Cierny and colleagues, the primary lesion in *medullary osteomyelitis* (type I) is endosteal and confined to the intramedullary (IM) surfaces of bone (e.g., a hematogenous osteomyelitis or an infection of an IM rod). *Superficial osteomyelitis* (type II) is a true contiguous-focus infection in which the outermost layer of bone becomes infected from an adjacent source, such as a decubitus ulcer or a burn. *Localized osteomyelitis* (type III) produces full-thickness cortical cavitation within a segment of stable bone. It is frequently observed in the setting of open fractures or when bone becomes infected from an adjacent implant. When the infected fracture does not heal and there is through-and-through disease of the hard and soft tissue, the condition is called *diffuse osteomyelitis* (type IV). Patients with posttraumatic osteomyelitis almost always have type III or type IV disease.

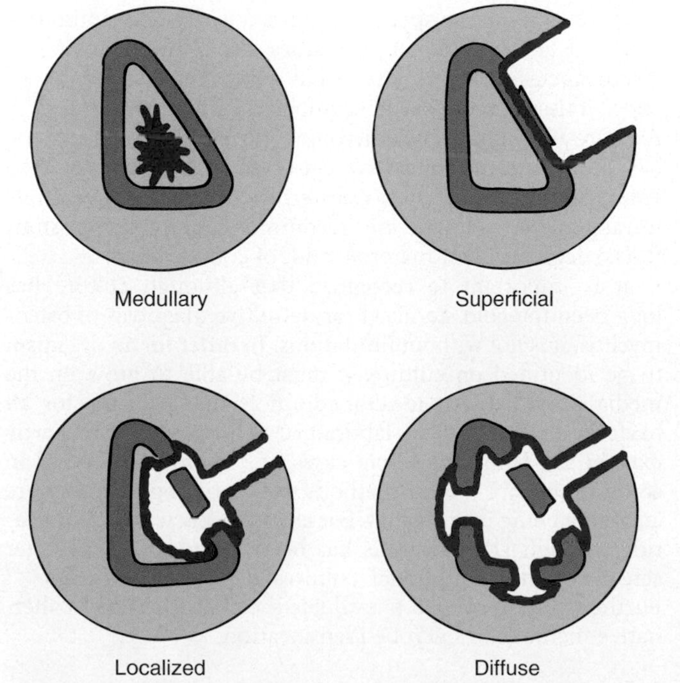

Figure 24-3. Anatomic types of osteomyelitis as they relate to the osseous location. *(Redrawn from Cierny G 3rd, Mader J, Penninck J: Adult osteomyelitis, Contemp Orthop 10(5):21, 1985.)*

The host condition portion of the Cierny-Mader classification stratifies patients according to their ability to mount an immune response and heal surgical wounds. A patient with a normal physiologic response is labeled an *A host,* a compromised patient a *B host,* and a patient who is so compromised that surgical intervention poses a greater risk than the infection itself is designated a *C host.* A further stratification is made in *B* hosts on the basis of whether the patient has a local (B^{L}), systemic (B^{S}), or combined ($B^{S,L}$) deficiency in wound healing. An example of a local deficit in wound healing would be venous stasis at the site of injury, whereas systemic deficits would include malnutrition, renal failure, diabetes, tobacco or alcohol use, or acquired immunodeficiency syndrome.

The physiologic classification also includes an assessment of the level of disability caused by the infection. This is an important variable in treatment planning for patients with compromised health. Although eradication of chronic osteomyelitis requires surgery, the morbidity and mortality risk associated with a major operation may outweigh the benefit if limited improvement in quality of life is expected.[89] Even though systemic spread of infection is a constant concern, antibiotic suppression of infection may be a reasonable goal for select patients.

Each classification system has strengths and limitations. They are all useful for communication and, to some extent, treatment planning. For chronic osteomyelitis, classification based on the route of inoculation is simple and easy to remember. The Cierny-Mader classification is more comprehensive and is more useful in terms of operative planning. However, as with all classification systems, it is impossible to capture the complexities of each individual with a few categories. Therefore, to optimize outcomes, it is necessary to follow a systematic approach, which is detailed in the next section, to gain a complete understanding of the patient's overall condition.

DIAGNOSIS

History

A detailed history not only facilitates making the diagnosis but also provides important information for planning treatment and predicting outcomes. Osteomyelitis should be suspected in anyone with bone pain who has a past history of trauma or orthopaedic surgery. Complaints often include persistent pain, erythema, swelling, and drainage of the involved area. Walenkamp and coworkers[93] described cyclical pain, increasing to "severe deep tense pain with fever," that often subsides when pus breaks through in a fistula. Although these symptoms are present for some, they certainly do not occur in everyone with the disease. Most often, symptoms are vague and generalized (e.g., "my leg is red and sore"), making it difficult to differentiate between cellulitis and a true bone infection.

In addition to patient symptoms, it is important to collect details regarding past trauma and surgery. In cases of prior trauma to the involved bone, it is important to establish the mechanism of injury and the treatment provided. If there was a previously diagnosed soft tissue or bone infection, the culture results should be reviewed along with previous antibiotics given. Furthermore, the ability of a host's soft tissues to heal and clear infection are largely dependent on the presence of comorbid conditions.[94] Vascular compromise, extremity edema, extensive scarring, and a history of radiotherapy impact soft tissue healing.[94] In addition, systemic factors including diabetes, poor nutritional status, chronic kidney disease, and immune deficiency may impact outcomes of surgery and must be considered in weighing the decision to attempt limb salvage versus amputation.

Physical Examination

Inspection of the soft tissues is the first step in a comprehensive physical examination. Erythema, open wounds, and draining sinuses strongly suggest an underlying infection. In the presence of exposed soft tissue or bone, the diagnosis is confirmed (Fig. 24-4). However, signs of osteomyelitis are often subtle. Fever is often absent and in cases of infected nonunions, the skin may appear benign.[95] Even small trivial-appearing skin lesions should be probed to determine depth, as a sinus tract extending to bone is pathognomonic for osteomyelitis (Fig. 24-5), The involved site should be palpated for tenderness, swelling, and structural abnormalities. Old fracture sites should be stressed and adjacent joints must be thoroughly examined. In addition, the length and alignment of the limb along with general functional limitations should be assessed.

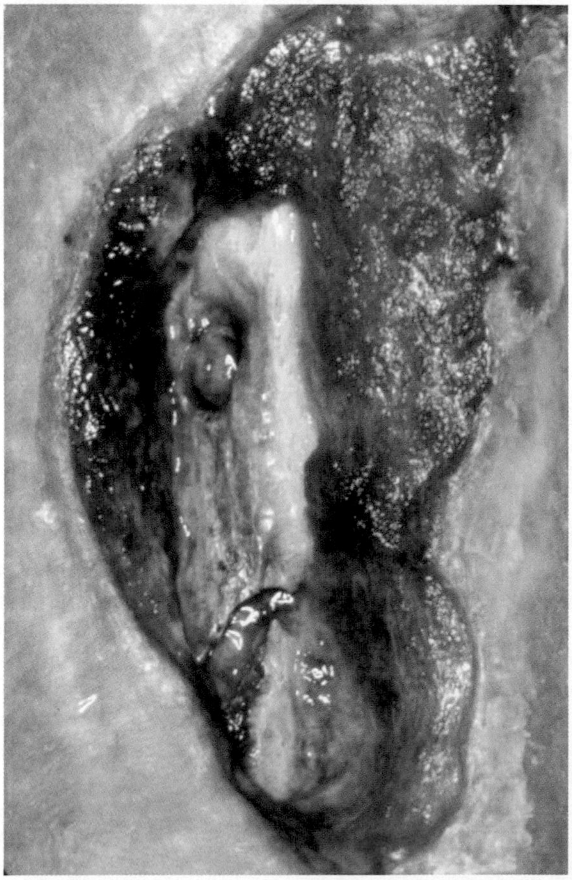

Figure 24-4. Exposed bone is an obvious sign that an underlying skeletal infection is present.

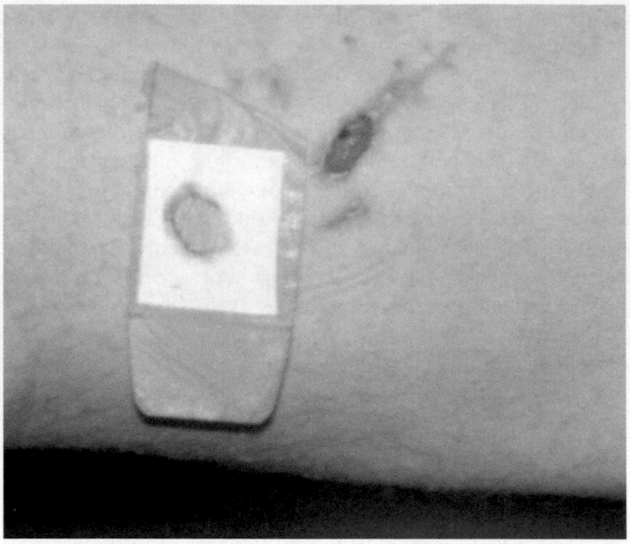

Figure 24-5. Even benign-appearing lesions must be carefully inspected and probed as is the case of this slow-draining sinus from a patient with osteomyelitis.

Cultures

Culturing drainage fluid and swabbing open wounds is often performed in the office setting. Although potentially helpful in identifying causative bacteria and guiding antibiotic choice, these results must be interpreted with caution, because such specimens often yield opportunistic organisms that have simply colonized the nutrient-rich exudate. In a prospective study[68] of 100 patients with chronic osteomyelitis, cultures taken from nonbone specimens agreed with bone cultures in only 30% of patients. Other studies also showed significant discrepancies in the results of cultures taken from drainage and soft tissue cultures when compared with bone cultures.[69,96] As a result, conclusive microbiologic diagnosis should be based on deep intraoperative cultures rather than needle or swab cultures taken in a nonsterile environment. Multiple intraoperative cultures are recommended including sinus tracts, deep purulent material, and, of course, bone.[34]

It is important to recognize that although culture has long been the gold standard for definitive diagnosis of osteomyelitis, it is not without limitations. In order for an organism to be identified on culture, it must be able to grow on the media provided. An ideal medium is not available for all bacteria in the clinical laboratory setting and may partly explain the culture-negative cases of osteomyelitis found in some studies.[19,68] Newer methods of identifying microbes are currently being investigated. For example, bacterial identification through DNA analysis has been found to have greater sensitivity than traditional cultures of infected wounds.[97,98] Further study is needed to evaluate the clinical utility of alternative methods of microbe identification.

Laboratory Values

White blood cell (WBC) counts, erythrocyte sedimentation rate (ESR), and C-reactive protein (CRP) levels have traditionally been part of the workup of any patient with suspected musculoskeletal infection. In an immunocompetent individual, elevated levels of these laboratory values are fairly sensitive indicators of some sort of acute infection. However, there is a paucity of studies showing a correlation between laboratory values and the presence of bone infection, although one group of investigators has shown CRP to be useful in the early detection of sequelae-prone acute osteomyelitis.[99] Most laboratory values are rather nonspecific to skeletal infection and, thus, add little to the clinician's ability to distinguish a superficial inflammatory process, such as a cellulitis, from a deeper, osteomyelitic one. Furthermore, although theoretically helpful in screening for an *acute* infection, the WBC count, ESR, and CRP are frequently normal in the setting of *chronic* osteomyelitis and, thus, are neither sensitive nor specific for it.[100]

Nutritional parameters, such as albumin, prealbumin, and transferrin, are helpful to obtain in the workup of a patient with suspected chronic osteomyelitis so that malnutrition can be identified and reversed before taking the patient to the operating room. Orthopaedic surgery patients who are malnourished have significantly higher infection rates than those who have a normal nutritional status.[101] Presumably, it would follow that patients who already have infection present would be more likely to respond to therapy if their nutrition were optimized beforehand.

Imaging

Diagnostic imaging plays an integral role in evaluating patients with known or suspected osteomyelitis, facilitating disease localization and preoperative planning. Early diagnosis is critical, allowing timely therapy and preventing many of the unfortunate complications.

Plain radiographs are the most appropriate initial imaging modality for patients with suspected or confirmed osteomyelitis.[18] Radiographs are inexpensive, readily available, and can reveal periosteal reaction, cortical erosion, endosteal scalloping and radiolucent or osteolytic lesions, as seen in Brodie abscess[18,102] (Fig. 24-6). Radiographs may demonstrate involucrum (layer of new living bone formed about necrotic bone), sequestrum (fragment of dead bone separated from viable parent bone by granulation tissue), and cloaca (opening in the involucrum through which granulation tissue and/or sequestra can be discharged), all hallmarks of subacute to chronic osteomyelitis.[103] Additional radiographic findings may indicate septic arthritis (loss of joint space and osseous erosions) and soft tissue infection (swelling, radiolucent streaks, and periostitis). However, radiographs have been shown to have a sensitivity and specificity of only 0.60 and 0.67, respectively, in diagnosing chronic osteomyelitis limiting their usefulness as an isolated study.[104] Other imaging modalities, namely magnetic resonance imaging (MRI) and nuclear scintigraphy, provide an accurate diagnosis at an earlier stage of disease.

The now widespread availability of MRI has greatly facilitated the diagnosis and localization of bone infection, particularly in the acute stage. MRI offers superior soft tissue contrast, delineating soft tissue infection and abscess as well as sinus tract communication with bone and/or joints. Abnormal bone marrow signal, manifesting as low signal on T1-weighted fast spin echo and high signal on T2-weighted images, is typical for acute osteomyelitis.[103] Subacute and chronic osteomyelitis have a more variable MRI appearance, although

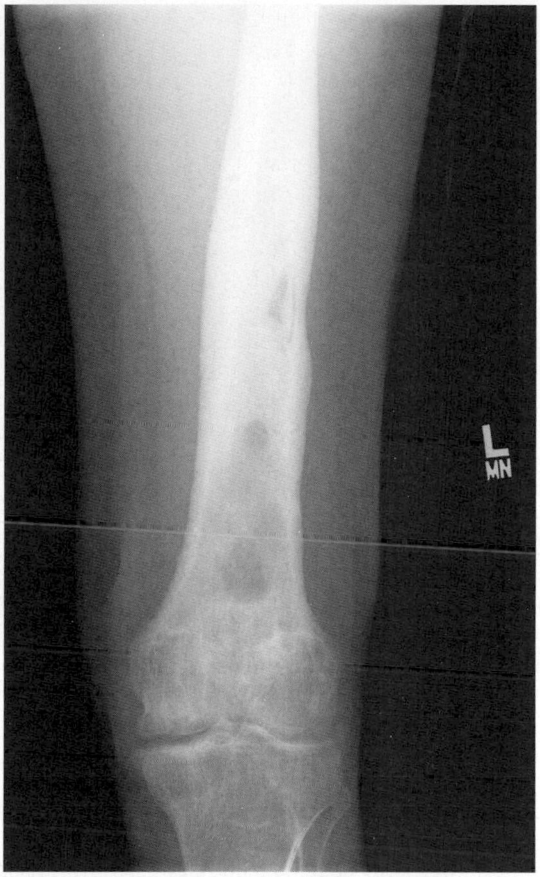

Figure 24-6. Osteomyelitis of the femur showing characteristic radiolucent lesions with cortical erosion and periosteal reaction.

chronic active cases do show similar signal characteristics.[103] Short tau inversion recovery (STIR) sequences show markedly increased fluid signal in areas of osteomyelitis and soft tissue infection.

Following IV administration of gadolinium contrast, areas of vascularized inflammatory tissue will enhance. Nonvascularized soft tissue abscesses will typically demonstrate peripheral and/or marginal enhancement. Brodie abscesses appear as well-defined regions of intraosseous low signal intensity on T1-weighted images with corresponding high-signal intensity on T2-weighted images; they may be further delineated with IV gadolinium contrast[103] (Fig. 24-7). Sequestra, although more clearly identified on computed tomography (CT), appear as regions of low to intermediate signal on both T1- and T2-weighted images and are notable for their lack of gadolinium enhancement. In cases of septic arthritis, inflamed synovium will enhance with gadolinium.[103] Despite the high sensitivity of MRI in identifying osteomyelitis, challenges remain. Distinguishing osteomyelitis from surrounding bone marrow edema remains difficult. Similarly, distinguishing soft tissue extension of infection from soft tissue edema is also a challenge. In cases of chronic osteomyelitis, differentiating active from inactive disease can be problematic. MRI resolution is also limited by metal artifact, making it less useful in cases of suspected periprosthetic infection.

The primary utility of CT in musculoskeletal infection is in delineating extent of osseous and soft tissue disease.[103] Many of the CT abnormalities in osteomyelitis are shared by both

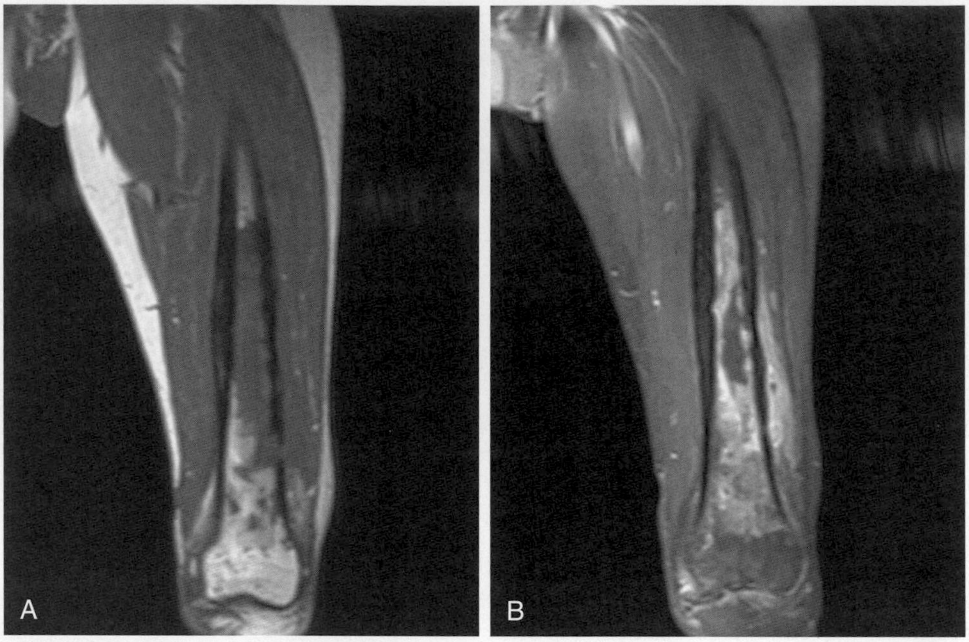

Figure 24-7. A, Coronal T1-weighted magnetic resonance imaging (MRI) with fat saturation showing low signal intensity in femoral diaphysis. **B,** Coronal T1-weighted MRI with fat saturation postcontrast showing enhancement of femoral diaphysis with nonenhancing abscess.

primary bone and metastatic tumors, including cortical bone destruction, new bone formation, and soft tissue mass. Gas within the medullary canal, best visualized with CT, is an uncommon but highly specific feature of osteomyelitis, analogous to the presence of gas within soft tissue abscesses.[103] CT may also reveal cortical sequestra and cloacae, as well as bone and soft tissue abscesses. In addition, CT is useful for gauging the amount of bony bridging in fracture healing to guide the timing of fixation removal.

Three-phase nuclear medicine bone scans using ^{99m}technetium (^{99m}Tc)-methylenediphosphonate (MDP) is a mainstay of musculoskeletal infection imaging, particularly for those patients *without* underlying bone disease, fractures, or orthopaedic prostheses.[103] ^{99m}Tc phosphonates are readily available. They provide a short physical half-life (6 hours) and a gamma energy of 140 keV, ideal for the gamma camera. Following injection, ^{99m}Tc-MDP flows through arteries and into capillaries, with leakage into the extracapillary space. Increased capillary permeability may be seen in infection, trauma, and tumors.[103] ^{99m}Tc-MDP also localizes to new bone formation, depositing in bone mineral and/or bone matrix. Increased tracer uptake on early blood flow and blood pool phases with absent or only mild uptake on the delayed phase is consistent with soft tissue infection. A fourth phase 24-hour scan may be helpful if the initial three-phase scan is nondiagnostic; increased uptake on all three or four phases of the bone scan is consistent with osteomyelitis.[103] It is important to note that three-phase bone scan positivity is nonspecific; that is, fractures, tumors, and other bone abnormalities may show a similar scintigraphic appearance (Fig. 24-8). Yet, in intact bone (i.e., normal radiographs), the sensitivity and specificity for osteomyelitis with three-phase bone scan is well over 90%.[105] In the presence of fracture or prior surgery, specificity drops substantially. Septic arthritis is characterized by hyperemia on early phase imaging and diffusely increased tracer uptake on delayed images. Again, these findings are nonspecific and may be seen with noninfectious inflammatory arthritis.[103]

Indium 111 (^{111}In)-labeled leukocyte scintigraphy is often used for confirmation or exclusion of musculoskeletal infection in patients with underlying bone disease and/or hardware. The radiotracer (labeled WBC) localizes to areas of infection rather than remodeled bone, as infection and/or abscess consists primarily of leukocytes.[106] The labeling process is labor intensive; roughly 50 mL of autologous blood is drawn into a syringe, red blood cells and platelets are separated, and

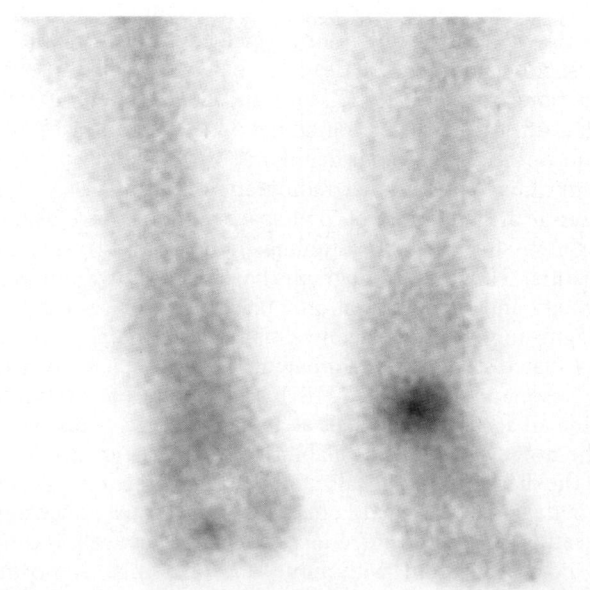

Figure 24-8. ^{99m}Technetium-methylenediphosphonate (MDP) showing increased uptake at the left ankle. On further imaging, this patient was found to have a fracture of the distal tibia.

leukocytes are then labeled with radiotracer and subsequently injected via a peripheral vein within 2 to 4 hours. Images are typically acquired 18 to 24 hours after radiotracer injection, allowing sufficient time for WBC localization and blood pool clearance.[106] Focal uptake greater than or equal to that in the liver or spleen is typical for an abscess. Potential sources for false-negative studies include nonpyogenic abscess, chronic low-grade infection, and vertebral osteomyelitis. False-positive results may be caused by healing fractures and surgical wounds. In cases where marrow distribution is not normal, that is, cases of previous disease, orthopaedic hardware or tumor, determining whether focal uptake represents infection versus atypical normal distribution is difficult. In these equivocal cases, combining the ^{111}In-labeled leukocyte study with a ^{99m}Tc sulfur colloid bone marrow study can improve specificity.[105,106] In the absence of infection, radiotracer distribution in the two studies is similar. If localized infection is present, osteomyelitis will appear as a photopenic defect on sulfur colloid owing to marrow displacement by underlying infection. Discordance between ^{111}In-labeled leukocyte and ^{99m}Tc sulfur colloid studies is consistent with osteomyelitis.[106,107]

There are disadvantages to using ^{111}In-labeled leukocytes. As ^{111}In is cyclotron produced, many hospitals, lacking facilities and personnel for radiolabeling, send the patient's blood to an outside commercial radiopharmacy.[106] The handling of patient's blood is also not without risk; misadministration to the wrong patient has unfortunately been reported. The rather long (18 to 24 hour) time delay between reinjection of labeled WBCs and imaging may be suboptimal for clinical decision making.[106] Also, the relatively high radiation dose to the spleen (the target organ) is of particular concern for pediatric patients, whose smaller blood volume distribution means a higher radiation dose.

Leukocyte labeling may be alternatively performed with ^{99m}Tc hexamethylpropyleneamine oxime (HMPAO) (Fig. 24-9). ^{99m}Tc-HMPAO offers a lower radiation dose and thus, allows a higher administered activity.[106] As it is a technetium-based compound, imaging also begins much sooner, typically

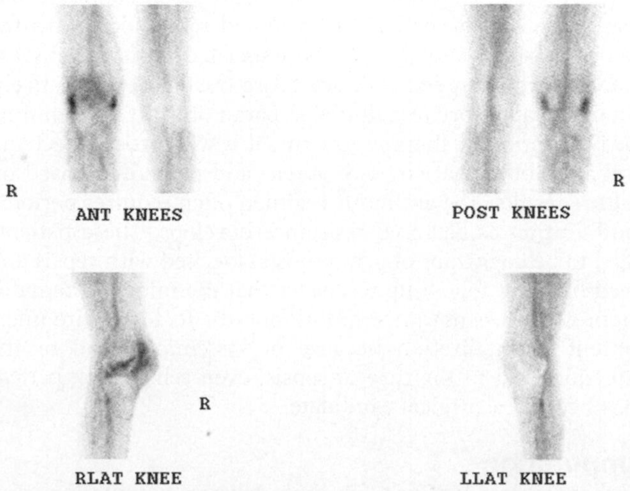

Figure 24-9. ^{99m}Technetium-tagged white blood cell (WBC) study shows an infected right knee prosthesis, and a noninfected left knee prosthesis. *ANT,* Anterior; *LLAT,* left lateral; *POST,* posterior; *RLAT,* right lateral. *(Image courtesy of Ronald J. Rosenberg, MD, FACNM, Director of Nuclear Medicine, Jefferson Radiology, PC.)*

1 to 2 hours after administration. Although this shortened examination time does provide images much sooner than with indium, the 18- to 24-hour window between injection and imaging with indium allows more time for leukocytes to migrate to sites of infection. Again, there are trade-offs. An important downside to using ^{99m}Tc HMPAO–labeled leukocytes is the inability to perform dual isotope imaging.[106]

Gallium 67 (^{67}Ga-citrate) scintigraphy is somewhat accurate for diagnosing low-grade, often indolent musculoskeletal infections, particularly vertebral osteomyelitis.[103] Similar to ^{99m}Tc-MDP, ^{67}Ga-citrate localizes to normal bone and will show greater accumulation at sites of increased bone turnover. ^{67}Ga-citrate images may be interpreted in conjunction with ^{99m}Tc MDP bone scans for better specificity; a positive dual isotope study will show either increased ^{67}Ga-citrate activity relative to technetium or dissimilar tracer distributions[106] (Fig. 24-10). Accuracy of such combined ^{67}Ga-citrate studies, however, remains inferior to dual isotope leukocyte imaging.

Positron emission tomography (PET) combined with CT holds great promise in the evaluation of osteomyelitis, offering both physiologic assessment of glucose metabolism and anatomic localization (Fig. 24-11). Briefly, the radiotracer fluorine 18 (^{18}F) fluorodeoxyglucose (FDG) is transported into cells by glucose transporters and phosphorylated by a hexokinase enzyme but not metabolized. The amount of cellular FDG uptake is related to both the number of glucose transporters and cellular metabolic rate.[108] Increased FDG accumulation in tumors, as well as sites of inflammation and infection, is caused by the greater number of glucose transporters in such diseased tissues. In the case of infection and inflammation, macrophages and leukocytes accumulate ^{18}F-FDG.[107] To minimize FDG uptake in normal tissue, patients will fast for at least several hours (typically overnight) prior to examination so as to reduce competition for glucose transporters.[108] While studies have shown the utility of PET for diagnosing osteomyelitis, FDG will also accumulate at sites of acute fracture, inflammatory arthritis, and healing bone following surgery. Moreover, because FDG accumulates in bone marrow, any condition that results in a hypercellular marrow state, such as those patients receiving granulocyte colony-stimulating factor (GCSF) following chemotherapy, will show elevated FDG activity. PET-CT has shown both high sensitivity and specificity for diagnosing spinal osteomyelitis.[108] PET-CT has not shown accuracy in differentiating loosening from infection in those with joint prostheses, not all too surprising when one considers that inflammation is present in both aseptic loosening and infection.[108] For these patients, dual isotope imaging with ^{111}In-labeled leukocytes and ^{99m}Tc sulfur colloid bone marrow scan remains the gold standard.[108,109]

MANAGEMENT

Overview

As discussed in the previous sections, osteomyelitis is a complex, multifaceted disease with highly varied presentation. Attempts at classification to guide treatment have been beneficial for communication, decreasing bias in research, and focusing treatment options. However, models have necessarily been simplistic and leave a broad area of judgment to the physician and patient in determining the most appropriate

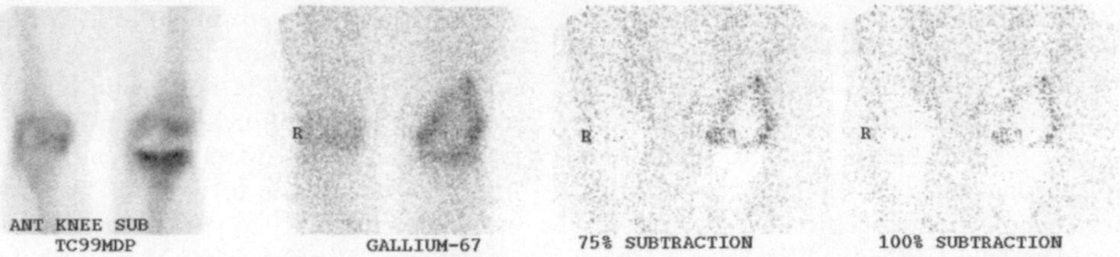

Figure 24-10. ^{99m}Technetium-methylenediphosphonate (^{99m}Tc-MDP) with gallium 67-citrate subtraction (*SUB*) shows increased uptake around left total knee arthroplasty with abnormal gallium excess on subtraction consistent with periprosthetic infection. *ANT,* Anterior. *(Image courtesy of Ronald J. Rosenberg, MD, FACNM, Director of Nuclear Medicine, Jefferson Radiology, PC.)*

intervention. As a result, we feel that the best management of chronic osteomyelitis involves a multidisciplinary approach incorporating the expertise of an orthopaedic surgeon, an infectious disease specialist, and in many cases, a plastic surgeon. For most of our patients, we also involve an internal medicine physician, nutritionist, wound care nurse, and physical therapist.

It is important to mention that given the challenge and extensive resources necessary for managing chronic osteomyelitis, prevention is obviously most desirable. Early administration of antibiotics along with prompt irrigation and débridement should be performed for all open fractures. Recent evidence has shown that early transfer to a definitive trauma center may be the most important factor in decreasing risk of infection following high-energy open fractures.[25]

The only definitive "cure" for osteomyelitis involves surgical elimination of all devitalized tissue. However, persistent infection with associated pain and chronic drainage are not absolute indications for surgery.[94] Before considering surgery, a few factors must be considered. First, one must assess the health status of the patient in terms of risk associated with major surgical intervention. The physiologic status of the patient not only influences whether or not surgery should be performed, but also what surgery is most reasonable. If the risk of surgery outweighs the risk of the disease, palliative treatment is most appropriate. For those considered safe to undergo surgery but presenting with multiple comorbidities, the ability to recover from multiple extensive surgeries and prolonged immobility, as is often necessary with limb salvage approaches, may be limited. However, if only a small area of débridement is needed, a surgical approach may still be recommended. Alternatively, in some patients, amputation may be desirable as it eliminates some of the risks associated with reconstruction and may allow a more rapid functional recovery.

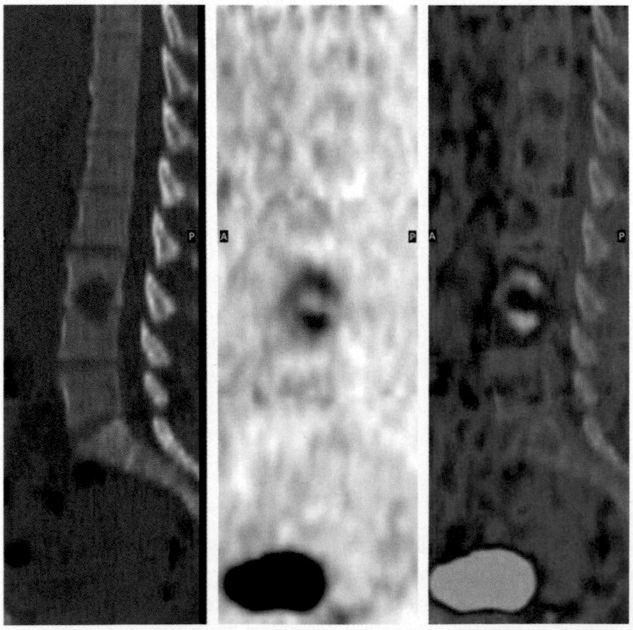

Figure 24-11. Positron emission tomography (PET)/computed tomography (CT) showing vertebral osteomyelitis involving the L3-L4 vertebral bodies. *(Image courtesy of Ronald J. Rosenberg, MD, FACNM, Director of Nuclear Medicine, Jefferson Radiology, PC.)*

Another critical factor to consider is the patient's goals. Even if limb salvage is feasible and the patient is healthy enough to undergo extensive surgical intervention, the patient may not wish to endure the multiple surgeries, physical and emotional hardship, and potential for failure in taking this route. As is shown in Figure 24-12, multiple treatment options must be considered for the patient with chronic osteomyelitis. These must be considered in the context of the individual patient to find the most appropriate intervention.

Suppressive Therapy

As has been discussed, chronic osteomyelitis can only be eradicated with surgical intervention. However, for a select group of patients, a palliative approach may be appropriate. The aim is not complete elimination of the infectious organisms, but rather, their suppression. This is typically reserved for patients in whom the morbidity and potential mortality of surgery is greater than the risk of chronic infection. It may also be chosen by patients who would rather deal with the recurrent signs and symptoms associated with the disease than undergo surgery. Even for those treated nonoperatively, obtaining appropriate cultures is paramount to determining the best antibiotic therapy. Treatment is with broad-spectrum oral antibiotics that cover *S. aureus* and is tailored based on culture results. The antibiotic regimen often requires periodic modification as bacterial resistance develops. These patients need to be cognizant of symptoms associated with sepsis and need frequent follow-up to ensure that the infection remains suppressed. It is not uncommon for patients to require intermittent hospitalization because of systemic spread of the infection, and in the case of sepsis, even a high-risk patient may become a surgical candidate.

Amputation

With improved options for limb salvage, amputation as a treatment for chronic osteomyelitis has dramatically decreased over the past 20 years.[110] Despite this trend, primary amputation rates are around 10% of patients with chronic osteomyelitis.[110] In most cases, these are performed for patients

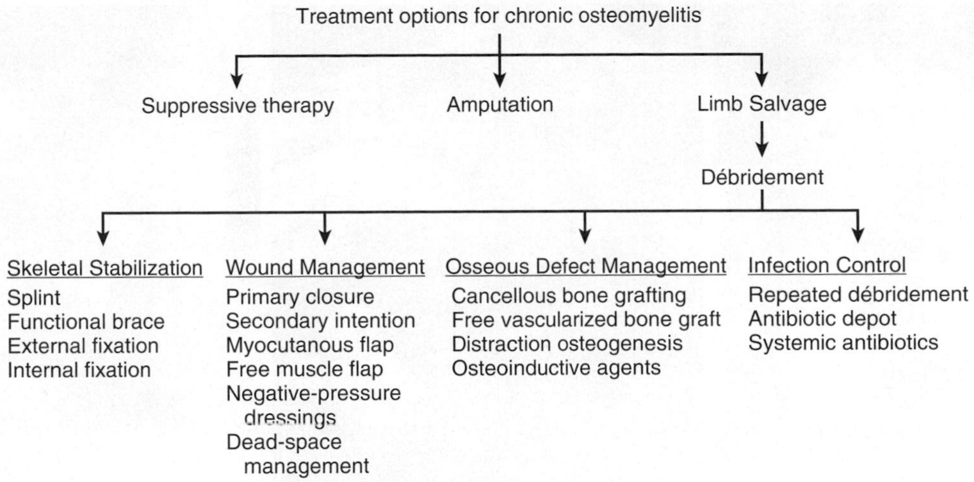

Figure 24-12. Treatment options algorithm.

who would be unable to tolerate the multiple surgeries and long rehabilitation associated with limb reconstruction. In addition, a small but substantial group of patients who attempt limb salvage will ultimately require amputation. However, amputation should not necessarily be viewed as a "bailout" procedure. Primary amputation along with modern prosthetic fitting and training can lead to a high level of function and relatively rapid recovery. Amputation is associated with shorter length of hospitalization, fewer operations, and quicker return to work compared to patients undergoing limb salvage.[111] Furthermore, in a recent study of combat-related extremity injuries, Doukas and colleagues[112] found, compared with limb reconstruction procedures, patients who had a limb amputation had a higher functional level, lower risk of post-traumatic stress disorder (PTSD), and were more likely to be engaged in vigorous sports.

Historically, at the time of amputation, little consideration was given for the postoperative recovery in terms of creating a stump favorable for prosthetic use.[113] It is now recognized that several variables have an impact on future function following limb amputation. The level of amputation is a key variable with above-knee amputations (AKAs) resulting in significantly greater energy expenditure, slower walking speed, shorter maximum walking distance, and greater pain compared with below-knee amputations (BKAs).[114-116] Through-the-knee amputations have also been used when the proximal tibia cannot be reasonably salvaged. These have had varied results in the literature, with some studies showing improved function and some showing worse function compared to AKA.[115,116] However, a consistent finding with through-the-knee amputations is difficulty with prosthetic fitting and pain with prosthetic use.[113,115,116]

In addition to the decision of which bone to amputate, the surgeon must consider the residual stump length and morphology. For example, if BKA is performed and too little tibia is left intact, the prosthetic socket may be too short for ideal function.[113] Conversely, if an amputation is performed immediately proximal to the ankle, it may be challenging to fit the prosthetic components between the stump and the prosthetic foot without creating a leg length discrepancy. Although standards, such as 15 cm distal to the tibial tubercle for BKAs have been described,[117] in many cases, a brief discussion with a prosthetist may facilitate an improved functional outcome.

Multiple types of soft tissue flaps can be used for stump coverage. For example, in BKAs, sagittal flaps, skew flaps, and the traditional long posterior flaps have each been described. In a Cochrane review,[118] no difference in outcomes were found between different flap types. However, a two-stage amputation, involving an initial guillotine followed by revision amputation, has resulted in improved outcomes for treatment of wet gangrene.[118] In a large retrospective database study, O'Brien and coworkers[119] found the overall failure rate for lower extremity amputations was 12.7% (12.6%, BKA; 8.1%, AKA; and 26.4%, transmetatarsal). Some of the factors associated with failure included emergency operation, sepsis, end-stage renal disease, obesity, and tobacco abuse.

Although multiple amputation options are available, BKA is most commonly used in our orthopaedic trauma population. The following is our technique and postoperative care.

Technique

For BKA (Fig. 24-13), we proceed systematically through each compartment of the lower leg, first dissecting the soft tissues of the anterior compartment and isolating the anterior tibial vessels and deep peroneal nerve. The vessels are clamped and the nerves resected as proximal as possible to avoid neuroma formation at the distal stump. Using a periosteal elevator, the periosteum of the tibia should be stripped distally from the planned level of transection. This process is continued posteriorly, carefully avoiding damage to the vessels of the deep posterior compartment. The fibula is then cleared of soft tissue a few centimeters proximal to the level of the planned tibial transection. Both the tibia and fibula are transected, usually with an oscillating or Gigli saw. The posterior tibial and peroneal vessels are then isolated and clamped and the tibial nerve is resected.

The soleus muscle in the superficial posterior compartment is then dissected away from the medial and lateral heads of the gastrocnemius to the level of the tibial stump and transected just distal to the clamped vascular structures. The posterior flap, which consists of the remaining gastrocnemius muscle, receives its blood supply from sural arteries coursing off the popliteal artery. The muscles of the lateral compartment are excised and the superficial peroneal nerve is resected. All vessels are ligated with vascular staples or suture. They are then transected in traction and allowed to withdraw into the

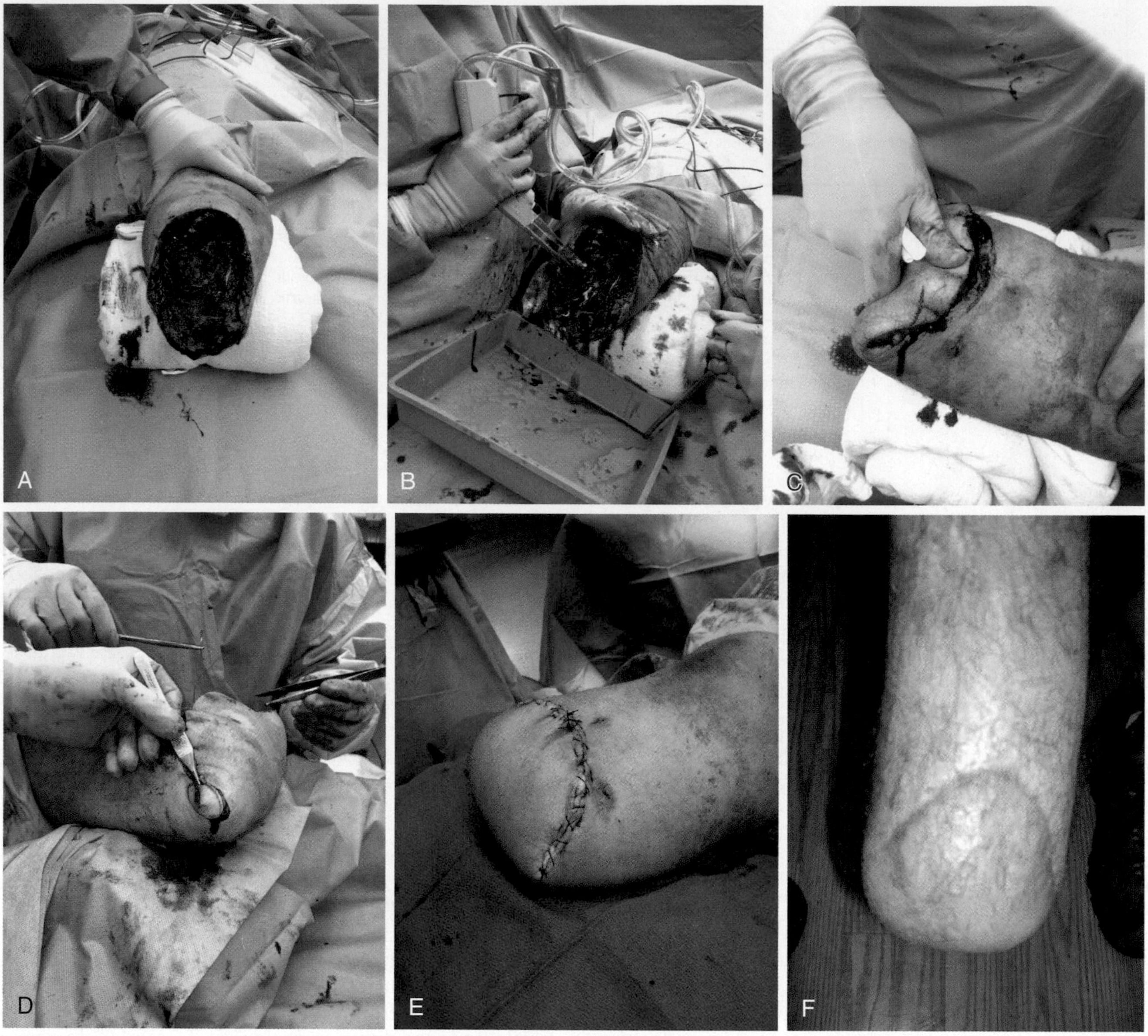

Figure 24-13. **A,** The limb is amputated leaving a posterior flap. **B,** The stump is thoroughly irrigated and then closed loosely with a drain in place. **C** through **F,** For the second stage, the incision is opened, skin edges are freshened, and dog ears are trimmed and the final closure is performed.

stump. The end of the tibia, especially the anterior portion that lies subcutaneously, is beveled and the sharp edges smoothed with a rasp. Finally the posterior flap is sutured to the anterior soft tissues, one to two drains are placed, and the skin is loosely approximated. In approximately 7 days, the second stage procedure is performed involving a repeat débridement, freshening of skin edges, and final closure.

Postoperative Care

During the first few postoperative days, physical therapy should be initiated to aid in transfers, bed mobility, and strengthening exercises. Non–weight-bearing ambulation with the aid of parallel bars, walkers, or crutches should begin soon thereafter. The patient is initially fit with a protective device (i.e., Nutmegger) to avoid soft tissue trauma to the stump and prevent knee flexion contractures (Fig. 24-14). When the sutures or staples have been removed, the patient is ready for use of a stump shrinker to mature the limb in preparation for prosthetic fitting. When the incision has healed, usually in 6 to 10 weeks, our prosthetist fits the patient with an initial prosthesis and prosthetic training with physical therapy begins.

Limb Salvage

As a testament to advances in bone infection care, outcomes of limb salvage protocols markedly improved over the past 20 years. As a result, technically demanding reconstruction procedures are being used in a wider range of patients with multiple comorbidities. Cierny[110] reported limb salvage attempts in 91% of his patients, including 63% of patients classified as B hosts. His overall success rate, defined as "infection-free, functional reconstruction at 2-year follow up," was 84% for limb salvage.

Deciding on a limb salvage approach is only the first of several difficult decisions in selecting the most appropriate

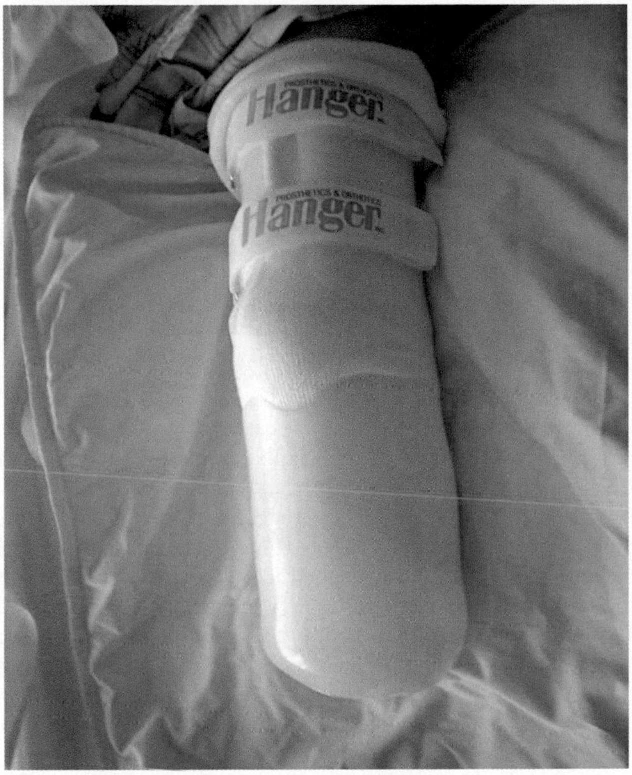

Figure 24-14. Nutmegger stump protector.

management of chronic osteomyelitis. In any limb salvage protocol, débridement is the first intervention. However, the next step is based on multiple factors including the extent of the disease process, the health and functional status of the patient, the resources available, and the skill set of the surgeons involved. Figure 24-12 shows several of the components to be considered in limb salvage surgery.

Débridement

"Make an incision or opening that will thoroughly uncover (saucerize) the infected area. ... Remove foreign material and dead or dying tissue as much as possible ... do not remove bony or soft parts that may contribute to repair. ... Fill cavity ..."[9]

Although this may look like the most recent guidelines for the treatment of chronic osteomyelitis, these excerpts were in fact taken from an article written by H. Winnett Orr in 1933. Although some of his recommendations on the management of bone infection are now outdated, his emphasis on thorough débridement and filling in of subsequent dead space are as relevant today as they were 85 years ago. Despite all the advances in medical technology over this time period, the quality of the surgical débridement remains the most critical factor in successfully managing chronic osteomyelitis.[120]

Even with detailed imaging techniques such as MRI, it is often difficult to assess the extent of osteonecrosis and infection preoperatively. Before making an incision, Walenkamp[100] supported the practice of injecting an obvious fistula with methylene blue dye to localize the focus of infection. In our practice, we found this approach to be beneficial in some cases to facilitate identification of all sinus tracts and quickly guide us to the involved area of bone (Fig. 24-15).

Once the area of necrosis is localized, débridement proceeds using a variety of instruments, such as curettes, rongeurs, and high-speed power burrs. The necrotic bone is excised until punctate haversian bleeding (paprika sign) is achieved. Stated simply, the goal of surgery is the complete excision of all dead or ischemic hard and soft tissues. If not removed, they would serve as a nidus for recurrent infection and cure would be impossible. Simpson and coworkers[121] examined the effect of resection area on outcomes of chronic osteomyelitis. After an average follow-up of 26 months, patients with wide excision of bone had no recurrence of osteomyelitis while those with a marginal excision had a 28% recurrence rate and those that underwent debulking and lavage alone had 100% recurrence within 1 year.

In addition to surgical excision of all necrotic tissues, the infected areas should be copiously irrigated. The ideal volume of fluid for irrigation is unknown, but 10 to 14 L have been recommended by some authors.[23,122] Traditionally, high-pressure, pulsatile lavage has been recommended for irrigation of infected wounds. Irrigation under pressure was believed to be beneficial in removing the highly adherent bacterial "slime" layer. However, several studies have provided evidence suggesting that pressurized irrigation may push bacteria deeper into soft tissues, the IM cavity, and cause injury to soft tissue and bone.[123-125] Muñoz-Mahamud and colleagues[126] showed no difference in the success rate of irrigation and débridement for orthopaedic implant infection when comparing high-pressure pulsatile lavage to low-pressure irrigation.

The addition of antiseptic agents, such as povidone-iodine and hydrogen peroxide, has not consistently shown benefit in increasing elimination of infection.[127] These agents have been shown to damage fibroblasts and potentially impair wound healing. As a result, they are not recommended for routine use in débridement for osteomyelitis. Similarly, the application of

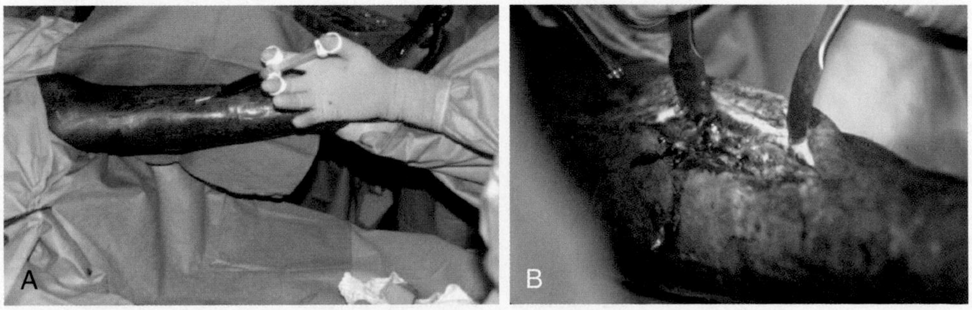

Figure 24-15. **A** and **B,** Methylene blue is injected into the sinus tract. Dissection is carried down to bone following the path of dye.

antibiotics to irrigant fluid has been studied. This has not been shown to be of substantial benefit and poses a risk of bacterial resistance and wound-healing complications.[127,128] In vitro evidence suggests that a 1% liquid soap solution may improve removal of adherent bacteria from bone without adverse tissue effect.[129,130] More research is needed to clarify the benefits and risks of different methods of irrigation. Currently, a large multinational study is underway examining the effects of pressure and soap additives to irrigation fluid for open fracture.[131] Based on currently available evidence, we recommend irrigation with 9 to 10 L of saline or a saline-soap solution under low pressure.

Although thorough débridement is necessary for eliminating all pathogenic bacteria, it is frequently not sufficient. Because of antimicrobial resistance factors, such as the formation of biofilm, persistent infection is unfortunately a fairly common occurrence. In a study of 53 patients who had positive cultures at the time of their initial débridement for chronic osteomyelitis of the tibia, 26% remained culture positive at the time of their second débridement.[132] To arrest this disease, therefore, multiple trips to the operating room for repeated débridement and a variety of reconstructive procedures are often necessary.

Skeletal Stabilization

H. Winnett Orr recognized the importance of post débridement immobilization in the treatment of chronic osteomyelitis.[6] He described this as the "method of immobilization and rest," and he emphasized maintaining length and position of long bones to allow healing. Unfortunately, the only available method in his time was splinting, which prevented regular wound inspection, and patients were forced to live with a pus-saturated splint that was only replaced when the smell became intolerable.[6]

Skeletal stability promotes revascularization, thus enhancing perfusion at the fracture site.[133] This improved blood flow may maximize the host's immune response, which allows it to resist infection at the fracture site more effectively.[134] In fact, in animal models of infected fractures, healing has been shown to correlate directly with the degree of fracture stability.[135]

Although splinting and casting may be used in some cases, other options are now available for maintaining proper skeletal alignment. Functional braces have been advocated for treatment of select fractures, including some type I and II open fractures.[136] Their use has also been described in infected nonunions.[137] Functional bracing has the advantage of allowing early weight-bearing. However, similar to rigid splints, functional bracing does not allow for regular wound inspection. As a result, its application in the treatment of chronic osteomyelitis is often limited by the concomitant soft tissue injury that must be addressed.

External fixation has several advantages for skeletal stabilization in the patient with chronic osteomyelitis. For one, external fixation poses minimal interference with appropriate soft tissue management (Fig. 24-16). In addition, minimal internal hardware is present to serve as a nidus for bacterial adherence. Furthermore, external fixation devices can be rapidly applied, which is obviously of benefit in the multiple-trauma patient with injuries in need of simultaneous treatment. Animal studies have shown an improved rate of fracture union in infected osteotomies treated with external fixation compared to internal fixation.[138] The Ilizarov method[139] is a frequently used form of external fixation in patients with chronic osteomyelitis. It has the advantage of allowing for controlled movement to allow correction of length as well as rotational, translational, and angular deformities. Although there are many drawbacks to the Ilizarov method, such as pain from the external fixator, frequent pin site infections, and a long period of time spent in the device (almost 9 months on average),[140,141] it has produced excellent outcomes in several studies.[141-146] What makes this mode of treatment even more valuable to patients is that it allows them to remain ambulatory throughout its duration.[140,147,148]

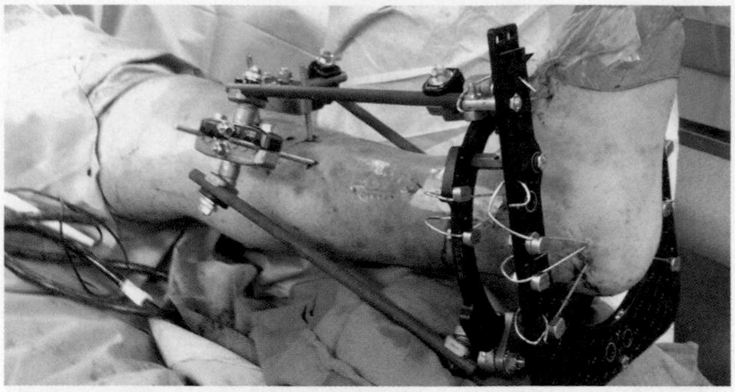

Figure 24-16. Jet X-Taylor Spatial Frame hybrid external fixator.

Internal fixation is rarely used for initial fracture stabilization in the presence of chronic osteomyelitis. However, treatment with an IM antibiotic-laden cement rod may be beneficial in select cases.[149] In the event of infected hardware, the decision to leave or remove the hardware depends on the condition of the bone. In the event of a fracture treated with internal fixation, the degree of union must be assessed. If greater than 50% union has occurred, it is reasonable to remove the hardware. However, if the fracture does not show evidence of healing and the hardware remains the primary stabilizer, the treatment decision is more challenging. If the infection has been present for a short duration, less than 6 weeks, or the bone defect involves an articular surface, the implant is typically left in place.[95] This requires regular follow-up to assess healing. Conversely, if the infection has been present for more than 6 weeks or the implant shows signs of failure, the hardware is typically removed, and the bone is stabilized with an external fixator.[95]

Skeletal Defect Management

Following excision of all devitalized tissue, it is common to find a skeletal defect. The goal of skeletal defect management is to eliminate dead space that may serve as a reservoir for bacterial growth and to provide the greatest potential for restoring bony stability. Several different approaches can be used to achieve this end and the choice is based on multiple variables including anatomic location, size of the defect, functional status of the patient, and the host's ability to recover from the surgery.

Bone reconstruction is generally part of a second-stage procedure, but good results have been reported when performed as a single-stage limb débridement and reconstruction.[150] One method of restoring skeletal defects involves application of osteoconductive, osteogenic, and/or osteoinductive material to the involved area. This is typically limited to defects less than 6 cm in size.[94] Papineau and colleagues[151] pioneered the technique of open cancellous autografting for bone lesions. This method, along with modifications of it, has been shown to have clinical success in 89% to 100% of patients with appropriate indications.[151-155]

Another option is demineralized bone matrix with or without the addition of bone morphogenic protein (BMP). BMPs are osteoinductive agents that stimulate osteoblast differentiation from mesenchymal precursor cells. They also promote bone matrix production and vascularization.[156] Two forms of BMP are commercially available: BMP-7 (also known as *osteogenic protein-1*) and recombinant human BMP-2 (rhBMP-2). Currently, high-quality clinical studies regarding the efficacy of BMP for treatment of appendicular skeleton defects remains limited.[156] In a group of grade III open fractures and nonunions included as part of a recent study,[157] 10 of 11 patients showed evidence of union with application of BMP-7. The remaining patient died of unrelated causes during the follow-up period. BMP-2 has been found to decrease the rate of nonunion, need for additional interventions, and allow faster bone and wound healing following open fractures.[158] Off-label use of rhBMP-2 for reconstruction of tibial defects has also been described, but further study is needed to determine its effectiveness for management of nonunions.[158]

Another option for management of larger skeletal defects involves acute shortening, with or without distraction osteogenesis. Acute shortening is used for long bone defects and simply involves bringing the débrided bone ends together. This necessarily results in a decreased limb length and as a result, a lengthening procedure is often necessary to maximize function. Ilizarov's method[139] of limb lengthening, along with later modifications of it, has been extensively used in limb reconstruction for osteomyelitis. This technique, as demonstrated in Illustrative Case 2 at the end of the chapter, involves applying a small wire-ringed external fixator to the extremity. The débrided bone ends are brought into close approximation. As callus forms, the bones are slowly distracted and new bone is allowed to fill the gap. The bone is lengthened at one-quarter of a millimeter every 6 hours. This method of distraction osteogenesis has been shown to be successful for limb reconstruction following treatment of osteomyelitis in several studies.[146,149,154,159,160] Some authors have also combined external fixation with an IM implant for tibia and femur bone defects.[149,160] This approach has shown a decreased rate of deformity and shortens the duration of external fixator use.[160]

Finally, vascularized free bone graft may be used to bridge the defect. Most commonly, a fibula graft is used. This approach is indicated for patients with defects larger than 5 to 6 cm.[161,162] Clinical studies have shown a success rate of 76% to 97%, but secondary surgeries are frequently necessary.[161,162] In addition to the complexity of the surgery, multiple potential complications including donor site morbidity, postoperative deformity, and stress fracture of the graft limit their use.[161]

Soft Tissue Coverage

Adequate soft tissue coverage is necessary to prevent recurrence of infection and promote bone healing. Similar to the management of skeletal defects, multiple factors must be considered in selecting the most appropriate intervention. These include the anatomic location of the lesion, the condition of the soft tissues at the time of débridement, the health of the host, and the resources available. For closure following débridement of infected bone and soft tissue, there are generally four approaches:

1. Direct skin closure (either at the time of the index procedure or in a delayed fashion)
2. Closure by secondary intention
3. Local myocutaneous flap coverage
4. Free muscle flap transfer[94,163]

Direct skin closure is possible in select cases in which the skin is well vascularized and able to be approximated without tension. In many cases, a second débridement is anticipated and a delayed primary closure may be performed if soft tissues are amenable.[94] This is typically performed within 7 days of the initial débridement. When the skin cannot be closed primarily, the wound must either be left open and allowed to granulate in, or soft tissues can be transposed. Allowing closure by secondary intention may be appropriate for certain patients in which soft tissue transpositions are unlikely to be effective or if the patient's comorbidities preclude additional surgery. However, this is associated with a higher risk of infection than tissue transposition procedures.[99] If closure by secondary intention is the goal, the treatment will usually involve wet-to-dry dressing changes or a negative-pressure dressing (i.e., wound vacuum-assisted closure [VAC]) (Fig. 24-17).

Use of well-vascularized soft tissue grafts is advantageous in most circumstances as it offers a new blood supply to the healing bone and decreases the risk of recurrent infection.[164,165] Local muscle flaps, which have the advantage of keeping the vascular supply intact, are almost always used if

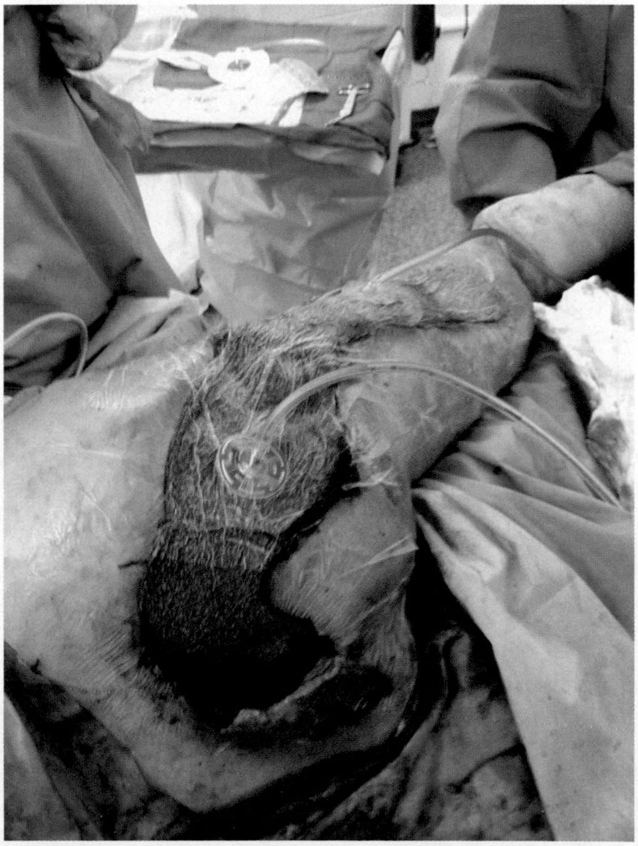

Figure 24-17. Wound vacuum-assisted closure (VAC) negative-pressure dressing.

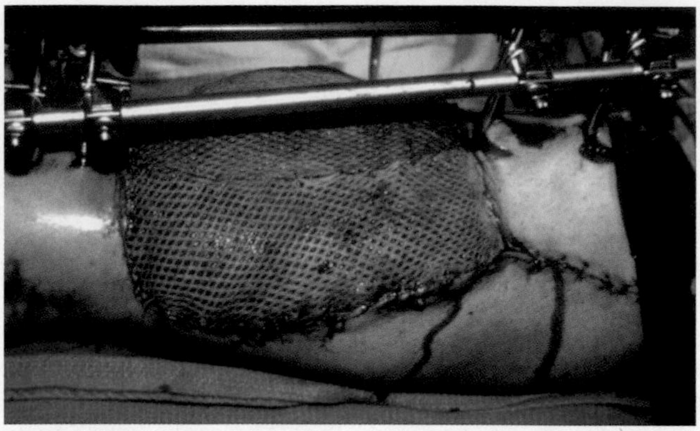

Figure 24-18. Large soft tissue defect following free flap coverage and split-thickness skin graft.

an adjacent muscle is available. In locations where local flap coverage is not possible, a transplanted flap is used. These so-called free flaps are usually from such donor muscles as rectus abdominis, latissimus dorsi, gracilis, and tensor fasciae latae[166] (Fig. 24-18).

It is difficult to study the isolated effect that the use of muscle transfers has had on clinical outcome. After all, this technique is almost always used in combination with several other therapeutic modalities, such as bone grafting, antibiotics, and, of course, débridement. Nonetheless, there is certainly a large amount of evidence that supports the use of muscle flaps as part of the therapeutic regimen.[166-169] Fitzgerald and colleagues[168] using either local or free flaps combined with thorough débridement and antibiotics, reported a 93% success rate in treating a sample of 42 patients with chronic osteomyelitis. These results demonstrated a significant improvement over previous treatment regimens that did not employ the use of muscle flap coverage. In another study, which retrospectively reviewed 34 patients with chronic osteomyelitis of the tibia, it was found that those who had received free muscle flap transfers as part of their surgical treatment were more likely to be drainage-free after more than 7 years of follow-up than patients who had received débridement alone.[169]

Hyperbaric oxygen therapy has been described as an adjunct to augment soft tissue healing and promote immune function.[16] In theory, increasing oxygen tension in compromised soft tissues may encourage local metabolic processes promoting fibroblastic and osteoblastic activity. In addition, hyperbaric oxygen may also enhance polymorphonuclear leukocyte activity promoting the clearance of infection.[87] However, there is a lack of solid scientific evidence to support the time and economic resources necessary for this intervention. Based on a systematic review of the literature, support for hyperbaric oxygen therapy for chronic osteomyelitis is limited to a few small case series.[170]

Infection Control

The surgical interventions described previously are designed to remove the bulk of microorganisms, promote blood flow to the area to facilitate resolution of infection, and cover the involved area to reduce the risk of recurrent exposure to pathogens. However, additional steps are frequently taken to facilitate eradication of infection and prevent recurrence. For this purpose, local and systemic antibiotics may be of advantage. Furthermore, because bacteria proliferate in spacious, warm, moist cavities, it is imperative that dead space created during débridement be eliminated. The bone grafting and soft tissue transfers help to decrease dead space, but in many cases supplementation is needed.

Numerous studies have shown that direct application of antibiotic solutions to a wound does not help to clear infection.[128,130] However, designs that allow elution of antibiotics over time have been found to be beneficial.[171,172] Most frequently, polymethylmethacrylate (PMMA) beads impregnated with antibiotics such as gentamicin, tobramycin, or vancomycin will be used for local infection control[163,173] (Fig. 24-19). This has been found to provide a local concentration that is many times higher than the MIC of bacteria and without systemic side effects.[163] The drug concentration achieved with local antibiotic depots has even been shown to interfere with biofilm formation and function, a benefit not seen with systemic administration.[174]

Although PMMA is the most widely used drug delivery system, it is nonabsorbable and, therefore, requires additional surgery for removal. A resorbable carrier with similar elution characteristics to PMMA would be of clear benefit, but clinical trials showing effectiveness of different delivery vehicles are limited.[175] In a small sample of patients, calcium sulfate beads impregnated with tobramycin or vancomycin have shown promising results.[171,176] Whatever the material, the antibiotic-laden beads are placed directly in the operative wound, which is then primarily closed. Unless the depot material is biodegradable, the antibiotic bead chains generally remain in the wound for approximately 4 weeks. Beads placed within the IM canal, however, should be removed sooner, within 2 weeks, before the layer of granulation tissue has formed, which would make removal difficult.[120]

Several clinical trials have supported the efficacy of local antibiotic bead implantation.[173,176-178] Even though the gentamicin concentration remains at sufficient levels for approximately 30 days after implantation, some skeptics may claim that beads are beneficial only insofar as they are able to fill dead space. Animal studies demonstrated the efficacy of antibiotic beads in eradicating osteomyelitis above and beyond placebo beads that have no antibiotic.[179] Thus, it appears that bead chains are helpful not only by serving as a temporary filler of dead space before reconstruction but also as an effective depot for the local administration of antibiotic.

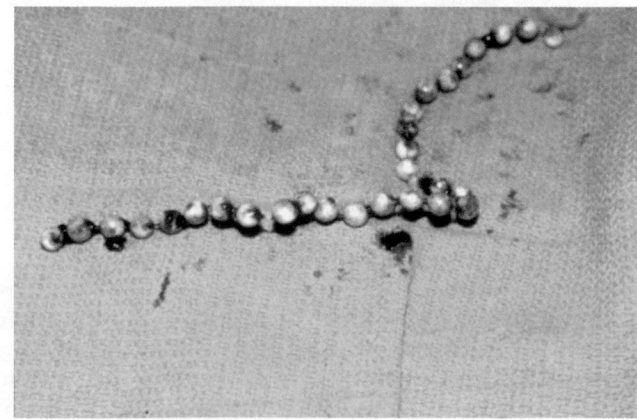

Figure 24-19. Polymethylmethacrylate (PMMA) antibiotic-impregnated beads.

Systemic Antibiotics

Although surgical débridement is the mainstay of chronic osteomyelitis treatment, systemic antibiotics play an important role in postoperative management. The choice of antimicrobial agent, route, and duration for the treatment of chronic osteomyelitis is often based on tradition and expert opinion.[180] A review of current literature provides limited insight due to the lack of quality randomized trials comparing various antibiotic regimens. In addition, there are multiple variables that influence the efficacy of an antibiotic. For example, the offending organisms must be susceptible, the patient must be able to tolerate the drug, and the antibiotic must be able to penetrate sufficiently to achieve the MIC in the surrounding tissues. Some studies have focused on the ability of an antibiotic to penetrate bone.[181] However, this feature is not relevant in osteomyelitis as the organisms hide in devascularized bone and are protected by a biofilm layer. The goal of systemic antibiotics is to eliminate infection in soft tissues surrounding the involved bone to prevent reinfection following thorough débridement. Achieving the MIC in the soft tissues is influenced by several factors including pharmacokinetics of the drug, serum concentration, and perfusion. Because of the many variables, in vitro models are poor predictors of an antibiotic's efficacy and cannot be used alone in guiding treatment.[181]

Four to six weeks of parenteral antibiotics are commonly recommended post débridement followed by a variable period of oral antibiotics.[181-183] The parenteral route has the advantage of 100% bioavailability. In addition, devitalized bone takes 3 to 4 weeks to revascularize after injury and therefore, a duration exceeding this seems reasonable. However, given the cost and inconvenience of parenteral antibiotics as well as the persistently high recurrence rate, the traditional recommendations have come under question.[183]

Many authors have described the outcomes of antibiotic treatment in managing patients with osteomyelitis, but there are few randomized trials comparing different antibiotic regimens.[180-183] Furthermore, conclusions drawn from studies are challenged by small sample sizes, heterogeneous patient populations, and various antibiotic choices. Lazzarini and colleagues,[180] performed a systematic review of 93 clinical trials, most of which were noncontrolled. Many of the studies did not provide clear criteria for diagnosis of osteomyelitis and more than half did not distinguish between classification of the disease, often including both acute and chronic cases. An additional problem was lack of any information on surgical treatment of the infection, which was absent in the majority of studies. Despite these limitations, the authors found the available literature suggests that oral or parenteral antibiotics may be equally effective due to similar "cure" rates in the various trials. Oral agents commonly used included β-lactams, cephalosporins, and fluoroquinolones. Of the oral agents, fluoroquinolones were found to have the most support for efficacy.

A systematic review of only randomized and quasi-randomized controlled trials, found little support for one antibiotic regimen over another.[183] Through meta-analysis of eight trials, including a total of 248 subjects, no difference in the final remission rate of osteomyelitis was found when comparing oral to parenteral antibiotics.[183] This suggests that given the convenience and decreased risk of catheter associate complications, oral antibiotics may be preferable. However, these results must be viewed with caution as the small number of subjects may not have allowed sufficient power to detect a difference. In addition, the rate of recurrence in long-term studies using only oral antibiotics has not been evaluated.

In multiple clinical studies, oral fluoroquinolones have been shown to achieve a 60% to 80% cure rate and trimethoprim-sulfamethoxazole (TMP-SMX) a 45% to 100% cure rate.[181] Based on pharmacokinetic and clinical data, Spellberg and Lipsky[181] suggest oral fluoroquinolones or TMP-SMX combined with rifampin are appropriate choices for empiric antibiotic treatment. For patients with gram-positive cocci on Gram stain, clindamycin is considered a reasonable alternative considering the potential resistance of staphylococci to fluoroquinolones. Oxacillin or cefazolin remain the drugs of choice for methicillin-sensitive *S. aureus* (MSSA). However, these are generalizations and once cultures are final, antibiotics should be tailored based on the specific sensitivities of the involved organisms.

Commonly used antibiotics for chronic osteomyelitis are shown in Table 24-2. It is our practice to use vancomycin and cefepime for the initial empiric coverage, changing to oral regimens consisting of dicloxacillin if we isolate oxacillin-sensitive *S. aureus* or to TMP-SMX, doxycycline, minocycline, or linezolid depending on the sensitivity pattern of the isolate. We often supplement any agent used in treatment with 1 to 2 months of rifampin.

For other staphylococci and gram-negative organisms, we choose an antibiotic on the basis of in vitro sensitivities, and supplement with rifampin if the organisms are found to be sensitive. Although commonly used for therapy of tuberculosis and of difficult-to-treat staphylococcal infections, rifampin is truly a broad-spectrum antibiotic, inhibiting the majority of bacteria of any genus. Rifampin has inherent antibiofilm activity, giving it a clear advantage in the treatment of chronic osteomyelitis.[184] Although a very active agent, it cannot be used as sole therapy because of a high spontaneous mutation rate in *Staphylococcus, Mycobacterium,* and presumably other species of bacteria. Patients treated with rifampin monotherapy for pyogenic infections can be expected to have active infections and rifampin-resistant bacteria within 1 week.[185]

The appropriate duration of systemic antibiotic therapy is not currently known. Interestingly, some of the best results reported in the literature are from a group who used antibiotics only perioperatively, coupled with aggressive débridement.[186] Given the high rate of recurrence of osteomyelitis, most surgeons and infectious disease specialists prefer an extended period of postoperative antibiotic therapy. Based on their review of currently available literature, Spellberg and Lipsky[181] recommend a duration of 8 to 16 weeks. Similarly, the Infectious Diseases Society of America recommends a minimum of 8 weeks of antibiotics for MRSA infection. This is consistent with our practice at the University of Connecticut Health Center, where we generally have our patients continue antibiotics until the operative site has healed completely.

ILLUSTRATIVE CASES

Case 1: Antibiotic Cement Rod

For infected nonunions in the presence of an IM nail, replacement of the device with an antibiotic cement rod is an option. This involves the following steps: (1) removing the nail, (2)

TABLE 24-2 *COMMONLY USED ANTIBIOTICS FOR TREATMENT OF CHRONIC OSTEOMYELITIS*

Antibiotic	Route	Dose/Frequency	Adverse Effects	Comments	Active Against MRSA
Initial Empiric Coverage					
Vancomycin	IV	15 mg per kg/12 h (adjusted based on weight, GFR, and trough levels)	Nephrotoxicity, ototoxicity, reversible neutropenia	Used in combination with cefepime for initial empiric coverage	XXXX
Cefepime	IV	1–2 g/8–12 h	Rare; colitis, anemia, neurotoxicity, cholestasis	Broad-spectrum bactericidal activity against many gram-positive and gram-negative bacteria, including *pseudomonas*	
Sensitivity Specific Coverage					
Cefazolin	IV	1–2 g/8 h	Rare; hypersensitivity reactions, dermatologic and GI disturbance	Effective against gram-positive bacteria	
Cephalexin	PO	500 mg–1000 mg qid; 1–2 gm bid	Rare; hypersensitivity reaction, dermatologic and GI disturbance	Effective against gram-positive bacteria; good oral bioavailability	
Ampicillin/ Sulbactram	IV	2 g:1 g/6 h	Rare; hypersensitivity reaction, dermatologic and GI disturbance	Broad-spectrum bactericidal activity against gram-positive, gram-negative, and anaerobic bacteria	
Piperacillin/ Tazobactam	IV	3.375 g/6 h	Rare; hypersensitivity reaction, dermatologic and GI disturbance	Broad-spectrum bactericidal activity against gram-positive, gram-negative, and anaerobic bacteria	
Imipenem/ Cilastatin	IV	500 mg/6 h	Eosinophilia, increase BUN/Cr, seizures	Effective against many gram-positive and gram-negative bacteria, including *Pseudomonas*	
Ertapenem	IV	1 g/day	Elevated LFTs, altered mental status, increased platelet count	Effective against many gram-positive, gram-negative, and anaerobic bacteria	
Daptomycin	IV	6 mg per kg/24 h	Insomnia, pharyngolaryngeal pain, peripheral neuropathy, rhabdomyolysis	Primarily effective against gram-positive bacteria	XXXX
Ciprofloxacin	IV/PO	500 mg/12 h	Tendon rupture, confusion in elderly	Broad spectrum against gram-positive and gram-negative bacteria; good oral bioavailability	
Doxycycline	IV/PO	100 mg/12 hours	Discoloration of teeth in children, hepatotoxicity, pericarditis	Broad coverage; good oral bioavailability	XX
Minocycline	IV/PO	100 mg/12 hours	Discoloration of teeth, vertigo	Broad coverage; may be effective for doxycycline-resistant MRSA; good oral bioavailability	XXX
Trimethoprim/ sulfamethoxazole	PO	800–160 mg/12 h	Agranulocytosis, TTP, ITP	Broad coverage; good oral bioavailability	XXX
Dicloxacillin	PO	250 mg/6 h	Rare: GI disturbance, anemia, elevated LFTs	Good gram-positive coverage; good oral bioavailability	
Clindamycin	IV/PO	450 mg/6 h	*C. diff.* colitis, fungal overgrowth	Effective against anaerobes and gram positive cocci; good oral bioavailability	X (if MRSA also sensitive to erythromycin)
Linezolid	IV/PO	600 mg/12 h	Lactic acidosis, optic neuritis, peripheral neuropathy, serotonin syndrome with serotonergic drugs	Good oral bioavailability; active against gram-positive bacteria, including MRSA and VRE	XXXX
Metronidazole	IV	Loading: 15 mg per kg; maintenance: 7.5 mg per kg/6 h	Disulfiram-like reaction to ethanol, metallic taste, ataxia	Anaerobic coverage	

bid, Twice daily; *IV,* intravenous; *mRNA,* messenger RNA; *MRSA,* methicillin-resistant *Staphylococcus aureus; PO,* orally; *qid,* four times daily; *rRNA,* ribosomal RNA; *VRE,* vancomycin-resistant *Enterococcus.*

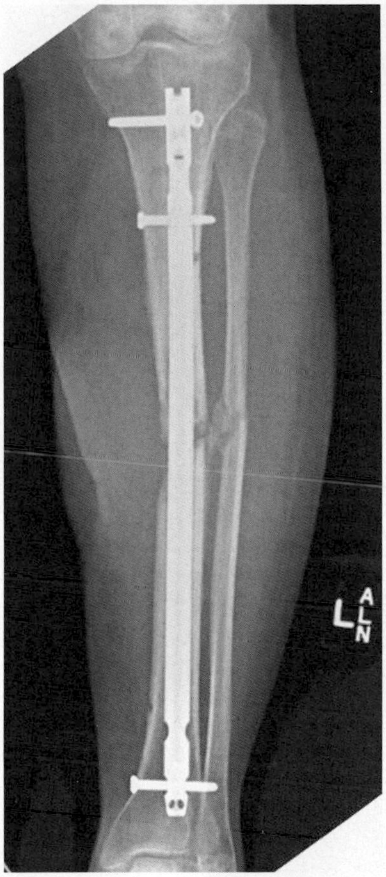

Figure 24-20. S.F.'s radiographs at time of referral to our bone infection clinic. She had an atrophic nonunion of her mid-diaphyseal tibia fracture status post exchange nailing.

reaming and irrigating the canal, (3) creating and introducing the antibiotic-laden cement rod, and (4) applying an external fixator. This technique is typically reserved for cases of minimal bone loss that have failed previous attempts at irrigation and débridement with exchange nailing as illustrated in the following example.

S.F. is a 41-year-old female involved in a motorcycle collision resulting in a grade IIIB open tibia fracture. She was initially treated with irrigation and débridement, placement of an IM nail, and soleus local muscle flap coverage. Her course was complicated by an infected nonunion with cultures positive for MSSA. She underwent multiple débridements with subsequent removal of the nail, placement of an antibiotic spacer, and application of an external fixator. She was treated with IV oxacillin for 6 weeks followed by oral minocycline. When clinical signs of infection resolved, she was treated with iliac crest bone grafting of the tibial nonunion and reinsertion of a tibial IM nail. However, her nonunion persisted and prompted referral to our service.

At the time of initial evaluation, S.F. was 1 year status post injury with a persistent tibia atrophic nonunion (Fig. 24-20). On examination, her previous incisions and pin tracts were healed but she had persistent tenderness at her fracture site and elevated inflammatory markers. Persistent IM osteomyelitis was suspected. We chose to remove the IM nail and introduce an antibiotic-impregnated cement rod. Figure 24-21 shows some of the key steps involved. First, the IM nail was removed and the canal was reamed and irrigated. Reamed material was collected for culture. The antibiotic-impregnated cement rod was created on the back table. We selected a 38-Fr chest tube to approximate the diameter of the nail. Cement was mixed with 2 g of vancomycin powder. The ball tip guidewire was cut to the appropriate size and placed into the tube to facilitate contouring of the rod. The antibiotic-laden cement was then injected into the tube and the tube and guide wire were bent to resemble the shape of the IM nail. The cement rod was then inserted. Finally an external fixator was applied for temporary skeletal stabilization. Her intraoperative cultures returned positive for MSSA. The infectious disease service was involved in the patient's care and based on their recommendations, she was treated with IV vancomycin for 6 weeks followed by oral cephalexin for 6 weeks.

After 4 months, laboratory tests including complete blood count (CBC), CRP, and ESR were ordered and remained within the normal range. A ^{99m}Tc bone scan with Ga subtraction study was performed showing no signs of active infection. The patient was brought back to the operating room for removal of the cement rod and external fixator. This was followed 2 weeks later by open reduction and internal fixation with application of a tibial plate along with application of cancellous bone chips, demineralized bone matrix, and rhBMP-2 to the tibial defect (Fig. 24-22). Cultures from this final operation were negative, but based on recommendations from the infectious disease service, she was maintained on cephalexin. She is presently recovering without signs of recurrent infection.

Case 2: Acute Shortening and Relengthening

The reconstructive strategy of acute shortening and limb relengthening consists of the following steps: (1) excising the necrotic bone and avascular scar, (2) applying the Ilizarov external fixator, (3) acutely shortening the limb by compression at the excision site, (4) making a corticotomy proximal or distal to the excision site, (5) providing soft tissue coverage if necessary, and finally (6) relengthening through the corticotomy site.

This technique, most effectively employed if the length of the necrotic bone is less than or equal to 4 cm, is illustrated by the case of J.S., a 27-year-old man who was referred to our clinic with chronic osteomyelitis and nonunion of his right tibia. Three years before, he had sustained a grade IIIB open fracture of his right tibial diaphysis in a motorcycle accident. At the time of the accident, he was initially treated with external fixation, which was later converted to an IM nail. In addition to the massive comminution and displacement of the fracture, his right leg sustained significant soft tissue damage secondary to the accident that required a gastrocnemius muscle flap with a split-thickness skin graft to cover the exposed bone adequately (Fig. 24-23). Unfortunately, J.S. developed signs of osteomyelitis including persistent pain, fever, and elevated inflammatory markers. The IM nail was removed and a second external fixator was applied (Fig. 24-24).

When the patient arrived at our clinic, he had no external fixator in place and the skin grafts were healing quite well (Fig. 24-25). He complained of pain with walking. On physical examination, the patient's right leg was in obvious varus. There was no erythema, fluctuance, or sinus tracts visible on the overlying skin. The gastrocnemius flap was pink, and the leg

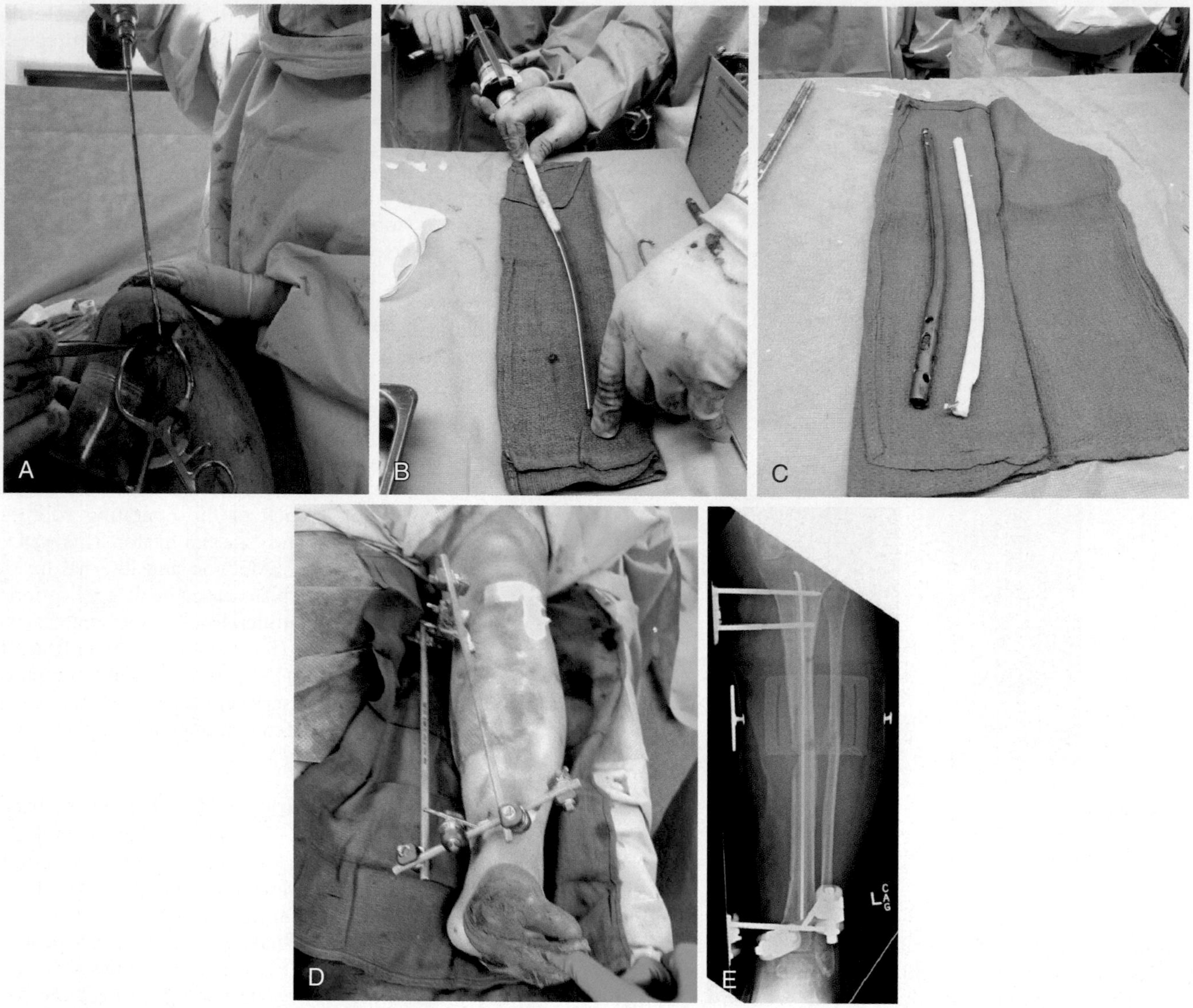

Figure 24-21. Placement of antibiotic-laden cement rod. **A,** After removing the tibial nail, the canal was reamed and irrigated. Reamings were collected for culture. A transverse incision was used because this was the location of a previous laceration and this incision was used for her previous tibial nailing. **B,** Cement was mixed with 2 g of vancomycin powder and injected into the chest tube approximating the diameter of the medullary canal. **C,** The rod is contoured to resemble the removed tibial nail and the plastic tube is cut longitudinally and removed. **D,** After inserting the cement rod, an external fixator is applied to provide temporary skeletal stabilization. **E,** Postoperative radiograph.

was neurovascularly intact with nearly full range of motion at the knee and ankle. Radiographic examination revealed a nonunion of the right tibia with approximately 25 degrees of varus and 30 degrees of dorsal angulation (Fig. 24-26). A bone scan was negative for active infection. At this point, a lengthy conversation was held with the patient and he elected for limb salvage surgery. J.S. was instructed to stop the oral antibiotics he had previously been prescribed (to optimize the yield of intraoperative cultures), and surgery was scheduled for a few weeks after this visit.

In the operating room, it was first important to determine how much tibial bone was involved in the disease process. To visualize the area in question, an incision was made lateral to the anterior muscle flap and dissection was continued down to the periosteum of the previous fracture site. Using a periosteal elevator to identify its cortices, the bone was found to be very sclerotic about 1.5 cm on either side of the nonunion. There was no evidence of frank pus. At this point, intraoperative biopsy specimens were obtained and sent for culture. Given the fact that the area of necrosis was limited, the decision was made to pursue a course of acute shortening followed by limb relengthening.

The next aspect of the surgery was thorough débridement of the sclerotic bone at and around the nonunion site. Using an oscillating saw, a 4-cm portion of the tibia and fibula that included the nonunion site was resected. The diaphyseal bone both proximal and distal to the débridement area was curetted to bleeding bone and irrigated with several liters of soap and saline. The bone ends were then reduced and the Ilizarov external fixator frame was applied. When the fixator was pinned to the proximal and distal portions of the tibia, rotational alignment was verified under fluoroscopy and the frame was secured. The bone ends were then placed under forceful compression. The final part of this operation was to

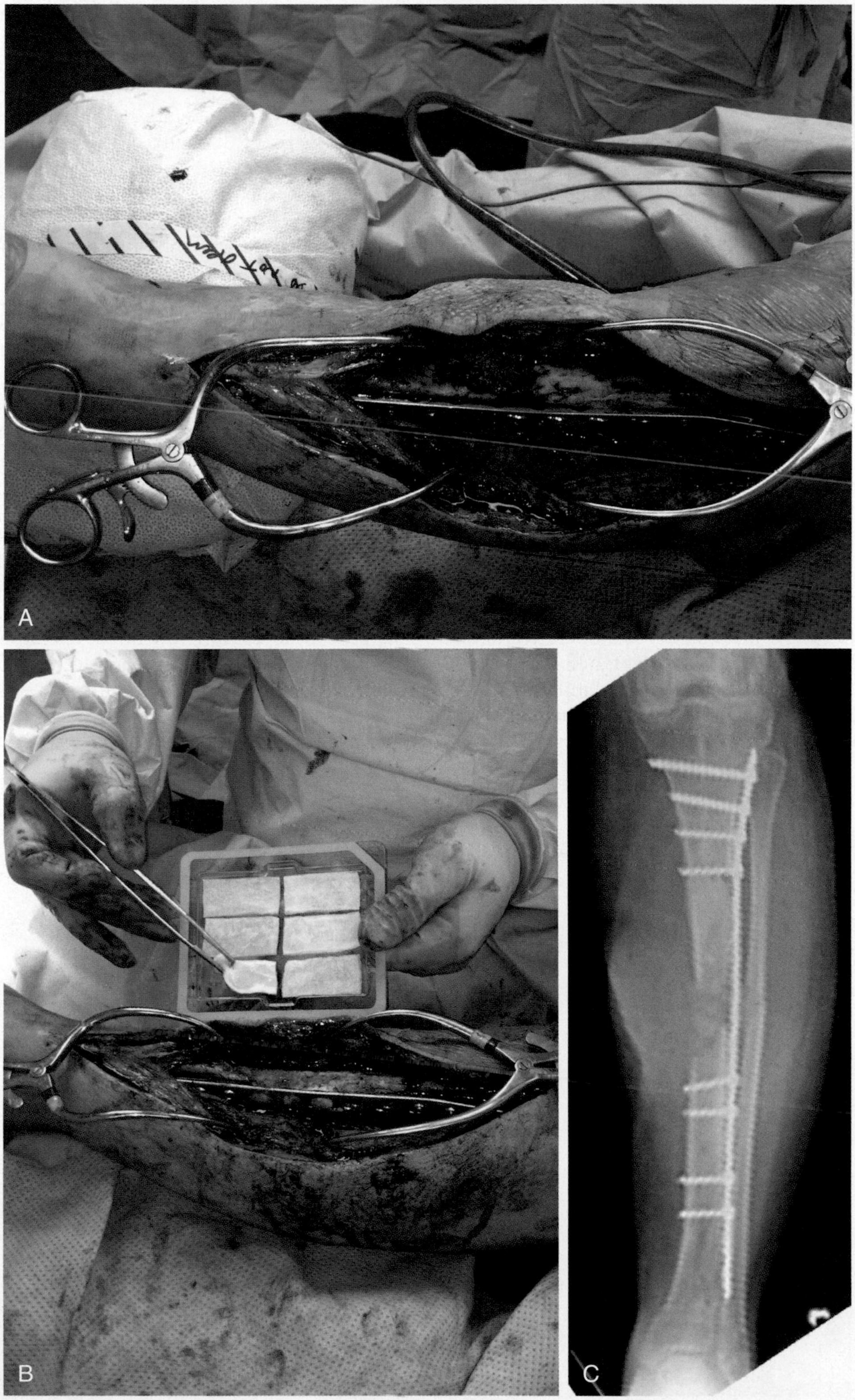

Figure 24-22. A, The tibial defect was thoroughly débrided and a 4.5-mm plate was used for fixation. Cancellous bone chips and demineralized bone matrix were applied to the defect. **B,** Recombinant human bone morphogenic protein-2 (rhBMP-2) (Infuse, Medtronic) was applied to collagen sponges and placed over the filled defect. **C,** Postoperative radiograph.

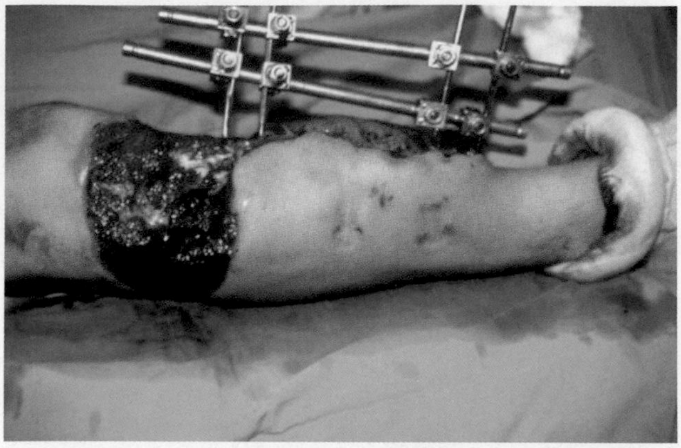

Figure 24-23. Massive soft tissue loss occurring at the time of initial injury. This was treated with an external fixator along with gastrocnemius flap and split-thickness skin graft.

make a metaphyseal corticotomy to allow subsequent limb relengthening.

The immediate postoperative course for J.S. was unremarkable. He received early mobilization from physical therapy with weight-bearing as tolerated on the right lower extremity. Before discharge from the hospital on postoperative day 3, the patient was instructed in how to lengthen the Ilizarov apparatus by approximately one-quarter of a millimeter four times a day starting 1 week after the operation. Although he was maintained with intravenous antibiotics during his brief hospital stay, J.S. was discharged home with oral antibiotics (a first-generation cephalosporin and rifampin) to which his intraoperative culture (*S. aureus*) would prove to be sensitive.

Three weeks postoperatively, the patient was ambulating on crutches without difficulty. Although the right leg was measured and found to be fully out to length approximately 4 months after the surgery, adequate fusion at the compression site remained problematic and the decision was made to augment the area with multiple half-pins and cancellous bone graft from the posterior iliac crest. After bone grafting, the patient did very well, and follow-up radiographs over the next several months showed increasing incorporation of the bone graft at the compression site as well as progressive lengthening and bone formation in the regenerate zone (Fig. 24-27).

Because Ilizarov external fixation allows early weight-bearing, J.S. remained active during the course of his treatment and continued to enjoy many of his favorite activities, including bow hunting (Fig. 24-28). Seven months after visiting our clinic, with radiographic evidence of excellent bone formation at both the proximal compression site and the distal regenerate zone, J.S. was brought back to the operating room to have the external fixator removed. He did extremely well in the months to follow, using only a right leg orthosis for support. One year after the initial operation, J.S. was found to have no leg length disparity and to be enjoying an extremely active life. Radiographic examination showed excellent leg alignment, with further callus formation at both the proximal and distal sites (Fig. 24-29).

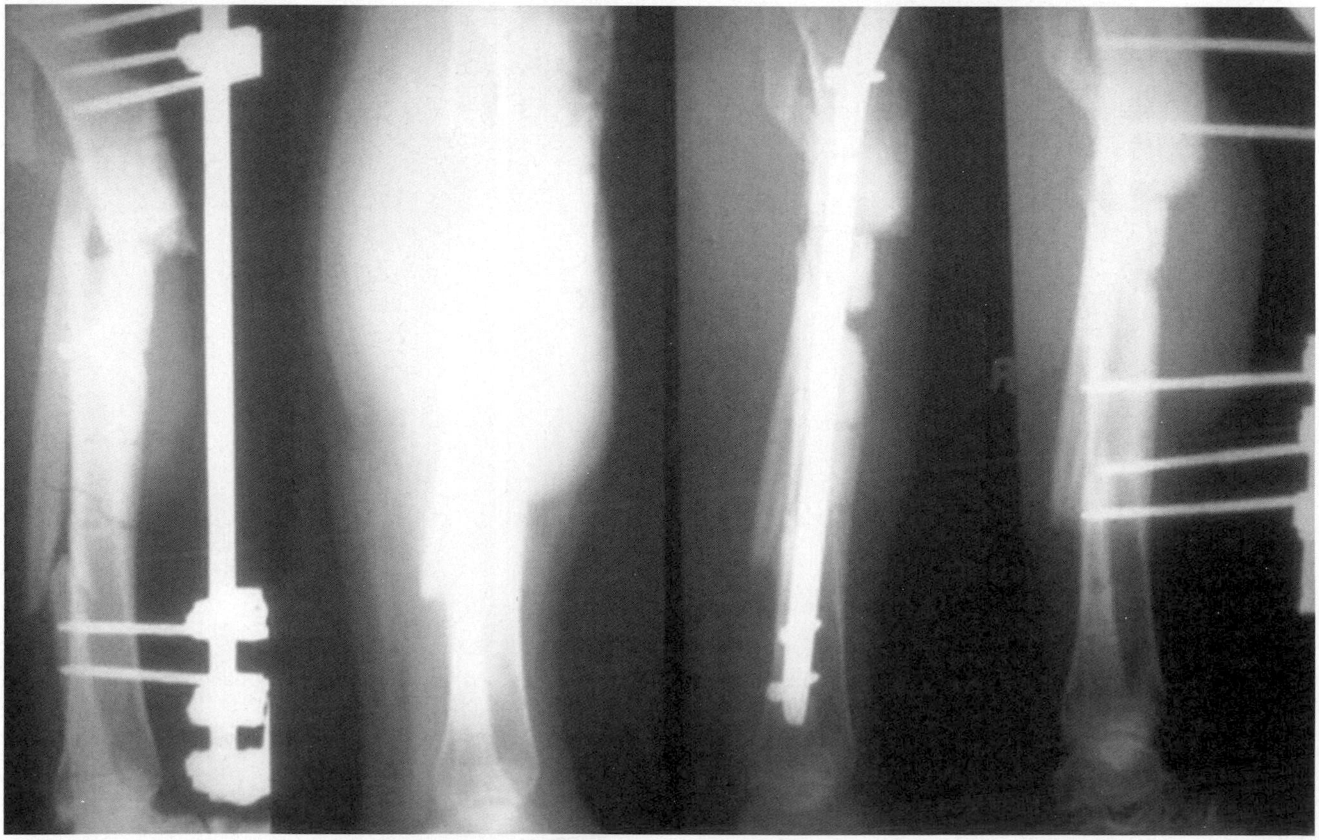

Figure 24-24. From left to right, initial treatment with external fixation, fixator "holiday," intramedullary nail placement, and finally removal of the nail and application of a second external fixator due to recurrent infection.

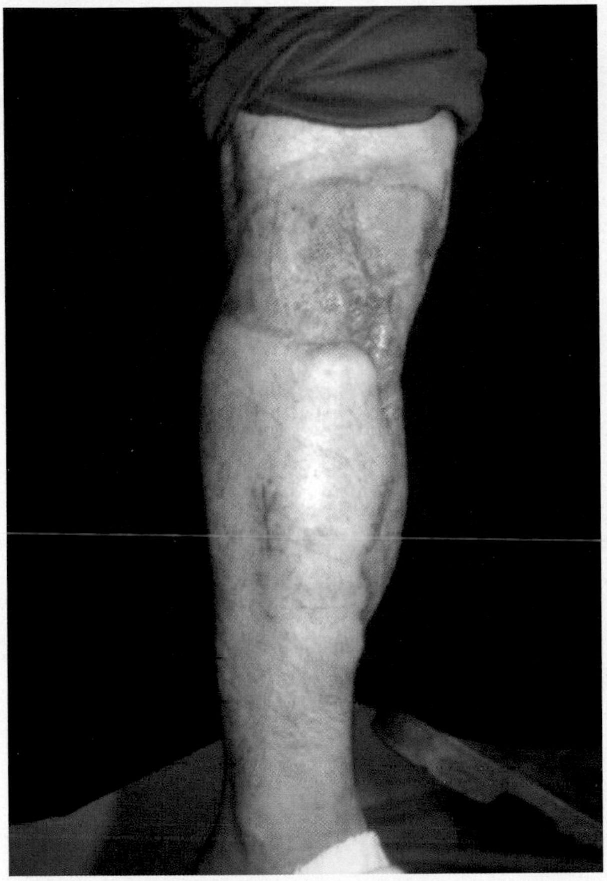

Figure 24-25. J.S. at the time of initial evaluation at our bone infection clinic.

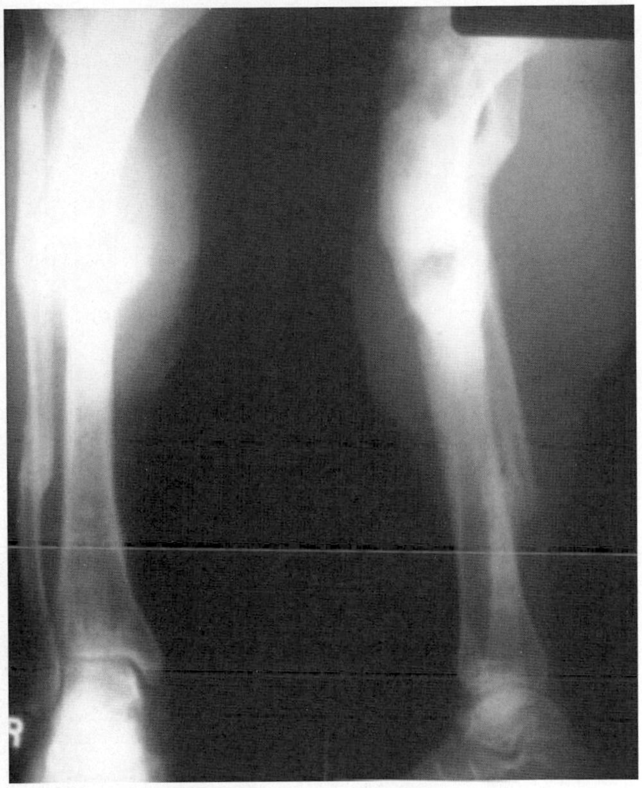

Figure 24-26. Radiographs showing nonunion of the tibia with varus and procurvatum deformity.

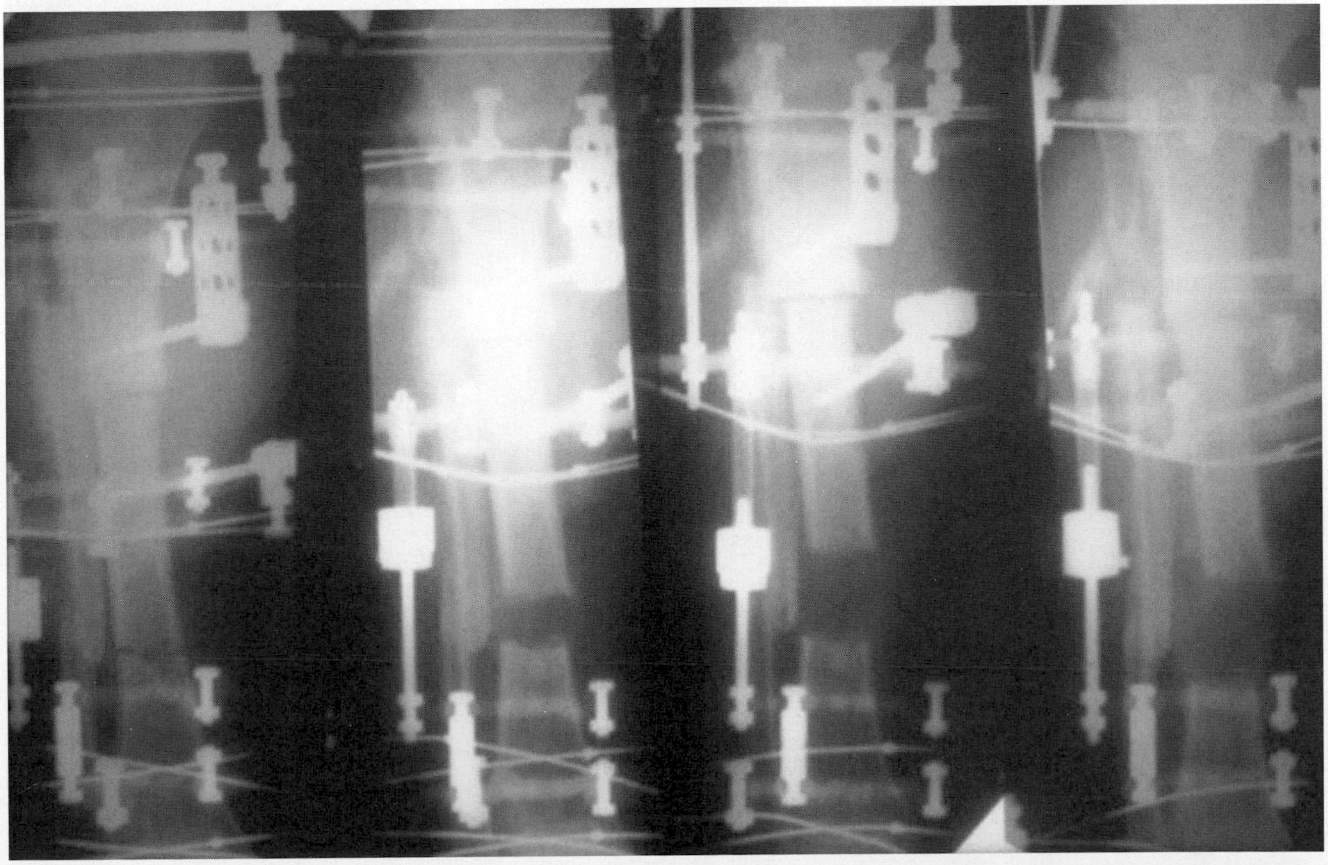

Figure 24-27. From left to right: acute shortening with application of Ilizarov external fixator. The proximal site was placed under compression and progressive lengthening occurred at the distal site.

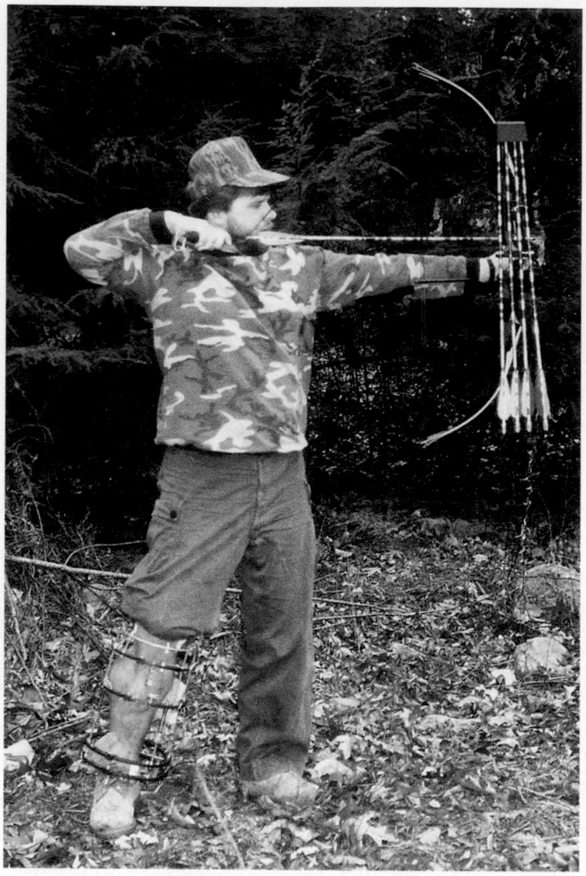

Figure 24-28. J.S. hunting with Ilizarov fixator in place showing that patients may remain active during their treatment.

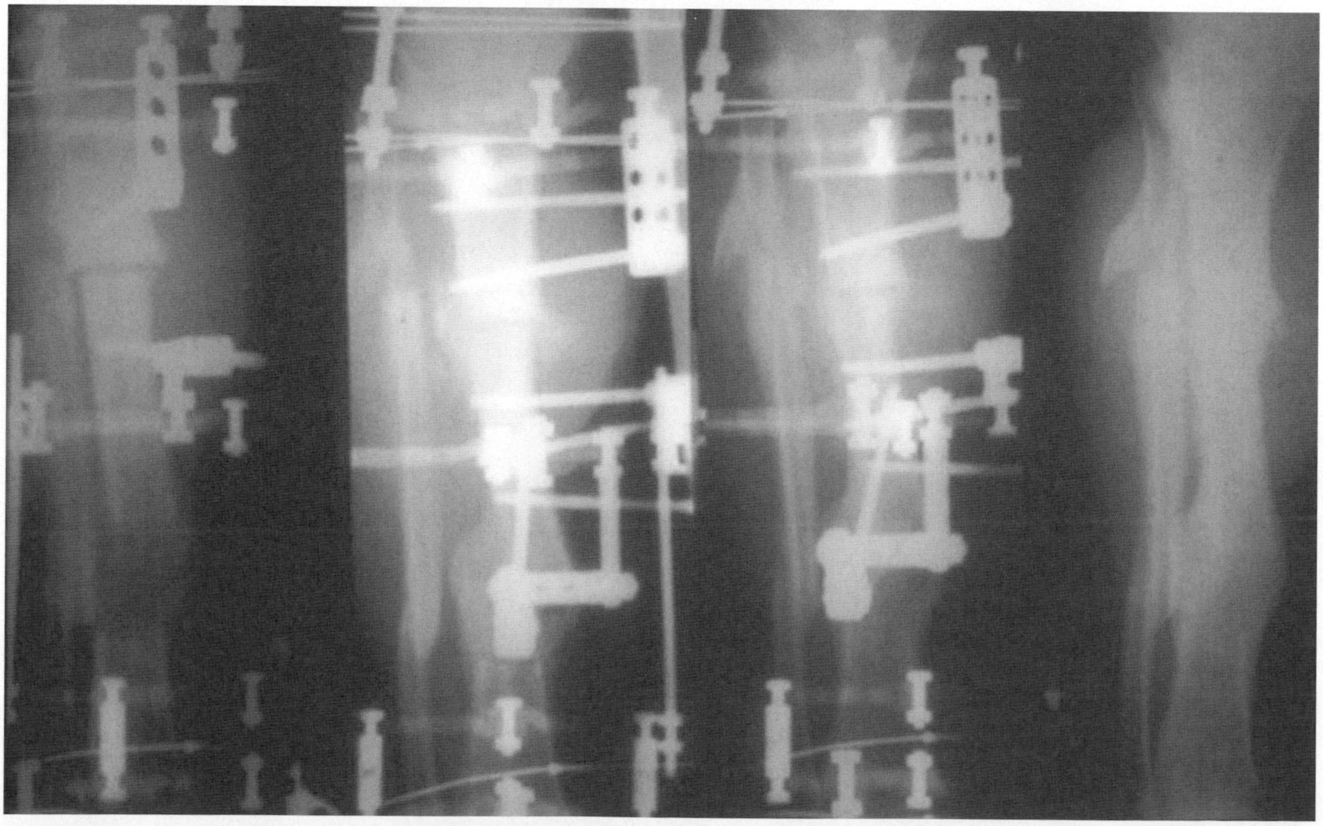

Figure 24-29. From left to right: progressive bone formation at both the proximal compression site and the distal regenerate zone. The last film was taken 1 year after the initial operation and 5 months following removal of the external fixator.

CONCLUSION AND FUTURE DIRECTIONS

Despite the rising prevalence of chronic osteomyelitis, great progress has been made over the past century in understanding the disease, achieving a rapid and accurate diagnosis, and providing potentially limb-sparing interventions. We have gained improved insight into the complexity of the biofilm communities and their mechanisms of antimicrobial resistance. We have improved access to advanced imaging including CT and MRI to allow diagnosis and localization of the infection. We have tested and improved our techniques of skeletal stabilization, soft tissue management, and discovered novel ways to control dead space while providing high local antibiotic concentrations. However, the battle has not been won and more challenges remain.

The evolution of bacteria with the adaptation of defense mechanisms against antimicrobials will be an ongoing challenge in the treatment of osteomyelitis. New antibiotics will need to be developed and used appropriately to maintain effectiveness. In addition, future research will need to focus on antimicrobial technology that allows bacterial cells living in biofilms and intracellularly to be targeted. Further, new antibiotic depots with similar elution characteristics to PMMA but that are incorporated into bone would limit the need for additional surgery for antibiotic bead extraction.

Another current challenge is correctly identifying the causative bacteria. Bone and soft tissue cultures are relied on as the gold standard in diagnosis of pathogens. However, the bacteria that grow on the standard culture plates are likely those that favor the media used (e.g., blood agar). Future development will include methods of identifying both free and adherent bacteria with alternative methods, such as molecular analysis, which may allow more accurate pathogen identification.

KEY REFERENCES

The level of evidence (LOE) is determined according to the criteria provided in the preface.

14. Lew DP, Waldvogel FA: Osteomyelitis. *Lancet* 364(9431):369–379, 2004. LOE III
19. Cierny G 3rd: Infected tibial nonunions (1981-1995). The evolution of change. *Clin Orthop Relat Res* 360:97–105, 1999. LOE III
20. Liu DS, Sofiadellis F, Ashton M, et al: Early soft tissue coverage and negative pressure wound therapy optimises patient outcomes in lower limb trauma. *Injury* 43(6):772–778, 2012. LOE III
23. Gustilo RB, Anderson JT: Prevention of infection in the treatment of one thousand and twenty-five open fractures of long bones: retrospective and prospective analyses. *J Bone Joint Surg Am* 58(4):453–458, 1976. LOE II
25. Pollak AN, Jones AL, Castillo RC, et al; LEAP Study Group: The relationship between time to surgical debridement and incidence of infection after open high-energy lower extremity trauma. *J Bone Joint Surg Am* 92(1):7–15, 2010. LOE III
34. Mouzopoulos G, Kanakaris NK, Kontakis G, et al: Management of bone infections in adults: the surgeon's and microbiologist's perspectives. *Injury* 42(Suppl 5):S18–S23, 2011. LOE V
66. Sheehy SH, Atkins BA, Bejon P, et al: The microbiology of chronic osteomyelitis: prevalence of resistance to common empirical anti-microbial regimens. *J Infect* 60(5):338–343, 2010. LOE IV
67. Wright JA, Nair SP: Interaction of staphylococci with bone. *Int J Med Microbiol* 300(2–3):193–204, 2010. LOE III
69. Patzakis MJ, Wilkins J, Kumar J, et al: Comparison of the results of bacterial cultures from multiple sites in chronic osteomyelitis of long bones. A prospective study. *J Bone Joint Surg Am* 76(5):664–666, 1994. LOE II
87. Mader JT, Shirtliff M, Calhoun JH: Staging and staging application in osteomyelitis. *Clin Infect Dis* 25(6):1303–1309, 1997. LOE V
89. Cierny G 3rd, Mader JT, Penninck JJ: A clinical staging system for adult osteomyelitis. *Clin Orthop Relat Res* 414:7–24, 2003. LOE V
95. Patzakis MJ, Zalavras CG: Chronic posttraumatic osteomyelitis and infected nonunion of the tibia: current management concepts. *J Am Acad Orthop Surg* 13(6):417–427, 2005. LOE V
102. Temkin S, Tisnado J, Montgomery DD: Plain radiographic evaluation of orthopedic infection: the initial step in imaging. *Techn Orthop* 26(4):233–237, 2011. LOE V
110. Cierny G 3rd: Surgical treatment of osteomyelitis. *Plast Reconstr Surg* 127(Suppl 1):190S–204S, 2011. LOE V
112. Doukas WC, Hayda RA, Frisch HM, et al: The Military Extremity Trauma Amputation/Limb Salvage (METALS) study: outcomes of amputation versus limb salvage following major lower-extremity trauma. *J Bone Joint Surg Am* 95(2):138–145, 2013. LOE III
116. Penn-Barwell JG: Outcomes in lower limb amputation following trauma: a systematic review and meta-analysis. *Injury* 42(12):1474–1479, 2011. LOE II
121. Simpson AH, Deakin M, Latham JM: Chronic osteomyelitis. The effect of the extent of surgical resection on infection-free survival. *J Bone Joint Surg Br* 83(3):403–407, 2001. LOE II
126. Muñoz-Mahamud E, García S, Bori G, et al: Comparison of a low-pressure and a high-pressure pulsatile lavage during debridement for orthopaedic implant infection. *Arch Orthop Trauma Surg* 131(9):1233–1238, 2011. LOE I
128. Anglen JO: Comparison of soap and antibiotic solutions for irrigation of lower-limb open fracture wounds. A prospective, randomized study. *J Bone Joint Surg Am* 87(7):1415–1422, 2005. LOE II
141. Dendrinos GK, Kontos S, Lyritsis E: Use of the Ilizarov technique for treatment of non-union of the tibia associated with infection. *J Bone Joint Surg Am* 77(6):835–846, 1995. LOE IV
156. Garrison KR, Shemilt I, Donell S, et al: Bone morphogenetic protein (BMP) for fracture healing in adults. *Cochrane Database Syst Rev* (6): CD006950, 2010. LOE I
167. Arnold PG, Yugueros P, Hanssen AD: Muscle flaps in osteomyelitis of the lower extremity: a 20-year account. *Plast Reconstr Surg* 104(1):107–110, 1999. LOE IV
178. Anagnostakos K, Wilmes P, Schmitt E, et al: Elution of gentamicin and vancomycin from polymethylmethacrylate beads and hip spacers in vivo. *Acta Orthop* 80(2):193–197, 2009. LOE III
183. Conterno LO, Turchi MD: Antibiotics for treating chronic osteomyelitis in adults. *Cochrane Database Syst Rev* (9):CD004439, 2013. LOE II

The complete References list is available online at https://expertconsult.inkling.com.

Chapter 25

Nonunions: Evaluation and Treatment

MARK R. BRINKER • DANIEL P. O'CONNOR

The following video is included with this chapter and may be viewed at https://expertconsult.inkling.com:

25-1. Plate osteosynthesis.

INTRODUCTION

Fracture nonunions may represent a very small percentage of the traumatologist's case load but can account for a high percentage of a surgeon's stress, anxiety, and frustration. A fracture nonunion may be anticipated following a severe traumatic injury, such as an open fracture with segmental bone loss, but may also appear following a low-energy fracture that seemed destined to heal.

Fracture nonunion is a chronic medical condition associated with pain, and functional and psychosocial disability.[1] Because of the wide variation in patient responses to various stresses[2] and the impact on the patient's family (relationships, income, etc.), these cases are often difficult to manage.

Some 90% to 95% of all fractures heal without problems.[3,4] Nonunions are the small percentage of cases in which the biological process of fracture repair cannot overcome the local biology and mechanics of the bony injury.

DEFINITIONS

A fracture is said to have "gone on to nonunion" when the normal biological healing processes cease to the extent that solid healing will not occur without further treatment intervention. The definition is subjective, with criteria that result in high interobserver variability.

The literature reveals a myriad of definitions of nonunion. For the purposes of clinical investigations, the U.S. Food and Drug Administration (FDA) defines a nonunion as a fracture that is at least 9 months old and has not shown any signs of healing for 3 consecutive months.[5,6] Müller's[7] definition is failure of a (tibia) fracture to unite after 8 months of nonoperative treatment. These two definitions are widely used, but their arbitrary use of a temporal limit is flawed.[8] For example, several months of observation are not required to declare a tibial shaft fracture with 10 cm of segmental bone loss to be a nonunion (i.e., an injury that will not heal without further intervention). Conversely, how does one define a fracture that continues to consolidate but requires 12 months to heal completely?[9]

We define **nonunion** as a fracture that, in the opinion of the treating physician, has a zero possibility of healing without further intervention. We define **delayed union** as a fracture, which in the opinion of the treating physician, shows slower progression to healing than anticipated and is at risk of nonunion without further intervention.

To understand the biological processes and clinical implications of fracture nonunion, an understanding of the normal fracture healing process is required.

FRACTURE REPAIR

Fracture repair is an astonishing process that involves spontaneous, structured regeneration of bony tissue and restoration of mechanical stability. The process begins at the moment of bony injury, initiating a proliferation of tissues that ultimately leads to healing.

The early biological response at the fracture site is an inflammatory response with bleeding and the formation of a fracture hematoma. The repair response is initiated by the presence of osteoprogenitor cells from the periosteum and endosteum and hematopoietic cells capable of secreting growth factors. Following solid fracture healing, bone remodeling progresses according to Wolff's law.[10-14]

The repair process, involving both intramembranous and enchondral bone formation, requires mechanical stability, an adequate blood supply, good bony contact, and the appropriate endocrine and metabolic responses. The type of healing is related to the extent of injury and the type of treatment (Table 25-1).

Healing via Callus

In the absence of rigid fixation, such as cast immobilization, stabilization of bony fragments occurs by periosteal and endosteal callus formation. If the fracture site has an adequate blood supply, callus formation progresses and increases the cross-sectional area at the fracture surface, which enhances fracture stability. Fracture stability is also provided by the formation of fibrocartilage, which replaces granulation tissue at the fracture site. Enchondral bone formation, in which bone replaces cartilage, occurs after calcification of the fibrocartilage.

Direct Bone (Osteonal) Healing

Direct osteonal healing occurs without external callus and is characterized by gradual disappearance of the fracture line over time. This process requires an adequate blood supply and absolute rigidity at the fracture site, most commonly accomplished via compression plating. In areas of direct bone-to-bone contact, fracture repair resembles cutting-cone type remodeling. In areas where small gaps exist between

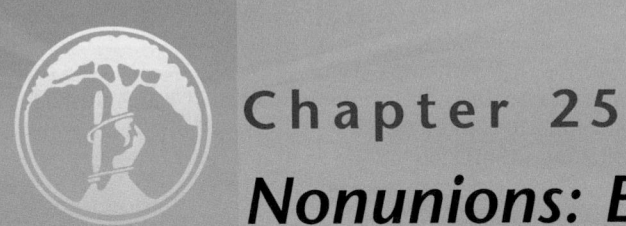

TABLE 25-1 *TYPE OF FRACTURE HEALING BASED ON TYPE OF STABILIZATION*

Type of Stabilization	Predominant Type of Healing
Cast (closed treatment)	Periosteal bridging callus and interfragmentary enchondral ossification
Compression plate	Primary cortical healing (cutting cone-type remodeling)
Intramedullary nail	Early: periosteal bridging callus Late: medullary callus
External fixator	Dependent on extent of rigidity Less rigid: periosteal bridging callus More rigid: primary cortical healing
Inadequate immobilization with adequate blood supply	Hypertrophic nonunion (failed enchondral ossification)
Inadequate immobilization without adequate blood supply	Atrophic nonunion
Inadequate reduction with displacement at the fracture site	Oligotrophic nonunion

fracture fragments, "gap healing" occurs via appositional bone formation.

Indirect Bone Healing

Indirect bone healing occurs in fractures that have been stabilized with less than absolute rigidity, including intramedullary nail fixation, tension band wire techniques, cerclage wiring, external fixation, and plate-and-screw fixation (when applied suboptimally). Indirect healing involves coupled bone resorption and bone formation at the fracture site. Healing occurs via a combination of external callus formation and enchondral ossification.

ETIOLOGY OF NONUNIONS

Predisposing Factors—Instability, Inadequate Vascularity, Poor Contact

The most basic requirements for fracture healing include: (1) mechanical stability, (2) adequate blood supply (i.e., bone vascularity), and (3) bone-to-bone contact. The absence of one or more of these factors predisposes the fracture to the development of a nonunion. The factors may be negatively affected by the severity of the injury, suboptimal surgical fixation, or a combination of injury severity and suboptimal surgical fixation.

Instability

Mechanical instability, excessive motion at the fracture site, can follow internal or external fixation. Factors producing mechanical instability include inadequate fixation (implants too small or too few), distraction of the fracture surfaces (hardware is as capable of holding bone apart as holding bone together), bone loss, and poor bone quality (i.e., poor purchase) (Fig. 25-1). An adequate blood supply with excessive motion at the fracture site results in abundant callus formation, widening of the fracture line, failure of fibrocartilage to mineralize, and ultimately failure to unite.

Inadequate Vascularity

Loss of blood supply to the fracture surfaces may arise because of the severity of the injury or because of surgical dissection. Several studies have shown a relationship between the extent of soft tissue injury and the risk of fracture nonunion.[15-17] Open fractures and high-energy closed injuries may strip soft tissues, damage the periosteal blood supply, and disrupt the nutrient vessels, impairing the endosteal blood supply.

Injury of certain vessels, such as the posterior tibial artery, may also increase risk of nonunion.[18] Vascularity may also be compromised by excess stripping of the periosteum as well as damage to bone and the soft tissues during open reduction and hardware insertion. Whatever the cause, inadequate vascularity results in necrotic bone at the ends of the fracture fragments, which often results in fracture nonunion.

Poor Bone Contact

Poor bone-to-bone contact at the fracture site may result from soft tissue interposition, malposition or malalignment of the fracture fragments, bone loss, and distraction of the fracture fragments (see Fig. 25-1). Whatever the cause, poor bone-to-bone contact compromises mechanical stability and creates a defect.

The probability of fracture union decreases as defects increase in size. The threshold value for rapid bridging of cortical defects via direct osteonal healing, the so-called osteoblastic jumping distance, is approximately 1 mm in rabbits,[19] but varies from species to species. Larger cortical defects may also heal, but at a much slower rate and bridge via woven bone. The "critical defect" represents the distance between fracture surfaces that will not be bridged by bone without intervention. The critical defect size depends on a variety of injury-related factors and varies considerably among species.

Other Contributing Factors

In addition to mechanical instability, inadequate vascularity, and poor bone contact, other factors may contribute to development of nonunion (Table 25-2). These factors, however, are not direct causes of nonunion, per se.

Infection

Infection in the zone of fracture increases the risk of nonunion.[17] Infection may result in instability at the fracture site as implants loosen in infected bone. Avascular, necrotic bone at the fracture site (sequestrum), common with infection, discourages bony union. Infection also produces poor bony contact as osteolysis at the fracture site results from ingrowth of infected granulation tissue.

Nicotine and Cigarette Smoking

Cigarette smoking adversely affects fracture healing. Nicotine inhibits vascular ingrowth and early revascularization of bone[20,21] and diminishes osteoblast function.[22-24] In rabbit models, cigarette smoking and nicotine impair bone healing in fractures,[25] in spinal fusion,[26,27] and during tibial lengthening.[28,29]

Delayed fracture healing and higher nonunion rates have been reported in patients who smoke.[30-35] Cigarette smoking

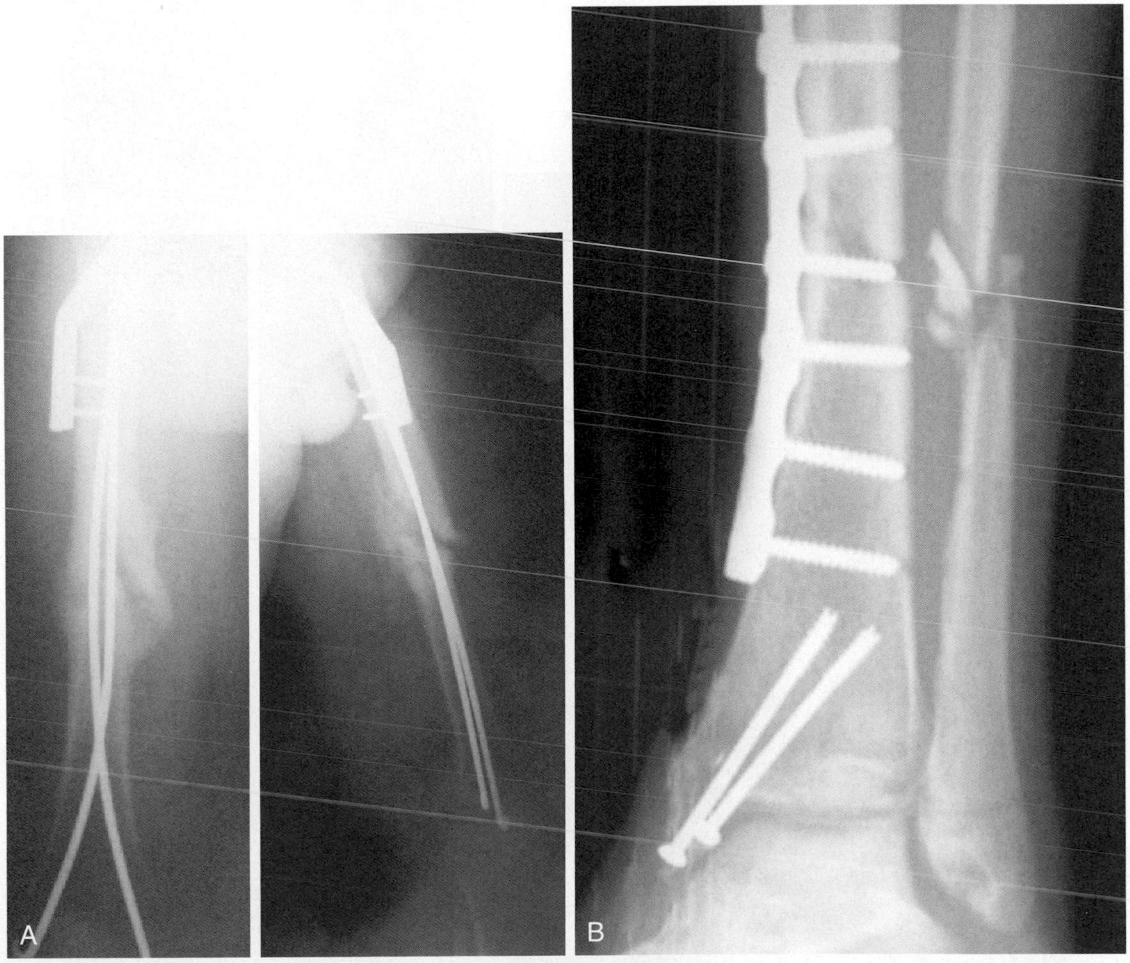

Figure 25-1. Mechanical instability at the fracture site can lead to nonunion. Mechanical instability can be caused by the following: **A,** Inadequate fixation: A 33-year-old man presented with a femoral shaft nonunion 8 months following inadequate fixation with flexible intramedullary nails. **B,** Distraction: A 19-year-old man with a tibia fracture treated with plate-and-screw fixation; this patient is at risk for nonunion because of distraction at the fracture site.

Continued

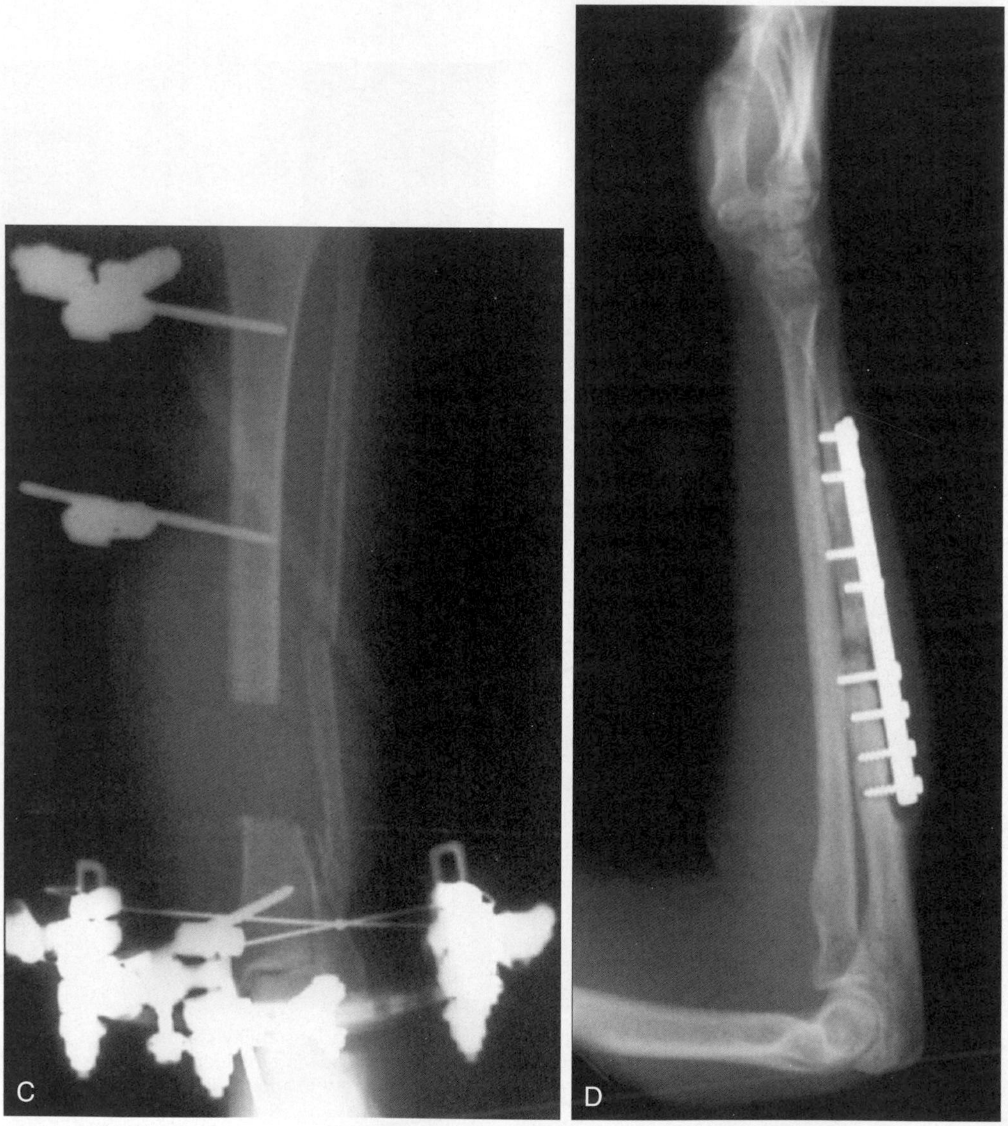

Figure 25-1, cont'd. C, Bone loss: A 57-year-old man presented with segmental bone loss following débridement of a high-energy open tibia fracture. **D,** Poor bone quality: A 31-year-old woman presented 2 years following open reduction internal fixation for an ulna shaft fracture; loss of fixation proved to be due to poor bone from chronic osteomyelitis.

TABLE 25-2 ETIOLOGY OF NONUNIONS

Predisposing Factors
Mechanical Instability
1. Inadequate fixation
2. Distraction
3. Bone loss
4. Poor bone quality
Inadequate Vascularity
1. Severe injury
2. Excessive soft tissue stripping
3. Vascular injury
Poor Contact
1. Soft tissue interposition
2. Malposition or malalignment
3. Bone loss
4. Distraction
Contributing Factors
Infection
Nicotine/cigarette smoking
Certain medications
Advanced age
Systemic medical conditions
Poor functional level
Venous stasis
Burns
Radiation
Obesity
Alcohol abuse
Metabolic and endocrine abnormalities
Malnutrition
Vitamin deficiencies

is also associated with osteoporosis and generalized bone loss,[36] so mechanical instability due to poor bone quality for purchase may play a role.

Certain Medications

A number of animal studies have shown that nonsteroidal antiinflammatory drugs (NSAIDs) negatively affect the healing of experimentally induced fractures and osteotomies.[37-45] Other animal studies have reported no significant effect.[46,47]

Delayed long-bone fracture healing has been documented in humans taking oral NSAIDs.[48-50] While this body of literature suggests that NSAIDs are a factor in delayed fracture healing, no consensus exists. Furthermore, the mechanism of action (direct action at the fracture site vs. indirect hormonal actions) remains obscure. Finally, whether all NSAIDs display similar effects and the dose-response characteristics of specific NSAIDs relative to delayed union or nonunion remain unknown.

Other medications have been postulated to affect fracture healing adversely, including phenytoin,[5] ciprofloxacin,[51] steroids, anticoagulants, and others.

Other Contributing Factors

Other factors that may retard fracture healing or contribute to fracture nonunion include advanced age,[5,31,52] systemic medical conditions (e.g., diabetes),[53,54] poor functional level with inability to bear weight, venous stasis, burns, radiation, obesity,[55] alcohol abuse,[53-55] metabolic bone disease,[56] malnutrition[57] and cachexia, and vitamin deficiencies.[58]

Rodent studies have shown that albumin deficiency produces a fracture callus with reduced strength and stiffness,[59] although early fracture healing proceeds normally.[60] Dietary supplementation of protein during fracture repair reverses these effects and augments fracture healing.[60,61] Protein intake in excess of normal daily requirements is unnecessary.[59,62]

EVALUATION OF NONUNIONS

No two patients with fracture nonunion are identical. The evaluation process is perhaps the most critical step in the patient's treatment pathway and is when the surgeon begins to form opinions about how to heal the nonunion. The goals of the evaluation are to discover the etiology of the nonunion and form a plan for healing the nonunion. Without understanding the etiology, the treatment strategy cannot be based on knowledge of fracture biology. A worksheet is an excellent method of assimilating the various data (Fig. 25-2).

Patient History

Evaluation begins with a thorough history, including the date and mechanism of the initial fracture, preinjury medical problems, disabilities, and associated injuries, as well as pain and functional limitations related to the nonunion. The specific details of each prior surgical procedure to treat the fracture and fracture nonunion must be obtained through the patient and family, the prior treating surgeons, and a review of all medical records since the time of the initial fracture.

Knowledge of prior operative procedures is critical for designing the right treatment plan. Ignorance of any prior surgical procedure can lead to needlessly repeating surgical procedures that have failed to promote bony union in the past. Worse yet, ignorance of prior surgical procedures can lead to avoidable complications. For example, awareness of prior external fixation is important when the use of intramedullary nail fixation is contemplated because of an increased risk of infection.[63-69]

The hospital records and operative reports from the time of the initial fracture may also be used to determine the condition of the tissues in the injury zone (open wounds, contamination, crush injuries, periosteal stripping, devitalized bone fragments, etc.) and the history of prior soft tissue coverage procedures.

The history should also include details regarding prior wound infections, including culture reports in prior medical records. Intravenous and oral antibiotic use should be documented, particularly if the patient remains on antibiotics at the time of presentation. Problems with wound healing and episodes of soft tissue breakdown should be noted, as should other perioperative complications (venous thrombosis, nerve or vessel injuries, etc.). Prior use of adjuvant nonsurgical therapies, such as electromagnetic field and ultrasound therapy should be described.

Finally, the patient should be questioned regarding other possible contributing factors for nonunion (see Table 25-2). The history of NSAID use should be obtained and their use should be discontinued. The pack-year history of cigarette smoking should be documented, and active smokers should be offered a program to halt the addiction, although it is unrealistic to delay treatment of a symptomatic nonunion until the patient stops smoking.

GENERAL INFORMATION

Patient Name: ______ Age: ______ Gender: ______

Referring Physician: ______ Height: ______ Weight: ______

Injury (description): ______

Date of Injury: ______

Mechanism of Injury: ______ Pain (0 to 10 VAS): ______

Occupation: ______ Was Injury Work Related?: Y N

PAST HISTORY

Initial Fracture Treatment (Date): ______

Total # of Surgeries for Nonunion: ______

Surgery #1 (Date): ______

Surgery #2 (Date): ______

Surgery #3 (Date): ______

Surgery #4 (Date): ______

Surgery #5 (Date): ______

Surgery #6 (Date): ______

(Use backside of this sheet for other prior surgeries)

Use of Electromagnetic or Ultrasound Stimulation? ______

Cigarette Smoking # of packs per day ______ # of years smoking ______

History of Infection? (include culture results) ______

History of Soft Tissue Problems? ______

Medical Conditions: ______

Medications: ______

NSAID Use: ______

Narcotic Use: ______

Allergies: ______

PHYSICAL EXAMINATION

General: ______

Extremity:

Nonunion: ______ Stiff ______ Lax

Adjacent Joints (ROM, compensatory deformities): ______

Soft Tissues (defects, drainage): ______

Neurovascular Exam: ______

RADIOLOGIC EXAMINATION

Comments ______

OTHER PERTINENT INFORMATION ______

NONUNION TYPE

______ Hypertrophic

______ Oligotrophic

______ Atrophic

______ Infected

______ Synovial Pseudarthrosis

Figure 25-2. Worksheet for patients with nonunions. *NSAID,* Nonsteroidal antiinflammatory drug; *ROM,* range of motion; *VAS,* visual analog scale.

Physical Examination

The general health and nutritional status of the patient should be assessed because malnutrition and cachexia diminish fracture repair.[57,59,62,70] Arm muscle circumference is the best indicator of nutritional status. Obese patients with nonunions have unique management problems related to achieving mechanical stability in the presence of high loads and large soft tissue envelopes.[71]

The skin and soft tissues in the fracture zone should be inspected. The presence of active drainage, sinus formation, and deformity should be noted. A neurovascular examination is performed to document vascular insufficiency and motor or sensory dysfunction.

The nonunion site should be manually stressed to evaluate motion and pain. Generally, nonunions with little or no clinically apparent motion have some callus formation and good vascularity at the fracture surfaces. Nonunions that display motion typically have poor callus formation, but may have vascular or avascular fracture surfaces. Assessment of nonunion site motion is difficult in limbs with paired bones in which one of the bones remains intact.

Active and passive motion of the joints adjacent to the nonunion, both proximal and distal, should be performed. Not uncommonly, motion at the nonunion site diminishes motion at an adjacent joint. For example, patients with a longstanding distal tibial nonunion often have a fixed equinus

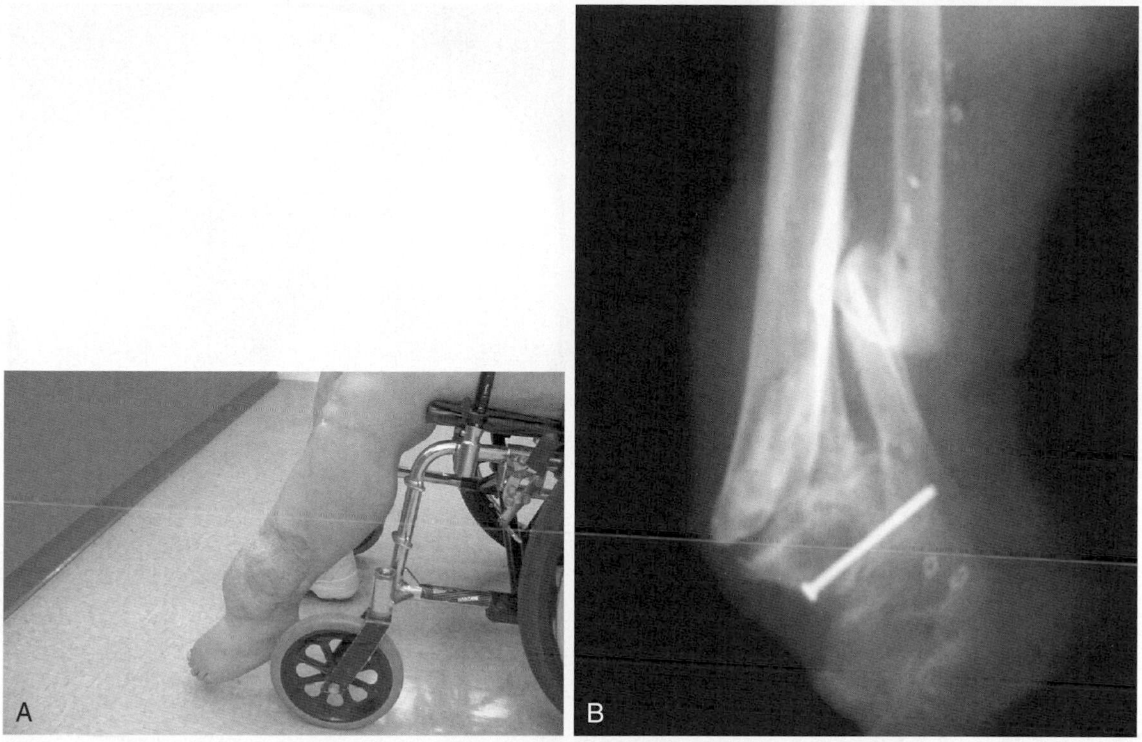

Figure 25-3. A 20-year-old young lady presented with a distal tibial nonunion 22 months status post a high-energy open fracture. **A,** Clinical photograph and (**B**) lateral radiograph showing apex anterior angulation at the fracture site resulting in the clinical equivalent of a severe equinus contracture.

contracture and limited ankle motion (Fig. 25-3). Similarly, patients with supracondylar humeral nonunions commonly have fibrous ankylosis of the elbow (Fig. 25-4). Such problems may alter both the treatment plan and the expectations for the ultimate functional outcome.

An interesting situation worth noting is the stiff nonunion with an angular deformity. These patients may present with a compensatory fixed deformity at an adjacent joint. The fixed deformity at the joint must be recognized preoperatively and the treatment plan must include its correction. Realignment of a stiff nonunion with a deformity without addressing an adjacent compensatory fixed joint deformity results in a straight bone with a deformed joint, thus producing a disabled limb. For example, patients who have a stiff distal tibial nonunion with a varus deformity often develop a compensatory valgus deformity at the subtalar joint to achieve a plantigrade foot for gait. On visual inspection, the distal limb segment appears aligned, but radiographs show the distal tibial varus deformity. To determine whether the subtalar joint deformity is fixed or reducible, the patient is asked to position the subtalar joint in varus (i.e., invert the foot). If the patient cannot invert the subtalar joint, and the examiner cannot passively invert the subtalar joint, the joint deformity is fixed. Deformity correction will therefore be required at both the nonunion site and the subtalar joint. Conversely, if the patient can achieve subtalar inversion, the deformity at the joint will resolve with deformity correction at the nonunion. In general, if the patient cannot place the joint into the position that parallels the deformity at the nonunion site, the joint deformity is fixed and requires correction. If the patient can achieve the position, the joint deformity will resolve with realignment of the long bone deformity (Fig. 25-5).

If bone grafting is contemplated, the anterior and posterior iliac crests should be examined for evidence (e.g., incisions) of prior surgical harvesting. For a patient who has had prior spinal surgery, determining which posterior crest has already been harvested may be difficult. In such a case, the posterior iliac crests may be evaluated via plain radiographs or computed tomography (CT) scan.

Radiologic Examination

Plain Radiographs

A review of the original fracture films reveals the character and severity of the initial bony injury. They can also show the progress or lack of progress toward healing when compared to the most recent plain radiographs.

Radiographs of the salient aspects of previous treatments will always tell the story of the nonunion to the astute observer. All prior plain films should be examined for the status of orthopaedic hardware (e.g., loose, broken, inadequate in size or number of implants) including removal or insertion on sequential films. The evolution of deformity at the nonunion site—whether a gradual process or single event, for example—should be evaluated via the series of prior radiographs. The presence of healed or unhealed articular, butterfly, and wedge fragments should also be noted. The time course of missing or removed bony fragments, added bone graft, and implanted bone stimulators should be reconstructed so that the healing response to each can be evaluated.

The nonunion is next evaluated with a series of new radiographs:

- An anterior-posterior (AP) and lateral radiograph of the involved bone including the proximal and distal joints

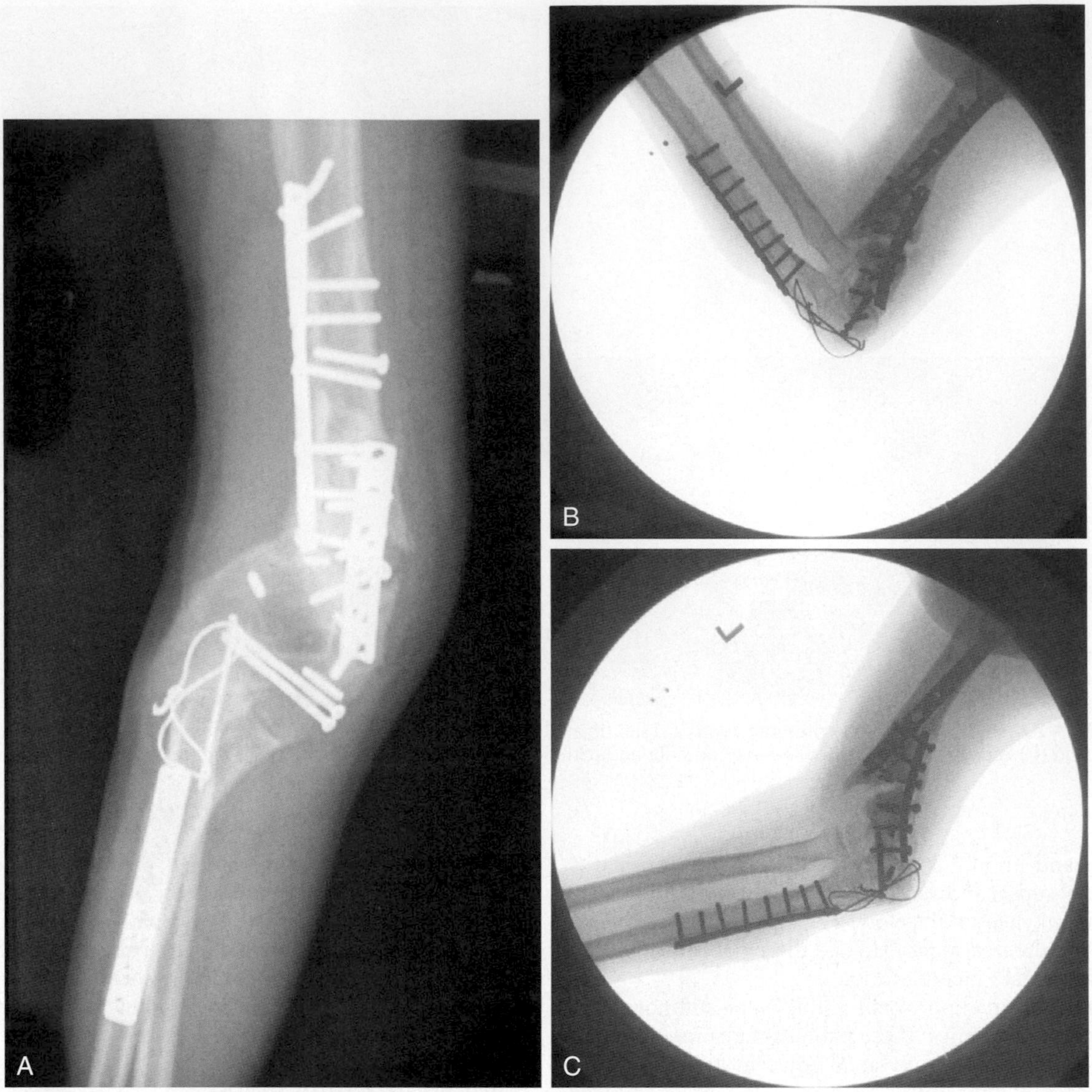

Figure 25-4. **A,** Anterior-posterior (AP) radiograph of a 32-year-old man who presented with a supracondylar humeral nonunion. On physical examination, it can be difficult to differentiate motion at the nonunion site and the elbow joint. This patient had very limited range of motion at the elbow but gross motion at the nonunion site. Cineradiography can be useful for evaluating the contribution of the adjacent joint and the nonunion site to the arc of motion. **B** and **C,** Cineradiography showing flexion and extension of the elbow, respectively, reveals that most of the motion is occurring through the nonunion site, not the elbow joint. This patient should be counseled preoperatively regarding elbow stiffness following stabilization of the nonunion.

- AP, lateral, and two oblique views of the nonunion site on small cassette films to improve magnification and resolution (Fig. 25-6)
- Bilateral AP and lateral 51-inch alignment radiographs for lower extremity nonunions for assessing length discrepancies and deformities (Fig. 25-7)
- Flexion/extension lateral radiographs to determine the arc of motion and to assess the relative contributions of the joint and the nonunion site to that arc

The current plain films are used to evaluate the following radiographic characteristics of a nonunion: anatomic location, healing effort, bone quality, surface characteristics, status of previously implanted hardware, and deformities.

Anatomic Location. Diaphyseal nonunions involve primarily cortical bone, whereas metaphyseal and epiphyseal nonunions largely involve cancellous bone. The presence of intraarticular extension of the nonunion should also be assessed.

Healing Effort and Bone Quality. The radiographic healing effort and bone quality helps to define the biological and mechanical etiologies of the nonunion. The assessment of healing includes evaluating radiolucent lines, gaps, and callus formation. The assessment of bone quality includes observing sclerosis, atrophy, osteopenia, and bony defects.

Radiolucent lines seen along fracture surfaces suggest regions that are devoid of bony healing. The simple presence of radiolucent lines on plain radiographs is not synonymous with nonunion, just as the lack of a clear radiolucent line does not confirm fracture union (Fig. 25-8).

Callus formation occurs in fractures and nonunions that have an adequate blood supply, but does not necessarily imply the bone is solidly uniting. AP, lateral, and oblique radiographs

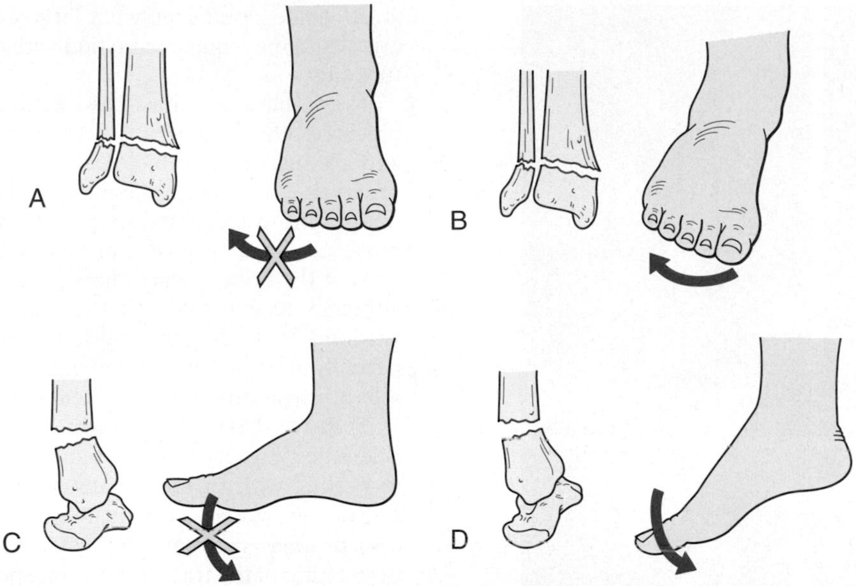

Figure 25-5. Angular deformity at a nonunion site, which is near a joint, can result in a compensatory deformity through a neighboring joint. For example, coronal plane deformities of the distal tibia can result in a compensatory coronal plane deformity of the subtalar joint. A deformity of the subtalar joint is (**A**) fixed if the patient's foot cannot be positioned into the deformity of the distal tibia, or (**B**) flexible if it can be positioned into the deformity of the distal tibia. Sagittal plane deformities of the distal tibia can result in a sagittal plane deformity of the ankle joint. A deformity of the ankle joint is (**C**) fixed if the patient's foot cannot be positioned into the deformity of the distal tibia or (**D**) flexible if it can be positioned into the deformity of the distal tibia.

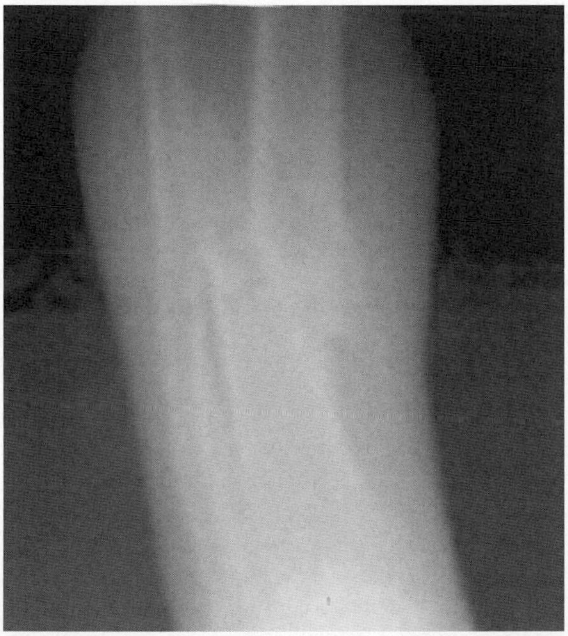

Figure 25-6. A nonunion is visualized better on small cassette views than on large cassette views (see Figure 25-7 for comparison).

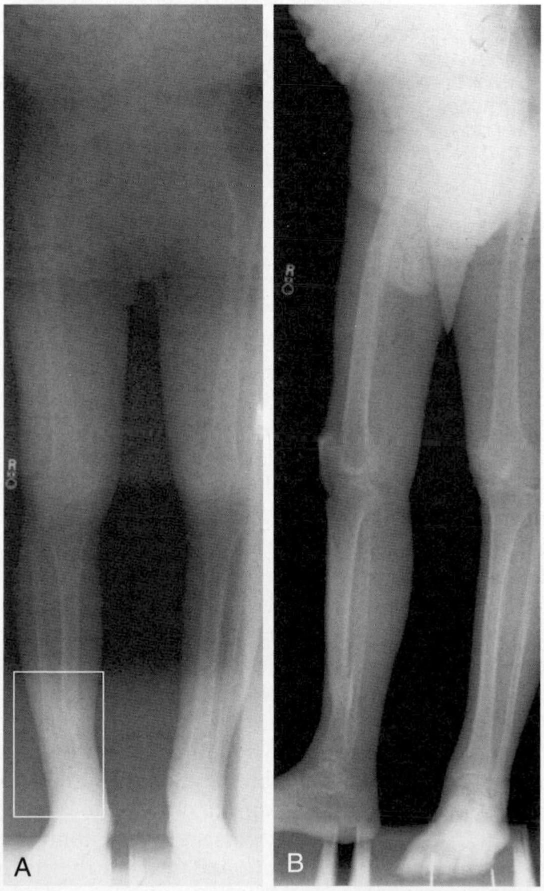

Figure 25-7. A 60-year-old man presented with a tibial nonunion and an oblique plane angular deformity as seen on the (**A**) 51-inch anterior-posterior (AP) alignment view and (**B**) 51-inch lateral alignment view.

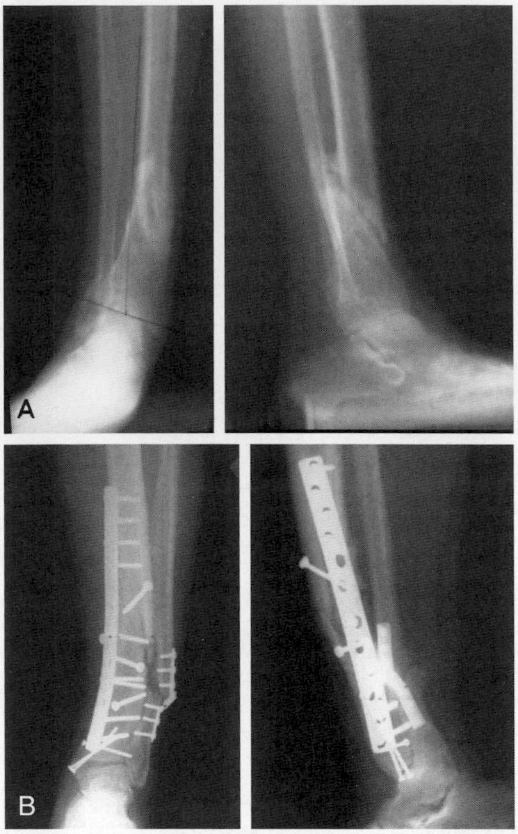

Figure 25-8. A definitive decision cannot always be made about bony union based on plain radiographs. **A,** This 88-year-old woman is 14 months status post a distal tibial fracture treated elsewhere with external fixation. Anterior-posterior (AP) and lateral radiographs are shown. Is this fracture healed or is there a nonunion? (See Figure 25-17.) **B,** This 49-year-old man presented 13 months status post open reduction internal fixation of a distal tibia fracture. Anterior-posterior (AP) and lateral radiographs are shown. Is this fracture healed or is there a nonunion? (See Figure 25-17.)

should be assessed for callus bridging the injury zone. All radiographs should be carefully checked for radiolucent lines so that a nonunion with abundant callus is not mistaken for a solidly united fracture (see Fig. 25-8).

Weber and Cech[72] have classified nonunions based on radiographic healing effort and bone quality into *viable nonunions,* which are capable of biological activity, and *nonviable nonunions,* which are incapable of biological activity.

Viable nonunions include *hypertrophic nonunions* and *oligotrophic nonunions.* Hypertrophic nonunions possess adequate vascularity and display callus formation. They arise because of inadequate mechanical stability with persistent motion at the fracture surfaces. The fracture site is progressively resorbed with accumulation of unmineralized fibrocartilage and displays a gradually widening radiolucent line with sclerotic edges. Capillaries and blood vessels invade both sides of the nonunion but do not penetrate the fibrocartilaginous tissue (Fig. 25-9).[73] As motion persists at the nonunion site, endosteal callus may accumulate and seal off the medullary canal, increasing production of hypertrophic periosteal callus. Hypertrophic nonunions may be classified as *elephant foot type,* with abundant callus formation, or *horse hoof type,* with less abundant callus formation. Oligotrophic nonunions have an adequate blood supply but little or no callus formation and arise from inadequate reduction with displacement at the fracture site.

Nonviable nonunions have inadequate vascularity, which precludes the formation of periosteal and endosteal callus, and are incapable of biological activity. The radiolucent gap observable on plain radiographs is bridged by fibrous tissue that has no osteogenic capacity. An *atrophic nonunion* is the most advanced type of nonviable nonunion. Classically, the ends of the bony surfaces have been thought to be avascular, although recent studies have questioned this conventional wisdom.[74,75] Radiographically, the fracture surfaces appear partially absorbed and osteopenic. Severe cases may have large sclerotic avascular bone segments or segmental bone loss.

Surface Characteristics. A nonunion's surface characteristics (Fig. 25-10) are prognostic in regard to its resistance to healing with various treatment strategies. Surface characteristics evaluated on plain radiographs include the surface area of adjacent fragments, extent of current bony contact, orientation of the fracture lines (shape of the bone fragments), and stability to axial compression (fracture surface orientation and comminution). The nonunions that are generally the easiest to treat have good bony contact and large, transversely oriented surfaces that are stable to axial compression.

Status of Previously Implanted Hardware. Plain radiographs reveal the status and stability of previously implanted hardware and the mechanical construct used to fixate the bone. Loose or broken implants denote instability at the nonunion site (i.e., the race between bony union and hardware failure has been lost)[7,76-81] that requires further stabilization before union can occur. Radiographs are also useful for planning any hardware removal needed to carry out the next treatment plan.

Deformities. Having assessed for clinical deformity via physical examination, plain radiographs are used to characterize further and more fully all associated deformities. Deformities are characterized by location (diaphyseal, metaphyseal, epiphyseal), magnitude, and direction and are described in terms of length, angulation, rotation, and translation.[82]

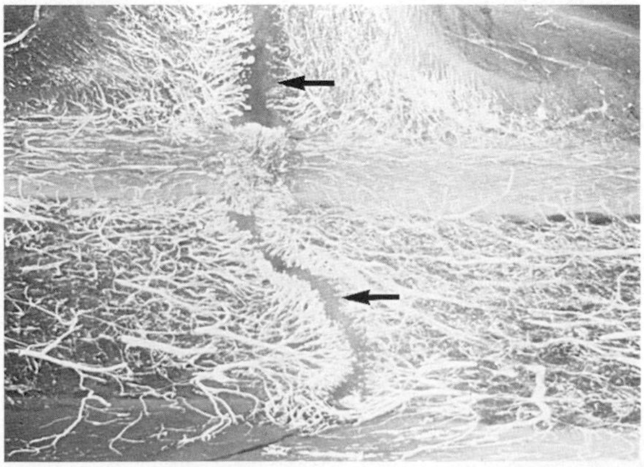

Figure 25-9. Microangiogram of a hypertrophic delayed union of a canine radius. Note the tremendous increase in local vascularity. The capillaries, however, are unable to penetrate the interposed fibrocartilage *(arrows). (From Rhinelander FW: The normal microcirculation of diaphyseal cortex and its response to fracture, J Bone Joint Surg Am 50A:78, 1968.)*

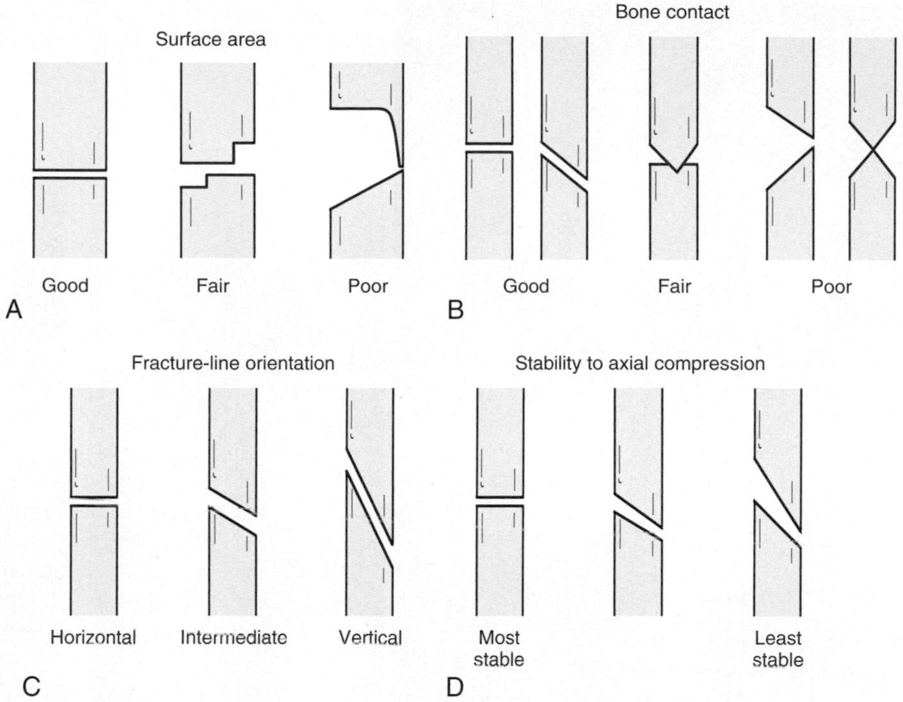

Figure 25-10. Surface characteristics at the site of nonunion. **A,** Surface area. **B,** Bone contact. **C,** Fracture line orientation. **D,** Stability to axial compression.

Deformities involving length include shortening and overdistraction. They are measured in centimeters on plain radiographs in comparison to the contralateral normal extremity, using an x-ray marker to correct for magnification. Shortening may result from bone loss (from the injury or débridement) or overriding fracture fragments (malreduction). Overdistraction may result from a traction injury or improper positioning at the time of surgical fixation.

Deformities involving angulation are characterized by magnitude and direction of apex of the angulation. Pure sagittal or coronal plane deformities are simple to characterize. Coronal plane angulation in the lower extremity commonly results in mechanical axis deviation of the extremity (Fig. 25-11). Varus deformities result in medial mechanical axis deviation, and valgus deformities result in lateral mechanical axis deviation.

Oblique plane angular deformities occur in a plane that is neither the sagittal nor the coronal plane and can be characterized using either the trigonometric method or the graphic method (see Fig. 25-11).[83-88]

Angulation at a diaphyseal nonunion is usually obvious on plain radiographs as divergence of the anatomic axes (mid-diaphyseal lines) of the proximal and distal fragments (see Fig. 25-11). The magnitude and direction of angulation can be measured by drawing the anatomic axes of the proximal and distal segments (see Fig. 25-11).

Angular deformities associated with nonunions of the metaphysis and epiphysis (juxtaarticular deformities) are less obvious and more challenging to evaluate as they cannot be characterized using the mid-diaphyseal line method. Recognition and characterization of a juxtaarticular deformity require using the angle formed by the intersection of a joint orientation line and the bone's anatomic or mechanical axis (Fig. 25-12). When the angle formed differs markedly from the contralateral normal extremity, a juxtaarticular deformity is present. If the contralateral extremity is also abnormal (e.g., bilateral injuries), published normal values are used for evaluation (Table 25-3).[85-87]

The center of rotation of angulation (CORA) is the point at which the axis of the proximal segment intersects the axis of the distal segment (Fig. 25-13).[82] For diaphyseal deformities, the anatomic axes are convenient to use. For juxtaarticular deformities, the axis line of the short segment is constructed using one of three methods: extension of the segment axis from the adjacent, intact bone if its anatomy is normal; comparing the joint orientation angle of the abnormal side to the opposite side if the latter is normal; or drawing a line that creates the population normal angle formed by the intersection with the joint orientation line.

The bisector is a line that passes through the CORA and bisects the angle formed by the proximal and distal axes (see Fig. 25-13).[82] Angular correction along the bisector results in complete deformity correction without introducing translational deformity.[83-87]

Rotational deformities associated with a nonunion may be missed on physical and radiologic examination. Accurate clinical assessment of the magnitude of a rotational deformity is difficult and plain radiographs offer little assistance. CT scanning is the best method of radiographic assessment of malrotation, as described in the next subsection.

Like angular deformities, translational deformities are characterized by magnitude and direction. The magnitude of translation is the perpendicular distance from the axis line of the proximal fragment to the axis line of the distal fragment.

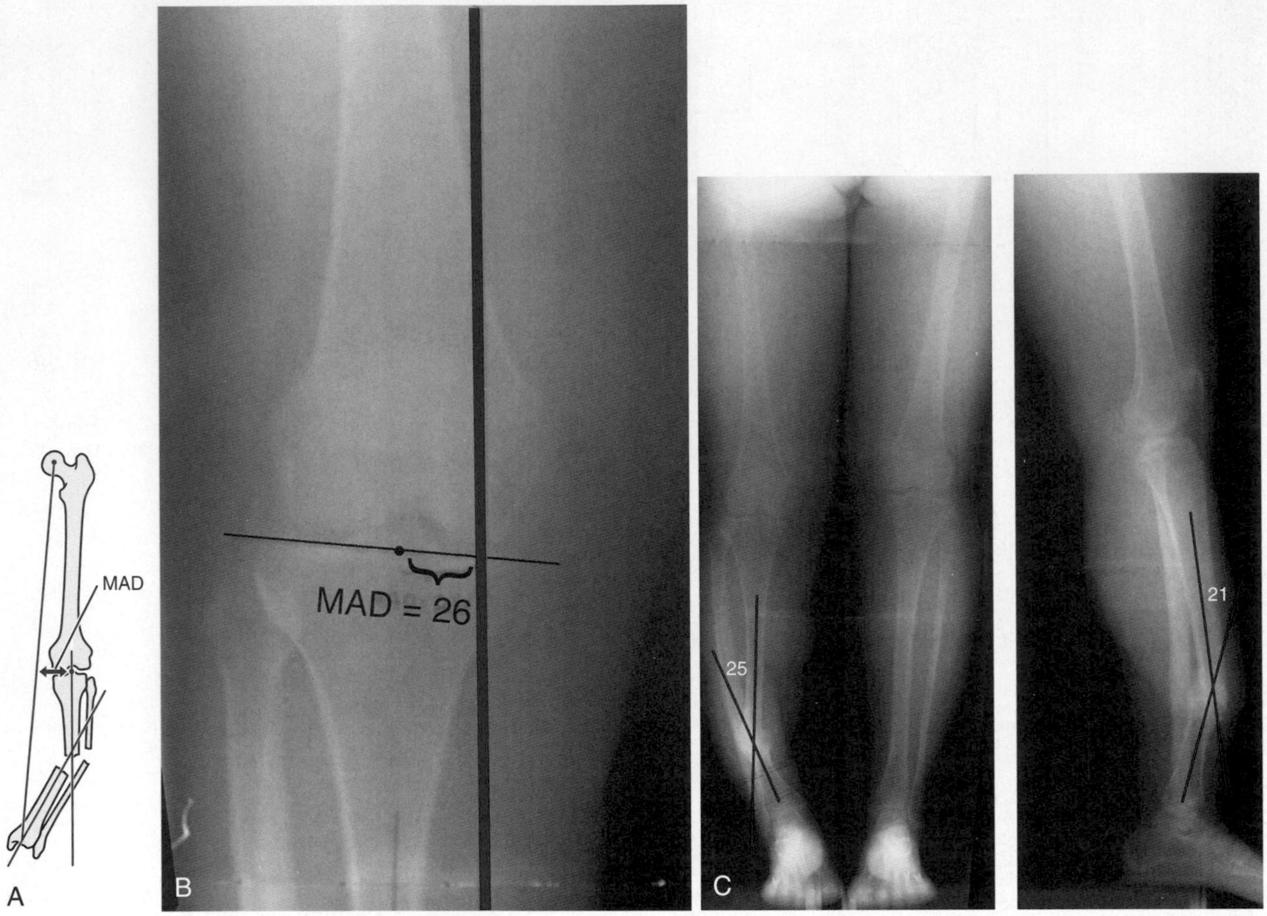

Trigonometric Method

Magnitude of oblique plane deformity =

$$\tan^{-1}\sqrt{\tan^2 \text{coronal deformity} + \tan^2 \text{sagittal deformity}}$$

$$\tan^{-1}\sqrt{\tan^2 25° + \tan^2 21°}$$

Solution = 31°

Orientation of oblique plane deformity =

$$\tan^{-1}\frac{\tan \text{sagittal deformity}}{\tan \text{coronal deformity}}$$

$$\tan^{-1}\frac{\tan 21°}{\tan 25°}$$

D

Solution = 39°

Graphic Method

Magnitude of oblique plane deformity =

$$\sqrt{\text{Coronal deformity}^2 + \text{Sagittal deformity}^2}$$

$$\sqrt{25^2 + 21^2}$$

Solution = 33°

Orientation of oblique plane deformity =

$$\tan^{-1}\frac{\text{Sagittal deformity}}{\text{Coronal deformity}}$$

$$\tan^{-1}\frac{21°}{25°}$$

E

Solution = 40°

Figure 25-11. A, In this example, there is a nonunion of the diaphysis of the tibia with a varus deformity resulting in medial mechanical axis deviation. Note the divergence of the anatomic axis of the proximal and distal fragments of the tibia. **B,** Close-up view of a section of an anterior-posterior (AP) 51-inch alignment radiograph of a 37-year-old woman with an 18-year history of a tibial nonunion. Note the medial mechanical axis deviation (MAD) of 26 mm. **C,** AP and lateral radiographs show a 25-degree varus deformity and a 21-degree apex anterior angulation deformity, respectively. **D,** Characterization of the oblique plane angular deformity using the trigonometric method. **E,** Characterization of the oblique plane angular deformity using the graphic method.

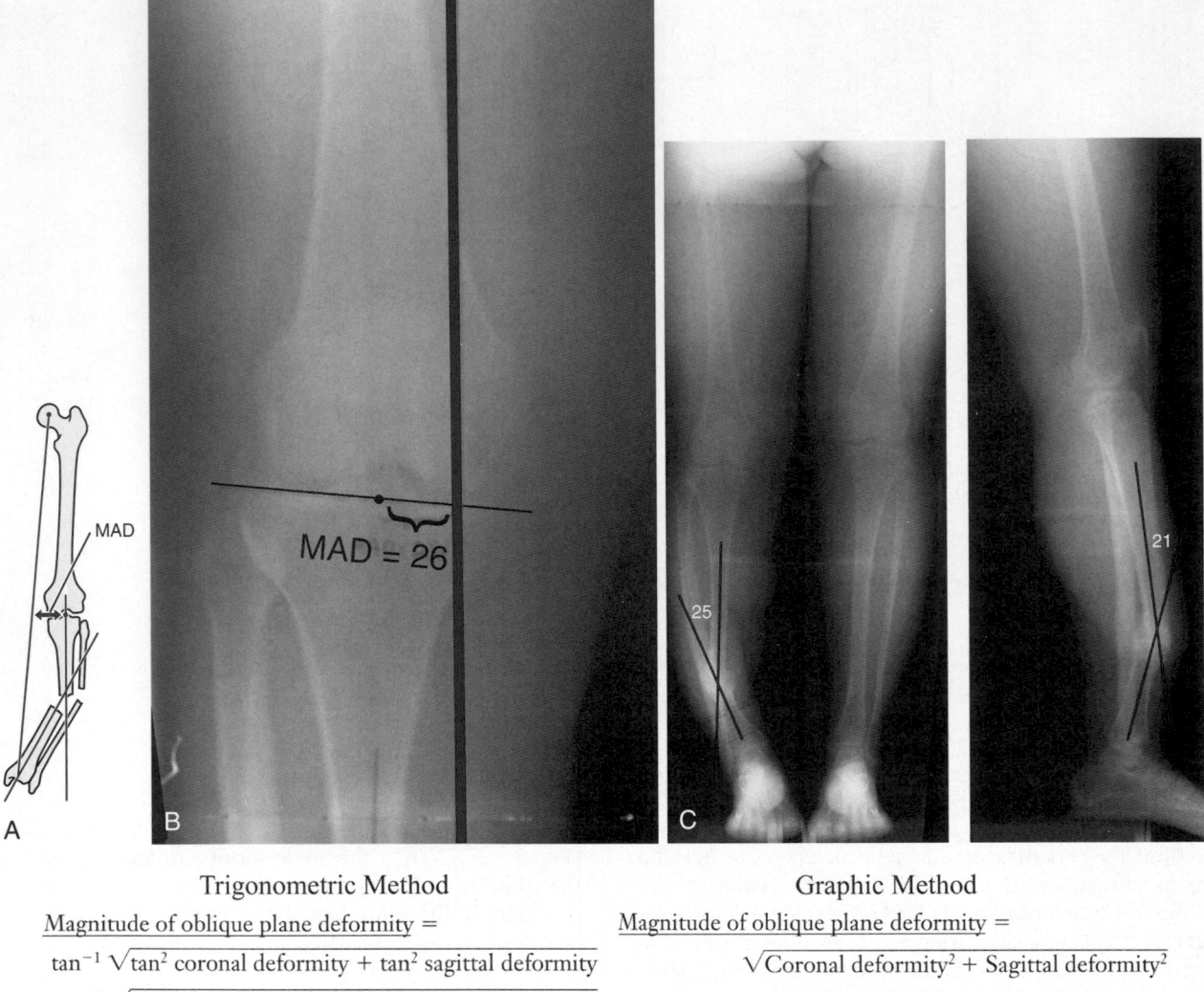

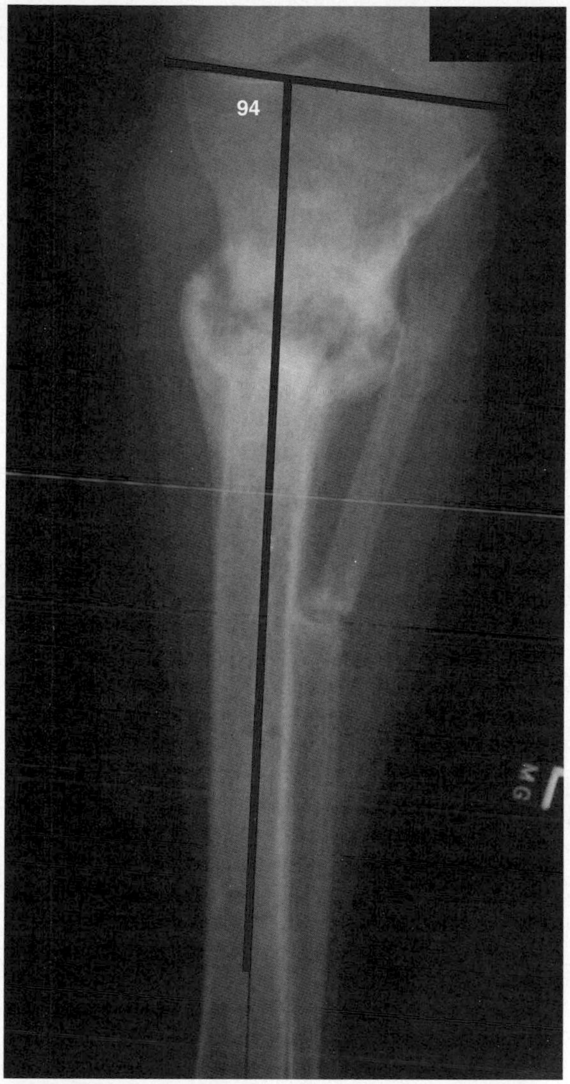

Figure 25-12. In this example, there is a nonunion of the proximal tibia with a valgus deformity resulting in lateral mechanical axis deviation. The proximal medial tibial angle of 94 degrees is abnormally high as compared to both the contralateral normal extremity and the population normal values (see Table 25-3).

With combined angulation and translation in which the fragments are not parallel, translation is measured at the level of the proximal end of the distal fragment (Fig. 25-14).[86]

When both angular and translational deformities are present, the CORA will be at different levels on the AP and lateral radiographs (Fig. 25-15). When the deformity involves pure angulation without translation, the CORA will be at the same level on both radiographs.

The radiographic evaluation should also identify any compensatory joint deformities adjacent to the nonunion. These compensatory deformities are not always clinically apparent. As previously stated, failure to recognize and correct the compensatory joint deformity leads to a healed, straight bone but suboptimal functional improvement.

Radiographic analysis should therefore be performed at adjacent joints for a nonunion with deformity. In particular, for a tibial nonunion with a coronal plane angular deformity, a compensatory deformity at the subtalar joint is not only common, but commonly missed. Varus tibial deformities result in compensatory subtalar valgus deformities, and valgus tibial deformities result in compensatory subtalar varus deformities. Compensatory subtalar joint deformities are evaluated using the extended Harris view of both lower extremities, which allows measurement of the orientation of the calcaneus relative to the tibial shaft in the coronal plane (Fig. 25-16).

Computed Tomographic Scanning and Tomography

Plain radiographs are sometimes insufficient to assess fracture healing. Sclerotic bone and orthopaedic hardware may obscure the fracture site, particularly in stiff nonunions or those well stabilized by hardware.[89] CT scans and tomography are useful in such cases (Fig. 25-17). CT scans can be used to estimate the percentage of the cross-sectional area that shows bridging bone (Fig. 25-18). Nonunions typically show bone bridging of less than 5% of the cross-sectional area at the fracture surfaces (see Fig. 25-18). Healed or healing fractures typically show bone bridging greater than 25% of the cross-sectional area. Serial CT scans may be used to evaluate the progression of fracture consolidation (see Fig. 25-18). CT scans are also useful for assessing intraarticular nonunions for articular step-off and joint incongruency.

Plain tomography helps to evaluate the extent of bony union when hardware artifact compromises CT images.

Rotational deformities may be accurately quantified using CT by comparing the relative orientations of the proximal and distal segments of the involved bone to the contralateral normal bone. This technique has been mostly used for femoral malrotation,[90-92] but may be used for any long bone.

Nuclear Imaging

Nuclear imaging studies are useful for assessing bone vascularity at the nonunion site, the presence of a synovial pseudarthrosis, and infection.

Technetium-99m-pyrophosphate ("bone scan") complexes reflect increased blood flow and bone metabolism and are absorbed onto hydroxyapatite crystals in areas of trauma, infection, and neoplasia. The bone scan will show increased uptake in viable nonunions because there is a good vascular supply and osteoblastic activity (Fig. 25-19).

A *synovial pseudarthrosis* (nearthrosis) is distinguished from a nonunion by the presence of a synovium-like fixed pseudocapsule surrounding a fluid-filled cavity. The medullary canals are sealed off and motion occurs at this "false joint."[72,93] Synovial pseudarthrosis may arise in sites with hypertrophic vascular callus formation or in sites with poor callus formation and poor vascularity. The diagnosis of synovial pseudarthrosis is made when technetium-99m-pyrophosphate bone scans show a "cold cleft" at the nearthrosis between hot ends of ununited bone (see Fig. 25-19).[93-96]

Radiolabeled (e.g., indium-111 or technetium-99m hexamethylpropyleneamine oxime [HMPAO]) polymorphonuclear neutrophils (PMNs) accumulate in areas of acute infection, so these scans are used for evaluating acute bone infection.

Gallium scans are useful for the evaluation of chronic bone infections. Gallium-67 citrate localizes to sites of chronic inflammation. The combination of gallium-67 citrate and technetium-99m-sulfa colloid bone marrow scans can clarify the diagnosis of a chronically infected nonunion.

TABLE 25-3 *NORMAL VALUES USED TO ASSESS LOWER EXTREMITY METAPHYSEAL AND EPIPHYSEAL DEFORMITIES (JUXTA-ARTICULAR DEFORMITIES) ASSOCIATED WITH NONUNIONS*

Anatomic Site of Deformity	Plane	Angle	Description	Normal Values (in degrees)
Proximal femur	Coronal	Neck shaft angle	Defines the relationship between the orientation of the femoral neck and the anatomic axis of the femur.	130 (range, 124–136)
		Anatomic medial proximal femoral angle	Defines the relationship between the anatomic axis of the femur and a line drawn from the tip of the greater trochanter to the center of the femoral head.	84 (range, 80–89)
		Mechanical lateral proximal femoral angle	Defines the relationship between the mechanical axis of the femur and a line drawn from the tip of the greater trochanter to the center of the femoral head.	90 (range, 85–95)
Distal femur	Coronal	Anatomic lateral distal femoral angle	Defines the relationship between the distal femoral joint orientation line and the anatomic axis of the femur.	81 (range, 79–83)
		Mechanical lateral distal femoral angle	Defines the relationship between the distal femoral joint orientation line and the mechanical axis of the femur.	88 (range, 85–90)
	Sagittal	Anatomic posterior distal femoral angle	Defines the relationship between the sagittal distal femoral joint orientation line and the mid-diaphyseal line of the distal femur.	83 (range, 79–87)
Proximal tibia	Coronal	Mechanical medial proximal tibial angle	Defines the relationship between the proximal tibial joint orientation line and the mechanical axis of the tibia.	87 (range, 85–90)
	Sagittal	Anatomic posterior proximal tibial angle	Defines the relationship between the sagittal proximal tibial joint orientation line and the mid-diaphyseal line of the tibia.	81 (range, 77–84)
Distal tibia	Coronal	Mechanical lateral distal tibial angle	Defines the relationship between the distal tibial joint orientation line and the mechanical axis of the tibia.	89 (range, 88–92)
	Sagittal	Anatomic anterior distal tibial angle	Defines the relationship between the sagittal distal tibial joint orientation line and the mid-diaphyseal line of the tibia.	80 (range, 78–82)

Anatomic Axes
Femur: Mid-diaphyseal line.
Tibia: Mid-diaphyseal line.
Mechanical Axes
Femur: Defined by a line from the center of the femoral head to the center of the knee joint.
Tibia: Defined by a line from the center of the knee joint to the center of the ankle joint.
Lower extremity: Defined by a line from the center of the femoral head to the center of the ankle joint.
(Normal values from Paley D, Tetsworth K: Mechanical axis deviation of the lower limbs: preoperative planning of multiapical frontal plane angular and bowing deformities of the femur and tibia, Clin Orthop Relat Res 280:65–71, 1992; Paley D, Tetsworth K: Mechanical axis deviation of the lower limbs: preoperative planning of uniapical angular deformities of the tibia or femur, Clin Orthop Relat Res 280:48–64, 1992.)

Other Radiologic Studies

Fluoroscopy and cineradiography (see Fig. 25-4) may be needed to determine the relative contribution of a joint and an adjacent nonunion to the overall arc of motion. Fluoroscopy is also helpful for guided-needle aspiration of a nonunion site.

Ultrasonography is useful for assessing the status of the bony regenerate during distraction osteogenesis. Fluid-filled cysts in the regenerate can be visualized and aspirated using ultrasound technology, thus shortening the time of regenerate maturation (Fig. 25-20). Ultrasonography can also confirm the presence of a fluid-filled pseudocapsule when synovial pseudarthrosis is suspected.

Magnetic resonance imaging (MRI) may occasionally be used to evaluate soft tissues and cartilaginous and ligamentous structures.

Sinograms may be used to image the course of sinus tracts in infected nonunions.

Angiography provides anatomic detail of vessels as they course through a scarred and deformed limb. While unnecessary in most patients presenting with a fracture nonunion, angiography is indicated if the viability of the limb is in question.[97]

Preoperative venous Doppler studies should be used to rule out deep venous thrombosis in patients with a lower extremity nonunion, who have been confined to a wheelchair or bedridden for an extended period. Intraoperative or postoperative recognition of a venous thrombus or an embolus in a patient who has not been screened preoperatively does not make for a happy patient, family, or orthopaedic surgeon.

Laboratory Studies

Routine laboratory work, including electrolytes and a complete blood count (CBC), are useful for screening general health. The sedimentation rate and C-reactive protein are useful in regard to the course of infection. If necessary, the nutritional status of the patient can be assessed via anergy panels, albumin levels, and transferrin levels. If wound healing potential is in question, an albumin level (≥3.0 g/dL preferred) and a total lymphocyte count (>1500 cells/mm^3 preferred) can be obtained. For patients with a history of multiple blood transfusions, a hepatitis panel and a human immunodeficiency virus (HIV) test may also be warranted.

When infection is suspected, the nonunion site may be aspirated or biopsied under fluoroscopic guidance. The aspirated or biopsied material is sent for a cell count and Gram stain, and cultures are sent for aerobic, anaerobic, fungal, and acid-fast bacillus organisms. To encourage the highest yield possible, all antibiotics should be discontinued at least 2 weeks prior to aspiration.

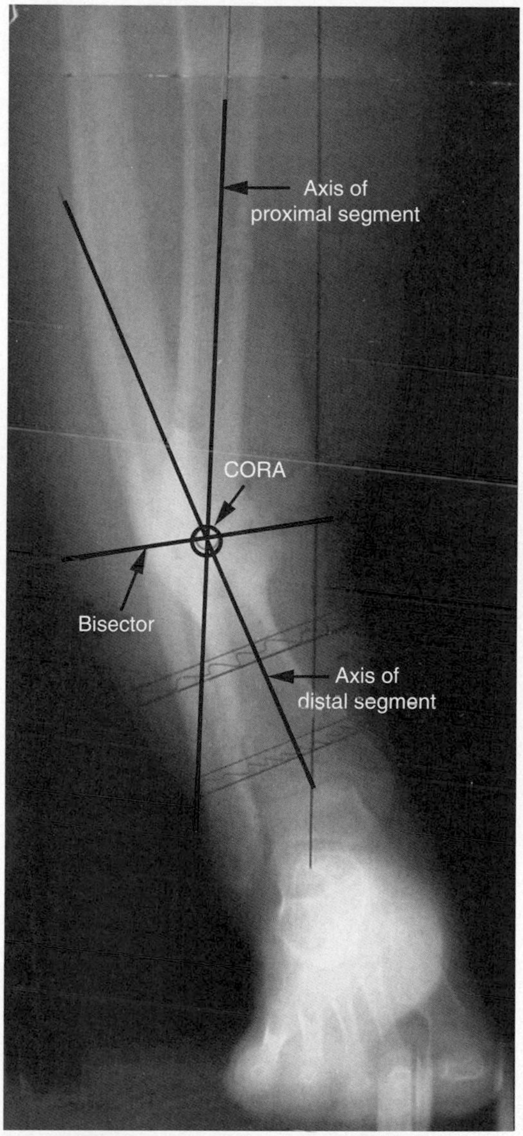

Figure 25-13. The same case shown in Figure 25-11 with a diaphyseal nonunion with deformity. The center of rotation of angulation (CORA) and bisector have been illustrated.

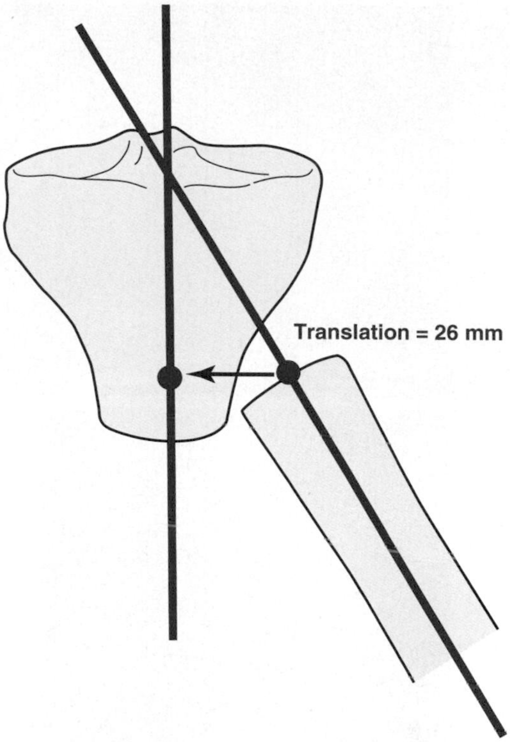

Figure 25-14. Method for measuring translational deformities. The magnitude of translation is measured at the level of the proximal end of the distal fragment.

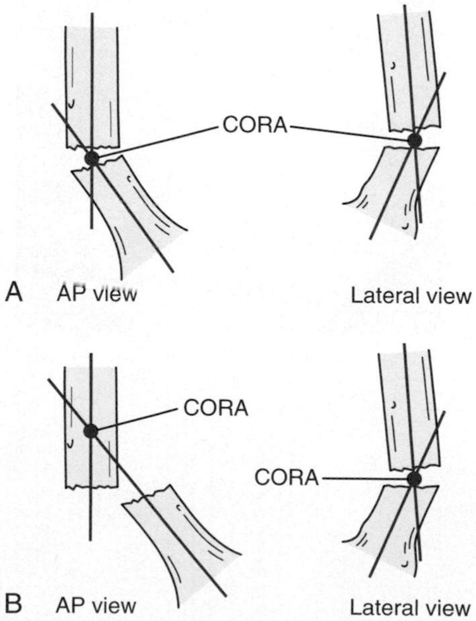

Figure 25-15. A, When the deformity at the nonunion site involves angulation without translation, the center of rotation of angulation (CORA) will be seen at the same level on both the anterior-posterior (AP) and lateral radiographs. **B,** When the deformity at the nonunion site involves both angulation and translation, the CORA will be seen at a different level on the AP and lateral radiographs.

Consultations

Many issues commonly accompany nonunion, including soft tissue problems, infection, chronic pain, depression, motor or sensory dysfunction, joint stiffness, and comorbid medical problems. A team of subspecialists are usually needed to assist in the care of the patient, beginning with the initial evaluation and continuing throughout the course of treatment.

A plastic reconstructive surgeon may be consulted preoperatively to assess the status of the soft tissues, particularly when the need for coverage is anticipated following serial débridement of an infected nonunion. Consultation with a vascular surgeon may be necessary if the viability (vascularity) of the limb is in question.

An infectious disease specialist can prescribe an antibiotic regimen preoperatively, intraoperatively, and postoperatively, particularly for the patient with a long-standing infected nonunion.

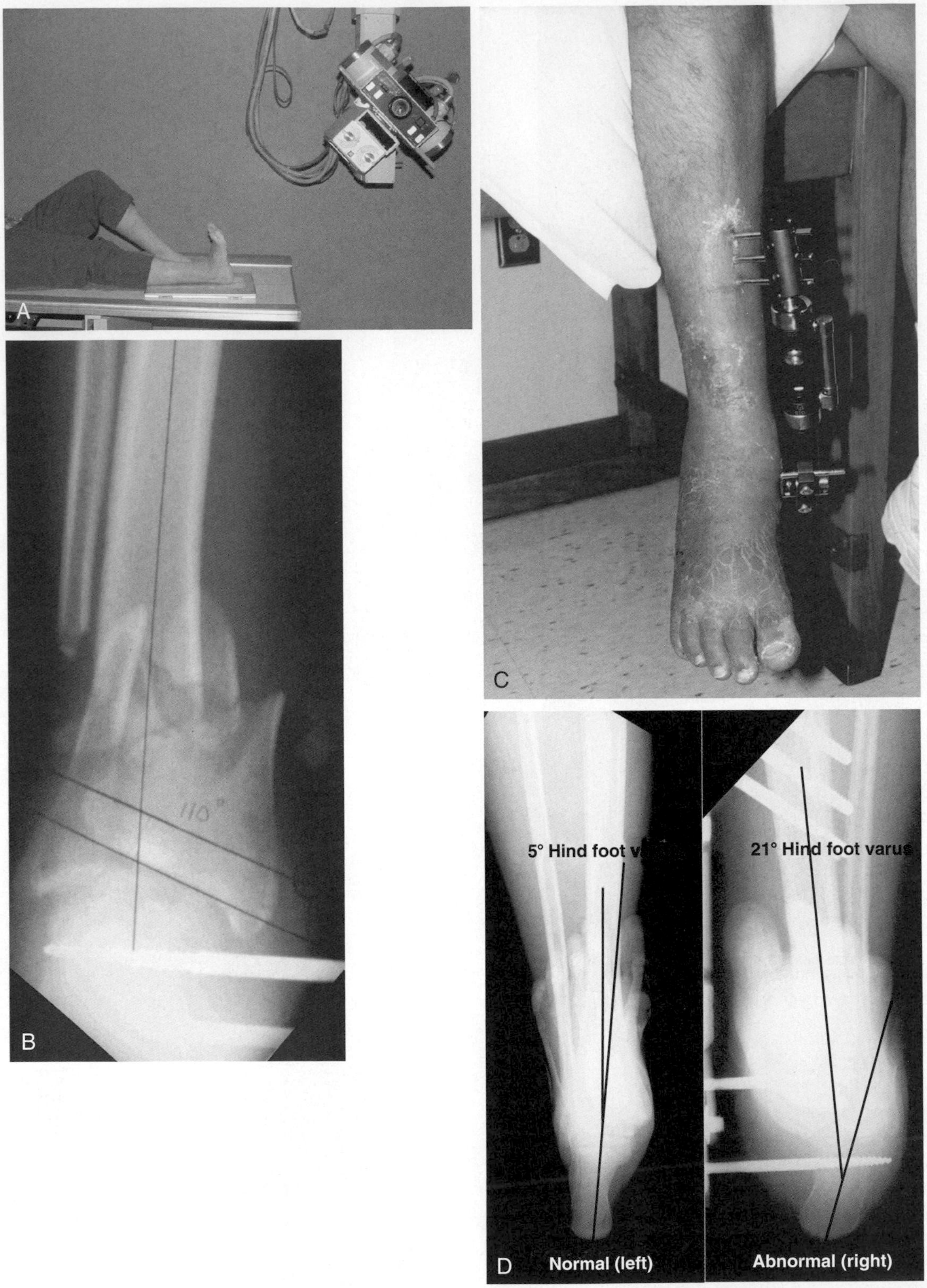

Figure 25-16. The extended Harris view is performed in order to image the orientation of the hind foot to the tibial shaft in the coronal plane. **A,** The patient is positioned lying supine on the radiography table with the knee in full extension and the foot and ankle in maximal dorsiflexion. The radiography tube is aimed at the calcaneus at a 45-degree angle with a tube distance of 60 inches. **B,** Anterior-posterior (AP) radiograph of the tibia shows a distal tibial nonunion with a valgus deformity. This patient had been treated with an external fixator at an outside facility. In an effort to correct the distal tibial deformity, the hind foot had been fixed in varus through the subtalar joint. **C,** On clinical inspection, this is not always obvious and can be missed. **D,** The extended Harris view of the normal left side as compared to the abnormal right side. Note the profound subtalar varus deformity of the right lower extremity. Both the distal tibial valgus deformity and the subtalar varus deformity must be corrected in this patient.

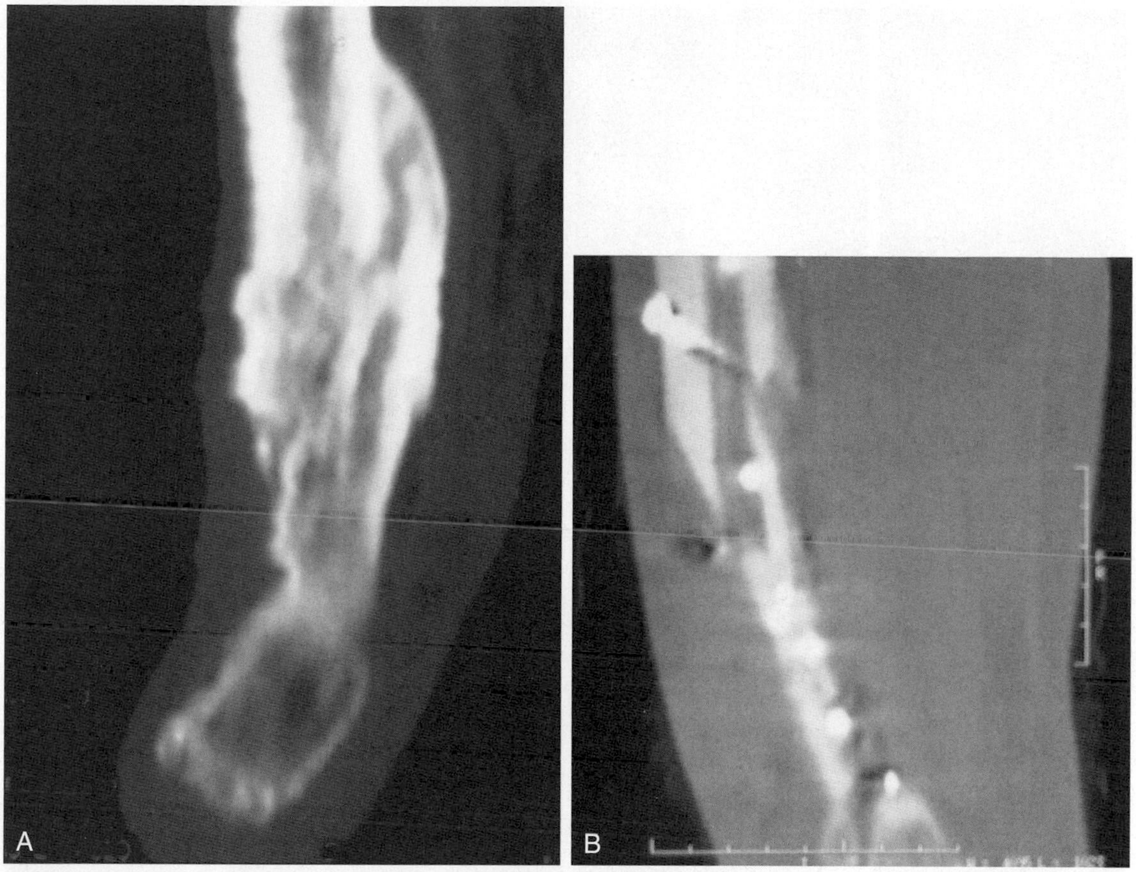

Figure 25-17. A, Computed tomography (CT) scan of the 88-year-old woman shown in Figure 25-8, *A* shows that this fracture is in fact healed. **B,** CT scan of the 49-year-old man shown in Figure 25-8, *B* shows that this fracture has gone on to nonunion.

Many patients with nonunions have dependency on oral narcotic pain medication. Referral to a pain management specialist is helpful both during the course of treatment and in ultimately detoxifying and weaning the patient off of all narcotics.[98-100]

Depression is common in patients with chronic medical conditions.[101-104] Patients with nonunions often have signs of clinical depression. Referral to a psychiatrist can provide great benefit.

A neurologist should evaluate patients presenting with motor or sensory dysfunction. Electromyography and nerve conduction studies can document the location and extent of neural compromise and determine the need for nerve exploration and repair.

A physical therapist should be consulted for preoperative and postoperative training with respect to postoperative activity expectations and the use of assistive or adaptive devices. The goals of immediate postoperative (inpatient) rehabilitation include independent transfers and ambulation, when possible. Outpatient postoperative physical therapy primarily addresses strength and range of motion of the surrounding joints, but may also include sterile or medicated whirlpool treatments to treat or prevent minor infections (e.g., external fixation pin sites).

Occupational therapy is also useful for activities of daily living and job-related tasks, particularly those involving fine motor skills such as grooming, dressing, and use of hand tools. Occupational therapy may also provide adaptive devices for activities of daily living during treatment.

A nutritionist may be consulted for patients who are malnourished or obese. Poor dietary intake of protein (albumin) or vitamins may contribute to delayed fracture union and nonunion.[57,59-62,70,105] A nutritionist may also counsel severely obese patients to reduce body weight. Obesity increases the technical demands of nonunion treatment and the risk of complications.[71]

Anesthesiologists and internists should be consulted during preoperative planning for the elderly or patients with serious medical conditions to decrease risk of intraoperative and postoperative medical complications.

TREATMENT

Objectives

Obviously, treatment is directed at healing the fracture. Healing, however, is not the only objective as a nonfunctional, infected, deformed limb with joint pain and stiffness will be an unsatisfactory outcome for most patients even if the bone heals solidly. Emphasis is, thus, on returning the extremity and the patient to the fullest function possible during and following treatment.

Treating a nonunion can be likened to playing a game of chess; it is difficult to predict the course until the process is

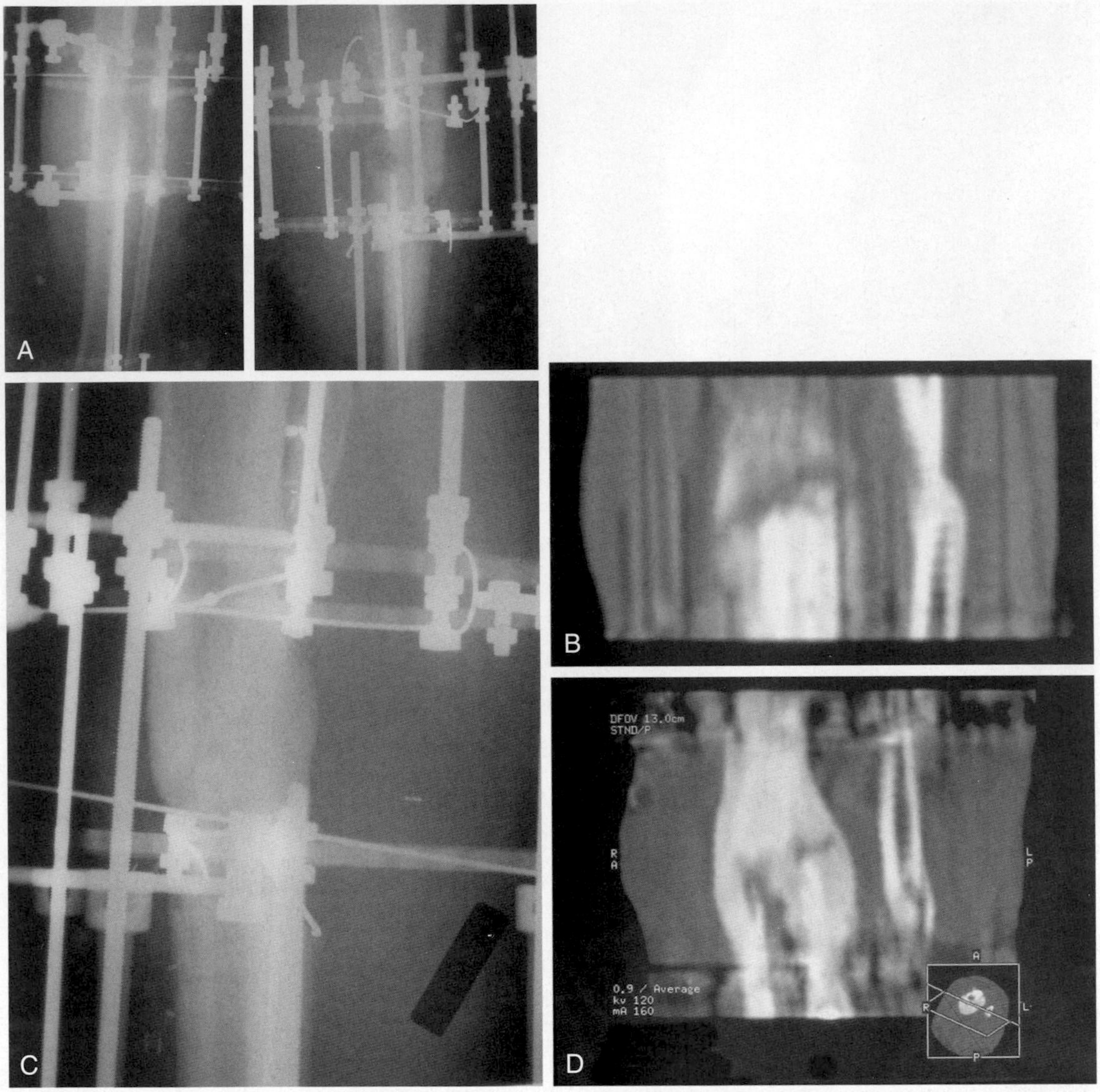

Figure 25-18. In addition to helping determine whether a fracture has united or has gone on to nonunion, computed tomography (CT) scans are a useful method for estimating the cross-sectional area of healing. In this case of an infected midshaft tibial nonunion, CT scanning is a useful method of estimating the progression of the cross-sectional area of healing over time. **A,** Radiograph of the tibia 4 months following injury. It is difficult to definitively say whether or not this fracture is healing. **B,** CT scan shows a clear gap without bony contact or bridging bone (0% cross-sectional area of healing). **C,** Radiograph 6 months later following gradual compression across the nonunion site. **D,** CT scan shows solid bony union (cross-sectional area of healing greater than 50% in this case).

underway. Some nonunions heal rapidly with a single intervention. Others require multiple surgeries. Unfortunately, the most benign-appearing nonunion occasionally mounts a terrific battle against healing. The treatment must, therefore, be planned so that each step anticipates the possibility of failure and allows for further treatment options without burning any bridges.

The patient's motivation, disability, social and legal issues, mental status, and desires should be considered before treatment begins. Are the patient's expectations realistic? Informed consent prior to any treatment is essential. The patient needs to understand the uncertainties of nonunion healing, time course of treatment, and number of surgeries required. No guarantees or warranties should be given to the patient. If the patient is unable to tolerate a potentially lengthy treatment course or the uncertainties associated with the treatment and outcome, the option of amputation should be discussed. While amputation has obvious drawbacks, it does resolve the medical problem rapidly and may, therefore, be preferred by certain patients.[106-110] It is unwise to talk a patient into or out of any treatment; this is particularly true for amputation.

When feasible, eradication of infection and correction of unacceptable deformities are performed at the time of nonunion treatment. When this is not practical or possible, the treatment plan is broken into stages with the following priorities:

1. Heal the bone.
2. Eradicate infection.
3. Correct deformities.
4. Maximize joint motion and muscle strength.

These priorities do not necessarily denote the temporal sequencing of surgical procedures. For example, in an infected

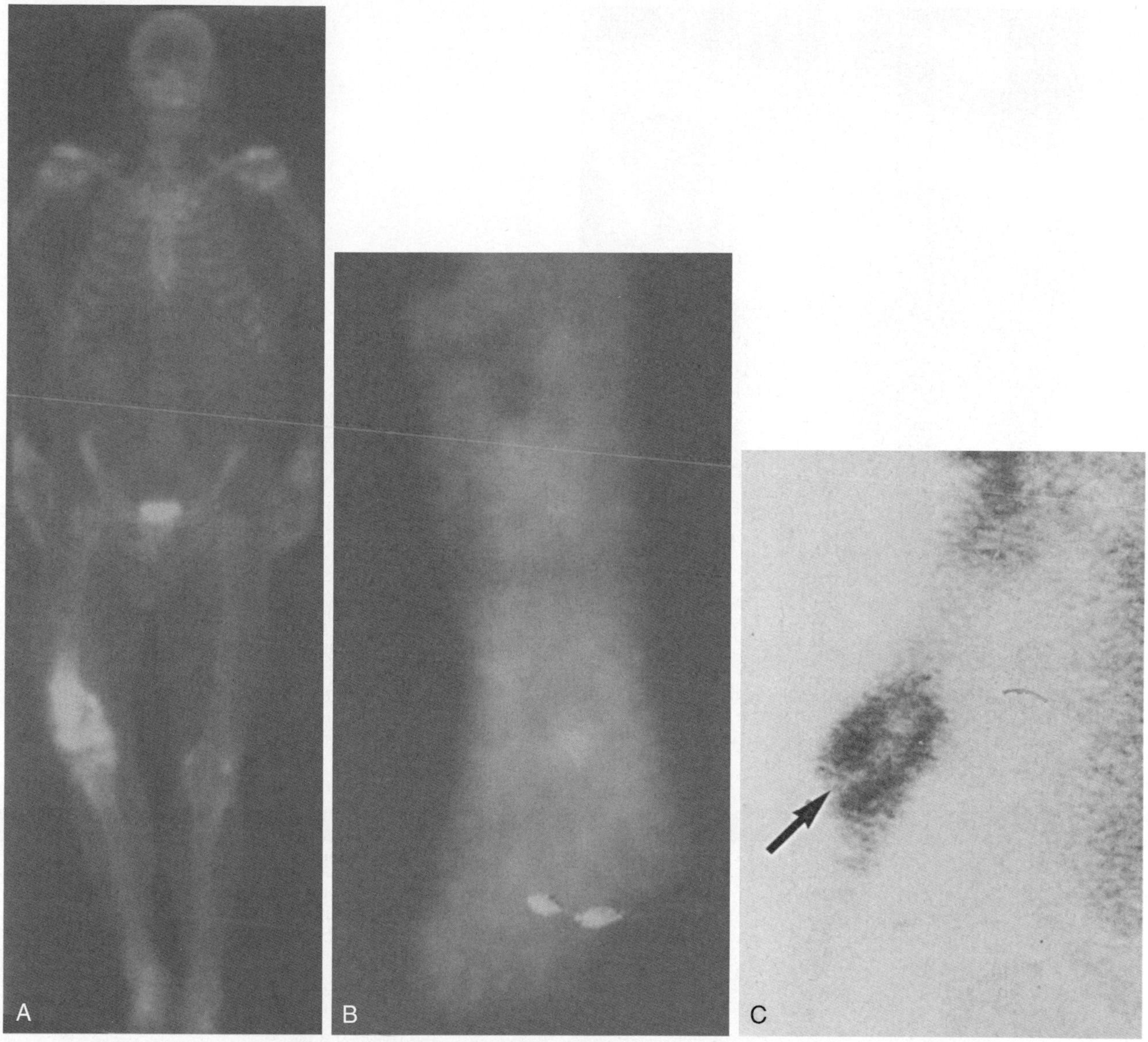

Figure 25-19. Technetium bone scanning of three different cases showing (**A**) a viable nonunion, (**B**) a nonviable nonunion, and (**C**) a synovial pseudarthrosis.

nonunion with a deformity, the treatment may begin with débridement to eliminate infection, but the overriding priority remains to heal the bone.

Strategies

The in-depth evaluation using the history and physical examination, radiologic examinations, laboratory studies, and consulting physicians provides for assessment of the overall situation. This assessment culminates in a treatment strategy specific to the patient's particular circumstances.

The choice of treatment strategy is based on accurate classification of the nonunion (Table 25-4). Classification is based on the nonunion type and treatment modifiers (Tables 25-5A and 25-5B).

Nonunion Type

The primary consideration for designing the treatment strategy is nonunion type (Fig. 25-21), which identifies the mechanical and biological requirements of fracture healing that have not been met. The surgeon can then design a strategy to meet the healing requirements.

Hypertrophic Nonunions. Hypertrophic nonunions are viable, possess an adequate blood supply,[73] and display abundant callus formation,[111] but lack mechanical stability. Providing mechanical stability to a hypertrophic nonunion results in chondrocyte-mediated mineralization of fibrocartilage at the interfragmentary gap (Fig. 25-22). Mineralization of fibrocartilage may occur as early as 6 weeks following rigid stabilization and is accompanied by vascular ingrowth into the mineralized fibrocartilage[111,112] (see Fig. 25-22). By 8 weeks following stabilization, there is resorption of calcified fibrocartilage, which is then arranged in columns and acts as a template for deposition of woven bone. Woven bone is subsequently remodeled into mature lamellar bone (see Fig. 25-22).[112]

Hypertrophic nonunions require no bone grafting.* The nonunion site tissue should not be resected. Hypertrophic

*References 10, 72, 77, 79, 81, 111, 113-117.

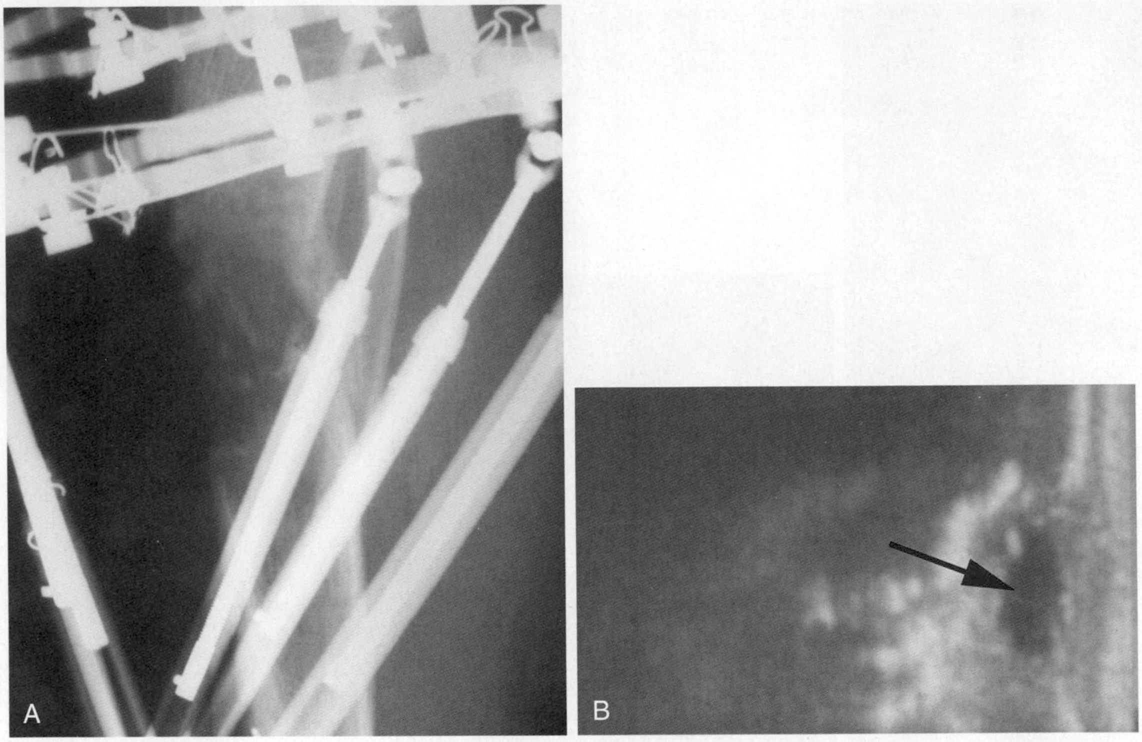

Figure 25-20. **A,** Radiograph of a slowly maturing proximal tibial regenerate. **B,** Ultrasonography shows a fluid-filled cyst *(arrow)*.

TABLE 25-4 *NONUNION TYPES AND THEIR CHARACTERISTICS*

Nonunion Type	Physical Examination	Plain Radiographs	Nuclear Imaging	Laboratory Studies
Hypertrophic	Typically do not display gross motion; pain elicited on manual stress testing	Abundant callus formation; radiolucent line (unmineralized fibrocartilage) at the nonunion site	Increased uptake at the nonunion site on technetium bone scan	Unremarkable
Oligotrophic	Variable (dependent on the stability of the current hardware)	Little or no callus formation; diastasis at the fracture site	Increased uptake at the bone surfaces at the nonunion site on technetium bone scan	Unremarkable
Atrophic	Variable (dependent on the stability of the current hardware)	Bony surfaces partially resorbed; no callus formation; osteopenia; sclerotic avascular bone segments; segmental bone loss	Avascular segments will appear cold (decreased uptake) on technetium bone scan	Unremarkable
Infected	Dependent on the specific nature of the infection: 1. Active purulent drainage 2. Active nondraining—no drainage is present but the area is warm, erythematous, and painful 3. Quiescent—no drainage or local signs or symptoms of infection	Osteolysis; osteopenia; sclerotic avascular bone segments; segmental bone loss	Increased uptake on technetium bone scan; increased uptake on indium scan for acute infections; increased uptake on gallium scan for chronic infections	Elevated erythrocyte sedimentation rate and C-reactive protein; white blood cell count may be elevated in more severe and acute cases; blood cultures should be obtained in febrile patients; aspiration of fluid from the nonunion site may be useful in the workup for infection
Synovial pseudarthrosis	Variable	Variable appearance (can appear hypertrophic, oligotrophic, or atrophic)	Technetium bone scan shows a "cold cleft" at the nonunion site surrounded by increased uptake at the ends of the united bone	Unremarkable

TABLE 25-5A ***TREATMENT STRATEGIES OF NONUNIONS BASED ON CLASSIFICATION: PRIMARY CONSIDERATION (NONUNION TYPE)***

	Treatment Strategy	
Classification	*Biological*	*Mechanical*
Hypertrophic		Augment stability
Oligotrophic	Bone grafting for cases that have poor surface characteristics and no callus formation	Improve reduction (bone contact)
Atrophic	Biological stimulation via bone grafting or bone transport	Augment stability, compression
Infected Draining-active Nondraining-active Nondraining-quiescent	Débridement, antibiotic beads, dead space management, systemic antibiotic therapy, biological stimulation for bone healing (bone grafting or bone transport)	Provide mechanical stability, compression
Synovial pseudarthrosis	Resect synovium and pseudarthrosis tissue, open medullary canals with drilling and reaming, bone grafting	Compression

nonunions want to heal and simply need a "push" in the right direction (Fig. 25-23). If the method of rigid stabilization involves exposing the nonunion site (e.g., compression plate stabilization), decortication of the nonunion site may accelerate bony consolidation. If the method of rigid stabilization does not involve exposure of the nonunion site (e.g., intramedullary nail fixation or external fixation), surgical dissection to prepare the nonunion site is unnecessary.

Oligotrophic Nonunions. Oligotrophic nonunions are also viable and possess an adequate blood supply, but display little or no callus formation, typically a result of inadequate reduction with little or no contact at the bony surfaces (Fig. 25-24). Therefore, treatment methods for oligotrophic nonunions include reduction of the bony fragments to improve bone contact; bone grafting to stimulate the local biology; or a combination of reduction of the bony fragments and bone grafting. Reduction of the bony fragments to improve bony contact can be performed with either internal or external fixation. Reduction is appropriate for oligotrophic nonunions with large, noncomminuted surface areas across which compression can be applied. Bone grafting is appropriate for oligotrophic nonunions that have poor surface characteristics and no callus formation.

Atrophic Nonunions. Atrophic nonunions are nonviable. Their blood supply is poor and they are incapable of purposeful biological activity (Fig. 25-25). While the primary problem is biological, the atrophic nonunion requires a treatment strategy that employs both biological and mechanical

TABLE 25-5B ***TREATMENT STRATEGIES OF NONUNIONS BASED ON CLASSIFICATION: TREATMENT MODIFIERS***

Anatomic Location Epiphyseal Metaphyseal Diaphyseal	See text for description of treatment modifiers.
Segmental Bone Defects	
Prior Failed Treatments	
Deformities Length Angulation Rotation Translation	
Surface Characteristics	
Pain and Function	
Osteopenia	
Mobility of the Nonunion Stiff Lax	
Status of Hardware	
Motor/Sensory Dysfunction	
Patient's Health and Age	
Problems at Adjacent Joints	
Soft Tissue Problems	
Metabolic and Endocrine Abnormalities	

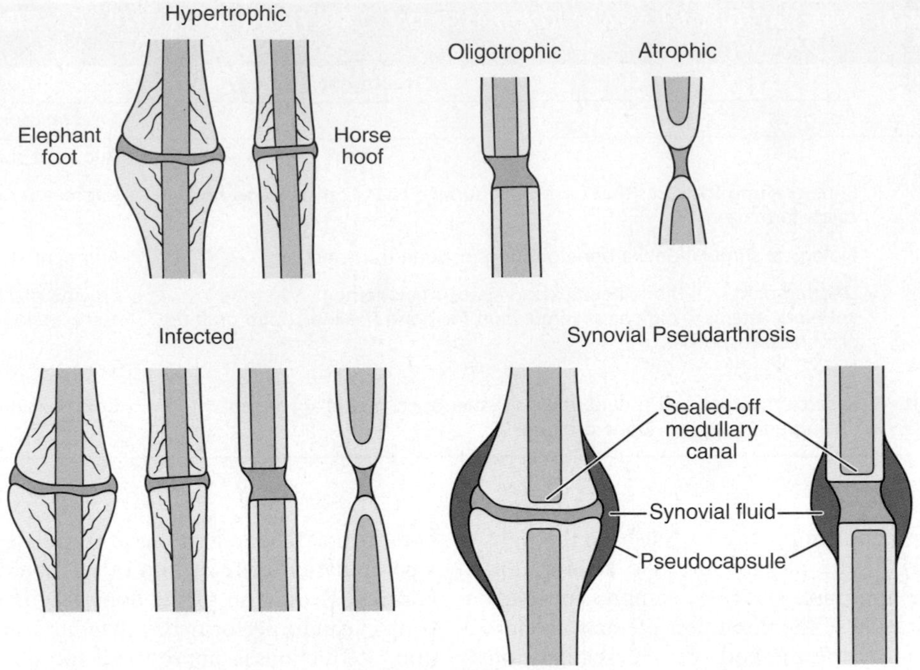

Figure 25-21. Classification of nonunions (nonunion types).

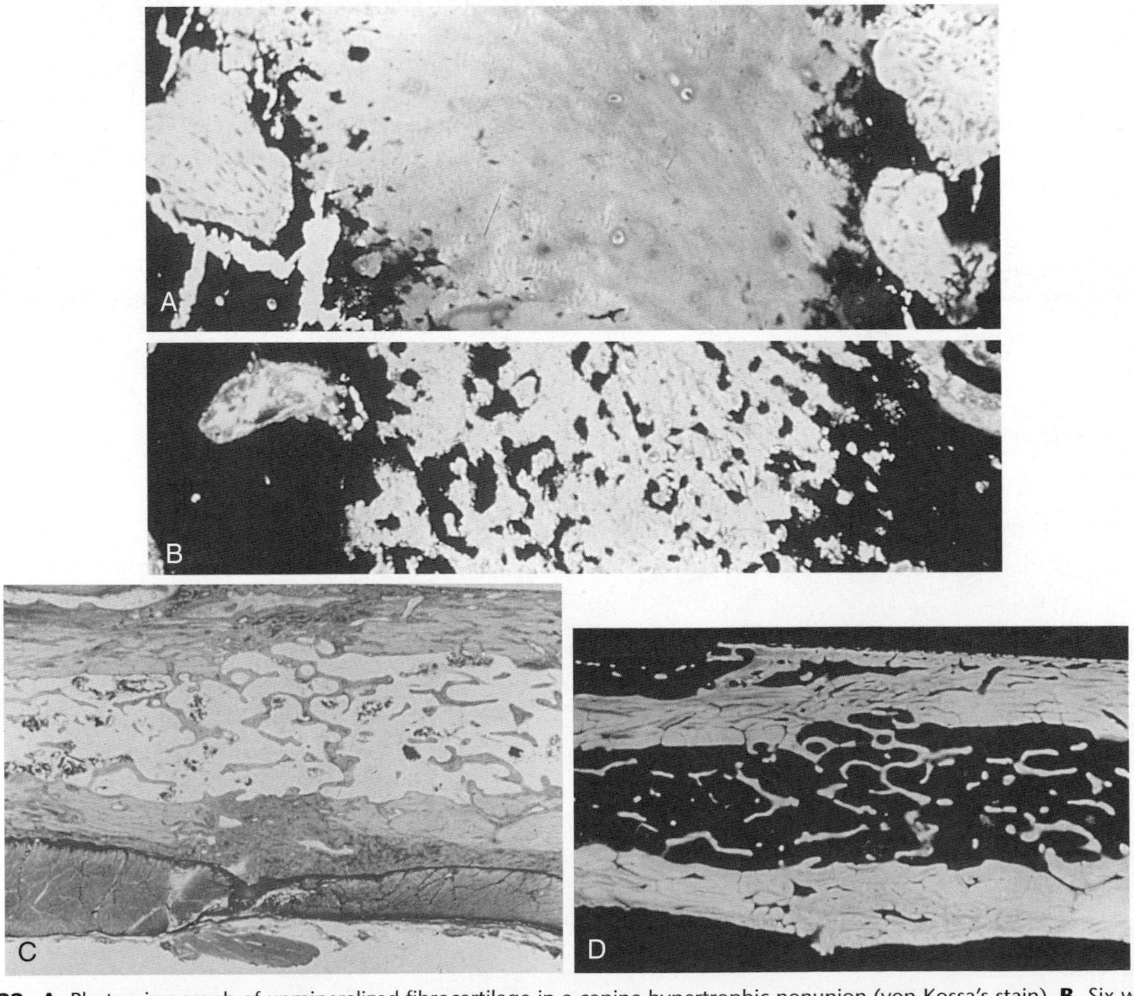

Figure 25-22. A, Photomicrograph of unmineralized fibrocartilage in a canine hypertrophic nonunion (von Kossa's stain). **B,** Six weeks following plate stabilization, chondrocyte-mediated mineralization of fibrocartilage is observed in this hypertrophic nonunion. **C,** This will go on to form woven bone, and will (**D**) ultimately remodel into compact cortical bone 16 to 24 weeks following stabilization. *(From Schenk RK: Histology of fracture repair and nonunion, Bull Swiss ASIF, October 1978.)*

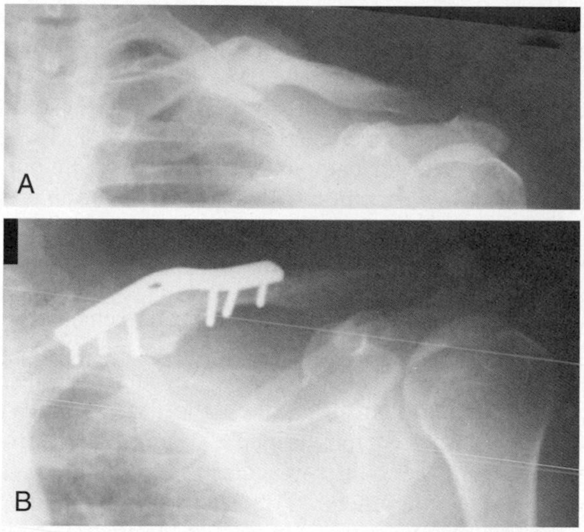

Figure 25-23. Plate-and-screw fixation of this hypertrophic clavicle nonunion led to rapid bony union. **A,** Radiograph shows a hypertrophic nonunion 8 months following injury. **B,** Radiograph taken 15 weeks following open reduction internal fixation (without bone grafting) shows complete and solid bony union.

techniques. Biological stimulation is most commonly provided by autogenous cancellous graft laid onto a widely decorticated area at the nonunion site. Small free necrotic fragments are excised and the resulting defect is bridged with bone graft; treatment of large bony defects is discussed later in the Segmental Bone Defects section. Mechanical stability can be achieved using either internal or external fixation, and the fixation method must provide adequate purchase in poor quality (osteopenic) bone.

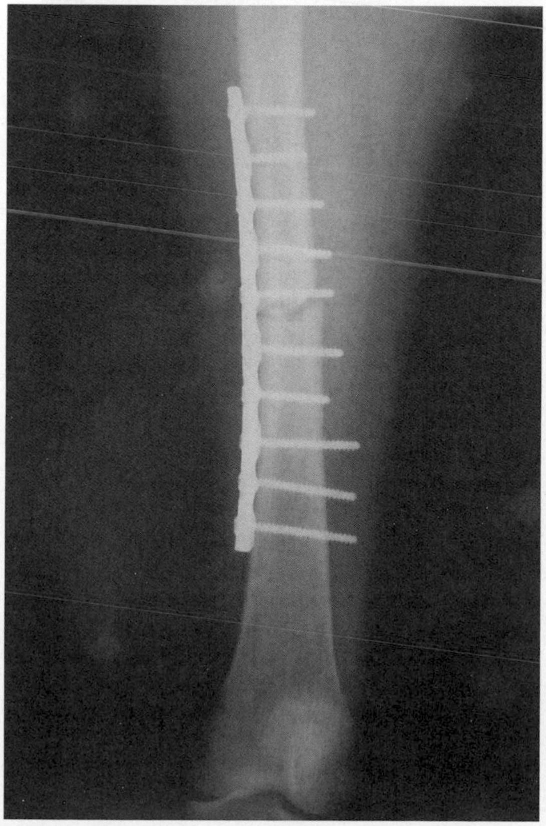

Figure 25-24. Oligotrophic nonunion of the femoral shaft referred in 21 months following failed treatment of the initial fracture with plate-and-screw fixation. Note the absence of callus formation and poor contact at the bony surfaces.

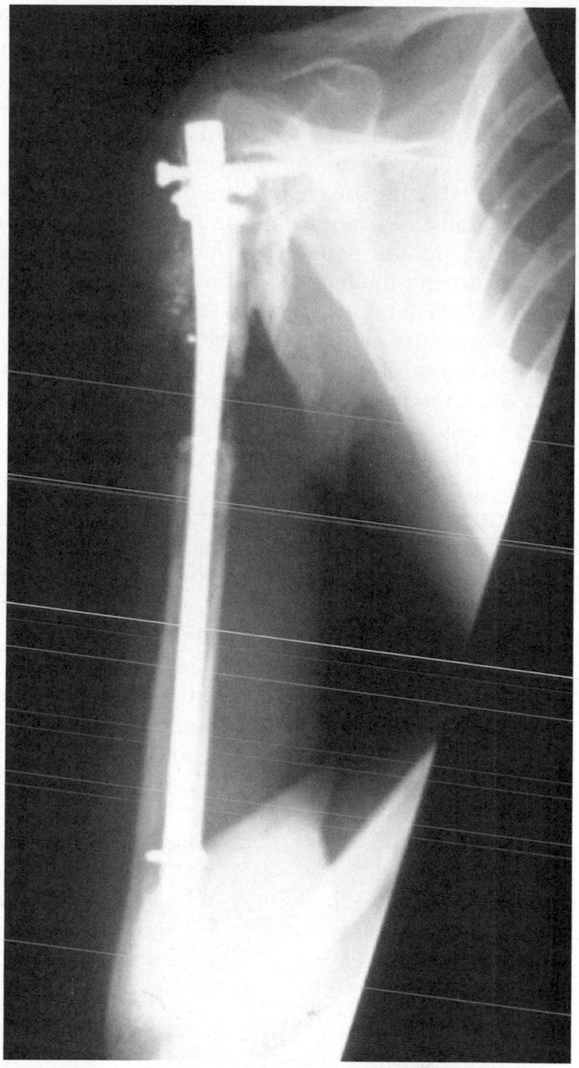

Figure 25-25. Atrophic nonunion of the proximal humerus. Note the lack of callus formation, the bony defect, and the avascular appearing bony surfaces.

When stabilized and stimulated, revascularization of an atrophic nonunion occurs slowly over the course of several months, as visualized radiographically by observing the progression of osteopenia as it moves through sclerotic nonviable fragments.[72,78]

No consensus exists regarding whether large segments of sclerotic bone should be excised from uninfected atrophic nonunions. Those who favor plate-and-screw fixation tend to retain large sclerotic fragments that revascularize over several months following rigid plate stabilization, decortication, and bone grafting. Those who favor other treatment methods tend to excise large sclerotic fragments and reconstruct the resulting segmental bony defect using one of several methods. Both of these treatment strategies result in successful union in a high percentage of cases. Our decision in these cases depends on the treatment modifiers, discussed in the next section.

Infected Nonunions. Infected nonunions pose a dual challenge: bone infection and ununited fracture. The condition is often further complicated by incapacitating pain (often with narcotic dependency), soft tissue problems, deformities, joint problems (contractures, deformities, limited range of motion), motor and sensory dysfunction, osteopenia, poor general health, depression, and a myriad of other problems. Infected nonunions are the most difficult nonunion type to treat.

The goals in treating infected nonunions are to obtain solid bony union, eradicate the infection, and maximize function of the extremity and the patient. Before starting a particular course of treatment, the length of time required, the number of operative procedures anticipated, and the intensity of the treatment plan must be discussed with the patient and the family. The course of treatment for infected nonunions is especially difficult to predict. The possibility of persistent infection and nonunion despite appropriate treatment should be discussed and the possibility of future amputation should be considered.

The treatment strategy for infected nonunions depends on the nature of the infection (draining, nondraining-active, nondraining-quiescent)[52] and involves both a biological and a mechanical approach.

Active Purulent Drainage. When purulent drainage is ongoing, the nonunion takes longer and is more difficult to heal (Fig. 25-26). An actively draining infection requires serial débridement. The first débridement should include obtaining deep cultures, including specimens of soft tissues and bone. No perioperative antibiotics should be given at least 2 weeks prior to obtaining deep intraoperative cultures. All necrotic soft tissues (e.g., fascia, muscle, abscess cavities, and sinus tracts), necrotic bone, and foreign bodies (e.g., loose orthopaedic hardware, shrapnel) should be excised.[118,119] The sinus tract should be sent for pathologic specimen to rule out carcinoma.[118] Pulsatile irrigation with antibiotic solution is effective in washing out the open cavity.

A dead space is commonly present following débridement. Initially, antibiotic-impregnated polymethylmethacrylate (PMMA) beads are inserted,[118] and a bead exchange is performed at each serial débridement. The dead space can subsequently be managed in a number of ways. Currently, the most widely used method involves filling the dead space with a rotational vascularized muscle pedicle flap (e.g., gastrocnemius or soleus[12,118]) or a microvascularized free flap (e.g., latissimus dorsi, rectus, others[120,121]). Another method involves open wound care with moist dressings, as in the Papineau technique,[76] until granulation occurs and skin grafting can be performed.

Bony defects following débridement can be reconstructed using bone grafting techniques, as discussed in the section on Segmental Bone Defects.

The consulting infectious disease specialist generally directs systemic antibiotic therapy. Following procurement of deep surgical cultures, the patient is placed on broad-spectrum

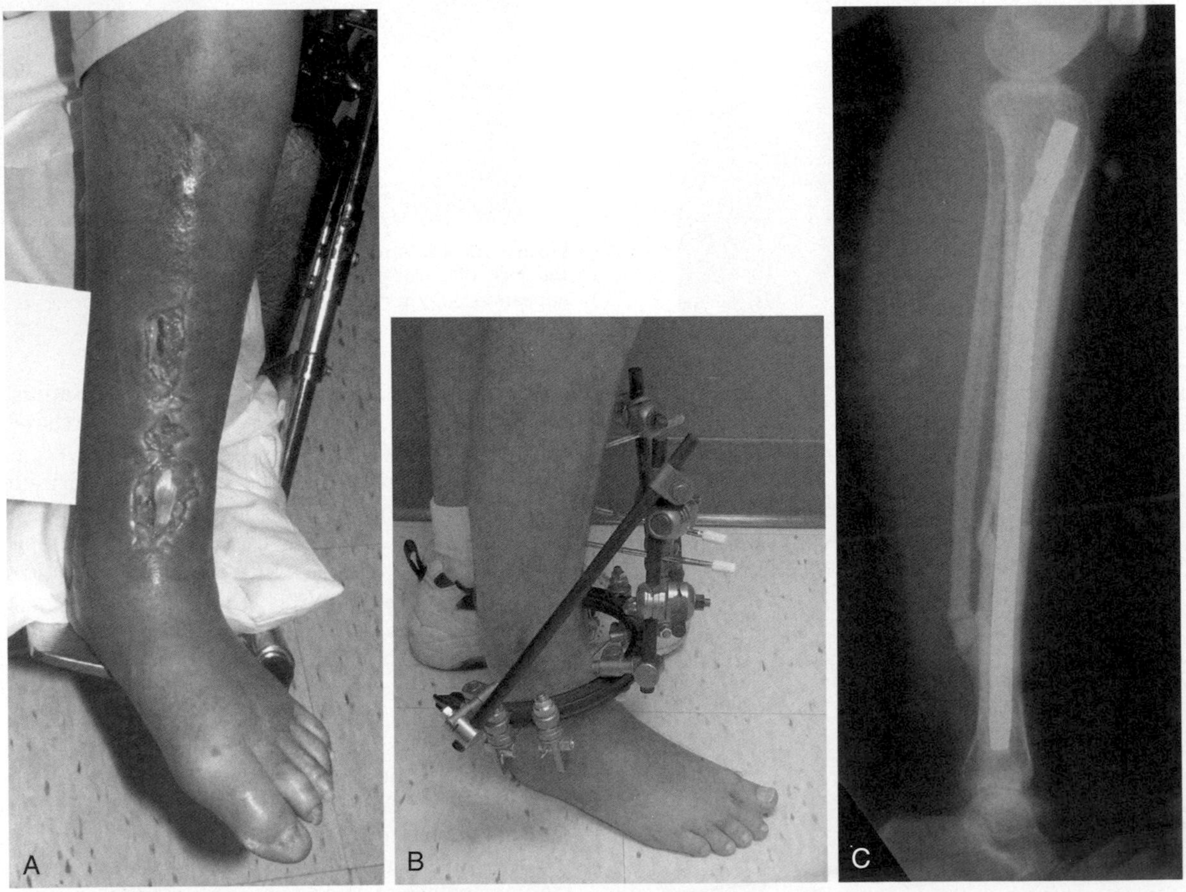

Figure 25-26. A, Clinical photograph of an actively draining infected tibial nonunion. **B,** Clinical photograph of a nondraining infected tibial nonunion. Note the presence of local swelling (there is also erythema) without purulent drainage. **C,** Radiograph of a nondraining quiescent infected tibial nonunion (this patient had a past history of multiple episodes of purulent drainage and during the workup, the gallium scan was noted to be positive).

intravenous antibiotics as the culture results are pending. When the culture results are available, antibiotic coverage is directed at the infecting organisms.

ACTIVE NONDRAINING. Nondraining infected nonunions present with swelling, tenderness, and local erythema (see Fig. 25-26). The history often includes episodes of fever. Treatment principles for these nonunions are similar to those described for actively draining infected nonunions: débridement, intraoperative cultures, soft tissue management, stabilization, stimulation of bone healing, and systemic antibiotic therapy. These cases typically require incision and drainage of an abscess and excision of only small amounts of bone and soft tissues. Nondraining infected nonunion cases may be managed with primary closure following incision and drainage or with a closed suction-irrigation drainage system until the infection becomes quiescent.

QUIESCENT. Nondraining-quiescent infected nonunions occur in patients with a history of infection but without drainage or symptoms for 3 or more months[52] or without a history of infection but with a positive indium or gallium scan (see Fig. 25-26). These cases may be treated like atrophic nonunions. With plate-and-screw stabilization, the residual necrotic bone may be debrided at the time of surgical exposure. The bone is decorticated and stabilized, and bone grafting may also be performed. If external fixation is used, the infection and nonunion may be treated with compression without open débridement or bone grafting.[122]

SYNOVIAL PSEUDARTHROSIS. Synovial pseudarthroses are characterized by fluid bounded by sealed medullary canals and a fixed synovium-like pseudocapsule (Fig. 25-27). Treatment entails both biological stimulation and augmentation of mechanical stability. The synovium and pseudarthrosis tissue are excised and the medullary canals of the proximal and distal fragments are drilled and reamed. The ends of the major fragments are fashioned to allow for interfragmentary compression with either internal or external fixation. Bone grafting and decortication encourages more rapid healing.

According to Professor Ilizarov, gradual compression alone across a synovial pseudarthrosis results in local necrosis and inflammation, ultimately stimulating the healing process.[122,123] In our hands, resection at the nonunion followed by monofocal compression or bone transport more reliably achieves good results.

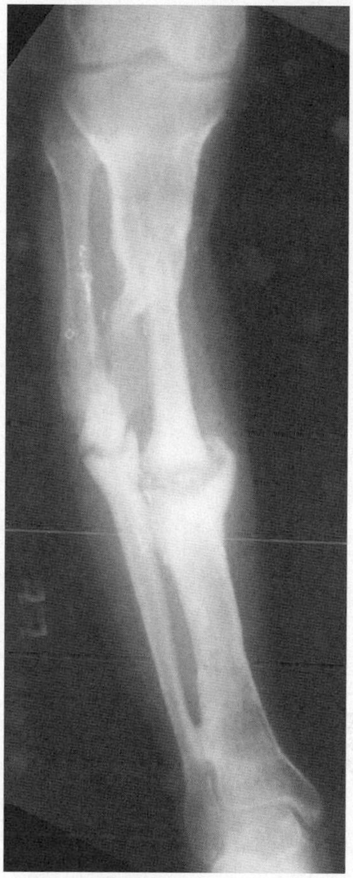

Figure 25-27. Plain radiograph of a tibial nonunion with a synovial pseudarthrosis.

Treatment Modifiers

The treatment modifiers (see Table 25-5B) provide a more specific classification of the nonunion and thus help to "fine-tune" the treatment plan.

ANATOMIC LOCATION. The bone involved and the specific region or regions (e.g., epiphysis, metaphysis, and diaphysis) defines the anatomic location of a nonunion.

EPIPHYSEAL NONUNIONS. Epiphyseal nonunions are relatively uncommon. The most common etiology is inadequate reduction that leaves a gap at the fracture site. These nonunions, therefore, commonly present with oligotrophic characteristics. The important considerations when evaluating epiphyseal nonunions are reduction of the intraarticular component(s) (eliminate step-off at the articular surface); juxtaarticular deformities (e.g., length, angulation, rotation, translation); motion at the joint (typically limited due to arthrofibrosis); and compensatory deformities at adjacent joints.

Epiphyseal nonunions are typically treated with interfragmentary compression using screw fixation, best achieved using a cannulated lag screw technique (overdrilling a glide hole) with a washer beneath the screw head. Previously placed screws holding the nonunion site in a distracted position should be removed.

Arthroscopy is a useful adjunctive treatment for epiphyseal nonunions (Fig. 25-28) to evaluate and reduce the articular step-off and place the cannulated lag screws percutaneously using fluoroscopy. The intraarticular component of the nonunion may be freshened up using an arthroscopic burr if necessary (typically not). Arthroscopy also facilitates lysis of intraarticular adhesions to improve joint range of motion.

Occasionally open reduction is required to reduce an intraarticular or juxtaarticular deformity. In such cases, the surgical approach may include an arthrotomy for lysis of adhesions.

METAPHYSEAL NONUNIONS. Metaphyseal nonunions are relatively common. In general, the nonunion type determines the treatment strategy.

Plate-and-screw stabilization provides rigid fixation and is performed in conjunction with bone grafting, except for hypertrophic nonunions (Fig. 25-29). Screw fixation alone (without plating) should never be used for metaphyseal nonunions.

Intramedullary nail fixation is another option (see Fig. 25-29). Because the medullary canal is larger at the metaphysis

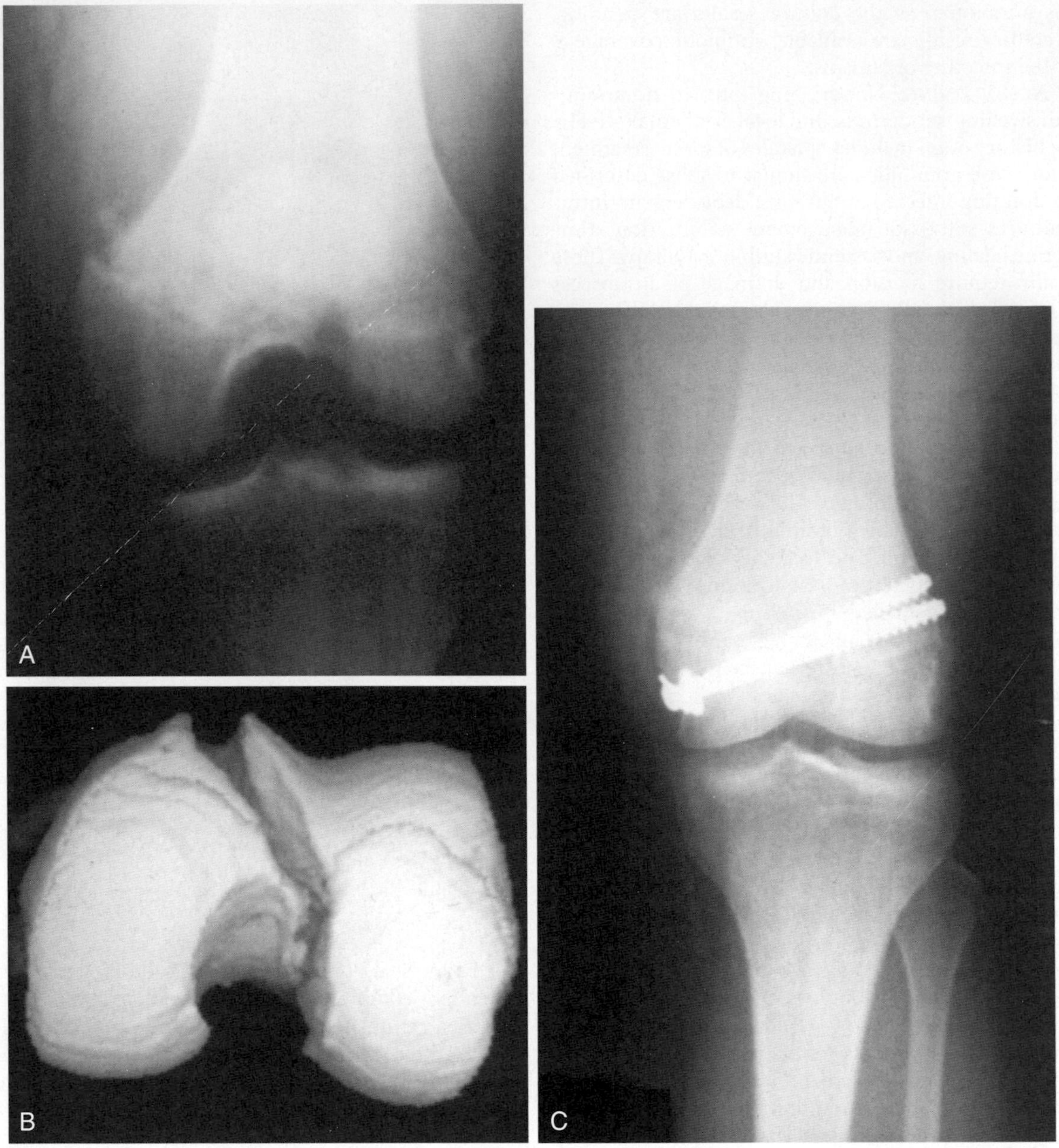

Figure 25-28. Epiphyseal nonunion (oligotrophic) of the distal femur in an 18-year-old who was referred in 5 months following injury. **A,** Preoperative radiograph. **B,** Preoperative computed tomography (CT) scan. **C,** Final result following arthroscopically assisted closed reduction and percutaneous cannulated screw fixation shows solid bony union.

than at the diaphysis, this method of fixation is predisposed to instability. Treatment of metaphyseal nonunions with nail fixation requires good bone-to-bone contact at the nonunion site; a minimum of two interlocking screws in the short segment (custom-designed nails can provide for multiple interlocking screws); placement of blocking (Poller) screws[124,125] to provide added stability (see Fig. 25-29); and intraoperative manual stress testing under fluoroscopy to ensure stable fixation.

External fixation may also be used to treat metaphyseal nonunions. Ilizarov external fixation is preferred because it offers enhanced stability and early weight-bearing (for lower extremity nonunions), as well as gradual compression at the nonunion site (see Fig. 25-29). Metaphyseal nonunions are particularly well suited for thin-wire external fixation because of the predominance of cancellous bone. For nonunions in the proximal humeral and proximal femoral metaphyses, internal fixation is generally preferable to external fixation because the proximity of the trunk makes Ilizarov frame application technically difficult.

Stable metaphyseal nonunions are frequently oligotrophic and typically unite rapidly when stimulated using conventional cancellous bone grafting or a percutaneous bone marrow injection. While both methods have a high rate of success, percutaneous marrow injection provides the benefits of minimally invasive surgery.[126]

The special considerations for metaphyseal nonunions are similar to those of epiphyseal nonunions and include juxtaar-

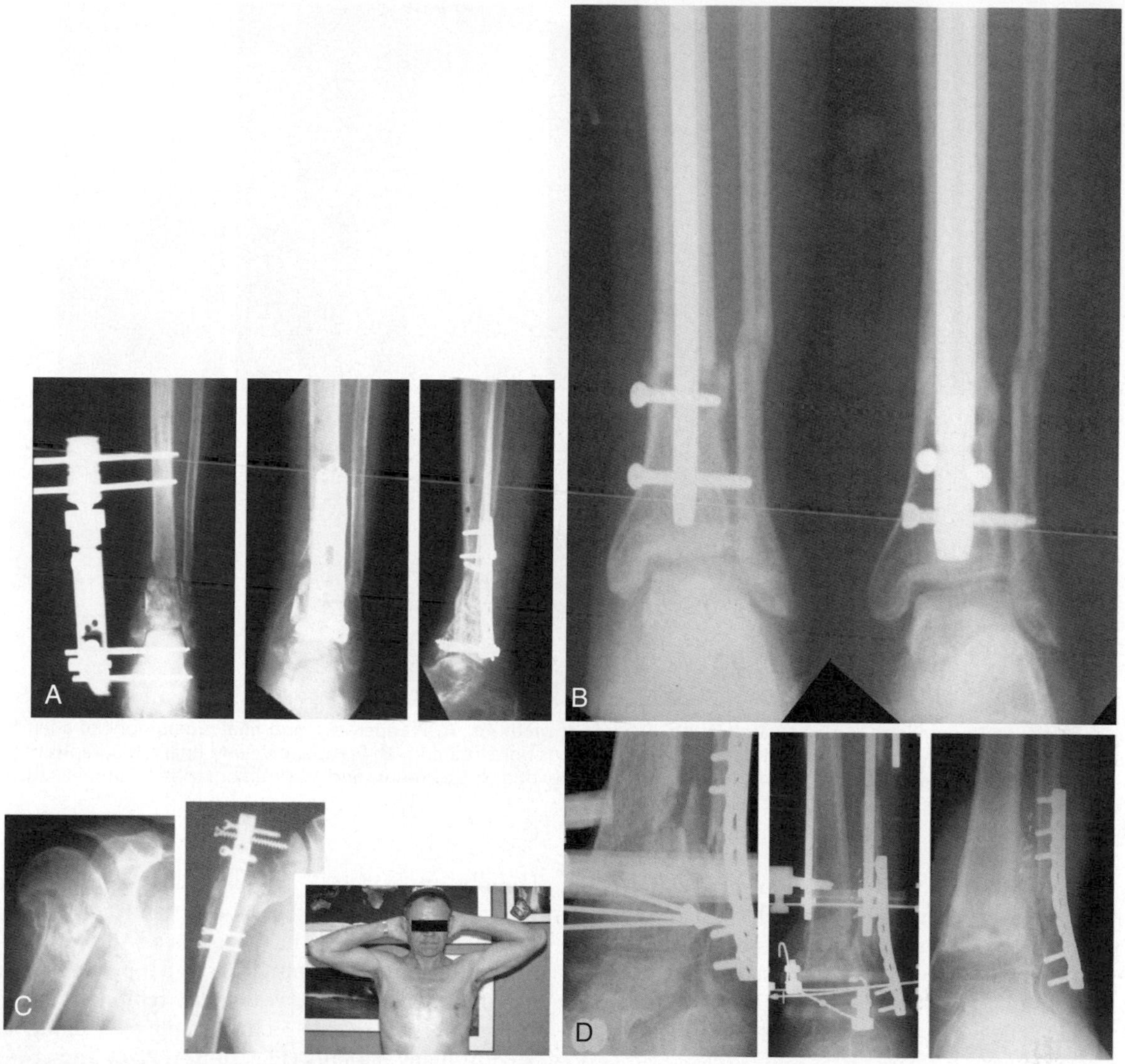

Figure 25-29. Metaphyseal nonunions can be treated using a variety of methods. **A,** Preoperative and final radiographs of an atrophic distal tibial nonunion treated with plate-and-screw fixation and autologous cancellous bone grafting. **B,** Preoperative and final radiographs of an oligotrophic distal tibial nonunion treated with exchange nailing. Note the use of Poller screws in the short distal fragment to enhance stability. **C,** Preoperative and final radiographs and final clinical photograph of a proximal metaphyseal humeral nonunion treated with intramedullary nail stabilization and autogenous bone grafting. **D,** Preoperative, during treatment, and final radiographs of a distal tibial nonunion treated using Ilizarov external fixation.

ticular deformities, motion at the adjacent joint, and compensatory deformities at the adjacent joints.

DIAPHYSEAL NONUNIONS. Diaphyseal nonunions traverse cortical bone and may be more resistant to union than metaphyseal and epiphyseal nonunions, which traverse primarily cancellous bone. Their more central location, however, makes diaphyseal nonunions amenable to many fixation methods (Fig. 25-30).

NONUNIONS TRAVERSING MORE THAN ONE ANATOMIC REGION. Nonunions traversing more than one anatomic region require a strategy for each region. In some cases, the treatment can be performed using the same strategy for each region. For example, a nonunion of the proximal humeral metaphysis with diaphyseal extension could be treated with a reamed intramedullary nail with proximal and distal interlocking screws. This single strategy provides mechanical stability and biological stimulation (reaming) to both nonunions. In other situations, several strategies must be used. For example, a nonunion of the distal tibial epiphysis with extension into the metaphysis and diaphysis could be treated using several strategies: cannulated screw fixation of the epiphysis, percutaneous marrow injection of the metaphysis, and Ilizarov external fixation stabilizing all three anatomic regions.

SEGMENTAL BONE DEFECTS. Segmental bone defects associated with nonunions may be a result of high-energy open fractures with bone lost at the accident, surgical débridement of devitalized bone fragments, surgical débridement of an infected nonunion, or surgical trimming at a nonunion site to improve surface characteristics.

Segmental bone defects may have partial (incomplete) bone loss or circumferential (complete) bone loss (Fig. 25-31). Treatment methods fit into three broad categories: static, acute compression, and gradual compression.

STATIC TREATMENT METHODS. Static treatment methods fill the defect between the bone ends. In static methods, the proximal and distal ends of the nonunion are fixed using

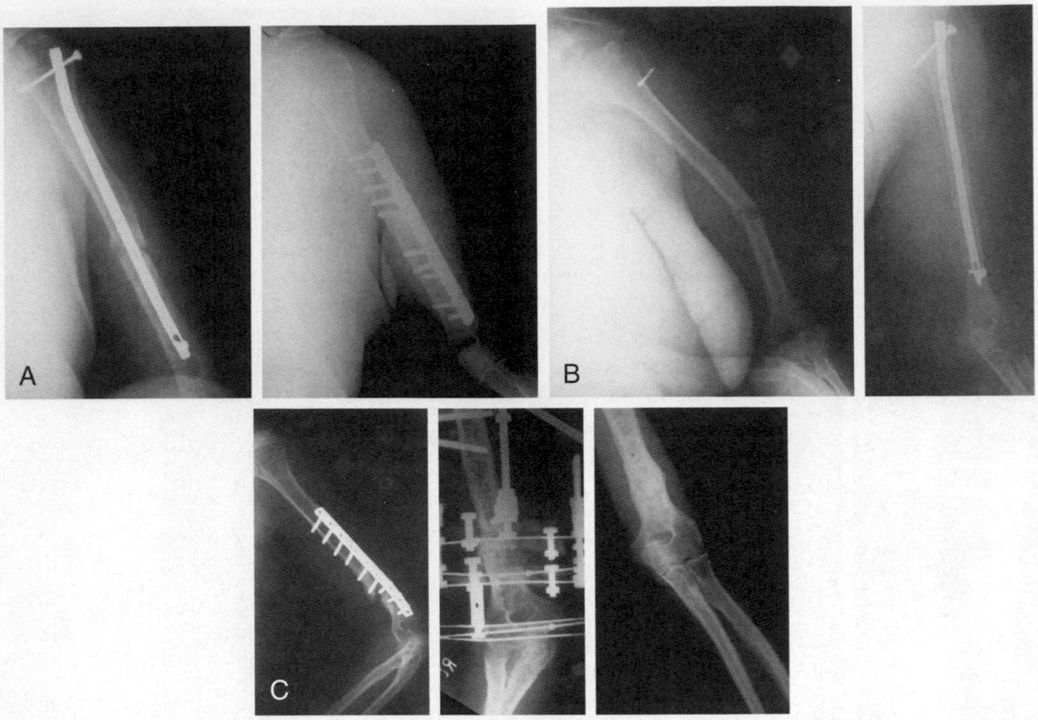

Figure 25-30. Diaphyseal nonunions can be treated using a variety of methods. **A,** Preoperative and final radiographs of a left humeral shaft nonunion treated with plate-and-screw fixation and autologous cancellous bone grafting. **B,** Preoperative and final radiographs of a left humeral shaft nonunion treated with intramedullary nail fixation. **C,** Preoperative, during treatment, and final radiographs of an infected humeral shaft nonunion treated using Ilizarov external fixation.

internal or external fixation, taking care to ensure that the bone is not foreshortened or overdistracted. Static methods for treating bone defects include autogenous cancellous bone graft, autogenous cortical bone graft, vascularized autograft, bulk cortical allograft, strut cortical allograft, mesh cage-bone graft constructs, synostosis, and Masquelet (induced-membrane) techniques.

Autogenous cancellous bone graft may be used to treat either partial or circumferential defects. The other methods are typically used to treat circumferential segmental defects. These methods are discussed in detail in the Treatment Methods subsection.

Acute Compression Methods. Acute compression methods obtain immediate bone-to-bone contact at the nonunion site by acutely shortening the extremity. Soft tissue compliance, surgical or open wounds, and neurovascular structures limit the extent of acute shortening that is possible. Some authors[122,127,128] have suggested that greater than 2 to 2.5 cm of acute shortening may lead to wound closure difficulties or kinking of blood vessels and lymphatic channels. In our experience, up to 4 to 5 cm of acute shortening is well tolerated in many patients (Fig. 25-32). Paley and coworkers have reported that acute shortening is appropriate for defects up to 7 cm in length.[129]

In the leg and forearm, the unaffected bone (e.g., fibula) must be partially excised to allow for acute compression of the ununited bone (e.g., tibia). Longitudinal incisions tend to bunch up when acute shortening is performed. An experienced plastic reconstructive surgeon is invaluable for the closure of these wounds. Transverse incisions are less difficult to close because they bunch up less when acute shortening is performed.

The bone ends should be fashioned to create opposing surfaces that are as parallel as possible. Flat cuts with an oscillating saw improve bone-to-bone contact but likely damage the bony tissues. Osteotomes, rasps, and rongeurs create less damage to the bony tissues but are less effective in creating flat cuts. No consensus exists regarding which method is best. We prefer to use a wide, flat oscillating saw and intermittent bursts of cutting under constant irrigation.

Acute compression methods provide immediate bone-to-bone contact and compression at the nonunion site, facilitating the initiation of healing. Acute compression with shortening also allows concomitant cancellous bone grafting of the decorticated bone at the nonunion site.

A disadvantage of acute compression of segmental defects is the functional consequences of foreshortening. In the upper

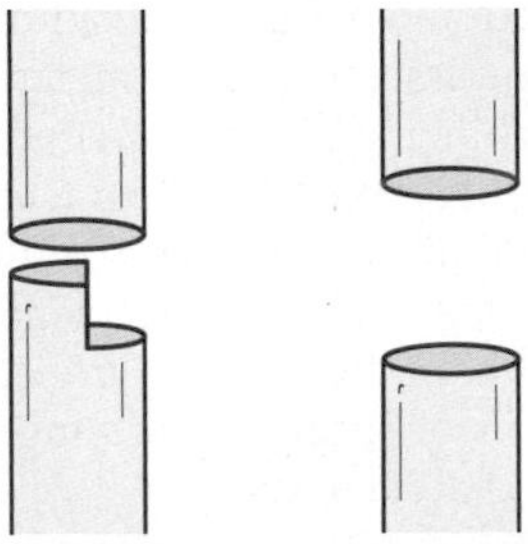

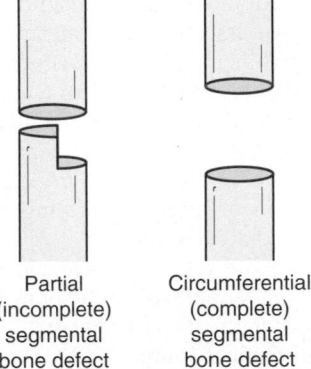

Figure 25-31. Segmental bone defects may be associated with either partial (incomplete) bone loss or circumferential (complete) bone loss.

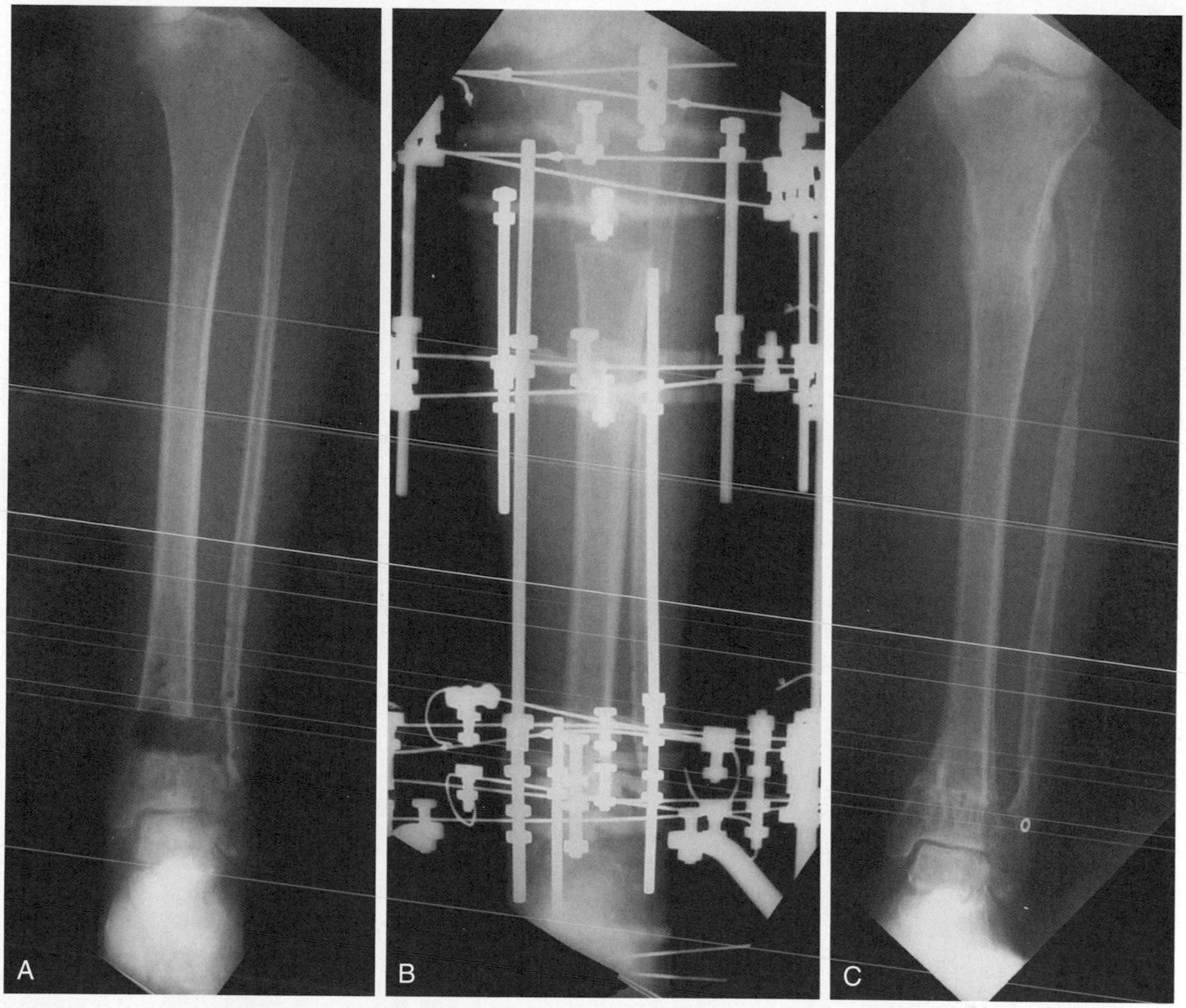

Figure 25-32. **A,** Circumferential (complete) segmental bone defect in a 66-year-old woman with an infected distal tibial nonunion on high-dose steroids for severe rheumatoid arthritis. **B,** Radiograph during treatment following acute compression (2.5 cm) using an Ilizarov external fixator and bone grafting at the nonunion site. **C,** Final radiograph shows a healed distal tibial nonunion and restoration of length from concomitant lengthening at a proximal tibial corticotomy site.

extremity, up to 3 to 4 cm of foreshortening is well tolerated. In the lower extremity, up to 2 cm of foreshortening may be treated with a shoe lift, many patients poorly tolerate a shoe lift for 2 to 4 cm of shortening, and most do not tolerate greater than 4 cm of foreshortening. Therefore, many patients undergoing acute compression concurrently or subsequently undergo a lengthening procedure of the same extremity or a foreshortening procedure of the contralateral extremity (see Fig. 25-32).

Acute compression is typically used to treat circumferential segmental defects. When using internal fixation devices, acute compression is most effectively applied by the intraoperative use of a femoral distractor or a spanning external fixator. When using plate-and-screw fixation, an articulating tension device may be used to gain further interfragmentary compression. Dynamic compression plates (DCPs; Synthes, Paoli, PA) may be used to provide further interfragmentary compression and rigid fixation. Oblique parallel flat cuts allow for enhanced interfragmentary compression via lag screws (Fig. 25-33). When using intramedullary nail fixation, acute compression across the segmental defect can also be applied intraoperatively using a femoral distractor or a spanning external fixator (Fig. 25-34). Compression can be applied using these temporary devices before or after nail insertion, but prior to static interlocking. In either case, the medullary canal should be over-reamed at least 1.5 mm larger than the nail diameter. When the nail is placed after compression (shortening), over-reaming permits nail passage without distraction at the nonunion site. When the nail is placed before compression, over-reaming allows the proximal and distal fragments to slide

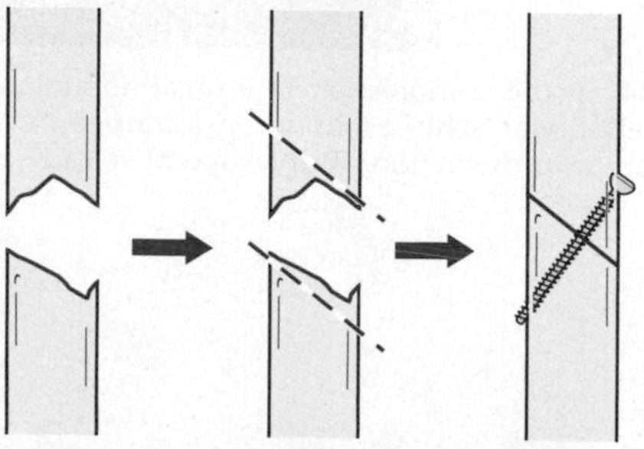

Figure 25-33. Oblique parallel flat cuts allow for enhanced interfragmentary compression via lag screw fixation when a segmental defect is treated with acute compression and plate stabilization.

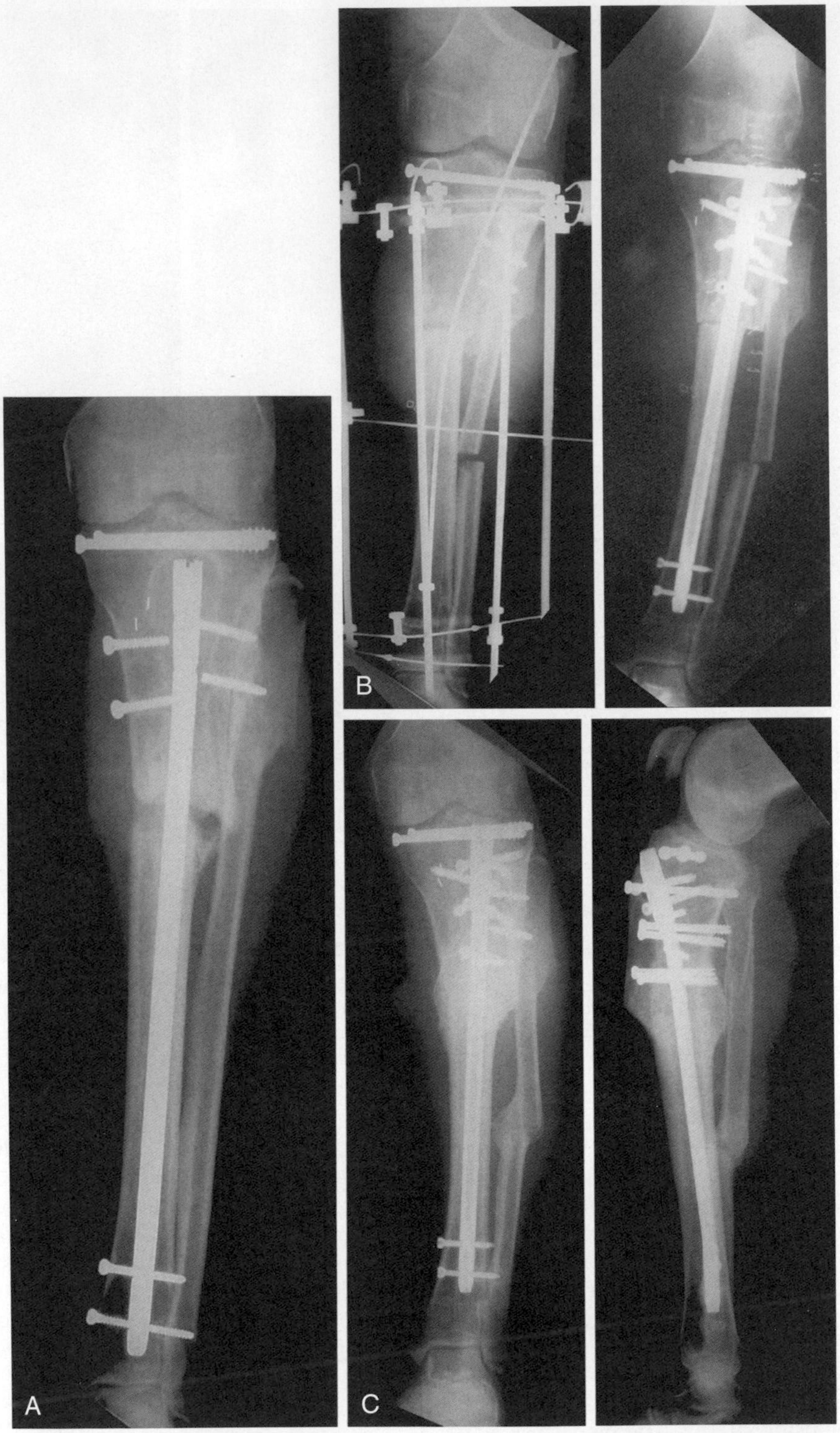

Figure 25-34. Acute compression of a tibial nonunion with a segmental defect using a temporary (intraoperative use only) external fixator. Definitive fixation was achieved using an intramedullary nail. Note the use of poller screws in the proximal fragment for enhanced stability. **A,** Radiograph on presentation. **B,** Intraoperative radiographs. **C,** Final result.

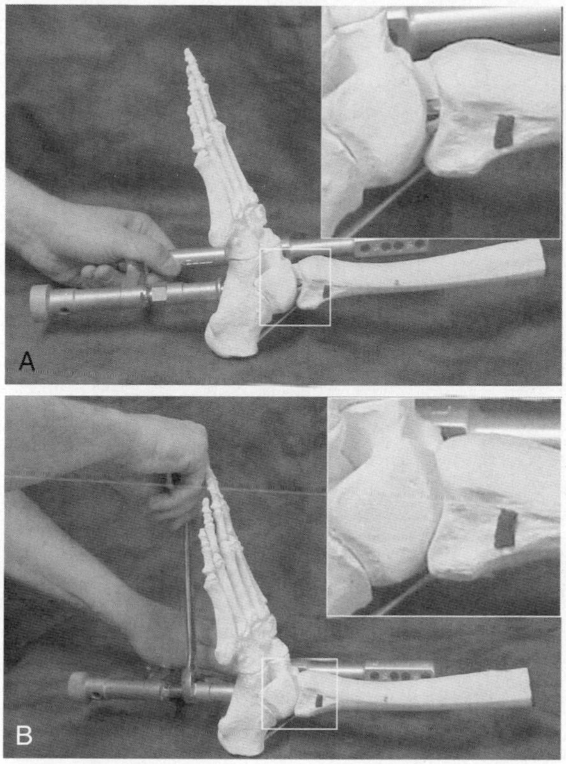

Figure 25-35. Some intramedullary nails allow for acute compression across a fracture site or a nonunion site. An example of such a nail is shown here. The Biomet Ankle Arthrodesis Nail (Warsaw, IN) is designed to allow for acute compression at the time of the operative procedure. **A,** Prior to compression. **B,** Acute compression being applied across the ankle joint using the compression device.

over the nail and compress without jamming on the nail. Prior to removal of the intraoperative compression device, the nail must be statically locked both proximal and distal to the nonunion site. Some intramedullary devices, such as the Ankle Arthrodesis Nail (Biomet, Warsaw, IN), allow for acute compression across the fracture or nonunion site during the operative procedure (Fig. 25-35). In our experience, nails that allow for acute compression, when available, are preferable to conventional nails for this specific type of treatment.

Acute compression can also be applied using an external fixator as the definitive mode of treatment. Transverse parallel flat cuts accommodate axial compression and minimize shear moments at the nonunion site. We favor the Ilizarov device when using external fixation for acute compression across a segmental defect. The Ilizarov frame can also restore limb length via corticotomy with lengthening at another site of the same bone (bifocal treatment).

Gradual Compression Methods. Gradual compression methods to treat a nonunion with a circumferential segmental defect include monofocal gradual compression (shortening) or bone transport. Both methods are most commonly accomplished via external fixation; again, we favor the Ilizarov device. Neither method is associated with the soft tissue and wound problems associated with acute compression. Monofocal gradual compression and bone transport, however, are both associated with malalignment at the docking site, whereas acute compression is not.

For monofocal gradual compression, the external fixator frame is constructed to allow for compression in increments of 0.25 mm (Fig. 25-36). Slow compression at a rate of 0.25 to 1.0 mm per day is applied in one or four increments, respectively. When a large defect exists, compression is applied at a rate of 1.0 mm per day; at or near bony touchdown, the rate is slowed to 0.25 to 0.50 mm per day. Compression in limbs with paired bones requires partial excision of the intact, unaffected bone.

For bone transport, the frame is constructed to allow a transport rate ranging from 0.25 mm every other day to 1.5 mm per day (Fig. 25-37). The transport is typically started at the rate of 0.50 to 0.75 mm per day in two or three increments, respectively. The rate is increased or decreased based on the quality of the bony regenerate.

When poor surface characteristics are present, open trimming of the nonunion site is recommended to improve the chances of rapid healing following docking. When trimming is performed during the initial procedure, the docking site can be bone grafted if the anticipated time to docking is approximately 2 months or less (e.g., 6-cm defect compressed at a rate of 1.0 mm per day). If the time to docking will be significantly greater than 2 months (for larger defects), two options exist. First, gradual compression or transport can be continued at a rate ranging from 0.25 mm per week to 0.25 mm per day after bony touchdown is seen on plain radiographs. Continued compression at the docking site is seen clinically and radiographically as bending of the fixation wires, indicating that the rings are moving more than the proximal and distal bone fragments. Second, the docking site can be opened when the defect is approximately 1 to 2 cm to freshen up the proximal and distal surfaces and bone graft the defect. Gradual compression or transport then proceeds into the graft material.

In our experience, continued compression without open bone grafting and surface freshening leads to successful bony union in many patients. Others believe that bone grafting the docking site significantly decreases the time to healing. A useful alternative to open bone grafting is percutaneous marrow injection at the docking site. We use this technique in patients who have one or two "contributing factors" (see Table 25-2) and are thus at increased risk for persistent nonunion. We reserve open bone grafting of the docking site for the following scenarios: patients with no radiographic evidence of progression to healing despite 4 months of continued compression after bony touchdown; patients with three or more "contributing factors" for nonunion who are therefore at very high risk of persistent nonunion at the docking site; and patients who require trimming of the bone ends to improve contact at the docking site.

Nonunions with partial segmental defects are not amenable to many of the treatment strategies that have been discussed. These defects are most commonly treated with a static method, such as autologous cancellous bone grafting and internal or external fixation. As the partial bone loss segment increases in length, the likelihood of bony union using conventional bone grafting techniques decreases. In cases of nonunion with a large (>6 cm) segment of partial (incomplete) bone loss, the treatment options are "splinter (sliver) bone transport" (Fig. 25-38), surgical trimming of the bone ends to enhance surface characteristics followed by an acute or gradual compression method, or strut cortical allogenic bone grafting.

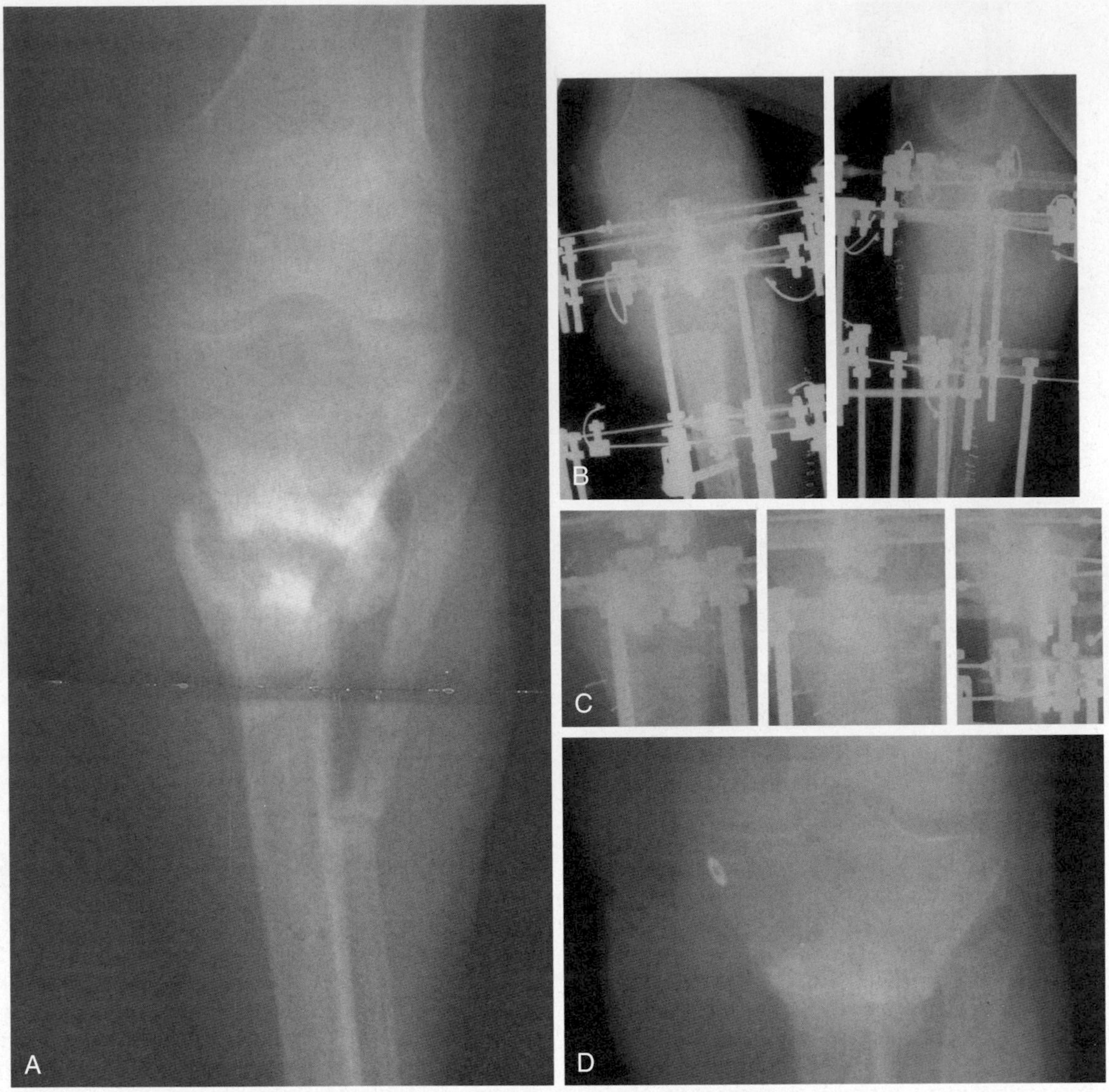

Figure 25-36. An example of a nonunion treated with gradual monofocal compression. **A,** Presenting radiograph of a proximal tibial nonunion in a 79-year-old woman with a history of multiple failed procedures and chronic osteomyelitis. **B,** Intraoperative radiographs following bone excision shows a segmental defect. **C,** Radiographs showing gradual compression at the nonunion site over the course of several weeks. **D,** Radiograph showing final result with solid bony union.

The diverse nature of nonunions with segmental bone defects makes synthesis of the literature quite difficult. A review of recent literature for treatment of complete segmental bone defects is shown in Table 25-6.[130-144] Our preferred methods are shown in Table 25-7.

Prior Failed Treatments. A nonunion's response (or lack thereof) to prior treatments provides insight into its character. Why did the prior treatments fail? Were the treatments appropriate? Were there any technical problems with the treatments? Were there any positive biological responses to any prior treatment? Did mechanical instability contribute to the prior failures? Did any treatment improve the patient's pain and function?

A prior treatment method that has provided no clinical or radiographic evidence of progression to healing should not be repeated unless the treating physician believes that technical improvements will lead to bony union. Repeating a prior failed procedure may be considered if the prior procedure produced a measurable clinical or radiographic improvement in the nonunion. For example, repeat exchange nailing of the femur can be effective in certain groups of patients,[34] but relatively ineffective in others.[145] Those who heal following serial exchange nailings show improvement following each procedure, whereas those whose nonunions persist show little or no clinical and radiographic response (Fig. 25-39).

The nonunion specialist must be part surgeon, part detective, and part historian. History has a way of repeating itself. Without a clear understanding and appreciation of why prior treatments have failed, the learning curve becomes a circle.

Deformities. The priority in patients who have a fracture nonunion with deformity is healing the bone. Healing the bone and correcting the deformity at the same time is not always possible. Will the effort to correct the deformity significantly increase the risk of persistent nonunion? If so, then

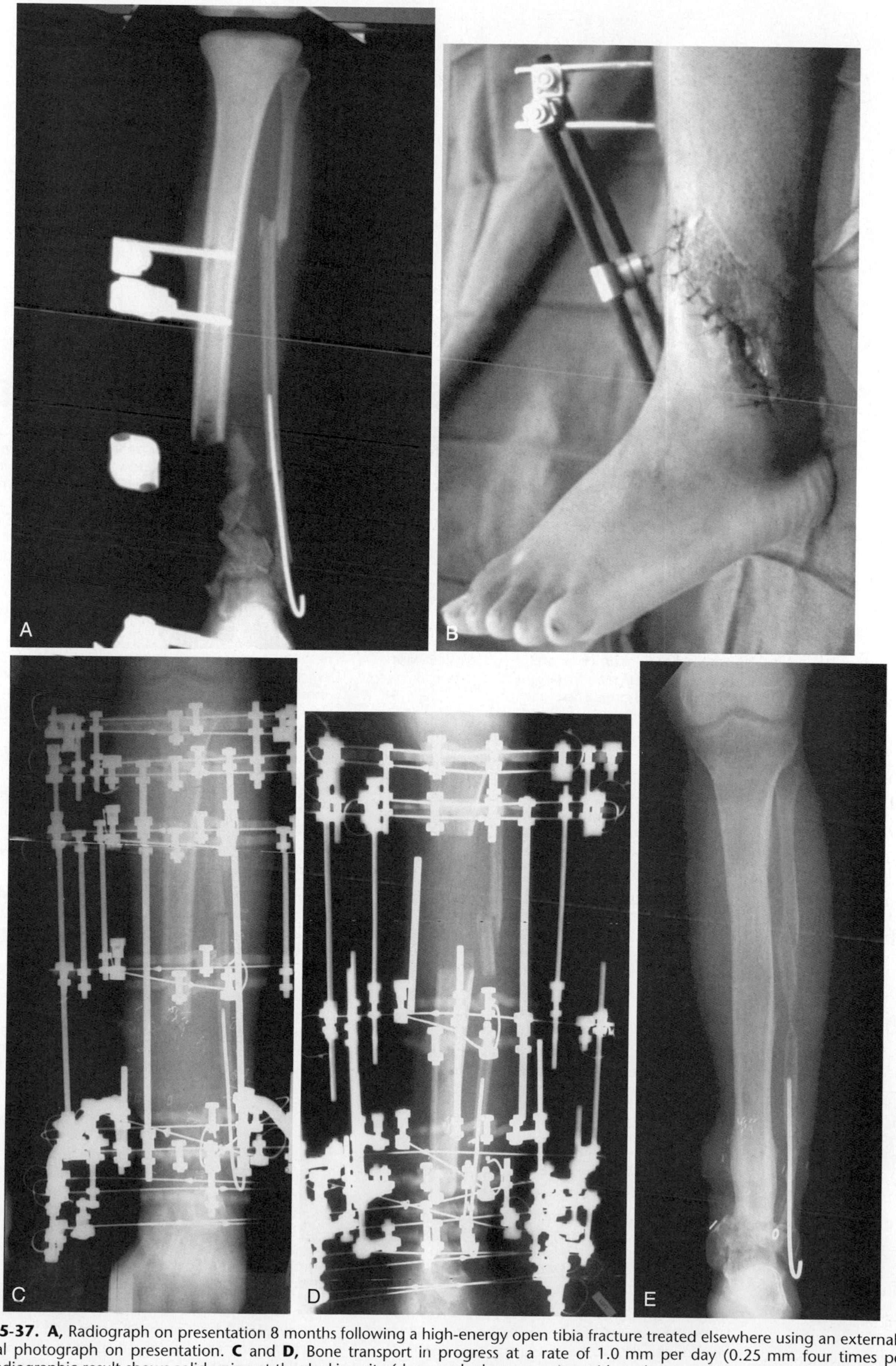

Figure 25-37. **A,** Radiograph on presentation 8 months following a high-energy open tibia fracture treated elsewhere using an external fixator. **B,** Clinical photograph on presentation. **C** and **D,** Bone transport in progress at a rate of 1.0 mm per day (0.25 mm four times per day). **E,** Final radiographic result shows solid union at the docking site (slow gradual compression without bone grafting resulted in solid bony union) with mature bony regenerate at the proximal corticotomy site.

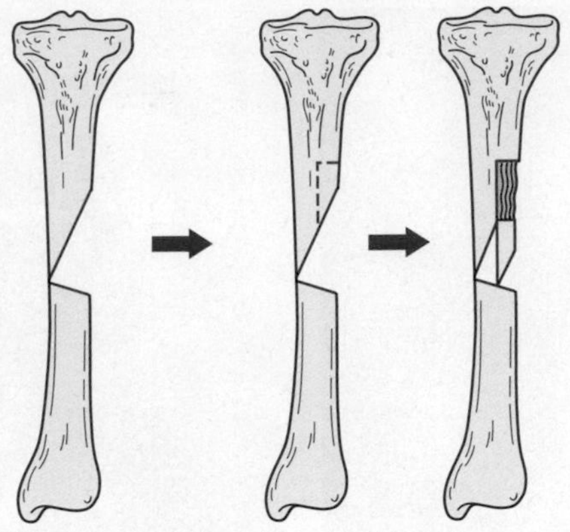

A B

Figure 25-38. A, Nonunion with a partial (incomplete) segmental defect. **B,** Splinter (sliver) bone transport can be used to span this defect.

TABLE 25-6 *REVIEW OF THE RECENT LITERATURE ON SEGMENTAL BONE DEFECTS*

Author	Patient Population	Findings/Conclusions
Cierny and Zorn, 1994	44 patients with segmental infected tibial defects; 23 patients were treated with conventional methods (massive cancellous bone grafts, tissue transfers, and combinations of internal and external fixation); 21 patients were treated using the methods of Ilizarov.	The final results in the two treatment groups were similar. The Ilizarov method was faster, safer in B-host (compromised) patients, less expensive, and easier to perform. Conventional therapy is recommended when any one distraction site is anticipated to exceed 6 cm in length in a patient with poor physiologic or support group status. When conditions permit either conventional or Ilizarov treatment methods, the authors recommend Ilizarov reconstruction for defects of 2 to 12 cm.
Green, 1994	32 patients with segmental skeletal defects; 15 were treated with an open bone graft technique; 17 were treated with Ilizarov bone transport.	The authors' recommendations are as follows: Defects up to 5 cm: cancellous bone grafting vs. bone transport. Defects greater than 5 cm: bone transport vs. free composite tissue transfer.
Marsh et al, 1994	25 infected tibial nonunions with segmental bone loss greater than or equal to 2.5 cm; 15 patients were treated with débridement, external fixation, bone grafting, and soft tissue coverage; 10 were treated with resection and bone transport using a monolateral external fixator.	The two treatment groups were equivalent in terms of rate of healing, eradication of infection, treatment time, number of complications, total number of operative procedures, and angular deformities after treatment. Limb length discrepancy was significantly less in the group treated with bone transport.
Emami et al, 1995	37 cases of infected nonunion of the tibial shaft treated with open cancellous bone grafting (Papineau, 1979) stabilized via external fixation; 15 nonunions had partial contact at the nonunion site, 22 had a complete segmental defect ranging from 1.5 to 3 cm in length.	All nonunions united at an average of 11 months following bone grafting. The authors recommend cancellous bone grafting for complete segmental defects up to 3 cm in length.
Patzakis et al, 1995	32 patients with infected tibial nonunions with bone defects less than 3 cm; all were stabilized with external fixation and were grafted with autogenous iliac crest bone at a mean of 8 weeks following soft tissue coverage.	Union was reported in 91% of patients (29 of 32) at a mean of 5.5 months following the bone graft procedure; union was achieved in the remaining 3 patients following posterolateral bone grafting.
Moroni et al, 1997	24 patients with nonunions with bone defects averaging 3.6 cm; 15 ulnar and 9 radial; all were treated with débridement, intercalary bone graft, and internal fixation with a cortical bone graft fixed opposite to a plate.	Union was reported in 96% of patients (23 of 24) at a mean of 3 months following surgery.
Polyzois et al, 1997	42 patients with 25 tibial and 17 femoral nonunions with bone defects averaging 6 cm; 19 (45%) patients had an active infection and 9 had a history of previous infection; all were treated with Ilizarov bone transport.	Union was reported in all patients (100%), although 4 (10%) patients required bone grafting of the docking site; all cases of infection resolved without further surgery; final leg length discrepancy was less than 1.5 cm in all cases.
Song et al, 1998	27 patients with tibial bone defects averaging 8.3 cm; 13 (48%) patients had an active infection; all were treated with Ilizarov bone transport.	Union was reported in all patients (100%), although 25 (96%) patients required bone grafting of the docking site; all cases of infection resolved without further surgery.

TABLE 25-6 *REVIEW OF THE RECENT LITERATURE ON SEGMENTAL BONE DEFECTS* (Continued)

Author	Patient Population	Findings/Conclusions
Atkins et al, 1999	5 patients with massive tibial bone defects; all were treated with Ilizarov transport of the fibula into the defect.	Union at the proximal and distal graft sites and hypertrophy of the graft was reported in all patients (100%).
Masquelet et al, 2000	35 patients with diaphyseal defects (27 in tibia) ranging from 4 to 25 cm; all were treated in two stages; first, a cement spacer was placed in the defect and retained for 2 months; second, the spacer was removed but the pseudosynovial membrane induced by the spacer was preserved in place and packed with cancellous autograft and the construct was stabilized with external fixation in the lower extremity and plating or nailing in the upper extremity.	Union was reported in 32 patients (91%) between 6 and 17 months with return to normal walking at an average of 8.5 months for lower extremity cases.
McKee et al, 2002	25 patients with infected nonunions (15 tibia, 6 femur, 3 ulna, 1 humerus) and associated bone defects averaging 30.5 cm were treated with tobramycin-impregnated bone graft substitute (calcium sulfate α-hemihydrate pellets).	Union and elimination of infection was reported in 23 of 25 (92%) patients, although 9 (39%) patients required autogenous bone grafting; three (12%) patients refractured, infection recurred in two (8%) patients, and nonunion persisted in 2 (8%) patients.
Ring et al, 2004	35 patients with nonunions of the forearm (11 ulna, 16 radius, 8 ulna and radius) with defects averaging 2.2 cm; 11 patients had a history of previous infection; all were treated with plate-and-screw fixation and autogenous cancellous bone grafting.	Union was reported in all patients (100%) within 6 months of surgery; 11 (31%) patients had unsatisfactory functional results due to elbow or wrist stiffness; 1 (3%) patient had a poor result due to deformity following bony union.
McCall et al, 2010	21 patients (15 tibia, 5 femur, 1 ulna) with defects ranging from 2 to 14.5 cm were treated with implantation of polymethylmethacrylate (PMMA) spacer for 4 to 6 weeks followed by reamer-aspirator-irrigator (RIA) bone graft and plating or intramedullary nailing.	Union was reported at an average of 11 months in 17 (75%) of 20 patients followed to treatment conclusion, although 7 (35%) required additional surgery (2 exchange nailing, 1 débridement and repeat RIA, 1 revision plating and cancellous autografting, 1 débridement and Ender rod fixation, 2 repeat débridements for infection).
Stafford et al, 2010	19 tibia and 8 femur nonunions with segmental defects ranging from 1 to 25 cm were treated with implantation of an antibiotic-impregnated PMMA spacer for 6 to 8 weeks followed by RIA bone graft and plating or intramedullary nailing.	Union was reported in 24 (89%) of the 27 injury sites within a year of the RIA surgery.
Karger et al, 2012	84 patients (61 tibia, 13 femur, 6 humerus, 4 forearm) with segmental defects ranging from 1 to 23 cm were treated in two stages; first, a cement spacer was placed in the defect and retained for 6 to 8 weeks; second, the spacer was removed while the induced pseudosynovial membrane was preserved and the space packed with cancellous autograft and stabilized with external fixation, plating, or nailing.	76 (90%) attained solid healing in an average of 14.4 months after implantation of the autograft; 14 of the 19 (74%) of the patients with tibial injuries required additional foot and ankle surgery for deformity or instability.

TABLE 25-7 *AUTHORS' RECOMMENDATIONS FOR TREATMENT OPTIONS FOR COMPLETE SEGMENTAL BONE DEFECTS*

Bone	Host	Segmental Defect	Recommend Treatment Options
Clavicle	Healthy or compromised	Less than 1.5 cm	Cancellous autograft bone grafting Skeletal stabilization
Clavicle	Healthy or compromised	1.5 cm or more	Tricortical autogenous iliac crest bone grafting Skeletal stabilization
Humerus	Healthy	Less than 3 cm	Cancellous autograft bone grafting vs. shortening Skeletal stabilization
Humerus	Healthy	3 cm or more	Bulk cortical allograft vs. vascularized cortical autograft vs. bone transport Skeletal stabilization
Humerus	Compromised	Less than 3 cm	Cancellous autograft bone grafting vs. shortening Skeletal stabilization vs. shortening
Humerus	Compromised	3 to 6 cm	Bulk cortical allograft vs. vascularized cortical autograft vs. bone transport Skeletal stabilization

Continued on following page

TABLE 25-7 *AUTHORS' RECOMMENDATIONS FOR TREATMENT OPTIONS FOR COMPLETE SEGMENTAL BONE DEFECTS* (Continued)

Bone	Host	Segmental Defect	Recommend Treatment Options
Humerus	Compromised	Greater than 6 cm	Bulk cortical allograft vs. vascularized cortical autograft Skeletal stabilization
Radius/Ulna	Healthy	Less than 3 cm	Cancellous autograft bone grafting vs. tricortical autogenous iliac crest bone grafting vs. shortening Skeletal stabilization
Radius/Ulna	Healthy	3 cm or more	Bulk cortical allograft vs. vascularized cortical autograft vs. bone transport vs. synostosis Skeletal stabilization
Radius/Ulna	Compromised	Less than 3 cm	Cancellous autograft bone grafting vs. tricortical autogenous iliac crest bone grafting vs. shortening Skeletal stabilization
Radius/Ulna	Compromised	3 to 6 cm	Bulk cortical allograft vs. vascularized cortical autograft vs. bone transport vs. synostosis Skeletal stabilization
Radius/Ulna	Compromised	Greater than 6 cm	Bulk cortical allograft vs. vascularized cortical autograft vs. synostosis Skeletal stabilization
Femur	Healthy	Less than 3 cm	Cancellous autograft bone grafting vs. bone transport vs. bifocal shortening and lengthening Skeletal stabilization
Femur	Healthy	3 to 6 cm	Bone transport vs. bifocal shortening and lengthening Skeletal stabilization
Femur	Healthy	6 to 15 cm	Bone transport vs. bulk cortical allograft Skeletal stabilization
Femur	Healthy	Greater than 15 cm	Bulk cortical allograft Skeletal stabilization
Femur	Compromised	Less than 3 cm	Cancellous autograft bone grafting vs. bone transport vs. bifocal shortening and lengthening Skeletal stabilization
Femur	Compromised	3 to 6 cm	Bone transport vs. bifocal shortening and lengthening vs. bulk cortical allograft Skeletal stabilization
Femur	Compromised	Greater than 6 cm	Bulk cortical allograft with skeletal stabilization vs. bracing vs. amputation
Tibia	Healthy	Less than 3 cm	Cancellous autograft bone grafting vs. bone transport vs. bifocal shortening and lengthening Skeletal stabilization
Tibia	Healthy	3 to 6 cm	Bone transport vs. bifocal shortening and lengthening Skeletal stabilization
Tibia	Healthy	6 to 15 cm	Bone transport vs. bulk cortical allograft Skeletal stabilization
Tibia	Healthy	Greater than 15 cm	Bone transport vs. bulk cortical allograft vs. synostosis Skeletal stabilization
Tibia	Compromised	Less than 3 cm	Cancellous autograft bone grafting vs. bone transport vs. bifocal shortening and lengthening Skeletal stabilization
Tibia	Compromised	3 to 6 cm	Bone transport vs. bifocal shortening and lengthening Skeletal stabilization
Tibia	Compromised	6 to 15 cm	Bone transport vs. bulk cortical allograft vs. synostosis Skeletal stabilization
Tibia	Compromised	Greater than 15 cm	Bulk cortical allograft with skeletal stabilization vs. synostosis with skeletal stabilization vs. bracing vs. amputation

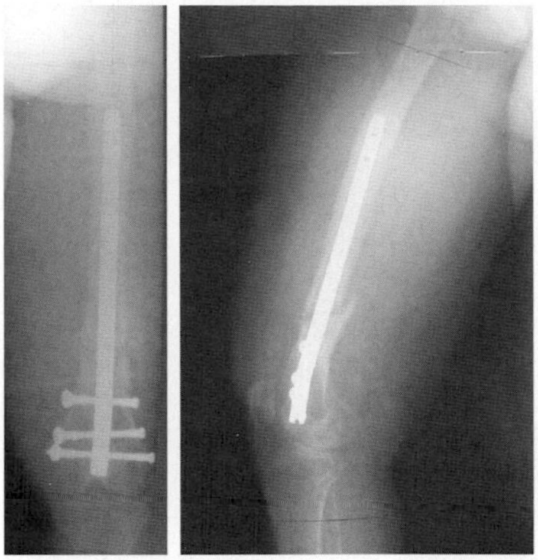

Figure 25-39. An example of a patient with a femoral nonunion that has failed multiple exchange nailings. This 51-year-old woman was referred in having failed three prior exchange nailing procedures.

treatment is planned to first address the nonunion and later address the deformity (sequential approach). If not, then both problems are treated concurrently. The extent of deformity that can be tolerated without correction varies by location and patient. Generally, if the deformity is anticipated to limit function following successful bony union, correction should be considered.

In our experience, most nonunions with deformity benefit from the concurrent treatment approach. Deformity correction often improves bone contact at the nonunion site and therefore promotes bony union. Certain cases, however, are better treated with a sequential approach: if the deformity is unlikely to limit function after successful bony union; if adequate bony contact is best achieved by leaving the fragments in the deformed position; or if soft tissue restrictions make the concurrent approach too complex.

Deformity correction can be performed acutely or gradually. Acute correction is generally performed in lax nonunions, particularly those with a segmental bone defect. Acute correction allows the treating physician to focus on healing the now-undeformed bone. With a large deformity, the ultimate fate of the soft tissues and neurovascular structures must be considered when acute deformity correction is contemplated.

Deformity correction of a stiff nonunion is more challenging. Acute correction typically requires surgical takedown or an osteotomy at the nonunion site. Both effectively correct the deformity, but damage the nonunion site and may impair bony healing. Gradual correction of a deformity in a stiff nonunion may be accomplished using Ilizarov external fixation. Correction of length, angulation, rotation, and translation may be performed in conjunction with compression or distraction at the nonunion site. The Taylor Spatial Frame (Smith and Nephew, Memphis, TN) has simplified frame preconstruction and expanded the combinations of deformity components that can be treated simultaneously (Figs. 25-40 to 25-43).[146]

Surface Characteristics. Nonunions that have large, transversely oriented adjacent surfaces with good bony contact are generally stable to axial compression and relatively easy to bring to successful bony union. By contrast, nonunions with small, vertically oriented surfaces and poor bony contact are generally more difficult to bring to bony union (Fig. 25-44).

Compression generally leads to bony union in nonunions when the opposing fragments have a large surface area. When the surface area is small, trimming of the bone ends may be necessary to improve the surface area for bony contact (Fig. 25-45). Similarly, transversely oriented nonunions respond well to compression. Oblique or vertically oriented nonunions have some component of shear, with the bones sliding past each other when subjected to axial compression. Use of interfragmentary screws with plate-and-screw fixation or steerage pins with external fixation minimizes these shear moments (Fig. 25-46; see Fig. 25-33).

Pain and Function. The "painless" nonunion is seen in three specific instances: hypertrophic nonunions, elderly patients, and Charcot neuropathy.

Some hypertrophic nonunions have relative stability and may not cause symptoms with daily activities unless the fracture nonunion site is stressed (i.e., running, jumping, lifting, or pushing). Painless hypertrophic nonunions occur mostly in the clavicle, humerus, ulna, tibia, and fibula. They are identified by a fine line of cartilage at a hypertrophic fracture site that is only visible on an overexposed radiograph. Subsequent tomograms or CT confirms the nonunion (Fig. 25-47).

Painless nonunions are also seen in the elderly, most typically involving the humerus, but occasionally in the proximal ulna, and less frequently in the femur, tibia, or fibula. Nonoperative treatment can be acceptable as long as day-to-day function is not affected. Nonoperative treatment should be considered in the elderly patient with multiple medical comorbidities that increase perioperative risks. In such cases, bracing or casting (Fig. 25-48), possibly including ultrasonic or electrical stimulation of the nonunion site, may be warranted.[147] Operative stabilization may be necessary if the patient's routine daily activities are impaired or if there is concern about the overlying soft tissues (Fig. 25-49).

Fracture nonunion in the presence of Charcot neuropathy can produce severely deformed and injured bones and joints that are relatively painless. These cases are usually treated nonsurgically with bracing unless the overlying soft tissues are jeopardized (see Fig. 25-49).

In all cases of painless fracture nonunion, the medical history, physical examination, and imaging studies should all be carefully considered when determining the treatment strategy. Operative intervention does not always improve the patient's condition and can result in serious problems. Simple, nonoperative treatment may control the patient's symptoms and maintain or restore function, thus providing a satisfactory outcome.

Osteopenia. Nonunions in patients with osteopenic bone are especially challenging. Osteopenia may be isolated to one bone, as with an atrophic or infected nonunion, or it may be general, as in osteoporosis or metabolic bone disease.

Intramedullary nailing is a good technique for osteopenic bone. Intramedullary nails function as internal splints and have beneficial load-sharing characteristics. Proximal and distal interlocking screws help maintain rotational and axial stability. Specially designed interlocking screws for purchase in poor bone stock are available. In cases requiring rigid fixation, an "intramedullary plate" construct can be achieved with a custom intramedullary nail and multiple interlocking screws (Fig. 25-50).

Plate-and-screw devices are prone to loosening in osteopenic bone where purchase at the screw-bone junction may be

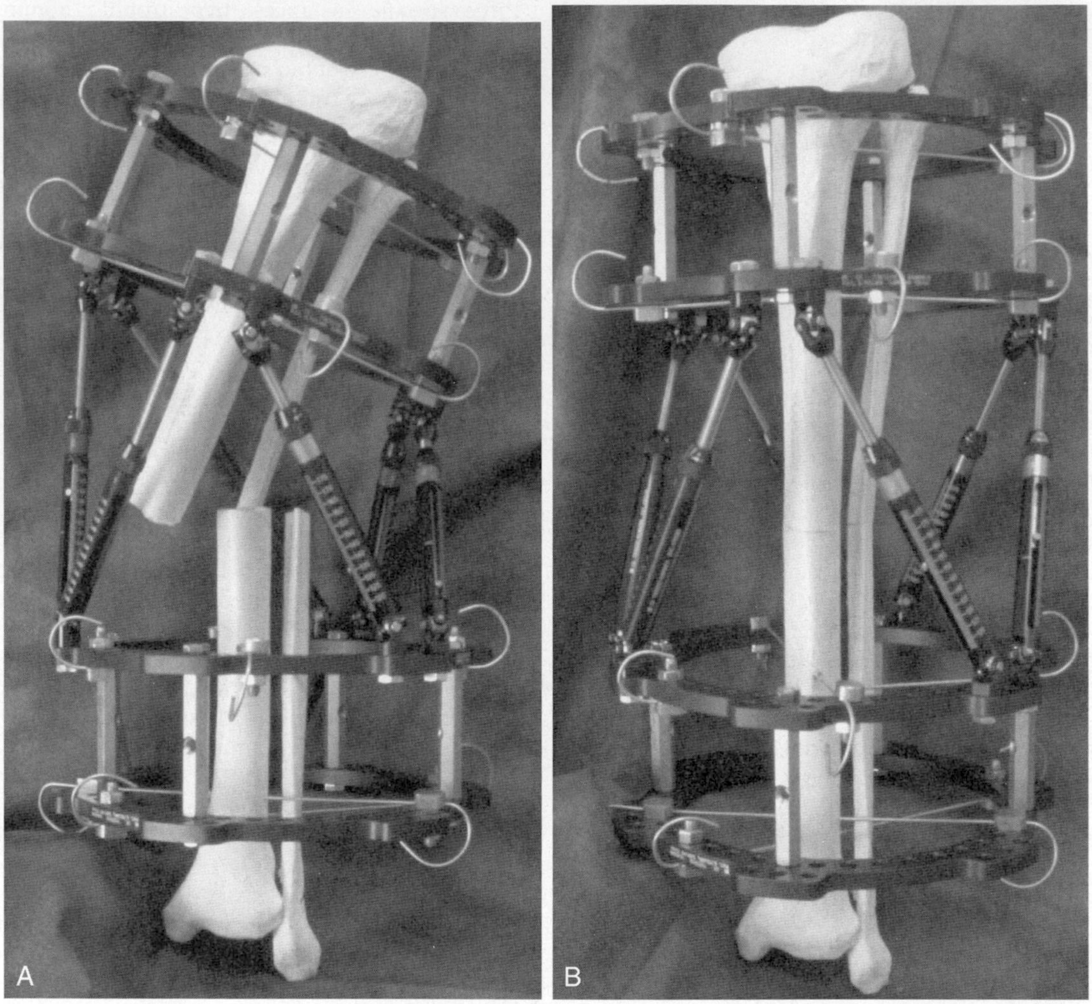

Figure 25-40. The Taylor Spatial Frame (Smith and Nephew, Memphis, TN) allows for simultaneous correction of deformities involving length, angulation, rotation, and translation. **A,** Saw bone demonstration of a tibial nonunion with a profound deformity. Note how the Taylor Spatial Frame mimics the deformity. **B,** Following deformity correction, accomplished by adjusting the Spatial Frame struts. The strut lengths are calculated using a computer software program provided by the manufacturer.

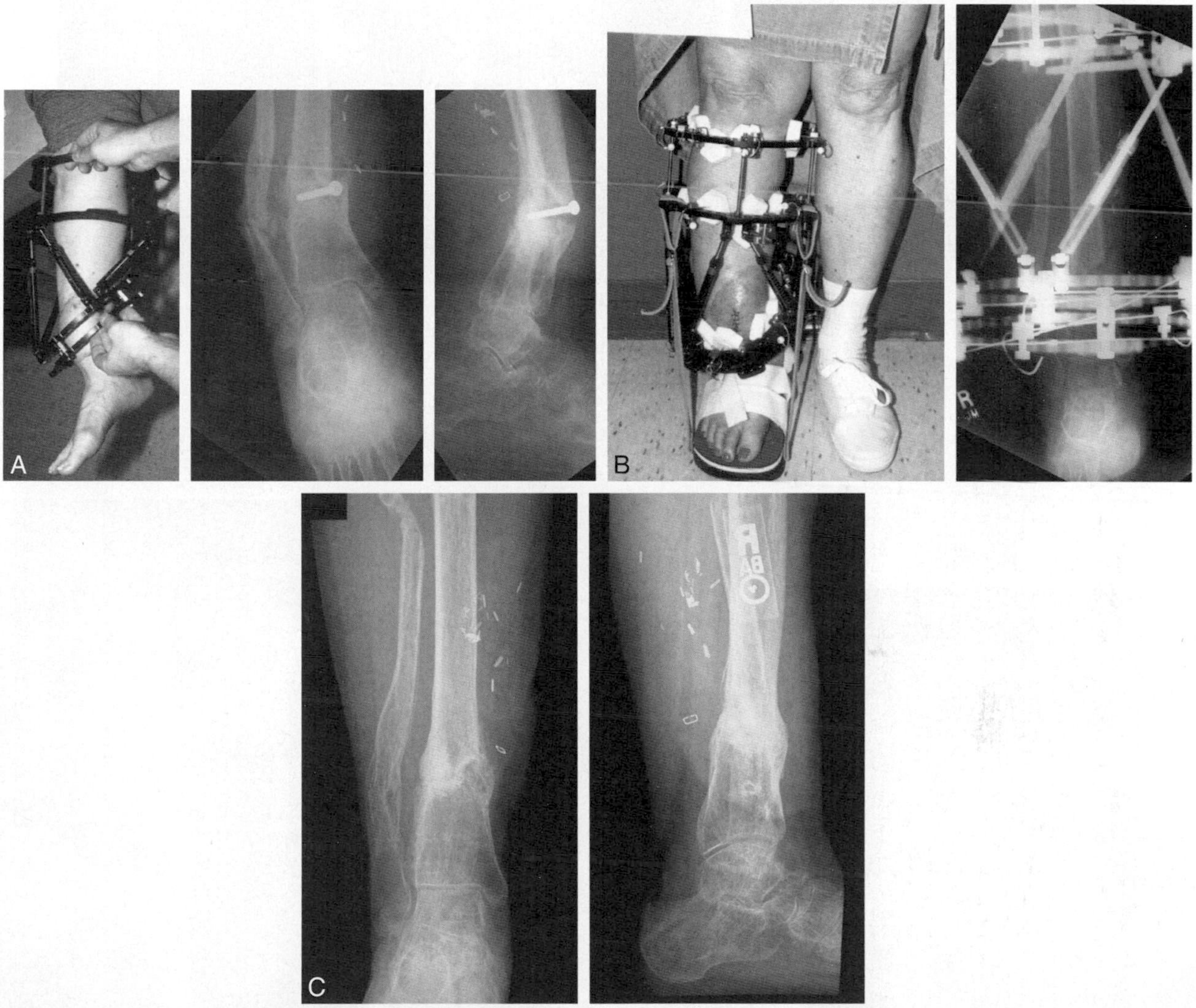

Figure 25-41. **A,** Preoperative clinical photograph showing frame fitting in the office, anterior-posterior (AP) radiograph, and lateral radiograph of a 58-year-old woman with a distal tibial nonunion with deformity referred in 14 months following a high-energy open fracture. **B,** Clinical photograph and AP radiograph during correction using the Taylor Spatial Frame. **C,** Final radiographic result.

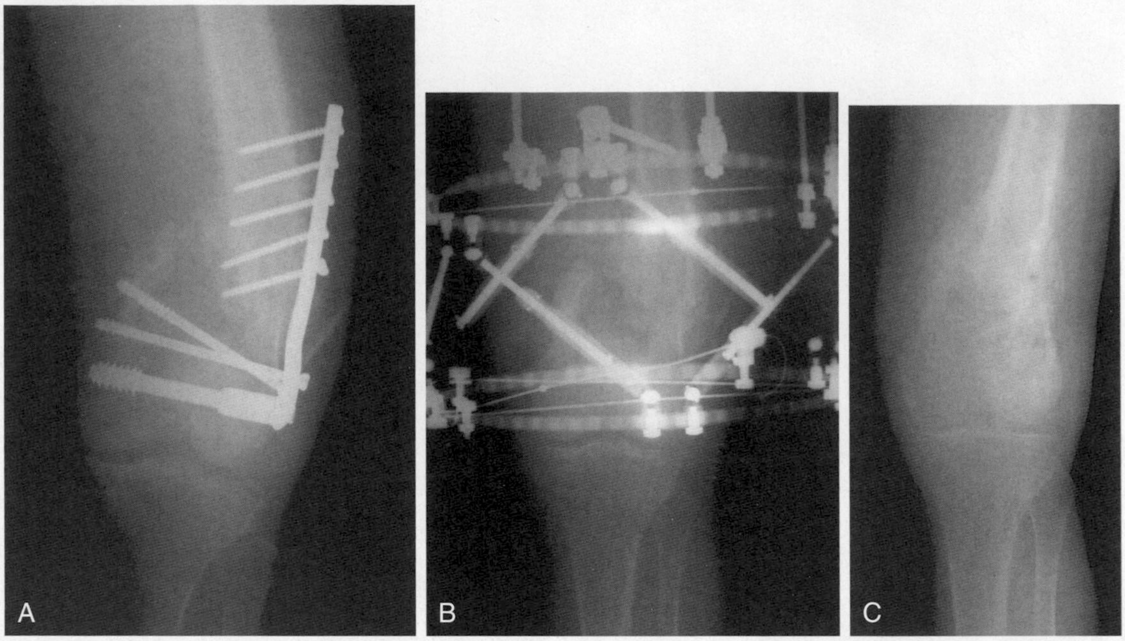

Figure 25-42. **A,** Preoperative radiograph of a 60-year-old man with a distal femoral nonunion with deformity referred in 6 months following open reduction internal fixation. **B,** Radiograph during correction using the Taylor Spatial Frame. **C,** Final radiographic result.

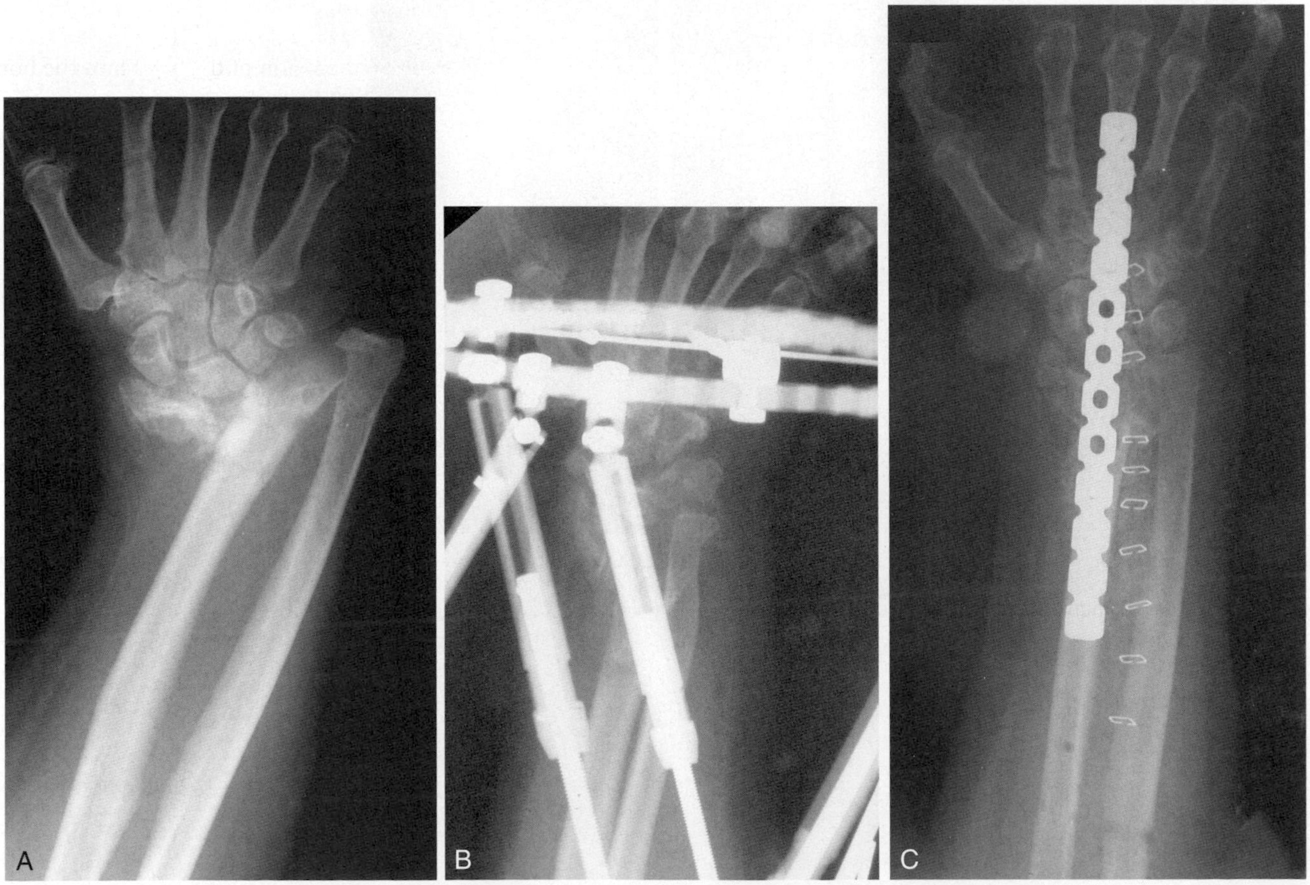

Figure 25-43. **A,** Preoperative anterior-posterior (AP) radiograph of a 73-year-old woman with a distal radius nonunion with a fixed (unreducible) deformity referred in 9 months following injury. **B,** AP radiograph during deformity correction using the Taylor Spatial Frame. **C,** Early postoperative radiograph following deformity correction and plate-and-screw fixation with bone grafting for a wrist arthrodesis.

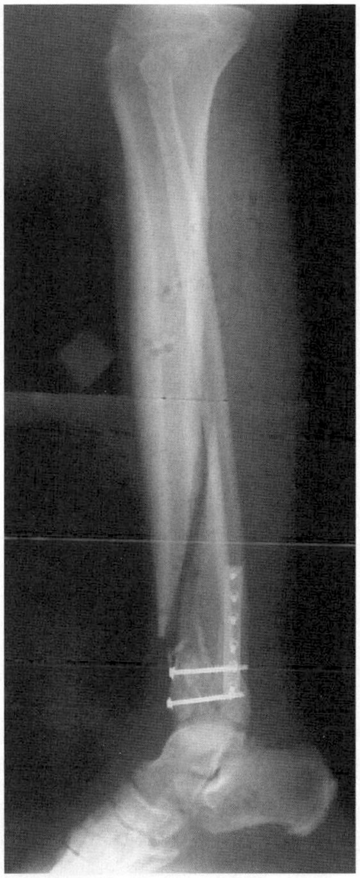

Figure 25-44. Lateral radiograph of the tibial nonunion of a 59-year-old man referred in 6 months following fracture. Nonunions such as this with vertically oriented surfaces and poor bony contact can be very challenging.

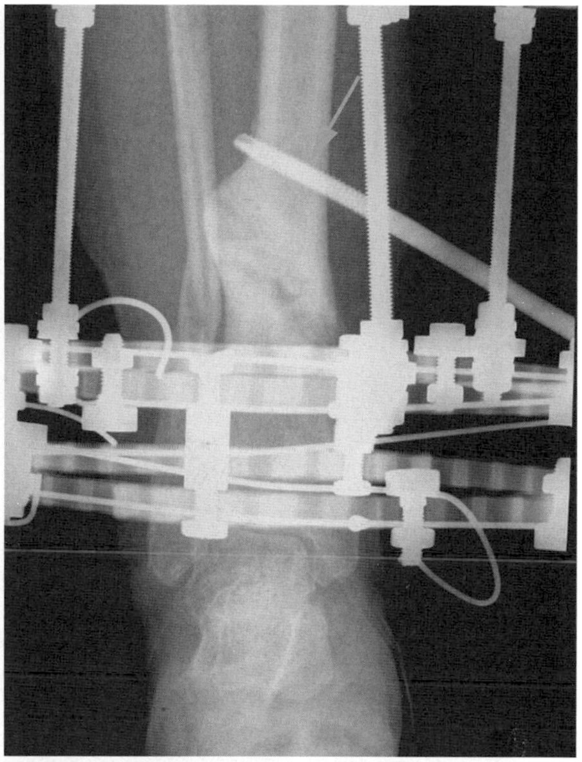

Figure 25-46. Steerage pins *(arrow)* enhance skeletal stabilization.

poor. Fixation may have to be augmented in such cases. Cortical allograft struts and bone grafting have been used to augment fixation of a standard compression plate in the treatment of osteopenic humeral nonunions.[148] Reinforcement of screw holes with PMMA bone cement (Fig. 25-51) is especially useful for nonunion of an osteopenic metaphysis. Locking plates greatly enhance fixation in osteopenic bone. Each screw acts as a fixed-angle device and distributes loads evenly across all screw-bone interfaces. Fixation is particularly enhanced with the use of diverging and converging locking screws.

The thin wires in Ilizarov external fixation provide surprisingly good purchase in osteopenic bone. Olive wires increase stability by discouraging translational moments at the wire-bone interface. A washer at the olive wire–bone interface distributes the load to prevent erosion of the olive into the bone.

Mobility of the Nonunion. A nonunion may be described as stiff or lax, based on the results of manual stress testing. A stiff nonunion has an arc of mobility of 7 degrees or less, whereas a lax nonunion has an arc greater than 7 degrees.[122,127]

Stiff hypertrophic nonunions may be treated using gradual compression, distraction, or sequential monofocal compression-distraction. Lax hypertrophic and oligotrophic

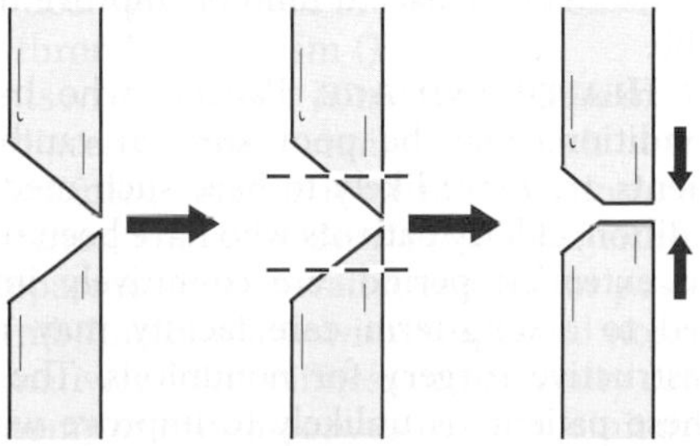

Figure 25-45. Trimming of the ends of the bone at a nonunion site may be used to improve the surface area for bony contact.

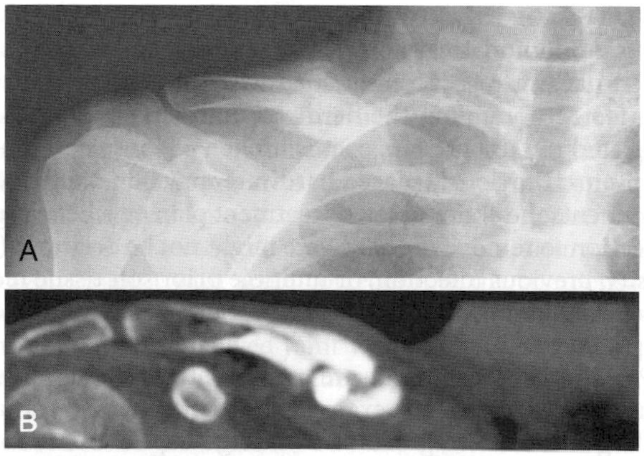

Figure 25-47. A, Anterior-posterior (AP) radiograph of a 17-year-old young man who presented 6 months following a clavicle fracture. He had been told by his prior treating physician that his clavicle was solidly healed. He had no complaints of pain. He was brought in by his mother who was concerned about the bump on his collarbone. **B,** Computed tomography (CT) scan confirms the diagnosis of nonunion.

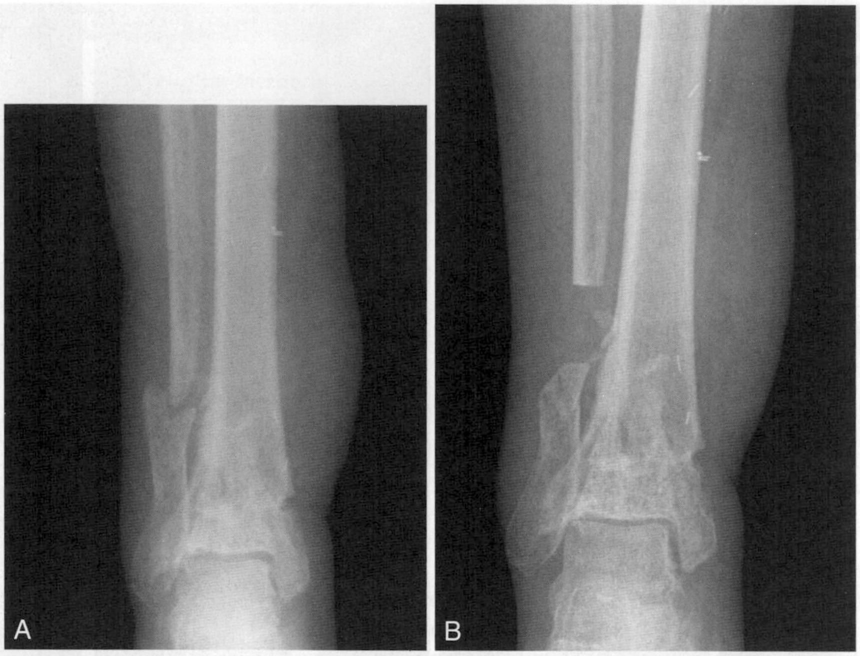

Figure 25-60. A, Presenting radiograph of a 70-year-old man who was referred in 28 months following a high-energy pilon fracture. The patient's primary complaint was pain over the fibula nonunion. Injection in this area with local anesthetic resulted in complete relief of the patient's pain. **B,** Final radiograph following treatment of the fibula nonunion via partial excision. The procedure resulted in complete pain relief.

shortening[151] and it results in rotational instability, although some intramedullary nails have oblong interlocking screw holes that prevent rotational instability (see Fig. 25-59). The technique may be useful for hypertrophic and oligotrophic nonunions of the lower extremity. Atrophic nonunions, infected nonunions, and synovial pseudarthrosis are best treated using other methods.

Dynamization of an external fixator involves removal, loosening, or exchange of the external struts spanning the nonunion. The method is most effective for lower extremity cases and is commonly used only after bony incorporation at the nonunion site is believed to be under way. Dynamizing an external fixator is therapeutic because axial loading at the nonunion site promotes further bony union. It is also diagnostic because an increase in pain at the nonunion site following dynamization suggests motion, indicating that bony union has not progressed to the extent presumed.

Excision of Bone. Excision of bone in the treatment of a nonunion falls into three distinct methods. The first method involves excision of one or more bone fragments to alleviate pain associated with the rubbing of the fragments at the nonunion site. Injection of local anesthetic into the nonunion site may suggest the extent of pain relief anticipated following bone excision (Fig. 25-60). Excision of bone will alleviate pain without impairing function at the fibula shaft[152] (assuming the syndesmotic tissues are competent) and the ulna styloid. Partial excision of ununited fragments of the olecranon and patella may be indicated in certain cases. Partial excision of the clavicle as a treatment for nonunion has been reported by Middleton and colleagues[153] and Patel and Adenwalla,[154] although we do not advocate this treatment option.

In the second method, excision of bone is performed on an intact bone to allow for compression across an ununited bone in limbs with paired bones. Most commonly, partial excision of the fibula allows compression across an ununited tibia in conjunction with external fixation or intramedullary nail fixation (Fig. 25-61).

The third method of bone excision is trimming and débridement to improve the surface characteristics (surface area, bone contact, and bone quality) at the nonunion site. This technique may be used for atrophic and infected nonunions and synovial pseudarthroses.

Screws. Interfragmentary lag screw fixation is effective for epiphyseal nonunions (see Fig. 25-28), patella nonunions[155] (Fig. 25-62), and olecranon nonunions.[156] Interfragmentary lag screw fixation may also be used with other forms of internal or external fixation for metaphyseal nonunions. Screw fixation alone is not recommended for nonunions of the metaphysis or diaphysis.

Cables and Wires. Cables or a cable-plates system can be used to stabilize a periprosthetic bone fragment that contains an intramedullary implant, thus eliminating the need for implants traversing the occupied medullary canal. This type of reconstruction is commonly performed with autogenous cancellous bone grafting, either with or without structural allograft bone struts (Fig. 25-63).

Tension band and cerclage wire techniques may also be used to treat nonunions of the olecranon and patella,[155] although we prefer more rigid fixation techniques.

Plate-and-Screw Fixation. The modern era of nonunion management with internal fixation can be traced to the establishment of the Swiss Arbeitsgemeinschaft für Osteosynthesefragen (AO) by Müller, Allgöwer, Willenegger, and Schneider in 1958. Building from the foundation of the pioneers that preceded them[113,157-164] and using the metallurgic skills of Swiss industries and a research institute in Davos, the AO Group developed a system of implants and instruments

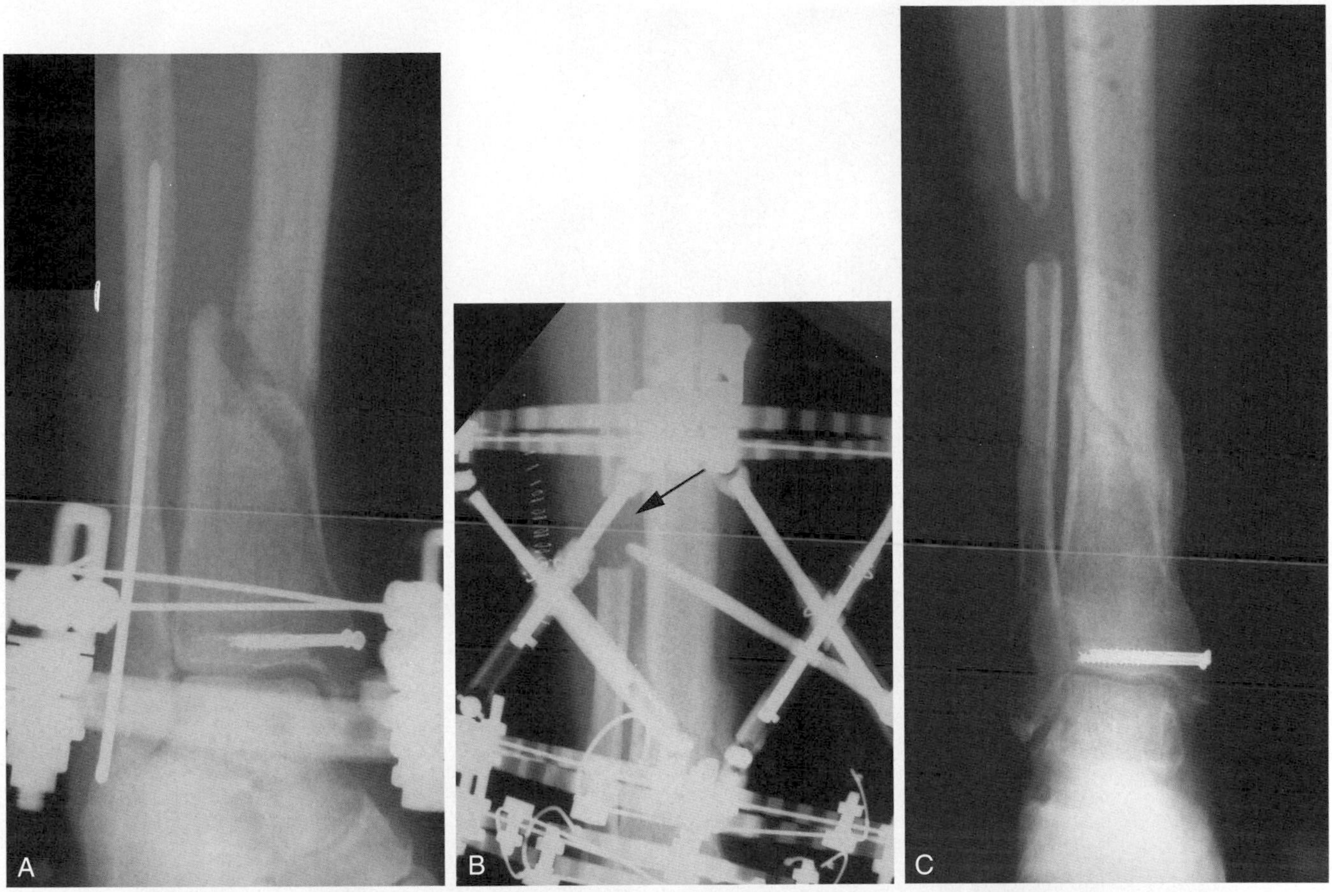

Figure 25-61. A, Presenting radiograph of a 42-year-old man who was referred in 5 months following a distal tibia fracture. **B,** The patient was treated with deformity correction and slow gradual compression using an Ilizarov external fixator. This required partial excision of the fibula *(arrow)*. **C,** Final radiographic result.

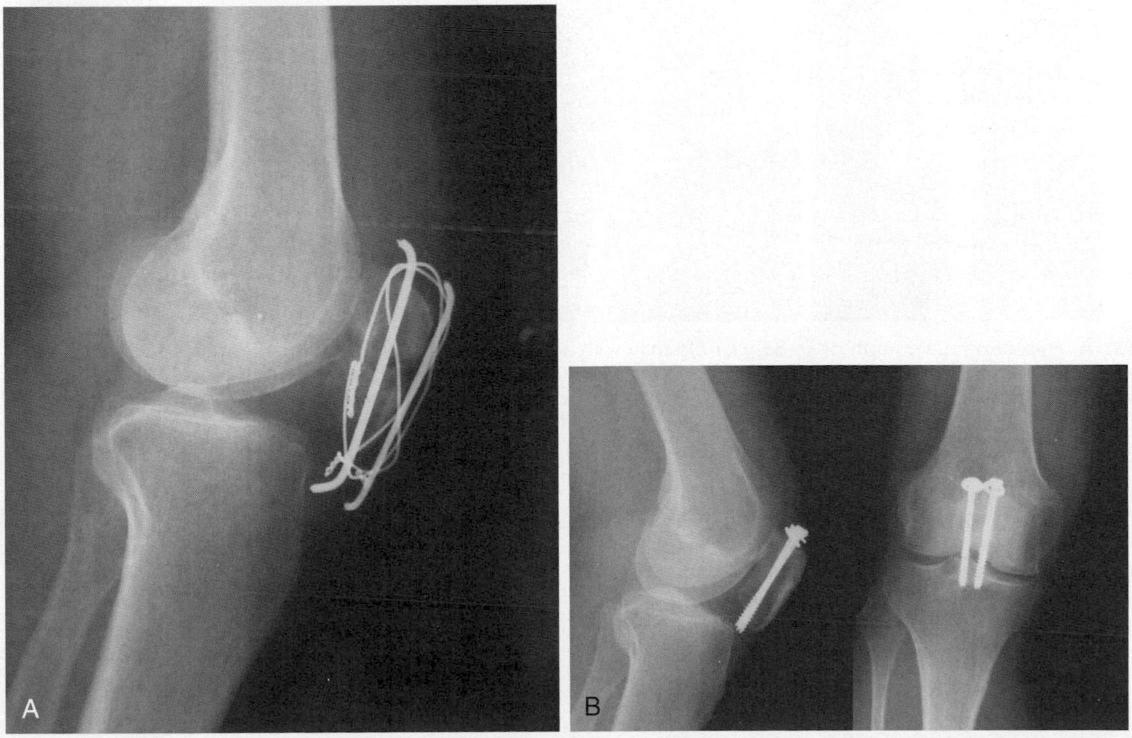

Figure 25-62. A, Presenting radiograph of a 55-year-old woman who was referred in with a patella nonunion having had four prior failed reconstructions. The patient was treated with open reduction and interfragmentary lag screw fixation. **B,** Final radiographic result shows solid bony union.

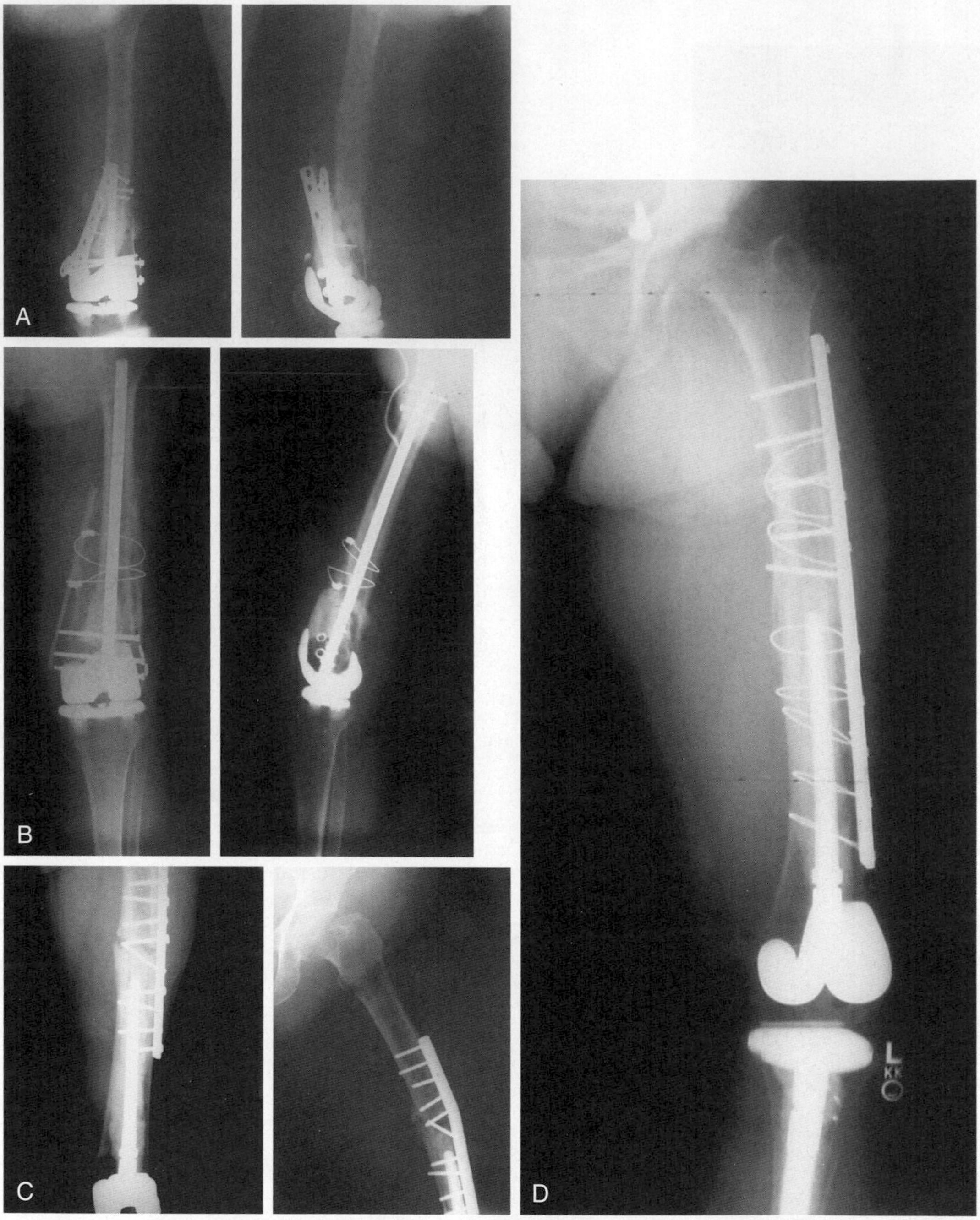

Figure 25-63. **A,** Presenting radiograph of an 83-year-old man with a periprosthetic fracture nonunion of the femur. The patient was treated with intramedullary nail stabilization with allograft strut bone graft with circumferential cable fixation. **B,** Final radiographic result shows solid bony union and incorporation of the allograft struts. **C,** Presenting radiographs of an 80-year-old woman who was referred in having failed multiple attempts at surgical reconstruction of a periprosthetic femoral nonunion. The patient was treated with plate stabilization with allograft strut bone graft with circumferential cable fixation. **D,** Final radiograph shows solid bony union.

still in use today and the most widely used modern concepts of nonunion treatment (Table 25-10).

Advantages of plate-and-screw fixation include rigidity of fixation; versatility for various anatomic locations (Fig. 25-64) (e.g., periarticular and intraarticular nonunions) and situations (e.g., periprosthetic nonunions); correction of angular, rotational, and translational deformities under direct visualization; and safety following failed or temporary external fixation. Disadvantages of the method include extensive soft tissue dissection; limitation of early weight-bearing for lower extremity applications; and inability to correct significant

TABLE 25-10 *AO CONCEPTS FOR NONUNION TREATMENT*
1. Stable internal fixation under compression
2. Decortication
3. Bone grafting in nonunions associated with gaps or poor vascularity
4. Leaving the nonunion tissue undisturbed for hypertrophic nonunions
5. Early return to function

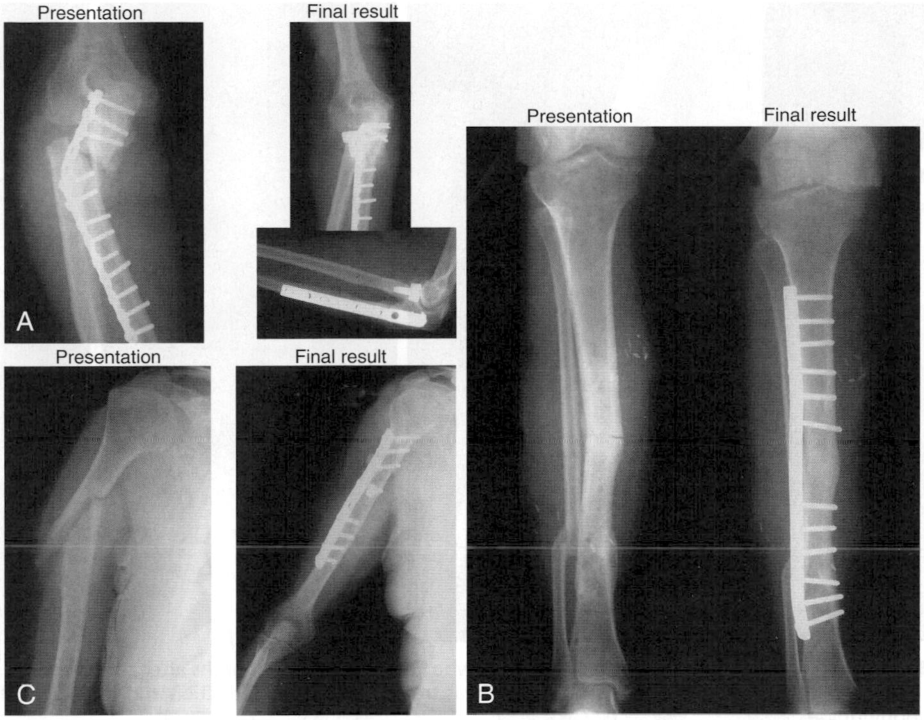

Figure 25-64. A, Presenting and final radiograph of a proximal ulna nonunion in a 60-year-old man referred in having failed three prior attempts at reconstruction. Blade plate fixation provided absolute rigid stabilization and in conjunction with autogenous bone grafting led to rapid bony union. **B,** Presenting and final radiograph of a tibial shaft nonunion that had failed treatment with an external fixator. Plate-and-screw fixation with autogenous bone grafting led to successful bony union. **C,** Presenting and final radiograph of a humeral shaft fracture that had failed nonoperative treatment and had gone on to nonunion. Plate-and-screw fixation with autogenous bone grafting led to successful bony union.

foreshortening from bone loss. Plate-and-screw fixation is applicable for all types of nonunions. In cases with large segmental defects, other methods of skeletal stabilization should be considered.

Many reports have documented success using plate-and-screw fixation for nonunions of the intertrochanteric femoral region,[165] femur,[166-168] proximal tibia,[169-171] tibial diaphysis,[172,173] distal tibial metaphysis,[174,175] fibula,[176] clavicle,[177-182] scapula,[183-185] proximal humerus,[186,187] humeral shaft,[93,188-191] distal humerus,[192-197] olecranon,[198] proximal ulna,[199] ulnar and radial diaphysis,[141] and distal radius.[200,201]

Locking plates use screws with threaded heads that lock into threaded screw holes on the corresponding plate. The locking of the screws creates a fixed-angle device, or "single-beam" construct, because no motion is allowed between the screws and the plate (Fig. 25-65).[202-204] The locked screws resist bending moments and, thus, resist progressive deformity during bony healing. A locking plate construct distributes axial load across all of the screw-bone interfaces, in contrast to traditional plate-and-screw constructs in which axial load is distributed unevenly across the screws.[203,204]

The bone fragments must be reduced prior to locking the locking plate, although newer designs include various adjunctive devices to assist in fracture reduction.[202,204] Care must also be taken to avoid leaving gaps at the nonunion site because the rigidity of the construct will maintain distraction.[204] Locking plates are considerably more expensive than traditional plates, and they should therefore be reserved for use in cases that are not amenable to traditional plate-and-screw fixation.[202]

The use of locking plates has been reported to be successful in the treatment of nonunions of the clavicle,[205] humerus,[206,207] femur,[208] and distal femur,[168] as well as in the treatment of periprosthetic femoral nonunions.[209]

Intramedullary Nail Fixation. Intramedullary nailing provides excellent mechanical stability to a fracture nonunion of a long bone previously treated by another method. Removal of a previously placed nail followed by placement of a new nail is exchange nailing, a distinctly different technique discussed later.

Intramedullary nail fixation is particularly useful for lower extremity nonunions because of the strength and load-sharing characteristics of intramedullary nails. Intramedullary implants are an excellent treatment option for osteopenic bone where purchase may be poor.

Intramedullary nail fixation as a treatment for nonunion is commonly combined with a biological method, such as open bone grafting, intramedullary bone grafting, or intramedullary reaming to stimulate biological activity at the nonunion site.

Hypertrophic, oligotrophic, and atrophic nonunions and synovial pseudarthroses may be treated with intramedullary nailing. Intramedullary nailing in cases with active infection has been reported,[210-213] but remains controversial. Because of the potential risk of seeding the medullary canal, and because safer options exist, we and others[214] generally recommend against intramedullary nailing in cases of active or prior deep infection.

Differing opinions also exist regarding intramedullary nailing in patients who have previously been treated with

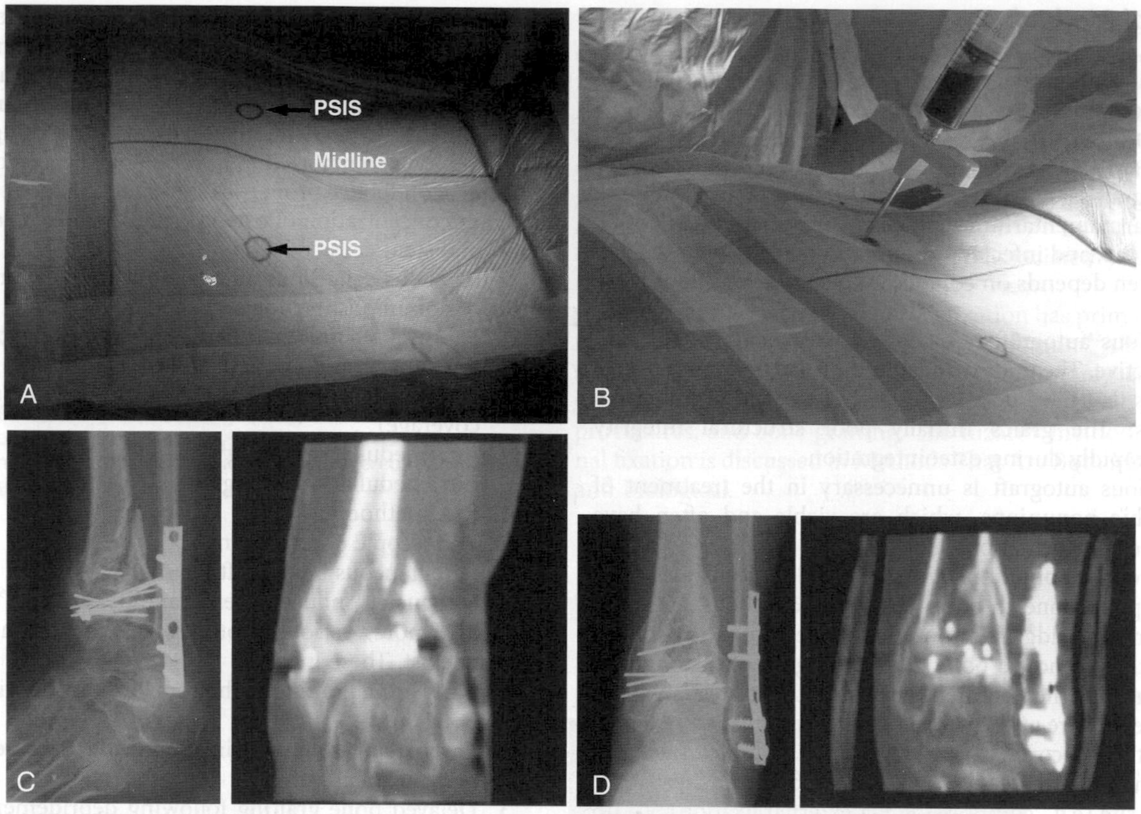

Figure 25-70. **A,** Clinical photograph showing the bony landmarks for harvesting bone marrow from the posterior iliac crest. *PSIS,* Posterior superior iliac spine. The patient has been positioned prone. **B,** Marrow being harvesting in 4-cc aliquots. **C,** Presenting radiograph and computed tomography (CT) scan of a 39-year-old woman referred in with a stable oligotrophic distal tibial nonunion. **D,** Radiograph and CT scan 4 months following percutaneous marrow injection shows solid bony union.

crest using a trochar needle.[126] We prefer the posterior iliac crest, an 11-gauge, 4-inch Lee-Lok needle (Lee Medical Ltd., Minneapolis, MN), and a 20-cc heparinized syringe (Fig. 25-70). Small aliquots are harvested to increase the concentration of osteoblast progenitor cells in each.[269] We harvest marrow in 4-cc aliquots, changing the position of the trochar needle in the posterior iliac crest between aspirations. Depending on the size and location of the nonunion site, we harvest 40 to 80 cc of marrow. Marrow is injected percutaneously into the nonunion site under fluoroscopic image using an 18-gauge spinal needle. The technique is minimally invasive, has low morbidity, and can be performed on an outpatient basis.[126] The technique works well for nonunions with small defects (<5 mm) that have excellent mechanical stability (see Fig. 25-70). Percutaneous marrow injection also enhances healing at the docking site in Ilizarov bone transport.

BONE GRAFT SUBSTITUTES. Bone graft substitutes, such as calcium phosphate, calcium sulfate, hydroxyapatite, and other calcium-based ceramics, may have a future role in the treatment of nonunions. Some of these materials may be impregnated with antibiotic and used to treat infected nonunions.[140,270] Some may be combined with autogenous bone graft to expand the volume of graft material.[271,272] To date, the efficiency and indications for these substitutes in the treatment of nonunions remains unclear.

GROWTH FACTORS. Ongoing research in the area of growth factors holds promise for advancement in the treatment of fracture nonunions.[273-278] This area is discussed in Chapter 4, Biology and Enhancement of Skeletal Repair.

DECORTICATION. Shingling[163,164,279] (Fig. 25-71) entails the raising of osteoperiosteal fragments from the outer cortex or callus from both sides of the nonunion using a sharp osteotome or chisel. Using an osteotome, thin (2 to 3 mm) fragments each measuring approximately 2 cm in length are elevated. The resulting decorticated region measures 3 to 4 cm in length on either side of the nonunion and involves approximately two-thirds of the bone circumference. The periosteum and muscle, which remain attached and viable, are then

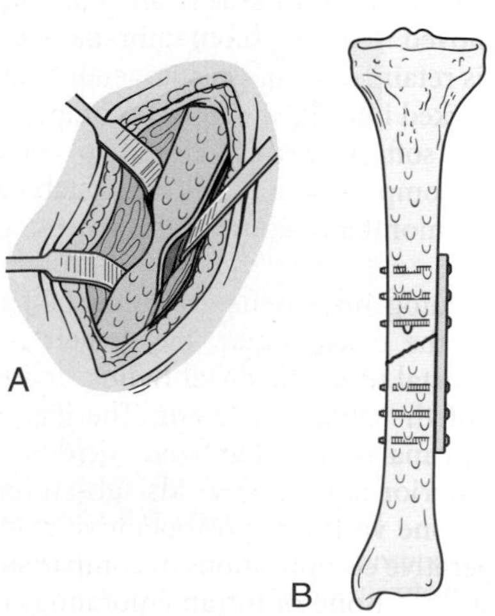

Figure 25-71. Decortication techniques. **A,** Shingling. **B,** Fishscaling (petaling).

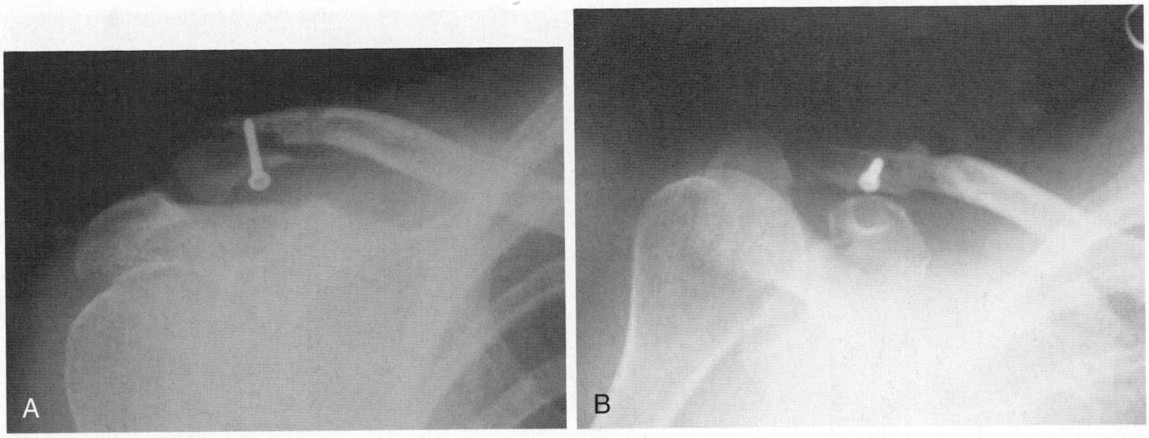

Figure 25-72. A, Presenting radiograph of a 40-year-old woman referred in 26 months following open reduction and internal fixation of a distal clavicle fracture. This patient did not wish any type of surgical intervention and, therefore, was treated with external electrical stimulation. **B,** Radiograph following 8 months of electrical stimulation shows solid bony union.

retracted with a Hohmann retractor. This increases the surface area between the elevated shingles and the decorticated cortex into which cancellous bone graft can be inserted.

If the bone is osteoporotic, shingling may weaken the thin cortex and should therefore be avoided. In addition, shingling should not be performed over the area of the bone fragments where a plate is to be applied. Petaling[280] or "fishscaling" (see Fig. 25-69) is performed with a tiny gouge. Once elevated, the osteoperiosteal flakes or petals resemble the petals of a flower or scales of a fish. Alternatively, a small drill bit cooled with irrigation can be used to drill multiple holes. Petaling or drilling is performed over a region 3 to 4 cm on either side of the nonunion. These techniques promote revascularization of the cortex, especially when combined with cancellous bone grafting.

Electromagnetic, Ultrasound, and Shock-Wave Stimulation. Electrical stimulation of nonunions by invasive and noninvasive methods has gained popularity since the 1970s[281-283] (Fig. 25-72). Devices available to treat nonunions via electrical stimulation are of three varieties: constant direct-current, time-varying inductive coupling (including pulsed electromagnetic fields), and capacitive coupling.[284-287] Direct current lowers the partial pressure of oxygen and increases proteoglycan and collagen synthesis.[287] Time-varying inductive coupling affects the synthesis and function of growth factors and other cytokines, particularly transforming growth factor-β (TGF-β), that modulate chondrocytes and osteoblasts.[285,287] Pulsed electromagnetic fields also induce messenger RNA (mRNA) expression of BMPs, producing an osteoinductive effect.[285] Capacitive coupling induces a bone cell proliferation that is thought to be related to the activation of voltage-gated calcium channels increasing prostaglandin E_2, cytosolic calcium, and calmodulin.[287]

Electrical stimulation does not correct deformities and usually requires 3 to 9 months of non-weight-bearing and cast immobilization, which may give rise to muscle and bone atrophy and joint stiffness. Electrical stimulation may be used to treat stiff nonunions without significant deformity or bone defect. The method is seldom effective for atrophic nonunions, infected nonunions, synovial pseudarthroses, nonunions with gaps of more than 1 cm, or lax nonunions.[287]

Ultrasound stimulates bone healing by affecting potassium ions, calcium incorporation in differentiating cartilage and bone cells, adenylate cyclase activity, and the activation of various cytokines.[287-289] Ultrasound therapy has been an Food and Drug Administration (FDA)-approved treatment for fracture healing since 1994, and the FDA-approved ultrasound for treatment of nonunions in February 2000.[287] Several studies of ultrasound therapy in the treatment of nonunion have reported bony union rates ranging from 85% to 91%.[288,290,291] Ultrasound may be used to treat stiff atrophic, oligotrophic, or hypertrophic nonunions that have no significant deformity.[289] Ultrasound is inappropriate for infected nonunions, nonunions with a large segmental defect, or lax nonunions.

High-energy extracorporeal shock wave therapy for nonunions has been reported by a number of investigators, with union rates exceeding 75%.[292-295] The technique may be more effective in pseudarthroses or nonunions showing uptake on technetium bone scan.[296] Atrophic nonunions may show no signs of healing until more than 6 months after the initial shock wave application.[295] It should not be used when the gap at the nonunion site is greater than 5 mm; when open physes, alveolar tissue, brain or spine, or malignant tumor are in the shock-wave field; or in patients with coagulopathy or pregnancy.[293]

Methods That Are Both Mechanical and Biological

Structural Bone Grafts. Several types of structural bone grafts are available, each with specific advantages and disadvantages (Table 25-11).

Vascularized autogenous cortical bone grafts provide structural integrity and living osseous tissue to the site of bony defects. Some vascularized grafts respond to functional loading via hypertrophy,[297,298] thus increasing in strength over time. Vascularized bone grafts may be obtained from several sites,[299-305] but the vascularized fibula is currently preferred because of its shape, strength, size, and versatility.[306-310]

Nonvascularized autogenous cortical bone grafts provide structural integrity using the patient's own tissue at the site of bony defects.

Bulk cortical allograft may be used to reconstruct large posttraumatic skeletal defects[311] (see Figs. 21-66 and 21-72).

TABLE 25-11 TYPES OF STRUCTURAL BONE GRAFTS

Type of Bone Graft	Potential Harvest Sites	Advantages	Disadvantages
Vascularized autogenous cortical bone graft	Fibula Iliac crest Ribs	• Immediate structural integrity • One-stage procedure • Potential for graft hypertrophy • Ability to span massive segmental defects	• Technically demanding • Propensity for fracture fatigue, particularly in lower extremity applications • Prolonged non–weight-bearing • Poorer results in patients with a history of infection[370] • Donor site morbidity: pain, neurovascular injury, joint instability or limited motion • Fixation problems when the defect is periarticular • Contraindicated for children
Nonvascularized autogenous cortical bone graft	Fibula Tibia Iliac crest	• Can be used to reconstruct large defects	• Prolonged non–weight-bearing • Prolonged support required in upper extremity applications • Donor site morbidity, including fracture for grafts from the tibia • Graft weakening during revascularization (years) • Propensity for fatigue fracture
Bulk cortical allograft	Virtually unlimited	• Less technically demanding than vascularized grafts • No donor site morbidity • Can be used in four ways: intercalary, alloarthrodesis, osteoarticular, or alloprosthesis	• Infection • Fatigue fracture • Nonunion at the host-graft junction • Disease transmission from donor to recipient
Strut cortical allograft	Virtually unlimited	• Versatility; may be used to treat partial (incomplete) segmental defects, complete segmental defects, augment fixation and stability in osteopenic bone, and augment stability in periprosthetic nonunions	• Infection • Fatigue fracture • Nonunion at the host-graft junction • Disease transmission from donor to recipient
Intramedullary cortical allograft	Virtually unlimited	• Used in long bone nonunions with osteopenia • Augments stability by acting like an intramedullary nail • Improves screw purchase: screws each traverse four cortices • Provides potential for intramedullary healing between host bone and allograft	• Infection • Fatigue fracture • Nonunion at the host-graft junction • Disease transmission from donor to recipient

Bone of virtually every shape and size is available from the bone bank, permitting reconstruction in most anatomic locations. Graft fixation may be achieved using a variety of methods. We prefer intramedullary fixation when possible because of its ultimate strength, load-sharing characteristics, and protection of the graft. Bulk allografts can be used in four ways: intercalary, alloarthrodesis (Fig. 25-73), osteoarticular, and alloprosthesis.

Infected nonunions may be treated with bulk allograft after the infected cavity has been debrided and sterilized. For infected nonunions with massive defects, we perform serial débridement with antibiotic bead exchanges until the cavity is culture negative. A custom-fabricated antibiotic-impregnated PMMA spacer is then implanted, and the soft tissue envelope is closed or reconstructed. At a minimum of 3 months, the spacer is removed and the defect is reconstructed using bulk cortical allograft (Fig. 25-74; see Fig. 21-66). Active infection is an absolute contraindication to bulk cortical allograft.

Strut cortical allografts may be used to reconstruct partial (incomplete) segmental defects, reconstruct complete segmental defects in certain cases, augment fixation and stability in osteopenic bone,[312] and augment stability in periprosthetic nonunions (see Fig. 25-63).

Intramedullary cortical allografts are typically used for long bone nonunions associated with osteopenia where the method of treatment is plate-and-screw fixation with cancellous autografting. The technique is particularly useful for humeral nonunions in elderly patients with osteopenic bone who have failed multiple prior treatments (Fig. 25-75).

MESH CAGE BONE GRAFT CONSTRUCTS. Mesh cage bone graft constructs may be used for treating segmental long bone defects.[313] The defect is spanned using a titanium mesh cage (DePuy Motech, Warsaw, IN) of slightly larger diameter than the bone. The cage is packed with allogeneic cancellous bone chips and DBM. This construct is reinforced by an intramedullary nail traversing the mesh cage bone graft construct.

EXCHANGE NAILING. Exchange nailing is a treatment method that is both mechanical and biological, which distinguishes it from intramedullary nailing, a purely mechanical method.[314]

TECHNIQUE. By definition, exchange nailing requires the removal of a previously placed intramedullary nail. With a nail

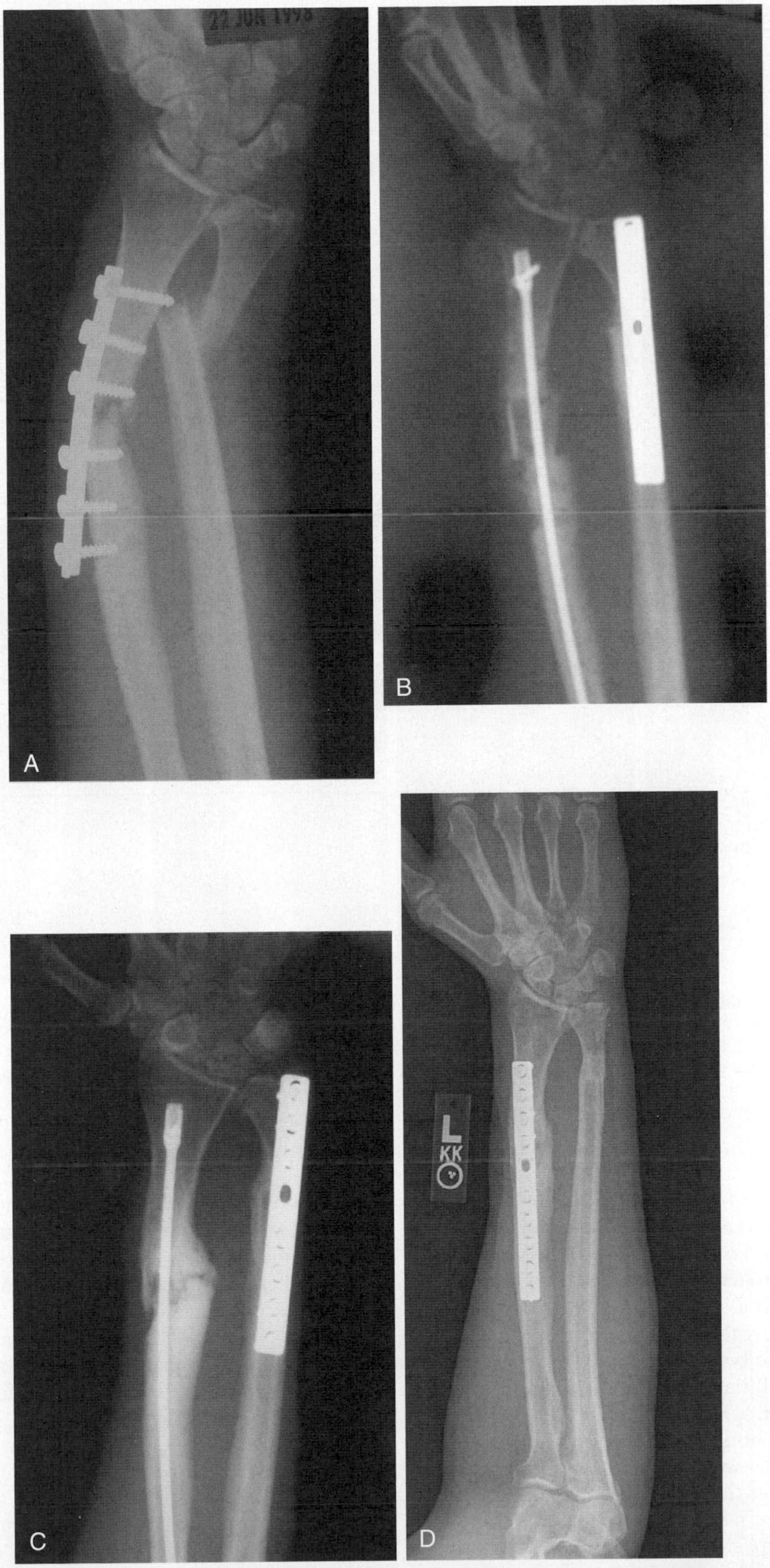

Figure 25-73. A, Presenting radiograph of a 45-year-old man referred in 7 months following open reduction and internal fixation of a both-bone forearm fracture. This patient had an open wound draining purulent material over the radius. The patient was treated with serial débridements and antibiotic beads. Following serial débridements, the patient was left with a segmental defect of the radius. **B,** Radiograph following placement of a bulk cortical allograft over an intramedullary nail and plate-and-screw fixation of the ulna. **C,** Follow-up radiograph at 11 months following reconstruction shows solid union of the proximal host-graft junction but a hypertrophic nonunion of the distal host-graft junction of the radius. The hypertrophic nonunion was treated with compression plating (without bone grafting). **D,** Final radiograph 14 months following compression plating shows solid bony union.

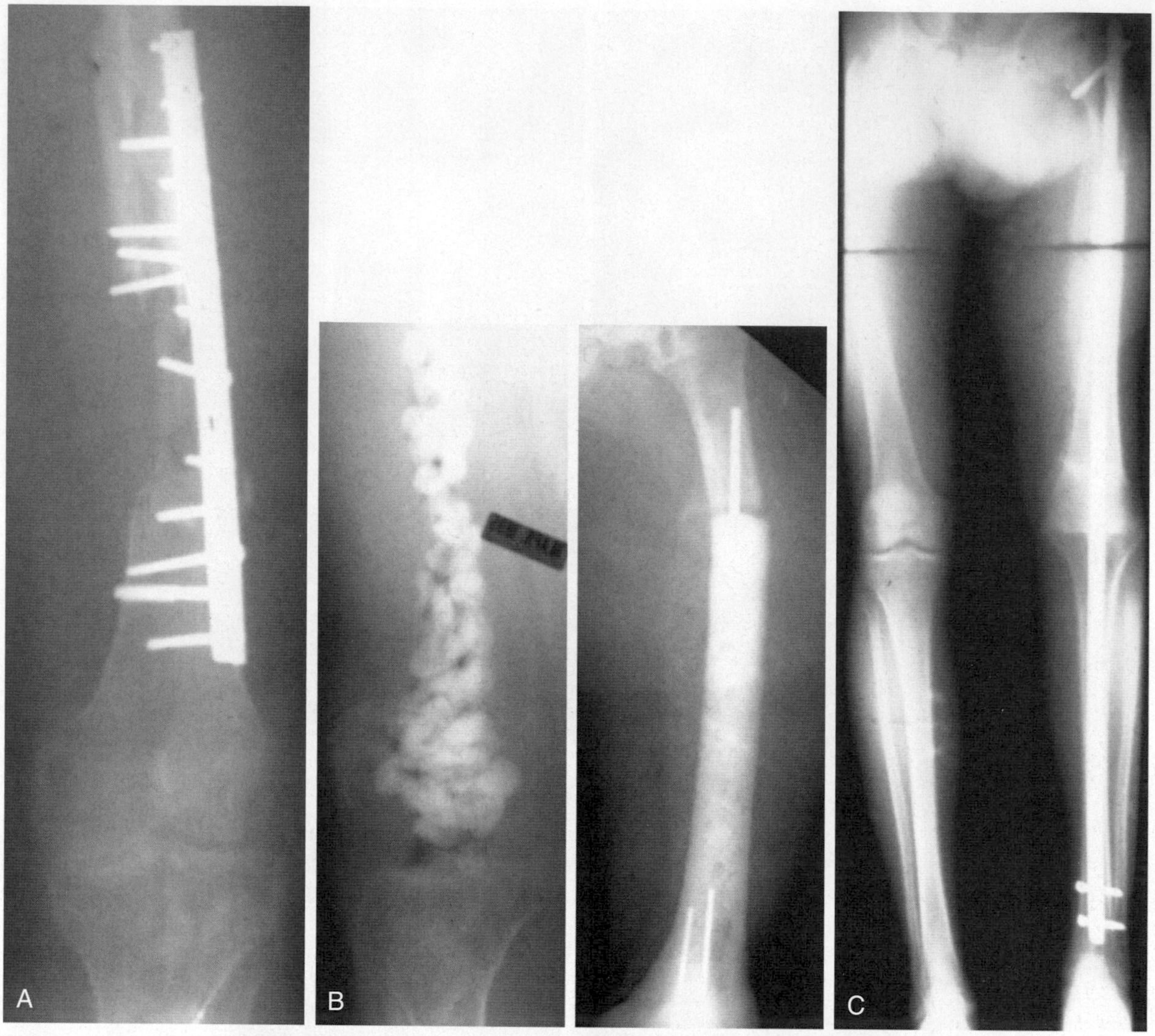

Figure 25-74. A, Presenting radiograph of a 25-year-old man treated with open reduction and internal fixation of an open femur fracture. The patient was referred in 16 months following the injury. Clinical examination revealed gross purulence and exposed bone at the nonunion site with global knee joint instability and an arc of knee flexion/extension of approximately 20 degrees. Aspiration of the knee yielded frank pus. **B,** Radiographs following radical débridement with placement of antibiotic beads and later an antibiotic spacer. **C,** Follow-up radiograph 6 years following alloarthrodesis using a bulk cortical allograft and a knee fusion nail shows solid bony incorporation. The patient is fully ambulatory without pain and has no evidence of infection.

already spanning the nonunion site, the problem of a sealed-off medullary canal is not an issue. Additionally, the medullary canal is already known to accept passage of an intramedullary nail, unless the nail has broken and there has been progressive deformity over time. Such a case may require extensive bony and soft tissue dissection at the nonunion site, so other treatment options may need to be considered.

Once the previous nail has been removed, the medullary canal is reamed with progressively larger reamer tips in 0.5-mm increments until bone is observed in the flutes of the reamers. As a general rule, we use an exchange nail that is 2 to 4 mm in diameter larger than the prior nail and over-ream 1 mm larger than the new nail. Reaming, therefore, typically proceeds to a reamer tip size 3 to 5 mm larger than the removed nail.

Following reaming, the larger diameter nail is inserted. We prefer to use a closed technique to preserve the periosteal blood supply and lessen the risk of infection. Provided that good bony contact exists at the nonunion site, we statically lock exchange nails, although many authors do not.[15,34,145,226,315] In most instances, we do not favor partial excision of the fibula with exchange nailing of the tibia because it diminishes stability of the construct.

Modes of Healing. Exchange nailing stimulates healing of nonunions by improving the local mechanical environment in two ways and by improving the local biological environment in two ways (Fig. 25-76).

The first mechanical benefit is that reaming to enlarge the medullary canal allows a larger diameter nail, which is stronger and stiffer and augments stability to promote bony union. The second mechanical benefit is that reaming widens and lengthens the isthmal portion of the medullary canal, which increases the endosteal cortical contact area of the nail.

The first biological benefit is that the reaming products act as local bone graft at the nonunion site to stimulate medullary healing. The second biological benefit is that medullary

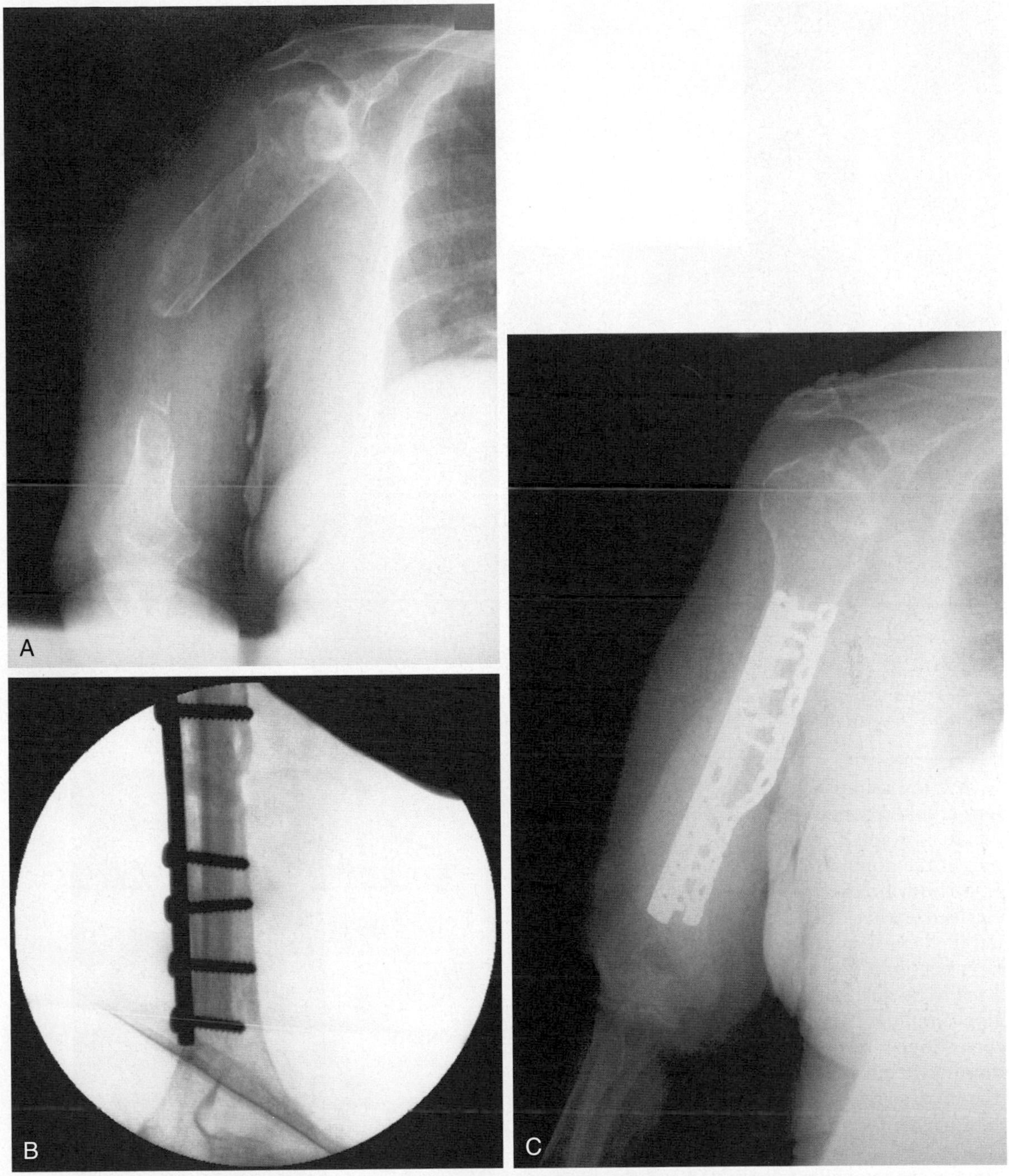

Figure 25-75. **A,** Presenting radiograph of an 83-year-old woman referred in 15 months following a humeral shaft fracture. The patient found this humeral nonunion very painful and quite debilitating. Because of the patient's profound osteopenia, she was treated with an intramedullary cortical fibular allograft and plate-and-screw fixation. **B,** Intraoperative fluoroscopic image showing positioning of the intramedullary fibula. **C,** Final radiograph 7 months following reconstruction shows bony incorporation without evidence of hardware loosening or failure. At follow-up, the patient was without pain, and had marked improvement in function.

reaming results in a substantial decrease in endosteal blood flow,[316-320] which stimulates a dramatic increase in both periosteal flow[321] and periosteal new bone formation.[322]

These mechanical and biological effects of exchange nailing make it applicable for both viable and nonviable nonunions.

Other Issues

Bone Contact. Exchange nailing is excellent when good bone-to-bone contact is present, but not when large partial or complete segmental bone defects exist. Because healing of nonunions with defects depends on many factors, it is difficult to determine which defects will unite with exchange nailing. Templeman and coauthors[315] advocate exchange nailing in the tibia when there is 30% or less circumferential bone loss. Court-Brown and coauthors[15] reported failures for exchange nailing in tibial nonunions when bone loss exceeded 2 cm in length and involved more than 50% circumferential bone loss. We have used intramedullary bone grafting[220] with excellent results during exchange nailing of long bones with defects, although the indications for this technique for nonunions are still evolving.

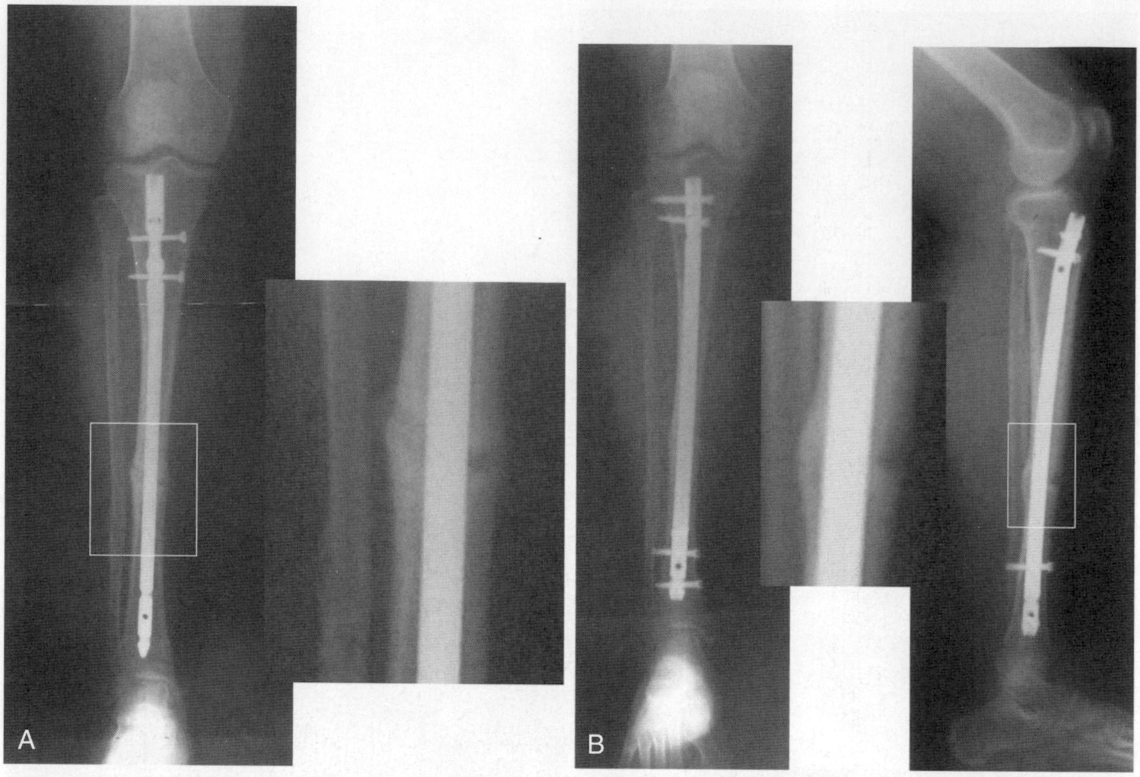

Figure 25-76. A, Presenting radiograph of a 51-year-old woman referred in 29 months following intramedullary nail fixation of an open tibia fracture. **B,** Five months following exchange nailing the tibia is solidly united.

Deformity. We are astonished by how a straight nail can result in a very crooked bone (Fig. 25-77). Deformity correction can be acute or gradual and can be performed during or after treatment of the nonunion. If deformity correction is to follow successful bony union, exchange nailing may be undertaken as described earlier. If the decision is to address the nonunion and the deformity concurrently, the deformity may be corrected either gradually or acutely. If acute deformity correction is felt to be safe, exchange nailing with acute deformity correction simplifies the overall treatment strategy. Acute deformity correction is relatively simple for lax nonunions. Stiff nonunions may require a percutaneously performed osteotomy and the intraoperative use of a femoral distractor or a temporary external fixator to achieve acute deformity correction. If the status of the soft tissues or bone favors gradual correction, then exchange nailing is rejected and the Ilizarov method is used.

Infection. Numerous authors have reported the use of intramedullary nail fixation for infected nonunions.[34,210-213,216,219] There is no consensus in the literature regarding the use of exchange nailing as a treatment for infected nonunions. For cases in which the injury has been previously treated with a method other than nailing, placement of an intramedullary nail can seed the entire medullary canal. The case of exchange nailing is entirely different. With an in situ intramedullary nail, the intramedullary canal is likely already infected, to some degree, along its entire length, and we are therefore not strictly opposed to exchange nailing of an infected nonunion (Fig. 25-78).

Exchange nailing for infected nonunions is best suited for the lower extremity in patients who are poor candidates for plate-and-screw fixation (osteopenia, multiple soft tissue

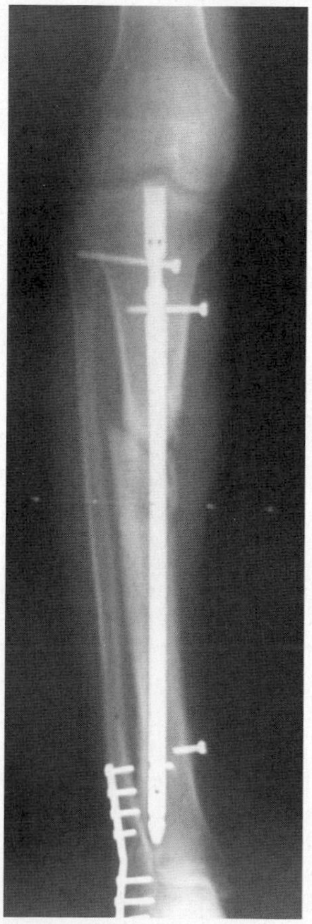

Figure 25-77. Presenting radiograph of a 22-year-old man referred in following multiple failed treatments of a tibial nonunion. Note that a very crooked bone can result despite the use of a straight nail.

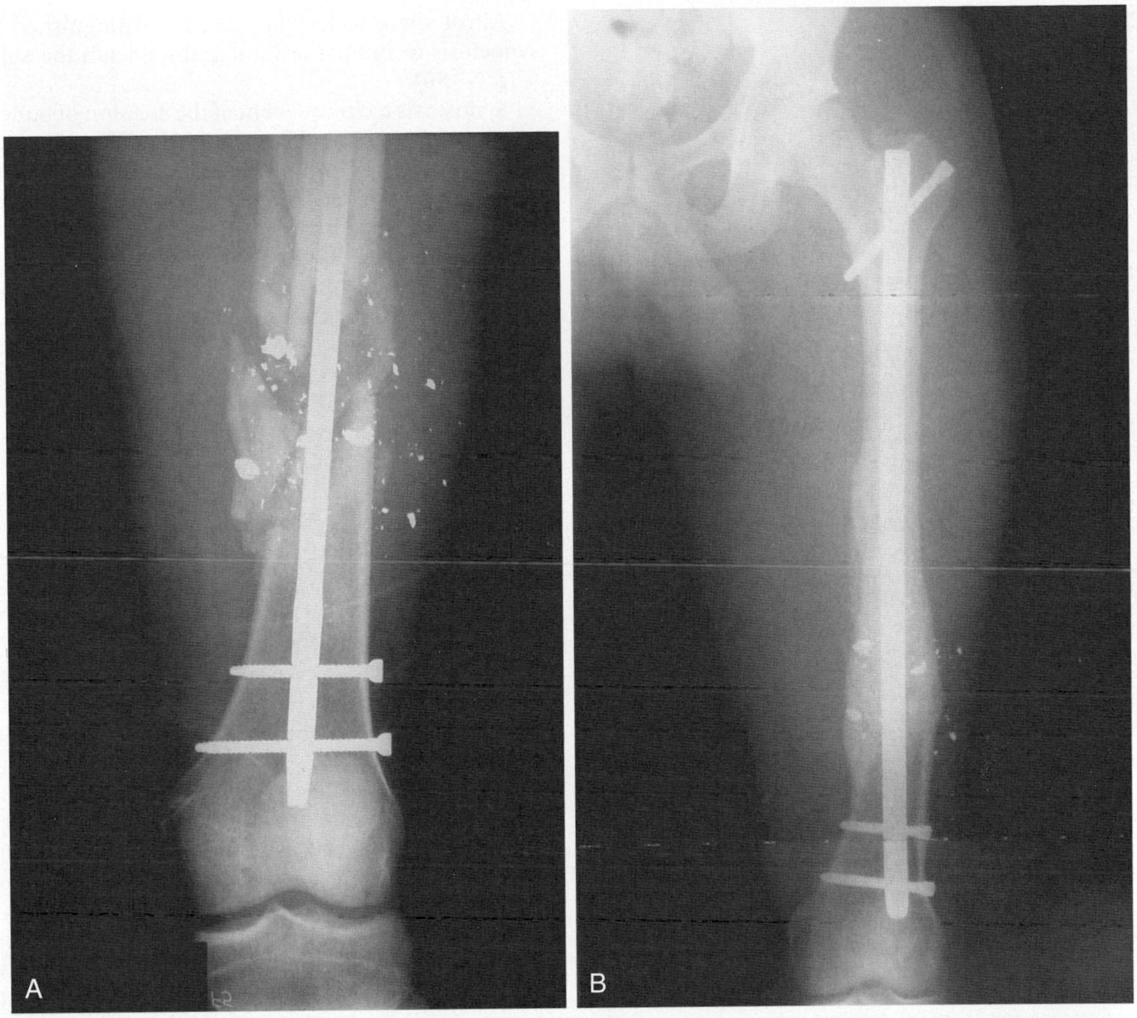

Figure 25-78. A, Radiograph of a 23-year-old man with an actively draining infected femoral nonunion resulting from a gunshot blast. This patient was treated with serial débridements followed by exchange nailing (with intramedullary autogenous iliac crest bone grafting) of the femoral nonunion. **B,** Follow-up radiograph 13 months following treatment shows solid bony healing. This patient has no clinical evidence of infection.

reconstructions, segmental nonunions) or external fixation (poor compliance or cognitive impairment), where the load-sharing characteristics of a nail may be of great benefit. When exchange nailing is used for infected nonunions, aggressive reaming of the medullary canal is a means of débridement. Reaming should use progressively larger reamer tips in 0.5-mm increments until the reamer flutes contain what appears to be viable healthy bone. All reamings should be sent for culture and sensitivity in cases of known or suspected infection. The medullary canal is irrigated with copious antibiotic solution and the larger diameter nail is placed. Serial débridement can be performed with an antibiotic-eluting nail being placed down the medullary canal at each operative session.

Literature Review for Exchange Nailing. The reported results for exchange nailing of uninfected tibial nonunions have been excellent. Court-Brown and coauthors[15] reported an 88% rate of union (29 of 33 cases) following a single exchange nailing of the tibia; the four remaining cases united following a second exchange nailing. Templeman and coauthors[315] reported a 93% rate of union (25 of 27 cases), and Wu and coauthors[323] reported a 96% rate of union (24 of 25 cases) with exchange nailing of the tibia.

The reported results for exchange nailing of femoral nonunions have been less consistent. Oh and coworkers[324] and Christensen[325] both reported a 100% union rate for aseptic femoral nonunions treated with exchange nailing, but Hak and coauthors[34] reported a union rate of 78% (18 of 23 cases), Banaszkiewicz and coauthors[326] reported a union rate of only 58% (11 of 19 cases), and Weresh and coauthors[145] reported only 53% (10 of 19 cases) united.[326] Recent technological advances allow intramedullary nailing to be used in the treatment of more comminuted and complex femoral fractures than had previously been possible. When these types of fracture go on to nonunion, they may not be appropriate for exchange nailing.[145,326]

The reported results of exchange nailing for humeral shaft nonunions are poor. McKee and coworkers[327] reported a 40% union rate (4 of 10 cases) for exchange nailing of humeral nonunions. Flinkkilä and coauthors[328] reported union in only 23% (3 of 13 cases) of humeral shaft nonunions treated with antegrade exchange nailing.

Summary. Based on the literature and our own experiences, the following comments and recommendations are offered:

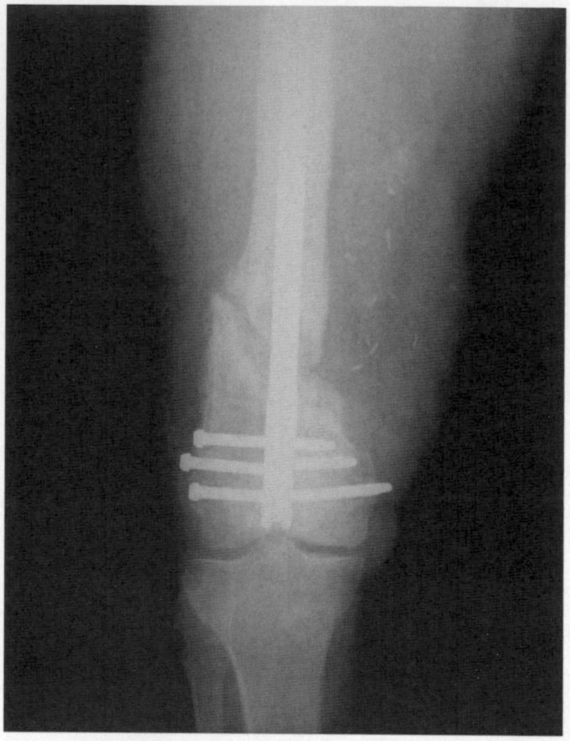

Figure 25-79. Radiograph of a 57-year-old man with a supracondylar femoral nonunion referred in having failed two prior exchange-nailing procedures. Exchange nailing is poor treatment method for nonunions in this region.

1. **Tibia**—Exchange nailing achieves healing in 90% to 95% of tibial nonunions.
2. **Femoral shaft**—Exchange nailing remains the treatment of choice for aseptic, noncomminuted nonunions of the femoral shaft, but the success rate is lower when nonunion follows intramedullary nailing of a comminuted or complex femoral shaft fracture.
3. **Supracondylar femur**—The supracondylar femur is poorly suited for stabilization of a nonunion with an intramedullary nail.[212] The medullary canal is flared in this region, resulting in poor cortical bone contact with the nail. Reaming during exchange nailing for nonunions of the supracondylar region may not increase periosteal blood flow or induce new bone formation. Other treatment methods should be utilized (Fig. 25-79).
4. **Humeral shaft**—Poor results have been reported for exchange nailing of humeral shaft nonunions.[327,328] Nail removal and plate-and-screw fixation with autogenous cancellous bone grafting is more effective. Ilizarov methods may be required for complex cases.

Synostosis Techniques. The leg and forearm benefit from structural integrity provided by paired bones, which permits the use of unique treatment methods for nonunions with bone defects. The literature regarding these methods is fraught with inconsistent and contradictory terms: fibula-pro-tibia, fibula transfer, fibula transference, fibula transposition, fibular bypass, fibulazation, medialization of the fibula, medialward bone transport of the fibula, posterolateral bone grafting, synostosis, tibialization of the fibula, transtibiofibular grafting, and vascularized fibula transposition.

All of these techniques can be distinguished as either a synostosis technique or local grafting from the adjacent bone (Fig. 25-80).

Synostosis techniques entail the creation of bone continuity between paired bones above and below the nonunion site. The bone neighboring the ununited bone unites to the proximal and distal fragments of the ununited bone such that the neighboring bone transmits forces across the nonunion site. From a functional standpoint, the limb becomes a one-bone extremity. Synostosis techniques do not necessarily rely on union of the original nonunion fragments to one another.

Many techniques have been described to create a tibiofibular synostosis for the treatment of tibial nonunions. Milch[329,330] described a tibiofibular synostosis technique for nonunion using a splintered bone created by longitudinally splitting the fibula, which could be augmented with autogenous iliac bone graft. McMaster and Hohl[331] used allograft cortical bone as tibiofibular cross-pegs to create a tibiofibular synostosis for tibial nonunion. Rijnberg and van Linge[332] described a technique to treat tibial shaft nonunions by creating a synostosis with autogenous iliac crest bone graft through a lateral approach anterior to the fibula.

Ilizarov[333] described the medialward (horizontal) bone transport of the fibula to create a tibiofibula synostosis for the treatment of tibial nonunions with massive segmental defects (see Fig. 25-80).

Weinberg and colleagues[334] described a two-stage technique for cases with massive bone loss. In the first stage, a distal tibiofibula synostosis was created; at least 1 month later, the second stage created a proximal tibiofibula synostosis.

The term "fibula-pro-tibia" sometimes describes a synostosis technique, but it is used inconsistently in the literature. Campanacci and Zanoli[335] described a fibula-pro-tibia tibiofibular synostosis technique using internal fixation to stabilize the proximal and distal tibiofibular articulations for tibial nonunions without large defects. Banic and Hertel[336] described a "double vascularized fibula" fibula-pro-tibia technique for large tibial defects in which the laterally grafted fibula with its intact blood supply creates a synostosis proximal and distal to the defect. By contrast, others[245,337] have described transference of a vascularized fibula graft into a tibial defect as a fibula-pro-tibia technique; transference does not create a synostosis. None of the techniques in the literature described as fibular transference, fibular transfer, fibular transposition, and tibialization refer to synostosis procedures.[138,297,307,338-341]

The synostosis method may also be used to treat segmental defects or persistent nonunions of the forearm (Fig. 25-81), most commonly when there is massive bone loss to both the radius and ulna.

Ilizarov Method. Ilizarov techniques for treatment of nonunions have many advantages (Table 25-12). The Ilizarov construct resists shear and rotational forces. The tensioned wires allow for the somewhat unique "trampoline effect" during weight-bearing activities. The Ilizarov method allows augmentation of the treatment as needed through frame modification. Frame modification generally is not associated with pain, does not require anesthesia, and can be performed in the office. Frame modification is not treatment failure; it is the need for continued treatment. Modifying other treatment methods, such as intramedullary nailing, requires repeat surgical intervention and is therefore considered treatment failure.

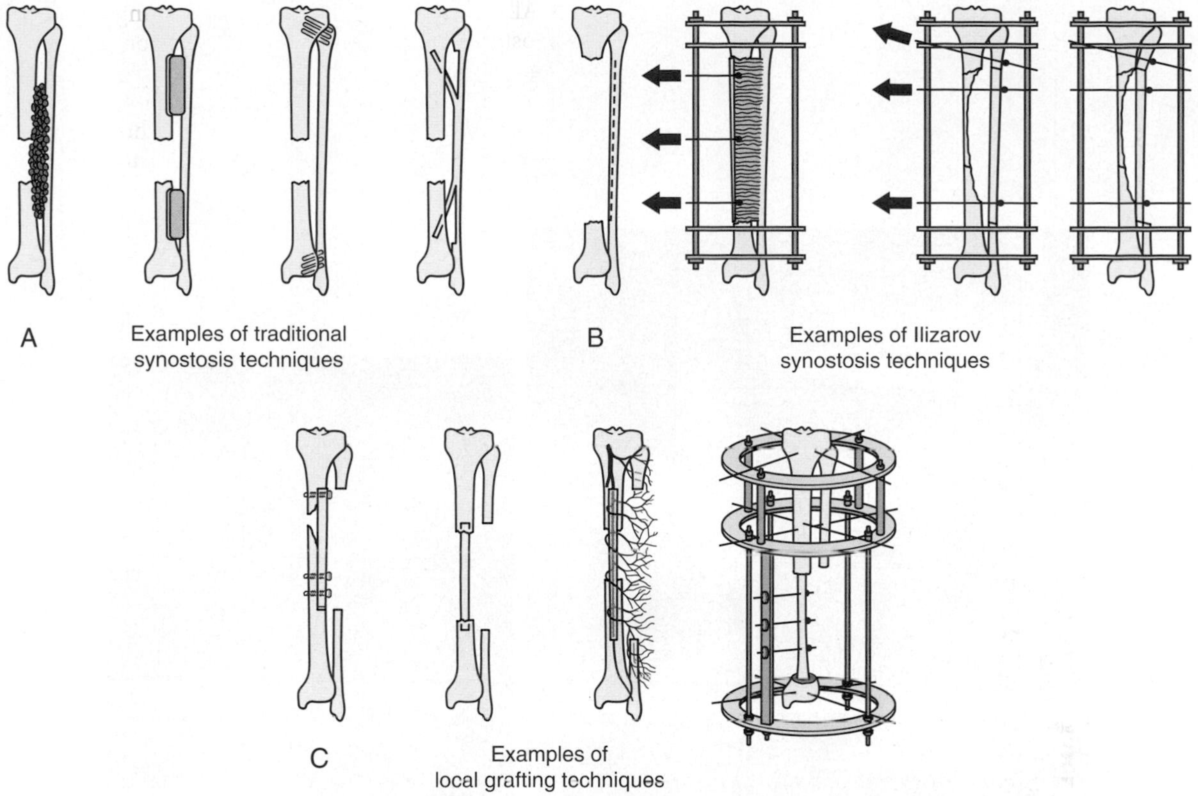

Figure 25-80. Illustration showing synostosis techniques for the tibia versus local bone grafting from the fibula.

The Ilizarov method is applicable for all types of nonunions, particularly those associated with infection, segmental bone defects, deformities, and multiple prior failed treatments. A variety of modes of treatment can be employed using the Ilizarov external fixator, including compression, distraction, lengthening, and bone transport. Monofocal treatment involves simple compression or distraction across the nonunion site. Bifocal treatment denotes that two healing sites exist, such as a bone transport where healing must occur at both the distraction site (regenerate bone formation) and the docking (nonunion) site. Trifocal treatment denotes that three healing sites exist, such as in a double-level bone transport (Table 25-13).

Compression (monofocal) osteosynthesis allows both simple compression and differential compression, which is used in deformity correction. The technique is applicable for hypertrophic nonunions (although distraction is classically used) (Fig. 25-82), oligotrophic nonunions (Figs. 25-83 to 25-85), and, according to Professor Ilizarov, synovial pseudarthroses.[122,127] Gradual compression is generally applied at a rate of 0.25 to 0.5 mm per day for a period of 2 to 4 weeks (see Figs. 25-81 and 25-82). Compression stimulates healing for most hypertrophic and oligotrophic nonunions. Compression is usually unsuccessful for infected nonunions with purulent drainage and intervening segments of necrotic bone. There is disagreement regarding compression as a treatment for atrophic nonunions.[149,342]

Slow compression over a nail using external fixation (SCONE) is a useful method for certain patients who have failed intramedullary nailing.[343-345] We have used this technique with great success in two distinct patient populations: patients who have failed multiple exchange femoral nailings (Fig. 25-86) and morbidly obese patients with distal femoral nonunions who have failed primary retrograde nail fracture fixation (Fig. 25-87).[343] The SCONE method is performed with percutaneous application of the Ilizarov external fixator. The method augments stability and allows for monofocal compression at the nonunion site once the nail is dynamized. The presence of the nail in the medullary canal encourages compressive forces while discouraging translational and shear moments.

Sequential monofocal distraction-compression has been recommended as a treatment for lax hypertrophic nonunions and atrophic nonunions. According to Paley,[149] "distraction disrupts the tissue at the nonunion site, frequently leading to some poor bone regeneration. This poor bone regeneration is stimulated to consolidate when the two bone ends are brought back together again."

Distraction is the treatment method of choice for stiff hypertrophic nonunions, particularly those with deformity (Fig. 25-88). Distraction of the abundant fibrocartilaginous tissue at the nonunion site stimulates new bone formation[149,333,346,347] and results in a high rate of healing.[346-348]

Sequential monofocal compression-distraction involves an initial interval of compression followed by gradual distraction for lengthening or deformity correction. This technique is applicable for stiff hypertrophic and oligotrophic nonunions, but is not recommended for atrophic, infected, and lax nonunions.[149,349]

Bifocal compression-distraction lengthening involves acute or gradual compression across the nonunion site with

Text continued on p. 715

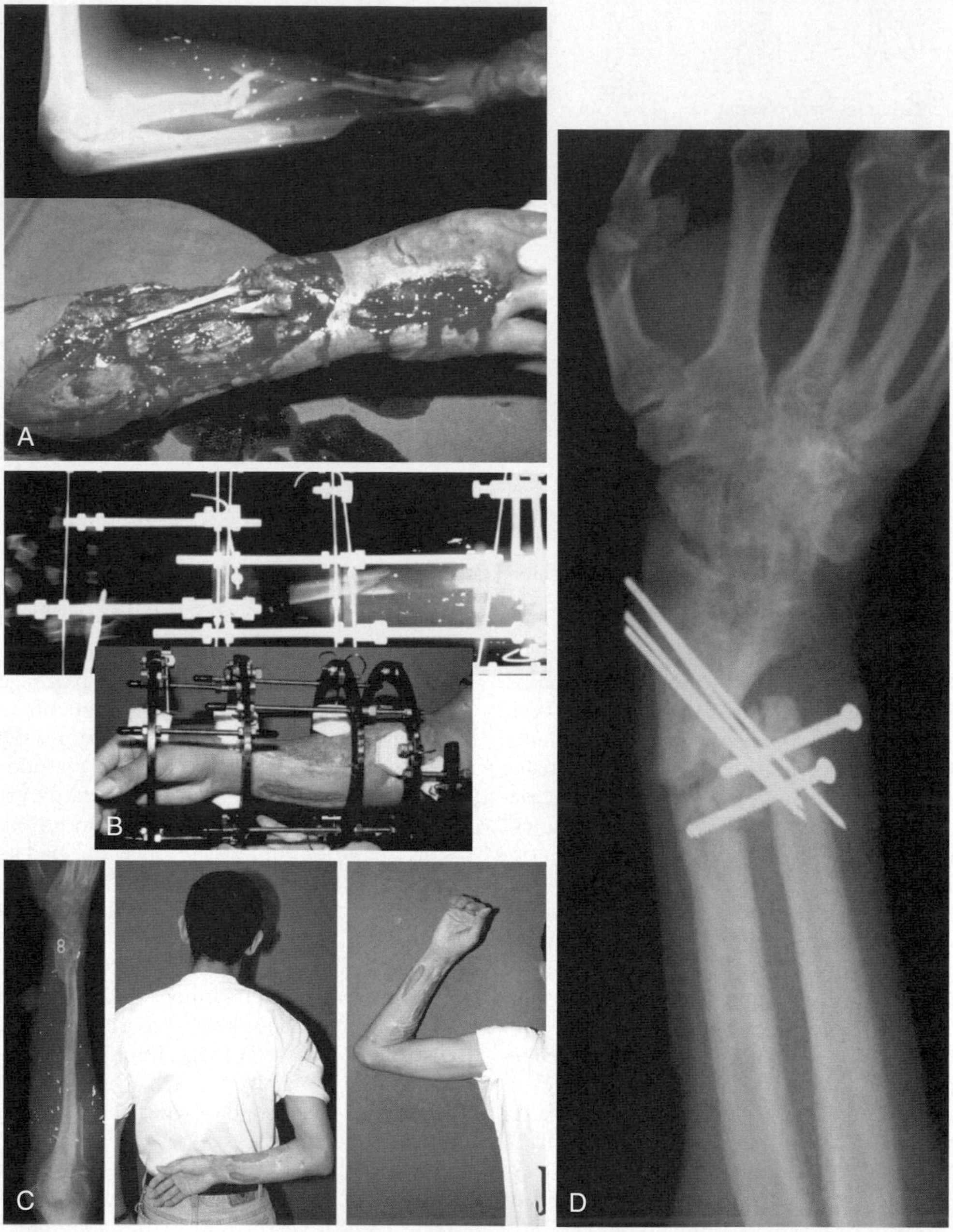

Figure 25-81. Two cases of forearm nonunions treated with synostosis. **A,** Presenting radiograph and clinical photograph of 32-year-old man referred with segmental bone loss from a gunshot blast to the forearm. **B,** Radiograph and clinical photograph of the forearm during bone transport of the proximal ulna into the distal radius to create a one-bone forearm (synostosis). **C,** Final radiograph and clinical photographs. **D,** Presenting radiograph of a 48-year-old man having failed multiple attempts at a synostosis procedure of the forearm.

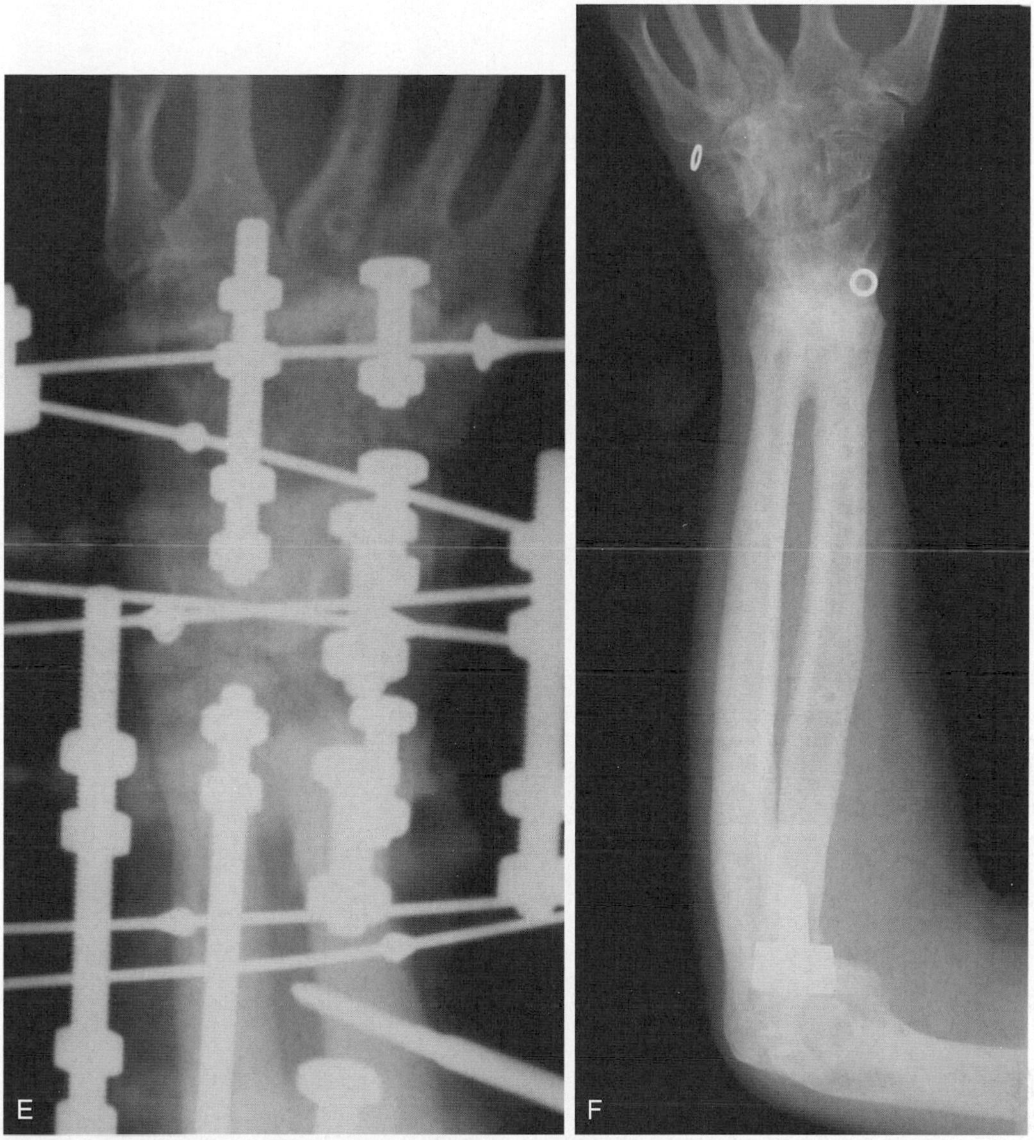

Figure 25-81, cont'd. E, Radiograph of the forearm during Ilizarov treatment with slow gradual compression. **F,** Final radiographic result shows solid bony union.

TABLE 25-12 *ADVANTAGES OF ILIZAROV TECHNIQUES*
1. Minimally invasive
2. Can promote bony tissue generation
3. Often require only minimal soft tissue dissection
4. Versatile
5. Can be used in the face of acute or chronic infection
6. Allow for stabilization of small intraarticular or periarticular bone fragments
7. Allow for simultaneous bony healing and deformity correction
8. Allow for immediate weight-bearing
9. Allow for early joint mobilization

TABLE 25-13 *ILIZAROV TREATMENT MODES*	
Monofocal	
	Compression
	Sequential distraction-compression
	Distraction
	Sequential compression-distraction
Bifocal	
	Compression-distraction lengthening
	Distraction-compression transport (bone transport)
Trifocal	
	Various combinations

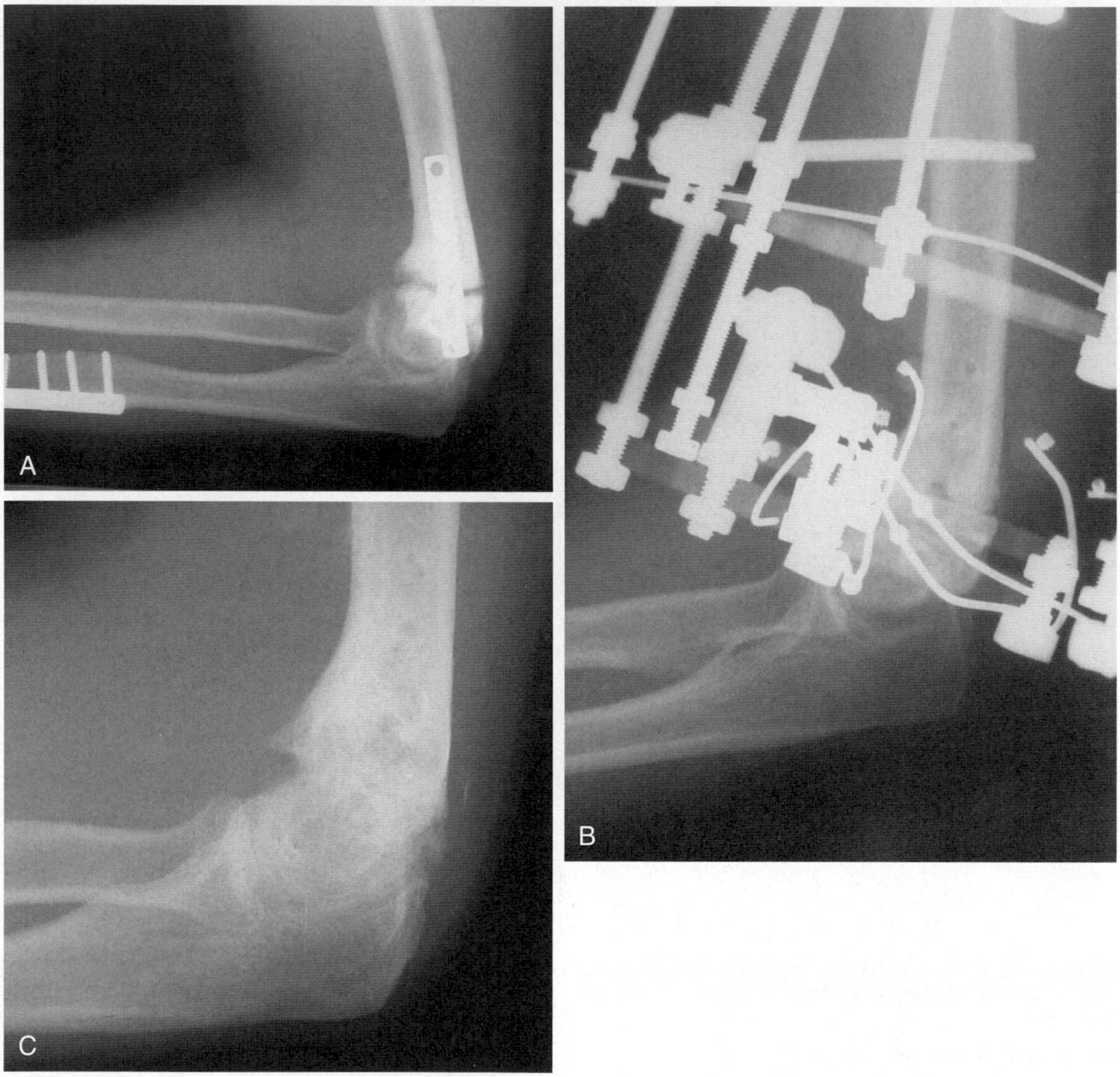

Figure 25-82. Ilizarov treatment of a hypertrophic distal humeral nonunion using gradual monofocal compression. **A,** Presenting radiograph. **B,** Radiograph during treatment using slow compression. Note the bending of the wires proximal and distal to the nonunion site indicating good bony contact. **C,** Final radiographic result shows solid bony union.

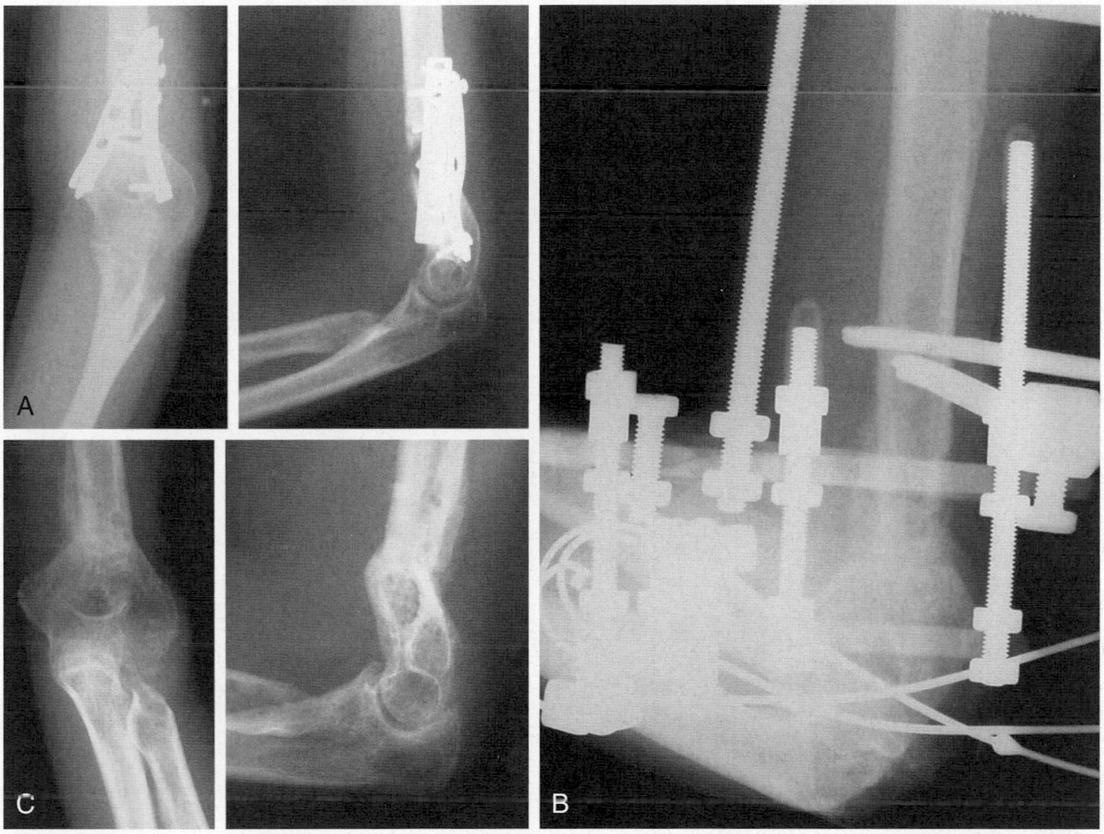

Figure 25-83. An example of an oligotrophic nonunion of the distal humerus treated with slow gradual compression using Ilizarov external fixation. **A,** Presenting radiographs. **B,** Radiograph during treatment using slow gradual compression. Note the bending of the wires indicating good bony contact. **C,** Final radiographic result shows solid bony union.

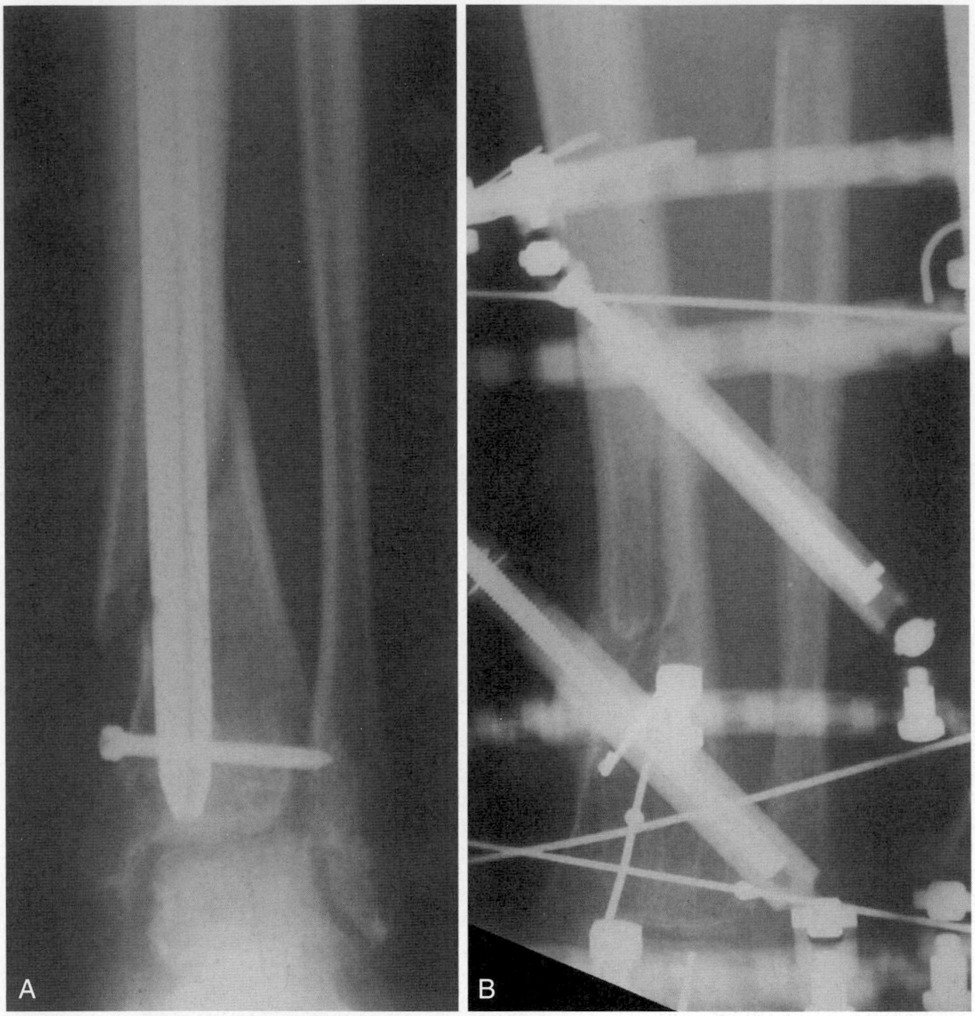

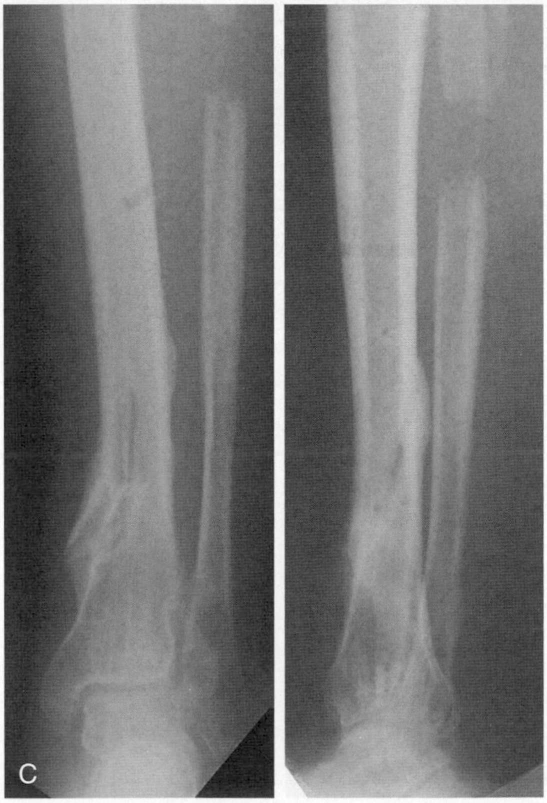

Figure 25-84. An example of an oligotrophic nonunion of the distal tibia treated with gradual deformity correction followed by slow gradual compression using Ilizarov external fixation. **A,** Presenting radiograph. **B,** Radiograph during treatment. **C,** Final radiographic result shows solid bony union with complete deformity correction.

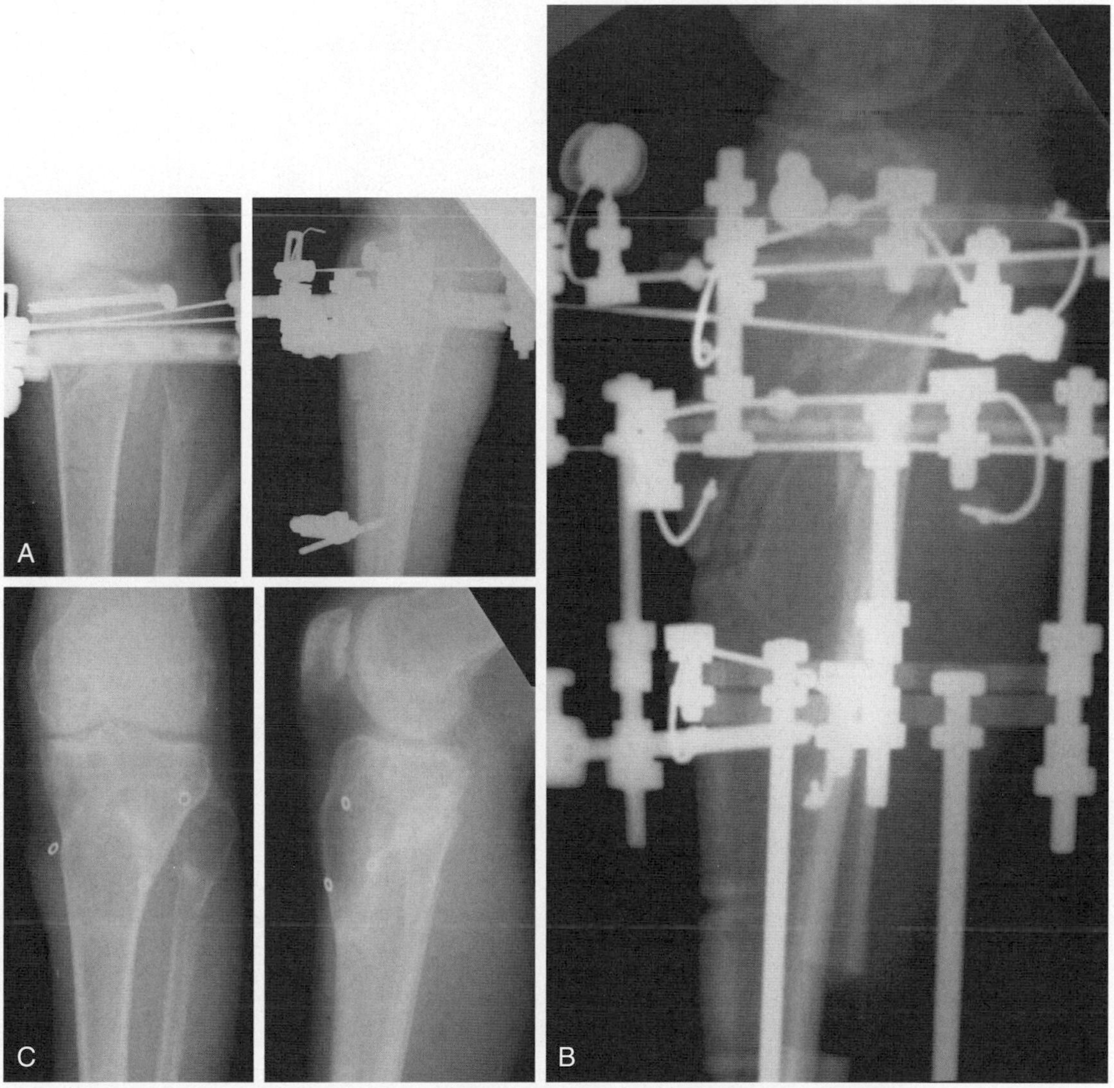

Figure 25-85. An example of an oligotrophic nonunion of the proximal tibial treated with slow gradual compression using Ilizarov external fixation. **A,** Presenting radiograph. **B,** Radiograph during treatment using slow gradual compression. **C,** Final radiographic result shows solid bony union.

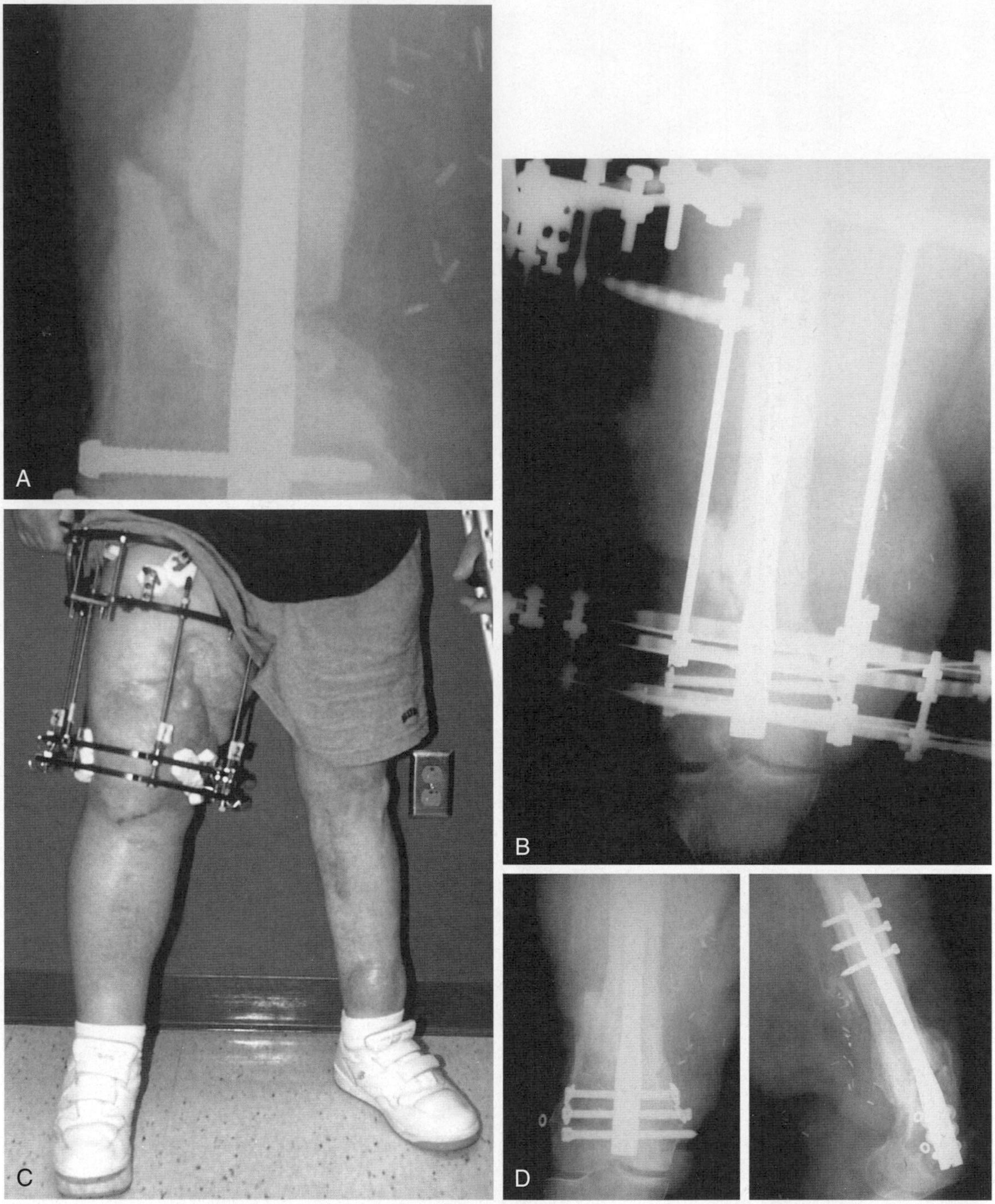

Figure 25-86. An example of successful treatment of a resistant femoral nonunion using the slow compression over a nail using external fixation (SCONE) technique. **A,** Presenting radiograph shows a femoral nonunion. The patient is a 67-year-old man who was referred in having failed two exchange nailings and two open bone graft procedures. **B,** Radiograph during treatment with slow compression over a nail using external fixation. **C,** Clinical photograph during treatment. **D,** Final radiographs show solid bony union.

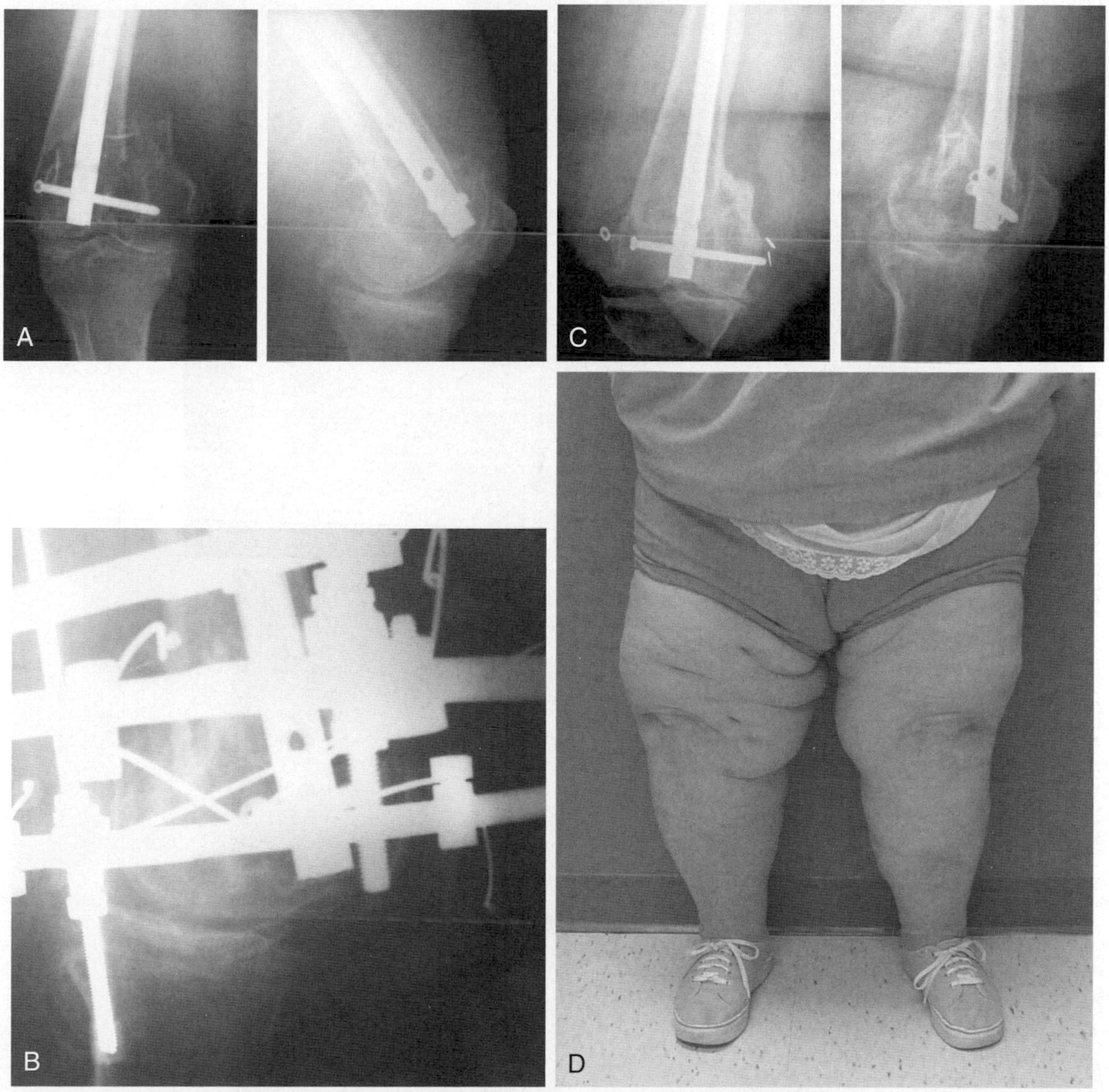

Figure 25-87. An example of successful treatment of a distal femoral nonunion in a morbidly obese elderly diabetic woman referred in 10 months following retrograde intramedullary nailing for a fracture. **A,** Presenting radiographs show a distal femoral nonunion. **B,** Radiograph during treatment with the slow compression over a nail using external fixation (SCONE) technique. **C,** Final radiographs show solid bony union. **D,** Clinical photograph following successful treatment.

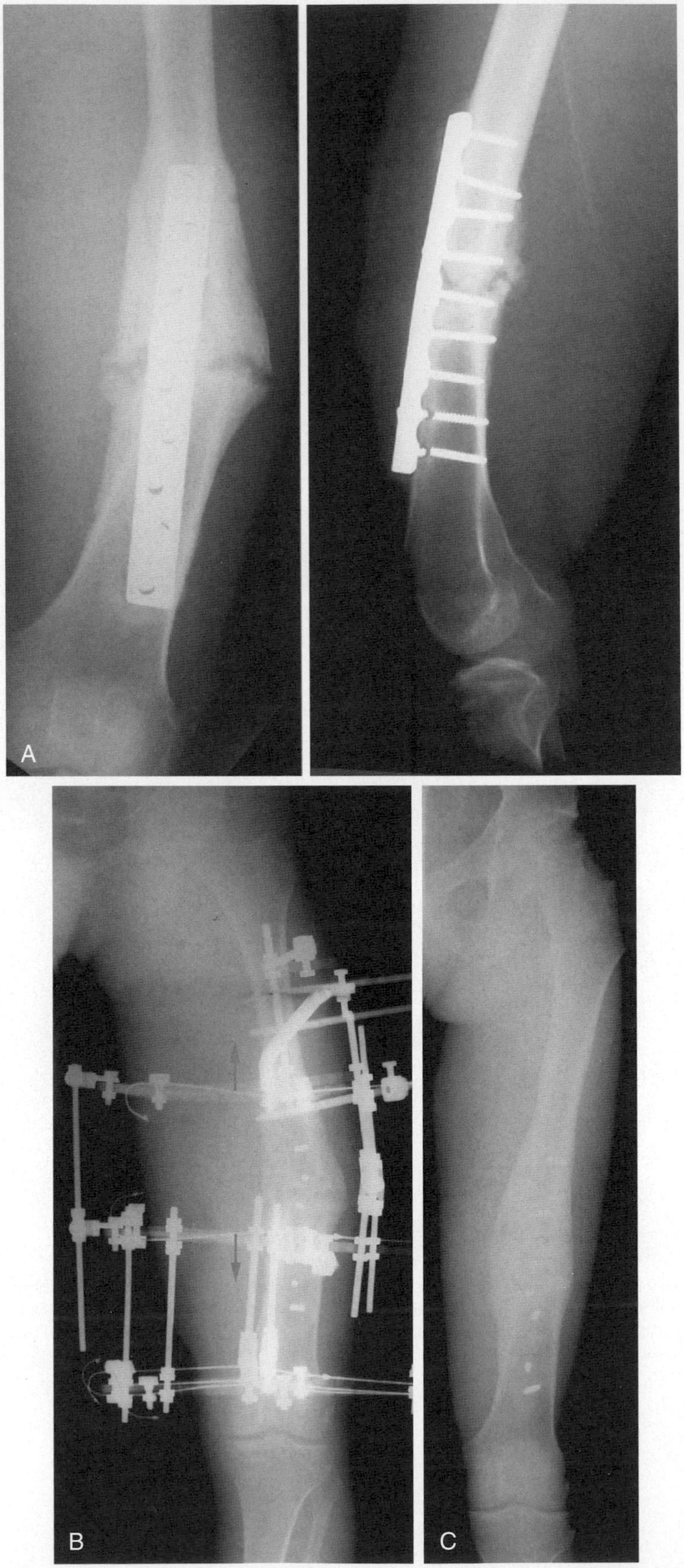

Figure 25-88. Treatment of a stiff hypertrophic nonunion of the femoral shaft using distraction. **A,** Presenting radiographs. **B,** Radiograph during treatment via distraction using the Ilizarov external fixator. Note that differential distraction also results in deformity correction. **C,** Final radiographic result shows solid bony union and deformity correction.

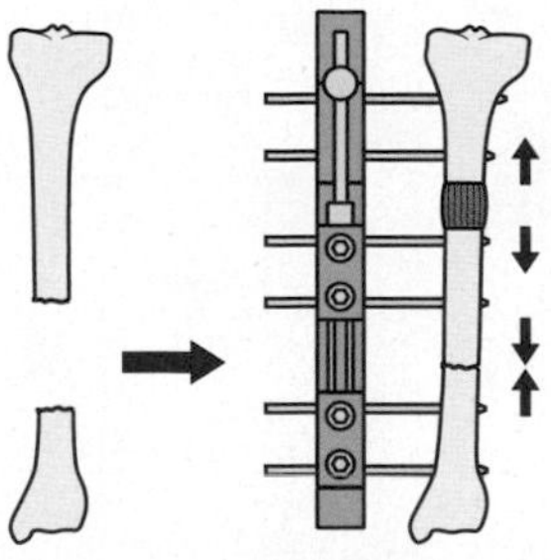

Figure 25-89. Compression-distraction lengthening.

lengthening through an adjacent corticotomy (Fig. 25-89). This method is applicable for nonunions associated with foreshortening and nonunions with segmental defects. Segmental defects may also be treated with bifocal distraction-compression transport (bone transport) (Fig. 25-90). This method involves the creation of a corticotomy (usually metaphyseal) at a site distant from the nonunion. The bone segment produced by the corticotomy is then gradually transported toward the nonunion site (into the bony defect). As the transported segment arrives at the docking site, compression is successful in many cases in obtaining union. Occasionally bone grafting with marrow or open bone graft is required.

Corticotomy and bone transport result in profound biological stimulation, similar to bone grafting. In a study of dogs undergoing distraction osteogenesis, Aronson[350] reported that blood flow at the distraction site increased nearly 10-fold relative to the control limb, peaking about 2 weeks after surgery. The distal tibia, remote from the distraction site, showed a similar pattern of increased blood flow. Consequently, bone transport can be useful in the treatment of atrophic nonunions.

The bone formed at the corticotomy site in lengthening and bone transport is formed under gradual distraction (distraction osteogenesis).[351-355] The tension-stress effect of distraction causes neovascularity and cellular proliferation. The method of bone regeneration is primarily via intramembranous bone formation.

Distraction osteogenesis depends on a variety of mechanical and biological requirements. The corticotomy/osteotomy must be performed using a low-energy technique. Corticotomy/osteotomy in the metaphyseal or metadiaphyseal region is preferred over diaphyseal sites. Stable external fixation promotes good bony regenerate. A latency period prior to initiating distraction of 7 to 14 days is recommended. The rate and rhythm of distraction is controlled by the treating physician, who monitors the progression of the regenerate on radiographs. The distraction phase classically is performed at a rate of 1.0 mm per day in a rhythm of 0.25 mm of distraction performed four times per day, although we typically begin distraction at 0.75 mm per day because some patients make bony regenerate more slowly. Following distraction, maturation and hypertrophy of the bony regenerate occur during the consolidation phase. The consolidation phase is generally two to three times as long as the distraction phase, but this varies widely.

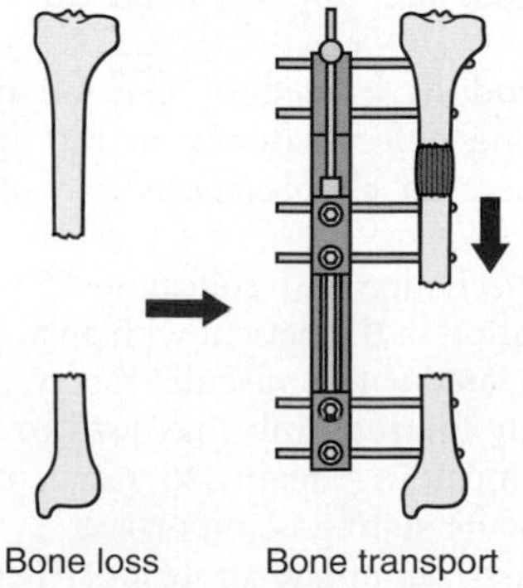

Figure 25-90. Distraction-compression transport (bone transport).

The treatment strategy for infected nonunions and nonunions associated with segmental defects depends on many factors (bone, soft tissue, and medical health characteristics). No clear consensus exists. Treatment options include conventional methods (resection, soft tissue coverage, massive cancellous bone grafting, and skeletal stabilization) and Ilizarov methods using one of two different strategies: bifocal compression-distraction (lengthening) or bifocal distraction-compression transport (bone transport).

A number of studies have compared these various methods. Green[131] compared bone grafting and bone transport in the treatment of segmental skeletal defects. For defects of 5 cm or less, he recommended the use of either technique, but recommended bone transport or free composite tissue transfer for larger defects. In a similar study, Marsh and coworkers[132] compared resection and bone transport to treatment with less extensive débridement, external fixation, bone grafting, and soft tissue coverage and found that the groups were similar in terms of healing rate, healing and treatment time, eradication of infection, final deformity, complications, and total number of operative procedures. The final limb length discrepancy was significantly less in the group treated with bone transport. Cierny and Zorn[130] compared conventional (massive cancellous bone grafts and tissue transfers) versus Ilizarov methods in the treatment of segmental tibial defects. The Ilizarov group averaged 9 fewer hours in the operating room, 23 fewer days of hospitalization, 5 months less of disability, and a savings of nearly $30,000 per case. Ring and coauthors[356] compared autogenous cancellous bone grafting versus Ilizarov treatment for infected tibial nonunions and concluded that the Ilizarov methods may best be used for large limb length discrepancy or for very proximal or distal metaphyseal nonunions. Paley and colleagues[129] concluded that acute shortening with subsequent relengthening has a significantly lower complication rate and less time in the external fixator than does bone transport for tibial defects, although both techniques provide excellent overall results. Mahaluxmivala and colleagues also recommended acute shortening with subsequent relengthening over bone transport because of shorter treatment time and fewer additional treatments (e.g., bone grafting) needed to achieve bony union.[357]

ARTHROPLASTY. In certain situations, joint replacement arthroplasty may be the chosen treatment method for a fracture nonunion. The advantages are early return to function with immediate weight-bearing and joint mobilization. The main disadvantage is the excision of native anatomic structures (bone, cartilage, ligaments, etc.). Arthroplasty as a treatment of nonunion is indicated in older patients with severe

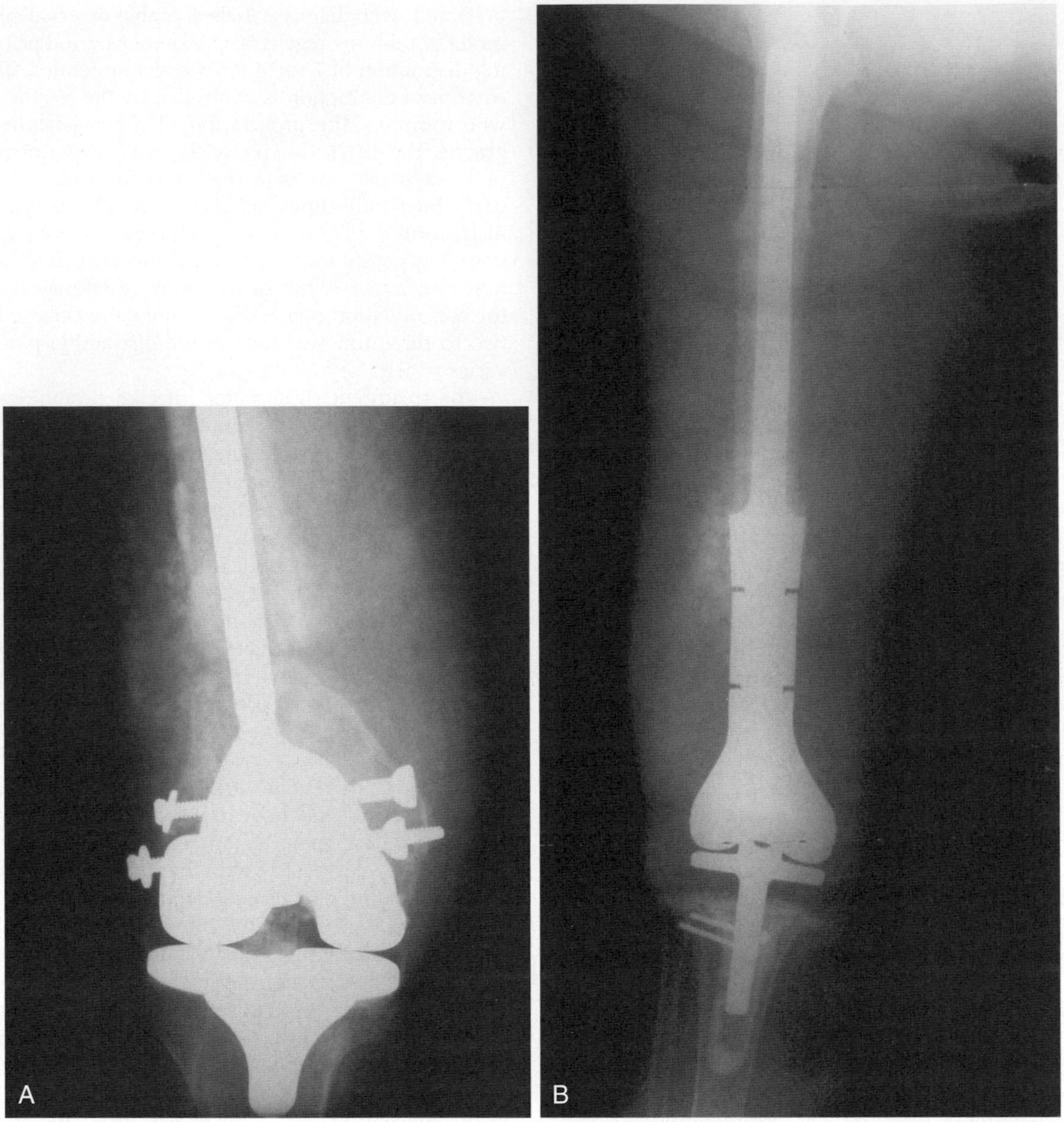

Figure 25-91. A, Presenting radiograph of an 82-year-old woman who was referred with a distal femoral periprosthetic nonunion. This patient had been wheelchair bound for 2 years and had had three prior failed attempts at nonunion treatment. **B,** Radiograph following joint replacement arthroplasty. The patient has had excellent pain relief and has resumed ambulation without the need for walking aids.

medical problems; long-standing resistant periarticular nonunions; periarticular nonunions associated with small osteopenic fragments; nonunions associated with painful posttraumatic or degenerative arthritis; or periprosthetic nonunions that either cannot be readily stabilized by conventional methods or have failed conventional treatment methods (Fig. 25-91).

Arthroplasty as a method of treatment for nonunion has been reported for the hip,[240,358,359] knee,[360-364] shoulder,[186,234,365,366] and elbow.[156,367]

Arthrodesis. Arthrodesis as a treatment method for nonunion is indicated for patients with previously failed (ununited) arthrodesis procedures (Fig. 25-92; Video 25-1); infected periarticular nonunions; unreconstructable periarticular nonunions in locations that are not believed to have good long-term result with arthroplasty (e.g., the ankle); unreconstructable periarticular nonunions in young patients who are not long-term candidates for arthroplasty; infected nonunions in which débridement necessitates removal of important articular structures (see Fig. 25-74); nonunions associated with unreconstructable joint instability, contracture, or pain that are not amenable to arthroplasty (see Fig. 25-74).

An alloarthrodesis procedure may be performed when a segmental bone defect extends to the epiphyseal region in a patient where an alloprosthesis is contraindicated (see Fig. 25-74).

Amputation. Lange and colleagues[368] published indications for amputation in the patient with an acute open fracture of the tibia associated with a vascular injury. Delay in amputation of a severely injured limb may lead to serious systemic complications, including death, so rapid, resolute decision making in the acute setting is important.

The decision to amputate or reconstruct a nonunion is a different matter. The patients do not present in extremis

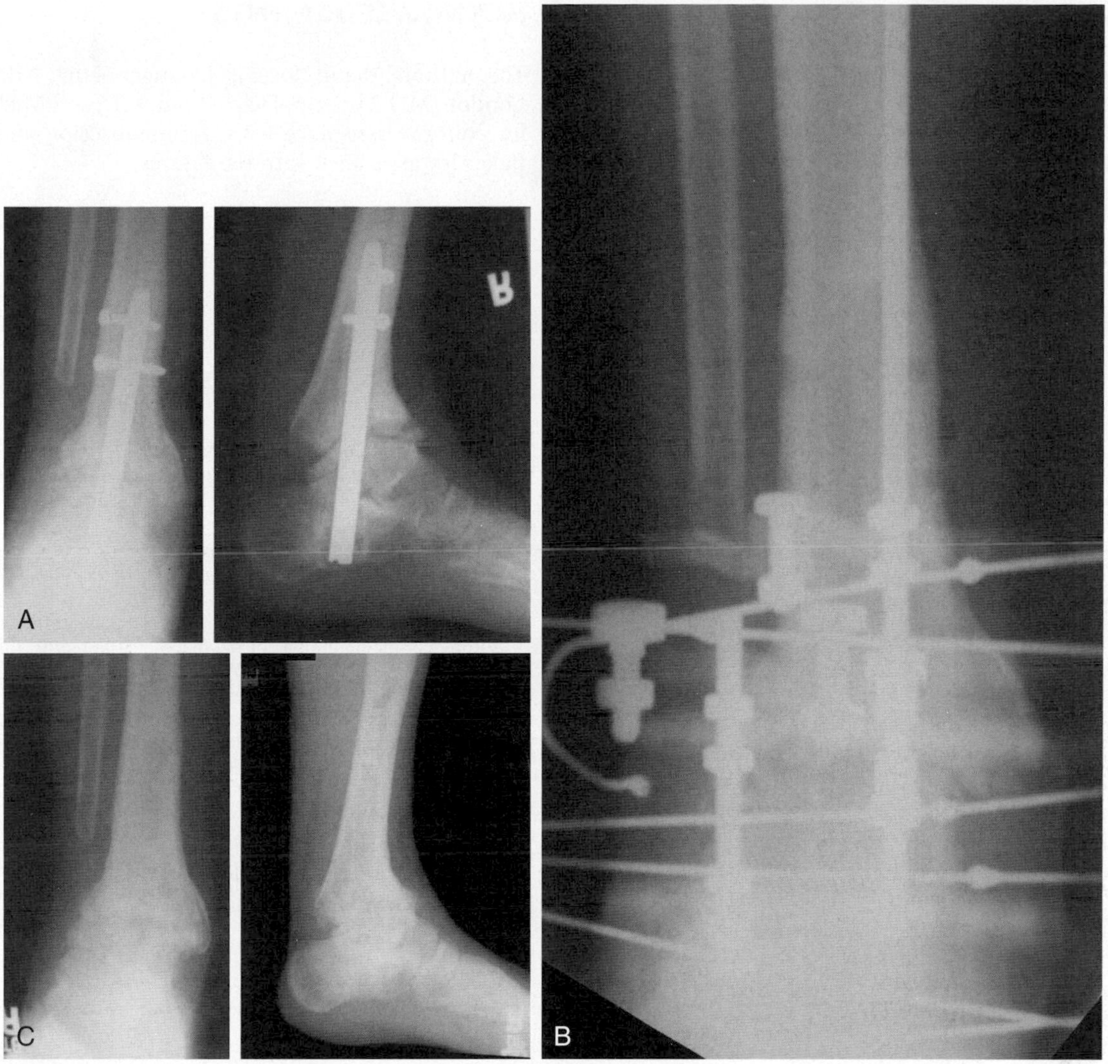

Figure 25-92. A, Presenting radiographs of a 25-year-old man who had had a total of 18 prior ankle operations and had had 5 failed prior attempts at ankle arthrodesis. **B,** The patient was treated with percutaneous hardware removal and gradual compression using an Ilizarov external fixator. The ankle joint was not operatively approached and no bone grafting was performed. **C,** Final radiographic result following simple gradual compression shows solid fusion of the ankle.

and have typically been living with the problem for a long time. In a study of quality of life in 109 patients with post-traumatic sequelae of the long bones, Lerner and colleagues[369] described the choice determinants in patients undergoing amputation:

1. Desire to discontinue treatment
2. Recommended by a doctor
3. Believed that they would never be cured

There are no absolute indications for amputation of a chronic ununited limb. Each case is unique and includes multiple complex issues, and treatment algorithms are usually not helpful.

Amputation of an ununited limb should be considered in several situations:

1. Sepsis arises in a frail, elderly, or medically compromised patient with an infected nonunion, such that there is concern about the patient's survival.
2. Loss of neurologic function (motor or sensory or both) is unreconstructable and precludes restoration of purposeful limb function.
3. Chronic osteomyelitis associated with the nonunion is in an anatomic area that precludes reconstruction (e.g., the calcaneus).
4. The patient wishes to discontinue medical and surgical treatment of the nonunion and desires to have an amputation.

All patients considering amputation for a nonunion should seek a minimum of two opinions from orthopaedic surgeons specializing in nonunion reconstruction techniques. Amputation should not be undertaken because the treating physician has run out of ideas, treatment recommendations, or stamina. Motivated patients who have a recalcitrant nonunion but wish to retain their limb can be referred to colleagues. Once a limb has been cut off, it cannot be put back on.

SUMMARY

The care of the patient who has a nonunion is always challenging and sometimes troubling. Because of the various nonunion types, and the constellation of possible problems related to the bone, soft tissues, prior treatments, patient health, and other factors, no simple treatment algorithms are possible. The care of these patients requires patience with the ultimate goal of bony union, restoration of function, and limited impairment and disability. An approach to the evaluation and treatment of these patients has been provided. A few simple axioms bear further emphasis.

The 10 Commandments of Nonunion Treatment

1. Examine thy patient and carefully consider all available information.
2. Thou shall learn about the personality of the nonunion from the prior failed treatments.
3. Thou shall not repeat failed prior procedures (those which have not yielded any evidence of healing effort) over and over and over again.
4. Thou shall base thy treatment plan on the nonunion type and the treatment modifiers, and not upon false prophecies.
5. Thou shall forsake the use of the same hammer for every single nail (the treatment of nonunions requires surgical expertise in a wide variety of internal and external fixation techniques).
6. Honor thy soft tissues and keep them whole.
7. Thou shall consider minimally invasive techniques (Ilizarov method, bone marrow injection, etc.), where extensive surgical exposures have failed.
8. Thou shall not take the previous treating physician's name or treatment method or results in vain, particularly in the presence of the patient. Honor thy referring physicians and keep them informed of the patient's progress.
9. Thou shall burn no bridges and shall leave thyself the option of a "next treatment plan."
10. Thou shall covet stability, vascularity, and bone-to-bone contact.

ACKNOWLEDGMENTS

The authors thank Joseph J. Gugenheim, MD, Jeffrey C. London, MD, Ebrahim Delpassand, MD, and Michele Clowers for editorial assistance with the manuscript, and Rodney K. Baker for assistance with the figures.

KEY REFERENCES

The level of evidence (LOE) is determined according to the criteria provided in the preface.

15. Court-Brown CM, Keating JF, Christie J, et al: Exchange intramedullary nailing. Its use in aseptic tibial nonunion. *J Bone Joint Surg Br* 77:407–411, 1995. LOE IV
56. Brinker MR, O'Connor DP, Monla YT, et al: Metabolic and endocrine abnormalities in patients with nonunions. *J Orthop Trauma* 21:557–570, 2007. LOE IV
84. Paley D, Tetsworth K: Mechanical axis deviation of the lower limbs. Preoperative planning of multiapical frontal plane angular and bowing deformities of the femur and tibia. *Clin Orthop Relat Res* 280:65–71, 1992. LOE V
130. Cierny G III, Zorn KE: Segmental tibial defects. Comparing conventional and Ilizarov methodologies. *Clin Orthop Relat Res* 301:118–123, 1994. LOE III
206. Ring D, Kloen P, Kadzielski J, et al: Locking compression plates for osteoporotic nonunions of the diaphyseal humerus. *Clin Orthop Relat Res* 425:50–54, 2004. LOE IV
256. Sagi HC, Young ML, Gerstenfeld L, et al: Qualitative and quantitative differences between bone graft obtained from the medullary canal (with a Reamer/Irrigator/Aspirator) and the iliac crest of the same patient. *J Bone Joint Surg Am* 94:2128–2135, 2012.
314. Brinker MR, O'Connor DP: Exchange nailing of ununited fractures. *J Bone Joint Surg Am* 89:177–188, 2007. LOE III

The complete References list is available online at https://expertconsult.inkling.com.

Chapter 26

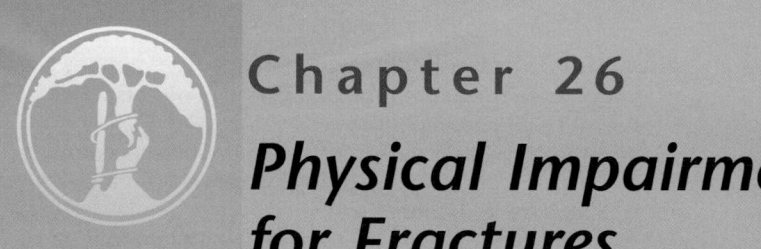

Physical Impairment Ratings for Fractures

THOMAS H. SANDERS • BRENT B. WIESEL • SAM W. WIESEL

Fractures account for only about 10% of all musculoskeletal traumatic injuries, but they cause a disproportionate amount of medical impairment. The costs of fracture care, including lost productivity, medical expenses, and disability payments, make this class of injury a significant burden both to employers and to society in general.

The role of physicians in the medical care of fractures is well established, but their job does not end when union has been achieved and rehabilitation is complete. Physician participation is equally vital in the impairment evaluation process. Many state and federal laws limit physician discretion in assigning permanent impairment ratings, and the physician is often caught between a desire to benefit the patient and the need to comply with these laws. This chapter presents some generic issues of impairment, reviews the epidemiology of fractures in the United States, and reviews the process of assigning an impairment rating.

GENERIC ISSUES OF DISABILITY AND IMPAIRMENT

Definitions

There is a certain amount of confusion about the role of the physician in determination of permanent disability and about the difference between impairment and disability. According to the sixth edition of the *Guides to the Evaluation of Permanent Impairment,* published by the American Medical Association (AMA), the following definitions apply[1]:

Impairment: a significant deviation, loss, or loss of use of any body structure or body function in an individual with a health condition, disorder or disease

Disability: activity limitations and/or participation restrictions in an individual with a health condition

Impairment rating: consensus-derived percentage estimate of loss of activity reflecting severity for a given health condition, and the degree of associated limitations in terms of activities of daily living (ADLs)

Determining the difference between disability and impairment is challenging, if not impossible. In some conditions, there is a predictable correlation between the injury and the expected degree of functional loss (complete spinal cord injury). In other conditions, it is harder to predict (radial nerve palsy after humerus fracture). Disability is dependent on a number of nonmedical factors, among them the patients' level of education, their work training and work history, their residual access to the workplace, and their socioeconomic background. Disability is context specific and can change over time. For example, an orthopaedic surgeon would be much more disabled by a finger amputation than an endocrinologist would be. If adaptations can be made to the work environment or task in question, a particular impairment may not limit an individual from performing the task. Physicians, in general, are considered experts only in the determination of impairment.

Impairment ratings enable the physician to estimate the quantitative losses to individuals as a result of their health condition, disorder, or disease. Impairment ratings are defined by anatomic, structural, and diagnostic criteria with which physicians are usually familiar. These ratings are determined by accepted diagnostic procedures. Most physicians, however, are not familiar with the full array of functional activities and participations that are required for comprehensive disability determinations. Impairment ratings are a physician-determined estimate that attempts to link impairment with a quantitative estimate of patients' functional losses in their personal world of activity.

A permanent impairment exists when the patient has reached maximal medical improvement yet a loss or derangement persists. Maximal medical improvement has been achieved when the injury or illness has stabilized and no material improvement or deterioration is expected in the next year, with or without treatment. Many jurisdictions require that a year elapse after the injury or most recent surgery related to the injury before determining that maximal medical improvement has been attained.

Role of the Physician

According to the AMA guidelines, determining whether an injury or illness results in a permanent impairment requires a medical assessment performed by a physician. The functions evaluated in determining permanent impairment are those that allow the individual to perform common ADLs, excluding work. These include self-care, communication, physical activity (including sitting, standing, reclining, walking, and stair climbing), sensory functions, nonspecialized hand activities, travel, sexual function, and sleep. Because musculoskeletal injuries account for the majority of impairment determinations, orthopaedists are frequently involved in this process.

Depending on local regulations, the physician determining impairment may be the treating physician with whom the patient has an established doctor-patient relationship or an independent physician who examines the patient only for the purposes of determining impairment and is not otherwise involved in the patient's care. In general, physicians acting as independent consultants for determination of impairment ratings do not establish a doctor-patient relationship with the patient being examined. If new diagnoses are uncovered during the course of an impairment evaluation, the physician has a medical obligation to inform the requesting party and the individual about the condition and advise the individual to seek appropriate medical treatment.

Third-Party Payers and the Workers' Compensation System

The concept of compensation for personal injuries is not a modern one. Historical evidence shows that social justice and compensation systems for injured parties have been around since recorded history. These systems attempted to legislate the exchange of money for losses resulting from personal injury.[2,3] The workers' compensation system in the United States was started in 1906 with the passage of the first law covering federal employees. By 1917, workers' compensation insurance was mandatory for a business to operate.[4]

Prior to the passage of the workers' compensation law, employees who were injured at work were required to sue and prove employer negligence to receive compensation. In essence, it is a form of insurance providing wage replacement and medical benefits to employees injured in the course of employment in exchange for mandatory relinquishment of the employee's right to sue for the tort of negligence. The workers' compensation system in the United States has evolved into a complex entity regulated by each state and representing approximately 1.5% of all employers' compensation expenditures.[4,5]

Impairment evaluations are most frequently requested by a third-party payer before settlement of a claim. The largest third-party payers are state workers' compensation boards, private insurance companies, the Social Security Administration, and the Department of Veterans Affairs.[6] Each of these groups has its own requirements for and definitions of impairment. Workers' compensation laws vary widely from state to state, and federal agency regulations are amended yearly. The agency requesting the impairment evaluation should specify which rules apply in the specific case, and the reviewing physician should abide by the specified rules. In some cases, older editions of the AMA guides have been incorporated in state laws, in which case, the appropriate edition must be consulted. Tort law (civil litigation or lawsuits) in some states does not specify any particular body of rules; in these cases, the evaluating physician has considerably greater freedom to describe and quantify a given impairment.

Correspondence is between the physician and the third-party payer. Updates should be in the form of letters mailed directly to the representative of the third-party payer. The patient should not act as an intermediary, although the patient's right to review his or her chart in the presence of the attending physician should always be honored.

Work Restrictions

In addition to assigning impairment ratings, the physician is often called on to give an estimate of residual work capacity. In this role, the physician is responsible for determining the level of physical activity that the patient can safely tolerate. The most widely accepted physical exertion requirement guidelines are those published by the Social Security Administration:

Very heavy work is that which involves lifting objects weighing more than 100 pounds at a time, with frequent lifting or carrying of objects weighing 50 pounds or more.

Heavy work involves lifting of no more than 100 pounds at a time, with frequent lifting or carrying of objects weighing up to 50 pounds.

Medium work involves the lifting of no more than 50 pounds at a time, with frequent lifting or carrying of objects weighing up to 25 pounds.

Light work involves lifting of no more than 20 pounds at a time, with frequent lifting or carrying of objects weighing up to 10 pounds.

Sedentary work involves the lifting of no more than 10 pounds at a time and occasional lifting or carrying of articles such as docket files, ledgers, or small tools.

TYPES OF DISABILITY

Temporary Total Disability

In general, a patient is judged temporarily totally disabled if, in the opinion of the treating physician, the patient is incapable of performing any job, for any reasonable period of time, during the course of a workday. Note that, by this definition, a patient's inability to perform his or her own job is not the primary issue. For example, a construction worker in a short arm cast for a distal radius fracture may well be incapable of his or her usual work but capable of sedentary or one-handed light work, so the worker is not totally disabled. Temporary total disability is also granted for patients whose pain is great enough to warrant regular narcotic use, whose mobility is so severely compromised as to make getting from home to the workplace unreasonably difficult, or who are hospitalized in an inpatient unit.

Patients are temporarily totally disabled from the moment of occurrence of a skeletal injury until they achieve a reasonable degree of mobility and independence, are able to perform their own ADLs to a reasonable degree, and are no longer dependent on narcotic analgesics. Obviously, patients who are hospitalized, are inpatients in a rehabilitation facility, or are homebound and require skilled nursing care are temporarily totally disabled. Patients who are dependent on crutches for ambulation are not necessarily totally disabled at all times unless they meet the other definitions of temporary total disability.

Periodic evaluation in the physician's office is necessary during the period of temporary total disability. Most state workmen's compensation laws mandate at least monthly visits during the period of temporary total disability, during which further documentation for ongoing temporary total disability status must be entered in the patient's record.

Temporary Partial Disability

Temporary partial disability begins with the termination of temporary total disability and continues until rehabilitation is complete and the patient is back to full activities with no restrictions or until a permanent impairment is assigned. During the period of temporary partial disability, the patient is allowed to return to the workplace with certain restrictions judged appropriate by the treating physician.

Once the period of temporary total disability is lifted, appropriate restrictions must be instituted by the physician. These may allow the patient to return to work in a light-duty situation in which the physical requirements of the job do not compromise healing or cause unacceptable discomfort. The physician is responsible for identifying the level of safe activity, which may be limited to sedentary work during the early recovery phase of an injury.

Patients recovering from back and neck injuries may benefit from a restriction on bending, twisting, stooping, lifting, and heavy overhead work. Upper extremity injury restrictions often include avoidance of heavy or repetitive use of the involved extremity. Restrictions after lower extremity injuries frequently include prohibitions against excessive walking, climbing, stooping, kneeling, running, and carrying.

Many employers and third-party payers publish and distribute forms with a listing of possible activities for the physician to check off. To the extent that the listed activities are of concern to the physician, these forms may be used, but it is often more useful for the physician to attach a note on letterhead stationery outlining the restrictions rather than to try to make his or her best judgment about appropriate restrictions fit within the confines of existing forms and classifications.

Periodic reevaluations of the patient's clinical status are made, usually at 2- to 6-week intervals. State law varies considerably on the issue of mandatory frequency of reevaluations during a period of temporary partial disability. In general, state laws permit somewhat longer intervals between clinic visits for patients with temporary partial disability than for those with temporary total disability, often between 4 and 8 weeks. Again, documentation in the record of the reason for ongoing temporary partial disability is important. Physician records and occasionally physician testimony are required for insurance payments for disability determination. It is worthwhile periodically to record range of motion, functional restrictions, medication use, and degree of autonomy with ADLs; these data can be used later to document the patient's degree of disability during any given period.

Temporary partial disability restrictions should be modified as the patient's symptoms warrant. This modification may require instituting greater restrictions and moving the patient back toward more sedentary activities if symptoms become excessive or gradual liberalization of activities as clinical status permits. Occasional periods of temporary total disability may be warranted, particularly after surgical procedures or operative manipulations of fractures.

Permanent Partial Disability

After maximal medical recovery has been achieved, the physician, possibly in cooperation with other occupational specialists, may be asked to recommend a permanent restricted activity level if the patient is unable to return to his or her original job. There are no widely accepted guidelines for determining the level of job restriction, but, in general, a patient who has any permanent partial impairment secondary to skeletal injury is unable to perform very heavy or heavy work safely.[7,8] If the permanent partial impairment is greater than 25%, most patients are unlikely to perform successfully in any but part-time or home-based occupations at the sedentary level. Between these two extremes, the physician must decide what a reasonable expectation is for the patient, taking into consideration the type of injury and impairment and the sorts of activities that are likely to exacerbate persistent pain. The physician may use functional capacity evaluations performed in conjunction with a physical therapist as an objective measure of particular activities that an individual patient is capable of tolerating.

As an example, a well-healed 10% compression fracture of the lumbar spine with some chronic back pain may result in a 5% permanent partial impairment. The patient is likely to have exacerbation of pain with bending, twisting, stooping, lifting of more than 20 pounds, or prolonged overhead work. He or she would be qualified for a job involving light work, with the restrictions specified previously.

The physician assigns impairment and specifies work restrictions, but the responsibility for finding an appropriate job lies with the patient or the third-party payer. With more aggressive job retraining and work hardening programs, patients with significant impairment are now returning to the workplace. When an injured individual is declared disabled from injury, it is almost always economically unfavorable both for the individual and for society as a whole.[9] If the physician performing the impairment evaluation is also the patient's treating physician, it is often worthwhile for the physician to work with the social worker, nurse, or occupational therapist representing the third-party payer to find an acceptable job for the patient or to encourage occupational retraining when appropriate.

EPIDEMIOLOGY OF FRACTURES IN THE UNITED STATES

Given the vast array of healthcare providers who care for musculoskeletal injuries in the United States, it is extremely difficult to accurately estimate the epidemiology of fractures. According to the National Center for Health Statistics and the Centers for Disease Control and Prevention (CDC), between 1999 and 2011, there were approximately 7.3 million physician visits per year for fractures of the extremities. Annually over that time, there was an average of 3.5 million emergency room visits and 867,000 hospitalizations for fractures of the extremities[10,11]

The U.S. Bureau of Labor Statistics tracks work-related injuries and resulting time away from work. In 2011, musculoskeletal disorders accounted for 33% of all injury and illness with 387,820 cases. Six occupations accounted for 26% of the musculoskeletal cases in 2011. nursing assistants, laborers, janitors and cleaners, heavy and tractor-trailer truck drivers, registered nurses, and stock clerks.[12] Heavy and tractor-trailer truck drivers required a median of 21 days away from work to recuperate compared to 11 days for all workers who sustained a musculoskeletal injury.

Approximately 90% of the musculoskeletal disorders are classified as sprains, strains, or tears. Fractures accounted for 8% of all injuries and illnesses to American workers. These types of injuries required more than three times the number of days to recuperate: 27 days compared with 8 days for all types of injuries and illnesses. Falls on the same level accounted for 33% of fractures and another 22% were the result of being struck by an object or equipment. Fractures of the hand accounted for 18% of the fracture cases and required a median of 11 days before returning to work. Ankle fractures, accounting for 12% of all fractures to workers, required a median of 42 days off of work. While accounting for smaller proportions of total cases, fractures, amputations, and multiple injuries with fractures each required a median of 25 days or more away from work to recuperate—more than three times the number of days for all types of injuries and illnesses.[12]

GUIDES FOR IMPAIRMENT DETERMINATION

Historical Perspective

Before the 1930s, in both the United States and Europe, arbitrary disability values were assigned for individual injuries. The entire disability determination process was performed by physicians, despite their lack of special training in social, economic, and occupational evaluation. This practice may have simplified rendering a judgment of disability, but it led to the awarding of the same compensation to individuals with markedly different degrees of residual disability.[6,13] Beginning in the 1930s, new systems of classifying residual deficits were introduced in the United States by individual authors in an effort to make the system of disability evaluation more equitable and objective.

Kessler described evaluation based on objective criteria such as range of motion in degrees and motor strength measured in foot-pounds.[13–15] McBride published a 10-point scale based on five anatomic and five functional criteria that, taken together, gave an estimate of overall impairment.[16,17] In an effort to reduce the influence of subjective and potentially biased data, Thurber published impairment scales based on range of motion alone.[18]

Development of the modern system for rating of permanent partial impairment by physicians began in 1956 with the introduction by the AMA of a series of guides designed to provide objective, reproducible impairment ratings.[19] These guides were intended to standardize evaluation of the result of industrial accidents for determining workers' compensation claims. The AMA series is now complete and is updated regularly. In addition to the guides for the spine and extremities, the AMA provides guides to the evaluation of other organ systems (e.g., neurologic, hematopoietic), but the evaluation of these systems is outside the area of training of orthopaedic surgery.

Numerous impairment guides are in use in the United States. Most states mandate the use of one particular set of guidelines for workers' compensation impairment determination. Some states create their own unique guidelines, which are based on a variety of practical, idiosyncratic, or occasionally political considerations. Increasingly, most states and the District of Columbia have adopted the guidelines published by the AMA. Most federal agencies concerned with impairment determination also use the AMA guides. More widespread use of the AMA guides seems to be leading to increasingly uniform and probably fairer impairment determinations across most jurisdictions.

In 2008, the AMA published the sixth edition of the *Guides to the Evaluation of Permanent Impairment*. This updated edition has been modified from previous editions. The rationale for this change from previous ratings methods is to standardize and simplify the ratings process, to improve content validity, and to provide a more uniform method that promotes greater inter-rater reliability and agreement.[1]

There are typically four considerations used to assess most cases of musculoskeletal impairment:

1. What is the problem (diagnosis)?
2. What difficulties does the patient report?
3. What are the examination findings?
4. What are the results of the clinical studies?

TABLE 26-1 *DEFINITION OF IMPAIRMENT CLASSES*

Functional Class	Impairment
0	No symptoms with strenuous activity (independent)
1	Symptoms with strenuous activity; no symptoms with normal activity (independent)
2	Symptoms with normal activity (independent)
3	Symptoms with minimal activity (partially dependent)
4	Symptoms at rest (totally dependent)

The upper extremity is divided into four regions: digits/hand, wrist, elbow, and shoulder. The lower extremity is divided into three regions: hip, knee and foot/ankle. The spine and pelvis are divided into four regions: cervical spine (occiput through T1), thoracic spine (T1 through T12), lumbar spine (T12 through S1), and pelvis (ilium, sacrum, and pubic rami).

The AMA guides rate impairment by a "whole person" concept. In this system, each part of the body is assigned a value reflecting the contribution of that part to the patient as a whole. The percentage each part contributes to the whole is based on the notion of function. Loss of function of the extremity is expressed as a percentage of the value of the extremity as a whole, and impairment to the whole person is calculated from this value. See tables for basic ratings of the upper and lower extremities and the pelvis and spine (Tables 26-1 to 26-4). While each bone and joint has a specific impairment rating defined by the AMA, in general, the upper extremities are valued at 60% of the whole person, the lower extremities at 40%. As an example, amputation at the wrist results in a 90% loss of function of the arm and a 54% impairment of the whole person.

The AMA guides historically relied solely on range-of-motion measurements for the determination of partial impairments of the spine and extremities, offering no consideration of pain, atrophy, shortening, and other subjective and objective data. Traditional range-of-motion–based estimates ignore causal issues and focus solely on measurable outcomes, specifically motion of local joints or spine segments. Diagnosis-related impairment estimates attempt to overcome

TABLE 26-2 *DEFINITION OF IMPAIRMENT CLASSES: LOWER EXTREMITY*

Class	Problem	Lower Extremity Impairment (%)	Whole Person Impairment (%)
0	No objective findings	0	0
1	Mild	1–13 LEI	1–5 WPI
2	Moderate	14–25 LEI	6–10 WPI
3	Severe	26–49 LEI	11–19 WPI
4	Very Severe	50–100 LEI	20–40 WPI

LEI, Lower extremity impairment; *WPI*, whole person impairment.

TABLE 26-3 *DEFINITION OF IMPAIRMENT CLASSES: UPPER EXTREMITY*

Class	Problem	Upper Extremity Impairment (%)	Whole Person Impairment (%)
0	No objective findings	0	0
1	Mild	1–13 UEI	1–8 WPI
2	Moderate	14–25 UEI	9–15 WPI
3	Severe	26–49 UEI	16–29 WPI
4	Very Severe	50–100 UEI	30–60 WPI

UEI, Upper extremity impairment; *WPI*, whole person impairment.

the inherent limitations of a one-dimensional motion-based estimating tool by focusing on the underlying diagnosis. For example, all patients with a calcaneus fracture and residual subtalar arthritis are grouped together for the purpose of impairment determination, leading to a more uniform and ultimately fairer determination than would be possible using range-of-motion measures alone. Another advantage of diagnosis-based impairment determinations is the reduced dependence on subjective or difficult to measure variables, such as range of motion, pain, weakness, or clumsiness.

The sixth edition of the guides incorporates functional assessment tools into its impairments ratings. While other body systems and conditions have well-documented grading schemes for correlating symptom severity with impairment, the musculoskeletal system has no such well-accepted, cross-validated outcome scale. There are a number of self-reported functional assessment tools used in orthopedics. The sixth edition of the guides uses the following:

- Spine: Pain Disability Questionnaire (PDQ)
- Upper Extremity: Shorter version of the Disabilities of the Arm, Shoulder, and Hand (DASH) questionnaire—the *Quick*DASH
- Lower Extremity: Lower Limb Outcomes Questionnaire

These self-reported outcome tests can be quickly and consistently administered in a physician's office. However, because results are based on self-report, manipulation is possible. As a result, the examiner must use the tools as just a part of his or her overall evaluation.

How to Perform an Impairment Evaluation

A final impairment rating cannot be made until the patient has reached maximal medical improvement (MMI). An impairment rating will be principally based on the diagnosis. The examiner will use the history, physical examination, imaging, and laboratory results to assign the patient to an impairment class. The "key" factors are what drive the assignment to the impairment class and ultimately determine the final impairment rating. To see the Generic Template for Impairment Classification Grids, see the sixth edition of the AMA *Guides to the Evaluation of Permanent Impairment* (2008, p 13, table 1-5).

Once assigned to a class, impairment ratings are further broken down into grades (A to E). By default, the impairment is assigned to the middle grade (C) within each class. The examiner then uses the history, physical, objective studies, and self-reported outcome tests, all "nonkey factors," to adjust the grade. For example, when evaluating a patient after an intraarticular distal tibia fracture, it is noted the patient has moderate to severe motion deficits and/or moderate malalignment. These "key" factors lead to an assignment to impairment class 2, defined as loss of 14% to 25% of lower extremity function and 6% to 10% of whole person function. The default grade is to "C," however after further evaluating the physical examination, imaging studies, self-reported outcome tests, and functional history—"nonkey factors"—the patient is assigned a grade of "E," the most severe grade available within impairment class 2. The final impairment rating is class 2, grade E, leading to a lower extremity impairment (LEI) of 25% and a whole person impairment (WPI) of 10%.

Each part of the body and each diagnosis has a unique grid with its own specific modifiers and impairment calculations. The exact formulas and methodologies in calculating the impairment rating for each of these can be found in the sixth edition of the AMA guidelines. Below are some examples which will hopefully clarify the process of assigning impairment ratings for fractures.

EXAMPLE 1. A 61-year-old woman slips on a wet floor at work and sustains a comminuted proximal humerus fracture for which she undergoes hemiarthroplasty. It is determined she has reached MMI. She complains of occasional shoulder pain, which minimally interferes with ADLs. Physical examination shows nearly full range of motion and good strength of the shoulder while radiographs confirm good placement of the implant. Her *Quick*Dash score is 23.

IMPAIRMENT RATING. Per the AMA guides, a diagnosis of shoulder hemiarthroplasty with normal motion is assigned to class 2 (14% to 25% upper extremity impairment [UEI], 8% to 15% WPI). She is automatically assigned to grade C; however, her minimal complaints in performing ADLs and good score on the self-assessment test, combined with her normal physical examination and radiographs combine to move her one grade down to grade B. This leads to a final impairment rating of class 2, grade B: 17% UEI, 10% WPI.

TABLE 26-4 *DEFINITION OF IMPAIRMENT CLASSES: SPINE AND PELVIS (BASED ON WHOLE PERSON IMPAIRMENT ONLY)*

Class	Problem	Cervical Spine (%)	Thoracic Spine (%)	Lumbar Spine (%)	Pelvis (%)
0	No objective findings	0	0	0	0
1	Mild	1–8	1–6	1–9	1–3
2	Moderate	9–14	7–11	10–14	4–6
3	Severe	15–24	12–16	15–24	7–11
4	Very severe approaching total functional loss	25–30	17–22	25–33	12–16

Example 2. A 68-year-old male executive fell at work and sustained a subtrochanteric fracture of the left femur, which was treated with open reduction and internal fixation. One year postoperatively, he has returned to work and golf, but must use a cane to walk and a cart for golf, neither of which he did before the accident.

Physical examination reveals an antalgic gait and the use of a 2.5-cm shoe lift on the left side. He has a 25-degree external rotation contracture. Radiographs show a fracture that has healed with 2.2 cm of shortening.

Impairment Rating. Diagnosis of "hip fracture malunion" is assigned to class 3 and a default grade of C (30% LEI, 12% WPI). Although his history reveals little trouble with ADLs and a return to golf, his physical examination reveals some significant deficits, which are confirmed on radiograph. Together, this leads to no further adjustment. Final impairment rating: class 3, grade C: 30% LEI, 12% WPI.

Example 3. A 34-year-old male is involved in a forklift accident. He sustained a complex pelvic ring fracture-dislocation for which he undergoes open reduction and internal fixation. After he has reached MMI, he is able to rise from a sitting position and walk with a walker. He has a 4-cm leg length discrepancy.

His functional assessment reveals a PDQ score of 134 (extreme disability) and radiographs reveal a sacroiliac joint with residual displacement and residual pubic diastasis.

Impairment Rating. Pelvic ring injury with severe complications leads to an assignment to class 4 with default to grade C (14% WPI). His poor score on the self-assessment test combined with limited physical examination and poor final results on radiograph lead to an increase to grade E. Final impairment rating: class 4, grade E: 16% WPI.

The validity of the AMA guides in assessing impairment after lower extremity fractures was validated in a study by McCarthy and colleagues.[20] They evaluated 302 patients 1 year after an isolated lower extremity fracture and found a mean residual impairment of 27%. The impairment rating calculated using the AMA guide correlated strongly with the performance of functional tasks. Interestingly, the correlation was highest when the impairment rating was based on strength evaluation instead of range of motion or diagnosis-related ratings.

Impairment and Fractures

Fractures cause several kinds of permanent changes, any of which may lead to a degree of partial impairment. In previous editions of *The Guides,* each element of fracture healing was considered separately in determining the overall level of impairment caused by a given injury. Issues such as handedness, infection, malunion, nonunion, limb length inequality, and intraarticular extension of a fracture would all add some incremental percentage of increased impairment to the total value. For example, a nonunion would add 5% to the total impairment value if asymptomatic and 10% if symptomatic, no matter where it was in the body. The previous convention for dealing with leg length discrepancy was to allow 5% permanent impairment for each half inch of shortening in excess of the half inch generally considered to be normal.[21] Thus, a leg length discrepancy of 2 inches after fracture would result in 15% limb impairment on the basis of this factor alone.

The sixth edition of *The Guides* no longer considers these factors separately but in the context of the overall injury. The diagnosis is the key to determining the level of impairment. The key and nonkey factors discovered through the history, physical, clinical studies, and functional assessment tools help to assign an impairment class and then a grade within each class. Previously, the fracture sequelae mentioned earlier would add a discrete value to the overall impairment. In the current system, they often will be enough to change a grade within impairment class (C to D or E). Sometimes, they are significant enough to change from one class into a more severe one (class 3 to class 4). For example, when considering impairment after a proximal tibial shaft fracture, malunions with angulation more than 20 degrees are automatically assigned to class 3 (26% to 49% LEI). A nonunion or an infection is placed into class 4 (50% to 100% LEI). These are obviously important factors in determining the final impairment, but only in the context of the diagnosis.

PREEXISTING CONDITIONS AND APPORTIONMENT

Preexisting medical conditions need to be apportioned before assignment of a scheduled loss-of-use rating. Apportionment is the process of dividing the degree of impairment detected at the time of examination between current and prior injuries or conditions. Apportionment generally implies a preexisting condition that has been made materially or substantially worse by a second injury or illness. Numerous methods can be used to assess apportionment, and no universal standard seems to have been adopted. The AMA guides recommend subtracting the WPI established for the preexisting condition from the current impairment rating. This recommendation clearly assumes that perfect, incontrovertible data exist about the preexisting condition, a circumstance rarely encountered. In most cases, a somewhat more arbitrary division is needed.

A reasonable starting place is a 50%-50% apportionment between preexisting and current causes unless objective new data show a worsening of the condition after onset of the current injury or illness. For example, a patient with a preexisting arthritic knee and a subsequent tibial plateau fracture on the affected side with subjective complaints of worsening symptoms after the fracture warrants an apportionment of 75% to the current injury and 25% to the preexisting condition. A patient with chronic low back pain made subjectively worse after a lifting injury warrants a 50%-50% apportionment in the absence of magnetic resonance imaging, electromyographic, or radiographic evidence of a new condition. If new test findings cannot be reliably assigned to the new or old injury or illness, the 50%-50% apportionment rule should be applied. The final determination of apportionment often comes down to the guidelines of the local jurisdiction and the physician's judgment.

Neurologic Injuries

The AMA guides outline appropriate standards for evaluating combined skeletal and neurologic injuries. If the impairment in an extremity is thought to result from an injury to the spine, the impairment guide to the spine should be used, as the final impairment value of the spine diagnosis considers the loss of extremity function. Impairments caused by peripheral nerve injuries are considered separately from other causes of joint dysfunction or pain. Sensory and motor deficits are also considered separately. As central nervous system injuries often lead to complex dysfunction of multiple organ systems (neurogenic bowel and bladder, sexual dysfunction) in addition to extremity myelopathy or paralysis, the neurologic WPI should be combined with the spine injury impairment.

Complex regional pain syndrome (CRPS), an occasional sequela of fracture, is also covered separately with its own diagnostic criteria and ratings. CRPS is a challenging and controversial topic and is difficult to diagnose. Legal issues and workers' compensation further cloud the majority of these cases.[22] In order for an impairment rating to be made for the diagnosis of CRPS, strict diagnostic criteria must be met. There must be:

- Continuing pain disproportionate to any inciting event
- Sensory, vasomotor, sudomotor, and trophic changes
- Radiographic signs
- No other diagnosis that better explains the signs and symptoms

Only once these criteria are met, can the diagnosis of CRPS be made and the impairment calculated.

Spine Fractures

Individual investigators have offered various schemes for determining impairment related to spinal fracture. Miller, for example, allowed 5% WPI for lumbar compression fractures up to 25%, 10% impairment for compression of 25% to 50%, and 20% impairment for lumbar compression fractures greater than 50%. He halved these values for fractures of the thoracic spine and allowed no impairment assignment for healed compression fractures of the cervical spine unless some other factor, such as nerve injury, is present.[21,23]

The AMA offers the most widely used spine impairment guidelines. As in other areas of the body covered previously, the final impairment rating is based on the diagnosis with the key findings placing the patient into an impairment class. At this point, other elements of the history, physical examination, clinical studies, and functional assessment tools will determine the grade within each class. The key elements when assessing a patient after spinal fractures are the amount of compression (less than 25%, 25% to 50%, or greater than 50%), residual deformity, and the presence of a radiculopathy at the appropriate level. If a spine fracture results in a more serious central nervous system deficit, then that impairment must be combined with the spine fracture impairment.

SUMMARY

Establishing a fair level of permanent partial disability after fracture requires the expertise of many professionals, including the orthopaedist, social worker, and vocational and rehabilitation therapists, as well as input from the patient and third-party payer. The evaluation of permanent partial impairment is the sole responsibility of the physician; this chapter is intended to evaluate some of the factors involved in making impairment determinations. By considering all the factors that contribute to the outcome of fracture care, a level of permanent impairment can be established that is fair to the patient. This impairment rating can then be used as one factor in determining a disability rating that is fair to the patient, the third-party payer, and society in general.

KEY REFERENCES

The level of evidence (LOE) is determined according to the criteria provided in the preface.

1. Rondinelli RD: *Guides to the evaluation of permanent impairment*, ed 6, Atlanta, GA, 2008, American Medical Association. LOE V
7. Wiesel SW, Feffer HL, Rothman RH: *Industrial low back pain: a comprehensive approach*, Charlottesville, VA, 1985, The Michie Company Law Publishers. LOE V
8. Wiesel SW, Feffer HL, Rothman RH: *Neck pain*, Charlottesville, VA, 1986, The Michie Company Law Publishers. LOE V
10. American Academy of Orthopaedic Surgeons: Hospitalizations, physician visits, and emergency room visits for fractures: 1999 to 2003. <http://www.aaos.org/wordhtml/research/stats/fracture_all.htm>. Accessed February 22, 2006. LOE IV
11. National Hospital Ambulatory Medical Care Survey: 2008 Emergency department summary. <www.cdc.gov/nchs/data/ahcd/nhamcs_emergency/2008_ed_web_tables.pdf>. Accessed March 3, 2014. LOE IV
12. U.S. Department of Labor, Bureau of Labor Statistics: Nonfatal occupational injuries and illnesses and illnesses requiring days away from work, 2012, November 26, 2013. <www.bls.gov/news.release/osh2.nr0.htm>. Accessed March 3, 2014. LOE IV
13. Kessler ED: The determination of physical fitness. *JAMA* 115:1940, 1591. LOE V
14. Kessler H: *Low back pain in industry*, New York, 1955, Commerce and Industry Association of New York. LOE V
15. Kessler HH: *Disability-determination and evaluation*, Philadelphia, 1970, Lea & Febiger. LOE V
20. McCarthy ML, McAndrew MP, MacKenzie EJ, et al: Correlation between the measures of impairment, according to the modified system of the American Medical Association, and function. *J Bone Joint Surg Am* 80:1034–1042, 1998. LOE II

The complete References list is available online at https://expertconsult.inkling.com.

a single area of medicine—venous thromboembolism (VTE)—will be reviewed.

In 2001, a single year after the publication of "To Err Is Human," AHRQ published a report entitled, "Making Health Care Safer: A Critical Analysis of Patient Safety Practices."[67] The focus of this report was to report the results of evidence-based reviews of patient safety practices that *could be readily implemented* to prevent potentially avoidable events. Many of these recommended practices ultimately became the basis of National Patient Safety Goals.[67] The top five recommendations from this work are:

1. Appropriate use of prophylaxis to prevent venous thromboembolism in patients at risk
2. Use of perioperative β-blockers in appropriate patients to prevent perioperative morbidity and mortality
3. Use of maximum sterile barriers while placing central intravenous catheters to prevent infections
4. Appropriate use of antibiotic prophylaxis in surgical patients to prevent perioperative infections
5. Asking that patients recall and restate what they have been told during the informed consent process

VTE measures were developed as a result of this recommendation. The National Consensus Standards for the Prevention and Care of Deep Vein Thrombosis (DVT) project between TJC and NQF formally began in January 2005. In 2006, NQF published "National Voluntary Consensus Standards for Prevention and Care of Venous Thromboembolism: Policy, Preferred Practices, and Initial Performance Measures."[67a] The initial recommendation was to assess every adult patient admitted to the hospital for the need for VTE prophylaxis. This was an initial National Patient Safety Goal for VTE prevention. Recent data suggest the overall use of VTE prophylaxis for high-risk in patients has increased since the implementation of VTE measures.

In the following years, the adoption of VTE prophylaxis has become so widely accepted the initial VTE patient safety goal has been retired. In its place several new VTE measures have been introduced.[68] Most of the surgically relevant VTE measures are incorporated into the SCIP measures. These include:

SCIP-VTE-1: Surgery patients with recommended venous thromboembolism prophylaxis ordered

SCIP-VTE-2: Surgery patients who received appropriate venous thromboembolism prophylaxis within 24 hours prior to surgery to 24 hours after surgery

SCIP-VTE-3: Intra- or postoperative pulmonary embolism (PE) diagnosed during index hospitalization and within 30 days of surgery (OUTCOME)

SCIP-VTE-4: Intra- or postoperative deep vein thrombosis (DVT) diagnosed during index hospitalization and within 30 days of surgery (OUTCOME)

Additional VTE measures apply more generally to nonsurgical patient populations of in patients. Altom and colleagues reviewed a large administrative data set of patients to assess the SCIP-VTE measures.[69] In a sample of more than 30,000 surgery patients, 89% of cases were found to follow SCIP-VTE measures. In this study, there was not an adverse impact of following the SCIP guidelines. Further investigation is needed to understand whether following SCIP guidelines reduces the incidence of VTE events. A DVT diagnosed following an elective hip or knee arthroplasty is now considered a never event by CMS.[68] At this time DVT following musculoskeletal trauma is not considered a never event.

Moving Toward High Reliability in Healthcare Delivery

Physicians provide the direction for our patients' healthcare when the patients are in hospital or ambulatory settings of care. Yet, paradoxically, the efforts to improve the delivery of healthcare have often been driven by elements in healthcare with frequently a minimal role for physicians. As a result, many physicians in practice and in training find themselves disconnected from the changes currently happening in healthcare. There are several key areas for all physicians to become familiar with regarding improving the delivery of healthcare.[53] These are (1) understanding process improvement methods, (2) embracing the culture of patient safety, (3) engaging in leadership in your practice locations, and (4) providing value in healthcare.[53]

Process improvement uses techniques to assess the process or flow of healthcare delivery with a goal of minimizing defects or errors that reach the patient.[52] These techniques are also known as *performance management*, or *quality improvement* among other names. Frequently, this work involves efforts to minimize variability in the processes in question. Many techniques used in high-risk industries to deliver high-quality and on-time service are being considered for use in healthcare, for example, techniques such as Six Sigma to analyze multifactorial processes that apply to frequently recurring tasks with a goal of improving the outcome of the task. Lean is a technique to eliminate unnecessary steps in recurring processes to allow greater efficiency with high quality. These are often data- and time-heavy processes that are frequently driven by hospital administrations.[52] Yet these techniques are also similar to those used by most physicians as the results are similar to the prospective clinical trials we use to develop evidence-based medicine recommendations.

Many situations in healthcare do not lend themselves to techniques such as Six Sigma, and a simpler, more nimble performance improvement technique can be valuable. One of the most common tools used is the Plan, Do, Study, Act (PDSA) cycle (Fig. 27-1).[70] When implementing a new process change, the results may not meet expectations. So it is safer, and more effective to test out improvements on a small scale before implementing them on a larger scale. Using PDSA cycles enables you to test out changes before wholesale implementation and gives stakeholders the opportunity to see if the proposed change will work. As with any change, ownership is key to implementing the improvement successfully. A range of colleagues can be involved in trying a process change on a small scale before it is fully operational. This technique is simple to use for situation-specific process improvements.

For surgeons, the daily work of learning the craft of surgery is a form of process improvement. We need to be mindful of the opportunities to improve patient care and have the vocabulary and techniques to advocate for these improvements.

Surgical patient safety has become a major focus in the past decade. In a recent review, Kuo and Robb report six critical elements of surgical safety (six C's), which are based on the most frequent causes of surgical harm and error reported to TJC Sentinel Event Database.[71] These surgical safety elements are: (1) communication, (2) consent, (3) checklists, (4) confirmation, (5) concentration, and (6) collection (of data). Knowledge and regular use of these six elements in orthopaedic surgical practice address the concerns identified in the AAOS

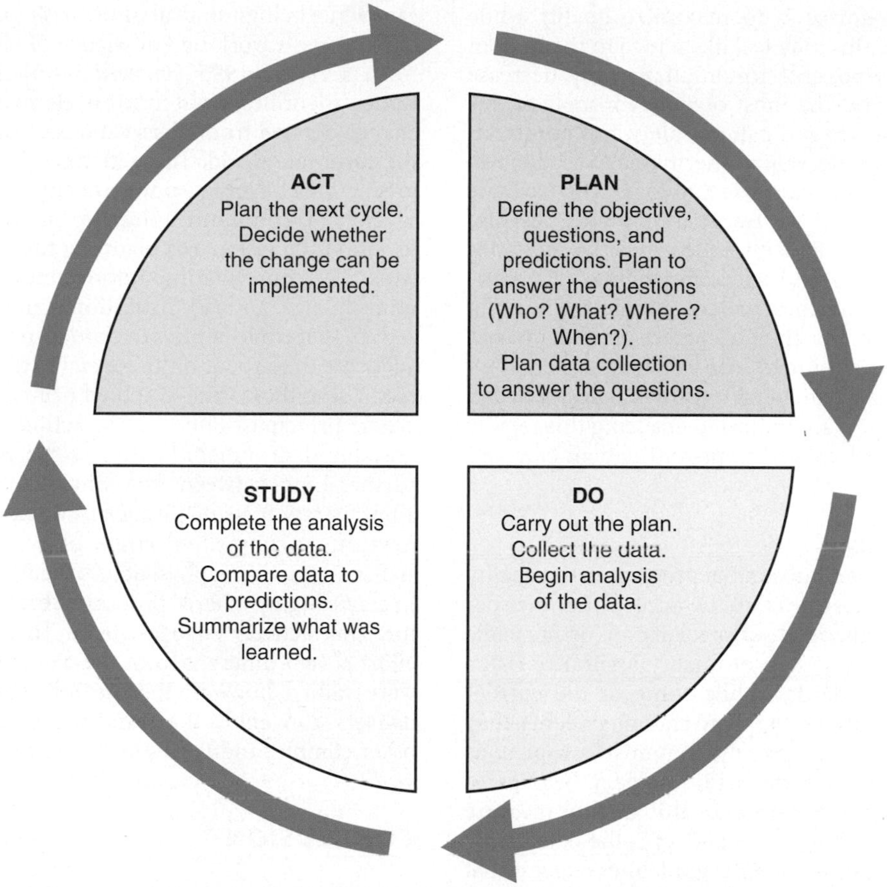

Figure 27-1. The four stages of the PDSA cycle: Plan—the change to be tested or implemented; Do—carry out the test or change; Study—interpret data before and after the change and reflect on what was learned; Act—plan the next change cycle or full implementation. *(Redrawn from UK National Health Service: Quality and service improvement tools: Plan, do, study, act (PDSA), NHS Institute for Innovation and Improvement 2008.* http://www.institute.nhs.uk/quality_and_service_improvement_tools/quality_and_service_improvement_tools/plan_do_study_act.html. *Accessed March 3, 2014. LOE V)*

2011 Surgical Safety Survey by reducing preventable surgical harm and improving orthopaedic surgical care.[71] At first, many of these elements may appear as unnecessary additions to the daily work of the surgeon. However, all of these are recommendations that have come from other industries that have learned to deliver highly reliable services or products in high-risk environments.

Poor surgical team communication can lead to unnecessary surgical harm. In one study, failures of communication in the operating room (OR) occurred in approximately 30% of team exchanges, and one-third of those failures resulted in effects that negatively impacted patient safety.[72] Similarly, poor communication is reported as an important cause of incorrect surgery.[73] Communication techniques, such as team briefings and debriefings, have improved surgical performance and safety.[74] Borrowing concepts of crew resource management from aviation, team briefings use checklists to confirm the care plan and allow for time to identify problems and knowledge gaps.

It is the role of the orthopaedic surgeon as the provider responsible for the patients' care to engage in the behaviors described by the six C's. This requires the orthopaedic surgeons to become leaders in their local environment to seek the best outcomes for our patients.[71]

Providing Value in the Delivery of Healthcare

Value-based healthcare comprises a theory and movement that has dominated healthcare reform recently including the Patient Protection and Affordable Care Act. The rising cost of healthcare for payers and patients has forced a need for greater accountability and transparency of value in healthcare. Value is defined simply as the benefit/cost of a treatment. The previous sections on quality have described in detail the numerator of this equation, both the definition and the reporting that allows transparency. Addressing the denominator requires critical evaluation of the resources we use to deliver healthcare through techniques such as cost-effectiveness analysis. Robert Kaplan and Michael Porter of Harvard Business School have highlighted the need for improvement in measuring costs before we can expect to effectively control them.[75]

Incentives to deliver value are at the center of payment reform. Episodic or bundled payments shift financial risk to the provider. This payment model is proposed to lead to greater coordination of care, reduced errors and readmissions, and more intensive management of the care pathway, all of which promise to result in cost reductions. Simultaneously, reforms such as tiering shift financial risk to the patient. This increased financial risk promises to accelerate the rise of consumerism in healthcare.

The goal of these reforms is to maximize quality while minimizing cost. While this may feel like a race to the bottom to minimize cost, it is possible to simultaneously decrease costs and increase quality. The most obvious example of this surrounds medical mistakes and patient safety, but numerous opportunities exist to create value. The increasing adoption and sophistication of information technology will facilitate innovative solutions to increase transparency and decrease the cost of providing care. Patients reflect positive opinions of both remote monitoring and teleconferencing.[76] Customized care, or care that matches patient characteristics and preferences, promises to match the correct treatment with the correct patient and eliminate low-value or unnecessary care.[77,78] Finally, physician leadership in care management and design, as well as advocacy, are critical to ensuring this rapidly evolving landscape moves toward improved patient care and superior value.

Surgeon Leadership

While recent years have seen substantial progress in the quality movement across healthcare, it could be argued that the specialty of orthopaedics and the subspecialty of orthopaedic trauma lag behind. The first step of quality assurance is the definition of quality standards. While some of the current "core measures" adopted by TJC apply to trauma patients, they do so with little specificity. Currently, the most conspicuous quality measure applied to orthopaedic surgery belongs to SCIP. While improved performance in this quality measure has been a major focus of both CMS and TJC, the data before and after the implementation of SCIP guidelines suggest that infection rates have actually increased in the total joint replacement population.[79] This finding should not serve as condemnation of the quality movement. There are numerous examples where consistently applying evidence-based care has led to dramatic improvements. Rather, this fact should serve as a reminder that quality criteria should be developed by those experienced in the field so that metrics are chosen than can improve care.[80]

It has long been acknowledged that among the myriad of complications that skeletal trauma patients are at risk for, thromboembolic disease and infection are among the most prevalent and most likely to result in significant morbidity. Despite this, guidelines and performance metrics in skeletal trauma have not been established for thromboembolic disease or infection prophylaxis. As holders of the public trust, it is the responsibility of the providers of skeletal trauma care to proactively address these issues while simultaneously being zealous advocates for existing quality and safety measures.

Establishing and expanding on a culture of safety and quality will not be easy, either nationally or locally, as this change is dependent on the collective action of many. Nationally, specialty societies will need to coalesce and become proactive in generating the evidence necessary to define "best practice." To be maximally effective, these practices should receive endorsement by recognized quality experts, such as the NQF, and hopefully consistently incorporated and measured by providers. At the local hospital level, orchestrating this change will also be difficult, as it requires careful nurturing of a culture of safety and high reliability. Taking an analogy from the corporate world, change initiatives of this magnitude fail to produce long-lasting change 80% of the time.[81] Recognizing the immense opportunity to improve the quality of trauma care while being mindful of this risk of failure should prompt one to have a working knowledge of change management.

In a classic 1995 *Harvard Business Review* article, John Kotter identifies eight critical elements to creating lasting change derived from observations of successes and failures in the corporate world. These include (1) establishing a sense of urgency, (2) forming a powerful guiding coalition, (3) creating a vision, (4) communicating the vision, (5) empowering others to act on the vision, (6) planning for and creating short-term wins, (7) consolidating improvements and producing still more change, and (8) institutionalizing new approaches.[82] He argues, that while failures in change management are common, adequate time spent on these eight steps largely mitigates this risk. Using these time-accepted principles IHI modified these classic principles into specific action items applicable to the hospital environment.[83] These steps include forming strong partnerships between key physician leaders and hospital administration, using physician champions to create and communicate a compelling vision of quality within the medical staff, and providing physicians the authority and responsibility to create highly reliable processes through a governance structure that actively engages them. This world of collaborative effort is very different from the one in which most physicians were trained; however, it is the only world in which healthcare delivery can enjoy the same degree of high reliability that other complex industries have realized.

CONCLUSION

In the last half century, the field of outcome measurement has evolved even more rapidly than the field of medicine itself. Rapidly changing from a dissemination of objective physical findings, patient-oriented measures now focus more heavily on the perceptions of the true customer—the patient. Scaling this focus on patient-centered outcomes has appropriately brought attention to the processes that support our care delivery. The changes necessary to transform healthcare into a highly reliable industry will not be accomplished without careful navigation of the change process by physicians heavily engaged in that vision.

KEY REFERENCES

The level of evidence (LOE) is determined according to the criteria provided in the preface.

11. Martin DP, Engelberg R, Agel J, et al: Comparison of the Musculoskeletal Function Assessment questionnaire with the Short Form-36, the Western Ontario and McMaster Universities Osteoarthritis Index, and the Sickness Impact Profile health-status measures. *J Bone Joint Surg Am* 79(9):1323–1335, 1997. LOE III
13. Dias JJ, Rajan RA, Thompson JR: Which questionnaire is best? The reliability, validity and ease of use of the Patient Evaluation Measure, the Disabilities of the Arm, Shoulder and Hand and the Michigan Hand Outcome Measure. *J Hand Surg Eur Vol* 33(1):9–17, 2008. doi: 0.1177/1753193407087121. PubMed PMID: 18332014. LOE III
28. Bergner M, Bobbitt RA, Kressel S, et al: The Sickness Impact Profile: conceptual formulation and methodology for the development of a health status measure. *Int J Health Serv* 6(3):393–415, 1976. LOE IV
29. Bergner M, Bobbitt RA, Pollard WE, et al: The Sickness Impact Profile: validation of a health status measure. *Med Care* 14:57–67, 1976. LOE IV
40. Castillo RC, MacKenzie EJ, Bosse MJ: Measurement of functional outcomes in the Major Extremity Trauma Research Consortium (METRC). *J Am Acad Orthop Surg* 20:S59–S63, 2012. LOE V
43. Brauer CA, Manns BJ, Ko M, et al: An economic evaluation of operative compared with nonoperative management of displaced intra-articular

calcaneal fractures. *J Bone Joint Surg Am* 87(12):2741–2749, 2005. LOE III
46. MacKenzie EJ, Jones AS, Bosse MJ, et al: Health-care costs associated with amputation or reconstruction of a limb-threatening injury. *J Bone Joint Surg Am* 89(8):1685–1692, 2007. LOE III
53. Chassin MR, Loeb JM: The ongoing quality improvement journey: next stop, high reliability. *Health Aff (Millwood)* 30(4):559–568, 2011. LOE V
59. Kohn LT, Corrigan J, Donaldson MS: *To err is human: building a safer health system*, Washington, D.C., 2000, National Academy Press, xxi, p 287. LOE III
71. Kuo CC, Robb WJ 3rd: Critical roles of orthopaedic surgeon leadership in healthcare systems to improve orthopaedic surgical patient safety. *Clin Orthop Relat Res* 471(6):1792–1800, 2013. LOE V
72. Lingard L, Espin S, Whyte S, et al: Communication failures in the operating room: an observational classification of recurrent types and effects. *Qual Saf Health Care* 13(5):330–334, 2004. LOE III

The complete References list is available online at https://expertconsult.inkling.com.

Chapter 28

Professionalism and the Economics of Orthopaedic Trauma Care

DOUGLAS R. DIRSCHL

INTRODUCTION

The practice of medicine is fundamentally and historically based in service; whether service to patients, service to communities, service to society, or service to one's partners and colleagues, the professional lives of physicians are linked to service. The professional lives of those doing orthopaedic fracture care are even more closely aligned to service, as the individuals treated have sustained painful injuries that cannot be scheduled or predicted. As such, the services of the orthopaedic fracture specialist also cannot always be scheduled or predicted, inculcating these individuals with an even higher service expectation than in many of their colleagues.

Whether written or unwritten, professional service is governed and shaped by contractual relationships. This chapter provides information on and explores three such relationships: that between an orthopaedic surgeon and his or her hospital and community related to providing orthopaedic care in the hospital emergency department; that between the medical profession and the federal government regarding obligations for the emergency medical treatment of patients; and that between an orthopaedic fracture surgeon and his or her group or hospital regarding the economic value of orthopaedic fracture care. While these three topics may seem unrelated, they are actually highly related, as all are matters of great importance to those in the practice of orthopaedic fracture care, all require knowledge that goes beyond the medical training received in residency and fellowship, and all involve relationships with colleagues, hospitals, and insurers. Understanding the issues, facts, perspectives, and considerations—from the perspectives of all involved in these matters—will better prepare orthopaedic fracture surgeons for a successful career and healthier relationships with their colleagues, hospitals, communities, and payers.

THE "ON-CALL" CONTROVERSY

Patients visiting a hospital emergency department (ED) expect to have 24-hour access to prompt, appropriate, and effective emergency musculoskeletal care. When local musculoskeletal care is "not available," patients are asked to go to (or are transferred to) another, often distant, location to receive care. When the care needed by the patient requires specialized expertise unavailable at the presenting hospital, the transfer of care is medically appropriate. Frequently, however, transfers occur for conditions that many would consider to be "routine" musculoskeletal conditions.

In a survey conducted by the American College of Emergency Physicians, three-quarters of ED medical directors reported that their hospitals have inadequate on-call specialist coverage.[1] In another survey, 42% of ED administrators felt that the lack of specialty coverage in the ED posed a significant risk to patients.[2] Providing care on an on call basis in a hospital ED has become unattractive to many specialists in critical disciplines, including orthopaedics.[3] Traditionally, ED call coverage was seen as an integral part of the profession of orthopaedic surgery. Orthopaedic surgeons were obligated, by hospital bylaws, to cover the ED for after-hours orthopaedic care; this coverage served the community and also provided a stream of patients for the orthopaedists' practices.

Subspecialization, the increased use of freestanding outpatient surgery centers, and managed care are among the factors that interrupted this traditional relationship. Subspecialty orthopaedic surgeons (e.g., hand, foot and ankle) have increasingly focused (and perhaps limited) their practices to their subspecialty area. Additionally, they perform the majority of their procedures in outpatient facilities that are often freestanding. Many of these individuals do not feel they require hospital privileges, as their patients rarely require hospitalization. With no hospital privileges, there is no need to meet the on-call obligations required of medical staff members. Additionally, their practices, being almost entirely elective and/or referral, do not rely heavily on the ED for patient referrals. Finally, many of these orthopaedists would argue that their subspecialty focus has resulted in them being "uncomfortable" treating orthopaedic injuries and conditions outside of their area of specialty; the hand surgeon might feel uncomfortable treating an ankle fracture or the total joint surgeon treating a distal radial fracture. The lack of reliance on a hospital setting allows these subspecialty orthopaedic surgeons to opt out of call responsibilities.

Without routine practice in the ED setting, the necessary skills to treat musculoskeletal conditions presenting in this setting do become less familiar to the orthopaedic surgeon, and it is true that the variety of musculoskeletal injuries seen in the ED is large. While the definitive surgical treatment, for example, of an anterior cruciate ligament (ACL) injury may be beyond the scope of practice of a total joint surgeon or of a proximal humeral fracture may be beyond the scope of practice for a foot and ankle surgeon, most musculoskeletal injuries do not require surgical treatment at all and almost none require emergent surgical care. The assessment and management of the vast majority of musculoskeletal injuries are required areas of education and skill development for all orthopaedic residency programs. Thus, the evaluation and initial bracing of the ACL injury, and the evaluation and initial splinting of the proximal humeral fracture should be within the skill sets of all those who have completed orthopaedic training. Because all board certified orthopaedic surgeons must demonstrate competence in the management of most urgent musculoskeletal conditions, it seems more likely that the problem of local ED access to orthopaedic care for simple injuries and to temporizing care for more serious injuries is more related to a lack of interest, rather than a lack of competence, on the part of the orthopaedic surgeons.

Many orthopaedists today are unwilling to provide ED coverage, citing conflicts with personal time and concerns about a reimbursement system that provides little or no compensation.[4] Managed care—particularly health maintenance organization (HMO) products and other so-called narrow networks—has altered the on-call relationship by insisting that patients receive specialty care from a narrow network of providers credentialed with that managed care plan. While these patients can generally obtain emergency care anywhere, they are required to see an in-network provider for any elective or semielective care; failure to do so results in increased out-of-pocket costs to the patient. An orthopaedic surgeon on call could be faced with a scenario where the patient for whom he or she is consulted for an ankle fracture requiring surgery is permitted to have a reduction and splinting performed in the ED by the on-call orthopaedist, yet might need to visit another orthopaedist for the surgery. These sorts of managed care relationships effectively reduced the stream of patients coming to one's practice from being on call for the ED. In many communities, orthopaedic surgeons became more reluctant to take call on this basis, arguing that the hassles and effort involved in call were not worth it if the definitive patient care was directed elsewhere by the managed care company.

Even among those orthopaedic surgeons interested in participating in ED call, the financial ramifications of doing so can create barriers. Appropriately capturing charges for care provided in the ED is not as easy as that delivered in one's office or in the operating room. In the office or the operating room (OR), most surgeons have an infrastructure that assists them in appropriate charge capture and coding, but surgeons typically lack such infrastructure for work they do in providing consultations and procedural care in the ED; it requires more organizational skill and attention to detail for surgeons to appropriately capture these billings than those from the office or the OR. Collecting payment for services provided in the ED may also be difficult, as emergency and trauma patients are more often uninsured than those seen in the office.[5] Additionally, the capture of accurate and appropriate insurance information from patients seen in the ED may or may not occur well; if these patients do not follow up in the surgeon's office, there may be no additional opportunity to obtain this information for appropriate billing. The argument can also be made that, in many cases, the orthopaedist is not only inadequately compensated for providing services in the ED, but also suffers financially by the ED patients—who are more likely to be uninsured—taking up follow-up appointment slots in the office, when these slots would have otherwise been filled by other patients from whom reimbursement might be received.

Perceptions and expectations for work–life balance have also changed the environment surrounding orthopaedic surgeons being on call. This is particularly true in smaller communities, which may have only a few orthopaedic surgeons on the hospital's medical staff. In past generations, being on call every third or fourth night was not unusual in these communities and was an expected part of being in the profession. This has changed, however, with physicians in all specialties (including orthopaedics) placing greater value on protecting personal and family time and being unwilling to be on call so frequently. This has left many smaller community hospitals in a conundrum: They do not have enough orthopaedic surgeons to provide full on-call coverage with a sustainable schedule, yet they do not have enough orthopaedic business in the community to attract enough orthopaedic surgeons to create a sustainable call schedule. Although some hospitals in such situations have found ways to maintain full coverage (payments for coverage, contracting with other groups, etc.), some have simply resigned themselves to the fact that they may not have 24/7 orthopaedic coverage for their ED.

Contributing to the problems associated with on-call trauma coverage by orthopaedic surgeons is what some have termed "the ongoing medical liability crisis."[6,7] The current liability system neither effectively compensates persons injured from medical negligence nor addresses system errors that, if corrected, could greatly improve patient safety and decrease medical errors. The current medical liability environment has had an adverse effect on those physicians willing to engage in high-risk situations, such as providing emergency care, and has served as a barrier for some who would provide emergency care in a different medicolegal environment.[8,9] In addition, liability risks are increased during the on-call hours because of the seriousness of the patient's emergency condition, in combination with streamlined after-hours staffing in most hospitals, decreased availability of specialized equipment and personnel, and fatigue associated with long working hours.

The lack of available and affordable medical liability insurance has led many physicians to change their practice patterns in ways that they believe decreases their liability exposure; this includes, for some, opting out of providing on-call services to an ED. All physicians have been affected by the medical liability crisis, but "high-risk" specialties (e.g., obstetrics, neurosurgery, and orthopaedic surgery) have been disproportionately affected.[10] This has, in many communities, forced patients to travel greater distances and wait longer to obtain care from these specialty services. Between 2003 and 2004, double- and triple-digit increases in medical liability premiums were seen across the country.[11] While liability rates stabilized to some extent between 2006 and 2008, the premiums remain exorbitant. Thus, declining payments from all sources, an increasing burden of uncompensated ED care, considerable medical liability costs, and the availability of new practice patterns are draining the pool of orthopaedic specialists willing and able to take ED call.

Adding to the complexity of the issues affecting surgeons willing to participate in ED call are a variety of "rumors" or misinformation. There are numerous commonly held misconceptions regarding the risk one assumes when caring for orthopaedic injuries in an ED setting.[12] Unfortunately, these misconceptions are widely held and are used to fuel the arguments for orthopaedic surgeons opting out of ED coverage, call, and caring for injured patients in the ED.

- *The uninsured are more likely to sue:* This is perhaps the largest myth, which is substantiated by the fact that some commercial malpractice insurance carriers advise physicians that their insurance premiums will decrease if the physicians will cease taking ED call.[13] A 1995 survey of physicians in California revealed that the majority did not treat Medicaid or uninsured patients because of the perceived risk of a lawsuit.[5] Burstin and colleagues, however, demonstrated on a review of claims in New York that the poor, young, and elderly are least likely to sue orthopaedic surgeons.[6] Medicare and Medicaid patients have also been shown to be less likely to sue than the general population,[14] and settlements when suits have been filed have been demonstrated to be 5 to 10 times greater for non-Medicaid insured patients.[15] A report by McClellan and colleagues also supports the finding that the uninsured are less likely to sue than are insured patients, possibly because they do not have easy access to legal representation.[16]

- *Trauma patients are more likely to sue their surgeon for their injuries:* The genesis of this misconception lay in the fact that many injured patients may be involved in litigation related to their injury and the treating surgeon may be called on to describe the patient's injuries, treatment, and prognosis, or even to serve as an independent medical expert. It is true that 5 of the 10 most prevalent orthopaedic conditions resulting in litigation are fractures.[17] However, most of these are claims for gross technical errors or failure to diagnose, and the rate of closed claims in these cases is lower than that in obstetrics-gynecology, family practice, and general surgery. In a review of 1452 closed malpractice claims, Studdert and colleagues found that 63% involved clear medical errors, and that 72% of patients with iatrogenic injury but no errors in judgment did not receive any monetary settlement.[18]
- *Unless they are experts in the patient's condition, surgeons will likely not meet the standard of care*: Although the term is mentioned frequently, most physicians poorly understand the term "standard of care." The legal definition of this term is "the level of care, skill, and treatment that, under the circumstances, is recognized as acceptable and appropriate by reasonably prudent similar healthcare providers."[19,20] The term is not intended to specify a single appropriate treatment in any given situation, but a range of treatments that are considered acceptable in the community and the setting in which the patient seeks care. The definition allows for variation by location and degree of training and experience; the level of care expected of an orthopaedic resident is different than that expected of an experienced surgeon, and that of a rural community orthopaedist is different than that of an urban trauma specialist.

The obstacles to achieving a successful plan for ED coverage by orthopaedists and orthopaedic subspecialties are daunting. Solutions must be tailor-made to meet the needs and optimize the resources of individual communities. The American Orthopaedic Association (AOA) recognized the significant crisis that exists in the provision of emergency musculoskeletal care. To uphold its commitment to patient access to high quality care and serve in a leadership capacity for the profession, the AOA established a Task Force on Emergency Department Call Coverage in 2008 under the aegis of its Orthopaedic Institute of Medicine (OIOM) to review the scope of this crisis, identify barriers impacting orthopaedic coverage in EDs across the United States, and propose solutions that can be adopted at the community level.

Based on survey results, peer-reviewed literature, expert opinion, and Task Force consensus, the following barriers to ED call coverage emerged: lifestyle and time away from family; poor reimbursement; increased liability risk; medical practice issues (e.g., disruption of elective practice, lack of inpatient practice); lack of comfort with skills needed for ED cases; and inadequacies of hospital emergency care resources. The Task Force felt that these barriers impact social, professional, and financial aspects of our current system and would require change at many levels to solve the problem and improve patient access to these services. Recommendations from the Task Force address these barriers with potential solutions, emphasize that most solutions must be individualized at the local level, and provide examples of a variety of solutions that have been successful in some communities.

The Task Force generated the following summary consensus statement:

Orthopaedic surgeons are ultimately the most qualified, capable, and cost-effective providers of musculoskeletal care. To help resolve the looming crisis in orthopaedic ED call coverage, the Orthopaedic Institute of Medicine Council recommends that in each community in the [United States], orthopaedic surgeons partner with hospitals and other stakeholders to discuss the issues, identify specific problems and local resources, and implement a solution that will ensure access for all patients to appropriate high quality emergency care for most musculoskeletal conditions. The solution in each community will be unique and determined by the identified issues that must be overcome in that community's medical environment. Modifications are also needed at the state, regional, and national levels to assist in removing barriers that are presently challenging access to emergency musculoskeletal care in many communities.[21]

The Task Force went on to recommend that solutions and alterations be enacted in eight key areas[21]:

1. *Delivery of Emergency Care:* Communities should ensure all patients have access to readily available orthopaedic surgical consultation in the ED by creating community-wide teams to assess needs for local services, and recommend and champion the solutions.
2. *Physician Leadership:* All orthopaedic surgeons should acknowledge a professional obligation to ensure that there is a system in their community to enable all patients to have access to timely and appropriate emergency musculoskeletal care. Orthopaedic professional organizations can support this goal by establishing professional guidelines specific to patient access to emergency musculoskeletal care.
3. *Education and Core Competency:* The orthopaedic profession should define core competences for the initial management of urgent and emergent musculoskeletal conditions and propose methods for maintaining these core competencies. The profession should continue to define minimal criteria for musculoskeletal emergency care and community care of transfers.
4. *Hospital Resources for Orthopaedic Emergency Care:* Hospitals should provide dedicated daily OR time for the management of musculoskeletal emergency cases

patient
EMTA
2. Physic
partic
on sele
on-call
patient
violatio
3. Physic
cannot
4. A recei
fer (i.e.
of care
transfe
transfe
the tra
EMTA
denied
capacit
EMTAL

The EMTA
institution ca
tion "after th
and involved
however, no
the EMTALA
that the EMT
tals and tha
advised to sir
with orthopa
is clearly lack

ECONOMI TRAUMA

Orthopaedic
than nearly al
within a mec
orthopaedic s
ing their relia
matologist ha
entities. The
and the hosp
depends, to a
surgeon, whic
private practi
hospital empl
contributes to
of orthopaed
obtain differe
solely to the
practice, that
or that of the

The financ
tologist on a
mented by Alt
that the additi
cially benefici
32% for the ex
gist, despite p
call. In this an

Chapter 29

*Psychological, Social, and Functional Manifestations of Orthopaedic Trauma and Traumatic Brain Injury**

PAUL E. LEVIN • ELLEN J. MACKENZIE • MICHAEL J. ROY • MICHAEL J. BOSSE • GEOFFREY S. F. LING

INTRODUCTION

Psychological stress is a normal human emotion associated with any disease. Most individuals confronting a diagnosis of a new disease are able to understand, accept, and move forward. Their ability to do this requires personal inner resources, as well as the support and understanding of their physicians, families, friends, and society. Musculoskeletal injuries often create a gamut of anxiety and fears related to future function and ability to remain active in everyday life. Among the many concerns are disabilities secondary to loss of a limb and unrepairable musculoskeletal injury, disfigurement secondary to the musculoskeletal injury, distress over finances and the ability to return to work, concerns about sexual function, and the ability to return to recreational activities. Patients frequently recover from the musculoskeletal injury uneventfully, but may never recover from the psychological comorbidity. Clinicians and researchers have considered psychological and physical injuries as distinct entities, but there is considerable evidence, both from military and civilian populations, that recovery from physical injuries is dramatically and adversely influenced by the presence of a variety of psychological and social comorbidities including depression, posttraumatic stress disorder (PTSD), or other psychiatric conditions.

It has become increasingly clear that as orthopaedic surgeons we must find a way to address the psychosocial needs of the patient and family so that we can do a better job of preventing a permanent disability and returning an individual to a fully functional member of society. Learning to actively seek out the concerns of our patients and families and validating and normalizing the common emotions associated with musculoskeletal injury creates a healthier psychological and social environment to assist recovery. Levin describes his daughter's fear of being able to ski again after major musculoskeletal trauma.[1] The fear, which was evident in his daughter's mood, was only identified by inquiring why she appeared concerned. She expressed a fear that she would never be able to ski again and her mood immediately improved when it was predicted that she would definitely be able to ski. Active involvement of a patient's family and friends during and after the hospitalization fills in the imperative psychosocial support that can only be supplied by an individual's "loved ones," and the orthopaedic surgeon should both encourage this involvement and guide the family in how they can be supportive.

The orthopaedic surgeon needs to be aware of numerous psychological and social sequelae associated with musculoskeletal injury, be able to recognize the symptoms and identify patients and family members in need of help from a professional mental health provider. This chapter will review our present understanding of the psychosocial comorbidities that are associated with musculoskeletal trauma and how these disorders can prevent a successful functional recovery from trauma. We will review the present state of our understanding of these common psychological comorbidities and strategies to treat these conditions, with particular attention paid to the role of the orthopaedic surgeon.

BIOMEDICAL VERSUS BIOPSYCHOSOCIAL MODEL OF MEDICINE

The biomedical model of disease is based on a generally accepted belief among both patients and physicians that symptomatology (pain, general malaise, fever, etc.) is related to an identifiable chemical, physiologic, or structural abnormality that may or may not be correctable. Initially, when a patient presents with acute orthopaedic trauma, this is a relatively straightforward exercise. The patient has a grade IIIB open tibia fracture and we are going to "cure" him or her by placing an intramedullary rod in his or her tibia and performing a gastrocnemius rotation flap and a split-thickness skin graft (STSG). Unfortunately, we have learned from the Lower Extremity Assessment Project (LEAP) and other studies, that individuals with seemingly similar musculoskeletal injuries can have very disparate recoveries.[2] We see the potential for disparate recovery among individuals with both severe as well as less severe injuries.

*The views expressed herein are solely the views of the authors and do not necessarily represent those of Uniformed Services University of the Health Sciences, the Department of Defense (DoD), or the U.S. government.

This observed dichotomy of successful treatment of an individual's disease (fracture) and recovery led Engel to the introduction of the biopsychosocial model and practice of medicine.[3-5] Engel believed that the biomedical model failed to recognize each patient's individuality and humanity. He observed that a patient's personality (individuality) along with the patient's social support structure dramatically affected recovery. We frequently discuss this philosophy when we acknowledge that the practice of medicine is "art not science." Clearly, science and scientific discovery comprise a major component in our dramatic successes in caring for the multiply injured patient. Despite this success, the failure to recognize human emotion and individuality can have a devastating effect on a person's recovery.

In the discussion that follows, we will focus on posttraumatic stress and depression, two common conditions that are associated with the aftermath of physical trauma. It is important to keep in mind, however, that most patients will not be diagnosed with either of these conditions, even in the face of significant physical injuries. However, studies have shown that even subclinical symptoms of emotional stress and anxiety, if not adequately addressed, can impact recovery. We will also review our rapidly expanding understanding of both mild traumatic brain injury (mTBI) and more extensive traumatic brain injury (TBI), which often accompany skeletal injury, especially in the military. It is important for the orthopaedic surgeon to understand how TBI can impact the functional recovery of their patients.

ANXIETY DISORDERS AND POSTTRAUMATIC STRESS

Acute anxiety symptoms are common following a physical injury and acute stress disorder (ASD) is among the first forms of psychological pathology diagnosable postinjury. It is characterized by a sense of numbing or detachment, restlessness, anxiety, irritability, problems focusing or concentrating, flashbacks, and sleep disturbance.[6] ASD is typically considered a short-term response to injury, with symptoms lasting between 2 and 30 days. A recent review of the literature found that signs and symptoms of ASD occurred in 23% to 45% of patents following physical trauma.[7]

The anxiety disorder spectrum includes generalized anxiety disorder (GAD), panic disorder with and without agoraphobia, PTSD, obsessive-compulsive disorder (OCD), social anxiety disorder, and specific phobias. Of these, GAD, panic disorder, and PTSD are most likely to be related to physical injury. Overall, anxiety disorders are perhaps even more common than depression, and total direct and indirect costs are similar to those associated with depression.

Generalized Anxiety Disorder and Panic Disorder

GAD has a prevalence of 4% to 6%.[8] The disorder features excessive anxiety and worry about a variety of events or activities over at least a 6-month period; difficulty exercising control over worrying; several symptoms associated with the anxiety, such as fatigue, irritability, restlessness, sleep disturbance, and difficulty concentrating; functional impairment; and the symptoms are not explained by the presence of another axis I disorder, another medical condition, or medication. GAD can be easily screened for, either by asking, "Are you bothered by nerves?," which had 100% sensitivity and 59% specificity in a study of primary care patients,[9] or with the two-item Generalized Anxiety Disorder scale (GAD-2). The GAD-2 had a sensitivity of 86% and specificity of 83% when using a cutoff score of 3, faring about as well as a GAD seven-item scale. Increasing its utility to the primary care physician, the GAD-2 is also effective at identifying other anxiety disorders: Using a cutoff of 2, its sensitivity was 91% for panic, 85% for social anxiety, 86% for PTSD, and 86% for any anxiety disorder.[10] The GAD-2 was recently combined with the two highly sensitive screening questions for depression regarding anhedonia and feeling down, depressed, or hopeless. The composite instrument, the four-item Patient Health Questionnaire (PHQ-4), was validated in more than 2000 primary care patients, and demonstrated a strong correlation with functional status, disability days, and health care utilization (Table 29-1).[11]

TABLE 29-1 *GAD-2 SCREEN FOR GENERALIZED ANXIETY DISORDER*

During the past month, have you been bothered a lot by:	
1. Nerves or feeling anxious or on edge?	
a. Not at all	(0)
b. Several days	(1)
c. More than half the days	(2)
d. Nearly every day	(3)
2. Worrying about a lot of different things?	
a. Not at all	(0)
b. Several days	(1)
c. More than half the days	(2)
d. Nearly every day	(3)

GAD-2, Two-item Generalized Anxiety Disorder scale.

Panic disorder can be one of the most frustrating of all medical conditions, with the average patient having been seen by many physicians and having had extensive testing including repeated "rule outs" for myocardial infarctions, Holter monitors, and invasive assessments, such as cardiac catheterization and esophagogastroduodenoscopy. In fact, panic disorder is associated with the highest utilization rates of medical services of all mental health problems. However, on identification of the correct diagnosis and initiation of effective treatment, these patients are often most amenable to successful treatment. Panic disorder is characterized by recurrent, unexpected panic attacks, which feature the abrupt onset of numerous somatic symptoms such as palpitations, sweating, tremulousness, dyspnea, chest pain, nausea, dizziness, and numbness. Symptoms typically peak within 10 minutes of onset and attacks usually have duration from 15 to 60 minutes. While as many as 30% of Americans may experience a panic attack during their lifetime, the prevalence of panic disorder is only 1% to 2%, as its diagnosis also requires that one or more of the attacks be followed by at least a month of persistent worry about having another attack, about the implications of the attack or its consequences, or a significant change in behavior related to the attacks.[12] Up to half of those with panic disorder also have agoraphobia, characterized by a fear of being in places from which escape might be difficult (e.g., in crowds, on a train or plane, on a bridge or in a tunnel). Individuals with agoraphobia either avoid such situations, or endure them with marked distress, even experiencing symptoms of panic.

Comorbid medical and/or psychiatric conditions are present in most patients with GAD. Panic disorder frequently coexists with major depression, GAD, PTSD, and/or other psychiatric disorders. GAD and panic disorders should be considered as primary diagnoses in the initial consideration of differential diagnoses, but the history and physical examination should also include consideration of hyperthyroidism, pheochromocytoma, Cushing syndrome, insulinoma, anemia, asthma or vocal cord dyskinesia, and cardiac conditions such as angina, mitral valve prolapse and atrial fibrillation or another arrhythmia, which all can mimic anxiety and panic disorders. Accordingly, symptoms that should be asked about, and carefully reviewed when present, include weight loss, heat intolerance, diaphoresis, headaches, lightheadedness, chest pain, palpitations, and dyspnea. Caffeine intake, as well as ingestion of drugs of abuse such as cocaine or amphetamines, should be assessed. Key physical examination elements include the vital signs, eye examination including an assessment of extrinsic ocular muscles and for exophthalmos, thyroid examination with a check for a bruit, cardiac and pulmonary examination, and assessment of the hair and skin. Laboratory testing need not be extensive—it should be guided by the findings on history and physical—but a complete blood count, serum chemistry panel, thyroid function tests, urinalysis, and electrocardiogram are prudent. Additional studies should not be routine, but may be necessary to rule out differential diagnoses depending on the presenting signs and symptoms.

Effective therapies are available for both GAD and panic disorder. Cognitive behavioral therapy (CBT) is the best evidenced nonpharmacologic therapy for these conditions, supported by many randomized controlled trials and several meta-analyses.[13,14] Several recent studies provide evidence that relatively brief courses of CBT, or even self-help CBT, is effective for GAD and panic disorder.[15-17] CBT seems to have a more durable effect, with lower relapse rates than pharmacologic therapy, and use of CBT in patients who failed pharmacologic therapy also showed significant efficacy.[18] However, there is good evidence that selective serotonin reuptake inhibitors (SSRIs) as well as venlafaxine are far superior to placebo in the treatment of both GAD and panic disorder, while pregabalin is also effective for GAD, and corresponding recommendations were recently made by an expert panel.[19] Among the anxiety spectrum disorders, there is stronger evidence that the combination of CBT and pharmacotherapy is superior to either alone for panic disorder, although there has been more recent evidence to suggest this may be a worthwhile approach for GAD as well.[13,20-22] Second-line therapies have been shown to have some utility but all have drawbacks, including tricyclic antidepressants such as imipramine (risk of fatal cardiac arrhythmias in overdose, as well as anticholinergic side effects), benzodiazepines (dependence and tolerance issues), and azaspirones such as buspirone (less compelling evidence, and relatively delayed onset of action).

Posttraumatic Stress Disorder (PTSD)

PTSD is unique among the anxiety disorders because it has a clear precipitant—exposure to a traumatic event, such as an industrial injury, motor vehicle or recreational accident, war, disaster, or an assault that involves an actual or threatened death or serious injury to one's self or others. PTSD is sometimes, but not always, preceded by acute stress disorder (ASD). ASD is characterized by symptoms that occur within 30 days of a traumatic experience, and when present, is not surprisingly associated with a higher risk of subsequent PTSD, with one study indicating that 78% of persons with ASD following a motor vehicle crash (MVC) met criteria for PTSD within 6 months.[23] The criteria for PTSD include disabling symptoms for at least 1 month in three different categories: reexperiencing the trauma (e.g., flashbacks, intrusive memories); avoiding thoughts, activities, people associated with the trauma (i.e., feeling emotionally "numb" about the traumatic event); and hyperarousal (e.g., irritability, difficulty concentrating, insomnia). PTSD was codified in the aftermath of the Vietnam War, but the symptoms and associated functional impairment it represents have been known for centuries. Homer depicts symptoms of this disorder in his account of Achilles in *The Iliad*, and hundreds of reports have appeared in the medical literature from the U.S. Civil War, both World Wars, and numerous other national and international conflicts. Most recently, PTSD has been well documented after the terrorist attacks of September 11, 2001,[24,25] Hurricane Katrina, and the wars in Iraq and Afghanistan.[26]

Although a majority of the general population has experienced trauma sufficient to induce PTSD, most of the exposed are resilient, so that the overall likelihood of developing PTSD after a traumatic event is estimated at 9% to 25%.[27-29] Community surveys identify a 2% to 5% point prevalence and an 8% to 12% lifetime prevalence for PTSD.[30-33] PTSD was documented in 39% of patients referred by their primary care providers for mental health services based on suspicion of depression or anxiety, but like most psychological disorders, PTSD often goes undiagnosed in primary care, and such patients often do not see mental health specialists.[34,35]

The gold standard instrument for the diagnosis of PTSD is the Clinician-Administered PTSD Scale (CAPS), but it is 17 pages long and must be administered by a professional, rendering it impractical for use in primary care.[36,37] The PTSD Checklist (PCL) is a 17-item screen, which can be self-administered (see Appendix, available online) and has had moderately good sensitivity and specificity,[38-40] but a newer, 4-item screen, the Primary Care PTSD (PC-PTSD), has fared at least as well in some studies,[41] using a cutoff of two or more positive replies (Table 29-2).

There have been several reports describing the prevalence of PTSD among persons who suffered physical injuries, in both military and civilian trauma populations. Rates vary considerably because of differences in how PTSD is measured, when it is measured, and the population being studied. Among

TABLE 29-2 *PC-PTSD*

Have you ever had any experience that was so frightening, horrible, or upsetting, that in the past month you:		
1. Have had nightmares about it or thought about it when you did not want to?	YES___	NO___
2. Tried hard not to think about it or went out of your way to avoid situations that remind you of it?	YES___	NO___
3. Were constantly on guard, watchful, or easily startled?	YES___	NO___
4. Felt numb or detached from others, activities, or your surroundings?	YES___	NO___

PC-PTSD, Primary Care–Posttraumatic Stress Disorder screen.

civilians, rates of PTSD following an MVC range from 6% to 54% (based on 51 prevalence estimates across 35 studies).[42] The National Study on the Costs and Outcomes of Trauma (NSCOT)[43] examined 1-year outcomes in 2707 trauma patients admitted to 69 hospitals across 12 states and found that 20.7% of patients with at least one injury with an Abbreviated Injury Scale (AIS) score of 3 or greater (associated with any injury mechanism) screened positive for PTSD (based on the PCL).[40] Relatively few studies have focused specifically on the prevalence of PTSD associated with musculoskeletal trauma.[44] In one of the more comprehensive of these studies, Starr[45] reported that 51% of 580 orthopaedic trauma patients admitted to two level I trauma centers met the criteria for the diagnosis of PTSD based on the revised Civilian Mississippi Scale for PTSD (measured at an average of 12 months postinjury).[46] The severity of injury does not appear to predict the development of PTSD. However, the type of trauma (e.g., physical assault vs. unintentional injury) as well as prior exposure to previous traumatic events has been shown to correlate with a higher likelihood of PTSD. Also, women are generally at higher risk of developing PTSD than men.

Recent data underscored the high prevalence of PTSD associated with combat duty in Iraq and Afghanistan.[26,47-53] Hoge and colleagues used the military version of the PCL[38] to estimate the prevalence of PTSD among U.S. Army infantry soldiers 3 to 4 months following their return from a year-long deployment to Iraq.[52] They found that 36.2% and 16.2% of injured soldiers with and without mTBI, respectively screened positive for PTSD. Using the same criteria as Hoge, Doukas and colleagues found that 17.9% of 324 service members who sustained a limb-threatening injury to the lower extremity screened positive for PTSD at an average of 38.6 months postinjury.[54] Rates of PTSD among service members and veterans are generally higher among those deployed versus not deployed, although there is evidence suggesting that exposure to specific combat experiences, rather than deployment alone, is more predictive of the development of PTSD symptoms.[55]

The risk of developing PTSD after physical injury in the combat setting is controversial. Some have argued that physical injury decreases the risk of PTSD because the physical injuries provide a focus for anxious energy and garners greater sympathy from others (social and psychological support). Physical injury often leads to evacuation from the battlefield and removes the injured from further threat or traumatization.[56] Studies that have found relatively low rates of PTSD in wounded service members have buttressed this perspective.[57] However, the presence of a significant physical injury is also an incessant reminder of the life-threatening circumstances that the service members are exposed to and this physical reminder of their prior circumstances may be a constant reminder leading to PTSD. Pathophysiologically, Koren and coworkers[56] hypothesized three potential mechanisms to explain why physical injury might increase the likelihood of PTSD. First, physical injury frequently increases activation of the hypothalamic-pituitary-adrenal (HPA) axis and related pathways. The HPA axis is altered in many PTSD patients, with studies documenting evidence such as lower baseline cortisol level,[58,59] although results have been decidedly mixed with regard to cortisol and PTSD. Second, physical injury may activate other key mediators that contribute to the development of PTSD, in that physical injury might stimulate additional pathways other than those initially stimulated by the trauma. Substance P, endogenous opioids, and proinflammatory cytokines all might contribute to the impact of physical trauma on psychological well-being, but further research is needed to explore this possibility. Third, injury might interfere with the body's attempts to recover from the trauma-induced alterations in such pathways. For example, physical injuries and PTSD-related nightmares interfere with sleep, thereby impairing both physical and psychological recovery.

Perception of a high degree of threat associated with the injury was an independent predictor of PTSD symptoms. A study of civilian MVC victims conducted diagnostic interviews at baseline as well as 1, 6, and 12 months later to assess independent predictors of the development of PTSD symptoms.[60] In this study, those with PTSD symptoms at 1 month actually had less severe injuries than those without PTSD symptoms. Somewhat surprisingly, there was no relationship between injury severity and PTSD at 6 and 12 months; however, coping style was a key modulator of the physical injury–PTSD link.[60] The strongest independent predictor of higher rates of PTSD symptoms was a coping style that relied on wishful thinking. Those engaging in wishful thinking tend to wish for a miracle, to want to change the circumstances or how they felt, or to pray that the situation would just go away. The researchers hypothesized that such individuals might get lost in such dreaming or fantasizing instead of developing more positive coping mechanisms. Coping mechanisms warrant study in other settings and with combat veterans to see if these findings can be replicated.

TRAUMATIC BRAIN INJURY AND POSTTRAUMATIC STRESS DISORDER

Many skeletal trauma patients also sustain a concomitant injury to the brain, although precise rates of co-occurrence are largely unknown. TBI can range from severe brain injuries with prolonged coma to a mild injury with no loss of consciousness and transient dazed feeling or confusion in the aftermath of a blow to the head. Differentiation of TBI severity remains a matter of considerable debate, but the DoD considers mTBI to include those with no more than 30 minutes loss of consciousness (LOC), moderate TBI including those with more than 30 minutes LOC but no more than 24 hours, and severe TBI limited to those with more than 24 hours LOC. Some reports claim more than 280,000 service members have experienced TBI in Iraq or Afghanistan, at least 80% of which are believed to be mild.[52] TBI is frequently labeled the "signature injury" of Operation Iraqi Freedom (OIF) and Operation Enduring Freedom (OEF).[61] The clinical presentations of mTBI and PTSD are often indistinguishable from each other, featuring impaired sleep, decreased concentration, and other symptoms. There is also evidence that these two disorders have some shared pathophysiology. The frequent co-occurrence of mTBI and PTSD, as well as the overlap in symptoms, has resulted in a growing controversy regarding the relationship between the two disorders and the implications for diagnosis and treatment, especially among veterans returning from OEF and OIF.[62,63] More research is clearly needed to better understand how mTBI impacts recovery from PTSD and how mTBI might influence the response to various therapies for PTSD.

A self-completed mail survey of 2235 U.S. military personnel returning from Iraq and Afghanistan reported that 12%

had a history consistent with mTBI, while 11% were positive for PTSD.[64] Even when overlapping symptoms were removed from the PTSD score, PTSD was more closely related to residual TBI symptoms than anything else. A similar pattern is found in survivors of MVCs, indicating that postconcussive symptoms of mTBI may be mediated by the interaction of neurologic and psychological factors.[6] Another study of MVC-related TBI found that 14% met criteria for ASD in the immediate aftermath of the TBI, and most of them went on to develop chronic PTSD, suggesting it was the psychological rather than physical impact that led to chronic symptoms.[23] Mild TBI spectrum is particularly difficult to define, as some of the persistent symptoms that have been attributed to mTBI, including headaches, dizziness, memory problems, irritability, and sleep problems, are often reported by those with PTSD and other psychological conditions, and those with persistent symptoms after TBI usually seem to meet criteria for a mood or anxiety disorder.

The diagnosis of mTBI is a clinical diagnosis that should be made by a neurologist or medical practitioner experienced with TBI. Evaluation should include a detailed history, physical and neurologic examination and, most importantly, an assessment of cognitive function. The decision to obtain neuroimaging is based on the level of suspicion of skull fracture or intracranial hemorrhage. Clinically available neuroimaging (computed tomography [CT] or magnetic resonance imaging [MRI]) is not adequate to rule out mTBI, which is a clinical diagnosis. If a patient has persistent altered mental status, LOC, abnormal Glasgow Coma Scale (GCS) score, focal neurologic deficit(s), or is clinically deteriorating, then neuroimaging should be obtained.

There is serious concern that reliance on self-reporting of symptoms to establish a diagnosis of mTBI is problematic and thus unreliable. This is both expected and obvious. After all, by definition, these patients are brain injured with alteration of consciousness and memory dysfunction. This is especially true of patients who suffer other severe injuries such as concomitant skeletal trauma. A recent report reviewed the reliability of mTBI diagnosis based on self-reported history of aberration of consciousness in patients suffering complex injuries requiring medical evacuation from the war theater.[65] Patients diagnosed with mTBI had normal neuroimaging, higher Injury Severity Scale (ISS) scores, and longer lengths of stay than those without mTBI. Patients with higher ISS scores and longer lengths of stay are more likely at the time of injury to require pain medication and suffer from hypoxia, hypotension, metabolic derangement, and other conditions that could affect awareness and consciousness. As these disorders can alter consciousness in the absence of TBI, their impact on the diagnostic criteria in patients with severe injuries, especially extremity trauma, cannot be ruled out, which renders the TBI diagnosis unreliable. The paradoxical finding that further supports this conclusion is that patients who reported LOC actually had a lower incidence of abnormalities on neuroimaging.

Findings from studies conducted at Walter Reed National Military Medical Center, have led to similar conclusions. In these investigations, self-report of feeling dazed or confused at the time of injury captures large numbers of individuals who experience PTSD and depression related to blast exposure regardless of whether there is any physical injury or PTSD. This is true also in civilian clinical practice. A study of hospitalized civilian trauma victims that compared 90 patients initially diagnosed with mTBI to 85 non–brain-injured trauma patients found identical rates of postconcussional syndrome (PCS) in both groups.[66] These results suggest no relationship between the diagnosis of mTBI and subsequent PCS symptomatology; moreover, the strongest predictor of PCS was in fact a prior mood or anxiety disorder, with an odds ratio of 5.76.

Although many patients will recover fully following mTBI, some may develop postconcussional disorder (PCD) or PCS. These have persistent symptoms analogous to psychological disorders. PCD was initially codified in the *Diagnostic and Statistical Manual of Mental Disorders,* Fourth Edition (DSM-IV) as an area requiring further research, with insufficient data to fully support it as a diagnostic entity.[67] PCD criteria require the history of a head trauma, followed by the onset of at least three of the following symptoms, which were not present prior to the trauma and have persisted at least 3 months: fatigue, headache, sleep disturbance, dizziness, irritability, anxiety or depression, personality changes, or apathy. By comparison, the World Health Organization's (WHO) *International Classification of Diseases,* Tenth Edition (ICD-10) includes criteria for PCS that are less restrictive, only requiring a history of TBI and three or more of the following eight symptoms: (1) headache, (2) dizziness, (3) fatigue, (4) irritability, (5) insomnia, (6) difficulty with concentration, (7) memory problems, and (8) intolerance of stress, emotion, or alcohol. Because PCD criteria require that the head trauma cause significant cerebral concussion, along with quantifiable impairment in memory or attention, it is not surprising that a study directly comparing the two sets of criteria in mTBI found that the ICD-10 criteria were met three times more frequently. However, neither set of criteria is ready for clinical use without further research. In fact, WHO[68] acknowledges in the description of PCS that

> *These symptoms may be accompanied by feelings of depression or anxiety, resulting from some loss of self-esteem and fear of permanent brain damage. Such feelings enhance the original symptoms and a vicious circle results. Some patients become hypochondriacal, embark on a search for diagnosis and cure, and may adopt a permanent sick role. The etiology of these symptoms is not always clear, and both organic and psychological factors have been proposed to account for them. The nosological status of this condition is thus somewhat uncertain. There is little doubt, however, that this syndrome is common and distressing to the patient. (p. 67)*

Perhaps as a result, most researchers continue to simply refer to the overall, albeit ill-defined, category of TBI, rather than using either PCS or PCD.

As the diagnosis of mTBI based on self-report is problematic, there is a broad effort to employ point-of-care screening tools. For these to be effective, it must first be recognized that most TBI patients are typically unaware that they are injured and thus do not seek medical attention. For this reason, it is incumbent on colleagues, leaders, coaches, and sideline officials to have heightened sensitivity that an individual may be at risk of having suffered an mTBI or concussion and to then institute screening, sometimes in the face of protestations by the victim that he or she is uninjured. There are a number of available point-of-injury clinical screening tools, such as the

Standardized Assessment of Concussion (SAC) and Sports Concussion Assessment Tool, version 3 (SCAT3).[69,70] The military uses the Defense and Veterans Brain Injury Center's (DVBIC) Military Acute Concussion Evaluation (MACE).[71,72] Embedded in the MACE is the SAC. The MACE collects history and symptoms and uses the SAC to test four cognitive domains: orientation, immediate recall, concentration, and memory. By regulation through the DoD Directive-Type Memorandum (DTM) 09-033, which is a general order that affects all service members, the MACE is administered to any service member to be at risk of having suffered an mTBI. "At risk" is defined as involvement in a vehicle blast event, collision, or rollover, presence within 50 meters of a blast (inside or outside of a vehicle), a direct blow to the head, or witnessed LOC.[73] If screening is positive, the victim is referred to an advanced medical provider for further evaluation and diagnosis.

Moderate to severe TBI is a life-threatening medical condition. Point-of-injury care is focused on the "ABCs" of airway, breathing, and circulation. A GCS score determination should be made. In the field, care focuses on maintaining oxygen saturation higher than 92%, partial pressure of oxygen (PO_2) higher than 60 mm Hg, partial pressure of carbon dioxide (PCO_2) at 40 mm Hg, and systolic blood pressure higher than 90 mm Hg.[74,75] Hyperventilation is reserved for those patients who are exhibiting clinical signs of cerebral herniation. Rapid transport to the nearest level 1 trauma center with neurosurgical and neurology critical care is essential. There, care is primarily dictated by neurology specialists if there is isolated TBI or with the general trauma surgery service if there are also complex injuries, including skeletal.

There is an elevated risk of developing depression or other psychiatric disorders among moderate to severe TBI survivors similar to that of other serious medical conditions, such as stroke or myocardial infarction. Several studies demonstrate that at least one-quarter to one-half of those with TBI have major depression.[76-78] However, moderate to severe TBI may, at least initially, provide some "protection" against the development of PTSD by obscuring the memory of the traumatic event. Further evaluation is necessary to better delineate the relationship between the severity of TBI and the risk of PTSD. In addition, it is important to emphasize the need for close attention to, and repeated formal assessment for, the potential evolution of PTSD symptoms as rehabilitation progresses and memory improves in individuals with moderate to severe TBI. A combination of serial neuropsychological testing, along with the use of validated instruments such as CAPS for PTSD, and Beck Depression Inventory or PHQ for depression, is advisable to best sort out improvement in TBI and potential onset of psychological disorders.

TBI and PTSD commonly occur together. Explosive blast patients who experience significant persistent and recalcitrant symptoms should have a thorough evaluation for PTSD and other psychological sequelae. This may be particularly beneficial to the individual patient, because there are specific treatments for PTSD, depression, and related conditions. Hoge and colleagues identified a significant association between mTBI and psychiatric symptoms, including PTSD in more than 40% of those who had LOC.[51] These investigators noted that the high rates of physical symptoms reported by soldiers could be attributed to PTSD and depression. When these conditions were included in the analyses, there was no direct relationship between mTBI and physical health problems except for headache. It should be noted that the diagnosis for mTBI in this study was based on self-reporting of alteration of consciousness.

Magnetic resonance spectroscopy (MRS) may be better than traditional MRI for identifying mTBI and differentiating it from PTSD. A study by Hetherington and colleagues[79] of veterans exposed to explosive blast and suffering persistent memory impairment associated with mTBI revealed decreased N-acetylaspartate (NAA)/choline (Ch) and NAA/creatinine (Cr) ratios in the anterior hippocampus when compared to patients exposed to blast but did not have these impairments. The hippocampus in affected TBI patients was also reduced in size. When compared to patients with PTSD, TBI patients had anterior hippocampus metabolic ratios that were significantly lower. PTSD patients exposed to blast had no difference in their anterior hippocampus NAA:Ch and NAA:Cr ratios when compared to blast-exposed patients who did not have PTSD. The metabolic ratios in the anterior hippocampus were also not different between blast patients with PTSD and PTSD patients who had no blast exposure. Furthermore, these metabolic ratios did not vary with patients diagnosed with depression or anxiety.

Proper clinical management for mTBI begins with immediately removing the victim from further play or activity. This is to avoid reinjury before the brain has adequately recovered. An injury during the vulnerable period results in further compromised autoregulation of cerebral blood flow, rapid development of cerebral edema, intracranial hypertension (elevated intracranial pressure), and neurologic deterioration to coma and, possibly, death.

Mild TBI treatment begins by allowing the patient to rest with minimal cognitive burden. Symptoms are managed using evidence-based clinical practice guidelines. Unfortunately, there is presently no clinically available pharmacologic agent that will facilitate or hasten the brain's recovery from TBI.

Return to work and type of work is guided by clinical improvement. The DoD DTM 09-033[72] and the American Academy of Neurology's 2013 sports concussion guidelines[80] each recommend that patients be prescribed rest without exposure to excess cognitive stimulation. Both physical and cognitive activities should be gradually increased as the patient tolerates, that is, without exacerbation of symptoms. When the patient can tolerate normal activities, then a provocative test can be performed. This provocative test is exertional physical activity (e.g., run) followed by cognitive testing. If the patient does not have symptoms recurrence and performs well on testing, then he or she may return to full play or work. Many states now have laws that require at least 24 hours' recovery and written permission from a neurologist or other medical practitioner skilled in managing concussion before return to play or work.

Treatment of mTBI is symptoms focused. In 2009, the U.S. Department of Veterans Affairs in conjunction with the DoD published a set of clinical practice guidelines for the management of concussion and mTBI. These are evidence-based recommendations for which pharmacologic and nonpharmacologic options are provided for each major symptom.[81] For example, headache is to be treated with acetaminophen or nonsteroidal antiinflammatory agents, insomnia with sleep hygiene and nonbenzodiazepine soporific agents acutely, dizziness with physical therapy, and so forth. The American

Academy of Neurology's guidelines[80] note that there is no specific treatment for accelerating or improving recovery from mTBI. The goals are to allow sufficient time for the brain to heal, to minimize risk of reinjury, and treat symptoms.

Recovery from mTBI is a gradual process with the majority of the cognitive recovery occurring in the first 6 months, and approximately 70% to 80% of individuals having few postinjury problems.[82] However, the remaining 20% to 30% have impaired function from residual symptoms that are usually psychiatric.[82] While depression, anxiety, and behavioral problems are commonly identified following TBI,[83,84] it is exceedingly difficult to discern whether persistent emotional and behavioral symptoms are directly related to the neurologic damage, a secondary reaction to the cognitive deficits of the injury, or a comorbid psychological complication of the trauma itself.[85]

Belanger and colleagues conducted a meta-analysis that raises doubts that persistent postconcussive syndrome symptoms are attributable solely to the injury.[86] This work revealed greater cognitive sequelae of mTBI in "convenience samples," that is, those seeking medical care for their symptoms, and those involved in litigation, as opposed to unselected or prospective samples. Litigation in particular was associated with stable or worsening cognitive function over time, which is perhaps not surprising; whether subconscious or not, functional improvement would presumably lessen reimbursement from pending litigation, serving as a disincentive to recovery.

In contrast, the investigators also found that studies with unselected populations or prospective designs had no evidence of residual neuropsychological impairment 3 months after their injury. In an exception, one longitudinal study of veterans compared long-term neuropsychological outcomes in those with self-reported mTBI after a motor vehicle accident, to those who had a motor vehicle accident without TBI, and another group who had not had an accident, at an average of 8 years after the accident.[87] Comprehensive neuropsychological testing identified no significant differences between the three groups, although the authors argued that minor, borderline differences on the Paced Auditory Serial Addition Test (PASAT) and California Verbal Learning Test (CVLT) suggested potential subtle attentional problems in the mTBI population. While this finding might indicate potential long-term adverse neuropsychological effects of mTBI, it is quite conceivable that such differences are entirely due to psychiatric comorbidity, which should be carefully assessed in any studies that evaluate the impact of mTBI. Regardless of the pathogenesis, it is clear that the residual emotional and behavioral changes have a significant impact on adjustment, including employment and social relationships.[88] Several factors influence this adjustment such as injury severity,[89] social support,[90] premorbid functioning,[91] and coping styles.[92] For example, coping strategies, such as avoidance, wishful thinking, worry, and self-blame, are associated with higher levels of depression and anxiety in TBI patients.[93-95] Coping strategies are an area that can be targeted for treatment intervention.[95]

There is an expectation that the military's social structure can assist soldiers who are struggling with poor concentration, attention, and memory. Having clear responsibilities, belonging to a group and a defined chain of command can provide needed support and structure to a recovering mTBI patient. However, the military can also be relatively unforgiving of mistakes, forgetfulness, or poor attention to detail, leading to soldiers receiving a counseling statement (i.e., an administrative warning) or an Article 15 (i.e., nonjudicial military discipline) for infractions related to their symptoms. This punitive response can lead to increased psychosocial stress, which exacerbates existing symptoms and may contribute to further maintenance of TBI symptoms. Rank structure can be an additional complication as military hierarchy demands more from those of higher rank. Anecdotally, some higher ranking soldiers have reported trying to "pass" as if they are not having difficulties in order to preserve pride and to meet expectations they believe are being placed on them. Intervention research may also need to include specific education for military leaders in how to handle TBI symptoms in the workplace as more soldiers resume their military duties.

Traumatic Brain Injury and Suicide

Suicide is tragic and represents a significant concern among TBI survivors. One study identified that 6.9% of patients who had a single TBI had suicidal ideation, a figure that rose to 21.7% among those who had sustained multiple TBIs.[96] This is in contrast to the non-TBI control group who had no suicidal thoughts. The multiple TBI group had higher rates of PTSD and depression, and depression severity was strongly associated with suicide risk. In contrast, however, another study of veterans with mTBI[97] did not identify an association between PTSD and suicide risk. Moreover, severe TBI was associated with lower suicide risk, as the duration of LOC was inversely correlated with suicidality,[98] presumably contributed to by both less memory of the trauma as well as less physical wherewithal to carry out a suicide attempt. Nevertheless, it is judicious to screen those with TBI, especially those with mTBI and/or symptoms of depression, and refer those with suicidal ideation to mental health professionals.

DEPRESSION

Depression plays a major role in the failure to achieve full functional recovery after trauma. High rates of depressive symptoms and major depressive disorder are commonly observed following physical injury and orthopaedic trauma. Depression is the second most commonly encountered condition in primary care, following hypertension. About one in six Americans will suffer an episode of major depression in their lifetime, and for most it will be a chronic disease, with a recurrence rate of 50% after their first episode, 70% after the second, and 90% after the third.[99] Depression may occur at any age, but the average age of onset is in the third decade of life.

To diagnose depression, ask about these nine symptoms:

- Depressed mood
- *S*leep disturbance
- Loss of *I*nterest or pleasure, that is, anhedonia
- Feelings of *G*uilt or worthlessness
- Low *E*nergy
- Poor *C*oncentration or memory
- *A*ppetite disturbance
- *P*sychomotor agitation or retardation
- *S*uicidal ideation

At least five of these symptoms must be present for most of the previous 2 weeks for a diagnosis of major depression. A popular mnemonic, SIG = E CAPS ("the prescription for

TABLE 29-3 *GUIDELINE FOR ADDRESSING DEPRESSIVE SYMPTOMS*

PHQ-9 Score	Action
1–4	None
5–9	Watchful waiting, with periodic screening
10–14	Treatment plan, considering counseling, follow-up, and pharmacotherapy
15–19	Immediate implementation of therapy
≥20	Pharmacotherapy and, if severe impairment or poor response to therapy, expedited referral to a mental health specialist

PHQ-9, Nine-Item Patient Health Questionnaire.

depressed patients is energy capsules") can be used to recall the eight other criteria that may accompany depressed mood.

Diagnosis can be further facilitated by the use of the Nine-Item Patient Health Questionnaire (PHQ-9) (see Appendix, available online).[100] The PHQ-9 is ideal for screening for depression, uniquely combining the following features:

- It is brief and compatible with time constraints.
- It is easy and inexpensive to administer.
- It makes accurate, validated diagnoses.
- The patient and provider are educated.
- It provides a score to connote severity and to facilitate longitudinal monitoring.
- Use has been associated with improved outcomes (in conjunction with provider education and mental health consultation).

Because the nine items are taken directly from the diagnostic criteria for major depression (see the bulleted list above), the instrument facilitates rapid diagnosis, with a cutoff score of 10 having 88% sensitivity and specificity for major depression. PHQ-9 scores correlate strongly with self-reported quality of life, interference of symptoms with usual activities, number of physician visits, and difficulties at work, at home, and with others.[100] Most valuable of all, the PHQ-9 score can be used as blood pressure or blood sugar are used to follow hypertension and diabetes mellitus, respectively, enabling a primary care provider to follow a patient's score to guide management as follows (see Table 29-3):

Although the full instrument takes less than a minute for most patients to complete, an even easier approach to initial screening is to start with only two of the items: (1) little interest or pleasure in doing things, and (2) feeling down, depressed, or hopeless. Since one of the two has to be positive to make a diagnosis of depression, this has high sensitivity, and a specific diagnosis can then be made with administration of the full instrument. In fact, even a single question, "Have you felt sad or depressed much of the time in the past year?" is nearly as sensitive (85%) and specific (66%) as more comprehensive questionnaires.[101]

The characteristics of this "diagnostic test" compare favorably with many tests commonly used by primary care providers to screen for cancer or heart disease.

Similar to what is seen with research on PTSD, different instruments and criteria have been used to assess for depression, which in part explains the disparate estimates of prevalence after physical injuries. One review reports depression rates of 28% to 42% in civilians experiencing physical injury.[7] Crichlow and colleagues[102] documented that 45% of 161 patients presenting to an orthopaedic trauma service had at least moderate symptoms of depression, including 3.7% with severe depression. In the LEAP study, 38% of 545 patients with lower extremity limb-threatening had moderate-to-severe depression, and an additional 19% had severe depression.[103] The prevalence of depression among service members and veterans has not been as thoroughly studied as has PTSD.[26,47-52,104] However, Hoge identified symptoms consistent with major depression in 13.0% of service members returning from Iraq or Afghanistan after an mTBI, versus 6.6% in those who were injured in the absence of a TBI.[52] Doukas and colleagues[54] reported that 39.6% of major extremity trauma patients injured in OIF/OEF screened positive for depressive symptoms, with 12.6% having a possible or probable diagnosis of major depression.

Depression is common following limb amputation, and a review of the literature found evidence for a bimodal peak.[105] Within 2 years following an amputation, individuals had depression rates ranging from 30% to 58%, a prevalence similar to that seen after severe medical complications such as heart attack and stroke. Individuals 2 to 10 years postamputation had depression rates similar to the general population, but those 10 to 20 years again manifest elevated rates of depression (22% to 28%), suggesting living with the amputation eventually had a wearying effect. Anxiety has been less carefully assessed after amputation, but it appears that high initial rates diminish within 2 years postamputation. Subsequent studies reaffirmed high prevalence rates for depression and anxiety following amputation,[106] especially in those with phantom or residual limb pain.[107] Horgan and MacLachlan[105] reported mixed results regarding an association between phantom limb pain and psychological conditions, with some evidence that depression is more common in those with persistent pain, corroborating an association previously seen between depression and chronic pain of diverse etiologies.

Traumatic loss of one or more limbs has been common in service members deployed to Iraq and Afghanistan. This is in part due to the nature of modern improvised explosive devices (IEDs), but it is also a credit to the success of protective measures that have left the torso relatively unscathed, as well as the quality of resuscitative care. Just as prior wars resulted in significant medical advances that benefited society at large, amputee care and the quality of prostheses has improved dramatically as a result of Herculean efforts to provide amputees with maximum function and mobility. Amputees are remaining on active duty and making valuable contributions to the war effort in ways that were inconceivable with prior wars. However, loss of a limb nevertheless profoundly influences one's self-image, and can be associated with psychological sequelae, as has been noted.

A number of cognitive factors that influence adjustment to amputation have been reported. Body image is a salient factor, whose study has been facilitated by the Amputation Related Body Image Scale, or ARBIS.[108] The ARBIS includes questions such as: "I avoided looking at my prosthesis" and "I thought that my prosthesis was ugly." Use of this instrument documented an association between adjustment to amputation and depressive symptoms; amputees' overall body image in fact predicts quality of life, depression, and self-rated health.[108] Factors closely linked with body image, such as self-consciousness and perceived stigma, also influence adjustment. Individuals with an amputation who report more public self-consciousness also note greater distress[106] and are at higher risk for functional disability.[109] Perceived stigma—believing that others hold negative attitudes toward you because of your disability—is also a risk for depression.[107] Individuals without disability have also been shown to exhibit behavioral avoidance when interacting with individuals with disabilities.[110]

Further research is needed to determine whether physically wounded service members have the same perceptions as civilian amputees. The acuity and severity of the trauma, need for immediate medical attention, frequent need for removal from imminent continuing danger, long-distance evacuation, and common need for multiple surgical procedures, all may impact one's body image during the initial adjustment period. However, proximity to other amputees in the context of the military medical setting may simultaneously help to normalize body image concerns and reduce stigma. Other factors may also be important in adjustment to amputation for military personnel. For example, concerns about independence and physical prowess may be more important than body image. Technological advances in prosthetics and rehabilitation, including the use of virtual reality, make it possible to better approximate prior levels of function, facilitating consideration of a much wider range of activities, including remaining on active duty. Striving for these goals with the benefit of the camaraderie and spirit inherent in the military environment may trump concerns about appearance. Alternatively, military service members may be more reluctant to acknowledge concerns about body image because of feelings of guilt or stigmatization. Future research is needed to better understand the significance of these and other factors contributing to adjustment to amputation, which can then enable corresponding therapeutic interventions.

Just as for TBI, coping styles greatly influence one's response to, and recovery from, amputation.[111,112] Livneh and coworkers[113] espouse a three-dimensional model: active/confronting approaches as opposed to passive/avoidant coping styles on the first axis, optimistic/positivistic coping versus pessimistic/fatalistic on the second, and social/emotional versus cognitive on the third axis. Each axis is best viewed as a spectrum, and some have more distinct differences than others.

Given that the first axis is the most sharply delineated, we focus on the importance of active versus passive coping style in understanding recovery from amputation. Active coping, planning, positive reframing, and acceptance are on the adaptive end, and alcohol and drug use, disengagement, self-criticism, and social withdrawal at the maladaptive end. Actively addressing problems is associated with improved psychosocial outcomes, whereas avoidance is associated with increased psychological distress and poor adjustment.[113] The need to identify positive aspects of coping was also highlighted by Dunn,[114] who characterized three cognitive coping styles: finding positive meaning in amputation, perceiving control over amputation, and adopting a positive outlook. All three had an inverse relationship with the level of depressive symptoms. The incorporation of these ideas into rehabilitation strategies may be beneficial.

Adjustment to amputation can also be viewed as a series of phases or stages.[115] The response to the loss of a limb has been described as paralleling the grieving process,[116] which Kübler-Ross famously divided into five stages. The initial stage is characterized by denial, in which individuals refuse to acknowledge that they have such a condition. This is followed by anger, when frustration with their condition may lead individuals to attack others. The third phase is bargaining, where individuals may offer to do something better in return for resolution or improvement in their condition. This is succeeded by depression, when hope is lost to some extent, and individuals become more passive about their condition. The final phase is acceptance, when individuals express acknowledgement of their condition and try to move on in as productive a manner as possible. Health care providers should not expect that all amputees will go through each stage, nor that the stages will necessarily occur in this exact order, but an understanding of these possible reactions may facilitate efforts to help amputees better cope with their loss of limb(s). It also provides a framework for explaining the pattern of anxiety and depression previously described in amputees, as bargaining or a more transitory phase of acceptance may explain improvements, whereas depression ensues in those for whom bargaining does not seem satisfactory, and gives way to hopelessness.

The Amputee Coalition of America similarly characterizes six key phases to recovery after amputation: enduring, suffering, reckoning, reconciling, normalizing, and thriving.[117] Enduring describes the individual getting through the surgery and pain. Suffering features questioning and experiencing emotions related to the loss. Reckoning involves coming to terms with the implications of the loss. The final three stages (reconciling, normalizing, and thriving) embody more positive aspects of change, including putting the loss in perspective, resetting priorities, and making the most of life. It is again important to emphasize that not all patients will experience every stage, and some may simultaneously experience features of more than one phase. Among the advantages of the Amputee Coalition model is that it (1) focuses on adaptive functioning; (2) provides specific behavioral descriptions of adjustment; (3) offers a mechanism for beginning to understand the emotions experienced by amputees; and (4) engenders hope for improvement in those still experiencing difficulties. However, it is a broad brush, and the individual physical and emotional circumstances of each amputee must be considered in developing specific, realistic, and attainable goals.

IMPACT OF PSYCHOLOGICAL COMORBIDITIES ON DISABILITY AND FAMILY FUNCTION

The studies cited earlier underscore the potential psychological impact of physical trauma, even when the actual physical insult is relatively minor in nature. General emotional stress and symptoms of ASD, PTSD, mTBI, and depression, in turn, have a profound impact on disability, return to work, health-related quality of life, and prolonged poor adjustment. Even subclinical levels of these conditions are related to poor health-related quality of life.[118-132]

The Trauma Recovery Project, a large, prospective epidemiologic study, was established to assess psychological and functional outcomes after significant physical trauma. Postinjury depression, PTSD, serious extremity injury, and length of stay in the hospital, were all found to be significantly associated with poor functional status at 6 months postinjury. The associations remained significant 12 and 18 months after injury in this study of 1048 trauma patients.[120,121] Another study found that PTSD was independently and inversely related to general health outcome 6 months after significant trauma, as measured on the well-validated Short Form-36.[123] At 12 months, the development of PTSD, depression, or substance abuse was associated with poorer work status, poorer general health, and overall satisfaction with recovery.[124]

Data from the LEAP study underscored the importance of this message for orthopaedic surgeons. The LEAP study[2,133] was designed to assess the outcomes of severe trauma below the knee, specifically comparing the results of limb salvage to amputation. In the design of the study, the investigators recognized the potential for factors outside of the surgeon's control to influence the recovery course. These included age, sex, race or ethnicity, education, income level, insurance status prior to the injury, work status, occupation, personality characteristics, social support, and self-efficacy. Additional items evaluated were the patient's self-rated health status and preinjury chronic medical conditions, exercise, smoking, and drinking habits. Receipt of injury compensation or litigation was also evaluated.

At 2 years postinjury, disability outcomes for the LEAP study cohort as a whole were poor as measured by the Sickness Impact Profile (SIP), a well-established measure of self-reported disability.[134] Forty-two percent of the patients had moderately severe to severe physical and psychosocial disabilities (i.e., SIP scores ≥10). Only 51% of those working preinjury had returned to work. Further follow-up at 7 months showed little improvement in overall outcomes; only 58% had returned to work and SIP scores were the same, and often worse, than at 2 years.[118,119]

What was most surprising about the results from the LEAP study were the few observable differences in outcome for those undergoing amputation versus limb reconstruction. Rather, it was other factors, over and above the decision to amputate versus reconstruct, that ultimately predicted who did poorly. These factors included rehospitalization for the treatment of a major complication; having less than a high school education; poverty; being nonwhite; having no insurance or Medicaid; having a poor social support system; having low self-efficacy; and smoking and involvement with the legal system. Self-efficacy, in particular, was a strong predictor of outcome. Self-efficacy refers to the confidence in being able to perform specific tasks or activities. Persons with low self-efficacy are more likely to disengage from the coping process because failure is expected.

Importantly, baseline measures of pain, acute anxiety, and depression (all assessed at 3 months following the injury) were highly significant predictors of a poor SIP disability at 2 and 7 years postinjury. It should be noted here that the high level of co-occurrence of psychological distress and pain has been well documented and several studies have suggested a strong link between pain in the early stages of recovery and subsequent psychological distress, including depression and PTSD.[135-138] The LEAP study also showed that in later phases of recovery, negative mood, and specifically anxiety, play a critical role in the persistence of pain long term.[139] Wegener and colleagues further examined the complex relationships among these variables and specifically looked at their impact on long-term functional outcomes.[140] He identified that the impact of pain on SIP functional outcome is primarily related to the influence of pain on depression and anxiety. This result supports the necessity of an integrated approach in addressing an individual's experiences of emotional distress in conjunction with our medical management of the patient's pain.

To further underscore the extent to which PTSD, depression, and pain drive disability following skeletal trauma, Castillo and colleagues[141] examined functional outcomes of the 429 U.S. service members who sustained a major lower or upper limb injury while serving in Afghanistan or Iraq. For the 10% of the patients with no pain, depression, or PTSD, outcomes (as measured by the Dysfunction Index of the Short Musculoskeletal Functional Assessment [SMFA])[142] are imperfect but less than one minimally clinically important difference (MCID) apart from population norms. In sharp contrast, the outcomes for patients experiencing high pain, depression, or PTSD were universally (255 out of 256 patients) very poor (i.e., greater than three MCIDs of population norms).

Effect on Family Members and Relationships

Although the tremendous impact that caring for injured family members and wounded soldiers has on families is well recognized, there is very little empirical research addressing the emotional impact that caring for an injured family member has on the remainder of the family. Several factors have the potential to increase stress reactions and affect coping resources in military families, in particular, disruption of family dynamics already induced by the deployment, the young age of many service members and their spouse (if married), and the loss of military environment and culture.[143] Although not explicitly limited to military families, one study of how having a father with PTSD has an impact on other family members was recently conducted in Bosnia and Herzegovina, where most of the male population fought in the civil war.[144] In comparison with control families, depression was more common in wives in the PTSD families. The effect of fathers with PTSD on their children was profound, resulting in them missing more school, being more easily upset, having greater eating and breathing problems, and experiencing more abdominal pain.

Indeed, it is well documented that PTSD symptoms compound difficulties in family adjustment following war zone deployments.[145,146] Additionally, the physical, cognitive, emotional, and behavioral changes experienced by physically wounded service members directly impact the family. For example, there are often changes in family roles, increased financial burden, loss of intimacy, and loss of employment due to changes in functioning.[147] Some unique aspects of military culture also have an influence on the impact that PTSD might have on families.

Large military communities such as Fort Bragg, North Carolina, and Fort Hood, Texas, can provide built-in support structures composed of other families who understand the impact of deployment-related stressors, but this is a trade-off because the posts are often far from their family of origin, diminishing that potential source of support. In fact, many families from remote posts such as Fort Riley, Kansas, have elected to return to their families of origin in instances where the military units deployed to Iraq for a year, and knew that they would be deployed again after only 1 year at home. The resulting prolonged geographic separation, wherein service members might only see their family for a month of vacation over a 3-year period, can greatly exacerbate intrafamily conflict, and may make it even more difficult for family members to appreciate the impact that physical or psychological injuries might be having on the life of a service member. Not surprisingly, divorce rates have been significantly higher in such instances. Significant physical injuries, such as moderate to severe TBI and amputation, may exacerbate matters if prolonged hospitalization and/or repeated surgical intervention is required, especially if performed at distant facilities, perpetuating the estrangement of service members and their families. Military medical centers do have some housing available for family members, including Fisher Houses specifically established for this purpose, but prolonged separation from home, school, and/or employment may not be practical for many families.

Dealing with moderate to severe TBI is especially challenging. Caregivers of persons with more severe TBI specifically have been found to demonstrate significant emotional distress in response to the traumatic injury.[148-150] Some family members already have a history of emotional distress and maladaptive family functioning prior to the impact of moderate to severe TBI.[151] Nevertheless, a focus on family adjustment is important as it correlates with the length and degree of recovery from the injury.[152] Basic education regarding symptoms of brain injury and an understanding of the emotional and behavioral consequences of moderate to severe TBI and how to manage them is extremely important, particularly in long-term management.[153,154] Specific educational elements geared toward children should be considered, and some, such as educational coloring books, have already been implemented by the military, although study of their efficacy would be useful. Without proper education, family members may personalize and blame the individual with any grade of TBI for symptoms such as frequent fatigue, lack of motivation, memory loss, or angry outbursts.

With regard to marital relationships, high rates of divorce and separation after moderate to severe TBI have been reported,[155] and as previously noted, marital problems are already a challenge for military families because of the high operations tempo in recent years. A variety of factors are associated with relationship satisfaction including the severity of the injury, the duration of the relationship, and time since injury. In a study examining relationships in the face of severe TBI, mood swings were a strong predictor in dissolution of the relationship.[156] Interventions oriented toward families have typically been educational, supportive, or therapy based, but there is little available evidence to document the effectiveness of such approaches.[151] There are some limited data to support the utility of educating family members regarding moderate to severe TBI and teaching behavioral management techniques for use with injured service members may also be effective,[152] but future research examining family interventions is warranted. We are currently working on an Internet-based intervention featuring educational elements targeted toward improving knowledge and generating behavioral changes in family members, using before and after testing to assess efficacy.

These results strongly support the need for clinicians to understand and proactively address both the physical injuries and the psychological disorders of their patients and their patient's families if they want to promote and achieve an optimal and successful recovery following orthopaedic trauma. Simply put, while physical injury adversely impacts psychological health, the converse is also true—psychological injury adversely impacts physical health and overall functional status. It is important for physicians to understand this two-way relationship, and address both body and mind in order to best care for their patients.

PREVENTION AND MANAGEMENT OF PSYCHOLOGICAL COMORBIDITIES

It is clear that when clinically diagnosed, PTSD and depression at the more severe end of the spectrum should be managed by an appropriate mental health professional. For less severe cases, there are effective approaches for these conditions as well as ASD, which can be initiated by other medical professionals. The literature is less clear regarding proven therapies for managing the sequelae of mTBI.

Treatment of Posttraumatic Stress Disorder

The most proven pharmacologic therapies for improving all categories of PTSD symptoms are SSRIs, but the best reported response rates are only 40% to 60%, and relapse after discontinuation of medication is common.[157-159] The α-blocker prazosin appears to reduce the frequency and intensity of intrusive nightmares.[160] Several forms of psychotherapy have at least moderate evidence to support their efficacy, including CBT, exposure therapy, cognitive processing therapy (CPT), narrative exposure therapy, and eye movement desensitization and reprocessing therapy.[161] Echoing previous reviews, an expert panel convened by the Institutes of Medicine concluded that CBT and exposure therapies are the only PTSD treatments with a sufficient evidence base to recommend them.[162] CBT characteristically includes elements of psychoeducation, controlled breathing and relaxation techniques, and cognitive restructuring. Exposure therapy helps individuals to confront stimuli (e.g., thoughts, images, objects, situations, or activities) associated with their traumatic experience through progressively more intense exposure, providing the therapist with opportunities to identify and neutralize behavioral cues; marginal exposure has been the most widely employed approach, whereby the therapist asks patients to recall their traumatic experience in progressively greater detail. This is often supplemented by in vivo exposure in which the patient confronts real-life circumstances that have been difficult because of precipitating memories or emotions related to prior trauma. Unfortunately, because avoidance is a cardinal feature of PTSD, a significant number are unwilling or unable to effectively engage in imagined exposure. Recent studies have shown some success in overcoming avoidance through the application of virtual reality, effectively immersing patients in an environment reminiscent of their trauma to facilitate recall.[163-165] There are multiple meta-analyses that indicate that CBT is effective not only for PTSD, but for all anxiety spectrum disorders.[166-168]

Treatment of Depression

The treatment of depression can be extremely challenging and frustrating for both the patient and provider, even without the comorbidity of skeletal trauma. In fact, comorbid depression dramatically increases the morbidity and mortality of common medical conditions such as diabetes mellitus and coronary artery disease. Primary care providers are often the

Adequately powered clinical trials are needed to examine the effectiveness and cost effectiveness of collaborative care models for skeletal trauma that incorporate strategies for improving patient self-efficacy and peer support that help patients recover without developing diagnosable psychiatric conditions. Development of brief instruments for screening patients at high risk of disability early in the acute phase of treatment would be helpful in directing resources where they are most needed. These instruments would not obviate the need to screen for conditions like PTSD and depression at follow-up (for which well-validated instruments already exist); rather they would assist in targeting interventions such as case management, peer support, and self-management that would benefit a broader group of individuals who do not screen positive for these conditions yet need the resources, support, and self-efficacy training to optimize their recovery. Finally, it will be important to find better ways to motivate patients and their families to take advantage of the support and resources made available to them. Although the stigma of the need for psychological support is less prevalent than in the past, many patients are often reluctant to avail themselves of psychosocial interventions because of a perceived weakness, stigma, or lack of self-awareness. The long-term impact of traumatic injury with threatened or actual loss of limb, career, and livelihood is invariably of great impact and duration. Mental health comorbidities frequently last well beyond the successful treatment of the musculoskeletal injuries. Ultimately, the necessity for ongoing treatment by a mental health professional may become of paramount importance to support psychological recovery to successfully restore function. Maintaining a well-integrated, holistic, multidisciplinary philosophy that considers the entire context of our patients, their families, and return to work and society is necessary to fully treat our patients.

KEY REFERENCES

The level of evidence (LOE) is determined according to the criteria provided in the preface.

1. [illegible]: The experience of an orthopaedic surgeon when the trauma hits home: observations and suggestions. J Bone Joint Surg Am 90(6):[illegible], 2008. LOE V
2. Bosse MJ, MacKenzie EJ, Kellam JF, et al: An analysis of outcomes of reconstruction or amputation after leg-threatening injuries. N Engl J Med 347(24):[illegible], 2002. LOE I
3. Engel GL: The clinical application of the biopsychosocial model. Am J Psychiatry [illegible]
4. [illegible]
5. Kroenke K, [illegible] primary care [illegible] Ann Intern Med 146[illegible]
26. Hoge CW, Castro CA, Messer SC, et al: Combat duty in Iraq and Afghanistan, mental health problems, and barriers to care. N Engl J Med 351(1):13–22, 2004. LOE II
42. Heron-Delaney M, Kenardy J, Charlton E, et al: A systematic review of predictors of posttraumatic stress disorder (PTSD) for adult road traffic crash survivors. Injury 44(11):1413–1422, 2013. LOE II
44. Aaron DL, Fadale PD, Harrington CJ, et al: Posttraumatic stress disorders in civilian orthopaedics. J Am Acad Orthop Surg 19(5):245–250, 2011.
45. Starr AJ, Smith WR, Frawley WH, et al: Symptoms of posttraumatic stress disorder after orthopaedic trauma. J Bone Joint Surg Am 86(6):1115–1121, 2004. LOE II
52. Hoge CW, McGurk D, Thomas JL, et al: Mild traumatic brain injury in U.S. soldiers returning from Iraq. N Engl J Med 358(5):453–463, 2008. LOE II
53. Grieger TA, Cozza SJ, Ursano RJ, et al: Posttraumatic stress disorder and depression in battle-injured soldiers. Am J Psychiatry 163:1777–1783, 2006. LOE II
54. Doukas WC, Hayda RA, Frisch HM, et al: The Military Extremity Trauma Amputation/Limb Salvage (METALS) study: outcomes of amputation versus limb salvage following major lower-extremity trauma. J Bone Joint Surg Am 95(2):138–145, 2013. LOE III
80. Giza CC, Kutcher JS, Ashwal S, et al: Summary of evidence-based guideline update: evaluation and management of concussion in sports: report of the Guideline Development Subcommittee of the American Academy of Neurology. Neurology 80(24):2250–2257, 2013. LOE II
103. McCarthy ML, MacKenzie EJ, Edwin D, et al: Psychological distress associated with severe lower-limb injury. J Bone Joint Surg Am 85(9):1689–1697, 2003. LOE I
115. Horgan O, MacLachlan M: Psychosocial adjustment to lower-limb amputation: a review. Disabil Rehabil 26(14–15):837–850, 2004. LOE III
119. MacKenzie EJ, Bosse MJ, Kellam JF, et al: Early predictors of long-term work disability after major limb trauma. J Trauma 61(3):688–694, 2006. LOE I
121. Holbrook TL, Hoyt DB, Stein MB, et al: [illegible] PTSD after major trauma: risk factors and functional outcome. J Trauma [illegible], 2001. LOE I
152. Rosenbloom BN, Khan S, McCartney C, et al: Systematic review of persistent pain and psychological outcomes following traumatic musculoskeletal injury. J Pain Res 6:39–51, 2013. LOE II
162. Berg AO, Breslau N, Goodman SN, et al: Treatment of posttraumatic stress disorder: an assessment of the evidence. Washington, DC, 2008, National Academies Press. LOE II
179. [illegible]: The Case for Patient-Centered Care in Orthopaedics. J Am Acad Orthop Surg [illegible], 2010.
180. Olson DP, Windish DM: Communication discrepancies between physicians and hospitalized patients. Arch Intern Med 170(15):1302–1307, 2010. LOE IV
195. Lorig KR, Holman HR: Self-Management Education: History, definition, outcomes, and mechanisms. Ann Behav Med 26(1):1–7, 2003.
196. Wegener ST, Mackenzie EJ, Ephraim P, et al: Self-management improves outcomes in persons with limb loss. Arch Phys Med Rehabil 90(3):373–380, 2009. LOE I
213. [illegible] perception of the [illegible] ICU [illegible]

The complete References list is available online at expertconsult.inkling.com.

SECTION TWO

Spine

EDITED BY PAUL A. ANDERSON

SECTION OUTLINE

Chapter 30

Imaging of Spinal Trauma

HUMBERTO ROSAS

INTRODUCTION

The imaging assessment of trauma patients has undergone a transformation over the past decade secondary to the development of multidetector-row computed tomography (MDCT), allowing faster image acquisition and the capability of multiplanar reformations. Historically, plain radiographs were the first-line modality in the evaluation of the spine with CT acting as a problem-solving tool in the evaluation of inadequately visualized segments of the vertebral column typically centered at the craniocervical and cervicothoracic junctions. Increased availability; advancement in technology allowing rapid, isotropic imaging with resulting high-resolution reformations and three-dimensional (3-D) reconstructions; and improved diagnostic accuracy have resulted in CT supplanting radiographs at trauma centers as the initial imaging study of the spine. An additional advantage is the capability of obtaining diagnostic images of the thoracic and lumbar spine after CT examinations of the chest, abdomen, and pelvis performed in the evaluation of visceral organ damage in polytrauma patients.

Currently patients often undergo several imaging studies in the evaluation of spine injuries, including radiographs, CT, and magnetic resonance imaging (MRI). Conservative estimates report that more than 1 million patients present to emergency departments (EDs) in the United States each year with blunt trauma and potential spine injury. Variability continues to exist regarding the appropriate imaging algorithm to adequately rule out spine injuries, resulting in overutilization of imaging resources at a cost of approximately $3.4 billion spent in the United States in the imaging assessment of the cervical spine alone.[1] This chapter reviews not only the imaging findings of spine trauma but also discusses the selection of the appropriate imaging modality and indications for imaging.

IMAGING SELECTION AND INDICATIONS

Optimizing imaging protocols requires identifying clinical risk factors with significant predictive value in determining if a spinal injury is present or absent. Imaging every blunt trauma patient is not a viable option because this would lead to unnecessary radiation exposure and undue costs to the health care system. To date, two prospective, observational cohort, multicenter trials have attempted to address the appropriate selection criteria for identifying trauma patients who require cervical spine imaging.

The protocols used to identify patients who require imaging are reviewed in Chapter 10. Briefly, patients can be divided into four groups: asymptomatic, temporarily nonassessable, symptomatic, and obtunded. The symptomatic and obtunded patients warrant further assessment for occult injuries with cross-sectional imaging. The decision of whether the temporarily nonassessable patient requires imaging depends on clinical circumstances. Traditionally, radiographs were the mainstay screening examination. Radiographs, however, have several limitations, particularly in patients with multisystem trauma who may be uncooperative, have concomitant injuries, are on a backboard, and have an overlying cervical collar in place. In this scenario, the radiographic examination is technically challenging, often resulting in poor study quality and requiring repeat imaging, leading to delays in management, increased radiation exposure, and incomplete evaluation of the entire spine. Missed injuries result from obscuration by the overlying soft tissues and overlap of bony structures, particularly at the craniocervical and cervicothoracic junctions; poor visualization of nondisplaced fractures, particularly those that involve difficult regions to assess radiographically such as the occipital condyles, atlas, axis, and lamina; and masking of underlying ligamentous injuries either from spontaneous reduction or stabilization after placement of a cervical collar.

The advent of MDCT has led to the replacement of radiographs in the primary screening of adult patients with suspected spine injuries.[2-4] CT, particularly in the evaluation of the cervical spine, has been shown to outperform radiographs regarding both speed of the examination and diagnostic accuracy.[5-8] CT-based protocols result in a reduction in trauma workup time and improved patient disposition from the trauma bay. A meta-analysis of seven studies by Holmes and colleagues comparing radiographs with CT revealed a pooled sensitivity of radiography for detecting cervical injuries of 52% as compared with 98% for CT.[9] Additionally, in patients stratified at a risk higher than 10% for spine fracture, CT is the preferred modality in regard to cost effectiveness and paralysis prevention.[10]

The current American College of Radiology recommendations based on a literature review of data on more than 72,000 adult patients with cervical trauma are to perform screening imaging with MDCT for patients with high-risk criteria based on the National Emergency X-Radiography Use Study (NEXUS) or the Canadian Cervical Rules (CCR). The NEXUS analyzed the clinical data and radiography in 34,069 blunt trauma patients, concluding that imaging of the cervical spine was unnecessary in the absence of posterior midline cervical tenderness or focal neurologic deficit in patients demonstrating a normal level of alertness, lack of clinical evidence of intoxication, or evidence of a distracting injury.[11] By applying these criteria, the sensitivity reported in adequately identifying patients at risk for a cervical spine fracture was 99.6%. The Canadian Cervical Spine (CCS) group used several criteria to deem patients at low risk for a cervical spine injury and safe to assess active range of motion.[12] First, the patient must be fully alert with a Glasgow Coma Scale score of 15. The second criteria include the absence of high-risk factors such as a fall from a height greater than 3 m or five stairs, an axial load to the head, a high-speed vehicular crash, a bicycle or motorcycle crash, the presence of paresthesias, or age older than 65 years. The third criteria include the presence of low-risk factors, including the absence of midline tenderness, ambulatory patients, delayed onset of neck pain, sitting position in the ED, and simple low-speed vehicular crash. Patients at low risk based on these criteria can be cleared clinically if they retain the ability to actively rotate their heads 45 degrees in both directions. The CCS group reported a sensitivity of 100% and a specificity of 42.5% in predicting the absence of a cervical spine injury in 8924 patients.

Similar recommendations for imaging of the thoracolumbar spine are advocated, although supportive literature currently is less definitive than that for the cervical spine.

Obtunded Patient

Controversy remains as to the appropriate imaging evaluation of obtunded trauma patients. Unrecognized injuries can result in devastating consequences, including paralysis and death.[13,14] The risk of neurologic sequelae is 10-fold greater in patients with occult cervical spine injuries compared with those whose injuries are identified on initial screening.[15,16] Conversely, unwarranted prolonged spinal immobilization has its own risks and complications, including pressure ulcers, venous thrombosis, and respiratory deterioration, as well as limits to mobility and central venous access sites.[17-19]

The vast majority of evidence indicates that the number of unstable cervical spine injuries is exceedingly low in the setting of a negative MDCT examination. Hogan and colleagues performed a retrospective study on 366 obtunded trauma patients who underwent MRI after negative CT scan findings on a 16-detector MDCT scanner.[20] The reported negative predictive value for ligament injury was 98.9% (362 of 3666) with none of the injuries involving more than one column or deemed mechanically unstable for a 100% negative predictive value for unstable cervical spine injuries. Como and colleagues prospectively studied 115 obtunded trauma patients with MRI after negative screening MDCT examination findings.[18] Acute injuries were found in six patients; however, the findings did not result in an alteration in management or require surgical intervention. Muchow and colleagues performed a meta-analysis determining the predictive value of MRI to evaluate cervical spine trauma. They found that there was a high false-positive rate, but the negative predictive value was 100%, indicating that negative MRI findings excluded possibility of cervical spine injury.[21] Despite several other studies demonstrating low false-negative rates and high sensitivity for MDCT, the subject of supplemental MRI remains a matter of debate because Menaker and colleagues concluded that negative MDCT findings are insufficient in this patient population. In this study group, 18 patients were found to have abnormalities on MRI after normal CT scans, 14 requiring extended collar immobilization and two necessitating surgery.[22] Further research regarding the need for additional imaging in the setting of negative CT examination findings, as well as the timing of supplemental imaging is required to optimize the treatment of these patients, avoid extended immobilization, and provide a cost-effective algorithm.

The Pediatric Patient

Concerns regarding the adverse health effects associated with radiation exposure have prompted further evaluation of imaging protocols and indications, particularly in the pediatric population.[23] Unfortunately, the national trend has been an exponential increase in use of CT examinations over the past 2 decades. Direct epidemiologic evidence has shown an increased risk of cancer after the organ dose delivered from common CT studies performed on two or three body parts (30–90 mSV).[24] In comparing single-detector CT examinations with radiographs of the cervical spine, Rybicki and colleagues found a 14-fold increase in radiation dose to the thyroid gland—26 mGy for CT compared with 1.8 mGy for radiography.[25] Muchow and colleagues estimated a lifetime increased relative risk of thyroid cancer of 25% in adolescent girls receiving a single screening cervical spine CT.[26]

The current recommendation for children younger than the age of 14 years is to perform radiographs rather than CT as the initial screening examination. The reasoning is that cervical spine injuries are relatively rare in this age group and commonly involve the upper cervical spine, a region that can be adequately evaluated with radiographs in children.[27] The same holds true for the thoracic and lumbar spine unless the patient has already undergone a CT examination of the chest, abdomen, and pelvis. In this scenario, CT reconstructions from the source data can be used. Cross-sectional imaging should be reserved as a supplement and problem-solving tool. Interestingly, a 2006 study evaluating 1692 pediatric trauma patients observed a substantial increase in use of CT (9%–21%) in this patient population based on alterations in hospital protocol during the two phases of the study without an increase in sensitivity in detecting spinal injuries.[28]

Although several studies have shown the NEXUS criteria to be reliable in children, a multicenter study of 12,537 pediatric trauma patients identified four predictors associated with a higher incidence of cervical spine injury: A GCS score of less than 14, Glasgow Coma Score EYE (GCS_{EYE}) score of 1, involvement in a motor vehicle crash, and age older than 2 years.[29] In these circumstances, CT may be the optimal initial imaging study. After age 14 years, the spine has developed fully; therefore, these patients should be treated in the same manner as adults. CT examinations, particularly in pediatric patients, should be optimized to reduce the radiation dose while maintaining image quality.[30] Dose reduction strategies include using automatic exposure control based on patient size and body habitus and tube current modulation.[31-33]

Geriatric Patient

Elderly patients present a diagnostic dilemma because fractures can be difficult to detect both clinically and with imaging because of underlying degenerative changes superimposed on osteopenia. The injury pattern also differs from the pattern in younger individuals with a higher proportion of injuries involving the upper cervical spine often caused by low-impact trauma such as a fall from standing height.[34]

Although studies have shown that clinical prediction rules developed for the adult population (NEXUS and CCR) can be applied to patients older than 65 years of age, the most important predictors of injury included neurologic deficit, head injury, and high-impact trauma.[35] CT remains the primary modality for assessing elderly patients suspected of having spinal trauma, but MRI may add vital information under certain circumstances. In equivocal cases in which a vertebra appears wedged without a discrete fracture line evident on CT and the patient is symptomatic at that level, MRI can help differentiate an acute from a chronic fracture by the presence of bone marrow edema.

Role of Magnetic Resonance Imaging

Magnetic resonance imaging is the modality of choice in the evaluation of the soft tissues, including the spinal cord, ligaments, intervertebral discs, musculature, and vasculature. MRI, however, is not well suited in the evaluation of osseous injuries, particularly those involving the posterior elements, because of the relative lack of cancellous bone in these structures. Improved sensitivities have been reported for injuries involving the vertebral body (37%–100%) compared with those involving the posterior elements (12%–45%). Although the sensitivity of MRI remains inadequate to replace CT in the evaluation of an osseous injury, the specificity is reported to be around 95%.[36-38] MRI is the preferred means to determine the acuity of osteoporotic fractures when indicated.

Debate continues, however, regarding MRI's role because of the lack of a standardized imaging protocol across medical centers, cost, difficulty in positioning patients with multisystem trauma within the bore, and evidence indicating that detection of occult injuries on MRI rarely results in alteration of medical management. After a normal CT examination, the incidence of abnormal MRI findings is approximately 15%, with only 0.3% of patients requiring the need for surgical intervention.[18,39,40]

Despite the small number of unstable cervical spine injuries detected with MRI in patients with normal CT examination findings, MRI is advocated in particular clinical circumstances, including in patients with neurologic impairment, progressive neurologic deficits, a change in neurologic status, or severe unexplained pain (Table 30-1).

In this patient population, unrecognized injuries identified on MRI examinations resulted in either urgent surgical intervention or prolonged collar immobilization. Menaker and colleagues performed a retrospective study on 203 patients, 18 of whom had injuries only detected with MRI, 16 of whom ultimately required a change in management.[22] MRI is ideally suited to diagnose and detect the presence of traumatic disc herniations, extramedullary hematomas, ligamentous injuries, and acute spinal cord injuries, as well as to characterize any associated central canal or foraminal stenosis.

TABLE 30-1 *INDICATIONS FOR MAGNETIC RESONANCE IMAGING*
Neurologic impairment
Progressive neurologic deficits
Change in neurologic status
Severe unexplained pain
Preoperative planning
Determine age of a fracture in patients with osteoporosis
Determine presence of a herniated disc in facet dislocation

Knowledge regarding the integrity of the ligamentous structures will aid in characterizing the extent of injury and potential for mechanical instability. MRI protocols use multiple sequences exposing differences in the hydrogen concentration of the soft tissues to allow for exquisite anatomic detail and identification of pathologic processes. Although the parameters vary widely depending on the field strength, coil design, and software capabilities of the MRI system, protocols should be tailored to provide sufficient clinical data in a timely fashion. Standardizing protocols and limiting imaging sequences reduce the time needed to perform exams in medically unstable patients.

Magnetic Resonance Imaging Protocols

Sagittal T2-weighted and proton density images delineate the ligaments from the surrounding soft tissues and bone, as well as areas of periosteal stripping or discontinuity. The ligaments appear as low signal intensity structures on all sequences because of a relative lack of mobile hydrogen atoms compared with the surrounding structures. Injuries are diagnosed by either identifying focal disruption of the ligament often with fluid seen tracking within the ligamentous gap or identifying attenuation of a ligament (Fig. 30-1). The ligamentous stump can have an associated avulsed fracture fragment as well. The accuracy of MRI in diagnosing a ligamentous injury varies among several studies with reported sensitivities ranging from 46% to 71% for the anterior longitudinal ligament, 43% to 93% for the posterior longitudinal ligament, 67% for the ligamentum flavum, 36% to 100% for the interspinous ligament, and 89% for the supraspinous ligament.[36,38,41-44]

The majority of MR protocols also include a sagittal T1-weighted sequence to delineate normal anatomy as well as assess the bone marrow, which should appear brighter than the adjacent intervertebral disc. Fracture lines will typically appear dark on the T1 sequences.

Other commonly used sequences include gradient echo sequences, short tau inversion recovery (STIR), and isotropic 3-D volumetric sequences such as vastly interpolated projection reconstruction (VIPR) imaging. Sagittal gradient echo sequences optimize detection of areas of hemorrhage caused by bloom artifact. This artifact is the result of susceptibility and dephasing on sequences that do not use a 180-degree radiofrequency refocusing pulse; the end result is that small areas of hemorrhage "bloom" and become more conspicuous to the reader. STIR sequences provide robust fat saturation and increased contrast between areas of edema and normal soft tissue as can be seen in cases of cord contusions or bone marrow edema surrounding fractures (Fig. 30-2). Isotropic 3-D volumetric sequences such as VIPR allow reconstructions in any imaging plane after a single acquisition. The literature to date, however, has not shown these additional sequences to provide information that would alter patient management.

Sagittal T2-weighted sequences also provide the highest correlation with patient prognosis in the setting of an acute spinal cord injury because the level of a cord laceration or transection or extent of edema and hemorrhage within the spinal cord can be determined.[45-47] In the acute or subacute period (1–7 days), edema is seen on the T2-weighted sequences as areas of hyperintense signal within the cord, and hemorrhage appears hypointense (Figs. 30-2 and 30-3). Four signal patterns have been described: normal, single-level edema, multilevel edema, and mixed hemorrhage and edema.[48] Patient

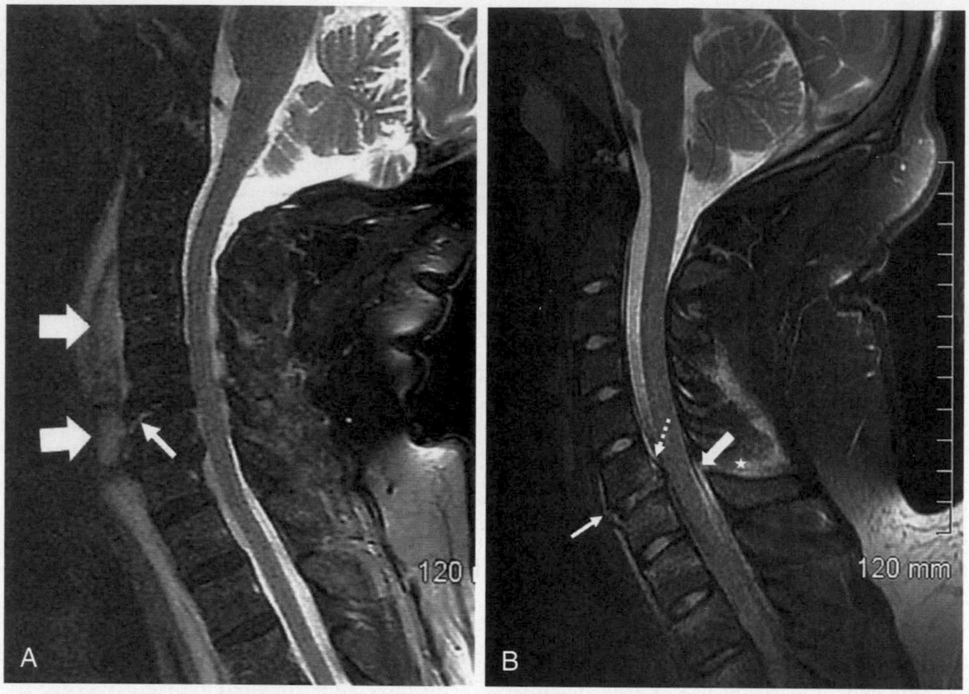

Figure 30-1. Sagittal T2-weighted magnetic resonance images demonstrating ligamentous injuries. **A,** Extension injury with discontinuity of the anterior longitudinal ligament (ALL) and fluid tracking through the torn portion of the ALL into the C5-C6 intervertebral disc space *(arrow)*. Formation of associated prevertebral soft tissue swelling and anterior hematoma *(thick arrows)* is noted. **B,** Flexion injury with disruption of the ALL *(arrow)* and ligamentum flavum *(thick arrow)*, stripping of the posterior longitudinal ligament *(dashed arrow)*, and hyperintense signal within the interspinous space *(star)* consistent with tearing of the interspinous ligaments.

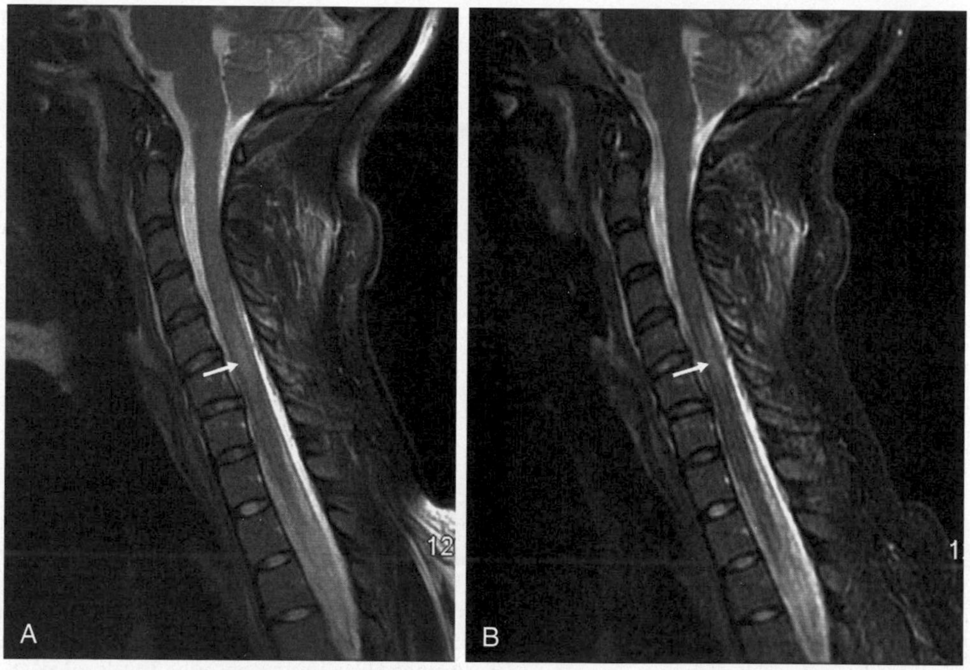

Figure 30-2. Mid sagittal T2-weighted fat saturation (**A**) and short tau inversion recovery (STIR) (**B**) images of the cervical spine after a flexion injury demonstrating focal hyperintense signal *(arrows)* within the central cord in keeping with edema. STIR sequences provide more robust fat saturation and increased soft tissue contrast accentuating regions of increased signal intensity.

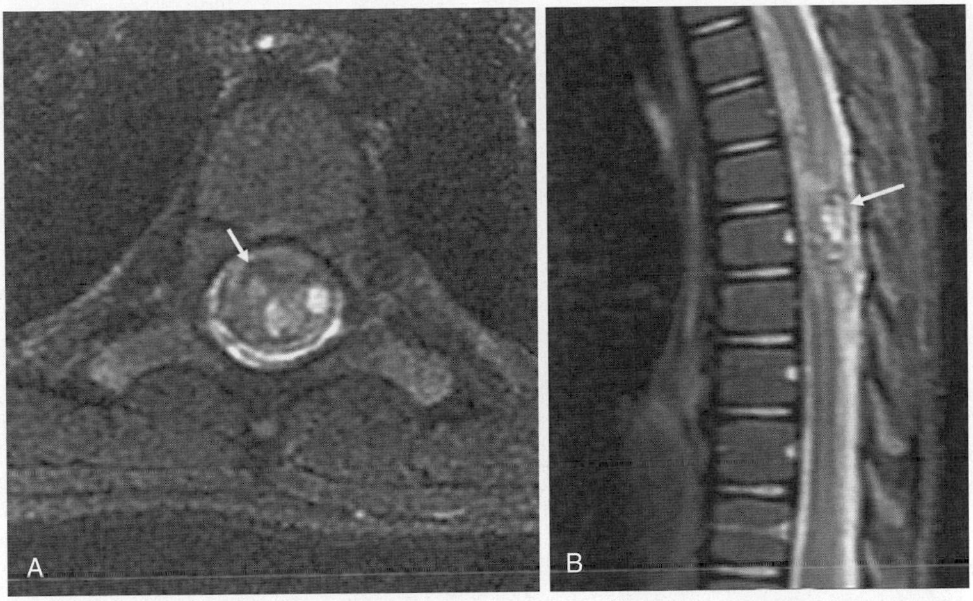

Figure 30-3. Severe traumatic cord injury of the thoracic spine. Axial (**A**) and sagittal (**B**) T2-weighted images reveal areas of mixed signal intensity within a partially transected thoracic cord. Areas of low signal intensity *(arrows)* represent areas of hemorrhage.

outcomes and the potential of restoring function directly relate to the MRI cord signal with patients recovering fully with normal signal characteristics on MRI regardless of initial neurologic status, but the most severe outcomes are associated with the hemorrhagic pattern. Interestingly, the greater extent and length of edema have been shown to lead to poorer average improvement; however, the same has not been shown with hemorrhage.[49-52]

Axial sequences, either T2 or T1 weighted, have not been found to have prognostic value but characterize clinically relevant lesions such as acute disc herniations and extramedullary hemorrhage, as well as assess with better accuracy the amount of cord compression, central canal stenosis, and foraminal stenosis (Figs. 30-4 and 30-5). The incidence of disc herniation on initial MRI approaches 36% with a higher proportion of concomitant injuries to the posterior ligament complex (64%) compared with the anterior longitudinal ligament (37%).[53-55] Doran and colleagues reported a high incidence of traumatic disc herniation in the setting of facet dislocations, both unilateral and bilateral.[56] The degree of canal stenosis, underlying cord signal changes, and evidence of impingement of the adjacent nerve roots must be documented, particularly in patients requiring surgical intervention, to optimize surgical treatment and neurologic recovery.

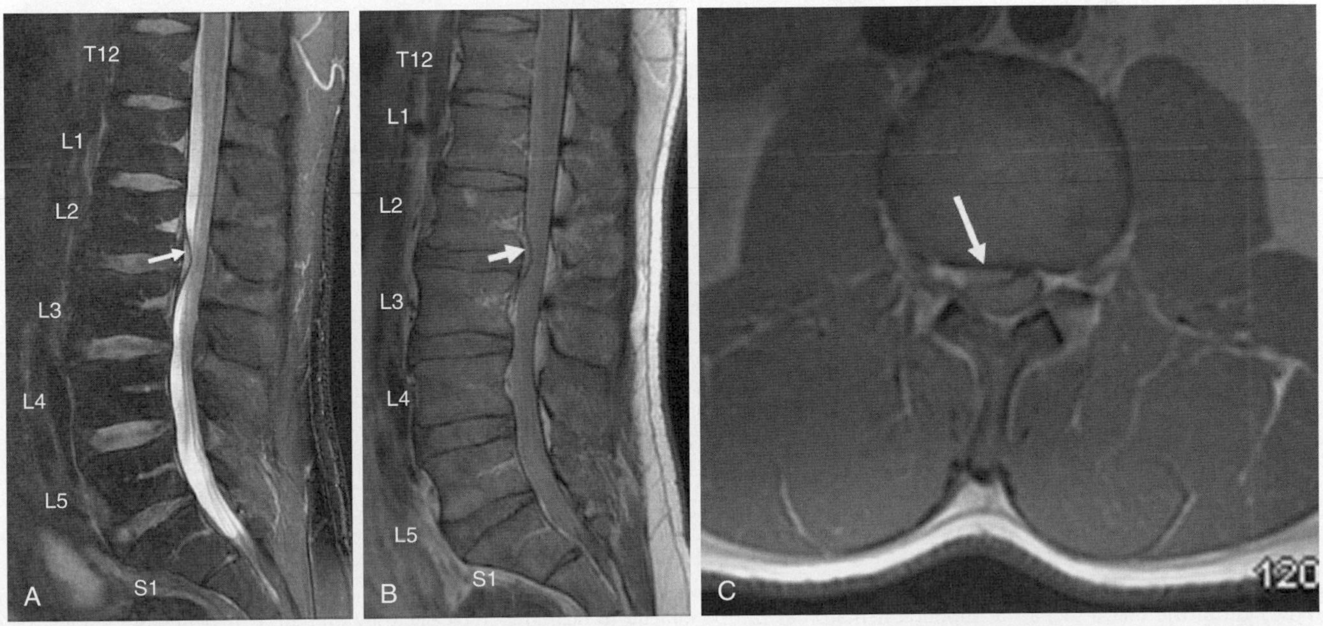

Figure 30-4. Acute epidural hematoma. Magnetic resonance images of the lumbar spine in a patient involved in a motor vehicle accident show an epidural hematoma anteriorly *(arrows),* which indents the thecal sac. The age of the blood products is determined by the signal characteristics, which are predominantly hyperintense in respect to the conus.

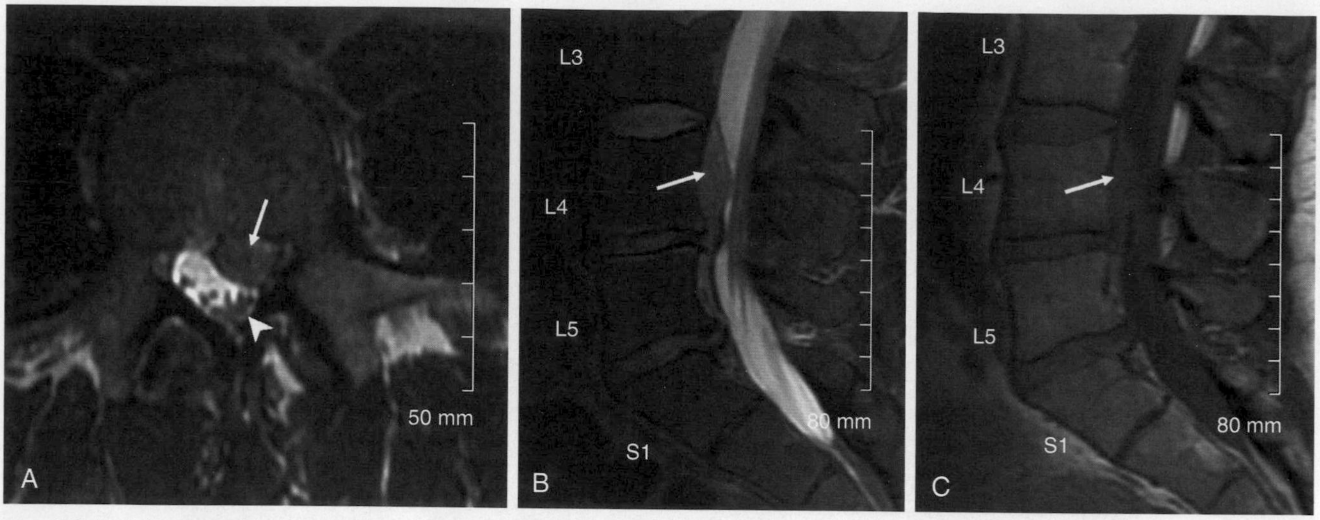

Figure 30-5. Subacute epidural hematoma. A large epidural hematoma *(arrow)* with internal intermediate signal intensity, isointense to the adjacent nerve roots, results in central canal stenosis and narrowing of the left lateral recess best depicted by the axial T2-weighted sequences (**A**). The hematoma not only indents the thecal sac but results in clumping of the traversing nerve roots *(arrowhead)*. **B,** Sagittal T2-weighted sequence. **C,** Sagittal T1-weighted sequence.

Optional coronal sequences can be obtained to aid in the evaluation of the craniocervical junction and characterize the alignment of dens and occipital condyle fractures.

Extramedullary hemorrhage is an uncommon consequence of spinal trauma occurring in approximately 1% to 2% of cases (see Figs. 30-4 and 30-5).[57] Epidural hematomas most commonly involve the cervical and thoracic spine and are thought to be venous in origin (see Figs. 30-4 and 30-5). Typically located dorsally because of the relationship of the dura ventrally with the posterior longitudinal ligament and local pooling within valveless, thin-walled dorsal epidural veins, it has been postulated that a sudden increase in intravenous pressure leads to rupture of these veins.[57] Younger patients and patients with fused spinal segments such as seen in ankylosing spondylitis and diffuse idiopathic skeletal hyperostosis (DISH) are at highest risk for the development of an epidural hematoma after a traumatic event.[57] Conversely, subdural hematomas more commonly occur ventral to the cord. The diagnosis can be difficult as the hematoma evolves over time (Figs. 30-6 and 30-7). In the hyperacute stage (1–6 hours), intact red blood cells contain oxyhemoglobin, which appears hyperintense on the T2-weighted sequences. At 1 to 3 days, oxyhemoglobin deoxygenates to deoxyhemoglobin with a paramagnetic effect, resulting in areas of hemorrhage appearing dark on the T2-weighted sequences compared with the spinal cord. Within 3 to 7 days, deoxyhemoglobin converts into intracellular methemoglobin, which remains dark on the T2-weighted sequences, but now appears bright rather than isointense on

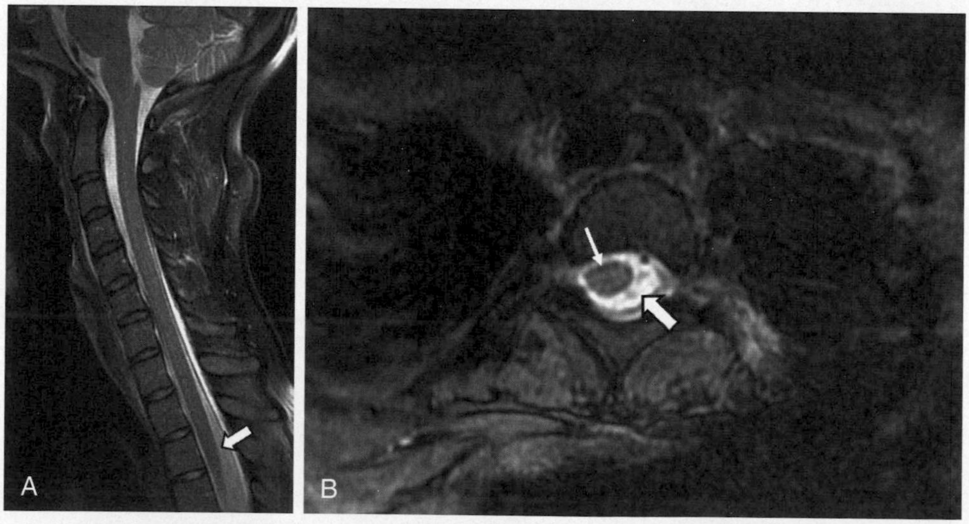

Figure 30-6. Subtle acute cervical subdural hematoma. Given similar signal characteristics to the subjacent cerebrospinal fluid and lack of compression of the thecal sac, acute subdural hematomas can be difficult to diagnose. Typically, they present as hyperintense lesions (block arrows on the sagittal (**A**) and axial (**B**) T2 fat-saturated sequences) within the dural sac silhouetting and typically displacing the adjacent spinal cord *(arrow)*. As evident on the axial T2-weighted sequence (**B**), the cervical cord is eccentrically located secondary to mass effect from the subjacent subdural hematoma. Lack of direct continuity with the adjacent osseous structures is another imaging clue to this diagnosis.

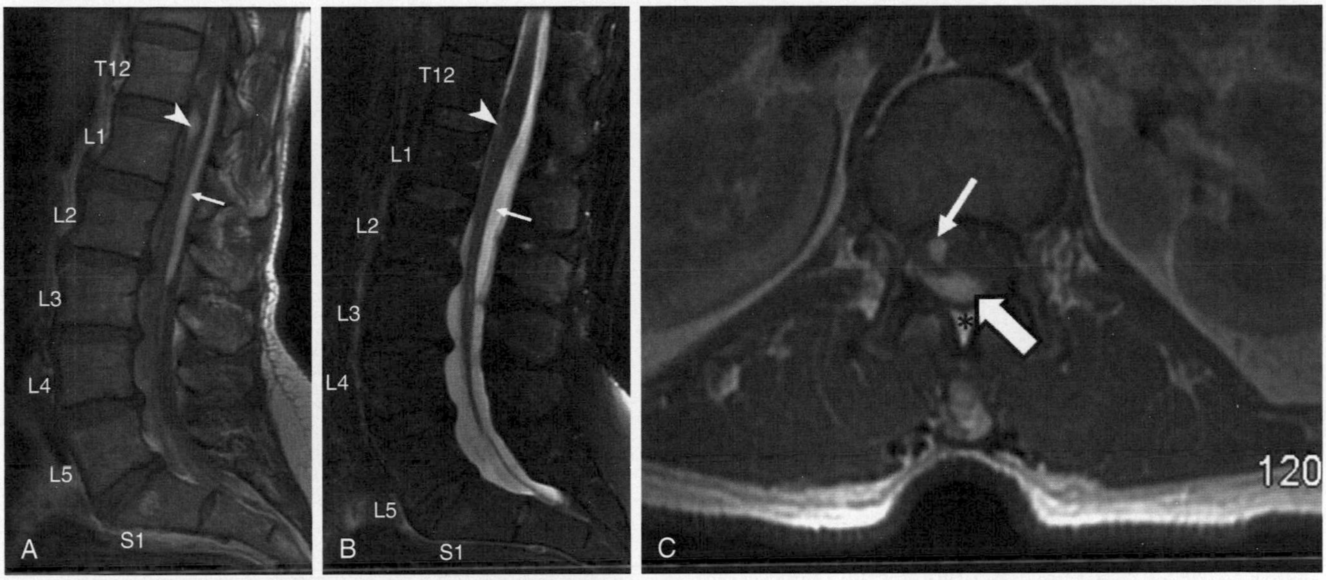

Figure 30-7. Sagittal T1- (**A**), sagittal T2- (**B**), and axial T1- (**C**) weighted sequences demonstrating a subdural hematoma *(arrows)*, which is clearly distinct from the epidural fat *(asterisk)*. In addition, intrathecal hemorrhage is seen involving the distal cord *(arrowheads)*. The blood products are hyperintense in signal compared with the adjacent cord.

the T1-weighed images.[58] Posterior fossa subdural hematomas are associated with craniocervical dissociation, which requires critical evaluation.

Although the research is lacking, based on the experience of several trauma centers, the optimal time interval between injury and MRI examinations is within 72 hours.[48,59] This recommendation is based on the natural progression of MR signal changes beyond this time interval. The length of cord edema increases by one vertebral level for each 1.2-day delay in imaging within the first 5 days. Single-level edema will progressively resolve within 3 weeks, and the initial hypointense signal of hemorrhage will transform to hyperintense signal between 1 to 2 weeks as deoxyhemoglobin is converted to extracellular methemoglobin. Additionally, soft tissue edema progressively resolves, resulting in reduced visibility of subtle ligamentous injuries.

Role of Flexion and Extension Views and Dynamic Fluoroscopy

The literature does not provide sufficient evidence to support the use of either flexion and extension views or dynamic fluoroscopy in the detection of cervical spine ligamentous injuries. Often the examination is inadequate with Bolinger and colleagues reporting visualization of the cervicothoracic junction in only 4% of fluoroscopic studies and Anglen and colleagues reporting 28% (236 of 837) of flexion and extension radiographs to be technically inadequate.[60,61] Duane and colleagues compared flexion and extension views with MRI in 271 patients.[62] Radiographs were nondiagnostic in approximately 30% of cases and did not facilitate treatment. Additionally, flexion and extension views resulted in increased cost and prolonged immobilization. A follow-up study showed that flexion and extension views failed to identify MRI-confirmed injuries. Freedman and colleagues concluded that the technique for flexion and extension views is unreliable and reported four false negatives in seven patients with injuries.[63] Furthermore, neurologic deficits have been described after dynamic fluoroscopy with the development of quadriplegia in one patient.[64] Given the low sensitivity for ligamentous injury detection, low rate of interpretable studies, high false-positive rates, and potential to induce neurologic deficits, the role of flexion and extension views or dynamic fluoroscopy is limited and should not be performed in obtunded patients.

Far less data are available concerning the indication for imaging the thoracolumbar spine with flexion and extension views; however, the same principles apply. In addition to low sensitivities, isolated unstable ligamentous injuries to the thoracolumbar spine are extremely rare in the absence of fractures. As is the case for the cervical spine, neurologic deficits indicate the need for imaging the symptomatic level with MRI.

IMAGING EVALUATION

A thorough understanding of normal anatomy, injury patterns, and subtle imaging signs of injury is essential to the evaluation of the spine and high diagnostic accuracy. Although many of the concepts detailed in following sections were developed in the interpretation of radiographs, they translate to CT and MRI. The concept of stability also plays a crucial role in spine imaging. Stability implies the ability to maintain normal alignment in response to physiologic loading and range of motion. Classification systems for predicting stability have been proposed over the years with the three-column theory of Denis being the most widely accepted.[65] The three-column theory divides the spine into anterior, middle, and posterior columns. The anterior column is composed of the anterior longitudinal ligament, the anterior two-thirds of the vertebral body and intervertebral disc, and the anterior annulus fibrosus. The middle column includes the posterior third of the vertebral body and intervertebral disc, as well as the posterior longitudinal ligament. Finally, the posterior column consists of the posterior elements: pedicles, lamina, ligamentum flavum, interspinous ligaments, supraspinous ligament, facet joints, and spinous processes. Disruption of two columns implies instability, and it is imperative to relay pertinent imaging findings to the referring physician regarding the extent of injury. As will be discussed further in the later sections, radiographic features of mechanical instability throughout the spine include translation of greater than 3 mm; vertebral body height loss of greater than 50%; kyphosis measuring more than 20 degrees; angulation greater than 11 degrees; and widening of the interspinous space, facet joints, intervertebral disc space, or interpedicular distance.

Cervical Spine

A systematic approach should be applied when evaluating either radiographs or cross-sectional imaging (MRI and CT) to detect subtle injuries. Radiographic assessment of the cervical spine includes standard three views (anterior-posterior [AP], lateral, and open mouth), although the vast majority of injuries are detected on the lateral view.[66] Given the inherent difficulty in visualizing the cervicothoracic junction secondary to obscuration by the overlying soft tissues and osseous structures, a swimmer's view is often necessary to demonstrate the anatomy to the T1 level. CT examinations should include reconstructions of the axial images in both the coronal and sagittal planes. Regardless of the modality, a checklist should be used when evaluating imaging studies to ensure high diagnostic accuracy. Each of the views will be discussed separately below, focusing on radiologic signs and measurements used in their interpretation.

Lateral View and Sagittal Computed Tomography Reconstruction

A review of the lateral cervical radiograph or sagittal reconstructions from a CT examination involves assessment of anatomic lines and relationships. For radiographs, the lateral projection provides the most informative view in the detection of cervical spine injuries, albeit with much lower sensitivities compared with CT. The following items should be assessed:

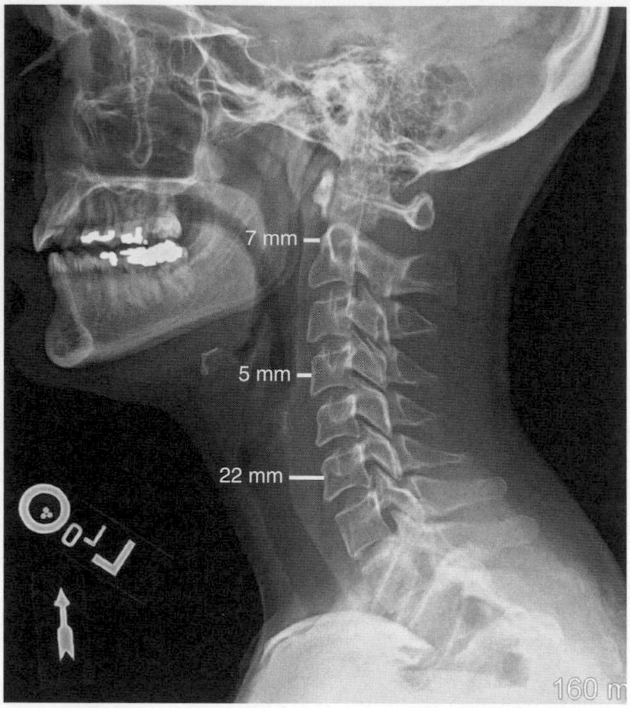

Figure 30-8. Normal width of the prevertebral soft tissues on a lateral radiograph.

- Focal prevertebral soft tissue swelling from soft tissue edema or hematoma may be indicative of an occult injury. The absolute measurement can vary based on head position, phase of inspiration, body habitus, and magnification. In adults, the normal width at the C3 and C4 levels is less than 5 mm (7 mm for C2), gradually increasing to 22 mm at the C6 level (Figs. 30-8 and 30-9). In children younger than 15 years of age, the prevertebral soft tissues should not exceed greater than two-thirds the width of the C2 body at the C3 and C4 levels or more than 14 mm at the C6 level.

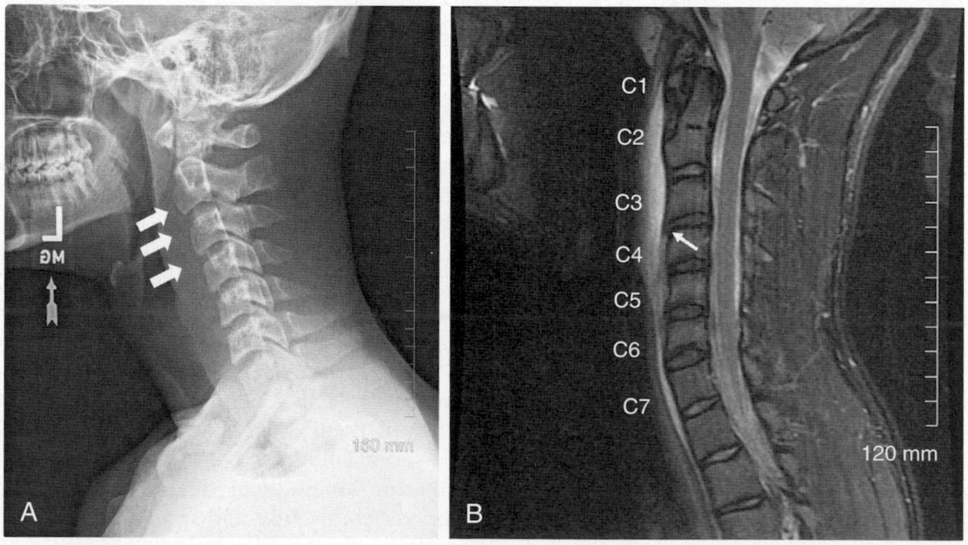

Figure 30-9. Prevertebral soft tissue swelling. **A,** Lateral view of the cervical spine demonstrates widening of the prevertebral soft tissues extending from C2-C5 and displacement of the upper airway. Corresponding magnetic resonance image (**B**) redemonstrates the prevertebral soft tissue swelling in addition to disruption of the anterior longitudinal ligament *(arrow)* at the C3-C4 level with a trace amount of associated anterolisthesis.

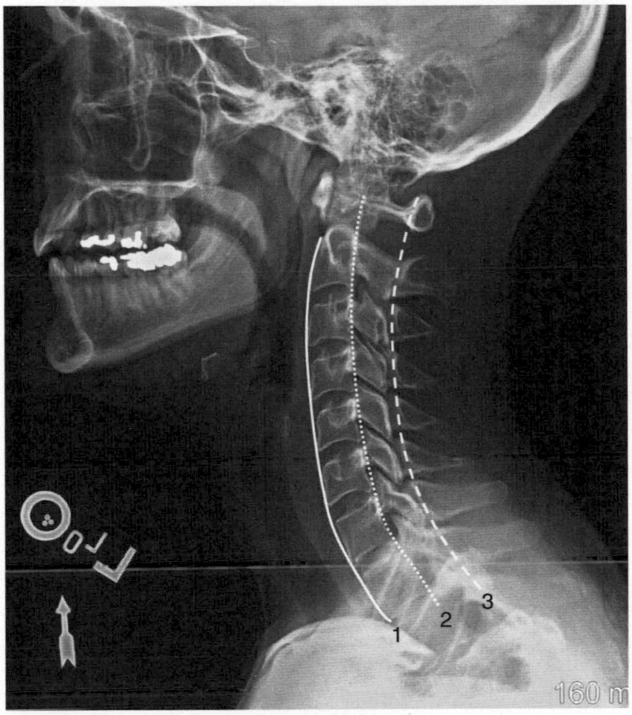

Figure 30-10. Normal lateral view of the cervical spine. Proper alignment is assessed by following three smooth, contiguous contour lines: *(1)* anterior vertebral line, *(2)* posterior vertebral line, and *(3)* the spinolaminar line.

- Alignment is evaluated by following three contour lines: the anterior vertebral line, the posterior vertebral line, and the spinolaminar line. A mild degree of translation of the vertebral bodies in either the anterior or posterior direction can occur normally with physiologic motion and should not exceed 2 mm (Fig. 30-10). The spinolaminar line, however, should be maintained regardless of positioning (see Fig. 30-11). Degenerative spondylolisthesis can occur in the geriatric population or patients with degenerative disease. C3-C4 and C4-C5 are the most commonly affected levels. The hallmark of this process is lack of pain and tenderness and associated facet degeneration.
- The atlantodental distance (ADI) normally measures up to 3 mm in adults and 5 mm in children. Although motion between the anterior arch of C1 and the dens can be present in children with flexion, this finding would be considered pathologic in adults. Widening of this space is associated with injuries to the transverse atlantal ligament and instability of the C1-C2 articulation (Fig. 30-12).[67]
- A confluence of radiographic shadows composed of the superior articular facet of C2, anterior and posterior vertebral cortex of C2, and transverse foramen form a corticated ring (Harris ring) superimposed over the C2 vertebral body on a true lateral view. Disruption of this composite ring shadow is associated with fractures, including atypical hangman's fractures and type III odontoid fractures (Fig. 30-13).[68]
- Malalignment of the atlanto-occipital articulation can be difficult to detect on plain radiographs. The Harris measurement has proven to be the most sensitive assessment of the anatomic relationship between the skull base and spine and is referred to as the atlanto-occipital dissociation rule of 12s. The measurements can be applied regardless of the degree of cervical flexion and extension. The rule states that the distance between the basion (inferior tip of the clivus) and tip of the dens or the horizontal distance between the basion and a vertical line drawn along and parallel to the posterior cortex of C2 should not exceed 12 mm (Fig. 30-14).[69,70]
- In the absence of degenerative disc disease, the intervertebral disc space should appear relatively uniform in height at all levels. Distraction of the vertebral bodies or focal diastasis involving either the anterior or posterior aspect of

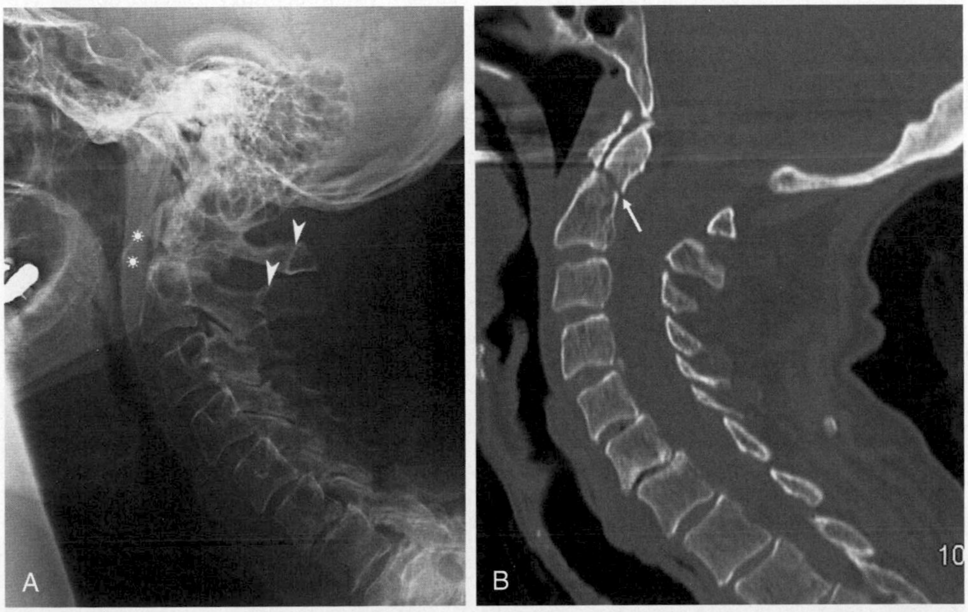

Figure 30-11. A, Prevertebral soft tissue swelling *(stars)* overlying the dens and C1 anterior tubercle indicating edema and hematoma formation. This in conjunction with offset of the spinolaminar line *(arrowheads)* is highly suspicious for an underlying fracture. **B,** Computed tomography examination confirms the presence of a fracture at the base of the dens *(arrow)* (type II fracture) barely discernible on the lateral radiograph (*arrow* in **A**).

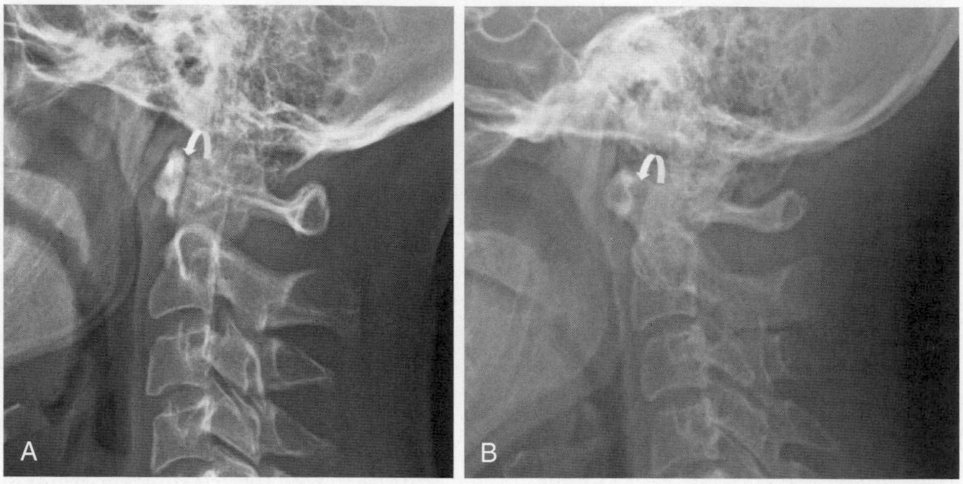

Figure 30-12. Atlantoaxial distance. Lateral coned-down views of the cervical spine demonstrate the normal anterior atlantodental distance (**A**) and mild diastasis (**B**) between the anterior process of C1 and the dens in a patient with a magnetic resonance imaging–proven injury to the transverse atlantal ligament.

the disc space suggests an underlying ligamentous injury (Fig. 30-15).

- On a perfectly positioned lateral view, the articular pillars should be superimposed. Differences in the amount of offset of the lateral masses between adjacent levels indicate abnormal motion along the longitudinal axis of the spine and a rotational injury such as a perched facet (see Fig. 30-15).
- The morphology of the vertebral body should be assessed with any discrepancy of 3 mm or greater in height when comparing the posterior and anterior margins of the vertebral body being suspicious for a compression fracture.
- Although the normal fanning of the spinous processes is not uniform, the interspinous distance (ISD) should never exceed 1.5 times the ISD of the adjacent levels (see Fig. 30-15).
- The epidural space should be analyzed on CT with soft tissue window setting to evaluate for epidural hematomas, which will demonstrate high attenuation or for the presence of a herniated disc, which typically has attenuation values similar to soft tissue. MRI may be indicated to further evaluate this especially in patients with ankylosing spondylitis.

Anterior-Posterior and Open-Mouth Views and Coronal Computed Tomography Reconstruction

Although studies have suggested that the AP view does not provide significant additional diagnostic information or improve sensitivities in the detection of cervical spine injuries, it does act as a supplement to the lateral view.[71] Normally on a true AP view or coronal CT reconstruction, the spinous processes form a continuous vertical line, and the cortices of the lateral masses demonstrate a smooth contiguous undulating surface (Fig. 30-16). Offset of the spinous processes, asymmetry in the intervertebral disc space, or differences in the width of the vertebral bodies between adjacent levels indicates a rotation injury. Lateral flexion type injuries resulting in compression of one of the articular pillars or asymmetric wedging of the vertebral body are often best visualized on the AP view. Sagittally oriented fractures through the vertebrae

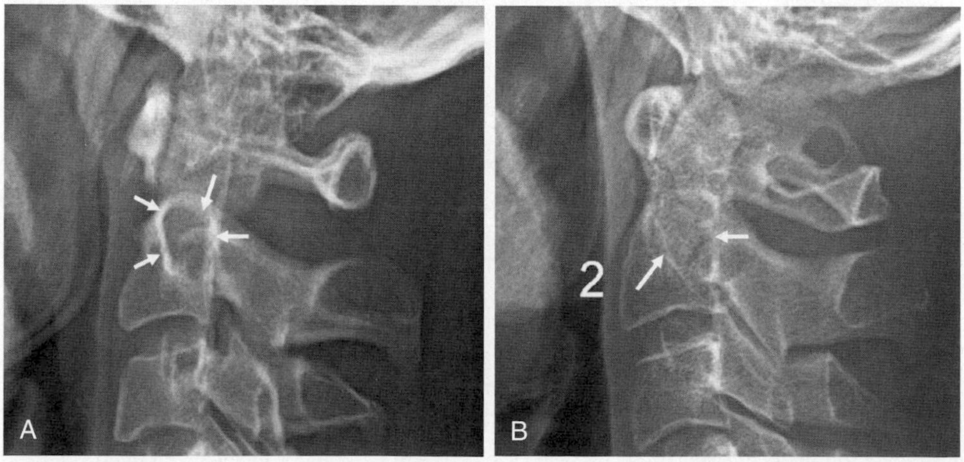

Figure 30-13. A, The C2 composite shadow *(arrows)* is composed of the superior articular facet of C2, anterior and posterior vertebral cortex of C2, and transverse foramen. The foramen transversarium interrupts the posterior inferior aspect of the ring. **B,** Subtle lucency traversing the anterior and posterior borders of Harris ring. A subsequent computed tomography scan confirmed a type III odontoid fracture.

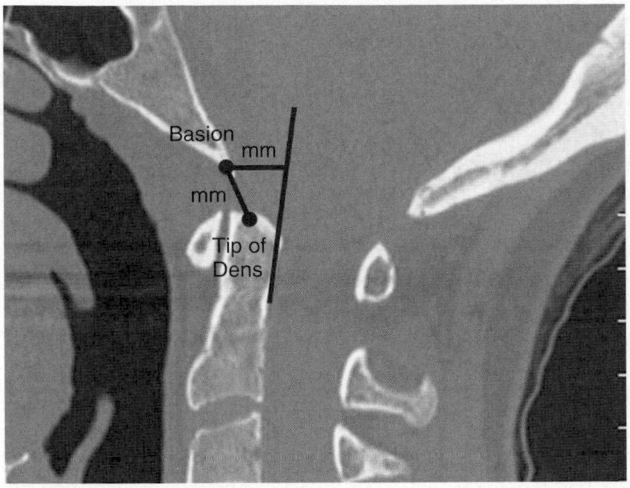

Figure 30-14. Normal atlanto-occipital anatomic relationship. The distance between the basion (inferior tip of the clivus) and tip of the dens or the horizontal distance between the basion and a vertical line drawn along and parallel to the posterior cortex of C2 should not exceed 12 mm.

and transversely oriented fractures of the lateral masses are often more conspicuous on the frontal view (Fig. 30-17).

The open-mouth view profiles the craniocervical junction and odontoid process, regions typically obscured on the AP view secondary to overlap from the facial bones and skull base. When performed properly, the lateral margins of the lateral masses of C1 and C2 should be aligned over one another. In the neutral position, the distance between the dens and medial border of the C1 lateral masses should be relatively equal (Figs. 30-18 and 30-19). Both improper position and injury may change this relationship and require further evaluation.

With C1-C2 rotation, the atlas moves as a unit, resulting in lateral offset of the lateral masses on one side and medial offset on the contralateral side. Despite this relationship, rotation, tilting, or torticollis can be difficult to distinguish from atlantoaxial rotatory subluxation radiographically. Either open-mouth views with the head turned 10 to 15 degrees to both the left and the right or dynamic CT can be performed to differentiate these two entities.[72] In rotatory subluxation, abnormal widening of the lateral atlantodental space remains fixed to one side. Bilateral offset of the articular pillars indicates a C1 ring fracture in adults (Jefferson fracture; see Fig. 30-19). Offset greater than 6 mm typically indicates a concomitant injury to the transverse ligament and instability. In children, mild bilateral offset is considered a normal anatomic variant attributed to discrepant growth of C1 and C2. The open-mouth view aids in the detection of not only C1 fractures and malalignment but fractures of the dens (Figs. 30-20 and 30-21) and lateral flexion fractures of the axis as well.

Thoracic and Lumbar Spine

Anterior-posterior and lateral radiographs are routinely ordered in the setting of acute trauma to the thoracic and lumbar spine with the swimmer's view used as a supplement to improve visualization of the upper thoracic spine and cervicothoracic junction. The same principles applied in the cervical spine can be used in the interpretation of imaging studies

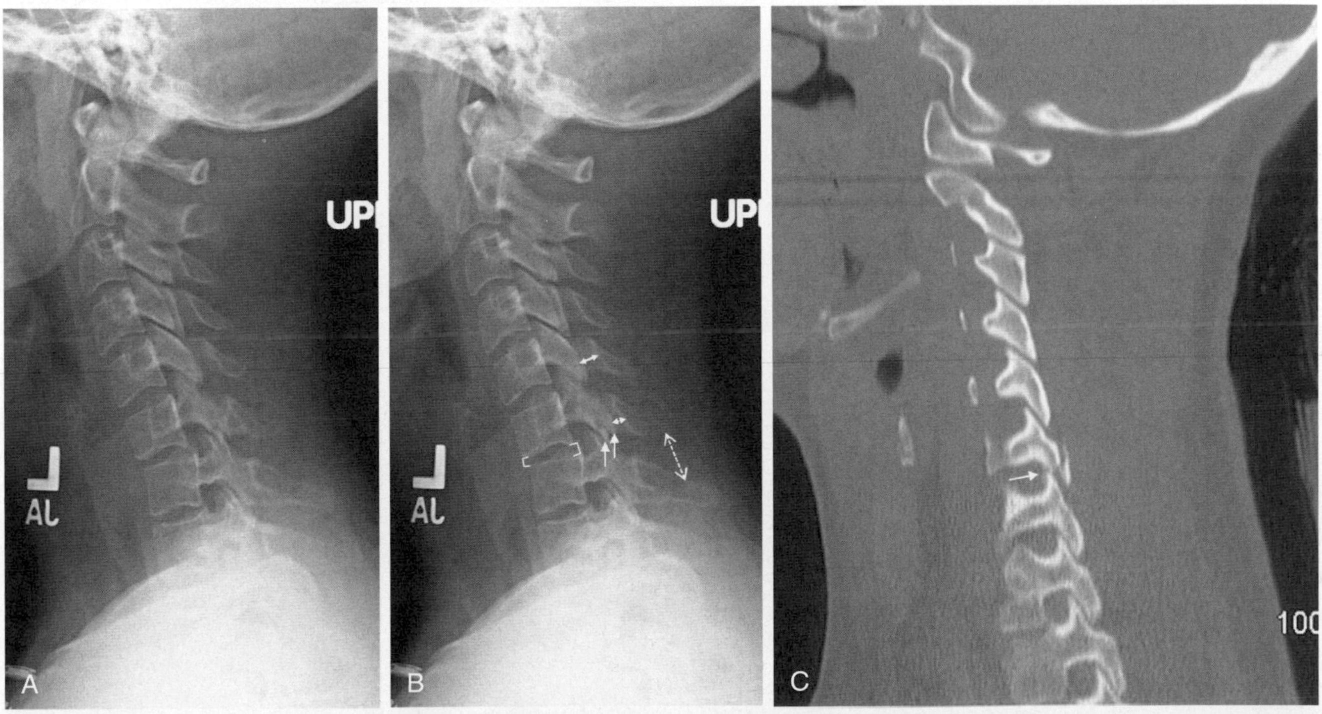

Figure 30-15. A and **B,** Lateral radiographs demonstrate several findings consistent with a flexion-rotation injury of the cervical spine. Asymmetry of the height of the intervertebral disc space *(brackets)*, widening of the interspinous space *(dashed double-headed arrow)*, and mild anterolisthesis of C5 on C6 is in keeping with a ligamentous injury secondary to a flexion type injury. Offset of the articular pillars of C5 *(arrows)* and a discrepancy in the distance between the posterior margins of the articular pillars and spinolaminar line *(double-headed arrows)* compared with adjacent levels indicate a rotational component. **C,** Computed tomography image confirming a unilateral, partially perched facet *(arrow)* in addition to a coronally oriented fracture through the posterior margin of the C6 lateral mass. Corresponding magnetic resonance imaging (see Fig. 30-1, *B*) illustrates the multiple associated ligamentous injuries in this patient.

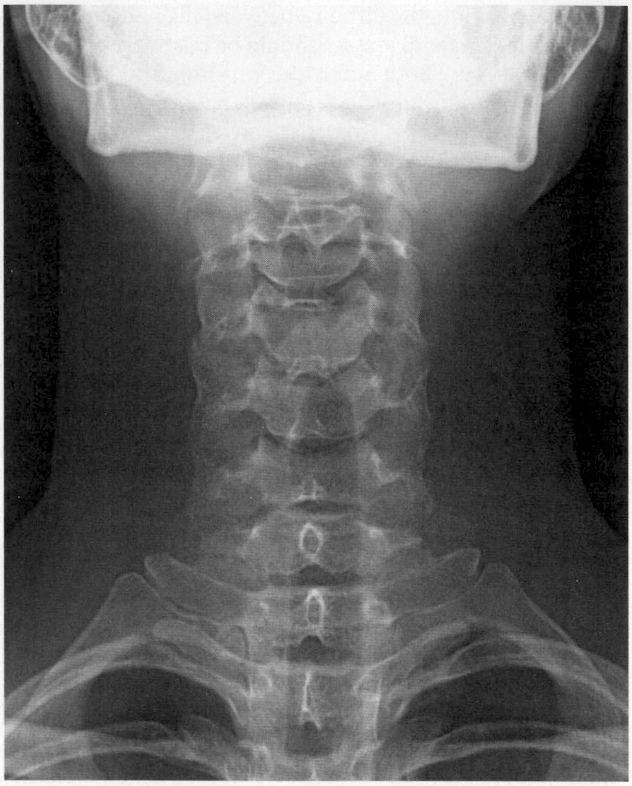

Figure 30-16. Normal anterior-posterior (AP) radiograph of the cervical spine. The lateral masses form a smooth undulating lateral border, the spinous processes are aligned vertically, and the spacing of the intervertebral discs and uncovertebral joints is uniform. The horizontal inclination of the facet joints precludes visualization on the AP view.

of the thoracolumbar spine, although the AP view plays a more prominent role. Focal prominence of the paraspinal structures on the AP view such as displacement of the paraspinal or mediastinal stripe can be seen secondary to hematoma formation subjacent to the site of fracture. Widening of the interpediculate distance suggests an underlying burst fracture, and diastasis of the interspinous space can be seen with severe flexion injuries disrupting the posterior ligamentous complex. As will be discussed, lateral translation and transverse process or rib fractures on the AP view combined with anterolisthesis on the lateral view indicates an unstable shear type injury.

Injury Patterns

Cervical Spine Injuries

Injuries of the vertebral column typically manifest in predictable patterns irrespective of location and are determined predominantly by the underlying mechanism of injury. Depending on the vector of the force applied, recognizable injury patterns cast what Daffner and colleagues referred to as a radiologic "fingerprint."[73] The five basic mechanisms include flexion, extension, rotation, shear, and axial loading. Although many injuries encompass a combination of forces, in general, a dominant force is usually discernible. Biomechanically, the vertebral column functions much like a single long bone, resulting in concomitant injuries at multiple levels in 10% to 25% of cases, requiring careful scrutiny for synchronous noncontiguous injuries at other levels.[73]

In evaluating the upper cervical spine, the most common sites of injury include the occipital condyles, the atlantoaxial and atlanto-occipital articulations, the dens, and the C1 arches. Occipital condyle fractures, although believed to be rare, are

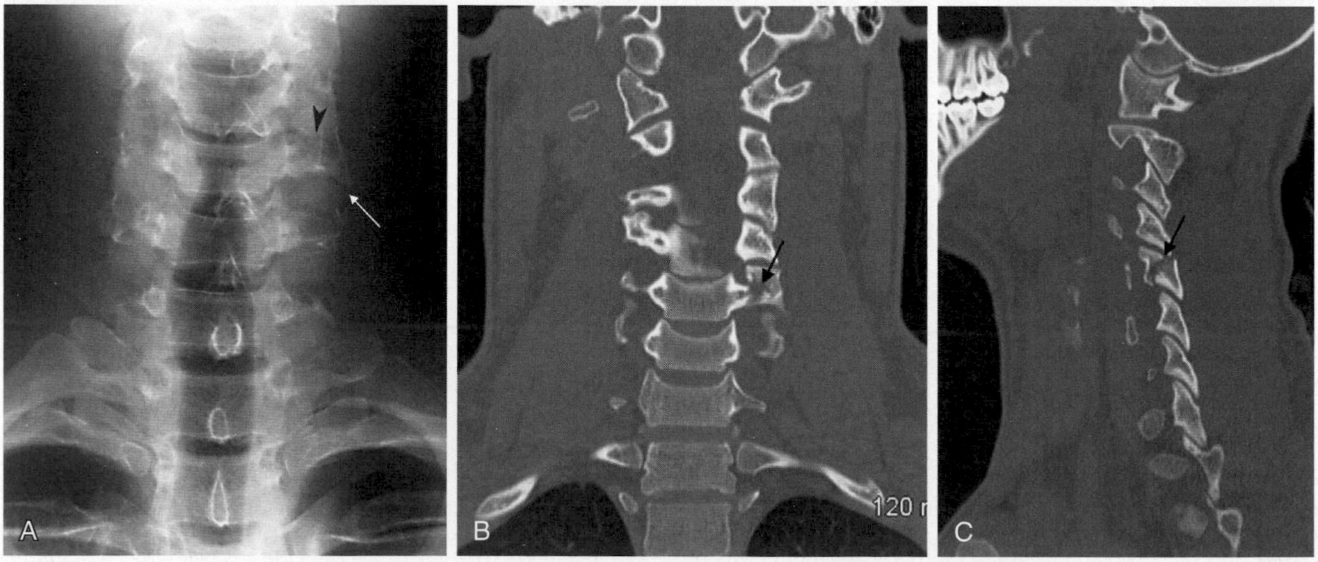

Figure 30-17. A, The anterior-posterior view shows loss of the typical smooth undulating left lateral border *(arrow)* and offset of the left C5-C6 facet joint. The facet articulation is well visualized, suggesting either diastasis of the joint or rotation of the articular mass. A subtle transversely oriented fracture of the lateral mass is evident *(arrowhead)*. The lateral view was radiographically normal. **B** and **C,** Computed tomography reconstructions confirm the lateral mass fracture *(arrow)* and slight diastasis and subluxation of the facet articulation.

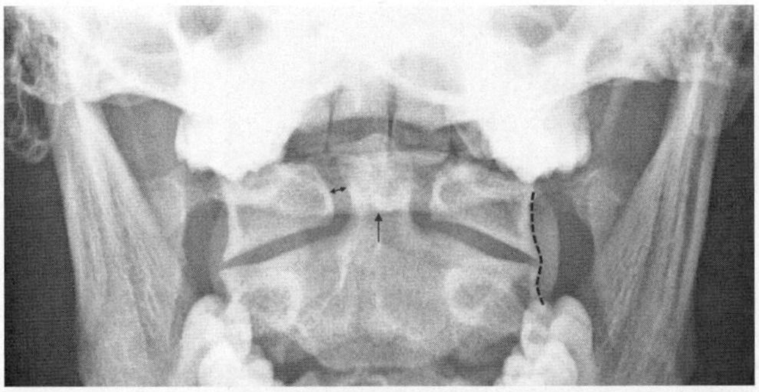

Figure 30-18. Normal open-mouth view. The lateral aspects of the articular masses of the atlas and axis are aligned *(dashed line).* The distance between the odontoid process and medial border of the C1 lateral masses is symmetric *(double-headed arrow).* A radiolucent Mach band traverses the dens created by overlap with the inferior surface of the posterior ring of C1 *(arrow).*

being diagnosed with increasing frequency with the advent of MDCT. Rarely detected on conventional radiographs, occipital condyle fractures can be easily diagnosed on high-resolution CT examination of the head and cervical spine, which must include images through the skull base. The most commonly used classification is the Anderson-Montesano system, which describes three patterns (Fig. 30-22).[74] Type I occipital condyle fractures represent stable nondisplaced fractures resulting from axial loading. Type II fractures are actually skull base fractures that extend either unilaterally or bilaterally into the occipital condyles or basion and are considered stable. Type III fractures represent the most common occipital condyle fracture with inferomedial displacement of an avulsed bone fragment originating from the attachment site of the alar ligament. The osseous fragment is typically displaced into the spinal canal or foramen magnum and should be considered an unstable injury until evidence otherwise.

Atlanto-occipital dissociation (Fig. 30-23) occurs after a shearing force, typically from direct trauma to the skull with the torso fixed in position or an opposing force acting on the torso. Disruption of the tectorial membrane and the important stabilizing ligaments between the skull and C2, the alar ligaments occurs, resulting in a high associated fatality rate caused by respiratory arrest from a stretch injury on the brainstem.[75] The frequency of this injury is higher in children because of the disproportionate size of the cranium. Type I injuries are the most common with the inciting force directed posterior to anterior disrupting the ligaments allowing for anterior translation and distraction of the skull in relation to C1. Type II injuries are caused by a distracting force with vertical diastasis between the occipital condyles and lateral masses of C1. Type III injuries are typically devastating because a posterior to anterior force on the cranium results in posterior translation and distraction at the craniocervical junction (Fig. 30-24). Craniocervical distraction type injuries can be elusive on imaging with the diagnosis relying on astute observation of anatomic relationships. The sensitivity of the basion to dens distance and the posterior axial line distance as described by Harris and colleagues (see Figs. 30-14 and

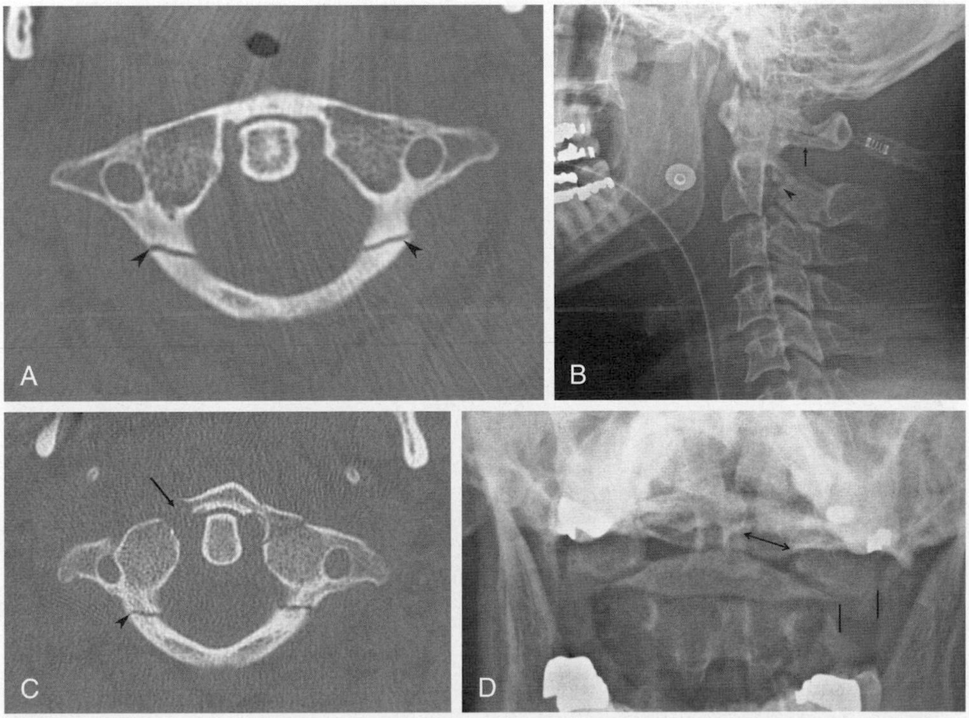

Figure 30-19. Atlas and Axis fractures. **A,** Nondisplaced fractures *(arrowheads)* involving the posterior arch of C1 bilaterally near the junction with the lateral masses. **B,** Lateral radiograph of the same patient demonstrating findings of an extension type injury with nondisplaced C1 fractures involving the posterior arch *(arrow)* and synchronous fractures of the pars interarticularis of C2 *(arrowhead).* **C,** Displaced Jefferson fractures with diastasis at the fracture site involving the anterior arch of C1 *(arrow)* and nondisplaced fractures of the posterior arch *(arrowhead).* **D,** Open-mouth view of the same patient shows widening of the lateral atlantoaxial space *(double-headed arrow)* and bilateral offset of the articular pillars (*lines* indicate the lateral border of the left lateral masses of C1 and C2).

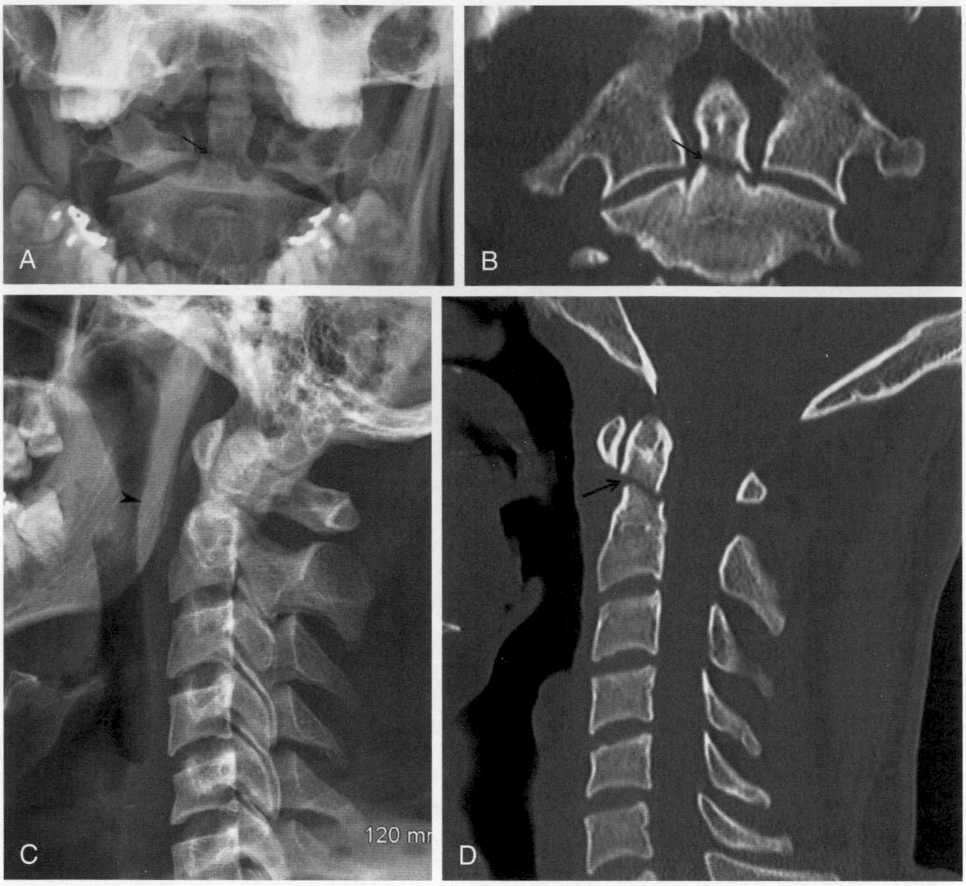

Figure 30-20. Type II dens fracture. Open-mouth view (**A**) and coronal computed tomography (CT) reconstruction (**B**) demonstrate a mildly displaced fracture *(arrows)* at the base of the dens above the level of the C2 lateral masses. **C,** Lateral radiograph of the cervical spine demonstrates focal prevertebral soft tissue swelling *(arrowhead);* however, the dens fracture is nearly imperceptible. Correlative sagittal CT reconstruction (**D**) clearly shows the fracture through the base of the odontoid process *(arrow).*

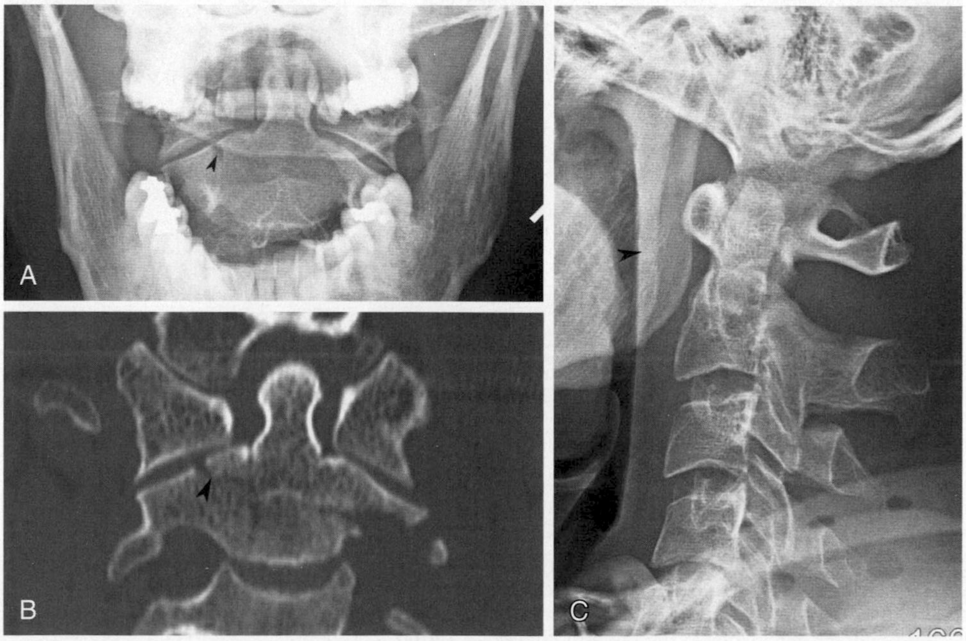

Figure 30-21. Type III dens fracture extending into the body of C2 *(arrowhead)* best visualized on the open-mouth view (**A**) and coronal computed tomography reconstruction (**B**). The lateral radiograph (**C**) shows associated prevertebral soft tissue swelling *(arrowhead).*

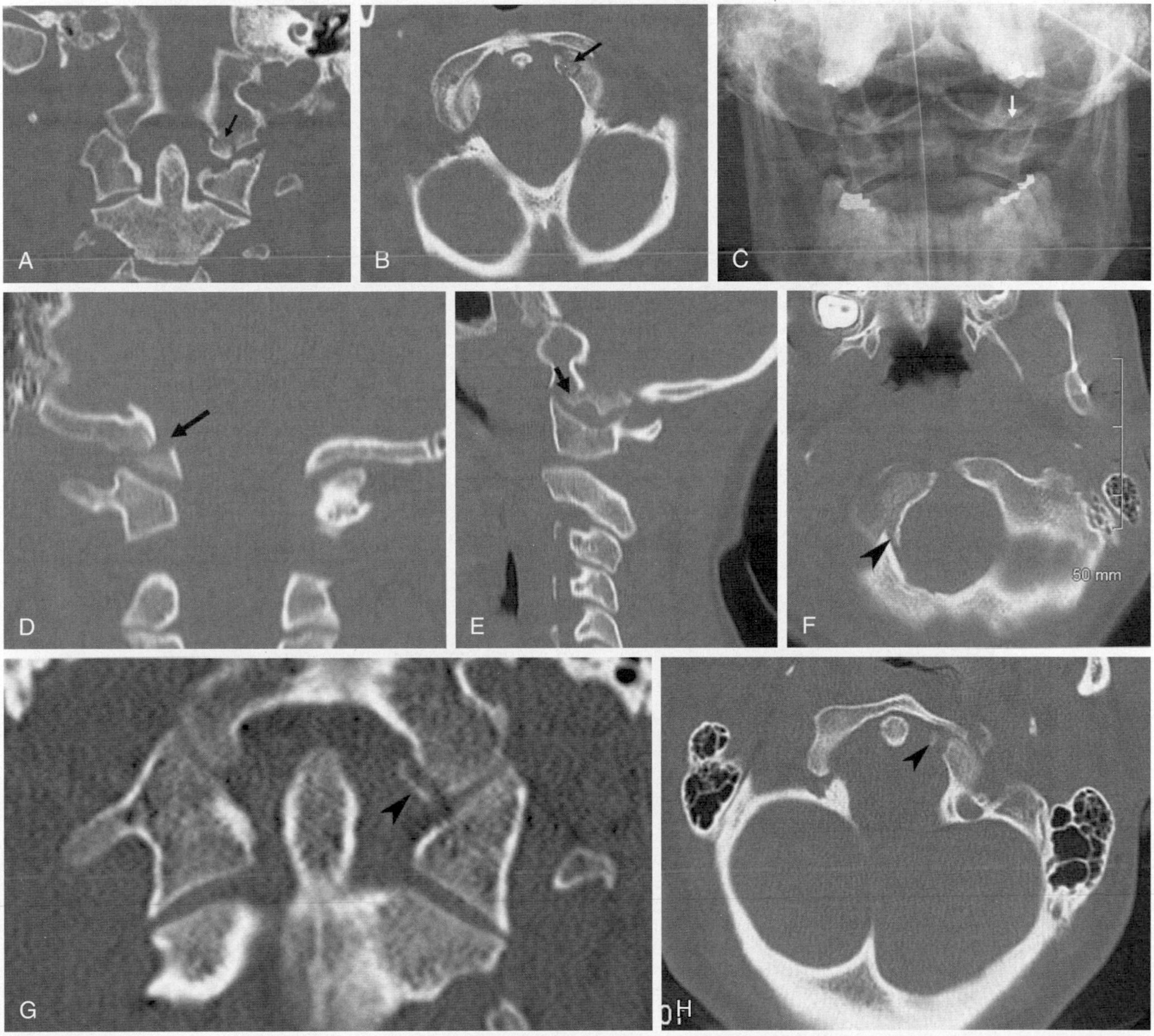

Figure 30-22. Occipital condyle fractures. **A** to **C,** Radiographically occult type I occipital condyle (OC) fracture *(black arrows).* Despite an adequate open-mouth view (**C**) and visualization of the left atlanto-occipital articulation *(white arrow),* the fracture line is not conspicuous. **D** to **F,** Type II OC fracture *(arrows)* with extension into the right skull base *(arrowhead).* **G** and **H,** Type III OC fracture with inferomedial displacement of an avulsed bone fragment originating from the attachment site of the alar ligament *(arrowhead).*

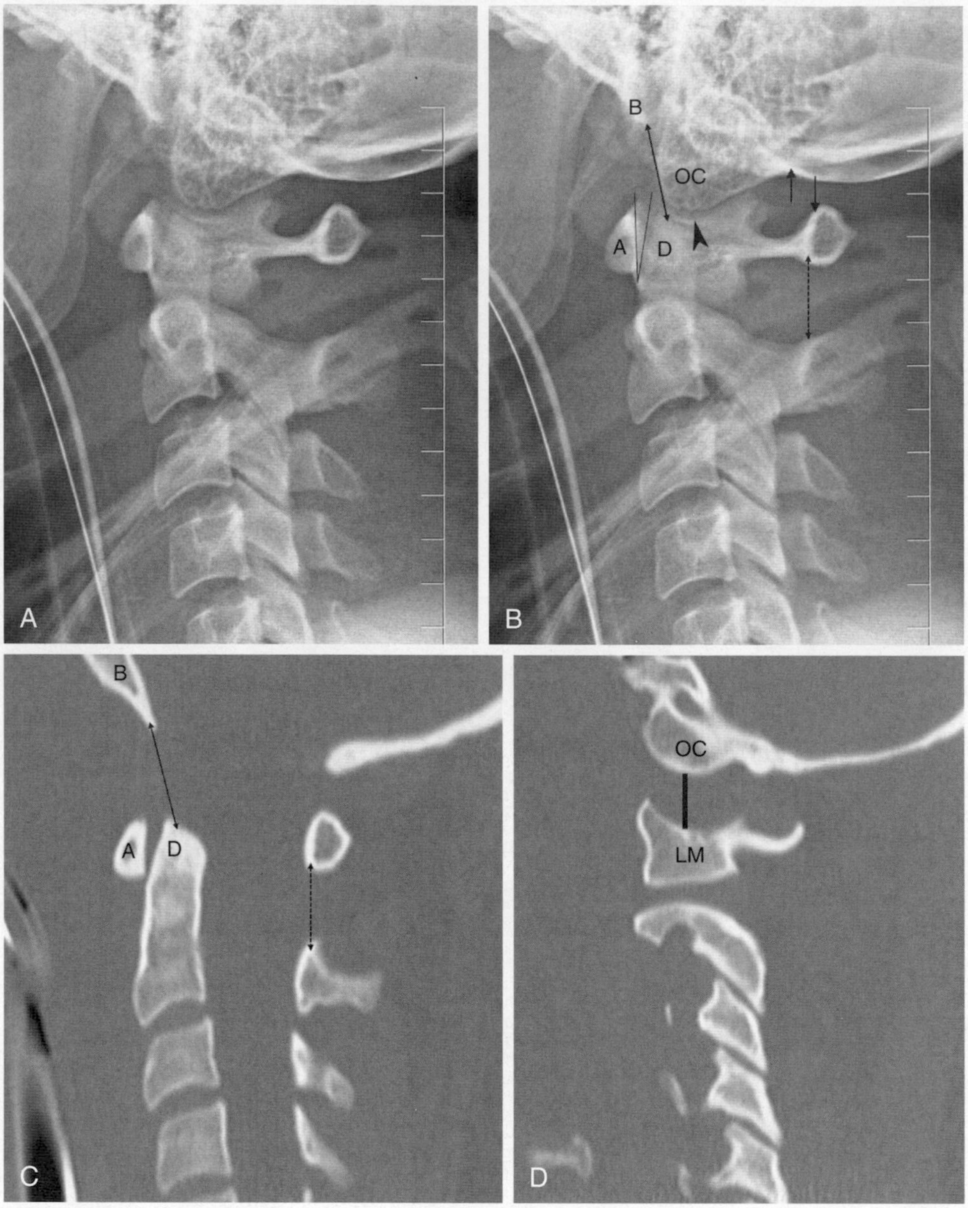

Figure 30-23. Craniocervical distraction injury. Nonannotated (**A**) and annotated (**B**) lateral radiographs of the cervical spine in a 28-year-old man involved in a motor vehicle accident shows a Type II atlanto-occipital dissociation with an elongated (>12 mm) basion–dens interval *(double-headed arrow).* Note the V sign with abnormal divergent alignment between the anterior arch of C1 and the odontoid process. The *dashed double-headed arrow* shows associated widening of the C1-C2 spinolaminar distance (>8 mm). The occipital condyles are displaced from the condylar fossa *(arrowhead)* of the atlas, and the posterior margin of the foramen magnum is anteriorly located relative to the C1 spinolaminar line *(arrows).* Computed tomography reformations (**C** and **D**) again demonstrate the radiographic findings and better depict the widening of the occipital cervical articulation. The sum of the distances between the midpoint of the occipital condyles and C1 condylar processes should not exceed 4 mm (sensitivity of 100%). A single unilateral measurement greater than 2 mm is also highly indicative of injury but is less sensitive compared with the sum. *A,* Anterior arch of C1; *B,* basion; *D,* dens; *LM,* lateral mass; *OC,* occipital condyle.

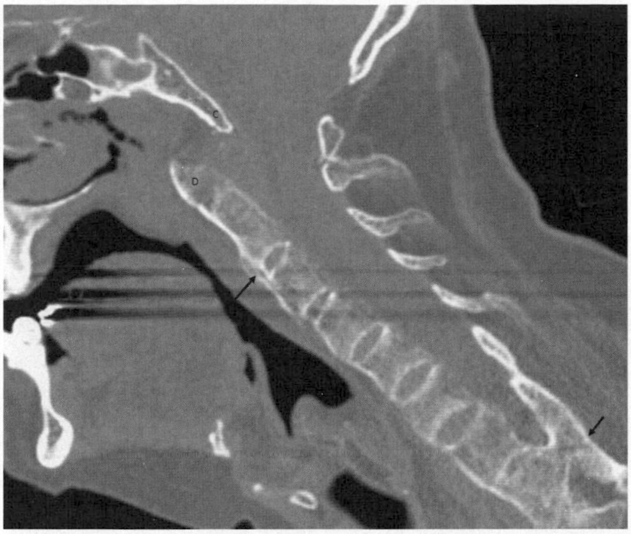

Figure 30-24. Type III craniocervical distraction injury with marked posterior displacement of the clivus (C) in respect to the dens (D) on this midsagittal computed tomography reformation. The patient has underlying ankylosing spondylitis with areas of osseous fusion marked by *arrows*.

30-23) approached 73% and 98%, respectively. More recently, Chang and colleagues described several additional CT measurements, including the midline occiput to spinolaminar line distance, sum of condylar displacement at the craniocervical articulation, midline C1-C2 spinolaminar line distance, and V-sign, which have potential in establishing the diagnosis of craniocervical distraction injuries with higher accuracy[76] (Figs. 30-23 and 30-25).

Rotational injuries typically occur in one of two locations, the thoracolumbar junction or the atlantoaxial region. Atlantoaxial dissociation (AAD) is a rare, typically purely ligamentous injury with the lateral masses of C1 perched over C2 (Fig. 30-26). Patients with Down syndrome, neurofibromatosis, Morquio syndrome, osteogenesis imperfecta, spondyloepiphyseal dysplasia, and chondrodysplasia punctata have a predisposition for this type of injury. The diagnosis is established by imaging demonstrating fixed rotation of C1 in respect to C2 regardless of head position, typically manifesting with irreducible offset of the lateral masses. The classification system is based on the amount and direction of displacement of C1 in relation to C2. Type I represents rotatory fixation without measurable increase in the ADI. In type II, ADI is less than 5 mm, and type III demonstrates greater than 5 mm of anterior translation of the atlas. Type IV is extremely rare with posterior displacement of the atlas.[77]

Fractures of the atlas (C1) are the consequence of either axial loading or hyperextension injuries. Compressive forces transmitted to C1 occur after an axial load to the vertex of the skull, typically resulting in fractures centered at the junction of the anterior and posterior arches of C1 with the lateral masses and commonly referred to as a "Jefferson" fracture (see Fig. 30-19). As discussed earlier, the open-mouth view demonstrates offset of the lateral masses of C1 in respect to C2 with injuries to the C1 ring; however, CT provides further characterization of the extent of injury. Eccentric loading and lateral tilt can lead to isolated fractures of the lateral mass of C1. In the setting of a hyperextension injury, either bilateral fractures of the posterior arch secondary to compressive forces or avulsion fractures of the anterior arch of C1 at the insertion of the longus colli muscles or ligamentous attachments to the skull base can be seen.

Odontoid fractures (Figs. 30-20, 30-21, and 30-27) are the result of multiple forces acting in unison. The Anderson-D'Alonzo classification system is commonly used to describe this type of injury.[78] A type I fracture is an avulsion off the tip of the odontoid process, which must be distinguished from a well-corticated ossification center residing superior to a rudimentary dens referred to as an os odontoideum. A transversely oriented fracture through the base of the dens is a type II fracture often diagnosed radiographically by identifying the fracture line or disruption of Harris ring. The dens is often posteriorly angulated or posteriorly displaced in respect to the C2 body with associated offset of the spinolaminar line between C1 and C2. A type III fracture courses into the C2 vertebral body. In type III fractures on the open-mouth or coronal CT section, the fracture line enters the atlantoaxial articulations, but in type II fractures, the fracture line does not involve this articulation.

A hangman's fracture (Fig. 30-28) is the colloquial name given to traumatic spondylolisthesis of C2 after a hyperextension and distraction injury such as with judicial hanging, although it can be associated with variable mechanisms.[79] The forced hyperextension is typically directed under the chin in circumstances of rapid deceleration of the head such as an unrestrained passenger's or driver's face striking the dashboard or windshield with the neck in the extended position. The force is transmitted through the weakest portion of C2, fracturing the pars interarticularis. Although an unstable injury, patients are typically neurologically intact because the fracture is decompressive with widening of the spinal canal. A classification system devised by Effindi and later modified by Levine and Edwards divides this type of injury into three types.[80] A type I injury is defined as bilateral nondisplaced isthmic fractures. Type II fractures include bilateral isthmic fractures, with greater than 3 mm of distraction across the fracture site, greater than 15 degrees of angulation at the fracture site, and an abnormal C2-C3 disc space secondary to associated ligamentous injuries with either anterior or posterior subluxation. A type III injury consists of a type II injury in addition to dislocation of the C2-C3 articular facet.

Hyperflexion and hyperextension injuries commonly involve the lower cervical spine with the extent of injury directly related to the degree and type of additional forces applied. Hyperflexion injuries account for 50% to 60% of all spinal column injuries. Pure flexion type injuries of the cervical spine include spinous process fractures (clay shoveler's fractures), anterior wedge compression fractures, isolated ligamentous injuries, and bilateral facet dislocation (Fig. 30-29). Flexion teardrop fractures and burst fractures occur with the addition of a compressive force such as axial loading.[81] The flexion teardrop fracture is a severe injury most commonly involving C5, which should not be confused with other less devastating triangular-shaped fractures emanating from the anteroinferior aspect of the vertebral body. Complete disruption of both the anterior and posterior ligamentous complex characterizes the imaging features with posterior displacement of the involved vertebra, narrowing of the posterior aspect of the disc space, and disruption of the posterior vertebral line in addition to the classic anterior teardrop-shaped

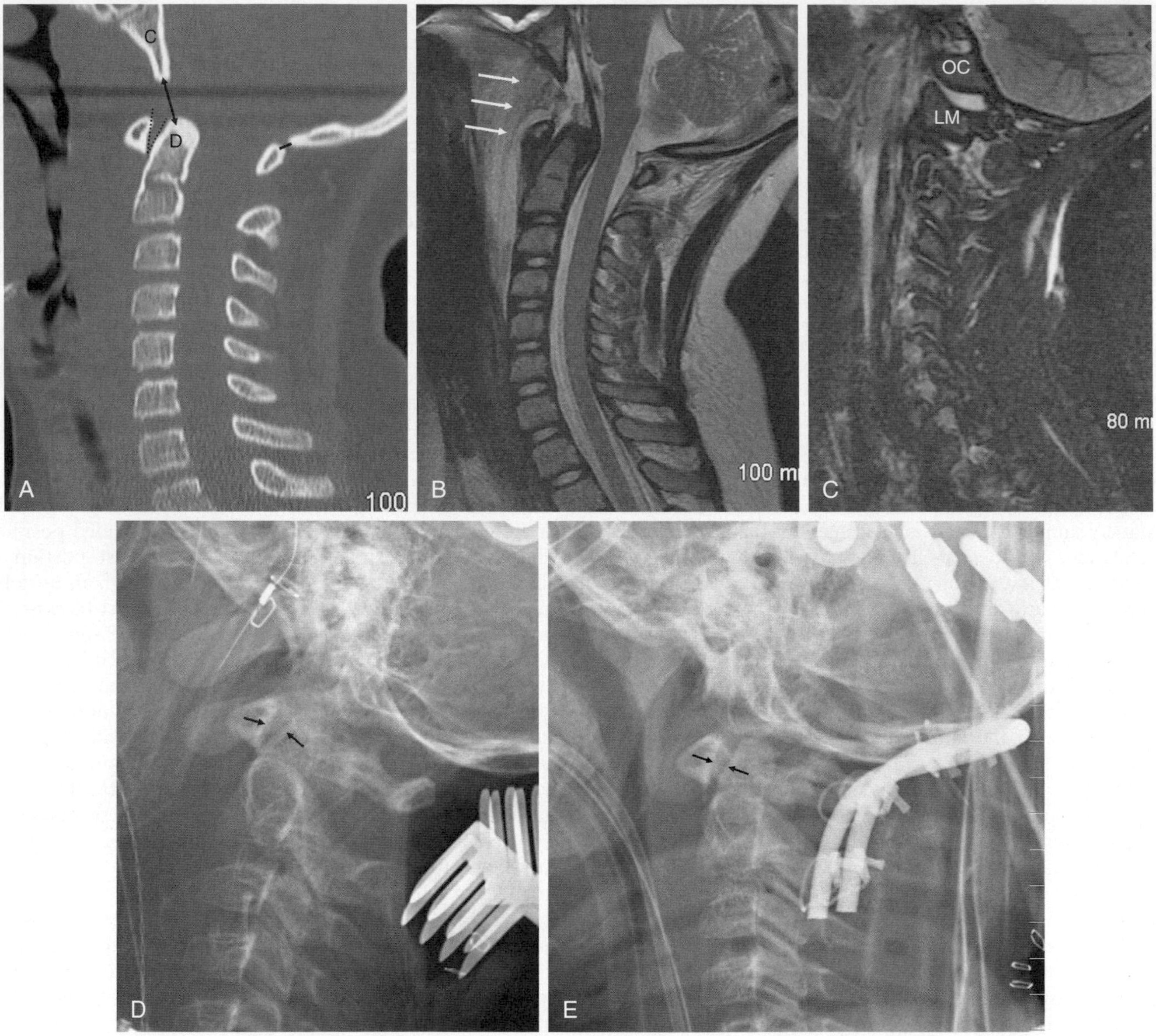

Figure 30-25. A, Midsagittal computed tomography reconstruction demonstrating the characteristic imaging findings of a type I atlanto-occipital dissociation with widening of the pre-dens angle resulting in a V sign, an elongated basion to dens interval *(double-headed arrow),* and a foreshortened (<6 mm) midline to occiput spinolaminar line *(line).* **B,** Sagittal T2-weighted magnetic resonance image (MRI) demonstrates similar findings in addition to extensive surrounding soft tissue edema *(arrow)* and disruption of the tectorial membrane and stabilizing ligaments. **C,** Off-lateral sagittal T2-weighted MRI illustrating anterior occipital condylar (OC) displacement in respect to the lateral mass (LM) of C1. **D,** Lateral radiograph showing abnormal divergent alignment between the anterior arch of C1 and the dens *(arrows).* **E,** Postreduction radiographs show the normal anatomic relationship restored between C1 and C2 with parallel contours *(arrows).*

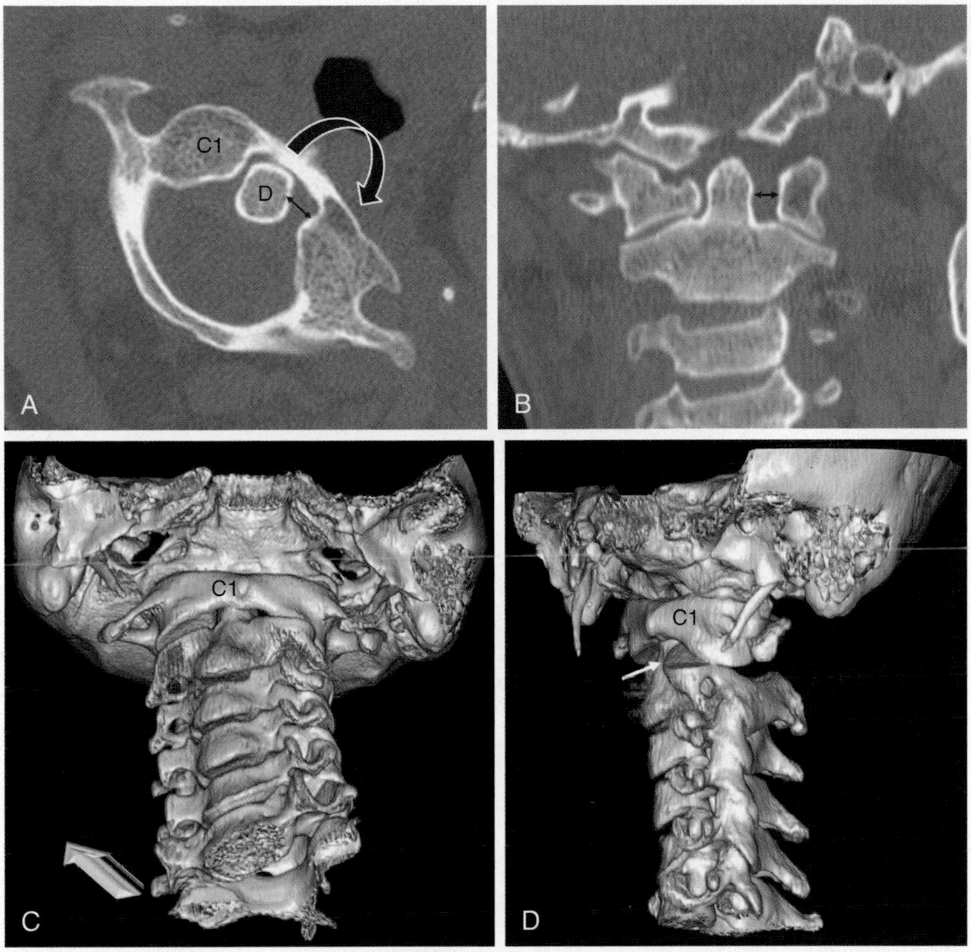

Figure 30-26. Type I atlantoaxial dissociation (AAD). **A,** Fixed rotation of C1 in respect to C2 is depicted on this axial computed tomography (CT) image. Widening of the lateral atlantodental space *(double-headed arrow)* on the left as well as clockwise rotation of C1 in respect to the dens (D) is a characteristic imaging finding. **B,** Coronal CT reconstruction demonstrates the eccentrically located dens and asymmetric widening of the lateral atlantodental space *(double-headed arrow).* **C,** Three-dimensional CT reconstruction shows C1 oriented anteriorly with the remainder of the cervical spine rotated approximately 45 degrees to the right. **D,** Offset of the lateral masses *(arrow)* with the lateral mass of C1 posteriorly subluxed and uncovering of the articular surface of the C2 lateral mass.

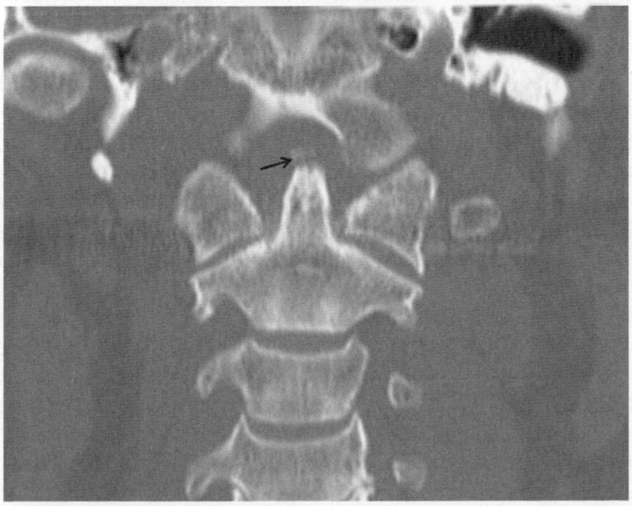

Figure 30-27. Rare type I odontoid fracture with avulsion of the tip of the dens *(arrow).*

fracture fragment (Fig. 30-30). Classically, patients present with neurologic symptoms consistent with acute anterior cord syndrome because the retropulsed posterior cortex may affect the anterior aspect of the spinal cord. Whereas rotational components and distraction lead to unilateral facet dislocations, lateral flexion injuries account for unilateral compression fractures of the vertebral bodies in addition to the aforementioned occipital condyle and odontoid fractures.

Accompanying the classic fractures and malalignment associated with hyperflexion injuries, other more subtle imaging findings include widening of the interlaminar, interfacet, or interspinous spaces (Fig. 30-31). Whereas anterior translation resulting from a hyperflexion injury typically disrupts the spinolaminar line, anterolisthesis in conjunction with hyperextension injuries generally maintains this alignment.[73]

Extension injuries are more common in the cervical spine compared with the thoracolumbar spine. Disruption of the anterior longitudinal ligament leads to widening of the

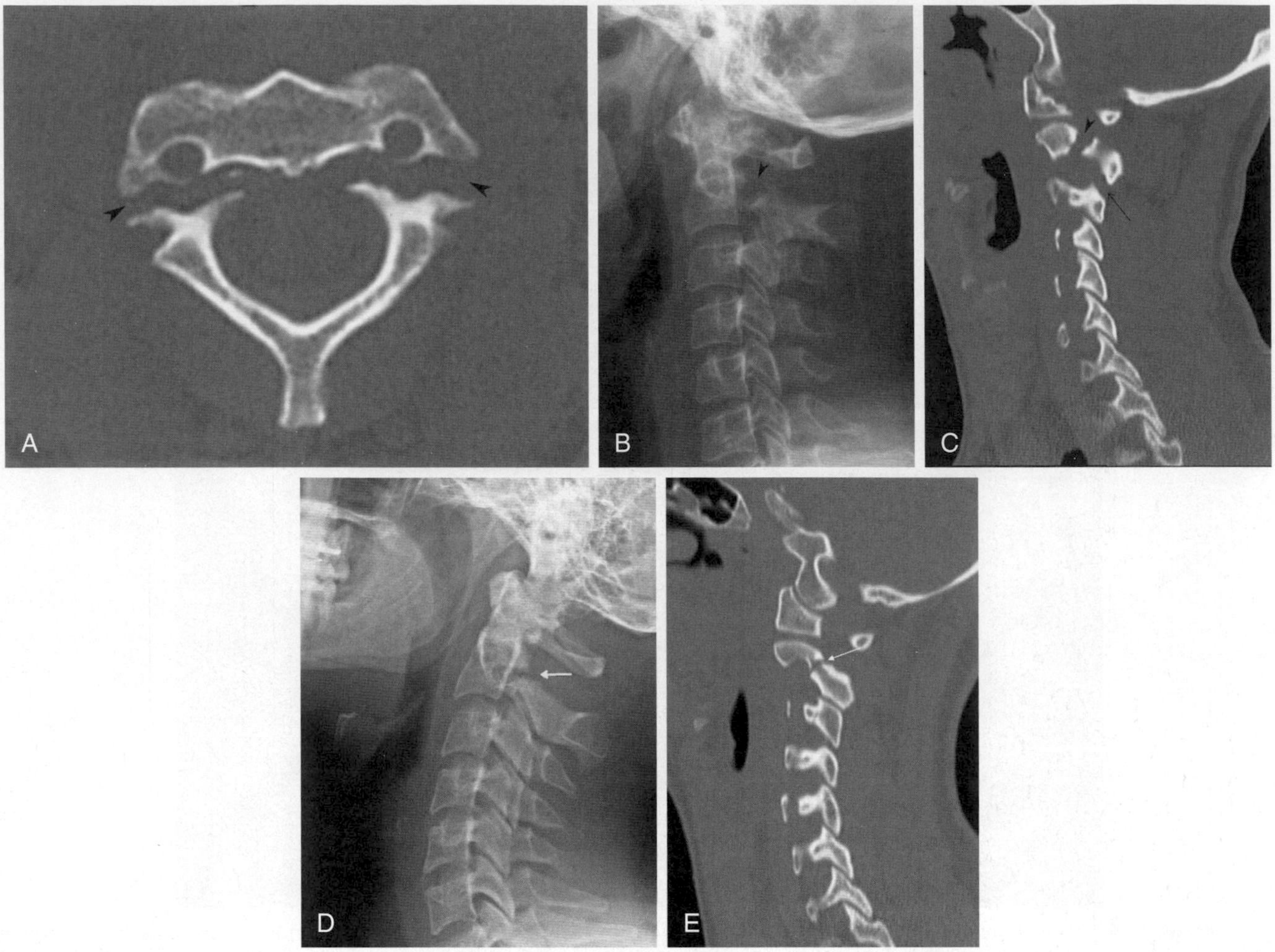

Figure 30-28. Hangman's fractures. **A** to **C,** Type II injury with displaced and angulated fractures through the pars interarticularis of C2 bilaterally *(arrowheads).* Diastasis across the C2-C3 facet joint is also noted *(arrow).* **D** and **E,** Type I injury with minimally displaced isthmic fractures *(white arrows).*

anterior intervertebral disc space (Fig. 30-32), which may be associated with vertebral fractures, avulsion fractures of the anteroinferior aspect off the vertebral body, or fracture-dislocations. The avulsion fractures tend to be small with the classic teardrop fracture involving C2 (Fig. 30-33) and the fragment being larger in height than width. Although retrolisthesis is typically seen with severe injuries, anterior subluxations may occur if the neural arch is fractured as with a hangman's fracture. Anterolisthesis after an extension injury can be distinguished from a flexion injury if the spinolaminar line and interlaminar distance are maintained.

Thoracic and Lumbar Spine

The type of injuries, mechanisms, and radiographic signs of instability are identical in the thoracolumbar spine as in the cervical spine. Flexion injuries such as compression fractures, burst fractures, facet dislocations, fracture-dislocations, and Chance fractures occur throughout the lumbar spine (Figs. 30-34 to 30-36). The majority of fractures are, however, centered at the thoracolumbar junction as the facet joints reorient from a coronal to a sagittal plane, in addition to the transition of a kyphotic curvature of the thoracic spine into a lordotic curvature of the lumbar spine placing the transition point as a site of mechanical vulnerability to any degree of motion. Although the mechanism of injury is similar to that of the cervical spine, shearing and rotatory injuries more commonly involve the lumbar spine and thoracolumbar junction. Shearing injuries have a unique imaging appearance demonstrating a greater degree of lateral translation and lateral dislocation in addition to concomitant rib and transverse process fractures.[82] The vertebra may have what has been described as a windswept appearance, particularly on axial CT images (Fig. 30-37). Because the surgical management requires reestablishing stability in multiple planes, distinguishing this type of injury from a burst fracture is imperative. Rotatory injuries result in severe fragmentation of the vertebral body, often with anterolisthesis and displacement of the facet joints (Fig. 30-38). The orientation of the displaced facet joints will reflect the direction in which the rotation occurred with one facet displaced anteriorly and the contralateral facet joint displaced posteriorly. A rotary array of the fracture fragments is characteristically seen on axial CT images. Similar to shearing injuries but unlike burst fractures, associated rib and transverse fractures occur with rotational injuries.

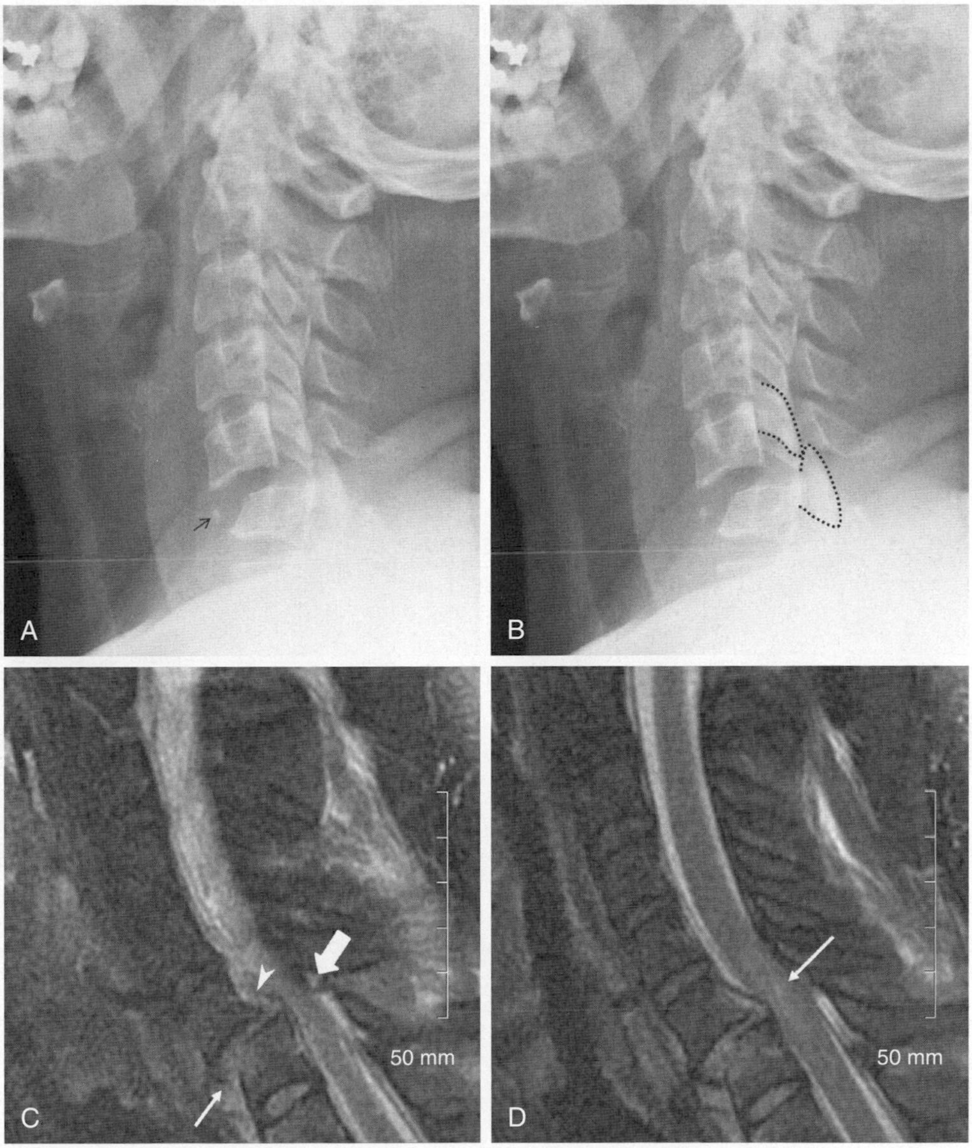

Figure 30-29. Severe flexion injury resulting in a bilateral facet dislocation. **A** and **B,** Lateral radiographs demonstrate bilateral facet dislocations (*dotted outline* in **B**), widening of the interspinous and interlaminar spaces, anterolisthesis of C5 on C6, and fracture of the anterior superior aspect of C6. **C,** Sagittal magnetic resonance image shows associated ligamentous injuries with disruption of the anterior longitudinal ligament *(arrow),* posterior longitudinal ligament *(arrowhead),* and ligamentum flavum (thick arrow). **D,** A cord contusion is seen at the C5-C6 level with central hyperintense signal intensity *(arrow).*

Spine Fractures in Patients with Preexisting Ankylosing Spinal Disorders

The ankylosed spine is susceptible to fracture after even minor trauma because of the altered biomechanical properties of a fused spine and forces directed on longer lever arms.[83,84] Despite low-impact trauma, poorer clinical outcomes occur in patients with ankylosed spines compared with the general trauma population. Unfortunately, even with modern imaging, the diagnosis is often delayed. Preexisting back pain may be difficult to distinguish from acute fracture pain because many patients, particularly with ankylosing spondylitis, do not present until abrupt neurologic symptoms occur, a phenomenon referred to as "the fatal pause."[85] The absence of major trauma, lack of awareness regarding these preexisting conditions, and vulnerability to unstable injuries superimposed on these injuries often being radiographically occult lead to a failure to diagnose or properly immobilize an unstable spine. Most of these fractures are caused by low-energy impact such as a fall from standing height and are typically localized to the cervical spine followed by the thoracic spine. The cervical region is predisposed to injury because of increased mobility, small vertebral bodies, oblique articular facets, and preexisting kyphotic deformity. Although fractures can occur through the intervertebral disc or vertebral body, Mac Millan and Paley reported independently that traumatic fractures in patients with partially fused segments of the spine tend to occur adjacent to the fused segment.[86,87] Increased risk of fracture instability has also been associated with a greater number of contiguously fused segments.

Patients with ankylosing spondylitis or DISH are particularly susceptible to extension injuries caused by a loss of elasticity and functional degradation of the ossified ligamentous

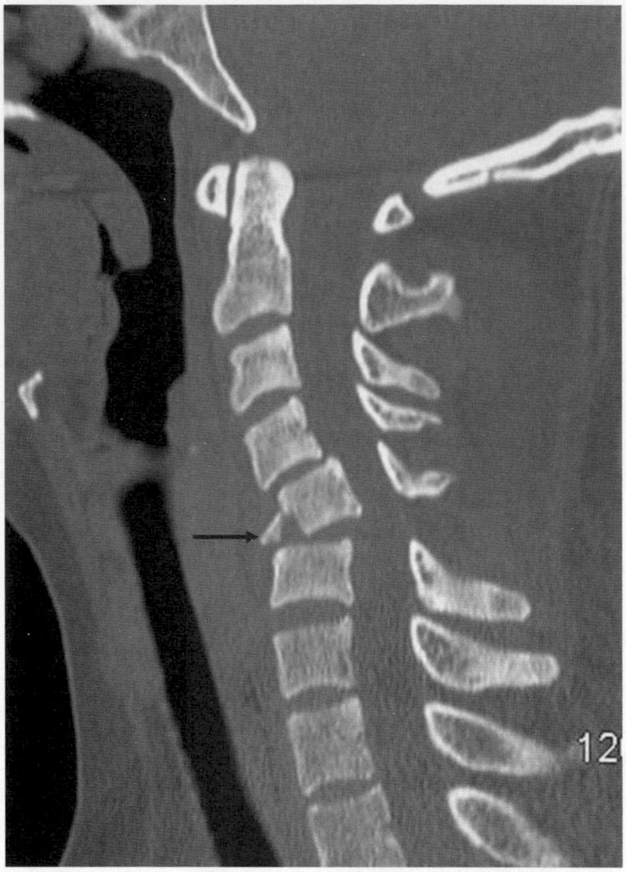

Figure 30-30. Flexion teardrop fracture of C5 with anterior displacement of a triangular-shaped fragment *(arrow)*, retropulsion of the vertebral body, and disruption of the posterior vertebral line.

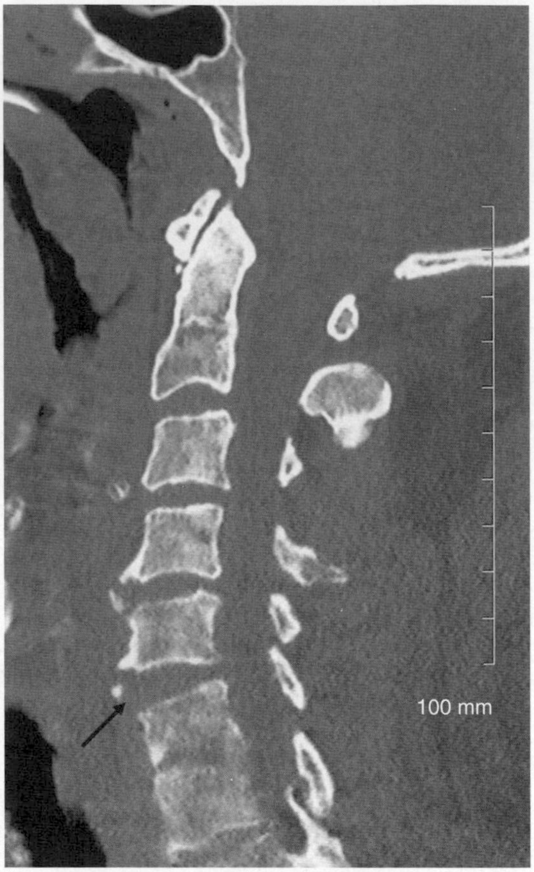

Figure 30-32. Sagittal reformatted computed tomography image demonstrates widening of the C5-C6 disc space anteriorly *(arrow)* and prevertebral soft tissue swelling consistent with a hyperextension injury.

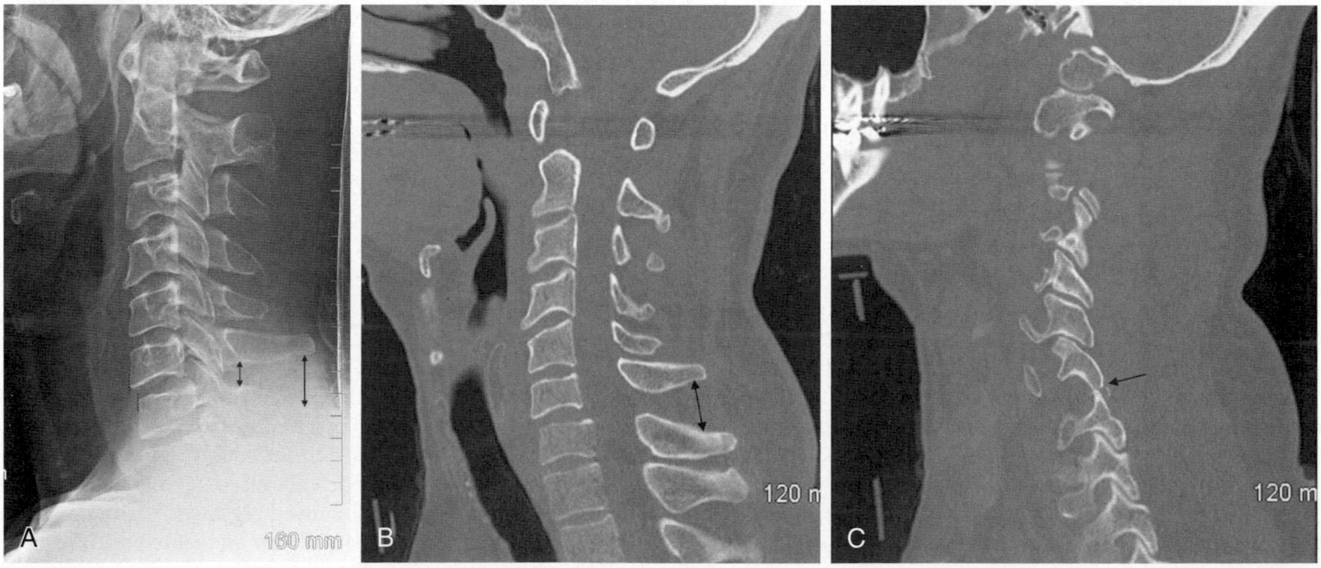

Figure 30-31. Subtle radiographic findings of a flexion injury. Lateral radiograph (**A**) and midsagittal computed tomography (CT) reconstruction (**B**) demonstrate findings of a flexion injury with disruption of the anterior vertebral line *(dashed lines),* slight diastasis of the posterior aspect of the intervertebral disc space, and widening of both the interlaminar and interspinous space *(double-headed arrows).* **C,** Off-lateral sagittal CT reconstruction shows the associated unilateral perched facet at C6-C7 *(arrow)* accounting for the radiographic findings.

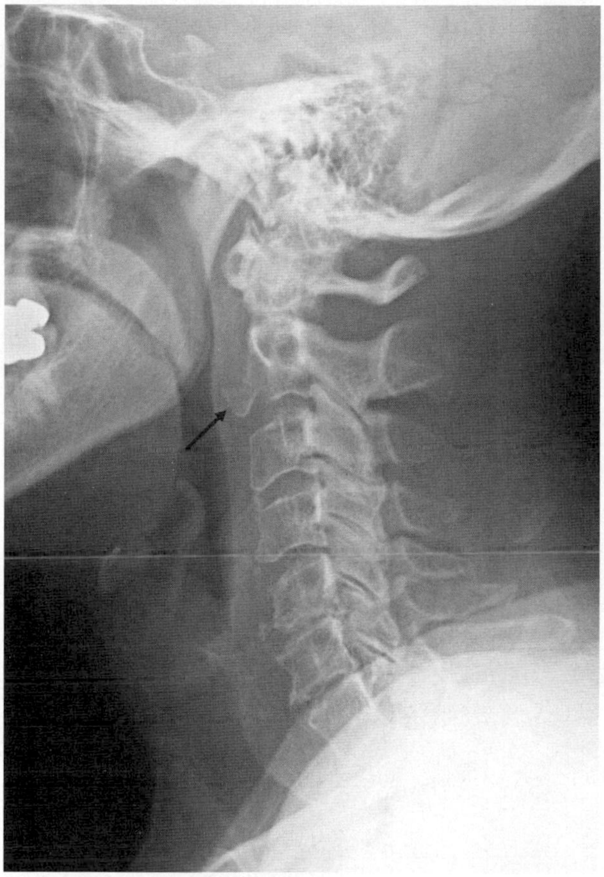

Figure 30-33. Lateral radiograph of the cervical spine demonstrating a C2 hyperextension teardrop fracture *(arrow)*. Subsequent magnetic resonance image showed normal appearing posterior longitudinal ligament, ligamentum flavum, and interspinous ligaments in keeping with an isolated hyperextension type injury.

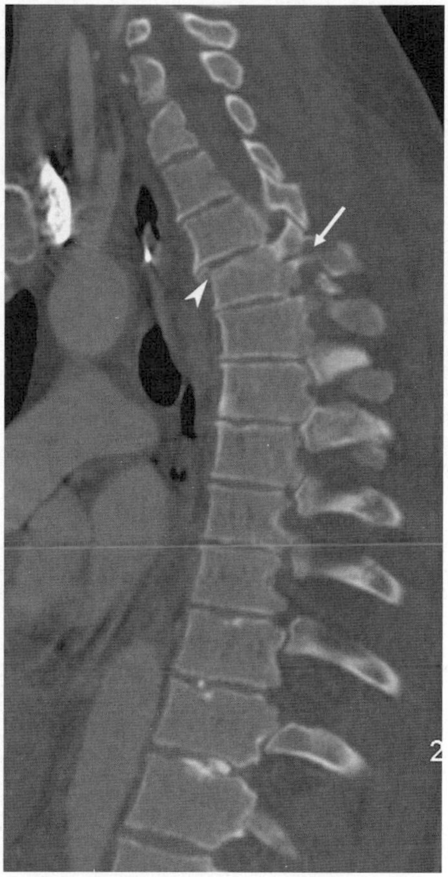

Figure 30-35. Chance fracture. Coronal reformatted computed tomography image of the thoracic spine demonstrates a horizontally oriented fracture of the vertebral body *(arrowhead)* with a split component extending into the posterior elements *(arrow)*.

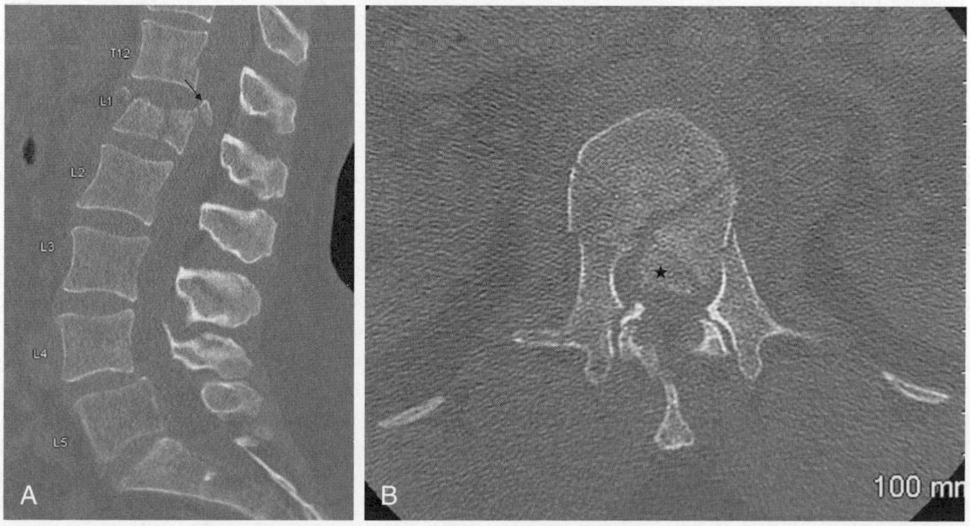

Figure 30-34. L1 burst fracture. **A,** Sagittal computed tomography (CT) reconstruction demonstrates involvement of both the anterior and middle columns with retropulsion of a fracture fragment into the spinal canal *(arrow)*. **B,** Axial CT image better defines the amount of central canal stenosis and size of the retropulsed fracture fragment *(star)*.

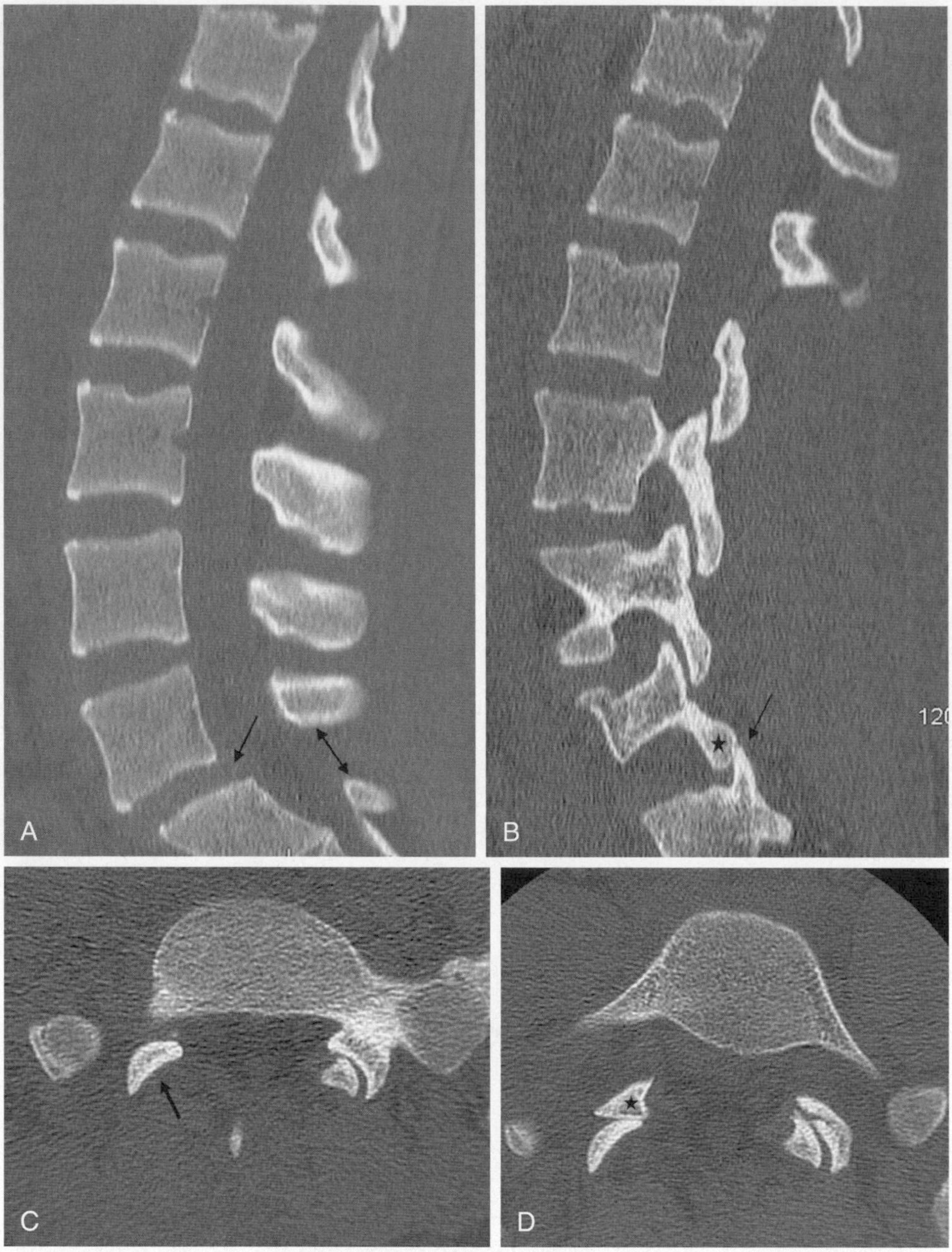

Figure 30-36. Unilateral facet dislocation. **A,** Midsagittal computed tomography (CT) image demonstrating secondary findings of a flexion rotation injury with anterolisthesis of L5 on S1 *(arrow)* and widening of the interspinous space *(double-headed arrow)*. **B,** Off-lateral sagittal CT reconstruction shows a perched facet with the inferior articular process of L5 *(star)* positioned anterior to the superior articular process of S1 *(arrow)*. **C** and **D,** Axial CT images show a "naked" facet on the right *(arrow)* and "reverse hamburger bun sign" with the inferior L5 articular process *(star)* located anterior to the superior articular process of S1, resulting in the convex portions of the articular processes to articulate. Notice the normal appearing contralateral facet joint for comparison.

complexes and disc spaces (Figs. 30-39 and 30-40).[87] The injuries commonly traverse all supporting ossified structures, often extending obliquely through the anterior longitudinal ligament into either the subjacent vertebra or posteriorly through the disc space resulting in marked instability.

Despite the extent of injury, radiographs are not uncommonly negative, potentially because of spontaneous reduction of the fracture or subluxation, overlap of preexisting osseous changes with the site of injury, generalized demineralization in patients with advanced disease, and failure to identify noncontiguous injuries (Fig. 30-40). It is this author's opinion a low threshold for obtaining spinal CT of the spine should be used in patients with fused spinal segments who have negative radiographs and a history of minor trauma. If the CT findings are negative, MRI is warranted in this high-risk population. Transfer and manipulation of these patients, particularly when positioning for imaging studies, should proceed with the utmost caution because of the highly unstable fracture configurations and potential to develop neurologic deficits.[88]

When interpreting CT examinations, attention to the surrounding soft tissues is imperative because rare associated complications such as aortic lacerations and tracheal injuries

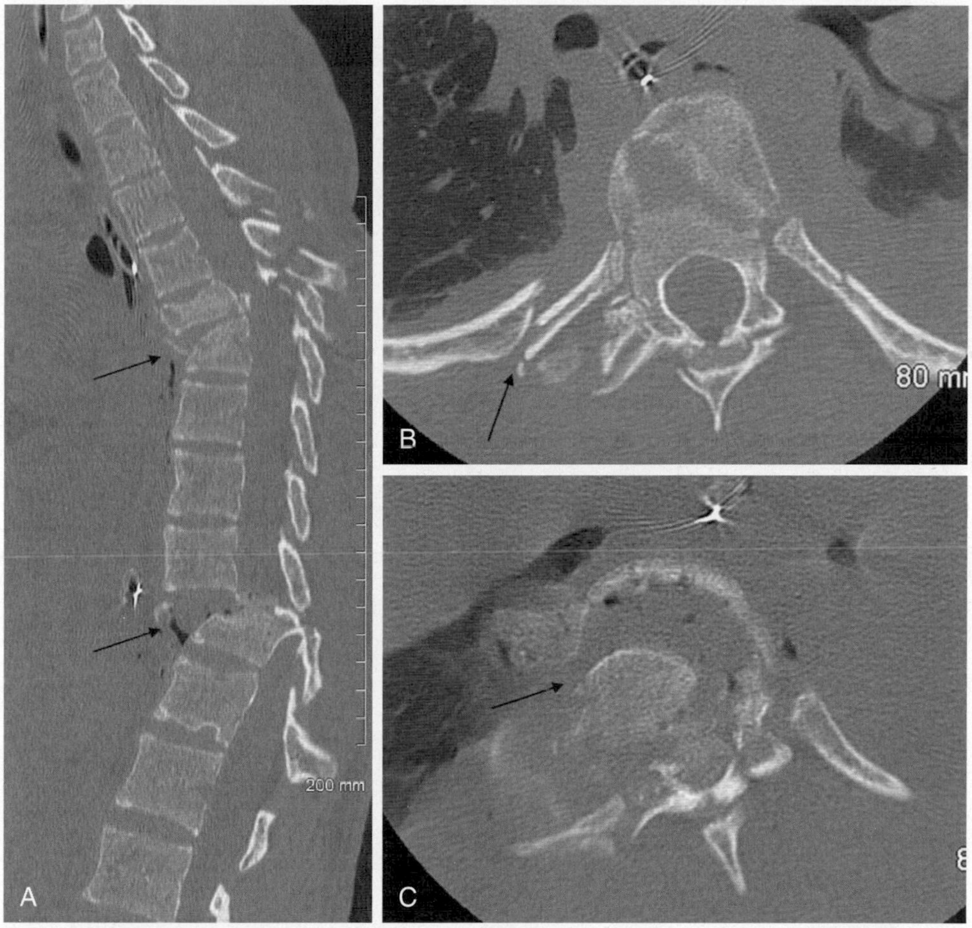

Figure 30-37. Shear injury. **A,** Sagittal computed tomography reconstruction shows findings of a flexion distraction type injury with vertebral body fractures *(arrows),* kyphosis, and anterolisthesis at the most caudal injury site secondary to perched facets. Burst fractures rarely dislocate, but shear injuries are typically associated with a component of either forward or lateral flexion. Other differentiating features from a burst fracture are rib (*arrow* in **B**) and transverse process fractures, as well as a linear oblique array (windswept appearance) of the fracture fragments as demonstrated in **C.**

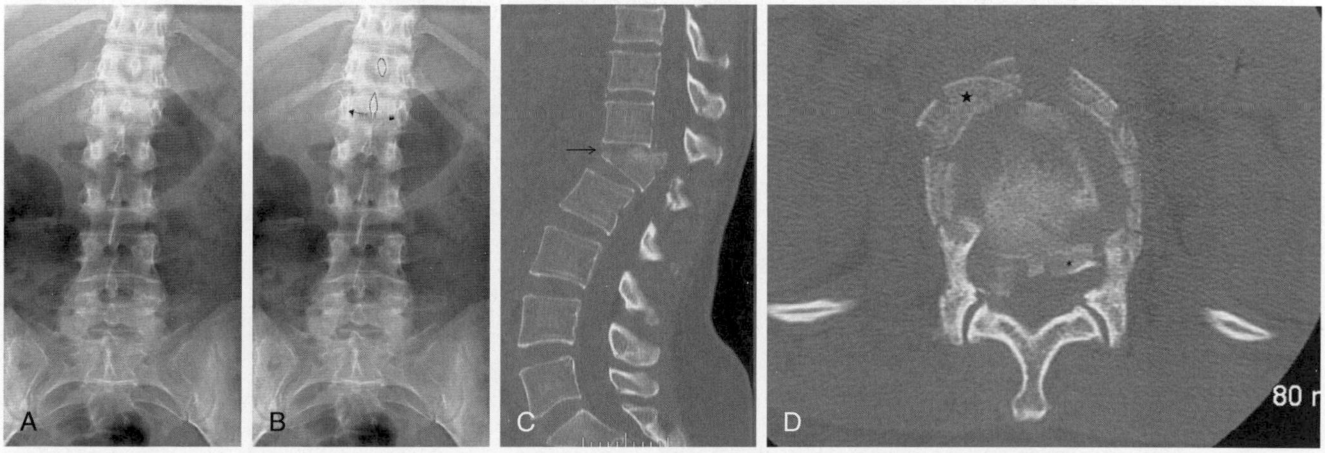

Figure 30-38. Rotational injury. **A** and **B,** Nonannotated and annotated anterior-posterior radiograph of the lumbar spine demonstrates secondary findings of a rotational injury with offset of the spinous processes (outlined) at the thoracolumbar junction. Widening of the interpedicular distance *(double-headed arrow)* indicates bursting of the L1 vertebral body. **C,** Sagittal computed tomography (CT) reconstruction demonstrates the L1 vertebral body fracture *(arrow)* and anterolisthesis of T12 on L1 secondary to perched facets. **D,** Axial CT images show the rotary array of fracture fragments with the anterior fragments rotated clockwise *(star)* and the posterior fragments rotated counterclockwise *(asterisk).*

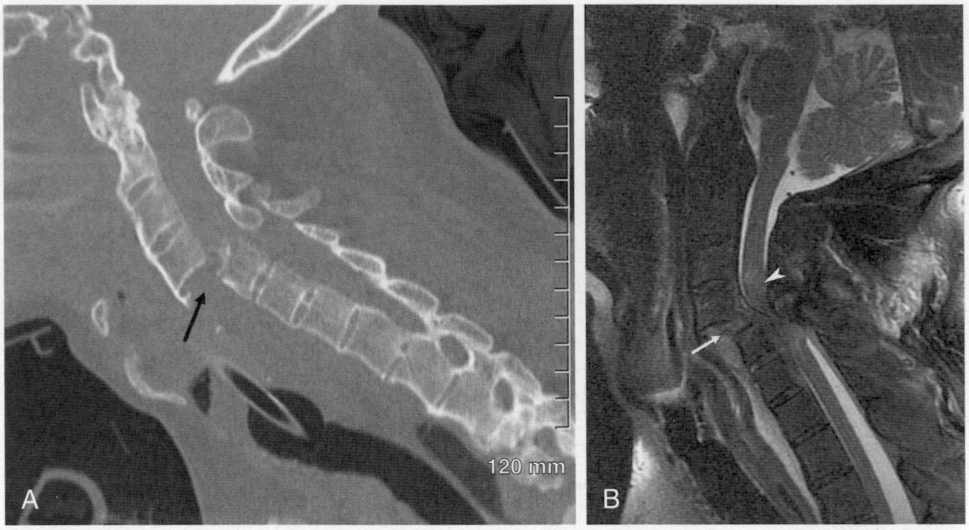

Figure 30-39. Spinal injury in the setting of underlying ankylosing spondylitis. **A,** Sagittal computed tomography image demonstrates a fracture *(arrow)* through the intervertebral C4-C5 disc and anterior displacement. **B,** Subsequent magnetic resonance imaging shows disruption through the bridging syndesmophytes *(arrow),* compression of the cervical cord, and cord edema *(arrowhead).*

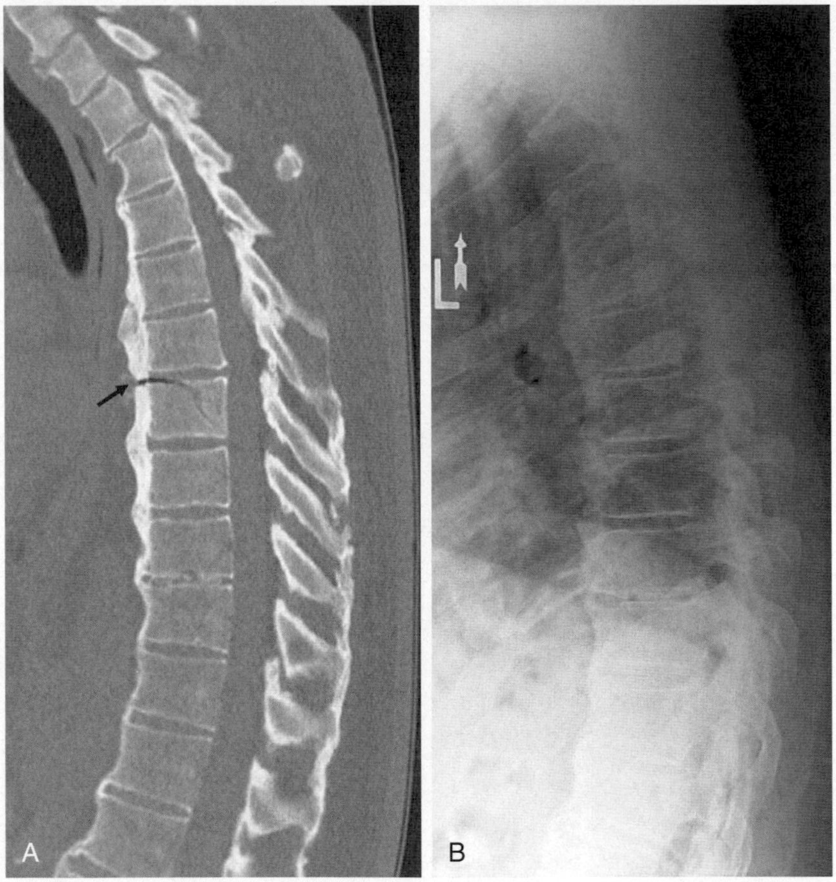

Figure 30-40. Diffuse idiopathic skeletal hyperostosis fracture. **A,** Sagittal computed tomography reconstruction demonstrates the characteristic flowing anterior ossification seen in patients with diffuse idiopathic skeletal hyperostosis and a transversely oriented fracture through the fused portion extending into the disc space and subjacent vertebral body *(arrow).* **B,** Lateral radiograph performed at the same time fails to show the unstable fracture.

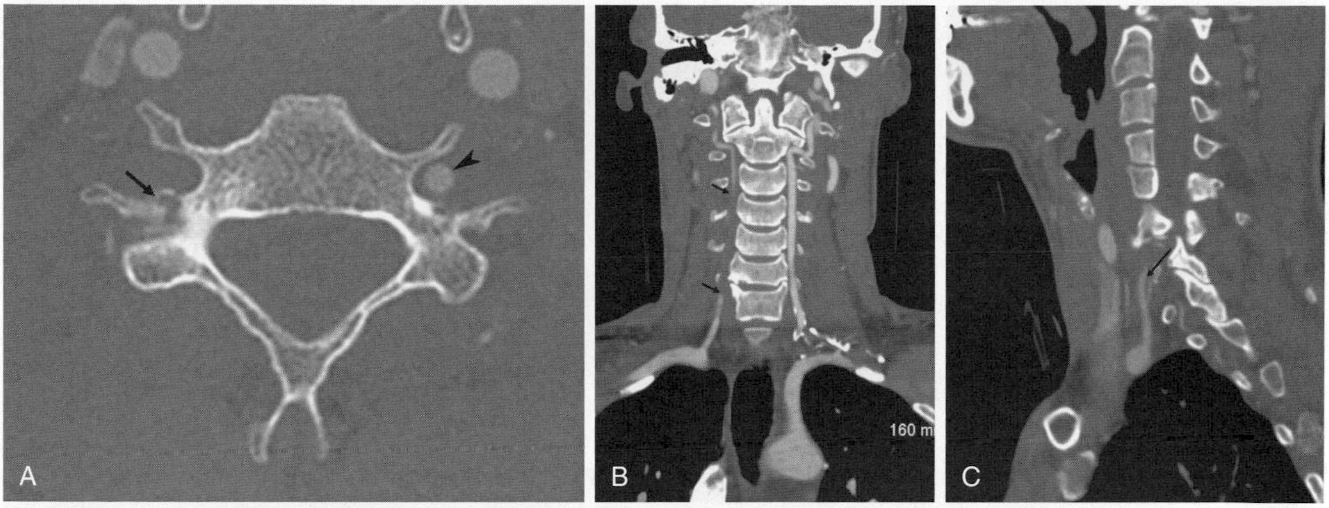

Figure 30-41. Computed tomography (CT) angiogram of a right vertebral artery injury after blunt trauma. **A,** Axial CT image demonstrates a fracture of the posterior tubercle of the right transverse process extending into the foramen transversarium *(arrow)*. Absence of contrast within the right vertebral artery is in keeping with an underlying vascular injury. Normal opacification of the left vertebral artery is seen *(arrowhead)*. **B,** Coronal reconstruction from a CT angiogram demonstrates segmental occlusion of the right vertebral artery (between the *arrows*) and normal-appearing left vertebral artery. **C,** Sagittal CT reformation shows a linear filling defect *(arrow)* within the proximal vertebral artery consistent with a dissection.

have been described in the literature. Any minor fracture in ankylosed spines should be considered as highly unstable.

Blunt Cerebrovascular Injuries

The true incidence of carotid and vertebral artery injuries after nonpenetrating trauma to the neck is unknown; however, these injuries are being reported with increased frequency because of the widespread availability of CT angiography (CTA) (Fig. 30-41) and its use as a screening examination for cerebrovascular injuries. Some estimate that 0.20% to 1.0% of blunt trauma patients have associated vascular injuries with an incidence of vertebral artery injuries between 17% and 46% in patients who sustain a cervical spine injury.[89-91] The rationale for early detection in asymptomatic patients stems from studies reporting significant improvement in neurologic outcomes upon early implementation of treatment, including anticoagulation and antiplatelet therapy.[92] Patients with these vertebral artery injuries are often asymptomatic upon presentation and may develop focal neurologic deficits unexplained by imaging up to 72 hours later (Fig. 30-42). Some reports claim an even further delay between the lucid interval and onset of neurologic symptoms of up to 3 months.[93]

Imaging of the vasculature is indicated in patients with fractures involving C1-C3; fractures coursing into the foramen transversarium or carotid canal; skull base fractures; Le Fort II or III facial fractures; severe chest injuries; malalignment of the cervical spine, particularly unilateral or bilateral facet dislocations; neurologic deficits unexplained by imaging, especially those involving the posterior circulation; and a GCS score of less than 6.[94-98] Cothren and colleagues. recommended screening patients who sustained one of the following types of injuries: (1) fractures extending into the foramen transversarium, (2) fractures involving one of the upper three cervical vertebrae, and (3) patients with subluxation. By using these guidelines, the authors calculated a theoretical detection rate of 93% of vertebral artery injuries.[99] Injuries to the vertebral artery generally involve the foraminal (V2) segment, which is vulnerable to damage because this portion is relatively fixed within the osseous canal of the transverse foramen. The types of vertebral artery injuries described include occlusion (88%), stenosis (8.5%), intimal flap or vessel irregularity (5.3%), dissection (4.3%), and (less commonly) pseudoaneurysms.[97,100-103]

Although historically conventional angiography has been the gold standard and is the most accurate method for the detection and characterization of injury as well as identification of collateral flow, limitations include invasiveness, potential complications, and logistic constraints in critically ill patients. Several authors have proposed reserving angiography for patients with equivocal or inconclusive imaging studies, in cases in which neuroradiology intervention is required, or if vascular injury is suspected based on clinical findings.[103-107] Magnetic resonance angiography (MRA) can be performed either with or without the administration of gadolinium contrast (Fig 30-42). The major drawback is the overestimation of stenosis or occlusion with MRA compared with other modalities. Furthermore, patients with indwelling or external ferromagnetic devices such as pacemakers, aneurysm clips, several types of external fixators, and ventilators are incompatible with the use of MRI. Multisystem trauma patients who may be hemodynamically unstable require the use of MR-compatible monitoring systems and present a challenge in performing acute cardiopulmonary resuscitation in a confined space and limited availability of nonferromagnetic equipment.

To date, despite the increased utilization of CTA as a screening examination for vascular injuries, the accuracy and diagnostic value remain to be determined. Advances in technology have led to fewer osseous artifacts with improved visualization of vertebral artery throughout its course. Conflicting results remain in the literature with sensitivities ranging between 41% and 97% and specificities of 86% and 100% being reported. Several studies have noted CTA to identify intimal flaps, stenosis, and pseudoaneurysms with a

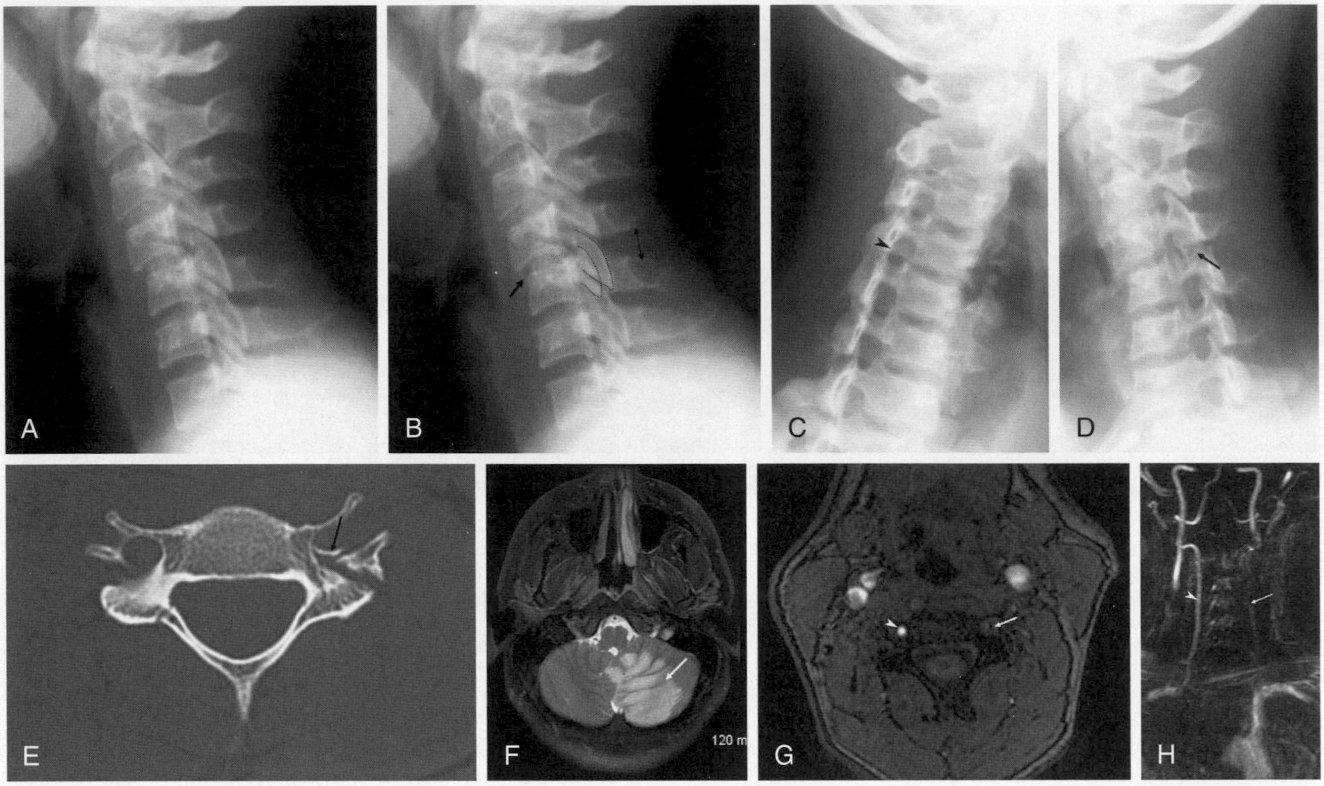

Figure 30-42. Delayed vascular injury after a motor vehicle accident. **A** to **D,** Lateral and oblique radiographs of the cervical spine show findings of a flexion rotation injury with anterolisthesis of C4 on C5 *(arrow),* offset of the C5 lateral masses *(dashed outline)* compared with normally opposed lateral masses at C4 and widening of the interspinous space *(double-headed arrow).* Oblique radiographs show a fracture through the superior articular process of C5 *(dashed arrow),* narrowing of the adjacent neural foramen, and mild anterior translation. The normal appearance of the foramen is seen on the contralateral side *(arrowhead).* The patient developed Wallenberg syndrome 1 week after the initial injury, which was undiagnosed. **E,** Axial computed tomography image demonstrates a fracture fragment displaced into the foramen transversarium *(arrow).* **F,** Brain magnetic resonance imaging confirmed a cerebellar infarct in the distribution of the left posterior inferior cerebellar artery *(arrow).* **G,** Axial image from a magnetic resonance angiogram (MRA) demonstrates an occluded left vertebral artery *(arrow)* and normal opacification of the right vertebral artery *(arrowhead).* **H,** Coronal image from an MRA shows occlusion of the left vertebral artery *(arrow).* The normal right vertebral artery is marked by the *arrowhead.*

comparable accuracy to conventional angiography and outperformance of MRA.[108-110]

Biffl and colleagues proposed a grading scale for vertebral artery injuries based on angiographic findings, which initially were developed and applied to blunt carotid artery injuries.[101,111] Grade I includes irregularity of the arterial wall, dissections, or intramural hematoma causing less than 25% luminal narrowing. Grade II results in luminal narrowing greater than 25% caused by intraluminal thrombus, dissection, or a raised intimal flap. Pseudoaneurysms are classified as grade III, and thrombosed vessels as grade IV. If the vessel is transected or an arteriovenous fistula is identified, it would represent a grade V injury. The grade, however, does not correlate with risk of cerebrovascular accident when evaluating the vertebral circulation, with grade II injuries having the highest association with ischemic events. The reported stroke rate in the setting of an injury to the posterior circulation is 24%. The same does not hold true for blunt carotid injury, with the incidences of stroke being 3%, 11%, 33%, 44%, and 100% for grade I to V injuries, respectively.[102,111]

Many trauma centers have adopted CTA as a screening tool for the detection of blunt cerebrovascular injuries despite the continued debate regarding its diagnostic accuracy. The institution of CTA-based screening protocols has been shown to reduce not only time to diagnosis but also stroke rates compared with digital subtraction angiography–based protocols. An average decrease of 2.65 hours in diagnosis and drop in stroke rate from 15.2% to 3.8% were reported by Eastman and colleagues.[112] Additionally, many of the earlier studies were performed in the era of single-detector CT scanners. The sensitivities and specificities reported have significantly improved when evaluating CTA performed with MDCT (16 slice or greater) scanners affording improved resolution, reduction in artifacts, and isotropic imaging, allowing reconstructions in any imaging plane without sacrificing resolution.

SUMMARY

Since its inception, CT imaging has played an integral role in diagnosing spinal injuries. The advent of multidetector technology allowed for faster isotropic, volumetric acquisition, affording the ability to construct high-resolution multiplanar reformations in any imaging plane, providing a faster and more accurate evaluation of the spine and obviating the need for radiographs in the majority of cases. MRI provides a valuable supplemental modality in evaluating the surrounding soft tissue structures or as a problem-solving tool in patients with unexplained symptoms or neurologic deficits. The extensive clinical and basic science research performed over the past 20 years has enriched our understanding of the mechanisms of injury, biomechanics of the spine, and imaging findings associated with spinal injury. Understanding and recognizing predictable patterns of injury allow for a more complete interpretation of the full extent of injury to guide medical management and improve diagnostic accuracy. Despite the advances, future work will rely on improving and optimizing imaging algorithms based on clinical factors as predictors of spinal injury, taking into account cost-effective analysis and risk stratification in addition to limiting overutilization and radiation exposure.

KEY REFERENCES

The level of evidence (LOE) is determined according to the criteria provided in the preface.

2. Bailitz J, Starr F, Beecroft M, et al: CT should replace three-view radiographs as the initial screening test in patients at high, moderate, and low risk for blunt cervical spine injury: a prospective comparison. *J Trauma* 66:1605–1609, 2009. LOE II
3. Como JJ, Diaz JJ, Dunham CM, et al: Practice management guidelines for identification of cervical spine injuries following trauma: update from the Eastern Association for the Surgery of Trauma practice management guidelines committee. *J Trauma* 67:651–659, 2009. LOE IV
4. Como JJ, Leukhardt WH, Anderson JS, et al: Computed tomography alone may clear the cervical spine in obtunded blunt trauma patients: a prospective evaluation of a revised protocol. *J Trauma* 70:345–349, discussion 9–51, 2011. LOE II
11. Hoffman JR, Mower WR, Wolfson AB, et al: Validity of a set of clinical criteria to rule out injury to the cervical spine in patients with blunt trauma. National Emergency X-Radiography Utilization Study Group. *N Engl J Med* 343:94–99, 2000. LOE I
12. Stiell IG, Wells GA, Vandemheen KL, et al: The Canadian C-spine rule for radiography in alert and stable trauma patients. *JAMA* 286:1841–1848, 2001. LOE I
21. Muchow RD, Resnick DK, Abdel MP, et al: Magnetic resonance imaging (MRI) in the clearance of the cervical spine in blunt trauma: a meta-analysis. *J Trauma* 64:179–189, 2008. LOE II
22. Menaker J, Philp A, Boswell S, et al: Computed tomography alone for cervical spine clearance in the unreliable patient—are we there yet? *J Trauma* 64:898–903, discussion 903–904, 2008. LOE III
23. Pearce MS, Salotti JA, Little MP, et al: Radiation exposure from CT scans in childhood and subsequent risk of leukaemia and brain tumours: a retrospective cohort study. *Lancet* 380:499–505, 2012. LOE II
26. Muchow RD, Egan KR, Peppler WW, et al: Theoretical increase of thyroid cancer induction from cervical spine multidetector computed tomography in pediatric trauma patients. *J Trauma Acute Care Surg* 72:403–409, 2012. LOE I
29. Pieretti-Vanmarcke R, Velmahos GC, Nance ML, et al: Clinical clearance of the cervical spine in blunt trauma patients younger than 3 years: a multi-center study of the American Association for the Surgery of Trauma. *J Trauma* 67:543–549, discussion 9–50, 2009. LOE III
31. Mulkens TH, Marchal P, Daineffe S, et al: Comparison of low-dose with standard-dose multidetector CT in cervical spine trauma. *AJNR Am J Neuroradiol* 28:1444–1450, 2007. LOE I
33. Singh S, Kalra MK, Thrall JH, et al: Automatic exposure control in CT: applications and limitations. *J Am Coll Radiol: JACR* 8:446–449, 2011. LOE IV
44. Haba H, Taneichi H, Kotani Y, et al: Diagnostic accuracy of magnetic resonance imaging for detecting posterior ligamentous complex injury associated with thoracic and lumbar fractures. *J Neurosurg* 99:20–26, 2003. LOE II
45. Andreoli C, Colaiacomo MC, Rojas Beccaglia M, et al: MRI in the acute phase of spinal cord traumatic lesions: relationship between MRI findings and neurological outcome. *Radiol Med (Torino)* 110:636–645, 2005. LOE I
51. Miyanji F, Furlan JC, Aarabi B, et al: Acute cervical traumatic spinal cord injury: MR imaging findings correlated with neurologic outcome—prospective study with 100 consecutive patients. *Radiology* 243:820–827, 2007. LOE I
60. Bolinger B, Shartz M, Marion D: Bedside fluoroscopic flexion and extension cervical spine radiographs for clearance of the cervical spine in comatose trauma patients. *J Trauma* 56:132–136, 2004. LOE II
62. Duane TM, Cross J, Scarcella N, et al: Flexion-extension cervical spine plain films compared with MRI in the diagnosis of ligamentous injury. *Am Surg* 76:595–598, 2010. LOE I
76. Chang W, Alexander MT, Mirvis SE: Diagnostic determinants of craniocervical distraction injury in adults. *AJR Am J Roentgenol* 192:52–58, 2009. LOE I
89. Bromberg WJ, Collier BC, Diebel LN, et al: Blunt cerebrovascular injury practice management guidelines: the Eastern Association for the Surgery of Trauma. *J Trauma* 68:471–477, 2010. LOE II
90. Cothren CC, Moore EE, Ray CE Jr, et al: Cervical spine fracture patterns mandating screening to rule out blunt cerebrovascular injury. *Surgery* 141:76–82, 2007. LOE II
92. Stein DM, Boswell S, Sliker CW, et al: Blunt cerebrovascular injuries: does treatment always matter? *J Trauma* 66:132–143, discussion 43–44, 2009. LOE III
97. Sliker CW, Shanmuganathan K, Mirvis SE: Diagnosis of blunt cerebrovascular injuries with 16-MDCT: accuracy of whole-body MDCT compared with neck MDCT angiography. *AJR Am J Roentgenol* 190:790–799, 2008. LOE I
98. Delgado Almandoz JE, Schaefer PW, Kelly HR, et al: Multidetector CT angiography in the evaluation of acute blunt head and neck trauma: a proposed acute craniocervical trauma scoring system. *Radiology* 254:236–244, 2010. LOE II
109. Goodwin RB, Beery PR 2nd, Dorbish RJ, et al: Computed tomographic angiography versus conventional angiography for the diagnosis of blunt cerebrovascular injury in trauma patients. *J Trauma* 67:1046–1050, 2009. LOE I
110. DiCocco JM, Fabian TC, Emmett KP, et al: Optimal outcomes for patients with blunt cerebrovascular injury (BCVI): tailoring treatment to the lesion. *J Am Coll Surg* 212:549–557, discussion 57–59, 2011. LOE III

The complete References list is available online at https://expertconsult.inkling.com.

Chapter 31

Pathophysiology and Emergent Treatment of Spinal Cord Injury

DAVINA V. GUTIERREZ • BASEM I. AWAD • MICHAEL P. STEINMETZ

INTRODUCTION

Traumatic spinal cord injury (SCI) is a potentially devastating event for individuals. Given the vast impact of SCI on individuals and society combined with the economic burden, it is clear that effective therapies are urgently needed. Because current treatment options are limited and provide either negative or modest effects, the development of new strategies to treat SCI are required.

A comprehensive understanding of SCI pathophysiology can lead to potentially promising treatment modalities. The current concepts of the injury pathophysiology indicate that the primary insult, typically caused by rapid spinal cord contusion with subsequent compression, can initiate a signaling cascade of neural damage and hypoxic sequelae known as the secondary injury. Preventing these secondary mechanisms offers the opportunity for neuroprotection and potentially supports reduced tissue destruction and improved neurological outcomes after initial spinal cord trauma.

A growing number of neuroprotective therapies have established some promise in preclinical experimental models. Concurrently, a rapid evolution of stem cell biology and application to treat SCI is occurring. Many of these experimental therapeutic strategies over the past 30 years have reached the point of translation into human evaluation and some have already gone into clinical trials. Despite their passage into clinical trials, evaluating the efficacy of suggested therapeutic strategies is still extremely challenging. The overall complexity is based on the infrequent nature of these injuries, heterogeneous clinical presentation, and the difficulty with classification and categorization of injuries.

In this chapter, we will focus on the pathophysiology of SCI and describe the most studied neuroprotective, neuroregenerative, and cell-based therapies used in SCI trials. Additionally, we will briefly review the current body of preclinical literature that might support the translation into human clinical trials.

SPINAL CORD INJURY EPIDEMIOLOGY: DEMOGRAPHICS AND BASELINE FEATURES

Data indicate that traumatic SCI is mostly prevalent among males aged 18 to 32 years and in developed countries, highly influenced by aging and elderly populations.[1] Global estimates conducted in 2007 report that approximately 133,000 and 226,000 incident cases of traumatic SCI occurred as a result of accidents and self-inflicted harm, respectively.[1] Gaining insight into the incidence and prevalence rates of SCI is crucial because of the large effect such an injury has on personal resources and the health care industry. Furthermore, the frequency of injury implies the necessity of enhanced prevention.

Published reports of SCI incidence within the United States describe 25 to 40 new cases per million each year.[1-4] Estimates reveal that SCI-related costs in the United States are about $9.7 million per year.[5,6] A multicenter, prospective study determined the spectrum, incidence, and severity of complications during initial hospitalization of patients with SCI and found that 79% of the patients included were male and of an average age of 44.6 years (range, 18 to 87 years).[7] Additionally, 25% of patients were 29 years or younger and 25% were older than 57 years.[7] Finally, the primary etiologies included falls (37%), motor vehicle accidents (28%), and sports or recreation (14%).[7] Of all injuries, 4% were caused by penetrating injuries.[7] Among persons involved in a review supplemented by inception cohort study, data found that the mean age of injury increased from 28.3 years during the 1970s to 37.1 years between 2005 and 2008 and directly reflects the overall increasing median age of the general U.S. population.[8,9]

A literature survey aimed at revealing data about the incidence, prevalence, and epidemiology of SCI concluded that the young, male patients were more likely paraplegic, complete or incomplete.[6] A review reported that 55.7% of new injuries enrolled in a combined U.S. data set since 2000 were injuries to the cervical spinal cord and that this percentage increased from 50.7% in the 1970s.[8,9] The increase in cervical injuries is directly influenced by higher rates in C1-C4 lesions, 12.3% to 27.2%, and to a doubling in the percentage of patients being discharged as ventilator dependent: 1.5% in the 1970s to 5.4% between 2000 and 2004.[9] The above-mentioned multicenter study indicated that of the participants recorded, the levels of injury were 78% for cervical, 18% for thoracic, and 4% for lumbar/sacral, and 1% were SCI without radiographic abnormality (SCIWORA).[7]

The preliminary neurological assessment on admission indicated a bimodal distribution of the American Spinal Injury Association (ASIA) grade of severity of neurological injury so that the incidence of grade A was 40% and that of grade D was 29%.[7] Not surprisingly, the severity of the injury is directly in proportion to a higher incidence of complications. Specifically, of the 126 patients with ASIA grade A, 106 (84.1%) incurred complications.[7] While an extensive amount of effort is focused on the prevention and treatment of acute events that are most ubiquitous among SCI populations, complications still arise. These include pneumonia, deep venous

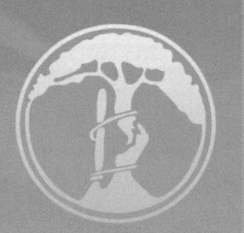

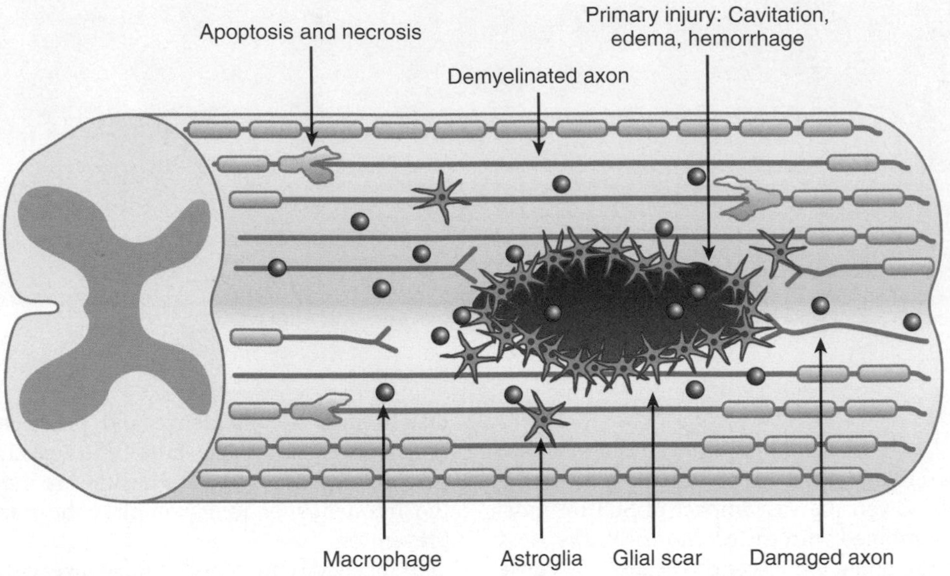

Figure 31-1. Pathophysiology of spinal cord injury (SCI). The diagram shows the pathological events occurring after SCI. The primary and secondary injury mechanisms involve hemorrhage, edema, inflammation, apoptosis, necrosis, excitotoxicity, blood vessel occlusion, ischemia and/or vasospasm, axonal demyelination, disruption of synaptic transmission, hypertrophic astrocytes and macrophages, which aid in the composition of the glial scar.

thrombosis (DVT), pleural effusion, severe bradycardia, shock, cardiac arrest, respiratory failure, septicemia, pulmonary embolus, and external events.[10-14] In particular, half of all complications occur within the first week of hospitalization and three-fourths within 2 weeks.[7] Since the 1970s, a remarkable amount of advancement has been achieved toward significantly diminishing the mortality rate during the first year after SCI.[9,15] Information relating to the gravity of particular impediments following SCI will definitely facilitate earlier recognition, effective treatment, and prevention.

THE PATHOPHYSIOLOGY OF SPINAL CORD INJURY: PRIMARY AND SECONDARY INJURY

In general terms, mechanical trauma to the spinal cord induces tissue necrosis and functional loss (Fig. 31-1). Any neurologic damage incurred at the moment of impact is the primary injury and occurs after concussion, contusion, laceration, transection, or intraparenchymal hemorrhage.[16] There are four characteristic mechanisms of primary injury: (1) impact plus persistent compression, (2) impact alone with transient compression, (3) distraction; and (4) laceration and transection (Table 31-1).[17] Out of those four, the most frequent mechanism of injury involves impact plus persistent compression.[17-19] The central gray matter is primarily damaged after the initial mechanical insult, while the peripherally located white matter is relatively spared.[17] Studies have suggested that irreversible damage to the gray matter transpires within the first hour after SCI, whereas the white matter is irreversibly damaged within 72 hours after SCI.[17,20]

Other pathophysiological events in the spinal cord that commence after the primary injury include hemorrhage, edema, disrupted microcirculation, local infarction (caused by hypoxia and ischemia), loss of autoregulation, vasospasm, neuronal damage, and disrupted nerve transmission.[16,17,21-23] Together, this interdependent cascade of systemic and cellular events initiated after the primary insult is referred to as the secondary injury and may occur within minutes after SCI (Table 31-2).[16,17,24] Mechanical disruption of the microvasculature sets in motion a series of pathways and interrelated processes that inevitably contribute to cellular necrosis and apoptosis within the spinal cord. These events can be further divided into (1) neurogenic shock, (2) vascular abnormalities, (3) free radical and lipid peroxidation, (4) excitotoxicity and electrolyte imbalance, (5) necrotic and apoptotic cell death, and (6) inflammatory and immunologic responses.

TABLE 31-1 *SUMMARIZED DESCRIPTION AND EXAMPLES OF THE PRIMARY MECHANISMS OF SPINAL CORD INJURY*

Primary Injury Types	Characteristics	Examples
Impact with constant compression	Most common; compression arising from fractures or ruptures	Burst fractures with retropulsed bone fragments compressing the cord; fracture-dislocations; acute disc ruptures
Impact alone	May involve transient compression	Hyperextension injuries as seen in patients with degenerative cervical spine disease
Distraction	Forcible stretching or shearing of the spinal column	Flexion, extension, rotation, or dislocation
Laceration/ transection	Varying degrees of injury, from minor injury to complete transection	Missile injury, sharp bone fragment dislocation, severe distraction

Source: *Adapted from Dumont RJ, Okonkwo DO, Verma S, et al: Acute spinal cord injury. Part I. Pathophysiologic mechanisms, Clin Neuropharmacol 24:254–264, 2001.*

TABLE 31-2 *SUMMARIZED DESCRIPTION OF THE SECONDARY INJURIES ASSOCIATED WITH SPINAL CORD INJURY*

Secondary Injury Events	Characteristics
Neurogenic shock	Bradycardia, hypotension, reduced peripheral resistance, decreased cardiac output, ischemia
Vascular disruption	Hemorrhagic and ischemic damage, disrupted microcirculation, hemorrhagic necrosis, vasospasm
Free radical generation and lipid peroxidation	Free radical production, oxidative stress, oxidation of proteins, lipids and nucleic acids, inactivation of mitochondrial respiratory chain enzymes, inhibited Na^+-K^+ ATPase, Na^+ channel inactivation
Excitotoxicity and electrolyte imbalance	Excessive release of glutamate, NMDAR and AMPAR activation, cytotoxic edema, intracellular acidosis, accumulation of intracellular Ca^{2+}
Necrotic and apoptotic cell death	Swelling, damaged organelles, lysis, cellular shrinkage, nuclear fragmentation
Inflammation and immunologic response	Neutrophil accumulation, macrophage and microglia migration, demyelination, wallerian degeneration, scarring, mitochondrial damage, cytochrome c release, caspase activation

Na^+-K^+ ATPase, Sodium- and potassium-activated adenosine triphosphatase.
Source: *Adapted from Dumont RJ, Okonkwo DO, Verma S, et al: Acute spinal cord injury. Part I. Pathophysiologic mechanisms, Clin Neuropharmacol 24:254–264, 2001; Kwon BK, Tetzlaff W, Grauer JN, et al: Pathophysiology and pharmacologic treatment of acute spinal cord injury, Spine J 4:451–464, 2004.*

Neurogenic shock is essentially inadequate tissue perfusion, resulting from paralysis of vasomotor input that ultimately produces deleterious disturbances of the balance between vasodilation and vasoconstriction.[17] Clinical characteristics include bradycardia, hypotension, and decreased cardiac output.[17,25] The resultant effects may result in further neurological damage if left unchecked. *Vascular insults* include hemorrhage and ischemia-reperfusion and are thought to be one of the most crucial features of secondary injury. Mechanical interruptions to the microvasculature, loss of microcirculation, and disrupted autoregulation produces petechial hemorrhage and intravascular thrombosis, which in combination with vasospasm of intact vessels and edema at the injury site, leads to local hypoperfusion and ischemia.[17,24,26] Postmortem studies of human spinal cords have reported a significantly higher amount of vascular perfusion in the gray matter than in the white matter and that this difference may be due to the disruption and/or thrombosis of the sulcal arterial network that supplies the gray matter.[24,27] Further exacerbating the microcircuitry injuries is the spreading of the damage beyond the initial site of injury into a wider zone of destruction. Eventually this ischemic damage spreads rostrally and caudally. Once this occurs, the amount of available oxygen decreases, anaerobic cellular respiration commences, and both lactic acid and free radicals are generated.[16,17,28,29] Oxygen-derived *free radicals* are produced during ischemia and are comprised of unpaired electrons. These molecules include superoxide, hydroxyl radicals, nitric oxide, and peroxynitrite oxidants; are highly reactive to lipids, proteins, and DNA; and contribute to oxidative stress.[17,24,30-32] Free radicals cause a progressive oxidation of fatty acids in cell membranes *(lipid peroxidation)* so that the oxidation process creates more free radicals to further propagate the reaction across the cellular surface.[24,33] During neurotrauma, the level of oxidative stress surpasses the normal level of protective cellular antioxidant capacity and leads to a net production of reactive molecules that progressively oxidize proteins, lipids, and nucleic acids.[17,29,34] Oxidative stress also negatively impacts significant mitochondrial respiratory chain enzymes, alters DNA and DNA-associated proteins, and inhibits sodium-potassium adenosine triphosphatase (Na^+-K^+ ATPase) that essentially precipitates metabolic collapse and cellular apoptosis and necrosis.[24,34]

While anatomically intact fiber tracts remain after SCI, there is still a loss of impulse conduction that has been attributed to modified intracellular and extracellular concentrations of key ions, biochemical derangements, and simultaneous fluid-electrolyte disturbances that inevitably lead to *excitotoxicity and electrolyte imbalance.*[16,17] To respond to the primary and secondary injuries, excitatory neurotransmitters are released but rapidly accumulate to toxic concentrations producing additional direct damage to spinal cord tissue.[17,24,35-38]

Specifically, glutamate is excessively released and quickly accumulates after SCI, activating ionotropic and metabotropic receptors such as *N*-methyl-D-aspartate (NMDA) and α-amino-3-hydroxyl-5-methyl-isoxazolopropionate (AMPA)/kainate receptors and inducing neuronal injury via excitotoxicity.[17,39,40] Glutamate-mediated NMDA receptor activation promotes extracellular calcium (Ca^{2+}) and sodium (Na^+) to move down a concentration gradient into the cell, where the levels of calcium are usually very low.[24] Changes in the intracellular concentrations of Na^+ and Ca^{2+} create profound physiological modifications and further damage such as cytotoxic edema, intracellular acidosis, activation of lytic enzymes, free radical production, inhibition of Na^+-K^+ ATPase activity, inactivation of membrane Na^+ channels, and dysregulation of mitochondrial oxidative phosphorylation.[17,24,34,41-43] An additional consequence of electrolyte imbalance includes augmented extracellular potassium (K^+) concentration, resulting in excessive neuronal depolarization, abnormal conduction, and possibly spinal shock.[17,44] Finally, magnesium depletion from intracellular stores can negatively impact glycolysis, oxidative phosphorylation, and protein synthesis.[17]

Necrotic and apoptotic cell death transpire after SCI and are prompted by ischemia, oxidative stress, and excitotoxicity.[45] Necrotic cell death arises after disrupted homeostatic mechanisms and leads to membrane and organelle damage, decreased adenosine triphosphate (ATP) generation, and passive cell swelling.[24] Conversely, apoptosis occurs when specific extrinsic or intrinsic traumas activate intracellular signaling cascades, activating caspase enzymes and dismantling of the cell.[24,46] Apoptosis has been shown to significantly contribute to SCI as it is found to influence neurons, oligodendrocytes, microglia, and possibly astrocytes.[17] Neuronal apoptosis contributes to cell loss and has obvious implications on outcome after SCI.[47] SCI-mediated neuronal apoptosis transpires extrinsically, mediated by the Fas ligand and receptor and/or inducible nitric oxide synthase production and intrinsically through direct caspase-3 proenzyme activation, mitochondrial damage, release of cytochrome c, and activation of the inducer caspase-9.[17,47-52]

After SCI, the inflammatory process is instantly activated and continues for several days postinjury. The *inflammatory and immunologic response* to injury within the central nervous system (CNS) is immensely varied when compared to other tissue because of the involvement of neutrophils, macrophage, T cells, cytokines, prostaglandins, and complement.[24,53] The response involves endothelial damage, the release of inflammatory mediators, changes in vascular permeability, development of edema, permeation of peripheral inflammatory cells, microglial activation, and phagocytosis of injured tissue.[16,23,54]

The functional significance of particular key immunological cells after SCI is controversial. Numerous investigations indicated that macrophage and/or microglia have positive contributions and detrimental consequences after injury.[55-61] Specifically, the activated microglia and monocytes represent the greater part of all inflammatory cells located at the injury site so that there is debate as to whether these cells help or hinder.[54,62-64] Clearly the inflammatory response is thought to be neurotoxic and neuroprotective, the early phases being injurious and the latter being protective.[24]

The grade of SCI is contingent on the extent of mechanical damage inflicted on the cord during the primary event but is also influenced by the secondary phase of injury. Additionally, the degrees of both primary and secondary injuries are directly influenced by the amount of energy delivered to the spinal cord at the moment of impact.[20,24] The extent of secondary injuries extends radially and longitudinally along the spinal cord in a rostral-to-caudal manner. The final outcome is central gray matter cavitation with loss of adjacent white matter tracts.[65,66] Numerous surgical and pharmacological strategies are now focused on stabilizing the injured cord and minimizing additional damage initiated by the secondary trauma.

IMMEDIATE THERAPEUTIC APPROACHES

The treatment of SCI focuses on minimizing secondary injury. This must begin immediately. Namely, focus should be on maintaining adequate tissue perfusion and oxygenation. Hypotension following traumatic injury has been noted to result in worse outcomes compared to a more normal blood pressure.[67-71] This may especially be true in patients presenting in spinal shock. There may be bradycardia, hypotension, and warm flushed extremities. Patients with cervical spinal cord injuries may present with reduced inspiratory and expiratory capacity. This may be caused by loss of accessory muscles for respiration and/or paralysis of the diaphragm. Either may result in hypoxia.

It is imperative that patients are managed in a setting where blood pressure and respiratory status may be monitored and also treated appropriately, namely an intensive care unit. Consideration should be given to early intubation, especially in those patients with high-cervical spinal cord injuries.[72] Early treatment of blood pressure should involve fluid resuscitation followed by pressor agents if needed. The choice of the agent to use is dependent on many factors and beyond discussion in this chapter. The goal should be to maintain mean arterial blood pressure greater than 85 mm Hg and continue this goal for at least 7 days postinjury. This recommendation is based on class III literature and is reported in the Guidelines for the Management of Acute Cervical Spine and Spinal Cord Injuries.[73]

Initial Closed Reduction

The authors believe that, at times, there should be an initial attempt at closed reduction of cervical spine dislocations. At times, closed reduction is skipped and the patient taken emergently to the operating room for open reduction and fixation. Closed reduction is most often used for unilateral and bilateral facet dislocations. Reduction appears possible in more than 80% of patients.[74,75] Authors have reported improved outcomes following urgent reduction; however, no class I or II data have been presented confirming these findings.

Early Decompression Surgery

The existing preclinical evidence supports that decompression surgery of the spinal cord after SCI attenuates secondary injury and improves neurological recovery.[76-78] This neuroprotective effect seems to vary inversely with the time elapsed from injury to decompression[77,78] and also the magnitude of compression. The impact of timing of decompression and stabilization following SCI has been difficult to establish in clinical trials. Vaccaro and colleagues published a randomized, prospective, controlled study on 64 patients with acute cervical SCI. Patients were randomized into either an early surgical decompression group (surgery performed <72 hours after SCI) or a late surgical group (surgery performed >5 days after SCI). The results showed that there was no significant benefit in terms of neurological or functional level in patients treated less than 72 hours compared to those treated more than 5 days after cervical SCI.[79] In contrast, a systematic review by LaRosa and colleagues reported that early decompression (within 24 hours after SCI) resulted in improved outcomes compared to both delayed decompression and conservative therapy.[80] In 2010, the Spine Trauma Study Group defined 24 hours as the cutoff to differentiate early versus late decompression surgery after SCI.[81] Recently, a multicenter prospective cohort study was conducted on 313 patients with acute cervical SCI. Of these, 182 underwent early surgical decompression (<24 hours after injury), while the remaining 131 patients underwent late surgery (>24 hours after injury).[82] Results demonstrated that 19.8% of patients treated with early surgery showed a grade II or higher improvement in the ASIA Impairment Scale at 6 months' follow-up compared to 8.8% in the late decompression group.

Therapeutic Hypothermia

Numerous clinical investigations have indicated that hypothermia is an effective neuroprotective treatment, shown to decrease pathophysiological complications associated with cardiac arrest, traumatic brain injury, stroke, aortic aneurysm, and neonatal hypoxic-ischemic encephalopathy.[83-87] Because of the benefits associated with this option, the potential application in SCI is now being examined. Specifically, hypothermia is known to decrease axonal swelling, lower tissue hemorrhaging and microglia accumulation, diminish oxidative stress, apoptosis, and reduce glutamate release so that SCI-induced ischemia may be treated in patients by cooling.[26,88-92] Studies have reported that systemic (surface and intravascular) hypothermia (89.6°–93.2° F [32°–34° C]) offers the most neuroprotective benefits that overcome harmful effects often associated with subphysiological temperatures.[93]

A retrospective analysis of 14 patients with acute cervical SCI graded as ASIA A, who received systemic hypothermia for 48 hours, found an associated conversion rate of 42.8% and specifically that 3 patients improved to ASIA grade B, 2 progressed to ASIA grade C, and 1 patient recovered to ASIA grade D.[93] Additionally patients exhibited respiratory and infectious complications but failed to demonstrate adverse effects such as coagulopathy, DVT, and pulmonary embolism in comparison to control patients.[93] A single case report described an NFL football player who sustained a C3-C4 fracture-dislocation, which resulted in an ASIA A SCI.[94] The individual underwent surgical decompression, intravenous methylprednisolone therapy, and systemic hypothermia and demonstrated significant and rapid neurologic improvement within weeks of the injury.[94] Furthermore, the patient eventually progressed to ASIA D. While the degree of contribution from hypothermia to recovery remains to be determined, these results demonstrate the need for additional preclinical and clinical investigations focused on hypothermia as a treatment for acute SCI. Recently, a meta-analysis of 16 publications sought to examine the efficacy of hypothermia on functional outcome, mean outcome, and variance and reported that regional cooling is neuroprotective when cord ischemia is present.[95,96] Overall, the authors suggest great translational potential for hypothermia and recommend further clinical studies.

Pharmacological Management: Methylprednisolone Sodium Succinate

One strategy that has been explored in an acute SCI environment is the use of corticosteroids. The application of these antiinflammatory agents originated more than 30 years ago and was based on findings that application reduced spinal cord edema.[97,98] The neuroprotective influences of corticosteroids include attenuated lipid peroxidation, inhibition of inflammatory cytokines, reduced calcium influx, reduced posttraumatic axonal dieback, and improved vascular perfusion.[99-102] Due to the accrual of promising preclinical data in animal models of SCI, the effectiveness of the corticosteroid methylprednisolone sodium succinate (MPSS) was examined in five prospective acute SCI trials in humans.[102,103]

The widespread use of MPSS in the clinical setting has been largely influenced by three large-scale prospective randomized double-blinded multicenter clinical trials reported as the North American Spinal Cord Injury Studies (NASCIS) I, II, and III. In brief, NASCIS I investigated the efficacy of 10 daily doses of either a moderate (1000 mg) or low (100 mg) dose of MPSS administered within 48 hours of SCI.[104] Data analysis indicated that there was no significant difference in the neurological outcomes between the two groups when examined at 6 weeks, 6 months, and 1 year.[104] Although neurological improvement showed no significant difference between the groups, wound infection, gastrointestinal (GI) hemorrhage, sepsis, pulmonary embolism, delayed wound healing, and death were all significantly higher for patients receiving the moderate dosage.[103] NASCIS II examined the difference between a high-dose application of MPSS (initial bolus of 30 mg/kg followed by a 23-hour infusion of 5.4 mg/kg per hour), naloxone (an opioid receptor antagonist), or placebo administered within 24 hours.[105,106] A post hoc analysis indicated that the group who received MPSS within 8 hours of injury demonstrated statistically significant sensory and motor recovery and that these improvements were visible at 1.5, 6, and 12 months postinjury.[105,106] The NASCIS III trial examined the efficacy of high-dose MPSS application (30 mg/kg bolus) for 48 versus 24 hours.[107,108] Data analysis indicated that patients had significant neurological functional recovery when they received MPSS within 3 to 8 hours and were treated for 48 hours; improvements were visible at 6 weeks and 6 months but not 1 year.[107,108]

The variability of clinical efficacy, as well as complications associated with and the propensity toward adverse effects have inevitably generated a great deal of controversy surrounding the use of MPSS in SCI cases. While MPSS is currently an accepted clinical option, there is still a need for additional neuroprotective agents with improved and consistent efficacy.

NEUROPROTECTIVE AND NEUROREGENERATIVE APPROACHES TO TREATING THE INJURED SPINAL CORD

Current medical and surgical interventions are currently focused on minimizing the extent of secondary injury and protecting the neural components that survived the primary mechanical injury. For example, postmortem studies of patients diagnosed as having "complete" injuries have indicated that the cord is rarely completely transected after blunt injuries.[24,109,110] While it is not known how much is remaining, intact spinal cord is needed to mediate significant distal neurologic function; data suggest that minimal motor function has been demonstrated in an incompletely paralyzed patient with around 7% of the normal number of axons below the level of injury.[24,110,111] Therefore, there is great potential in the idea that some progress toward neuroprotection and preservation after SCI may somehow significantly impact functionally relevant neurological recovery.

Monosialotetrahexosylganglioside

Gangliosides are sialic acid-containing glycosphingolipids that are abundant in the outer surface of neuronal membranes. A number of experimental CNS injury studies indicated that the systemic administration of monosialotetrahexosylganglioside (GM-1) resulted in neuroprotective effects that included neural repair, functional recovery, inhibition of excitotoxicity, and prevention of apoptosis.[112-114] A single-center prospective double-blinded randomized trial of SCI patients administered 100 mg of intramuscular GM-1 for 30 days reported statistically significant improvement in ASIA motor score for the treatment group.[115] These positive results prompted a prospective clinical trial that randomized 797 patients into placebo, low-dose GM-1 (300 mg loading dose, followed by 100 mg/day for 56 days) or high-dose GM-1 (600 mg loading dose, followed with 200 mg/day for 56 days).[116] Data indicated that the experimental group did not demonstrate statistically significant recovery at 26 weeks but analysis did suggest a trend toward improved motor and sensory scores and augmented bowel and bladder function.[24,116] These improvements were especially evident in patients with incomplete spinal cord injuries and suggest that there may be a potential benefit for subjects living with incomplete paraplegia.

Minocycline

Minocycline is a tetracycline family derivative that is often employed in the treatment of acne and rosacea and has been demonstrated as being neuroprotective in animal models of stroke, Parkinson disease, Huntington disease, amyotrophic lateral sclerosis (ALS), and multiple sclerosis.[102,117] Additionally, a multitude of studies have shown that minocycline lessens secondary injury and supports functional recovery in animal models of SCI.[118-121] The range of activities include inhibition of microglial activation and proliferation, decreased excitotoxicity, stabilization of mitochondria, reduced apoptosis, neutralization of free oxygen radicals, inhibition of nitric oxide synthase, decreased inflammation, and Ca^{2+} chelation.[117,122]

Taking the preclinical findings into consideration, a phase II placebo-controlled randomized trial of minocycline in acute SCI was conducted. In brief, patients who presented within 12 hours in injury were stratified into three groups according to their severity, and were given intravenous administration of minocycline for 7 days.[122] Data analysis indicates that patients treated with minocycline demonstrated 6 points greater motor recovery than the placebo group but that no difference was evident for thoracic SCI.[122] A change of 14 motor points was detected in patients with cervical injury and with cervical motor-incomplete injuries; results approached significance.[122]

While the clinical data do not report statistically significant results, improvements in motor output suggest a potential therapeutic advantage. Furthermore, minocycline possesses pharmacological and mechanistic promise that supports additional efficacy investigations.

Cethrin

Rho guanosine triphosphatase (GTPase) is one of five members of the Ras superfamily that primarily functions as a molecular modulator of signal transduction pathways in eukaryotic cells.[123] In general, the Rho family regulates numerous actin-mediated processes that include morphogenesis, endocytosis, phagocytosis, and motility.[123] Within the nervous system, Rho family members are essential components of axonal growth and guidance.[124] Rho activation mediates neuronal responses to repulsive cues, induces growth cone collapse and neurite retraction so that inhibition of Rho support axonal growth.[124] Experimental investigations have indicated that Rho activity is increased following SCI in neurons, astrocytes, and oligodendrocytes and suggests that Rho signaling influences SCI pathophysiology such as neuronal apoptosis and glial plasticity.[124-126] Because Rho is involved in an inhibitory signaling cascade that supports growth cone collapse and inhibition of neurite and axonal outgrowth, discovering a pharmacological means to inhibit Rho activation may prevent the downregulation of axon regeneration.

A phase I/II clinical trial compared the effectiveness of a single dose (0.3, 1, 3, 6, and 9 mg) of Cethrin on neurological improvement in patients with thoracic and cervical SCI.[127] Patients received Cethrin within 1 week of injury during a decompression surgery and delivery was as follows: Cethrin was combined with a fibrin sealant and directly applied to the dura mater at the injury site.[127] Data indicated that 66% of patients with cervical SCI, who received a dose of 3 mg, improved from ASIA grade A to ASIA grade C or D and that only 6% of those with thoracic SCI demonstrated similar recovery.[127] These encouraging findings support the use of Cethrin as a safe and effective means to promote functional recovery after SCI.

Autologous Macrophage

Activated autologous macrophage was the first cellular substrate transplanted into patients after SCI.[102] This study was based on an early animal model of SCI whereby the ex vivo activation of autologous macrophage, injected into the injured spinal cord, promoted the functional recovery and augmented the synthesis of beneficial trophic factors.[128] An early clinical trial enrolled eight patients with complete SCI and transplanted the macrophage within 14 days of injury.[129] The investigation reported improvement from ASIA grade A to ASIA grade C in 3 of 8 patients.[129] A phase II randomized controlled multicenter trial expanded this study to 43 patients with either cervical or thoracic SCI and did not reveal statistically significant functional recovery between the two groups.[130] Therefore, the data indicate that the application of autologous incubated macrophage to the injured spinal cord was not an effective therapeutic option.

Riluzole

An extensive array of data has demonstrated that voltage-gated sodium channels become constitutively activated during the secondary injury cascade.[131] Amplified intracellular sodium (Na^+) levels induce cellular swelling, intracellular acidosis, increased calcium influx, and glutamate excitotoxicity.[132-134] To target the neuronal ionic imbalance, pharmacological therapies have focused on inhibiting Na^+ channel activation. By using various Na^+ channel antagonists, preclinical studies have displayed neural tissue preservation and behavioral improvement following SCI.[135-138]

Of particular interest to both preclinical and clinical SCI studies is riluzole, a neuroprotective agent approved for the treatment of ALS patients.[139] Experimental investigations have indicated that riluzole-treated animals exhibit significant tissue preservation and improved neurobehavioral outcomes when compared to control animals.[140] The promising preclinical data coupled with the clinical efficacy of ALS treatment has prompted a prospective, multicenter phase I trial by the North American Clinical Trials Network (NACTN) to establish the pharmacokinetics and safety of riluzole treatment on acute SCI.[141] The trial enrolled 36 patients (ASIA grades A through C) and was designed as a single-arm, open-labeled, matched comparison study that had an end point follow-up set to 6 months with neurological, functional, and pain assessments continued out to 12 months postinjury.[138] In brief, patients received their first dose of riluzole (50 mg) within 12 hours of injury and were administered treatment every 12 hours for 2 weeks.[138] Data indicate that the most significant mean motor score improvements were present in grade B patients.[141] Additionally, pinprick scores were 10 points higher for riluzole-treated patients compared to registry participants.[141] While the pilot data suggest a beneficial trend on motor function, additionally studies (phase II trial) are needed to completely define neurological outcomes.

Improving Axonal Conduction in the Injured Spinal Cord

Fampridine

A traditional viewpoint of myelin is that it plays a significant role in signal transduction so that any mechanical insult likely decreases conduction velocity. Following SCI, although some nerve fibers remain uninterrupted across the injury, there is an overall redistribution of sodium (Na^+) and potassium (K^+) channels across the axon caused by myelin disruption. Reports indicate that 6 to 8 weeks following SCI, voltage-gated K^+ channels demonstrate altered distribution on axons following demyelination.[142] Specifically, rapidly activating K^+ channels that were once obscured by myelin show increased activity, drive the membrane potential close to the K^+ equilibrium potential, and support blockade of axonal conduction.[143]

To inhibit the exposed fast K^+ channels on demyelinated axons, researchers have used 4-aminopyridine (4-AP) to promote the facilitation of axonal conduction, broaden action potentials, and augment synaptic transmission.[144-146] Laboratory investigations have shown that 4-AP treatment improves conduction in rat spinal nerve roots,[147,148] supports conduction in demyelinated rat sciatic nerves,[149] and promotes functional motor behavior in a chronic SCI model.[145] Together these studies demonstrate that 4-AP application not only suppresses fast-acting K^+ channels but also improves conduction along demyelinated axons after SCI.

The success of the in vitro studies prompted investigators to determine if 4-AP enhances motor function and sensation in the clinical setting after injury. An early clinical trial examining the efficacy of 4-AP in chronic SCI patients revealed neurological improvements that included increased motor control and sensory ability and reduced chronic pain and spasticity after application.[150] These advancements lasted 48 hours postinfusion and prompted studies aimed at using sustained release 4-AP. An oral fampridine-SR (sustained release 4-AP) exploratory trial demonstrated that treating patients with incomplete SCI resulted in improved sensory scores, augmented motor function, and decreased spasticity.[151] While variations in the amount and frequency of fampridine delivery have generated additional clinical studies, data suggest that patients receiving drug treatment demonstrate functional improvement.[152,153]

CELL-BASED THERAPIES FOR SPINAL CORD INJURY

Cellular transplantations for the management of SCI have been the subject of interest for many recent preclinical studies, because their therapeutic effects are multifactorial and promising for neural plasticity and repair. Various cell types have the potential to promote axonal growth, myelin formation, synaptic reconnection, trophic factor secretion, lesion modification, glial scar degradation, and removal of inhibitory signaling. In the following paragraphs, we will address the potential benefits of the most widely studied cells that include: Schwann cells (SCs), olfactory ensheathing cells (OECs) bone marrow stromal cells (BMSCs), and neural stem/progenitor cells (NSPCs).

Schwann Cells

It has been well established that following SCI, endogenous SCs invade and migrate into the spinal cord.[154-156] Additionally, it has been recognized that transplanted SCs can also facilitate the invasion of host SCs into the injured spinal cord.[157,158] Preclinical studies showed that the incoming SCs myelinate or ensheathe large numbers of regenerated axons within the contusion cavity.[159] Interestingly, this phenomenon is not exclusive to animal models in that large numbers of SCs and their associated axons have been found in chronic, human SCIs.[155,160] Since then, the efficacy of transplanted SCs has been widely investigated after SCI.

A number of previous studies clearly established that SCs are able to act as both trophic and physical substrates. SCs can facilitate the regeneration of sensory axons from the dorsal root ganglia, as well as propriospinal axons adjacent to the injury site. However, studies demonstrated that SCs alone are not sufficient to promote regeneration of the corticospinal tracts, nor do they permit axons that enter spinal cord grafts to exit and reenter the host spinal cord.[161] Consequently, co-treatment and combinational strategies have been developed to help in functional axonal regeneration through the lesion site and to enhance plasticity and recovery, such as neuroprotective agents, chondroitinase ABC, cell substrates, and enhanced or growth factor expression.[162-165]

Clinical translation emphasizes the need for a preclinical demonstration of behavioral benefits with human SCs. However, it is notable that human SCs have been reported in only two preclinical rodent studies and both were in thoracic full transection SCI models.[161,166,167] In one study, the authors stated a significant behavior benefit in the Basso, Beattie, and Bresnahan (BBB) scale and the incline plane test.[167] However, the SCs were applied in conjunction with a Matrigel and guidance channel that are presently not approved by the Food and Drug Administration (FDA).[167]

Considering the ethical and immunological compatibility facts that surround the use of fetal tissue as a source for SCs, an autologous transplantation approach is appealing to eliminate these concerns. However, an autologous approach necessitates sacrificing a peripheral nerve, and a number of weeks are needed to amplify the cells to fill the large cystic cavities that are usually seen in the injured spinal cords.[168,169] To avoid harvesting a peripheral nerve from an injured patient, alternative sources of SCs from postnatal skin or adult bone marrow have recently been pursued in preclinical settings. Both studies showed significant improvement on the BBB scale, suggesting that alternative sources can be effective and potentially less invasive sources of autologous SCs.[157,170]

Despite the lack of preclinical studies using the human SCs, two clinical trials have been published recently using the autologous human SCs. In 2008, Saberi and colleagues reported the results of four patients with chronic thoracic SCI who underwent autologous SCs transplantation. No detrimental effect was reported.[171] In 2013, Yazdani and colleagues published a series of eight patients who received autologous SCs in combination with BMSCs. No adverse effect or functional improvements were detected during a 2-year follow-up period.[172] In the meantime, both trials are considered a promising move toward more clinical applications of SCs.

Olfactory Ensheathing Cells

OECs surround the axons of sensory neurons of the olfactory bulb, as well as in the nasal olfactory mucosa. OECs have the ability to facilitate a lifelong proliferation capacity as they normally mediate the transition between axons in the peripheral nervous system (PNS) olfactory mucosa and their synapses in the CNS olfactory bulb.[173] Additionally, OECs can promote axonal regeneration through the lesion site and facilitate axonal reentry at the graft-host border. The mechanism behind this response is debatable in that OECs possibly migrate with the growing axons, thereby preventing the axons from recognizing the nonpermissive environment.[174] Another potential mechanism involves the capability of OECs to decrease the host astrocyte response and chondroitin sulphate proteoglycan expression after SCI.[156,175]

Indeed, isolation of OECs showed heterogeneity in morphology, antigen expression, and function between cells of different origins.[176-178] The adult human olfactory mucosa, unlike other mammals, is not contiguous but randomly distributed with respiratory mucosa in the upper nasal cavity.[179,180] Consequently, olfactory mucosa biopsies from adult humans will almost always contain respiratory epithelium.[181] Additionally, because the trigeminal nerve innervates the olfactory and respiratory mucosa as well as olfactory bulb, it is possible that OEC preparations may also contain SCs from the trigeminal nerve.[182] This heterogeneity and potential contamination applying to OEC isolation requires very strict standards and protocols to purify the cells before experimental and clinical application.[181] Based on the literature, OECs derived from the olfactory bulb of adult rodents are the most commonly studied cells in preclinical settings, compared to OECs derived from the lamina propria of the olfactory mucosa. Most of these studies employed the sharp SCI models that are clinically less relevant compared to blunt contusion injury models (as reviewed in 2011 by Tetzlaff and colleagues).[161]

Interestingly, in 2000, Ramon-Cueto and colleagues reported that OECs can promote regeneration in corticospinal axons and improve motor behaviors after 3 and 7 months post thoracic cord transection.[183] Although a few additional studies used OECs alone in more clinically relevant thoracic contusion injury models, none of them showed behavioral benefits.[156,184,185] However, the combination of OECs with SCs appears to promote behavior benefits.[184] Behavior recovery was also reported when the adult bulb-derived OECs were transfected to express brain-derived neurotrophic factor (BDNF) and neurotrophin-3 (NT-3).[186]

However, preclinical animal studies showed inconsistent OEC regeneration capacity (within olfactory mucosal grafts) in independently replicated experiments.[165,187] Feron and colleagues published a clinical trial using autologous, nasal biopsied OECs from patients with complete thoracic paraplegia. Twelve to twenty million cells were injected directly into the injured cord. Patients were assessed postsurgery with no adverse outcomes and no changes in magnetic resonance imaging (MRI) at 1 year.[188] Patients were further evaluated at 3 years with a variety of outcome measures. No alterations in MRI were detected and there were no adverse outcomes, such as loss of function or neuropathic pain.[189]

Additionally, three more clinical trials have been published using olfactory mucosa OECs[190-192] but showed mixed results and outcomes. Taken together, these reports indicate that the clinical application is relatively safe with indications that it may improve outcomes.

Bone Marrow Stromal Cells and Mesenchymal Stem Cells

Perhaps, BMSCs are the most widely studied stem cells in preclinical settings and most applied in human transplantation. The stromal cells are isolated and separated from the hematopoietic cell fraction of the bone marrow. Therefore, BMSCs are typically a crude mixture of stromal cells that support the growth of hematopoietic stem cells and mesenchymal stem cells. Although mesenchymal stem cells can be separated from the rest of hematopoietic cell fraction by adherence to plastic or using additional markers, this heterogeneity can explain the variable results among different laboratories.[161] In 2005, Neuhuber and colleagues implanted human BMSCs from four different donors in hemisected rats and showed highly variable behavior outcomes.[193]

Both rodent and human BMSCs have been studied extensively in SCI models and have demonstrated some behavioral efficacy. However, these beneficial effects were mainly referred to the indirect environmental modification rather than direct differentiation of BMSCs to neurons or oligodendrocytes. Although neurogenesis is possible in vitro,[194] there is a debate whether this occurs in vivo to produce behavioral benefits.[195,196] Several studies reported more tissue sparing, as well as reduced apoptosis, inflammation, and demyelination after the transplantation of BMSCs.[197-202] Despite these findings, the exact mechanism by which BMSCs provide tissue sparing, neuroprotection, and improvement in behavior outcomes is still unknown.

Several clinical trials have been published using a mixture of BMSCs and hematopoietic (mononuclear) cells.[203-207] Although most of these studies used uncharacterized mixtures of cells and were not controlled, they reported modest functional recovery, improved quality of life, and no significant adverse effects with up to a 4-year follow-up period. Finally, it appears that we still need to understand more about the cell sourcing, selection criteria, and the mechanism by which BMSCs function.

Neural Stem and Progenitor Cells

NSPCs are multipotent cells naturally present in the fetal and adult neural tissue.[208,209] Self-renewing NSPCs primarily reside in the subventricular zone lining the lateral ventricles of the forebrain, the hippocampal dentate gyrus, and the periventricular region of the spinal cord.[210-213] NSPCs can also be derived from embryonic stem cells or induced pluripotent stem cells.[214-216] However, transplantation of embryonic stem cell–derived neural cells has ethical concerns and the possibility of tumorigenesis due to the incomplete differentiation of pluripotent cells.[217] Human NSPCs typically have been isolated from the fetal brain and spinal cord of aborted fetuses[218] and from adult surgical brain biopsy and postmortem tissue.[219-220] Recently, Mothe and colleagues isolated and cultured multipotent NSPCs from the adult human spinal cord of organ transplant donors, and reported cell differentiation into neurons and glia following transplantation in rats with SCI.[221] To date, autologous sources of adult NSPCs are unavailable, so patients who received NSPCs should require immunosuppressive drugs.

Most experimental studies involving NSPC transplantation into SCI models have shown modest behavior efficacy; however, the exact mechanism behind functional recovery has not been completely defined.[161] Previous studies showed that the grafted NSPCs have been differentiated primarily into astroglial cells with some oligodendrocytes but rarely neurons.[161] Macias and colleagues reported that astrocytic differentiation of grafted NSPCs has been associated with the development of allodynia in SCI animals.[222] Recently, several strategies have been used to promote the differentiation of NSPCs into a specific lineage, either in vitro, before transplantation, or concurrently between transplanted NSPCs and growth factors or lineage-specific determinants.[223-225]

From a translation perspective, there is an ongoing phase I/II clinical trial in Switzerland involving purified human neural stem cells generated from the brain of an aborted human fetus. The cells are injected directly into the spinal cord rostral and caudal to the injury site. However, the short-term data from the first patient cohort has not been published yet.[217] Recently, Neuralstem Inc. started a phase I clinical trial in the United States using human fetal neural stem cells for the treatment of chronic SCI. Patients will receive six direct intraspinal injections. Patients will receive a follow-up for 60 months to assess graft survival into the transplant using MRI, pain, infection, motor function, and quality of life. To date, there is no published data on the safety or efficacy of these transplantations.[217]

COMBINATORIAL PRECLINICAL INVESTIGATIONS

A number of impediments prevent recovery and regeneration after SCI and include upregulated inhibitory molecules, deficient neurotrophic support, and low intrinsic capabilities for axonal regrowth in damaged neurons.[226,227] Specific groups of inhibitory molecules include myelin-associated proteins and chondroitin sulfate proteoglycans (CSPGs) that function to prevent axon regeneration and plasticity.[228] Regeneration and sprouting are blocked when the myelin-associated inhibitory molecules, Nogo-A, myelin-associated glycoprotein, myelin glycoprotein, versican, semaphorins, and ephrins are concentrated to the injury site.[229-232] Numerous studies have attempted to circumvent these obstacles and strategies have included Nogo-A inhibition, CSPG digestion, neurotrophin application, rehabilitation, bridge grafts, and cell transplantations.[163,226,233-239] While these interventions have elicited promising outcomes, none of the individual approaches have completely restored functional output. Therefore, it is critical that a novel therapeutic method not only targets the multitude of cellular and molecular events that collectively hinder plasticity and regeneration but also creates an environment that permits axonal growth and sprouting after SCI.

Specifically, there is a trend toward establishing a combinatorial approach to SCI to ensure increased effectiveness in physiological restoration. For example, Schnell and colleagues sought to examine if an intrathecal application of anti-Nogo-A monoclonal antibody (Nogo-Ab), long-term administration of the neurotrophic factor neurotrophin-3 (NT-3), and viral delivery of the NMDA-NR2d subunit could promote the regeneration of functional synaptic connections after a spinal cord hemisection injury.[227] Data suggest that the combined Nogo-A antibody, neurotrophin-3, and NMDA-NR2d subunit treatment generated more robust electrophysiological (synaptic transmission), anatomical (sprouting, axonal growth, and establishment of a synaptic detour around the injury), and behavioral (locomotor output) results when evaluated against the components individually or in pairs.[227] Another study examined the potential of chondroitinase ABC (ChABC) and neurotrophin NT-3 treatment combined with increased NR2d expression in promoting axonal sprouting and behavioral recovery after hemisection.[226] Investigators focused on the primary mechanisms of each therapy that include CSPG digestion, reducing the inhibitory environment, enhanced neurotrophin concentration, and promotion of novel synaptic connections.[226] Although data indicated that each therapeutic contributed to functional recovery, the additive results of combining all agents together overwhelmingly suggest that this is the most effective means to promote the formation or strengthening of spinal circuits and support functional recovery.[226] Finally, data found that the combined therapeutic approach using ChABC and anti-Nogo antibody (ATI-335) to treat a spinal cord lesion elicited substantial functional restoration and augmented axonal regeneration and sprouting that was more significant than individual application.[228] Together these data clearly demonstrate the potential of combined treatments in regeneration, sprouting, and behavioral recovery.

CONCLUSIONS

Although emerging evidence from SCI preclinical studies show considerable promise, objective standards are still required to meticulously assess these preclinical therapeutic agents to facilitate more clinically relevant translation. Current available treatment modalities for SCI provide at best modest efficacy. Hence, considering the SCI pathophysiology and multifactorial nature of secondary events is crucial. The combinational therapies with a multifaceted mode of neuroprotection, regenerative, and rehabilitative approaches seem to exhibit greater efficacy than individual therapies. Cell transplantation strategies have enormous therapeutic potential, although it is difficult to make definitive conclusions from the published studies because varying controlled and noncontrolled proposals were used. Some of these cell therapies lacked reporting of preclinical data for the method in which the cells were employed. Therefore, a more inclusive understanding of the complex biologic processes and potential strategies are still highly required. Finally, a comprehensive communication and cooperation between clinicians, researchers, and the public is paramount to develop highly effective therapies and treat SCI.

KEY REFERENCES

The level of evidence (LOE) is determined according to the criteria provided in the preface.

6. Wyndaele M, Wyndaele JJ: Incidence, prevalence and epidemiology of spinal cord injury: what learns a worldwide literature survey? *Spinal Cord* 44:523–529, 2006. LOE I

73. Walters BC, Hadley MN, Hurlbert RJ, et al: Guidelines for the management of acute cervical spine and spinal cord injuries: 2013 update. *Neurosurgery* 60(Suppl 1):82–91, 2013. LOE I

74. Anderson GD, Voets C, Ropiak R, et al: Analysis of patient variables affecting neurologic outcome after traumatic cervical facet dislocation. *Spine J* 4:506–512, 2004. LOE III

82. Fehlings MG, Vaccaro A, Wilson JR, et al: Early versus delayed decompression for traumatic cervical spinal cord injury: results of the Surgical Timing in Acute Spinal Cord Injury Study (STASCIS). *PLoS One* 7:e32037, 2012. LOE I

83. Bernard SA, Gray TW, Buist MD, et al: Treatment of comatose survivors of out-of-hospital cardiac arrest with induced hypothermia. *N Engl J Med* 346:557–563, 2002. LOE I

103. Hurlbert RJ: Methylprednisolone for acute spinal cord injury: an inappropriate standard of care. *J Neurosurg* 93:1–7, 2000. LOE II

104. Bracken MB, Collins WF, Freeman DF, et al: Efficacy of methylprednisolone in acute spinal cord injury. *JAMA* 251:45–52, 1984. LOE I

105. Bracken MB, Shepard MJ, Collins WF, et al: A randomized, controlled trial of methylprednisolone or naloxone in the treatment of acute spinal-cord injury. Results of the Second National Acute Spinal Cord Injury Study. *N Engl J Med* 322:1405–1411, 1990. LOE I

107. Bracken MB, Shepard MJ, Holford TR, et al: Administration of methylprednisolone for 24 or 48 hours or tirilazad mesylate for 48 hours in the treatment of acute spinal cord injury. Results of the Third National Acute Spinal Cord Injury Randomized Controlled Trial. National Acute Spinal Cord Injury Study. *JAMA* 277:1597–1604, 1997. LOE I
108. Bracken MB, Shepard MJ, Holford TR, et al: Methylprednisolone or tirilazad mesylate administration after acute spinal cord injury: 1-year follow up. Results of the third National Acute Spinal Cord Injury randomized controlled trial. *J Neurosurg* 89:699–706, 1998. LOE I
115. Geisler FH, Dorsey FC, Coleman WP: Correction: recovery of motor function after spinal-cord injury–a randomized, placebo-controlled trial with GM-1 ganglioside. *N Engl J Med* 325:1659–1660, 1991. LOE I
116. Geisler FH, Coleman WP, Grieco G, et al: The Sygen multicenter acute spinal cord injury study. *Spine (Phila Pa 1976)* 26:S87–S98, 2001. LOE I
122. Casha S, Zygun D, McGowan MD, et al: Results of a phase II placebo-controlled randomized trial of minocycline in acute spinal cord injury. *Brain* 135:1224–1236, 2012. LOE I
127. Fehlings MG, Theodore N, Harrop J, et al: A phase I/IIa clinical trial of a recombinant Rho protein antagonist in acute spinal cord injury. *J Neurotrauma* 28:787–796, 2011. LOE II
129. Knoller N, Auerbach G, Fulga V, et al: Clinical experience using incubated autologous macrophages as a treatment for complete spinal cord injury: phase I study results. *J Neurosurg Spine* 3:173–181, 2005.
130. Lammertse DP, Jones LA, Charlifue SB, et al: Autologous incubated macrophage therapy in acute, complete spinal cord injury: results of the phase 2 randomized controlled multicenter trial. *Spinal Cord* 50:661–671, 2012.
141. Grossman RG, Fehlings MG, Frankowski RF, et al: A prospective, multicenter, phase I matched-comparison group trial of safety, pharmacokinetics, and preliminary efficacy of riluzole in patients with traumatic spinal cord injury. *J Neurotrauma* 31(3):239–255, 2014. doi: 10.1089/neu.2013.2969. [Epub 2013 Oct 11].
151. Potter PJ, Hayes KC, Segal JL, et al: Randomized double-blind crossover trial of fampridine-SR (sustained release 4-aminopyridine) in patients with incomplete spinal cord injury. *J Neurotrauma* 15:837–849, 1998. LOE I
171. Saberi H, Moshayedi P, Aghayan HR, et al: Treatment of chronic thoracic spinal cord injury patients with autologous Schwann cell transplantation: an interim report on safety considerations and possible outcomes. *Neurosci Lett* 443:46–50, 2008. LOE II
190. Lima C, Pratas-Vital J, Escada P, et al: Olfactory mucosa autografts in human spinal cord injury: a pilot clinical study. *J Spinal Cord Med* 29:191–203; discussion 204–196, 2006. LOE II
205. Saito F, Nakatani T, Iwase M, et al: Spinal cord injury treatment with intrathecal autologous bone marrow stromal cell transplantation: the first clinical trial case report. *J Trauma* 64:53–59, 2008.
206. Saito F, Nakatani T, Iwase M, et al: Administration of cultured autologous bone marrow stromal cells into cerebrospinal fluid in spinal injury patients: a pilot study. *Restor Neurol Neurosci* 30:127–136, 2012. LOE II
207. Yoon SH, Shim YS, Park YH, et al: Complete spinal cord injury treatment using autologous bone marrow cell transplantation and bone marrow stimulation with granulocyte macrophage-colony stimulating factor: Phase I/II clinical trial. *Stem Cell* 25:2066–2073, 2007. LOE II

The complete References list is available online at https://expertconsult.inkling.com.

Chapter 32

The Timing of Management of Spinal Cord Injuries

KRISTIAN DALZELL • ARIA NOURI • MICHAEL G. FEHLINGS

INTRODUCTION

Spinal cord injury (SCI) is a devastating event for the affected individual who may, as a result, develop significant motor, sensory, and autonomic deficits. These losses often translate into significant functional impairments and substantially affect both the quality of life and life expectancy of patients. In addition, SCI patients may have a profound effect on, and place a significant burden on, their families and society. Indeed, according to the Centers for Disease Control and Prevention (CDC), in the United States, the average medical cost of SCI ranges between $15,000 and $30,000 per year with an estimated lifetime cost of $500,000 to more than $3 million, depending on the severity of injury (http://www.cdc.gov/traumaticbraininjury/scifacts.html).

Injury to the spinal cord may occur anywhere along its course and the site of injury will largely determine the level of postinjury function as well as influencing the risk of developing postinjury complications. Ultimately, the level of function attained after SCI is fundamentally dictated by the age of the patient, preexisting comorbidities, the etiology and extent of the SCI, as well as the timing of spinal cord decompression. Commonly, however, the management of SCIs is further complicated by accompanying associated injuries to the appendicular skeleton related to the mechanism of injury (e.g., motor vehicle accidents [MVAs], falls, and blunt trauma). Such injuries can influence the timing of surgical decompression of the spinal cord and thereby significantly affect the overall level of functional recovery.

This chapter will review the issue of timing of decompression and surgical fixation of the injured spinal column in patients with a SCI. In the discussion, we will consider the initial management of the patient from the time of injury and how management in this early period presents an opportunity to profoundly influence the ultimate neurological recovery and functional outcome. At the center of this discussion will be the recently published Surgical Timing in Acute Spinal Cord Injury Study (STASCIS) trial results.[1] Although the period from initial injury to definitive hospital management is often considered separate, it is important to emphasize that there are many opportunities, even at this stage, to influence the ultimate outcome in both positive and negative ways.

Later in the chapter, we will also discuss focused considerations of surgical timing in patients with SCI in the setting of multitrauma and thoracic SCI, as well as controversies surrounding the timing of management of patients with a traumatic central cord injury. In addition, the evidence for the current recommendations will be explored.

Finally, we will discuss evolving and exciting new treatment strategies that have the potential to be translated into clinical practice. As will be seen throughout the chapter, however, substantial research remains to be done in all of these areas and much of the current medical practice remains at the discretion of clinical experience.

EPIDEMIOLOGY

Incidence

Incidence rates of SCI provide an opportunity to assess the efficacy of prevention strategies as well as technologies such as seatbelts, airbags, and impact-reduction technologies aimed at decreasing the occurrence of such injuries. Wyndaele and Wyndaele[2] attempted to investigate the incidence around the world via a literature survey looking at data from 1995 onward; however, the analysis of their findings was limited by the lack of uniformity in methodologies used by various authors. Nevertheless, their estimated incidence of SCI globally was between 10.4 and 83 per million inhabitants per year. Tetraplegia constituted one-third of these injuries and half the SCI injuries were complete lesions. The mean age was 33 years old and males outnumbered females by 3.8 : 1.[3-4] It is worthy of note that the age distribution of traumatic SCI appears to be bimodal, with peaks in young adulthood attributable most notably to MVAs, and in elderly patients aged 65 years and older attributable chiefly to falls.[3]

Although a lack of concrete incidence rates does not affect the management of medical intervention, its scarcity hinders the evaluation of preventive measures aimed at reducing traumatic SCI rates. Furthermore, data that are available are likely to underrepresent the actual incidence rates of SCI due to the nature of the traumatic events resulting in these injuries, which carry a high prehospital fatality rate.[3] Indeed, Wilson and colleagues[4] state that, in the Canadian population, an additional 20% of traumatic SCI patients die before arrival to the hospital.

Prevalence

Prevalence rates are difficult to determine from the available literature.[2] It is believed that there are currently 2.5 million individuals living with SCI (International Campaign for Cures of Spinal Cord Injury Paralysis website: http://campaignforcure.org). Wyndaele and coworkers[2] reported the results of four studies from Australia, Sweden, Finland, and the United States indicating a prevalence rate in these countries between 223 and 755 per million, with higher rates seen in the United States and Australia. It is important to note that these data do not necessarily reflect the prevalence in developing countries, and the populations of Europe, United States, and Australia only constitute approximately 20% of the world's population. Therefore the true global prevalence of SCI remains unknown. The prevalence of SCI is an important statistic as it gives an indication of the burden of SCI on health care and social security resources. Calculations by O'Connor[5] forecast an increase in incidence and prevalence of SCI with more cases seen in the elderly and a profound increase in the number of patients with incomplete tetraplegia. Again the data available for these calculations are scarce and the true global prevalence is unknown.

There are significant and increasing costs associated with SCI, and there are indications that these costs are rising. This was recently highlighted by Baaj and colleagues in a cost analysis demonstrating a significant increase in the cost from $500 million in 1997 to $1.3 billion in 2006, an increase of 160%.[6]

SPINAL CORD INJURY PATHOMECHANICS: CURRENT OPINION

During a traumatic event involving the spine, numerous anatomical changes may occur including fracture of bony structures, as well as dislocation of facet joints that compress and/or damage the cord or are involved in disrupting sufficient arterial perfusion. The severity of these changes and the time to medical intervention dictate the extent of neurological and functional loss.

There is a widely held belief by most surgeons treating spinal injuries that ongoing compression of the spinal cord should be addressed as a matter of high priority and urgency.[7] Central to this widely held opinion is a relatively recent appreciation that the initial traumatic event is only partially responsible for the total impact of an SCI that determines long-term functional recovery.

Traumatic SCI can be broken down into two stages of injury: primary injury resulting from the insult of the traumatic event, and secondary injury that represents the cascade of inflammatory and biochemical events subsequent to the primary injury resulting in tissue damage (see Fig. 32-3, *A*). If left unchecked and uncorrected, secondary injury will progress and cause significantly more tissue damage and neuronal loss than initially incurred from the primary mechanical insult. Secondary injury involves a perpetuating process of ischemia, edema, increased excitatory amino acids, and lipid peroxidation[8] (Fig. 32-1).

In a recent systematic review,[9] it was concluded, based on assimilating the available preclinical and clinical literature combined with a modified Delphi process, that decompression via surgery should be performed within 24 hours when medically feasible. This is also reflected in the results of the STASCIS trial,[1] two studies of international spinal surgeon opinions,[7,10] and a study currently underway in which the timing of early decompression is defined as less than 12 hours.[11] The latter study is attempting to address the potential biases of a prospective observational multicenter comparative cohort study by applying a rigorous and well-defined protocol. These authors have published their study protocol and intended analysis methods. The planning and organization along with accurate power calculations is likely to yield a highly significant contribution to the growing body of knowledge regarding timing of decompression and stabilization in SCI.

Preclinical and Clinical Evidence

A considerable body of preclinical data has now been accrued regarding the timing of decompression of acute SCIs. In these preclinical studies, a variety of animal models and compression models have been employed. A recent high-quality study[12] employed a dog model comparing (1) intravenous (IV) methylprednisolone and decompression at 6 hours, (2) IV saline and decompressive surgery at 6 hours, or (3) IV methylprednisolone alone. The surgically treated animals experienced significantly better neurological recovery at 2 weeks postinjury than the nonsurgically treated animals, independent of steroid administration.

In a recent systematic review of the evidence available for preclinical data, Furlan and colleagues[9] state there is a biological rationale to support early decompression of the spinal cord. In addition, the evidence suggests that early decompression is safe and feasible. These authors identified 19 preclinical studies of sufficient quality to be included in the review. Eleven of these studies indicated a time-dependent effect of spinal cord compression on the behavioral recovery, spinal cord blood flow disturbances, electrophysiological recovery, and histopathological characteristics of the lesion.

TREATMENT STRATEGIES AND TIMING

Treatment of the patient with an acute SCI begins at the scene of the injury. Early emergency treatment of the patient is a vital step in limiting further primary and secondary SCI. The medical management of the patient, with particular attention to cardiopulmonary resuscitation, is central to this aim. The maintenance of adequate blood pressure and oxygenation gives the delicate spinal cord tissue the greatest chance of avoiding or minimizing secondary injury.

Accepted and well-practiced protocols to avoid further SCI in the process of retrieval and transportation should be employed and regularly scrutinized. The American Association of Neurological Surgeons and Congress of Neurological Surgeons (AANS/CNS) Joint Guidelines Committee introduced the updated Guidelines for the Management of Acute Cervical Spine and Spinal Cord Injury in 2013.[13,14] This publication gives an extensive and up-to-date review of the accepted guidelines for the management of patients with acute SCI (Table 32-1).

In addition to the acute emergent care of the patient with SCI, there has been a focused attempt to find treatment strategies that not only limit the degree of primary injury, but also potentiate the chances of recovery through repair and regenerativion. This has not been a simple process and the task of unraveling this complicated problem has been made more difficult by the variability in the quality of research on this topic. Long-held beliefs based on anecdotes and opinions have been difficult obstacles to approach and overcome.

Efforts by investigators to demarcate early and late surgical treatment into time frames have been hindered by the incongruence of findings between them with regard to outcome. However, considering practicality as well as current evidence, including that of the STASCIS trial, it seems most reasonable to define early and late surgical decompression as less than 24

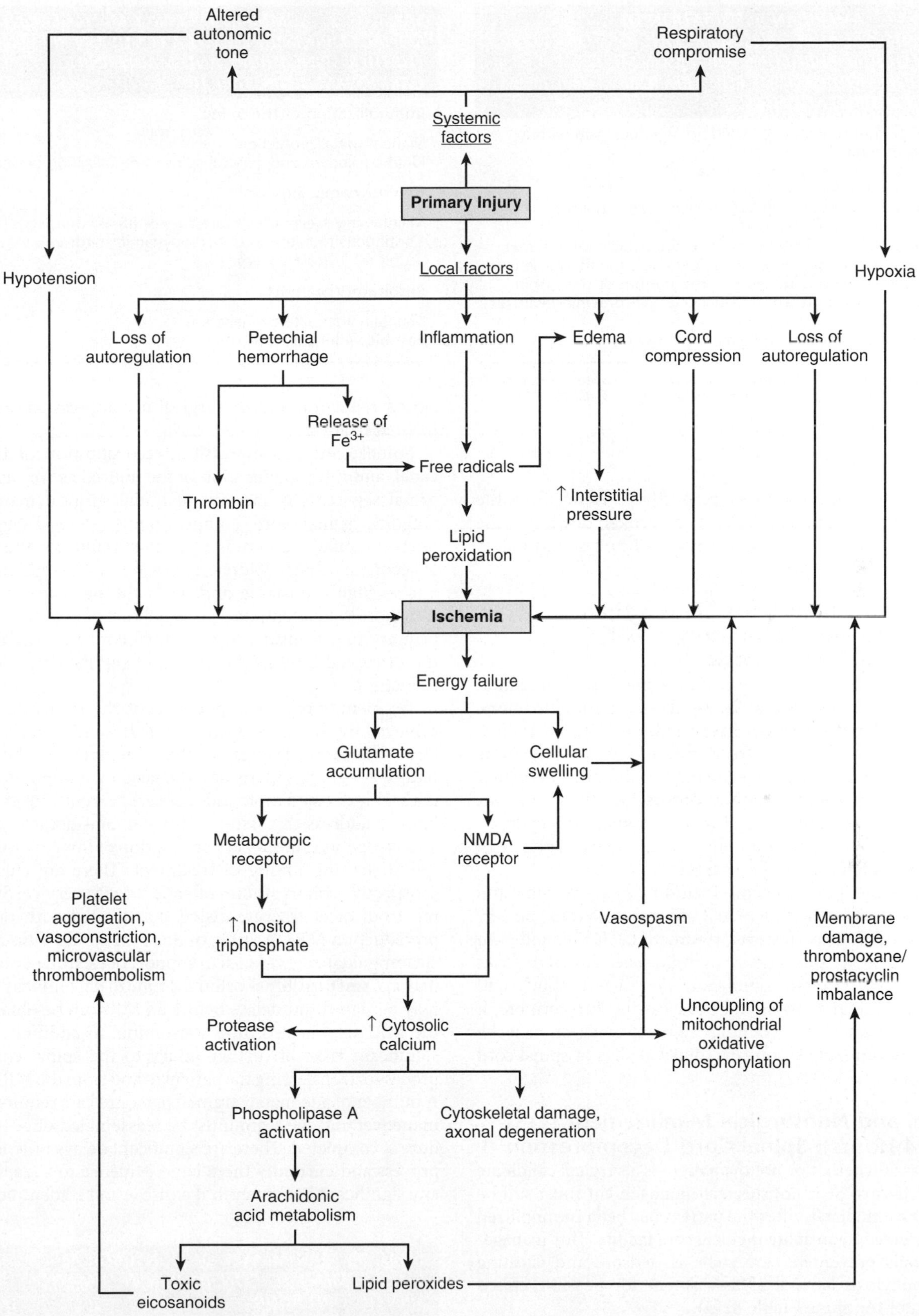

Figure 32-1. The pathophysiological process underlying traumatic spinal cord injury. *NMDA, N*-methyl-D-aspartate acid. *(Source: From Amar AP, Levy ML: Pathogenesis and pharmacological strategies for mitigating secondary damage in acute spinal cord injury, Neurosurgery 44:1027–1039,1999, Fig. 1.)*

TABLE 32-1 AMERICAN ASSOCIATION OF NEUROLOGICAL SURGEONS AND CONGRESS OF NEUROLOGICAL SURGEONS JOINT COMMITTEE GUIDELINES: INDICATIONS FOR CERVICAL SPINE IMMOBILIZATION

1. Spinal pain or tenderness, including any neck pain with a history of trauma
2. Significant multiple system trauma
3. Severe head or facial trauma
4. Numbness or weakness in any extremity after trauma
5. Loss of consciousness caused by trauma
6. If mental status is altered (including drugs, alcohol, trauma) and no history is available, or the patient is found in a setting of possible trauma (e.g., lying at the bottom of stairs or in the street); or the patient experienced near drowning with a history or probability of diving
7. Any significant distracting injury

Source: *From Theodore N, Hadley MN, Aarabi B, et al. Prehospital cervical spinal immobilization after trauma, Neurosurgery 72:22–34,2013, doi:10.1227/NEU.0b013e318276edb1.*

TABLE 32-2 SUMMARY OF EARLY MANAGEMENT OF SPINAL CORD INJURY WITH A FOCUS ON PREVENTING FURTHER SPINE INJURY AND MAINTAINING CARDIOVASCULAR STABILITY

Immobilization of the Spine
Manual spinal protection Rigid backboard and cervical spine immobilization device.
Hemodynamic Support
Maintaining mean arterial pressure of 85–90 mm Hg Continuous monitoring of hemodynamic status in intensive care unit for at least a week
Respiratory Support
Maintain adequate oxygenation Possible ventilatory intubation

hours and more than 24 hours, respectively. Henceforth, the timing of management of SCI has been broken down into the following: within the first hour, within 24 hours, and longer than 24 hours after injury.

Early Management (Less Than 1 Hour): Maintaining and Optimizing Physiological Homeostasis

It is clear that first aid is the primary medical intervention that needs to be employed at the site of any traumatic injury. If significant blunt trauma is suspected, or localized trauma involving the spine has occurred, immobilization of the spine must be performed to stabilize the patient and prevent further injury. Depending on the tools at disposal on the scene, this may either be achieved through manual spinal protection, or utilization of a cervical immobilization device along with placing the patient on a rigid backboard.

The assessment of vital signs, including hemodynamic and respiratory status, as with any first aid response must be performed expeditiously. However, traumatic SCIs demand even more vigilance in this regard as high-level spinal injuries frequently present with significant neurogenic shock and accompanying hypotension and bradycardia. Furthermore, if SCIs are suspected, maintaining high oxygenation may be crucial in minimizing secondary injury at sites of spinal cord compression (Table 32-2).

Surgical and Nonsurgical Management (Less Than 24 Hours): Spinal Cord Decompression

Regardless of whether or not the patient is a surgical candidate for correction of SCI, nonsurgical management must still be employed immediately after the patient has been immobilized and transferred to an acute medical care facility. This management entails preventive care such as bedsore and Cushing ulcer prophylaxis as well as assessment for possible closed reduction of the spine (Table 32-3).

The emphasis of treatment beyond stabilizing the patient is on spinal cord decompression. Imaging via magnetic resonance imaging (MRI) or computed tomography (CT) to evaluate the extent of injury generally precedes any intervention and allows for the assessment of potential candidacy for closed reduction and/or surgical decompression and instrumented fixation.

Spinal cord decompression, reconstitution of the spinal canal, and rigid stabilization of the injured as well as unstable spinal segments is the aim of initial surgical management. Ongoing spinal cord compression from a disrupted and unstable spinal segment is a potent stimulus for the initiation of secondary injury. More often than not, the injured segment is also highly unstable and, with the need to transfer and transport the patient, there is a real risk of ongoing additional primary injury insults to the spinal cord through motion at the disrupted level in the setting of significant canal volume reduction.

As mentioned, decompression of the spinal cord can be achieved by closed or open means. If a unilateral or bilateral facet dislocation is present, then attempts may be made to reduce this by closed means. The need for a prereduction MRI is a highly debated topic and there are currently no clear guidelines to address this issue.[15] This is a considerable gap in the knowledge, as unnecessary acquisition of imaging would critically delay the timing of treatment. There are currently no prospective cohort studies of patients with cervical SCI resulting from facet fracture-dislocation treated with or without prereduction MRI. A study of this type would ultimately offer clearer guidance, evidence in support of treatment recommendations, and possibly shorten the time to decompression. There may be significant delays before an MRI can be obtained, and the MRI scan is also time consuming. In addition, there are significant risks of further injury to the spinal cord in the process of transferring the patient to and from the MRI scanner. A number of adequately trained personnel are required for this maneuver and the team must be reassembled once the procedure is completed. There are significant delays inherent in this process and currently there is no evidence to suggest there is any significant benefit even if a disc lesion is identified.

TABLE 32-3 SUMMARY OF NONSURGICAL MANAGEMENT TO CONSIDER IN TRAUMATIC SPINAL CORD INJURY

- Cushing ulcer (stress ulcer) prevention
- Bedsore prevention
- Hemodynamic support
- Closed reduction
- Thromboprophylaxis

There is also currently no prospective comparative study of closed reduction versus anterior decompression and stabilization for patients with MRI-documented herniated discs in association with unreduced cervical fracture-dislocation injuries. A study of this type would provide class II medical evidence in support of a treatment recommendation.

If closed reduction fails, there is a complex fracture pattern, disc or bone material in the canal, or other circumstances that preclude closed reduction, then proceeding to open reduction is indicated.

The role of early reduction of facet joint dislocation is difficult to investigate and is not amenable to investigation with a randomized clinical trial. There are case reports in the literature that do give some insight into the potential benefit of undertaking early closed reduction. Collision sports are associated with traumatic cervical injuries and, in particular, facet dislocations resulting in SCI.[16] In 2011, Newton and colleagues reported on a series of patients who sustained cervical spine dislocations playing rugby. Thirty-two patients presented with complete paralysis. Eight patients had reductions performed within 4 hours and, of these, five patients made a full recovery. In the patients who underwent reduction after 4 hours, only one made recovery that was considered useful. The subgroup of patients with SCI secondary to facet dislocation has been recognized as a possible cohort with significant recovery potential.[16]

A recently published multicenter cohort study[17] demonstrated that patients with facet dislocation in association with SCI presented with a greater severity of neurological deficit and the injuries were associated with a higher energy mechanism. Bilateral facet dislocation was associated with a more profound neurological deficit than unilateral facet dislocation as reflected in the American Spinal Injury Association (ASIA) impairment scale grade and ASIA motor score (Table 32-4).[18] At 1 year, with baseline neurological differences taken into account, patients with facet dislocation and SCI experienced a smaller amount of motor recovery compared with patients without facet dislocation. Moreover, patients with SCI associated with facet dislocation also had a longer duration of hospital stay and these outcomes occurred despite having decompression performed significantly sooner than patients without facet dislocation (25.1 hours vs. 41.3 hours, respectively).[17] Ongoing investigation by these authors is also taking place to determine the relationship between time to reduction in patients with facet dislocation and SCI and neurological recovery.[17]

The greatest evidence for early surgical decompression, being defined as before 24 hours, has emerged from the STASCIS trial. Its implications are discussed further in the next section.

TABLE 32-4 ***AMERICAN SPINAL INJURY ASSOCIATION IMPAIRMENT SCALE***

A	Complete: No motor or sensory function is preserved in the sacral segments S4-S5.
B	Incomplete: Sensory but not motor function is preserved below the neurological level and includes the sacral segments S4-S5.
C	Incomplete: Motor function is preserved below the neurological level, and more than half of key muscles below the neurological level have a muscle grade less than 3.
D	Incomplete: Motor function is preserved below the neurological level, and at least half of key muscles below the neurological level have a muscle grade of 3 or more.
E	Normal: Motor and sensory function are normal.

Source: *From American Spinal Injury Association (ASIA): International Standards for Neurological Classification of Spinal Cord Injury (ICOS), revised April 2011. http://www.asia-spinalinjury.org/elearning/ISNCSCI_Exam_Sheet_r4.pdf. Accessed April 9, 2014.*

Surgical and Nonsurgical Management (More Than 24 Hours)

Regardless of the timing of spinal decompression, patients generally remain in a critical condition with 4.4% to 16% of SCI patients succumbing to their injuries before hospital discharge.[19] Furthermore, the median hospital stay after SCI is 67 days.[19]

As is indicated in the previous section, surgical decompression of the spinal cord should be performed within 24 hours after injury. Although timely management has been supported by the STASCIS trial and is the aim of treatment, in reality, many patients are operated on after this time period. In a study by Tator and colleagues in 1999, the authors demonstrated that 24% of patients with SCI were treated within 24 hours of injury and 40% had surgery by 48 hours.[20]

With regard to closed reduction, in 2003, O'Connor and colleagues[21] noted that the procedure was unsuccessful after 5 days (to 2 weeks) in all of their five patients. Although this suggests a decrease in the likelihood of a successful closed reduction if delayed, class I and II evidence does not exist to support the supposition that early closed reduction leads to improved neurological outcome.

It is recommended by the AANS that a patient maintain a mean arterial pressure of 85 to 90 mm Hg for the first 7 days to maintain adequate vascular perfusion to the spinal cord. If volume replacement is inadequate in achieving this, the use of vasopressors is indicated.[22] SCI patients should also be monitored in the intensive care unit (ICU) for at least 7 to 14 days after their injury as ICU stay has been associated with less morbidity and mortality as well as improved neurological recovery.[22]

In the ICU, the focus of treatment of SCI patients pertaining to the nervous system is that of neuroprotection and prevention of secondary injury. The use of glucocorticoids has been studied by a number of investigators. Although limited benefits have been demonstrated in the National Acute Spinal Cord Injury Study (NASCIS) trials, their administration beyond 8 hours after injury remains largely unsupported. It is also worthy of note that patients who received corticosteroids in the NASCIS II and III trials suffered higher rates of complications, including pulmonary embolisms, pneumonia, gastrointestinal (GI) disturbances, sepsis, and wound infections.[19] Indeed, in the most recent joint AANS/CNS guidelines, the following is stated: "Methylprednisolone in the treatment of acute human SCI is recommended as an option that should only be undertaken with the knowledge that the evidence suggesting harmful side effects is more consistent than the suggestion of clinical benefit."[23]

Evidence from STASCIS

On the basis that ongoing compression of the spinal cord leads to further injury due to secondary mechanisms, the largest prospective multicenter cohort trial to date was undertaken to investigate the relative effectiveness of early (<24 hours) versus late (≥24 hours) decompression surgery with respect to neurological outcome at 6 months posttraumatic SCI.[1] The relationship between the timing of surgery and inpatient hospital complications and mortality were assessed.

Six institutions specializing in the care of patients with SCI took part in the study. Data regarding baseline neurological function, timing to decompression, and ASIA impairment Scale (AIS) were collected for analysis in 313 study participants. Enrollment in the study required adequate imaging in the form of plain radiograph, CT, and MRI scans of the cervical spine. The presence of cervical spinal cord compression between C2 and T1 demonstrated on MRI or CT myelography was required for inclusion in the study and was assessed by a validated method as previously described by the authors.[24]

The results of this study report that in the 182 patients who underwent surgery, surgery in the "early" group was performed at a mean of 14.2 ± 5.4 hours compared to surgery at 48.3 ± 29.3 hours in the late group ($P < 0.01$). There was no significant difference between genders in the two study groups but the early group was younger ($P < 0.01$). In addition to the significant difference in age, the early group presented with more profound neurological deficits ($P < 0.01$) with more AIS grade A and B in the early group. There was no significant difference in the etiology of the SCI between the groups. The early group was significantly more likely to receive steroids than the late group.

The outcome measure for this study was the change in AIS grade from presentation to 6 month follow-up. The odds of at least a two-grade AIS improvement were 2.8 times higher among the early surgery group and the odds of a one-grade improvement were 1.4 times higher in the early group. This effect persisted after multivariate analysis taking into account the administration of steroids and the differences in neurological status between the two groups seen at presentation. Significant neurological improvement has been defined by the GM-1 ganglioside (Sygen) trial, the largest therapeutic trial in SCI, as at least two-grade improvement in AIS at 6 months follow-up postinjury.[1,21]

Both groups experienced similar rates of at least one complication (24.2%–30.5%) and rates of early mortality (within 30 days) with one death in each group. Three deaths occurred in the early group after 30 days postinjury secondary to cardiorespiratory complications.

FOCUSED CONSIDERATIONS

Traumatic Central Cord Syndrome[3-4,22-24]

The classic central cord injury is a clinical entity that occurs through an extension mechanism in the setting of degenerative changes in the cervical spine and culminates in rapid canal narrowing.[2,24-27]

In patients age 50 years or older, there are degenerative changes that involve the uncovertebral joints, the intervertebral disc, and the ligamentum flavum. The force extension movement of the cervical spine causes further rapid narrowing of the canal and compresses the spinal cord. This leads to compression of the white matter of the cord secondary to central hematomyelia of the gray matter. A second, younger group of patients, typically younger than 50 years of age, has been identified with the constellation of symptoms and signs that are typical of a central cord injury. This group differs from the older patient group in that a more forceful etiology is present and the predisposing degenerative changes are absent. The more forceful etiology may result in fracture and instability that is often absent in the elderly degenerative group. A third younger group has also been identified with a nontraumatic etiology associated with an acute cervical central disc herniation.

The pathophysiology of traumatic central cord syndrome (TCCS) remains controversial primarily due to a scarcity of literature on the topic. Schneider and colleagues, in their 1954 publication, suggested that the site of injury is centrally located in the cord; however, indications from histological studies have suggested damage to the lateral corticospinal tract and related this to the predominate upper extremity pathological manifestation.[30] Accordingly, in light of the fact that much remains unknown about the pathomechanics, management of TCCS remains based on clinical experience more so than on evidence-based medicine.

A recent systematic review by Dahdaleh and coworkers[36] looked at literature evaluating the timing for surgical treatment of TCCS patients. Their results yielded only a few papers that investigated the effects of surgical timing. Although in 2002, Guest and colleagues[7,29,33a] indicated that patients treated within 24 hours or less fared better than those who were operated on more than 24 hours after injury, other authors, including Stevens and colleagues in 2010, Anderson and colleagues in 2012, and Arabi and associates in 2011, did not find a significant difference between these time groups. However, it is worthy of note that the surgical indications for patients encompassed different etiological reasons for TCCS between authors, including fractures, acute disc herniations, acute stenosis as well as dislocations, and therefore, the results have limited generalizability. It would seem reasonable to assume that patients would benefit from surgical treatment within 24 hours as was shown in the STASCIS trial if the cause of TCCS is significantly traumatic. Indeed, patients who present with acute symptoms due to hyperextension injury or exacerbation from long-standing degenerative causes may not achieve the same benefits from early surgery (≤24 hours) as those who experienced a more acute traumatic event; however, given the current literature, this remains speculative. Despite this, there are indications that younger patients achieve better outcomes than older patients after surgery.

At the present time, all studies that have sought to investigate surgical timing, as well as the benefits of surgical intervention in general over conservative management for subpopulations of patients with TCCS, are retrospective in nature and present, at best, class III evidence to support their findings. Accordingly, for the time being, evidence with regards to surgical timing in TCCS is insufficient to steer clinical practice.

Thoracic Spinal Cord Injury[8,30]

It is well recognized that a difference in the level of injury in the cervical and lumbar spinal cord can have a profound influence on the ultimate level of functional recovery obtained. Less has been published on the mechanism of injury, the level of injury, and the timing of decompression or the effects of these factors on functional outcome from thoracic SCI. In 2012, Bransford and colleagues[34] performed a systematic review and critical appraisal to address these issues. The authors identified three registry studies and seven retrospective cohort studies that satisfied the inclusion criteria. The level of evidence was generally considered to be poor quality (level of evidence III). There is a paucity of epidemiological data on the mechanisms, both traumatic and nontraumatic, of thoracic SCI. Pulmonary trauma is often associated with thoracic level injuries, and these may have an effect on the rate and extent of recovery due to influences on total ICU stay and ventilator requirements.[31] Similar results are reflected in the epidemiological data available from Australia.[32]

In the United States, the most common etiology of thoracic SCI in 2010 was vehicular accident (41%) followed by violence-related injuries (27%), falls (19%), and sports-related injuries (3%). The estimated life expectancy for those surviving at least 24 hours varied depending on the age at injury. Life expectancy for those aged 20 years was 77% of normal life expectancy compared with 40.2% for those aged 80 years at the time of injury.[1] This compares to a life expectancy of 61% to 68% and 16% to 25% for 20- and 80-year-olds, respectively, for injuries in the C1 through C8 region.

The timing of treatment and its influence on recovery and outcome in thoracic SCI has not received the same degree of attention and research as cervical SCI.[7,10,33] In 2006, Schinkel and colleagues published the results of their level of evidence III retrospective registry study comparing recovery and outcome data in three groups. In this study, a control group ($n = 93$), an early surgery group receiving treatment within 72 hours ($n = 156$), and a late surgery group receiving treatment after 72 hours ($n = 49$) were compared. In all categories, the early surgery group fared significantly better than the late surgery group with regard to ventilator dependence ($P = 0.02$), ICU stay ($P = 0.001$), hospital length of stay ($P = 0.048$), mortality ($P < 0.05$), and lung failure ($P = 0.016$).[35]

In 2010, Frangen and associates demonstrated that in patients with severe thoracic spine injuries, surgery was safe and prevented complications.[38] These authors demonstrated shorter periods of ventilator support, fewer pulmonary complications, shorter ICU and hospital stays, and faster recoveries in patients undergoing early surgical decompression and stabilization.

Multitrauma Patients with Spinal Cord Injury

The chief concern during the initial management of patients with potential cervical spinal injuries is that neurological function may be impaired as a result of pathological motion of the injured vertebrae. It is estimated that 3% to 25%[16,35] of SCIs occur after the initial traumatic insult, either during transit or early in the course of management.

The dilemma in managing patients with unstable spine injuries, with or without associated SCI and significant multitrauma, is a difficult problem to resolve. The constellation of injuries, comorbidities, age, and other factors unique to each patient means this question must be wrestled with on every new presentation. There are some basic principles that can be followed as the prioritization of care evolves. The initial Advanced Trauma Life Support and Early Management of Severe Trauma (ATLS/EMST) principles that are started at the scene of the injury should be followed and advanced on presentation to the treating facility. There will potentially be a combination of hypovolemia and hypotension secondary to long bone, pelvic, and intraabdominal trauma; neurogenic shock; and potentially cardiogenic shock secondary to cardiac contusion or significant preexisting cardiac comorbidities. Significant pulmonary contusion can contribute to this difficult situation and impair adequate oxygenation of fragile neural tissues as well. It is imperative that all individuals involved in the care of trauma patients are cognizant of the potential for SCIs.[16,32,36]

The particular problem with this patient population fundamentally lies with their prerequisite for stabilization and evaluation, including vital imaging, for the plethora of possible life-threatening comorbidities. Ultimately, these factors contribute to a significant delay in treatment of potential SCI simply due to the nature of their injury. As discussed earlier, there may be a potential to shorten the time of intervention if medical imaging is found to be insignificant in improving prognosis for patients who may benefit from closed reduction of SCIs; however, such research remains to be conducted.

OUTCOMES RELATED TO SPINAL CORD TRAUMA

Wilson and colleagues, in a 2012 systematic review, identified the clinical predictors of neurological and functional outcome (Fig. 32-2) as well as survival (Table 32-5).[45] These authors examined the basic clinical elements that are routinely collected at initial presentation and included neurological examination characteristics, demographics, and injury mechanism and etiology.

Complications related to SCI were also assessed by a subanalysis of the STASCIS trial results by Wilson and colleagues in 2013.[17,37] Results of logistical multivariate analysis indicated that "severe initial AIS grade ($p < 0.01$), a high-energy injury mechanism ($p = 0.07$), an older age ($p = 0.05$), the absence of steroid administration ($p = 0.02$), and the presence of comorbid illness ($p = 0.02$) were associated with a greater likelihood of complication development during the period of acute hospitalization." Of particular note is the finding that absence of

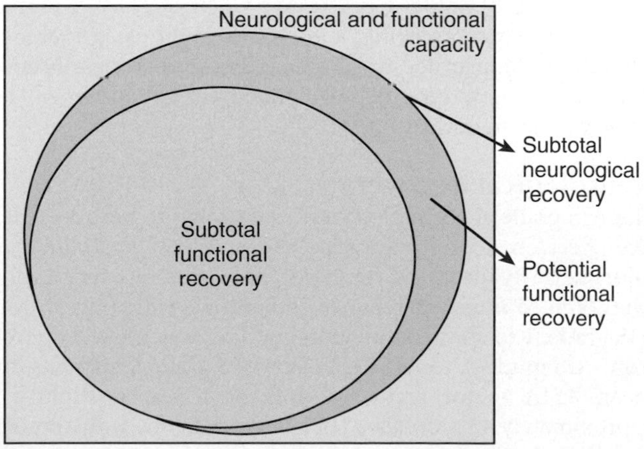

Figure 32-2. A conceptual illustration demonstrating the relationship between neurological and functional recovery in patients with traumatic spinal cord injury (SCI). The *entire box* represents full neurological and functional capacity. Subtotal neurological recovery represents the amount of neurological recovery a patient attains after treatment for traumatic SCI. Subtotal functional recovery illustrates that functional outcome is limited by neurological recovery. The *light purple region* represents the potential area of functional recovery that can be garnered up to the limit of neurological recovery.

TABLE 32-5 *PREDICTORS OF OUTCOME OF ACUTE SPINAL CORD INJURY IN THE ACUTE HOSPITAL SETTING*

Functional recovery	The degree of neurological injury, level of SCI, reflex pattern, as well as age, have been identified as consistent predictors of functional outcome.
Neurological recovery	The degree of neurological injury (assessed via ASIA scale, Frankel grade, or injury completeness), level of injury, and the presence of a zone of partial preservation have been identified as consistent predictors of neurological outcome.
Survival	The degree of neurological injury, level of SCI, age, as well as the presence of multisystem trauma in higher-energy injury mechanisms, have been identified as consistent predictors of survival.

ASIA, American Spinal Injury Association; *SCI,* spinal cord injury.
Source: *Data from Wilson JR, Cadotte DW, Fehlings MG: Clinical predictors of neurological outcome, functional status, and survival after traumatic spinal cord injury: a systematic review, J Neurosurg Spine 17(1 Suppl):11–26, September 2012 Sep. doi:10.3171/2012.4.AOSPINE1245.*

corticosteroid use was related to more complications, as previous findings have reported the contrary.

Functional Recovery

The optimal level of functioning a patient with a SCI achieves is related to the spinal level and the extent of injury. Significant functional abilities can be maintained with preservation of even one functioning spinal level.[17,38] In order to accurately assess recovery, a reliable and valid assessment must be conducted at presentation to establish a baseline and repeated as recovery progresses.

A potential source of error exists in conducting testing and scoring of sensory and motor function. To address this, ASIA published the International Standards for Neurological Classification of Spinal Cord Injury (ISNCSCI).[17,39,40] Formal training in scaling, scoring, and classification using ISNCSCI has been demonstrated to significantly improve classification skills and is now considered a mandatory requirement for clinical trials investigating SCI.[19,41]

Neurological Recovery

The AIS grade at admission has been shown to have a predictive effect on neurological recovery at 1 year postinjury. As injury severity increases, the expected level of recovery diminishes. Ten to fifteen percent of individuals will convert from AIS grade A to an incomplete injury and only 2% will convert from AIS grade A to AIS D.[20,42] For AIS grade C patients, the mean ASIA motor recovery score at 1 year postinjury is approximately 43 points for tetraplegic patients, with approximately 70% converting to AIS grade D or E.[21,43] More limited gains are seen in AIS grade D patients with only 4% converting to AIS grade E at 1 year after injury.

The neurological level of injury at the time of admission is also predictive of outcome. Cervical SCIs demonstrate a 9.6 point increase in ASIA motor score 1 year after AIS grade A SCI, compared to a 2.6 point average improvement seen in thoracic and lumbar complete lesions. However, due to the difficulties in motor testing for the thoracic levels between T2 and T9, the ASIA motor scores are unlikely to fully capture the full extent of spinal cord recovery.[15,42]

Functional recovery is similarly affected by the level and extent of injury found at initial admission following SCI and is essentially a product of neurological recovery. The chances of walking at 1 year after complete paraplegia is 5%, and 0% in complete tetraplegics, in spite of 10% converting to motor incomplete.[22,44]

Survival

Patients with SCI frequently succumb to their injuries prior to arrival at the hospital. Often this is directly the result of the significant trauma sustained from the cause of injury, such as MVA. However, at other times, death at the scene is related to high-level SCIs, cardiovascular instability, or respiratory compromise.[22,45] Indeed, mortality rates are highest immediately postinjury and within the first hours. This rate then drops precipitously after admission to the hospital.[19,46]

Survival following SCI has improved over the last 3 to 4 decades. In 1970 to 1971, 38% of individuals died prior to reaching the hospital[1,47]; however, this percentage improved to 15.8% by 1997 to 2000.[24,48] More recently, Varma and colleagues reported early mortality rates of 13% in their series with a median of 12 days until death occurred.[49] In this large retrospective study, they also reported the adjusted odds of early mortality following traumatic SCI. These included

- Increased age, older than 20 years of age (odds ratio [OR], 1.2; $P < 0.0001$)
- Male gender (OR, 1.6; $P = 0.016$)
- One or more comorbidities $P < 0.0001$
- Concomitant severe systemic injuries (Injury Severity Scale [ISS] > 15) (OR, 1.9; $P = 0.012$)
- Concomitant traumatic brain injury (OR 3.7; $P < 0.0001$)

EVOLVING AND FUTURE TREATMENT STRATEGIES

Although a number of treatment strategies for improving outcomes after traumatic SCI remain the subject of current investigation, there are no recommended therapeutic agents available at this time. There are, however, efforts to improve treatment via alternative means, including therapeutic hypothermia and cellular transplantation (including stem cells).

Although current evidence is insufficient to support the use of therapeutic hypothermia, a recent phase 1 trial wherein patients were systemically cooled to 33 °C (91.4 °F) and matched with controls, demonstrated a beneficial effect of cooling and has merited further exploration of this treatment option.[50] The underlying therapeutic mechanism of this technique is based on the thought that cooling will slow secondary injury; therefore, it is reasonable to assume that the efficacy of cooling is time dependent, with earlier cooling likely garnering greater benefits.

Conversely, cellular transplantation remains in its infancy and, although a number of different studies have been conducted, they are challenging to interpret collectively based on their early investigative nature. Having said this, however, they present an exciting opportunity for regenerative potential in the future, likely to be used in conjunction with pharmacological and surgical treatments.

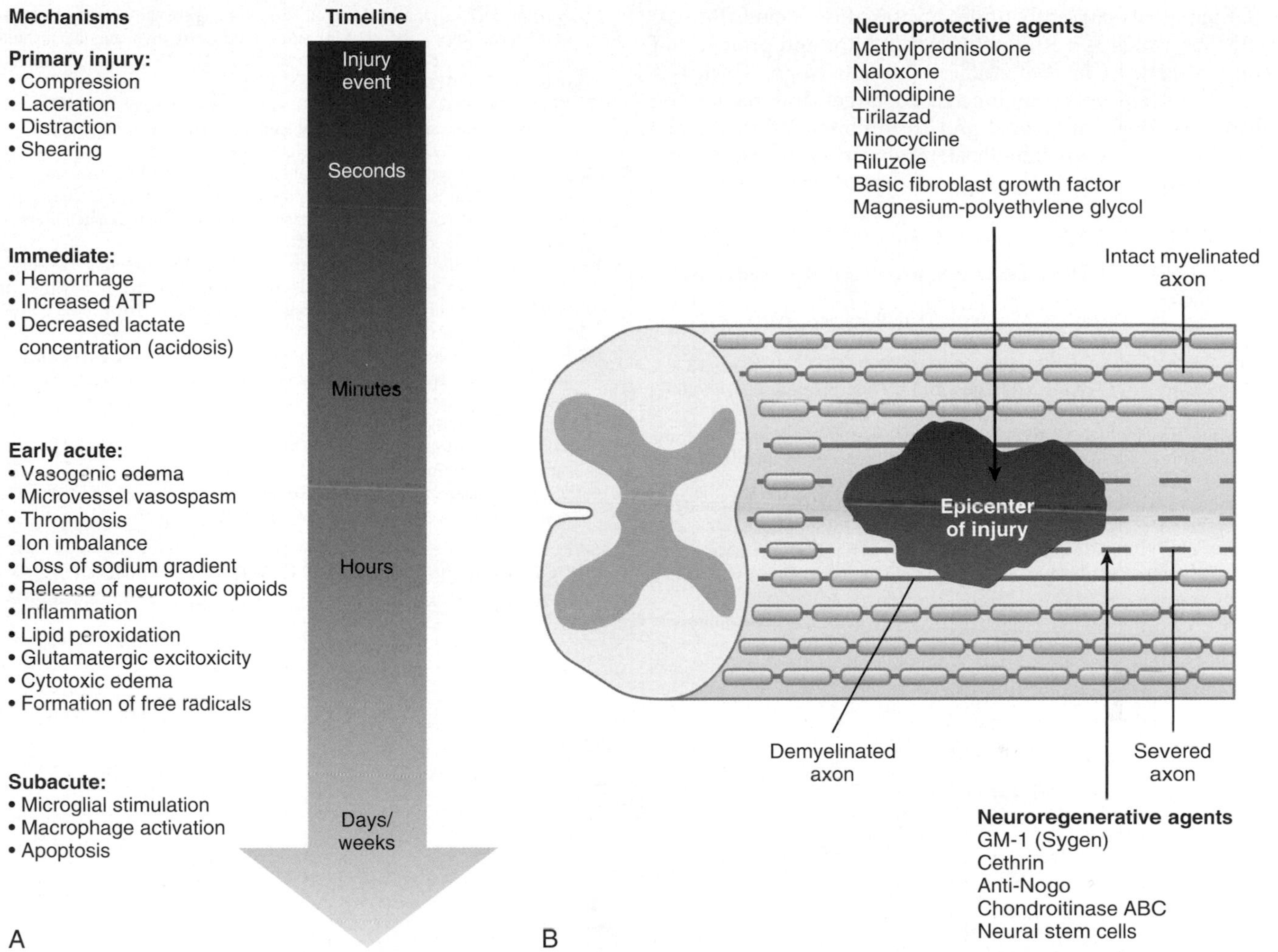

Figure 32-3. A, Primary and secondary mechanisms of injury determining the final extent of spinal cord damage. The primary injury event starts a pathobiological cascade of secondary injury mechanisms that unfold in different phases within seconds of the primary trauma and continuing for several weeks thereafter. **B,** Longitudinal section of the spinal cord after injury. The epicenter of the injury progressively expands after the primary trauma as a consequence of secondary injury events. This expansion causes an increased region of tissue cavitation and, ultimately, worsened long-term outcomes. Within and adjacent to the injury epicenter are severed and demyelinated axons. The neuroprotective agents listed act to subvert specific secondary injuries and prevent neural damage, while the neuroregenerative agents act to promote axonal regrowth once damage has occurred. *ATP,* Adenosine triphosphate. *(Source for B: From Wilson JR, Forgione N, Fehlings MG: Emerging therapies for acute traumatic spinal cord injury, CMAJ 185(6):485–492, 2013.)*

Pharmacological and biological treatment options in traumatic SCI are being investigated in two capacities: (1) neuroprotective agents to limit the secondary injury associated with the cascade of events that follow the injury, including cellular membrane disruption, inflammation, and apoptosis; and (2) neuroregenerative agents aiming at promoting and supporting repair and regeneration of axons, as well as the supporting cellular matrix (Fig. 32-3).

In a 2013 review on emerging therapies, Wilson and associates discussed five therapeutic agents that were investigated in phase III clinical trials; four of these are considered neuroprotective, and a single one, GM-1 ganglioside, is considered neuroregenerative.

Neuroprotective Agents

These include methylprednisone, naloxone, tirilazad, and nimodipine. None of these have been shown to improve outcome, with the exception of methylprednisolone when instituted before 8 hours; however, even this remains controversial. It is worthy of note that these drugs did show preclinical efficacy, and, therefore, the limited amount of negative results have not yet definitively precluded their utility.

Other drugs in earlier states of investigation include riluzole, minocycline, and basic fibroblast growth factor. Whereas the mechanism of neuroprotection in minocycline remains unknown, both riluzole and basic fibroblast growth factor are believed to exert their neuroprotective function by reducing glutamate-mediated excitotoxicity, albeit by different pharmacological mechanisms.

Neuroregenerative Agents

GM-1 ganglioside (Sygen), the only neuroregenerative agent to date to have been assessed in phase III trials, has been shown in laboratory studies to augment axonal regeneration after injury. However, in a single randomized controlled study of 760 subjects, no marked neurological improvement was observed at 6 months as defined by an increase of two grades on the Benzel scale.[22,21]

Other agents currently under investigation include BA-210 (Cethrin), which is a Rho pathway inhibitor and promoter of axonal growth in *in vivo* studies; and anti-Nogo, which is a monoclonal antibody engineered to target and reduce the function of Nogo, an axonal growth inhibitor. While BA-210 (Cethrin) has shown beneficial results in early trials, anti-Nogo remains in the early stages of clinical investigation.[22]

KEY REFERENCES

The level of evidence (LOE) is determined according to the criteria provided in the preface.

1. Fehlings MG, Vaccaro A, Wilson JR, et al: Early versus delayed decompression for traumatic cervical spinal cord injury: results of the Surgical Timing in Acute Spinal Cord Injury Study (STASCIS). Di Giovanni S, ed. *PLoS One* 7(2):e32037, 2012. doi: 10.1371/journal.pone.0032037.t007. LOE II
4. Wilson JR, Singh A, Craven C, et al: Early versus late surgery for traumatic spinal cord injury: the results of a prospective Canadian cohort study. *Spinal Cord* 50(11):840–843, 2012. doi: 10.1038/sc.2012.59. LOE II
7. Fehlings MG, Rabin D, Sears W, et al: Current practice in the timing of surgical intervention in spinal cord injury. *Spine* 35(Suppl 21):S166–S173, 2010. doi: 10.1097/BRS.0b013e3181f386f6. LOE: This reference represents the introduction to a series of systematic reviews whose evidence may vary.
9. Furlan JC, Noonan V, Cadotte DW, et al: Timing of decompressive surgery of spinal cord after traumatic spinal cord injury: an evidence-based examination of pre-clinical and clinical studies. *J Neurotrauma* 28(8):1371–1399, 2011. doi: 10.1089/neu.2009.1147. LOE III
16. Newton DD, England MM, Doll HH, et al: The case for early treatment of dislocations of the cervical spine with cord involvement sustained playing rugby. *J Bone Joint Surg Br* 93(12):1646–1652, 2011. doi: 10.1302/0301-620X.93B12.27048. LOE IV
17. Wilson JR, Vaccaro A, Harrop JS, et al: The impact of facet dislocation on clinical outcomes after cervical spinal cord injury. *Spine* 38(2):97–103, 2013. doi: 10.1097/BRS.0b013e31826e2b91. LOE II
24. Rao SC, Fehlings MG: The optimal radiologic method for assessing spinal canal compromise and cord compression in patients with cervical spinal cord injury. Part 1. An evidence-based analysis of the published literature. *Spine* 24(6):598–604, 1999. LOE III
26. Lenehan B, Fisher CG, Vaccaro A, et al: The urgency of surgical decompression in acute central cord injuries with spondylosis and without instability. *Spine* 35(Suppl 21):S180–S186, 2010. doi: 10.1097/BRS.0b013e3181f32a44. LOE III
34. Bransford RJ, Chapman JR, Skelly AC, et al: What do we currently know about thoracic spinal cord injury recovery and outcomes? A systematic review. *J Neurosurg Spine* 17(Suppl 1):52–64, 2012. doi: 10.3171/2012.6.AOSPINE1287. LOE III
45. Wilson JR, Cadotte DW, Fehlings MG: Clinical predictors of neurological outcome, functional status, and survival after traumatic spinal cord injury: a systematic review. *J Neurosurg Spine* 17(Suppl 1):11–26, 2012. doi: 10.3171/2012.4.AOSPINE1245. LOE II

The complete References list is available online at https://expertconsult.inkling.com.

Chapter 33

Craniocervical Injuries

33A Occipital-Cervical Spine Injuries

RICHARD JACKSON BRANSFORD • MARK W. MANOSO • CARLO BELLABARBA

Injuries to the occipital-cervical spine largely fall into two broad categories, (1) atlanto-occipital dissociations (AODs) or craniocervical dissociations (CCDs) and (2) occipital condyle fractures. Historically, the term AOD has been used; however, because these injuries can involve the occipital–C1 articulation, the C1–C2 junction, or a combination of the two, the term CCD is probably better because it is more accurate and encompassing. By pure terminology, AOD is a type of CCD, yet there are other patterns of CCD that really would not fall into the pure definition of AOD.

These injuries involve trauma to the complex articulation, including the occipital bone, the occipitoatlantal articulation, the atlas, the axis, and the ligaments that span from the axis to occiput. The susceptibility of the cervicocranium to injury is related to (1) the large lever arm induced by the mass and immobility of the cranium combined with (2) the relative freedom of movement more caudally with reliance on ligamentous structures rather than on intrinsic bony stability for the maintenance of craniocervical alignment. This functional unit is maintained by highly specialized bony segments connected via a complex ligamentous system whose vulnerability to injury may compromise the structural integrity of the craniocervical junction. Injury to the craniocervical junction is almost always caused by high-energy trauma and is frequently associated with other injuries, including closed head injuries, facial fractures, and either associated atlas or axis fractures or subaxial spine injuries. Craniocervical injuries with associated high cervical spinal cord injuries are thought to account for 10% to 25% of traffic fatalities.[1,2]

Certainly, within these injuries there is a spectrum of instability, ranging from very stable nonoperative injuries such as isolated, nondisplaced occipital condyle fractures to highly unstable injuries with severe spinal cord injuries such as widely distracted CCDs. Increasing awareness of these injuries and use of routine computed tomography (CT) has resulted in earlier diagnosis and more appropriate, aggressive management, thus allowing an increasing number of these patients to survive. Despite the evolution of learning and improvement in management, cases of catastrophic failure to diagnose and subsequent neurologic deterioration still occur even in experienced trauma centers.[3,4]

The goal of this chapter is to review the anatomy and methods of diagnosis to identify the wide spectrum of injuries that occur at the occipital cervical junction. Current classifications will be discussed as well as operative and nonoperative management and outcomes of treatment.

ANATOMY

The skull base, atlas, and axis comprise the three bony components of the upper cervical spine and form an integrated functional unit. The five unconstrained joints of the upper cervical spine rely primarily on an intact, multilayered ligamentous system for stability. This unique anatomic arrangement allows the upper cervical spine to contribute a substantial portion of neck motion.

Occiput

The occiput forms the major portion of the foramen magnum (Fig. 33A-1, *A*). From the anterolateral aspect of foramen magnum, the occipital condyles project caudally on each side to form convex bony surfaces that articulate with the matched concave superior articular facet of the atlas with a joint capsule and synovial joint (Fig. 33A-1, *B*). These bony protuberances are semilunar in shape, forming almost a 180-degree arc when viewed sagittally. From the anterior view, they are wedge shaped with increased extension medially tapering off more laterally. The geometry of the occiput as it articulates with C1 allows the condyles to move like a rocking chair within the C1 lateral masses. Posteriorly, on the inside of the skull along the midline, the internal occipital crest extends toward the transverse sulcus and is the key location for occipital fixation.[5] Just lateral and ventral to the occipital condyles is the hypoglossal foramen through which cranial nerve XII descends. Given the close proximity of cranial nerve XII, it is prone to injury with fractures of the occipital condyle and AODs and with C0–C1 transarticular screw fixation. The ventral aspect of foramen magnum is bounded by the basion, which is the caudal extent of the clival plate. The dorsal boundary of foramen magnum is the opisthion.

Atlas

The atlas is a complicated ring-shaped structure allowing for a critical link between the occiput and the axis. The ring is formed from large lateral masses connected together by thin ventral and dorsal arches (Fig. 33A-1, *C*). The lateral masses viewed anteriorly are trapezoidal in shape to match the occipital condyles, essentially narrow medially and project out to a thickened lateral aspect similar to a bowtie. Lateral to the lateral mass is a foramen through which the vertebral arteries pass as they course rostrally from C2 to wrap posteriorly over the C1 arch and enter the foramen magnum to form the basilar artery. Just anterior to the C1 ring lies the internal

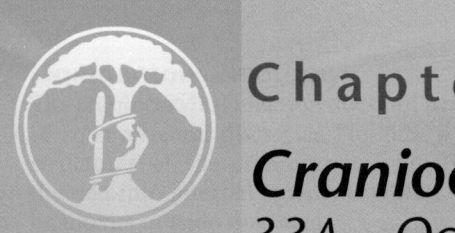

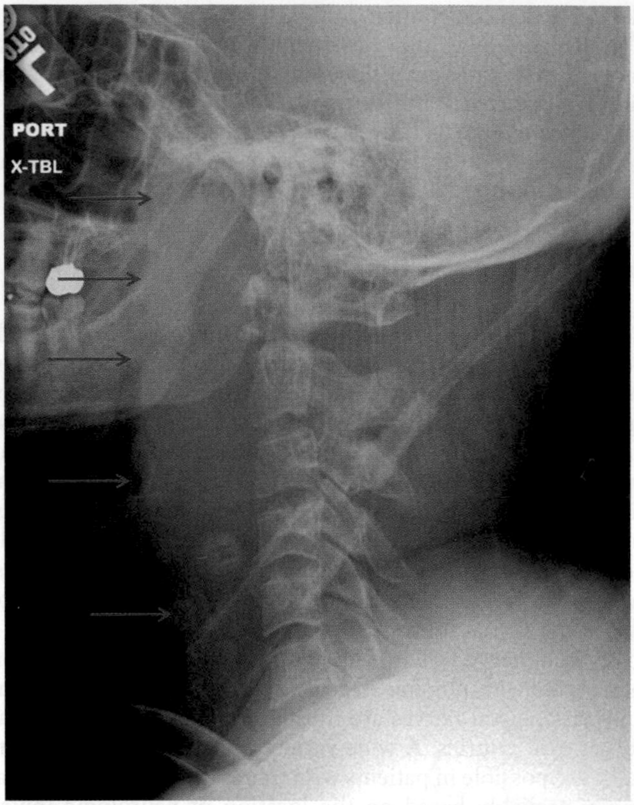

Figure 33A-2. Lateral trauma supine radiograph demonstrating significant anterior soft tissue swelling in the setting of a craniocervical dissociation. Also note the anterior horizontal fracture through the C1 ring.

the occipital condyles and the neural arch of the axis, thus reducing the diagnostic value of such radiographs.[16,17]

A high degree of emphasis has been placed on interpretation of screening lines on lateral radiographs to warn of the possibility of AOD.[18-20] Prevertebral soft tissue swelling on the lateral cervical radiograph may be present[19] (Fig. 33A-2). The Powers BC/AO ratio, which compares the distance between the basion and posterior arch of the atlas (BC) with the distance between the anterior arch of atlas and the opisthion (AO), has poor reliability[21] as does the atlanto-odontoid-basion distance, initially described by Wholey and colleagues.[22] Harris and colleagues refined the Basion-Dens interval (BDI) and added the basion-axis interval (BAI).[16,17] Both the BAI and the BDI should remain 12 mm or less in 95% of adults ("rule of 12s") (Fig. 33A-3). Although indicative of AOD if positive, 35% of patients may have normal BAIs and BDIs and still have an AOD.[4] Thus, the Harris lines are not completely reliable and seem to have much higher specificity than sensitivity in detecting occipitocervical dissociation.

As implied earlier, radiographic representation of the craniocervical distance also varies with age. Kaufman and colleagues[18] proposed measuring the actual distance between the articular surfaces of the occiput and the superior facet of the atlas on a lateral cervical spine radiograph. These authors held 5 mm as the maximum distance. However, obliquity and rotatory malposition of the head by even a few degrees, as well as mastoid process overlap, can make this measurement attempt challenging, if not nearly impossible. Using a cohort of 16 pediatric patients with AOD and a comparison group of 138 intact patients the authors identified significant false-positive rates for other screening tests, such as Sun's, Harris', Wholey's, and Powers'.[23-25]

Computed Tomography

Computed tomography is the imaging modality of choice in high-risk trauma patients. Helical imaging with sagittal and coronal reformats have been shown to be timely, cost effective, and more sensitive and specific in high-risk patients, particularly at the craniocervical junction. Three-dimensional image reformations, obtained from fine-cut CT scans, are rarely clinically useful but may assist with interpretation of more unusual upper cervical injury patterns. The potential for harmful effects of radiation from diagnostic CT, particularly to the thyroid, should be considered.

Occipital condyle fractures are rarely visualized on plain radiographs and are almost always diagnosed from head or cervical spine CT. Reformations of the atlanto-occipital articulation in the coronal and sagittal planes are essential to determine their stability. Displacement may indicate

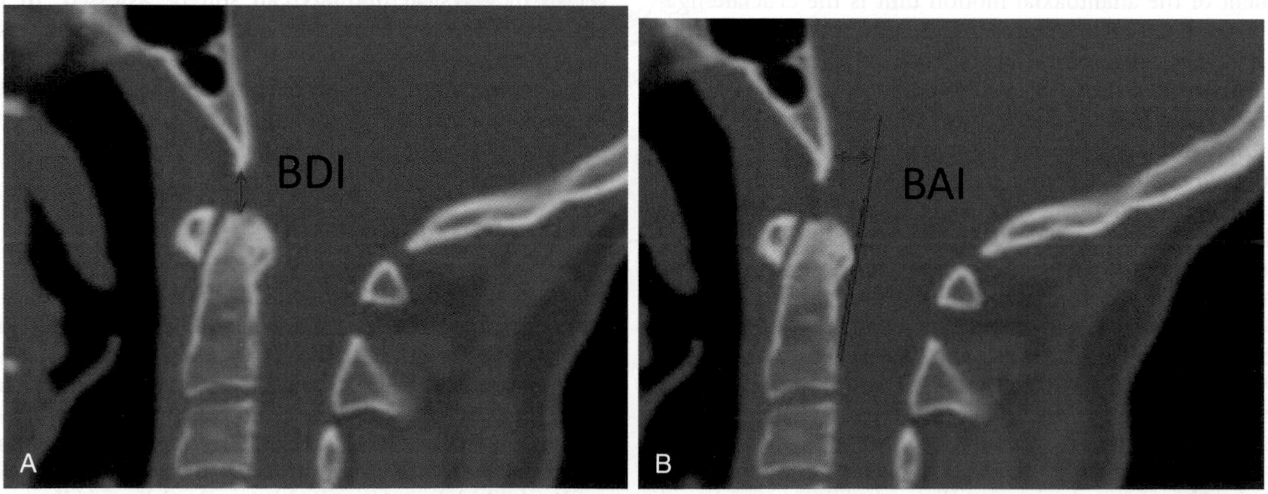

Figure 33A-3. **A,** Harris lines demonstrating the BDI, which should be less than 12 mm. **B,** Harris lines demonstrating the basion-axis interval (BAI), which should be less than 12 mm. A value of more than 12 mm on either one of these is highly suggestive of a craniocervical dissociation.

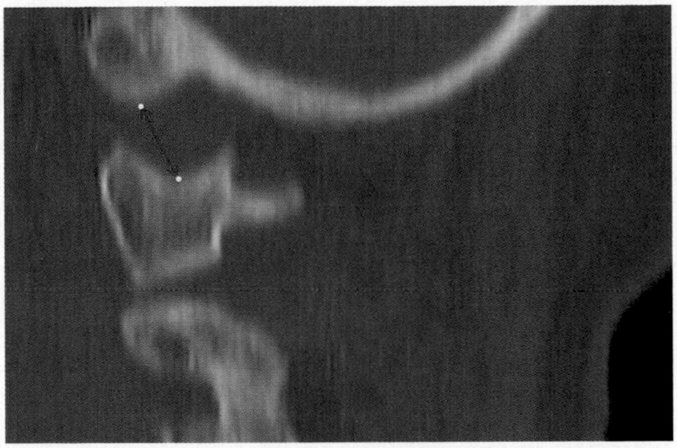

Figure 33A-4. Parasagittal computed tomography reformat demonstrating incongruent occipital–C1 joint in a case of craniocervical dissociation.

instability caused by rupture of the internal craniocervical ligaments.

Interpretation of the CT scan is critical to the timely diagnose of CCDs. Occipital condyle fractures and other fractures of C1 and C2 may be intrinsically unstable but also may portend a much more serious injury such as CCD.

One of the primary advantages of CT imaging over plain radiographs is that parasagittal and coronal CT images can be used to directly assess the congruency of the occipitocervical junctions. Subluxation or distraction can therefore be directly identified rather than relying on indirect measurement via radiographic lines (Fig. 33A-4). Pang and colleagues reported an average craniocervical interval (CCI) of 1.28 mm in normal children 0 to 18 years of age with a high degree of conformity between left- and right-sided measurements. None of the CCIs exceeded 1.95 mm.[26] In adults, gapping of more than 2 mm between the occipital condyles and C1 lateral masses indicates craniocervical instability. The coronal reformats are also useful to assess widening either between the occiput and C1 (Fig. 33A-5) or between C1 and C2 (Fig. 33A-6). Certain fracture patterns may also be suggestive of distraction such as type I odontoid fractures caused by alar ligament avulsions or type III occipital condyle fractures, also caused by alar ligament avulsions. A horizontal cleavage fracture of the anterior C1 ring has been implicated as having a distractive injury pattern that is associated with AODs[27] (Fig. 33A-7).

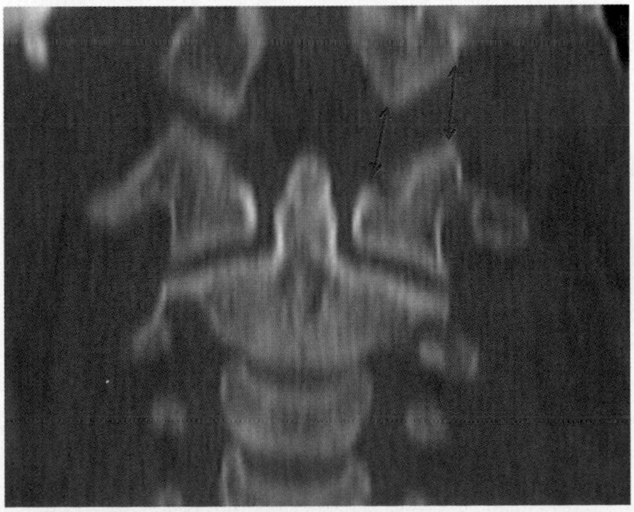

Figure 33A-5. Coronal computed tomography reformat demonstrating widening of the occipital–C1 joint (particularly on the left side) in a case of craniocervical dissociation.

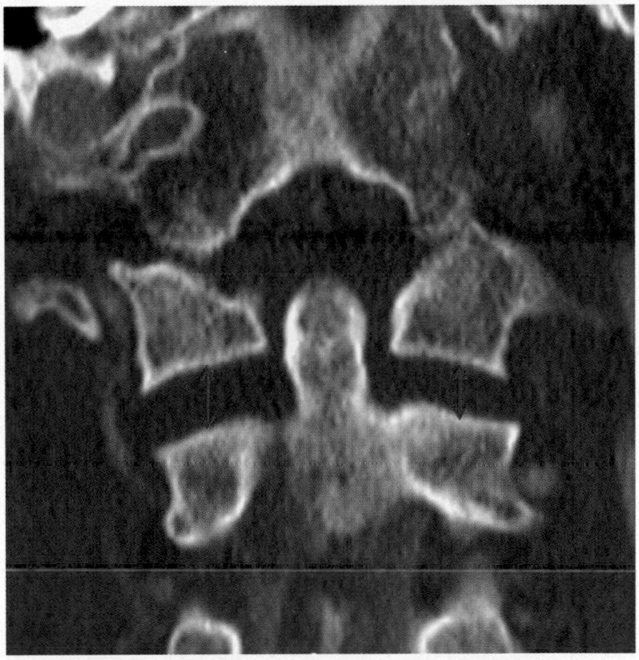

Figure 33A-6. Coronal computed tomography reformat demonstrating widening of the C1–C2 joints in the case of a craniocervical dissociation.

Magnetic Resonance Imaging

If magnetic resonance imaging (MRI) is indicated, it is imperative to communicate to the radiologists the goal of the MRI so that it is protocoled appropriately. An MRI examination geared specifically toward the craniocervical junction will be more sensitive than a standard cervical spine MRI. In the setting of trauma, the fat suppression sequences and coronal sections are the most helpful. An MRI is indicated either in the presence of neurologic injury to assess spinal cord injury or to aid in the diagnosis of an AOD. Indicators of a highly unstable injury include significant prevertebral soft tissue swelling, increased joint edema at the occipitocervical joints or C1–C2, tectoral membrane disruption, subarachnoid hemorrhage, and ligamentous injury to the alar ligaments.[26] MRI may be overly sensitive and must be interpreted in light of the mechanism and CT findings.

Traction Test

The traction test is a unique dynamic examination used to help to determine whether a CCD actually exists when CT, MRI, and all other tests are equivocal. There is no other spine trauma situation in which it is used, and even in the realm of CCD, its utility is quite limited because most injuries are delineated with CT imaging either alone or combined with MRI. In the few cases in which CT and MRI are not diagnostic, a radiographic traction test can be performed.[3,28,29] Greater than 2 mm of distraction between the occiput and C1 or between C1 and C2 is indicative of an unstable injury (Fig. 33A-8). The

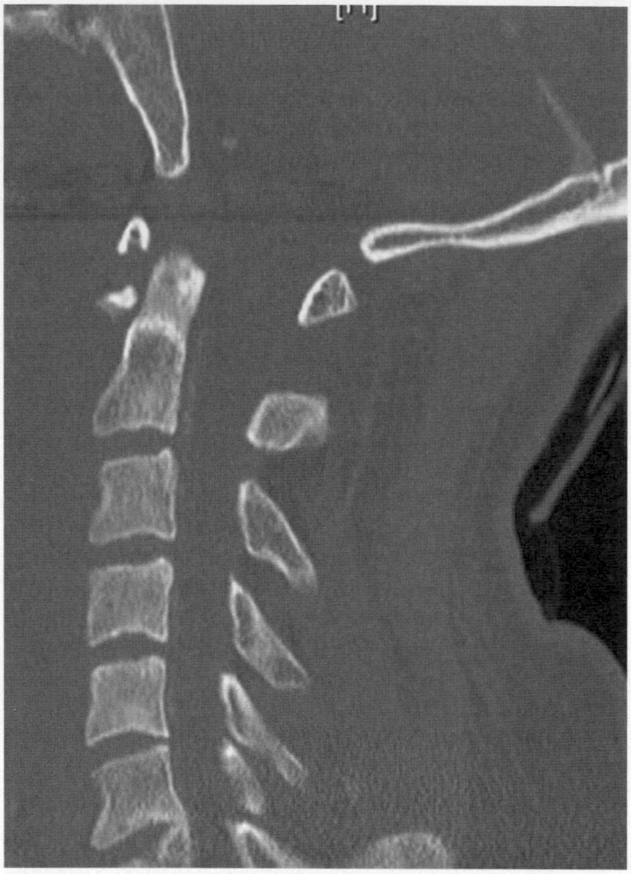

Figure 33A-7. Midsagittal computed tomography reformat demonstrating horizontal fracture through the anterior C1 ring not uncommonly associated with craniocervical dissociations.

amount of weight required for traction testing has not been well defined, although cadaveric studies suggest that the craniocervical traction test reliably demonstrates instability and requires no more than 5 to 10 lb of traction to yield a positive result when the alar ligaments, the tectoral membrane, and the joint capsules are disrupted.[10] In the authors' experience, the primary role of traction testing has been to confirm that there remains sufficient ligamentous integrity of the craniocervical junction to proceed with nonoperative treatment in situations in which imaging studies have shown some worrisome features for craniocervical instability (e.g., degree of joint subluxation) but other findings (e.g., extent of soft tissue swelling) have been less convincing. Our experience has been that traction testing has served to decrease our diagnosis of occipitocervical dissociation in situations when the diagnosis would otherwise have been made if based on strict interpretation of static imaging parameters, thus saving patients from the morbidity of an unnecessary occipitocervical fusion.

OCCIPITAL CONDYLE FRACTURES

Mechanism of Injury

Occipital condyle fracture can occur via a variety of mechanisms, which are illustrated in the classification. The three primary mechanisms involve impaction or axial loading, distraction with avulsion, or direct blows to the head with associated skull fractures that may then extend to the occipital condyle.

Classification and Management

The most commonly used classification is the three-part classification described by Anderson and Montesano in 1988[30] (Fig. 33A-9). Type I fractures are caused by impaction or axial load. Frequently, these are comminuted in nature.

Type II injuries are skull-based fractures that extend into the occipital condyle. Type III injuries are avulsion injuries with the alar ligaments "pulling off" a bony piece of the occipital condyle typically because of distraction. These injuries may potentially be unstable and associated with a CCD.

Imaging

These injuries are frequently missed on plain radiographs, although, on occasion, an open-mouth odontoid view can demonstrate an occipital condyle injury. With the increased use of CT scans, these injuries are more readily identified. Typically, they are more easily identified with coronal CT reformats (Fig. 33A-10).

Management

The management of occipital condyle fractures has been widely discussed[31,32] and is largely dependent on whether there is associated CCD. Craniocervical instability is identified when

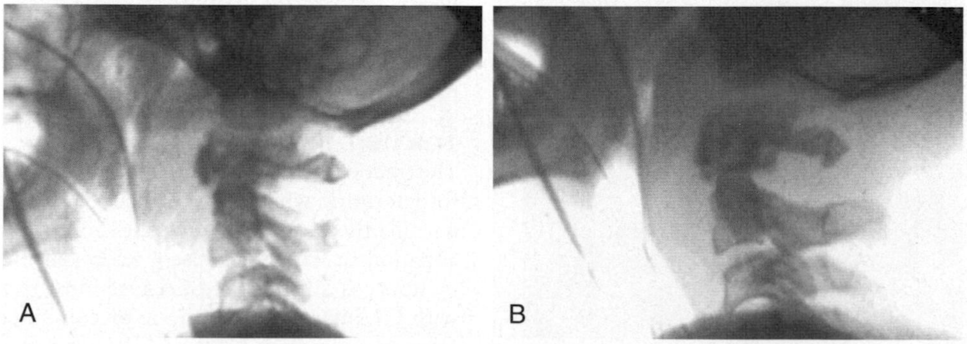

Figure 33A-8. A, Baseline fluoroscopy test of a patient suspected of having an unstable craniocervical dissociation but well reduced on computed tomography and indeterminate magnetic resonance imaging. **B,** Fluoroscopy films of same patient with 10 lb of traction demonstrating distraction between the occipital condyles and the C1 joint. After this positive traction test result, this patient underwent occiput to C2 instrumented fusion.

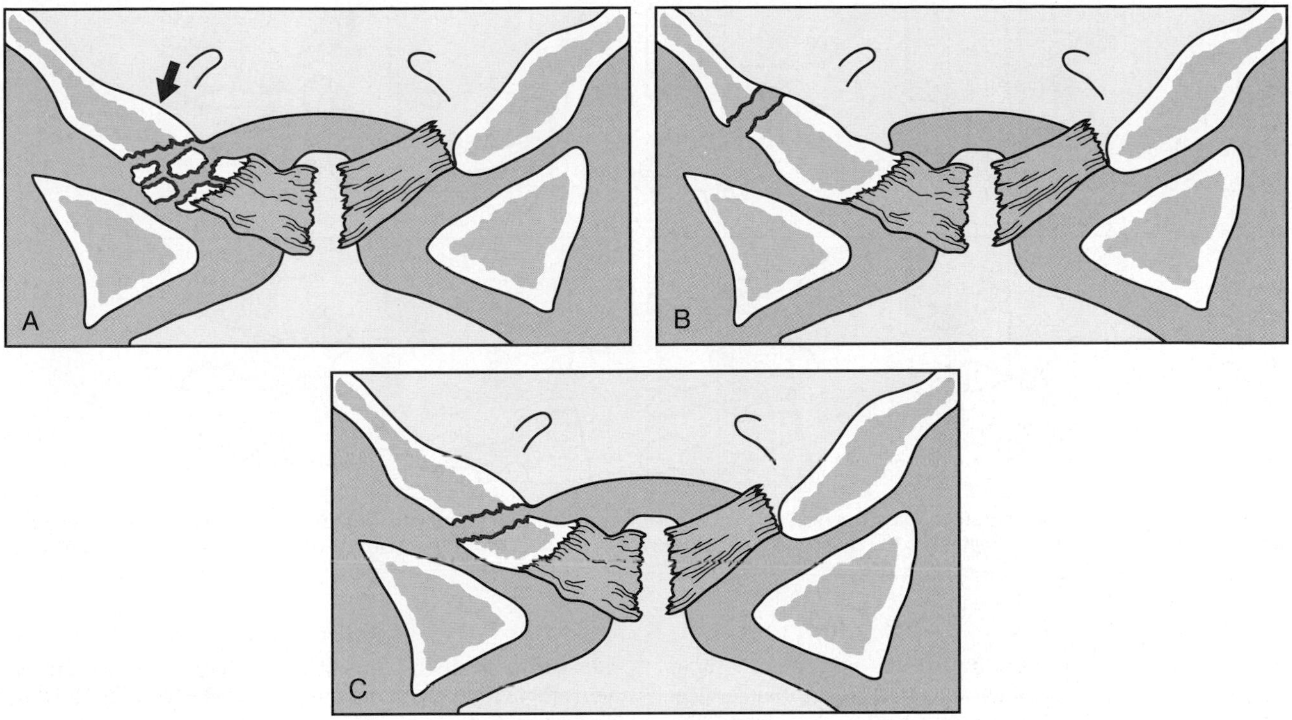

Figure 33A-9. A, Type I fracture with axial load through the occipital condyle with impaction. **B,** Type II fracture, which is an extension of a basilar skull fracture into the occipital condyle. **C,** Type III fracture, which is a distractive mechanism with avulsion of the occipital condyle via the alar ligament. *(From Anderson PA, Montesano PX: Morphology and treatment of occipital condyle fractures, Spine (Phila Pa 1976) 13(7):731–736, 1988.)*

there is displacement of the occipital condyles and C1 lateral masses or by a positive traction test result. Type I injuries can be treated conservatively because they are stable injuries with minimal risk of displacement or neurologic injury. Surgery is not recommended, but even the use of various external orthoses has not been proven to make a difference in outcome.

The management of type II injuries is based on the extent of the skull fracture and underlying head injury rather than on the less relevant occipital condyle injury. In most cases, treatment will consist of hard collar. Rarely, the entire occipital condyle may be sheared off the skull, resulting in the need for occipitocervical stabilization.

If a type III injury is identified or suspected, an MRI of the craniocervical junction can help assess the degree of instability and help ascertain the presence or absence of an associated CCD. If a CCD is not present, then a hard collar can be used, although no studies comparing nonoperative treatment methods are available. Type III fractures with CCD are managed by occipitocervical fusion.

Outcomes and Associated Injuries

Hanson and colleagues retrospectively reviewed 95 patients with 107 occipital condyle fractures.[33] According to the Anderson classification, there were 3, 23, and 65 cases of type I, II,

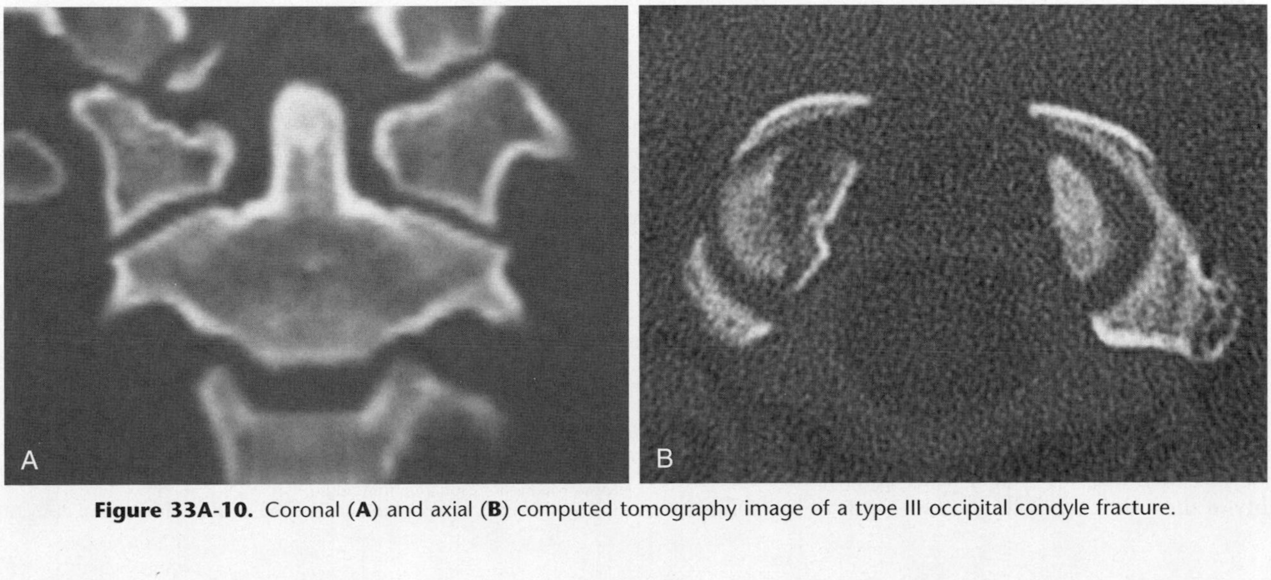

Figure 33A-10. Coronal (**A**) and axial (**B**) computed tomography image of a type III occipital condyle fracture.

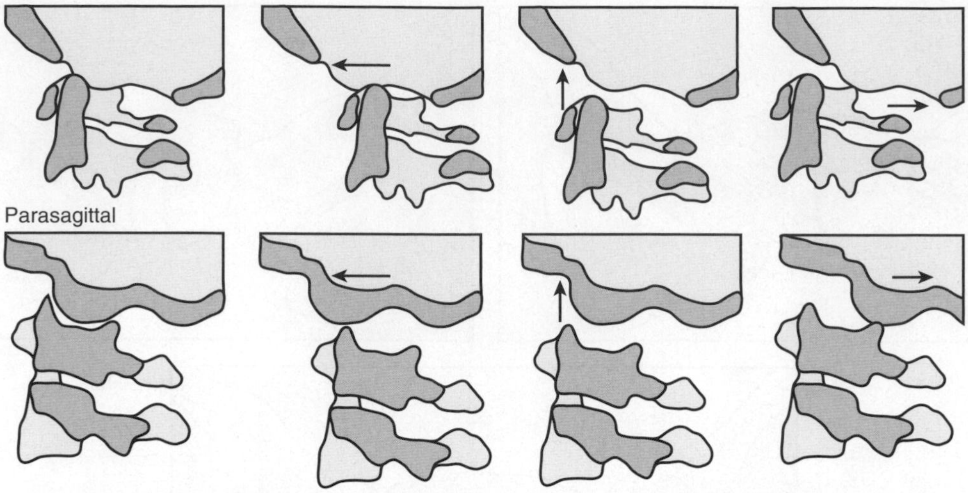

Figure 33A-11. The classification described by Traynelis and colleagues.[36] From left to right, normal without craniocervical dissociation, anterior, distractive, and posterior. *(From Traynelis VC, Marano GD, Dunker RO, et al: Traumatic atlanto-occipital dislocation. Case report, J Neurosurg 65(6):863–870, 1986.)*

and III, respectively. Unilateral injury was present in 77% of cases. More than one-third of patients had additional cervical spine fractures. Twelve patients had craniocervical instability and were treated surgically. Thus, only 18% with avulsion injuries had associated unstable craniocervical dissociations. Long-term results were related to associated traumatic brain injury (TBI) rather than the occipital condyle fracture itself.

Another retrospective review looked at 100 patients having 106 occipital condyle fractures.[34] TBI was present in 56 percent of patients. Unilateral injuries occurred in 94% of this group. Three patients were treated surgically, all of whom had atlanto-occipital dislocation associated with occipital condyle fracture. At follow-up, no patients treated nonoperatively developed late instability or required other treatment. The treatment algorithm suggested in this study supports that stable injuries without displacement can be treated in a rigid collar for 6 weeks. For cases with mild displacement, a halo orthosis may be beneficial. Occipitocervical fusion was performed in the three patients with associated CCD.

CRANIOCERVICAL DISSOCIATIONS

Historical Perspective

Craniocervical dislocations occur in 0.67% to 1.0% of all acute cervical spine injuries and are present in 8% of victims of fatal motor vehicle accidents.[21,34,35] Craniocervical injuries are now recognized as a spectrum of injury patterns with varying degrees of stability.

Classification

Traynelis and colleagues identified three craniocervical dissociation patterns based on the direction of displacement[36] (Fig. 33A-11). This system is limited because the extreme instability of AOD injuries renders the position of the occiput relative to the neck arbitrary and more dependent on external positioning forces, and there is an absence of a severity component of the injury.

A useful classification system must quantifiably assess the stability of the craniocervical junction. Signs of instability are translation or distraction of more than 2 mm in any plane,[9] neurologic injury, or concomitant cerebrovascular trauma.[37,38] The problem lies in segregating patients with minimally displaced (≤2 mm) craniocervical injuries who can be treated nonoperatively versus those with highly unstable but partially reduced injuries who require operative stabilization in spite of misleading well-aligned static images. The Harborview craniocervical injury classification attempts to identify the severity of the traumatic disruption in a three-tier system analogous to that of basic ligamentous extremity injury[29] (Table 33A-1). Type I injuries are isolated structural injuries and can be treated nonoperatively; these include unilateral type III occipital condyle injuries or isolated alar ligament tears. A type III injury is a complete disruption of all interconnecting ligaments with obviously unacceptable instability; patients are subclassified on the basis of whether they survive for at least 24 hours from the time of their injury.

The type II injury, which is a craniocervical disruption with borderline radiographic screening values, is inherently unstable but may be missed on cursory evaluation or even difficult

TABLE 33A-1 *HARBORVIEW CLASSIFICATION OF CRANIOCERVICAL DISSOCIATIONS (CCDs)**

Stage	Description of Injury
1	MRI evidence of injury to craniocervical osseoligamentous stabilizers Craniocervical alignment within 2 mm of normal Distraction of 2 mm or less on provocative traction radiograph
2	MRI evidence of injury to craniocervical osseoligamentous stabilizers Craniocervical alignment within 2 mm of normal Distraction of more than 2 mm on provocative traction radiograph
3	Craniocervical malalignment of more than 2 mm on static radiographic studies

MRI, Magnetic resonance imaging.
*Stages 2 and 3 represent injuries defined as true craniocervical dissociations.

to categorize as unstable based on careful review of the imaging. Clinical evaluation of these patients is often unhelpful because the lesser degree of displacement usually equates to the absence of neurologic deficits. Incomplete, type II stable injuries of the craniocervical junction can have similar degrees of displacement as partially reduced yet highly unstable injuries. The differentiation between the two is a primary challenge to timely recognition of craniocervical dissociation. The authors have found dynamic traction testing to be a useful diagnostic aid in the accurate categorization of these patients with type II injuries (see Fig. 33A-8).

Imaging

Studies have suggested that a delay in diagnosis may result in secondary neurologic deterioration in patients with these potentially life-threatening injuries.[2-4,36,39] Although the advent of a systematic head and neck CT protocol has likely contributed to the reduction of missed craniocervical injuries, improved education and awareness of these injury types among survivors of high-energy trauma has probably played a greater role.[3,4]

In summary, the diagnosis of CCD is often missed on plain radiographs with sensitivity ranging from 0.57% to 0.76%.[40] The inclusion of the upper cervical spine in routine head CTs obtained for the assessment of the obtunded patient can reveal the presence of a suboccipital hematoma, which may be indicative of CCD.[41] The inclusion of the foramen magnum in routine cranial CT scans has also increased the rate of detection of occipital condyle and type I odontoid fractures, which may be an indicator for a CCD as well.[33,42] Definitive CT scan of the cervical spine should include reformatted views, including sagittal and coronal views, especially of the transition zones.[43-45] If there are questionable findings but the diagnosis is still in question, MRI may be warranted.[46-48] MRI can aid in identifying ligament injuries, intramedullary changes, and hematoma formation in the epidural or paravertebral spaces.[49-52] In the rare cases of demonstrated cord disruption, MRI may play an important role in the discussion of life-prolonging interventions.[53] Despite the availability of definitive diagnostic testing, patients with CCD continue to be subject to critical delays in timely diagnosis with diagnostic delays as long as 2 years having been reported.[54]

The prognosis of patients with CCD appears to be related to the severity of the initial neurologic findings. If patients survive CCD, there appears to be a trend toward improvement neurologically with some patients even returning to normal but most having long-term residual neurologic deficits.[3]

Neurologic Issues

Neurologic injuries are commonly associated with CCD but can vary widely and can range from quadriplegia with lack of respiratory drive ("pentaplegia") to a perplexing variety of incomplete cervicomedullary injury syndromes and isolated cranial nerve injuries, such as the cruciate paralysis of Bell and the Wallenberg syndrome.[55-57]

Vascular Injuries

Vascular injuries are not infrequent with upper cervical spine trauma, although the incidence remains unclear and depends on the diagnostic modalities used.[37,58] The prospect of concurrent vascular damage commonly dictates CT or MRI-based angiography. Vertebral artery disruption should be considered in any distractive upper cervical spine injury, such as CCD. Lesions include vasospasm, intimal tears, thrombosis, dissection, and pseudoaneurysmal dilatation. In a retrospective study of 29 patients having CCD managed operatively, 15 patients (52%) had 30 blunt cerebrovascular injuries, including 16 vertebral artery and 14 carotid injuries. Three of the 15 had a stroke.[59] Thus, although there is minimal literature with respect to vascular injuries, these are high-mechanism, distractive injuries and appear to have a relatively high rate of vertebral artery and carotid artery injuries. It is therefore ideal to try to obtain either a CT angiogram or other vascular study in these patients.

Associated Injuries

Associated injuries are common in patients with CCD, including subaxial cervical spine and axis fractures in up to 50% of cases.[3] Neurologic injuries occur in 70% to 100% of survivors, including incomplete and complete spinal cord injury, TBI, Wallenberg syndrome, and cranial nerve injury. Cranial nerve injuries have been reported to include V, VI, VII, IX, X, XI, and XII.[26,60]

Nonoperative Management

The emphasis on initial management is clearly focused on assuring the best possible chance for patient survival. The Advanced Trauma Life Support (ATLS) principles remain unchallenged in their role of following a principled resuscitation and diagnostic pathway.[19] After establishing vital functions, particularly of the airway, efforts are directed at timely injury recognition and providing protection of the cervical spine. For a patient with a diagnosed CCD, any nonoperative care initially provides temporary stabilization as a bridging measure until definitive care can be rendered. The patient's head should be immobilized using sandbags, tape, or special head holders while radiographic evaluation is being completed. Skeletal traction is to be avoided. Realignment with a halo vest has been suggested as preferable for acute temporary stabilization but may be inadequate to immobilize severe instability and may have an undesired distractive effect.[61-63] Accompanying resuscitation efforts include vasopressor support for suspected neurogenic shock and emergent assessment for potential intracranial trauma.

A halo vest can also be considered in adult patients with minimal instability (Stage I CCD) and Stage II CCD who have a negative traction test result.[61,64] Closed reduction and external immobilization of unstable AODs generally does not lead to a satisfactory outcome because these are typically ligamentous injuries with minimal healing potential. Anatomic alignment is also difficult to maintain over time.

Unlike adults, children seem to have a greater inherent capacity to achieve a stable atlanto-occipital segment through a fibrous ankylosis with nonoperative care.[65-67] Nonsurgical management in children has the advantage of avoiding surgical injury to the growth centers and disruption of normal craniocervical junction development. More recently, authors have recommended early surgery because of concern for the failure of any nonsurgical measures to provide sufficient stability to this inherently unstable region.[68-70] van de Pol and colleagues reported on a patient with AOD who sustained a recurrent dislocation while in a halo vest.[62] Halo vest wear can aggravate respiratory compromise in a susceptible patient.[64] There continues to be considerable controversy as to optimal management in the pediatric population, partly driven by the variable degree of instability.

Operative Management

Surgical craniocervical stabilization is indicated for all patients with an atlanto-occipital joint displacement of greater than 2 mm on static imaging studies or with provocative traction testing or in the presence of neurologic injury.[3,28,71] In the context of a polytraumatized patient, stabilization is performed as soon as medically possible to prevent further neurologic deterioration.

Anesthetic Principles

Manual inline traction, awake fiberoptic intubation, and transnasal intubation are recommended as adjuvant techniques to establish formal airway access for patients with a known CCD while minimizing the potential for secondary injury displacement.[72] An unstable upper cervical spine fracture-dislocation requires atraumatic endotracheal airway access with minimal manipulation. Awake fiberoptic intubation and positioning of a patient allows for clinical neurologic monitoring.

Premature extubation can lead to airway obstruction and a need for emergent reintubation.[73] Assessment of airway swelling before postoperative extubation and a low threshold for delaying extubation until swelling has diminished are important early postoperative management issues. Temporary loss of a patient's gag reflex should also be taken into consideration in the initial postoperative phase as a means of minimizing the risk of aspiration.

Generally, these patients should have a mean arterial pressure maintained above 85 mm Hg to maintain cord perfusion, particularly in those with known spinal cord injuries.

Monitoring

Electrophysiologic neuromonitoring can be used as an alternative to awake positioning and frequently is the only option because many of these patients arrive intubated, sedated, and in critical condition. Prepositioning signals with motor evoked potentials (MEPs) and somatosensory evoked potentials (SSEPs) are obtained for baseline analysis and followed by repeat studies immediately after positioning. Neuromonitoring is then continued throughout the operative case. These are highly unstable injuries; therefore, any change in signal should prompt an assessment to confirm no change in alignment.

Positioning

Prone positioning of the intubated patient is performed with Mayfield tongs or a halo on an operating table suitable for spine surgery, allowing full image-intensifier access. The authors' preferred table is the prone Jackson table. Prone positioning should be performed cautiously, and fluoroscopy should be available to immediately assess alignment. Vertical distraction and subluxation may occur after prone positioning. Reverse Trendelenburg positioning should be avoided because it produces a distraction force between the fixed cranium and the cervical spine.

The head should be positioned in neutral alignment and held rigidly. Sagittal plane alignment should be checked by calculation of the occipitocervical angle. This is the angle formed between the McGregor line (hard palate to occiput) and the inferior end plate of C2.[74] Normal occipitocervical angles range from 10 to 20 degrees. The simpler, as yet scientifically unvalidated, seemingly reliable technique used at the authors' institution is to align the posterior angle of the mandible with the anterior cortex of C2 (Fig. 33A-12). This has proven to be a successful technique with good outcomes and no cases of significant occipitocervical flexion-extension malalignment. Malalignment of the craniocervical junction can result in airway obstruction, dysphagia, dysphonia, vascular injuries,[75-77] and difficulty viewing the horizon or the ground.

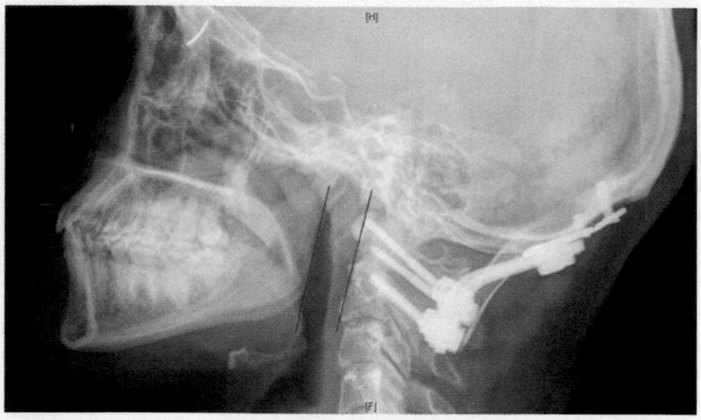

Figure 33A-12. Postoperative lateral radiograph demonstrating the roughly parallel lines extending up the angle of the posterior mandible and the anterior body of C2. This is a simple intraoperative guide to try to re-create the normal physiology with an occipitocervical fusion.

Approach and Technique

Craniocervical dissociations are most effectively treated through a posterior approach. Following a midline longitudinal incision, the midline intermuscular plane is developed, allowing subperiosteal exposure of the posterior elements. The incision is extended rostrally to the inion to expose the occiput. Care must be taken in working along the occipital–C1 junction as well as the C1–C2 junction to avoid inadvertent durotomy. The atlas should be dissected in a subperiosteal plane, keeping in mind the course of the vertebral artery on the superior aspect of the posterolateral arch. The large, bifid spinous process of the axis is a helpful orientation aid during the early dissection. The C2–C3 interspinous ligament should be preserved if the intended fusion will not extend below C2.

If screw fixation of the axis with pedicle, pars, or transarticular screws is desired, visualization of the superior and medial walls of the C2 pedicles as a reference point is recommended, which requires dissection of the atlantoaxial membrane off the superior lamina of the axis.[78,79] Exposure of the C1–C2 facet joints may be necessary for a formal arthrodesis of this motion segment, for instance, in the absence of an intact posterior arch of C1.[80] This dissection can result in considerable hemorrhage if meticulous care is not used because of the overlying extensive epidural venous plexus. To facilitate exposure, the C2 nerve root is reflected cranially. When denuding or decorticating the atlantoaxial joint, the vertebral artery's course immediately lateral to the joint should be taken into account.[81]

Occipital Plating

Current constructs bridge the occipitocervical junction via contoured rods that connect to an independently placed

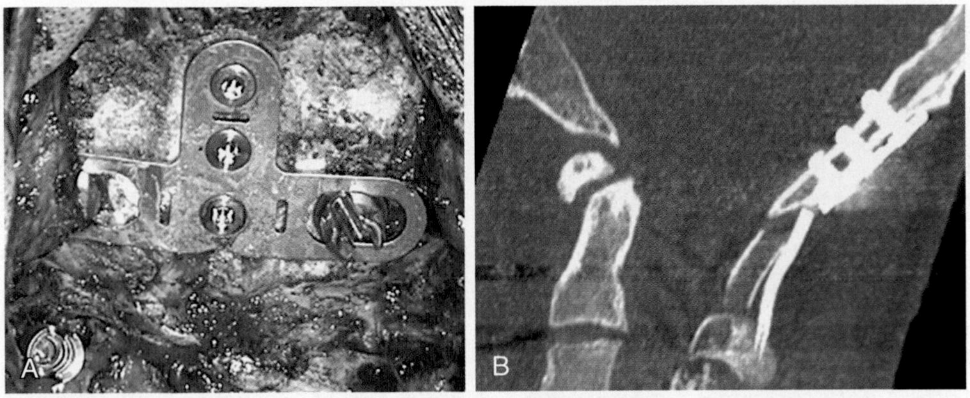

Figure 33A-13. A, Intraoperative photograph demonstrating placement of an occipital plate secured to the midline keel of the occiput in a patient with a craniocervical dissociation variant and Klippel-Feil syndrome. The rods have not yet been placed to secure the occiput to the C1 and C2 segmental screws. **B,** Postoperative sagittal reformatted computed tomography scan demonstrating location of screws in the midline keel in the same patient.

occipital plate secured with locking screws. An occipital plate can be applied to the midline of the occiput, where the thick midline keel provides the greatest resistance to pullout (Fig. 33A-13). The plate is then attached independently to the atlantoaxial screws with a contoured rod. This stepwise mode of instrumentation increases the ease of occipitocervical instrumentation and provides a powerful tool for reduction and manipulation.[82-84]

A complete understanding of occipital anatomy is essential to optimize screw safety and fixation. The thickest occipital portion is typically located in the midline at the superior nuchal line, and it has been reported to measure up to 17.5 ± 3 mm.[85] Drilling above the level of the inion should be avoided to avoid hardware prominence and possible injury to the transverse sinus or its confluence with the sagittal sinus with potentially fatal consequences to the patient.

C1 Screw Options

C1 screw fixation is not always necessary in the management of CCDs because the C1 vertebra can often be spanned with instrumentation crossing from the occiput to C2. However, C1 screws can provide additional stability and routine use is the authors' preference. The C1 lateral mass screw placement as originally described by Goel and colleagues[86] and modified by Harms and Melcher[81] uses a starting point on the posterior aspect of the C1 lateral mass proper, caudal to the prominence where the posterior arch meets the lateral mass (Fig. 33A-14). Access to this starting point requires dissection through the extensive overlying venous plexus, which may lead to problematic bleeding,[87] and requires retraction[81] or transection of the C2 root,[87] either of which may result in occipital numbness and dysesthesias. The authors prefer a C1 screw starting point that is somewhat more rostrally located, at the more readily accessible junction of the posterior arch and lateral mass,[88] which minimizes the need for dissection through the previously mentioned venous plexus and the likelihood of injury to the C2 root (Fig. 33A-15). This modification is not a viable option in all patients, and individual anatomy must be assessed before surgery on CT parasagittal imaging.

Blunt dissection of the C1 posterior arch is carried laterally to the junction of the arch with the lateral mass. This dissection is performed in a strictly subperiosteal manner over the superior aspect of the arch to avoid injury to the vertebral artery. Before placement of instrumentation, one can typically palpate the medial and lateral borders of the lateral mass and the C1–C2 joint, allowing for safe placement of a lateral mass screw. For orientation purposes, the exposure of the pars interarticularis of C2 also helps serve as a general guide to the appropriate starting point for C1 lateral mass screw placement.

A true lateral fluoroscopic view of C1 is then obtained and used to guide a bicortical channel with a drill bit starting approximately 2 mm lateral to the junction of the lateral mass with the posterior arch of C1, generally just medial to where the posterior arch narrows at the vertebral artery sulcus. Creating a bony concavity with a burr is advisable to prevent the drill bit from migrating along this relatively narrow and convex bony ridge. The drill is directed bicortically in the true sagittal plane toward the middle of the anterior margin of C1 on lateral fluoroscopy. This starting point and trajectory help avoid the vertebral artery foramen, the spinal canal, and the atlanto-occipital joint. Rocha and colleagues reported that the width of the C1 lateral mass ranges from 7.7 to 12.8 mm.[89] In general, excellent purchase can be achieved,

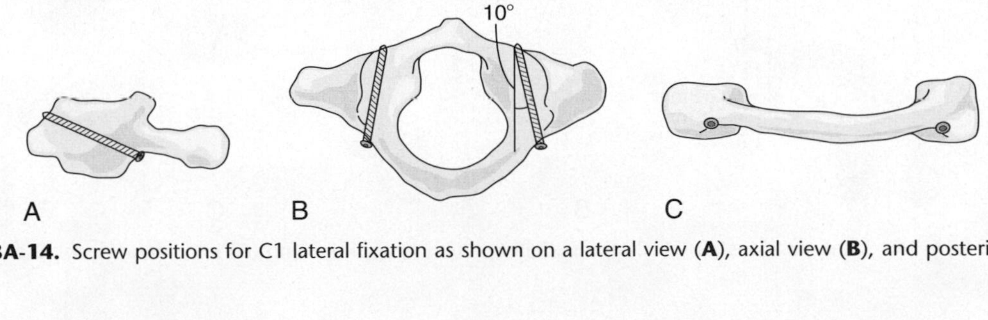

Figure 33A-14. Screw positions for C1 lateral fixation as shown on a lateral view (**A**), axial view (**B**), and posterior view (**C**).

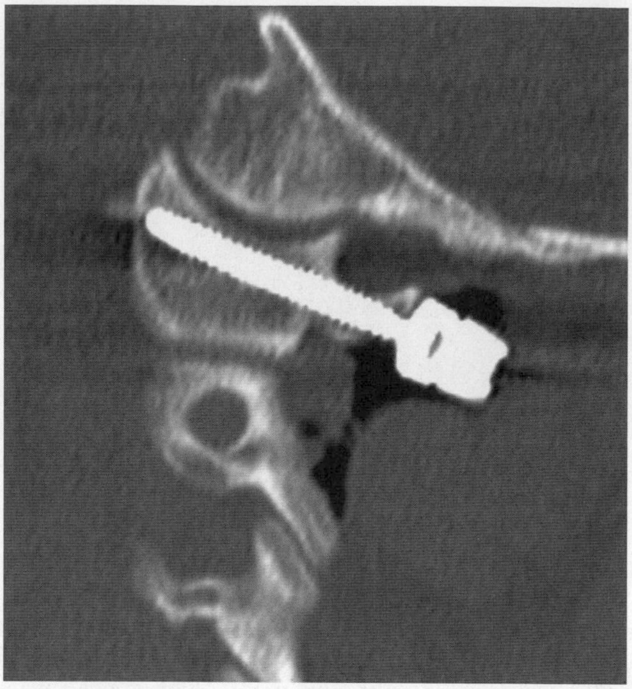

Figure 33A-15. Postoperative parasagittal computed tomography reformat demonstrating the "ridge" starting point for a C1 lateral mass screw, which starts on the posterior lamina and is more caudal to that described by Goel and Laheri[86] and Harms and Melcher.[81]

even in elderly patients with osteoporosis, with screws measuring 22 to 30 mm in length. A bicortical 3.5- or 4.0-mm screw is then placed.

Another potential technique to gain purchase to C1 is with transarticular screws, which allow for fixation to C1 and C2 with the same screw. The nuances of this technique are described in the section on C2 screw options.

C2 Screw Options

Recent advances in anatomic understanding and modern day instrumentation now allow for four primary types of screw fixation to C2: (1) transarticular screws, (2) pedicle screws, (3) pars screws, and (4) translaminar screws. With the advent of many C2 options, the surgeon can tailor the choice based on the patient's anatomy as interpreted on CT scan to use the safest technique and minimize screw-related complications.

Transarticular C1–C2 screws offer a stiff form of atlantoaxial stabilization complex and were the first screw-based fixation strategy developed for instrumentation of the atlantoaxial complex.[90,91] This procedure is technically challenging and requires congruous atlantoaxial joint reduction. The presence of anatomic variants, such as the medial vertebral artery coursing across the C2 segment or skeletal dysplasia, can pose significant obstacles to safe completion of this procedure.[92,93] Other complications include injury to the ICA and the hypoglossal nerve. Because both the hypoglossal nerve and the ICA lie anterior to the lateral portion of the C1–C2 facet joint, they are at risk of penetration with anterior screw insertion.[94,95] Careful evaluation of the preoperative CT scan is critical to determine the suitability of this technique. Furthermore, the necessary screw trajectory may be blocked by patient body habitus or by the head and neck position required for acceptable fracture alignment. If safe placement of transarticular screws appears doubtful, then other C2 fixation techniques should be considered.

To prevent spinal canal penetration, the medial wall of the isthmus of the axis is visualized and palpated with a neural elevator. Two small paramedial incisions are then made at the cervicothoracic junction to allow the appropriate trajectory of percutaneous drilling and screw placement through a cannulated obturator and drill guide. The starting point for transarticular screws is located in the medial to central third of the inferior articular process of the axis. Drilling with a long Steinmann pin or guide wire for a cannulated screw system is then performed under lateral C-arm guidance, with a 45- to 60-degree vertical inclination trajectory aiming for the mid to upper third of the anterior tubercle of the atlas. Intraarticular passage of the drill or guide wire can be ascertained by direct inspection of the joint. A medial angulation of 0 to 15 degrees is desirable to achieve optimal C1 lateral mass purchase while avoiding an excessively lateral course that may result in vertebral artery[78] and hypoglossal nerve injury[96] (Figs. 33A-16 and 33A-17). Hypoglossal nerve injury can also be avoided by minimizing the extent to which the drill tip penetrates the anterior cortex of the C1 lateral mass or the placement of excessively long screws, the avoidance of which also prevents ICA injury.[79,97] Cadaveric and radiographic studies have shown

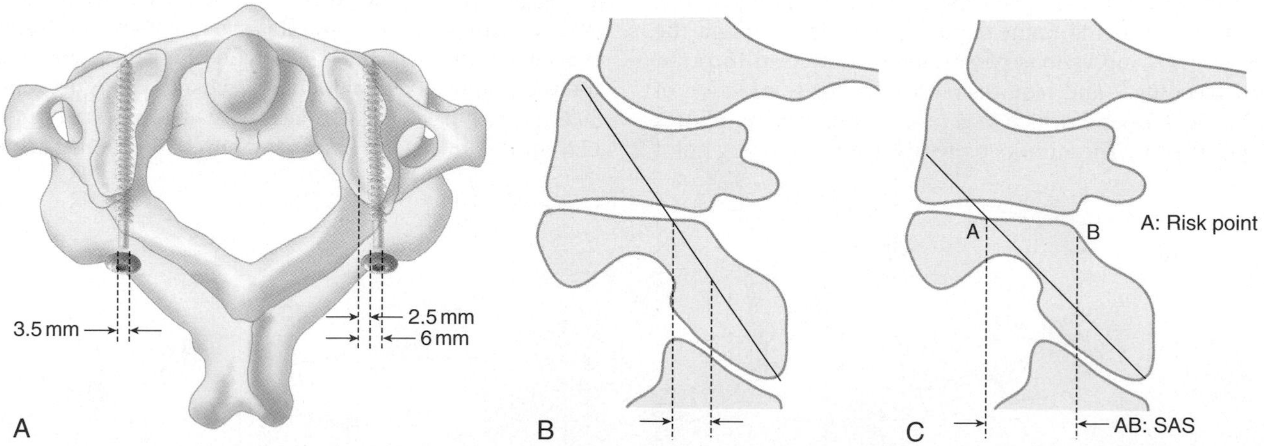

Figure 33A-16. Screw positions for C1–C2 transarticular screws in axial drawing (**A**) and lateral views (**B** and **C**).

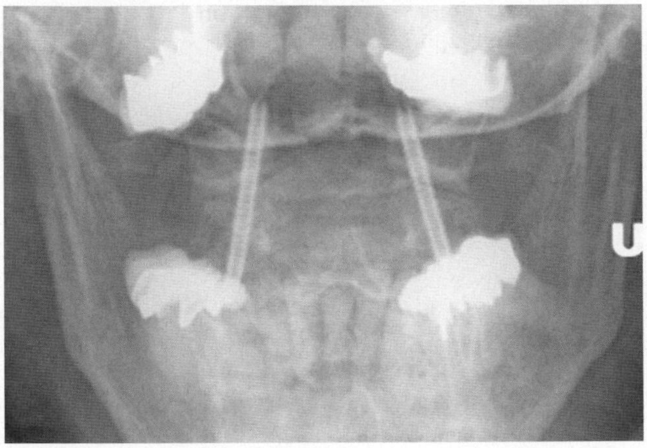

Figure 33A-17. Open-mouth radiograph demonstrating transarticular screws at C1–C2.

that the anterior cortex of the lateral mass becomes engaged when the screw tip lies an average of approximately 6 to 7 mm posterior to the anterior tip of the arch of C1 on lateral radiographs.[96] If a vertebral artery injury is suspected with the placement of the first screw, a contralateral transarticular screw should not be placed.

C2 "pars" screw and "pedicle" screw terminology are frequently used interchangeably, but in reality, the trajectories are quite different, and many screw placements are a combination of pars and pedicle screw with respect to anatomic placement. In general, men have larger C2 pedicle dimensions than women, and men are more likely to safely accommodate C2 pedicle screws.[98,99] The trajectory of the C2 pedicle screw is much less cephalad and more medially angulated than the transarticular screw (Fig. 33A-18). However, not all C2 pedicles have sufficient bone stock for screw placement with 9% of patients reportedly having inadequate anatomy that precludes the safe placement of C2 pedicle screws.[100] The C2 pedicle screw tends to be less technically demanding than a transarticular screw and does not require anatomic C1–C2 alignment before placement.

Complications can be minimized by meticulously coagulating the venous plexus above the C2 pedicle and inferior to the C2 nerve root and by medially palpating the pedicle wall. The drill or Kirschner wire is aimed in line with the directly visualized pedicle, and the medial cortex is protected to allow safe drilling and screw placement.

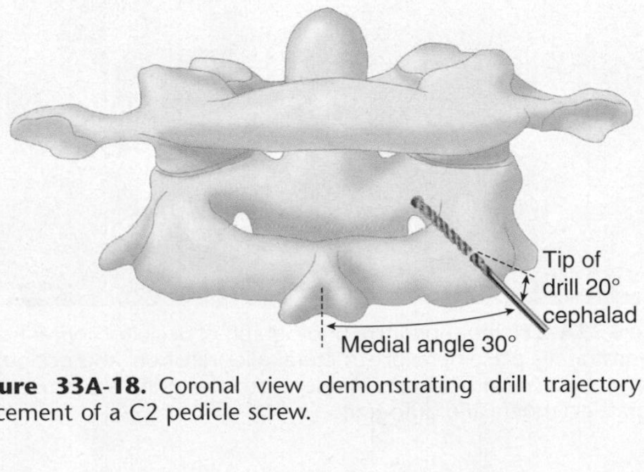

Figure 33A-18. Coronal view demonstrating drill trajectory for placement of a C2 pedicle screw.

C2 pars screws follow a different trajectory than C2 pedicle screws. The trajectory is quite similar to the transarticular screw with a low starting point and minimal medial angulation. The screw tip is intended to end superior to the transverse foramen above the vertebral artery and stop short of the C1–C2 joint (Fig. 33A-19). The C2 pars screw typically averages 24 to 28 mm in length and is the authors' preferred technique for C2 fixation. The pars screw may be used when the anatomy of the pedicle or the vertebral artery precludes safe placement of transarticular or C2 pedicle screws. For instance, in the case of an unfavorably large and medial vertebral artery foramen, a shorter pars screw can be placed that stops short of the posterior margin of the vertebral foramen.

When placing C2 pedicle and pars screws, the C2 lateral mass is cleared of soft tissue to its lateral border and rostrally up onto the pars. A blunt elevator is used to palpate along the medial border of the pedicle to visualize the trajectory of the screw and to ensure that there is no medial cortical violation. A C-arm is helpful in determining the depth of drilling and in achieving an optimal angle. A more medial trajectory is typically required than that used with transarticular screws—approximately 20 to 25 degrees for C2 pedicle screws versus approximately 10 degrees for pars interarticularis screws. Anticipated screw lengths range between approximately 22 and 30 mm.

The translaminar technique for C2 fixation in which screws are placed in the lamina of C2 starting from the contralateral spinolaminar junction can be used as an alternative to the previously described methods[101] (Fig. 33A-20). The translaminar technique is a viable option for C2 fixation, particularly in patients with anatomy unsuitable for C2 pedicle screws or transarticular screws or in patients in whom there is already a vertebral artery injury. The C2 translaminar construct has proved to be biomechanically sound in stabilizing the atlantoaxial joints.[102,103] The C2 lamina is the largest in the cervical spine and all elements at risk are visualized directly during insertion, which allows for relatively safe placement.

The first step in C2 translaminar screw fixation is to dissect the lamina. Preoperative imaging is essential to assess dimensions, optimal placement, and anticipated screw lengths. The entry point is located lateral to the spinous process at the spinolaminar junction. A blunt dissector is placed along the medial wall of the lamina in a trajectory aimed toward the lateral mass between the anterior and posterior cortices of the lamina. Although not essential, subperiosteal dissection along the caudal margin of the C2 lamina allows for palpation of the anterior cortex of the lamina to assist with screw trajectory and identify anterior cortical penetration of a drill bit or screw into the spinal canal. Anticipated screw lengths measure 25 to 35 mm. Careful planning is required to avoid screw abutment in the posterior aspect at the junction of the laminae near the spinous process. Ideally, one screw is inserted inferior and is aimed slightly superiorly, and the contralateral screw is begun more superiorly and is aimed slightly inferiorly into the lamina.

Cable Options

Early techniques that used stand-alone onlay bone grafting progressed to include posterior wiring, which provided stability.[104,105] Pseudarthrosis rates of up to 23% have been reported with onlay grafting and nonrigid fixation (wiring) methods.[104-108] An 89% fusion rate has been reported using

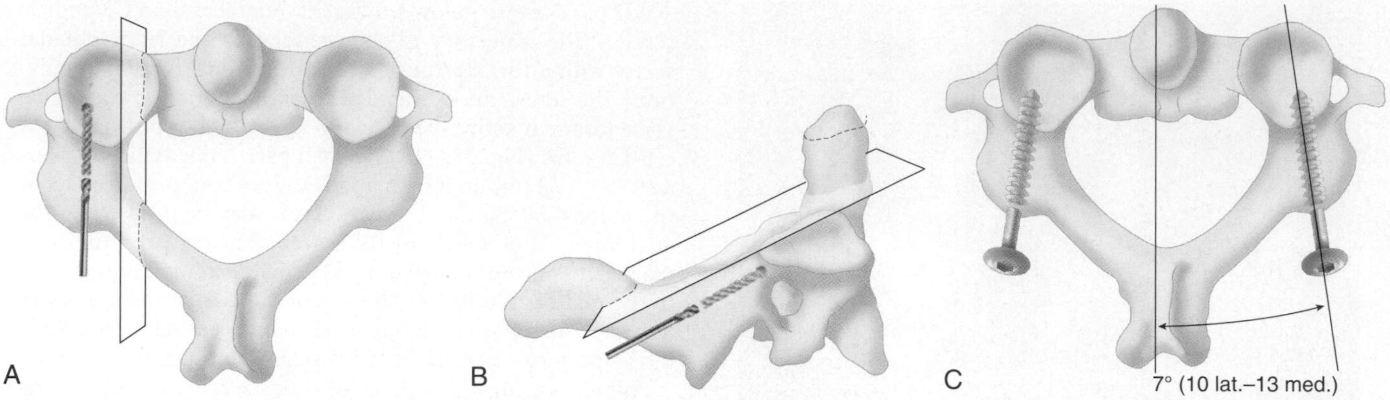

Figure 33A-19. **A,** Axial view demonstrating drill trajectory of C2 pars screw. **B,** Lateral view demonstrating trajectory of C2 pars screw. **C,** Axial view demonstrating the position of screws within the pars of C2.

onlay grafting alone, which eliminates hardware-associated complications but requires the use of aggressive postoperative immobilization techniques, including recumbency and skull-tong traction, a Minerva jacket, and a halo.[109] Onlay structural autograft with cerclage wire alone resulted in comparatively improved fusion rates[105] but had the disadvantage of requiring more comprehensive postoperative external immobilization. It was complicated by wire breakage in 78% of patients[110] and late fracture of the graft in up to 15% of patients.[111] The next advance was the development of semirigid fixation using rod-and-wire techniques.[112-114] In this construct, contoured U-shaped rods, which substituted for the onlay bone graft, were secured to the occiput with threaded wires and linked to sublaminar wires in the suboccipital spine. Wiring techniques have given way to the mechanically superior screw–plate constructs described earlier.

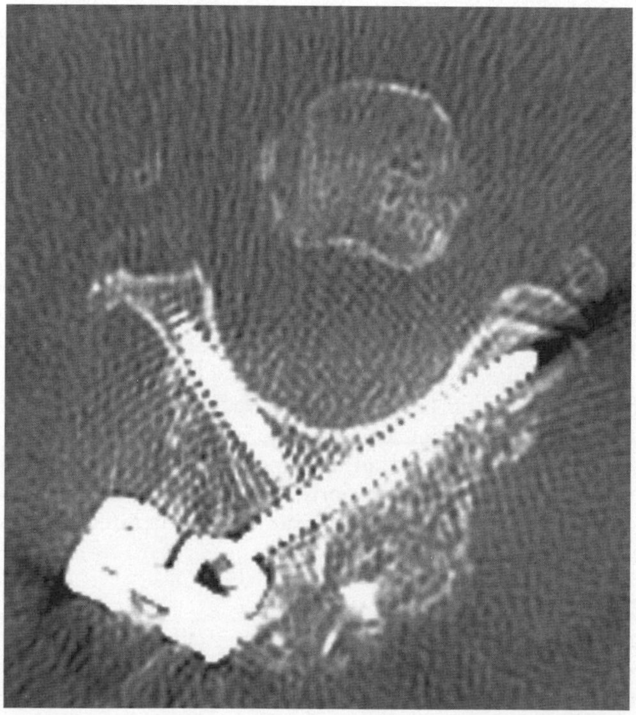

Figure 33A-20. Postoperative axial computed tomography scan demonstrating placement of translaminar screws.

Typically in today's era, cables are used less frequently because rod–screw constructs are more stable and allow for more reliable fusions. Cables may still be indicated in very young children who are not suitable for screw fixation. Cables can, however, be helpful to aid in securing structural allografts or autografts and to add additional stability.

Bone Graft Options

The authors' preferred approach is to combine a rigid posterior segmental fixation construct with a structural tricortical iliac crest allograft or autograft that is secured to the occiput and the upper cervical spine as an adjunct to the internal fixation (Fig. 33A-21). The bone graft is attached to the craniocervical junction after decortication and placement of rigid internal fixation devices. This graft is fashioned to cradle the occiput and straddle the C2 spinous process. Allograft extenders or morselized autograft can aid in fusion as well as fill the voids around the structural graft. In a recent review of 48 patients with operatively managed CCDs, there were no cases of pseudoarthrosis using structural grafts in concert with allograft extenders and local autograft.[3,4]

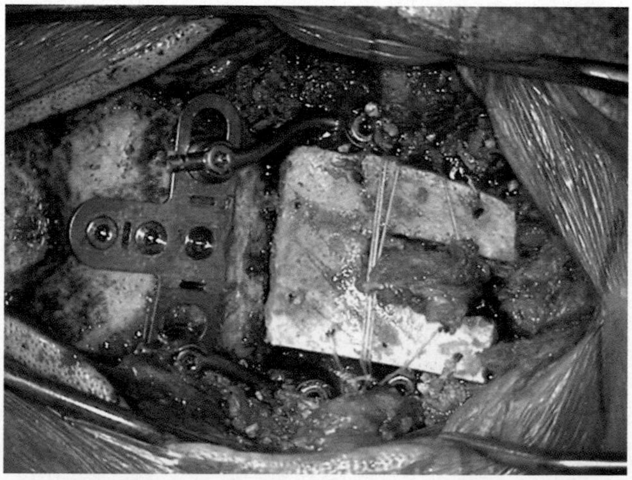

Figure 33A-21. Intraoperative photograph of occipitocervical fusion demonstrating placement of structural allograft from the occiput to C2 and secured with sutures. Underneath the graft is a mixture of allograft extenders and autograft.

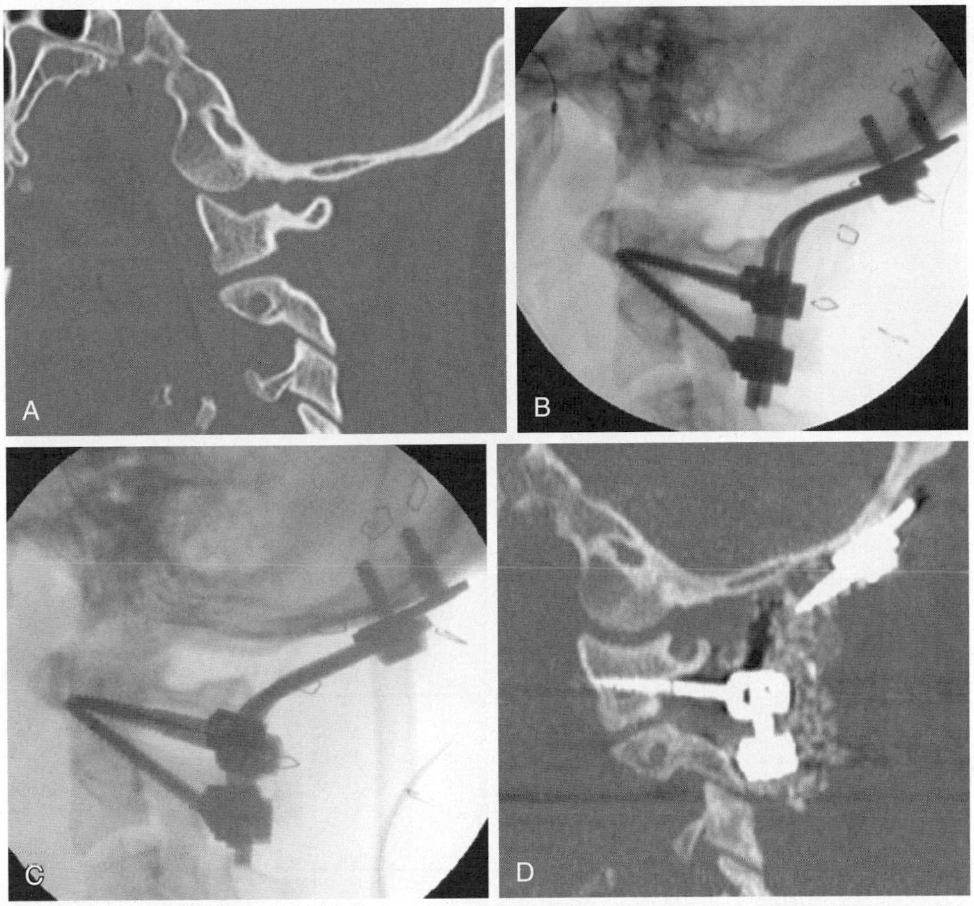

Figure 33A-22. A, Initial sagittal computed tomography (CT) reformat demonstrating subluxation of occipital–C1 joint consistent with craniocervical dissociation. **B,** Intraoperative fluoroscopy view demonstrating appropriate placement of occipitocervical instrumentation but distracted occipital–C1 joint. **C,** Intraoperative fluoroscopy view demonstrating reduced occipital–C1 joint after rods have been recontoured and replaced. **D,** Postoperative sagittal CT reformat demonstrating reduction of the occipital–C1 joints.

Reduction and Postoperative Care

After all screws and the occipital plate have been placed, it is imperative to make sure that the occipital–C1 joints and C1–C2 joints are reduced (Fig. 33A-22). This can be difficult to ascertain with C-arm imaging alone, but it is imperative to restore physiologic alignment. One must also ensure appropriate upper cervical flexion-extension alignment as has been previously discussed.

The authors tend to obtain a postoperative CT scan to ensure accurate screw placement and to ensure reduction. Typically, most patients with reasonable bone quality can be managed postoperatively in either a rigid collar or with no immobilization at all. External immobilization should rarely be required beyond 2 to 3 months after surgery. When discontinuing external immobilization, regardless of treatment form, the stability of the injury should be reassessed with flexion–extension and open-mouth odontoid radiographs.

Outcomes and Complications

Most occipitocervical dissociations are fatal. The outcome of survivors depends on (1) the type and severity of associated injuries, particularly closed head injuries; (2) the severity of neurologic injury; and (3) the timeliness with which the diagnosis of AOD is recognized and can be operatively stabilized. In Bellabarba and colleagues' initial case series, 13 of 17 (76%) patients had at least a 24-hour delay in diagnosis, and five (38%) of these patients deteriorated neurologically before diagnosis compared with no deterioration in the four patients who had been diagnosed without delay. In the follow-up to this series, the delay in diagnosis was decreased to only five of 31 (26%), yet the one patient who had a neurologic deterioration was the only one in whom there had been a delay in diagnosis of over 48 hours. Although the improvement in diagnostic delays (26% vs. 76%) resulted in a much lower missed injury rate (3% vs. 29%), long-term neurologic outcomes were more dependent on the severity of the presenting neurologic injury, which was much worse in the latter group, and suggests that more severely neurologically impaired patients are surviving AODs in greater numbers.[3,4]

Logic dictates that survivors have less displaced or even spontaneously reduced injuries, and neurologic deficits in survivors are likely to be less severe. Partly because of these reasons and despite substantial advances in neuroimaging, occipitocervical dissociations continue to be frequently missed. Early recognition and timely fixation of these injuries improves outcome by protecting against neurologic deterioration. Delayed diagnosis in these highly unstable injuries has been associated with secondary neurologic deterioration and possibly death in up to 75% of patients.[3,115,116] These unacceptably high numbers underscore the importance of

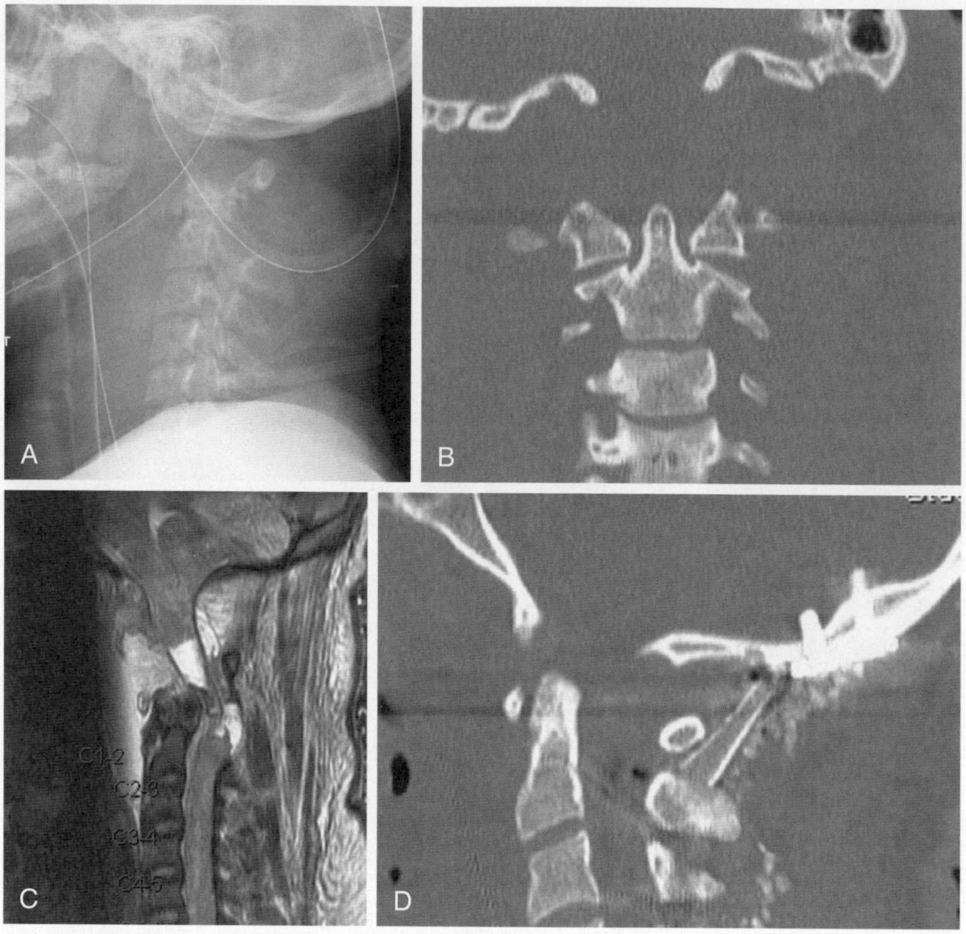

Figure 33A-23. A, Cross-table trauma lateral of a 16-year-old young man with a severe craniocervical dissociation (CCD) with 4 to 5 cm of distraction with complete spinal cord injury and cord transection who survived and underwent operative management and lived for about 12 months before succumbing to pulmonary complications. **B,** Coronal reformat computed tomography (CT) scan demonstrating significant distraction. **C,** Sagittal T2 magnetic resonance image demonstrating CCD with cord transection at C2. **D,** Postoperative sagittal CT reformat after reduction and occipitocervical instrumented fusion.

improving our current cervical spine trauma screening measures.

Although many of these patients have significant neurologic deficits at admission, the prognosis is better than many other neurologic injuries. In a series of 17 patients, the American Spinal Injury Association (ASIA) motor score improved from 43 to 79, and the number of patients with useful motor function (ASIA grade D or E) increased from 7 (41%) before surgery to 13 (76%) after surgery.[3,4] With ever increasing improvement in care starting at the scene of the trauma, more patients are surviving injuries that historically certainly would have been fatal. This has led to patients with severe injuries surviving yet with devastating neurologic injuries, adding a whole new level of ethical challenges as well (Fig. 33A-23).

CONCLUSIONS

Craniocervical injuries are caused by high-energy trauma. Careful assessment is required to avoid delayed or missed diagnosis. Unfortunately, these remain common and can result in significant morbidity or death. The best diagnostic test is the CT scan with sagittal and coronal reformats. Occipital condyle fractures are mostly stable and can be treated with a cervical orthosis. The avulsion type (type III) injuries may be associated with atlanto-occipital instability requiring surgical treatment. Craniocervical instability or dissociation is classified by the amount of displacement. Patients with small amounts of displacement (<2 mm) that are stable to traction may be treated nonoperatively. Patients with more than 2 mm displacement or atlanto-occipital dislocations should undergo posterior occipitocervical fusion with instrumentation.

Great strides have been made in the reconstruct stability at the occipitocervical junction. Modern rigid craniocervical fusion techniques using screw and plate constructs with structural graft has nearly resolved the issue of pseudarthroses and loss of fixation associated with wire contructs.[3,4,108,117] Potential technical problems include malreduction, which may result in neurologic worsening, and possible penetration of the inner cortex of the skull, which can lead to injury to neural or vascular structures. The bigger challenge in treating survivors of craniocervical dissociation lies in recognizing their often radiographically subtle yet highly unstable injuries and maintaining sufficient stability to protect neurologic function during the initial preoperative treatment phase, which includes the requisite resuscitation and multisystem evaluation in these universally polytraumatized patients.

KEY REFERENCES

The level of evidence (LOE) is determined according to the criteria provided in the preface.

3. Bellabarba C, Mirza SK, West GA, et al: Diagnosis and treatment of craniocervical dislocation in a series of 17 consecutive survivors during an 8-year period. *J Neurosurg Spine* 4(6):429–440, 2006. LOE IV
4. Bellabarba C, Bransford RJ, Chapman JR: Timing to Diagnosis and Neurological Outcomes in 48 Consecutive Craniocervical Dissociation Patients. *Spine J* 11(Suppl 10):S57–S57, 2011. LOE III
25. Pang D, Nemzek WR, Zovickian J: Atlanto-occipital dislocation. Part 1. Normal occipital condyle-C1 interval in 89 children. *Neurosurgery* 61(3):514–521, discussion 521, 2007. LOE IV
26. Pang D, Nemzek WR, Zovickian J: Atlanto-occipital dislocation. Part 2. The clinical use of (occipital) condyle-C1 interval, comparison with other diagnostic methods, and the manifestation, management, and outcome of atlanto-occipital dislocation in children. *Neurosurgery* 61(5):995–1015, discussion 1015, 2007. LOE III
27. Vilela MD, Bransford RJ, Bellabarba C: Horizontal C-1 fractures in association with unstable distraction injuries of the craniocervical junction. *J Neurosurg Spine* 15(2):182–186, 2011. LOE IV
30. Anderson PA, Montesano PX: Morphology and treatment of occipital condyle fractures. *Spine (Phila Pa 1976)* 13(7):731–736, 1988. LOE IV
32. Maserati MB, Stephens B, Zohny Z, et al: Occipital condyle fractures: clinical decision rule and surgical management. *J Neurosurg Spine* 11(4): 388–395, 2009. LOE IV
33. Hanson JA, Deliganis AV, Baxter AB, et al: Radiologic and clinical spectrum of occipital condyle fractures: retrospective review of 107 consecutive fractures in 95 patients. *Am J Roentgenol* 178(5):1261–1268, 2002. LOE IV
36. Traynelis VC, Marano GD, Dunker RO, et al: Traumatic atlanto-occipital dislocation. Case report. *J Neurosurg* 65(6):863–870, 1986. LOE IV
59. Kazemi N, Bellabarba C, Bransford R, et al: Incidence of blunt cerebrovascular injuries associated with craniocervical distraction injuries. *Evidence-Based Spine-Care Journal* 3(4):63–64, 2012. LOE IV
71. Chaput CD, Torres E, Davis M, et al: Survival of atlanto-occipital dissociation correlates with atlanto-occipital distraction, injury severity score, and neurologic status. *J Trauma* 71(2):393–395, 2011. LOE IV
75. Miyata M, Neo M, Fujibayashi S, et al: O-C2 angle as a predictor of dyspnea and/or dysphagia after occipitocervical fusion. *Spine (Phila Pa 1976)* 34(2):184–188, 2009. LOE IV
77. Bagley CA, Witham TF, Pindrik JA, et al: Assuring optimal physiologic craniocervical alignment and avoidance of swallowing-related complications after occipitocervical fusion by preoperative halo vest placement. *J Spinal Disord Tech* 22:170–176, 2009. LOE IV
88. Bransford RJ, Freeborn MA, Russo AJ, et al: Accuracy and complications associated with posterior C1 screw fixation techniques: a radiographic and clinical assessment. *Spine J* 12(3).231–238, 2012. LOE III
98. Bransford RJ, Russo AJ, Freeborn MA, et al: Posterior C2 instrumentation: accuracy and complications associated with four techniques. *Spine (Phila Pa 1976)* 36(14):E936–E943, 2011. LOE III

The complete References list is available online at https://expertconsult.inkling.com.

33B Atlas Fractures and Atlantoaxial Injuries

JOHN C. FRANCE • CARA L. SEDNEY

INTRODUCTION: SCOPE AND PURPOSE

The atlas (C1) has a unique anatomy and as a result, its injuries are considered separately from those of other cervical vertebrae. Similarly the relationship between the atlantoaxial articulation differs from the levels caudal to it in the subaxial spine, so the effects of injury to this area will also be considered in this chapter.

Injuries to the C1 ring are frequently associated with injury at the cephalad or caudal levels. Thus, whenever an injury is noted, one must carefully assess the occipitocervical junction, the axis, and subaxial vertebrae. When concomitant injuries occur, it is often the injury to those adjacent levels that dictates treatment. For example, a fracture of the posterior arch of the atlas is often seen with odontoid fracture, but it is the location and displacement of the odontoid fracture that would determine whether operative or nonoperative treatment is warranted. The fracture of the posterior arch of the atlas would only play a role in operative decision making because the posterior arch would not be available as a point of fixation. This chapter will discuss injuries to the C1 ring and atlantoaxial instability.

The atlantoaxial articulation plays an important role in rotational mobility of the cervical spine and is subject to rotary dislocations, which will be covered here. Also the ligamentous support, in particular the transverse ligament, is critical in maintaining stability as the C1 ring rotates about the odontoid process.[1] Injury to the transverse ligament can result in abnormal anterior atlantoaxial translation putting the spinal cord at risk. Injury to the transverse ligament can occur in isolation or in conjunction with atlas fractures, although traumatic rupture of the transverse ligament leading to atlantoaxial instability is rare.[2-4] These injuries are commonly fatal, but, if the patient survives there is almost always some degree of spinal cord injury.[5-8] They represent a diagnostic challenge, even postmortem when minimal signs of trauma are evident.[9] These injuries are more frequently seen in older patients with posttraumatic instability developing in the fifth decade of life and beyond.[10,11]

MECHANISM OF INJURY AND BIOMECHANICS

Most upper cervical injuries are the result of automobile accidents or falls.[12-17] The predominant mechanism of injury is usually forced flexion or extension secondary to unrestrained deceleration forces and from cranial impaction resulting in axial loading to the atlas.

Jefferson initially described the bursting type of atlas fracture,[18] which is an axial loading injury. With an axially directed force, the occipital condyles are driven into superior articular

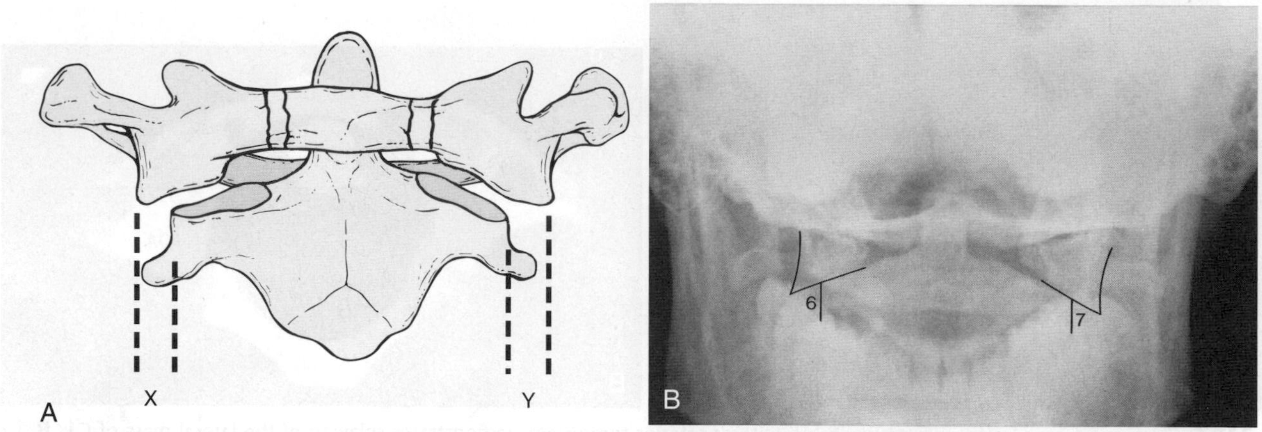

Figure 33B-7. **A,** Atlantoaxial offset. If X + Y is greater than 6.9 mm, transverse atlantal ligament rupture is implied. **B,** Admission open-mouth plain film view demonstrating the method for determining total lateral translation. 6, 6 mm offset; 7, 7 mm offset. *(Source: From Levine AM, Edwards CC: Treatment of injuries in the C1-C2 complex, Orthop Clin North Am 17:31–44, 1986.)*

Associated disruption of the posterior longitudinal ligament (PLL) (tectorial membrane) can lead to instability with this variant.[64] In the absence of associated atlanto-occipital or atlantoaxial instability, the treatment is rigid collar immobilization.

5. Lateral mass fractures are generally the result of combined axial loading and lateral compression. If severe enough, the occipital condyle can settle onto the lateral mass of C2, creating a cock-robin deformity. Unilateral lateral mass sagittal split fractures have been described by Bransford to occur and led to late cock-robin deformity, significant loss of neck rotation, and severe neck pain that required traction and occipitocervical fusion, even in the face of an intact transverse atlantal ligament.[65]
6. Transverse process fractures may be unilateral or bilateral, resulting from an avulsion with lateral bending. These are usually considered benign injuries when in isolation but may be associated with vertebral artery injury.
7. Inferior tubercle avulsion fractures are thought to be avulsion injuries of the longus colli muscle caused by hyperextension of the neck. Nonoperative treatment is recommended.

Anterior and posterior ring fractures by themselves are considered stable patterns but they are often associated with fractures at other levels that will determine overall stability. Lateral mass compression fractures are also usually stable but have to be evaluated in context of other potential injuries. The unilateral and bilateral lateral mass fractures can be stable or unstable depending on the degree of displacement. If enough displacement exists, it is implied that a greater soft tissue disruption occurred, especially the transverse ligament, which could allow the lateral mass to extrude laterally and the occipital condyle to settle caudally onto the C2 superior facet with axial loading. The amount of lateral displacement is measured between the lateral borders of the C1 and C2 lateral masses on a coronal view (Fig. 33B-7). For the unilateral lateral mass separation, stability has not been well defined. The concern with the unilateral injury is that it will gradually displace laterally as the occipital condyle settles with gravity onto the C2 superior articular facet. There are no established criteria via classification to predict which of these fractures are unstable and at risk for this type of displacement and which will remain stable.

Atlantoaxial rotary subluxations were classified by Fielding and associates[30] (Fig. 33B-8). This classification takes into account the integrity of the transverse ligament and the

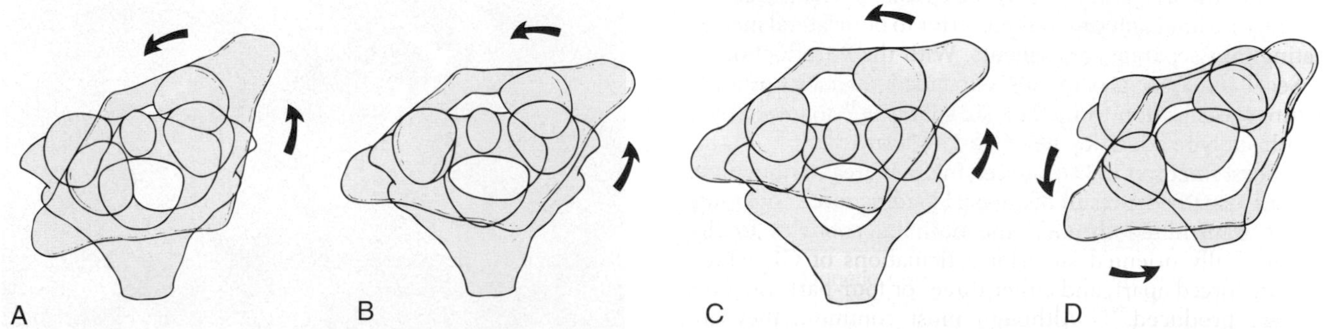

Figure 33B-8. Drawings showing the four types of rotatory fixation. **A,** Type I: rotatory fixation with no anterior displacement and the odontoid acting as the pivot. **B,** Type II: rotatory fixation with anterior displacement of 3 to 5 mm and one lateral articular process acting as the pivot. **C,** Type III: rotatory fixation with anterior displacement of more than 5 mm. **D,** Type IV: rotatory fixation with posterior displacement.

position of the facet joints. It was expanded on by Levine and Edwards to include frank rotatory dislocation (type V).[17]

Type I rotatory fixation, the most common, was seen in 47% of Fielding and associates' series and occurs within the normal range of motion.[30] The transverse ligament is intact and acts as the pivot point with anterior subluxation of one facet and posterior subluxation of the contralateral facet. Type II rotatory fixation occurred with an associated deficiency of the transverse ligament and 3 to 5 mm anterior displacement of the atlas. It was the second most common injury (30%) and occurs with unilateral anterior displacement of one lateral mass of the atlas when the opposite intact joint acted as a pivot. Type III rotatory fixation was seen with greater than 5 mm anterior displacement of the atlas on the axis and occurs with both transverse ligament and secondary stabilizer (alar ligaments, apical ligament, facet capsules) insufficiency. Both lateral masses of the atlas were subluxed anteriorly, one more than the other, thus producing the rotated position. Type IV rotatory fixation, the most uncommon, was observed when there was posterior displacement of the atlas on the axis due to a deficient dens. Type V, frank rotatory dislocation, may also be seen, although it is extremely uncommon.[17,66] The cause of this injury in adults is almost universally associated with trauma involving a flexion-rotation mechanism of injury. The atraumatic form in adults is very rare. Many different causative theories have been proposed, including effusion of the synovial joint producing attenuation of the ligaments,[67] facet synovial fringes from inflammation blocking atlantoaxial reduction,[68] rupture of one or both of the alar ligaments and transverse ligament,[69] or hyperemic decalcification with loosening of the ligaments.[70] Muscle spasms in addition to a combination of any of the aforementioned possibilities may also play a role.[71,72] More recently, Fielding and colleagues noted that this injury is occasionally associated with lateral mass articular fractures and that muscle spasms occur secondarily as a result of inflammation.[30] They postulated that ligament and capsular contractures result in a fixed deformity.

MANAGEMENT

Atlas Fractures

Emergent Treatment

The initial management strategy as with any cervical injury is to maintain stability and address any neurological deficits with appropriate spinal cord injury protocols while managing the basic trauma concerns such as airway management, and so forth. Most patients with isolated atlas fractures are neurologically intact and the focus of treatment is the fracture itself. A rigid collar is satisfactory initial immobilization unless the C1 ring injury is part of other complex cervical injuries.

Indications for Definitive Care

Definitive care will be dictated by the degree of stability and associated injuries. In the face of combined atlas and axis fractures, the axis fracture usually guides the treatment. Most isolated atlas injuries heal with conservative nonoperative treatment.[73] As is true for other spine fractures, it is important to assess atlas fracture stability when deciding treatment, which in the case of isolated atlas fractures is largely determined by the integrity of the transverse atlantal ligament. The goal of treatment would be to avoid progressive neurologic deficit (which would be a rare occurrence), avoid a cock-robin deformity or torticollis, and minimize late pain. These fractures tend to heal well with immobilization so the goal is to maintain alignment while healing occurs.

Bursting atlantal fractures have been categorized by Spence and colleagues into stable and unstable based on the integrity of the transverse ligament as determined radiographically.[22] In their classic study, the atlantoaxial offset was measured in experimentally produced burst fractures. On an open-mouth odontoid film, burst fractures in which the transverse ligament remained intact produced an atlantoaxial offset of less than 5.7 mm, whereas those associated with rupture of the transverse ligament produced an atlantoaxial offset greater than 6.9 mm (see Fig. 33B-7). It should be noted that Spence's rule is an attempt to identify integrity of the transverse atlantal ligament, the direct evaluation of which was previously described using MRI. Heller and colleagues reported that because of radiographic magnification, the cutoff for stability should be increased to 8.1 mm.[74] Spence's rule works well for establishing stability for the true Jefferson fracture, which disrupted the atlas ring anteriorly in two places and posteriorly in two places allowing the left and right lateral masses to separate in a bursting pattern. For the unilateral fracture that results from an axial load with lateral tilt, this formula may not work. Only one of the lateral masses displaces, but it can move far enough laterally to allow the ipsilateral occipital condyle to subside onto the superior facet of axis resulting in a torticollis deformity. The initial lateral offset of the unilateral C1-C2 lateral masses may not be greater than 6.9 mm but would be considered an unstable pattern because of the progressive deformity that results.

The "odontoid–lateral mass interspace" was evaluated by Sutherland and coworkers, who noted that asymmetry can occur in the neutral position and that the interspace tended to increase with ipsilateral rotation of the head.[75] Stability can also be assessed with evaluation of the ADI in lateral flexion and extension radiographs (Fig. 33B-9). In normal individuals, the maximum ADI should be less than 3 mm in adults and less than 5 mm in children.[50,51,54] In the case of a unilateral lateral mass or comminuted fracture, there may be significant lateral offset on one side only; this can allow the occipital condyle to displace vertically and create late pain and deformity. When this is recognized, operative treatment should be considered early, but in the absence of deformity can also be considered late for resultant arthrosis with pain. Inferior tubercle avulsion fractures typically involve a transverse fracture of the inferior pole or midportion that usually results from a distraction mechanism with neck hyperextension. This occurs at the attachment site of the longus colli muscle and is thought to be mechanically stable.[76]

Levine and Edwards devised a treatment algorithm for atlas fractures depending on the atlantoaxial offset.[77] For atlas fractures that show 2 to 7 mm of combined lateral mass, halo vest immobilization for 3 months is appropriate. However, for fractures with an offset greater than 7 mm, they recommend an initial period of axial traction for 4 to 6 weeks followed by 1 to 2 months of halo vest wear. Prolonged traction may not be well tolerated and direct osteosynthesis techniques allowing more immediate mobilization of the patient may be preferred and will be described later. In either case, after 3 months of immobilization, the stability of the atlantoaxial articulation should be verified with lateral flexion-extension films. Any

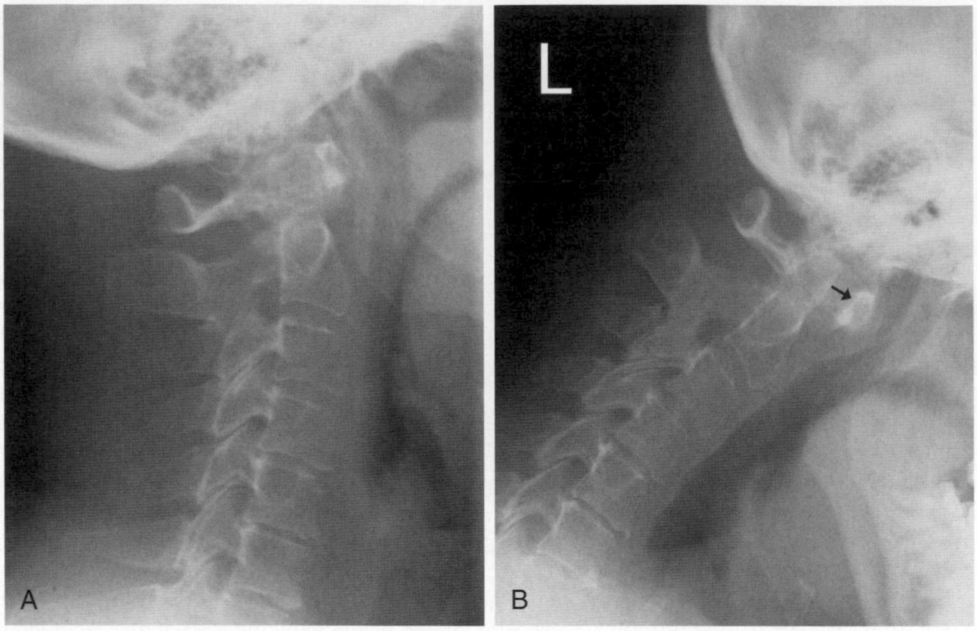

Figure 33B-9. A, An extension lateral radiograph with normal atlantodens interval (ADI) followed by a widened ADI on flexion as indicated by the *arrow* (**B**).

significant instability (ADI >5 mm in adults, >4 mm in children) at that point warrants posterior C1-C2 fusion. In addition to Levine and Edwards, other authors reported a very low incidence of residual instability with the use of this algorithm.[17,22,41,62,78-80] As shown by Fielding and coworkers, the ADI increases to approximately 5 mm when the transverse ligament is transected alone, and the alar ligaments, the apical ligament, and facet capsules are left intact.[50] This may explain the low incidence of residual instability that presumably results from intact secondary stabilizers.[17,78] Thus, the axial compression-type injury described here is not nearly as unstable as a hyperflexion-type atlantoaxial dissociation. The latter type injury results in tearing of the accessory ligaments, including the alar and apical ligaments and facet capsule, along with the transverse ligament, which is the reason for its instability.

Nonoperative Treatment

The majority of C1 ring injuries can be treated nonoperatively. Simple, uncomplicated arch fractures, minimally displaced burst and lateral mass fractures (combined atlantoaxial offset of <5.7 mm), and transverse process fractures can be reliably managed with halo or semirigid collar immobilization until union occurs.[17,81] The anterior or posterior arch fractures, if isolated, are managed in a rigid collar for 6 weeks, then assessed for stability with flexion-extension radiographs. Nondisplaced bilateral or unilateral lateral mass fractures are also managed in a hard collar for 6 to 12 weeks. Displaced bilateral or unilateral lateral mass fractures, if deemed stable, are treated nonoperatively. The historical treatment for the displaced burst fractures has been halo immobilization for 12 weeks, but in recent years, there has been some shift toward rigid collars for 12 weeks.[79] Another option in the past was traction for 4 to 6 weeks to aid reduction and gain early healing then conversion to halo immobilization for the remainder of 12 weeks' overall treatment. Surgical management or rapid mobilization in the halo vest is preferred over prolonged immobilization if deemed unstable.

Surgical Treatment

Surgical treatment options of displaced unstable atlas fractures include traction reduction followed by posterior fixation-fusion of C1-C2 with transarticular screw (Fig. 33B-10) fixation, C1-C2 fixation using a variety of techniques,[82-84] or occipitocervical fusion to span the injury.[85,86] Recently, with the increasing familiarity of C1 lateral mass screws, the fracture can be repaired more directly with bilateral lateral mass screws in C1 and a rod to reconnect them to each other (osteosynthesis), avoiding fusion across motion segments (Fig. 33B-11).

Surgical Anatomy. The atlas is a bony ring with two enlarged lateral masses and two thin arches connecting them. Mechanically, the superior and inferior articular facets lie anterior to the posterior facets of the subaxial spine. The superior articular surfaces face upward and medially to receive the occipital condyles of the skull, which face laterally. The inferior articulating surfaces face downward and slightly medially and rotate on the corresponding anteriorly placed superior facets of the axis. The posterior arch consists of a modified lamina with a posterior tubercle that gives attachments to the suboccipital muscles. The anterior arch connects the lateral masses and has a tubercle on which the longus colli muscles insert.

Understanding the bony anatomy of the C1 ring, particularly the lateral masses, is critical for screw placement. In addition, the surgeon must know the relationship of the vertebral artery to the C1 ring to avoid injury. The vertebral artery exits out of the C1 foramen transversarium and lies directly on the superior surface of the posterior C1 arch within a groove while traveling medially and then turns superiorly to enter the foramen magnum. Its course through the C2 foramen can vary significantly and be at risk during screw insertions, and, thus,

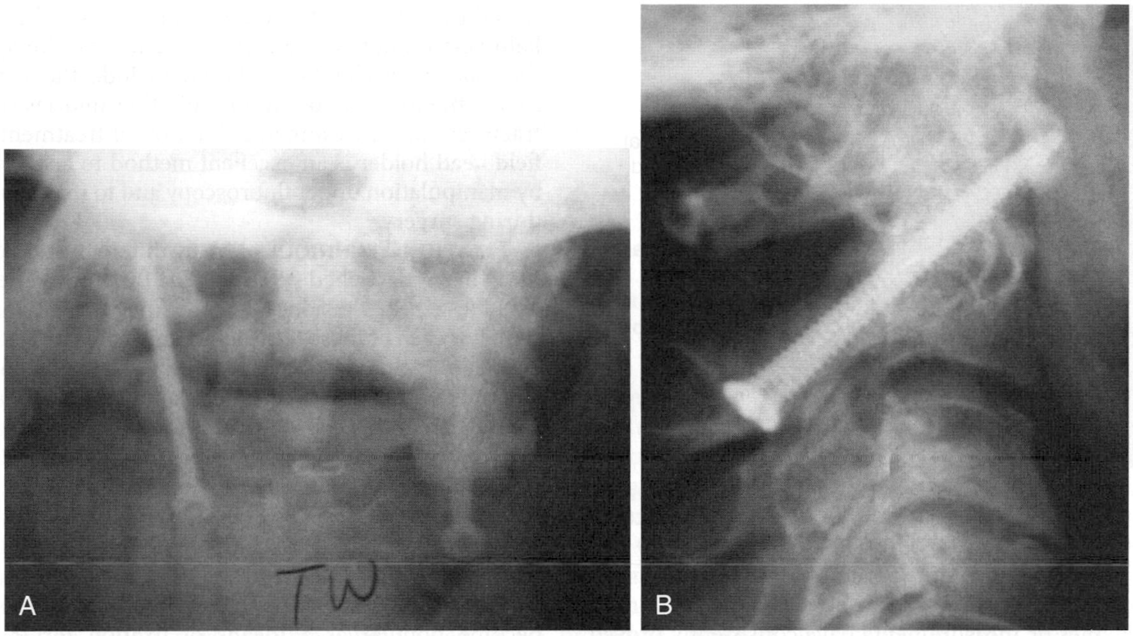

Figure 33B-10. Open-mouth odontoid view (**A**) and lateral view (**B**) of C1-C2 transarticular screws. *(Courtesy Robert McGuire, MD, Mississippi University.)*

should be studied for each individual patient. The carotid artery courses along the anterolateral aspect of the C1 lateral mass. A preoperative CTA can be useful to define any vascular injury that could affect your choice of screw placement as well as in defining the arterial anatomy as described earlier. Vital neurologic structures are in close proximity to the atlanto-occipital joint. Within the base of the occipital condyle lies the hypoglossal canal and the hypoglossal nerve (cranial nerve XII). Just lateral to the occipital condyle and posterior to the carotid canal is the jugular foramen that contains cranial nerves IX through XI.[87] The jugular foramen lies in close proximity to the hypoglossal canal within 3 mm on the extracranial side and 7 mm on the intracranial side[88] (Fig. 33B-12). There is also a venous plexus at the insertion point for a C1 lateral mass screw. The C2 nerve root exits directly medial to the lateral mass under the arch of C1 and must be mobilized or transected to access the screw starting point.

Positioning Techniques. Proper patient positioning is crucial to optimize the likelihood of success for a surgical technique and to avoid patient harm. No accepted method ensures proper alignment, and the exact positioning performed will depend on the type of fixation planned. Positioning for occipito-cervical fusion focuses on a physiologic amount of flexion to enable forward gaze without impairing swallowing or airway functions. The positioning should be inspected both clinically and radiographically. No specific

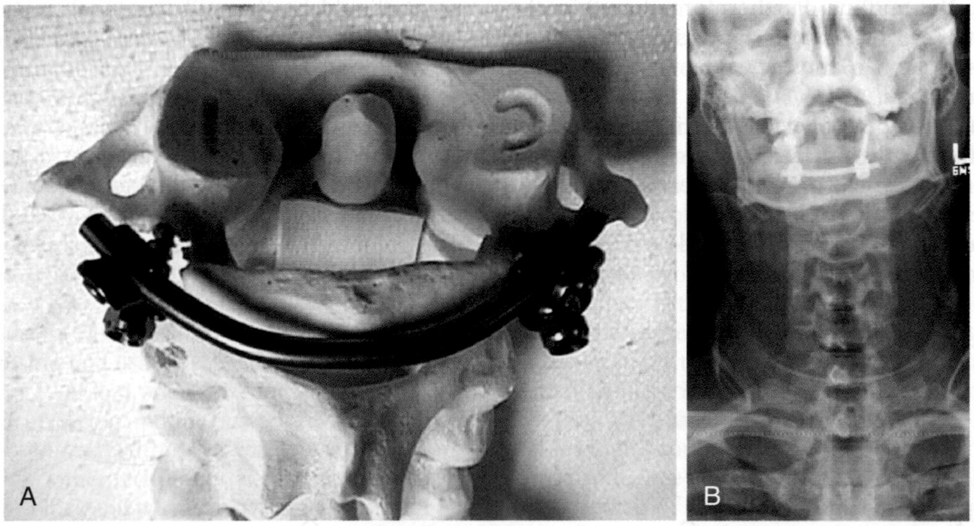

Figure 33B-11. A, saw bones demonstration of using C1 lateral mass screws and transverse connecting rod to reduce a classic Jefferson fracture, thus achieving direct fracture healing and avoiding a fusion. *(Courtesy Jens Chapman, MD, University of Washington.)* **B,** Postoperative anteroposterior view of C1 osteosynthesis.

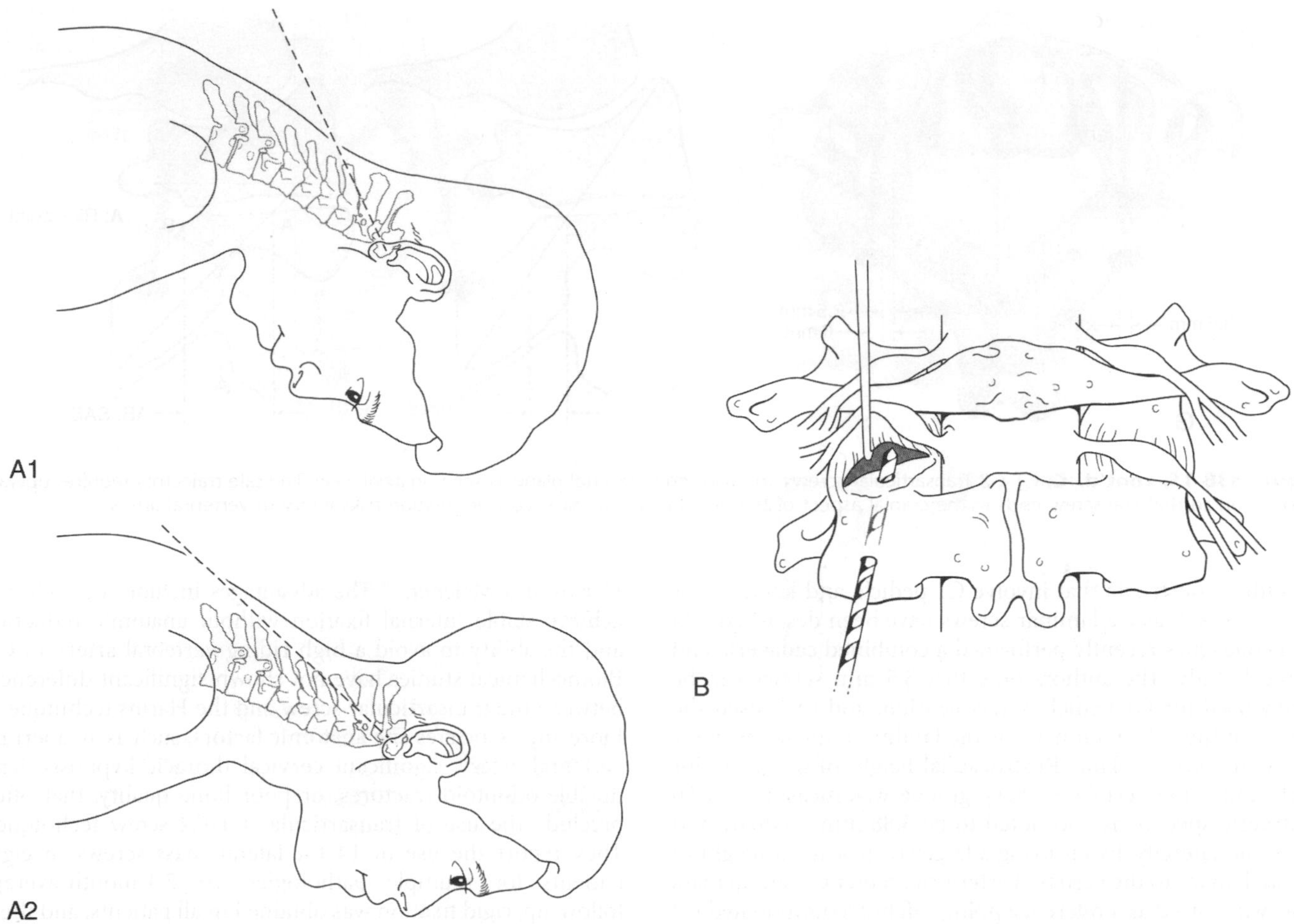

Figure 33B-17. Magerl method of fixation with transarticular C1-C2 screws. The patient is placed prone and the head immobilized with Mayfield skull tongs. The position of the neck needed for reduction of the deformity influences the exposure. **A1,** If the head can be flexed forward, the transarticular screws can be placed through the same posterior incision; however, if extension is needed to maintain the reduction of C1 (**A2**), a shorter incision is needed for exposure of the posterior elements of C1-C2, and the drill bit and instrumentation are passed into the wound through percutaneous incisions. **B,** The medial wall of the C2 pedicle should be exposed to aid in orienting the direction of the drill. The starting point for drilling is just medial to the edge of the facet joint and the inferior margin of the lamina of C2. Progress of the drill bit across the C1-C2 facet should be monitored using lateral image intensification for cephalad-caudal trajectory and direct visualization of the pars to assess medial-lateral trajectory. *(From Levine AM, Eismont FJ, Garfin SR, et al., editors: Spine trauma, Philadelphia, 1998, Saunders, pp 274, 275.)*

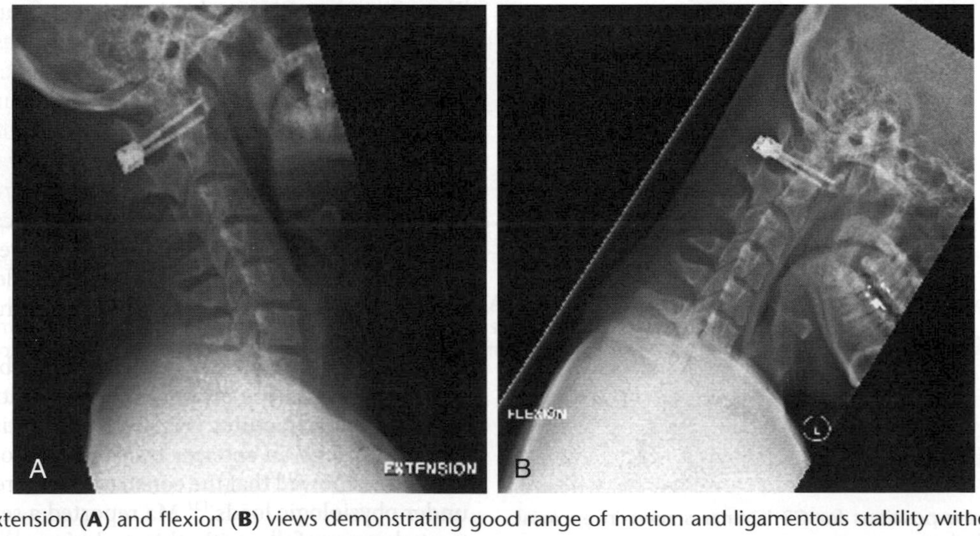

Figure 33B-18. Extension (**A**) and flexion (**B**) views demonstrating good range of motion and ligamentous stability without subluxation after C1 osteosynthesis.

the high complication rate of transoral surgery, two other studies[134,135] performed posterior C1 osteosynthesis with bilateral lateral mass screws connected via a rod under compression with good clinical outcomes. Late subluxation caused by ligamentous instability have not been seen in those authors' experience.

The technique of posterior direct osteosynthesis is done through a traditional posterior midline approach, with exposure similar as described previously (taking care for the vertebral artery along the superior aspect of the ring of C1). C1 lateral mass screws are placed as previously described and a horizontal rod connects them under compression (see Fig. 33B-11). Bransford and coworkers have demonstrated a small series of cases with good outcome on follow-up and preservation of motion.[65]

Pitfalls and Avoidance of Complications. Pitfalls lie in the placement of screws and in achieving an adequate fusion. Screw starting points should be selected with care and confirmed with radiography to avoid injury to the vertebral artery or high cervical cord. Trajectory should be similarly confirmed by radiography, with the use of a stab incision to the side of the incision for more lateral trajectory of C2 pedicle screws if needed, or inferiorly to enable dropping of the hand for C1-C2 transarticular screw placement. Preoperative CT or CTA should be studied before surgery to identify any bony abnormalities that would lend preference for one screw type over another. The preoperative CTA should also be used to assess the location of the internal carotid artery with respect to C1, as Currier and colleagues have reported a case of internal carotid artery injury during C1 screw placement, with a subsequent radiographic anatomic study confirming close proximity and laterality of the carotid to C1 resulting in a moderate risk of carotid injury in 48% of patients and a high risk in 12%.[136,137] In these cases, unicortical fixation or alternative techniques should be considered. Strong consideration should be made for the use of autograft to encourage bony fusion, which may be difficult to achieve.

Management of Intraoperative Problems. If in the course of drilling, tapping, or screw insertion, a vertebral artery injury is recognized, then the ipsilateral screw may be placed to tamponade the bleeding; however, the contralateral screw should not be inserted to avoid a potentially deadly bilateral vertebral artery injury. Consideration should be made for a postoperative angiogram to rule out pseudoaneurysm formation that could require embolization.

Postoperative Care and Rehabilitation. Postoperative care centers on encouraging fusion. Smoking cessation is encouraged. Osteoporosis should be investigated and treated if discovered. A cervical collar may be worn for comfort or to encourage fusion per surgeon preference. Although controversial, Jeanneret and Magerl[83] did not recommend postoperative immobilization when C1-C2 TAS is augmented with sublaminar wiring. In the event that wiring is not used in addition to screw placement and posterior fusion, immobilization with a semirigid collar brace has been recommended.[138]

Atlantoaxial Injuries and Transverse Atlantal Ligament Injuries

Emergent Treatment

The emergent treatment of atlantoaxial injuries is similar to that mentioned earlier for atlas fractures. Airway management and maintenance of stability are the main concerns.

Indications for Definitive Care

Treatment of atlantoaxial instability depends to some degree on whether the transverse ligament injury is a midsubstance tear or an avulsion of the ligament from the C1 lateral mass. However, most authors agree that nonoperative management is not indicated and that reduction followed by posterior fusion is the treatment of choice.[4,10,11,50,139] The time at which surgery should be performed to optimize outcome is unclear.

Nonoperative Treatment

Nonoperative treatment is generally not recommended for this injury unless it is a nondisplaced avulsion injury.

Surgical Treatment

The time at which surgery should be performed to optimize outcome is unclear. Because axial rotation is the major motion that occurs at the C1-C2 articulation, it would seem that a fusion that resists this type of motion is most appropriate. The various surgical options for posterior C1-C2 arthrodesis are the same as in atlas fractures mentioned earlier.

Surgical Anatomy. The atlantoaxial articulation comprises three joints: the paired lateral atlantoaxial facet joints and the central atlantoaxial joint. The lateral atlantoaxial facet joints are covered by thin, loose capsular ligaments that accommodate the large amount of rotation at this level. The central atlantoaxial joint, making up the ADI, is the articulation of the odontoid process with the posterior aspect of the C1 anterior arch. The crucial stabilizing structure is the transverse atlantal ligament, which essentially serves to harness the atlas to the dens of the axis. This ligament originates from two internal tubercles on the posterior aspect of the anterior arch of C1 and functions to stabilize the dens against the anterior arch of the atlas during rotation and translation. The paired alar ligaments attach to tubercles on the lateral rim of the foramen magnum and provide additional stability to the occipitoatlantal articulation. The apical dental ligament runs from the tip of the odontoid process to the ventral surface of the foramen magnum and is only a minor stabilizer of the craniocervical junction.[5,140]

Positioning Techniques. Positioning is done similarly to that described for atlas fractures, with utmost care to maintain proper alignment due to the extreme instability of some of these injuries. A Mayfield head holder works well to position and hold it rigidly. The positioning can be performed under lateral fluoroscopy to assure safety and proper alignment.

Surgical Approach. The surgical approach is the same as described earlier for atlas fractures.

Reduction Techniques. A recent case report discussed a patient with traumatic anterior atlantoaxial dislocation in whom atlantoaxial vertical dissociation developed after Gardner halo skull traction with 4.02 lb (1.5 kg). In addition to monitoring the C1-C2 LMI, the occiput-to-C1 interval should be observed during traction reduction. Furthermore, the closed-reduction attempt should be done only in a patient who is alert and oriented enough to cooperate with sequential neurologic exams. Some authors report, however, that longitudinal instability usually occurs with atlantoaxial dissociation and that longitudinal traction should be avoided altogether.[141,142]

Fixation Techniques. Biomechanical studies have shown that rigid fixation with Magerl's TAS or Harm's technique of C1 lateral mass and C2 pedicle screws are preferable.[109,143,144]

Pitfalls and Avoidance of Complications. Avoidance of complications is similar to those described earlier for atlas fractures.

Management of Intraoperative Problems. Management of intraoperative problems is similar to that described earlier for atlas fractures.

Postoperative Care and Rehabilitation. Postoperative care and rehabilitation is similar to that described earlier for atlas fractures.

Atlantoaxial Rotatory Subluxations and Dislocations

Emergent Treatment

Emergent treatment for rotary subluxations and dislocations is similar to that described earlier for atlas fractures.

Indications for Definitive Care

Although atlantoaxial rotatory instability in children usually responds to either immobilization or combined traction and immobilization,[145] only a few case reports describe this in adults.[146,147] In children, the most important factor in determining the efficacy of nonoperative management is the duration of rotatory subluxation, and similar experience in adults has been reported by Castel, who notes difficulty in reducing a dislocation, which occurred 4 weeks previously.[147]

Nonoperative Treatment

A recent adult case report noted a rugby player presenting with a 4-week history of torticollis who was treated with halo traction for 10 days followed by gentle manipulation. The transverse ligament at that time was noted to be intact and the patient was treated in a Minerva jacket for 6 weeks, after which no rotatory instability was noted with dynamic CT studies.[147] Closed manual reduction has also been described in the pediatric age group,[148] and in several adult cases.[149,150]

Nonoperative treatment for atlantoaxial rotary subluxations would require an intact transverse atlantal ligament and includes immobilization in a halo for several months.[42] Nonoperative treatment for traumatic atlantoaxial dislocations is not recommended.

Surgical Treatment

Surgical treatment is similar to that described earlier for atlas fractures and transverse ligament injuries with posterior C1-C2 arthrodesis. Specifically in the instance of posterior dislocations, several cases of irreducible lesions have been reported, which required subsequent anterior transoral or retropharyngeal decompression via odontoidectomy to achieve open reduction, followed by posterior stabilization via the techniques described earlier.[26]

Surgical Anatomy. Surgical anatomy is similar to that described earlier for atlas fractures.

Positioning Techniques. Positioning techniques are similar to those described earlier for atlas fractures.

Surgical Approach. The posterior surgical approach is similar to that described earlier for atlas fractures.

Reduction Techniques. Levine and Edwards advocate manipulation for acute cases due to trauma. Traction should be applied to the patient while he or she is awake, and because the reduction can usually be heard and palpated transorally, topical anesthetic should be applied to the posterior pharynx. A halo should be applied if the injury is stable.

Fixation Techniques. Arthrodesis as described earlier for atlas fractures. Arthrodesis can be done in situ and should be reserved for those cases that involve instability, neurologic involvement, or failure to maintain reduction.[17]

Pitfalls and Avoidance of Complications. Avoidance of complications is similar to that described earlier for atlas fractures

Management of Intraoperative Problems. Management of intraoperative problems is similar to that described earlier for atlas fractures.

Postoperative Care and Rehabilitation. Postoperative care and rehabilitation is similar to that described earlier for atlas fractures.

COMPLICATIONS

Because of the close proximity of critical structures to the high cervical levels, the possible complications from surgery in this area are significant and have been mentioned previously. Vertebral artery injury from a laterally misplaced screw can lead to brainstem or posterior circulation strokes, which may be devastating if collateral flow is inadequate. Medial displacement of a screw into the canal may lead to spinal cord injury or cerebrospinal fluid leakage. The usual complications of any surgery, including the risk of anesthetic induction as well as infection, are applicable to surgeries in this area. The thin occipital skin and the use of cervical collars postoperatively may predispose some patients, such as the elderly, to erosion of occipito-cervical hardware through the skin.

OUTCOME

Many patients with fractures of the atlas have long-term clinical complaints of scalp dysesthesias, neck pain, and decreased range of motion.[62,77] The incidence of these long-term complications increases with involvement of the lateral masses, as well as with other injuries to the occiput or C1-C2 articulation.[151] Other reported complications include nonunion.[62] A single study of 47 patients who underwent surgery for atlantoaxial dislocation from a variety of etiologies demonstrated achievement of pain relief in 95% of patients; however, only a very small subset of these patients had atlantoaxial dislocation caused by trauma, and therefore, these results may not be generalizable to patients with a traumatic injury.[152] A recent retrospective long-term analysis noted significantly lower quality of life in those patients with Jefferson fractures greater than 7-mm displacement as well as in those individuals with associated injuries.[153] This could suggest that more aggressive surgical management of these injuries may result in better long-term outcomes; however, no current literature exists on this topic.

META-ANALYSES AND SYSTEMATIC REVIEWS

A number of meta-analyses and systematic reviews have been conducted on these topics; however, firm information on isolated C1 injuries is still limited. Longo and colleagues performed a systematic review of treatment in halo vest immobilization for upper cervical spine injuries, although specific information for isolated C1 fractures is difficult to glean from this study.[154] A systematic review of the complications of upper cervical spine trauma in elderly patients was also conducted by Jubert and colleagues; however, this mainly represents C2 fracture data.[155]

GUIDELINES

Guidelines for the treatment of isolated fractures of the atlas in adults, as well as combination fractures of the atlas and axis in adults, were produced in 2002 and updated in 2013; however, because of insufficient evidence, only treatment options (level III evidence) are described.[156,157]

COST-EFFECTIVENESS

There have been no systematic assessments of cost-effectiveness between or among the various treatment options for these injuries.

CONCLUSION

Injuries to the atlas and atlantoaxial joint have the potential for acute catastrophic neurologic compromise as well as chronic disability. Although relatively rare in younger patients in clinical practice, these injuries are more common among elderly osteoporotic patients. Although similar in their mechanism of injury patterns, each specific injury requires a unique treatment algorithm to optimize outcomes. Many of the injuries may be treated conservatively; others, however, require a more aggressive surgical approach. Because of the rarity of some of these injuries, recommendations for treatment are often difficult.

KEY REFERENCES

The level of evidence (LOE) is determined according to the criteria provided in the preface.

1. Dickman CA, Sonntag VK: Injuries involving the transverse atlantal ligament: classification and treatment guidelines based upon experience with 39 injuries. *Neurosurgery* 40:886–887, 1997. LOE IV
18. Jefferson G: Fracture of the atlas vertebra. Report of four cases and a review of those previously recorded. *Br J Surg* 7:407–422, 1920. LOE IV
22. Spence KF Jr, Decker S, Sell KW: Bursting atlantal fracture associated with rupture of the transverse ligament. *J Bone Joint Surg Am* 52:543–549, 1970. LOE IV
57. Radcliff K, Sonagli MA, Rodrigues LM, et al: Does C1 fracture displacement correlate with transverse ligament integrity? *Orthop Surg* 5:94–99, 2013. LOE V
65. Bransford R, Chapman JR, Bellabarba C: Primary internal fixation of unilateral C1 lateral mass sagittal split fractures: a series of 3 cases. *J Spinal Disord Tech* 24:157–163, 2011. LOE IV
156. Ryken TC, Hadley MN, Aarabi B, et al: Management of acute combination fractures of the atlas and axis in adults. *Neurosurgery* 72:151–157, 2013. LOE III
157. Ryken TC, Hadley MN, Aarabi B, et al: Management of isolated fractures of the atlas in adults. *Neurosurgery* 72:127–131, 2013. LOE III

The complete References list is available online at https://expertconsult.inkling.com.

33C C2 Fractures

CHRISTIAN W. MÜLLER • SEBASTIAN DECKER • JOHN C. FRANCE • RYAN T. GOCKE • CHRISTIAN KRETTEK

INTRODUCTION: SCOPE AND PURPOSE

Fractures of the axis are diverse with several patterns having varying prognoses and include odontoid or dens fractures, traumatic spondylolisthesis of the axis, better known as the hangman's fracture, and poorly characterized axis body fractures. Fractures of the odontoid process are frequently spine injuries, occurring in 10% to 20% of all cervical spine injuries.[1,2] The atlantoaxial articulation provides important stability for the upper cervical spine; fractures of the odontoid result in spine instability with potential for spinal cord injuries. Moreover, fatal injuries can occur on this level,[3,4] although fatal traumatic quadriplegia due to an odontoid fracture is a rare phenomenon.[5] Hangman's fractures or traumatic spondylolisthesis represent distinct fractures of the axis and account for 4% to 7% of all cervical fractures.[6]

In Western civilization, there is a growing incidence of odontoid fractures compared to all spinal fractures. This is attributed both to the increase of the elderly population in Western society and technological advancements and availability of imaging modalities such as computed tomography (CT) or magnetic resonance imaging (MRI).[7] Radiographic visualization of the cervical spine using plain radiographs and CT scans results in a sensitivity of up to 100% for detecting cervical spine injuries.[8,9] In the elderly, C2 fractures typically result from simple falls, whereas in the younger population, high-energy trauma, such as motor vehicle accidents, leads to C2 fractures. Many patients sustain distracting injuries, which may mask the correct diagnosis.[10,11]

This chapter will summarize injuries of the axis and treatment options. Finally, detailed descriptions of surgical procedures will be presented.

maintains a minimal physiologic space between the atlas and the odontoid, the atlantodens interval (ADI). The ADI is 3 mm or less in adults and 5 mm or less in children. Enlargement indicates loss of integrity of the transverse atlantal ligament with resulting instability (see Fig. 33B-3). The articular capsular ligaments are thin and do not provide much stability. As shown in a biomechanical cadaveric study, the ligamentous upper cervical spine is stronger in extension than in flexion.[22]

During rotational movement, the atlas rotates around the dens with a range of motion of approximately 40 degrees. Flexion and extension between the atlas and the axis is limited to 20 degrees; lateral bending is limited to 5 degrees.[12] At least 50% of the rotational range of the cervical spine occurs on this level and the atlantoaxial articulations have little inherent stability. In a recent biomechanical study, stiffness of the cervical spine was shown to increase during maturation while the range of motion decreased.[23]

The mechanisms of injury for odontoid fractures are widely unknown but are most likely a combination of forces including hyperflexion, lateral bending, rotation, and extension. Although multiple injury patterns can result in traumatic spondylolisthesis, hyperextension and axial load are thought to be a major cause in type I and II injuries, whereas flexion forces are more likely to result in type IIA and III injuries.[10,24-26] In the elderly who sustain atlas fractures from falls from standing height, the mechanism is usually hyperextension, and the dens may have preexisting bony erosion from degenerative disease, which may have predisposed the patient to fracture.

EVALUATION

Clinical Assessment

The assessment of the cervical spine is very important for triage and initiation of further diagnostics, especially radiologic imaging. However, clinical tests, especially examining the axis, are not available. The cervical spine should be considered as a whole while symptoms at the level of C2 are suspicious for axis injuries. The protocols to evaluate the cervical spine after trauma are reviewed in Chapter 10.

During inspection, different aspects should be carefully considered. Open fractures of the axis are extremely rare. Nonetheless, soft tissue damage should be noted, including contusions of the head, especially the occiput and the front, as head impacts indicate strain of the cervical spine, too. These may give evidence as to the mechanism of injury. The spine contours should be analyzed for kyphosis or gibbus deformity. However, kyphosis and gibbus can be present in different diseases, for example, ankylosing spondylitis. After severe injuries, deviation of spinous processes that are usually located in a median sagittal line may be observed.

On structural damage, the head and cervical spine are often held in relieving posture. Fractures of the upper cervical spine can be accompanied with rotatory displacement or torticollis.

Immediate sudden neck pain after trauma is suspicious for injuries of the cervical spine, especially if associated with tenderness directly on top of the spinous processes. This has to be differentiated from muscle pain after distortion with compression pain of the muscles only, which is located more laterally. Moreover, facet joints have to be palpated and analyzed for tenderness. Pain on axial load indicates bony injuries and, if located in upper cervical spine levels, can be an indicator of C2 fractures. The pain is often referred in the distribution of the greater occipital nerve and thus patients complain of occipital headache.

Dislocated cervical spine injuries can result in complete tetraplegia. However, incomplete neurologic deficits can be subtler and have to be searched for by thorough neurologic examination, especially of the arms. Missing anal sphincter reflexes indicate complete paraplegia. Incomplete paraplegia goes along with retaining functions.

As fractures of the axis, especially odontoid fractures, often occur in the elderly, palpation and range of motion have to be interpreted with caution as symptoms can be caused by other diseases. Neurologic pathologies, for example, dementia can be misleading. Moreover, especially in the elderly, fractures can be completely asymptomatic. Physicians should be alert whenever the mechanism of injury can result in cervical spine fractures in these situations. As fractures of the axis must not be missed, radiologic diagnostics should be applied liberally if clinical examination cannot exclude severe injuries and the mechanism of injury is suspicious for any injury. Rihn and Harris summarized details as to the detailed clinical examination of the cervical spine.[27]

Imaging

The imaging of the spine is described in Chapter 30. Evaluation of axis fractures requires both lateral and open-mouth views if plain radiographs are used. However, CT has more sensitivity and provides a more complete understanding of the fracture morphology. Other contiguous and noncontiguous fractures are common with axis fractures, and therefore, complete imaging of the spine is required. MRI is rarely required to evaluate axis fractures. CT angiography may be warranted when there is atlantoaxial displacement between or fractures involve the foramen transversarium.

Radiologically, odontoid fractures can be assumed if a fracture line is visible or the dens is dislocated, which often results in asymmetry of the dens in between the occipital condyles. Lateral tilting of the dens is suspicious for a type III fracture if no other fracture is visible. In healthy individuals, the odontoid angle is not less than 87 degrees; however, in type III fractures, angulation up to 67 degrees has been noted. The altered odontoid angle may be the only radiologic sign of a fracture.[28] On lateral views, the ADI can be evaluated.

In a retrospective study of confirmed cases of odontoid fractures, Ehara and colleagues found that in 47 out of 50 cases (94%), plain radiographs disclosed the fracture. Initial cross-table lateral view alone showed the fracture in 43 cases. In the remaining four cases, routine plain films revealed the fracture: open-mouth view in three cases and lateral skull view in one case.[9]

Furthermore, CT allows precise analysis of the fracture morphology. Thin CT slice thickness should be used to avoid missing transverse fractures.[29] Modern multidetector helical CT obtains volumetric data so that reconstruction can be formatted with equal spatial resolution in all three planes, allowing more precision of the extent of comminution.[30] Interobserver reliability is increased in CT compared to plain films as demonstrated by Barker and colleagues.[31] Bono and colleagues analyzed the interobserver and intraobserver reliability of angulation and displacement measurements for

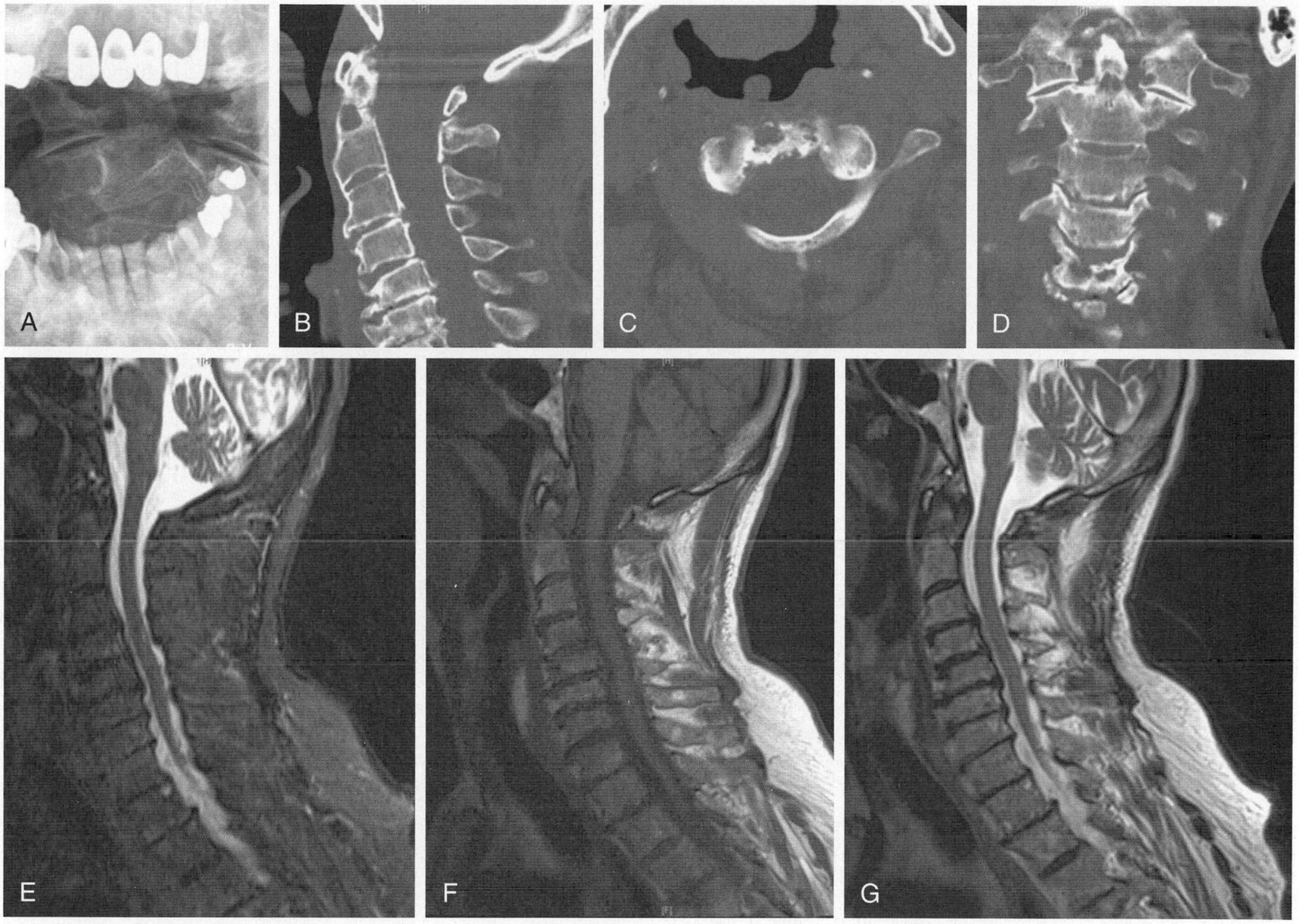

Figure 33C-5. An 81-year-old male suffered from slight tenderness of the upper cervical spine after a car accident. He did not have any complaints before and no previous injury was reported. Radiographic diagnostics revealed a type II odontoid fracture that directly crossed a large cyst at the base of the dens (**A–D**). Only a small hematoma and edema were shown in computed tomography (CT) scan and magnetic resonance imaging (MRI) (**B–G**). Due to the age and nondisplacement, rigid collar immobilization was applied only.

odontoid fractures, as well as traumatic spondylolisthesis, and compared results from plain films and CT. Intrarater analysis demonstrated high reproducibility; however, interobserver evaluation was poor. The authors stated that radiographic measurements for C2 fracture are of moderate reliability with only limited agreement.[32] Additionally, CT and lateral plain films provide essential information about the integrity and rigidity of the subaxial levels. CT also allows estimation of bone quality useful for surgical planning.

Retropharyngeal soft tissue swelling or hematoma formations at the craniocervical region are indicators of probable injury. In geriatric patients, erosions in the dens or remote fractures may be present and can be discriminated by identification of a hematoma as a sign of a fresh fracture and by critical analysis of the fracture lines. In difficult cases, MRI can be used to determine fracture. Moreover, MRI provides information about integrity of ligaments, especially interspinous ligaments and the anterior longitudinal ligament that may be helpful in evaluating stability (Fig. 33C-5). Lateral flexion-extension cervical spine radiography has been proposed in order to determine stability of dens fractures.[33]

Hangman's fractures can usually be diagnosed on the lateral view. Hematoma formation between the axis and the trachea indicate rupture of the anterior longitudinal ligament, which occurs in type IIA and III fractures. Three-dimensional (3-D) imaging is essential in the analysis of hangman's fractures as well. CT scans reveal extent of dislocation, rotational deformity, and intraarticular fractures.[32] MRI is needed infrequently to examine intervertebral discs and ligaments.[34]

DIAGNOSIS AND CLASSIFICATION

Odontoid Fracture

Anderson and D'Alonzo introduced the most common classification for odontoid fractures in 1974 and divided them into types I through III depending on the location of the fracture line (Fig. 33C-6).[35]

Type I fractures are rare and account for approximately 1% of odontoid fractures.[36] They represent avulsion fractures of the alar or apical ligaments at the tip of the odontoid process. The most likely mechanism of injury of a type I fracture is traction in the coronal plane of the alar ligaments and may therefore represent an occipito-cervical dissociation.[37,38] Type I odontoid fractures have to be differentiated from a congenital nonunion of the tip of the odontoid, an ossiculum terminale, which, however, is a rare phenomenon that usually does not need any specific therapy.[39] Nevertheless,

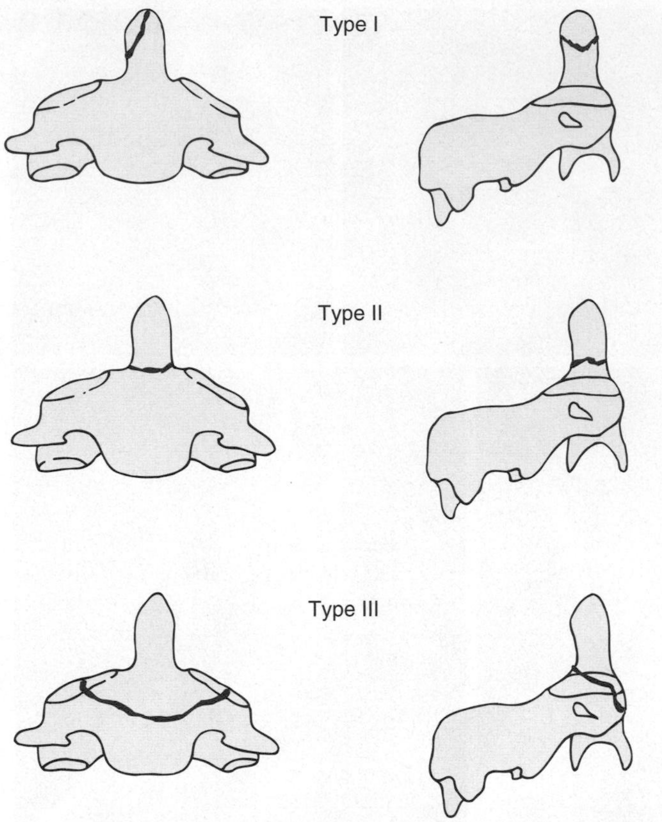

Figure 33C-6. Three types of odontoid fractures as seen in the anteroposterior *(left)* and lateral *(right)* planes. Type I is an oblique fracture through the upper part of the odontoid process itself. Type II is a fracture at the junction of the odontoid process and the vertebral body of the second cervical vertebra. Type III is really a fracture through the body of the atlas. *(Redrawn from Anderson LD, D'Alonzo RT: Fractures of the odontoid process of the axis, J Bone Joint Surg Am 56:1663–1674, 1974.)*

cases of instability have been reported that required fixation.[40] Moreover, ossifications of the ligaments near the apex of the odontoid can sometimes resemble type I fractures.[41,42]

Type II fractures are located at the junction of the odontoid base and the C2 vertebral body and have the highest incidence among odontoid fractures accounting for 65% to 74% of all odontoid fractures.[35,43] Eysel and Roosen subclassified type II fractures with respect to the orientation of the fracture line to facilitate decision making whether ventral or dorsal fixation is more advisable. Type IIA fractures present horizontally, type IIB fractures present with a fracture line extending from superior-anterior to inferior-posterior, and type IIC fracture lines extend from superior-posterior to inferior-anterior. Type IIC fractures are the most unstable. Eysel and Roosen recommended anterior screw fixation for types IIA and IIB fractures, whereas C1/C2 posterior fusion was recommended for type IIC fractures.[44]

Type III fractures according to Anderson and D'Alonzo present with a fracture line that passes through the cranial cancellous vertebral body. Although the classification introduced by Anderson and D'Alonzo is commonly used, controversy exists as to the distinction between type II and type III fractures.

Grauer and colleagues modified the classification by Anderson and D'Alonzo to aid in surgical decision making. They distinguished between those fractures that do not involve the superior articular facet of C2 (type II) and those that do involve the superior articular facet (type III). Type II fractures were divided into nondisplaced fractures (type IIA), anterior-superior to posterior-inferior and displaced transverse fractures (type IIB), and anterior-inferior to posterior-superior or comminuted fractures (type IIC). They recommended external immobilization in type IIA fractures, anterior screw fixation in type IIB fractures, and posterior atlantoaxial fusion in type IIC fractures.[45] Hadley and coworkers called a comminuted type II fracture, type IIA, which had a much poorer prognosis for healing nonoperatively.

Distinction of type II from type III fractures can be difficult and interpretation of plain films and CT scans vary between physicians. Barker and colleagues analyzed the interobserver and intraobserver reliability of the Anderson and D'Alonzo classification with special regard to type II and type III fractures comparing plain films and CT. Both neuroradiologists and spine surgeons participated in the study. Interobserver and intraobserver reliability was better with CT scan than with plain films. Nevertheless, the overall interobserver reliability was moderate. The authors pointed out that the lack in reproducibility and reliability might have affected the classification of odontoid fractures in previously published studies and might therefore have affected study results.[31]

Traumatic Spondylolisthesis (Hangman's Fracture)

The traumatic spondylolisthesis of the axis is classically characterized by bilateral fracture through the C2 pars interarticularis. This injury pattern has been described as the result of judicial hanging since the late nineteenth century, but Schneider in 1965 first coined the phrase "hangman's fracture" for the radiographic appearance of the injury regardless of its actual cause.[46-48] In fact, judicial hanging usually results in hyperextension and distraction with complete disruption of the C2-C3 disc space and associated ligaments between them.[47,49,50] However, the bilateral fractures through the C2 pars interarticularis observed with hanging can also occur after falls and motor vehicle accidents from various combinations of extension, axial compression, and flexion and cause different degrees of disc disruption.[51-53] In motor vehicle accidents, traumatic spondylolisthesis of the axis was reported half as commonly (a reported incidence of 27%) as odontoid fracture.[54] In fatal motor vehicle accidents, only occipitoatlantal dislocations were more common.[55] Interestingly, only a minority of judicial hangings actually result in a bilateral fracture through the C2 pars interarticularis. An anatomic study including 34 victims of judicial hanging revealed only three typical hangman's fractures and three other fractures of the axis.[56,57]

The anatomic nomenclature must be kept in mind when describing these injuries. Although the pars interarticularis of the axis and the pedicle of the axis are, strictly speaking, two distinct anatomic structures, the two terms have been used interchangeably in the literature. As with most injuries of the upper cervical spine, traumatic spondylolisthesis tends to produce acute decompression of the neural canal and neurologic involvement is relatively uncommon in survivors (seen in 6% to 10%).[48,55,58-60] However, reports of atypical hangman's fractures that involve the posterior C2 vertebral body have shown the potential for spinal canal compromise with displacement of the vertebral body fragment into the spinal canal

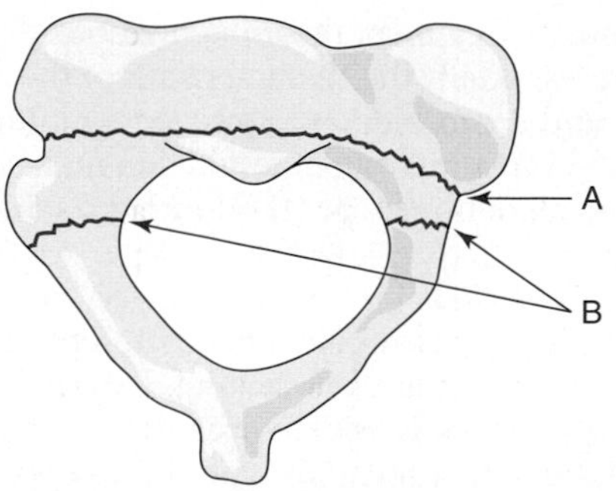

Figure 33C-7. The atypical hangman's fracture line (**A**) leaves the canal circumferentially intact and puts the spinal cord at risk if displaced, whereas the typical hangman's fracture (**B**) displaces the vertebral body anteriorly and its corresponding posterior element posteriorly, thus creating increased space for the spinal cord.

(Fig. 33C-7).[61] Some case reports of these injuries describe closed reduction and halo vest immobilization (HVI) with subsequent neurologic deterioration because of development of a large epidural hematoma.[62] Craniofacial trauma is very common with these injuries; moreover, vertebral artery and cranial nerve injuries have also been reported. Associated cervical spine injuries with C2 traumatic spondylolisthesis almost always involve the upper three cervical vertebrae.[59,60,63]

Stability of this injury has been shown to be related to the integrity of the ligaments and disc between the C2-C3 bodies and can be determined radiographically.[55,64] The most common classification was published first by Effendi and modified by Levine (Fig. 33C-8).[64,65] The classification system takes into account both angulation of the dens and displacement of the C2 body in relation to the C3 body. The integrity of the C2-C3 discoligamentous complex (disc, anterior longitudinal ligament, posterior longitudinal ligament) is considered based on the radiographic findings.

Type I fractures are nondisplaced and show no angulation and have less than 3 mm of displacement (Fig. 33C-8, *A*). They usually result from a hyperextension and axial loading force that fractures the neural arch through the pars and there is minimal disruption to the C2-C3 disc.

Type II fractures present with significant translation and some angulation (Fig. 33C-8, *B*). They usually result from a hyperextension and axial load (as seen with type I injuries) followed by flexion and compression. The combined forces result in disruption of the posterior longitudinal ligament and disc in a posterior-to-anterior direction and may have a compression fracture of the C3 anterior-superior end plate.

Type IIA fractures show slight or no translation but severe angulation of the fracture fragments (Fig. 33C-8, *C*). This fracture pattern is seen with flexion and distraction and results

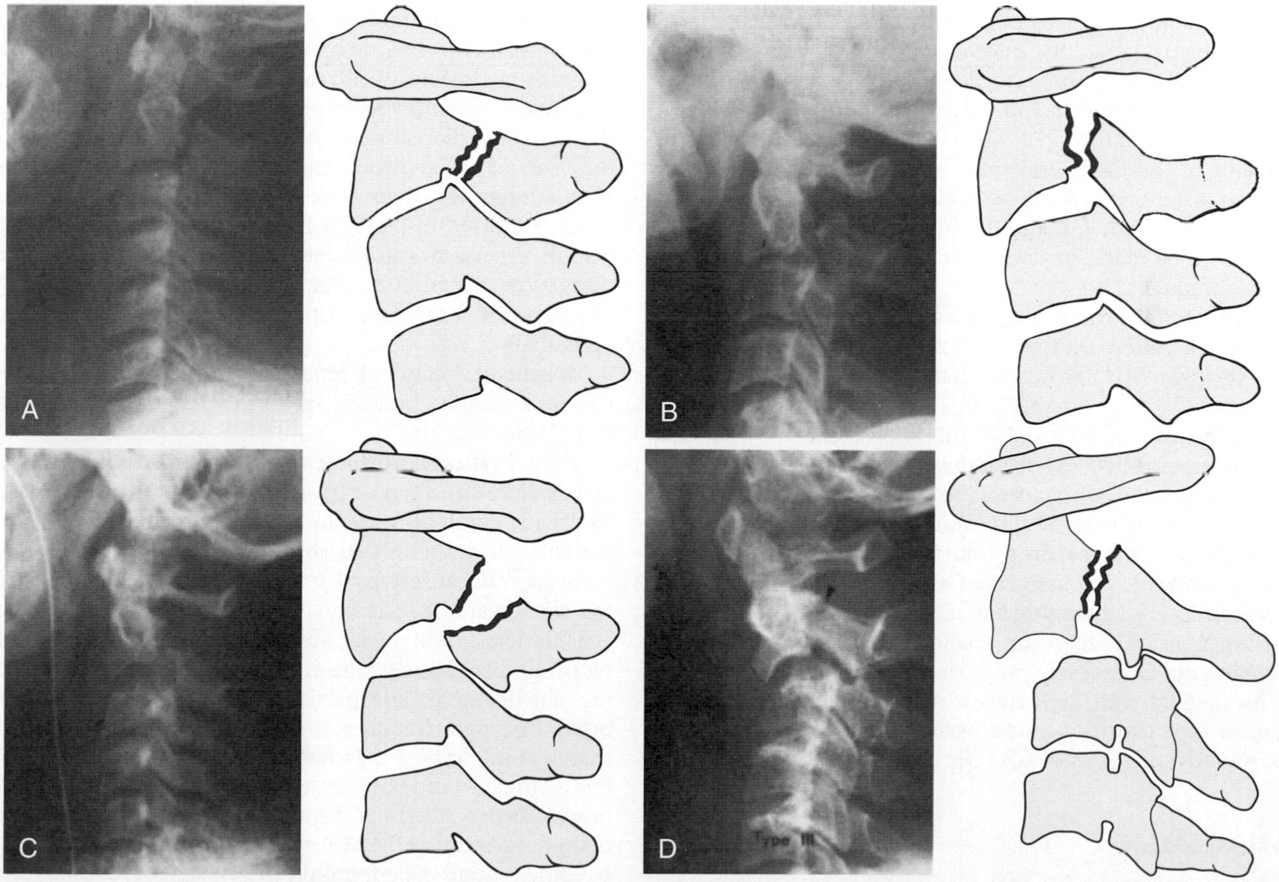

Figure 33C-8. Classification of traumatic spondylolisthesis of the axis. **A,** Type I injuries have a fracture through the neural arch with no angulation and as much as 3 mm of displacement. **B,** Type II fractures have both significant angulation and displacement. **C,** Type IIA fractures show minimal displacement, but severe angulation is present. **D,** Type III axial fractures combine bilateral facet dislocation between C2 and C3 with a fracture of the neural arch of the axis. *(Source **A–C:** From Levine AM, Edwards CC: The management of traumatic spondylolisthesis of the axis, J Bone Joint Surg Am 67:217–226, 1985; **D:** From Levine AM, Edwards CC: Treatment of injuries in the C1-C2 complex, Orthop Clin North Am 17:42, 1986.)*

in a vertical tear of the posterior longitudinal ligament and the disc.

Type III fractures have a concomitant unilateral or bilateral C2-C3 facet dislocations (Fig. 33C-8, *D*). The spinal canal is narrowed in this pattern and spinal cord injury is more likely than other hangman's type fracture. This pattern is thought to result from flexion and compression resulting in complete disruption of the discoligamentous complex.

Generally speaking, type I fractures are thought to be stable because of an intact C2-C3 discoligamentous complex; types II, IIA, and III are unstable because of disruption at the C2-C3 interspace. In their series of 131 patients, type II fractures were the most common and seen in 56% of patients, followed by type I injuries, type III, and type IIA, which accounted for 29%, 10%, and 6% of patients, respectively.[64]

Josten advocated that type II hangman's fractures represent a very heterogeneous group and divided these fractures into those with intact anterior ligaments (so-called Josten type 2) and those with ruptured anterior ligaments (so-called Josten type 3), whereas a locked dislocation constituted a Josten type 4 fracture.[66]

Atypical C2 Fractures (Corpus Fractures)

Lateral mass fractures of the C2 vertebra are rarely reported and have a mechanism of injury similar to those causing lateral mass fractures of the atlas. Axial compression and lateral bending forces combine to compress the C1-C2 articulation and result in a depressed fracture of the articular surface of C2. Patients generally have a history of pain without neurologic deficit. Plain radiographs may be unremarkable, although anteroposterior and open-mouth views sometimes demonstrate lateral tilting of the arch of C1 and asymmetry of the height of the C2 lateral mass. If lateral mass fracture is suspected, CT of the area is helpful to more clearly delineate the injury. A search for additional fractures in the cervical spine should be made, as concomitant injuries of the cervical spine are frequent.[67]

Benzel classified these "corpus fractures" according to their predominant pattern as type 1 (coronal), type 2 (sagittal), or type 3 (horizontal).[68] However, combinations and variations are common.[69]

Small avulsion fractures of the anterior-inferior corner of the axis, so-called extension teardrop, tend to be stable injuries, associated with an extension-type mechanism and without associated neurologic injury. They are distinct from lower cervical spine teardrop injuries resulting from flexion, which are unstable and associated with neurologic injury 75% of the time. A distinguishable radiographic feature of extension-type (C2) teardrop fracture is anterior rotation of the fragment. Conversely, a flexion-type teardrop fracture remains aligned with the anterior margin of the spine. A C2 extension-type teardrop fracture can be associated with traumatic spondylolisthesis of C2 (Fig. 33C-9).[70,71]

MANAGEMENT

Odontoid Fractures

Introduction

The treatment of odontoid fractures remains controversial with both surgical and nonsurgical methods being recommended. Morbidity is high, especially in the elderly, following either treatment. Treatment recommendations depend on the fracture type, especially the characteristics of the fracture line, patient age, and comorbidities. However, a multicenter study showed, that no treatment at all resulted in no healing in all of 18 type II and all of three type III odontoid fractures.[43]

Treatment Options

Definitive evidence-based guidelines as to optimal treatment for odontoid fractures are still lacking. External immobilization for 6 to 8 weeks is widely accepted for type I and III fractures. Optimal treatment for type II fractures is most controversial. Most authors prefer surgical treatment, but here, too, controversy exists as to which technique should be used.[72] Nondisplaced or minimally displaced type II injuries can be managed by closed reduction and external HVI, especially in younger patients. Patients presenting with re-displacement following reduction, inadequate reduction, or delayed (approximately 2 weeks) presentation after injury should be treated operatively.[73] Fusion rates of posterior C1-C2 fixation are excellent, but fixation is associated with 50% loss of atlantoaxial rotation. Theoretically, anterior screw fixation preserves atlantoaxial rotation motion. In an in vitro biomechanical study of halo vest and odontoid screw fixation of type II dens fracture spinal motions with the dens screw alone could not be differentiated from physiologic limits[74]; however, a CT study by Jeanneret and colleagues showed decreased atlantoaxial mobility after screw fixation of the odontoid in 8 out of 13 patients at examinations 7 to 82 months after injury.[75] Furthermore, this technique requires closed reduction and is not technically feasible in all cases. Konieczny reported a new treatment algorithm for type II and III fractures: In accordance with earlier studies, fractures were classified as stable if they had an initial displacement of less than 5 mm and initial angulation of less than 11 degrees on the CT scans as well as anteroposterior displacement of less than 2 mm on lateral flexion-extension sagittal radiographs. Stable odontoid fractures were treated in a collar for 12 weeks. Unstable fractures as well as stable fractures with neurologic deficits were treated operatively.[33]

In general, treatment depends on type of fracture, stability, risk of nonunion, biologic age of the patient, and comorbidities (Table 33C-1).

Type I Odontoid Fractures. Most type I fractures are nondisplaced and can be treated nonoperatively unless associated with craniocervical instability. In stable type I injuries, patients are immobilized in a rigid or semirigid collar for 6 weeks.[35] Because type I fractures are avulsion fractures of the alar or apical ligaments, the integrity of the atlantodens articulation should not be affected. Nevertheless, some authors reported disruption of the occipital portion of at least one of the alar ligaments and partial rupture of the tectorial membrane in type I fractures.[76,77] This questions whether type I fractures might be a manifestation of occipital-cervical instability, which would be an indication for surgery. Detailed diagnostics as described in Chapter 33A should be performed, as missed occipital-cervical instability may be fatal. Soft tissue swelling around the odontoid can be a sign of subluxation and, therefore, instability.[37]

Type II. Optimal treatment for type II fractures remains controversial and treatment options include hard collars, HVI, or surgery with anterior screw fixation or posterior fusion. Type II fractures are at the highest risk for nonunion

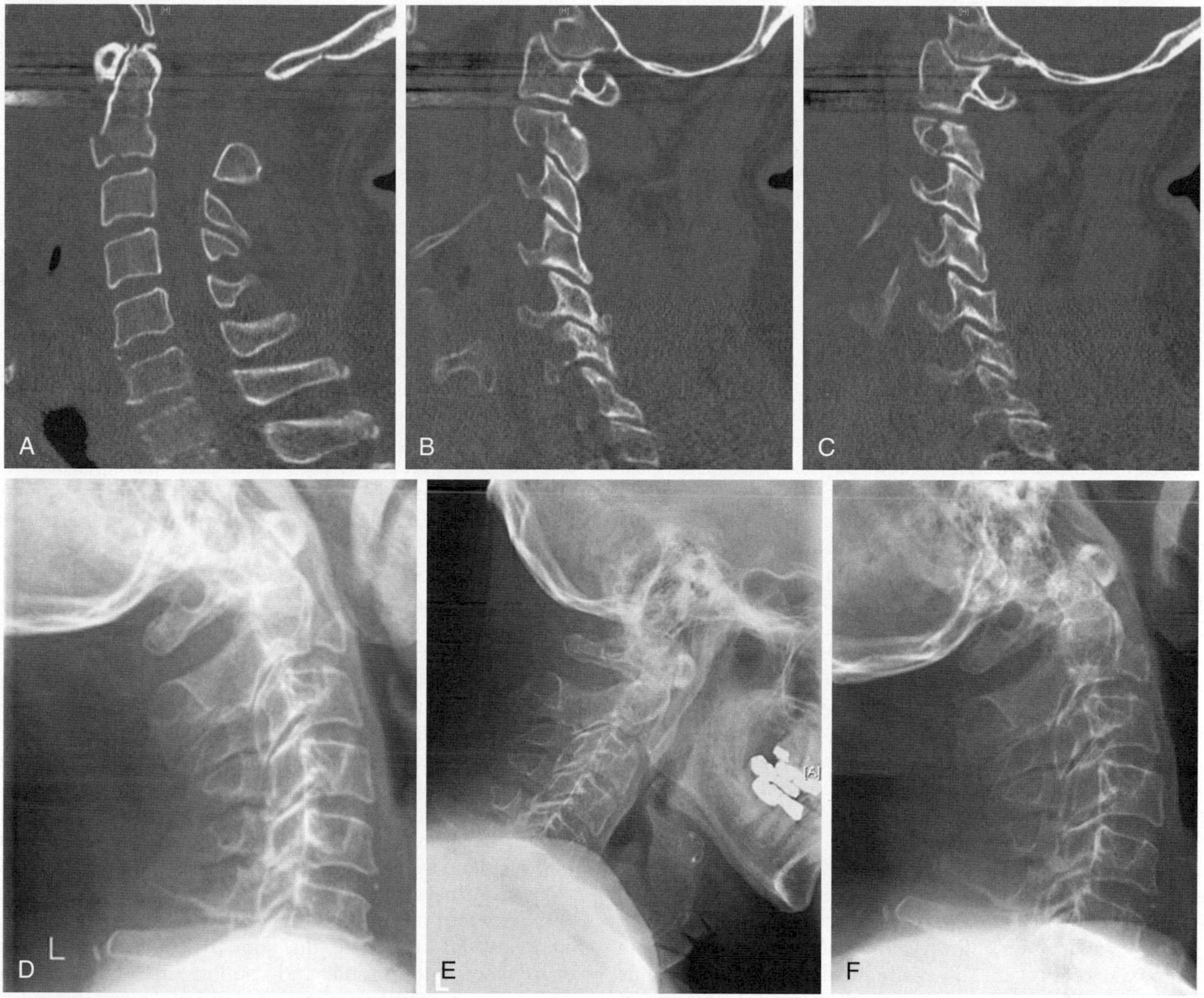

Figure 33C-9. A 59-year-old restrained car driver who crashed into a truck and sustained a teardrop fracture of C2. Additional injuries were traumatic brain injury type II with subarachnoid bleeding, fracture of the skull, fracture of the os sphenoidale, open fracture of the maxilla, multiple soft tissue wounds, and a fracture of the first lumbar vertebra. Halo vest immobilization was applied for 6 weeks followed by 4 weeks of semirigid collar immobilization. **A–C,** Acute fracture is demonstrated. Ten weeks after injury, the fracture was healed in plain radiographs (**D**) and stable in flexion (**E**) and extension (**F**) films.

TABLE 33C-1 *TREATMENT OPTIONS FOR ODONTOID FRACTURES*

	Treatment	Indications
Type I	Hard collar	No craniocervical displacement
	Occipital-cervical fusion	Associated craniocervical dissociation
Type II	Hard or soft collar	Geriatric fracture
	Halo vest	Nondisplaced fractures (<5 mm)
	Odontoid screw	High risk for nonunion (displaced, angulated)
		Nondisplaced in polytrauma patient
		Cannot tolerate halo vest
	Posterior C1-C2 fusion	Displaced type II, especially elderly
		Associated injuries, such as C1 ring fractures, C2 body fractures
		Displaced type II when odontoid screw not possible, e.g., barrel chest, fracture comminution
Type III	Halo vest	Displaced but reducible fracture
	Hard or soft collar	Nondisplaced fracture
		Geriatric fracture
	Internal fixation	Osseous instability in extension-flexion radiographs

with the incidence being up to 85% in the elderly when treated nonoperatively.[78]

Risk Factors for Nonunion. Odontoid fracture healing depends on various factors such as age as well as reduction and stabilization.[79-81] Clark and White found that displacements greater than 4 to 5 mm and angulation greater than 10 degrees were associated with nonunions in type III fractures in 40% and 22% of cases, respectively; 48 patients with type III fractures and various treatments were analyzed.[43] Moreover, external factors such as smoking affect healing through a decreased blood flow. Elderly patients, as well as people suffering from osteoporosis, tend to have a higher risk of nonunion.[82,83] Posterior displacement, as well as delayed treatment, result in higher rates of nonunion.[81]

Greene and colleagues analyzed the integrity of the transverse atlantal ligament using MRI in patients suffering from odontoid fractures. Disruption was associated with acute or delayed instability. Therefore, authors recommend surgical treatment in case of transverse atlantal ligament rupture.[84] However, analysis of the transverse atlantal ligament depends on the quality of the MRI as shown by Schmidt and coworkers who compared 1.5 and 3 tesla MRI for its evaluation.[85] Anterior screw fixation in these cases might be relatively contraindicated as to the potential risk for rotational instability and C1-C2 posterior stabilization providing better mechanical stability should be favored.[86,87]

Nonoperative Care. Nonoperative treatment is most effective using the halo vest, although, as many patients, such as the elderly, poorly tolerate this immobilization method, simpler methods such as soft and hard collar and cervicothoracic braces are likewise recommended.

Odontoid Screw

Advantages and Disadvantages. Anterior screw fixation can be performed via a limited anterior approach with little dissection of muscles. As this procedure results in a direct reduction and fixation of the fracture, rotational motion of the atlantoaxial joint is generally maintained. The patient remains in supine position, which can be advantageous in cases of comorbidities or accompanying injuries. However, reduction can be difficult and impede the ideal trajectory for drilling and inserting the screw. Proper intraoperative imaging with preferably two image intensifiers is mandatory.

Indications and Contraindications. Anterior screw fixation is well indicated in younger patients with fair bone quality and reducible fractures without gross comminution. Relative contraindications are conditions in which primary fracture healing is doubtful, as in delayed surgery, comminuted fractures and other fracture types in which a lag screw effect cannot be achieved, such as type IIC fractures according to Eysel and Rosen, or with severe osteoporosis. Absolute contraindications are irreducible fractures or fractures that can only be reduced in flexion, severe thoracic kyphosis, barrel chests, or stiff cervical spines that impede drilling and screw positioning.[78,88-90] However, in our own clinical practice, a large majority of young or older aged patients is successfully managed with anterior screw fixation (Fig. 33C-10).

Posterior C1-2 Fusion

Advantages and Disadvantages. Depending on the fixation techniques, posterior fusion does not necessarily require closed reduction beforehand. Basically all fracture types can be addressed. However, exposure of the dorsal aspects of C2 and C1 requires detachment of muscles and can result in significant intraoperative bleeding. Posterior fusion leads to significant reduction of rotational motion of the cervical spine.

Indications and Contraindications. In comparison to anterior screw osteosynthesis, the main indications for posterior C1-C2 fixation are comminuted fractures, severe osteoporosis, irreducible fractures, and pseudarthrosis, as well as most cases in which anterior screw osteosynthesis is contraindicated.[33,91-93]

Data comparing anterior screw fixation and posterior fusion are lacking. No guidelines exist as to when to use which technique and clinical results seem to be similar, although fusion rates are greater after posterior fixations compared to anterior screw fixation. Posterior fusion after posterior C1-C2 stabilization was documented in 96% to 100% of patients.[43,94-96] Different techniques are available including the Gallie, Magerl, and Harms techniques.[97,98] Lin and colleagues compared the Gallie and Harms techniques for the treatment of type II and III fractures. Fusion time was equal for both treatment protocols.[99]

Aryan and colleagues published a study on 102 patients with upper cervical spine instability caused by chronic type II odontoid fractures in 48 of these cases. They performed posterior C1-C2 screw fixation using the Harms technique as well as a modification of it. Nonunion occurred in two cases (2%).[100]

Type III. Type III odontoid fractures, too, have been treated both surgically and nonsurgically. They account for up to 30% of all odontoid fractures.[101] While there is a consensus that treatment is necessary, data on the outcome without external immobilization or surgery are rare. Without treatment, nonunion rates up to 100% have been observed.[43] Treatment options include external immobilization in collars as well as halo vests or Minerva jackets. Fusion rates using halo vests or Minerva jackets are 81% to 100%, whereas most authors report union rates higher than 90%.[43,101-107] However, complications related to this kind of immobilization have to be taken into account and comfort in daily life is poor. Alternatively, rigid or nonrigid cervical collars have been applied for immobilization. In the few series, healing rates up to 100% have been reported; however, adequate evidence is missing.[43,103,105,108] Operative intervention with posterior cervical fixation for type III fractures has also been performed with union rates of 97% to 100%. While healing rates are excellent, complications including death occurred in up to 4% of cases.[43,103,105,109] Anterior screw fixation can also be performed with union rates up to 100% being reported.[103,109] Overall, nonunions are rare in type III injuries. For significantly displaced fractures, authors recommend reduction and halo immobilization, whereas nondisplaced fractures might be treated in a rigid collar. However, some physicians also recommend C1-C2 posterior arthrodesis in cases of 5 mm or more of vertical displacement. Type II fractures according to the Grauer classification have been shown to heal well after screw osteosynthesis (Fig. 33C-11).[110-112]

Geriatric Odontoid Fractures. Odontoid fractures in the elderly are associated with significant morbidity and mortality similar to that following hip fracture. Treatment is therefore being intensively examined. Risks associated with surgery or prolonged immobilization, however, have to be assessed individually. Medical comorbidities and associated injuries have to be taken into consideration. Stable nonunions might be acceptable in patients with otherwise limited activities.[113]

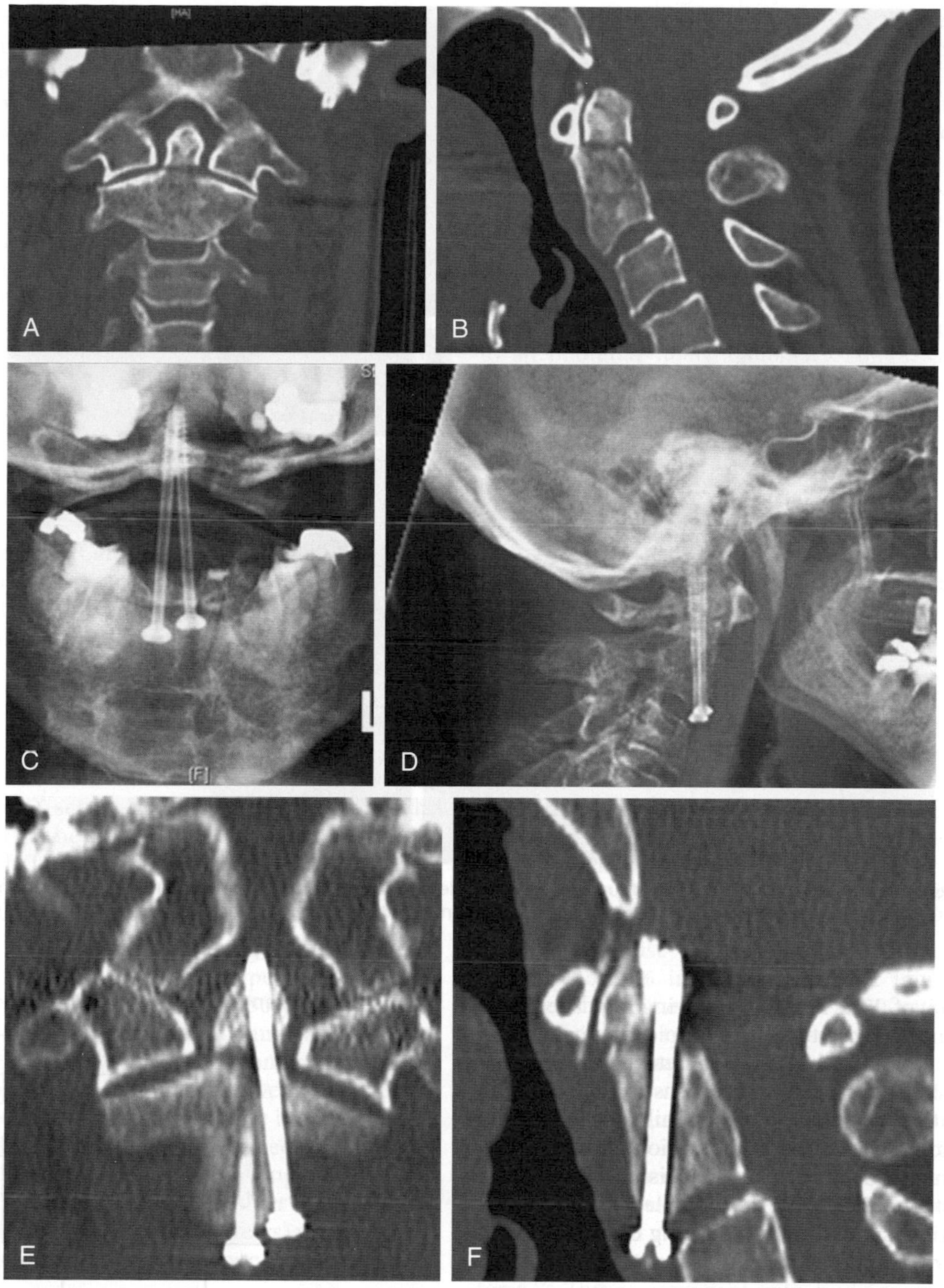

Figure 33C-10. A through **F,** A 61-year-old female presented with a nonunion 12 months after anterior screw fixation of a type II odontoid fracture caused by a riding accident. Moreover, she suffered from an atlas arch fracture that did not heal either. The direction of the screws for osteosynthesis of the dens was very posterior. No secondary dislocation was observed. The patient still suffered from pain 1 year after injury. We recommended revision surgery; however, the patient refused.

As type II dens fractures often occur in the elderly, Börm and coworkers analyzed the effect of age on fusion after anterior screw fixation in a case-control study. They stated that union rates were similar in people aged older or younger than 70 years.[114] Chapman and colleagues recently published that surgical treatment for type II odontoid fractures in the elderly did not negatively impact survival; instead, long-time survival tended to be better in the surgically treated group; 322 patients were included in this retrospective study.[115] Anterior screw fixation results in comparable cervical spine function levels in young people and the elderly; however, surgical complication rates and mortality were higher in the elderly.[116] Smaller studies on nonrigid or semirigid stabilization with collars showed controversial results. Chaudhary and colleagues reported that six of nine patients treated with a rigid collar for minimally or nondisplaced type II odontoid fracture were fused at a mean follow-up of 5 months, whereas seven of eight patients were fused in the surgical group.[117] Contrarily, Molinari and colleagues found radiologic evidence of osseous union using plain radiographs in only 2 out of 34

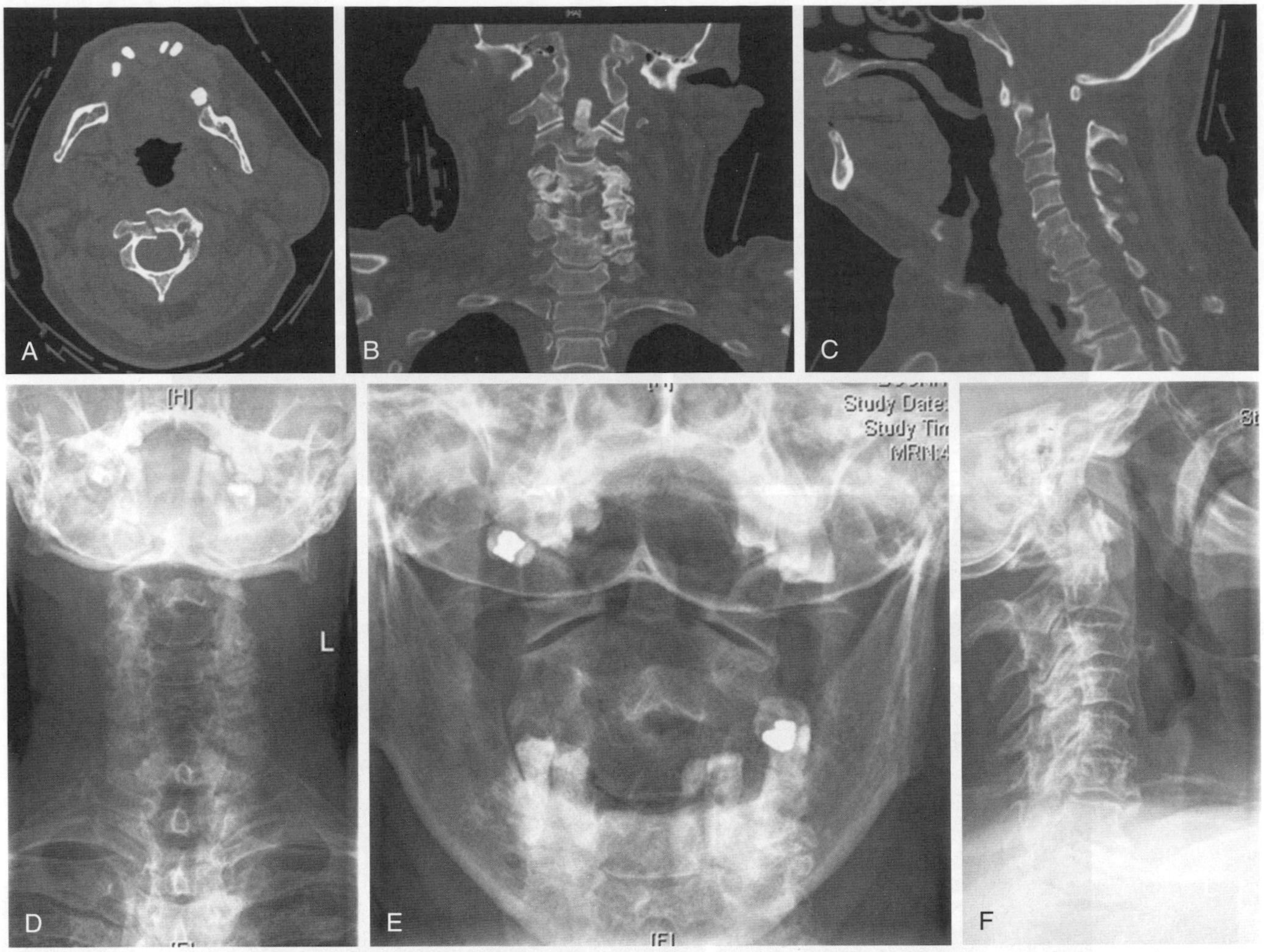

Figure 33C-15. A 74-year-old geriatric male patient suffering from an atypical C2 corpus fracture involving the C2 articular process. The patient was treated with closed reduction and halo vest immobilization for 6 weeks followed by a soft collar for another 6 weeks. The halo had to be revised after 1 week due to loosening. No further complications occurred. No pain was observed after 3 months; however, motion was limited. Overall mobility of the patient was equal to preinjury. **A** through **C,** The acute fracture is seen. **D** through **F,** Plain films at 5 months' follow-up.

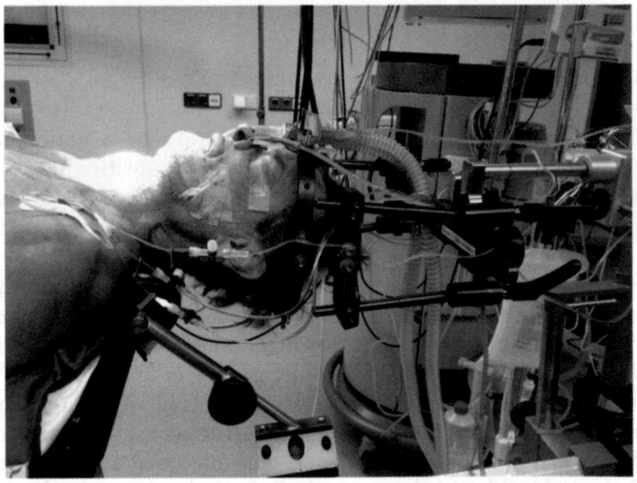

Figure 33C-16. A halo ring is applied and connected to a reductioning and positioning system. Reduction is maintained and might even be adapted during the procedure.

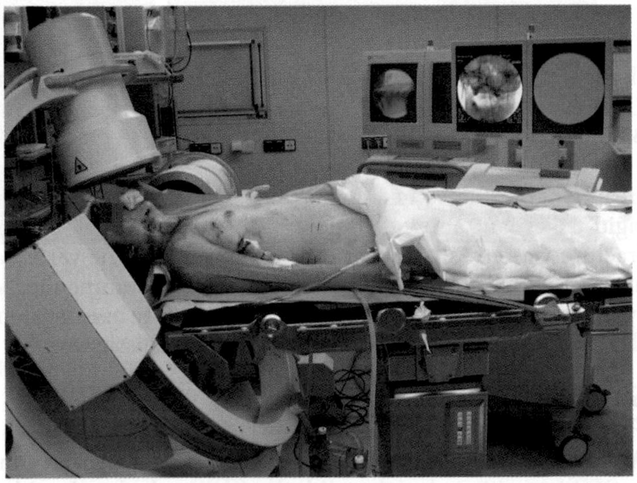

Figure 33C-17. Two image intensifiers are installed as shown in order to have biplanar views during drilling and screw insertion.

Posterior Procedures. For a posterior approach, the patient is placed in a prone position. The table is brought into a reverse Trendelenburg position to decrease bleeding. Reduction is performed and slight traction is applied with any of the means mentioned earlier. Ocular compression has to be prevented. The arms are gently tucked to the sides. It can be helpful to rotate the operating table, so that the anesthesiology team is located at the foot of the patient.[98] The patient's neck, occiput, and, if applicable, the iliac crest are prepped in a standard manner.

Surgical Approach

Anterior Approach to C2. The anterior retropharyngeal approach needed for fixation of C2 fractures is similar to the anterior approach to the subaxial cervical spine (see Chapter 34). For anterior screw osteosynthesis, reduction should be performed before draping. For screw osteosynthesis, we prefer a right-sided approach if the surgeon is right-handed. For screw osteosynthesis we prefer a transverse skin incision at the level C5-C6. The superficial platysma muscle is incised in the same direction. Occasionally, cervical veins need to be ligated. Palpating the pulse of the carotid artery, blunt dissection is carried out until the hard surface of the subaxial spine is palpated. The carotid sheath is retracted laterally, the trachea and esophagus are retracted medially using a radiolucent retractor. Subperiosteal dissection is carried out until the C2-C3 disc is reached. Full exposure of the disc is not mandatory for simple screw fixation.

For discectomy and anterior C2-C3 fusion, a more extensile approach including exposure of the superior laryngeal nerve is needed. A radiolucent Hohmann retractor can be placed above the C2-C3 level for better overview.

The complications from these approaches are related to soft tissue structures in the neck. Problems with swallowing or breathing can occur because of retropharyngeal edema or hematoma formation especially in the elderly. Nerve dysesthesias can involve the greater auricular, hypoglossal, facial, recurrent laryngeal, and spinal accessory nerves.[171]

At the conclusion of the procedure, platysma muscle and skin are closed in layers, the latter using resorbable intracutaneous sutures.

Posterior Approach. The patient's hair is shaved up to two fingerbreadths above the posterior occipital protuberance. After standard skin preparation and draping, a longitudinal midline skin incision is made over the craniocervical junction. With meticulous hemostasis, the upper cervical spine is exposed, paying close attention to the midline raphe. This technique helps to prevent excessive hemorrhage. It is crucial to bear in mind that the vertebral vessels lie on the superior aspect of the posterior arch of C1 approximately 1.5 to 2.0 cm lateral to the midline. Attempts have been made to reduce intraoperative blood loss. Some surgeons advocate the use of an "ultrasonic scalpel," but, so far, trials supporting its effectiveness are missing.[172] Cho and colleagues published the application of a thrombin-soaked absorbable gelatin compressed sponge at the end of posterior cervical spinal surgery resulting in significantly decreased postoperative drain output and consequent hospital stay.[173]

Other Approaches. Very rarely in fracture treatment and mainly when anterior decompression is required, a lateral or transoral approach can be advisable to gain a full anterior exposure of the C2 body. These approaches are described in Chapter 33B.

Reduction and Fixation Techniques

Fixation options are manifold. Some advantages favor the use of anterior techniques. Muscle dissection is negligible compared to dorsal approaches. Furthermore, flexion of the neck is sometimes necessary for certain posterior techniques, but may result in fatal cord damage. In the presence of a failed posterior stabilizing technique, anterior techniques may be the surgeon's only option. Finally, although neurologic compromise is rare in C2 fractures, an anterior approach allows acute decompression of the spinal canal when needed. Conversely, literature on optimal biomechanical properties, in both anterior and posterior stabilizing techniques, favors dorsal fixation techniques. A recent cadaveric study analyzed the biomechanical stability of different fusion techniques including anterior cervical plating, anterior transarticular stabilization (TAS), posterior rod-screw construct, and posterior TAS. The posterior rod-screw construct was found to have the highest biomechanical stiffness, followed by posterior TAS, anterior TAS, and finally, anterior cervical plating.[174,175]

Anterior Screw Fixation of the Dens. Nakanishi and colleagues first described the anterior screw fixation of the dens. This technique avoids extensive dissection of muscles and preserves atlantoaxial motion. The main indications are Anderson type II odontoid fractures that present with a horizontal (Grauer type IIA) or oblique (type IIB) fracture line, as well as "shallow" or "rostral" type III fractures. The procedure is technically demanding and success requires several prerequisites. Short-necked patients, patients with stiff cervical spines, thoracic kyphosis, barrel-chested habitus, and fracture configurations that can be held reduced only while in flexion create difficulty with drill and screw trajectory and should make the surgeon opt for another treatment method.[111]

Patient positioning is critical, as just described. The fracture must be reducible and preferably reduced prior to draping.

After gaining access through a standard C5-C6 anterior approach, the ALL is split longitudinally over the body of the axis. Using fluoroscopy, drill holes are made starting at the anteroinferior aspect of C2 toward the cranial tip of the dens. Care must be taken to start within the C2-C3 disc to get into the inferior aspect of the C2 body and avoid starting on the anterior portion of the body, which can lead to screw cutout. Drill trajectory should be checked in both planes and, after gauging depth and tapping the hole, a small-fragment (3.5 mm) lag screw is inserted (Fig. 33C-18). It is important to achieve a lag screw effect by drilling over the proximal cortex or using a partially threaded screw (in this case one must be certain that the threads do not span the fracture site). Alternatively, a guide wire can be placed first, drilled over and followed by a cannulated screw. Another technical variation is the use of double-threaded compression screws.[112,176,177]

If the obliquity of the fracture is from posterior-cephalad to anterior-caudal (Grauer type IIC, opposite the usual obliquity), this technique is relatively contraindicated because the fracture will displace anteriorly and inferiorly as the screw is tightened. Endoscopically assisted anterior screw fixation has also been used. In this technique, authors used a 10-mL polyethylene syringe as a tubular retractor and a 2-cm skin incision.[178] Furthermore, the introduction of computer

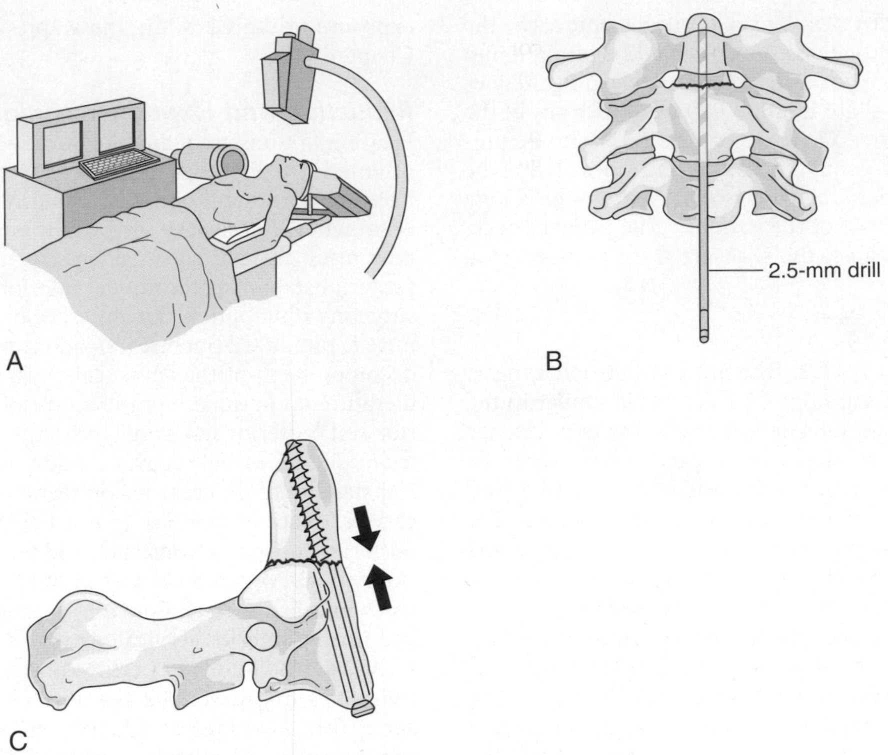

Figure 33C-18. **A,** Patient positioning for anterior odontoid screw fixation. Screw positions shown in anteroposterior (**B**) and lateral (**C**) views.

navigation prompted a cadaveric comparison of standard fluoroscopy with fluoroscopy-based computer navigation. The study showed no difference in accuracy of screw placement or procedural time, but radiation exposure was less with virtual fluoroscopy.[179] Postoperatively, semirigid collar immobilization is recommended for 6 to 8 weeks.

Ongoing debate exists as to whether one or two screws should be implanted during anterior screw fixation. Biomechanical studies do not reveal significant differences in stiffness between a single or dual screws but that either technique only provides about 50% the stability of a healthy odontoid.[180-182] McBride and coworkers treated 12 cadaveric odontoids (six in each group) with either one 4.5-mm cannulated Herbert screw or two 3.5-mm Arbeitsgemeinschaft für Osteosynthesefragen (AO) cannulated screws. Torsional stiffness was found to be greater with the Herbert screw, sheer stiffness showed no statistical difference.[180] Healing rates do not appear to differ between single and dual screws, but complication rates may. In a systematic review, Patel and colleagues found surgical complication rates to be 8.6% and 14.7% for one versus two screws, respectively. They attributed the higher complication rate to the difficulties in inserting two screws in a triangular pattern compared to only one.[183,184] Moreover, insertion of two 3.5-mm screws has been found feasible in only 65% of patients because of small diameters of the dens in CT measurements.[185] They confirmed results from an earlier study, which, looking at adult odontoid morphology, found that the average transverse outer diameter was 10.4 mm (ranging from 8.2 to 13.2 mm) and that the average transverse inner diameter was 7.2 mm (ranging from 4.4 to 11.0 mm) measured in CT scans.[186] As clinical comparisons are sparse, a recent retrospective analysis looked into osseous union 3 months postoperatively using a CT scan. Osseous union was achieved in 9 of 15 patients treated with two screws and in 0 of 3 patients treated with a single screw (Fig. 33C-19).[187]

Anterior Transarticular C1-C2 Screw Fixation. Anterior transarticular C1-C2 screw fixation has stability comparable to posterior C1-C2 fixation and is mainly indicated in odontoid fractures type II of the elderly who exhibit either significant arthritis of the C1-C2 joint or an accompanying fracture of the atlas ring. Another indication is failed anterior screw fixation of the dens, if no further reduction is needed. The limitation of this technique is the difficulty of performing arthrodesis.

The surgical approach is the same as described earlier for odontoid screw. The anterior exposure should allow for a good visualization of the laterally placed C1-C2 joint. A curette is used to denude the cartilage of the atlantoaxial joints under fluoroscopic control. The starting points for the C1-C2 screws are located undersurface of the overhanging lip of the lateral mass of C2. The direction of the screws is some 25 degrees lateral into the lateral mass of C1, which can best be judged by use of the image intensifiers in both planes. Guide wires followed by cannulated screws are helpful in achieving adequate positioning. Alternatively, starting points can be chosen at the midpoint of the C2 body in the transverse plane and the respective medial thirds of the C1-C2 facets in the sagittal planes. The screws should then be angulated laterally in the coronal plane approximately 30 to 35 degrees to allow for perpendicular screw placement across the facet joints. Additional anterior screw fixation of the dens as described earlier, if applicable, will contribute to the biomechanical stability.[188-191]

Anterior Discectomy and Fusion. Unstable traumatic spondylolisthesis with disruption of the ALL (Effendi and Levine types IIA and III) may be rarely treated with anterior

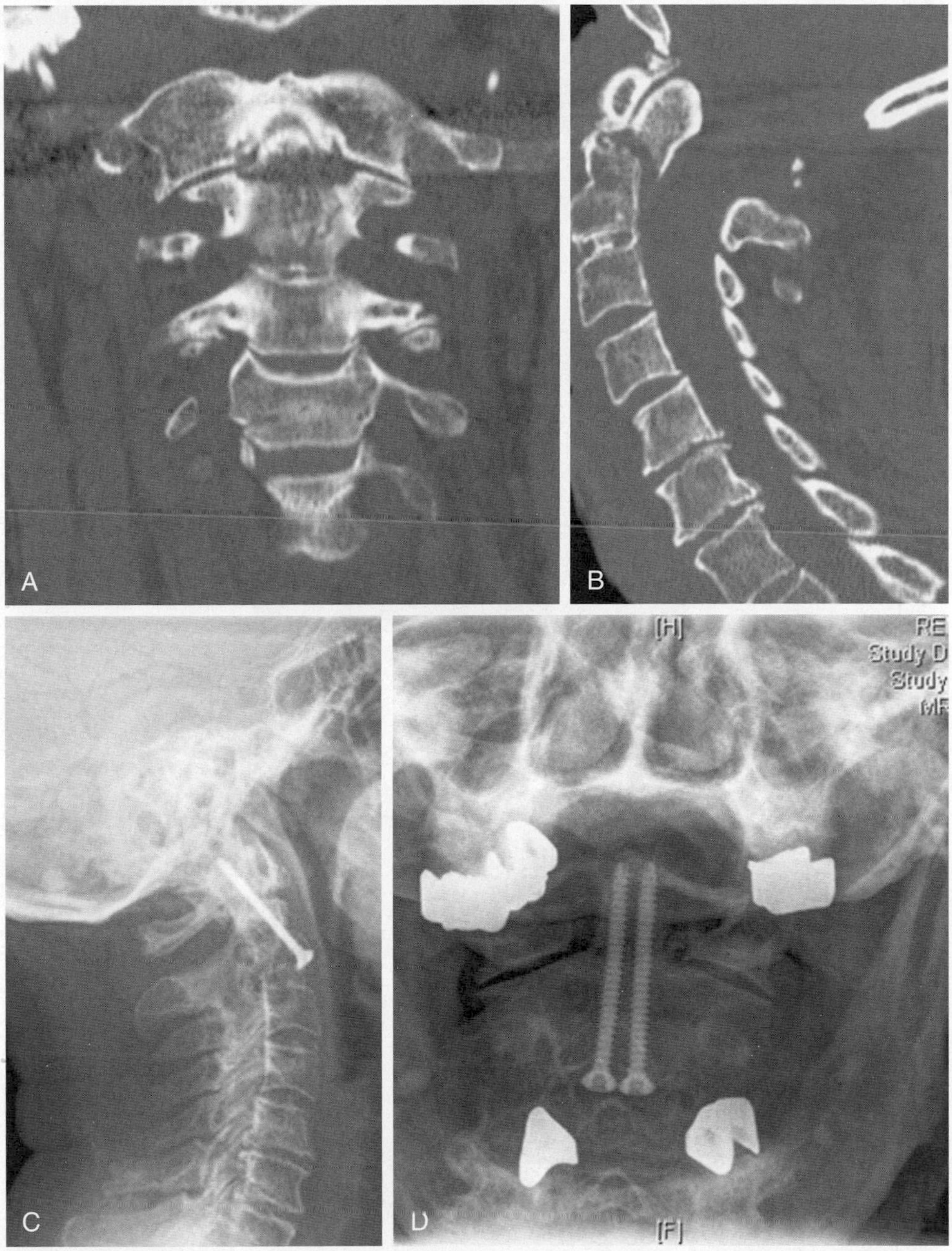

Figure 33C-19. A and **B,** A 72-year-old woman with a posteriorly displaced type II odontoid fracture as well as a C1 arch fracture after a simple fall with her head hitting a wardrobe. Anterior screw fixation was performed and semirigid immobilization was applied for 6 weeks. At 3 months' follow-up, she was totally satisfied with only the flexion being slightly limited. **C** and **D,** Plain films document anatomic reduction without signs of secondary displacement or screw loosening.

discectomy and fusion. This technique uses a standard anterior approach and is conducted in the same manner as in the subaxial cervical spine (Fig. 33C-20).

Posterior C2 Pedicle Screw Fixation ("Judet"). This technique was first described by Robert Judet in 1962. Its main indication is fixation of displaced hangman's fractures Effendi type II. However, it can be used in type III hangman's fractures, if it is combined with an additional fixation of the C2-C3 segment.

It is paramount that the fracture be reduced prior to draping. The patient is put in a prone position with any of the traction aids mentioned earlier. Usually, a slight extension will lead to reduction, which has to be checked with lateral fluoroscopy. The posterior arch of C2 is exposed via a limited dorsal midline approach. The insertion point of the screw lays halfway 2 to 3 mm lateral to the junction between the C2 lamina and the inferior facet, and 2 to 3 mm cephalad to the C2-C3 facet joint. We use a 2.5-mm oscillating drill with a protective sleeve. The screws are predrilled some 20 degrees in a medial direction and 25 degrees upward as seen on lateral fluoroscopy. It is better to err in the medial rather than the lateral direction because the medial aspect affords more room before the cord is encountered as opposed to the position of the vertebral artery laterally. The screw length, usually 30 to 35 mm, is measured by use of a depth gauge. A 3.5-mm small fragment cortex screw or lag screw is inserted

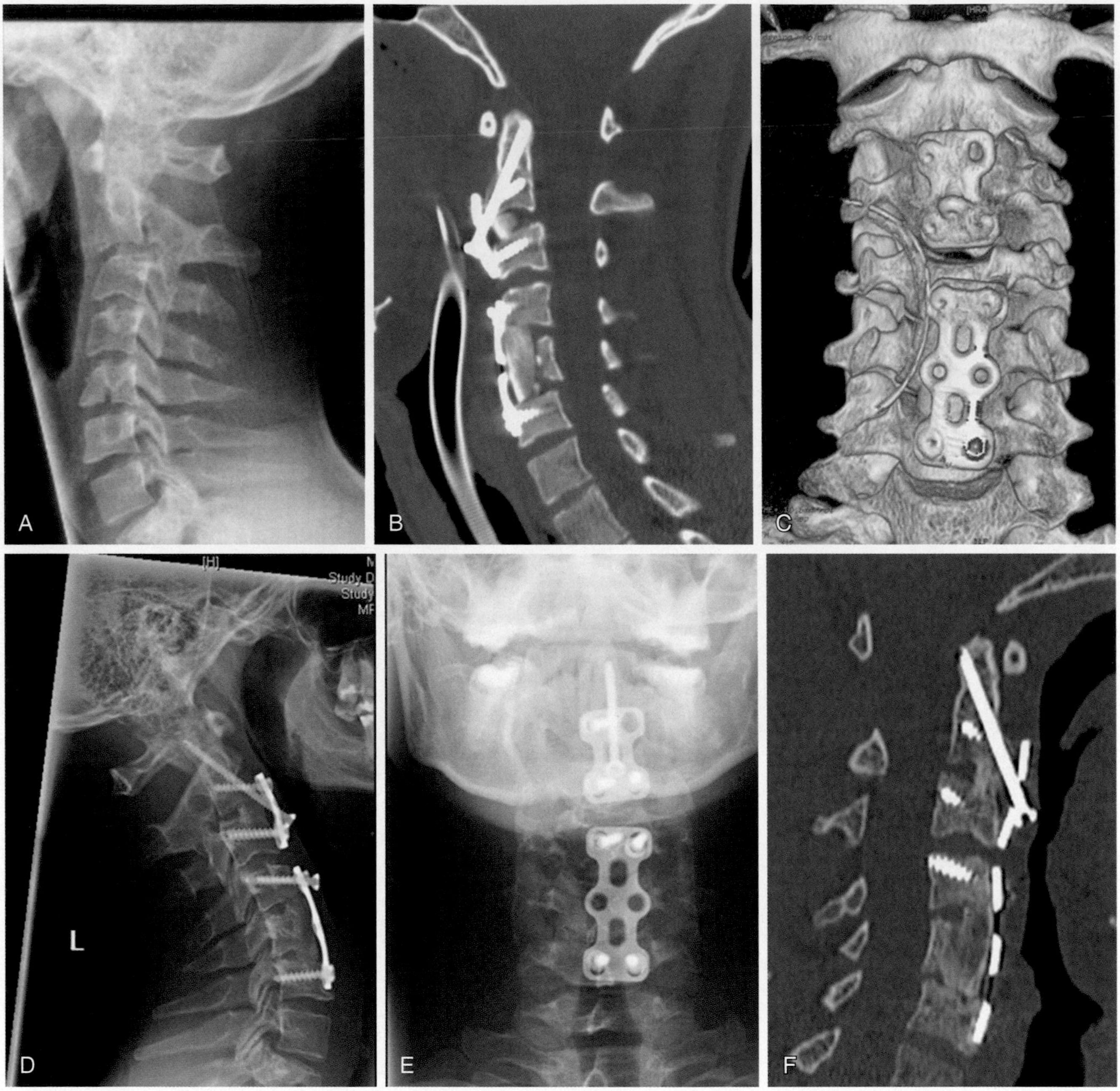

Figure 33C-20. This 21-year-old man jumped headfirst into a boat and suffered from an Effendi type II fracture with unilateral dislocation of C2-C3. Moreover, he suffered from a discoligamentous injury of C5-C6 and split fracture of C5. Anterior surgery was performed with anterior C2-C3 discectomy and fusion as well as anterior C4-C6 fusion with interposition of cortical bone from the iliac crest. **A,** The first radiograph obtained in the emergency unit. **B** and **C,** Postoperative computed tomography (CT) scans 1 day after injury. **D** through **F,** Results at 6 months with achieved fusion without secondary dislocation.

after tapping the cortex at the entry point (see Fig. 33C-14). Postoperatively, a nonrigid collar is advised for 6 to 8 weeks. This technique provides good stability and spares fixation of a motion segment. However, it places the vertebral artery at risk; therefore, one has to envision its actual course by CT or MRI scans.[192,193]

Posterior C1-C2 Screw-Rod Fixation ("Harms Construct"). Harms and colleagues first described this technique, which achieves fixation of the C1-C2 segment by connecting C2 pedicle screws as described earlier and C1 lateral mass screws by use of a polyaxial screw-rod system. Indications in the treatment of C2 fractures are reverse oblique odontoid fractures (Grauer IIC), Anderson type II odontoid fractures in patients in whom anterior approach is not feasible, as well as delayed surgery in displaced odontoid fractures, and nonunions and malunions of the odontoid.

Reduction can be performed intraoperatively; nevertheless, intraoperative traction can be helpful in order to facilitate visualization of the entry points. As described by Harms, the cervical spine is exposed subperiosteally from the occiput to C3-C4. The C1-C2 complex is exposed to the lateral border of the C1-C2 articulation. Bleeding typically arises from dissection around the epidural venous plexus along the C1-C2 joint. The dorsal root ganglion of C2 is retracted in a caudal

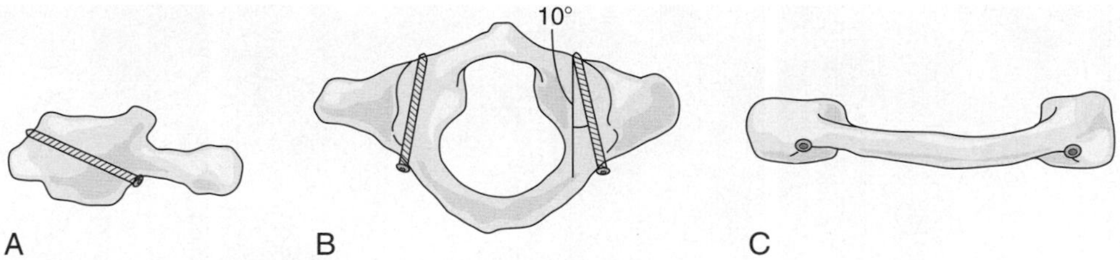

Figure 33C-21. Screw positions for C1 lateral fixation as shown on a lateral view (**A**), axial view (**B**), and posterior view (**C**). The two alternative starting points are noted.

direction to expose the entry point for the C1 screw, which is in the middle of the junction of the C1 posterior arch and the midpoint of the posterior inferior part of the C1 lateral mass. This entry point is marked with a 1- to 2-mm high-speed burr to prevent slippage of the drill point. The pilot hole is then drilled in a straight or slightly convergent trajectory in an anterior-posterior direction and parallel to the plane of the C1 posterior arch in the sagittal direction, with the tip of the drill directed toward the anterior arch of C1. The drilling is accomplished with guidance from intraoperative landmarks, preoperative fine-cut axial CT images, and lateral fluoroscopic imaging (Fig. 33C-21). It should stop 3 mm before the anterior tubercle as seen on the lateral projection. The length of the screw is measured with a small depth gauge. The hole is tapped and a 3.5-mm polyaxial axon screw, which features an unthreaded distal portion, is inserted bicortically into the lateral mass of C1. The unthreaded portion minimizes any chance of irritation to the greater occipital nerve and allows the polyaxial portion of the screw to lie above the posterior arch of C1. The C2 pedicle screws are placed as described earlier ("Judet") and 3.5-mm rods are used to connect the polyaxial C1 and C2 screws on both sides. Prior to this, additional reduction maneuvers can be carried out. For a definitive fusion, C1 and C2 are decorticated posteriorly, and cancellous bone taken from a small incision in the posterior iliac crest can be placed over the decorticated surfaces of C1 and C2.

Although technically demanding, this technique provides the highest degree of stability and nonunions are rare. Again especially, the exact course of the vertebral artery has to be envisioned for drilling and screw placement (Figs. 33C-22 and 33C-23).[98,171,193,194]

Posterior Transarticular C1-C2 Screw Fixation ("Magerl"). Magerl and Jeanneret first described this technique of fixation with transarticular C1-C2 screws. Basically, the indications are the same as for posterior C1-C2 screw-rod fixation. However, biomechanical stability is inferior in comparison to screw-rod fixation as described earlier; therefore, nowadays this technique is rarely chosen in the treatment of C2 fractures.

The patient is placed prone and the head is immobilized with any of the traction aids described earlier. Surgical approach and entry point are identical to the description of the C2 pedicle screw. For a transarticular screw, the angle is more relatively parallel to the body, again judged by the lateral fluoroscopy, and is extended across the C1-C2 articulation aiming at the cephalad end of the anterior arch of C1 (Fig. 33C-24). Preoperative CT is essential in determining that there is adequate room within the pars for the screw to pass safely above the vertebral artery. Frequently, this procedure is combined with a fusion, according to Gallie, or posterior wiring (Fig. 33C-25). The most feared of complications in posterior screw placement at the level of C1 and C2 is an injury of the vertebral artery. If in the course of drilling, tapping, or screw insertion, bleeding from the vertebral artery occurs, the other screw should not be inserted to avoid a potentially deadly bilateral vertebral artery injury. The screw on the side of the injury should still be inserted and may help control bleeding. Consideration should be made for a postoperative angiogram to rule out pseudoaneurysm formation that could lead to embolization.[97,193,195]

Anatomic contraindications to TAS placement include pathologic destruction or collapse of C2, an aberrant vertebral artery anatomy or a large vertebral artery groove with a secondarily narrow C2 isthmus (20% of cases), or cranial assimilation of C1. A recent cadaveric study of the axis showed that the isthmus size and width were not symmetrical in 41% of the specimens, and, as demonstrated in other studies, 20% of the specimens revealed a C2 isthmus diameter that was smaller than that of the 3.5-mm screw.[196] Because some patients have unilateral anomalies that prevent bilateral TAS placement, one study looked at the outcomes with the use of a unilateral TAS. At a mean follow-up of 31 months, the authors in this study reported solid fusion in 18 of 19 patients (Fig. 33C-26).[197]

META-ANALYSES AND SYSTEMATIC REVIEWS

In 2008, a Cochrane review on surgical versus conservative management for an odontoid fracture was published.[198] The authors searched multiple databases and reference lists of publications and clinical trial registries. They did not identify any studies that met their inclusion criteria. The review content has been updated in September 2010.

Nourbakhsh and coworkers conducted a meta-analysis to evaluate healing rates of surgical and nonoperative treatments for acute type II odontoid fractures. Twenty-six studies, all of class IV evidence, were included. They reported fusion success for (1) patients younger or older than 45 to 55 years or (2) patients with fracture displacement of 4 to 6 mm or by the direction of displacement. No information is given on how and when fusion was confirmed. The authors found a statistically significantly higher fusion rate for operative management compared with external immobilization (85% vs. 60%, $P = 0.01$) for patients older than 45 to 55 years. However, the overall fusion rate was more than 80% for patients younger than 45 to 55 years, regardless of treatment modality, and no significant differences were observed between surgically and nonsurgically treated patients (89% and 81%, respectively;

COST-EFFECTIVENESS

To date, there is no data published on cost-effectiveness.

CONCLUSIONS

C2 fractures put patients at risk of significant morbidity. Although conservative treatment has prevailed for a long time, during the last two decades more refined surgical techniques and instrumentations have evolved. Surgical therapy has become more popular and provides excellent results in many cases. However, adequate randomized controlled trials on treatment and outcomes of C2 fractures are lacking. Surgical fixations require sound knowledge of the inherent risk of the procedures, as well as excellent 3-D imaging of the individual anatomy of the patient for exact planning. Image-guided intraoperative navigation might play a greater role in the future. Odontoid fractures more and more occur in the growing elderly population. Comorbidities and individual level of activities might influence decision making and conservative treatment will still remain a valuable option in many cases.

KEY REFERENCES

The level of evidence (LOE) is determined according to the criteria provided in the preface.

31. Barker L, Anderson J, Chesnut R, et al: Reliability and reproducibility of dens fracture classification with use of plain radiography and reformatted computer-aided tomography. *J Bone Joint Surg Am* 88(1):106–112, 2006. LOE II
35. Anderson LD, D'Alonzo RT: Fractures of the odontoid process of the axis. *J Bone Joint Surg Am* 56(8):1663–1674, 1974. LOE IV
45. Grauer JN, Shafi B, Hilibrand AS, et al: Proposal of a modified, treatment-oriented classification of odontoid fractures. *Spine J* 5(2):123–129, 2005. LOE III
64. Effendi B, Roy D, Cornish B, et al: Fractures of the ring of the axis. A classification based on the analysis of 131 cases. *J Bone Joint Surg Br* 63(3):319–327, 1981. LOE II
65. Levine AM, Edwards CC: The management of traumatic spondylolisthesis of the axis. *J Bone Joint Surg Am* 67(2):217–226, 1985. LOE IV
82. Lewis E, Liew S, Dowrick A: Risk factors for non-union in the non-operative management of type II dens fractures. *A NZ J Surg* 81(9):604–607, 2011. LOE IV
108. Müller EJ, Schwinnen I, Fischer K, et al: Non-rigid immobilisation of odontoid fractures. *Eur Spine J* 12(5):522–525, 2003. LOE IV
115. Chapman J, Smith JS, Kopjar B, et al: The AOSpine North America geriatric odontoid fracture mortality study: a retrospective review of mortality outcomes for operative versus non-operative treatment in 322 patients with long-term follow-up. *Spine (Phila Pa 1976)* 38(13):1098–1104, 2013. LOE III
116. Platzer P, Thalhammer G, Ostermann R, et al: Anterior screw fixation of odontoid fractures comparing younger and elderly patients. *Spine (Phila Pa 1976)* 32(16):1714–1720, 2007. LOE III
117. Chaudhary A, Drew B, Orr RD, et al: Management of type II odontoid fractures in the geriatric population: Outcome of treatment in a rigid cervical orthosis. *J Spinal Disord Tech* 23(5):317–320, 2010. LOE IV
119. Osti M, Philipp H, Meusburger B, et al: Analysis of failure following anterior screw fixation of type II odontoid fractures in geriatric patients. *Eur Spine J* 20(11):1915–1920, 2011. LOE III
123. Smith JS, Kepler CK, Kopjar B, et al: Effect of type II odontoid fracture nonunion on outcome among elderly patients treated without surgery: based on the AOSpine North America geriatric odontoid fracture study. *Spine (Phila Pa 1976)* 38(26):2240–2246, 2013. LOE II
131. Platzer P, Thalhammer G, Sarahrudi K, et al: Nonoperative management of odontoid fractures using a halothoracic vest. *Neurosurgery* 61(3):522–529, discussion 529–530, 2007. LOE IV
145. Li XF, Dai LY, Lu H, et al: A systematic review of the management of hangman's fractures. *Eur Spine J* 15(3):257–269, 2006. LOE III
146. Longo UG, Denaro L, Campi S, et al: Upper cervical spine injuries: indications and limits of the conservative management in halo vest. A systematic review of efficacy and safety. *Injury* 41(11):1127–1135, 2010. LOE III
199. Nourbakhsh A, Shi R, Vannemreddy P, et al: Operative versus non-operative management of acute odontoid type II fractures: a meta-analysis. *J Neurosurg Spine* 11(6):651–658, 2009. LOE III

The complete References list is available online at https://expertconsult.inkling.com.

Chapter 34

Subaxial Cervical Spine Trauma

LOUIS F. AMOROSA • ALEXANDER R. VACCARO

INTRODUCTION

The subaxial cervical spine is composed of C3 through C7 vertebrae. Epidemiologic studies have shown cervical spine fractures or dislocations to occur in 2% to 3% of trauma patients.[1,2] However, injuries to the subaxial cervical spine account for 65% of all cervical spine fractures and more than 75% of dislocations, with C6 being the most commonly fractured subaxial vertebra and C5 to C6 being the most commonly dislocated level.[3]

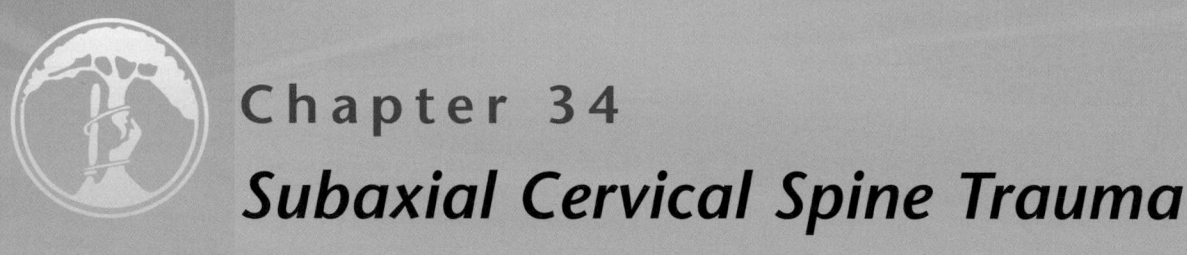

Historically, debate has existed on the proper classification and treatment of subaxial cervical spine injuries.[4] Little evidence existed for the best form of treatment for subaxial cervical spine injuries; however, more recent evidence-based classification and treatment systems have brought us closer to a more systematic way of evaluating and treating subaxial injuries. This chapter provides an understanding of different types of subaxial cervical spine trauma as well as evidence-based methods of treating them.

ANATOMY

Osseous Structures

The osseous anatomy of the subaxial cervical spine is relatively constant, with the exception of C7, a transitional vertebra at the cervicothoracic junction. The posterior vertebral body ventrally, the pedicles laterally, and the laminae posteriorly form the boundaries of the spinal canal (Fig. 34-1). Each vertebral body has an endplate superiorly and inferiorly. As the superior endplate extends from midline laterally, it slopes upward to form the uncinate process. The uncovertebral joint of Luschka is formed by the concave uncinate process of the inferior vertebra with the convex lateral inferior endplate from the suprajacent vertebral body. This is an important landmark when performing anterior discectomy or corpectomy.

The transverse process extends from the pedicle laterally and anterior to the lateral mass. Unique to the cervical spine, within the transverse processes, is located the foramen transversarium through which the vertebral artery typically ascends beginning at C6. This particular anatomic feature allows for safe placement of pedicle screws into C7, which is discussed in detail later in the chapter.

Another feature of the vertebrae unique to the cervical spine is the lateral mass. The lateral mass forms the dorsal surface of the vertebra lateral to lamina. The lateral mass superiorly is bordered by the superior articular facet and inferiorly by the inferior articular facet. The subaxial cervical facets are oriented like shingles on a house. That is, the inferior articular facet of the cephalad vertebra is dorsal to the superior articular facet of its infrajacent vertebra (Fig. 34-2).

The lamina borders the lateral mass medially, which then slopes posteromedially, converging with the contralateral lamina to form the spinous process. Cervical spinous processes are often bifid except for C7. C7 typically has the most prominent spinous process of the subaxial cervical spine and is usually an easily palpable landmark.

Nonosseous Structures

The intervertebral disc borders the respective endplates of the superior and inferior vertebrae. It contributes significantly to stability of the vertebral disc motion segment. The nucleus pulposus is at the center of the disc and surrounding the central pulposus is the tougher fibrous annulus fibrosus.

Anterior elements are the anterior longitudinal ligament (ALL), intervertebral disc, vertebral body, intertransverse ligament, and posterior longitudinal ligament (PLL).[5] The ALL runs longitudinally along the entire length of the spine anterior to the vertebrae or vertebral bodies. The ALL along with the anterior vertical fibers of the annulus fibrosus serve as important restraints to hyperextension. These anterior annular fibers typically fail in extension before the failure of the stronger ALL.[6,7]

The PLL runs longitudinally along the posterior aspect of the vertebral bodies the entire length of the spine.[5] Because of its more posterior location, the PLL resists flexion moments with strength similar to the ALL.[8] The PLL thins laterally, and the posterior annular fibers are relatively weak compared with anterior annular fibers at the same level, which likely contributes to the relatively common occurrence of disc protrusions and herniations in this region[9] (Fig. 34-3).

The posterior elements are defined as the structures posterior to the PLL.[5] These include the facets, laminae, and spinous process, as well as the associated soft tissue structures, which include the ligamentum flavum, facet capsules, and interspinous and supraspinous ligaments. The ligamentum flavum extends from the anteroinferior surface of one lamina to the superoposterior surface of the inferior lamina. Although elastic in young people and resistant to flexion, with the aging process, the ligamentum hypertrophies and stiffens and may be a source of posterior impingement with anterior distraction injuries.

The cervical facet capsules in this region are patulous and do not restrict motion until extremes of flexion are reached.[10,11] However, adjacent joints and capsules of levels not being fused should not be disrupted during posterior surgical exposures because this risks adjacent-segment instability.

The ligamentum nuchae is a triangular fibrous membrane that overlies the supraspinous and interspinous ligaments and runs between the external occipital protuberance of the skull and the spinous process of C2 and C7. When the ligamentum nuchae was resected in a cadaveric model, cervical

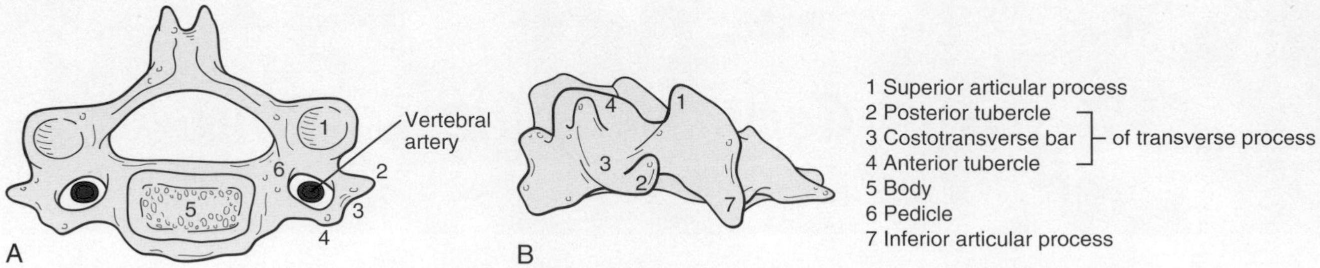

Figure 34-1. Osseous anatomy of the subaxial cervical spine. **A,** Typical vertebral body viewed from above. **B,** Viewed from the left side. Cervical pedicles *(6)* are very short and extend at a medial angle from the superior articular process *(1)*. The lateral mass (consisting of the superior *[1]* and inferior *[7]* articular processes] is rhomboid in shape when viewed from the lateral view. The superior surface of the vertebral body *(5)* is raised at the posterolateral corners to form the uncovertebral joints.

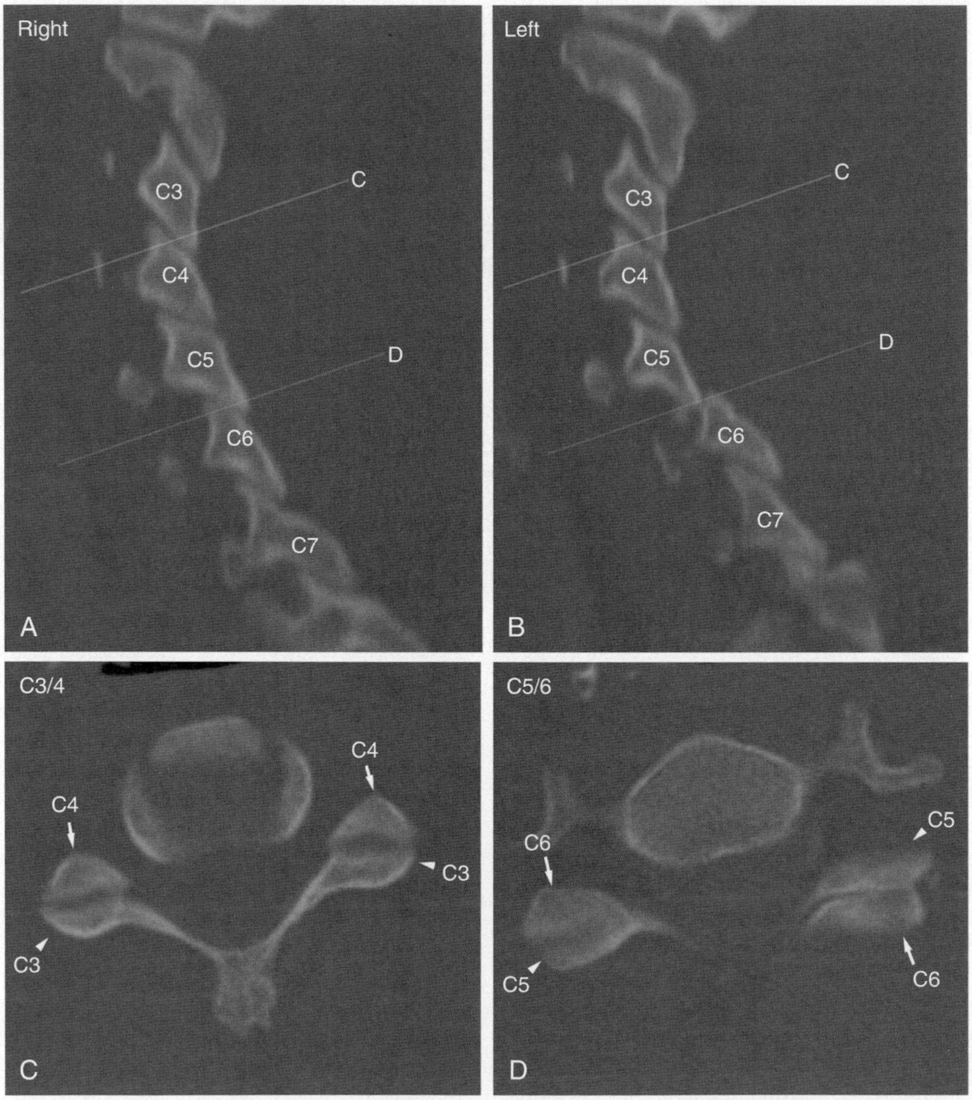

Figure 34-2. Shingling of the facets in the subaxial cervical spine. The rhomboid-shaped facets overlap in a "shingling" pattern in the subaxial cervical spine. This is well visualized in the sagittal computed tomography reconstructions of the right (**A**) and left (**B**) facets. Note the left-sided C5 to C6 facet fracture-dislocation (**B**). On the axial cuts of the normal C3 to C4 level (**C**), note the shingling pattern of the facets, the superior facet of C4 is anterior to the inferior facet of C3. At the level of the injury, note that the right-sided facets have maintained their alignment, with the superior facet of C6 being anterior to the inferior facet of C5 (**D**). However, on the left, the C5 inferior facet is anterior to the C6 superior facet.

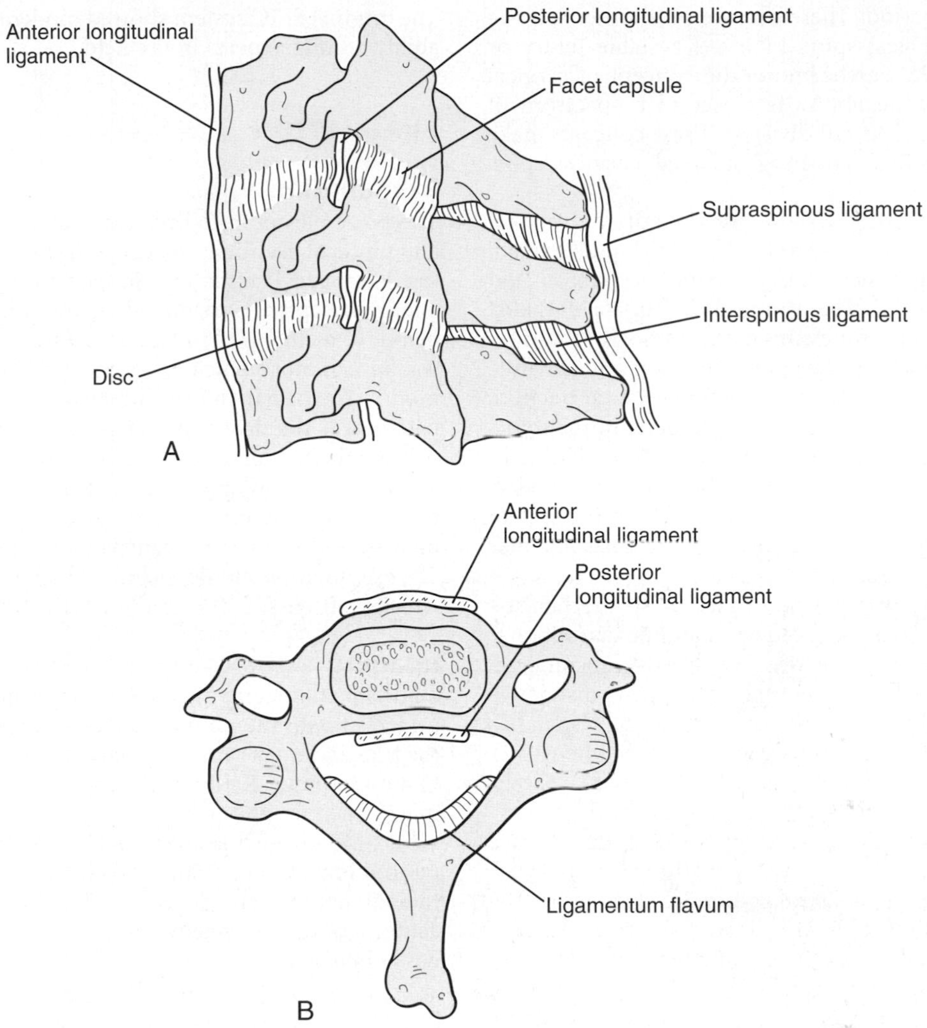

Figure 34-3. Ligamentous anatomy of the subaxial cervical spine when viewed from lateral (**A**) and from above (**B**).

spine stiffness decreased by 27%, and flexion increased by 28% indicating the importance of this structure as a stabilizing force.[12] The ligamentum nuchae, infraspinous ligaments, and supraspinous ligaments are restraints to flexion and fail at the lowest forces in biomechanical cadaveric studies.[11]

BIOMECHANICS

The Concept of Biomechanical Stability of the Cervical Spine

Under normal physiologic conditions, the human cervical spine is extremely mobile, allowing a high degree of flexibility and rotational movement. However, the same reasons that the cervical spine is so mobile also contribute to its susceptibility to indirect injury mechanisms. Most motion in the cervical spine is caused by occipito-cervical (O-C1) and atlantoaxial motion (C1–C2). In vitro cadaveric studies have demonstrated each level of the normal subaxial cervical spine contributes 8 to 10 degrees of flexion and 3 to 5 degrees of axial rotation.[5] In vivo magnetic resonance imaging (MRI) studies of healthy volunteers have found between 1.5 and 4.6 degrees of axial rotation at each subaxial level[13] and lateral bending at each level to be between 1.9 and 5.7 degrees.[14] C2 to C3 has the most lateral bending at about 5 degrees; however, this is not significantly different than at other cervical levels.[15]

White and Panjabi defined spinal instability as "the loss of the ability of the spine under physiologic loads to maintain its pattern of displacement so that there is no initial or additional neurological deficit, no major deformity, and no incapacitating pain."[5] Therefore, according to this definition, the spine is stable if it can withstand loads during normal activity without severe pain, neurologic deficit, or major deformity. Much of the stability of the subaxial spine is based not on osseous structures but on the ligaments that hold them in place. This explains why dislocated facets are considered unstable even after closed reduction. The ligaments holding them in place have been disrupted and are not expected to heal with the strength needed to maintain stability.

Quantifying Instability

In the absence of obvious dislocation or subluxation, destabilizing injuries in the subaxial spine are often subtle. Spinal imaging, whether plain radiographs, computed tomography (CT) scan, or MRI, is often static. These imaging studies do not show the spine under conditions of motion, loading, or at the moment of injury. Flexion and extension lateral radiographs are effective at showing instability but are not indicated in the acute injury period. Therefore, we need other ways of deciding when a cervical spine injury is a stable injury or whether it is unstable. Furthermore, the concept of cervical spine stability versus instability is closer to a spectrum of stability rather than a clear-cut division. These concepts make diagnosing and effectively treating subaxial cervical spine injuries challenging.

Several different scoring systems for quantifying cervical spine instability have been introduced. White and Panjabi introduced a scoring system based on biomechanical and radiographic studies.[5,16-18] The White and Panjabi checklist assigns points based on competence or disruption of the anterior and posterior ligaments, the amount of static and dynamic displacement based on a "stretch test" using cervical traction, the neurologic status of the patient, the diameter of the spinal canal, and the anticipated loads on the spine. A total score of 5 or more points constitutes an unstable subaxial cervical spine injury.[5] The clinical utility and reliability of the system has been called into question and, furthermore, does not offer treatment recommendations.

The Allen and Ferguson system is based on six mechanistic patterns along with substages based on anatomic disruption.[19] The major patterns are compressive flexion, vertical compression, distractive flexion, compressive extension, distractive extension, and lateral flexion. The Allen-Ferguson system has been shown to have poor interobserver reliability when all 21 phylogenies are used[20,21] and only moderate interobserver reliability when only the six basic phylogenies are used.[20,21]

The Cervical Spine Injury Severity Score is based on a scoring system for the four columns of the cervical spine: anterior, posterior, and two lateral columns[22] (Fig. 34-4). The anterior column includes the ALL, vertebral body, and PLL. The posterior column includes the laminae, spinous processes, ligamentum flavum, and nuchal attachments. A visual analog scale from 1 to 5 is used to assess each of the four columns with increasing scores for increasing displacement or disruption. The sum of scores can range from 0 to 20, with scores greater than 7 indicating the recommendation for surgical treatment of the injury (Fig. 34-5). Studies have shown high intraobserver and interobserver reliability with use of the Cervical Spine Injury Severity Score at all levels of training and experience.[23,24] Although the Cervical Spine Injury Severity Score is useful for quantifying stability, it does not offer a classification system for injuries.

The Subaxial Cervical Spine Injury Classification (SLIC) system is based on three different parameters: the injury morphology, the neurologic status of the patient, and the integrity of the discoligamentous complex (DLC).[21] Morphology is divided into no abnormality, compression, burst, distraction injury, and a rotational or translational injury (Table 34-1). The DLC includes the intervertebral disc, ALL and PLL, ligamentum flavum, interspinous ligament, supraspinous ligament, and facet capsules and can be classified as intact, indeterminate, or disrupted based on MRI interpretation. The neurologic status is divided into intact, nerve root injury, complete cord injury, incomplete cord injury, or continuous cord compression in the setting of a neurologic deficit. Points are assigned for each of these descriptions, and total points are summed; the higher the points, the more severe the injury. Multiple injuries are individually scored and not cumulative. The total score helps to guide operative versus nonoperative treatment with higher points indicating the need for surgery. The original SLIC system showed moderate interobserver reliability among experts in the field.

EVALUATION

Examination

The principles of initial patient evaluation, including history and physical examination, cervical spine immobilization, and the Advanced Trauma Life Support protocol, are discussed in another chapter. Understanding the injury mechanism may help give a clue to the likely structures injured. If the patient was in a motor vehicle accident (MVA), the most common mode of subaxial injury, the evaluator should know if the patient was the driver, passenger, in the front seat, passenger seat, seatbelted, in a head-on collision, rear-ended, T-boned, at high speed, low speed, or ejected from the vehicle. In addition to fully understanding the injury mechanism, the assessment should decipher relevant patient factors and comorbidities. The examination should include a full neurologic examination, which is discussed in detail in another chapter.

Imaging

Static spinal imaging seen with radiographs and CT scan may underestimate the amount of displacement that occurred at the time of injury caused by the elastic recoil of the intact soft tissue anatomy.[25] Radiographs and CT may give clues to severe injury such as pretracheal edema, but often these clues are subtle. MRI, which is often challenging to obtain in the acute period in severely injured patients, and flexion-extension radiographs, which also cannot be obtained normally in the acute period, are usually the most useful indicators of soft tissue injury.

DIAGNOSIS AND CLASSIFICATION

One of the challenges of subaxial cervical spine injuries is the nomenclature associated with the various injury patterns. Many classification systems have been introduced with varying degrees of acceptance or reliability.[26] The Spine Trauma Study Group recently introduced a method of standardizing with the Subaxial Cervical Injury Description System (SCIDS).[27] The SCID system is meant to complement the SLIC system. The SCID defines 11 distinct injury types (Table 34-2). The SCID system had 56.4% interrater agreement and 72.8% intrarater agreement. Using the SCID system as a common language and the SLIC system to decide on treatment helps to create a more common language and should lead to a more systematic approach of classification and treatment of subaxial injuries. The Spine Trauma Study Group has also begun to introduce specific treatment algorithms based on systematic literature reviews for some of these injuries, which are discussed later in this chapter.[28]

MANAGEMENT

General Management Considerations

Basic principles of treating subaxial cervical spine injuries are to prevent further neurologic injury, reduce fractures or dislocations, and provide stability to the spinal column.

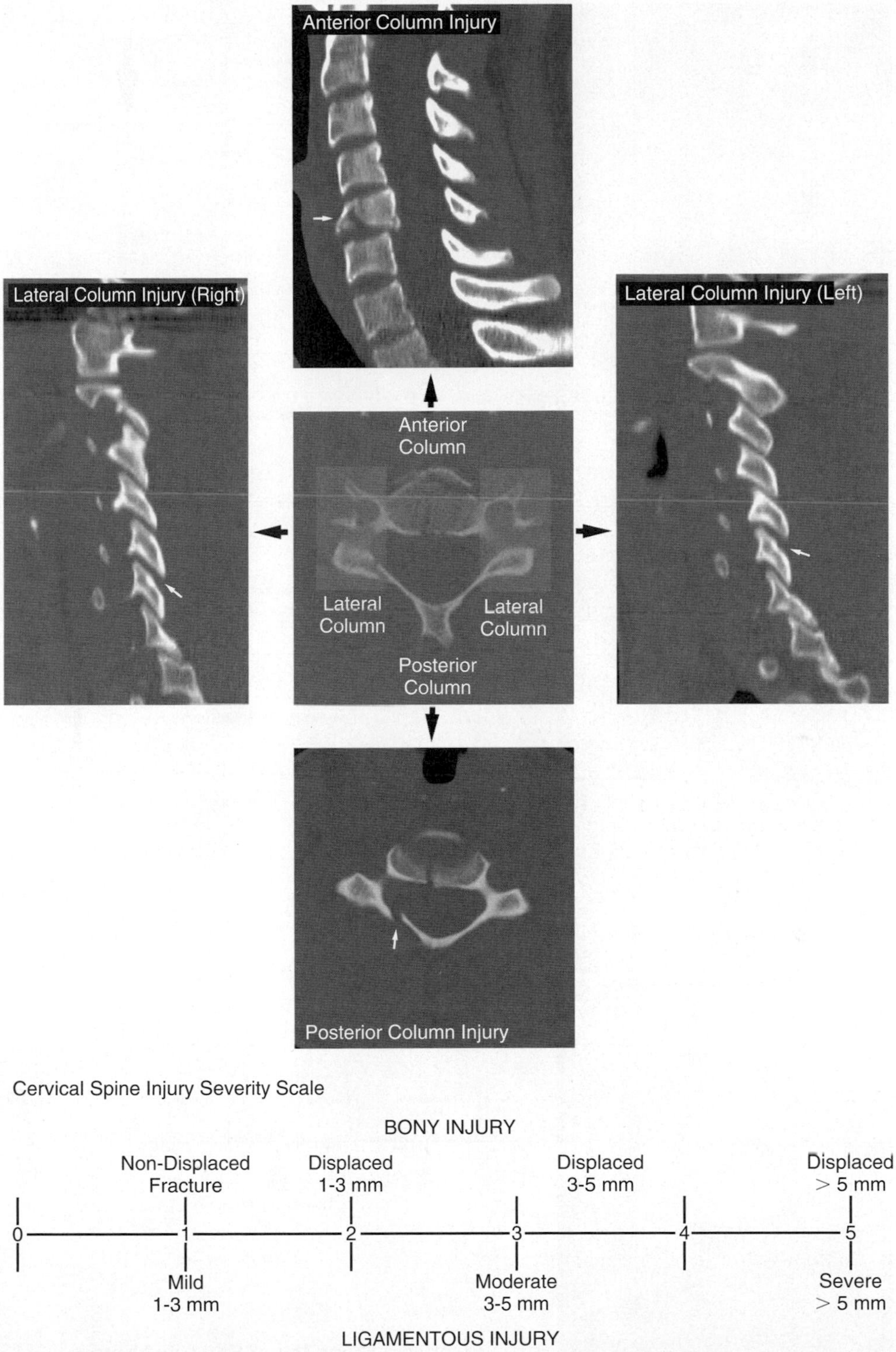

Figure 34-4. The Cervical Spine Injury Severity Score. This algorithm can be used to quantify the mechanical stability of the injury with the goal of deciding on the need for operative treatment. The cervical spine is divided into four columns (anterior, posterior, and two lateral columns), and the severity of injury to each column is assessed using whatever imaging modalities are available (e.g., plain film radiography, computed tomography, magnetic resonance imaging). The severity of the bony or ligamentous injury to each column is then assigned a number according to the analog scale shown below the films, with 0 being uninjured, and 5 being the most severely injured. The sum of the scores for each of the four columns then represents the Cervical Spine Injury Severity Score.

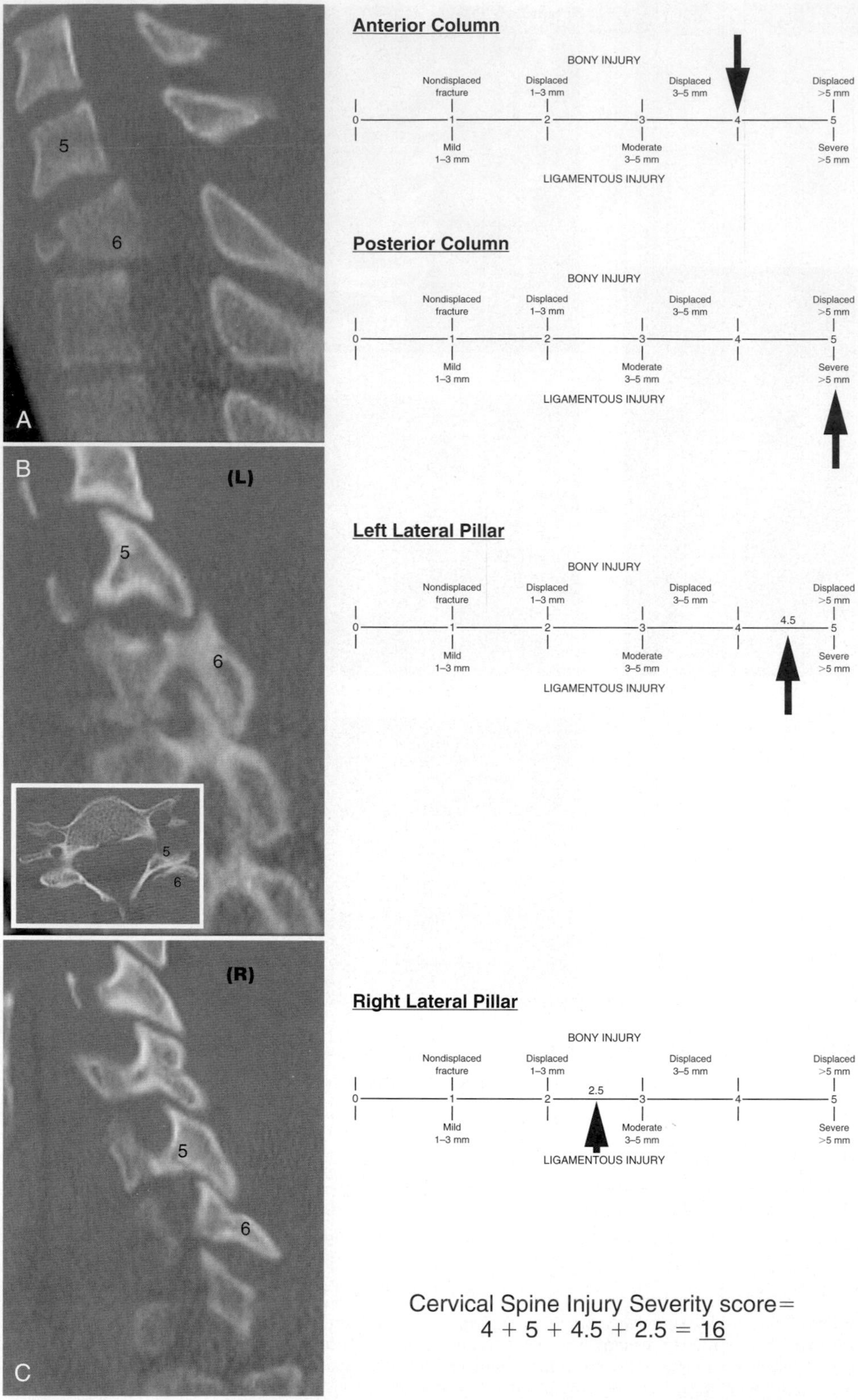

Figure 34-5. Application of the Cervical Spine Injury Severity Score. This patient presents with a flexion teardrop fracture. The midsagittal computed tomography reformat (**A**) shows a fracture of the anterior body of C6, retrolisthesis of the C6 body into the spinal canal, and wide separation of the C5 and C6 spinous processes. Based on this, the anterior column injury was graded a 4, and the posterior column injury graded a 5. The left sagittal reformat (**B**) with axial cut *(inset)* shows the C5 to C6 facet dislocation, giving the left lateral pillar a score of 4.5. The right sagittal reformat (**C**) shows diastasis of the C6 to C7 facet, giving the right lateral pillar a score of 2.5. The sum of these four pillars is the Cervical Spine Injury Severity Score; in this case, it is 16. Scores greater than 7 indicate sufficient instability to warrant surgical stabilization.

TABLE 34-1 *SUBAXIAL INJURY CLASSIFICATION SCALE**

	Points
Morphology	
No abnormality	0
Compression	1
Burst	+1 = 2
Distraction (e.g., facet perch, hyperextension)	3
Rotation or translation (e.g., facet dislocation, unstable teardrop, or advanced-stage flexion compression injury)	4
Discoligamentous complex	
Intact	0
Indeterminate (e.g., isolated interspinous widening, MRI signal change only)	1
Disrupted (e.g., widening of disc space, facet perch or dislocation	2
Neurologic status	
Intact	0
Root injury	1
Complete cord injury	2
Incomplete cord injury	3
Continuous cord compression in setting of a neurologic deficit (neuro modifier)	+1

*Scores less than 4 indicate nonoperative treatment. Scores greater than 4 indicate operative treatment. If injuries exist at more than one level, the Subaxial Cervical Spine Injury Classification score should be calculated at each level and each injury scored separately (i.e., the scores are not additive). Compression injury includes compression fractures, burst fractures, sagittal or coronal plane fractures of the vertebrae, flexion teardrop fractures, and nondisplaced or minimally displaced lateral mass and/or facet fractures. Distraction injury includes anterior distraction injuries. Translation/Rotation injury includes unilateral and bilateral facet fracture-dislocations, floating lateral mass fractures, and bilateral pedicle fractures.

MRI, Magnetic resonance image.

From Vaccaro AR, Hulbert RJ, Patel AA, et al; Spine Trauma Study Group: The subaxial cervical spine injury classification system: a novel approach to recognize the importance of morphology, neurology, and integrity of the disco-ligamentous complex, Spine 21:2365–2374, 2007, Table 1.

If a neurologic deficit exists, the determination needs to be made as urgently as possible whether or not a continuous source of compression exists and whether it is from fracture fragments, dislocation or subluxation, or epidural hematoma. The timing of decompression and whether or not pharmacologic agents are indicated is discussed in depth in Chapter 31.

The injury pattern will help determine the degree of mechanical stability and, along with the SLIC score, can help determine whether the injury merits operative treatment. With more unstable injuries, surgical fixation is indicated, but stable injuries can generally be managed nonoperatively. Any subluxation or dislocation in general should be reduced. Whether or not these should be reduced closed or open depends on patient factors and the presence of a neurologic deficit. This is discussed later in the chapter in more detail.

Important patient factors other than neurologic status to consider when deciding on treatment include the presence of other injuries; noncontiguous spinal injuries; and comorbidities such as heart disease, chronic obstructive pulmonary disease, and other diseases in which the patient may be at high risk for adverse events. Diabetes and smoking increase nonunion and infection risk. Body habitus may also influence the management decision. Polytraumatized patients are at greater risk of aspiration pneumonia, decubitus ulcers, urinary tract infection, deep venous thrombosis, pulmonary embolus, and

TABLE 34-2 *THE SUBAXIAL CERVICAL INJURY DESCRIPTION SYSTEM*

Injury Type (Name)	Definitions (Description)
Spinous process fracture	Fracture that detaches a portion of the spinous process or the entire spinous process from the cervical lamina
Isolated lamina fracture	Fracture that extends through the lamina medial to the facet joint or lateral mass and lateral to the base of the spinous process. No subluxation or kyphosis is present in this injury pattern.
Unilateral facet dislocation	Disruption of a single facet joint in which the inferior articular process of the cranial vertebra has translated anterosuperiorly over the superior articular process of the caudal vertebra
Bilateral facet dislocation	Disruption of both facet joints in which the inferior articular processes of the cranial vertebra have translated anterosuperiorly over the superior articular processes of the caudal vertebra. This pattern of injury may be associated with comminution or fracture of the facet joint complex. Perched facets, in which the tip of the inferior articular process abuts the superior articular process, qualify as dislocations as long as there is no articular surface apposition.
Facet subluxation	Misalignment of two adjacent vertebrae resulting in less than full apposition of facet articular surfaces (unilateral or bilateral)
Flexion teardrop fracture	Vertebral body fracture characterized by a triangular or quadrangular bone fragment derived from the anteroinferior vertebral body. Coexistent anterior cranial-caudal vertebral body height loss must also be present.
Lateral mass fracture	Fracture of any portion of the lateral mass complex, including the articular processes and the pedicle. This categorization includes the so-called "floating lateral mass," in which ipsilateral fractures of the lamina and pedicle result in superior and inferior articular processes that are in discontinuity with the native vertebrae.
Compression fracture	Vertebral body fracture with loss of craniocaudal height. No involvement of the posterior cortical margin and no translation or rotational deformity are allowed.
Burst fracture	Vertebral body fracture with loss of craniocaudal height and involvement of the posterior cortical margin. This fracture pattern is often associated with retropulsion of bone fragments into the spinal canal.
Anterior distraction injury	Bone, ligament, or disc injury that results in craniocaudal distraction of the anterior disc space to a greater extent than the posterior disc space. By definition, this injury pattern represents disruption of the anterior tension band.
Transverse process fracture	Fracture along any portion of the transverse process, including fractures that extend into the foramen transversarium.

From Bono CM, Schoenfeld A, Gupta G, et al: Reliability and reproducibility of subaxial cervical injury description system: a standardized nomenclature schema, Spine (Phila Pa 1976) 36(17):E1140–E1144, 2011, Table 2.

other complications from prolonged intensive care unit stays. Therefore, operative management, which immediately provides internal mechanical stability to allow for greater mobilization, may decrease the burden of injury in the acute period.

Principles of Nonoperative Management

A variety of cervical orthoses are available, each of which has varying capacity to stabilize the spine. The most basic difference between the different options is that some are cervical orthoses alone that only brace the neck itself, and others are cervicothoracic braces that extend the brace to the thorax. Chapter 39 is devoted to cervical and cervicothoracic braces in more detail.

When a cervical orthosis is used as definitive treatment, upright radiographs should be obtained with the orthosis in place to ensure proper alignment is maintained. If there is significant displacement seen with the orthosis, operative management should be considered. Patients should be followed with serial radiographs beginning approximately 7 to 14 days after the injury to assure that the orthosis is fitting properly and to verify that halo pins if used are not loose or infected. Radiographs are obtained every 4 weeks up until approximately 12 weeks postinjury at which time flexion and extension lateral plain radiographs are obtained to make sure healing has occurred. If failure occurs any time in the course of nonoperative treatment, operative treatment should be considered.

Principles of Operative Management

For unstable subaxial cervical spine injuries, operative management is indicated in anyone medically stable enough to undergo surgery. Operative management allows for direct decompression of the spinal cord, anatomic reduction and realignment, rigid stabilization, and bone grafting to promote fusion. The timing of surgical intervention is discussed in Chapter 32 but early fixation of an unstable cervical spine injury with a neurologic deficit not only potentially improves neurologic recovery but likely decreases the complication rate in the acute hospitalization period.[29]

MANAGEMENT OF SPECIFIC INJURIES

Flexion Teardrop Fracture

The teardrop fracture is a "vertebral body fracture characterized by a triangular, or quadrangular, bone fragment derived from the anteroinferior vertebral body. Coexistent anterior cranial-caudal vertebral body height loss must also be present."[27] Flexion teardrop fractures are most commonly caused by MVAs or by diving into shallow water. They have also been associated with American football spearing injuries.[30]

Flexion teardrop fractures occur with the head flexed and an obliquely downward axial force concentrated on the anterosuperior vertebral body. With increasing loading force, the anterior column fails in compression, with the fracture propagating through the caudal disc space and into the posterior column. The posterior elements may become distracted and eventually disrupted with fracture or ligamentous disruption (or both). The involved vertebra essentially is split into a caudal segment composed of the teardrop component anteroinferiorly and a cephalad segment composed of the posterosuperior aspect of the intact vertebral body and the posterior elements (Fig. 34-6). Although the anterior fracture is typically the most obvious radiographic finding, the integrity of the ligamentous complex posteriorly determines the stability of the injury.

Definitive Treatment of Teardrop Fractures

Nonoperative Treatment. Teardrop fractures with displacement or neurologic injury meet the criteria for operative treatment based on the SLIC system. Nondisplaced teardrop fractures may not represent the true amount of displacement that occurred at the time of injury. If after examining advanced imaging studies, the DLC is considered intact and the patient is neurologically intact, nonoperative treatment is appropriate with a hard cervical orthosis with close radiographic follow-up to ensure alignment is maintained. Typically, the orthosis is used for 10 to 12 weeks at which time flexion-extension lateral radiographs are obtained to ensure healing and stability. A halo vest may also be used in the absence of posterior ligamentous disruption with close attention to potential halo vest complications.

Operative Treatment. Teardrop fractures with neurologic injury, vertebral displacement, or disruption of the DLC are unstable injuries and require operative treatment. If displacement and concomitant spinal cord injury exists, initial awake closed reduction using Gardner-Wells tongs and 10 lb of traction with increasing weight under radiographic control should be attempted. If complete reduction is achieved and no residual spinal cord compression exists, posterior-only stabilization with lateral mass screws and rods can be performed alone.[31] A recent study described anterior discectomy of the involved caudal disc space and fusion to the infrajacent level with the use of an anterior locking plate.[32] This treatment was successful in 20 of 21 patients who healed with a mean loss of cervical lordosis of 2.6 degrees.

If after awake closed reduction, there remains any retrolisthesis, anterior corpectomy with strut grafting and plating may be performed to decompress the spinal cord and provide anterior column support. Teardrop fractures with DLC disruption or facet fracture or dislocation posteriorly may also benefit from posterior fixation after the anterior corpectomy and grafting. Circumferential fusion may provide the most biomechanically stable construct, although clinical evidence is lacking.[33]

Fisher and colleagues retrospectively compared the results of halo vest immobilization versus anterior corpectomy and plating in 24 and 21 patients, respectively, who had unstable teardrop fractures.[34] At final follow-up, the halo group had 11.4 degrees of kyphosis versus 3.5 degrees in the corpectomy group, a statistically significant difference. The halo group also had five failures, four of whom required surgery, but the corpectomy group had no failures, demonstrating the superiority of surgical management of these injuries.

Compression Fracture

Compression fractures are "vertebral body fracture with loss of craniocaudal height. No involvement of the posterior cortical margin and no translational or rotational deformity are allowed."[27] Although common in the thoracic and lumbar regions of the spine in individuals with osteoporosis, compression fractures in the cervical spine are less common. Typically, when they occur in the cervical spine, compression fractures

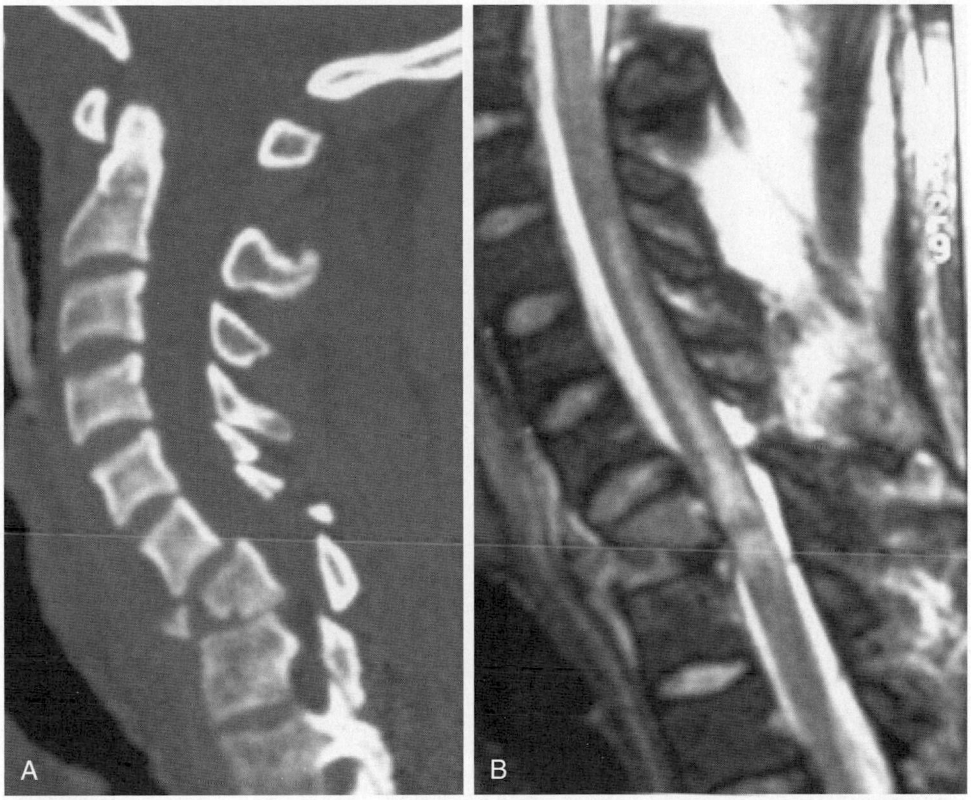

Figure 34-6. Force propagation in a flexion teardrop fracture. **A,** The coronal fracture line separates the anteroinferior vertebral body (the teardrop component) from the remaining posterosuperior body. The fracture can propagate posteriorly through the spinal cord and posterior column, causing disruption of the ligamentous complex or fracture, as seen here. **B,** Magnetic resonance image demonstrates spinal cord injury caused by fracture and compression from posteriorly displaced vertebral body of C7 and malaligned spinal column.

are caused by low-energy mechanisms in individuals with osteoporosis or those with metabolic bone disease. Compression fractures can also occur in conjunction with a flexion-distraction injury mechanism and facet fracture-dislocation. When cervical compression fractures occur from a high-energy mechanism, an MRI should be obtained to evaluate the status of the DLC to ensure that the facet joints did not sublux or dislocate and spontaneously relocate.

Definitive Treatment

An isolated vertebral compression fracture with minimal loss of height or kyphosis should be treated with a rigid cervical collar for approximately 10 weeks with radiographic follow-up to ensure that alignment does not worsen. A metabolic bone disease consult should be obtained if warranted. Multiple cervical compression fractures may result in a progressive kyphotic deformity. With significant deformity affecting quality of life, surgical realignment procedures can be considered.

Burst Fractures

Burst fractures are defined as "vertebral body fracture with loss of craniocaudal height and involvement of the posterior cortical margin. This fracture pattern is often associated with retropulsion of bone fragments into the spinal canal."[27] The mechanism of injury is initially pure axial loading. With severe injury and axial loading, eventually the subaxial spine will buckle and flex or extend, which may cause fracture of the posterior elements or ligamentous disruption, respectively. The most severe burst fractures with retropulsion have a high likelihood of spinal cord injury.

Treatment Recommendations of Burst Fractures

Treatment is dictated by the severity of the injury and the neurologic status of the patient. Most patients with burst fractures with retropulsion have a neurologic deficit. Without retropulsion or neurologic deficit, the patient may be managed nonoperatively with a rigid external cervical orthosis with close radiographic follow-up to ensure maintenance of alignment and no kyphotic collapse (Fig. 34-7).

With retropulsion and neurologic deficit, surgery is indicated based on the SLIC scoring system. The posterior elements may also be injured, and MRI and CT should be analyzed for disruption of the DLC. Surgery should involve direct decompression of the spinal cord via an anterior corpectomy, strut grafting, and plating. Biomechanical cadaveric studies have shown that this method of fixation provides adequate stability in this injury pattern; however, if there is evidence on MRI of posterior ligamentous disruption, consideration should be given to combined anterior and posterior fixation[35] (Fig. 34-8).

Clinically, in a retrospective study comparing halo immobilization or skull traction with anterior corpectomy and plating in patients with flexion teardrop or burst fractures, operatively treated patients were significantly more likely to recover at least one grade of motor function and had a mean

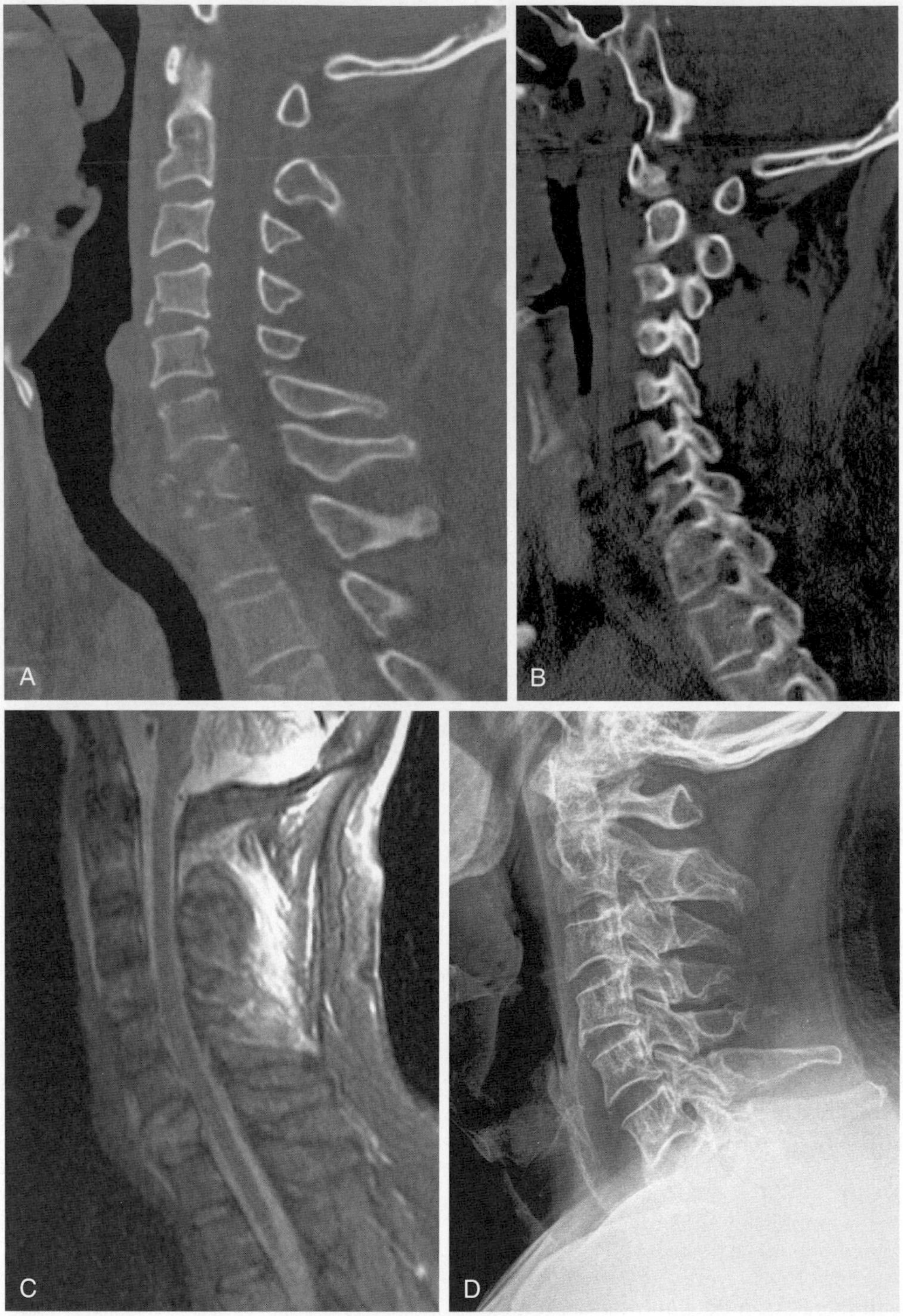

Figure 34-7. A, A 49-year-old man involved in motor vehicle accident with multiple cervical spine fractures, including a C2 fracture, antero-inferior endplate fracture of C4, and burst fracture to C7 (Subaxial Cervical Spine Injury Classification [SLIC] morphology = 2). The patient was neurologically intact (SLIC neuro = 0). The sagittal computed tomography (CT) scan shows minimal retropulsion of the C7 vertebral body. **B,** Parasagittal CT scan revealed the facet joints to be reduced. **C,** Magnetic resonance image showed retropulsion of the C7 body without cord edema. The posterior ligamentous complex was intact (SLIC DLC = 0; total SLIC score: 2 + 0 + 0 = 2 → nonoperative). **D,** The patient was treated nonoperatively with cervical orthosis; at 22 months after the injury, all fractures had healed, and no kyphotic deformity was present.

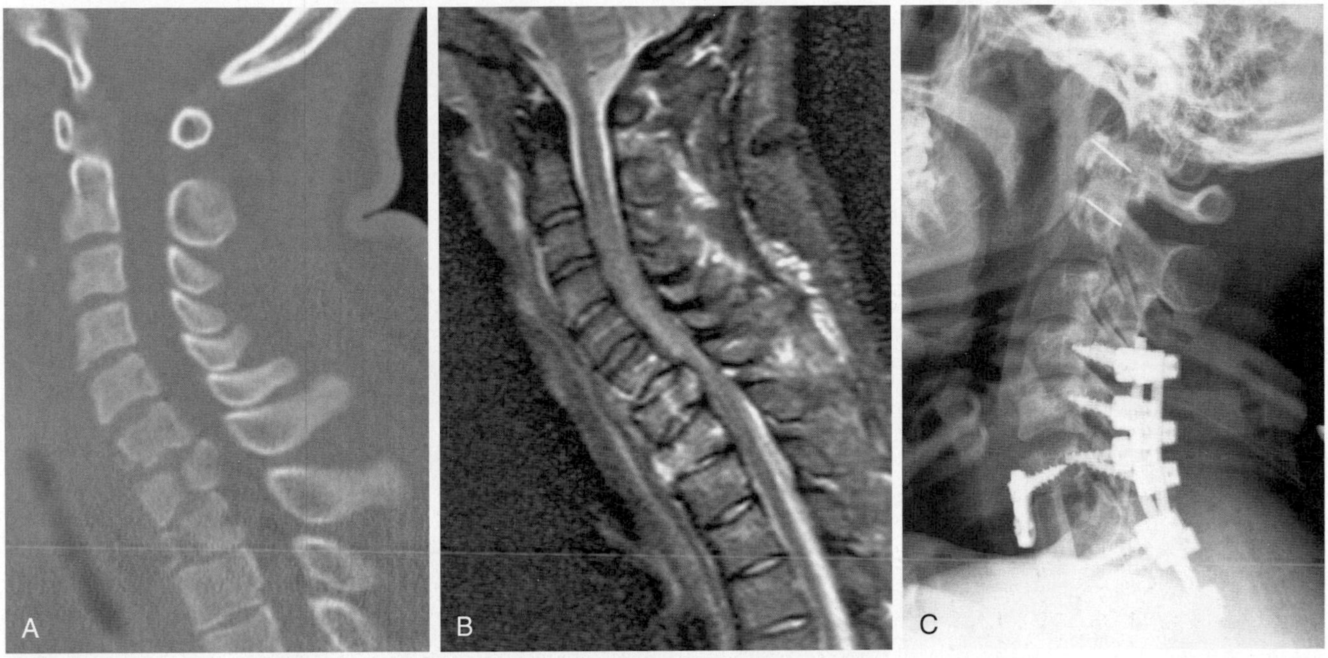

Figure 34-8. A, A 19-year-old woman was ejected from a vehicle and sustained a complete spinal cord injury at the level of C6 and multiple fractures, including a C6 compression fracture (Subaxial Cervical Spine Injury Classification [SLIC] morphology = 1), C7 burst fracture (SLIC morphology = 2), and T1 compression fracture. **B,** Magnetic resonance image shows spinal cord injury, retropulsion of the C7 vertebral body, and disruption of the posterior ligamentous complex (SLIC: 2 + 2 + 2 = 6 → operative). **C,** The patient underwent decompression through an anterior approach on the night of her injury with C7 corpectomy and partial T1 corpectomy with strut allograft and buttress plate. She then underwent posterior stabilization and fusion at a later time when more stable to prevent kyphotic collapse.

lordosis of 2.2 degrees versus a mean kyphosis of 12.6 degrees in the nonoperatively treated group.

Facet Subluxation, Unilateral Facet Dislocation, Bilateral Facet Dislocation, and Facet Fractures

Facet subluxations, unilateral facet subluxations, and bilateral facet dislocations will be discussed as a group because the structures injured, the injury mechanisms, and general treatment guidelines are similar and are typically discussed together. Facet subluxations are "misalignment of two adjacent vertebrae resulting in less than full apposition of facet articular surfaces (unilateral or bilateral)."[27] Unilateral facet dislocations are "disruption of a single facet joint in which the inferior articular process of the cranial vertebra has translated anterosuperiorly over the superior articular process of the caudal vertebra."[27] Bilateral facet dislocations are defined as "disruption of both facet joints in which the inferior articular processes of the cranial vertebra have translated anterosuperiorly over the superior articular processes of the caudal vertebra. This pattern of injury may be associated with comminution, or fracture, of the facet joint complex. Perched facets, in which the tip of the inferior articular process abuts the superior articular process, qualify as dislocations as long as there is no articular surface apposition."[27]

These injuries all share a similar flexion injury mechanism either from a sudden deceleration in a MVA or a fall onto the head in which the head flexes. The center of rotation of the flexion moment is anterior to the vertebral body, such that the posterior elements of the spine become distracted and fail. There is frequently a concomitant compressive force to the subjacent vertebral endplate.

Unilateral Facet Dislocations

Cadaveric studies have shown that unilateral facet dislocations are created when the neck was flexed and bent laterally with subsequent axial torque.[36] Another study showed that pure distraction applied unilaterally coupled with axial rotation creates enough force to cause a unilateral facet dislocation without the addition of a separate flexion moment.[37] A cadaveric study of nine specimens in which unilateral facet dislocations or fracture-dislocations were created found upon postinjury dissection facet capsular tears and annular disruption in all specimens.[38] In eight specimens, the ligamentum flavum was injured, and the interspinous and supraspinous ligaments were stretched in three and four specimens, respectively, but never completely torn. Disruption of the annulus accounts for acute traumatic disc herniation with potential neurologic deficit that is often associated with these injuries.

Without CT scan, unilateral facet dislocations can be missed because often spinal malalignment is subtle (Fig. 34-9). On CT, a unilateral facet dislocation demonstrates a rotational deformity with reversal of the normal position of the superior and inferior facets at the dislocated level (Fig. 34-10). The axial CT will show the inferior dislocated facet of the cephalad vertebrae lying anterior to the superior facet of the caudal vertebrae. Sagittal CT scan will also reveal the typical appearance of the completely dislocated or perched inferior facet sitting anteriorly or on top of the caudal superior articular facet.

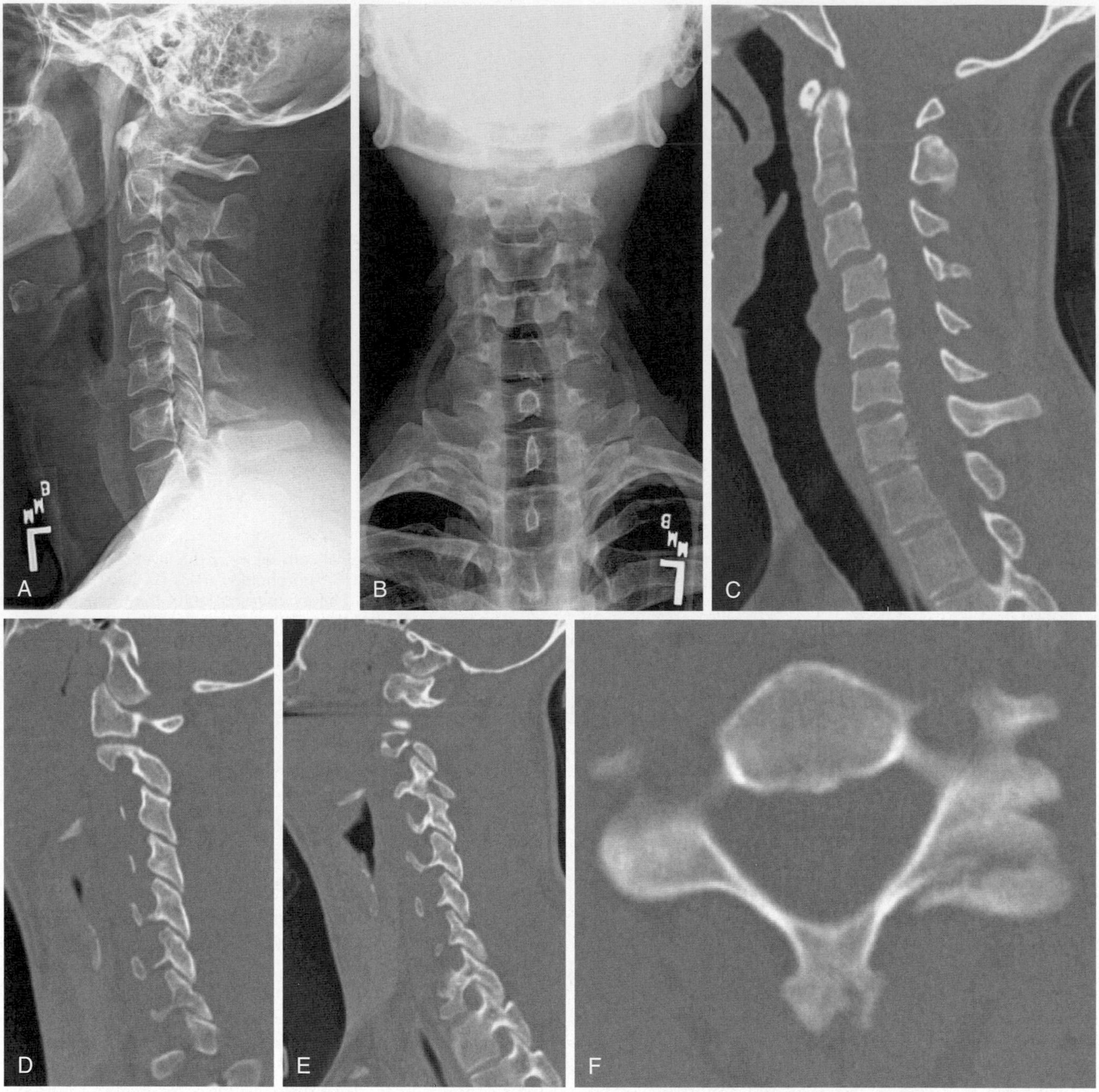

Figure 34-9. A 35-year-old man involved in motor vehicle accident. **A,** Lateral injury radiograph shows anterolisthesis of C3 on C4 and a "bowtie" appearance of the facet at this level. **B,** On the anterior-posterior view, there is loss of the spinous process at the rotated level because it is not an orthogonal view due to the rotation of the injured level. **C** and **D,** Computed tomography (CT) scan reveals unilateral facet fracture dislocation on the left and uninjured contralateral side (**E**). Axial CT scan demonstrates the rotational nature of the injury in which only one side is disrupted (**F**).

Bilateral Facet Dislocations

Bilateral facet dislocations have 50% or greater anterior translation of the dislocated vertebral body. Bilateral facet dislocations with only mild displacement on static imaging studies often underestimate the degree of displacement at the moment of injury.

Pure distraction and flexion is likely to produce a pure dislocation of the facets (Fig. 34-11). However, in actual real-life high-energy traumas such as MVAs, multiple force vectors can occur concurrently. The flexion-distraction mechanism, combined with torsion, lateral bending, compression, or translation, may produce various combinations of fractures or dislocations (or both) of unilateral or bilateral facets[39] (Fig. 34-12). Often the superior facet of the caudal vertebra is fractured and displaced into the foramen by the inferior facet of the cephalad vertebra. Patients may have a nerve root injury caused by the fracture impinging on the nerve root in the neuroforamen. Laminae and spinous process fractures may also occur concurrently with this injury.

Magnetic resonance imaging is the best study to elucidate the full extent of soft tissue injury associated with facet injuries. In a retrospective study of 48 patients with unilateral (25

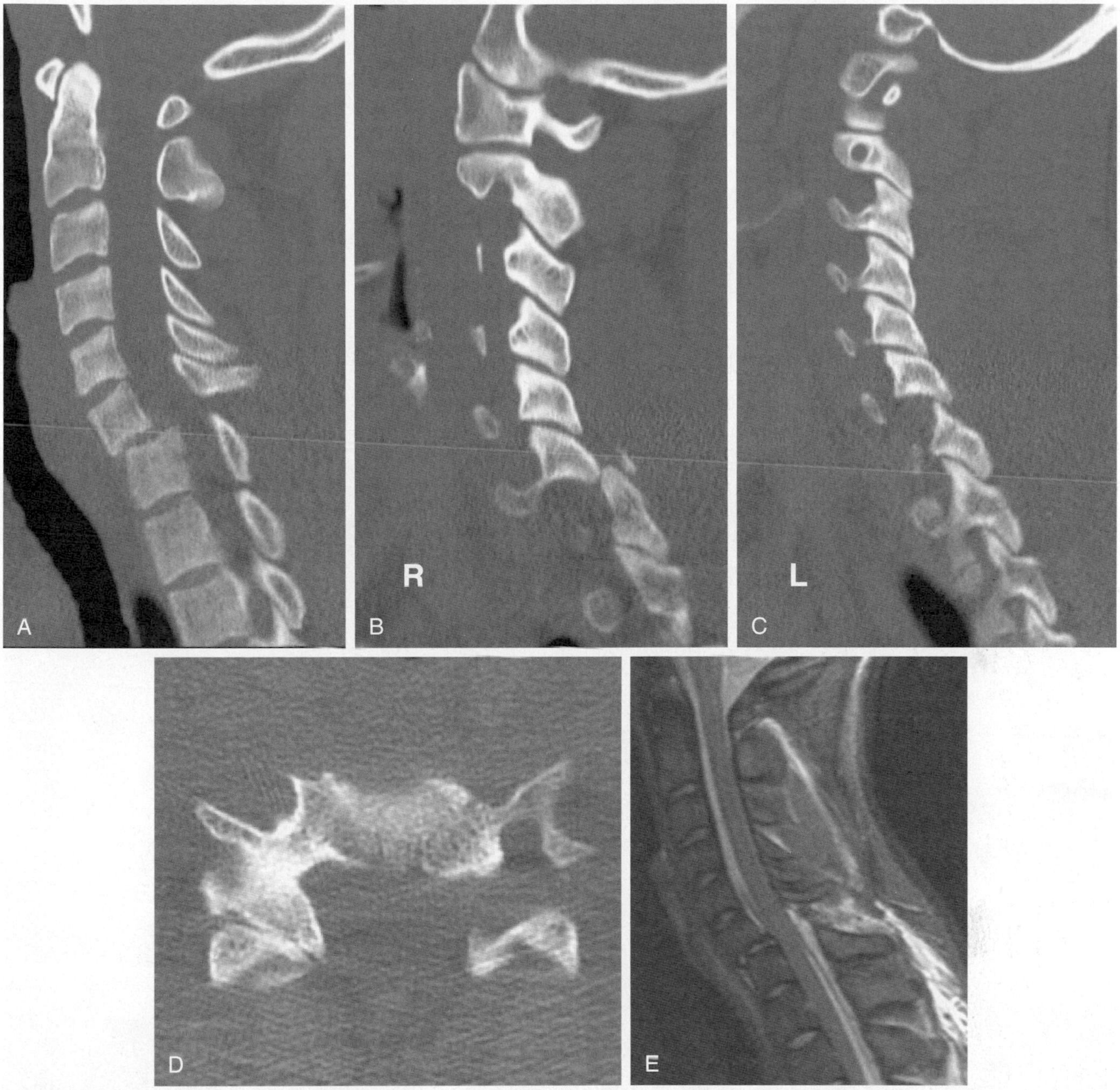

Figure 34-10. A, A 21-year-old male rugby player was injured in a game and complained of neck pain and paresthesias in the arms but was neurologically intact (Subaxial Cervical Spine Injury Classification [SLIC] neuro = 0). Computed tomography (CT) scan shows C6 to C7 bilateral facet injuries with a dislocated facet and an associated fracture (**B**) and a contralateral facet subluxation (**C**) (SLIC morphology = 4). **D,** Axial CT scan shows complete dislocation of the unilateral facet. **E,** Magnetic resonance image shows anterolisthesis with disruption of the discoligamentous complex (SLIC DLC status = 2). The patient was close reduced while awake and subsequently underwent posterior fixation and fusion (total SLIC score = 0 + 4 + 2 = 6 → operative).

patients) or bilateral (23 patients) facet injuries, the authors found high rates of disruption to the posterior ligamentous complex (posterior muscles, interspinous and supraspinous ligaments, ligamentum flavum, and facet capsules).[40] Disc herniations occurred in 56% of unilateral facet dislocations and 82.5% of bilateral facet dislocations. Another study of 30 bilateral facet dislocations found the ALL to be disrupted 27% of the time and the PLL to be disrupted in 40% of cases; however, disc disruption occurred in 90% of these injuries.[41] The study also found that when compared with findings at surgery, MRI was accurate in diagnosing 24 of 26 ligamentous disruptions.

Treatment Recommendations

Treatment recommendations for bilateral dislocation injuries depend on the severity; whether a dislocation or fracture-dislocation is present; the status of associated surrounding soft tissue structures, specifically the DLC; and the neurologic status of the patient.

Disc Herniations and the Reduction of Facet Dislocations

Perhaps the most controversial aspect of treating subaxial cervical spine trauma is the treatment of facet dislocations in the

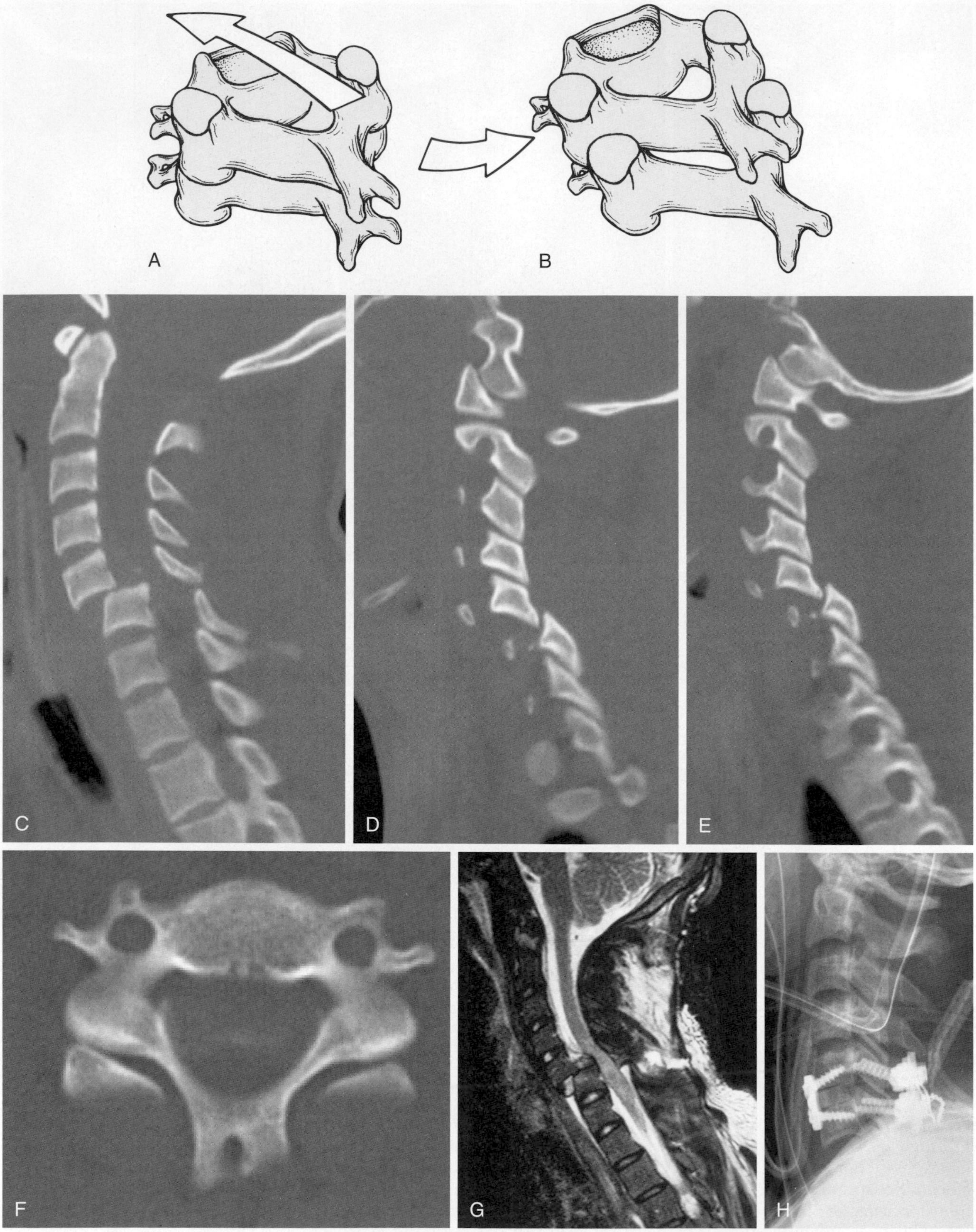

Figure 34-11. Bilateral facet dislocation mechanism. With sufficient forward flexion with distraction (**A**), both facets can dislocate (**B**). With lesser distraction and more forward translation, the facets can fracture. **C** and **D,** A 29-year-old woman with bilateral facet dislocation after a motor vehicle accident with incomplete spinal cord injury (Subaxial Cervical Spine Injury Classification [SLIC] neuro = 4 [3 + 1 {neuro modifier for continuous cord compression}]). **E,** Axial computed tomography scan shows the inferior facet of the superior vertebra completely dislocated anteriorly to the superior facets of the caudal vertebra (SLIC morphology = 4). **F,** Magnetic resonance image shows a large traumatic disc herniation (SLIC DLC status = 2). Circumferential stabilization of bilateral facet dislocations offers the most rigid stability to prevent deforming forces due to discoligamentous disruption from causing late kyphotic collapse and resultant deformity (total SLIC score = 4 + 4 + 2 = 10 → operative) (**G** and **H**).

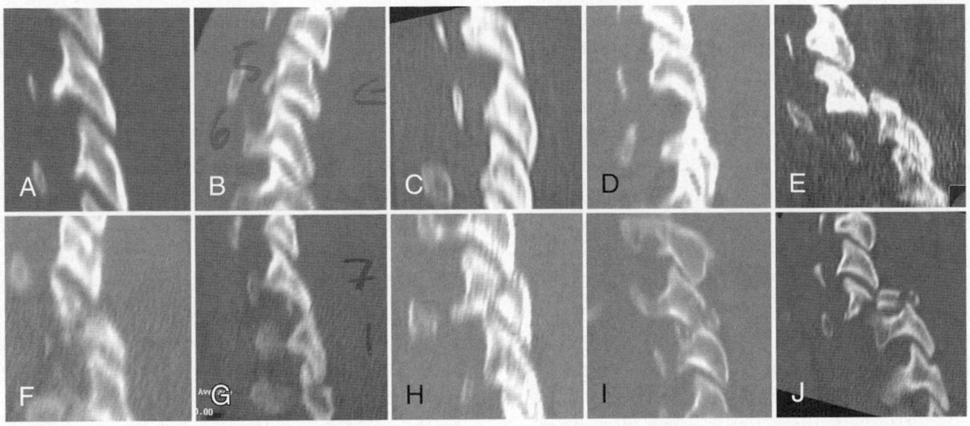

Figure 34-12. Different facet injuries that may result from various combinations of flexion, compression, and rotation. Different configurations of facet injuries can occur, depending on the extent and timing of the forces acting on the spine at the time of injury. The top row (**A–E**) demonstrates a spectrum of purely ligamentous injuries, starting from the normally aligned facet (**A**). The facet capsule may be disrupted with subtle widening (**B**), and greater soft tissue disruption leads to facet subluxation (**C**), perching (**D**), and frank dislocation (**E**). The bottom row (**F–J**) demonstrates various fracture patterns. Most commonly, the superior facet is fractured and pushed forward into the foramen (**F**). Superior facet fracturing can be associated with facet subluxation or dislocation as well (**G**). Less commonly, the inferior facet is fractured, a pattern that may be associated with extension injuries and that often compromises the ability to place screws into this segment (**H**). Both the inferior and superior facets may be fractured (**I**). Finally, significant comminution of the facet (**J**) may preclude stable screw fixation at this level.

presence of a traumatic disc herniation. With reduction of the dislocation, there is a risk of displacing a traumatic disc herniation further into the spinal canal (Fig. 34-13). This was illustrated by Eismont and colleagues, who reported a 33-year-old patient who became quadriplegic after open reduction of a bilateral facet dislocation from a herniated disc behind the C6 body, which required anterior discectomy and fusion.[42] Much debate exists surrounding both closed and open reduction of these injuries and the risk of causing a spinal cord injury or worsening the neurologic status of the patient with the reduction maneuver.

Disc herniations can be difficult to define, especially in the presence of dislocation. Vaccaro and colleagues defined a traumatic disc herniation to be present when material with signal intensity consistent with disc protrudes posteriorly to the posterior cortical line of the inferior vertebral body.[43] Others have defined disc herniation in the setting of facet dislocation as any ventral spinal cord or nerve root compression caused by disc material.[44,45] The presence of a neurologic deficit on presentation has been shown to correlate strongly with the presence of a disc herniation.[45,46] The rate of reported disc herniation in the presence of facet dislocation varies considerably ranging from 18% to 62% with higher rates for bilateral than unilateral dislocation.[43-46]

Whether or not to obtain a MRI before attempting reduction is controversial. In a retrospective study of 11 patients

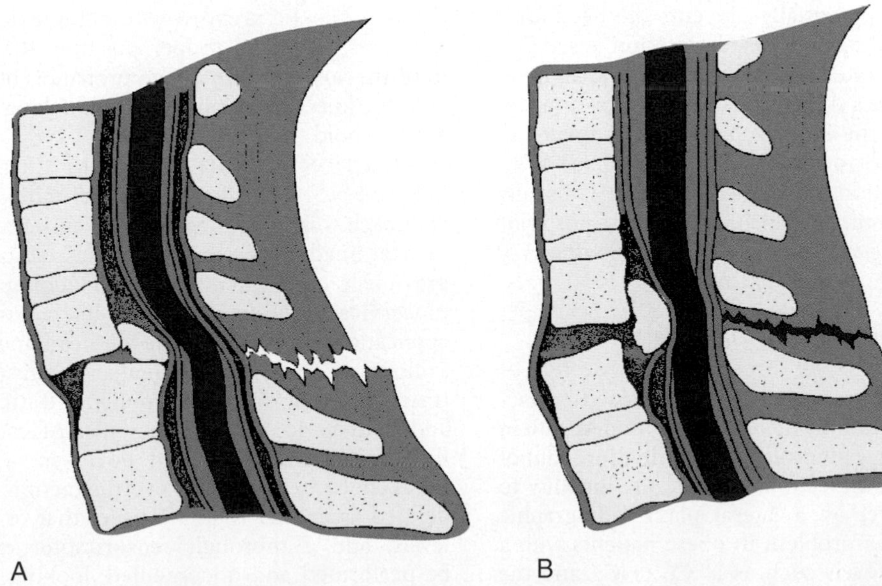

Figure 34-13. A, A disc herniation associated with unilateral or bilateral facet dislocation. **B,** There is a risk of worsening of neurologic deficit or paralysis if the disc flips back into the spinal cord instead of reducing into the disc space with the closed reduction of the dislocation.

with unilateral or bilateral facet dislocations, nine of whom had neurologic injury, all had prereduction MRI.[43] Postreduction MRI revealed three additional herniations and worsening of one of the two prior herniations. No patient sustained worsening of neurologic status. The study suggests that the presence of a disc herniation does not preclude an attempt at closed reduction if the patient is awake, alert, and cooperative.

In a complete spinal cord injury, the benefit of rapid reduction and indirect decompression of the spinal cord would seem to outweigh the knowledge gained from a MRI. In a neurologically intact patient with a facet dislocation, the knowledge gained from prereduction MRI may or may not be of particular benefit and may also dissuade the treatment team from performing the reduction closed if a disc herniation is present.

In a patient presenting with an incomplete neurologic deficit, the most likely cause of the deficit is a disc herniation.[45,46] Realigning the spine needs to be weighed against the risk of causing the disc to retropulse into the spinal cord, further worsening the neurologic status of the patient. If MRI can be obtained rapidly as is often now the case in spinal cord injury and trauma centers, it is acceptable to obtain a prereduction MRI, although a traumatic disc herniation does not necessarily preclude a safe and successful closed reduction in an awake and alert patient.[43] In awake and alert patients who have a complete spinal cord injury (American Spinal Injury Association [ASIA] type A), prereduction MRI can be bypassed given the risk–benefit analysis of realigning the spine in a timely fashion in a patient with minimal risk of worsening the neurologic condition.

To date, no permanent neurologic deficit has ever been reported in an awake and alert patient undergoing closed reduction of a cervical facet dislocation. An awake, alert, and cooperative patient can safely undergo attempted closed reduction in a closely monitored environment. If the patient is obtunded or if a reliable neurologic examination cannot be obtained, closed reduction should not be attempted. In awake patients, closed reduction offers the potential for earlier decompression of the spinal cord.

Closed reduction also potentially prevents the need for a multistage surgical procedure. If a disc herniation is seen on MRI, a logical alternative to closed reduction is first an anterior procedure to perform a discectomy followed by a posterior procedure to reduce the facet dislocation and finally an anterior procedure to perform a fusion of the disc space. With a successful closed reduction, only one procedure is usually necessary, an anterior decompression and fusion or a posterior fusion. This avoids prolonged operative time and blood loss in patients who are typically polytraumatized.

Technique of Closed Reduction of a Cervical Facet Dislocation

Contraindications. Contraindications to closed reduction of cervical facet dislocations include an obtunded patient or one in whom a reliable neurologic examination cannot be obtained. Other contraindications include the inability to visualize the affected level on a lateral plain radiographic image. This is most often a problem in obese patients with a thick neck and at lower levels such as at C6 to C7 and the cervicothoracic junction. These patients require a MRI to rule out disc herniation followed by open reduction. Fractures at other levels of the spine, specifically the upper cervical spine, should be ruled out because they can displace with traction. Although a fractured facet at the injured level is not an absolute contraindication, it may make the chances of a successful closed reduction less likely.[47,48] Unilaterally dislocated facets in some series have been shown to be more difficult to reduce than bilaterally dislocated facets, although this is not a contraindication to an attempt at closed reduction.[49] A stiffening spine disease such as ankylosing spondylitis (AS) is also a relative contraindication to cervical traction unless a form of traction such as bivector traction is used to realign the cervical spine rather than to reduce a dislocated facet.

Positioning. The setting for closed reduction should be in a highly monitored environment. The procedure can be performed in an emergency trauma room, the intensive care unit, or an operating room (OR). Intravenous analgesia and a mild sedative that can be titrated will calm the patient and also have an effect to relax tense and spastic neck muscles, making the reduction easier to obtain. Close monitoring of the airway and respiratory status is essential, and therefore an anesthesiologist may be required.

The patient is placed in the supine position on a bed or stretcher. The reverse Trendelenburg position is used to counteract the pull of increasing weight applied cranially. A roll can be placed between the scapulae and the shoulders taped to the foot of the bed to better visualize the lower cervical spine and provide countertraction.

Pin Insertion. Stainless steel Gardner-Wells tongs are preferred as traction weights of greater than 80 lb can cause MRI compatible tongs to disengage from the skull. Local anesthesia is injected into the skin at the site of pin placement, approximately 1 cm above the pinna and in line with the external auditory meatus. Because exaggerating the deformity is necessary to loosen or disengage the dislocated facet or facets, placing the pins slightly posterior to the external auditory meatus may create more of a flexion moment. The pins must be below the equator of the skull; otherwise, they risk disengagement through cephalad creep from the skull with application of weight. Shaving is not normally performed, although the pins may be covered with bacitracin ointment or the skin may be prepped with chlorhexidine as prophylactic measures. When in proper position, the pins are tightened until the spring strain gauge protrudes outward 1 mm, flush with the knob of the pin. The side locking nuts are then tightened to hold the pins in place.

Traction Weight. An initial traction weight of 5 lb followed by 10 lb is begun. Lateral radiographs are obtained after each weight application. The entire cervical spine should be examined closely on the lateral radiograph to assess for previously undetected injuries, including injuries to the craniocervical junction, which may distract with minimal weight application. The position of the head and neck on the plain radiograph should be evaluated to ensure that the proper traction vector is being applied. At this point, weight is added in 5- to 10-lb increments. At each weight increase, the following steps should be taken: a lateral radiograph is taken to examine for overdistraction of all disc spaces, defined as greater than 1.5 times that of adjacent uninjured levels, and a thorough sensorimotor examination should be performed and documented, looking for any changes in neurologic status that may have occurred with increased weight applied.

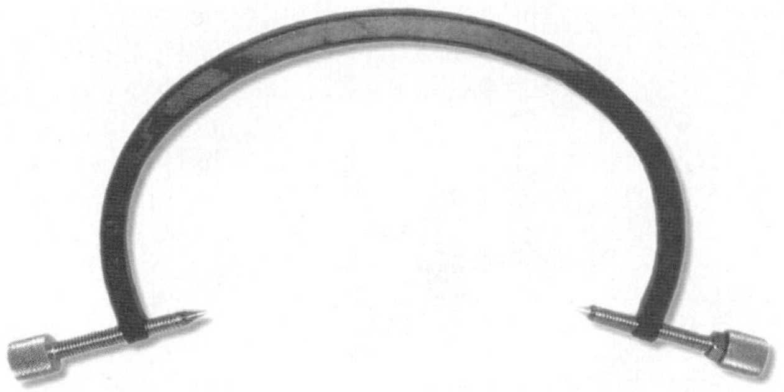

Figure 34-14. Gardner-Wells tongs.

With increasing traction and distraction, the dislocated inferior facet of the upper vertebrae should become distracted enough to minimize or remove the presence of bony impingement between itself and the superior articular facet of the lower vertebrae. The final stage of the reduction can be accomplished by lowering the height of the traction pulley or by placing an interscapular bump beneath the patient. Either of these maneuvers should create an extension vector, which allows the facets to return back into proper alignment, with the inferior facet of the cephalad vertebrae lining posterior to the superior facet of the caudal vertebrae. Unilateral facet dislocations, because of the more complex coupled forces involved with the injury mechanism, may be more difficult to reduce with longitudinal traction alone. In these instances, a lateral bending and derotation maneuver may be performed by an individual experienced in the technique. To accomplish this, the physician places his or her hands around the traction tongs with the thumbs above the traction pin against the sides of the skull with the second through fifth finger tips applied to the back of the cervical spine. At the time of facet perch, a downward force is applied to the located facet, and a gentle axial distraction and rotational moment is applied to the dislocated facet in the direction needed for reduction. This maneuver is followed again by lowering the height of the traction pulley or by placing an interscapular bump beneath the patient (Figs. 34-14 to 34-17).

If in-line traction does not result in reduction, maneuvers that involve accentuating or exaggerating the deformity to disengage the locked facets may be required. This is accomplished by arranging the traction pulley in such a way that the vector of pull results in a flexion moment to the cervical spine, allowing the dislocated facets to disengage. Up to 30 to 45 degrees of head flexion may be necessary to disengage the facets.

After the reduction has been attained, the traction weights may be gradually decreased to approximately 15 to 25 lb followed by a confirmatory lateral radiograph. If subluxation recurs, a higher weight may be necessary to maintain the reduction. At this point, while an assistant maintains in-line manual traction, the stainless steel Gardner-Wells tongs used for the reduction may be switched to MRI-compatible tongs in anticipation of obtaining a MRI or a halo vest can be applied until definitive operative stabilization. A MRI is obtained as soon as possible afterward to evaluate for any compressive lesions such as a traumatic disc herniation, whether or not one was obtained before the reduction.

There exists no evidence-based recommendation on the maximum weight to be applied before deciding that the dislocation is irreducible. As long as the patient can tolerate the procedure and remains neurologically stable while at the same time the cervical spine radiographically appears to demonstrate no deleterious effect of traction, increasing weight of up to 140 lb has been reported to successfully reduce facet dislocations safely.[50]

In the event of neurologic deterioration, the traction should be removed slowly, and the reduction maneuver should be reversed if performed (i.e., the extended cervical spine should be again gently flexed until function improves). An emergent MRI should be obtained to evaluate possible causes of neurologic deterioration, and the OR should be notified for emergent decompression, open reduction, and stabilization. In addition to disc herniation as a possible cause, other causes that have been reported for neurologic decline during or soon after closed reduction include epidural hematoma,[51] disrupted ossification of the posterior longitudinal ligament (OPLL),[52] ligamentum flavum infolding,[53] and preexisting cervical stenosis exacerbated by traction and manipulation.[54] In summary, closed reduction of cervical facet dislocations in awake, alert, and cooperative patients should be attempted in a closely monitored environment with an experienced treatment team.

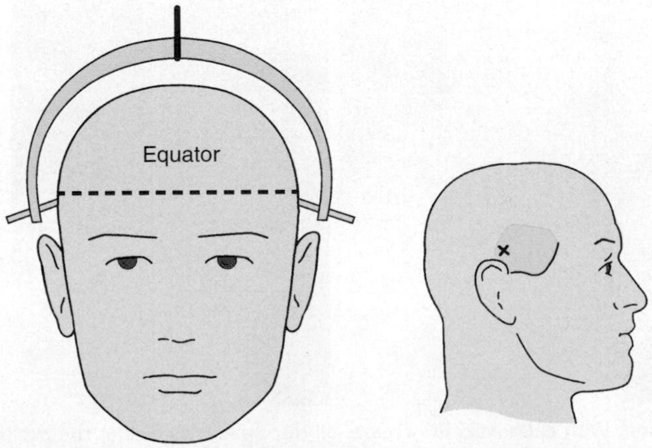

Figure 34-15. The pins are located above the pinna in line with the external auditory meatus below the equator of the skull.

Definitive Treatment of Unilateral and Bilateral Facet Fractures and Dislocations

The SLIC score may be used to help guide operative versus nonoperative treatment. If operative treatment is necessary, various surgical options can be used. Surgical treatment options depend on the severity of the injury, the presence of a neurologic deficit, and the location of the spinal cord or nerve root compression.

Unilateral Facet Dislocations

Unilateral facet dislocations and unilateral facet fracture-dislocations benefit from operative stabilization. An anterior stabilization or posterior stabilization procedure may be effective unless there is a superior endplate fracture of the lower involved vertebrae, and then a posterior or circumferential procedure is recommended (Fig. 34-18).

Clinical outcome studies have found that allowing a unilateral facet dislocation to heal in the dislocated position results in a higher incidence of long-term pain and

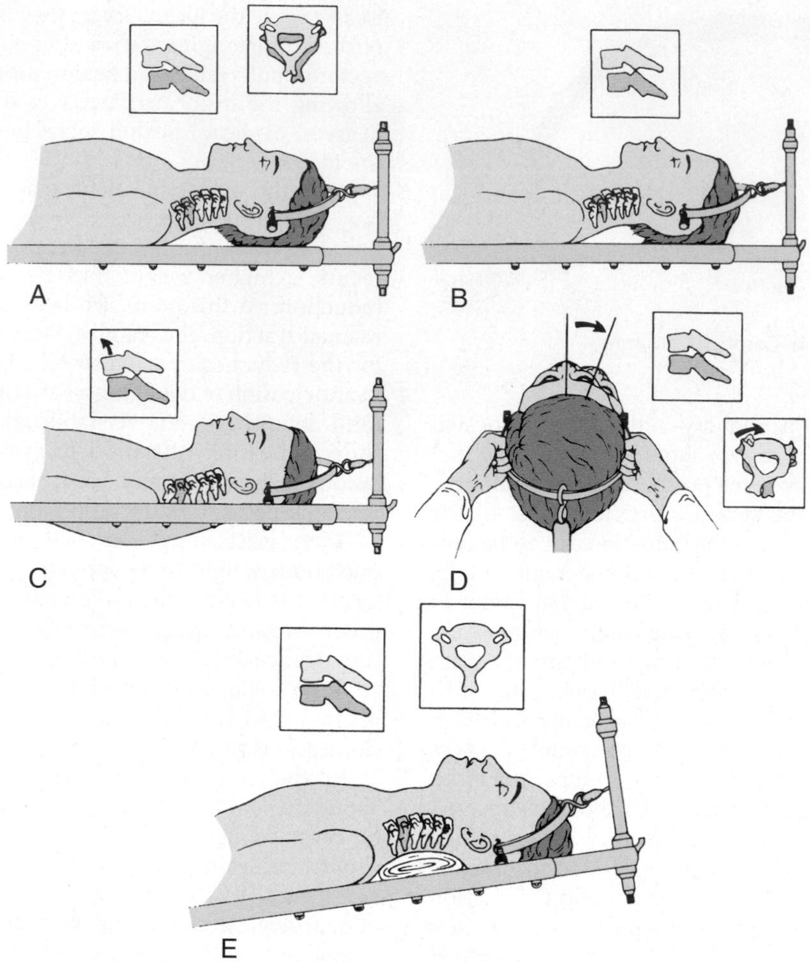

Figure 34-16. The patient should be awake, alert, and cooperative. **A,** Traction is applied in line with the spine. **B** and **C,** With each progressive weight increase, a neurologic examination should be performed to monitor for any changes in status, and lateral radiograph should be obtained to monitor the effect of traction on the injured level as well as all disc spaces and occipitocervical junction. **D,** As the facets become distracted enough to reduce, a flexion moment is applied to unlock bilateral dislocations or a combination of lateral bend and rotation is used to unlock unilateral dislocations. **E,** After reduction is achieved, traction weight is gradually lowered to 15 to 25 lb and the neck kept in extension to hold the facets reduced.

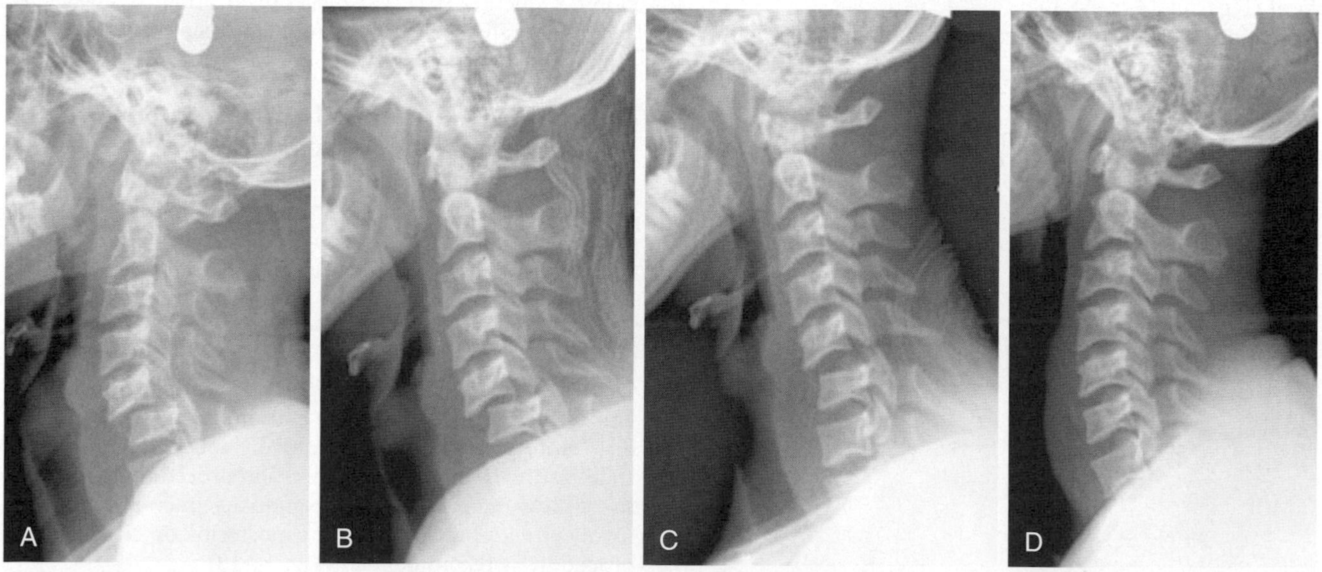

Figure 34-17. Awake closed reduction of a bilateral cervical facet dislocation. With each weight increase, all disc spaces as well as the occipitocervical junction should be examined closely to ensure no occult injuries and sensorimotor examination performed. The vector of traction weight should be with the head slightly flexed to exaggerate the injury mechanism. With increasing weight, the facet becomes unlocked. **A,** No weight added. **B,** Thirty lb of weight. **C,** Sixty lb of weight with the locked facets cleared. **D,** After the locked facets are cleared, the neck should be extended to relocate the dislocated facets. Weight is gradually then removed back down to 15 to 25 lb of weight, ensuring no subluxation or redislocation with serial radiographs with each decrease.

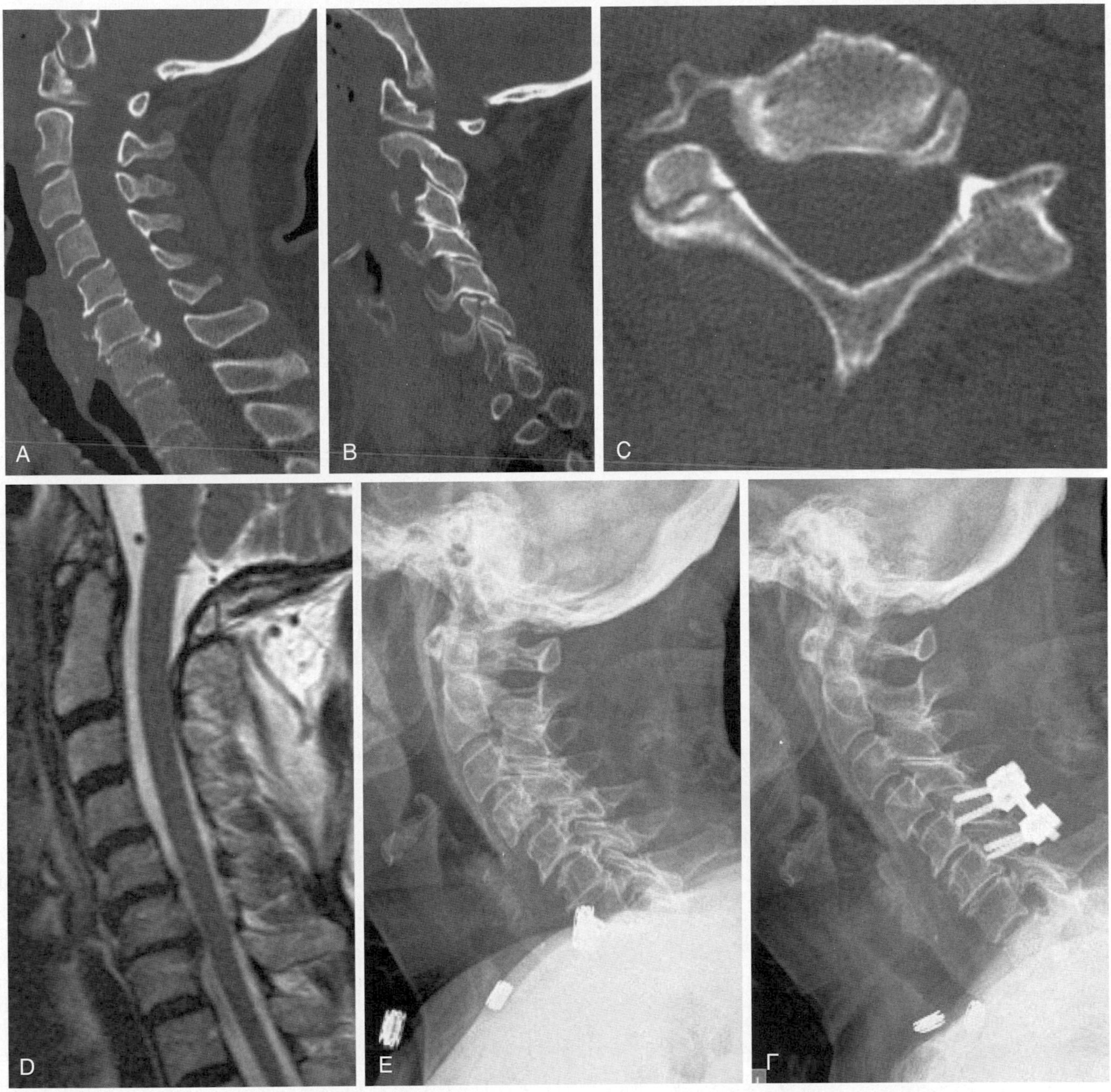

Figure 34-18. Failure of nonoperative treatment of a unilateral facet fracture. **A** to **C**, An 83-year-old woman fell down a staircase, sustaining multiple facial fractures and a nondisplaced unilateral facet fracture of the superior articular facet of C6 measuring 10 mm from the tip of the facet. She was neurologically intact. **D,** Magnetic resonance imaging revealed no new cord compression, and the posterior ligamentous complex appeared intact. **E,** The patient underwent surgery for her facial fractures and after surgery complained of new paresthesias in the bilateral upper extremities. Upright lateral radiographs revealed anterolisthesis of C5 to C6 of 5 mm. **F,** She underwent posterior stabilization and fusion from C5 to C6.

disability.[55,56] Halo vest immobilization is better used for upper cervical spine injuries and does not offer enough stability to adequately treat unstable subaxial injuries definitively. Unacceptably high failure rates of halo vest immobilization for subaxial cervical spine dislocations and fracture-dislocations have historically been reported.[57-59]

Surgical treatment of unilateral facet fractures and fracture-dislocations can involve either an anterior discectomy and fusion or posterior cervical stabilization and fusion. Clinical outcomes have found anterior surgery to be adequate to attain fusion in these injuries. A prospective randomized trial found a 100% fusion rate in the anterior group versus 89% in the posterior group at 12 months after surgery, although this was not a statistically significant finding, with no difference in functional outcome scores.[60] A retrospective study found 15 of 17 patients with unilateral facet fractures or dislocations fused with anterior surgery alone.[61] Another retrospective study of 25 patients with unilateral facet fracture-dislocations, 21 of whom were treated with anterior discectomy and fusion, found a 100% fusion rate.[62] Furthermore, anterior surgery offers the benefit of direct spinal cord decompression if there is an associated disc herniation present.

Bilateral Facet Dislocations

Bilateral facet fractures or dislocations require operative stabilization. Multiple cadaveric studies have demonstrated superior biomechanical stability of posterior fixation with lateral mass screws over anterior discectomy and fusion with a plate in this injury pattern.[35,63,64] However, clinical results have been surprisingly satisfactory with anterior discectomy and fusion with modern plate technology. If a disc herniation and neurologic deficit are present after closed reduction, then standard recommendations are an anterior discectomy and fusion followed preferably by a posterior stabilization procedure.

If the dislocation is irreducible by closed means, then the posterior approach should be used to openly reduce the facet dislocation in the absence of a traumatic disc herniation. Open reduction techniques of reducing facet dislocations and realigning the spine via the posterior approach include placing towel clamps or tenaculums on the involved spinous processes and applying a kyphosing moment to disengage the facets followed by a gentle distraction and realignment maneuver to position the inferior facet of the superior vertebra dorsal to the superior articular facet of the inferior vertebra (Fig. 34-19).

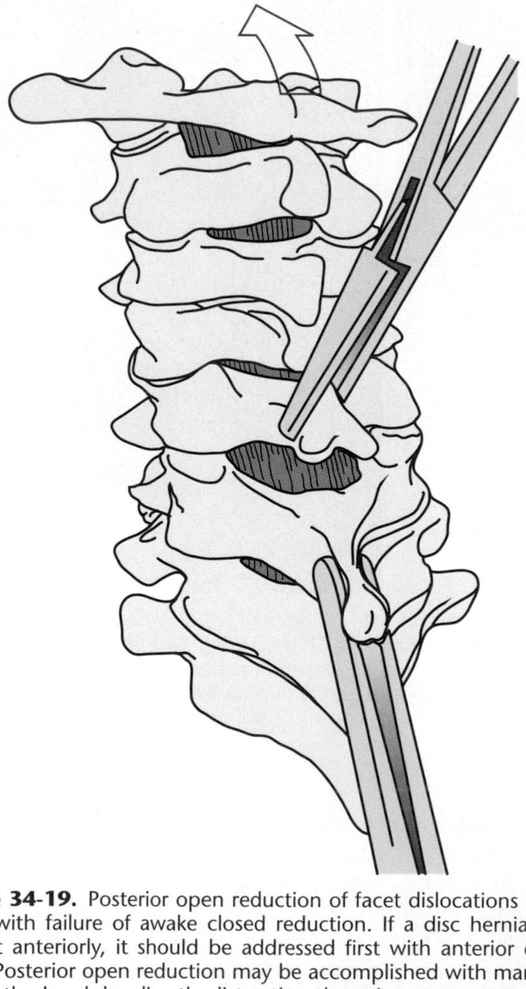

Figure 34-19. Posterior open reduction of facet dislocations is indicated with failure of awake closed reduction. If a disc herniation is present anteriorly, it should be addressed first with anterior discectomy. Posterior open reduction may be accomplished with manipulation of the head; by directly distracting the spinous processes of the involved levels with bone tenaculums or clamps; by using an elevator to lever the dislocated facet posteriorly; or by burring away part of the superior facet of the inferior vertebrae, which is the posterior block to reduction and realignment. *(Redrawn from Albert TJ, Vaccaro AR: Spine surgery: tricks of the trade, 2009, Fig. 6-1, p 13.)*

This may be assisted by the use of an elevator between the dislocated facet or facets and levering the dislocated inferior facet or facets dorsally. The head, which is typically held in position by Mayfield tongs, can be flexed to accentuate the deforming force, allowing for more distraction across the dislocation. Additionally, the caudal superior articular facet may be burred down, allowing the dislocated cephalad inferior articular facet to realign into its normal dorsal position.

In reduced bilateral dislocations, either anterior or posterior surgery can be performed. The advantages of an anterior approach are the ability to address traumatic disc herniation in one stage, avoidance of prone positioning in spinal cord injury patients, and less blood loss. Furthermore, if the posterior approach is used in fracture-dislocations, often one or both sides of the injured level need to be bypassed to allow for stable screw fixation, an issue that may be avoided with the anterior approach. The posterior approach offers stronger fixation, the ability to reduce facet dislocations, and more reliable fusion success. In a randomized study by Brodke and colleagues, no differences were observed between anterior and posterior instrumentation for unstable cervical spines.[31] An alternative is to perform a combined approach to minimize the potential for early or late surgical failure.

Clinical evidence for the use of an anterior-only approach in bilateral facet dislocations and fracture-dislocations varies. A retrospective study was performed of 22 patients with bilateral facet fracture-dislocations who underwent preoperative reduction and then anterior discectomy and fusion.[65] Although there was one instrumentation failure, all 22 patients successfully fused with the anterior procedure alone. Others have reported higher failure rates of anterior surgery alone.[61,66] The presence of an endplate fracture or facet fracture-dislocation may be a contraindications to anterior-only treatment in bilateral facet injuries.

If an anterior approach is chosen for a bilateral facet fracture-dislocation, it is important not to place an interbody graft that overdistracts the joint. Overdistraction with a graft that is too large can result in a neurologic deficit or worsening of a preexisting neurologic deficit. It is better to use an appropriately sized interbody graft followed by a posterior stabilization procedure in the setting of significant instability at the level of the dislocation.

When an anterior approach is used in a case of unreduced bilateral facet dislocation, the discectomy can be performed followed by an attempted open reduction and realignment of the spine. If a large disc herniation is present posterior to the vertebral body, it may be necessary to perform a partial corpectomy to remove all of the disc material. After the disc is removed, an open reduction can be performed anteriorly using several methods. This may involve skull traction under plain radiography or lateral fluoroscopy or by using Caspar pins or minilaminar spreaders alone or in combination to gently distract the vertebral bodies followed by a realignment maneuver.[67] This may involve placing the Caspar pins in the respective vertebral bodies in a divergent trajectory and using the minilaminar spreader to distract the interspace as the Caspar pins are brought together to disengage the facets followed by a rotational maneuver to accomplish a reduction.

If open reduction is unsuccessful after anterior discectomy, the patient should then be turned prone and a posterior open reduction performed along with fixation. Finally, the patient

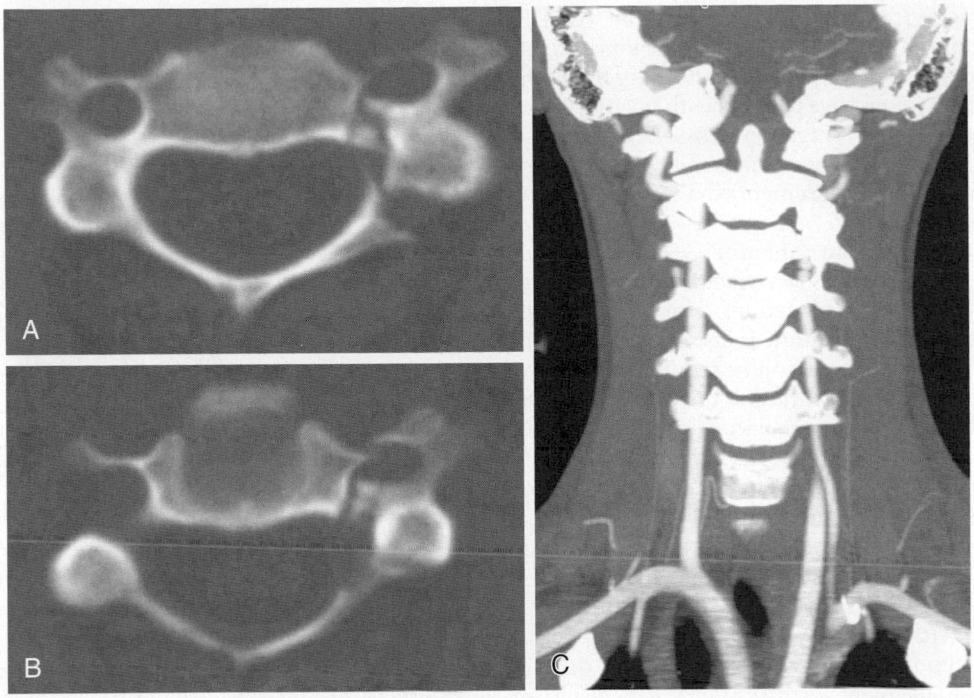

Figure 34-20. Floating lateral mass at C3 sustained in motor vehicle accident. This is a rotational mechanism and has the potential to destabilize both C2 to C3 and C3 to C4. Operative fixation for the floating lateral mass fractures is indicated. **A,** Axial computed tomography (CT) scan shows fractured lamina. **B,** Another CT slice shows the fractured pedicle and the fracture extending into the foramen transversarium. **C,** There is also an associated focal dissection of the left vertebral artery at the injury level, although the vessel remained patent above, and the patient was asymptomatic.

should be returned to the supine position, the anterior wound reopened, and an interbody graft placed into the disc space followed by an anterior plate to provide the necessary anterior column support.

Biomechanical evidence supports combined anterior-posterior fixation followed next by posterior only and then anterior-only fixation as the most rigid forms of stabilization for these injuries. Retrospective clinical evidence to support both methods is available. However, no high-level clinical evidence exists to support one method over the other.

Lateral Mass Fractures

The Spine Trauma Study Group has defined lateral mass fractures as a "fracture of any portion of the lateral mass complex, including the articular process and the pedicle. This categorization includes the so-called 'floating lateral mass,' where ipsilateral fractures of the lamina and pedicle result in superior and inferior articular process fractures that are in discontinuity with the native vertebrae"[27] (Fig. 34-20). They likely occur from a combination of extension, lateral compression, and rotation of the cervical spine, and the fracture line can extend into its superior or inferior facet (or both), the foramen transversarium, transverse process, ventrally into the pedicle, or dorsally into the lamina.[19,68] Lateral mass fractures often appear to be benign injuries, typically nondisplaced or minimally displaced, and the fracture may disguise an injury to the soft tissue. MRI is always indicated to fully evaluate the state of the soft tissues because subtle radiographic and CT findings often mask a disruption of the DLC in this injury pattern.[69]

Authors have classified different types of lateral mass fractures. Kotani and colleagues reported on 23 patients with lateral mass fractures and classified them into four distinct patterns: 11 with separation (floating lateral mass); four with comminution; five with split injuries in which there is a coronal split fracture, resulting in the superior articular facet of the caudal vertebrae to telescope or invaginate into the cephalad fractured lateral mass; and two with traumatic spondylolysis caused by bilateral pars fractures.[70] In a similar classification, Lee and Sung reported on a retrospective series of 27 patients with lateral mass fractures and classified them into four patterns: 16 had a unilateral spondylolisthesis, five had separation (essentially a floating lateral mass), four had a comminution, and two had a split lateral mass.[71]

Treatment Recommendations

Lateral mass fractures that are isolated, nondisplaced, and without disruption of the DLC can be conservatively treated with an external orthosis. Close radiographic follow-up is necessary to ensure that no displacement occurs. However, floating lateral mass fractures in which the lateral mass is fractured anteriorly at the pedicle and posteriorly at the lamina represent an unstable rotational injury to the facet joint, which even if not initially displaced, have a high propensity to displace, resulting in instability to both the cephalad and caudal interspaces. As such, these fractures typically are best managed with operative fixation.

Few studies have examined clinical outcomes of lateral mass fractures. In a retrospective study by Lifeso and Colucci, nonoperative treatment and posterior fixation had high failure rates, but patients with anterior discectomy and fusion went on to stable healing and improved neurologic status.[68] In another retrospective study of 19 patients with subaxial fractures and dislocations, four were in patients with floating lateral mass fractures. All four patients were treated with a two-level anterior cervical discectomy and fusion (ACDF) with a structural allograft and plate.[72] Three of the four patients had fusion and had little pain or disability after surgery. In the study of Lee and Sung, four of five patients with floating lateral mass fractures treated with a single-level ACDF failed treatment because of adjacent-segment instability or malalignment; therefore, the authors recommended a two-level ACDF for these injury patterns.[71]

The considerations for an anterior versus posterior approach for a floating lateral mass fracture are similar to those for facet fractures and dislocations. However, whether or not anterior or posterior fixation is used, in the case of floating lateral mass fractures, the injury requires a two level stabilization, which essentially bridges the fractured level and potentially the unstable cephalad and caudal levels. Depending on the presence of a disc herniation, the patient's status, and specific injury characteristics, anterior or posterior approaches can be used. Contemporary thought, however, is to strongly consider a circumferential approach to minimize the potential for early or late failure.

Anterior Distraction Injury

The Spine Trauma Study Group defined an anterior distraction injury as "bone, ligament, or disc injury that results in craniocaudal distraction of the anterior disc space to a greater extent than the posterior disc space. By definition, this injury pattern represents disruption of the anterior tension band."[27]

Anterior distraction injuries are caused by an extension mechanism which causes disruption of the anterior column in the form of ALL and anterior annulus or ALL and transverse vertebral body fracture. An anterior osteophyte may also avulse from the anterior inferior vertebral body, often referred to as an "extension teardrop" fracture. The distraction injury may then propagate posteriorly, causing compressive fractures to the posterior elements or disrupting the posterior ligamentous complex, causing a highly unstable both-column spinal injury.

Anterior distraction injuries typically occur in two distinct patient populations. They can be caused by high-energy mechanisms in younger patients. In elderly patients with cervical spondylosis, AS, or diffuse idiopathic skeletal hyperostosis (DISH), a low-energy mechanism, such as a ground-level fall or a blow to the face or forehead, can result in an anterior distraction injury, destabilizing the cervical spine and causing incomplete or complete quadriplegia. A retrospective study of 112 elderly patients with ankylosed spines who sustained this injury found the 1-year mortality rate was 32%, and spinal cord injury was present in 58% of patients.[73] Elderly patients without ankylosed spines but with cervical spondylosis also may sustain this injury pattern. This is a common scenario in the setting of a central cord syndrome in which the anterior distraction mechanism can cause a pincer-like mechanism of spinal cord injury caused by canal narrowing between the posterior disc–osteophyte complex and in-buckled ligamentum flavum even without frank disruption of the anterior column (Figs. 34-21 and 34-22).

The spine is ankylosed or essentially fused in patients with AS and DISH, and it acts more like a long bone, such as the femur, resulting in a fracture between two long lever arms. Even in the absence of significant displacement, fractures in these patients are considered highly unstable and prone to displacement with movement. Due to the long lever arms

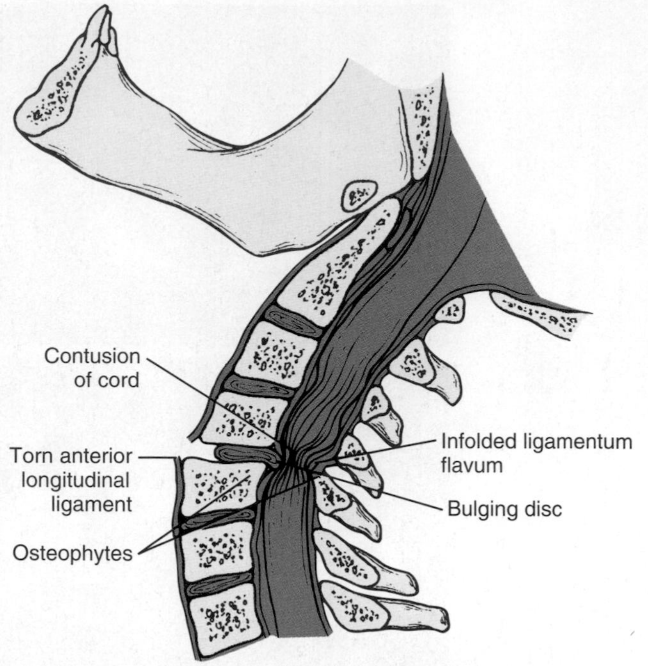

Figure 34-21. The anterior distraction injury can result in a "pincer-like" compression injury to the spinal cord. The spinal cord is compressed by both the disc or disc–osteophyte complex anteriorly as well as the infolding of the ligamentum flavum posteriorly.

above and below the fracture because of the fused spine, initial nondisplaced or minimally displaced fractures can easily become displaced with resultant catastrophic neurologic injury. Often because of the diffuse arthritis as well as extreme cervicothoracic kyphosis prevalent in some of these patients, it may be difficult to recognize nondisplaced and potentially highly unstable fractures[74] (Fig. 34-23). Therefore, any elderly patient with AS or DISH who presents with neck pain even after a minor trauma should be presumed to have an unstable cervical spine fracture until proven otherwise with CT and MRI. CT, including sagittal and coronal reconstructions, should be examined closely for fractures. MRI should also be obtained to examine for bone or soft tissue edema, which may be the only clue to an injury. An epidural hematoma and concomitant neurologic deficit, which is associated with spinal fractures in the setting of an ankylosed spine, may be the most obvious imaging finding of an injury.[75,76] Furthermore, the identification of an injury in the cervical spine should prompt advanced imaging studies of the entire spine because these patients are predisposed to noncontiguous fractures in other regions of the spine[77] (Fig. 34-24).

Treatment Recommendations for the Nonankylosed Spine

Patients presenting with anterior distraction injury through bone alone without displacement based on CT or discoligamentous disruption on MRI can be treated nonoperatively with an external orthosis.

In the setting of a stable spine and a neurologic deficit, which is common in the setting of a central cord syndrome in elderly patients with a spondylotic spine, surgery is often considered. The hyperextension injury, although not causing enough trauma to destabilize the spine, causes a pincer-like mechanism of spinal cord compression by either disc material

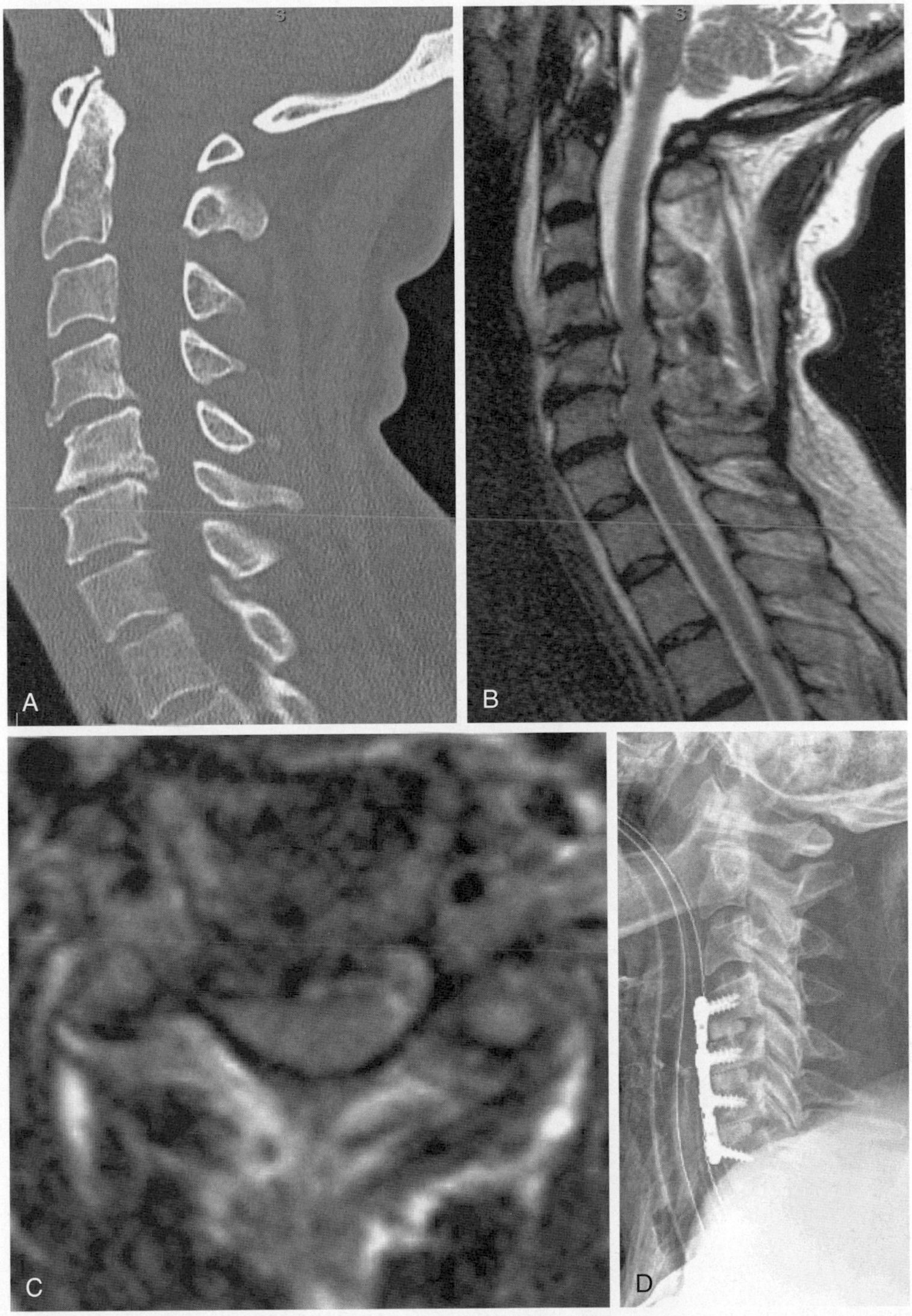

Figure 34-22. Extension distraction injury in the spondylotic spine. A 55-year-old woman sustained a ground-level fall onto her face and presented with a central cord syndrome with bilateral upper extremity pain, weakness, and numbness (Subaxial Cervical Spine Injury Classification [SLIC] neuro = 3). **A,** Sagittal computed tomography scan reveals multilevel spondylosis and an avulsed C4 anteroinferior vertebral body osteophyte ("extension teardrop"), suggesting an anterior distraction injury (SLIC morphology = 3). **B** and **C,** Magnetic resonance imaging reveals multilevel cervical spondylosis and severe stenosis with myelomalacia suggestive of spinal cord injury from C4 to C7 (SLIC DLC status: = 1). **D,** The patient underwent anterior cervical discectomy and decompression at these levels and subsequently recovered neurologic function (total SLIC score = 3 + 3 + 1 = 7 → operative).

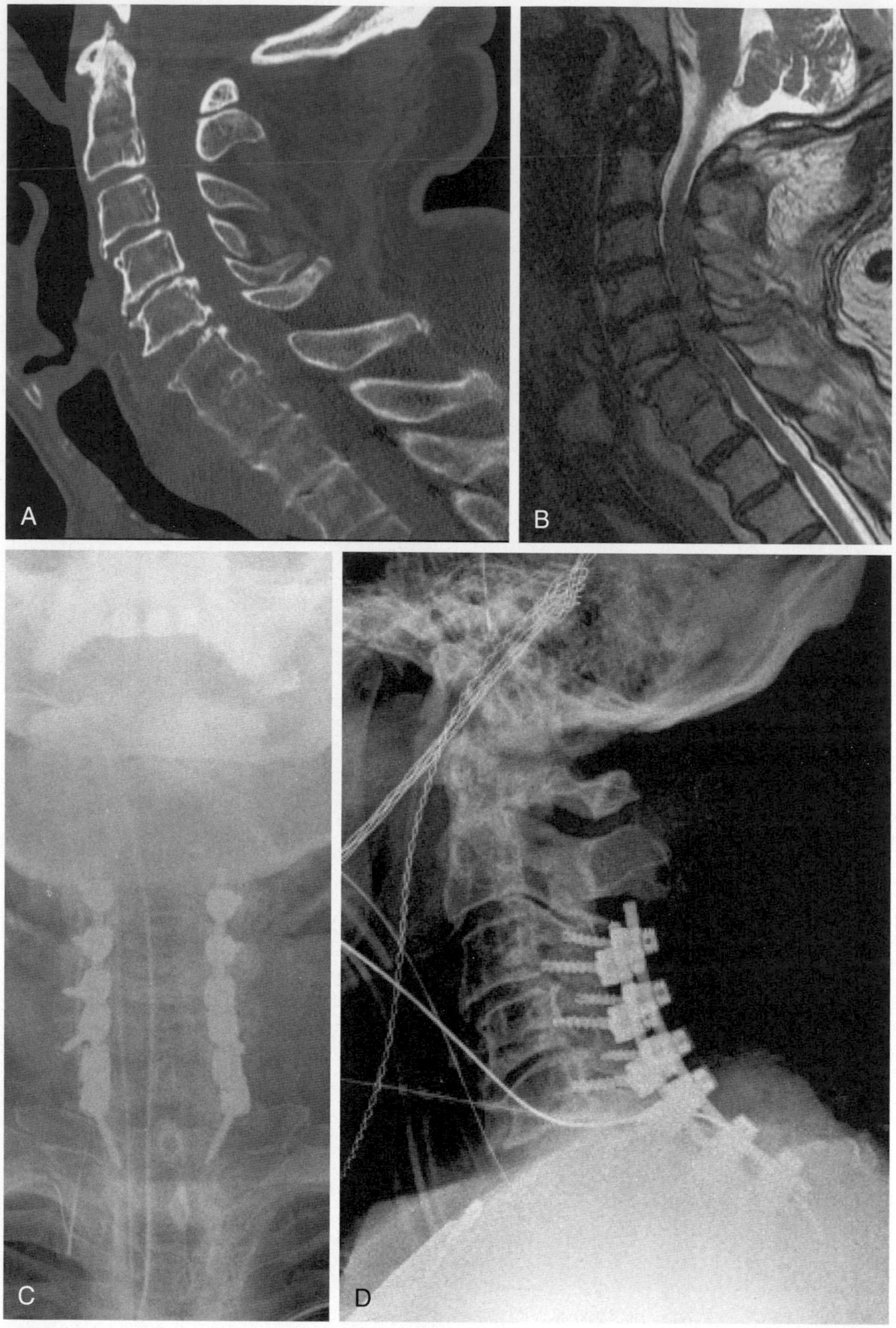

Figure 34-23. An 81-year-old man presented after a fall complaining of neck pain and weakness in the bilateral upper extremities (Subaxial Cervical Spine Injury Classification [SLIC] neuro = 3). **A,** A computed tomography scan reveals partially ankylosed spine with anterior distraction injury at C6 to C7 (SLIC morphology = 3). **B,** Sagittal magnetic resonance image reveals severe stenosis with disc space disruption at C6 to C7 (SLIC DLC = 2). **C** and **D,** The patient subsequently underwent posterior cervical decompression and fusion from C3 to T1 with resolution of weakness in the arms (total SLIC score = 3 + 3 + 2 = 8 → operative).

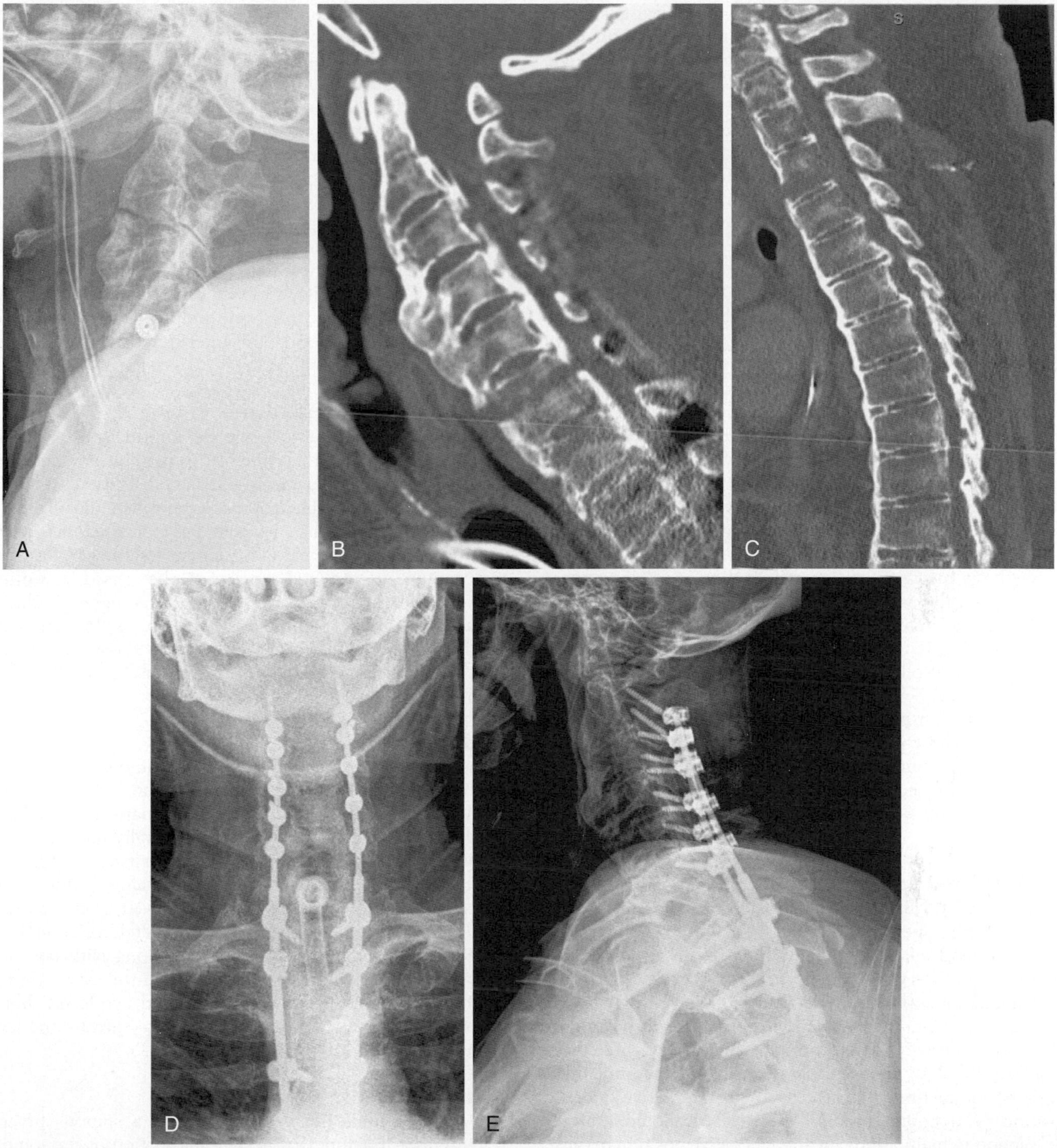

Figure 34-24. Noncontiguous injury in anterior distraction injuries. A 67-year-old man with diffuse idiopathic skeletal hyperostosis was an unrestrained driver in a motor vehicle accident and presented with a complete spinal cord injury (American Spinal Injury Association [ASIA] class A) at the C4 level. **A,** Lateral cervical spine radiograph reveals a transverse fracture through C3. **B,** A sagittal cervical computed tomography (CT) scan reveals an additional transverse fracture through C6. **C,** A sagittal thoracic CT scan reveals another transverse fracture through T3. **D** and **E,** The patient was subsequently treated with posterior stabilization and fusion from C2 to T6.

or infolding of the ligamentum flavum. There exists controversy on whether or not surgical decompression versus nonoperative treatment results in any difference in neurologic outcomes. No prospective randomized study has yet to be performed that compares nonoperative to operative decompression, or for that matter, timing of operative decompression, in patients who present with traumatic central cord syndrome without spinal instability. However, a systematic review of the existing literature found that there may be some neurologic benefit for early surgical decompression (less than 24 hours) in patients with a neurologic deficit (ASIA class C or worse) in those with spinal stenosis from preexisting spondylosis without fracture instability.[78]

For anterior distraction injuries in which there is evidence of ligamentous injury without neurologic deficit, operative treatment may be indicated depending on what structures are disrupted. For example, if only the ALL or the anterior part of the disc spaced is ruptured, nonoperative treatment with an external orthosis or halo immobilization may be considered. The patient should be followed closely with radiographs to ensure alignment is maintained. However, if the posterior annulus and PLL are disrupted, then even if there is no displacement, likely there is enough ligamentous instability to merit operative stabilization. The presence of translation or retrolisthesis merits operative stabilization. Anterior discectomy and fusion is usually recommended. Circumferential fusion should be considered with anterior distraction injuries with retrolisthesis.

Vaccaro and colleagues reported on a retrospective series of 24 patients with anterior distraction injuries. Eight patients were treated with halo vest immobilization, and 16 patients were treated surgically. A recognized challenge of the halo was the inability to control progressive displacement and kyphosis.[79] Injuries treated with anterior decompression and fusion had good clinical and radiographic success.

Treatment Recommendations for the Ankylosed Spine

Patients with AS or DISH who sustain anterior distraction injuries require operative treatment. Cervical immobilization should be used with caution in patients with a high degree of preexisting cervicothoracic kyphosis because standard rigid collars force the neck into extension, which may aggravate displacement. Neurologic decline and death have been reported because of inadvertent rigid collar placement in these patients.[80] Rather than extending the neck, it is recommended to place padding under the head to support the native kyphotic position.[81] If traction is used preoperatively, it should be bivector traction to maintain the head in its native position because normal single-vector traction will cause the neck to extend. Halo vest immobilization may also be used to immobilize the neck before surgery, although halo vest immobilization as definitive treatment in elderly patients with ankylosed spines has been associated with a high mortality rate caused by aspiration.[82] The anesthesia team should be involved early on because these patients are at increased risk of airway compromise caused by fracture displacement and increasing soft tissue edema.[83]

Posterior stabilization two or three levels above and below the injury is recommended for these patients. Anterior reconstruction may be performed in addition to restore the anterior tension band but is rarely needed. A retrospective study of 36 patients with AS who underwent operative stabilization found that five of 10 patients who underwent an anterior-only procedure experienced implant failure and required revision to a combined anterior and posterior stabilization procedure.[84] A retrospective study of 112 patients in which 58 were treated with posterior fixation only found that none failed and all healed.[73] Of seven patients treated with anterior-only fixation, one failed. The authors recommended that at least three levels cephalad and caudad to the fractured level should be instrumented posteriorly to prevent failure. Thus, the evidence suggests that long-segment posterior-only fixation may be adequate to stabilize these injuries in this patient population. However, if there is a large fish-mouth open deformity at the fractured level, anterior interbody grafting to provide anterior column support and restore the anterior tension band should be considered.

Isolated Lamina Fracture

The Spine Trauma Study Group defines an isolated lamina fracture as a "fracture that extends through the lamina medial to the facet joint/lateral mass and lateral to the base of the spinous process. No subluxation or kyphosis should be present in this injury pattern."[27] Isolated laminar fractures in the absence of associated posterior element fractures or ligamentous rupture are rare and are likely to be caused by a direct blow or extension injury (Fig. 34-25). A radiographic clue to an isolated laminar fracture in the absence of CT scan is disruption of the spinolaminar line on the lateral radiograph. This should prompt advanced imaging studies to better characterize the injury.

Treatment

Patients with isolated laminar fractures without an associated neurologic deficit or ligamentous injury can be treated with a rigid cervical collar alone. Case reports have described isolated laminar fractures that displace ventrally into the spinal canal, causing spinal cord injury.[85,86] In this instance, posterior decompression is indicated. Laminectomy alone is not recommended because it destabilizes the involved levels and may result in postlaminectomy kyphosis. Therefore, concurrent stabilization is typically recommended along with posterior decompression to remove fragments from the canal. Usually the fractured level should be bridged, and two levels should be stabilized—one level caudad to the fracture to one level cephalad.

Spinous Process Fracture

The Spine Trauma Study group defines a spinous process fracture as a "fracture that detaches a portion of the spinous process, or the entire spinous process, from the cervical lamina."[27] The classic spinous process fracture is the so-called "clay shoveler's fracture," which occurs in the lower cervical and upper thoracic levels, typically C6, C7, or T1, and was first described in 1940 in Australian miners who experienced a pop and pain in the neck and upper back as the clay they were shoveling remained stuck to their shovels.[87] Clay shoveler's fractures are thought to be avulsion injuries of the spinous process from the pull of the supraspinous ligament. These also commonly occur with MVAs and during athletic events (Fig. 34-26).

Isolated spinous process fractures are typically benign injuries treated with immobilization. Advanced imaging studies

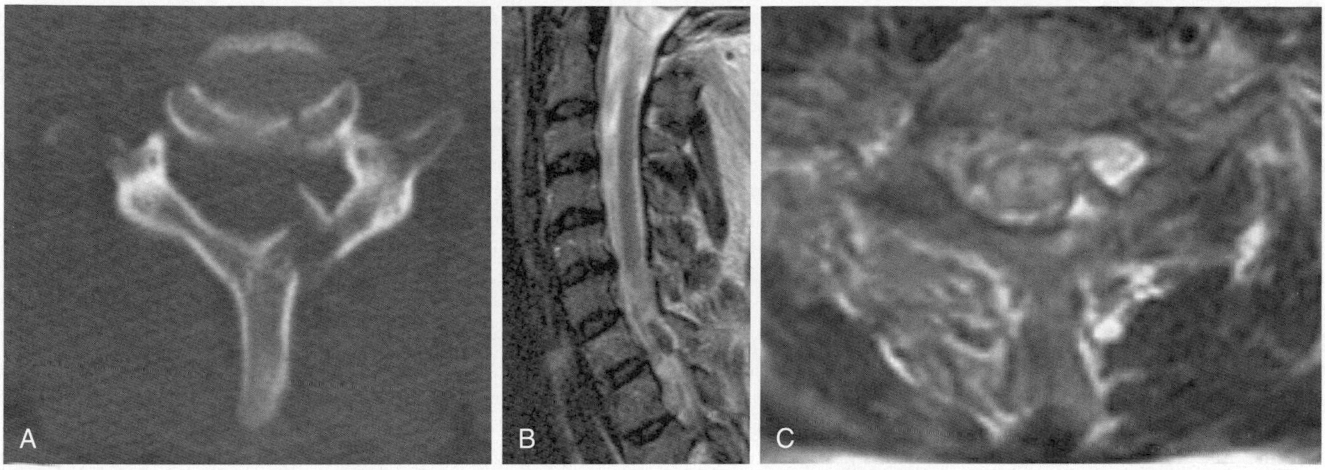

Figure 34-25. Isolated lamina fracture. A 37-year-old man was brought to the emergency department after being assaulted with a baseball bat with an incomplete spinal cord injury at the C7 level (Subaxial Cervical Spine Injury Classification [SLIC] neuro = 4 {3 + 1 {neuro modifier}}). **A,** A computed tomography scan revealed a lamina fracture of C7 with a nondisplaced sagittal fracture line extending into the vertebral body anteriorly (SLIC morphology = 0). **B** and **C,** Magnetic resonance imaging revealed the fractured lamina displaced into the canal with massive spinal cord edema extending cephalad and caudal to the fracture (SLIC DLC = 0). He underwent a posterior decompression and fusion with a partial laminectomy of C6 and T1 and complete laminectomy of C7 with stabilization and fusion from C5 to T2 (total SLIC score = 4 → ± operative intervention; operative intervention was performed given that there was a direct source of continued compression on the spinal cord).

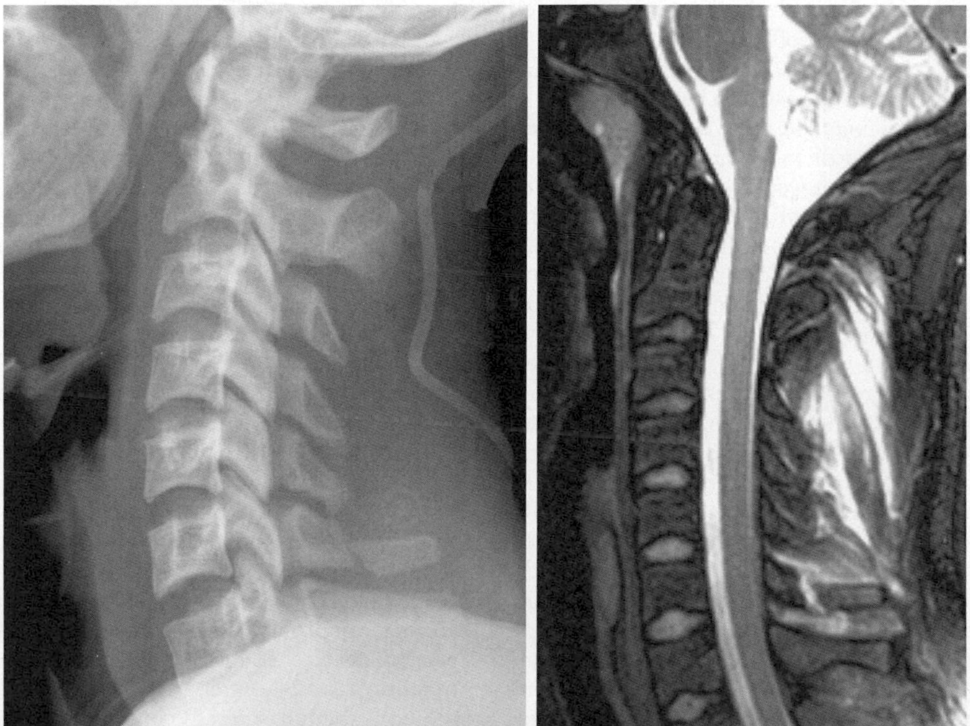

Figure 34-26. Typical C6 spinous process avulsion fracture seen on a lateral radiograph (**A**) and magnetic resonance image (**B**) of a 21-year-old man after a motor vehicle accident with only neck pain (Subaxial Cervical Spine Injury Classification [SLIC] neuro = 0; morphology = 0; discoligamentous complex = 0; total SLIC score = 0 → nonoperative). Classically called a "clay-shoveler's fracture," this injury most commonly occurs at C6, C7, and T1.

should be obtained to evaluate for soft tissue injury or other fractures in the cervical spine sustained during the trauma. The typical clay shoveler's fracture is oriented perpendicular to the axis of the spinous process and directed inferiorly. However, a subtle radiographic finding, referred to as a spinolaminar breach, in which the fracture obliquely extends into the lamina, has been associated with delayed instability and a neurologic deficit.[88] Radiologic evidence of a spinolaminar breach should prompt MRI to examine the status of the posterior ligamentous complex.

Treatment

Isolated spinous process fractures without any associated instability can be managed with an external orthosis and symptomatic analgesia for 8 to 10 weeks with radiographic follow-up to ensure healing. When no longer painful, the patient can be returned to full activities after appropriate rehabilitation.

Transverse Process Fracture

The Spine Trauma Study Group defines a transverse process fracture as a "fracture along any portion of the transverse process, including fractures that extend into the foramen transversarium."[27] Transverse process fractures occurring in conjunction with other cervical spine injuries are relatively common. Isolated transverse process fractures at C7 have been postulated to occur in MVAs with modern shoulder belt usage in which rapid deceleration causes an oblique hyperflexion moment.[89] In a prospective study of blunt trauma victims, 76 patients had subaxial spine injuries.[90] Forty-nine patients had a transverse process fracture, 21 of whom had isolated transverse process fractures. C7 was the most commonly injured. The authors followed a protocol in which patients with isolated transverse process fractures were treated with no restrictions in movement and no immobilization. In the 14 patients available for follow-up at a mean of 2.3 years, high patient satisfaction, low Neck Disability Index scores, and normal range of motion were obtained, with no adverse events related to the transverse process fracture.

The main concern with an isolated transverse process fracture that extends into the foramen transversarium is injury to the vertebral artery. At the most commonly fractured level, C7, the vertebral artery normally has not yet entered the foramen transversarium. In a retrospective study, 11 of 60 (18%) transverse process fractures were isolated injuries; the remaining 49 (82%) were in conjunction with other cervical fractures.[91] In 47 of 60 transverse process fractures (78%), the fracture extended into the foramen transversarium. Vertebral angiography was performed in eight patients with transverse process fractures extending into the foramen transversarium. In seven of these eight patients, there was evidence of vertebral artery occlusion or dissection. Two of these seven patients developed symptoms consistent with a vertebral-basilar artery stroke. Four of the seven patients with vertebral artery occlusion were managed with 6 weeks of Coumadin.

Definitive Treatment

Isolated transverse process fractures likely do not require immobilization, although a soft or rigid collar for 10 to 14 days along with oral pain medication may help relieve symptoms. Typically, follow-up flexion extension dynamic plain radiographs are obtained at this time to rule out delayed instability. Transverse process fractures in combination with other injuries to the subaxial spine require whichever treatment is appropriate for that particular injury; however, no specific surgical treatment is needed to address the transverse process fracture.

In the presence of neurologic deficit, MRI followed by MR or CT angiography should be done to evaluate for nerve root avulsion or vertebral artery injury. Typically, vertebral artery injuries require anticoagulation therapy and further diagnostic evaluation such as vertebral angiography.

Surgical Techniques

Approach. Multiple factors should be considered when choosing the surgical approach. Both anterior and posterior approaches have distinct advantages and disadvantages. In most situations, the pathology itself will dictate which approach is most appropriate. This typically is determined by the location of spinal cord compression and deformity or displacement. The approach used should be able to most directly decompress the spinal cord and restore spinal alignment. However, certain factors should also be considered such as the ability of the fractured level to accept instrumentation. For example, if there is a facet dislocation at C5 to C6 but there is also a superior endplate fracture of C6, this would put an anterior discectomy and bone grafting at greater risk of graft subsidence and failure. Therefore, a posterior C5 to C6 fusion would be a better alternative in this situation. Alternatively, if there is a C5 to C6 fracture-dislocation with a comminuted C6 lateral mass, it may be easier to achieve stable fixation anteriorly; otherwise, C6 would need to be bypassed posteriorly, necessitating extension of the fusion to an uninjured C7 level posteriorly. If a floating lateral mass fracture is present in this situation, it is recommended to fuse to C7 regardless of the approach because of the potential for failure if a standalone anterior C5 to C6 fusion is performed.

The anterior approach has several advantages. It allows for direct decompression of ventral pathology, restores the anterior weight-bearing column, has a significantly lower infection rate, and avoids further trauma to neck muscles. In polytrauma patients or noncontiguous spinal injuries, the anterior approach avoids the risks of turning the patient prone, and anesthesia has better control of the airway. Disadvantages of the anterior approach include the potential for suboptimal biomechanical stability and the difficulty of directly restoring alignment of the cervical spine. The anterior approach also risks exacerbating anterior soft tissue edema present from the injury and may result in further soft tissue trauma to the esophagus, larynx, and trachea. In elderly patients, swallowing and airway problems are common postoperatively and may necessitate tracheotomy and percutaneous endoscopic gastrostomy tube placement. In patients with quadriplegia, pulmonary function is already compromised because of intercostal muscle dysfunction and an inability to clear secretions, which can be exacerbated by esophageal dysmotility brought on by anterior cervical surgery.

The posterior approach has several advantages. Biomechanically, posterior fixation restores the posterior tension band of the posterior ligamentous complex and therefore better resists kyphotic forces. Two stiff rods placed posterolaterally better resist axial rotation and lateral bending than anterior fixation in biomechanical testing.[92] Comparing fusion rates between anterior and posterior approaches in a group of 52 randomized patients who did not require a reduction- or decompression-specific approach, Brodke and colleagues found a 90% fusion rate with an anterior approach versus 100% in the posterior approach, although this was not statistically significant.[31]

Other advantages of the posterior approach include its extensile nature, which allows multiple levels to be easily decompressed and stabilized and, if necessary, extended to the thoracic spine. It is technically easier to restore the normal cervical lordosis through the use of screw rod constructs and manipulation of the head. Translational deformities such as posterior facet subluxations and dislocations can be directly reduced using the posterior approach. The posterior approach does not increase anterior soft tissue edema, thereby minimizing any compromise to airway and swallowing capability.

Disadvantages of the posterior approach again include positioning prone polytrauma injured patients. There is also a higher risk of wound complications as well as greater risk of violating adjacent uninjured facets, thus increasing the risk of adjacent-segment degeneration and instability.

Circumferential fusion enables stabilization of both columns of the cervical spine. Providing anterior column support to buttress axial load and restoring the tension band of the posterior column make for the most biomechanically stable construct.[33,93] Highly unstable injuries merit circumferential fixation. Typically, the anterior approach is used first to initially decompress and stabilize the spine, at which point the patient can be more safely turned prone for posterior fixation. Certain injury patterns also may merit circumferential fusion such as a traumatic disc herniation with facet dislocation irreducible by closed means. Some authors recommend circumferential fusion for patients with AS who sustain anterior distraction injuries through both columns of the spine.[94] More evidence is needed before use of circumferential fusion can be definitively recommended algorithmically.

Surgical Anatomy. Preoperative CT scan and MRI should always be analyzed closely to identify dysplastic or dysmorphic vertebrae and anomalous vascular paths. A review of 1000 cervical MRIs noted severe aberrancy of the carotid artery in 2.6% of patients, most commonly in elderly women with kyphosis.[95] Other studies using CT angiography have demonstrated an anomalous course of the vertebral artery in 5.75%[96] and 5.1% of cases.[97] A study of 222 cadaveric specimens found an anomalous course of the vertebral artery in 2.7% of cases.[98]

The Lateral Mass. The lateral mass is typically used for fixation of screws from the posterior approach at the C3 through C6 levels. The articular facets border the lateral mass superiorly and inferiorly. Medially, the lateral mass meets the axilla between it and the lamina. Laterally, the lateral mass borders soft tissues (Fig. 34-27). From the lateral view, the lateral mass has a rhomboid-shaped appearance. From cephalad to caudad in the cervical spine, the slope of the articular facets becomes steeper and the lateral mass thinner.[99,100] At C7, the lateral mass is the thinnest but also typically the vertebral artery has not entered the foramen transversarium at this level, and therefore, C7 pedicle screws (instead of lateral mass screws) are generally a stronger method of fixation[101] (Fig. 34-28).

Directly anterior to the ventral surface of the lateral mass lies the corresponding nerve root, within 0.3 to 2.3 mm anterior to the cortex.[102] Anterior to the nerve root lies

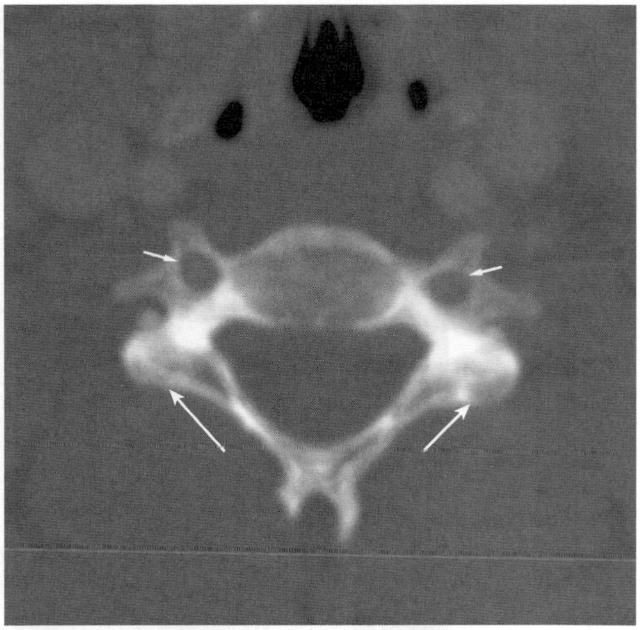

Figure 34-27. Relationship between the foramen transversarium and the lateral mass. From the posterior approach, the surgeon is able to see and feel the posterior surface of the lateral mass *(large arrows)*. In the placement of lateral mass screws, it is important to aim up and outward, away from the foramen transversarium and path of the vertebral artery *(small arrows)*.

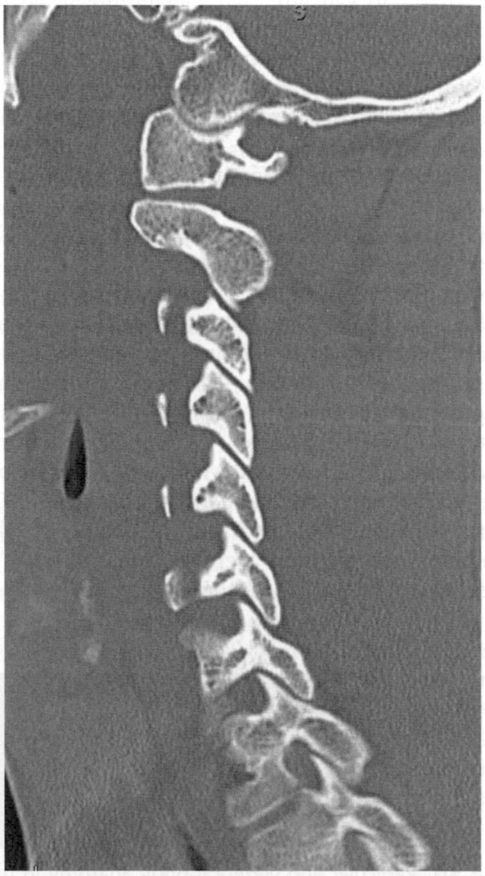

Figure 34-28. As one descends from cephalad to caudad, the facets become thinner and steeper, making it difficult to obtain adequate fixation in C7, which is one of the reasons why pedicle screws are typically preferred to lateral mass screws at this level.

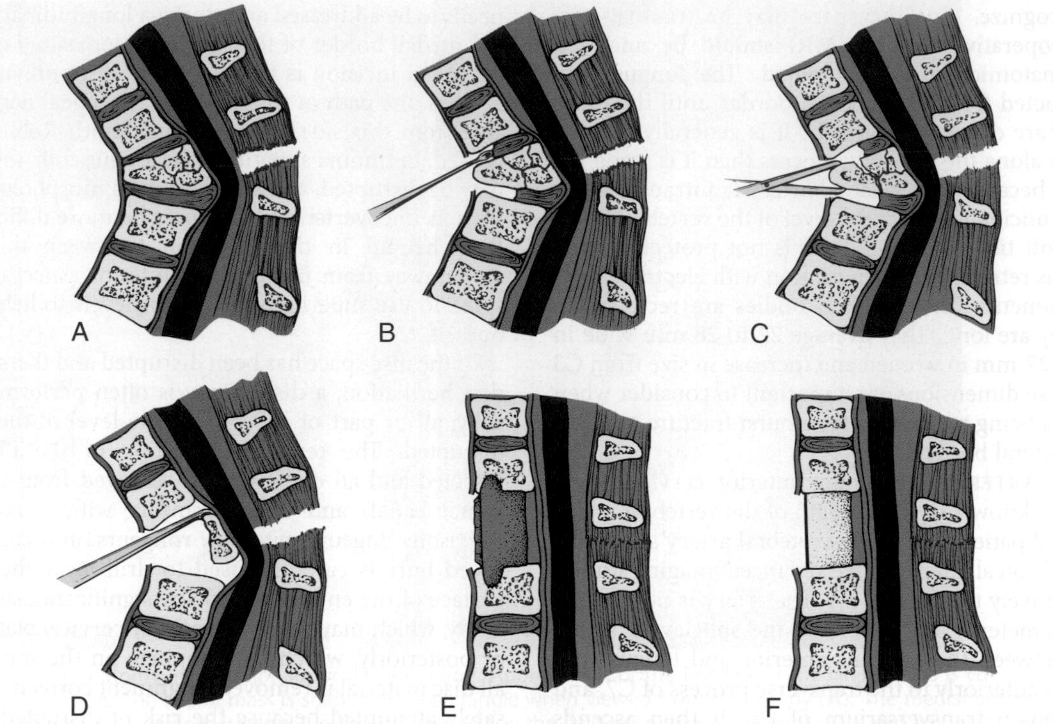

Figure 34-31. Technique of anterior corpectomy. This is an illustration of a burst fracture with posterior ligamentous disruption (**A**) and the extent of kyphosis is exaggerated (typically this would be realigned with traction or extension of the head). The discectomies are performed first (**B**), and then the vertebral body is removed with a burr and rongeur (**C**). The bone can be saved for reinsertion with a reconstruction cage or allograft fibular if autograft iliac crest bone graft is not being used. The entire vertebral body is removed (**D**) as far posteriorly as the posterior longitudinal ligament, which may be disrupted from the injury as well. The spine is realigned (**E**) and strut bone graft placed (**F**), usually then followed by anterior buttress plating.

especially in the setting of trauma, although fusion rates have been shown to be comparable with both.[115] The plate should be as short as possible and the screws placed at an angle away from the involved disc and directed medially. Violation of adjacent levels may increase the risk of adjacent-segment degeneration. A lateral radiograph is taken to ensure proper implant placement.

When placing screws into the anterior vertebral body, proper location, length, and orientation should be carefully considered. Preoperative CT scans should be analyzed to measure the depth of the vertebral body because there can be a significant amount of variability. In men, midsagittal depth averages 17 to 18 mm and 15 to 16 mm in women.[112] Two screws per vertebral level are routinely placed through a plate. They should be unicortical and converge medially, typically 14 to 16 mm in length. Screws should be directed medially and away from the endplate. Directing the screws laterally risks cortical penetration and foramen transversarium violation. Directing the screws away from the endplate in the sagittal plane has been shown to be biomechanically more stable than screws parallel to the endplate. However, the screws should not be at so steep an incline as to violate the adjacent uninvolved endplate and disc space, which would increase the risk of adjacent-segment degeneration.

Endplate anatomy is important to consider when placing interbody grafts to decrease the risk of graft subsidence and fusion failure (Fig. 34-33). The superior endplate is thicker than the inferior endplate. Whereas the superior endplate is also thicker posteriorly than it is anteriorly, the inferior endplate is thicker anteriorly and thinner posteriorly.[110,116] The peripheral aspects of the endplates also have higher bone mineral density than the central zone of the endplate.[117] This has important ramifications when placing an interbody graft. Grafts that sit on the thick endplates are less likely to subside, especially in osteoporotic bone. It is thus important while performing endplate carpentry to not only use a high-speed burr to remove cartilage but also to ensure that the endplate is wide enough to accommodate a graft and that the endplate is flat enough such that the entire graft surface area makes direct contact with the endplates, including laterally on a thicker endplate mantle, which decreases the risk of subsidence. Placing the interbody implant with a gap between it and the endplate increases the likelihood of fusion failure. Another technical error is to burr overly aggressively with resultant violation of the endplates such that cancellous bone is exposed. This increases the risk of graft subsidence and failure. After irrigation and hemostasis is obtained, a drain is placed and the wound closed.

Posterior Stabilization and Decompression

Posterior stabilization is indicated when multiple levels of the spinal cord need to be decompressed and for destabilizing posterior column injuries that cannot be reduced or stabilized in a closed manner. Posterior fixation also offers better biomechanical fixation of the spine because a lateral mass screw–rod construct restores the tension band of the disrupted posterior ligamentous complex and may be performed in conjunction with an anterior approach.

After fiberoptic intubation, the head is stabilized with Mayfield tongs, and the patient is carefully turned prone

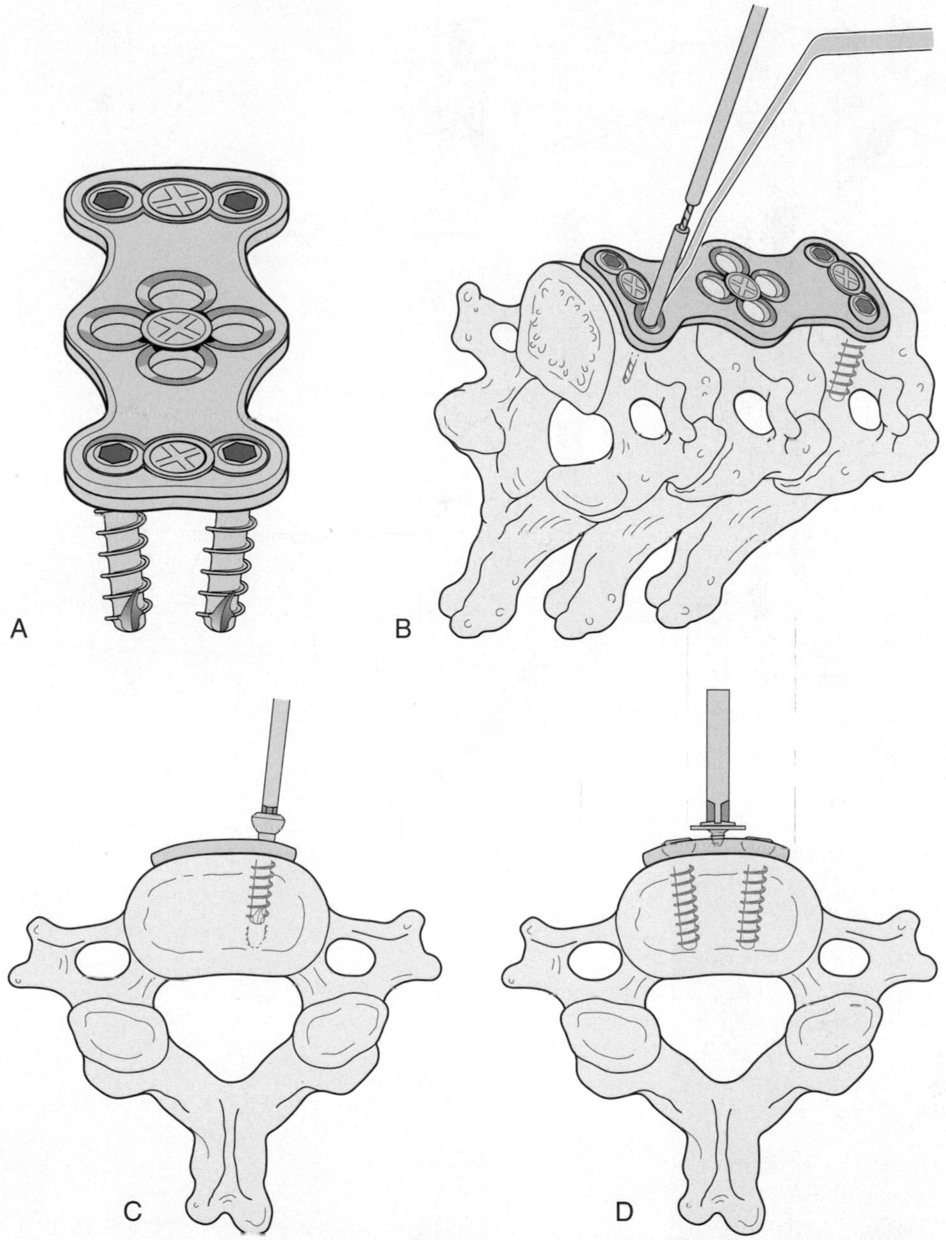

Figure 34-32. Anterior cervical buttress plating. **A,** Contemporary plating systems prevent the screws from backing out from the plate. The screw either locks rigidly to the plate, or the system allows for limited rotational or translational motion between the screw and plate for "dynamization" of the graft. **B,** Screws should be unicortical and drilled to a predetermined distance. **C,** The screw is placed unicortically directed slightly medially. **D,** In some systems, a locking screw prevents the screw from backing out.

while the surgeon controls the head and cervical spine. After proper positioning is achieved, the head can be secured to the bed with the Mayfield tongs and head holder. An alternative is using a turning frame where traction can be maintained throughout the turning process. A lateral radiograph is obtained to assure best possible alignment. The skin is then prepared with chlorhexidine antiseptic.

A midline incision is used and the fascia split at the ligament nuchae. In fractures and dislocations, the spinous process or laminae may be fractured, and dissection should proceed cautiously to avoid iatrogenic dural or spinal cord injury. When exposing the lateral masses, it is important not to disrupt adjacent facet capsules that are not planned for fusion.

From the posterior approach, irreducible facet dislocations or subluxations can be reduced directly using various maneuvers. These include release of the head hold and manual traction on the neck while visualizing the reduction openly, traction manipulation of the spinous process with towel clamps or tenaculums, and unlocking the dislocated facet by levering it dorsally with an elevator. Throughout these reduction maneuvers, changes in neuromonitoring should be followed closely for deterioration. If the above options fail, removing a portion of the superior facet of the jumped inferior vertebrae will allow the cephalad dislocated facet to be more easily reduced into position.

After the reduction has been achieved, instrumentation is placed. If a pure ligamentous injury occurred, it is usually only

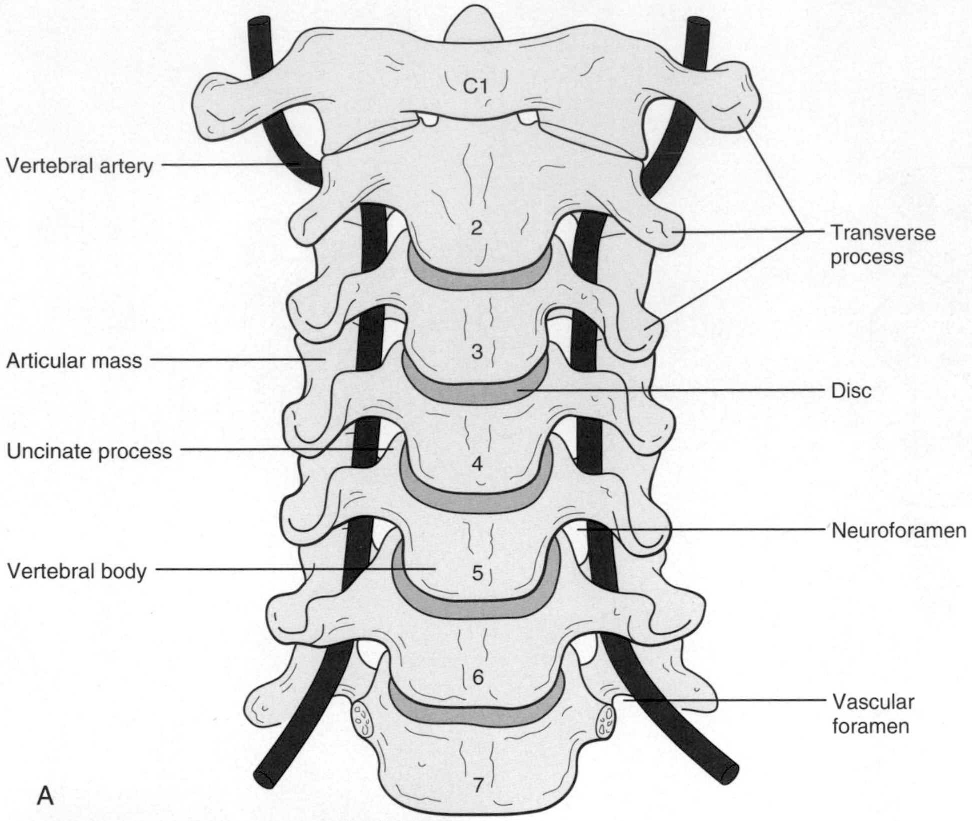

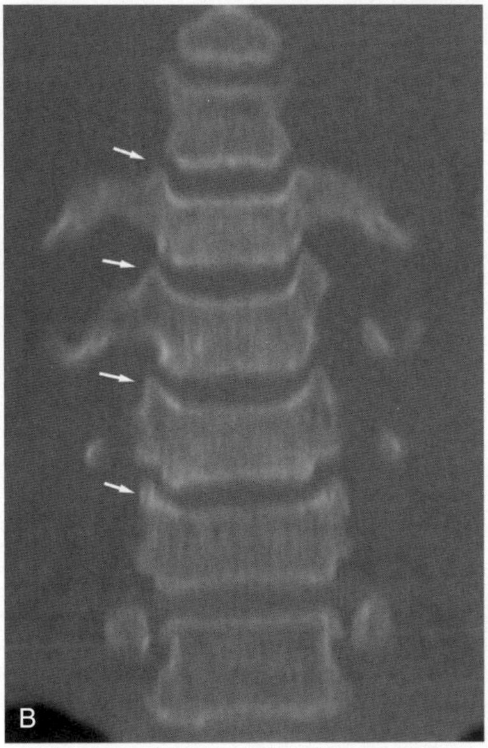

Figure 34-33. When viewed from the anterior approach (**A**), the uncinate processes at the posterolateral corners of the superior endplates are important landmarks for defining the lateral borders of the disc space. On the coronal computed tomography reconstruction (**B**), the uncinate processes *(arrows)* form the uncovertebral joint with the convex undersurface of the suprajacent vertebral body.

necessary to instrument and fuse the two involved levels. However, if a facet fracture has occurred, this level should be bypassed, and instrumentation should be placed at the levels cephalad or caudal to the fractured level.

Lateral mass screws are typically used from C3 through C6 and pedicle screws at C2, C7, and below. Pedicle screws, which are longer and enter the vertebral body, offer better biomechanical fixation by providing support to the anterior and posterior spinal columns. Typically, screw holes are created before decompression because this prevents an aberrant drill from injuring the exposed spinal cord, and the spinous process can be used as a landmark for proper trajectory when drilling

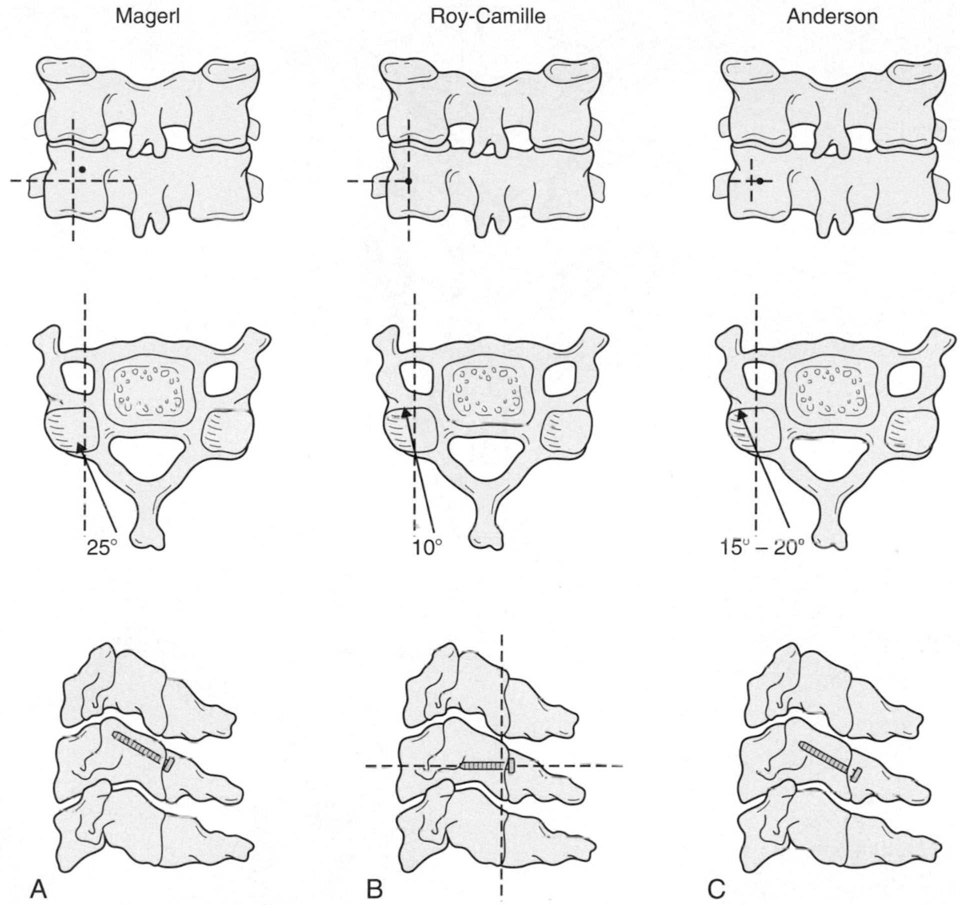

Figure 34-34. Lateral mass anatomy and techniques for placing lateral mass screws. Several techniques have been described to guide safe placement of screws. In the Magerl technique (**A**), the starting point is 1 to 2 mm medial and cephalad to the center of the lateral mass and angled 25 degrees outward and 30 degrees upward, parallel to the facet joint. In the Roy-Camille technique (**B**), the starting point is the center of the lateral mass, and the screws are directed straight forward and 10 degrees outward. In the Anderson technique (**C**), the starting point is 1 to 2 mm medial to the center of the lateral mass and angled 15 to 20 degrees outward and 20 to 30 degrees upward.

lateral mass holes. The cartilage of the facet joints planned for fusion should be burred at the time of screw cannulation. Screws are not actually placed until after the laminectomy because they typically obstruct burring for the laminectomy.

Several different methods of lateral mass fixation have been described. Roy-Camille used the starting point as the center of the lateral mass with the drill oriented perpendicular to the posterior aspect of the spine and 10 degrees laterally in the transverse plane.[118] Magerl, Anderson, and An later modified lateral mass screw placement by aiming the screw laterally and cephalad, such that its tip lies in the upper outer quadrant of the lateral mass when viewed from directly posteriorly, which is considered the "safe zone," with the lowest risk of vertebral artery and nerve root injury.[103] Magerl recommended starting the drill hole 2 to 3 mm medial and superior to the center of the lateral mass angling 30 degrees cephalad and 25 degrees laterally.[119] Anderson recommended a starting point 1 mm directly medial to the midpoint of the lateral mass with the screw angled 30 to 40 degrees cephalad and 10 degrees laterally.[120] An also recommended a starting point 1 mm medial to the lateral mass center with the drill angled 15 degrees cephalad and 30 degrees laterally[121] (Fig. 34-34). This is one reason why the screw holes are drilled before laminectomy—to use the spinous process as a trajectory landmark (Fig. 34-35).

Studies have shown that bicortical lateral mass fixation may risk penetration of the foramen transversarium as well as nerve root injury.[122] Furthermore, biomechanical studies have found equivocal results testing pullout strength between bicortical and unicortical lateral mass fixation.[123,124] Typically, unicortical screws of 14 to 16 mm in length in a normal adult spine directed to the upper outer quadrant of the lateral mass are used.

To place lateral mass fixation, the borders of the lateral masses are identified, and the center is located. Starting 1 to 2 mm medial to the point, a small hole is made with a 1- to 2-mm burr. After this starting hole is burred, the hole is drilled to the desired screw length in the proper upward and outward trajectory. To aid in outward trajectory of the drill guide, the drill can be laid against the spinous process, which, in the absence of significant deforming trauma, falls within the proper outward or lateral trajectory angle. The angle should be parallel to the facet articulation and outward 10 to 20 degrees. An adjustable stopped drill allows for control depth until desired length is achieved. Bilateral screw purchase is not always needed but is helpful in patients with osteoporosis or ankylosed spines. After all screws are placed, the facet joints are decorticated, and bone graft material is placed.

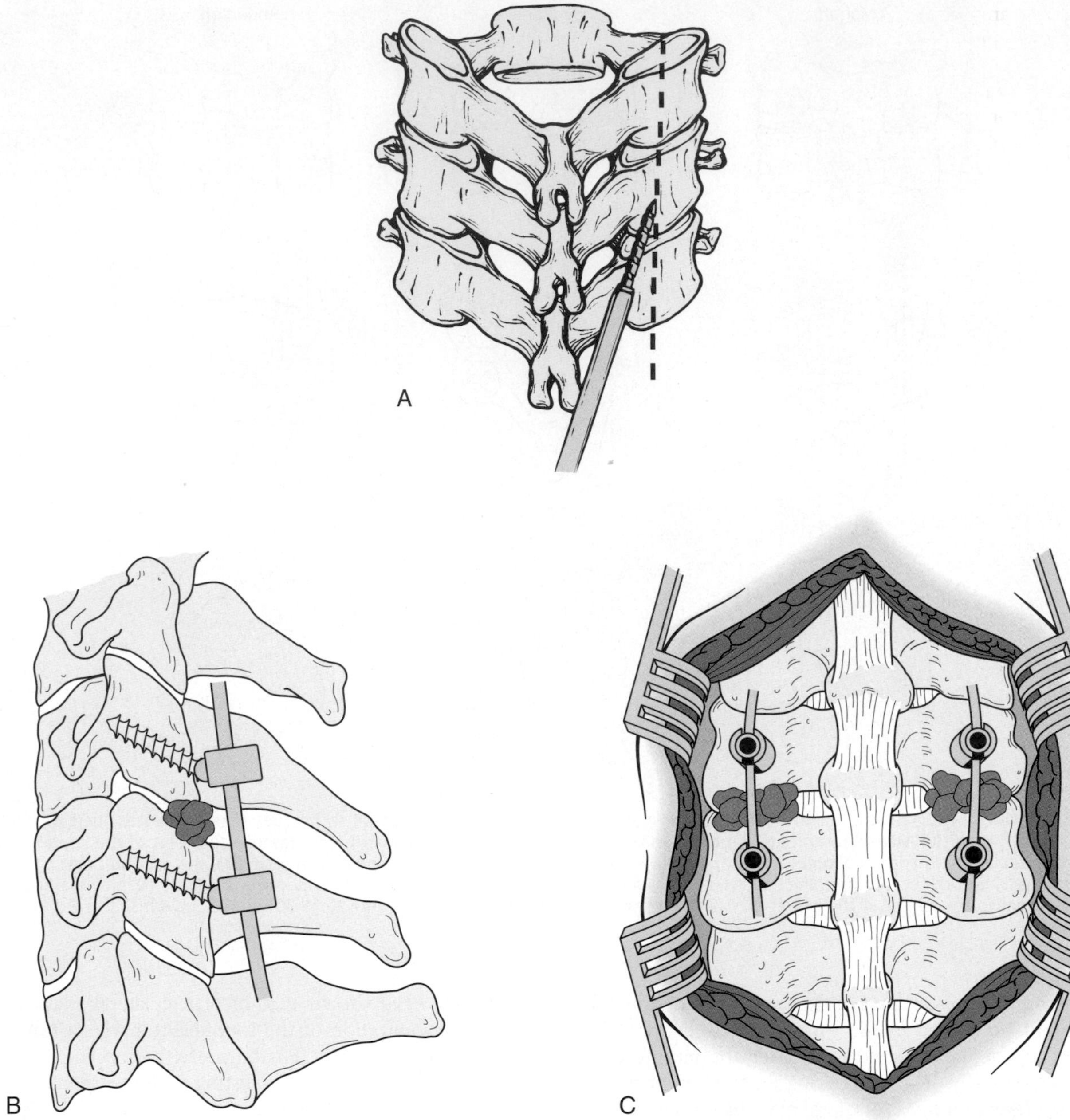

Figure 34-35. Technique for lateral mass screw insertion. To aid in proper outward trajectory, resting the drill against the spinous process at the correct starting point typically gives a good trajectory (**A**). The drill's upward trajectory should ideally be in line with the upward slope of the facet joints at that level (**B**). The facet joints should be burred out and bone graft placed into the space to promote fusion at the levels being instrumented (**C**).

Cervical pedicle screw fixation at subaxial levels other than C7 is technically challenging and in general is not recommended. The C7 vertebra is transitional with anatomic features resembling both lower cervical and upper thoracic vertebrae. The lateral masses at this level are thinner and the facet joints steeper in the sagittal plane making lateral mass fixation poor compared with the other subaxial levels, especially when a construct ends at this level.[125] The vertebral artery at this level has not usually entered the foramen transversarium yet and is not immediately lateral to the pedicle as it is at higher levels. Therefore, cervical pedicle screws at C7 are often the recommended form of fixation. Because topographical landmarks at C7 can be variable, we recommend performing a laminoforaminotomy with a burr and small Kerrison rongeur, at which time the C7 pedicle can be palpated with a right-angled nerve hook to verify its superior, medial, and inferior borders before cannulation.[126] The preoperative CT scan should be examined closely to verify the angle of the pedicle in the transverse plane, which is on average 33 degrees at this level.[104] Lateral fluoroscopy is typically not useful at this level because of the shoulders blocking adequate visualization of the pedicle.

A laminectomy can be performed at multiple levels of the cervical spine (Fig. 34-36). A high-speed burr is used to perform the laminectomy slightly medial to the convergence of the lateral mass and the lamina. Both outer and inner cortices of the laminae are burred away in a controlled fashion. A towel clamp is used to maintain gentle, continuous upward pressure on the spinous processes, while a 1-0 Kerrison rongeur or a scalpel is used to gently cut the ligamentum flavum away from the spinal cord. The removed spinous processes and laminae can be ground and used for local bone graft, placed laterally to the rods and within the decorticated facet joints. The screws are placed into the previously cannulated holes. The head can be placed into the appropriate amount of lordosis by manipulating the Mayfield head holder gently while visualizing the spinal cord. The rods are then contoured and placed appropriately.

The wound is irrigated. Hemostasis is achieved. Bone graft is placed. A deep drain is placed gently along the midline over

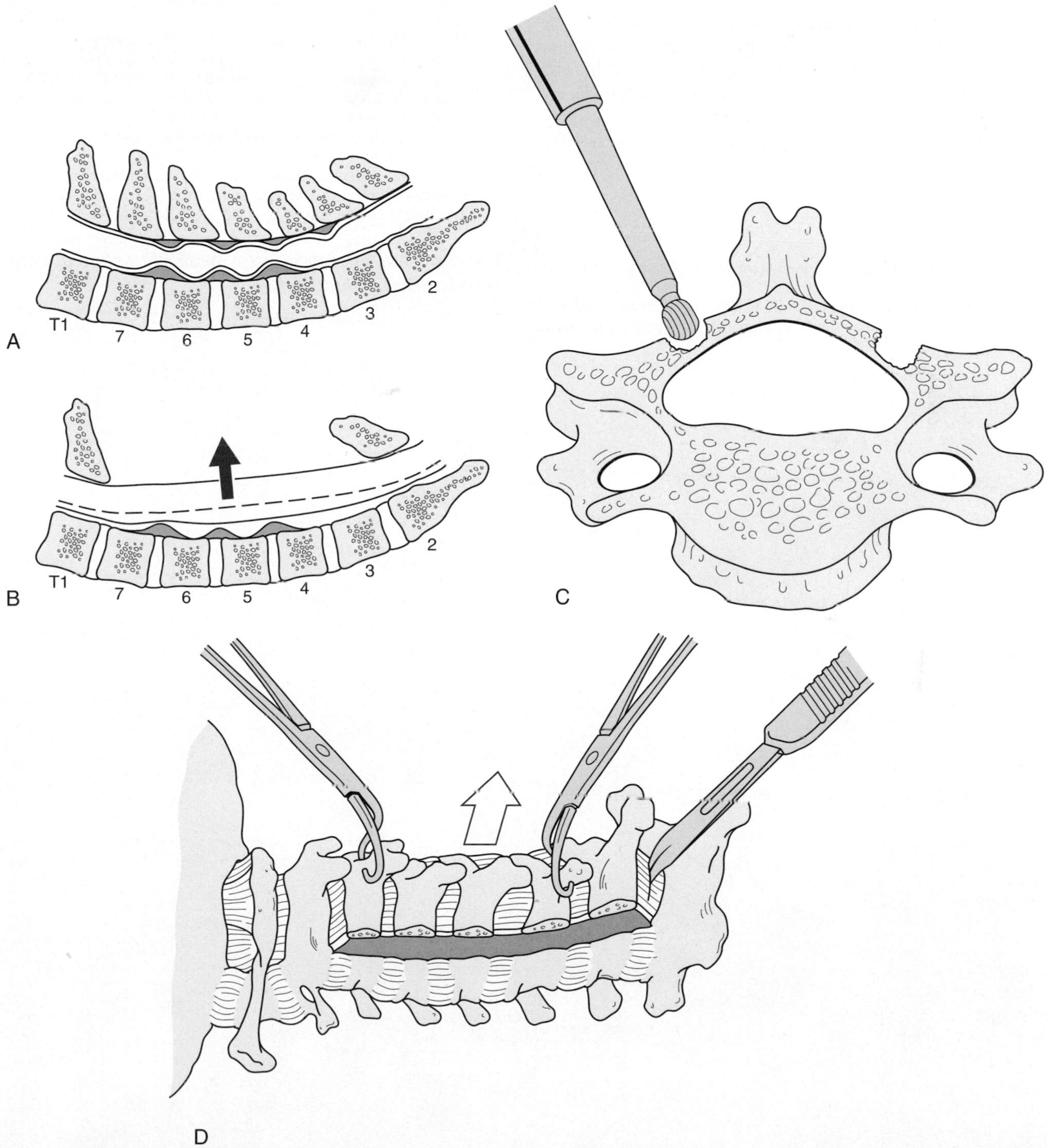

Figure 34-36. Posterior laminectomy-decompression, which is always performed with posterior stabilization to prevent postlaminectomy kyphosis. **A,** With multilevel stenosis and posterior spinal cord impingement, laminectomy may be indicated. If there is ventral pathology as well, after the laminectomy is performed, the spinal cord tends to drift posteriorly away from the anterior source of compression (**B**). The laminectomy is performed by burring troughs along the lateral borders of the lamina (**C**) followed by upward gentle pressure and separating the ligamentum flavum from the spinal cord with either 1-0 Kerrison rongeur or a scalpel (**D**).

the spinal cord. The wound is closed in multiple layers. The divided paraspinal muscles and ligamentum nuchae should be repaired at closure to prevent a web-necked deformity and disabling neck extensor muscle disability. A lateral radiograph is taken to ensure adequate reduction and screw placement.

SUMMARY

Injuries to the subaxial cervical spine commonly occur in trauma. There is a wide variety of injury patterns. It is important to consider not only the bony injury but also the soft tissue injury and neurologic status of the patient when deciding on treatment. New classification systems and increasingly better evidence with regard to treatment and outcomes offer promise that a more systematic evaluation and treatment of these injuries is on the horizon.

KEY REFERENCES

The level of evidence (LOE) is determined according to the criteria provided in the preface.

1. Hasler RM, Exadaktylos AK, Bouamra O, et al: Epidemiology and predictors of cervical spine injury in adult major trauma patients: a multicenter cohort study. *J Trauma Acute Care Surg* 72:975–981, 2012. LOE II
20. Stone AT, Bransford RJ, Lee MJ, et al: Reliability of classification systems for subaxial cervical injuries. *Evid Based Spine-Care J* 1:19–26, 2010. LOE V
21. Vaccaro AR, Hulbert RJ, Patel AA, et al: The subaxial cervical spine injury classification system: a novel approach to recognize the importance of morphology, neurology, and integrity of the disco-ligamentous complex. *Spine* 32:2365–2374, 2007. LOE V
23. Anderson PA, Moore TA, Davis KW, et al: Cervical spine injury severity score. Assessment of reliability. *J Bone Joint Surg Am* 89:1057–1065, 2007. LOE V
28. Dvorak MF, Fisher CG, Fehlings MG, et al: The surgical approach to subaxial cervical spine injuries: an evidence-based algorithm based on the SLIC classification system. *Spine* 32:2620–2629, 2007. LOE V
29. Fehlings MG, Vaccaro A, Wilson JR, et al: Early versus delayed decompression for traumatic cervical spinal cord injury: results of the Surgical Timing in Acute Spinal Cord Injury Study (STASCIS). *PLoS One* 7:e32037, 2012. LOE I
31. Brodke DS, Anderson PA, Newell DW, et al: Comparison of anterior and posterior approaches in cervical spinal cord injuries. *J Spinal Disord Tech* 16:229–235, 2003. LOE II

The complete References list is available online at https://expertconsult.inkling.com.

Chapter 35

Thoracolumbar Fractures

35A Classification

ANDREI F. JOAQUIM • ALPESH A. PATEL

INTRODUCTION

The thoracolumbar spine represents the most common site of fractures in the spine.[1] It is comprised of injuries to the thoracic spine (T1-T10), thoracolumbar junction (T11-L2), and lumbar spine (L3-L5).

Classification of spinal injuries is a critical step. It provides a common language for identification and comparison of injuries. This common language is fundamentally important in clinical care, education, and research as it allows for valid comparisons between physicians, institutions, and nationalities in the treatment of thoracolumbar spine trauma (TLST).

An ideal classification system must be precise, accurate, and valid. Precision or reliability refers to the ability of repeat application of the classification to the same condition with similar results. It is commonly evaluated with the percent of agreement. Accuracy is the truth to which, compared to a reference standard, the classification defines the image. Sensitivity, specificity, and positive and negative predictive values are measures of the accuracy. Besides precision and accuracy, a measurement must be valid in the clinical context to be useful. A classification must also be predictive of the patient's outcome and aid in the comparison of potential forms of treatment.

HISTORICAL REVIEW

In 1934, Böhler grouped spine fractures into five injuries according to their morphology, based on plain radiographs.[2] In 1949, Nicoll proposed a classification of thoracic and lumbar fractures into four types: (1) anterior edge fracture, (2) lateral edge fracture, (3) fracture dislocation, and (4) isolated fractures of the neural arch.[3] The author postulated that fracture stability was associated with the integrity of the interspinous ligament. Fractures, therefore, could be labeled as stable or unstable based on their integrity. This concept was critically important as it was the first description of the role of the posterior ligamentous complex (PLC) in spinal stability.

In 1970, Holdsworth introduced a new classification scheme based on the concept of columns.[4] He proposed that there were two columns responsible for vertebral stability: an anterior column, composed by the vertebral body, intervertebral disc, and anterior and posterior longitudinal ligaments; and a posterior column, composed by the facet joints, interspinous, supraspinous, and yellow ligaments. He also stated that spinal stability required the integrity of the posterior column. Four basic mechanisms of injuries were described: compression, flexion, extension, and flexion-rotation. Holdsworth also described the term "burst" as a fracture secondary to axial overload with consequent herniation of the nucleus pulposus into the superior vertebral endplate. He considered this injury stable.

In 1977, Louis modified Holdsworth's concept of two columns to three columns: one anterior and two posterior.[5] The anterior column was formed by the vertebral body and disc, whereas the two posterior columns were formed by the facet joints and ligaments of each side. He also proposed that the lamina and the pedicles were responsible for additional stabilization of the vertebrae. Another important point in the Louis system was the graduation of the stability based on a nominal system; he postulated that there were degrees of instability, within a continuum between a stable and an unstable injury. Based on morphologic and mechanical criteria, values were attributed to injuries: 2 points for loss of substance in the columns; 1 point for vertical spine injuries; 0.5 point for incomplete injuries of the pedicles, vertebral body, or lamina; 0.25 point for fractures in the transverse or spinous process. Injuries with 2 or more points were considered unstable. For the first time, treatment was proposed based on a numerical score.

In 1983, based on evaluation of 100 cases of thoracolumbar fractures using then newly available computed tomography (CT), McAfee and colleagues proposed six different injuries.[6] They also proposed that burst fractures can be stable when anterior and middle columns fail because of a compressive load with no loss of integrity of the posterior elements and unstable when the posterior elements are disrupted. This disruption can lead to failure in compression, lateral flexion, or rotation, but most likely results in posttraumatic kyphosis and the development of neurologic symptoms.

In 1983, Denis modified the column models proposed by Holdsworth and Louis.[7] The spine was again divided into three columns: (1) an anterior column (anterior half of the vertebral body and intervertebral disc, within the anterior longitudinal ligament); (2) a middle column (posterior half of the vertebral body and intervertebral disc plus the posterior longitudinal ligament); and (3) a posterior column (supraspinous, interspinous, and yellow ligament plus the facet joints) (Fig. 35A-1). In his theory, Denis proposed that an isolated posterior injury would not compromise stability. Injury to two columns would be necessary to make the spine "unstable." Denis also classified spinal injuries in two groups: major and minor. This latter minor group includes transverse and spinous process fractures, as well as pars interarticularis fractures. Major injuries were then classified in five types: A, B, C, D, and E. The burst fracture concept was redefined as an injury to the anterior and middle columns and classified as unstable, as two columns

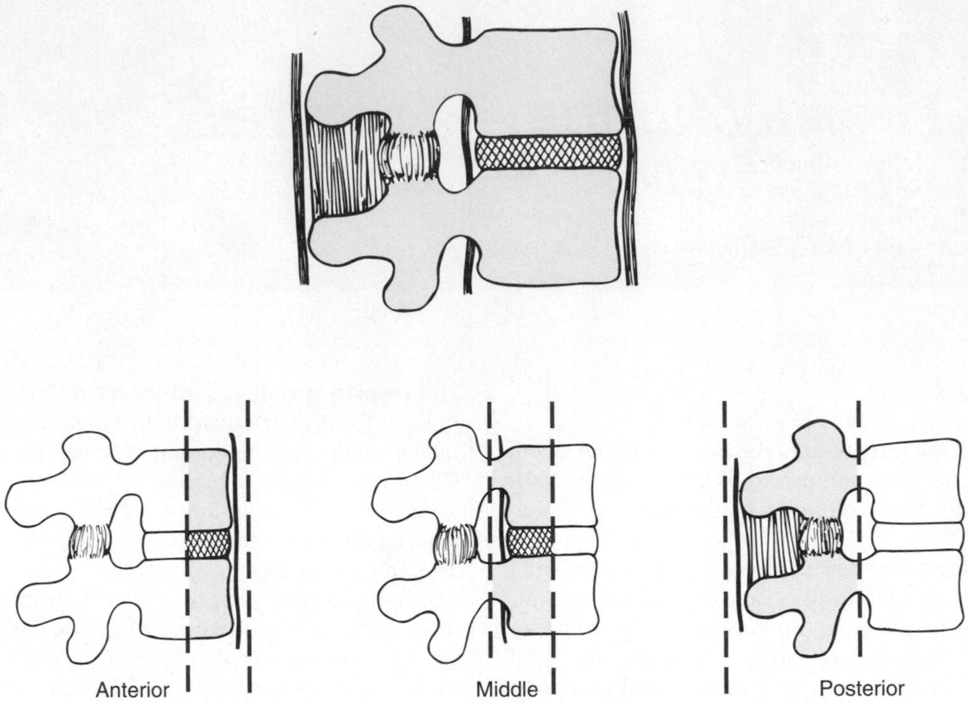

Figure 35A-1. Denis' three-column model of the spine. The middle column is made up of the posterior longitudinal ligament, the posterior annulus fibrosus, and the posterior aspects of the vertebral body and disc.

were injured. Although widely used, the Denis system was criticized for not being comprehensive, for having low reliability and reproducibility, and for the theoretical nature of the middle column, in that it is not an anatomic entity and, therefore, characterization of middle column injuries remained difficult.[8,9]

In 1990, White and Panjabi defined spinal injuries based on the concept of stability, which is the ability of supporting elements of the spine to resist physiologic loads so as to prevent neurologic injury, deformity, or pain.[10] This descriptor provides continuing clarity of the clinical definition of spinal stability and remains a critical determinant of treatment.

McCormack and colleagues proposed a point system in 1994 known as *load-sharing classification* (LSC) to distinguish three-column spinal fractures according to the amount of damaged vertebral body, the spread of the fragments, and the amount of corrected kyphosis after short-segment instrumentation.[11] Their system was an attempt to predict screw breakage in short-segment reconstruction and to identify spinal fractures requiring additional anterior reconstruction.

The classification system developed by Magerl and coworkers, also known as the *Arbeitsgemeinschaft für Osteosynthesefragen (AO) Classification of Fractures* (Table 35A-1), is probably the most widely discussed system in 1990s and early 2000s.[9] It was a pathomechanistic classification based on a review of 1445 plain radiograph fractures. The system considered prognostic aspects regarding healing and patient recovery. Injuries are primarily classified according to the main mechanism of injury as type A (axial force injuries, including compression and burst fractures), type B (distraction), and type C (rotational).

Type A: Injuries secondary to compression fractures, in the vertebral body, such as compression and burst fractures, without injury to the PLC. Small bone injury in the posterior elements can be present.

Type B: Injuries resulting in transverse disruption, with anterior or posterior distraction.

Type C: The most severe injuries, with anterior and posterior element disruption and rotation.

These injuries are then subclassified into detailed and numerical groups and subgroups, with more than 50 subtypes. The severity of the cases increases from A to C, also increasing incrementally according to groups and subgroups.

The Magerl system is frequently criticized for its high degree of complexity, decreasing its reliability, and also for not considering the neurologic status in the decision-making process.[12,13] Although beneficial for research, these factors limit its application in clinical practice and education. It is also important to mention that the system was proposed based on plain radiographs, without considering the potential benefits of modern high-resolution CT scanning with reconstruction and magnetic resonance imaging (MRI) in defining spinal injuries. Even considering its potential pitfalls, the AO system is still used worldwide.

TABLE 35A-1 ***MAGERL CLASSIFICATION OF SPINE INJURIES (AO CLASSIFICATION SYSTEM)***

Type	Characteristic
Type A	Compression and burst fractures (no PLC injury)
Type B	Anterior and/or posterior element injuries with distraction (vertical forces)
Type C	Anterior and posterior element injuries with rotation

PLC, Posterior ligamentous complex.
Source: *Magerl F, Aebi M, Gertzbein SD, et al: A comprehensive classification of thoracic and lumbar injuries, Eur Spine J 3:184–201, 1994.*

THORACOLUMBAR INJURY CLASSIFICATION SYSTEM

Considering this entire historical context, in 2005 the Spine Trauma Study Group proposed a new system to help surgeons classify and treat thoracic and lumbar spine fractures.[13] The system is based on three major descriptors, all of them associated with the treatment and prognosis of these injuries: (1) injury morphology, (2) integrity of the PLC, and (3) neurologic status.

The system is known as Thoracolumbar Injury Classification System and Severity Score (TLICS) and was developed to help surgeons guide treatment (Table 35A-2). According to the obtained score, conservative or surgical treatment can be proposed. Its main advantage is its quantification of the neurologic status and also its assessment of the integrity of the PLC and the effect of these critical factors on the decision-making process.

After all individual characteristics are classified and scored, the summation of each variable leads to a final score. When three or fewer points are obtained, conservative treatment is proposed. Five or more points suggest that surgical treatment is probably the best treatment option. Patients with four points can be treated conservatively or surgically, according to surgeon's preference. Other variables can also influence the final treatment option, such as body habitus, obesity, comorbidities, patient age, systemic injuries, patient preference, institutional or health system capacity, among many others (Figs. 35A-2 and 35A-3).

TLICS has been well accepted by the scientific community. Some studies suggested good reliability and reproducibility, and also attest that it is an important tool for medical education.[14-18]

TABLE 35A-2 *THORACOLUMBAR INJURY CLASSIFICATION SYSTEM AND SEVERITY SCORE (TLICS)*

Variable	Points
Injury Morphology	
Compression	1
Burst	+1
Translation/rotation	3
Distraction	4
Neurologic Status	
Intact	0
Nerve injury	2
Cord, conus medullaris	
Incomplete	3
Complete	2
Cauda equina	3
PLC Integrity	
Intact	0
Indeterminate*	2
Injured	3

PLC, Posterior ligamentous complex.
*Indeterminate status is attributed to patients without evident disruption on computed tomography (CT) scan reconstructions (without clear dislocation) but with suggested ligamentous injury at the short tau inversion recovery (STIR) or T2-weighted magnetic resonance imaging (MRI) sequence.

UPDATED AO CLASSIFICATION

Vaccaro and colleagues as the AOSpine Spinal Cord Injury and Trauma Knowledge Forum recently published an updated thoracolumbar (TL) spine injury classification system.[19] The new AOSpine TL injury classification system, similar to the TLICS system, defines three basic parameters: morphologic classification of the fracture, neurologic status, and clinical modifiers. Fracture morphology is defined as type A (compression injuries), type B (tension band injuries), and type C (translation/displacement). Neurologic status is defined as N0 (intact), N1 (transient deficit, resolved), N2 (radiculopathy), N3 (incomplete spinal cord or cauda equina injury), and N4 (complete spinal cord injury, American Spinal Injury Association [ASIA] grade A). Finally, two clinical modifiers were reported: M1, fractures with indeterminate injury to tension band; and M2, patient-specific comorbidities. Fracture morphology is further defined by subgroups of A0 to A4 and B1 to B3 (Table 35A-3).

The authors reported overall moderate-to-fair interobserver reliability and substantial-to-excellent intraobserver reliability. With the addition of the morphology subtypes, however, reliability decreased. The new AO system has not been tested outside of the describing authors and, therefore, its generalizability to other surgeons, residents, and students remains unknown. Furthermore, the new system has not been clinically validated in patient care. Future studies may address these informational gaps, providing a more complete assessment of the new system.

RELIABILITY OF CLASSIFICATION SYSTEMS

Reliability refers to the extent to which repeated measurements of the same situation agree with each other. Potential sources of variation include the patient, the physician, and the radiologic instrument used (such as CT scan vs. MRI). The variability of the physician can be divided into intrarater (when the reliability is accessed by the same physician) or interrater (when accessed by a different health care provider). As a practical point of view, interrater reliability is the most important evaluation to consider a classification system reproducible and potentially useful.

Reliability is generally measured by Cohen's kappa coefficient, a statistical instrument to quantify agreement. Generally, the magnitude of the agreement is classified according to the kappa value (Table 35A-4). Table 35A-5 presents the reliability of the most useful classification systems.

MORPHOLOGY AND CLASSIFICATION SYSTEM

Morphology is one of the most crucial characteristics in a classification system for traumatic spine injuries. Some basic morphologic characteristics can be easily described, such as fracture line description and vertebral displacement. Some fracture morphologies are related to spinal instability and can

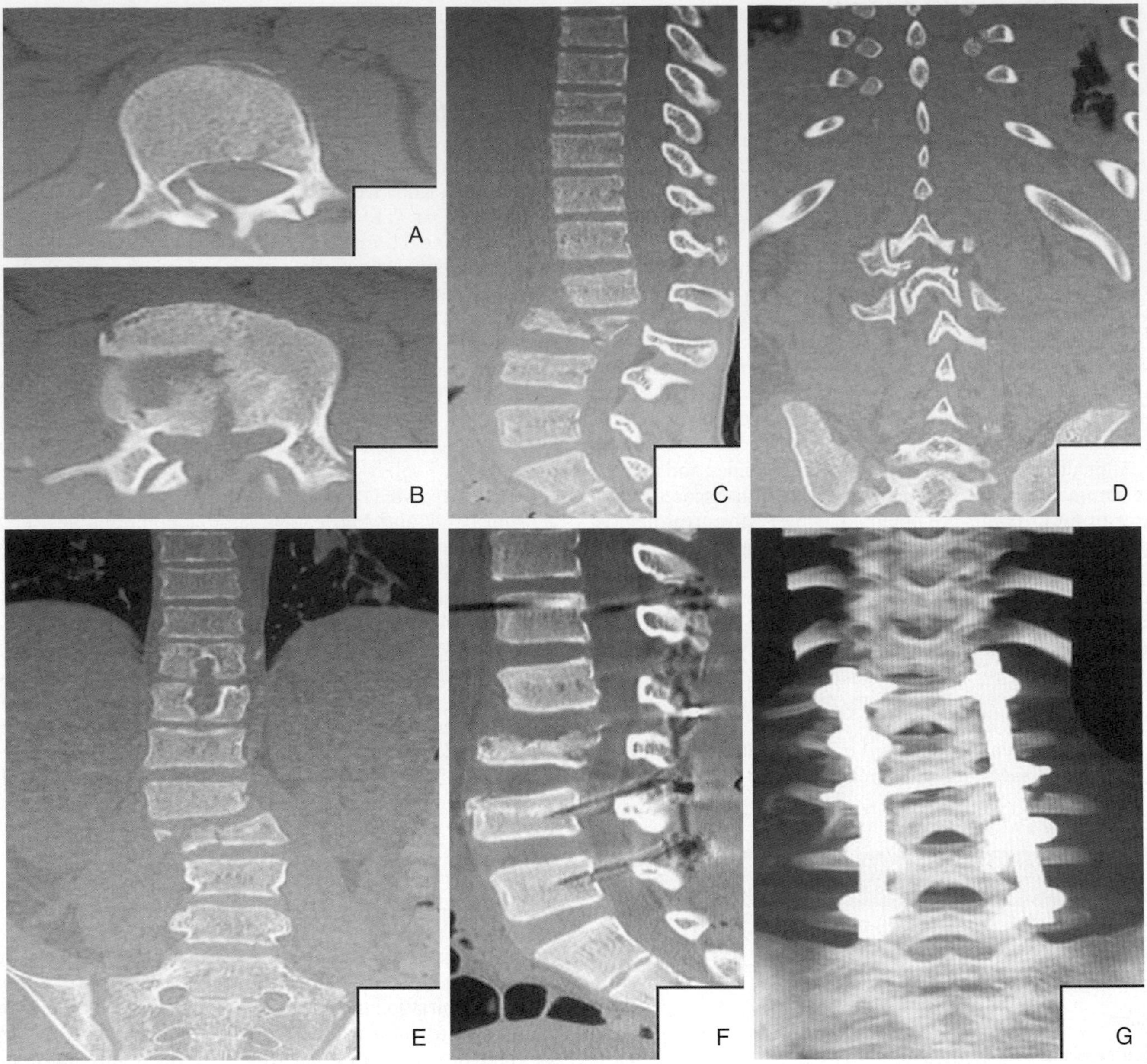

Figure 35A-2. A 22-year-old man presented after a car accident and an L3 translational injury with no neurologic status. **A** and **B,** Axial computed tomography (CT) scan showing vertebral body and laminar fracture. A sagittal (**C** and **D**) and coronal (**E**) CT scan reconstruction showing a rotational injury between L2 and L3, with spinal translation in both planes. Diastasis of facet joints can be seen (**D**). This injury can be classified as type C, according to the Arbeitsgemeinschaft für Osteosynthesefragen (AO) classification system. Applying the Thoracolumbar Injury Classification System and Severity Score (TLICS), we have 3 points for morphology plus 3 points for posterior ligamentous complex (PLC) plus 0 for neurologic status, giving a total of 6 points. Surgical treatment was proposed, with L1 to L5 posterior instrumentation, as shown in **F** and **G.**

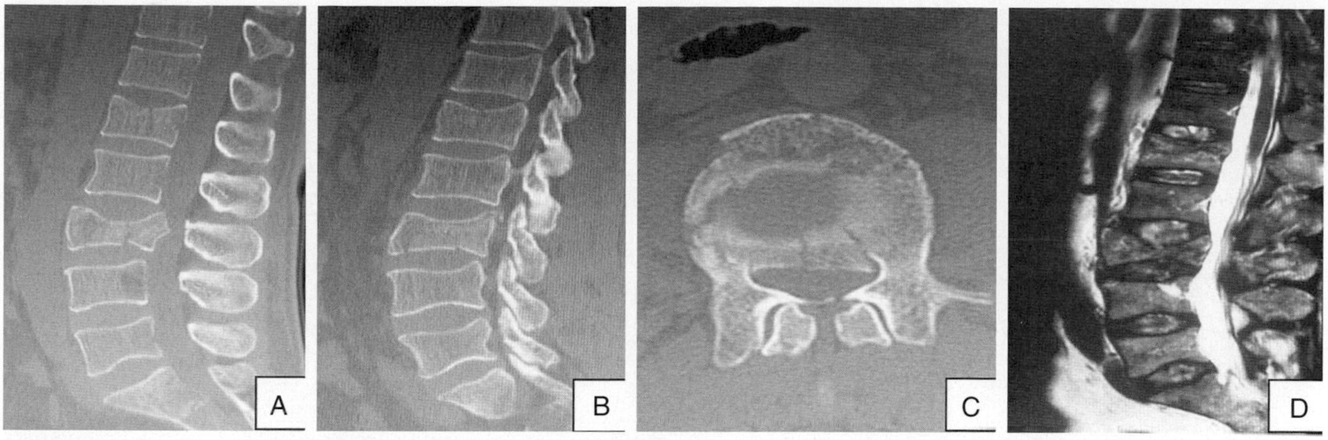

Figure 35A-3. A 57-year-old man sustained a fall from a height with an L1 compression and an L3 burst fracture. **A** and **B,** There is no facet joint diastasis or any rotation or distraction evident in sagittal computed tomography (CT) reconstruction. **C,** An axial CT scan of L3 showing injury of the posterior body wall and canal compression. **D,** A sagittal T2-weighted magnetic resonance imaging (MRI). There is no posterior ligamentous complex (PLC) injury based on CT and MRI. The patient was neurologically intact. L1 and L3 are Arbeitsgemeinschaft für Osteosynthesefragen (AO) type A injuries (compression and burst fractures). The Thoracolumbar Injury Classification System and Severity Score (TLICS) for L1 fracture is 1 point for morphology plus 0 for PLC plus 0 for neurologic status, giving a total of 1 point. The TLICS for L3 was 2 points for morphology plus 0 points for PLC plus 0 for neurologic status, giving a total of 2 points. The patient was successfully treated nonsurgically.

TABLE 35A-3 *SUMMARY OF THE NEW AOSPINE THORACOLUMBAR TRAUMA CLASSIFICATION SYSTEM*

Fracture Morphology	
A	*Compression*
A0	No injury/process fracture
A1	Wedge/impaction
A2	Split/pincer
A3	Incomplete burst
A4	Complete burst
B	*Tension Band Injuries*
B1	Posterior transosseous disruption
B2	Posterior ligamentous disruption
B3	Anterior ligamentous disruption
C	*Translation/Displacement*
Neurologic Status	
N0	Intact
N1	Transient, resolved
N2	Radiculopathy
N3	Incomplete spinal cord or cauda equina injury
N4	Complete spinal cord injury (ASIA grade A)
Clinical Modifiers	
M1	Indeterminate tension band
M2	Patient-specific comorbidities (AS, DISH, osteopenia, etc.)

AS, Ankylosing spondylitis; *ASIA,* American Spinal Injury Association; *DISH,* diffuse idiopathic skeletal hyperostosis.

TABLE 35A-4 *MAGNITUDE OF AGREEMENT ACCORDING TO COHEN'S KAPPA COEFFICIENT*

Kappa Value	Magnitude of the Agreement
<0	Chance
0.01–0.20	Slight
0.21–0.40	Fair
0.41–0.60	Moderate
0.61–0.80	Substantial
0.81–0.99	Almost perfect

TABLE 35A-5 *INTERRATER RELIABILITY OF THE MOST COMMON CLASSIFICATION SYSTEMS ACCORDING TO COHEN'S KAPPA COEFFICIENT IN DIFFERENT STUDIES*

System		Interrater Reliability Range (Kappa Score)
Dennis System	For major fracture subtype	0.52–0.60
	For entire classification system	0.39–0.45
Magerl System	For the three main types	0.33–0.42 (studies using plain radiographs, CT, or MRI)
TLICS	Morphology	0.608
	PLC status	0.641
	Neurologic status	0.91
	Total score	0.576–0.74
Updated AO		
	Type A	0.72
	Type B	0.58
	Type C	0.70

AO, Arbeitsgemeinschaft für Osteosynthesefragen; *CT,* computed tomography; *MRI,* magnetic resonance imaging; *PLC,* posterior ligamentous complex; *TLICS,* Thoracolumbar Injury Classification System and Severity Score.

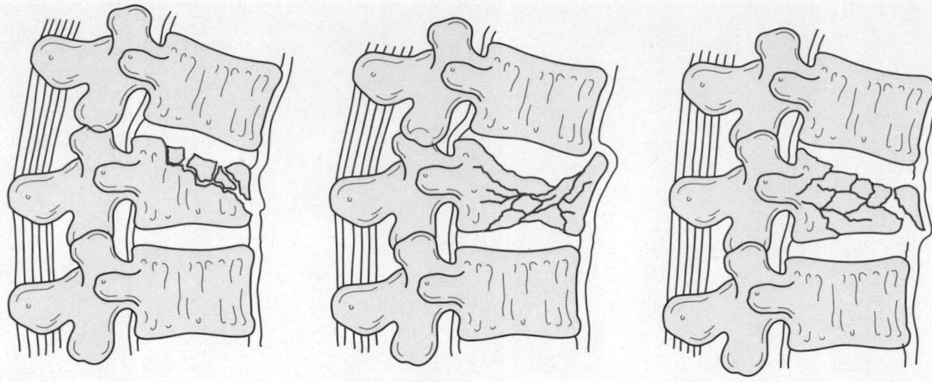

Figure 35A-4. Comprehensive classification of type A spinal injuries. The three categories of type A fractures include impaction injuries *(A1)*, of which wedge fractures are most commonly seen; split fractures *(A2)*, of which the pincer fracture is the typical injury; and the burst fracture *(A3)*. *(Redrawn by permission from Gertzbein SD: Classification of thoracic and lumbar fractures. In Gertzbein SD, editor: Fractures of the thoracic and lumbar spine, Baltimore, 1992, Williams & Wilkins.)*

guide treatment. Morphology characteristics are generally used indirectly to describe the severity of a spinal injury. The main morphology described in thoracolumbar trauma are briefly presented in the following sections.

Compression Fractures

Compression fractures are generally considered stable injuries; they exhibit minimal body height loss (<10%) and kyphosis (<25 degrees) (Fig. 35A-4). By definition, compression fractures do not involve the posterior wall of the vertebral body. Compression fractures most commonly involve the superior and anterior endplate resulting in vertebral body wedging. Other patterns are the anterior body only, the pincer fracture where a fracture line divides the anterior and posterior vertebral body, and less commonly, an inferior endplate fracture. An important component of compression fractures is the maintenance of the posterior osseous ligamentous complex.

Burst Fractures

Burst fractures are characterized by fractures and loss of height of the anterior and posterior portions of the vertebral body. The hallmark of the burst fracture is the retropulsion of the posterior wall and canal compromise. This may lead to neurologic deficits. Centrifugal extrusions of the bone fragments are generally presented. The pedicles are expanded apart, which is best seen as widening of anteroposterior or coronal plane reconstructions. Like compression fractures, several patterns of body and posterior involvement have been described that might affect treatment decisions. Most commonly, the superior endplate is fractured, whereas a more unstable injury is when the fracture comminution extends to involve both superior and inferior endplates.

Magerl and colleagues proposed that burst fractures have an intact PLC. However, the authors of TLICS proposed that some burst fractures can have PLC injury, having an increasing risk of instability. Burst fractures can be associated with laminar and spinous process fractures.

Perhaps the greatest impact the TLICS system can have is in the evaluation and treatment of burst fractures. The TLICS system does not account for some classically described characteristics of burst fractures. Factors such as loss of vertebral body height, segmental kyphosis, and canal compromise, despite their widespread use, have no evidence to support their importance in managing patients without neurologic deficits. Studies have examined the impact of these classic radiographic measures on patient outcome and have shown no relationships with only neurologic function consistently predicting patient outcomes.[20-22] As an example, kyphosis greater than 30 degrees and/or 50% of vertebral body height loss were indirect radiologic measures of PLC disruption, such as substantial canal compromise.[23,24] Based on these historical analyses, Radcliff and coworkers studied the relation of loss of vertebral body height, kyphosis, and canal compromise observed on CT scan with the PLC status according to MRI findings.[25,26] They reported that these factors did not correlate with PLC injury and the MRI should be used when there is clinical concern. However, there is lack of consistent evidence on the utility of MRI in the evaluation and management of spinal fractures. As such, despite the proven utility of the TLICS system, the controversy regarding the treatment of burst fractures remains, especially in the evaluation of the PLC status.[27] Over time, with additional evidence and clinical utilization of the TLICS system, consistency in the treatment of stable burst fractures can be achieved with the betterment of patient treatment and outcomes.

Flexion-Distraction Injuries

Flexion-distraction injuries are a flexion injury of the spine, characterized by a compression injury to the anterior portion of the vertebral body and a transverse fracture through the posterior elements of the vertebra and the posterior portion of the vertebral body (Fig. 35A-5).

The mechanism of injury is rotation about a fulcrum located within the vertebral body, so that the middle and posterior columns fail in tension and the anterior column fails in compression. Its association with extreme forward flexion in automotive accidents results in the literature name of "seat-belt" fractures. The Chance fracture variant occurs when all three columns fail under tension often involving only bony structures (Fig. 35A-6). Various patterns of flexion-distraction and Chance fractures have been described and are differentiated by combinations of bony, soft tissue, and facet articulation involvement.

Many abdominal injuries especially bowel perforation were described in association with flexion-distraction injuries and lead to a high level of suspicion in patients with this injury morphology.

Hyperextension Injuries

Hyperextension injuries can present with anterior column disruption through the disc or the vertebral body, secondary to severe spine hyperextension. These injuries are frequently described in patients with diffuse idiopathic skeletal hyperostosis (DISH) and ankylosing spondylitis (AS) and are considered unstable. They can have or not have PLC involvement, increasing the degree of instability. Sometimes it is possible to see a fracture line crossing the syndesmophytes of the ankylosed spine.

Fracture-Dislocation

Fracture-dislocations are the most severe spinal cord injuries and are commonly associated with neurologic deficits. These injuries have vertebral body displacement, complex fractures, and joint subluxation and rotation, in a multitude of patterns with displacement beyond the normal range (Fig. 35A-7). Compression and burst fractures can be found in association with this complex group of injuries.

CONCLUSIONS

The use of classification systems is to provide taxonomy for communication and to guide treatment. In clinical practice, the fracture pattern is assessed and a morphologic name is associated. This is important as each morphologic type may have its own treatment paradigm. Then the severity of injury is determined using systems such as AO and TLICS or for burst fractures, the McCormack system. This is important as injuries vary in the severity even when having the same morphologic type. In the following chapters in this section, the treatment of the various fracture types is discussed.

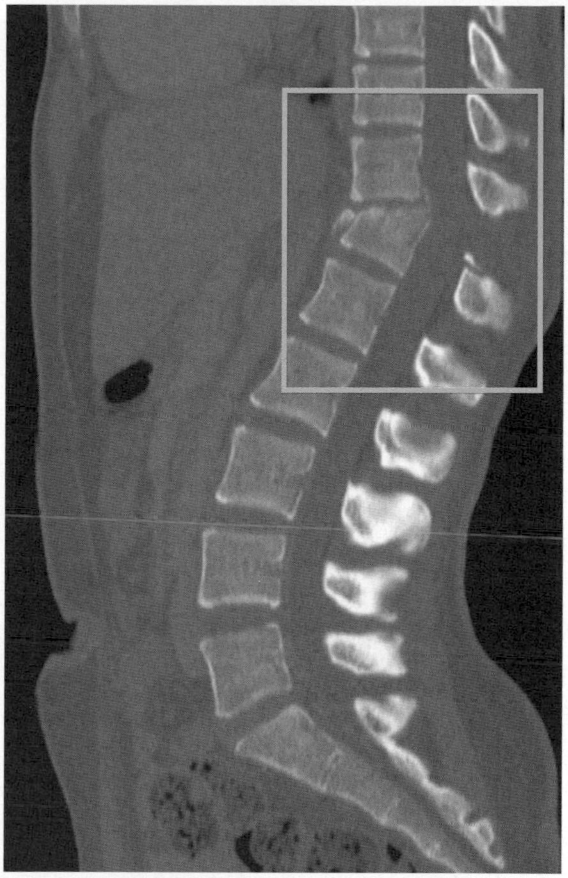

Figure 35A-5. Flexion-distraction injury at T11-T12 demonstrates small anterior compression injury but wide posterior splaying consistent with posterior distraction.

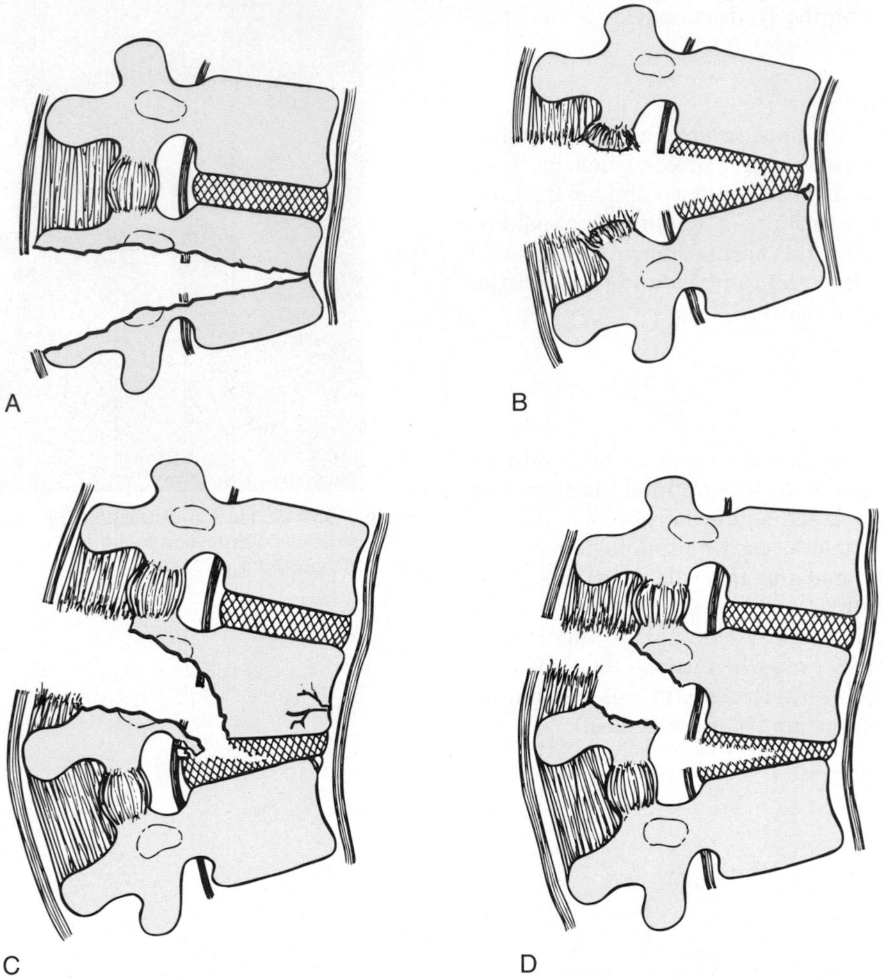

Figure 35A-6. Denis' classification of flexion-distraction injuries. These may occur at one level through bone (**A**), at one level through the ligaments and disc (**B**), at two levels, with the middle column injured through bone (**C**), or at two levels with the middle column injured through ligament and disc (**D**).

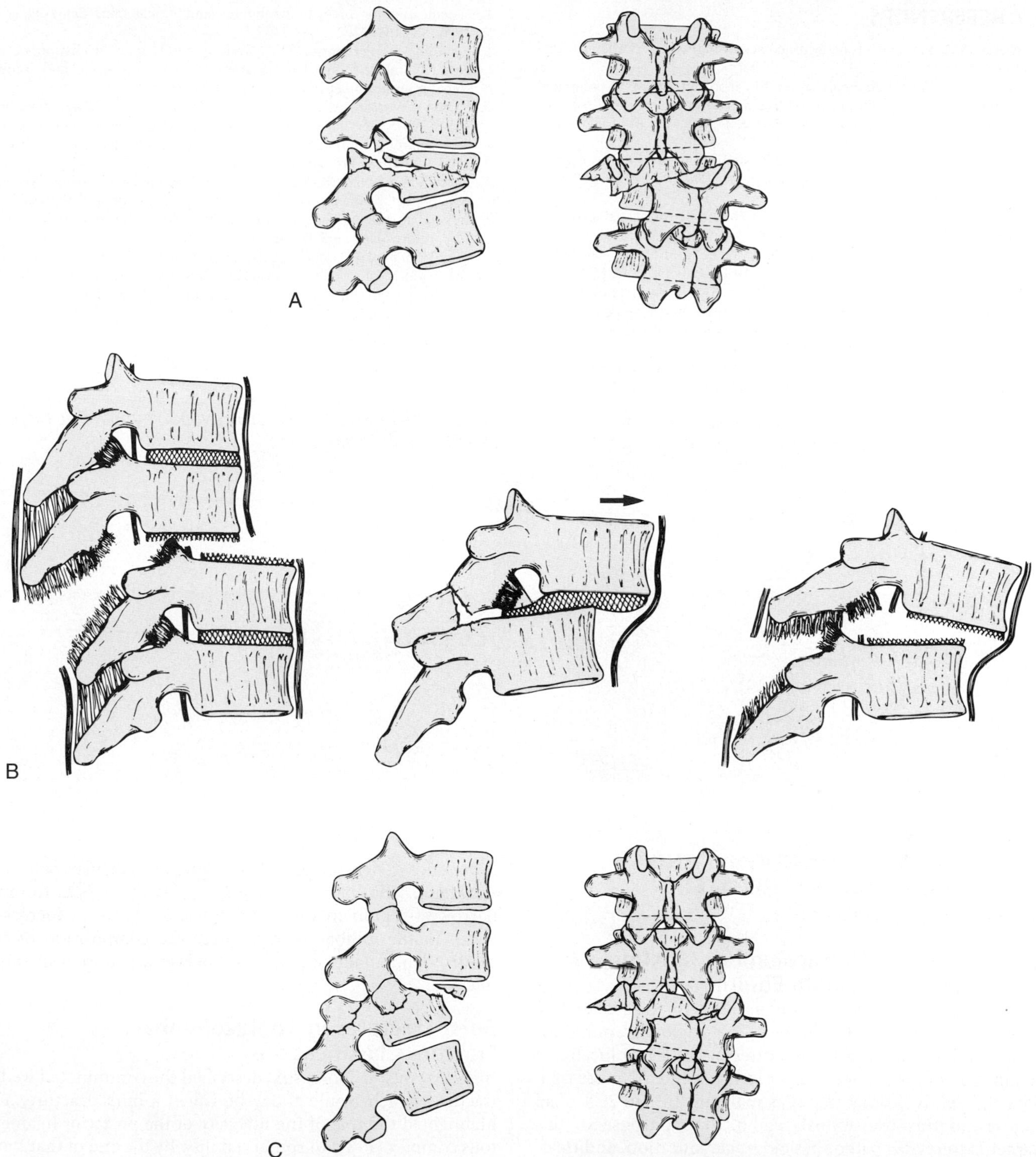

Figure 35A-7. Denis' classification of fracture-dislocation of the spine. **A,** Type A is a flexion-rotation injury, occurring either through bone or through the disc. There is a complete disruption of all three columns of the spine, usually with the anterior longitudinal ligament remaining the only intact structure. Commonly, this is stripped off the anterior portion of the vertebral body below. These injuries are usually associated with fractures of the superior facet of the more caudal vertebra. **B,** Type B is a shear injury. The type that produces anterior spondylolisthesis of the more cephalad vertebra usually fractures a facet, but the type that causes a posterior lithiasis of the more cephalad vertebra normally does not cause a fracture of the facet joint. **C,** Type C is a bilateral facet dislocation. This is a flexion-distraction injury but with disruption of the anterior column in addition to the posterior and middle columns. This disruption through the anterior column may occur through either the anterior intervertebral disc or the anterior vertebral body.

KEY REFERENCES

The level of evidence (LOE) is determined according to the criteria provided in the preface.

6. McAfee PC, Yuan HA, Fredrickson BE, et al: The value of computed tomography in thoracolumbar fractures: an analysis of one hundred consecutive cases and a new classification. *J Bone Joint Surg Am* 65:461–473, 1983. LOE II
7. Denis F: The three column spine and its significance in the classification of acute thoracolumbar spinal injuries. *Spine (Phila Pa 1976)* 8:817–831, 1983. LOE III
9. Magerl F, Aebi M, Gertzbein SD, et al: A comprehensive classification of thoracic and lumbar injuries. *Eur Spine J* 3:184–201, 1994. LOE II
11. McCormack T, Karaikovic E, Gaines RW: The Load-Sharing classification of spine fractures. *Spine (Phila Pa 1976)* 19:1741–1744, 1994. LOE II
13. Vaccaro AR, Lehman RA, Hulbert PA, et al: A new classification of thoracolumbar injuries: the importance of injury morphology, the integrity of the posterior ligamentous complex, and neurologic status. *Spine (Phila Pa 1976)* 30:2325–2333, 2005. LOE II
14. Koh YD, Kim DJ, Koh YW: Reliability and validity of Thoracolumbar Injury Classification and Severity Score (TLICS). *Asian Spine J* 4:109–117, 2010. LOE I
15. Lewkonia P, Paolucci EO, Thomas K: Reliability of the thoracolumbar injury classification and severity score and comparison with the Denis classification for injury to the thoracic and lumbar spine. *Spine (Phila Pa 1976)* 37:2161–2167, 2012. LOE I
16. Joaquim AF, Fernandes YB, Cavalcante RC, et al: Evaluation of the Thoracolumbar Injury Classification System in thoracic and lumbar spinal trauma. *Spine (Phila Pa 1976)* 1:33–36, 2011. LOE I
17. Patel AA, Vaccaro AR, Albert TJ, et al: The adoption of a new classification system: time-dependent variation in interobserver reliability of the thoracolumbar injury severity score classification system. *Spine (Phila Pa 1976)* 32:E105–E110, 2007. LOE III
26. Radcliff K, Klepler CK, Rubin TA, et al: Does the load-sharing classification predict ligamentous injury, neurological injury, and the need for surgery in patients with thoracolumbar burst fractures? Clinical article. *J Neurosurg Spine* 16:534–538, 2012. LOE I
27. van Middendorp JJ, Patel AA, Schuetz M, et al: The precision, accuracy and validity of detecting posterior ligamentous complex injuries of the thoracic and lumbar spine: a critical appraisal of the literature. *Eur Spine J* 22(3):461–474, 2013. LOE III

The complete References list is available online at https://expertconsult.inkling.com.

35B Treatment of Thoracolumbar Burst Fractures

PHILIPPE PHAN • POLINA OSLER • KIRKHAM BERWICK WOOD

ANATOMY, CLASSIFICATIONS, AND RADIOLOGIC FINDINGS RELATED TO BURST FRACTURES

Anatomy of the Thoracolumbar Junction, Spinal Cord, and Cauda Equina

The thoracolumbar junction is typically defined as extending from T10 through L2 (inclusive). This region accounts for more than half[1] of all spinal fractures because it is located at the junction of the mobile lumbar lordosis and the more rigid thoracic kyphosis. Burst fractures make up 10% to 20% of all fractures in this transitional region.[2] The purpose of this chapter is to review pathophysiology, classification, and treatment of thoracolumbar burst fractures.

Unique to this region is also the transition from a spinal cord and the conus medullaris (upper motor neuron) to the cauda equina (lower motor neuron). The conus medullaris usually starts at T11 and ends around the L1 to L2 disc space. When it extends lower into the lumbar spine, it is often associated with a hypertrophic filum terminale and tethering of the spinal cord. In traumatic situations, the level of the injury and its localization with respect to the level of conus medullaris determines the degree of neurologic damage. As an example, a severe burst fracture at T12 might have elements of upper motor cord level injury (bowel and bladder dysfunction) and lower motor neuron pathology (lumbar radicular pain and weakness). The space available for the cord changes from its narrowest region in the midthoracic spine to an increased width in the lumbar region where the composition of the cauda equina made of peripheral nerves are more resilient to injuries.

Burst Fractures in Thoracolumbar Fracture Classifications

In 1943, Watson-Jones[3] first described the comminuted wedge fracture, which would today be called a burst fracture, and highlighted the role of the integrity of the posterior ligamentous complex (PLC) in spinal stability. By the end of that same decade, Nicoll's classification of thoracolumbar spine trauma further described the morphology of fractures based on a review of injuries sustained by coal miners.[4] It defined stability using an anatomic classification based on four specific structures: the vertebral body; the disc; the intervertebral joints; and most important, the interspinous ligaments (ISLs). It was not until 1970 that Holdsworth.[5] semantically distinguished "wedge compression fractures" from "compression burst fractures," but in his classifications, both fracture types were stable.

By the 1980s, the term *burst fracture* was defined in Denis' classification as one of the four main categories of thoracolumbar injuries.[6,7] His classification divides the spine into three columns with an emphasis on the middle column, which comprises the posterior vertebral body, posterior disc, and posterior longitudinal ligament. Mechanical instability was defined when two of the three columns were disrupted; therefore, all burst fractures were considered unstable according to this scheme. Denis' classification also defined neurologic instability when a neurologic deficit occurred in the setting of a spinal fracture.

The evolution in describing burst fractures is highlighted by the difficulty so many authors had in assessing its stability, which ultimately should guide treatment. Therefore, based on 100 computed tomography (CT) examinations of thoracolumbar injuries, McAfee and colleagues[8] further classified them into six categories, including distinct categories for stable and unstable burst fractures. That classification emphasized the role of the PLC (including the facet joints) as a major factor in fracture stability.

McCormack and colleagues have described the load-sharing classification for burst fractures. It is theorized and proven practically that the vertebral bodies' ability to share load depends on the degree of comminution. In this system, the degree of comminution, fracture fragment displacement, and deformity are each graded 0 to 3 points and summed. Higher scores indicate greater instability and a greater likelihood of failure of short segment fixation. The system has been shown to have good interobserver and intraobserver reliability.[9] In an effort to guide management, the Spine Trauma Study Group developed the Thoracolumbar Injury Classification and Severity Score (TLICS; Table 35B-1),[10] which considers burst fractures as an intermediate severity fracture pattern based on radiographic appearance. Surgical recommendations for burst fracture are then guided by both neurologic status and the integrity of the PLC as many classifications have suggested in the past for burst fracture. That classification has demonstrated good intrarater and interrater reliability[11] and validity[11,12] and will therefore be the basis for the treatment of thoracolumbar fractures in this chapter.

TABLE 35B-1 *THORACOLUMBAR INJURY CLASSIFICATION AND SEVERITY SCORE**

Injury Characteristic	Qualifier	Score
Injury Morphology		
Compression	— Burst	1 +1
Rotation and translation	—	3
Distraction	—	4
Neurologic Status		
Intact	—	0
Nerve root	—	2
Spinal cord, conus medullaris	Incomplete Complete	3 2
Cauda equina	—	3
Posterior Ligamentous Complex Integrity		
Intact	—	0
Suspected or indeterminate	—	2
Disrupted	—	3

*Score <4 degrees, nonsurgical; 4 degrees, nonsurgical or surgical; and >4, surgical.
PLC, Posterior ligamentous complex.

Radiologic Findings of the Burst Fractures

Radiographic findings of a burst fracture on an anterior-posterior (AP) radiograph or coronal CT reconstruction are an increase in the interpedicular distance compared with the level above or below and a decrease in vertebral height. On the lateral radiograph or sagittal CT scan, findings can include a decrease in vertebral height, lack of definition of the contour of the cortices of the vertebral body with retropulsion of the posterior cortex into the spinal canal, local kyphosis around the fractured vertebra, and an increase in the interspinous distance (Fig. 35B-1, *A*). An increase in the interspinous distance should increase the level of suspicion for disruption of the PLC. Comparing this interspinous distance between supine and upright images may identify a functionally incompetent PLC. CT scans are used to further detail the fracture pattern and assess instability (widening of the facet joint) and canal compromise at the level of injury (Fig. 35B-1, *B*).

The Posterior Ligamentous Complex

As originally defined by Holdsworth,[5] the PLC is generally defined by five components at the level involved: the supraspinous ligament (SSL) and ISL, the ligamentum flavum (LF), and the right and left facet capsules.[13] Vacarro and colleagues.[14] also added the thoracolumbar fascia as part of the PLC. Determination of PLC integrity, however, remains a topic of controversy despite its central role in management determination.

Physical examination may help in the assessment of the integrity of the PLC. Severity of pain, on palpation of the spinous processes, presence of hematoma, or identification of gaps between them are indicators of disruption of the PLC. Further simple logrolling and assessing pain response can help measure stability of the fracture.

Radiologic imaging has proven helpful but, unfortunately, not definitive in all cases. Vacarro and members for the Spine Trauma Study Group[15] extracted 12 criteria considered important to evaluate PLC disruption on magnetic resonance imaging (MRI) from the published English literature since 1949. Those criteria were posterior edema on short tau inversion recovery (STIR) MRIs; disrupted PLC components (i.e., LF, ISL, or SSL) on MRI; focal kyphosis without vertebral body injury; interspinous spacing greater than that of the level above or below on an AP plain radiograph; palpable interspinous defect on examination; focal posterior tenderness on examination; diastasis of the facet joints on radiograph, MRI, or CT; avulsion fracture off the superior or inferior aspect of contiguous spinous processes; history of the injury mechanism; more than 50% compression of the anterior vertebral body on lateral plain radiographs without fracture of the posterior wall on CT scan; and vertebral translation (Fig. 35B-2). Twenty-eight surgeons returned the survey, and more than half ranked "vertebral body translation" as the most important factor followed by increased interspinous spacing and diastasis of the facet. Although Denis and the Arbeitsgemeinschaft für Osteosynthesefragen (AO) classification rely mainly on bony morphology from radiographs and CT scans, the emphasis on the role of the PLC to spinal instability has led to the

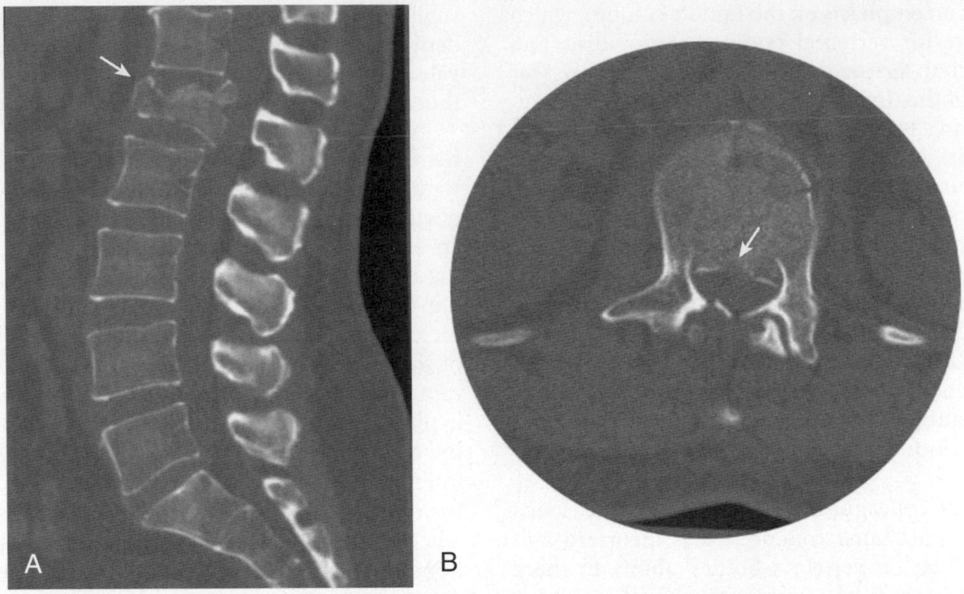

Figure 35B-1. Lateral (**A**) and anterior-posterior (**B**) plain radiograph views of the lumbar spine showing an L1 burst fracture *(small arrow)* with retropulsion of bone into the spinal canal *(large arrow).*

inclusion of MRI as part of spinal fracture evaluation. MRI was often considered a critical modality to evaluate PLC integrity.[16,17] In that study, disrupted PLC components (i.e., LF, ISL, or SSL; "black stripe") on T1-weighted sagittal MRI was the fourth most important factor in evaluating PLC disruption. However, MRI findings should be considered with caution. Vaccaro and colleagues[14] have highlighted low-specificity values for detecting ISL and SSL injuries on MRI, suggesting a large proportion of false-positive injuries on MRI compared to preoperative surgical findings. Thus, despite the central role of PLC integrity in the evaluation and decision making for thoracolumbar spine injuries as suggested by the TLICS, there remain few strict criteria or clear definition in defining a PLC injury, and the exact prognosis associated with PLC injuries related to radiographic, neurologic, and patient-reported outcomes has yet to be defined.[15]

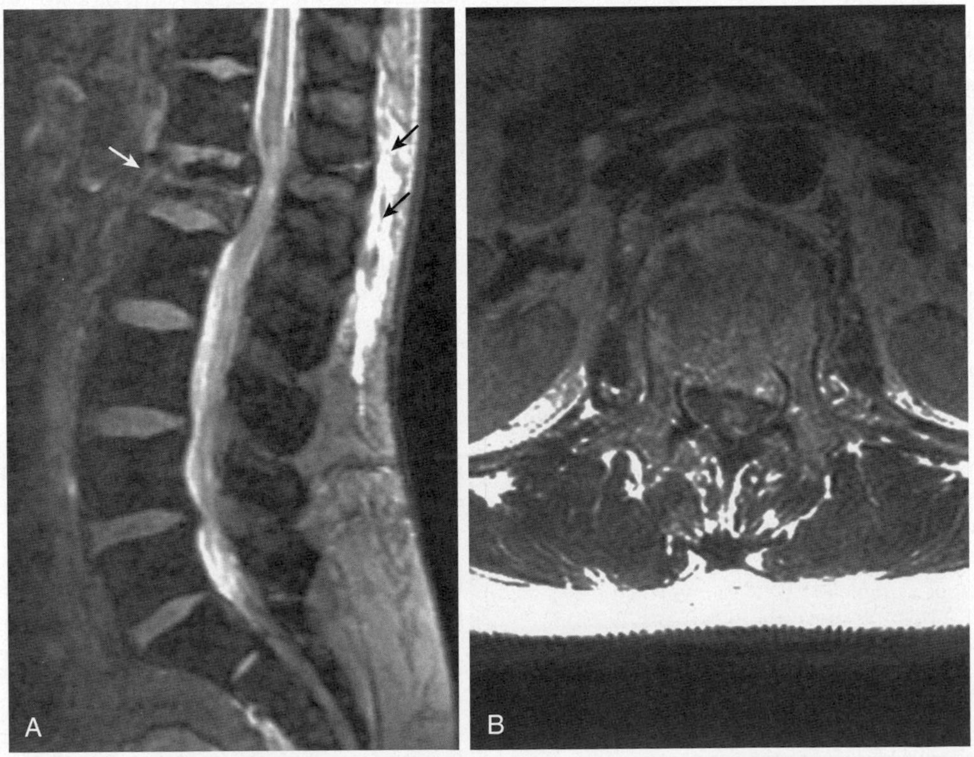

Figure 35B-2. Sagittal (**A**) and axial (**B**) T2-weighted magnetic resonance imaging views of the lumbar spine showing the L1 burst fracture *(white arrow)* with compression of the spinal cord at the same level with surrounding regions of increased signal intensity corresponding to the surrounding edema *(black arrows).* The degree of the canal narrowing can readily be seen on the axial image on the *right*.

TREATMENT

Nonoperative Treatment

Indication

In a stable burst fracture (without significant PLC disruption) and absence of a neurologic deficit, nonoperative treatment is the treatment of choice. In a randomized controlled trial (RCT) of 47 consecutive patients with stable burst fractures without neurologic deficit, Wood and colleagues[2] found no major long-term advantage when comparing operative treatment with nonoperative treatment based on radiographic criteria, Short Form 36 (SF-36), and Owestry questionnaires, but more frequent complications and greater cost were found in the operative group. Those findings were not reproduced in a later RCT with 34 patients; Siebenga and colleagues[18] found that for stable burst fracture without neurologic deficit, short segment stabilization provided less kyphotic deformity, better functional outcomes, and higher return to original work than in the nonoperative group. They concluded that in addition to fracture stability and neurologic findings, treatment should also take into consideration the amount of deformity and patient preference with respect to complication risks (Fig. 35B-3).

Bracing

Traditionally, stable thoracolumbar burst fractures have been treated with a custom thoracolumbar spinal orthosis (TLSO) or a hyperextension brace such as a Jewett brace. Thoracic burst fractures from T5 to T10 may be treated similarly. Upper thoracic burst fractures from T1 to T5 are treated with a TLSO with neck extension.

The use of bracing may not always be necessary, however. Two recent RCTs compared bracing with no bracing in patients with stable burst fractures at the thoracolumbar junction.[19,20] These studies found that bracing had no effect on pain, radiologic results, or functional outcome.[19,20] In our opinion, bracing is still considered for lower lumbar fractures (rigid lumbosacral orthosis [LSO]), stable thoracolumbar fractures with intractable pain or concern for patient compliance (rigid TLSO), and a lower thoracic fracture at risk of kyphosis (orthosis with upper trunk support such as a Jewett brace or a rigid TLSO with neck extension).

Activity

When the patient is able to stand, an upright radiograph should be taken to ensure that upright loading at the fracture site does not produce an increased deformity. When conservative treatment is chosen, ambulation should be initiated as early as possible to avoid complications associated with bed rest (deep venous thrombosis leading to pulmonary embolism, pneumonia, or decubitus ulcers). In the first 3 to 6 months, activity with risks (manual labor, prolonged seating, impact sports, bending or heavy lifting) should be avoided. A progressive increase in activity with the above restrictions is allowed with close follow-up at 1, 4, 8, and 12 weeks. Patients are warned to seek attention if there is the development of weakness or numbness or changes in bowel or bladder function. During follow-up visits, close attention is paid to the deformity at the fracture site. If there is an increase in the deformity (kyphosis >30 degrees or scoliosis >10 degrees), intractable pain or neurologic symptoms, surgery may be considered. When there is radiographic evidence of fracture

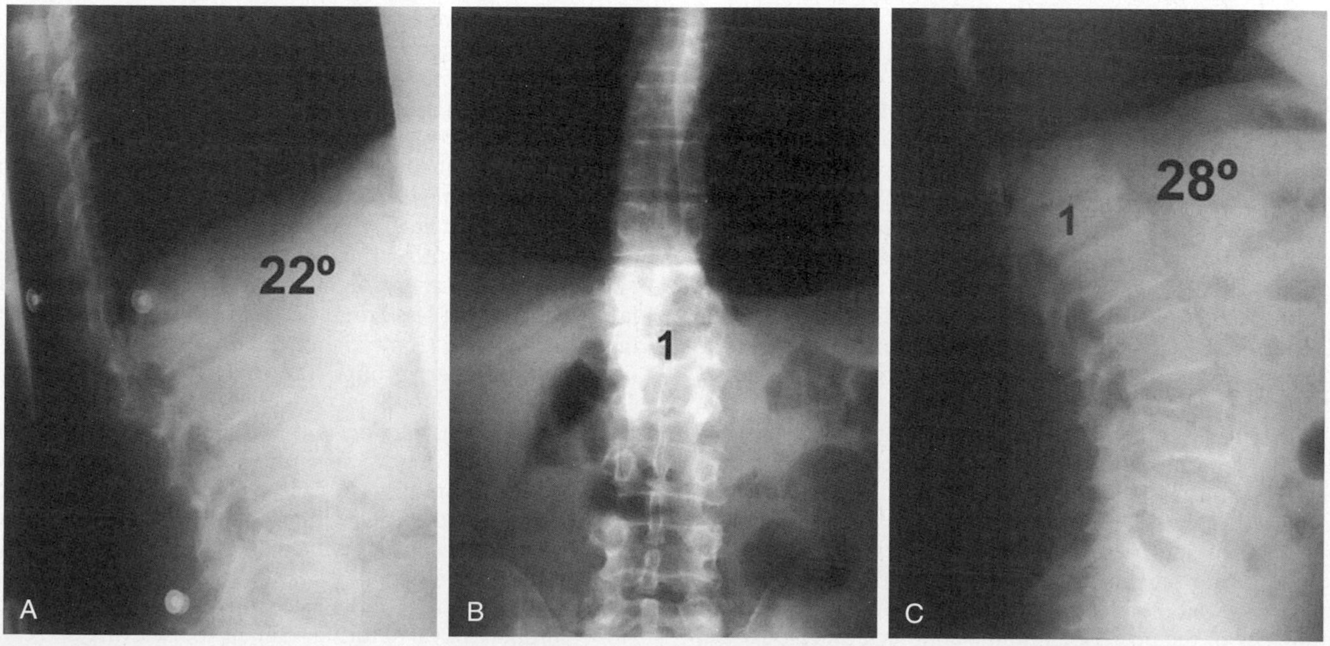

Figure 35B-3. Lateral and anterior-posterior (AP) plain radiographs of the thoracolumbar spine of a patient with an L1 burst fracture, which was treated nonoperatively with a thoracolumbar orthosis. **A,** Lateral plain radiograph made with patient in a thoracolumbar orthosis at the time of discharge from the hospital, demonstrating a 22-degree kyphosis. **B** and **C,** AP and lateral views, respectively, of the same patient taken 36 months after the injury, demonstrating progression of the deformity to 28 degrees of local kyphosis. *(Figure reproduced with permission from Wood K, Buttermann G, Butterman G, et al: Operative compared with nonoperative treatment of a thoracolumbar burst fracture without neurological deficit. A prospective, randomized study, J Bone Joint Surg Am 85(5):773–781, 2003.)*

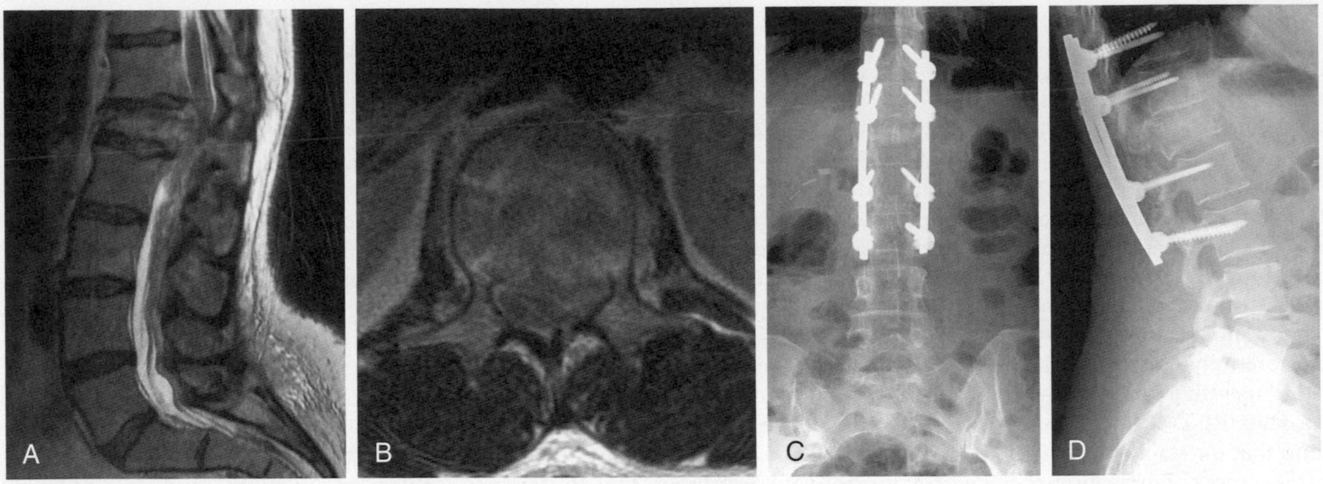

Figure 35B-4. Sagittal (**A**) and axial (**B**) views of the T2-weighted magnetic resonance image of a 51-year-old woman who fell after completing a ski jump and sustained a severe burst fracture of L1 with disruption of both endplates, 20 degrees of local kyphosis, and 65% canal compromise caused by bony retropulsion. She was neurologically intact. Postoperative anterior-posterior (**C**) and lateral (**D**) radiographs show restoration of sagittal alignment with fixation and posterolateral fusion from T11 to L3.

healing, flexion and extension radiographs are taken to exclude motion at the fracture site.

Geriatric Considerations

Senile fractures from osteoporosis in elderly patients should also be closely monitored with frequent radiologic examinations in the first month because they are at higher risk of kyphosis deformity leading to neurologic compromise. Patients and family members should be warned to watch neurologic function closely. Assessment of osteoporosis is recommended to limit further fractures (particularly the spine, hip, wrist, and shoulder) and pharmacologic treatment is implemented if needed.

Surgical Treatment of Burst Fractures

Surgical Indication

Surgical treatment of thoracolumbar burst fractures is indicated when there is evidence or risk of neurologic worsening or stability compromise. For this reason, the TLICS uses neurologic status and two factors influencing stability (injury morphology and PLC integrity) as components influencing surgical decision. The approach and surgical technique to use should take into consideration three main criteria:

1. The fracture pattern
2. The ability to decompress neural elements (based on fracture pattern and age of the fracture)
3. The presence of PLC lesions

Other indications for surgical treatment are when associated with multiple injuries or in those who cannot be managed with an orthosis such as very obese individuals.

Burst fractures can be treated with an anterior, posterior, or combined approach for decompression and instrumentation. Posterior spinal instrumentation at the thoracolumbar junction is well established and has its advantages, including familiarity of the posterior midline approach; the lack of pulmonary, visceral, and vascular structures; and the ability to relatively safely reexplore the surgical site if necessary. In most acute cases, decompression and stabilization can be achieved from a posterior approach with limited associated comorbidities (Fig. 35B-4). Posterior instrumentation also permits stabilization of the posterior elements when the PLC is torn. Limitations of the posterior approach are that the decompression is indirect (usually achieved from reduction of bony fragments by tension of the posterior longitudinal ligament and ligamentotaxis) or, alternatively, by the need to mobilize the dural sac to achieve proper decompression. Further hardware failure and reoperations are common, especially when the vertebral bodies have more severe injury and comminution.

In the past, fusion was routinely performed in conjunction with posterior instrumentation for burst fractures. Fusion-less fracture care has the advantage of minimizing stiffening of spinal segments while still providing stabilizing forces while the fracture heals. This can be performed using an open or minimally invasive technique. In most cases, hardware is removed 9 to 12 months later. Dai and colleagues reported the results of a randomized trial comparing fusion with no fusion after instrumentation for thoracolumbar burst fractures.[21] At 5 to 7 years of follow-up, they found no difference in clinical and radiologic outcomes between the two groups. Tian and colleagues performed a meta-analysis of four studies comparing fusion with no fusion.[22] The fusion-less group had shorter operative times, but no difference in clinical results or complications were present between groups. Radiologic results favored the fusion-less group that had less postoperative vertebral height loss. Complications and hardware failure were not different between groups. The topic is discussed further in Chapter 35E.

Anterior reconstruction with instrumentation can overcome some of the limitations of the posterior approach when direct visual decompression can be achieved, particularly in the case of subacute or chronic fracture in which the bony fragments can only be mobilized with difficulty. Also, the anterior approach allows application of a large distractive force to be applied, restoration of the mechanical integrity of the anterior column, removal of torn or damaged discs, direct decompression of the spinal canal, potential avoidance of iliac crest harvesting, and frequently fusion of fewer levels of the spine.

The combined anterior approach is often indicated for the more severe fractures with neurologic deficits. If a posterior fusion did not result in complete decompression then an anterior decompression should be considered. Similarly, if adequate stability was not achieved after posterior instrumentation and patients are at risk or are developing kyphosis, then anterior reconstruction should be considered. For highly unstable burst fractures treated initially anteriorly, posterior instrumentation should be considered.

In a neurologically intact patient with burst fractures, anterior or posterior approaches have proven to be equivalent for radiographic and patient-reported functional outcomes in a series by Wood and colleagues.[23] Similar results were found in an RCT from Lin and colleagues[24] for burst fractures with neurologic deficit in which radiologic and motor score improvement did not show any significant difference between the two approaches. However, different rates of complications were reported in the two RCTs. Wood and colleagues[23] found that the anterior approach had fewer complications and reoperation; in their series, 17 complications were seen in their posterior group with hardware removal of painful instrumentation in nearly one-third of those patients. To the contrary, Lin and colleagues[24] have suggested that posterior approach would lead to less blood loss, shorter operative times, and better pulmonary function postoperatively.

Currently, there is limited consensus about the effect of timing of surgery on neurologic recovery. Clinical judgment should be taken into consideration, and, in general, spinal care should be handled after the treatment of life- and limb-threatening injuries.

The Anterior Thoracolumbar Approach with Corpectomy and Instrumentation

SURGICAL INDICATION, ADVANTAGES, AND LIMITATIONS. The anterior thoracolumbar retroperitoneal approach is most commonly indicated for burst fractures between T10 and L3, which can also benefit from direct anterior decompression. Other indications include a large retropulsed fragment with marked canal compromise (>50%) and incomplete neurologic deficit and anterior comminution and kyphosis less than 30 degrees requiring additional anterior column support. After a posterior stabilization, an anterior approach should be considered when there is suboptimal neural recovery resulting from inadequate canal (Fig. 35B-5).

The main advantages of the anterior thoracolumbar approach are the possibility to directly visualize the fracture, directly decompress the spinal cord from the side of the pathology, and reconstruct the anterior column. This reconstruction is thought to allow a better correction of the kyphotic deformity than posterior approach.[25] The main limitation of this approach is that it only addresses the ventral or compression side of the spine. Therefore, an additional posterior approach may be required for stabilization in cases in which the PLC and its tension band effect are lost.

For burst fractures of T10 and above, anterior decompression and fusion are performed using a transthoracic approach usually from the right side. A video-assisted transthoracic (VATS) approach may minimize pulmonary injury but is technically demanding and application of instrumentation is challenging.

SURGICAL TECHNIQUE: ANTERIOR

POSITIONING. For fractures below T12, a left-sided approach with the patient positioned in a right lateral decubitus position is preferred to avoid retraction of the liver and damage to the frail vena cava. Patients are positioned in a lateral decubitus position (Fig. 35B-6). After the patient is positioned, attention is given to check all pressure points, particularly the brachial plexus, under an axillary roll. The elbows and knees are protected with gel pads to protect the ulnar and common peroneal nerves, respectively. The patient might be positioned with the thorax and abdomen leaning slightly forward to allow abdominal contents to fall forward during the exposure. Some surgeons prefer straight lateral positioning to maintain orientation of the vertebral body during the instrumentation. To improve exposure, the fracture level can be placed over the table break and, depending on fracture stability and neurologic involvement, the table can be broken to raise the vertebra of concern into the operative field. At the time of fixation, it is necessary to level the table to avoid the introduction of scoliosis deformity.

For lower thoracic injuries, a transthoracic approach is used. Intubation is performed with a double-lumen tube that allows deflation of the right lung during surgery. The patient is positioned in the left lateral decubitus position with the right side up (Fig. 35B-6, *B*). Similar precautions to protect neurovascular structures are carried out as described earlier.

LANDMARK, INCISION, AND APPROACH. The incision is based on the vertebra affected. Given the cephalocaudal direction of the ribs, the incision should be made on the rib one to two levels above the region of interest. For example, to treat a L1 burst fracture, the incision should be centered on the 11th or 12th rib. The incision follows the ribs on its whole length. After skin incision, the abdominal muscle layers are transected in line with the rib in the following order from posterior to anterior: latissimus dorsi and external oblique; serratus posterior inferior and internal oblique, transversus abdominis, sacrospinalis, and multifidus.

The rib is then dissected subperiosteally, and particular care is given to use an elevator circumferentially, particularly to avoid damage to the subcostal neurovascular bundle. The rib is cut anteriorly at the cartilaginous junction and posteriorly close to the rib head. A self-retaining retractor is then placed. When the 12th rib is excised, its tip is at the junction of the transversalis fascia, pleura, and diaphragm, which facilitates the identification of the retroperitoneal space and dissection of the pleura, which is reflected upward while the quadratus lumborum is retracted downward. Above the 12th rib, the pleural space is accessed through a small incision, which is extended in line with the incision while protecting the underlying structures.

When necessary, the diaphragm is detached from its insertion above the arcuate ligament, leaving 2 cm of the periphery to aid repair at closure. To facilitate closure, it is recommended to leave suture tags of different colors along the diaphragm incision.

In the retroperitoneal space, the peritoneum, retroperitoneal fat, and kidneys are reflected anteriorly to expose the quadratus lumborum and the psoas muscle overlying the vertebral bodies. A malleable retractor can be used to protect and maintain the viscera anteriorly. The psoas is dissected from anterior to posterior of the lateral aspect of the vertebral body until the base of the pedicle is palpated and the ventral neural foramen exposed. In the case of a transthoracic decompression, after the rib is removed, the pleura is opened, and the lateral aspect of the vertebral bodies is exposed. The right lung can then be deflated.

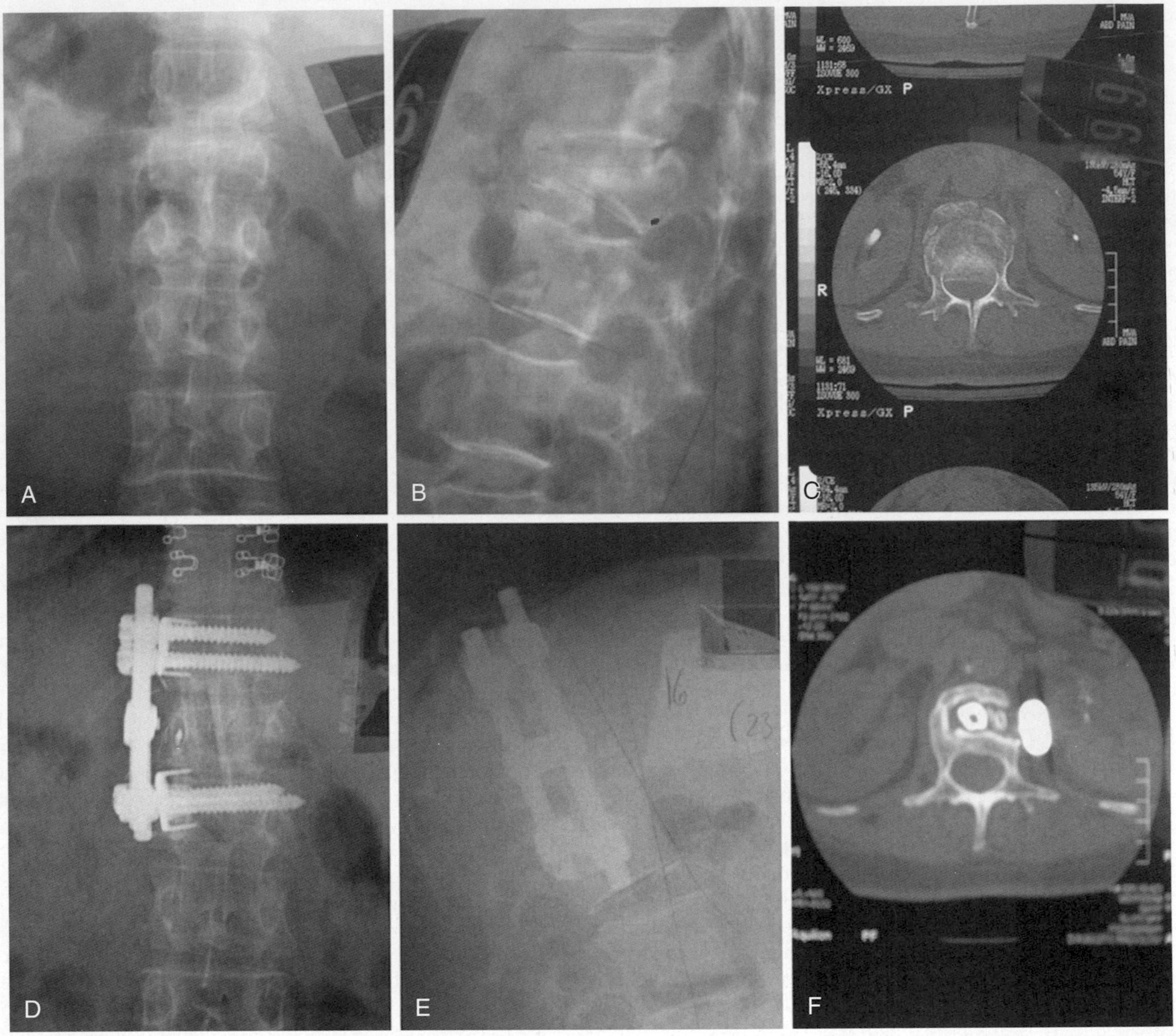

Figure 35B-5. Anterior-posterior (AP) (**A**) and lateral (**B**) plain radiographs of a 54-year-old woman who was involved in a roll-over motor vehicle accident with a sustained burst fracture at L1. Axial computed tomography (CT) reconstruction (**C**) shows the appearance of the burst fracture with bone retropulsion resulting in 55% canal occlusion. The *bottom row* shows the postoperative appearance of the injury: AP (**D**) and lateral (**E**) plain radiographs of the lumbar spine taken 2 years after the surgical stabilization show maintenance of correction. Axial CT reconstruction (**F**) at 2 years after surgery shows only modest 5% residual canal occlusion. *(Reproduced with permission from Wood KB, Bohn D, Mehbod A: Anterior versus posterior treatment of stable thoracolumbar burst fractures without neurologic deficit: a prospective, randomized study, J Spinal Disord Tech 18(suppl):S15–S23, 2005, Fig. 1, A-F.)*

The fractured vertebral body is then localized based on the surrounding hematoma and the deformity and confirmed by an intraoperative radiograph (Fig. 35B-6, *C*). Upon confirmation of the adequate level, the fractured and adjacent levels are exposed by releasing the overlying pleura followed by isolation and ligation of the segmental arteries, which allows the great vessels to be mobilized and facilitates a safe approach to the contralateral side if needed.

Corpectomy and Decompression. After adequate exposure is completed, discectomies are performed between the vertebra of interest and the adjacent levels (Fig. 35B-6, *D*). The corpectomy can be started using the pedicle as a guide for the posterior margin and the depth of the discectomy for the contralateral border. Using osteotomes or chisels, the middle and anterior vertebral body is resected about 1 cm anterior to the pedicle base (Fig. 35B-6, *E*). The bone from the corpectomy is kept for bone grafting. After an adequate corpectomy is achieved to the contralateral wall and pedicle, decompression of the dural space is performed. The posterior wall is first thinned using a high-speed diamond burr and curettes and Kerrison rongeurs then complete the decompression which should span between the disc spaces and from ipsilateral pedicles to contralateral pedicles (Figs. 35B-6, *F* to *H*).

Instrumentation and Fixation. After the corpectomy, the overall alignment is checked and reduction maneuvers applied as needed with manipulation of the spine from external pressure or distraction within the corpectomy site applied with a laminar spreader or using an expandable cage mechanism. Alternatively, the instrumentation can be used as sites for distractors to regain lordosis and vertebral height (Fig. 35B-7, *A* and *B*). Tricorticate iliac crest, allograft femurs or humeri, titanium mesh cage, and expandable cages are possible options to provide anterior support or fusion. When using cages, vertebral corpectomy bone graft is placed in the cage while structural bone graft from rib resections can be used to bridge both endplates longitudinally. Superior and inferior endplates are prepared using a curette or a burr to promote bleeding and vascular supply to the graft, but attention should be taken not to compromise the mechanical support of the endplates, which can lead to graft impaction and kyphosis. Additional support with internal fixation can be provided with transvertebral screws and rods or plates (Fig. 35B-7, *C* to *F*). Screws are placed laterally toward the contralateral side with care to not injure the visceral and vascular structure. The endplates and vertebrae posterior walls are used as guides for screw orientation. Precise measurement of the screw length when the opposite cortex is breached with the ball-tip probe is essential. Upon placement of one or two screws in each of the adjacent vertebrae, one or two rods or a plate is placed and gentle compression can be applied to secure the anterior graft or cage in place.

Closure and Postoperative Course. Before closure, thorough hemostasis is ensured and, if possible, the pleura is repaired over the hardware. A chest tube is placed under direct visualization and the diaphragm os closed following the suture stitches left upon opening. The abdominal musculature is closed in multiple layers.

Postoperative clinical and radiographic monitoring of the chest guide the timing of the removal of the chest tube when there is no evidence of pneumothorax and when drainage has subsided. Postoperative ileus is common and a nasogastric tube is placed as needed.

Postoperatively, a thoracolumbar orthosis may be used up to 12 weeks. Its use is at the surgeon's discretion depending on the level of instability, bone quality, the addition of posterior fixation, and patient compliance. Standing radiographs of the thoracolumbar spine are taken when the patient is able to stand to ensure construct integrity under physiologic loads. Ambulation is initiated postoperatively as early as possible, but physical therapy typically begins months after surgery when a successful fusion seems likely.

Complications from Anterior Thoracolumbar Approach. Complications can be grouped into three categories, surgical approach, decompression, and structural integrity.[26,27]

Early complications related to the approach include pneumothorax, atelectasis, pneumonia, ileus, infection, nerve injury (particularly genitofemoral nerve and nerve root from the lumbar plexus), and visceral and vascular lesions. During decompression, particular care must be taken not to injure the dural sac. If a spinal fluid leak is noted from iatrogenic manipulation or secondary to the trauma, early repair should be attempted. If this fails, cerebrospinal fluid (CSF) drainage via a lumbar drain is recommended. In thoracic cases, the negative pleural pressure keeps CSF leaks from sealing; therefore, lumbar drainage should be considered.

Late complications include incisional hernia. Other late complications are related to disruption of the structural integrity of the construct from bone and bone–instrument failure or pseudarthrosis, which have both been described

Text continued on p. 932

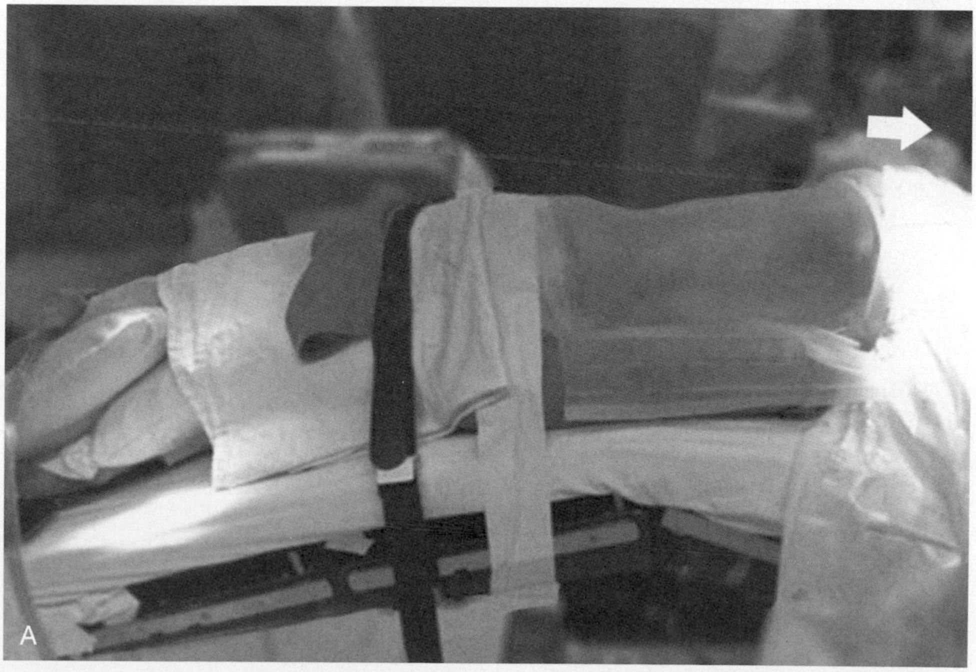

Figure 35B-6. A, Positioning of the patient for the anterolateral approach. The *arrow* points toward the head of the patient. The patient is positioned on the right side, and the left side is exposed and prepared for the approach. This allows the surgeon to avoid damaging the liver during the approach to the spine. Technique of anterior transthoracic corpectomy and fusion.

Continued

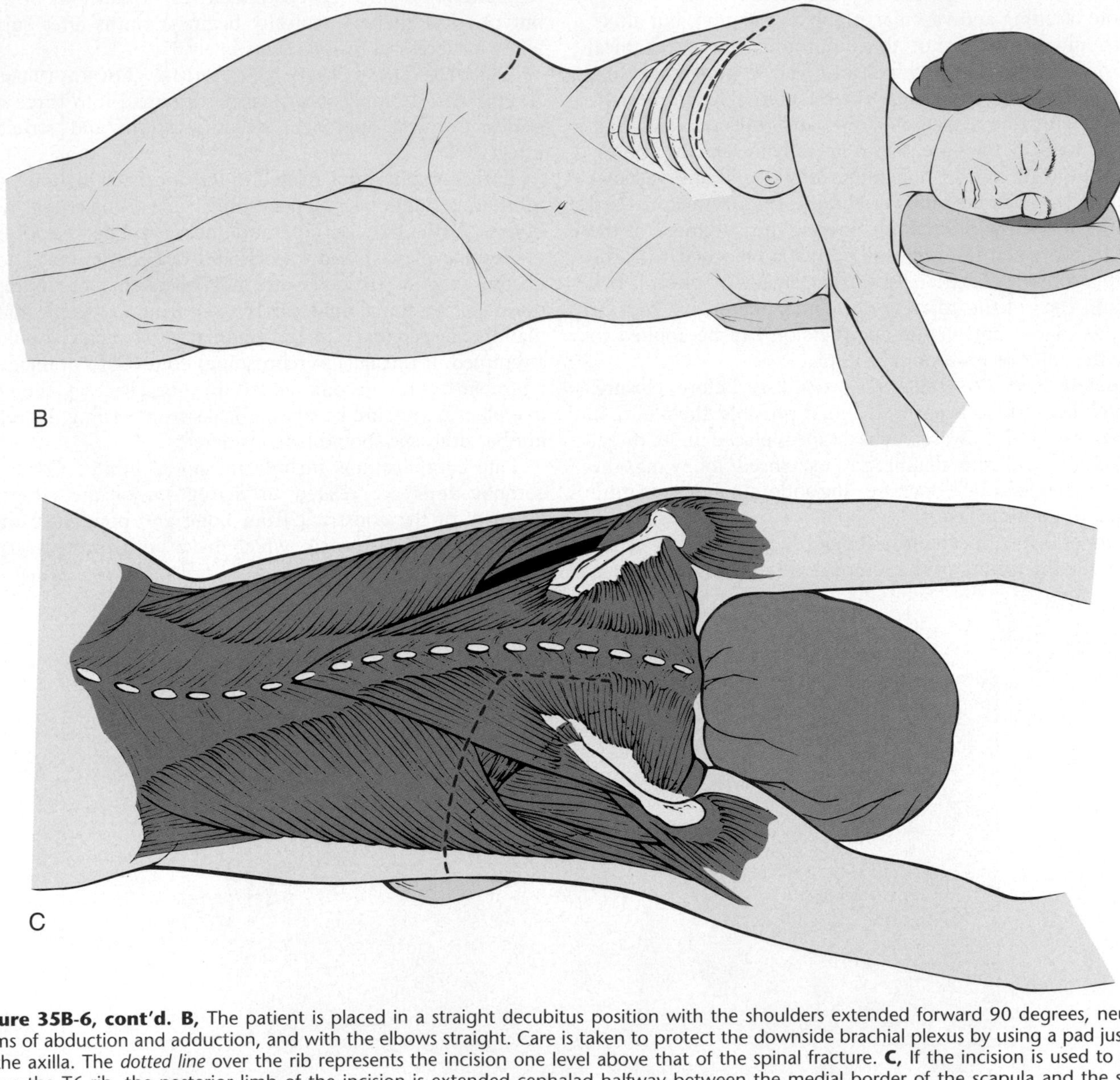

Figure 35B-6, cont'd. B, The patient is placed in a straight decubitus position with the shoulders extended forward 90 degrees, neutral in terms of abduction and adduction, and with the elbows straight. Care is taken to protect the downside brachial plexus by using a pad just distal to the axilla. The *dotted line* over the rib represents the incision one level above that of the spinal fracture. **C,** If the incision is used to expose above the T6 rib, the posterior limb of the incision is extended cephalad halfway between the medial border of the scapula and the spinous processes. All of the intervening muscles down to the chest wall are divided and tagged for later repair.

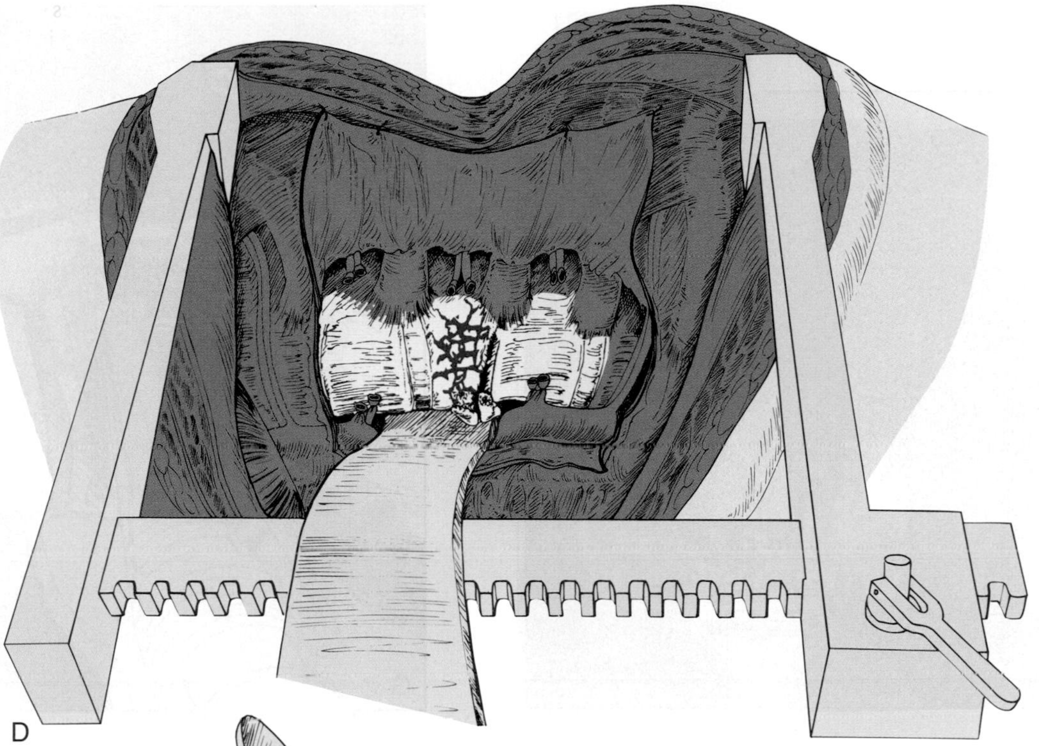

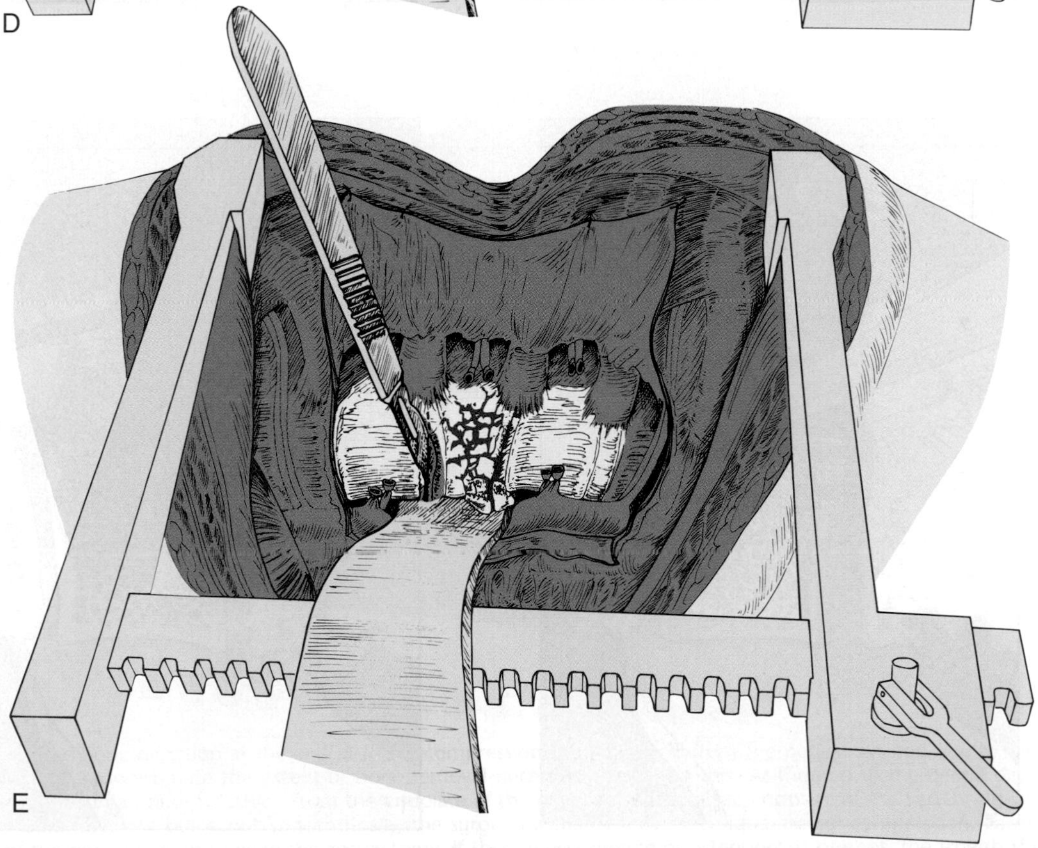

Figure 35B-6, cont'd. D, After the thoracic cavity has been entered, the self-retaining chest retractor is inserted. The parietal pleura is incised halfway between the anterior great vessels and the posterior neural foramina, and the segmental vessels are ligated at this same level. The vertebra to be excised as well as one vertebra above and one vertebra below are exposed. Extraperiosteal dissection provides the best plane. A malleable retractor is placed on the opposite side of the spine and connected to the self-retaining chest retractor with a clamp. This malleable retractor serves to protect the great vessels during the vertebral corpectomy. **E,** A scalpel and rongeur are used to remove the discs above and below the level of the vertebral fracture. *Continued*

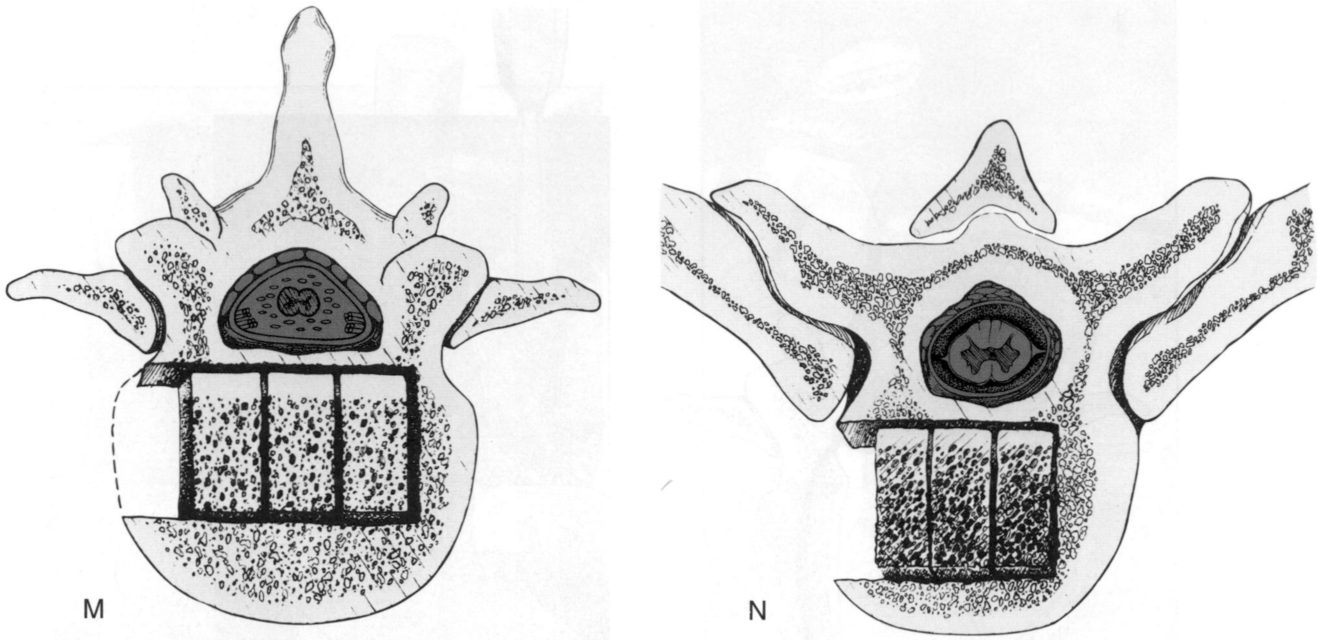

Figure 35B-6, cont'd

between 5% and 10%. The frequency of those complications has lessened over the years with the evolution of modern rigid spinal instrumentation, including addition of fixation to the corpectomy graft.

SURGICAL TECHNIQUE: POSTERIOR

The technique of posterior instrumentation for burst fractures is described in Chapter 35C.

OUTCOME

Nonoperative Treatment versus Operative Treatment for Thoracolumbar Fractures without Neurologic Deficit

In the thoracolumbar burst fractures without neurologic deficit, a meta-analysis from Gnanenthiran and colleagues[28] retrieved four major trials[2,18,29,30] for a total of 79 randomized patients (41 with operative treatment and 38 with nonoperative) with a mean follow-up time from 24 to 118 months. No differences in pain, Roland Morris Disability Questionnaires scores, or return to work rates were present between operative and nonoperative groups. At approximately 4 years, the operative group had an improvement in kyphosis from baseline by 1.8 degrees with a mean of 11 degrees, as opposed to a kyphosis of 16 degrees with a worsening of 3.3 degrees in the nonoperative group. Although the amount of correction was significantly different between the treatments, the final degree of kyphosis was not. Operative treatment was also associated with higher complication rates and costs. There was also no association found between kyphosis and pain. Return to work rate were 67% for the nonoperative group compared with 70% in the operative group, a statistically insignificant difference.

Comparison of Anterior and Posterior Approach

Wood and colleagues[23] conducted a prospective randomized study comparing anterior versus posterior treatment of stable thoracolumbar burst fractures without neurologic deficit or loss of structural integrity of the PLC. Thirty-eight patients had a minimum 2-year follow-up, 18 had posterior spine fusion and 20 had an anterior approach. Although lengths of hospital stay and operating times were similar, blood loss was higher in the anterior group, but significantly more adverse events (instrumentation removal, wound dehiscence, instrumentation, or bone failure) were observed in the posterior group. Clinical results between the two groups were similar and demonstrated good pain reduction based on visual analog scale (VAS) scores, improvement in disability score (RMFDS) to 8.3 for posterior group and 8.9 for the anterior group, and ability to return to work after 6 months of 44% for the posterior group and 55% for the anterior group. The study concluded that anterior surgery might lower complications and prevent additional surgeries.

Lin and colleagues[24] also conducted a prospective randomized study comparing anterior versus posterior treatment of thoracolumbar burst fractures but included patients with neurologic deficits and unstable fracture patterns. A total of 64 patients were recruited and equally distributed in comparable group for baseline characteristics. At a minimum of 2-year follow-up, all patients achieved adequate solid fusion and significant neurologic improvement independent from the approach used. In that study, it was found that the posterior approach was associated with less blood loss, complications, shorter operative time, and better postoperative pulmonary function. Although it is often believed that an anterior approach provides a better decompression from direct visualization, this study demonstrated that the posterior approach provided as good a decompression and neurologic improvement while having fewer perioperative complications.

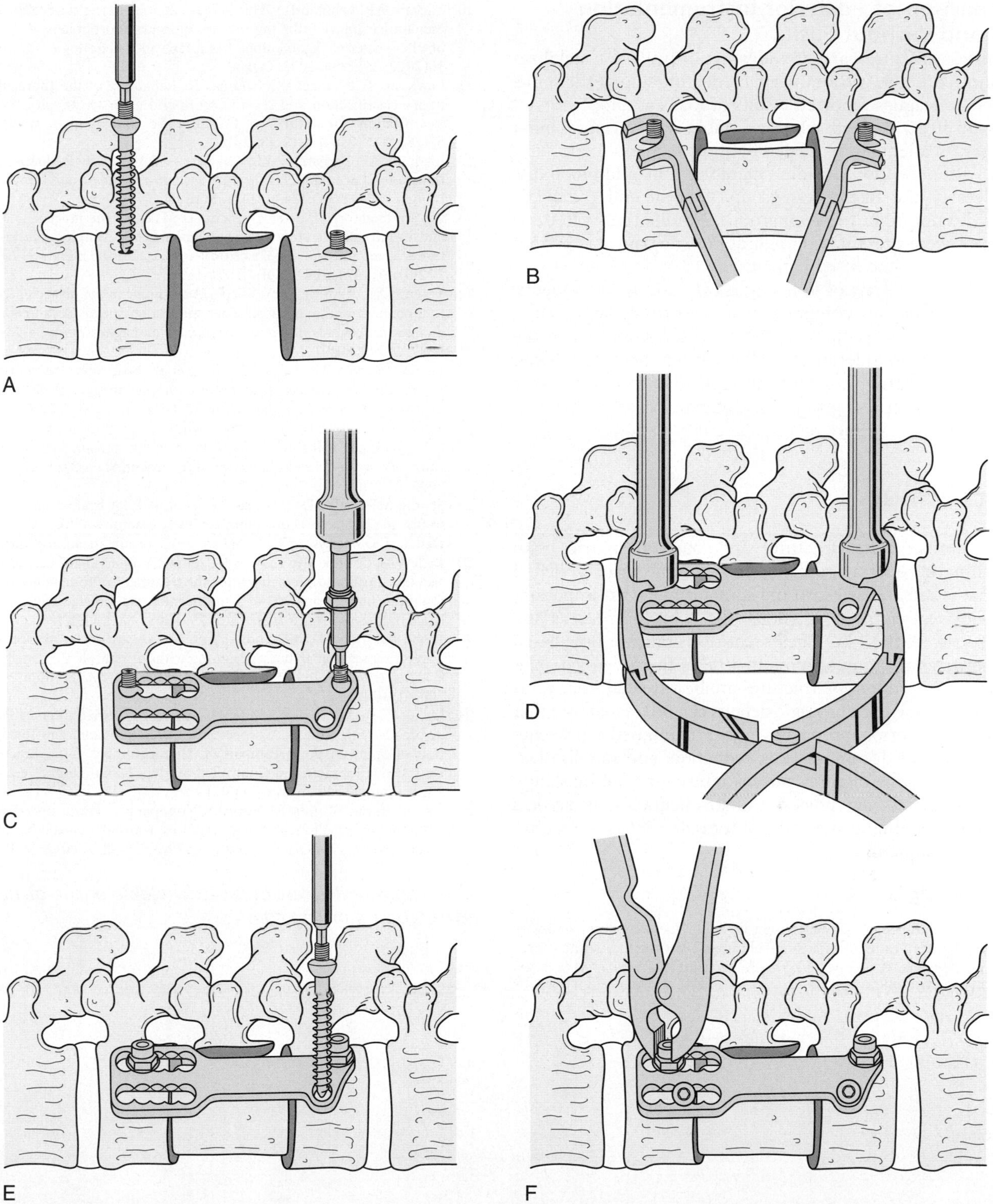

Figure 35B-7. Technique for anterior spinal instrumentation after corpectomy. **A,** After using a depth gauge directed on the exposed vertebral body, appropriately sized screw lengths are selected to engage the opposite cortex of the vertebral body. The bolts are placed parallel to the adjacent endplate to avoid intrusion into the disc space above and below the corpectomy site. **B,** Distraction is applied against the bolts, allowing easy insertion of the strut graft into the corpectomy site. **C,** Determination of proper length of plate via a template is important to avoid impingement of the superior or inferior disc space. Locking nuts are applied and provisionally tightened. **D,** Compressive forces are applied and locking nuts are tightened firmly. **E** and **F,** Finally, two anterior screws are placed, and the nuts are crimped down, preventing possible backing out or loosening. *(Redrawn with permission from Zdeblick TA: Z-Plate-ATL Anterior Fixation System: Surgical Technique. Sofamor Danek Group, Inc. All rights reserved.)*

Comparison of Posterior Instrumentation with and without Fusion

Fusion-less fracture care provides opportunity for stabilization and reduction without permanent stiffening of the spine. Dai and colleagues reported results of RCTs at 5 to 7 years of follow-up in 73 patients who had stable-type vertebral burst fractures.[21] Patients were treated by short segment instrumentation with or without fusion. Operating time and blood loss were less in the fusion-less group. Clinical and radiologic results did not differ between groups. No differences in complications were present, although donor site pain was present in two-thirds of the fused patients.

In a meta-analysis of four studies including 220 patients, Tian and colleagues compared fusion to fusion-less instrumentation for thoracolumbar burst fractures. Similar to the results by Dai, no difference at follow-up was present between groups.[22] Operating time and intraoperative blood loss were less in the fusion-less group. No differences were present in rates of hardware failure or surgical complications.

CONCLUSIONS

Thoracolumbar burst fractures are common injuries with the hallmark being a fragment from the posterior vertebral wall that is retropulsed into the spinal canal. Two important factors drive treatment decisions: the neurologic status and the integrity of the PLC. Treatment decisions are now based on a new classification scheme that takes these two variables into account. Stable-type fractures are best treated nonoperatively. Patients with neurologic deficits can be treated by either anterior or posterior approaches or even combined approaches with the goal of decompression, reduction, and stabilization. For other unstable fractures, posterior instrumentation should be performed. When posterior instrumentation is used, a fusion-less technique may be appropriate, but this requires further investigation.

KEY REFERENCES

2. Wood K, Buttermann G, Butterman G, et al: Operative compared with nonoperative treatment of a thoracolumbar burst fracture without neurological deficit. A prospective, randomized study. *J Bone Joint Surg Am* 85(5):773–781, 2003. LOE II
10. Vaccaro AR, Lehman RA, Hurlbert RJ, et al: A new classification of thoracolumbar injuries: the importance of injury morphology, the integrity of the posterior ligamentous complex, and neurologic status. *Spine* 30(20):2325–2333, 2005. LOE V
11. Lewkonia P, Paolucci EO, Thomas K: Reliability of the thoracolumbar injury classification and severity score and comparison with the Denis classification for injury to the thoracic and lumbar spine. *Spine* 37(26):2161–2167, 2012. LOE III
12. Joaquim AF, Fernandes YB, Cavalcante RAC, et al: Evaluation of the thoracolumbar injury classification system in thoracic and lumbar spinal trauma. *Spine* 36(1):33–36, 2011. LOE III
13. van Middendorp JJ, Patel AA, Schuetz M, et al: The precision, accuracy and validity of detecting posterior ligamentous complex injuries of the thoracic and lumbar spine: a critical appraisal of the literature. *Eur Spine J* 22(3):461–474, 2013. LOE III
14. Vaccaro AR, Rihn JA, Saravanja D, et al: Injury of the posterior ligamentous complex of the thoracolumbar spine: a prospective evaluation of the diagnostic accuracy of magnetic resonance imaging. *Spine* 34(23):E841–E847, 2009. LOE II
17. Lee JY, Vaccaro AR, Schweitzer KM, et al: Assessment of injury to the thoracolumbar posterior ligamentous complex in the setting of normal-appearing plain radiography. *Spine J* 7(4):422–427, 2007. LOE V
18. Siebenga J, Leferink VJM, Segers MJM, et al: Treatment of traumatic thoracolumbar spine fractures: a multicenter prospective randomized study of operative versus nonsurgical treatment. *Spine* 31(25):2881–2890, 2006. LOE II
19. Shamji MF, Roffey DM, Young DK, et al: A Pilot Evaluation of the Role of Bracing in Stable Thoracolumbar Burst Fractures Without Neurologic Deficit. *J Spinal Disord Tech* Aug 18, 2012. [Epub ahead of print]. LOE I
20. Bailey CS, Dvorak MF, Thomas KC, et al: Comparison of thoracolumbosacral orthosis and no orthosis for the treatment of thoracolumbar burst fractures: interim analysis of a multicenter randomized clinical equivalence trial. *J Neurosurg Spine* 11(3):295–303, 2009. LOE I
23. Wood KB, Bohn D, Mehbod A: Anterior versus posterior treatment of stable thoracolumbar burst fractures without neurologic deficit: a prospective, randomized study. *J Spinal Disord Tech* 18(Suppl):S15–S23, 2005. LOE II
24. Lin B, Chen Z-W, Guo Z-M, et al: Anterior Approach Versus Posterior Approach with Subtotal Corpectomy, Decompression, and Reconstruction of Spine in the Treatment of Thoracolumbar Burst Fractures: A Prospective Randomized Controlled Study. *J Spinal Disord Tech* June 1, 2011. [Epub ahead of print]. LOE I
28. Gnanenthiran SR, Adie S, Harris IA: Nonoperative versus operative treatment for thoracolumbar burst fractures without neurologic deficit: a meta-analysis. *Clin Orthop Relat Res* 470(2):567–577, 2012. LOE II

The complete References list is available online at https://expertconsult.inkling.com.

35C Identification, Classification, Mechanism, and Treatment of Thoracolumbar Fracture-Dislocations

JOHN R. DIMAR II • PAUL C. CELESTRE • ASHISH UPADHYAY • NANDITA DAS

Thoracic and upper lumbar spine injuries are among some of the most common types of spinal injuries. Fracture-dislocations of the thoracolumbar spine have long been recognized as potentially unstable spine injuries that often present with significant neurologic injury. These injuries are generally a result of high-energy trauma, such as high-speed motor vehicle accidents, falls from heights, and occupational injuries, and are frequently associated with polytrauma. Caring for patients who have undergone such traumatic spinal fractures is challenging because a majority of these patients also have concomitant polytrauma with injury to other organ systems. Commonly associated injuries that occur with fracture-dislocations include closed head injuries, pulmonary contusions, splenic and hepatic lacerations, bowel injuries, vascular injuries, long bone fractures, and neurologic injuries. Because spinal fracture-dislocations have the potential to be highly unstable, these injuries require diligence in providing safe transport to the emergency department; rapid and precise diagnosis; and, when the patients are medically stable, emergent surgical reduction, decompression, and primary stabilization to prevent secondary neurologic injury. Flexion-distraction injuries, commonly referred to as Chance fractures, are a unique subset of high-energy thoracolumbar spine injuries. These injuries commonly result from rapid deceleration during motor vehicle accidents. Chance injuries are unstable and commonly require surgical stabilization.

Proper determination of the mechanism of injury is very important for appropriate surgical management of the patient. To expedite the treatment of traumatic injuries to the spine, various spinal injury classification systems have evolved over time, and each generation of spinal trauma surgeons has refined and modified the systems to describe the most commonly recognized fracture patterns.[1-14]

CLASSIFICATION

Fracture-Dislocations

Fracture-dislocations of the thoracolumbar spine result from high-energy injuries. Most commonly, the rostral vertebra is translated anteriorly on the caudal vertebra, but it is not unusual to see injury patterns that include retrolisthesis or lateral translation. Although they can be classified by direction of dislocation, this is arbitrary and practically makes little difference in regard to treatment. They are devastating spinal injuries that are frequently accompanied by a complete neurologic deficit. Fracture-dislocations of the spine inherently disrupt all three columns and are thus unstable and treated with surgery.

Flexion-Distraction Injuries

Two definitions of flexion-distraction injuries have been recently proposed and evaluated for reliability.

Definition A: Flexion-distraction injuries involve an axis of rotation anterior to the anterior longitudinal ligament as opposed to flexion-compression injuries that involve an axis of rotation within the vertebral body

Definition B: Flexion-distraction injuries are any injuries in which there is disruption of the posterior ligamentous complex (PLC) but no retropulsion of the vertebral body into the canal (i.e., there can be some vertebral compression as long as it is not associated with retropulsion, which would make it a flexion-compression injury).

In the study survey, 67% of the treating physicians agreed to definition B, and the remaining 33% agreed to definition A. In reality, these are similar injury patterns that both include disruption of the PLC. The more recent classification systems strongly suggest that these unstable injuries require immobilization or an open reduction, instrumentation, and fusion to restore alignment and prevent secondary neurologic injury. Here it is important to understand that the mechanism of injury will frequently guide the surgical planning. These definitions may be inadequate and truncated because these injuries have long been postulated to represent a continuum of a flexion and distraction moment where the PLC fails followed by the disruption of the facets, posterior longitudinal ligament, the disc, anterior longitudinal ligament, and finally displacement of the superior vertebral body on top of the other that often injures the spinal cord or cauda equina. Additionally, other forces can be part of the injury, including rotation, coronal angulation, extension, and compression, with the latter causing concurrent fracturing of the body.

Another pattern similar to flexion-distraction injuries is the eponymous Chance fracture. In this injury, an extreme distraction moment imparted to the thoracolumbar spine results in the fracture line extending from the posterior spinouts process through the pedicles, vertebral body, and anterior longitudinal ligament.[3] The injury usually involves primarily bone, but varying amounts of posterior ligamentous and discoligamentous injury may be present.

ASSESSMENT OF SEVERITY OF INJURY

White and Panjabi[15] described the instability of the spine as follows: "Inability of the spine, under physiologic loads, to maintain the relationships between the vertebrae so that there is neither initial nor subsequent neurological deficit, deformity and/or pain." In the clinical setting, this is hard to apply and therefore other methods to quantify the severity of injury have been developed.

Vaccaro and the Spine Trauma Study Group (STSG) combined the morphologic parameter of the spinal injury with the integrity of the PLC and the degree of neurologic injury into a novel classification system known as the Thoracolumbar Injury Classification and Severity (TLICS) system.[16] Because the integrity of the PLC, which is poorly visualized on computed tomography (CT) scanning, plays a key role in fracture evaluation using the TLICS system, the authors recommended the use of magnetic resonance imaging (MRI) studies to evaluate the integrity of the PLC. The goal of this novel classification system is to predict which fractures are unstable and require surgical stabilization. The system requires the surgeon to grade the fracture and assign points by evaluating three key components of the injury: neurologic status, fracture morphology, and integrity of the PLC (Fig. 35C-1).

At least two or three additional points are assigned to the total tally for any patient having a partial spinal cord injury or with cauda equina syndrome. This is then combined with the fracture morphology points, and the points are determined by evaluating the status of the PLC. Based on this system, any fracture scoring 5 points or above requires consideration for surgery, score of 4 is equivocal, and scores of 3 or less should receive nonoperative treatment. In the case of grading fracture-dislocations, which are inherently unstable, the system reliably grades the injury with a minimal score of 5 to 6 points and generates a surgical recommendation. The system is quick and intuitive to use and can provide a useful algorithm to formulate a potential treatment plan. The TLICS classification scheme assigns 7 points to Chance fractures, not including any points for neurologic deficits: 4 for pattern of injury and 3 for disruption of the PLC; thus according to the TLICS system, all Chance fractures meet operative criteria.

The TLICS has been evaluated and shown to have good to excellent interobserver reliability.[16] Owing to its intuitive classification algorithm and ease of use, it has become commonly used among current spinal trauma surgeons.[17]

MECHANISMS OF INJURY

Studies have shown that the direction of the force applied to the spine will directly determine the fracture pattern and consequently impact the level of stability. The focus of this

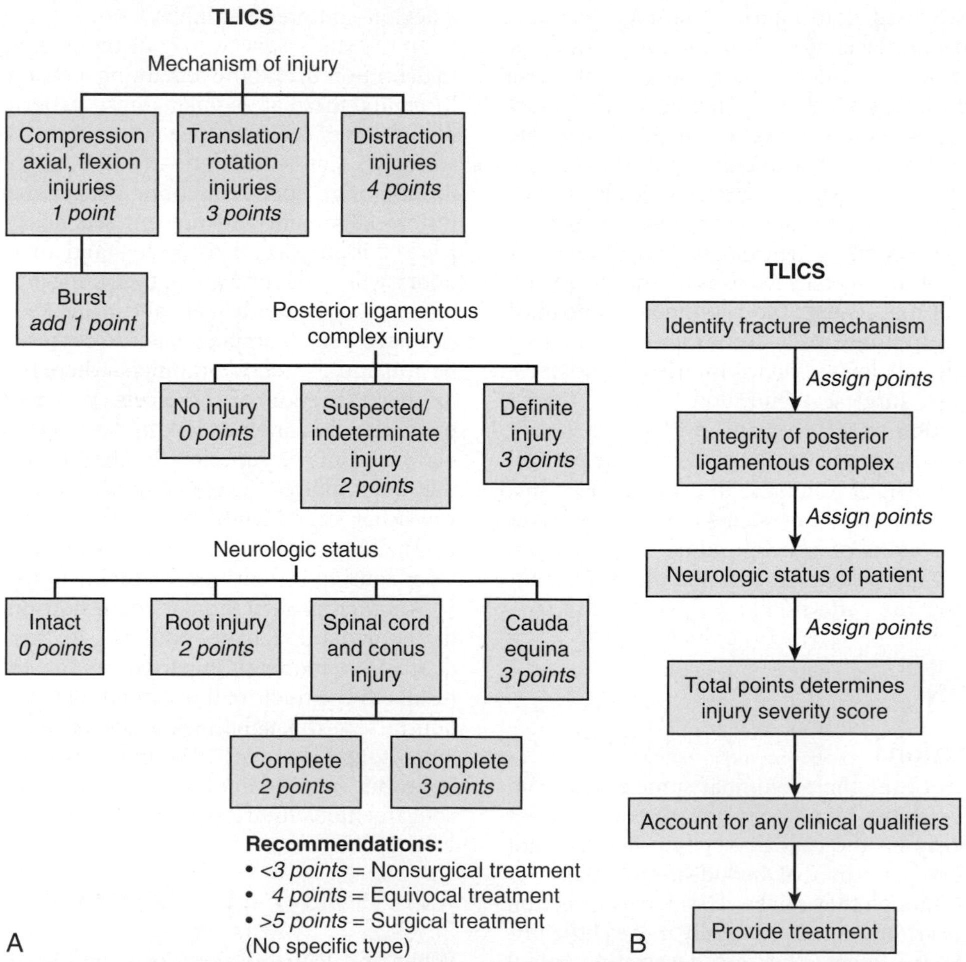

Figure 35C-1. A, Schematic Vaccaro Thoracolumbar Injury Classification and Severity (TLICS) three-part spine fracture classification system, which includes the mechanism of injury, the neurologic status, and the status of the posterior ligamentous complex. The total point tally guides the treatment decision. This is the first system to incorporate the neurologic status to determine surgical indications. **B,** TLICS classification flow chart. *(From Vaccaro A, Zeiller SC, Hulbert RJ, et al: The thoracolumbar injury severity score: a proposed treatment algorithm, J Spinal Disord Tech 18:209–215, 2005, Figs. 2, 3, and 4.)*

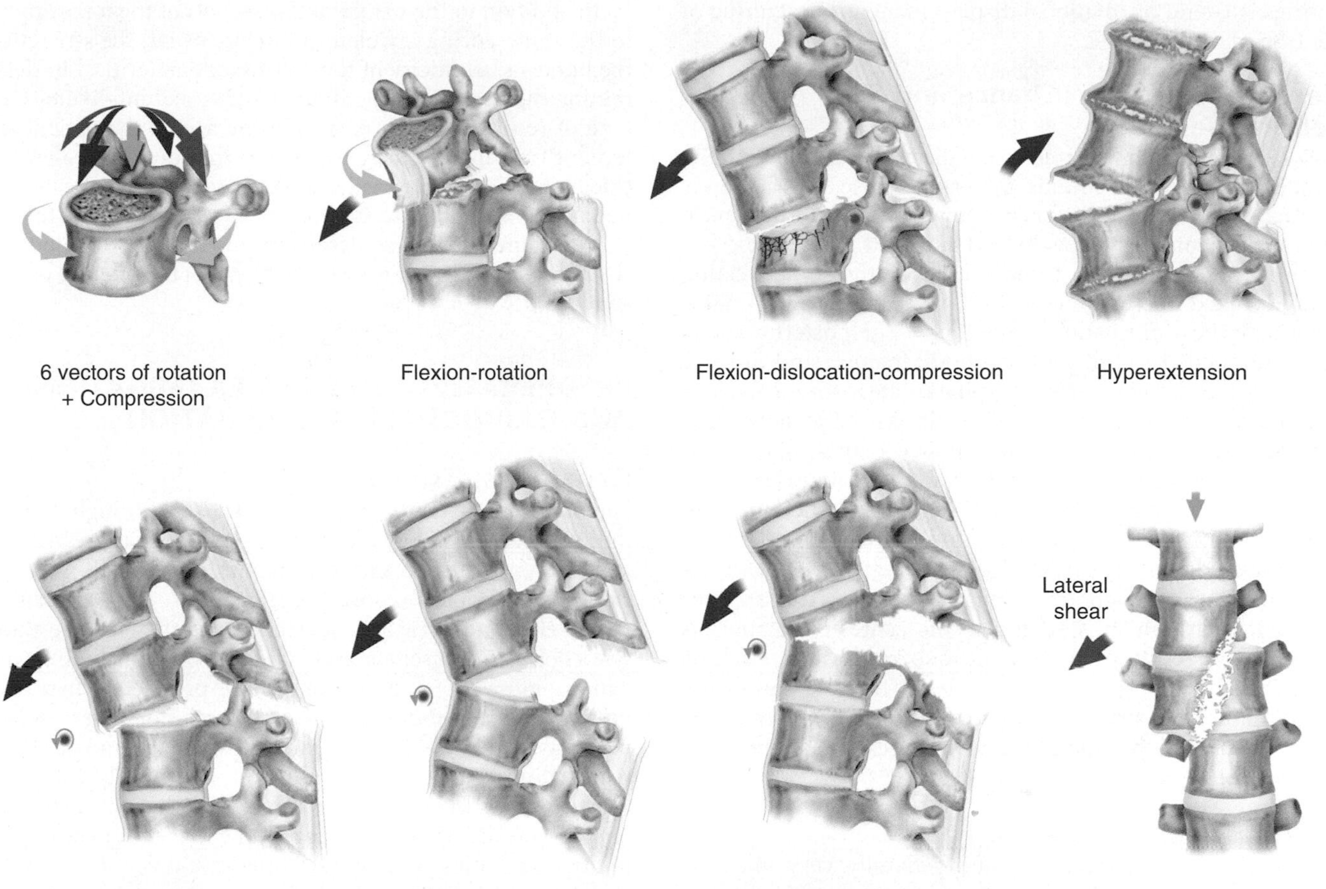

Figure 35C-2. Illustrations of injury patterns. These mechanisms generally describe the direction of the deforming force. It is important to understand that every injury is unique and may consequently have fractures that combine features of the commonly recognized injury patterns. Unfortunately, when these fractures occur in the thoracolumbar spine, they may render it mechanically unstable, thus carrying a significant risk of having a concurrent neurologic injury.

discussion on the mechanism of injury is limited to flexion, flexion rotation, lateral shear, extension, and distraction forces, which, when severe enough, have the potential to disrupt the structural integrity of the spine, causing a fracture-dislocation. Thoracolumbar fracture-dislocations are generally thought to result from the acute transition of the rigid thoracic spine to the more mobile lumbar spine. White and Panjabi reported that in a cadaveric evaluation of the spine, the flexion and extension ranges of motion in the lower thoracic spine increase from 5 to 12 degrees from T6 to T7 to T12 to L1 compared with the lumbar spine, which averages 15 degrees.[15] They also demonstrated that the axial rotation and lateral side bending of the thoracic spine is greater than that of lumbar spine because of the coronal orientation of the facets compared with the more sagittal lumbar facet joints.[15]

This mismatch in the range of motion and the rigidity of the thoracic spine secondary to rib buttressing compared with the lumbar spine makes the thoracolumbar junction susceptible to fractures when a severe and violent flexion, extension, rotational, or shear force occurs during high-energy trauma. This ultimately results in the force of the injury being concentrated at the thoracolumbar junction, producing a variety of fracture patterns that can render the spine unstable and subject the spinal cord and cauda equina to risk of injury. As a result of these biomechanical effects, almost 50% of all vertebral body fractures and 40% of all spinal cord injuries are concentrated at the thoracolumbar junction.[18] The mechanisms that can create an unstable thoracolumbar fracture by exceeding the age-determined inherent range of motion and stability of the thoracolumbar spine include *flexion, flexion-compression, flexion-rotation, flexion-distraction, extension, lateral shear or slice,* and *compression* (Fig. 35C-2).

Flexion Injuries

Flexion injuries to the spine are the easiest to understand because they occur with pure violent flexion force moments and are frequently combined with some degree of axial loading. Flexion injuries result in compression and burst fracture patterns of injury and may not include disruption of the PLC.

Flexion-Rotation Injuries

Flexion-rotation injuries occur after rotational forces are applied simultaneously with flexion moment to the thoracolumbar spine, resulting in the complete disruption of all of the PLC and extension through the anterior disc and vertebral body. These injuries are often associated with facet fractures, are highly unstable, and can progress to a complete disassociation of the involved spinal segments. They carry a high likelihood of a complete neurologic injury.[19] The hallmark of these injuries is lateral or rotational displacement and fracturing of the transverse processes.

Flexion-Distraction (Chance and Seat Belt Injuries)

Two types of flexion-distraction injuries are described. The Chance fracture is a unique pattern because it is a purely distractive injury.[3] The seat belt injury pattern is prototypical of the mechanism and has helped clarify the actual mechanism of these injuries as being caused by the spine rotating around a fixed fulcrum anteriorly (e.g., a lap belt) and sustaining a hyperflexion rotational moment.[20] The posterior spinal processes, pedicles, and vertebral body fracture and displace as they fail under tension as the spine rotates around an anterior fulcrum while the anterior longitudinal ligament often remains intact. The force of this injury may also result in numerous severe intraabdominal soft tissue injuries.[20,21] In the more common flexion-distraction injury, the center of spinal rotation is within the vertebral body. The posterior elements, including the pedicle, posterior longitudinal ligament, and posterior disc annulus, fail in tension. The anterior vertebral body, which is ventral to the center of rotation, is compressed, resulting usually in a compression fracture. Alternatively, with greater force, a burst fracture can occur. Thus, the flexion-distraction injury has tensile failure of the posterior and middle columns and compressive failure of the anterior column.

Lateral Shear Injuries

Lateral shear injuries are rare and generally very unstable. They are often associated with other fracture patterns, including flexion-rotation and lateral compression, thus creating very complex injuries. These injuries often involve a combination of the facet fractures, have oblique fractures through the vertebral body or a bursting component, can displace in any direction, and have a high association with concurrent complete neurologic injury. They are often associated with severe polytrauma, including the chest and abdomen.

Extension Injuries

Extension injuries are usually a result of a forceful extension force that is applied to a rigid spine and often occurs at the apex of the thoracic kyphosis after a fall backward or a forceful blow to the back of a spine.[19] This results in the disruption of the anterior spurs and ossified disc along with potential fracturing of the posterior facets and other ossified structures, creating a traumatic osteoclasis or "traumatic osteotomy" of the spine. Depending on the rigidity of the spine, these injuries may be stable if the posterior elements are intact or grossly unstable if both the anterior and posterior spinal columns are autofused such that translation occurs, resulting in neurologic injury. The injury is often dramatically discovered with lateral radiographs or after sagittal CT scans that reveal significant opening of the anterior disc space after the patient is lying on the examination table, which hyperextends the spine. The rigidity observed in these patients is often due to either ankylosing spondylitis or degenerative spondylosis typified by diffuse idiopathic skeletal hyperostosis (DISH). Patients with either condition may sustain catastrophic neurologic injury caused by fracture displacement or delayed deterioration if not accurately diagnosed and treated in a timely manner.[21]

In addition to the nature and direction of the force applied to the spine during a violent traumatic event, the strength of the bone and elasticity of the soft tissues are critical in determining the severity of the injury. Additional modifiers to the type of resultant fracture include the age of the patient, the level of fracture, the degree of comminution, the presence of osteoporosis and osteomalacia, the development of avascular necrosis, and damage to supporting structures such as the ribs and sternum. Preexisting deformity, including spondylolisthesis, kyphosis, and scoliosis, can also impact the fracture pattern and stability.

PREOPERATIVE PHYSICAL EXAMINATION AND RADIOGRAPHIC EVALUATION

General Assessment

Spinal trauma patients, particularly those with high-energy–induced fracture-dislocations of the spine, often present with acute polytrauma and therefore require a thorough multispecialty assessment. Because these patients often present in shock, either hemorrhagic or neurogenic, they require extensive efforts to resuscitate and stabilize them, including intubation, intravenous fluids or blood products, chest tube placement, intraabdominal assessment (for liver, spleen, pancreas, and bowel injury), and long bone splinting or external fixation. The trauma evaluation is critically important because more than half of patients with flexion-distraction injuries of the thoracolumbar spine have intraabdominal injuries, including hollow viscus perforations.[22] This number may be even higher in the pediatric population.[23] An acute abdomen secondary to undetected intraabdominal injury is associated with significant morbidity and mortality. It is recommended that a general assessment of the patient's overall mental functioning (Glasgow Coma scale[24]), polytrauma status (Injury Severity score[25,26]), neurologic status (American Spine Injury Association [ASIA],[27-29] International Standards for Neurological Classification of Spinal Cord Injury[24,30]), and comorbidities (Charleston Co-morbidity Index[31]) be conducted. Although plain radiographs of the chest, abdomen, pelvis, spine, and long bones remain useful, most trauma centers now use more advanced imaging such as CT scanning and MRIs of targeted areas. This is particularly true for obtunded patients in whom a rapid CT scan of the chest, abdomen and pelvis, and total spine is required to rule out any unknown injuries.

Physical Examination

Physical examination in the conscious patient should include evaluation of the entire spine from the occiput to the sacrum for any points of tenderness, painful gaps or step-offs between the spinous processes that may be indicative of ligamentous injury, subcutaneous bruises or contusions, subcutaneous air, and the general alignment of the spine. In flexion-distraction type injuries soft tissue injuries can be detected by noting hematoma, significant paraspinous tenderness, and palpation of gaps between spinous processes. In fracture-dislocations a gibbous deformity and step-off between spinous processes are palpable.

The neurologic examination includes a complete assessment of the motor strength, sensory examination, proprioception, and rectal tone. If the patient is in spinal shock, the anal wink and bulbocavernosus reflex are less relevant for the prognosis of the injury because most of these patients should have had emergent reduction and stabilization of their spine within 72 hours of the injury. The ASIA standards for the neurologic examination are used to guide physicians through a complete neurologic examination.[27-29]

Radiographic Examination

A CT or plain radiographs are used to identify injury as discussed in Chapter 30. Fracture-dislocations by definition have translation of the cephalad vertebrae compared with the adjacent caudal vertebrae. The facet articulations are dislocated and in many cases have associated fractures. The displacement can be from 10% to complete spondyloptosis. The posterior elements are always disrupted. When other force vectors were present, varying amounts of axial rotation, lateral subluxation, or scoliosis may be present.

Fracture-dislocations are easy to recognize on CT and are always unstable; therefore MRI is, in general, not useful to aid treatment. MRI may be indicated to assess neurologic injury, especially if it does not correlate to the level of bony injury. In flexion-distraction injuries, MRI can help determine the severity of injury to the PLC that may guide treatment.

TREATMENT CONSIDERATIONS

The goal of surgery is the restoration and maintenance of normal anatomic alignment, prevention of neurologic deterioration, promotion of fracture healing, and restoration of useful function.

Spinal Cord Injuries

Spinal cord injuries are common in fracture-dislocations and less so with flexion-distraction injuries. The management of patients with associated spinal cord injuries includes correction of anemia, oxygenation, and maintenance of mean arterial pressure to a minimum of 80 mm Hg as described in Chapter 31. The use of prophylactic steroids in spinal cord injury remains controversial because some studies have shown marginal improvement of neurologic function, but others have shown a significant increase in complications after their use. The authors generally do not recommend their use in thoraco lumbar spine trauma because of their potential side effects.[32-35]

The identification of any neurologic function below the level of the injury, including sensory or motor function or sensory sparing of the perineum, particularly if there is progressive return of function after injury, is a strong indication for immediate open reduction, decompression, and stabilization to maximize the chance of neurologic recovery. The prognosis for recovery varies depending on at what level the fracture-dislocation occurs and how severe the initial displacement and compression was that injured the spinal cord or cauda equina. A partial or complete spinal cord injury carries a worse prognosis for recovery, but a patient with contusion at the level of the conus medullaris may present with deceptively normal motor examination findings because the patient may only have loss of sensation of the perineum. Bladder function is difficult to evaluate initially because most patients will already have a urinary catheter inserted as part of the initial polytrauma management. A cauda equina injury, in which there may be variable loss of neurologic function, has the best chance of recovery after surgical stabilization of a fracture-dislocation. It is the authors' opinion that incomplete spinal cord injury requires expedited treatment at all levels of care, including transport and surgical intervention, to maximize neurologic recovery, but truly complete injuries do not require emergent treatment in fracture-dislocations.

The timing of surgery in thoracolumbar trauma is driven by two major factors. The first is to maximize neurologic recovery by early decompression and stabilization. This restores intramedullary blood flow and reduces secondary spinal cord injury. Early treatment is supported by preclinical data that have been supportive of early decompression for incomplete neurologic injuries.[36] The second reason for early surgery is to reduce complications, hospital stays, and overall costs. Cengiz and colleagues[37] reported a randomized trial comparing early surgery (within 8 hours of injury) and late surgery (after 3 days). They found improved neurologic outcomes, shorter hospital stays, and fewer systemic complications in the early treatment group. Other noncontrolled trials exclusive of patients with neurologic injury similarly show decreased postoperative ventilator requirements, decreased time in intensive care unit and hospital stays, lower pulmonary complications in thoracic injuries, and a trend toward fewer systemic complications[38-41] with early surgery.

The authors' treatment algorithm for patients with spinal cord injuries is based on the patient's overall medical status and neurologic examination. The ASIA system is most useful for grading and communicating a patient's neurologic status. In the authors' opinion, the patients requiring the most urgent surgical intervention are those with a documented progression of their neurologic injury or an incomplete neurologic injury (i.e., ASIA B, C, and D). Patients with incomplete injuries should be taken to surgery urgently, preferably in less than 6 hours after injury, to prevent a possible progression of their neurologic injury caused by secondary injury. Patients with complete spinal cord injuries (ASIA A) as well as those with normal neurologic examination findings (ASIA E) are taken to surgery when medically stabilized. Obtunded patients who are not able to cooperate with a neurologic examination are commonly encountered and should be treated as if they present with an incomplete injury unless there is MRI evidence of spinal cord transection. ASIA A patients must be counseled that neurologic recovery is unlikely and that surgery is being performed to stabilize the spine and facilitate rehabilitation rather than to reverse their spinal cord injury.

GENERAL APPROACH

After a thorough physical examination and radiographic assessment of the spine, the authors find the TLICS classification[14] useful in determining both the classification of the fracture and the treatment plan. Injuries with TLICS scores of 5 or greater are treated surgically and those with scores of 3 or less are treated nonoperatively. A TLICS score of 4 requires individualized treatment.

Nonoperative Care

The vast majority of thoracolumbar compression and burst fractures are treated in a brace. Low-energy injuries, such as osteoporotic compression fractures and low-energy compression or burst fractures that do not show disruption of the PLC, can be treated in a thoracolumbar spinal orthosis (TLSO) brace. Typically, patients are braced for 2 to 3 months and then gradually weaned out of the brace as their symptoms improve. Upright radiographs in the brace are essential before the patient is discharged from the hospital to ensure there is no significant instability or kyphosis, and follow-up radiographs are typically taken at 2, 6, and 12 weeks and again at 6 months from injury.

TREATMENT OF SPECIFIC INJURY TYPES

Fracture-Dislocations

All thoracolumbar fracture-dislocations are highly unstable and should be treated surgically. The most commonly used approach is posterior in which open reduction can be achieved along with simultaneous transpedicular fixation. Neurologic decompression is indicated if there are comminuted fragments of bone or ligamentum flavum infolding causing residual stenosis. In most instances, the canal stenosis resolves with reduction of the fractured spine and restoration of the normal spinal canal diameter. A laminar fracture occasionally will entrap the nearby dura mater, leading to an inadvertent durotomy that requires repair. The authors recommend stabilization of the spine with segmental pedicle screws or hook fixation with a minimum of two levels above and below the injury. Three levels should be considered in severely destabilized spines and those that have adjacent levels of injury where fixation might be compromised.

If a residual incomplete neurologic injury pattern persists after posterior stabilization, a postoperative MRI or CT myelogram is indicated to identify any canal compromise. If severe enough, an anterior decompression to remove any residual anterior bony fragments that are still causing significant spinal cord or conus medullaris compression is indicated. An anterior reconstruction may also be indicated to restore the anterior column if a severe concurrent bursting component exists, creating a loss of anterior column support.

Chance and Flexion-Distraction Injuries

Chance and flexion-distraction injuries generally occur in a younger patient population and surgery should be reserved for fractures that cannot be successfully reduced with hyperextension bracing or casting. The authors recommend bracing or casting for skeletally immature patients. In adults, these fractures are treated surgically with posterior reduction and instrumentation (Fig. 35C-3). Particularly in the case of bony Chance injuries, a fusion is not needed after reduction and short segment compressive hook or pedicle instrumentation suffices because the bony structures will generally heal and the instrumentation can be removed 1 year later. However, certain seat belt injuries can be profoundly devastating and follow high-energy decelerating injuries because the seat belt lies above the pelvis and over the abdomen. Because of this position, the severe hyperflexion force of rotation is usually focused at the L3 vertebra, which serves as the center of rotation of the spine. These injuries may be severe enough that they completely disrupt the spinal integrity; avulse the cauda equina; and cause concurrent serosal tearing, liver and spleen lacerations, bowel rupture and entrapment, and vascular intimal tearing or aortic rupture. It is critical that when corrective surgery is done in these severe seat belt injuries that a vascular and general surgeon be available to be part of the surgical team in case some of these severe associated injuries are unmasked during open reduction.[20,42] These injuries often require open reduction and fixation if there is more than 20 degrees of kyphosis, a concurrent neurologic injury, or a ligamentous-type injury pattern in adults (Fig. 35C-4). Usually a short segment instrumentation with or without fusion using a tension band construct consisting of interspinous wiring, compression hooks, or a pedicle screw–rod construct combined with supplemental bracing will suffice. In cases of severe disassociation of the spine, rigid fixation is mandatory.[20]

Distraction Injuries

Fractures combined with significant distraction injuries are fortunately rare and are very unstable. They generally do not require a true reduction maneuver because they are so globally unstable that they often reduce by postural correction with careful placement on the operating table. A word of caution: grossly unstable distraction injuries should not be placed on a Wilson frame because they may further distract because of an unrecognized complete decoupling of the spinal segments, resulting in neurologic injury (Fig. 35C-5). Generally, a temporary rod and subsequent compression will help to decrease any segmental kyphosis and distraction seen through the injured segment. If the distraction is severe enough in the thoracic spine, the pleural space may be violated, resulting in lung herniation, and in the lumbar spine, the psoas muscle and retroperitoneum may be exposed. Similar to patients with Chance and seat belt injuries, there may be concurrent abdominal injuries, including bowel injury with entrapment, liver, spleen, and vascular injury.[42]

Lateral Shear or Slice Injuries

Occasionally, fracture-dislocations that involve lateral shear or posterior translation are encountered after high-energy injuries (Fig. 35C-6). All of these injuries should be considered highly unstable. They cannot always be reduced with simple reduction techniques because of bony comminution, vertebral body displacement, and obscured anatomy. Intraoperative fluoroscopy and CT scanning are useful to aid in reduction for these multiplanar injuries. For these patients, in addition to all of the various previously described techniques, the authors recommend placement of pedicle screws three levels above and below the fracture. Subsequently, four temporary rods may be placed in each segment. Rod holders along with compression and distraction clamps can now be used to move either the upper or lower section as a unit to reduce the fracture-dislocation. These injuries are commonly associated with fractures of the posterior elements, paraplegia secondary to cord transection, and resultant traumatic durotomies.[19]

Hyperextension Injuries

The focus of treatment of extension injuries should be to reverse the injury by first kyphosing the spine, preferably by postural reduction on a Wilson frame with serial radiographs, fluoroscopy, or intraoperative CT scanning (Fig. 35C-7). Great diligence in transferring the patient into the prone position is also required so that no translation of the ankylosed segments occurs, causing neurologic injury. For the same reason neuromonitoring, including motor evoked potentials (MEPs) and somatosensory evoked potentials (SSEPs), is also essential during positioning and surgery to

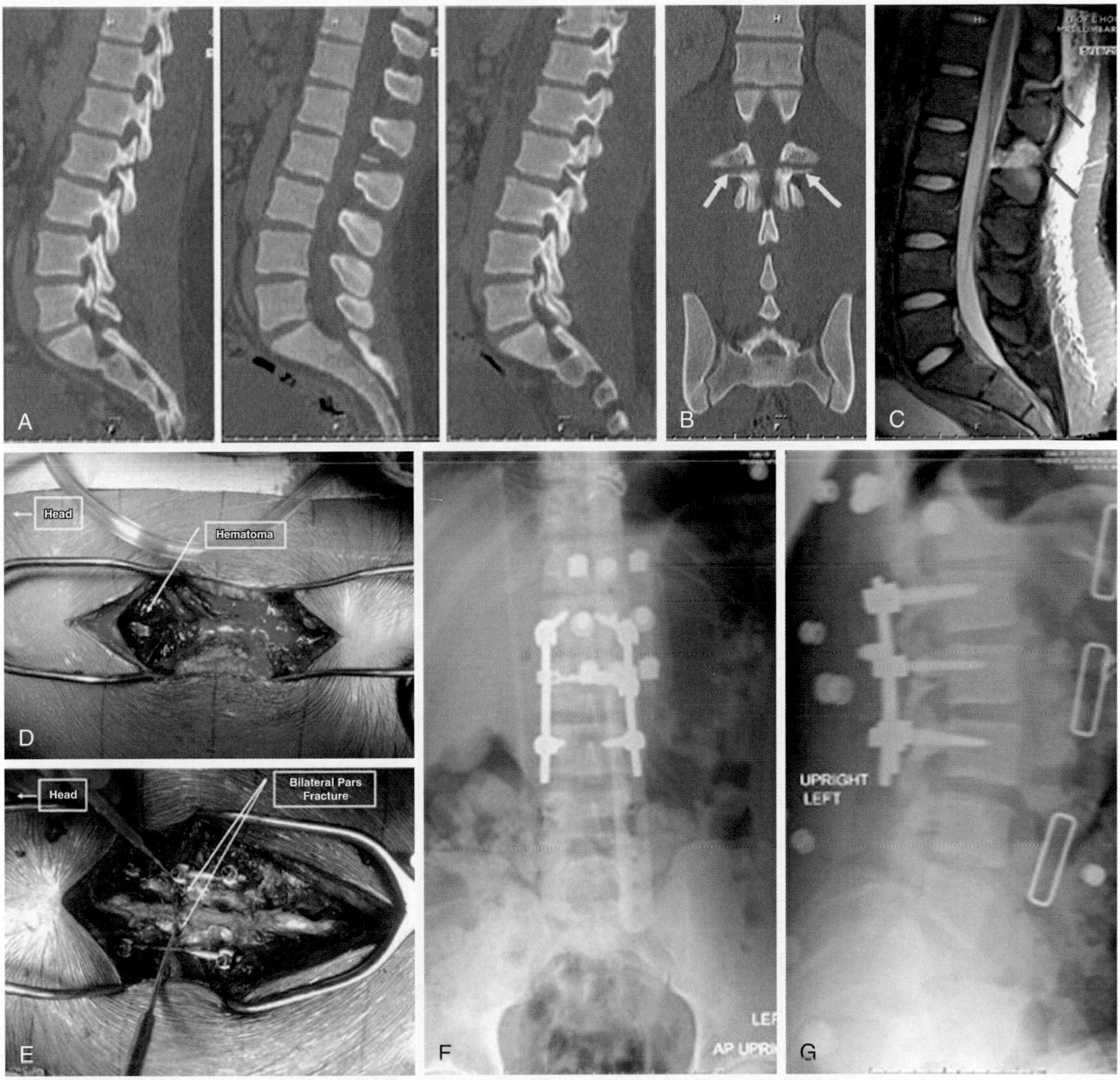

Figure 35C-3. This 17-year-old young man lost control of his motorcycle and slid under a guard rail. The patient was found to have an open femur fracture and a L2 Chance fracture, American Spine Injury Association (ASIA) E. The femur fracture was treated with an intramedullary nail. **A,** Sagittal computed tomography images showing fractures of L2 pedicle. **B,** Coronal view showing the same. **C,** Sagittal magnetic resonance image showing a posterior ligamentous injury. **D** and **E,** Intraoperative view showing ligament injury and pars interarticularis fractures. **F** and **G,** Anterior-posterior and lateral postreduction radiographs.

alert the surgeon to problems caused by positioning. Because the posterior structures are frequently intact, a gradual reduction of the anterior opening of the vertebral bodies can be accomplished by restoring the spine to its preexisting sagittal alignment. This can be done surgically by contouring the rod after pedicle screw placement to estimate the amount of preexisting kyphosis that was present before the injury and any residual need for correction can be done with in situ rod benders. A longer construct in ankylosing spondylitis is recommended because the coexisting osteoporosis in these patients may lead to early failure at the bone–screw interface and loss of correction. Posterior compression, particularly with hook constructs, should be avoided because it will result in opening of the anterior fracture and possible translation of the segments, resulting in canal compromise and neurologic injury. If canal stenosis is noted before surgery or neurologic deterioration occurs during surgery, a concurrent decompression can be done.

SURGICAL TECHNIQUE

Anesthetic Considerations

Successful treatment of these unstable injuries requires a clear preoperative plan, an operating room team that includes a surgical technician familiar with the instrumentation, a

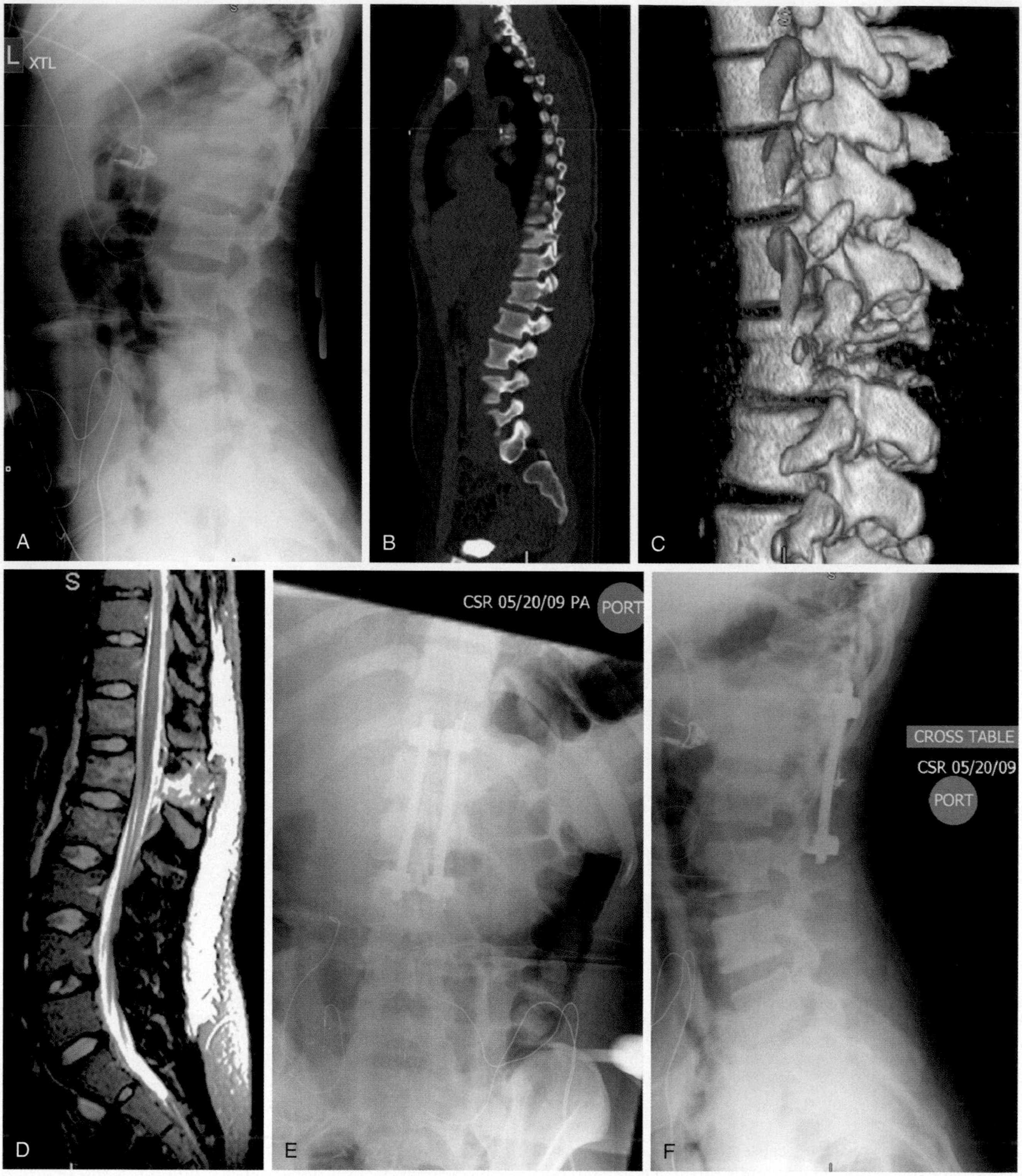

Figure 35C-4. This 17-year-old female restrained driver lost control of her car, running into a tree head on. Trauma workup revealed a left clavicle fracture, fractured ribs, and an L1 fracture. On examination, her injury is American Spine Injury Association (ASIA) E, and she has severe back pain, ecchymosis, and local kyphosis noted in the midback. **A,** Lateral radiograph showing L1 process splaying. **B,** Sagittal computed tomography (CT) scan showing the L1 body fracture. **C,** Three-dimensional CT scan showing an L1 posterior process gap. **D,** Magnetic resonance image showing posterior ligaments ruptured. **E** and **F,** Anterior-posterior and lateral postoperative radiographs showing the tension band hook system.

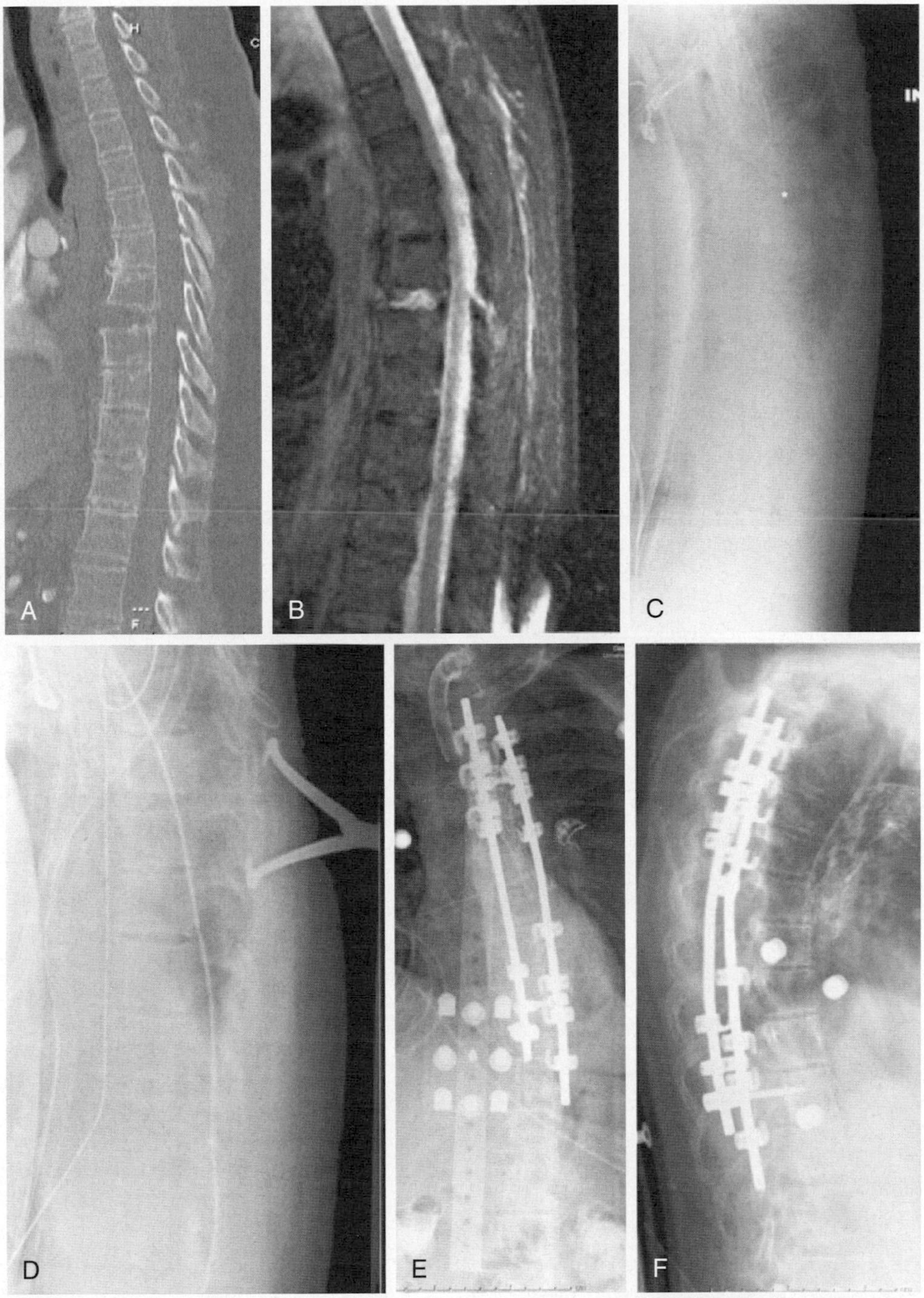

Figure 35C-5. **A** and **B,** Sagittal computed tomography and short tau inversion recovery (STIR) magnetic resonance image scan demonstrating T7 to T8 distraction injury in a 71-year-old woman after a motor vehicle accident. Her injury is an American Spine Injury Association (ASIA) E. **C,** Intraoperative radiograph demonstrating distraction through the fracture after the patient was placed on a Wilson frame. Somatosensory evoked potentials (SSEP) and motor evoked potentials (MEP) signals were lost. **D,** Intraoperative radiograph after application of AO large tenaculum with return of SSEP and MEP signals. **E** and **F,** Final anterior-posterior and lateral radiographs. The patient had a complete neurologic recovery.

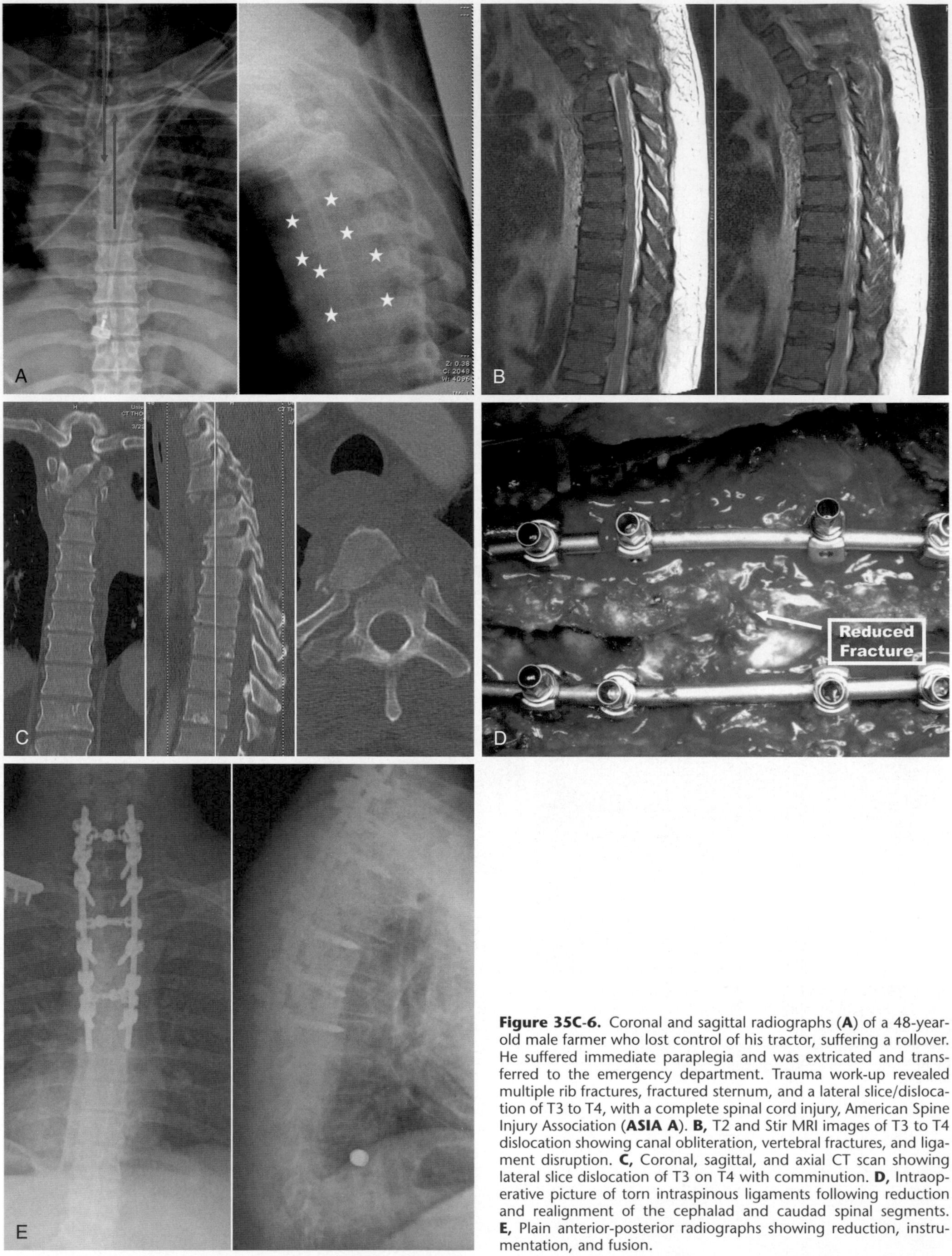

Figure 35C-6. Coronal and sagittal radiographs (**A**) of a 48-year-old male farmer who lost control of his tractor, suffering a rollover. He suffered immediate paraplegia and was extricated and transferred to the emergency department. Trauma work-up revealed multiple rib fractures, fractured sternum, and a lateral slice/dislocation of T3 to T4, with a complete spinal cord injury, American Spine Injury Association (**ASIA A**). **B,** T2 and Stir MRI images of T3 to T4 dislocation showing canal obliteration, vertebral fractures, and ligament disruption. **C,** Coronal, sagittal, and axial CT scan showing lateral slice dislocation of T3 on T4 with comminution. **D,** Intraoperative picture of torn intraspinous ligaments following reduction and realignment of the cephalad and caudad spinal segments. **E,** Plain anterior-posterior radiographs showing reduction, instrumentation, and fusion.

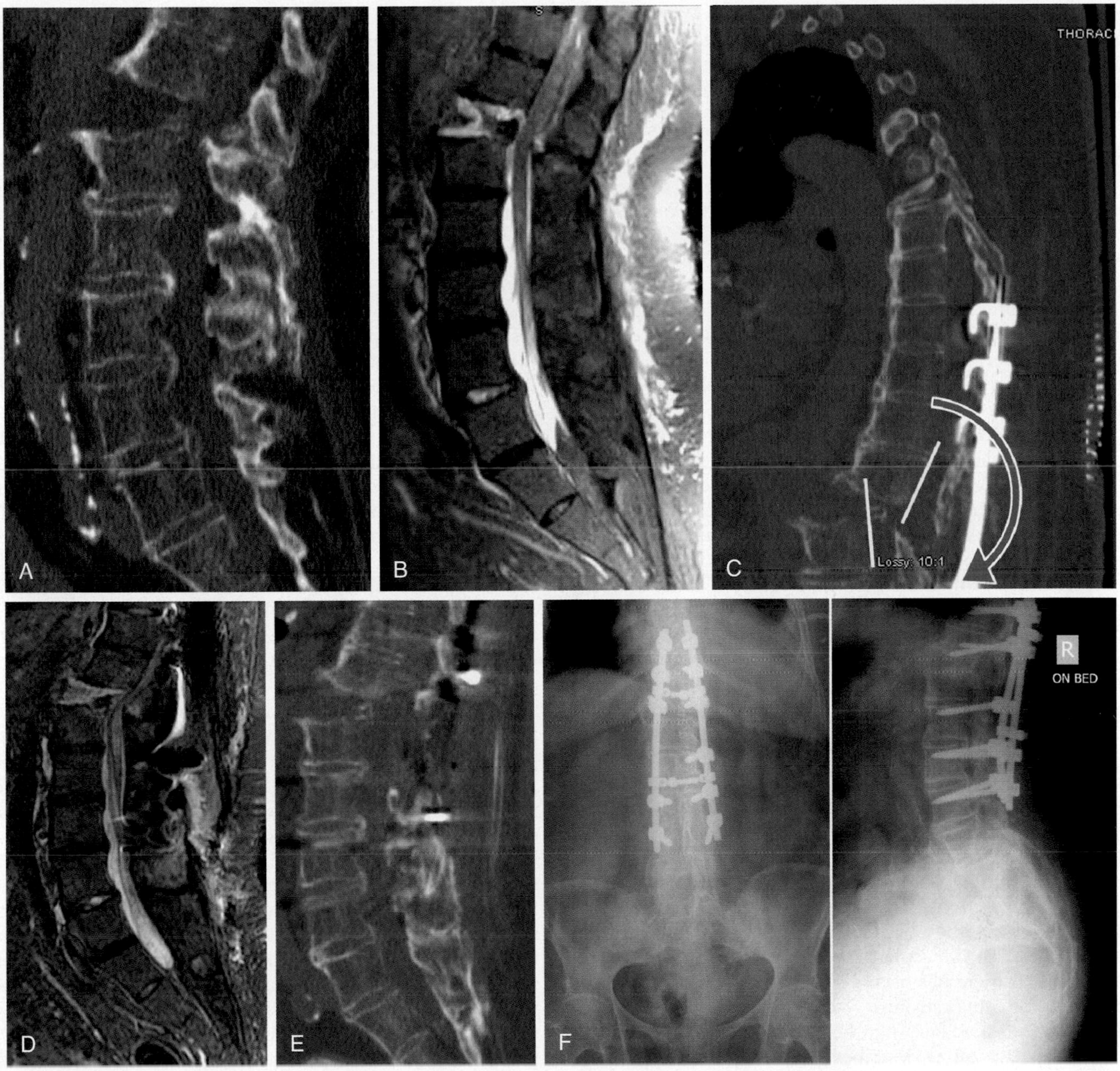

Figure 35C-7. Sagittal computed tomography (CT) (**A**) and T2-weighted magnetic resonance images (MRIs) (**B**) of a 57-year-old morbidly obese woman after a fall, American Spine Injury Association (ASIA) E with a T12 to L1 hyperextension injury through an ankylosed spine. The patient was treated with bed rest for 14 days before being transferred from an outside hospital. Postoperative sagittal (**C**) CT and T2-weighted MRI images (**D**) after posterior instrumentation with an all-hook construct. The patient was noted to have postoperative neurologic decline, and these repeat images demonstrate accentuation of the deformity and increased cord compression. **E,** The patient was taken back to the operating room on an emergent basis, and her construct was revised to an all pedicle screw construct. A postoperative sagittal CT (**F**) demonstrates improved canal clearance, and the patient was noted to have resolution of her neurologic deficits.

neurologic monitoring technician, a nurse, and an anesthesiologist familiar with total-intravenous anesthetic (TIVA) techniques. In incomplete injuries, TIVA facilitates neurologic monitoring, including MEPs and SSEPs, and intraoperative electromyographic (EMG) testing to confirm pedicle screw placement in the lumbosacral spine. The authors recommend these three modalities for all patients except those that are known to be ASIA A. In cases that may involve extended operative times or multiple spinal segments, consideration of the use of the cell-saver or various pharmacologic agents to decrease blood loss may be useful.[43,44]

Positioning

A patient with an unstable kyphotic fracture-dislocation deformity is positioned on a Jackson Spine Table (Mizuho OSI, Union City, CA) with six-post support consisting of chest pads, anterior-superior iliac spine pads, and thigh pads, which help reduce the inherent kyphosis in fracture-dislocations by reversing the injury mechanism. Conversely, a Wilson frame should be used in extension fracture-dislocation to restore the "normal" excessive kyphosis of the ankylosed spine, thus reducing the fracture by reversing the hyperextension mechanism that caused the displacement.

Exposure

A midline skin incision is followed by a posterior subperiosteal exposure of the spine, including at least two pedicles or levels above and below the injured segment. In the lumbar spine, the medial half of the transverse process should be exposed to facilitate pedicle screw insertion via anatomic landmarks, but it is unnecessary to perform a complete exposure of the lateral gutter because the fusion will take place through the facets. Facet joints are then removed with a rongeur, a 1-cm osteotome, or a high-speed drill. Care should be taken to preserve and save all local bone for later bone grafting. A single intraoperative lateral radiograph should be obtained after placing a sharp awl into a pedicle to serve both as a marker for levels as well as the sagittal orientation of the pedicle. Localization of the fracture location is critical because intraoperative radiographs are often of poor quality, particularly with fracture-dislocations of the upper thoracic spine, and anatomic identification of the fracture is often difficult because of multiple posterior spinous process fractures that obscure the actual fracture level.

Fracture Reduction

Reduction of a fracture-dislocation can be achieved through a combination of techniques with positioning on the table being foremost. Before open reduction, any facet fracture fragments, laminar bone, or infolding ligamentum flavum that is in the spinal canal should be removed to avoid entrapment after reduction. If the facets are dislocated and do not spontaneously reduce, then reduction can be achieved by several methods, including partial resection of the facets or leverage with a Penfield probe. Towel clips can be placed into the spinous process of the adjacent segments to gently distract the spine and elevate the cephalad vertebrae to reduce the facet dislocation. If there has been a simultaneous rotational force applied to the spine causing a flexion-rotational dislocation, a unilateral dislocated facet may be present that can be reduced in a similar fashion as described previously. However, these injuries frequently involve more severe trauma and may be very difficult to reduce because of entrapped soft tissue, neural elements, disc material, and bony fragments that may require removal for a successful reduction of the injury. Many surgeons prefer to place temporary rods into the pedicle screws above and below the fracture in various fashions so they can be gripped with rod instruments and manipulated to achieve reduction.

After reduction is achieved, the alignment can be maintained by the application of a large bone tenaculum or towel clamp around the spinous processes. The use of an 18-gauge cerclage wire through the spinous process above and then underneath the spinous process below the injured level followed by the gradual tightening of the wire is also useful in reducing a fracture-dislocation of the thoracolumbar spine and for holding the initial partial reduction. Alternatively, placement of rods (normal anatomic contour) into the lower (caudad) pedicle screws and subsequent reduction of the rod into the proximal (cephalad) screws with a combination of a rocker, vertical mechanical rod–screw head reducer, or rod holder can pull the proximal spine out of kyphosis and reduce the fracture. Placement of reduction screws is another option to reduce the spine dorsally but is generally unnecessary and costly.

Instrumentation

Posterior stabilization is the treatment of choice for flexion-distraction injuries and fracture-dislocations of the thoracolumbar spine. Contemporary pedicle screw fixation allows for rigid stabilization in all directions of the thoracolumbar spine, particularly in rotation when compared with hook constructs. Pedicle screws allow for the reduction of a fracture-dislocation, restoration of normal sagittal alignment, and reconstitution of the posterior spinal tension band. This leaves sufficient room for a large bony surface for fusion and gives the surgeon the option to perform a laminectomy for neurologic decompression, if indicated. Pedicle screw insertion can be assisted by instant digital plain radiographs, fluoroscopic guidance, intraoperative computerized tomography (CT) combined with image guidance, and in the lumbar spine using running EMG pedicle probe stimulation followed by post pedicle screw placement EMG re-stimulation. In areas obscured by the shoulders, particularly in the T1 to T6 area, only a posterior-anterior (PA) radiograph may be useful. The use of intraoperative CT scanning may also be useful in identifying the appropriate levels and confirming pedicle screw or iliac screw positioning.

Pedicle screws are inserted in a standard fashion at least two levels above and below the fracture, according to the preoperative template. In our institution, pedicle screws are placed with one of three methods: freehand, fluoroscopy, or with image guidance. The freehand method is used most frequently and uses a bone awl or pedicle finder probe that has been placed into a pedicle adjacent to the fracture using anatomic landmarks. A single intraoperative lateral radiograph is taken to determine the level as well as the sagittal angulation of the pedicles. Subsequently the screws are placed using anatomic landmarks, and final PA and lateral radiographs are taken to confirm adequate hardware position. Rarely do we use fluoroscopy to identify small pedicles or intraoperative CT scanning combined with image guidance. Frequently, it is possible to achieve interfragmentary fixation of the fracture posterior elements with a 30-mm pedicle screw if the fracture-dislocation contains a burst component.[45] In patients with poor bone quality or those that are ASIA A, it may be desirable to achieve three levels of fixation above and below the fracture or use additional hooks to supplement the pedicle fixation because the lamina may be stronger.

Generally, at least two levels above and below the fracture are required to ensure stabilization of the spine in these unstable injuries and, if there is any question of stability or simultaneous fracturing of the posterior elements, more levels need to be included in the construct, particularly when treating rotational dislocations (Fig. 35C-8). After the fracture is reduced, fine tuning of the reduction can be accomplished by several methods, including in situ rod bending and compression of the construct, which can selectively shorten either side of the spine to correct any coronal imbalance or can globally shorten the entire posterior column to restore additional normal sagittal alignment through the instrumented segments (Fig. 35C-9).

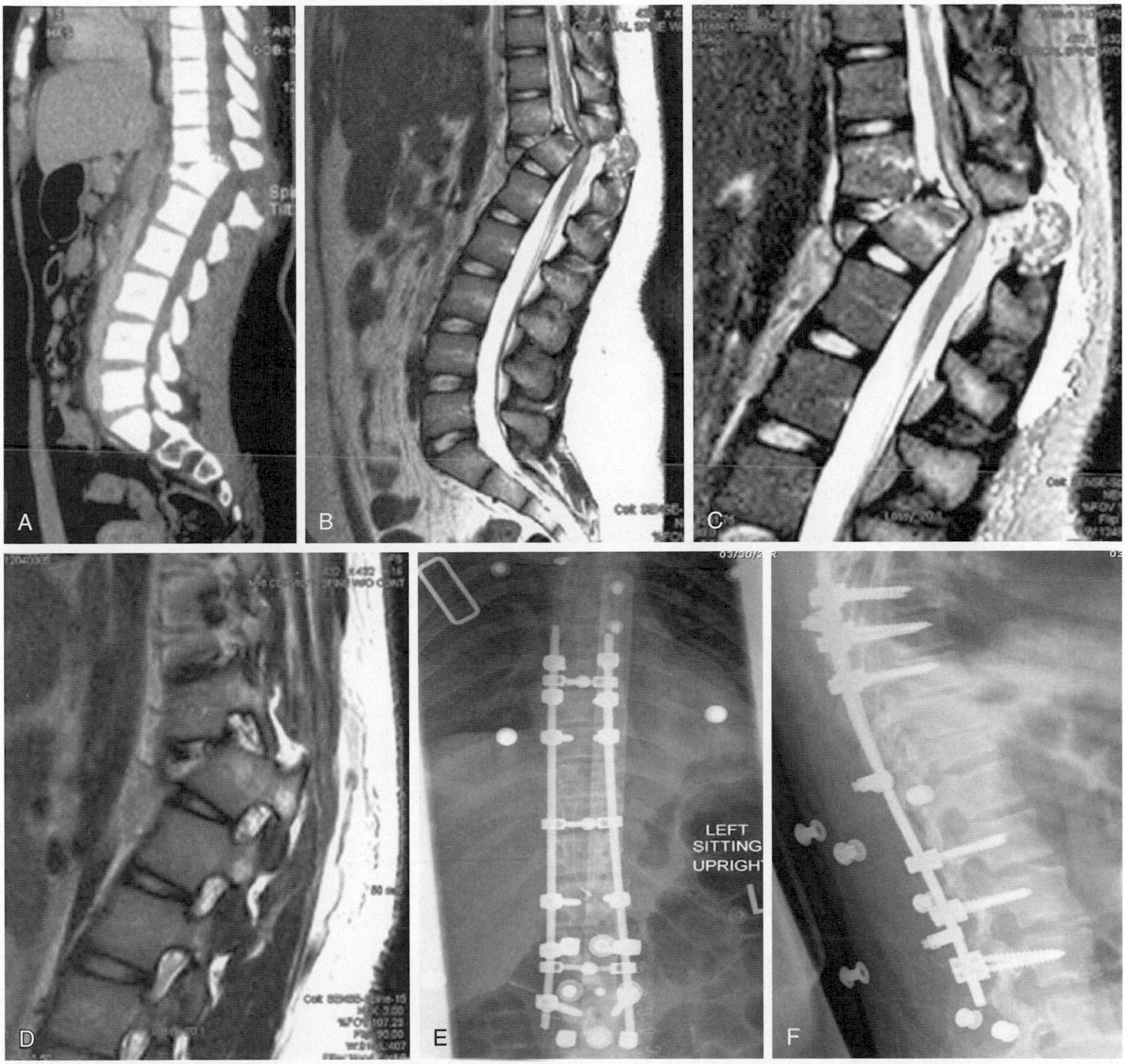

Figure 35C-8. This 16-year-old young woman was involved as a passenger in a motor vehicle accident after her sister lost control. She was wearing a seat belt. She was transported to the emergency department complaining of severe TL back pain, lower extremity weakness, and numbness. Her injury was American Spine Injury Association (ASIA) C. **A,** Sagittal computed tomography scan. **B,** Sagittal magnetic resonance images showing complete disruption of ligaments. **C,** Intraoperative view showing complete disruption of the posterior ligamentous complex. **D,** Intraoperative view demonstrating fracture reduction and instrumentation. **E** and **F,** Anterior-posterior and lateral radiographs showing final reduction.

Fusion

Although some authors[46] do not advocate that a concurrent fusion be done with spine fracture fixation, it is our opinion that because of the risk of neurologic injury in fracture-dislocations, there is an absolute need for long-term stability; therefore, a fusion is indicated in the majority of cases. The fusion bed is prepared by thoroughly decorticating the facets, lamina, and posterior spinous processes using an osteotome or high-speed burr and saving all autogenous bone.

In the majority of patients, posterior iliac crest bone graft is harvested through a 6- to 8-cm separate vertical incision over the posterior iliac crest while an oblique incision should be avoided to prevent injury to the clunneal nerve that passes over the iliac crest. If the fusion is extended below L3, then the iliac crest can be approached subcutaneously through the same incision. Allograft cancellous chips or demineralized bone matrix can be used primarily as a bone graft extender in patients with longer fusions in which insufficient local or iliac bone graft is obtained.[47] Among high-risk patients (those older than 65 years of age, smokers, and those diagnosed with osteoporosis or other comorbidities), the "off-label" use of recombinent bone morphogenic protein-2 (rhBMP-2) is occasionally used as an adjunct to healing but only after an extensive discussion with the patient and family regarding the risks and benefits.[48]

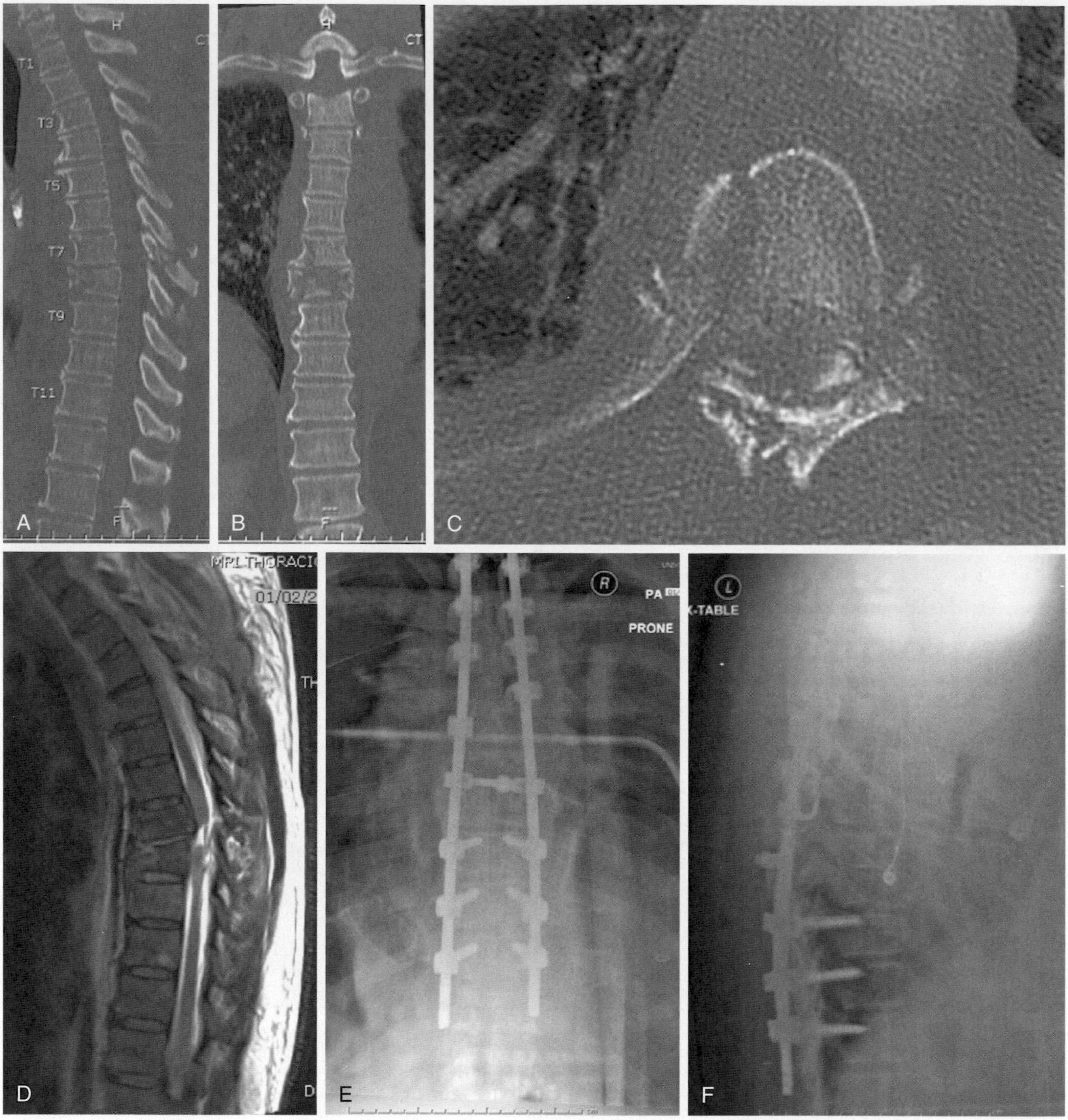

Figure 35C-9. A 63-year-old man after a high-speed motor vehicle accident resulting in an unstable fracture-dislocation at T8. The injury was American Spine Injury Association (ASIA) A with extensive bruising and degloving of the back and pneumothorax. **A,** Sagittal computed tomography (CT) scan showing spinous process fractures demonstrating disruption of the posterior column. Coronal (**B**) and axial (**C**) CT scan images showing the extensively disrupted anterior and middle columns. **D,** T2-weighted magnetic resonance image shows extensive ligamentous edema in the interspinous ligaments and subfascial hematoma along with disruption of the spinal cord. **E** and **F,** Postoperative anterior-posterior and lateral radiographs showing segmental instrumented stabilization of the fracture-dislocation with a pedicle screw below the injury and hooks above it.

Wound Closure

Wound closure is done in layers starting with the deep fascia, which is closed using #1 Vicryl in an interrupted figure-of-8 fashion. A deep drain is placed except in the setting of cerebrospinal fluid leak. The subcutaneous layer is closed over a drain with interrupted buried simple 2-0 Vicryl sutures and a running 3-0 Monocryl and Dermabond. The superficial drain is attached to bulb suction while the deep drain is kept to gravity. They are both removed on postoperative day 3 or when their output is less than 30 cc per 8 hour shift.

Postoperative Care

At our institution, postoperative care consists of bracing for 3 months in a TLSO; treatment with calcium citrate (1.2 g) and vitamin D (2000 units); serial radiographs; and outcome measures at 6 weeks, then at 3, 6, 12, and 24 months if the patients consent.

COMPLICATIONS

The treatment of spinal fractures that require surgical stabilization, particularly those with a coexistent spinal cord injury, frequently have associated trauma to numerous other skeletal sites and organ systems that compounds patient recovery.[25,37,49-52] The presence of concurrent chronic illnesses has also been shown to significantly increase the chance of developing posttraumatic complications.[4] The synergistic effect of any preexisting comorbidities, polytrauma, and the need for extensive surgery required in stabilizing any long bone fractures and the unstable fracture-dislocation of the spine frequently leads to a high incidence of complications.[49,52,53] Complications can occur during all three major phases of treatment: preoperatively, perioperatively, and postoperatively. Complications that may occur during any phase include progressive neurologic deficit, hypotension, infection, deep vein thrombosis, pulmonary embolus, pneumonia or respiratory failure, myocardial infarction, urinary tract infections, and cerebrovascular accidents.[41,49-51,53-56] Perioperative complications specifically related to surgery include blood loss, spinal fluid leaks, spinal cord or nerve root injury, major vascular injury, instrumentation misplacement, and retroperitoneal or pleural violation. These complications are so prevalent that one study showed a 79% incidence of total complications.[57] Also, there may be severe soft tissue injuries that need to be addressed at the time of surgery, including skin, fascial, and muscle tears, with degloving skin injuries representing one of the most difficult treatment issues because of their propensity to develop infections or necrosis.

Intraabdominal Injuries

Intraabdominal complications can occur in any fracture-dislocations of the spine but are commonly associated with a seat belt injury or a Chance fracture. The associated injuries include serosal tearing, a duodenal injury resulting in a fistula, ruptured gallbladder and spleen, liver laceration, pancreatitis, hollow viscus rupture (66%),[42] transection of jejunum, small bowel perforation, or entrapment between the vertebrae and a major vessel injury.[20,23] The *seat belt sign* (i.e., transverse low anterior abdominal bruising from a lap belt) has been found to be highly predictive of an abdominal injury (85%) and subsequent need for laparotomy (70%).[58] These injuries may be identified with an abdominal CT scan or peritoneal lavage. When considering surgical stabilization, it is very important to have a general or vascular surgeon on standby in case some of these intraabdominal injuries are present.[20]

Dural Tears

Traumatic durotomies are frequently encountered in the setting of high-energy injuries such as flexion-distraction injuries or fracture-dislocations of the thoracolumbar spine. Complete absence of the dura with exposed neural elements may also be encountered. It is the authors' experience that traumatic durotomies are rarely amenable to primary repair. We regularly treat these with a combination of fibrin glue, fat, or muscle grafts and synthetic dural graft material. Iatrogenic durotomies are commonly reparable and all attempts should be made to obtain a primary watertight closure. Subarachnoid drainage using a lumbar drain and postoperative Trendelenburg positioning are options to help decrease hydrostatic pressure on the repair or patch. We do not routinely use subfascial drains in the setting of traumatic durotomies that cannot be repaired primarily.

Neurologic Complications

Neurologic injury can occur because of the initial injury or as part of the treatment process. The immediate impact of the injury itself can produce neurologic deficits as part of either a concussive or a disruptive effect. This results in the patients presenting initially with neurologic deficits, the severity and pattern of which depends on the anatomic parts of the nervous system involved, ranging from single nerve root involvement to complete spinal cord injury. The severity of neurologic injury has been shown to have a direct correlation with local and systemic complications even after the surgical stabilization of these injuries.[40] Whether or not a delayed neurologic deterioration is considered a complication is debatable, but progression can occur after the initial injury from a compressive effect of the fractured fragments, soft tissues, or a developing hematoma. This group comprises about 3.4% of patients admitted after spinal trauma and has a much better prognosis if surgical reduction, decompression, and stabilization are carried out.[59] As previously stated, the effect of timing of surgery on the neurologic outcome continues to be debated with the consensus being that the initial neural axis injury level and motor score are the most predictive of neurologic outcome,[60] and at the very least early surgery will decrease the chance of a secondary neurologic injury from an inadvertent mobilization injury on the hospital floor. Evacuation of hematoma or corpectomy done through an anterior approach and laminectomy through a posterior approach are the methods most commonly used for achieving decompression of the neural structures. Indirect reductions of the fractures or dislocations using instrumentation are also used for the same purpose. A very small number of patients may develop late neurologic deterioration caused by a progressive deformity after nonoperative treatment.

The most preventable neurologic complication is the one that occurs from the surgical treatment itself. This can happen from the direct injury caused by surgical instruments or the stabilizing instrumentations such as hooks and screws, the reduction maneuver, an expanding epidural hematoma, loss of fixation leading to instability, and spinal cord ischemia resulting from vascular compromise. Continuous and careful intraoperative and postoperative monitoring, early detection, and appropriate quick intervention are key factors in the prevention and treatment of this complication.

It is imperative to always use intraoperative neurologic monitoring to identify a potential neurologic complication during surgery. MEP, SSEP, and EMG modalities should be regularly used to monitor the spinal cord and nerve root function. Any deterioration in the signals should alert the surgeon to inform the anesthesia team to immediately evaluate the patient for hypotension and hypothermia and to take corrective measures. If this is ineffective, then the instrumentation should be loosened or removed. Instrumentation may cause additional neurologic injury by narrowing the spinal canal and causing cord compression or impinging the exiting nerve roots. This impingement can occur at the time of insertion, during distractive or compressive maneuvers, or after loss of fixation from the bone. Improved placement of pedicle screws to avoid the risk of neurologic injury can be facilitated by proper training, using a continuous running EMG probe during pedicle screw placement, and the use of fluoroscopy.[61] Navigated pedicle screw insertion using the O-arm (Medtronic, Memphis, TN) or other similar technologies are a major advancement in the accurate placement of the pedicle screws.[32,62]

Occasionally, postoperative neurologic deterioration can occur because of loss of fixation that results in the recurrence of the traumatic deformity and neurologic compression. This can be prevented by periodic radiographic evaluations in the postoperative period, thus facilitating the early detection of the loss of fixation and preventing the development of late deformity. The loss of fixation by the pedicle screws can lead to penetration into the central spinal canal or the lateral recess, leading to neurologic compromise. This should be immediately addressed with the removal of the offending screw and by providing additional fixation points. Long-term monitoring of the reduction and status of the fracture healing should continue until solid fusion or healing is confirmed.

Postoperative Infections

Perhaps one of the most devastating postoperative complications is the occurrence of a postoperative infection, which can occur in up to 10% of patients in reported series.[63] The key to preventing postoperative infections is having well-developed perioperative protocols. These protocols should require precise presurgical planning, including preoperative antibiotic showers when feasible, a thorough preoperative skin preparation and use of adhesive antibacterial membrane, perioperative antibiotics, meticulous soft tissue care, rapid and efficient surgery to minimize operative time, pulsatile lavage, frequent loosening and repositioning of the retractors to prevent myonecrosis, instillation of vancomycin powder directly into the wound when indicated, and a tight closure of the fascia and skin. Vancomycin powder has been shown to dramatically lower the infection rate and should be used in all high-risk surgical stabilizations.[64,65] Postoperative infections generally occur within 2 to 3 weeks after the index surgical spine procedure and may present with drainage, fever, an elevated sedimentation rate, and elevated C-reactive protein (CRP). An MRI can be useful in identifying the extent of the infection.[66] Superficial infections (above the fascia) can be treated with local wound care, packing, and oral or intravenous outpatient antibiotics. However, meticulous wound examination needs to be done to rule out any possibility of the existence of a deep wound infection that requires serial and aggressive wound debridement.[67,68] Adjuncts to surgical debridement include perioperative antibiotics, irrigation, vancomycin powder or tobramycin bead placement into the wound. Consultation with an infectious disease specialist is highly recommended. When dealing with complex soft tissue problems, such as degloving injuries, the involvement of a plastic surgeon is recommended, particularly when vacuum-assisted closure is implemented to stimulate the formation of granulation tissue and wound cleansing.[69-71]

Prompt diagnosis and treatment of patients who develop deep infections optimizes treatment success and will generally clear an early-onset infection. Although early treatment allows for the retention of the spinal instrumentation, a delay in open debridement or inadequate oral antibiotic treatment often leads to a chronic infection requiring instrumentation removal or exchange.[70]

Other Complications

There are numerous other complications, most of which are not unique to traumatic injuries to the spine and can also occur during surgery and in the postoperative period. Pulmonary complications secondary to prolonged mechanical ventilation may result in pneumonia and eventually the need for a tracheostomy. Although rare, thrombophlebitis and pulmonary embolus, which have incidences of 15% and 0.5% to 2.7%, respectively, may also occur and require therapeutic anticoagulation or inferior vena cava filter placement.[72-74]

After severe polytrauma, patients with spinal injuries may experience acute renal failure after an acute hypotensive episode caused by blood loss or neurogenic hypotension (because of a loss of sympathetic tone), which causes acute tubular necrosis and may require temporary dialysis. In cases of either a complete thoracolumbar level spinal cord injury or a conus medullaris injury, the patient may also develop a neurogenic bladder that requires a urology consultation for bladder training and intermittent bladder catheterization. Patients with neurogenic bladders have frequent urinary tract infections that eventually lead to renal failure, urosepsis, and death. Finally, long-term monitoring of renal function and rapid treatment of urinary tract infections is critical because renal failure was once the leading cause of death (40%) in spinal cord injury patients before routine antibiotic availability, which reduced the urologically related deaths to 2.8%.[75]

Decubitus ulcers are common after thoracolumbar fracture-dislocations because of the high frequency of a concurrent neurologic injury resulting in a loss of protective sensation. These ulcers commonly occur on the sacral and ischial tuberosities, occiput, olecranon, and other bony prominences. They are frequently preventable by providing proper sitting and wheelchair cushioning such as gel pads, foam or air cushions, and the proper education of the patient to perform periodic weight shifts using the upper extremities to prevent skin ischemia.[76] When ulcers occur, they are a costly and time-consuming problem that results in a serious morbidity to the patient. They can form quickly and need aggressive wound care and protection of the area to allow healing so that a full skin thickness ulcer with bony involvement and osteomyelitis does not develop. A full-thickness ulcer with underlying bony involvement requires complex reconstruction using multiple débridements and skin and myocutaneous flaps. A well-trained nursing staff or dedicated care team is critical to preventing this complication.

The presence of chronic painful dysesthesia has a reported incidence of 60% to 80% with 40% of those demonstrating severe enough pain to affect their activities of daily living. The onset of post-traumatic spinal cord dysesthesia can occur within weeks to years following the injury and is more common in older patients and with thoracic spinal cord injuries than with cervical injuries.[77] The symptoms can be treated with gabapentin (Neurontin), pregabalin (Lyrica), baclofen, antidepressants, anticonvulsants, opioids, clonidine, and sodium and potassium channel blockers.[78,79]

CONCLUSION

Fracture-dislocation injuries of the spine are major traumatic injuries that occur in many patterns and are frequently associated with neurologic injury. Because these injuries to the thoracic and lumbar spine result in displacement of the vertebrae, they will almost certainly render the spine unstable because of the disruption of the spine's critical stabilizing structures. Additionally, fracture-dislocation injuries to the spine are frequently associated with injuries to multiple organ systems, and early surgery has been shown to improve numerous nonneurologic outcome parameters, including the ability to safely mobilize the patient and decrease the intensive care stay, hospital stay, hospital costs, and the incidence of pneumonia in thoracic fractures. Treatment by modern surgical intervention protocols also provides immediate reduction and long-term stabilization of these injuries and protects the patient from any secondary neurologic injury. When these surgical techniques are combined with modern neuromonitoring modalities, versatile pedicle instrumentation systems, bone graft materials and substitutes, and precise intraoperative guidance systems, the surgical interventions can be effective in treating these complex and unstable injuries.

KEY REFERENCES

The level of evidence (LOE) is determined according to the criteria provided in the preface.

14. Vaccaro A, Zeiller SC, Hulbert RJ, et al: The thoracolumbar injury severity score: a proposed treatment algorithm. *J Spinal Disord Tech* 18:209–215, 2005. LOE III
16. Vaccaro A, Baron EM, Sanfilippo J, et al: Reliability of a novel classification system for thoracolumbar injuries: the Thoracolumbar Injury Severity Score. *Spine* 31(11 Suppl):S62–S69, 2006. LOE III
37. Cengiz S, Kalkan E, Bayir A, et al: Timing of thoracolumbar spine stabilization in trauma patients; impact on neurological outcome and clinical course. A real prospective (RCT) randomized controlled study. *Arch Orthop Trauma Surg* 128(9):959–966, 2008. LOE II
38. Bellabarba C, Fisher C, Chapman JR, et al: Does early fracture fixation of thoracolumbar spine fractures decrease morbidity or mortality? *Spine* 35(9):S138–S145, 2010. LOE IV
39. Rutges J, Oner FC, Leenen LP: Timing of thoracic and lumbar fracture fixation in spinal injuries: a systematic review of neurological and clinical outcome. *Eur Spine J* 16(5):579–587, 2007. LOE IV
40. Dimar J, Carreon LY, Riina J, et al: Early versus late stabilization of the spine in the polytrauma patient. *Spine* 35(21 Suppl):S187–S192, 2010. LOE III
57. Dimar J, Fisher C, Vaccaro A, et al: Predictors of complications after spinal stabilization of thoracolumbar spine injuries. *J Trauma* 69(6):1497–1500, 2010. LOE III
60. Kingwell S, Noonan VK, Fisher CG, et al: Relationship of neural axis level of injury to motor recovery and health-related quality of life in patients with a thoracolumbar spinal injury. *J Bone Joint Surg Am* 92(7):1591–1599, 2010. LOE III

The complete References list is available online at https://expertconsult.inkling.com.

35D Fractures of the Low Lumbar Spine

ADRIENNE MORAFF • DAVID M. PRIOR • TIMOTHY MOORE

Fractures of the lower lumbar spine present unique challenges in diagnosis, initial management, and long-term outcomes. Differences in anatomy, biomechanics, and neurologic elements at this level all contribute to a picture distinct from fractures in other areas of the spine. Proper management of these injuries requires thorough knowledge of these attributes and the corresponding differences in the way these fractures must be evaluated and treated.

Low lumbar spine fractures, starting at L3 and ending at the L5 to S1 disc, are often discussed together with fractures of the thoracolumbar junction. The thoracolumbar junction is a transition point between the largely immobile thoracic spine, stabilized by the rib cage, and the much more mobile lumbar spine. Fractures of this area are common because energies unable to overcome the bony stabilization forces in the thoracic spine cause enough deformation and tension at the flexible junctions of L1 or L2 to cause the cortical bone and ligamentous complexes to fail.

The low lumbar spine is distinct from the thoracolumbar junction because it represents a mobile, flexible, lordotic segment of the spine (Table 35D-1). Structural components most often fracture at the junction between the mobile and immobile, or flexible and inflexible, as seen in the thoracolumbar junction. In contrast, L3 and L4 fall in the center of this highly flexible region of the spine and thus are less likely to fracture when traumatic forces are applied to the spine. On the caudal end of the low lumbar spine, the transition of L5 into the immobile sacrum is protected by a large iliolumbar ligamentous complex that provides unique stability not seen in the thoracolumbar junction. Fractures in this area of the spine are much less frequent and display specific patterns of injury. As such, the classification systems standardized for the

TABLE 35D-1 *UNIQUE DISTINCTIONS BETWEEN LOW LUMBAR AND THORACOLUMBAR INJURIES*

Thoracolumbar	Low Lumbar
Anatomic	
Kyphotic alignment	Lordotic alignment
Tolerates further kyphosis	Kyphosis poorly tolerated
Facet orientation coronal plane	Facet orientation sagittal plane
Smaller bodies and discs	Larger bodies and discs
Spinal cord, conus, and cauda equina	Cauda equina and exiting nerve roots
Smaller canal diameter and cross-sectional area	Greater canal diameter and cross-sectional area
Biomechanical	
Weight-bearing line anterior to spine	Weight-bearing within vertebral body
Motion in all three planes	Motion more limited to flexion-extension
Higher flexion bending loads	More axial and extension bending loads
Surgical Consideration	
Small pedicles	Large pedicles
Increased risk of neurologic injury	Lower risk of neurologic injury
Fusion tolerated	Fusion poorly tolerated
Anterior approaches accessible	Anterior approaches less accessible

thoracolumbar junction may not be applicable in the low lumbar spine. Treatment algorithms developed for the thoracolumbar junction similarly are not necessarily applicable to the low lumbar spine and care must be taken to tailor treatment appropriately.

Injuries to the low lumbar spine occur much less frequently than other areas of the spine. Fractures of L3 to L5 account for 4% of all spine fractures[1] compared with thoracolumbar junction fractures (T12–L2), which account for approximately 60% of all spine fractures as detailed in previous chapters.[2]

Quality literature is lacking in directing treatment for low lumbar injuries. Historically, operative treatment has often been perceived too risky with many complications and often avoided in neurologically intact patients. Neurologically intact patients with low lumbar fractures have often been treated with benign neglect. Chronic pain and deformity have been acceptable outcomes in times past with surgery reserved for injuries with significant vertebral body comminution and neurologic deficits. Modern posterior spinal instrumentation allows a safe approach to correct sagittal and coronal plane deformities and decompression if needed while protecting the neurologic elements. The added risks of a transperitoneal or retroperitoneal approach can usually be avoided using new techniques that allow reconstruction of the anterior and middle columns posteriorly. These newer fixation techniques have changed many institutions' approaches to the management of these fractures with greater emphasis on operative correction of severe deformity if present.

Low lumbar fractures are distinct from injuries to the thoracolumbar junction. The most important difference is in the ability to tolerate focal kyphosis. Focal kyphosis is tolerated in the thoracolumbar junction because the sagittal plane deformity can be "hidden" by compensation in the upper thoracic and low lumbar spines. Focal kyphosis is not well tolerated in the low lumbar spine. A minimal sagittal plane deformity in this area disrupts the overall sagittal alignment and mechanics of the spine as a unit. The pelvis attempts to decrease the sacral inclination by turning the sacrum more vertically, necessitating the hips to hyperextend. The deformity is akin to a "flat-back" deformity and positive sagittal balance. The ability of the fractured vertebral body to maintain sagittal alignment is paramount in determining treatment for low lumbar fractures. Because of this intolerance to focal kyphosis, the accepted (but not clinically validated) parameters for deformity acceptance in the thoracolumbar spine of 30 degrees of focal kyphosis and 50% loss of height[3] do not pertain to fractures of the low lumbar spine.

The anatomy of the low lumbar spine is made up of the individual bony elements, intervertebral discs, ligamentous complexes, and overall arrangements of the elements in situ. Sagittal balance is vital for normal function, particularly in the lumbar spine. Net sagittal balance is determined by the concert of all the above components. The bony anatomy is determined by the fixed kyphosis of the thoracic spine (15–49 degrees[4]). Because the thoracic spine structure is fixed by the rib cage, it is a relative constant and determines the lordotic nature of the more flexible cervical and lumbar spines. The normal curvature of the spine transitions from lordosis in the cervical spine, to kyphosis in the thoracic spine, back to lordosis in the lumbar spine (Fig. 35D-1). Lordosis in the lumbar spine is created by the anterior orientation of the superior endplate of the sacrum in the sagittal plane, necessitating anterior angling of the superior lumbar segments. The intervertebral discs at this level are greater in height anteriorly than posteriorly, which supports the lordotic curve to the apex at L3. The importance of maintenance of the appropriate degree of curvature in the spine to prevent pain and loss of function is apparent at every spinal segment. Loss of lordosis in the lumbar spine is a source of potentially disabling pain because the axial loading forces of the spine become abnormally distributed more anteriorly along the vertebral bodies rather than primarily over the middle column in the normal lumbar spine. Loss of curvature produces shear stress over the disc spaces and increases strain on the posterior ligamentous complexes (PLCs) and the posterior longitudinal ligament. Restoration and maintenance of lordosis in low lumbar fractures is vital to successful management of these injuries. Posttraumatic "flat-back" deformity can be a cause of significant morbidity in the form of pain and need for surgical correction.[5]

Axial load, or the forces exerted vertically downward by the action of gravity on the body, is greatest in the low lumbar spine. The vertebral bodies are correspondingly larger, as are the intervertebral discs. This distributes the load over a larger weight-bearing surface, decreasing the percentage of compression borne by a given area of vertebral body compared with other areas of the spine. In the normal alignment, the weight-bearing line falls anterior to thoracolumbar junction but posterior or within the body of the low lumbar fractures. This decreases bending moments in the low lumbar fractures and makes these patients somewhat less likely to develop

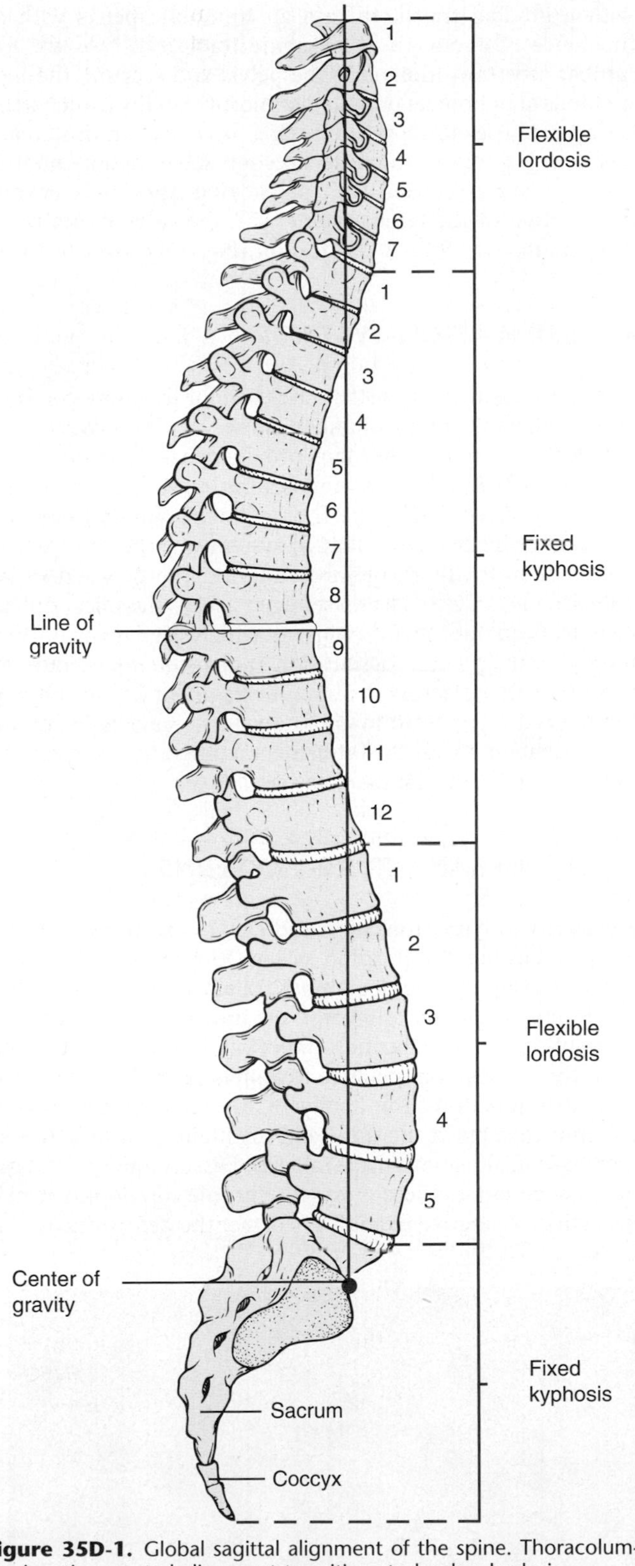

Figure 35D-1. Global sagittal alignment of the spine. Thoracolumbar junction neutral alignment transitions to lumbar lordosis.

progressive kyphosis. Furthermore, the decreased bending moments reduce stress on pedicle screws, so fixation can often be obtained using a single level above and below.

A unique advantage in the low lumbar spine is the larger diameter of the pedicles. This makes instrumentation safer and allows the use of larger screw diameters, achieving stronger fixation with lower risk of screw failure. Risk of further neurologic damage from surgery is lower because the cauda equina and exiting nerve roots are more tolerant than spinal cord. However, fusion in the lumbar spine is much less tolerated and should be avoided as much as possible. Furthermore, intervertebral disc injuries, which are a major but poorly recognized component of thoracolumbar injuries, are likely more significant in the lower lumbar spine than at higher levels.

The structure of L5 in relation to the rest of the axial spine bears mentioning separately. As previously mentioned, structural components tend to fail at the junction of immobile and mobile segments. The sacrum just below L5 is highly immobile within the pelvis. Rather than being a vulnerable stress point, as seen in the thoracolumbar junction, the variable placement of L5 below the pelvic brim and ligamentous attachments to the ilium protect it from injury. Because it is below the pelvic brim, L5 is shielded from most direct blows that might cause structural failure. The iliolumbar ligaments, attaching at the large transverse processes of L5, further stabilize this level. These anatomic characteristics protect the lumbosacral junction from the vulnerability to fracture under stress as seen in the thoracolumbar spine.

The neural elements of the spinal cord at the lower lumbar level are also different from the rest of the spine. The spinal cord ends in the conus medullaris at approximately L1 in a normal spine. The conus contains the anterior horn cells for bladder and bowel function and the bulbocavernosus reflex. Below the conus lies the cauda equina, or terminal nerve roots of the spinal cord. The cauda equina is entirely composed of lower motor neuron fibers, all with synapses in the conus medullaris. As a result, injuries to the neural elements in the low lumbar spine usually involve the lower motor neurons of the cauda equina only, with correspondingly better chance for recovery compared with upper motor neuron injury in the spinal cord (Fig. 35D-2).

The diameter and cross-sectional area of the spinal canal in the lumbar spine are smaller than in the cervical spine but larger than in the thoracic spine. In the thoracic spine, the spinal canal averages $17.2 \times 16.8\ mm^2$ and contains a spinal cord measuring approximately $86.5\ mm^2$ or about 50% of the canal area. In the lumbar spine, the canal is larger, usually greater than 100 mm, and the mobile roots of the cauda equina occupy a small percentage of the overall area.[6] The canal at this level is wedge shaped with the point of the wedge oriented posteriorly, its sides formed by the lamina, allowing L5 to exhibit the widest spinal canal dimension.[7] The comparative excess space for the neurologic elements explains the tolerance against neurologic injury that this area of the spine exhibits.[8]

UNIQUE BIOMECHANICAL FEATURES

The motion of any segment of the spine is controlled by the orientation of the facet joints. Except at L5 to S1, the low lumbar facet joints lie in the sagittal plane with convex inferior facets seated within concave superior facets. This arrangement allows for flexion and extension. Less shingling and greater space between the posterior elements of adjacent lumbar levels contribute to this freedom of motion in extension. Because of the slight lateral-facing orientation, there is some

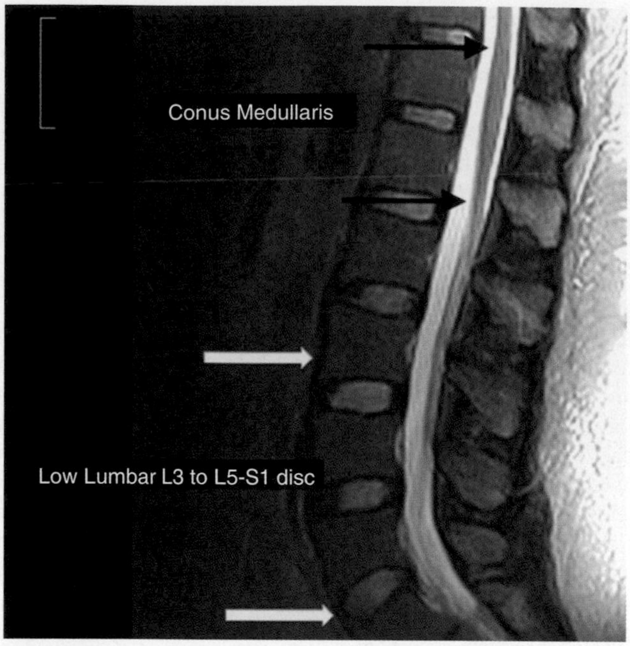

Figure 35D-2. Sagittal T2-weighted magnetic resonance image of lumbar spine. The conus medullaris variably ends at the L1 to L2 level. The cauda equina exits below the conus, often allowing more canal disruption without neurologic damage in low lumbar injuries.

degree of lateral bending but to a lesser degree compared with flexion and extension. Because the inferior facet joints are bounded in the horizontal plane by the superior facet joints of the vertebrae below it, the amount of rotation in the lumbar segment is very limited.[9]

The low lumbar spine is distinct from the thoracolumbar junction in the distribution of physiologic stresses. The thoracolumbar junction is a critical transition between the thoracic spine, immobilized and stabilized by the rib cage, and the mobile lumbar spine. Basic fracture biomechanics dictate that structural elements fail at the junction between high stability and lower stability, making this area particularly vulnerable to failure under stresses. This is reflected in the incidence of thoracolumbar fractures which make up 60% of all spine fractures. In contrast, the low lumbar region is a flexible segment with a gradual transition into an immobile pelvis with an incidence of about 4% of all spine fractures.[1,10] As the low lumbar area transitions into the pelvis and sacrum, the ligamentous attachments provide significant stability, which make isolated injuries to L5 very rare. If a force acts on this area, it has to be significant to create a recognizable injury. Often L5 fractures are associated with pelvic ring injuries or involve dissociation of the lumbar spine with the sacrum and pelvis as in traumatic L5 to S1 dislocation (Fig. 35D-3).

CLASSIFICATION SYSTEMS

Multiple classification systems are used for the more common and predictable thoracolumbar spine.[11-16] These have been detailed in Chapter 35A. Many providers use these same classification schemes for low lumbar injuries. At the time of this manuscript preparation, the Thoracolumbar Injury Classification and Severity Score (TLICS) system was the most widely used system for thoracolumbar trauma. The new Arbeitsgemeinschaft für Osteosynthesefragen (AO) classification has recently been published[14] and is not widely used thus far. What these thoracolumbar classification systems *do not* account for is focal kyphosis across the fracture fragment or the ability of the injured segment to maintain lordosis. As detailed earlier in this chapter, this is the fundamental difference between low lumbar and thoracolumbar injuries.

LOW LUMBAR INJURY PATTERNS

For clarity of communication and lack of an appropriate low lumbar–specific classification system, the same fracture patterns affecting the thoracolumbar spine can be applied to the low lumbar segments. However, the integrity of the posterior elements may not be the most important factor in determining operative versus nonoperative treatment, as it is in the thoracolumbar junction. The ability of the anterior and middle columns to support the spine and maintain lordosis is fundamental in dealing with these injuries. Disruption of this sagittal balance either acutely or as a chronic development may necessitate operative fixation to correct the deformity.

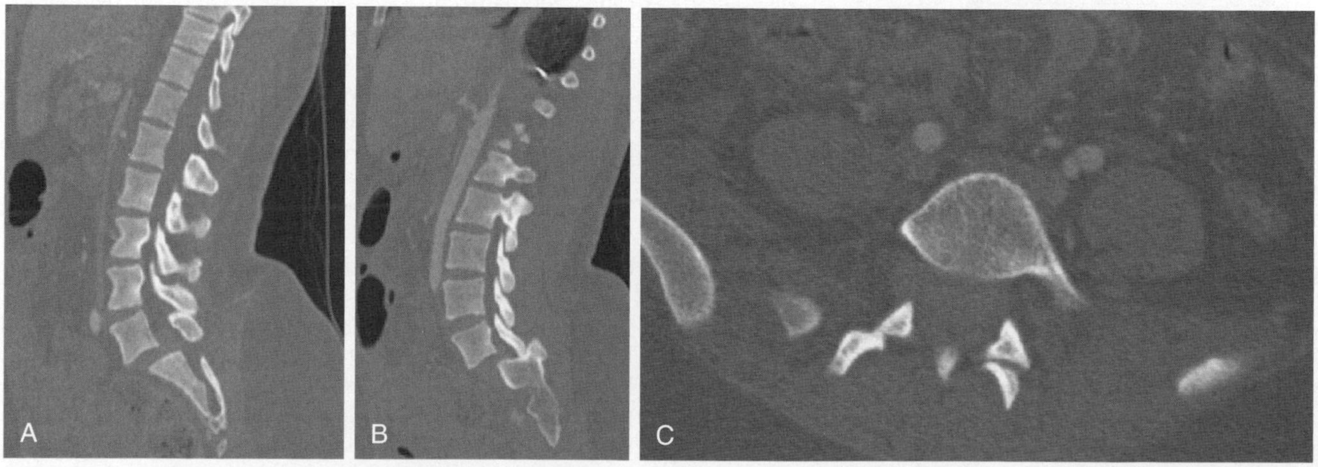

Figure 35D-3. **A,** Sagittal midline computed tomography (CT) scan of 22-year-old patient who was run over and dragged by a motor vehicle shows anterior translation of L5 on S1. **B,** Sagittal CT scan in the plane of articulation confirms L5 to S1 facet dislocation. **C,** Axial CT scan shows dislocation of L5 to S1 with dislocated and locked facet joints.

The terminology of "compression," "burst," "flexion-distraction," "Chance," and "fracture-dislocation" can help us understand low lumbar injuries.[18] In 2002, Anderson[17] reported on 54 patients, 25 with compression fractures, 21 burst fractures, three flexion-distraction fractures, and five fracture-dislocations within the lower lumbar spine. Thirty-four of the patients were neurologically intact, 17 were incomplete, and three were complete neurologic injuries. Recently, Lehman and colleagues[20] reported thoracolumbar and low lumbar burst fractures sustained by officers in military combat. Of the 32 patients sustaining burst fractures, 19 were in the low lumbar spine. One patient sustained noncontiguous burst fractures in the thoracolumbar and low lumbar area. Of the 19 low lumbar burst fractures, 10 sustained neurologic injury, two of which were complete injuries. The authors believed the body armor changed the body mechanics, thus lowering the transition zone from the thoracolumbar area to the lower lumbar area.[20]

In addition to the bony injuries, several injury patterns involve the paraspinous musculature, ligamentous structures, and bony avulsions that should be considered as well. L5 transverse process fractures in vertical shear pelvic injury patterns are indirect evidence of iliolumbar ligament compromise and should be treated accordingly (Fig. 35D-4). Additionally, multiple transverse process fractures may be indicative of more high-energy injuries. Nerve root avulsions may happen concordantly with transverse process fractures and must be evaluated with physical examination findings, imaging, and intraoperative exploration when necessary. Spinous process widening or avulsions can be indicators of PLC compromise.

Disc herniation in the adult population at the time of traumatic injury can occur and cause neurologic compromise. Decompression by removal of herniated disc fragments usually is sufficient to decompress the neural elements. In contrast, pediatric and adolescent patients may sustain endplate avulsions because the ligamentous attachments in this population are stronger than their bony elements (Fig. 35D-5). These avulsions may also cause neurologic compromise and should be treated with excision.

Compression Fractures

Fractures involving the superior endplate of the vertebral body are much more common in the thoracolumbar spine than in the low lumbar area. Close follow-up is necessary for these injuries to ensure that the patient does not develop focal kyphosis across the segment. These fractures have the capability of creating significant sagittal plane deformity and may lead to chronic low back pain when they occur in the low lumbar area. In contrast to compression fractures sustained in younger populations, compression fractures in elderly adults may occur with minimal trauma and be progressive. It is important to recognize that complete compression of the anterior column with posterior column involvement and neurologic compromise may occur months after injury, necessitating close follow-up for all low lumbar fractures treated nonoperatively.[20] Close attention should be paid to the PLC when high-energy injuries cause compression fractures. This pattern of injury occurs often as a flexion moment across the fulcrum of the middle column, causing compression in the anterior column and tension on the posterior column. The posterior column distraction injury may not be readily identifiable on computed tomography (CT) because it does not evaluate the ligamentous complex well. A high index of suspicion is necessary to critically evaluate alignment seen on plain radiographs and CT. Signs such as significant kyphosis greater than 30 degrees and widening of the interspinous process distance on plain radiographs or CT should prompt consideration of further evaluation for ligamentous injury by magnetic resonance imaging (MRI) (Fig. 35D-6).[20,21]

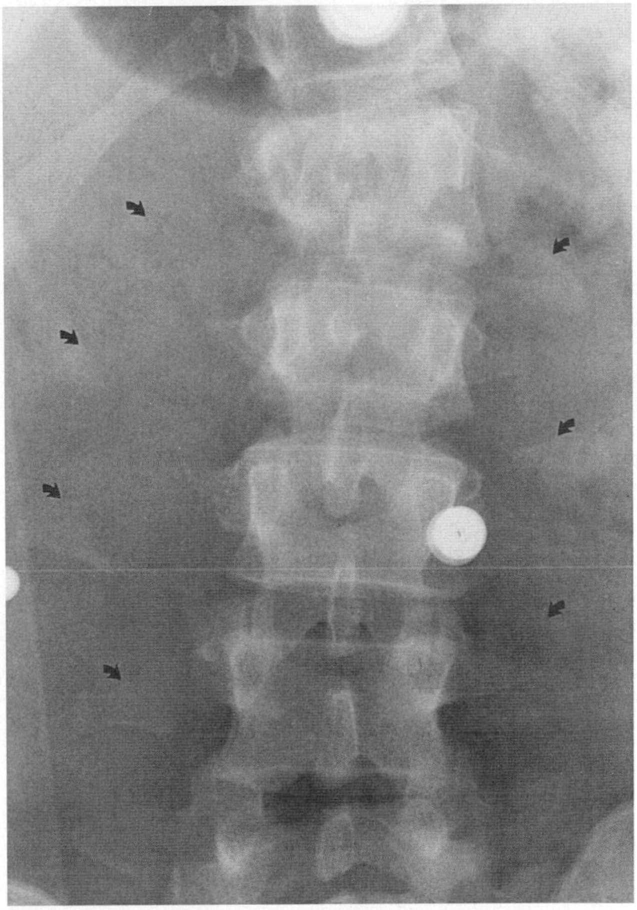

Figure 35D-4. Multiple transverse process fractures *(arrows)* seen on plain radiograph in a 24-year-old man involved in a motor vehicle collision.

Burst Fractures

By definition, burst fractures involve both the anterior and middle columns and are caused by a combination of flexion and axial loading. In Denis type A fractures, the predominant injury pattern is one of axial compression with significant vertebral body height loss and minimal kyphosis. The posterior vertebral body relationship with the pedicle may be compromised as well, and pedicle fractures are common in this injury pattern. Denis A fracture patterns are more common higher in the lumbar spine and occur more frequently at L2 and L3. Denis type B burst fractures have more of a flexion moment at the time of injury and represent a different type of injury pattern. These occur more commonly in the lower lumbar vertebrae, L4 and L5. They are characterized by a more pronounced kyphosis and height loss within the anterior column. Additionally, there is often a posterior-superior vertebral body "culprit" fragment retropulsed within the spinal

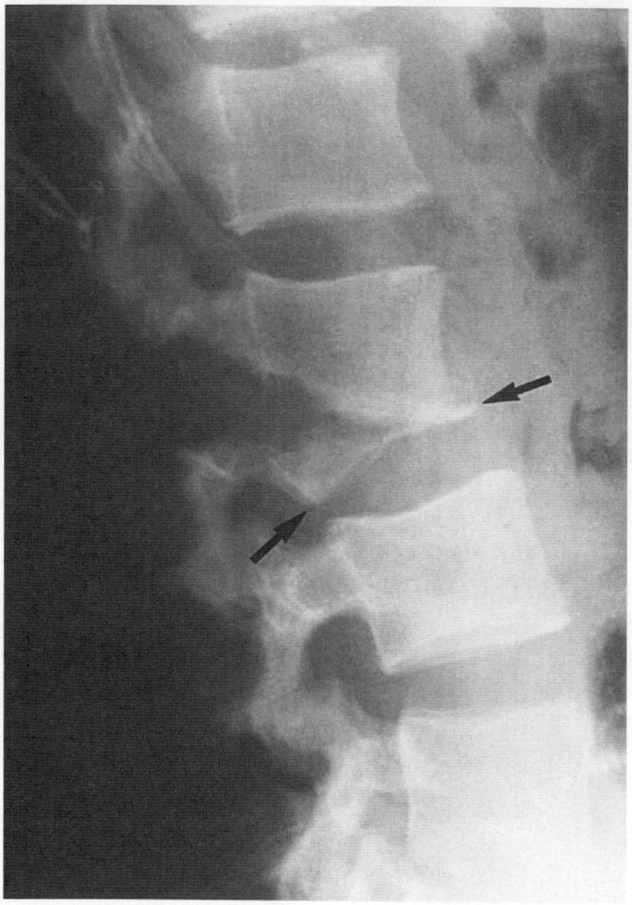

Figure 35D-5. Plain radiograph of an adolescent girl who sustained endplate avulsion fractures *(arrows)* of L3 from a flexion-distraction type injury.

canal that can create neurologic compromise as well.[20] As detailed earlier, there is a greater tolerance of the more voluminous spinal canal at the level of the lumbar spine to accommodate the fragment without creating a neurologic deficit. The neuroanatomy of the cauda equina also allows for more canal involvement without creating a neurologic deficit. Compared with the thoracolumbar area, these fractures often do not cause significant neurologic injury. Because of this, these fractures have often been treated by nonoperative means but often lead to significant morbidity secondary to loss of sagittal alignment and gross instability across the fracture segment. Pedicle fractures tend to be more common in the low lumbar area when there is a Denis type A burst pattern. Although a pedicle fracture may be tolerated in the thoracic and thoracolumbar area, close attention must be given to a pedicle fracture in the low lumbar area and avoidance of significant unilateral collapse, which can lead to posttraumatic coronal malalignment or significant subluxation of the fracture segment. Another feature common to burst-type injuries is a vertically oriented greenstick fracture of the spinous process or lamina. These frequently occur with dural tears, and often spinal nerve roots may be incarcerated within the greenstick fracture, necessitating decompression and release, as well as dural repair.[20]

Application of the TLICS system to management of low lumbar burst fractures may not appropriately represent their severity and risk for sagittal malalignment. If a burst fracture occurs in the thoracolumbar region with significant canal compromise, it is more likely to create a neurologic injury than in the low lumbar area. This increases the score of the fracture because the TLICS takes this into account and scores more highly when a neurologic injury has occurred. The same amount of canal compromise might not create a neurologic injury in the low lumbar area, but the injured osteology may

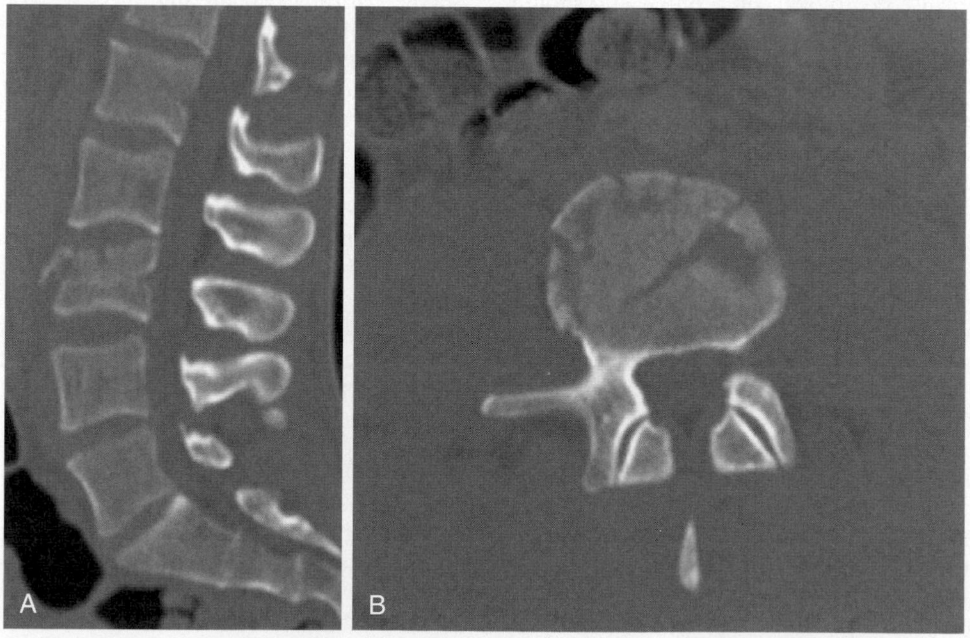

Figure 35D-6. Sagittal (**A**) and axial computed tomography scans (**B**) of a 27-year-old man involved in a motorcycle crash showing L3 compression fracture involving the superior endplate only.

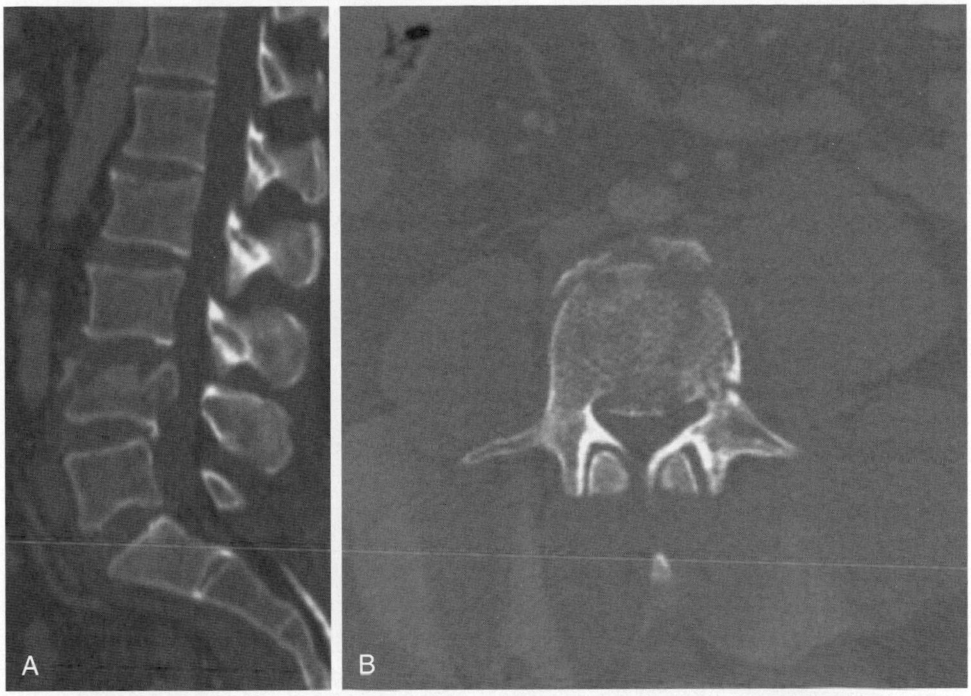

Figure 35D-7. Sagittal (**A**) and axial (**B**) computed tomography scans of a 47-year-old patient involved in a motorcycle crash showing an L4 burst fracture with left pedicle fracture.

not be competent enough to maintain the segment's alignment under physiologic loading. A severely comminuted L4 burst fracture in a neurologically intact patient might only score a 2 with the TLICS system but lead to progressive kyphosis and a flatback deformity if treated without surgical stabilization (Fig. 35D-7).

Flexion-Distraction (Chance) Fractures

Three major variants of flexion-distraction injuries occur in the lower lumbar spine. Purely bony injuries, first categorized by Chance in 1948, are often seen with the upper spine flexing over a fixed lumbopelvic junction. The injury extends from anterior to posterior through the vertebral body, into the pedicles, and exits the spinous process. This injury pattern is considered a relatively stable one and neurologic compromise is infrequent. Another variant involves facet joint subluxation or dislocation with anterior translation of the cephalad spinal segments. Significant neurologic compromise can follow injuries of this type depending on the magnitude of translation of one spinal segment with respect to adjacent segments. A third variant involves both bony and soft tissue elements and disruption of the PLC.

Flexion through the anterior and middle columns with distraction through the posterior elements can create an unstable segment with the ability to fall into focal kyphosis. In the thoracolumbar area, these injuries are often treated with surgery, but the natural progression in the low lumbar area is not well known. With injury to the low lumbar segments, there is more compensation within the anterior and middle columns without compromise to the posterior osteoligamentous complex (Fig. 35D-8). Relative sparing from neurologic injury must be weighed against progressive kyphosis and loss of sagittal plane alignment when considering nonoperative treatment measures.

Fracture-Dislocations

Fracture-dislocations are high-energy injuries that disrupt both the bony and ligamentous restraints of the motion segment (Fig. 35D-9). In the lower lumbar segments and especially through L5, these injuries are often associated with pelvic ring disruptions and fractures involving the superior articular processes of S1. These injuries usually require operative intervention to reduce the dislocation and segmental instrumentation to maintain the reduction. No matter where it occurs in the spine, this fracture pattern often involves devastating neurologic injury.

Shear Injuries

Significant multiplanar stress must be applied to the spinal column to sustain shear type injuries (Fig. 35D-10). Additionally, underlying conditions such as ankylosing spondylitis and diffuse idiopathic skeletal hyperostosis (DISH) may predispose to this type of high-grade injury pattern (Fig. 35D-11). Characteristically, this involves considerable translation in both coronal and sagittal planes. Disruption of all three columns occurs and must be taken into consideration when deciding on operative treatment. Shear-type injuries are highly unstable and not usually amenable to nonoperative measures.[20]

ASSESSMENT

Full Trauma Assessment

The evaluation of any trauma patient should follow the algorithms outlined by the Advanced Trauma Life Support protocol as discussed in Chapter 10. Immediate evaluation of airway, breathing, circulation, disability, and exposure are accomplished quickly by an experienced trauma team. The

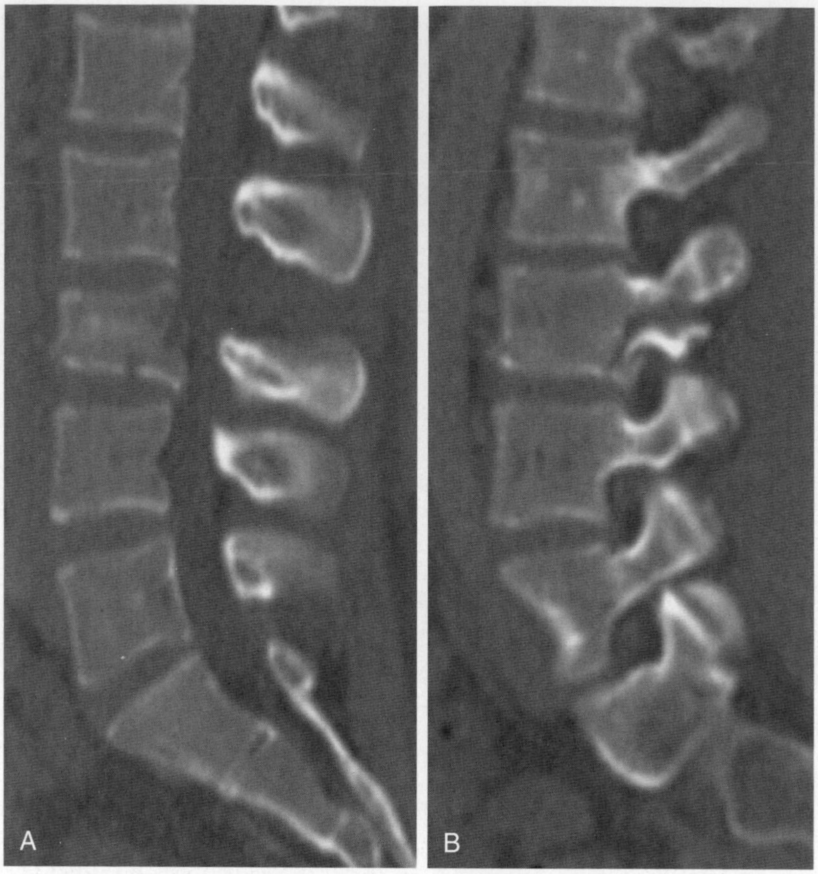

Figure 35D-8. A, Sagittal computed tomography (CT) scan of a 26-year-old patient involved in an all-terrain vehicle crash showing flexion and compression of the anterior column with distraction through the middle and posterior columns. **B,** Sagittal CT in plane of pedicles shows distraction to pedicle and extending into the vertebral body.

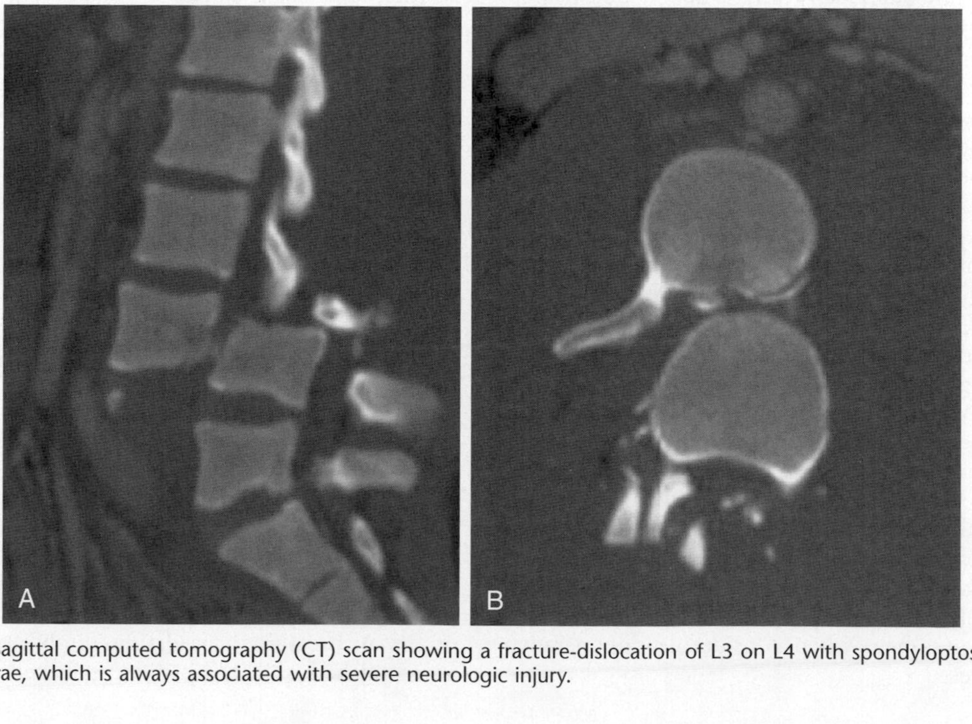

Figure 35D-9. A, Sagittal computed tomography (CT) scan showing a fracture-dislocation of L3 on L4 with spondyloptosis. **B,** Axial CT scan showing two vertebrae, which is always associated with severe neurologic injury.

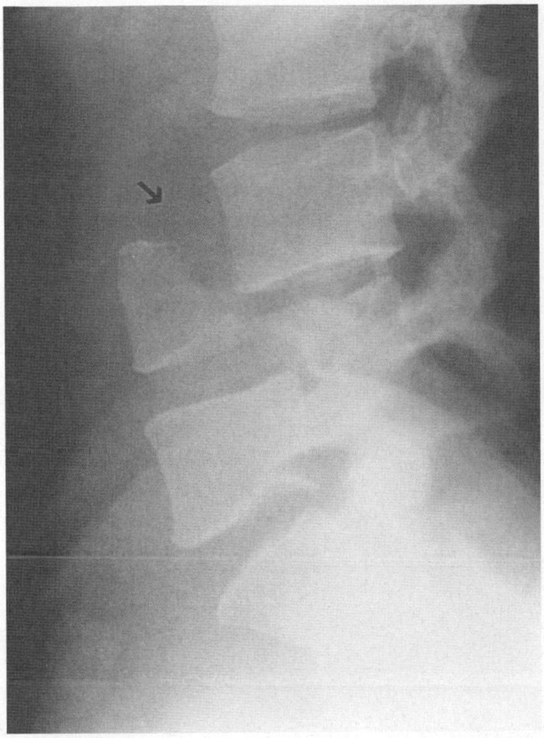

Figure 35D-10. Plain film demonstration of a high-grade shear mechanism of injury with axial and sagittal plane translational deformity *(arrow)* with three-column involvement.

secondary survey includes a full physical examination, including examination of the back and a complete neurologic assessment.

Key findings on physical examination include injuries with documented association with spinal fractures, including intraperitoneal free fluid and fractures of the rib, long bones of the lower extremity (femur, tibia), calcaneus, or pelvis.[17] Examination of the back should include the entire spine from the cervical spine to the sacrum and coccyx. With inline stabilization of the cervical spine, logrolling of trauma patients is imperative to assess for soft tissue integrity, tenderness, crepitus, step-off, and gross malalignment of the spine. Low lumbar injuries, especially at L5, may be associated with a degloving injury, the so-called Morel-Lavallee lesion, which may complicate any planned surgery and can be associated with considerable blood loss. Radiographic artifact needs to be ruled out in all trauma patients when considering surgical stabilization of apparent injuries.[22]

Examination

Neurologic Status

A full neurologic examination should be completed on admission as soon as the condition of the patient permits it. Complete documentation of motor function in major motor nerve root distributions in both upper and lower extremities should be performed when possible. Pinprick sensation in all major dermatomes as well as the perianal region should be performed. The bulbocavernosus reflex represents S4 and S5 and is most often spared even in the presence of complete cord injury more cephalad. In the absence of this reflex, spinal shock is likely present, a transient condition lasting usually 24 to 48 hours, with return of the bulbocavernosus reflex signaling its end. However, absence of this reflex in patients with low lumbar fractures indicates impairment of the cauda equina. Full evaluation of patients who are unconscious, intoxicated, demented, or otherwise unable to fully cooperate with the examination poses a difficult challenge. A high level of clinical suspicion for spinal cord injury is required in these patients. Reassessment should take place frequently in the first 48 hours of admission, as well as whenever there is a significant change in the clinical status of the patient. It is vital to obtain an accurate neurologic assessment because this will be a primary factor in the management of the patient. Patients with neurologic injury or patients who demonstrate deterioration on the neurologic examination should undergo decompression as soon as they are stable enough to permit surgery. Patients who are neurologically intact should be closely monitored for development of new neurologic symptoms.

In general with spinal trauma, neurologic injury is often caused by direct injury to the spinal cord. This is not normally seen in low lumbar fractures because the conus medullaris lies at L1. The cauda equina is the continuation of the cord from L2 and below. As a result, almost all neural injuries secondary to fractures of the low lumbar spine are peripheral nerve injuries. Compression of the cauda equina may present with motor or sensory deficits, as well as urinary and fecal incontinence or retention, saddle anesthesia, and low back pain that radiates down one or both legs. Complete injuries are rare at this level given the relative tolerance of lumbar nerves to injury compared with the spinal cord and the space within the spinal canal, which is widest at this level. Overall incidence of neurologic injury with lower lumbar spine trauma ranges from 47% to 76% in recent studies. The prognosis for improvement of neurologic injury is also comparatively better than for cord injuries. Injury may occur secondary to compression by fracture fragments or by traction on the nerve root, the latter of which may produce radiculopathy on the contralateral side to any fragments within the spinal canal.

American Spinal Injury Association Scale

Multiple systems are used to classify injury to the spinal cord. Isolated nerve root injuries should be described by the affected level and appropriate laterality.

The level of neurologic injury is defined as the most caudal segment of the spinal cord with fully intact motor and sensory function bilaterally. The American Spinal Injury Association (ASIA) motor score is based on manual muscle testing. Ten muscles are used to score motor function, five in the upper extremities and five in the lower extremities. Each muscle is scored out of 5 bilaterally, giving a total possible score of 100 for motor. Sensation is determined in each dermatome and graded as absent, impaired, or normal, with particular attention to sacral (S4–S5) sparing.

The ASIA impairment scale is a modification of the Frankel scale used to classify severity of neurologic injury (Fig. 35D-12). It is less useful in lower lumbar fractures because it does not take into account bladder and bowel impairment.

IMAGING

Radiographs

Radiographs play an increasingly small role in the initial evaluation of these injuries, with most patients undergoing CT as

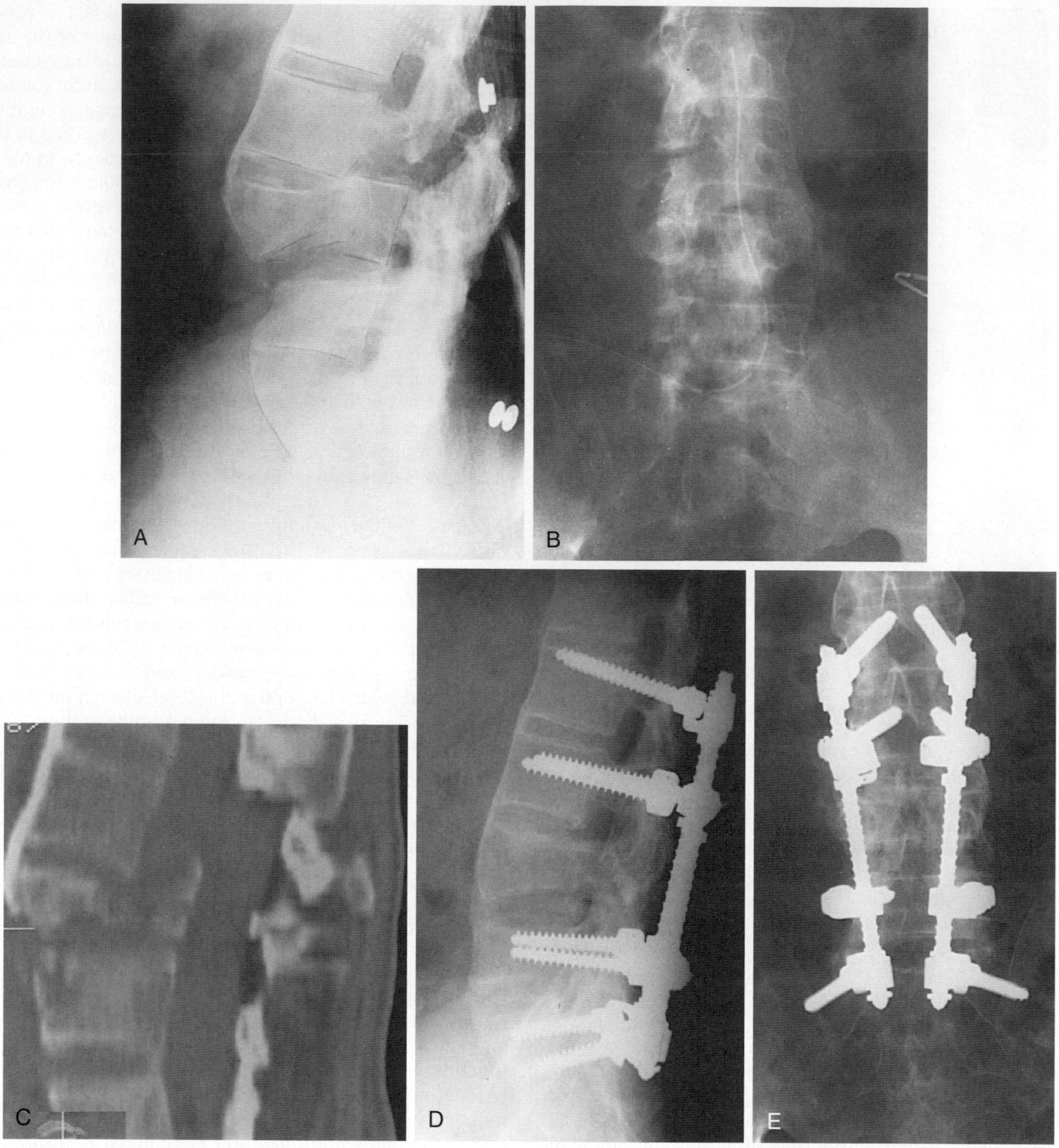

Figure 35D-11. Demonstration of a high-grade shear injury in a 31-year-old man with ankylosing spondylitis with subsequent instrumented fusion and correction of traumatic deformity.

a screening study. Anterior-posterior and lateral weight-bearing, standing radiographs of all low lumbar fractures should be obtained during the hospital evaluation if nonoperative treatment is selected. This gives the provider a "baseline" to compare future radiographs against and helps to determine stability. Stable injuries show no change from supine radiographs. Occult unstable fractures upon application of the axial load associated with weight-bearing will show an increase in these parameters on standing radiographs. This can often change the treatment of the injury.

Computed Tomography

Multidetector CT has supplanted plain film radiographs as the most diagnostically relevant medium to define bony injury in the lower lumbar spine.[23] It also better delineates canal compromise from retropulsed fracture fragments. It should be noted that attempting to obtain CT or MRI imaging on a hemodynamically unstable patient is contraindicated. When imaging is emergently necessary and it is unsafe to perform advanced imaging, plain radiographs should be used to screen the patient for injury. Further radiographic evaluation can

ASIA IMPAIRMENT SCALE

☐ **A = Complete:** No motor or sensory function is preserved in the sacral segments S4–S5.

☐ **B = Incomplete:** Sensory but not motor function is preserved below the neurological level and includes the sacral segments S4–S5.

☐ **C = Incomplete:** Motor function is preserved below the neurological level, and more than half of key muscles below the neurological level have a muscle grade less than 3.

☐ **D = Incomplete:** Motor function is preserved below the neurological level, and at least half of key muscles below the neurological level have a muscle grade of 3 or more.

☐ **E = Normal:** motor and sensory function are normal.

CLINICAL SYNDROMES

☐ Central Cord
☐ Brown-Sequard
☐ Anterior Cord
☐ Conus Medullaris
☐ Cauda Equina

Figure 35D-12. The American Spinal Injury Association (ASIA) impairment scale.

wait until immediate threats to life have been adequately managed.

Magnetic Resonance Imaging

Magnetic resonance imaging is an important imaging modality to aid in decision making in two areas. First is to evaluate the posterior osteoligamentous structures.[24-27] Some indirect evidence of ligamentous compromise can be determined based on the amount of displacement, kyphosis, and height loss on other imaging modalities but MRI is the most sensitive and specific. Additionally, MRI can offer information regarding nerve root and cauda equina compression as well as associated disc herniation. It is not the most expedient imaging modality, however, and its judicious use should be dictated by the ability to alter or augment surgical planning and not be ordered reflexively.

MANAGEMENT

Immediate

The first step in management is maintenance of airway, breathing, and circulation by a well-trained trauma team. Patients with airway compromise from injury or an inability to protect their airway secondary to mental status should be intubated in the trauma bay. Pulmonary compromise from chest injuries, including pneumothorax, flail chest, or lung parenchymal injury, should be managed by the trauma team as soon as the primary assessment has been completed. Hemodynamically compromised patients should be aggressively resuscitated with fluids and blood products, with judicious administration of intravenous (IV) fluids in the presence of neurogenic shock. Sources of bleeding should be rapidly identified and managed by an experienced trauma team surgeon. Significant displacement such as in the case of complete spondyloptosis may benefit from emergent closed reduction maneuvers.

Goals of Management

The basic goals of management of low lumbar fractures are the same as for any other type of spinal injury: decompression if indicated, restoration of anatomic alignment, stabilization, and prevention of further neurologic injury. In addition, preservation of motion segments and maintenance of sagittal balance are imperative when treating lower lumbar fractures. It is important to remember that the trauma patient may have multiple life-threatening injuries whose importance may supersede even their neurologic injury. Up to 50% of patients with L5 burst fractures had associated injuries to the thorax, pelvic ring, and extremities.[28] Surgery, however necessary, is taken by the body as a traumatic event that can be equivalent to any trauma experienced in the field, with violation of the protection of skin from outside elements, blood loss, and damage to internal organs and body systems, as well as significant hemodynamic changes. Collaboration with a well-trained trauma team and appropriate timing are essential for the success of any operation performed.

Nonoperative Treatment

There are currently no accepted guidelines for the management of low lumbar fractures. Nonsurgical management with careful follow-up should always be considered in a neurologically intact patient with a stable injury pattern (Table 35D-2). If decompression is not a management concern, the physician must consider stability of the injured segment and its ability to maintain neutrality or lordosis for the long-term functionality of the spinal unit. This is where experience and judgment combine with contemporary literature and outcomes to formulate appropriate treatment plans on a case-by-case basis. For example, an L3 burst fracture will require different management than an L5 pincer fracture with a Denis zone II sacral fracture. In addition, the age and activity level of the patient should always be considered when offering treatment for low lumbar burst fractures and maintaining motion segments becomes paramount in dealing with these injuries compared with thoracolumbar levels.

When considering nonsurgical treatment, the physician needs to focus on the potential for progressive sagittal deformity that can occur frequently in these injuries. Nonoperative treatments consist of observation, bracing, bed rest, and postural reduction. Soon after patients are mobilized, standing radiographs are obtained to determine the injury's behavior under physiologic stresses. Increased kyphosis may indicate

TABLE 35D-2 *INDICATIONS FOR NONOPERATIVE TREATMENT*	
Neurologic	Intact Isolated root injury
Fracture patterns	Transverse process Spinous process Compression fractures Stable burst fractures Bony Chance Bony flexion-distraction

an unstable fracture that requires alternative treatment such as stabilization.

Typical injury patterns amenable to nonoperative means are transverse process and spinous process fractures. In addition, compression fractures without significant kyphotic deformity and burst fractures without high-grade deformity or neurologic deficit may also be treated nonoperatively. Early mobilization may take place in patients with transverse or spinous process fractures or those with compression fractures once adequate pain control is achieved. Many low lumbar burst fractures can be treated nonoperatively. Those most amenable to nonoperative care have little kyphotic deformity, intact PLC, and a vertebral body that is not comminuted. Chance-type and flexion-distraction injuries that are primarily bony patterns and either have little kyphosis or can be reduced can be treated successfully nonoperatively.

Bracing has not been shown to affect the outcome in nonsurgical management of thoracolumbar fractures[29-31] but has not been studied specifically in low lumbar injuries. If bracing is used for injuries of L4 and lower spinal segments, the addition of a thigh cuff to limit hip flexion can decrease shear and flexion across the low lumbar segments. Thoracolumbar spinal orthosis (TLSO) bracing may diminish intersegmental motion within the lumbar spine and this may be improved with use of thigh extension. Paradoxically, increased motion has been shown below L4 with traditional TLSO immobilization, so thigh extensions should be used in these cases. Additionally, there may be a role for Risser casting in the pediatric population for bony Chance-type fractures as well.

Surgical Treatment

Surgical treatment involves all of the basic principles of treatment as with any other area of the spine:

1. Decompression of neural elements
2. Restoration of anatomic alignment
3. Stabilization
4. Prevention of further neurologic injury.

In addition, important considerations within the relatively mobile lumbar spine should include

1. Preservation of motion segments
2. Avoidance of complications

Decompression of low lumbar segments can be done almost exclusively through a posterior approach. Often restoration of the anterior column, if needed, can be performed more effectively under the same anesthesia or staged anterior transperitoneal or retroperitoneal approach.

When dealing with a patient with a significant low lumbar fracture, the basic principles of the TLICS[13] system can be useful, particularly in facilitating communication among providers regarding varying injuries. The TLICS does, however, have some shortcomings when dealing with lower lumbar injuries (Table 35D-3). For example, the anterior column can be significantly disrupted without causing a neurologic deficit or disruption of the posterior osteoligamentous complex, which would cause an L4 burst fracture to score low (2) on TLICS and encourage nonsurgical management. If, during close follow-up, the provider sees significant focal kyphosis and disruption of global sagittal alignment, (s)he should consider surgical stabilization to restore and maintain lumbar lordosis and global sagittal alignment despite the low TLICS score. In addition, delay of operative treatment by 6 weeks or more may be difficult from an anterior-only or posterior-only approach as some healing of the traumatic injury has occurred with residual deformity of both the anterior and posterior columns.[20] If surgery is being considered, some differences between treating thoracolumbar and low lumbar fractures are summarized in Table 35D-1.

TABLE 35D-3 *SURGICAL CONSIDERATIONS BETWEEN THORACOLUMBAR (T10–L2) AND LOW LUMBAR (L3–L5/S1) FRACTURES*

Factors Affecting Surgery	TLICS (T10–L2)	Low Lumbar (L3–L5/S1 Disc)
Posterior column	XXXX	XX
Vertebral body comminution	XX	XXXX
Kyphosis	X	XXXX
Neurologic injury	XXX	X
Fusion	XX	X

TLICS, Thoracolumbar Injury Classification and Severity Score; *X,* minimal importance; *XXXX,* maximal importance.

The timing of such surgery remains a topic of debate. It is the authors' recommendation that significant acute neurologic deficit associated with low lumbar fractures should be decompressed as soon as possible. Data concerning cauda equina compression in trauma is scarce, but early decompression has been shown to be safe and reduce length of stay and postoperative respiratory morbidity in patients with cervical and thoracolumbar spinal cord injuries.[32-40] Furthermore, there is good evidence that decompression of cauda equina syndrome from disc herniations and hematomas must be performed within 24 to 48 hours to achieve optimal results. Neurologic compression comes in many forms in the lower lumbar spine: from retropulsed fragments in the case of burst fractures, from traction injuries caused by fracture-dislocations, and from incarcerated nerve root injuries in the case of laminar fractures.[41] Decompression has been shown to be safe for acute neurologic deficit, and some studies show improved neurologic recovery.[6,7,10,17,42] The decompressive procedure usually warrants stabilization to prevent further neurologic injury and provide an optimal environment for fracture healing. This is achieved with instrumentation with or without fusion.

Decompression

Within the lumbar spine, unique characteristics make decompression approaches more straightforward than other areas of the spine but also have some challenges as well. Indirect decompression methods such as ligamentotaxis through the posterior elements are difficult to achieve in a hyperlordotic segment of the spine and, as such, are less successful than direct decompression. Laminectomy and dural repair are warranted in the case of incarcerated nerve roots in greenstick fractures. Rarely is laminectomy alone sufficient for decompression of retropulsed fragments in the presence of neurologic compromise and either mobilization of the thecal sac with direct posterior decompression or direct decompression anteriorly should be performed.[33] In the presence of retropulsed fragments in a burst fracture without neurologic compromise, no formal decompression is necessary because the natural course of these injuries is for the body to resorb much of the fragmentation that is compressing the thecal sac.[43]

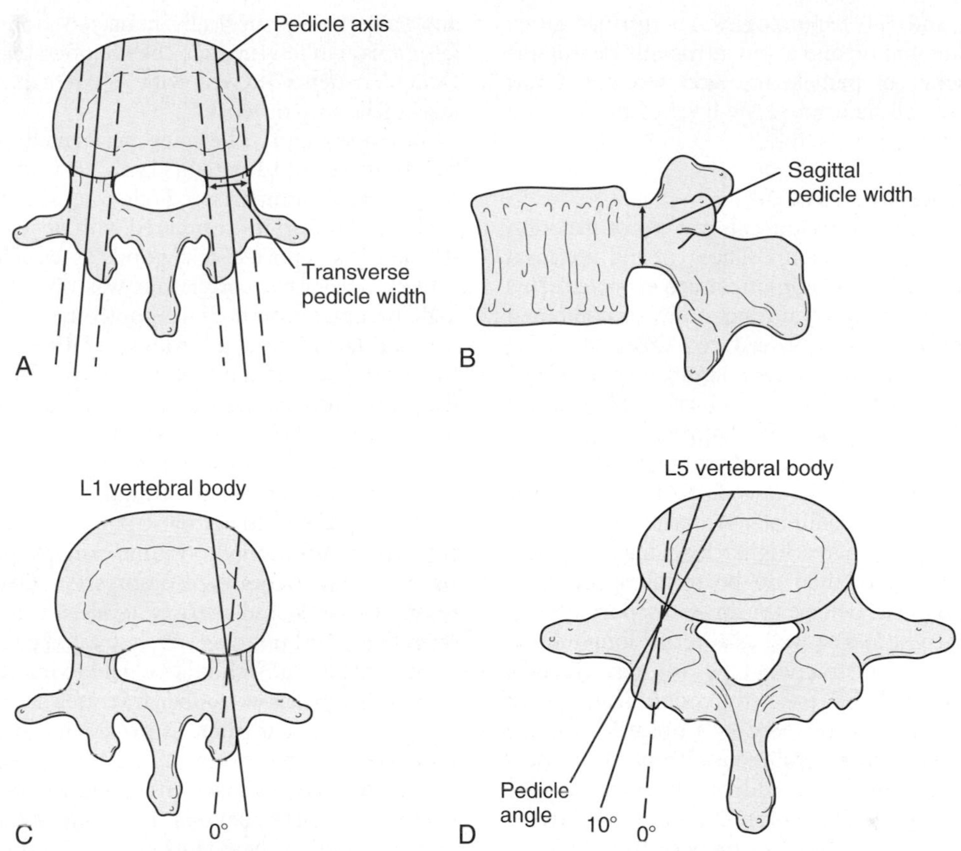

Figure 35D-13. Pedicle screw orientation of the lower lumbar spine follows predictable anatomic patterns of increasing pedicle width and medial inclination from L2 to L5.

Restoration of Alignment

The unique characteristic of low lumbar injuries is the intolerance of these segments to focal kyphosis. Most spine traumatologists feel a goal of treatment is to maintain lordosis or at least neutral sagittal alignment across the injured segment. It is becoming more accepted that fractures that create overall sagittal alignment issues may be ones to consider offering the patient surgical stabilization even in the face of no neurologic injury. This is due to the more complete understanding of the concept of global sagittal alignment as well as regional sagittal balance in affecting clinical outcomes.[44]

Posterior Instrumentation

Modern posterior segmental instrumented constructs afford sufficient stability to maintain alignment depending on the pattern of injury. Additionally, given the relative tolerance of the dura and spinal nerve roots to mobilization at this level, indirect and direct decompressions can be performed from posterior-only approaches. Critical attention needs to be focused on whether or not to perform a fusion, the number of instrumented and fusion levels, and the need to cross the sacroiliac joint for stability to the pelvis. In a study comparing short segment instrumentation and concomitant fusion versus no fusion, Wang and colleagues[46] demonstrated improved functional outcomes, less donor site morbidity, and improved sagittal profile in patients treated by instrumentation without fusion rather than with fusion. If the decompression portion of the procedure requires significant bony removal, a fusion procedure should be considered to stabilize the posterior column of the spine. Fusion in general does not prevent postoperative loss of correction in sagittal profile, however.[45]

Additionally, posterior approaches obviate the morbidity associated with operating in the peritoneal cavity as well as retroperitoneal extracavitary approaches. Long segment constructs are not well tolerated in the lumbar spine and may not be necessary to restore stability to the PLC. They can precipitate later degenerative changes in the remaining uninvolved lower lumbar segments. Additionally, posterior approaches afford the opportunity for percutaneous fixation, which holds added benefit of decreased surgical site morbidity and diminished blood loss despite an initially steeper learning curve. Some reduction and restoration of alignment may be achieved through posterior constructs with distraction and reduction techniques.[10] However, one should expect some postoperative loss of correction with both posterior-only and posterior and anterior combined constructs.

Robust posterior segmental instrumentation may be achieved with modern pedicle screw and rod constructs (Fig. 35D-13). Cobalt–chrome rods of 5.5 mm or greater diameter and monoaxial and polyaxial pedicle screws with outer thread diameters of 6.5 and 7.5 mm may be used in adult lumbar trauma with excellent corrective abilities. Cobalt–chrome rods are significantly stiffer and resist kyphotic tendencies. Long-term follow-up is needed to evaluate for potential future loss of correction or maintenance of lumbar lordotic alignment. Distraction and compression maneuvers are combined to correct both coronal and sagittal plane deformities at the time of instrumentation. Intraoperative neuromonitoring as well as use of fluoroscopy and CT technologies can further guide placement of instrumentation and avoid iatrogenic neurologic injury. In the presence of pedicle fracture, screw and rod instrumentation may still be used at the level of the fracture in the lumbar spine.[20]

Anterior Column Reconstruction

In low lumbar fractures, anterior column reconstruction should be considered if significant collapse of the vertebral body and loss of overall sagittal alignment are expected. This can be done by a posterior-only, anterior-only, or combined (often staged) posterior-anterior procedures. Often the polytrauma status of the patient precludes a large anterior or retroperitoneal approach. Compared with anterior and posterior combined approaches, posterior-only approaches may not afford the same long-term correction of traumatic deformity and may lead to loss of lordosis as well as spinal stenosis requiring later surgical procedures.[46] Anterior approaches to the lower lumbar spine have a higher learning curve and more associated morbidities than do posterior approaches. Some spine traumatologists believe the anterior approach can address significant height loss as well as anterior longitudinal ligament disruptions in distraction-type injuries directly. Anterior approaches should be reserved for significant loss of anterior height that cannot be restored by a posterior pedicle screw construct. These can be combined with posterior percutaneous or open procedures that address concomitant PLC disruption and posterior neural compression. Alternatively, anterior and posterior stabilization can be performed in multiple staged procedures. Associated visceral organ injuries in high-grade distraction type injuries oftentimes prevent anterior approaches to the lumbar spine. Expandable cages as well as femoral allograft secured by plates or screws may be used in anterior constructs to restore lordotic alignment. Plate constructs can be beneficial in treatment of pathology from a lateral approach at the level of L3 to L5 and anteriorly at L4 to S1.[20]

Maintenance of Alignment

In the presence of high-grade burst fractures or significant disruption of the anterior column, posterior-only constructs may not produce sufficient long-term correction of deformity and should be supplemented by addition of anterior cage or strut grafting and appropriate anterior fixation.[20] This does not mean that all injuries to the lumbar spine require both anterior and posterior approaches and many injuries may be treated without the morbidity of anterior approaches through pedicle screw and rod constructs. Examples of this include bony and ligamentous flexion-distraction injuries as well as fracture-dislocations and shear injuries. Whenever possible, motion segments should be preserved but not at the expense of compromising stability.

Outcomes

A study by Dai and colleagues in 2002 compared operative and nonoperative management for 54 patients with L3 to L5 fractures. All patients with neurologic compromise or potential mechanical instability were offered surgery if their condition permitted it. Surgical fixation was performed with Harrington or Luque rods or transpedicular screw and rod constructs. Conservatively treated patients underwent bed rest and bracing. No neurologic deterioration was observed in any patient. The surgically managed group had significantly less pain on follow-up than the nonoperatively treated patients. Overall, patients did well, with 76% returning to their previous level of activity or work.[19]

Kaminski and colleagues performed posterior operative stabilization on 10 patients with L5 fractures. There was no nonoperative comparison. Follow-up showed an initial loss of lordosis of 8 degrees compared with postoperative alignment. All patients reported fair, good, or excellent outcomes and activity levels. No correlation was observed between radiologic parameters and clinical outcomes.[28,47]

Long-term follow-up from several studies on lower lumbar fractures demonstrate that neurologic decline is rare, and, in fact, some recovery is expected. In the case of a single nerve root injury, complete recovery, even in nonoperative cases, can occur.[17,28,48] Loss of lordosis resulting in flatback deformity and even kyphosis can occur in higher grade injuries, leading to deformity-related lower back pain that may require surgical correction. Additionally, trauma can precipitate lumbar stenosis, which may require decompression. Overall, a high rate of return to work and activity level can be expected in both operatively and nonoperatively treated patients.[17,49]

Special attention should be paid to management of L5 fractures among the low lumbar fractures. If the patient is neurologically intact and there is no significant pelvic ring injury, regardless of how comminuted the vertebral body is, these injuries tend to heal fairly predictably with progressive ambulation with assisted devices. The ligamentous stability afforded by the iliolumbar ligaments and the location below the pelvic brim provide additional stability not seen at L3 and L4. Several studies have shown good outcomes from nonoperative management of L5 fractures, including burst fractures. The spinal canal is the widest at L5, providing a larger potential buffer zone against neurologic injury. Butler and colleagues in 2007 reviewed 14 cases of neurologically intact, isolated L5 burst fractures treated either with bed rest and bracing or operatively with pedicle screw fixation at the level above and below the fracture.[7] The study was not matched for severity of injury, with operative cases tending to have more severe deformity preoperatively. At the time of follow-up, patients in the operative group had a 19% loss of vertebral body height and 11 degrees of kyphosis. The conservatively managed group had 15.7% loss of height and 10.4 degrees of kyphosis. Most important, the nonoperative group reported less pain and fewer activity restrictions than the surgically managed patients. There was no correlation in the study between the degree of anatomic derangement and clinical outcomes. The study was limited by small sample size but provides evidence to support its recommendation that patients with L5 burst fractures with mild to moderate deformity, minimal canal compromise, and without neurologic deficit can be managed with bed rest with or without bracing.[7]

Treatment of Specific Injury Patterns

Transverse Process, Spinous Process, and Endplate Fractures

In the presence of minor trauma and maintained global sagittal balance, these injuries may be treated nonoperatively with analgesics, external immobilization for comfort, and early mobilization. Unrecognized posterior ligamentous injuries can occur and should be evident on standing flexion-extension plain radiographs and treated with external immobilization or surgical fixation if advanced kyphotic deformity persists. Avulsion fractures of endplates in the pediatric population with neurologic compromise should be surgically decompressed.[20]

Compression Fractures

Careful differentiation between compression fractures and burst fractures must be performed, usually with the aid of CT scan. Isolated anterior column injuries may be treated conservatively with analgesics and external orthoses. Fractures of L4 and below require thigh extension to immobilize the motion segments at the lumbosacral junction. Flexion-extension radiographs should be obtained after bony consolidation to evaluate for residual instability. In the case of elderly patients with compression fractures from minor trauma, additional evaluation and treatment of osteopenia and osteoporosis should be performed in concert with medical specialists. These injuries in isolation rarely require surgical treatment unless they acutely progress to involve significant deformity. Vertebroplasty is highly effective in osteoporotic fractures that are symptomatic after 3 weeks of conservative care.

Burst Fractures

Acute surgical indications for burst fractures include central compression with greater than 50% canal compromise or with neurologic deficit from retropulsed fragments, greater than 25 degrees of kyphosis, and incarcerated nerve roots with concomitant dural tear in the case of laminar fractures. Without significant vertebral body comminution or kyphotic deformity, posterior-only approaches may be used to decompress an instrument from one level above to one level below the site of injury (Fig. 35D-14). Pedicle screws at the injury level may additionally be used but might need to be diminished in length if there is significant pedicle compromise (Fig. 35D-15). Fractures that demonstrate a high magnitude of kyphotic deformity or significant height loss and vertebral body comminution should be supported with anterior cage and plate-type constructs to restore anterior column height and stability.

Restoration of lordosis may be performed through several techniques (Fig. 35D-16). The best technique is simple postural reduction during prone position. Using hip extension and bolsters under the chest can achieve lordotic reduction. Utilization of precontoured rods may assist in adding lordosis to a construct. The use of monosegmental screws and proper rod contour can be effective tools to reduce kyphosis and recreate lordotic alignment.[50,51]

Posterior exposure of burst fractures should be performed in standard fashion with care taken to avoid violation of the facet capsules of adjacent segments that are not included in the instrumented portion of the operation to preserve motion segments (Fig. 35D-17). If laminar fractures or spinous process fractures are found on imaging or during initial exposure, decompression of any entrapped nerve roots and dural repair should be performed before any attempts at fracture reduction to avoid further iatrogenic neurologic injury. Every effort should be made to preserve the adjacent interspinous and supraspinous ligaments to avoid hypermobility at uninstrumented segments.

Flexion-Distraction Injuries

Bony Chance fractures that maintain their alignment are amenable to nonoperative treatment. They should be managed with TLSO and careful, close clinical and radiographic follow-up to ensure no progressive deformity or neurologic deficit develops. For PLC disruptions and Chance injuries involving soft tissue structures, posterior-only instrumentation constructs are appropriate and may be performed open or percutaneously with or without fusion. Facet dislocations require some form of reduction, as well as stabilization with instrumentation and fusion. In addition to bony injury, there is also usually an associated disc injury in facet dislocations, and undue compression posteriorly should be avoided to prevent further injury. Although the reduction is being performed, preservation of the facets should be of the utmost importance because they contribute greatly to the overall stability of the spine. When simple PLC disruptions occur, it is possible to stabilize the spine by instrumenting only two segments. With further disruption and displacement, as well as with injury to the pedicle, additional levels may need to be instrumented.

All low lumbar fracture-dislocations should be managed operatively. Usually reduction is achieved by postural means or by direct manipulation of the two vertebrae. Unless there is comminution, a single-level instrumentation with fusion is adequate. For comminuted fractures or those with significant displacement, multiple levels of fixation may be required. In this case, we recommend fusion only of the dislocated segment and then rod removal at a later date.

Complications

Neurologic Deterioration

Unstable injury patterns may lead to iatrogenic neurologic injury during patient transport or transitioning to and from the operating table and vigilance is necessary to ensure inline stabilization of patients and appropriate transport measures. Undue stress on neurologic elements may be caused by reduction maneuvers intraoperatively and can be avoided with careful decompression before any reduction maneuvers are performed and, additionally, using intraoperative multimodal neuromonitoring. Inadequate stabilization of unstable injuries may lead to late-onset neurologic deterioration and require further surgical procedures.

Nonunion

Meticulous decortication of all areas to be fused must be carried out. In addition, rigid fixation constructs are required to maintain a biomechanical environment suitable for bony healing. Patients must be counseled on the increased risk of nonunion if they smoke or use other tobacco-containing products. Bone graft supplementation should be appropriately used at the levels to be fused posteriorly as well as posterolaterally along the transverse processes in posterior fusion constructs.

Loss of Correction

It is essential to preserve motion segments in the lower lumbar spine if at all possible but not at the expense of compromising construct stability. Often, anterior and posterior combined constructs are necessary to attain and maintain satisfactory correction. Loss of correction ultimately may result even in these cases but is lessened greatly with close attention to detail by creating a rigid construct and bolstering the biologic environment for healing. Flatback deformity is a known entity after lower lumbar fractures treated both surgically and non-

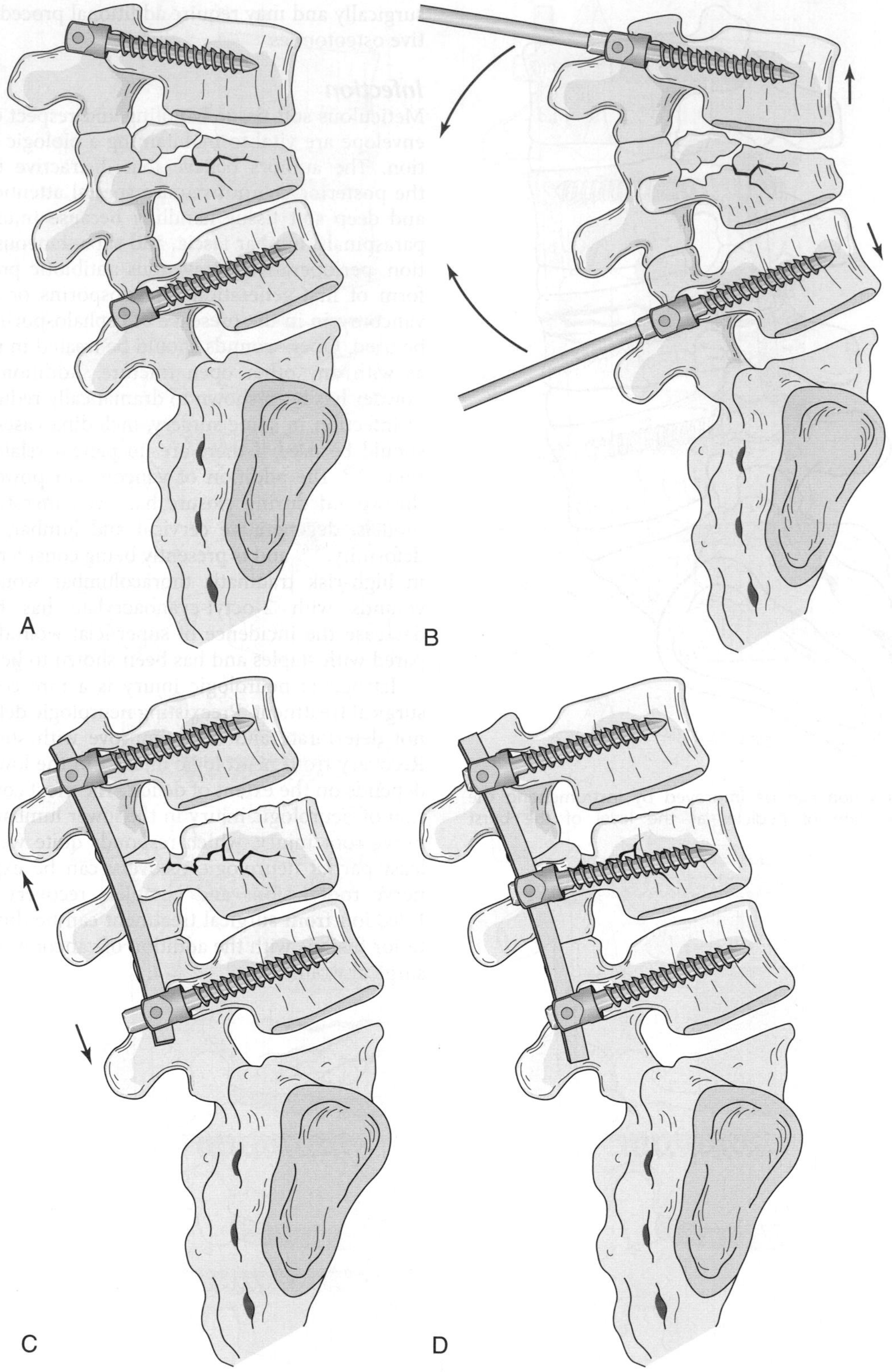

Figure 35D-16. Reduction maneuvers in instrumented posterior constructs for lower lumbar injuries.

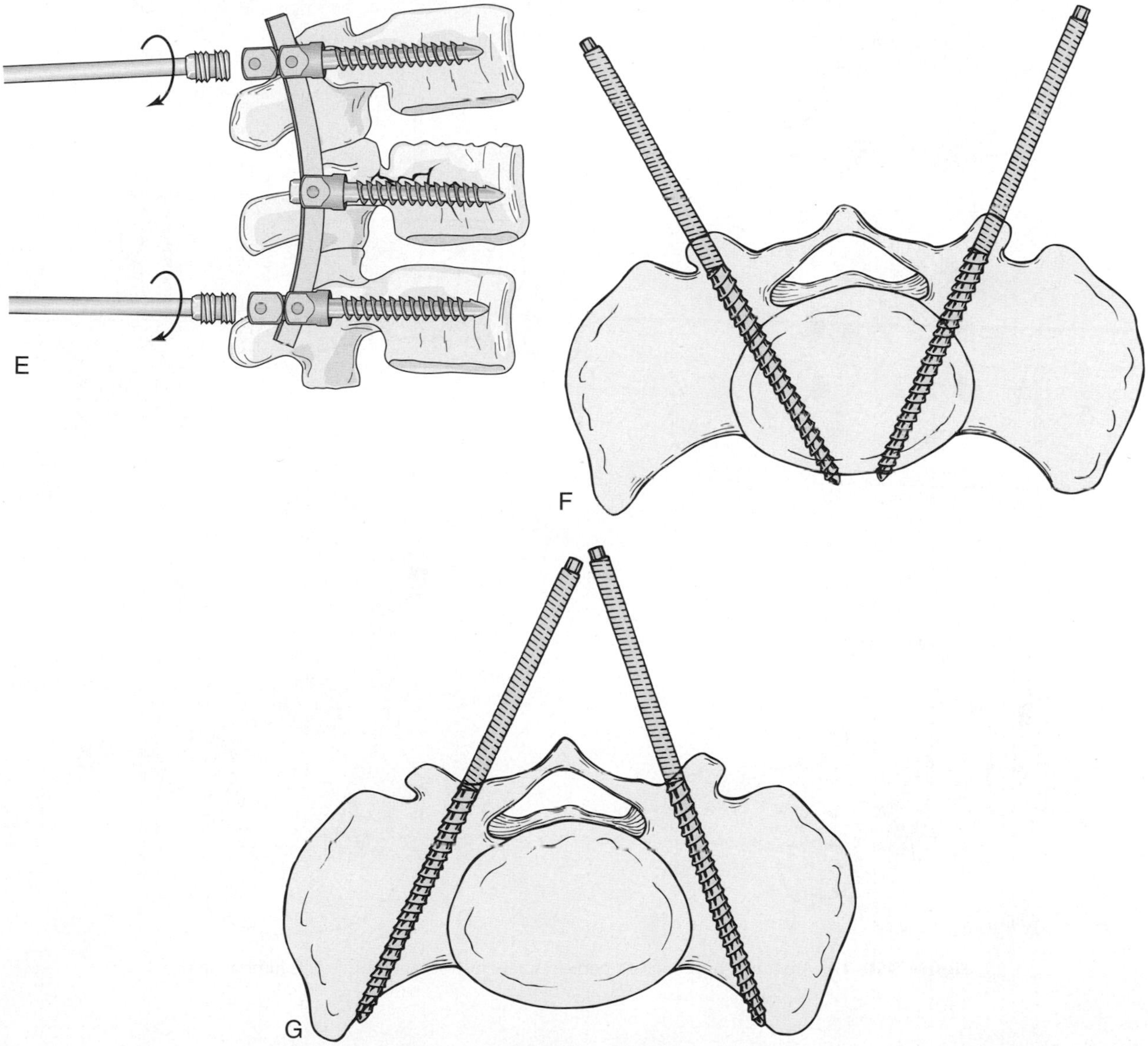

Figure 35D-16, cont'd

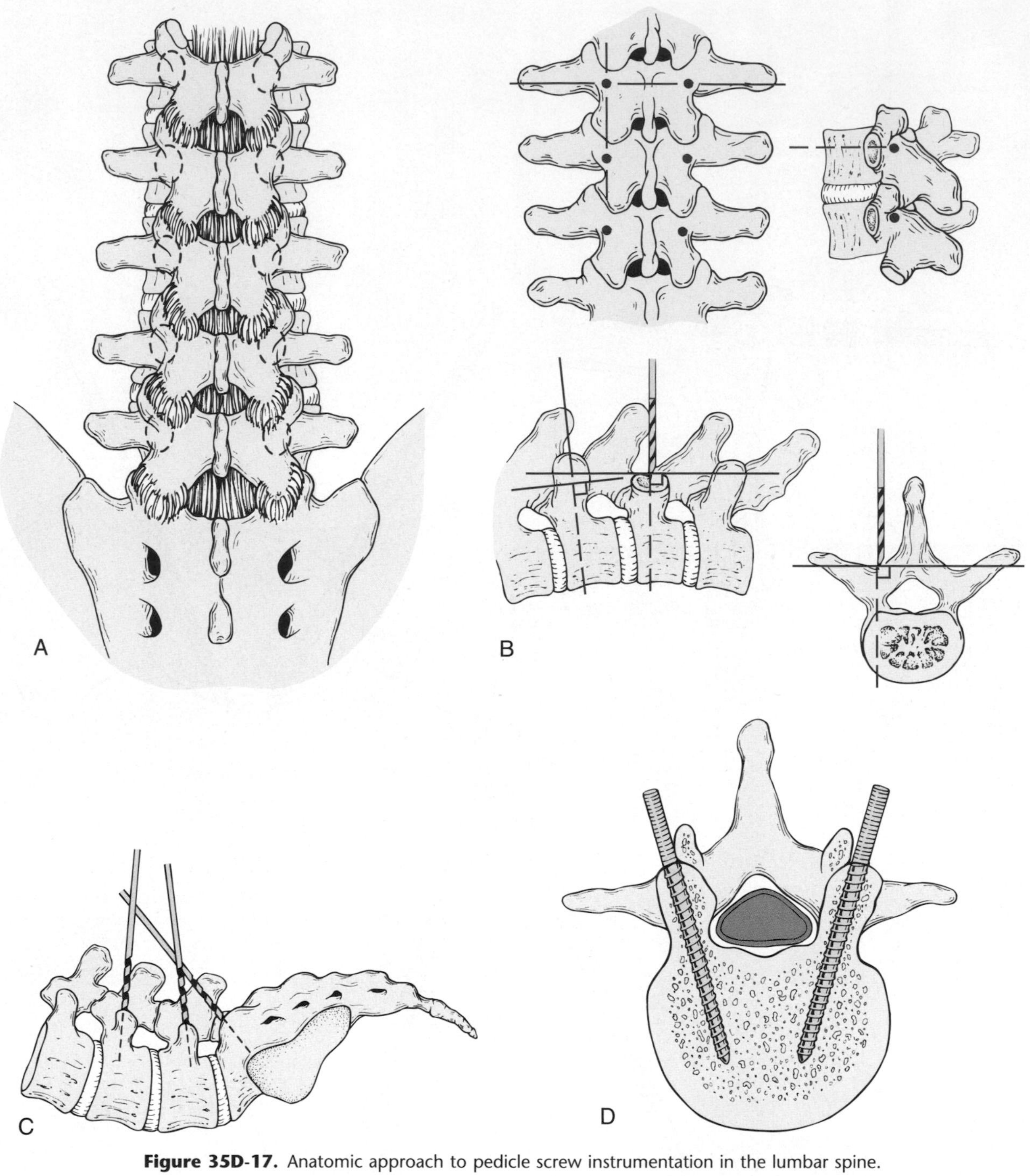

Figure 35D-17. Anatomic approach to pedicle screw instrumentation in the lumbar spine.

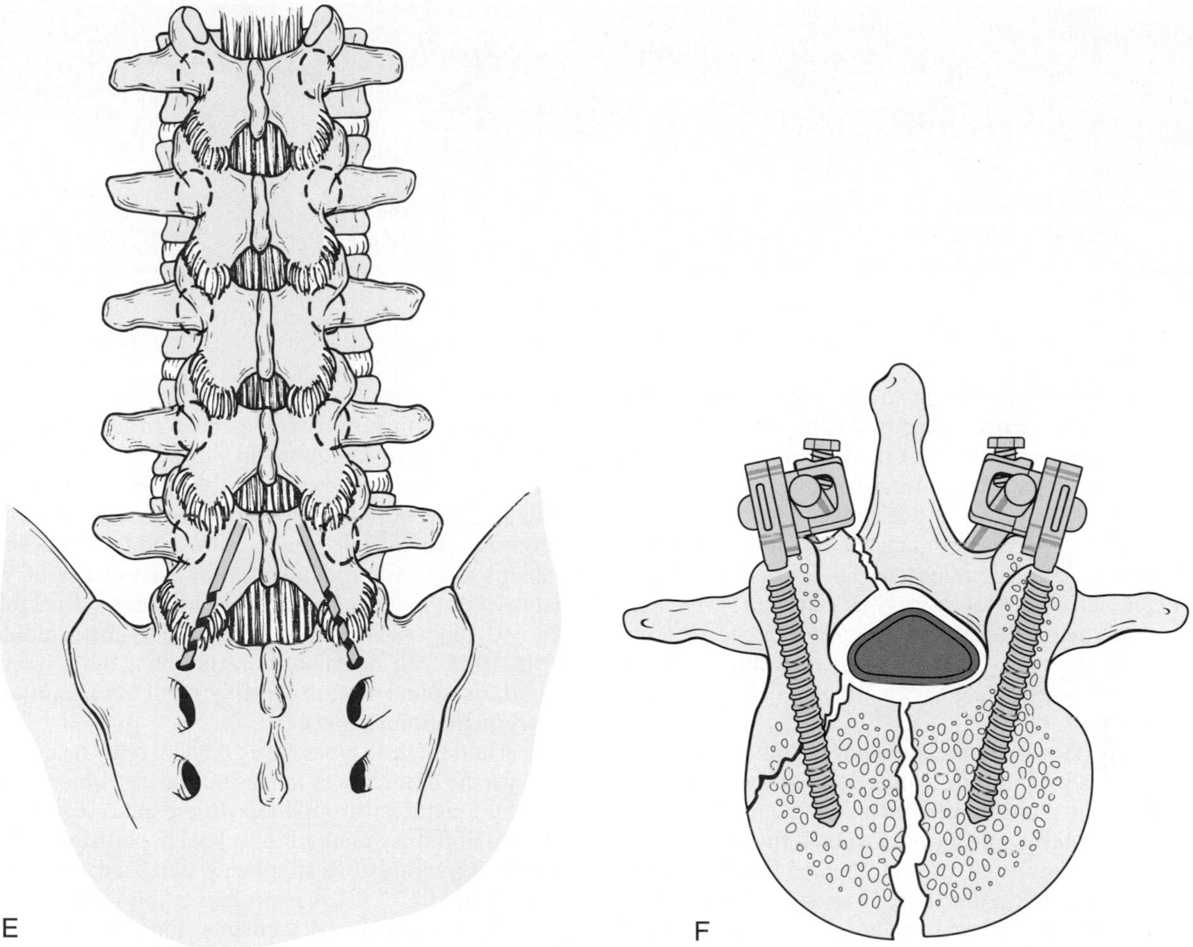

Figure 35D-17, cont'd

KEY REFERENCES

The level of evidence (LOE) is determined according to the criteria provided in the preface.

29. Pizones J, Izquierdo E, Sánchez-Mariscal F, et al: Sequential damage assessment of the different components of the posterior ligamentous complex after magnetic resonance imaging interpretation: prospective study 74 traumatic fractures. *Spine* 37(11):662–667, 2012. LOE II
31. Bailey C, Urquhart J, Dvorak M, et al: Orthosis versus no orthosis for the treatment of thoracolumbar burst fractures without neurologic injury: a multicenter prospective randomized equivalence trial. *Spine J* [Epub 2013 Oct 31]. LOE II
32. Shamji M, Roffey M, Young D, et al: A pilot evaluation of the role of bracing in stable thoracolumbar fractures without neurologic deficit. *J Spinal Disord Tech*, Aug 18, 2012. [Epub ahead of print]. LOE II
35. Wilson JR, Singh A, Craven C, et al: Early versus late surgery for traumatic spinal cord injury: the results of a prospective Canadian cohort study. *Spinal Cord* 50(11):840–843, 2012. LOE II
36. Fehlings MG, Vaccaro A, Wilson JR, et al: Early versus delayed decompression for traumatic cervical spinal cord injury: results of the Surgical Timing in Acute Spinal Cord Injury Study (STASCIS). *PLos One* 7(2): e32037, 2012. LOE II
46. Wang ST, Ma HL, Liu CL, et al: Is fusion necessary for surgically treated burst fractures of the lumbar spine? *Spine* 31(23):2646–2652, 2006. LOE II
52. Jindal N, Sankhala SS, Bachhal V: The role of fusion in the management of burst fractures of the thoracolumbar spine treated by short segment pedicle screw fixation: a prospective randomised trial. *J Bone Joint Surg Br* 94(8):1101–1106, 2012. LOE II
54. Korovessis P, Baikousis A, Zacharatos S, et al: Combined anterior plus posterior stabilization versus posterior short-segment instrumentation and fusion for mid-lumbar (L2-L4) burst fractures. *Spine* 31(8):859–868, 2006. LOE II
56. Ando M, Tamaki T, Yoshida M, et al: Surgical site infection in spinal surgery: a comparative study between 2-octyl-cyanoacrylate and staples for wound closure. *Eur Spine J* 23(4):854–862, 2014. LOE II
62. Gans I, Dormans JP, Spiegel DA, et al: Adjunctive vancomycin powder in pediatric spine surgery is safe. *Spine* 38(19):1703–1707, 2013. LOE II
64. Tubaki VR, Rajasekaran S, Shetty AP: Effects of using intravenous antibiotic versus only local intrawound vancomycin antibiotic powder application in addition to intravenous antibiotics on postoperative infection in spine surgery in 907 patients. *Spine* 38(25):2149–2155, 2013. LOE II
65. Martin JR, Adoqwa O, Brown CR, et al: Experience with intrawound vancomycin powder for spinal deformity surgery. *Spine* 39(2):177–184, 2014. LOE II

The complete References list is available online at https://expertconsult.inkling.com.

35E New Concepts in the Management of Thoracolumbar Fractures

ERIC J. BELIN • JOHN NEAL VI • OLIVER TANNOUS • PAUL A. ANDERSON • SETH K. WILLIAMS • STEVEN C. LUDWIG

Thoracolumbar injuries can be generally categorized as stable or unstable. Whereas most stable fractures are treated with bracing, unstable fractures are best treated surgically. A small group of injuries, in particular burst fractures in neurologically intact patients, present a decisional dilemma because controversy exists concerning injury stability and the need to treat with surgery. Surgery is not trivial because the typical treatment consists of a spinal fusion that can span several segments above and below the injury level. Modern pedicle screw constructs have allowed a movement toward short segment fusions but may be associated with increased kyphosis and hardware failure.

New thoughts about the management of spinal trauma are aimed at minimizing the physiologic burden and complications of surgery in multiply injured patients and decreasing the negative long-term effects of a spinal fusion. Another method is to not only limit the number of fused segments but also to avoid fusion altogether. Thus, spine fracture care becomes more aligned with extremity care in which the goal is to internally stabilize segments to allow bony healing. In tandem with this concept, minimally invasive spinal instrumentation has become mainstream and is being applied to fracture care. These minimally invasive techniques involve less blood loss and potentially less surgical time than open techniques, thus decreasing the physiologic burden of surgery to the polytraumatized patient. This has allowed the concept of "damage control orthopaedics," now widely applied in cases of pelvis and extremity trauma, to be applied to spine trauma. Fusionless instrumentation, minimally invasive instrumentation, and damage control orthopaedics may have developed independent of one another, but these new concepts in thoracolumbar trauma management are intimately related.

FUSIONLESS SPINE TRAUMA CARE

Fusionless instrumentation is performed to stabilize the fracture but without a fusion being performed. The benefits are obvious: temporarily stabilize the spine to achieve and maintain reduction to allow for fracture healing without permanent stiffening from a spine fusion. Although this technique is now commonly associated with minimally invasive surgery, its use was established with more traditional open techniques.[1-5] Preservation of motion segments by avoiding fusion is a well-known tenet of fracture care. Before the advent of pedicle screw instrumentation Harrington rods were used which required instrumentation two or three levels above and below the injury site. To avoid long segment fusions, a "rod long, fuse short" method was used that required local fusion at the injury site and subsequent rod removal 1 year later.[6] Dekutoski and colleagues performed a retrospective review of 30 patients at a mean 34 months of follow-up who were treated with the rod long, fuse short technique. The unfused segments regained 5 to 6 degrees of flexion-extension motion after hardware removal, and overall results were good to excellent in all patients. Kyphosis did increase by an average of 9 degrees between immediate postoperative imaging to final follow-up.[7] Ko and colleagues performed fusionless instrumentation on 60 patients with unstable thoracolumbar burst fractures and found that spinal motion and alignment were maintained after instrumentation removal.[8]

Certain fracture types have excellent bony healing potential and are the best choices for fusionless instrumentation (Table 35E-1). Fractures through ankylosed spine segments such as in cases of diffuse idiopathic skeletal hyperostosis (DISH) and ankylosing spondylitis, after being stabilized, have been found to heal rapidly.[9,10] If the instrumentation is performed exclusively across ankylosed segments, there is arguably no role for performing a fusion. In these cases, there is no need to remove the hardware because the instrumented segments are already fused. This is the best indication for fusionless instrumentation. Flexion-distraction and Chance-type fractures with predominantly bony injury patterns also heal rapidly and are good candidates for fusionless instrumentation (Fig. 35E-1). Grossbach and colleagues compared 11 patients with flexion-distraction injuries treated by fusionless technique with 29 patients who underwent open fusion. There were no differences in clinical and radiologic outcomes, but there were shortened operative times and blood loss. This may be useful in children who readily heal posterior ligamentous complex injuries, although this concept has not been objectively evaluated.[11,12]

Burst fractures disrupt the intervertebral disc and have varying degrees of vertebral body comminution. In highly comminuted fractures or those with severe vertebral body wedging, reduction may be difficult to achieve with posterior

TABLE 35E-1 *INDICATIONS FOR FUSIONLESS OR MINIMALLY INVASIVE FRACTURE INSTRUMENTATION*
Ankylosing spondylitis
Diffuse idiopathic skeletal hyperostosis
Bony Chance-type fractures
Flexion-distraction injuries
Burst fractures
Multiple-level spine fractures
Adjunct to anterior decompression and fusion

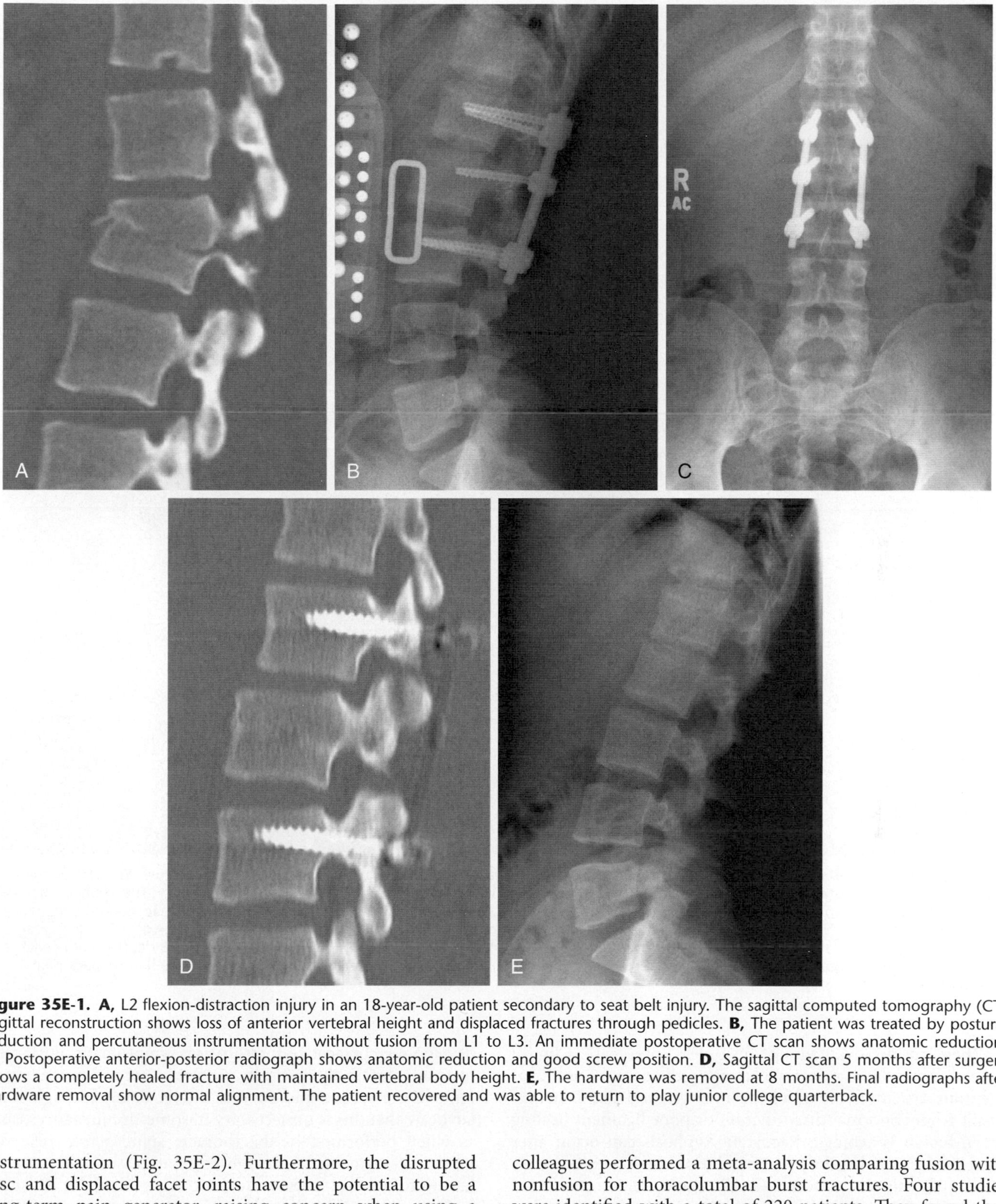

Figure 35E-1. **A,** L2 flexion-distraction injury in an 18-year-old patient secondary to seat belt injury. The sagittal computed tomography (CT) sagittal reconstruction shows loss of anterior vertebral height and displaced fractures through pedicles. **B,** The patient was treated by postural reduction and percutaneous instrumentation without fusion from L1 to L3. An immediate postoperative CT scan shows anatomic reduction. **C,** Postoperative anterior-posterior radiograph shows anatomic reduction and good screw position. **D,** Sagittal CT scan 5 months after surgery shows a completely healed fracture with maintained vertebral body height. **E,** The hardware was removed at 8 months. Final radiographs after hardware removal show normal alignment. The patient recovered and was able to return to play junior college quarterback.

instrumentation (Fig. 35E-2). Furthermore, the disrupted disc and displaced facet joints have the potential to be a long-term pain generator, raising concern when using a fusionless technique. However, several studies indicate that burst fractures may be treated successfully by this technique. Dai and colleagues reported 5- to 7-year results of a randomized trial of posterior short segment instrumentation with and without fusion for stable burst fractures at the thoracolumbar junction. They found little difference in clinical and radiographic outcomes between the two groups.[1] Tian and colleagues performed a meta-analysis comparing fusion with nonfusion for thoracolumbar burst fractures. Four studies were identified with a total of 220 patients. They found that patients treated without fusion had shorter operative times and less blood loss, although the second procedure of hardware removal was not included in their analysis. Radiologic results were not different between the two groups except for greater vertebral height loss after instrumentation in the fusion group. No difference in clinical outcomes or instrumentation failure was present between groups.[5]

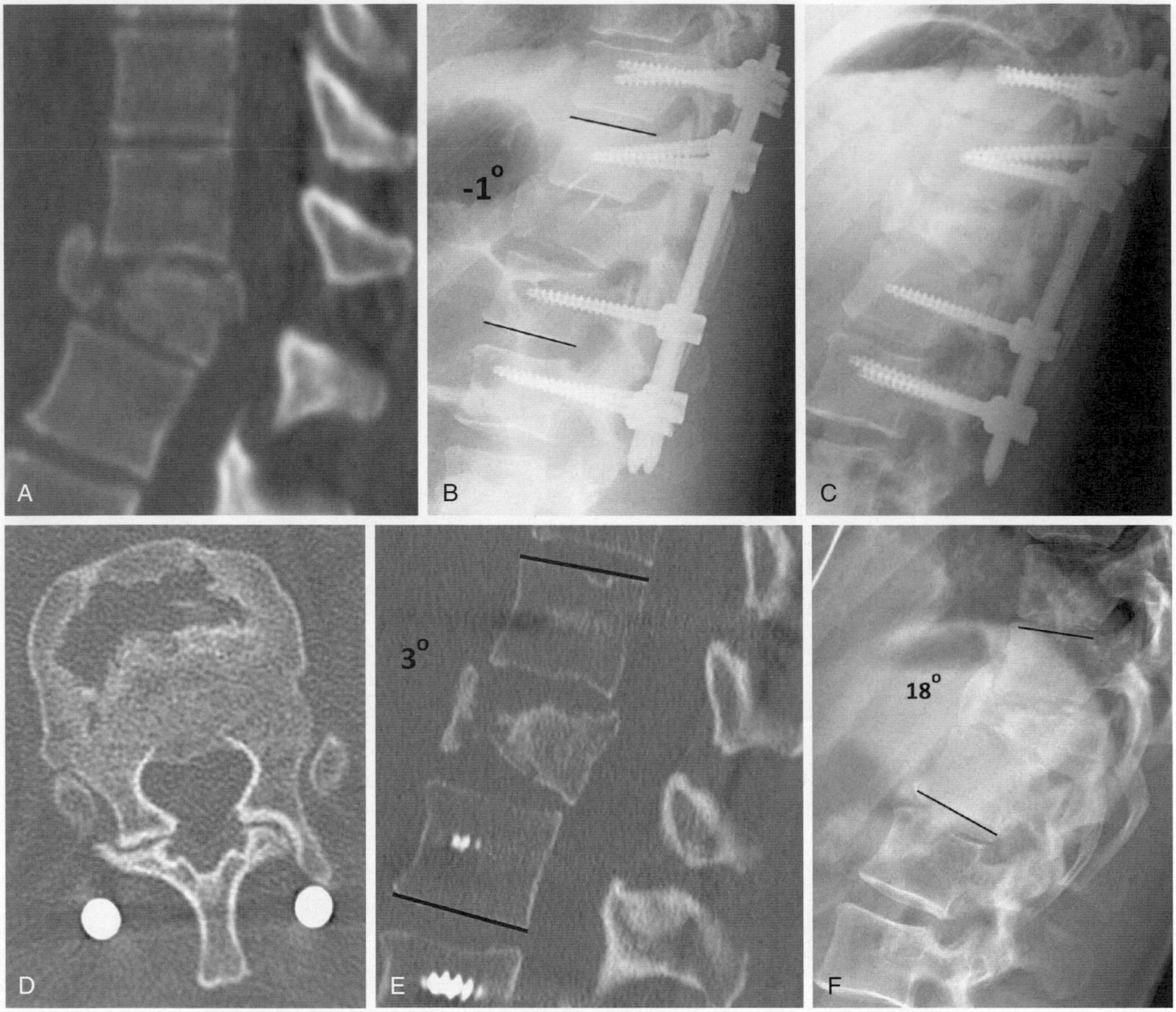

Figure 35E-2. A, Sagittal computed tomography (CT) scan of a 38-year-old woman who sustained a T12 burst fracture. She was treated with closed reduction, percutaneous instrumentation without fusion from T10 to L2. **B,** Postoperative lateral radiograph. The kyphosis has been reduced but without expansion of the vertebral body. **C,** Lateral radiograph taken 1 year after surgery. The patient had good maintenance of alignment. **D,** Sagittal CT scan at 1 year demonstrates poor healing of center of body where discs have herniated. **E,** Axial CT scan 1 year after surgery shows a central void but healing laterally. Her hardware was removed at this time. **F,** Kyphosis increased to 18 degrees with collapse of T12 into L1 likely because of the lack of intervertebral disc of T12 to L1, which had herniated into the body of L1. She had no back pain 1 year after hardware removal.

There are disadvantages of fusionless spine care. Clinical success depends on primary healing of the osseous and ligamentous structures, including the intervertebral disc. Pain may result from abnormal disc function or poor ligament healing when fusion is avoided. Recurrent kyphosis can occur after hardware removal or the instrumentation can loosen or break. Facet arthrosis is a concern. Gardner and Armstrong found autofusion in only two of 75 facet joints traversed by rods but not fused after rod long, fuse short treatment of lumbar burst fractures.[13] Kahanovitz and colleagues, however, warned that stabilization using Harrington rods across a mobile facet joint might lead to osteoarthrosis based on a canine study and biopsy of eight human facet joints obtained during hardware removal.[14,15] It is unknown whether this applies to pedicle screw fixation and earlier instrumentation removal or if the development of facet joint arthrosis is symptomatic. Fusionless instrumentation theoretically requires a second procedure to remove the screws and rods at a later date, although some advocate that this is unnecessary in some circumstances, such as when performed in the thoracic spine across relatively immobile segments. Although costs are associated with the hardware removal, patients tolerate this well, and it is usually performed in our institutions as an outpatient.

MINIMALLY INVASIVE STABILIZATION WITH PERCUTANEOUS INSTRUMENTATION

Successful reports of fusionless spine care emerged during the time that percutaneous pedicle screw instrumentation was

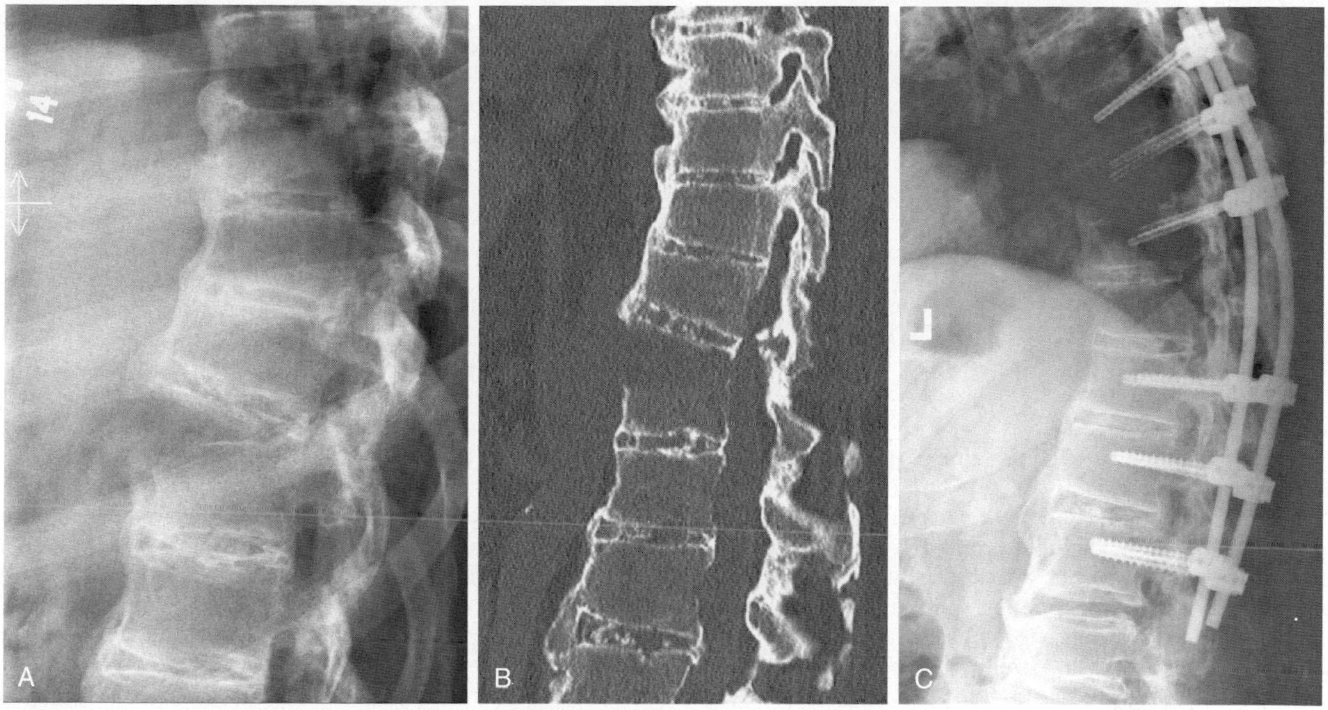

Figure 35E-3. **A,** A 45-year-old man with ankylosing spondylitis sustained an extension type fracture. Lateral radiograph shows anterior distraction of T11 to T12. **B,** Sagittal computed tomography scan shows severe distraction injury. **C,** The patient was treated by closed reduction using postural reduction and bolstering to achieve reduction and then percutaneous instrumentation three levels above and below the fracture site.

becoming prevalent for degenerative conditions. The natural progression of fusionless spine care was instrumentation with percutaneous rather than open techniques. The same construct is placed as in open techniques but with muscle splitting rather than muscle stripping as is necessary with an open approach. There are two ways to perform minimally invasive stabilization, either with paired parasagittal Wiltse-style approaches or through multiple small incisions made just large enough to accommodate the screws. The objective of minimally invasive stabilization is to stabilize the spine injury while minimizing blood loss, surgical time, and complications such as surgical site infection, with the overall goal of decreasing the physiologic burden of surgery. When it is believed that an arthrodesis is appropriate, facet fusions can be performed through the same percutaneous incisions used for the screws, although percutaneous instrumentation is most commonly applied without adjunctive fusion.

The indications and construct length for percutaneous stabilization are almost identical to those of open instrumentation. Possible contraindications include incomplete neurologic injury with the need to directly decompress the spinal cord or nerve roots, fracture-dislocations in a neurologically intact patient with risk for neurologic deterioration without an open direct reduction, and delayed fixation in cases in which postural reduction cannot be expected to restore spinal alignment. As with open fusionless techniques, percutaneous instrumentation is ideally suited to fractures across ankylosed spine segments (Fig. 35E-3) and flexion-distraction injuries with a primarily bony component (see Fig. 35E-1). Unstable burst fractures in a neurologically intact patient are another appropriate indication. Multiple-level fractures are also good candidates for minimally invasive instrumentation because, compared with the open technique, percutaneous instrumentation over multiple segments should be possible with much less blood loss and surgical time and avoids a long fusion and the potentially long-term deleterious consequences associated with this, such as loss of spine flexibility and adjacent segment deterioration. Multiply injured patients with stable thoracolumbar fractures can be difficult to manage with orthoses, especially when pelvic, abdominal, or chest trauma makes bracing impractical. Percutaneous stabilization may enable immediate patient mobilization, avoidance of skin breakdown from the orthosis, and ease of nursing care. Consideration can be given to percutaneous stabilization in fracture-dislocations with complete neurologic injury, with the goal of restoring stability and indirectly decompressing the spinal canal. It is also possible in cases that require a direct decompression to place the instrumentation percutaneously several levels above and below the level of injury and locally decompress the spinal canal through a small midline incision. This is particularly useful in cases of ankylosing spondylitis.

Grossbach and colleagues reported a retrospective cohort analysis comparing open versus percutaneous techniques for treatment of flexion-distraction injuries. They found no differences in clinical or radiographic outcomes but had shorter operative times and less blood loss using the percutaneous techniques. No differences were present between groups in adverse events.[16] Similar findings were reported by Wang and colleagues,[17] Wild and colleagues,[18] Palmisani and colleagues,[19] and Lee and colleagues.[20] Ni and colleagues[21] successfully treated 36 patients with burst fractures using percutaneous instrumentation with an operative time averaging 78 minutes and an average blood loss of 75 mL. In the authors' experience, this is typical for short segment constructs. Percutaneous pedicle screw placement using fluoroscopic techniques has been shown to have a high accuracy rate in the trauma setting.[22-24]

Several authors have reported percutaneous balloon-assisted reduction techniques with or without vertebral body augmentation.[25-31] This can be used with open surgery or as an adjunct to percutaneous pedicle screw instrumentation. The idea is to aid with reduction and provide anterior column support without adding additional surgical physiologic burden. The role for this technique has not been clarified.

SURGICAL TECHNIQUE: PERCUTANEOUS INSTRUMENTATION

Positioning

Successful treatment of thoracolumbar injuries depends on maintenance of neurologic function and restoration of spinal alignment and stability. Postural reduction is usually successful in restoring spinal alignment, although rod contouring can be used in young patients with excellent bone quality.[32] In patients with ankylosed spine segments, a Wilson frame may best accommodate preexisting kyphosis. Otherwise, a Jackson frame is appropriate, with pillows placed underneath the thighs to allow for restoration of lumbar lordosis. The computed tomography (CT) scan is carefully reviewed before surgery, and the pedicles are measured for diameter and length at each of the planned instrumentation levels.

Screw Starting Point

Anterior-posterior (AP) fluoroscopy is the primary imaging modality for safe minimally invasive pedicle cannulation. Biplanar fluoroscopy may be used but crowds the field and is typically reserved for cases with difficulty obtaining reliable AP views, such as in obese patients and when there are advanced degenerative changes. The pedicles are visualized on a true AP intraoperative fluoroscopic image, with the endplates of the vertebral body perpendicular to the floor (Fig. 35E-4, *A*). It is important that the vertebra of interest is centered on the fluoroscopic image. In general, the superior aspect (12 o'clock) of the pedicle should overlie the cranial endplate and the lateral pedicle border should overlie the lateral aspect of the vertebral body. After a true AP image has been obtained, Kirschner wires (K-wires) are laid over the skin horizontally and vertically across the center of the pedicles, where lines are drawn (Fig. 35E-4, *B*). The intersection of the lines represents the approximate start point for the pedicle screws (Fig. 35E-4, *C*). The typical incision is made approximately 1 cm lateral to the lateral border of the pedicle or 2 cm lateral at L5 and S1 because of a more oblique screw trajectory.

To reduce intraoperative blood loss, the predicted screw trajectory is first infiltrated with 5 to 7 mL of local anesthetic with epinephrine on a spinal needle. An incision is then made through skin and subcutaneous tissues and then a fascial incision made slightly medial to the skin incision to accommodate the oblique screw trajectory.

Pedicle Cannulation

The CT scan should be reviewed to plan the screw diameter, length, and trajectory. Particular attention should be paid to the L5 and S1 trajectory which, when compared with the higher lumbar and thoracic pedicles typically requires a slightly more lateral starting point with a more oblique lateral-to-medial trajectory. A Jamshidi needle is introduced into the incision and placed under AP fluoroscopy at the lateralmost border of the pedicle in the sagittal plane and the middle of the pedicle in the axial plane, corresponding to the 3 o'clock and 9 o'clock positions of the pedicle, respectively (Fig. 35E-4, *D*). The Jamshidi needle is advanced a few millimeters such that it is anchored in bone and a pen mark is placed on the needle measured 20 mm from the skin. The typical pedicle is approximately 20 mm in length, so the Jamshidi needle is advanced to a depth of 20 mm as determined by the pen mark becoming flush with the skin. The pedicle is cannulated under AP fluoroscopy with the Jamshidi needle advanced with a mallet in a lateral-to-medial trajectory. A fluoroscopic image obtained after approximately 10 mm of advancement should show the tip of the Jamshidi needle in the center of the pedicle (Fig. 35E-4, *E*). As long as a true AP fluoroscopic view has been obtained, the lateral view will later show a proper cephalad-caudal trajectory. At 20 to 25 mm of advancement, the tip of the Jamshidi needle should be at the medial border of the pedicle on the AP view (Fig. 35E-4, *F*). If the needle is medial to the pedicle border at this depth, a medial pedicle breach is likely present.

Lateral fluoroscopy is then used to finalize the appropriate cephalad-caudal direction with the Jamshidi needle advanced approximately 10 mm into the vertebral body. A guide wire is introduced through the cannulated Jamshidi needle and advanced into the vertebral body and positioning is again confirmed with AP and lateral imaging (Fig. 35E-4, *G*). Before moving to the next level, sponges can be packed into the incisions to control bleeding and the K-wires are held out of the way with hemostats.

All other pedicles are cannulated similarly and then the pedicles are tapped over the K-wires. Tapping does not need to extend past the pedicle (20 mm) into the vertebral body, which will help prevent pulling out the K-wire as the tap is removed. The K-wire should be closely monitored to prevent this.

Screw Insertion

Screw length can be determined from preoperative imaging or intraoperative measurements. The screws are inserted at their respective levels with lateral fluoroscopy used to confirm appropriate insertion depth with care taken not to advance the K-wire beyond the anterior vertebral body cortex (Fig. 35E-4, *H*). After screws are inserted, the K-wires are removed. If the pedicle screw heads are offset in height on the lateral view, rod passage and final set screw tightening may be difficult and could result in pullout of one or more of the screws. Depending on the system used, the screw is either attached to a removable tower system, or reduction tabs extend from the screw heads themselves and are broken free after final set screw tightening.

Rod Insertion

The rod length is determined by direct measurement or by placing a rod in place and checking fluoroscopically. If desired, the rod should have a lordotic contour to aid reduction. However, with poor bone quality, care should be taken to contour the rod appropriately so as not to place excessive stress through a particular screw. The rod is passed percutaneously, preferably in a cephalad-to-caudal direction to prevent

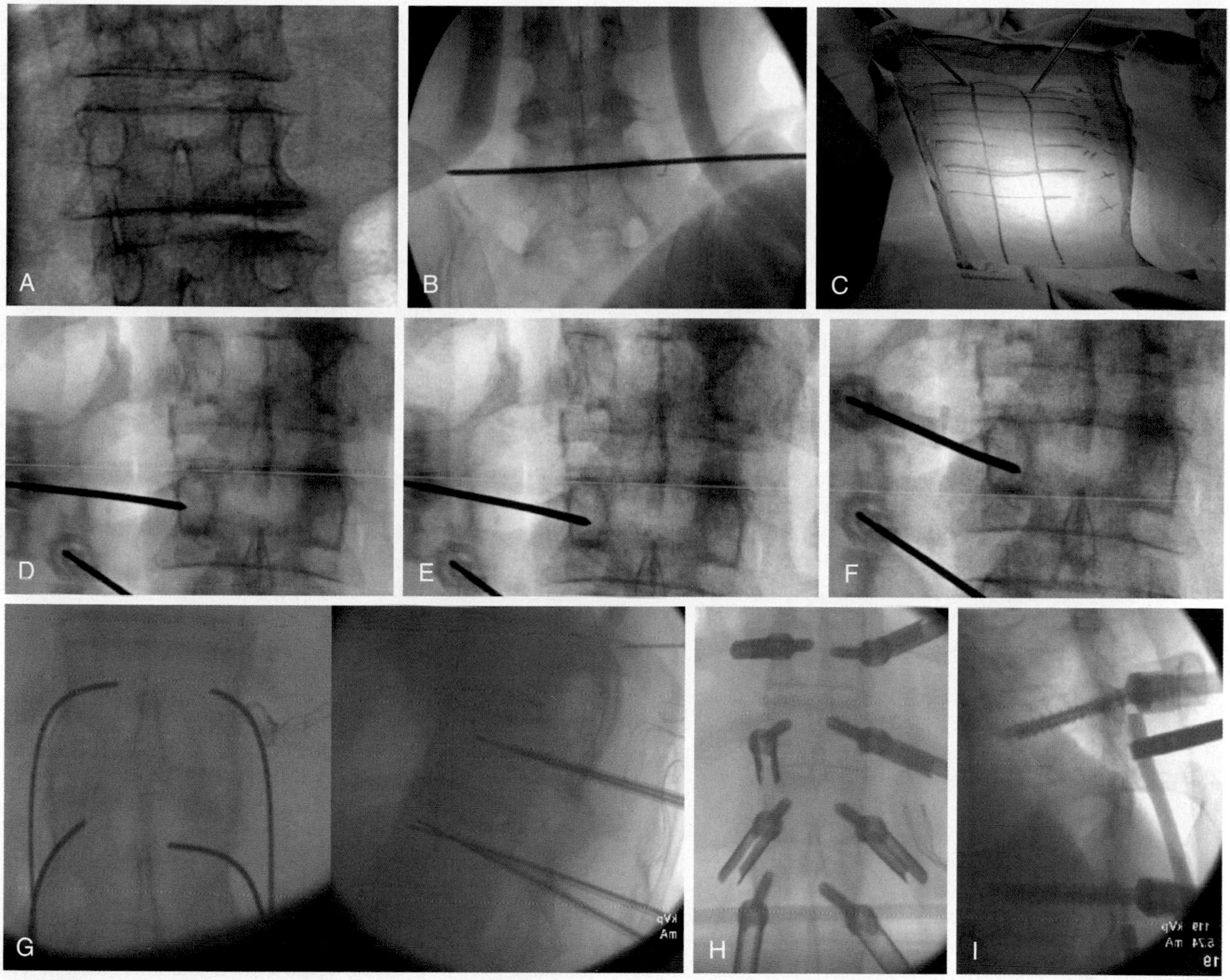

Figure 35E-4. A, Anterior-posterior (AP) fluoroscopic image showing that the x-ray beam is parallel to the superior endplate and that the superior edge of the pedicles is aligned so that it appears to just touch the superior endplate. **B,** A K-wire is positioned along the superior edge of the L5 pedicle. **C,** Methodically, a vertical lines is drawn 1 to 2 cm lateral to all planned instrumented pedicles and horizontally at each level along the cranial aspect of the pedicle. **D,** A Jamshidi needle is placed at the 9 o'clock position of the left pedicle. **E,** The Jamshidi needle is advanced 10 mm and is not seen to be in middle of the pedicle. **F,** The Jamshidi is now advanced 20 cm and is located just at the posterior vertebral body margin (not shown). On the AP image, the needle is seen to be just at the medial pedicle border, indicating that it is not penetrating into the spinal canal. **G,** Placement of guide pins; AP *(left)* and lateral *(right)* images. **H,** AP fluoroscopic image after screw placement before rod passage. **I,** The rod was passed from caudal to cranial because of severe kyphosis. To aid reduction of the rod, the proximal incision was enlarged, and the rod is being manipulated with regard to the rod holder.

the possibility of the rod passing under the lamina, but depending on the sagittal rod contour, it may be advisable to pass the rod in a caudal-to-cephalad direction. There may be difficulty in passing the rod over long segments, especially when there is excessive kyphosis as in cases of ankylosing spondylitis or when the thoracolumbar region requires a lordotic rod contour at one end and a kyphotic contour at the other end of the rod (Fig. 35E-4, *I*). To simplify matters, small incisions may be made along the rod pathway and the rod tip intermittently controlled directly using a Kocher or a low-profile rod holder. Set screws are then placed and final tightening performed.

Reduction Technique

In most cases, reduction is achieved by postural means. This can be aided by hip hyperextension or bolstering the chest to induce lordosis. Kyphosis is common in patients with ankylosing spondylitis and a Wilson frame may be useful under these circumstances. In patients with good bone quality, contouring the rod to assist with reduction is possible, but this should be done with caution to avoid screw pullout. Some minimally invasive pedicle screw systems allow compression across the screws to further induce lordosis, although this reduction does not seem to be as powerful as when performed with an open technique. In facet dislocations, a small midline incision can be used to expose the injured site to allow manual manipulation of the vertebrae to achieve reduction, with the instrumentation placed percutaneously.

Wound Closure

Wound closure is then performed. It is usually not necessary to close fascia because a subcutaneous stitch followed by two simple nylon skin sutures is usually sufficient. The exception is at the lordotic L4 to S1 levels, where a single longer incision is usually used to place multiple screws because of screw head convergence at the skin. In this circumstance fascial closure is recommended.

Facet Joint Fusion

If facet joint fusion is planned as part of the percutaneous instrumentation procedure, dilators are placed over the K-wires before tapping and screw placement. The dilators are used to create a field to perform the facet fusion. When used in a wanding-type fashion, the dilators act to clear the overlying soft tissue from the facet joint. After the appropriate sized dilator is placed over the facet joint, the surgeon should assess that the optimal facet joint visualization has been obtained. This requires angling the tube cranially and medially to center it over the facet joint. Electrocautery is used to clear the facet joint of overlying soft tissue and capsule. This material is removed with a pituitary rongeur. After the facet joint is cleared of overlying soft tissue and adequately visualized, a high-speed cutting burr is introduced into the tube. Lateral view intraoperative fluoroscopy can be obtained with the burr in place to confirm correct placement at the facet joint. The facet joint is then decorticated with the high-speed burr. Bone graft material of the surgeon's choice is introduced through the dilator and packed around the facet. The dilator tube is removed, the pedicle is then tapped, and the screw is inserted over the K-wire. This procedure is performed in sequence bilaterally at all facet joints to be addressed.

DAMAGE CONTROL SPINE SURGERY

Damage control orthopaedics was developed as part of the treatment of extremity injuries in multiply injured patients. Injury results in a systemic inflammatory response that in severe cases can lead to multiple organ damage. The inflammation is followed by an antiinflammatory response. The antiinflammatory response may become so severe as to induce an immunocompromised state that further increases the risk of infection and poor healing. The important factors involved with the inflammatory response are cytokines, leukocytes, and endothelium. These responses are normal and the effects vary depending on the severity of the trauma and the intrinsic responses of the host. In less severe cases, the inflammatory response is well tolerated and the patient rapidly improves unless further injuries occur. A surgery performed at this stage can reestablish the inflammatory response at even greater levels than initially occurred, which can ultimately lead to acute respiratory distress syndrome or multisystem organ failure. This has been termed the secondary injury or "hit." Strategies to avoid this have been shown to reduce mortality and morbidity in the treatment of extremity trauma.

Damage control spine surgery has the same goals as that of general trauma orthopaedics: to control hemorrhage, manage soft tissue injury, and provisionally stabilize fractures without creating a second hit. In addition, in the spine, achieving reduction of dislocations, correcting malalignment to maximize neurologic recovery, and stabilizing the injury to allow for unrestricted nursing care and patient mobilization are early goals. These goals need to be balanced against the possibility of causing a secondary insult by performing a spine surgery; therefore, minimally invasive techniques and fusionless surgery are well suited to this treatment paradigm.

The role and effectiveness of damage control spine surgery have little evidence basis. The following are general concepts for management of critically injured patients who meet criteria for damage control orthopaedics. In patients with unstable cervical spine fractures, dislocations, or spinal cord injuries, reduction should be considered with tong traction unless there is a contraindication. If surgery is required to reduce a dislocation or decompress an injured spinal cord, then an anterior approach is preferred because it minimizes further muscle trauma and avoids the prone position that may be poorly tolerated. In the thoracolumbar spine, unstable injuries can be treated using postural reduction techniques and stabilization with percutaneous instrumentation. When necessary, the fracture site can be separately approached through a small midline incision to allow for a safe direct reduction and decompression. Although in some cases this is the definitive treatment, in other cases, the goal is to provide only provisional fixation. Further surgery to improve fixation, perform fusion when deemed appropriate, or further decompress the neural elements would be delayed until the patient is physiologically stable. In general, anterior approaches should be avoided, although one exception may be a mini-open retroperitoneal or extrapleural lateral approach to focally decompress the spinal canal provided the surgeon has experience with this technique.

Stahel and colleagues reported a prospective cohort study comparing spine damage control with delayed posterior stabilization (>24 hours) in 114 multiply injured patients. Further reconstructive spine surgeries were delayed for at least 72 hours. They found that the spine damage control group had significantly fewer complications, shorter intensive care unit stays, and a shorter overall hospitalization length of stay. The authors recommended establishing a standardized spine damage control protocol to provide a safe and efficient treatment strategy.

CONCLUSION

Fusionless spinal instrumentation, percutaneous pedicle screw and rod placement, and damage control spine surgery have become interrelated and are increasingly meaningful for thoracolumbar trauma treatment. Fracture stabilization with percutaneous techniques has become so safe and effective, with minimal physiologic burden to the patient, that there is even some risk of inappropriate expansion of surgical indications. This speaks to the success of these concepts and techniques, but care must be taken in the decision-making process. There is a deficiency in the literature, but with increased interest and study, the proper indications will become clearer.

KEY REFERENCES

The level of evidence (LOE) is determined according to the criteria provided in the preface.

1. Dai LY, Jiang LS, Jiang SD: Posterior short-segment fixation with or without fusion for thoracolumbar burst fractures. a five to seven-year prospective randomized study. *J Bone Joint Surg Am* 91(5):1033–1041, 2009. LOE I
3. Wang ST, Ma HL, Liu CL, et al: Is fusion necessary for surgically treated burst fractures of the thoracolumbar and lumbar spine?: a prospective,

randomized study. *Spine (Phila Pa 1976)* 31(23):2646–2652, discussion 2653, 2006. LOE I

5. Tian NF, Wu YS, Zhang XL, et al: Fusion versus nonfusion for surgically treated thoracolumbar burst fractures: a meta-analysis. *PLoS One* 8(5): e63995, 2013. LOE I
10. Westerveld LA, Verlaan JJ, Oner FC: Spinal fractures in patients with ankylosing spinal disorders: a systematic review of the literature on treatment, neurological status and complications. *Eur Spine J* 18(2):145–156, 2009. LOE III
13. Gardner VO, Armstrong GW: Long-term lumbar facet joint changes in spinal fracture patients treated with Harrington rods. *Spine (Phila Pa 1976)* 15(6):479–484, 1990. LOE III
14. Kahanovitz N, Arnoczky SP, Levine DB, et al: The effects of internal fixation on the articular cartilage of unfused canine facet joint cartilage. *Spine (Phila Pa 1976)* 9(3):268–272, 1984.
16. Grossbach AJ, Dahdaleh NS, Abel TJ, et al: Flexion-distraction injuries of the thoracolumbar spine: open fusion versus percutaneous pedicle screw fixation. *Neurosurg Focus* 35(2):E2, 2013. LOE III
18. Wild MH, Glees M, Plieschnegger C, et al: Five-year follow-up examination after purely minimally invasive posterior stabilization of thoracolumbar fractures: a comparison of minimally invasive percutaneously and conventionally open treated patients. *Arch Orthop Trauma Surg* 127(5):335–343, 2007. LOE III
22. Heintel TM, Berglehner A, Meffert R: Accuracy of percutaneous pedicle screws for thoracic and lumbar spine fractures: a prospective trial. *Eur Spine J* 22(3):495–502, 2013. LOE II

The complete References list is available online at https://expertconsult.inkling.com.

Chapter 36

Fractures in the Ankylosed Spine

MICHAEL FINN • RAMESH KUMAR

INTRODUCTION

Ankylosing spinal conditions are a group of disorders that lead to progressive bony fusion of the axial skeleton, resulting in a "stiff spine." The two distinct clinical entities most relevant to the spine surgeon are diffuse idiopathic skeletal hyperostosis (DISH) and autoimmune spondyloarthropathies, a group of disorders characterized by immunologically mediated spondylosis, of which ankylosing spondylitis (AS) is prototypical. Although unique in many ways, both disorders lead to discoligamentous ossification of the mobile spine, and consequently, place patients at high risk for spinal fracture. The changes associated with these disease processes also predispose those who are injured to a higher rate of neurologic deficit than fractures seen in the general population. Fractures in this patient population present a particular challenge for the practicing spine surgeon as patients tend to have highly unstable fractures and significantly altered spinal biomechanics. The optimum management of fractures and associated pathologies in these patients is complex and the topic of much debate. The authors review the clinical characteristics, epidemiology, pathophysiology, fracture types, and treatment of patients with DISH and AS.

DIFFUSE IDIOPATHIC SKELETAL HYPEROSTOSIS

Clinical Characteristics

DISH is a seronegative osteoarthritis characterized by widespread ligamentous ossification and calcification. When initially described, it was thought to affect only the axial skeleton; however, it may diffusely involve the entire musculoskeletal system.[1-4]

DISH causes ossification of the anterior longitudinal ligament and adjacent paraspinal soft tissues. This leads to formation of the characteristic "flowing" syndesmophytes that bridge multiple vertebral bodies, but leave the intervertebral spaces relatively intact. Original radiographic criteria required involvement of at least four contiguous vertebrae[5]; however, more recent criteria require only three contiguous vertebrae in the presence of peripheral enthesophytes.[6] DISH most commonly affects the thoracic spine and favors the right side. It may also involve the cervical[7,8] and lumbar spine.[9] Involvement at these levels more commonly involves the lower cervical and upper lumbar regions and has been known to cause cervical myelopathy,[10] lumbar stenosis,[11] and oropharyngeal dysphagia due to esophageal compression by osteophytes.[12-14]

DISH is commonly asymptomatic or minimally symptomatic. Presenting symptoms may include decreased range of motion and stiffness of the spine. In advanced cases, immobility of the spine may be severe and lead to kyphotic postural abnormalities reminiscent of AS.[15] Syndesmophytes may lead to a variety of compressive syndromes including dysphagia, respiratory failure, and lumbar radiculopathy.

The diagnosis is based on radiographic findings: (1) flowing calcification and ossification along the anterolateral aspects of at least four contiguous vertebral bodies with or without associated localized point excrescences at the intervening vertebral body-disc junctions; (2) a relative preservation of intervertebral disc height in the involved vertebral segments and the absence of extensive radiographic changes of "degenerative" disc disease, including vacuum phenomena and vertebral body marginal sclerosis; (3) absence of apophyseal joint bony ankylosis and sacroiliac joint erosion, sclerosis, or bony fusion (Table 36-1).[5]

The syndesmophytes are horizontally oriented and hyperostosis is heaviest just anterior to the disc space and lightest just below and above the site of vertebral body attachment. Within the cervical spine, there may be hyperostosis around the atlantoaxial joint and occiput, as well as ossification within the posterior longitudinal ligament and ligamentum nuchae.[16] Ossification within the lumbar spine involves mainly the anterior longitudinal ligament, however, unlike in thoracic spine, ossification here equally affects the right and left sides.

The effect of DISH on bone mineral density (BMD) has been heavily investigated. Initial studies with dual-energy x-ray absorptiometry (DXA) scan showed a significantly higher body BMD in patients with DISH compared to controls.[17-18] One study concluded that this finding may even decrease the fracture risks in patients with DISH.[18] However, more recent studies have found that DXA significantly overestimates the BMD in patients with DISH.[19,20] This is thought to be due to the contribution of ossification of the anterior longitudinal ligament as measurements on the right side of the spine were significantly higher than those taken on the left.[20] More recent studies using quantitative computed tomography (CT) have shown no significant differences in body BMD between patients with DISH and control subjects.[21]

Epidemiology

As opposed to AS, DISH is a disease of the aging population. An autopsy study found an incidence of 28% with an average age of 65 years old.[9] Other studies based on radiographic criteria have found an increasing incidence of the disease after the age of 50 years,[22] with the highest prevalence being in patients older than the age of 70 years.[23] It affects males more commonly than females and may have some genetic predisposition as whites have been found to be more commonly affected in the U.S. population[24] and prevalence in Koreans and African blacks is quite low.[22,25] As DISH is associated with age, diabetes, and obesity, its prevalence can be expected to

TABLE 36-1 *RADIOGRAPHIC CRITERIA FOR DIAGNOSIS OF DIFFUSE IDIOPATHIC SKELETAL HYPEROSTOSIS*

I.	Presence of flowing calcification and ossification along the anterolateral aspects of at least four contiguous vertebral bodies with or without associated localized pointed excrescences at the intervening vertebral body–disc junctions.
II.	Relative preservation of intervertebral disc height in the involved vertebral segments and the absence of extensive radiographic changes of "degenerative" disc disease, including vacuum phenomena and vertebral body marginal sclerosis.
III.	Absence of apophyseal joint bony ankylosis and sacroiliac joint erosion, sclerosis, or bony fusion.

Source: From Resnick D, Niwayama G: Radiographic and pathologic features of spinal involvement in diffuse idiopathic skeletal hyperostosis (DISH), Radiology 119(3):559–568, 1976.

increase as societies Westernize and life expectancies increase.[26,27] An increasing prevalence of DISH along with advancements in radiographic imaging may also lead to a higher incidence of fractures in this patient population.

Etiology and Pathophysiology

The pathogenesis of aberrant bone formation seen in DISH is still largely unknown. As opposed to AS, the incidence of human leukocyte antigen B27 (HLA-B27) positivity is low in DISH. Several metabolic derangements have been associated with DISH. These include dyslipidemia, hyperuricemia, oral vitamin A therapy, diabetes mellitus, hypertension, hyperinsulinemia, obesity, elevated growth hormone, and insulinlike growth factor 1 (IGF-1) levels.[28-34] Patients with DISH have also been found to be at higher risk for the development of metabolic syndrome, cardiovascular disease, and stroke.[35,36]

Spinal Fractures in Diffuse Idiopathic Skeletal Hyperostosis

Patients with DISH are at risk for vertebral column fractures as discoligamentous supporting structures become ossified and the spine becomes rigid. Increased disease burden leads to increased fracture risk, as the spine loses its soft structural supports and takes on the characteristics of a long bone with long lever arms. As segments become rigid and fuse, the length of the lever arm grows, putting more stress on adjacent nonfused levels and predisposing them to fracture. The creation of lever arms also increases the drive for fracture displacement and, thus, the risk of neurologic injury after fracture.

The cervical spine is the most common site of fracture, with most injuries occurring between the C5 and C7 levels.[37-40] The frequency of fractures decreases down through the thoracic and into the lumbar spine. Hyperextension is the most common fracture mechanism, accounting for injury in up to 89% of patients compared with 2.4% in the general population.[37,38,41] Other mechanisms causing fracture include compression and rotation with flexion rarely representing a traumatic fracture mechanism.[38,39] Fractures are generally unstable as they typically involve both the anterior and posterior elements of the spinal column. The majority of fractures in DISH occur through the vertebral body, as opposed to through the disc space, which is more typical in AS.[38-40] The discrepancy between these two fracture patterns is likely due to the lack of apophyseal joint ankylosis and relative preservation of intervertebral disc anatomy seen in DISH. Although BMD is relatively well preserved in DISH, the pattern of ossification likely also contributes to the unique fracture pattern seen. Verlaan and colleagues quantified the volume of the anterolateral ossification mass (ALOM) seen in DISH. They found that the ALOM volume was lowest at the mid-vertebral level and highest at the mid-intervertebral disc space.[42] This relative lack of bone density at the mid-third of the vertebral body may represent a biomechanically weak point at higher risk for fracture.

The mechanism of injury leading to fracture in patients with DISH is often subtle. The majority of patients will have low-energy impacts leading to unstable fractures.[38,43,44] The most common mechanism in several case series is a fall from standing.[38] Oftentimes, patients are unable to recall any causative traumatic event. Unfortunately, this leads to a much higher rate of delayed diagnosis than the general population. Caron and coworkers found that nearly 20% of patients with ankylosing spinal disease, including DISH, experienced a delay in diagnosis, and this delay was associated with an 81% likelihood of decline of neurologic function.[37] In a series of 8 cases of patients with DISH and fracture, Paley and colleagues found that diagnosis was delayed in 3 of 8 patients.[45] The cause for this delay is multifactorial. First, the patient may only have minimal symptoms at the time of trauma and may not present for medical evaluation. Second, the index of suspicion for the assessing physician may be low as these patients often present with unimpressive mechanisms and symptoms. Third, radiographic evaluation of fractures in an ankylosed spine is difficult, resulting in subtle, but unstable, fractures going unnoticed on plain radiographic evaluation. Both CT scanning and magnetic resonance imaging (MRI) are essential in the evaluation of patients with DISH as they have a much higher sensitivity for the detection of fractures than plain radiographs. Specifically, T2-weighted MRIs can often detect marrow edema, indicating an occult fracture that was otherwise not seen. As mentioned before, fractures are most commonly transvertebral, but may involve the intervertebral disc space and often span all three columns of the spine. Transdiscal fractures can be identified by widening of the intervertebral space, which may be accompanied by a tear within the anterior longitudinal ligament. Transvertebral fractures most often present as a lucency across the vertebral body on CT with associated marrow edema near the fracture site on MRI, although this edema may be lacking in certain cases. These fractures are almost always accompanied by disruption of the posterior osteoligamentous structures. Patients with DISH present with nonhealing fractures that display evidence of pseudarthrosis. This is evident as osteolysis with occasional sclerosis and vacuum phenomenon involving the intervertebral space, endplates, and vertebral bodies adjacent to the fracture site. This process can mimic infectious spondylodiscitis.[16,46] Patients have also been known to present with a fluid collection within the fracture site on T2-weighted MRI after hyperextension injury, which may be misleading for an infectious or neoplastic etiology.[47]

Despite the prevalence of low-energy injuries in patients with DISH, the incidence of significant neurologic injury is very high. In a series of 33 patients with DISH and cervical spine trauma, Bransford and colleagues found the incidence of spinal cord injury to be 76%, of which 28% of these were

TABLE 36-2 *COMMON SERONEGATIVE SPONDYLOARTHROPATHIES AND THEIR RELATIVE PREVALENCE*

Spondyloarthropathy	Prevalence (%)
Ankylosing spondylitis	0–10
Reactive arthritis	1–7
Psoriatic arthritis	0.02–0.2
Enteropathic arthritis	10–15% of patients with Crohn disease/ulcerative colitis
Undifferentiated spondyloarthritis	Undetermined

Source: From Zochling J, Smith EU: Seronegative spondyloarthritis, Best Pract Res Clin Rheumatol 24(6):747–756, 2010.

complete.[44] Westerveld performed a literature review including 55 cases of DISH with fracture and found the rate of neurologic injury at time of admission was 40%, and 14% of patients went on to develop neurologic dysfunction at some later point in time.[38] Numerous other case reports have been published showing catastrophic neurologic injury even after minor trauma.[8,48] This high rate of neurologic injury is relatively proportional to the rate of unstable spinal column fractures seen in this population. This is complicated by the fact that many of these unstable fractures are not diagnosed at initial encounter and a potentially preventable neurologic injury occurs in a delayed fashion. Another contributing factor may be the frequency in which epidural hematomas are associated with fracture[49] in this patient population. Caron and colleagues described an incidence of 7% of patients with DISH/AS having epidural hematomas associated with their fracture.[37] Some have speculated that this might be secondary to an increased likelihood of bleeding from the cancellous bone in these patients,[50] although this has been debated.[51] The severity of instability has been correlated with the length of the ankylosed spinal segment, that is, patients with longer ankylosed segments are prone to more severe spinal cord injury.[40]

ANKYLOSING SPONDYLITIS

AS is a systemic inflammatory disease characterized by inflammation of multiple articular and paraarticular structures resulting in bony ankylosis. AS is the third most common chronic arthritis in the United States[52] and the most common of the seronegative spondyloarthropathies (Table 36-2).[53]

These arthritides are typified by sacroiliac and multijoint inflammatory changes but are seronegative for rheumatoid factor. Other seronegative arthritides include reactive arthritis (Reiter disease), psoriatic spondyloarthropathy, and enteropathic spondyloarthropathies (associated with inflammatory bowel diseases). Although AS and DISH have many features in common regarding spinal biomechanics, they represent very unique disease processes. (See Table 36-3 for a list of similarities and differences between DISH and AS.)

Clinical Characteristics

Sacroiliitis is the hallmark of AS and the presenting manifestation in the majority of patients who typically complain of morning stiffness with lower back and sacral pain that classically improves with activity. In the early stages of the disease, patients may also complain of mild constitutional symptoms associated with a systemic inflammatory process including low-grade fever, malaise, and loss of appetite.[53] In time, lower back pain progresses to involve the rib cage, the thoracic spine, and the cervical spine.[54] Chronic inflammation leads to ossification of affected joints and ligaments,[55] and with advanced disease the spine becomes ankylosed and is rendered completely rigid, and effectively functions as a long bone or "bamboo spine" housing the spinal cord.[56] Normal spinal curvature is lost and replaced by a fixed hyperkyphosis which can, in severe cases, significantly impair the patient's vertical gaze as the head is fixed in a downward position. This pattern of ascending involvement is characteristic, but atypical patterns, more commonly seen in women, are also observed. Peripheral joint involvement is a less common manifestation and is seen mostly in chronic progressive disease. The hips are the most commonly affected joint (50% of patients) and the joint most often requiring surgical intervention. The glenohumeral and knee joints are also frequently affected (30%), whereas the joints of the hands, wrists, and feet are only occasionally involved. In addition to joint disease, 25% to 40% of AS patients suffer from a number of extraarticular manifestations.[53] These occur more commonly in patients with the HLA-B27 allele and include the cardiovascular (aortitis, cardiomyopathy, pericarditis, cardiac conduction defects), pulmonary (restrictive ventilation, apical pulmonary fibrosis, pulmonary cavitation), renal (amyloidosis with renal failure) and visual systems (uveitis). With the exception of uveitis,

TABLE 36-3 *DIFFERENCES AND SIMILARITIES BETWEEN DIFFUSE IDIOPATHIC SKELETAL HYPEROSTOSIS AND ANKYLOSING SPONDYLITIS*

Feature	DISH	AS
HLA-B27 association	Rare	Common
Age of symptom onset	>50 years	2nd to 3rd decade of life
Pain	Variable	Common
Extraaxial manifestations	Common	Common
SI joint erosion	Absent	Common
Spinal mobility	Decreased	Decreased
Postural abnormalities	Rare	Common (severe kyphosis)
Syndesmophyte orientation	Horizontal	Vertical
Apophyseal joint involvement	Limited	Ankylosed
Disc space involvement	None	Common
Common fracture mechanism	Hyperextension	Hyperextension
Common fracture type	Transvertebral	Transdiscal

AS, Ankylosing spondylitis; *DISH*, diffuse idiopathic skeletal hyperostosis; *HLA-B27*, human leukocyte antigen B27; *SI*, sacroiliac.
Source: From Olivieri I, D'Angelo S, Palazzi C, et al: Diffuse idiopathic skeletal hyperostosis: differentiation from ankylosing spondylitis, Curr Rheumatol Rep 11(5):321, 2009.

which affects up to 20% of patients,[57] these extraarticular manifestations are rare. The natural history of the disease is benign in most cases with greater than 90% of patients remaining functionally active over a follow-up period of 35 years in one study.[58] Approximately two-thirds of these patients, however, suffered from lifelong back problems. Prognosis can be predicted by the degree of progression in the first 10 years, with slower progression predictive of a more benign course.

Epidemiology

Symptomatic onset usually occurs between the ages of 15 and 35 years with an average age of 28 years. Only 10% of patients are younger than 15 years and only 5% are older than 50 years at disease onset.[59] AS has a prevalence of approximately 1 to 1.5%[60,61] in the white population, but its prevalence varies by region, ethnic group, and sex.[62] Although early studies reported an overwhelming 10:1 male predominance, more recent studies indicate that there is less gender disparity with a ratio closer to 2 to 3:1.[63,64] Although the overall pattern of disease expression is similar, females tend to be diagnosed later in life and have milder spinal disease.[65,66]

Etiology and Pathophysiology

An association between the development of AS and the presence of the HLA-B27 antigen, an allele of the major histocompatibility complex, was first described in 1973 by two independent groups.[67,68] Calin reported that 90% of U.S. whites with AS tested positive for the HLA-B27 antigen.[71] However, because only 6% to 7% of those with the HLA-B27 antigen develop AS, with an approximately equal portion developing another spondyloarthropathy,[53] the antigen is thought to only enhance genetic susceptibility, perhaps interacting with other genetic loci or an environmental trigger.[69] The infectious agent, *Klebsiella pneumoniae,* has been suspected as a possible trigger.[70] Additionally, while the presence of the HLA-B27 antigen is highly associated with disease development in whites, the same does not hold true for African Americans and Japanese.[71] There additionally appears to be a familial association of the disease, with relatives of those affected being 11 to 29 times more likely than nonrelatives to develop the disease. HLA-B27 positive relatives of those affected are afflicted with the disease 20% of the time.[62]

The primary pathophysiology of AS involves infiltration of T cells and macrophages into the attachment sites of ligaments, tendons, and joint capsules where they release cytokines including interleukin-1B (IL-1B), tumor necrosis factor-α (TNF-α) and interferon-γ (IFN-γ).[72] This inflammation causes cortical bone erosion and induces new bone formation. The initial erosive changes are well demonstrated on plain radiograph with the characteristic "Romanus lesion" caused by cortical erosions at the corners of the vertebral bodies with a reactive sclerosis. A similar process occurs in the peripheral joints, where a proliferative synovitis invades subchondral bone and cartilage, leading to ossification and bony ankylosis. It is unknown what triggers ossification of these joints as the exact molecular and cellular mechanisms of this process are poorly understood.[53,55,73]

Spinal Fractures in Ankylosing Spondylitis

AS patients are predisposed to spinal fractures for several reasons. Osteoporosis is a frequent complication of AS, affecting 19% to 62% of patients.[74,75] Its severity is largely correlated with other indices of disease severity such as patient age, male gender, peripheral joint involvement, degree of spinal fusion, and disease duration. The origins of osteoporosis can be attributable to several factors, including inflammatory mediators such as TNF-α and IL-6, immobility, and support provided by extraspinal bone.[53,76] Decreased BMD in AS patients is largely confined to the axial skeleton and can be difficult to measure using traditional DXA techniques secondary to obscuration of the vertebral body by aberrant bony formations. More accurate assessment can be obtained using newer quantitative CT scanning or DXA scanning of the lateral portion of the L3 vertebral body.[74] Nonetheless, decreased BMD in the peripheral and axial skeleton has been shown to be associated with vertebral body fractures in AS.[77] Moreover, osteoporosis significantly increases the risk of vertebral compression fracture in these patients.[74]

Other reasons that predispose AS patients to fracture is loss of flexibility and ability to absorb impact.[78] Patients with total spinal involvement are at the greatest risk of fracture.[79,80] Overall AS patients have a four- to sevenfold increase in the incidence of spinal fracture when compared with the general population.[81,82] Furthermore, a recent epidemiologic study showed, for reasons thus far unclear, that the frequency of fracture in patients with AS is increasing.[83] Even minimal trauma, including patient transfers, intubation, chiropractic manipulation, and ground-level falls can cause severe fractures in affected patients.[51,84-86] Also, patients with AS have kyphotic deformities that affect their balance making them more likely to fall. Further, the head and face being forward of the trunk creates a point of contact creating an extension force.

Fractures in this population are classically transdiscal,[87] but commonly involve the vertebral body as well.[37] Axial hyperextension is the most common mechanism of injury followed by flexion, rotational, and compression type injuries.[38] The cervical spine is most frequently fractured.[37,38] Diagnosis is delayed in up to 85% of cases as the patients' primary symptom is pain and many of these patients have a long history of chronic back pain.[88-90] Similar to DISH, fractures in AS carry a significantly higher degree of morbidity than those in the nonankylosed patient. Of those fractures that are brought to clinical attention, approximately 60% are complicated by an associated neurologic injury, which is roughly three times the rate in patients without this disorder.[73,80] The rate of neurologic injury appears to be similar for both thoracic and cervical spine fractures.[91] Furthermore, vertebral fractures in this population are associated with a mortality of up to 30%.[73,80] Noncontiguous fractures occur in up to 20% of cases, which can be easily overlooked unless careful scrutiny is given to the entire spinal column.[92] Because of the high risk of overlooking fractures in this population, any new complaint of pain in a patient suffering AS must be treated as a fracture until proven otherwise.

Prognosis of Fractures in Ankylosed Spines

There are several reasons, which apply to both AS and DISH, for why these patients have such high levels of morbidity. Often there is a delay in diagnosis and there is a lack of effective nonoperative treatment. The fused spine creates enlarged lever arms, which concentrate force on the weakest area of the spine, often across the fused intervertebral disc space. When a fracture does occur, it is often a three-column injury affecting the complete diameter of the spinal column[78] and is further rendered unstable by the ossification and loss of supporting ligamentous structures. Especially in AS, there is a high frequency of epidural hematoma associated with fractures.[93] Fractures occurring in the middle of long fused segments have poor healing capacity and if treated incorrectly at onset will develop kyphosis and late neurologic deficits.

TREATMENT OF DIFFUSE IDIOPATHIC SKELETAL HYPEROSTOSIS AND ANKYLOSING SPONDYLITIS

Fractures in DISH and AS are a unique therapeutic challenge for the practicing spine surgeon (Table 36-4). Multisegmental autofusion changes spinal biomechanics to a setting in which the spine acts similar to a long bone with long lever arms acting over the area of fracture, increasing the moment arm forces seen at the fracture site thereby increasing the risk of displacement. This is accompanied by a high rate of kyphotic postural deformities and poor bone quality in many patients. These factors combine to elevate risk at every potential point in treatment from selecting an adequate orthotic to positioning the patients for surgery to safely intubating.

To further complicate therapeutic decision making, patients with DISH and AS have a high incidence of concurrent medical comorbidities. Cardiac disease is statistically the most common of these; however, many of these patients have pulmonary disease, hypertension, and diabetes mellitus.[39,44] These factors contribute to an elevated mortality rate of up to 32% in one series of patients with DISH or AS who suffered fractures.[37] Interestingly, patients treated nonoperatively may have higher mortality rates, with pulmonary complications being the most common complicating factor.[38]

Although impaired mobility in nonoperatively treated patients may predispose to a number of complications, there is no randomized controlled trial evaluating operative versus nonoperative therapy and these data may be the result of a selection bias. As would be expected, severity of neurologic injury also correlates with mortality.[44] There is no consensus on the management of spine fractures in patients with DISH and AS and treatment methods vary widely in the published literature. *More recently because of the high incidence of progressive neurologic deterioration in cases treated nonoperatively, we and others recommend surgical stabilization for most patients with fractures in ankylosed spines.*

TABLE 36-4 *CHALLENGES IN THE MANAGEMENT OF PATIENTS WITH FRACTURES AND ANKYLOSED SPINES*

Diagnosis	Low clinical suspicion due to low energy mechanisms Difficulty interpreting radiographic imaging Presence of noncontiguous fractures
Biomechanics	Long lever arms predispose to fracture displacement Loss of elasticity and energy absorption Preexisting kyphotic deformity
Nonoperative treatment	Skin breakdown Presence of kyphotic deformity Frequent loss of reduction
Surgical management challenges	Airway difficulties Loss of reduction during positioning Osteoporosis Obscure landmarks
Complications	Epidural hematoma Wound infection Hardware failure Cardiopulmonary events

Nonoperative Treatments

Nonoperative treatment modalities typically consist of immobilization of the fractured area. This can be accomplished with bed rest or external orthotics ranging from soft braces to rigid external fixators (e.g., halo fixation). There are significant risks associated with attempting to treat these fractures in this manner. Bed rest is associated with significant morbidity, including the risk of deep venous thrombosis (DVT), pulmonary embolism (PE), pneumonia, insulin resistance, and wound breakdown.[94] While bed rest may be the best option for patients with significant multisystem injuries who are unable to withstand surgery, it is not recommended in those with acceptable surgical risks.

The utilization of external orthoses can be considered as hyperostosis is a disease that may also lead to reliable bony fusion with external immobilization alone. However, the majority of fractures in DISH are highly unstable and at significant risk for displacement. Studies examining the use of external orthoses in this setting have been sporadic and poorly controlled, but do echo the poor outcomes when examined collectively.

Outcomes of Nonoperative Treatment

Westerveld and colleagues reviewed a series of 400 patients in which 46% were treated with external immobilization including traction, halovest, cervical collar, brace, and bedrest.[38] They found that surgical treatment led to improved neurologic function when compared with conservative therapy. Caron and coworkers reviewed 112 patients with AS and DISH with fractures, of whom 18% were treated definitively with external immobilization. None of the patients braced had significant changes in angulation, translation, or distraction from their spinal fracture. They found a mortality rate of 55% in patients who underwent external immobilization alone compared to 23% in the surgically treated group.[37] Other series have demonstrated a high rate of osteolysis and progressive neurologic injury with nonsurgical treatments.[45,95]

Other authors have advocated nonoperative management, citing cases of adequate reduction obtained with traction and sufficient maintenance of alignment being held with external fixation (collars, halos, etc.) for fusion to occur without further neurologic compromise.[96,97] There are several caveats, however, to conservative nonoperative treatment. Immobilization alone is often inadequate because of the unusual degree of instability associated with these fractures.[98] Neurologic deterioration has been reported to occur subsequent to the application of traction[99] and halo devices.[100] It may also predispose patients to pulmonary compromise and decline.[39] Additionally, fixed postural abnormalities in these patients make the application of external fixation devices difficult and, at times, dangerous as they may hold these patients against their preinjury alignment and contribute to further injury.

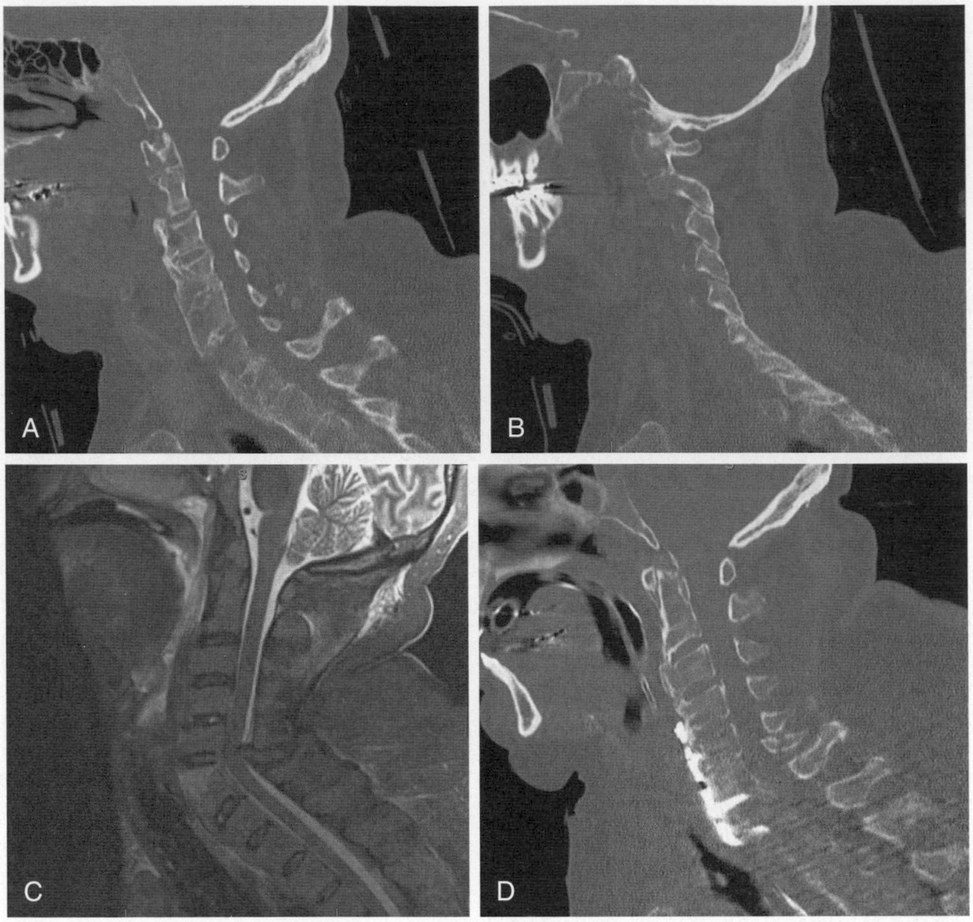

Figure 36-1. Mid-sagittal (**A**) and sagittal reformatted C-spine computed tomography (CT) scan (**B**) demonstrating fracture through C6 vertebral body in a 55-year-old female with neck pain after an in-hospital ground-level fall. The patient was admitted for multiorgan failure and acute respiratory distress syndrome. She was neurologically intact and treated in a C-collar. **C,** Magnetic resonance imaging (MRI) showing dislocation of fracture after emergent intubation performed with inline cervical traction. Patient developed left hemiparesis after intubation. **D,** Postoperative CT demonstrating anterior fixation and reduction of fracture. The patient's frail medical condition precluded posterior fixation.

A final cautionary note must be given to the utilization of external orthotics in patients with fixed spinal deformities. Most noncustom external orthotics are designed to adapt to spines that possess relatively normal contours. In patients with significant postural abnormalities, such as those with the profound cervical-thoracic kyphosis often seen in DISH and AS, the utilization of a normal collar may act to displace the fracture and may lead to neurologic injury.[101] A halo may be used to better maintain the patient's unique position and reduce the risk of fracture displacement. Halo utilization, however, is also fraught with significant risks including pin-site infection, fracture displacement, impaired mobilization, falls, and the development of nonunions.[102,103] In general, we find that the role of external immobilization in DISH and AS to be of somewhat limited utility, although its use may be considered for the treatment of stable fractures not involving all three columns of the spine. Significant deformity including angulation and subluxation due to fracture should be viewed as a relative contraindication to the use of external immobilization alone, unless a palliative course of therapy is being pursued.

Surgical Treatment

We favor an aggressive therapeutic approach, favoring surgical fixation due to the high rate of unstable injuries seen in this population and significant risk of neurologic deterioration without fixation. When surgical intervention is undertaken for these fractures, the spine surgeon must be aware of all the pitfalls unique to this patient population and take preemptive steps to reduce their risk.

Anesthetic and Positioning Considerations

Intubation, transferring, and positioning must be undertaken carefully as there is a substantial risk of exacerbating existing neurologic injury or creating new fractures with these maneuvers[51] (Fig. 36-1). Intubation should be discussed with the anesthesiology team prior to commencement. Patients with cervical fractures should be maintained with inline cervical stabilization with care taken not to extend the neck during intubation. This may require awake intubation with fiberoptic bronchoscope[104] or intubating laryngeal mask.[105] Patients with DISH and no fracture still present a challenge for securement of the airway. The horizontally oriented syndesmophytes commonly seen in DISH predispose these patients to airway compression with subsequent laryngeal edema and airway compromise.[106]

Posteriorly oriented cervical syndesmophytes can lead to neurologic compression and injury with hyperextension of the neck. Positioning is a vulnerable time in which further

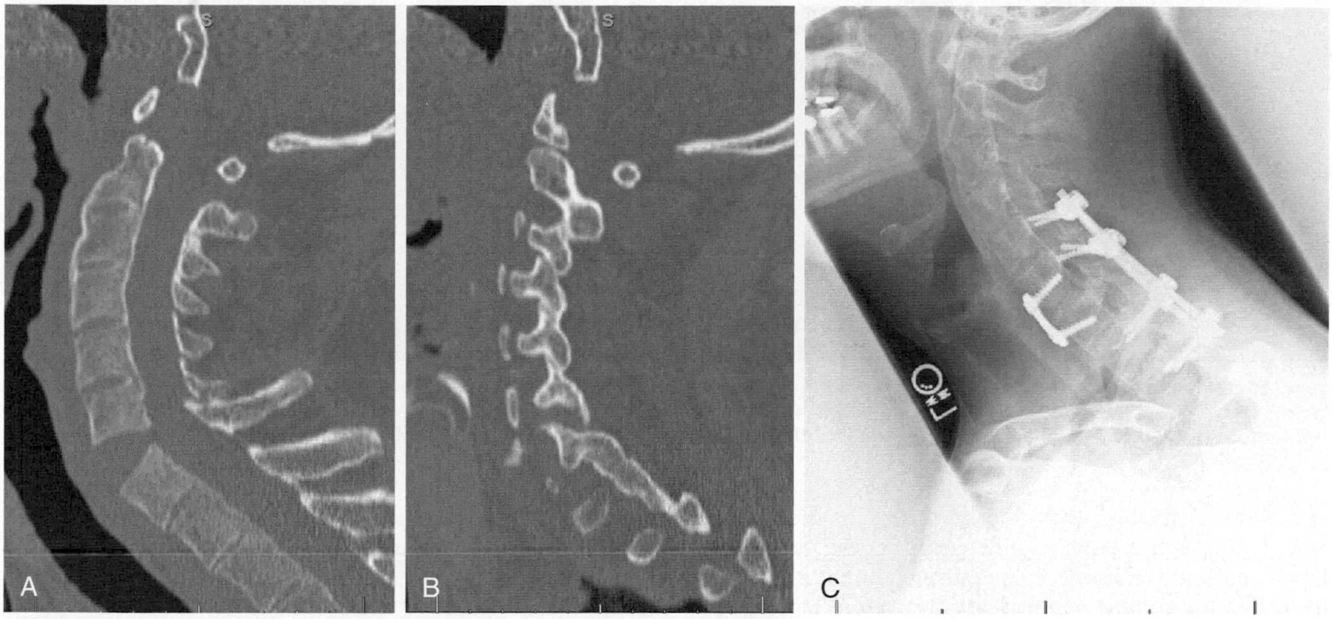

Figure 36-2. Sagittal reformatted computed tomography (CT) scan (**A** and **B**) demonstrating fracture through an ankylosed C6-C7 disc space in a 39-year-old involved in a motor vehicle accident. **C,** Postoperative radiograph demonstrating anterior and posterior fixation. The patient recovered without neurologic deficit.

neurological injury may occur. Poor bone quality and altered spinal biomechanics predispose these patients to fracture during even routine positioning.[107] When using a posterior approach, extreme caution must be taken to prevent further dislocation at the fracture site when turning the patient prone. Using a rotating Jackson table for prone positioning reduces spinal range of motion when compared with traditional manual techniques and may add an additional layer of safety.[108] In the prone position, the head must be rigidly immobilized in a Mayfield or halo fixator to maintain anatomic alignment.

In patients with fracture-dislocations, we typically attempt reduction under live fluoroscopic visualization as ossification and fracture of supporting ligaments lends greater than normal instability to the injured area. The use of neurologic monitoring may be considered in patients without complete neurologic injuries. Ensuring stable neurologic potentials before and after positioning can reassure the surgeon of the safety of positioning.

Principles of Surgical Treatment

The goals of surgical intervention are to stabilize the spine and decompress affected neural elements. Firm guidelines for surgical treatment of these fractures are lacking but a common-sense approach based on fracture type, alignment, and neurologic compromise should be applied. Surgery should be performed at the earliest safe convenience given the high rate of neurologic deterioration associated with fractures. Several authors advocate for a posterior only[37,109] or combined anterior-posterior surgical approach.[110] Patients with acute fractures who present without neurologic deficit and who are in good alignment may undergo posterior fusion only.

Fractures in DISH and AS patients should be treated as if they are "long bone fractures." We recommend that posterior instrumentation extends multiple levels above and below the site of fracture, with or without decompression. Caron and colleagues found no fixation failure with fusion of three levels above and below.[37] As the spine is already rigid in these patients, longer constructs do not compromise mobility and offer greater strength of fixation.

Most patients can be treated by a posterior approach only. An anterior or anterior-posterior approach may be warranted for poor bone quality or need for ventral cord decompression. The anterior approach is difficult and instrumentation is usually inadequate due to poor bone quality.

Fracture reduction can be challenging. Care must be taken not to overcorrect the sagittal balance in these patients. Overcorrection of a preexisting kyphotic deformity may lead to points of structural weakness prone to hardware failure as well as neurologic compromise. At times, posterior fixation alone may be inadequate as it may be difficult to obtain complete apposition of the anterior elements of the spine. Although this theoretically may predispose to pseudarthrosis, in our experience the anterior defect remodels with bone.

Indications for anterior or a 360-degree approach (Fig. 36-2) include significant posterior displacement of the vertebral body resulting in continued neural compression, the presence of a symptomatic disc herniation, or inability to obtain multilevel posterior spinal fusion due to fracture at several levels or some other anatomical variation.

Fixed deformity and the inability to flex and extend the fused spine can make exposure difficult (Fig. 36-3).[73] While deformity correction can be undertaken at the time of fracture treatment,[111] caution must be exercised as complications, including nonunion and vertebral artery injury, may result.[78,112] Normal anatomic landmarks can be dramatically altered, and once the spinal levels of interest are exposed, special care must be taken to avoid surgical complications. Taggard and Traynelis recommend the placement of short (13 mm) lateral mass screws in the cervical spine to avoid nerve root injury should the trajectory be poor secondary to an obscured entry point.[113] Posterior cervical fixation is undertaken with lateral mass and

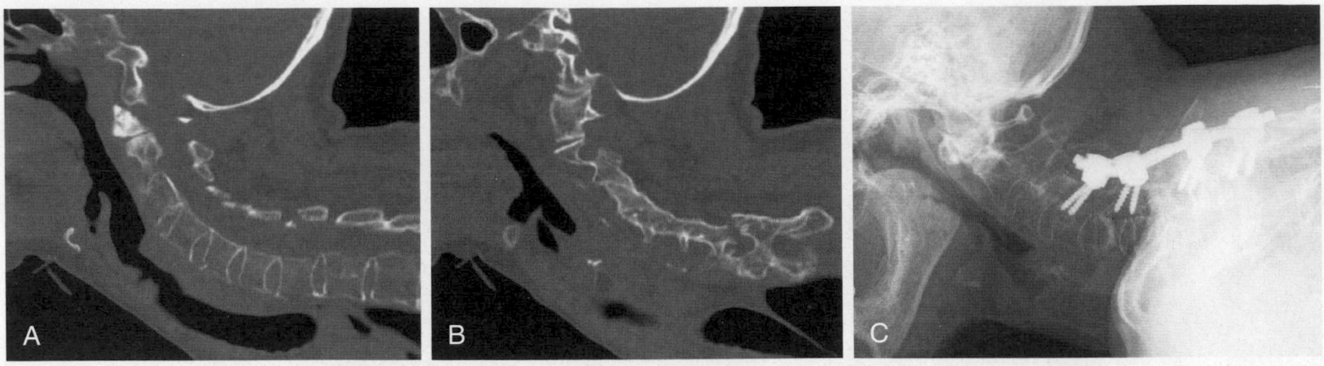

Figure 36-3. Sagittal (**A**) and parasagittal computed tomography (CT) scan (**B**) demonstrating a fracture through the anterior and posterior elements of C7 in a 77-year-old female with severe kyphotic and lordotic deformities of the spine who presented with neck pain after a low-speed motor vehicle accident. The patient underwent posterior spinal fusion (**C**) and was able to mobilize in the immediate postoperative period.

thoracolumbar fixation with pedicle screws in the standard manner, although anatomic differences in the fused spine warrant caution.[113] Careful preoperative planning is needed to understand the unique surgical anatomy. Other specific pitfalls include ossified ligaments and osteoporotic bone which may make spine decompression and the use of strut grafts difficult.[73] Finally, frequent arachnoid diverticula may predispose to postoperative spinal fluid leak.[51,114]

Complications of Surgical Treatment

Operative and medical complications are invariably high in this patient population and range from 33% to 84%.[37,39,44] Common complications include aspiration pneumonia, respiratory failure, and DVT.[38] The rate of postoperative hardware failure varies. Anterior fusion alone should be approached cautiously as one series found a 50% implant failure rate.[115]

Bransford and colleagues reported only one construct failure in a series of 33 patients.[44] Likewise, other series report a relatively low rate of construct failure.[37,39] Reoperation for wound infection and suboptimal positioning of hardware is also noted, but does not appear to be elevated compared to the general population.

Surgical Outcomes

Despite these complications, neurologic recovery is significantly higher in surgically treated patients.[38] Furthermore, the rate of adverse events and mortality appears to be much higher in patients treated conservatively compared to surgically treated patients.[38] Overall, approximately 50% experience some improvement in neurologic function following injury while as many as 35% may make a complete recovery.[51,78,90,91]

Special Considerations

Pseudarthroses also demand the attention of the spinal surgeon. Pseudarthroses present with increased back pain and neurologic deficit that is often radicular (Fig. 36-4).[116] Pseudarthroses occurring at the intervertebral disc space are believed to be the result of a trauma that was often trivial and unrecognized.[116,117] Fracture through the ossified intervertebral disc must be combined with posterior element instability (e.g., fracture through or nonfusion of the facets).[118] The resulting instability results in progressive osteolysis of the vertebral bodies with adjacent sclerosis. More severe cases evolve to overt instability with subluxation and thecal sac compression.[116,118] These lesions can be difficult to distinguish from infection or neoplastic infiltration on imaging; however, a history of trauma combined with a lack of enhancement and presence of posterior element mobility support the diagnosis.[116] Surgery is the best treatment of these lesions as 40% of patients fail conservative treatment.[118] Progressive neurologic deficit, pain, and subluxation are indications for surgery, which can often be undertaken via a posterior approach.[51] Neural element compromise mandates decompression, and severe instability with three-column disruption mandates posterior and anterior fusion with excision of the pseudarthrosis and anterior graft placement.[51]

Spinal stenosis is a relatively infrequent comorbidity in AS, affecting 3 out of 105 patients in one series.[73] It may occur secondary to anterior compression from syndesmophytes, posterior ligamentous proliferation, and ossification, or it may be coincidental.[51,119,120] These patients may be treated with posterior decompressive laminectomies as in other cases of spinal stenosis. More importantly, spinal stenosis must be suspected in all AS patients who are undergoing spinal procedures for other reasons and care must be taken when performing laminectomies in these situations.[51]

AS patients may also occasionally suffer from instability at the C1-C2 joint, which may consist of rotary and anterior atlantoaxial subluxation.[121] Such instability is estimated to affect 1% to 2% of patients[122,123] and appears to be more common in those with long-standing severe disease, although it has been reported as an initial manifestation of AS.[124] The etiology of this instability is thought to be twofold with subaxial fusion resulting in increased physical stress across a joint that may already have added ligamentous laxity and bony erosions secondary to the disease process itself.[125] Although both surgical[125] and nonsurgical treatments[51] have been proposed, we feel that C1-C2 fusion via either a transarticular screw or Harms fixation after adequate reduction, should be the mainstay of treatment. We have also successfully used odontoid screw fixation in patients with odontoid fracture to preserve motion about the atlantoaxial joint, which in many cases is the only mobile joint remaining in patients with severe disease (Fig. 36-5).

CONCLUSION

AS and DISH are complex disease processes with significant implications for the spine surgeon. Spine fractures in these

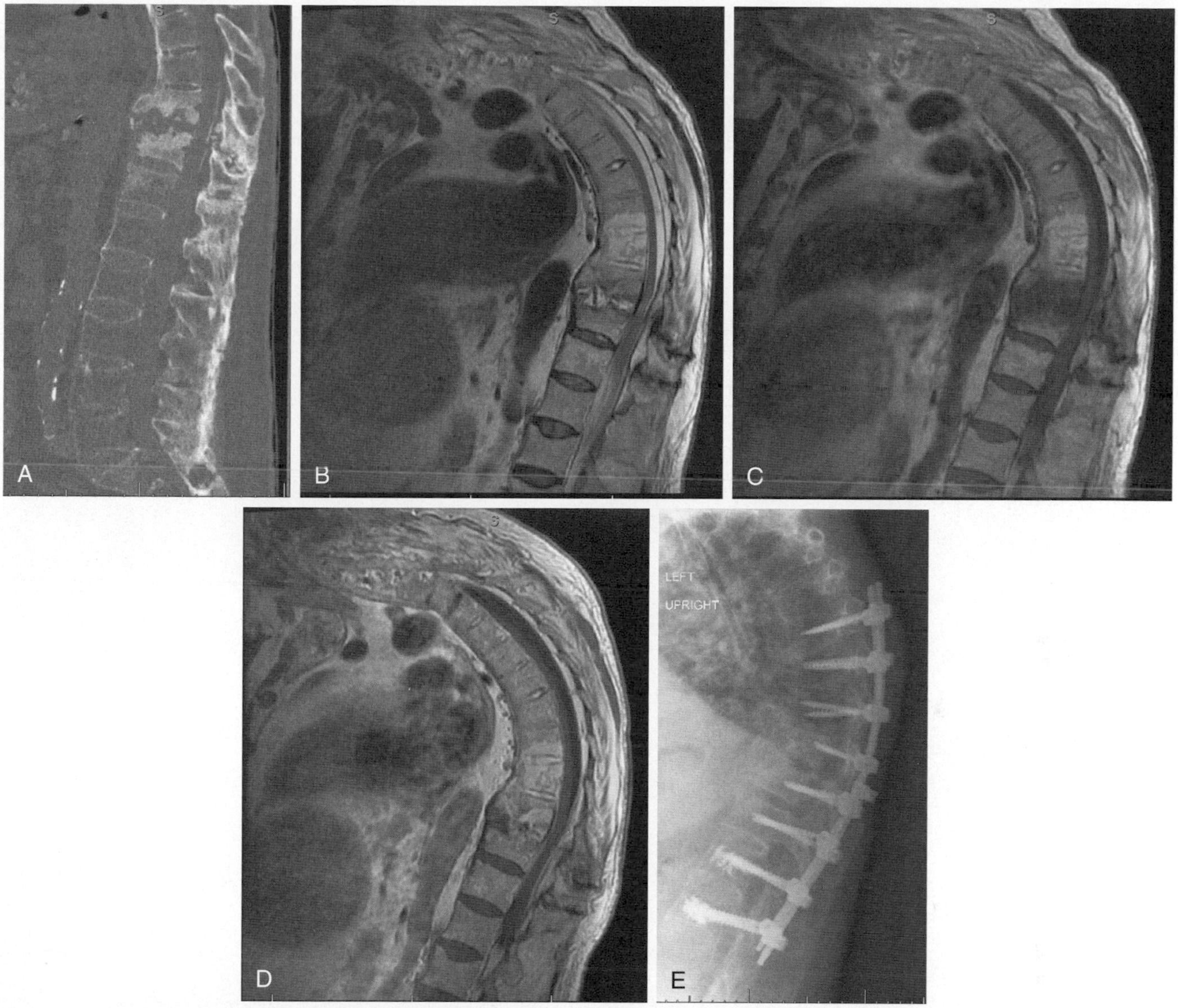

Figure 36-4. Sagittal reformatted computed tomography (CT) scan (**A**) and magnetic resonance imaging (MRI) T2 (**B**), T1 (**C**), and postcontrast (**D**) of a 74-year-old male with a 1-year history of back pain and 6 months of increasing paraparesis after a ground-level fall. Patient underwent needle-guided biopsy, which did not reveal infection. Patient underwent T7-L2 posterior spinal fusion with Smith-Peterson osteotomies at T10-T11 (**F**). Reactive fibrous tissue was noted at pseudoarthrotic level.

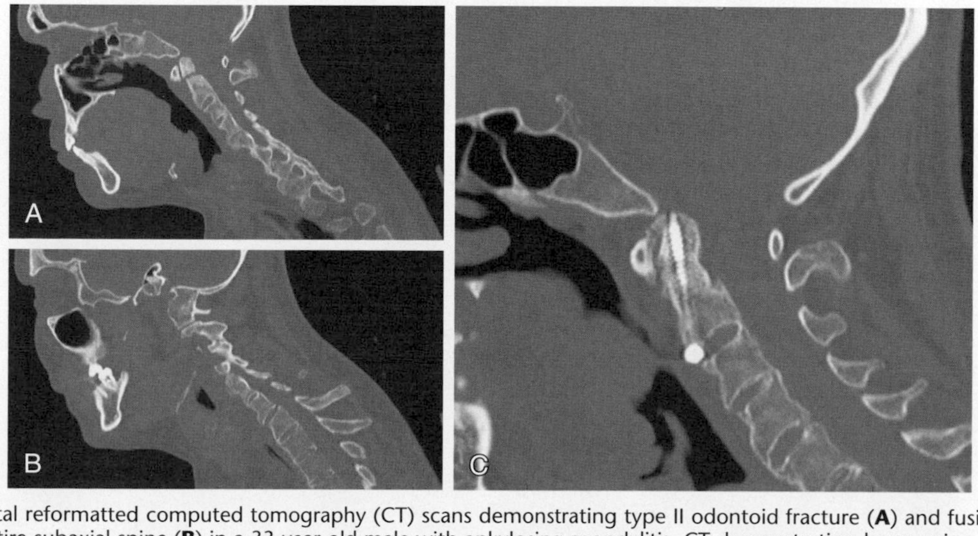

Figure 36-5. Sagittal reformatted computed tomography (CT) scans demonstrating type II odontoid fracture (**A**) and fusion of the occiput to C1 as well as the entire subaxial spine (**B**) in a 33-year-old male with ankylosing spondylitis. CT demonstrating bony union of odontoid fracture after odontoid screw placement (**C**). Motion of the atlantoaxial joint, the patient's only remaining mobile segment, was preserved.

patients carry a significantly higher morbidity and mortality than those in the general population. Treatment of these fractures is a contentious issue with a paucity of data available to compare the outcomes of those treated surgically versus those treated conservatively. We prefer aggressive surgical management of spinal fractures in these patient populations as we have experienced rapid mobilization and definitive fracture fixation without a large degree of surgical morbidity.

KEY REFERENCES

The level of evidence (LOE) is determined according to the criteria provided in the preface.

2. Resnick D, Shaul SR, Robins JM: Diffuse idiopathic skeletal hyperostosis (DISH): Forestier's disease with extraspinal manifestations. *Radiology* 115(3):513–524, 1975. LOE III
37. Caron T, Bransford R, Nguyen Q, et al: Spine fractures in patients with ankylosing spinal disorders. *Spine* 35(11):E458–E464, 2010. LOE III
38. Westerveld LA, Verlaan JJ, Oner FC: Spinal fractures in patients with ankylosing spinal disorders: a systematic review of the literature on treatment, neurological status and complications. *Eur Spine J* 18(2):145–156, 2009. LOE III
42. Verlaan JJ, Westerveld LA, van Keulen JW, et al: Quantitative analysis of the anterolateral ossification mass in diffuse idiopathic skeletal hyperostosis of the thoracic spine. *Eur Spine J* 20(9):1474–1479, 2011. LOE II
44. Bransford RJ, Koller H, Caron T, et al: Cervical spine trauma in diffuse idiopathic skeletal hyperostosis: injury characteristics and outcome with surgical treatment. *Spine* 37(23):1923–1932, 2012. LOE III
81. Weiss RJ, Wick MC, Ackermann PW, et al: Increased fracture risk in patients with rheumatic disorders and other inflammatory diseases—a case-control study with 53,108 patients with fracture. *J Rheumatol* 37(11):2247–2250, 2010. LOE III
83. Robinson Y, Sanden B, Olerud C: Increased occurrence of spinal fractures related to ankylosing spondylitis: a prospective 22-year cohort study in 17,764 patients from a national registry in Sweden. *Patient Saf Surg.* 7(1):2, 2013. LOE III
113. Taggard DA, Traynelis VC: Management of cervical spinal fractures in ankylosing spondylitis with posterior fixation. *Spine* 25(16):2035–2039, 2000. LOE III

The complete References list is available online at https://expertconsult.inkling.com.

Chapter 37

Osteoporotic Spinal Fractures

JASON W. SAVAGE • PAUL A. ANDERSON

INTRODUCTION: SCOPE AND PURPOSE

Osteoporosis is a common disease that is characterized by structural deterioration of bone architecture and manifests itself as fragility fractures occurring at multiple skeletal sites, most commonly involving the spine, hip, or wrist.[1,2] It is increasingly recognized that osteoporosis is an important health problem because of the large affected population and the devastating impact of osteoporotic fractures on patient morbidity and mortality, as well as on societal costs.[3] The purpose of this chapter is to highlight the clinical and socioeconomic concerns of osteoporotic spine fractures and to give an overview of nonoperative and operative treatment for patients who sustain these injuries.

The prevalence of osteoporosis in the United States is estimated to increase from approximately 10 million to more than 14 million people in 2020.[2,4] Using the World Health Organization's definition of osteoporosis, a bone mineral density (BMD) more than 2.5 standard deviations below the mean in young, normal people, approximately 30% of postmenopausal white women in the United States have osteoporosis.[5] Prevalence rates are lower when bone density is assessed at a single skeletal site, and it is estimated that 16% to 20% of this population has osteoporosis of the lumbar spine.[5] Historically, fragility spine fractures in men were thought to be uncommon. However, recent population-based studies show an unexpectedly high frequency of vertebral fractures in men.[3,6-11] It is now estimated that men account for more than 25% of the burden of osteoporosis-related fractures in the United States.[2]

Cooper and colleagues reported that the overall age- and sex-adjusted incidence of vertebral fractures to be 117 per 100,000[7] and that altogether, 25% of women 50 years of age or older had one or more vertebral fractures.[3] This rate is consistent with the 20% reported in an Australian population,[12] 21% reported in a random sample of 70-year-old Danish women,[13] and the 24% documented among elderly white women from other longitudinal studies.[10] The U.S. population 50 years of age and older is predicted to increase by 60% between 2000 and 2025, eventually reaching 120 million people,[14] which will undoubtedly cause a rise in the number of people affected by osteoporotic fractures.

Unlike fractures of the hip and forearm, spine fragility fractures are often not associated with a fall or trauma. It is estimated that only 30% of osteoporotic vertebral fractures come to clinical attention,[7,15-17] and many are incidentally found on routine imaging studies. Unfortunately, many of these patients present with a substantial increase in back pain that often causes significant morbidity. Even if the acute pain of a spinal fragility fracture subsides, many patients develop irreversible spinal deformity, usually an increase in kyphosis, that is associated with significant health consequences, including decreased physical functioning (sarcopenia) and health-related quality of life (HRQOL),[18,19] chronic back pain,[16] impaired balance, and increased subsequent falls.[20] Another concerning finding is that patients who have one or more vertebral fracture at baseline are five times more likely to develop another spinal fragility fracture compared with patients without prevalent vertebral fracture at baseline.[21]

For most patients, pain and its effect on physical function are the leading cause of morbidity associated with these fractures. A recent prospective observational study showed that radiographically detected vertebral fractures were associated with long-term substantial increases in back pain and back-related disability compared with before fracture.[16] After adjustments for covariates, women with a fracture had a 2.4 times higher risk for increased back pain compared with women without a fracture during the 4-year follow-up period. Furthermore, the annual rate of days of bed rest was nine times higher in women with a first incident fracture, and the rate of limited activity days was approximately twice has high compared with the control group.[16] Based on their data, the authors estimated an additional 10 days per year of limited activity because of back pain in the fragility fracture group. This is comparable to the days of limited activity for patients with diabetes (15 days), ischemic heart disease (15 days), and arthritis and rheumatism (7 days).[22]

Osteoporotic fractures have a significant impact on HRQOL.[18] Hallberg and colleagues found that HRQOL was significantly lower for all domains, physical and mental, at the 3- and 24-month follow-up after osteoporotic fractures in women 55 to 75 years of age. Moreover, vertebral fractures have a considerably greater and more prolonged impact on HRQOL than hip, forearm, and humerus fractures.

Osteoporotic spine fractures are also associated with an increased risk of death.[23-26] Lau and colleagues reviewed Medicare claims from 1997 through 2004 and found that the overall mortality rate after a vertebral fracture was twice that of the matched control participants.[27] The survival rates after a fracture diagnosis, as estimated with the Kaplan-Meier method, were 53.9%, 30.9%, and 10.5% at 3, 5, and 7 years, respectively, and were significantly lower compared with control participants. The mortality risk was greater for men than women, and the overall difference in mortality was greatest when the patients were younger at the time of fracture. Kado and colleagues showed that women with at least one new fracture have an age-adjusted 32% increased risk of death compared with those without incident vertebral fracture.[28] They concluded that this increased risk of death is explained in large part by associated weight loss and markers of decreased physical function. Mortality risk is 25% greater after spine fracture than hip fracture.[29]

Osteoporosis, and in particular osteoporotic spine fractures, has a great socioeconomic impact and therefore has become an important public health problem and concern. In 2005, fragility fractures in the United States resulted in 2.5 million medical office visits, 430,000 hospital admissions, and 180,000 nursing home admissions.[1] Their direct cost was $17 billion.[1,30] The projected increase in the elderly U.S. population will likely cause this economic burden to significantly increase over the next several decades. Therefore, healthcare professionals need to focus on identifying patients at risk for osteoporosis and use evidence-based treatment strategies to prevent fractures in an ultimate effort to decrease the morbidity and mortality associated with these fractures. In select patients who fail nonoperative treatment, surgical intervention may be indicated.

MECHANISM OF INJURY AND BIOMECHANICS

There is a general loss of bone mass with age; therefore, osteoporosis represents an extreme form of the normal aging process. The clinical manifestation of osteoporosis is fracture of the axial or appendicular skeleton (or both). Although extremity fractures are usually related to falls, approximately half of spinal fragility fractures are "spontaneous" without a traumatic event.[31] A fracture occurs when the forces applied to the vertebrae exceed its strength. Therefore, factors related to skeletal fragility and spinal loading play important roles in their development.[32]

In general, the ability of cortical bone to resist fracture deteriorates with aging. Several studies have indicated that although the elastic properties of cortical bone decrease modestly with age, the strength and toughness decrease more substantially.[31] The porosity of cortical bone increases significantly with aging, and porosity is negatively correlated with bone material properties.[33] This leads to a loss of stiffness, strength, and toughness. Unlike the appendicular skeleton, which is composed primarily of cortical bone, the axial skeleton or vertebral column is predominantly trabecular in nature. The mechanical properties of trabecular bone (modulus and strength) are most affected by apparent density, or bone mass. The apparent density of trabecular bone decreases markedly with aging in both men and women. The loss of bone mass is the most significant contributor to an increase in fracture risk, but there are also changes in the microarchitecture, tissue properties, and levels of microdamage that significantly affect the strength of the vertebra. Increasing bending forces from kyphosis may significantly increase fracture risk in osteoporotic patients.

The compressive strength of vertebral trabecular bone decreases by approximately 70% from 25 to 75 years of age.[34] There is a reduction in the thickness and number of individual trabeculae, which leads to microstructural damage and weakening of the trabecular bone. Further, horizontal trabeculae are preferentially lost. This results in a more anisotropic structure, which has a greater susceptibility to fracture. Transverse trabeculae are preferentially thinned and perforated while the remaining vertical trabeculae maintain their thickness. This structure is likely to be more susceptible to buckling under normal compressive loads and has a decreased ability to withstand unusual or off-axis loads.[35]

Other age-related changes contribute to spinal fragility fractures, including intervertebral disc degeneration and changes in neuromuscular function. The intervertebral discs play an important role in distributing forces that are transmitted to the vertebral bodies. With increasing age, the intervertebral disc is subject to the degenerative cascade, including dehydration of the nucleus pulposus, fibrosis of the annulus, and osteophyte formation, which disables the disc to distribute compressive forces evenly. As a result of this altered stress distribution, the anterior vertebral body is stress shielded during normal erect posture but severely overloaded when the spine is flexed.[36] Therefore, the anterior vertebral body becomes vulnerable to osteoporotic fracture. It is important to note that altered stress distribution is also often caused by spinal fusion procedures. The abnormal stress that is placed at the adjacent level leads to an increased risk of developing an osteoporotic fracture at the adjacent segment.

Significant changes in neuromuscular function also play a role in the development of osteoporotic spine fractures. Muscular strength decreases 24% to 36% by the age of 70 years,[37] and these changes in force production could detrimentally change the loading of the spine because antagonist muscle contraction is key for maintaining stability of the spine during flexion and extension.[38] This reduction in intrinsic spine stability may contribute to poorer balance and postural stability, which may further contribute to falls that lead to fractures.[32] Osteoporotic patients have associated sarcopenia, correction of which offers a management opportunity.

EVALUATION

Patients who sustain osteoporotic spine fractures often present to their primary care doctors or emergency departments complaining of acute-onset back pain. A thorough spine and neurologic examination should be performed, and the entire spinal column should be palpated and inspected for areas of tenderness to palpation, as well as focal abnormalities (i.e., palpable step-offs between the spinous processes). A detailed motor and sensory examination should be documented, and the presence of any pathologic reflexes should be elicited (hyperreflexia, clonus, Babinski sign, and so on). It is rare for these patients to sustain a neurologic injury, but in such cases, an accurate motor and sensory level and degree of injury (American Spinal Injury Association Grade A–E) needs to be clearly defined.

DIAGNOSIS AND CLASSIFICATION

Upright biplanar plain radiographs of the spine should be the first imaging modality used to evaluate patients with a suspected osteoporotic spine fracture. An anteroposterior (AP) and lateral radiograph should be taken of the suspected area of injury based on the physical examination. If a fracture is present, the degree of vertebral body collapse and presence of focal or global deformity should be noted. A computed tomography (CT) scan should be used if the radiographs are equivocal or more detail is needed to help determine treatment. CT is much more sensitive and specific in detecting spinal column injuries compared with plain radiographs. If CT has been performed, an estimation of bone mineral density (BMD) can be made by determination of Hounsfield units, which can easily be measured using the CT software.[39] Finally, magnetic resonance imaging (MRI) is used to determine, if necessary, the acuity of the fracture, or in the presence of neurologic compression.

MANAGEMENT

The majority of patients having osteoporotic spine fractures are initially treated nonsurgically, with the use of analgesics, a brief period of bed rest, initiation of osteoporosis medication, bracing, and physical therapy.[40,41] It is important to mobilize these patients as quickly as possible and limit the amount of narcotic pain mediation used. In a select group of patients, cement augmentation procedures or more invasive surgical interventions may be warranted.

Cement Augmentation: Vertebroplasty and Kyphoplasty

Cement augmentation of painful osteoporotic compression fractures is the percutaneous stabilization of vertebral bodies with polymethylmethacrylate (PMMA) and more recently other ceramic alternatives. It is a common procedure with as many as 75,000 being performed annually in the Medicare population in the United States. Two techniques are widely used, vertebroplasty and kyphoplasty. Vertebroplasty was initially described for the treatment of aggressive hemangioma of the lumbar spine. It is performed through a needle, which is inserted via a transpedicular approach into the vertebral body. Liquid cement is installed under pressure to fill the fractured vertebral body, which rapidly polymerizes. Improvement in kyphotic angulation, if any, is obtained by prone positioning in extension. Kyphoplasty attempts to reduce the wedge-shaped vertebrae and thus improve kyphotic angulation by expansion of the compressed verbal body using an inflatable balloon. After vertebral body expansion, cement augmentation is performed.

Indications

The indications and timing of cement augmentation are poorly delineated, leading to variations in use and in outcomes, raising concern that the procedure is overused. This controversy was further escalated with publication of two randomized controlled trials (RCTs) that reported that vertebroplasty was no better than sham treatment.[42,43] These results led to editorials in lay and peer-reviewed journals of its unproven efficacy and to withdrawal of coverage in North America as well as other countries.[44]

The common indication is patients with painful osteoporotic compression fracture that fails to improve with time and nonoperative management.[45] The time between fracture and consideration of cement augmentation is controversial. Most authors suggest a minimum of 3 weeks of nonoperative care, although the usual duration of symptoms of osteoporotic vertebral compression (OVC) fracture is 2 to 3 months. Another indication is in patients hospitalized for pain and functional impairment secondary to osteoporotic fractures.[46] In these patients, cement augmentation can afford rapid improvement and has been shown to be cost effective. Other indications are in painful primary bone tumors such as aggressive hemangioma and giant cell tumors and lytic metastatic tumors with fracture or pending fracture. Finally, cement augmentation is indicated in patients with painful nonunion of a vertebral fracture, so-called Kummel disease.[47]

Contraindications for cement augmentation include asymptomatic patients, history of vertebral osteomyelitis, allergy to bone fillers or opacification agents, uncorrected coagulopathy, or for prophylaxis. Relative contraindications are radicular pain, bone retropulsion against neural structures, greater than 70% collapse, multiple pathologic fractures of diffuse disease, and lack of surgical backup to manage complications.

Patient Selection

Because back pain is common and associated with other diseases of aging, the pain must be correlated to the fracture. Localized tenderness at the fracture site is most often present, although referred pain patterns such as low back pain for a T12 or L1 lesion can be confusing. Confirmation that a new fracture is present by a MRI, bone scan, or from serial images should be established. MRI is excellent to determine fracture acuity, pattern, and identification of adjacent occult fractures. MRI findings include increased signal intensity in the body on T2 and short tau inversion recovery (STIR) images and decreased signal on T1.

Several fracture patterns pose difficulties for cement augmentation. Kummel disease is a fracture nonunion in which a fluid-filled cleft is created within the vertebral body. Cement placement can be challenging because containment may be lacking when vertebral height has been lost.[48] Vertebra plana occurs when more than 70% height has been lost. This is also technical challenging, but Young and colleagues have had satisfactory outcomes in such cases, although cement leakage is more common.[49] Burst fractures or those with defects in the posterior vertebral body wall are at higher risk for cement migration into the spinal canal. Hartmann and colleagues, however, have shown that kyphoplasty is safe and feasible in 26 patients who had burst-type fractures.[50] In these cases, kyphoplasty may be preferred over vertebroplasty to limit extravasation of cement. Other important considerations are the degree of kyphotic deformity and osteoporosis. When severe in both cases, failure may occur to either new fractures or refracture of cement at the index level.

Vertebroplasty Technique

Anesthesia and Patient Positioning. Vertebroplasty is performed under local anesthesia and conscious sedation. Because the patient is in a prone position, careful monitoring is needed to assess the airway, ventilation, and pain. The procedure may be done in a radiology suite or operating room. The patient lies on radiolucent bolsters, which can provide some lordosis. The use of two orthogonal C-arm fluoroscopy units, obtaining simultaneous AP and lateral images facilitates the procedure. After positioning, AP radiographs are checked to ensure that the spine is squarely positioned, noting that the spinous process is exactly between the pedicles.

Pedicle Insertion. In the lumbar spine, a transpedicular approach is used to gain access to the vertebral body. In the thoracic spine, this approach may be used if possible, but if the pedicle is too small, then a lateral extrapedicle approach will be required. The goal is to place a coaxial 8-, 10-, or 11-gauge needle down the pedicle into the fractured body below the endplate or fracture. The starting point for needle insertion is the upper outer margin of the pedicle. Using biplanar fluoroscopic control, the needle should pass into the pedicle aiming medially and caudally. On the AP view, the needle should not appear medial to the pedicle until it is positioned into the vertebral body, which occurs after 15 mm of depth. The needle is advanced until its tip is about 1 cm from the anterior cortex. On the lateral view, the needle position will vary depending on fracture morphology. The goal is to use the remaining cortical margins to "contain" the cement to avoid extravasation. The process is repeated on the opposite side. After proper needle position is ensured, the inner trocar is removed, and the cement can be inserted.

Cement Application. The bone cement is mixed and contains barium to aid radiographic analysis. The viscosity will affect the distribution into the trabecular patterns of the vertebral body and the risk of extravasation. In general, as viscous a material as possible is injected at a slow rate under biplanar radiographic visualization. Proprietary devices are available that pressurize the cement, forcing it into the vertebral bodies. Most commonly, 2 to 3 cc of cement is inserted into each side. The trocar is replaced until the cement polymerizes, and then the needle is removed. During cement installation, imaging is critically assessed for extravasation (Fig. 37-1). Extravasation will limit the amount of cement that can be placed. Common areas of extravasation are lateral, intradiscal, and anterior. Extravasation posteriorly requires aborting the procedure.

Postoperative Care. After polymerization the patient can be mobilized without bracing or restrictions of activity. However, osteoporotic patients with or with vertebroplasty are at risk for new fracture, and medical management of this condition is an essential component of vertebroplasty care.

Kyphoplasty

Kyphoplasty is the elevation of the endplate using a balloon tamp or other mechanical devices. In addition to expanding the vertebral body, it corrects wedging of the vertebrae, reduces the kyphotic deformity, and creates a void where bone void filler can be installed. This void allows use of more viscous bone filler installed under lower pressure that theoretically may lessen risk of extravasation.

Technique. The patient is positioned as described earlier for vertebroplasty. Although classically done under general anesthesia, kyphoplasty may be done with local anesthesia and conscious sedation. An 8- to 11-gauge coaxial needle is placed into the pedicle directed into the vertebral body. The needle is located just anterior to the base of pedicle on the lateral view. The trochar is removed, and a small Kirschner wire (K-wire) is advanced into the body and directed to within 1 cm of the anterior vertebral body. The coaxial needle is removed, and a large working cannula is inserted over the K-wire until it is just inside the vertebral body. A drill is then used to create a path in the body to within 1 cm of the anterior cortex. The balloon tamp can now be inserted through the working cannula into the body and is positioned to be anterior to the posterior vertebral body wall. The process is repeated on the opposite side.

The balloons are expanded using radiopaque solution, and the pressure is monitored. Biplanar radiographs are monitored for balloon position and the degree of correction of the deformity. Balloon expansion continues until correction is obtained, the maximum pressure is reached, or the balloon contacts the cortical margins. The balloons are then deflated and removed and replaced by cannulas filled with cement. Using hand pressure, the cement is installed into the vertebra by insertion of an obturator into the cannulas. During installation, biplane images are scrutinized for extravasation. Most commonly, 2 to 3 cc of bone filler is installed per side. After bone void filler installation, the obturators are inserted into the cannulas until polymerization has occurred. The cannulas may then be removed.

Modifications of Cement Augmentation. Many modifications to simplify and reduce the risk of cement augmentation have been proposed. In biomechanical studies, comparison of a single-side approach versus bilateral pedicle approaches has shown that more cement can be placed using bilateral techniques but that stiffness and failure strength are not clinically significantly different. This is true for both vertebroplasty and kyphoplasty. In a cohort studies, Chen and colleagues and Wang demonstrated similar pain relief and radiographic outcomes between unilateral and bilateral kyphoplasty approaches.[51,52] To provide better distribution of cement with a unilateral approach, a more lateral starting point can be used, which allows greater medial angulation. Alternatively, curved cannulas have been developed to allow unilateral cement placement. A unilateral approach decreases time, costs, and radiation exposure.

The volume of cement will change the biomechanical properties of the repaired vertebral body. Because the vertebral bone volume varies among individuals and by anatomic level (T1–L5), the absolute amount of cement that should be used cannot be stated. Mean bone volumes of intact bodies range from about 10 mm^3 at upper thoracic vertebrae to 35 mm^3 in the lower lumbar vertebrae. The amount of "fill," percent bone volume of fractured vertebrae, appears to give best clinical results. Nieuwenhuijse and colleagues reported that responders to vertebroplasty had greater fill of up 22% than nonresponders, who had only 15%.[53] They recommended that optimal results are obtained when the fill is 24% of the fractured vertebral body. Depending on the severity of the fracture and the fracture type, this is 3 to 4 mm^3. Increasing cement volume increases biomechanical stiffness but also the chance of extravasation and possible adjacent-level fracture.

Radiographic morphology has an effect on specific cement techniques, indications, and outcomes. Decreased BMD reduces resistance to cement flow and possibly leads to more risk of extravasation. Furthermore, the construct is more at risk to fail because of further compression locally or at adjacent levels. This emphasizes the importance of medical management of metabolic bone disease. The presence of an intervertebral cleft most commonly occurs at the thoracolumbar junction and is an indication an unstable fracture, which often will be associated with pain. Radiographically, there is severe collapse with presence of gas inside the body and/or associated disc space. Supine and upright radiographs show significant change in height and angulation, indicating instability. MRI will show dark lines on T1 and fluid cavities of T2 and STIR sequences. In a cohort study by Nieuwenhuijse and colleagues, patient-reported outcomes were similar between patients with and without clefts, but pain relief occurs more slowly in these patients, and cement extravasation is more likely.[53] Severe compression fractures or so-called vertebra plana produce technical difficulties to the delivery of cement. Modified techniques are needed that require the needle to be placed in a more caudal direction and use of bilateral approaches. Pain relief appears satisfactory in these severe cases, but the incidences of cement leakage and refracture are higher.[54] With severe collapse, the posterior wall can be

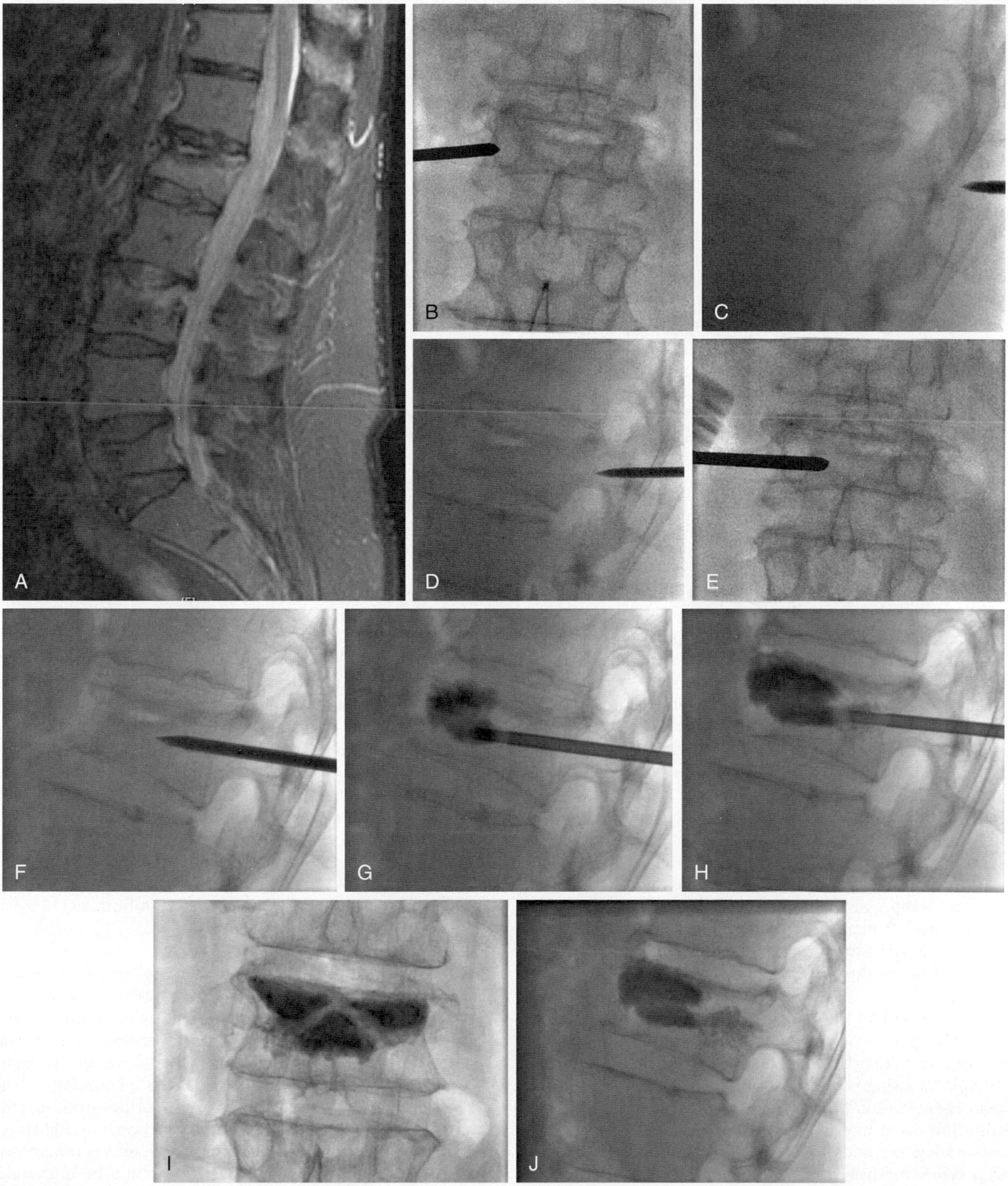

Figure 37-1. A 71-year-old man with an L3 osteoporotic compression fracture who had debilitating back pain despite 3 weeks of adequate nonoperative conservative care. **A,** Sagittal sequence in magnetic resonance imaging demonstrating the acute L3 compression fracture. **B** to **J,** The technique of performing a vertebroplasty. **B** to **F,** Appropriate placement of the trochar needle through the pedicle and into the vertebral body on biplanar fluoroscopy. **G** to **J,** Injection of cement into the vertebral body.

retropulsed into the canal with or without neurologic change. In the presence of neurologic deficits, cement augmentation should not be undertaken without adequate decompression. In patients with pain and these burst-type fractures, the use of cement augmentation is controversial. Hartmann and colleagues reported excellent outcome in 26 patients with burst-type fractures and no cement leakage into the spinal canal.[50] Although kyphosis and vertebral body height correction was achieved initially, this was lost in most patients because of subsidence during follow-up.

Cement Formulations. Polymethylmethacrylate- and calcium phosphate (CaP)–based cement are commonly used for cement augmentation. Recently, chemical modifications of PMMA have improved rheology properties to optimize fluid flow through the needle and to change the rate of polymerization, thus reducing temperature. A simple method to reduce the exothermic reaction is to cool the monomer with ice before mixing. In general, the use of a more viscous cement is preferable to avoid extravasation. Other formulations in testing are nanosphere particles and other compounds that may have a biologic effect on bone cells to increase bony attachment and therefore stability. Clinical outcomes showing advantages of these alternatives over PMMA are lacking. Cortoss is an approved methyl-methacrylate compound with radiopaque bioglass ceramic particles having material properties close to bone. In a randomized controlled trial, Cortoss did not show any significant improvement over standard PMMA.[55]

Calcium phosphate cements have been approved for bone void fillers and are widely used in orthopaedic trauma and tumor reconstruction. They are intriguing bone fillers because they have the capacity for resorption and remolding and have a minimal exothermic reaction. Their use in vertebroplasty has been slow in North America because animal studies have shown that one formulation fragments after installation, resulting in embolization and hemodynamic collapse. Although used outside the United States, these compounds need critical evaluation for safety before use in osteoporotic fractures.[56] Another concern is the biomechanical performance. CaP cement is a ceramic compound having excellent compressive strength but limited torsional and shear strength.[56] Blattert and colleagues compared CaP with PMMA for the treatment of osteoporotic burst-type fractures and found that a third of patients treated by CaP had structural failure.[57]

Expansion Devices. Correction of vertebral wedging and kyphotic deformities are additional goals, which may have long-term benefits. Classically, this is accomplished with kyphoplasty using an inflatable balloon. Improvements in kyphotic angulation (3 degrees) and anterior vertebral height restoration occur after kyphoplasty compared with vertebroplasty. Other methods to expand the body include titanium and polymer meshes that maintain correction after expansion and contain the injected cement. Curved probes that can directly manipulate the endplate have been proposed as well as polymeric expandable devices. These devices are either not approved by the Food and Drug Administration or have not been systematically studied to demonstrate their safety and effectiveness.

Biopsy. Bone biopsy may be obtained during cement augmentation with a low risk and with adequate samples for pathologic diagnosis being obtained in more than 90% of cases.[58] Routine biopsies have shown a small incidence (2%–10%) of undiagnosed malignancy, especially multiple myeloma and lymphoma, and if histomorphometry is performed, a high incidence of osteomalacia secondary to vitamin D deficiency.[59,60]

In patients having known malignancy, the incidence of neoplasm findings on biopsy is greater than 50%.[58] Currently, most authors do not recommend routine biopsy and use it only when there is clinical suspicion or in patients with a history of malignancy.

Cement Augmentation in Spinal Metastasis

Bone metastasis with resultant fractures occurs in 8% to 14% of cancer patients, most commonly in breast, prostate, lung, and thyroid cancers. In addition, multiple myeloma is associated with osteoporosis and spinal fracture in up to 24%.[61] Pain from vertebral fractures can significantly reduce quality of life. The goal of management of pathologic spinal fractures is to prevent neurologic deterioration, palliate pain, and maintain function. Nonoperative treatments include pain management with opioids and other analgesics, bracing for oncology patients, radiotherapy, and chemotherapy or hormonal therapy. Bracing is poorly tolerated in oncology patients. Prevention of further fractures can be accomplished with intravenous administration of bisphosphonate medications such as zoledronate.

For painful metastatic fractures that do not respond to nonoperative management, cement augmentation can be considered. In an RCT, Berenson compared nonoperative treatment with kyphoplasty in patients with painful metastatic fractures.[61] They found at 1 month significantly greater pain relief, overall function, and HRQOL in the kyphoplasty group. No difference in adverse events was present between the groups. Comparison of vertebroplasty with kyphoplasty for the management of metastatic lesions does not show any difference, although only cohort studies are available. Cement augmentation in metastatic lesions requires special consideration. Defects in the vertebral body wall increase the likelihood of cement extravasation. Embolism of tumor displaced during cement installation has been shown to occur in animal models, but there have been no reports in humans.[62]

Surgical Intervention

As discussed in the previous section, cement augmentation (vertebroplasty or kyphoplasty) is warranted for palliative reasons but is not indicated for patients with neurologic deficits. Some fracture types and clinical situations may warrant more aggressive surgical intervention. Generally speaking, this is limited to situations when there is a neurologic deficit from retropulsed bone within the canal or progressive deformity that causes significant pain and functional disability. Any reconstructive surgery in osteoporotic patients is fraught with potential complications and therefore should be undertaken after careful patient selection and only after full informed consent.

In patients with neurologic deficits, there are several approaches to decompress the canal and provide stability to the compromised vertebral column. However, each patient should be approached individually, and there is no exact algorithm for the surgical management of these patients. The advantages of anterior surgery are the direct resection of the retropulsed bony fragment and subsequent decompression of the canal, as well as reconstruction of the weight-bearing anterior column. However, an anterior approach is not well tolerated in elderly patients who often have significant comorbidities. Furthermore, short-segment anterior fixation is often not adequate in osteoporotic patients. Therefore, a posterior approach is favored in these elderly patients with neurologic deficit from osteoporotic spine fractures.

Posterior decompression and stabilization with instrumentation is commonly used in fragility fractures with neurologic involvement (Fig. 37-2). A circumferential decompression can be performed from a posterior approach. Transpedicular access to the posterior vertebral body allows the surgeon to adequately decompress the retropulsed fragment and avoids the morbidity associated with an anterior approach. The

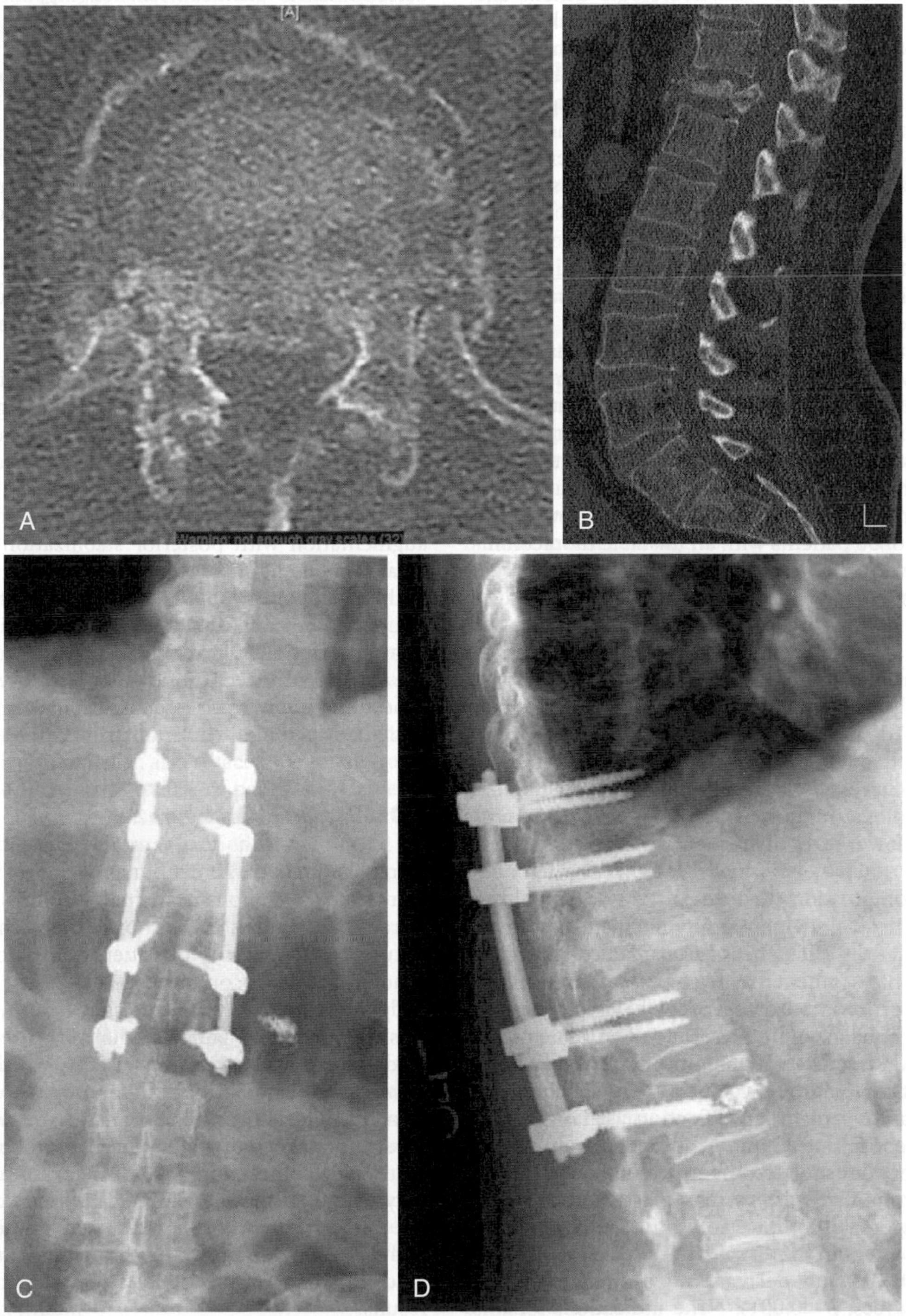

Figure 37-2. A 61-year-old man with a T12 osteoporotic burst fracture resulting in an incomplete spinal cord injury (American Spinal Injury Association Grade C). **A** and **B,** Computed tomography images demonstrating the T12 burst fracture with approximately 50% canal compromise from the retropulsed fragment. The patient underwent a T11 to L1 decompression and T10 to L2 posterior spinal fusion with instrumentation and had significant improvement in his lower extremity motor strength postoperatively. **C** and **D,** AP and lateral x-ray demonstrating wide central decompression from T11-L1 with T10-L2 posterior pedicle screw stabilization and spinal fusion with locally obtained autograft and allograft. Overall alignment is improved with extension positioning on open jackson OR table.

META-ANALYSIS AND SYSTEMATIC REVIEWS

Anderson performed a meta-analysis of six RCTs comparing cement augmentation with nonoperative treatment showing significant improvement in all outcomes, including pain relief, function, and HRQOL in the vertebroplasty group.[77] Secondary fracture risk was identical between the groups. The results were robust, but significant heterogeneity was present, indicating that important differences between studies were present that affected results. These differences included indications, timing, technical factors, and patient comorbidities.

GUIDELINES

The American Academy of Orthopaedic Surgery (AAOS) published evidence-based guidelines for the treatment of symptomatic osteoporotic spinal compression fractures in 2011 (www.aaos.org/research/guidelines/SCFguideline.asp).[80] Based on two prospective RCTs in 2009,[42,43] the AAOS recommended "against vertebroplasty for patients who present with an osteoporotic compression fracture. …" The utility and validity of these guidelines have been questioned because of recently published data. A meta-analysis by Anderson and colleagues[77] provides strong evidence in favor of cement augmentation in the treatment of symptomatic vertebral compression fracture (VCF). To our knowledge, there are no guidelines for the treatment of patients with osteoporotic spine fractures associated with neurologic injury or significant misalignment.

COST EFFECTIVENESS

In 2005, spine fragility fractures in the United States resulted in 2.5 million medical office visits, 430,000 hospital admissions, and 180,000 nursing home admissions.[1] Their direct cost was $17 billion, which is clearly a socioeconomic concern. Unfortunately, the cost effectiveness of various treatment modalities, including cement augmentation, is not clearly defined at this point in time, and further studies are needed.

CONCLUSION

Osteoporotic spine fractures are associated with significant morbidity and an increased risk of death. These fractures often cause a significant amount of pain and therefore are associated with functional disability and a decreased quality of life, as measured by HRQOL measures. In general, patients who sustain an osteoporotic spine fracture are 2.5 times more likely to experience significant back pain and have 10 days of limited activity caused by back pain compared with control participants. HRQOL scores in patients with spinal fragility fractures are significantly lower for all domains (physical and mental) and likely have a considerably greater and more prolonged impact on quality of life than hip, forearm, and humerus fractures. Several studies have shown a significant increase in risk of death in patients who sustain osteoporotic spine fractures. The treatment of osteoporotic spine fractures is predominately nonoperative, with the exception of the presence of neurologic injury or disabling pain (Fig. 37-3). Therefore, healthcare

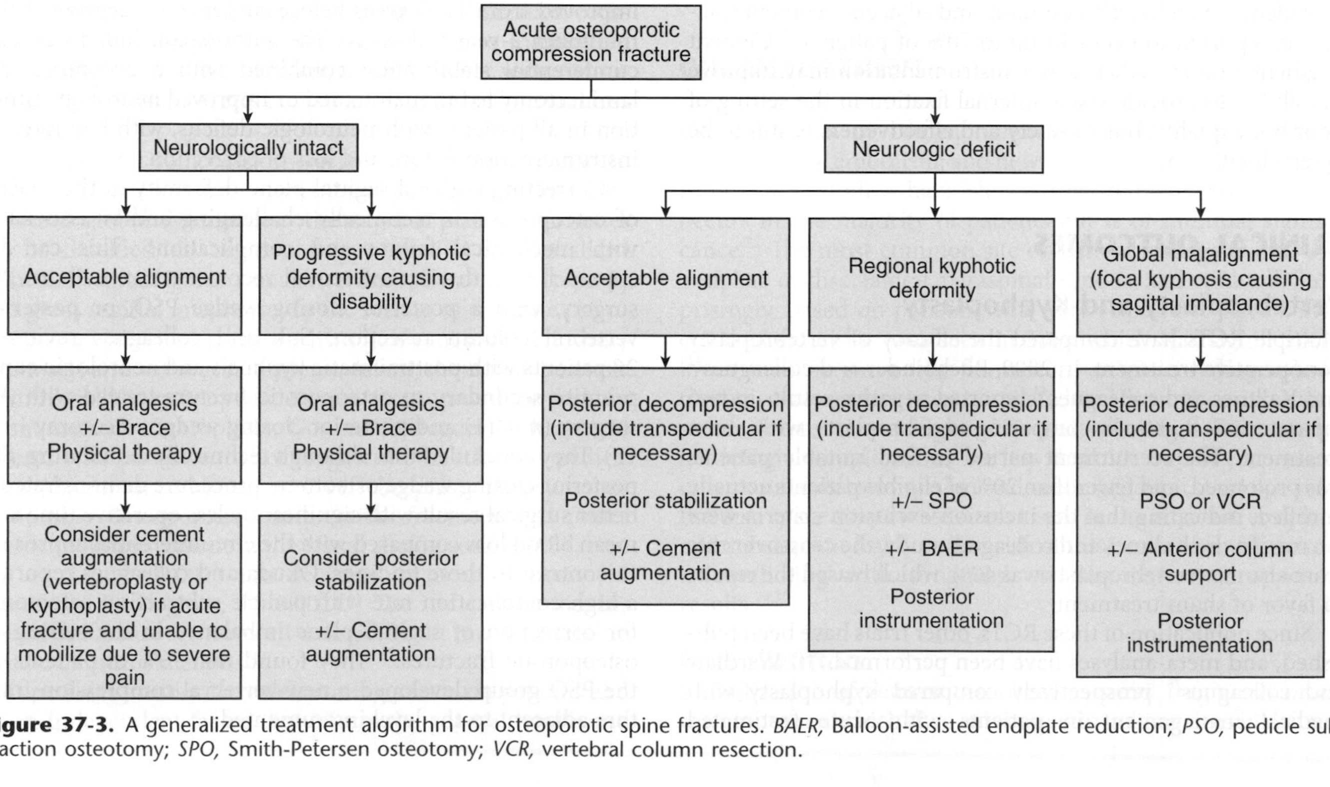

Figure 37-3. A generalized treatment algorithm for osteoporotic spine fractures. *BAER,* Balloon-assisted endplate reduction; *PSO,* pedicle subtraction osteotomy; *SPO,* Smith-Petersen osteotomy; *VCR,* vertebral column resection.

professionals need to focus on identifying patients at risk for osteoporosis and optimize the nonoperative treatment for these patients in an ultimate effort to decrease the morbidity and mortality associated with these fractures.

KEY REFERENCES

The level of evidence (LOE) is determined according to the criteria provided in the preface.

1. Eckman EF: The role of the orthopaedic surgeon in minimizing mortality and morbidity associated with fragility fractures. *J Am Acad Orthop Surg* 18:278–285, 2010.
18. Hallberg I, Rosenqvist AM, Kartous L, et al: Health-related quality of life after osteoporotic fractures. *Osteoporos Int* 15:834–841, 2004. LOE II
23. Edidin AA, Ong KL, Lau E, et al: Mortality risk for operated and nonoperated vertebral fracture patients in the Medicare population. *J Bone Miner Res* 26:1617–1626, 2011. LOE II
27. Lau E, Ong K, Kurtz S, et al: Mortality following the diagnosis of a vertebral compression fracture in the Medicare population. *J Bone Joint Surg Am* 90:1479–1486, 2008. LOE II
42. Buchbinder R, Osborne RH, Ebeling PR, et al: A randomized trial of vertebroplasty for painful osteoporotic vertebral fractures. *N Engl J Med* 361:557–568, 2009. LOE I
43. Kallmes DF, Comstock BA, Heagerty PJ, et al: A randomized trial of vertebroplasty for osteoporotic spinal fractures. *N Engl J Med* 361:569–579, 2009. LOE I
77. Anderson PA, Froyshteter AB, Tontz WL Jr: Meta-analysis of vertebral augmentation compared to conservative treatment for osteoporotic spinal fractures. *J Bone Miner Res* 2012. LOE II
78. Wardlaw D, Cummings SR, Meirhaeghe JV, et al: Efficacy and safety of balloon kyphoplasty compared with non-surgical care for vertebral compression fracture (FREE): a randomized controlled trial. *Lancet* 373:1016–1024, 2009. LOE I
79. Farrokhi MR, Alibai E, Maghami Z: Randomized controlled trial of percutaneous vertebroplasty versus optimal medical management for the relief of pain and disability in acute osteoporotic vertebral compression fractures. *J Neurosurg Spine* 14:561–569, 2011. LOE I

The complete References list is available online at https://expertconsult.inkling.com

Chapter 38

Avoiding Complications in Spine Trauma Patients

GEORGE M. GHOBRIAL • SHANNON HAN • JAMES S. HARROP

INTRODUCTION

Complications and adverse events in the management of spinal trauma can occur in any organ system. Avoidance and prevention of these complications requires multidisciplinary knowledge in spinal cord medicine. Unfortunately, there is no consensus in the literature regarding the true incidence of complications, which have been reported between 10% and 20%.[1] Nasser and colleagues[2] reported the incidence of complications in a systematic review. They reviewed 105 articles including 79,471 patients, of whom 13,067 had a complication for an overall incidence of 16.4% per patient.[2] Interestingly, in a similar comparison in the thoracolumbar literature, complications were more than double when compared to cervical (17.8% vs. 8.9%, respectively). This topic is important because of the increased growth of case volume, use of new technology in the field of spine surgery, and severity of complications.[3]

Complications are categorized into three general divisions for simplicity: the preoperative, intraoperative, and postoperative. This provides a simple and logical method to analyze prevention and management paradigms. Preoperative complications refer to early patient evaluation, assessments, decision making, and timing of treatment. Intraoperative decision making refers to complications related to surgical technique, approach, and risk. Postoperative decision making refers to both perioperative management and outpatient management. These arbitrary delineations in complication management are often ambiguous in outcome reports. For example, the definition of the postoperative time period that constitutes or determines when a postoperative event is attributed to the surgical procedure varies (Table 38-1). This lack of standardization can result in misleading data that prevents the direct comparison among studies.

Another important attribute of complications is their severity. Lebude and coworkers[4] graded severity complications into major or minor categories. The definition of a major complication is that which produces a permanent detriment or that which requires reoperation. This definition intends to include all adverse events in a perioperative period of 30 days. Minor complications were defined as causing transient detrimental effects including medical adverse events. Other systems for spine surgery grade severity using four to six categories.[5] Rampersaud and colleagues developed the Spine Adverse Events Severity System (SAVES); validation studies on the use of this tool supports author claims of its simplicity in capturing spine-specific events commonly missed by hospital metrics.[6-8]

The most common area of study regarding adverse events in spinal surgery is understanding the true incidence and prevalence. However, the scope of this chapter will be primarily focused on the identification and prevention of complications at the various stages of care as related to the spine trauma patient.

PREOPERATIVE

Preoperative Evaluation and Decision Making

Patients who are injured and in severe pain or who have a spinal cord injury (SCI) are willing to undergo a procedure with a higher complication rate.[9] It is, therefore, important that the spine surgeon provide the best estimation of the complication rate, numerical risk of most commonly encountered complications for a procedure, as well as a "likelihood of success." Specific goals of surgery must be addressed and the patient's objectives must match that of the surgeon to ensure the greatest patient satisfaction. Bono and colleagues[9] in a preoperative questionnaire asked patients to score leg and back pain on a scale of 0 to 10. These same patients were then asked to list acceptable scenarios of complications that were presented. A multivariate analysis showed that patients with high-intensity low back pain (LBP), history of prior spinal injections, high educational status, white race, occupation, and a history of nonspinal surgery were indicators of patients with the greatest acceptance of a complication.[9]

Complications with Preoperative Cervical Collar Management

The use of cervical collars is common in suspected spinal trauma patients, as it is suspected that up to 25% of SCIs are caused by pathologic motion of injured cervical vertebrae segments after the initial time of injury.[10] The American Association of Neurological Surgeons (AANS)/Congress of Neurological Surgeons (CNS) cervical spine guidelines state that there is insufficient evidence for the use of cervical collars for the prevention of additional injury.[11-13] However, when any spine trauma is suspected and there is a mechanism that could potentially have caused a cervical injury, then cervical immobilization is reasonable.[14,15] Prolonged use of a hard cervical collar, however, can cause skin breakdown and ulceration. This is especially true in patients who are cognitively impaired or are in intensive care units (ICUs). An effort to clear the spine as outlined in Chapter 10 with a goal to remove the collar as early as possible should be performed. Geriatric patients with type II odontoid fractures are common where

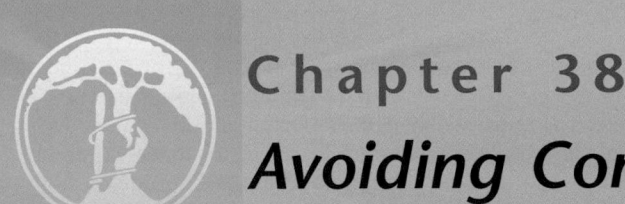

TABLE 38-1 *SUMMARY OVERVIEW OF COMPLICATIONS*

Preoperative	Intraoperative	Postoperative
Early patient evaluation Surgical decision making Timing of treatment Preoperative radiographic assessment	Surgical technique (durotomy, wrong-level surgery, instrumentation complications) Approach Graft-site complications Use of rhBMP-2 Use of neurophysiologic monitoring	Defining postoperative period Surgical site infection Antimicrobial prophylaxis Decubitus ulcers Pneumonia DVT

DVT, Deep venous thrombosis; *rhBMP-2,* recombinant human bone morphogenetic protein-2.

prolonged treatment with a hard cervical collar has inconsistent results. Skin problems are frequent and efficacy is questionable. Prolonged collar use is needed and subsequent skin breakdown becomes a common finding because of pressure ulcers from long-term collar use.[16] Many surgeons argue for early operative intervention in this population to encourage early mobilization and not require prolonged immobilization in a collar. The Arbeitsgemeinschaft für Osteosynthesefragen (AO) Spine Odontoid Fracture Study, a retrospective review of operative versus nonoperative treatment for type II odontoid fractures, reported that treatment with rigid cervical collars resulted in a higher mortality rate than operative treatment.[17]

Preoperative Timing

The timing of surgical intervention after a traumatic spinal cord injury has been controversial. Research into the timing of surgery has been slowed because of the lack of standardized definition. Widely quoted studies defined "early" as surgery performed within 72 hours or after 5 days illustrating the variability in the term "acute." In these studies, no statistical difference was found with regard to hospital length of stay or neurologic improvement by American Spinal Injury Association (ASIA) grade between groups.[18] Recent literature prospectively compared neurologic outcomes by the ASIA Impairment Scale (AIS) between patients with SCI treated earlier or later than 24 hours. This multicenter, international study group reported that early surgical stabilization for acute traumatic SCI resulted in a greater chance of improvement of AIS by 2 points at 6 months with an odds ratio of 2.8.[19]

One subset of patients for which it has been even more difficult to determine a benefit is those with central cord syndrome. Timing for surgery of central cord syndrome is more controversial. Because of the relatively older age group, higher frequency of spontaneous improvement, and its lack of homogeneous pathologies of SCI, many studies have excluded central cord syndrome from timing studies.[20]

Steroids in Spinal Cord Injury: Indications and Potential Complications

The use of methylprednisolone was recommended for acute traumatic SCI within 8 hours of onset by the second National Acute Spinal Cord Injury Study (NASCIS-2).[21-23] In the NASCIS-2 study, Bracken and coworkers reported that there was a neurologic benefit at 6 and 12 months in the methylprednisolone groups who were at the risk for pneumonia and sepsis.[24] There is still much debate on this topic, but given the minimal benefit reported in this study and potential complications, numerous surgeons have stopped using these medications.[25] The most recent 2013 guidelines by the AANS/CNS Joint Section have for the first time discouraged the use of methylprednisolone in SCI.[26] Regardless, the perceivable benefit is outweighed by the added morbidity of its use.

Preoperative Nutritional Status

Nutrition and metabolic requirements during acute traumatic injuries and wound healing are much greater than baseline. Klein and colleagues[27] retrospectively reviewed 27 patients who underwent lumbar spinal surgery for vertebral osteomyelitis finding that a significant proportion (24/26) of the chronically malnourished had postoperative complications. Further, in the same study of 114 patients who underwent lumbar decompressive surgery, poor nutritional status was a factor in 11 of 13 (85%) postoperative infections encountered. It is, therefore, important to maximize nutrition and initiate enteral nutrition as soon as safely possible to enhance wound healing in spinal injured patients.

Obesity

Although malnourishment is an independent risk factor for infection, obesity is also a concern for increased morbidity. Weight loss has always been a recommendation for patients with symptomatic spinal disease but not relevant in spinal trauma. This is important as there is a significant contribution of obesity to morbidity. In a retrospective review, Patel and colleagues[28] found that increasing body mass index (BMI) correlated with a risk for significant perioperative complications. However, these conclusions have been contradicted by a prospective study that found that BMI did not correlate with the incidence of minor or major perioperative complications.[29]

Prognostic Implications of Diagnosis

Further preoperative considerations by the surgeon regarding risk of complications should be associated with the patient's diagnosis and treatment. Yadla and coworkers[30] found in a review of 248 consecutive spinal surgery patients that there was a higher likelihood of adverse events when the patient had a diagnosis of infection or neoplasm in the thoracolumbar spine, rather than degenerative disease or trauma alone. However, this difference was not statistically significant, most likely because there were too few participants. In the literature, patient populations who undergo operations for the treatment of infection and neoplasm have generally had an overall higher complication rate.[1,31]

INTRAOPERATIVE MANAGEMENT

Neurophysiologic Monitoring

The literature supports the use of electrophysiologic monitoring for spine deformity cases.[32] However, these benefits are less precise in the treatment of degenerative cases or trauma cases. In a survey of spine surgeons, the majority reported they used somatosensory evoked potential (SSEP) monitoring for spinal surgery, in addition to other neurophysiologic modalities.[33] In

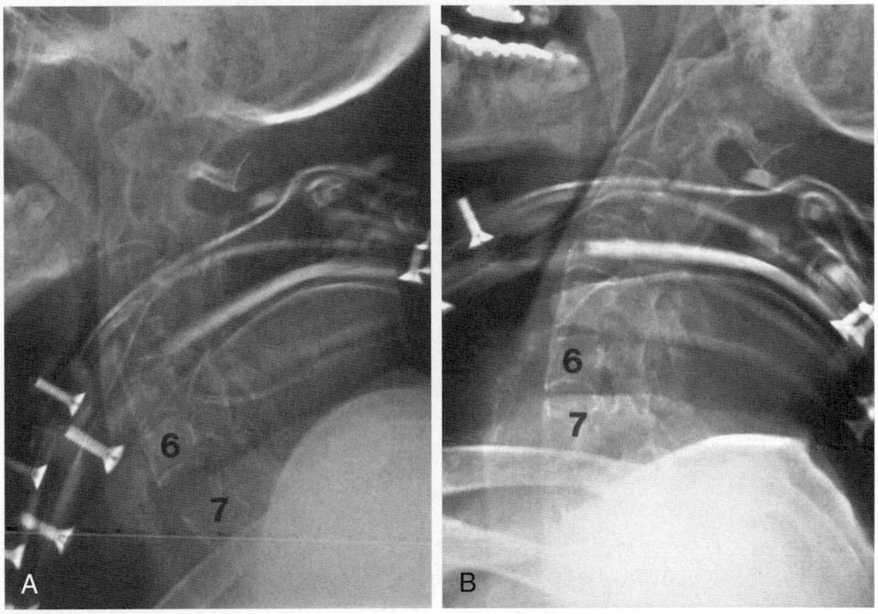

Figure 38-1. Lateral intraoperative radiographic localization is vital in identifying cervical vertebrae. Keep in mind preoperative lateral imaging is important to give the surgeon an idea of the inconsistencies in identifying lower cervical spine segments.

this study, the presence of fellowship training was highly correlative with the use of neurophysiologic modalities. In addition, the use of motor-evoked potentials were frequently used for the surgical decompression of myelopathic patients.

A position statement by the American Society of Neurophysiologic Monitoring said that multimodality neurophysiologic monitoring and the pedicle screw stimulation technique is not proven to reduce neurologic injury by prospective, randomized controlled trials (RCTs), but is an effective technique.[34] Similarly, Resnick and colleagues in a statement for AANS/CNS Joint Section on Spine and Peripheral Nerve Disorders said that the pedicle screw stimulation technique is one diagnostic measure that can enhance the accuracy of pedicle screw placement. More than 1000 papers were reviewed spanning a decade of practice, concluding that due to the lack of prospective, randomized data there is no evidence to support the use of this procedure as a measure to significantly improve patient outcomes.[35] The difficulty of determining if a technique and its improvements translate to improved outcomes is ongoing.

Preoperative and Intraoperative Imaging

Preoperative imaging is of great importance for adequate localization of the disease, characterization with a spinal pathology, and, particularly, for localization in the operative suite (Fig. 38-1). Intraoperative localization is important to limit the possibility of wrong level surgery. This requires appropriate imaging review, knowledge of regional anatomy, and correlation with the patient's clinical symptoms. This is particularly concerning for the physician given the medicolegal implications, in addition to the emotional and medical cost to the patient.[36] In a AANS/CNS spine section survey, as many as 50% of respondents in an anonymous survey reported at least one wrong-level surgery during the course of their careers.[37] From the data collected, the prevalence of wrong-site surgery was estimated at 1 in 3110 surgical cases, with approximately 70% occurring in the lumbar region and a 17% incidence of legal settlement.[37]

Despite the use of intraoperative radiographic localization to confirm the operative level, errors persist. Malpositioning of pedicle screws still occurs, despite the use of intraoperative imaging (Fig. 38-2). Segmental anomalies must be identified preoperatively and a common scheme for identification of the relevant anatomy must be used by the surgeon, cosurgeon, and radiologist. Examples of segmental anomalies that are fairly common include a lumbarized sacrum, sacralized fifth lumbar vertebrae, and six lumbar vertebra.[38] Even in the thoracic and

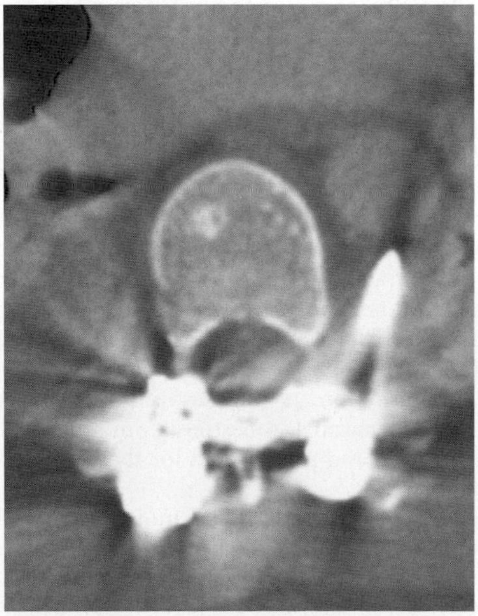

Figure 38-2. Computed tomography (CT) scans of the thoracic spine demonstrating laterally positioned screw. In the proximity of the thoracic aorta, preoperative measurement and limitation of the left pedicle screw to not exceed the distance from starting point to the aorta is important, since even in the presence of intraoperative fluoroscopy, malpositioning of the pedicle screws may occur.

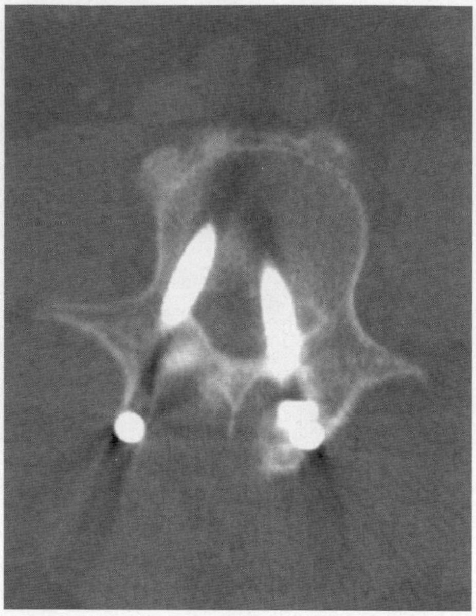

Figure 38-3. Computed tomography (CT) scans of the lumbar spine demonstrating a medial pedicle breach. Neurophysiologic stimulation, in situ palpation of the medial pedicle wall with a probe, and intraoperative fluoroscopy are all intraoperative tools to avoid this complication.

cervical spine, presence of anomalies such as a cervical rib or the absence of a pair of thoracic ribs, although rare, have been reported.[39] It is important to realize that the radiologist typically localizes thoracic pathology numbering from C2. This is not possible in the operating room (OR) because fluoroscopy techniques typically cannot visualize through the upper thoracic spine (Fig. 38-3). Thus, levels should be labeled preoperatively from scout images obtained showing the entire neuraxis. The use of intraoperative computed tomography (CT) or image navigation may aid in correct identification of levels if in doubt and to assess hardware position.

Intraoperative Blood Loss

Intraoperative blood loss should be limited, along with the use of blood products, which should be available for spine procedures, without exceptions. Tse and coworkers[40] recommend a variety of measures to limit blood loss and to limit intraoperative transfusions: discontinuation of antiplatelet agents more than 1 week prior to elective surgery, proper positioning to lower venous pressure, intraoperative red-blood-cell salvage, and even preoperative blood self-donation are some recommended techniques. Further communication with the OR personnel (anesthesia, nursing, etc.) about potential bleeding and preparation for these events can limit morbidity.

Aminocaproic acid, an antifibrinolytic agent, has seen increased off-label use for the reduction of blood loss for prolonged spinal surgeries, particularly for deformity correction. In their RCT, Berenholtz and colleagues[41] saw a 30% decrease in postoperative blood transfusions and a 1-day ($P < 0.05$) decrease in ICU length of stay in the group treated with aminocaproic acid. Although the majority of results are supportive,[42] there is conflicting evidence in the literature in more "routine" spinal surgeries.[43]

Incidental Durotomy

Incidental spinal durotomy is a leading cause of medical malpractice in spine surgery.[44] Takahashi and coworkers[44] in a review of 1014 consecutive cases found an incidence of 4% incidental durotomy in nonrevision spinal cases. That incidence ranged from 2% in single-level lumbar discectomy to an incidence as high as nearly 19% in the presence of juxtafacet cysts. Durotomy occurrence in revision surgery, because of the difficulty with variable anatomy, is even greater.[45]

Incidental durotomy should be managed with a watertight primary dural closure when possible. Some surgeons advocate the use of fibrin glue as reinforcement, followed by 24 to 48 hours of flat bed rest, to limit cerebrospinal fluid (CSF) pressures while the dura heals. Another technique is the use of lumbar drains to divert spinal CSF and provide a decreased pressure gradient. In trauma with a high-velocity mechanism, major dural injuries can occur, for example, as with a lumbar burst fracture. Repair can be provided by duraplasty with synthetic dural grafts. More novel repairs have been reported, involving a posterior transthecal approach to first repair the ventral dural tear, provide cauda equina decompression, followed last by posterior duraplasty.[46]

Recombinant Human Bone Morphogenetic Protein-2

Carragee and colleagues,[47] in a review of industry-sponsored recombinant human bone morphogenetic protein-2 (rhBMP-2) publications, estimated a 10% to 50% incidence of adverse events, depending on approach and dosages used. In fact, use of rhBMP-2 in anterior cervical fusion cases have had over a 40% risk of adverse events,[47-49] the most concerning of which includes severe soft tissue swelling and airway compromise. Additionally, ectopic bone formation, fever, inflammation, radiculitis, osteolysis, and prolonged pain have also been associated with its use. Carragee and colleagues[47] also highlighted the higher rate of retrograde ejaculation in males who had rhBMP-2 during one- and two-level anterior lumbar interbody fusions from L4 to S1.[50,51] However, some authors have publications that disagree with these findings. In addition, rhBMP-2 is a growth factor and its potential for inducing oncologic effects is not known. Caution should be used when it is utilized with patients having a history of cancer. It is rarely needed in spinal trauma patients as they likely have already induced a brisk inflammatory response and high levels of bone morphogenic protein (BMP) cytokines.

Pulmonary Complications

Pulmonary complications after SCI are common and can lead to mortality and morbidity as well as prolonged hospitalization. Aarabi and coinvestigators[52] sought to define predictors of pulmonary complications in SCI and found that the severity of overall injury was the chief predictor of pulmonary complications. In 178 complete cervical spinal cord patients, Aarabi and coworkers found a statistically significant relationship between age, prior preexisting medical and pulmonary conditions, higher cervical level of injury and the need for a tracheostomy and risk of pulmonary complication.[53] As expected, all of the 19 patients with C2 and C3 injuries required a tracheostomy.[54] SCI results in significant impairment of ventilation. These patients will initially have stable pulmonary function but will weaken and tire over time requiring respiratory support. This is especially true in those with higher levels of

SCI. Anticipation of this deterioration and early tracheostomy may reduce subsequent pulmonary complications. As previously mentioned, the use of methylprednisolone in acute traumatic SCI has an elevated risk of pneumonia versus the minimal potential benefit of improved neurologic outcome as presorted by the NASCIS-2 study. In summary, SCI patients with multiple systemic injuries and pulmonary complications can quickly become critical if not treated aggressively.

POSTOPERATIVE MANAGEMENT

Surgical Site Infection

Surgical site infection has emerged as one of the most prevalent of surgical complications, despite numerous prophylactic measures. Commonly recognized risk factors include advanced age, obesity, diabetes, smoking, malnutrition, radiation, prior spinal surgery, prior spinal infection, use of instrumentation, graft placement, and postoperative hematoma.[27,55]

Kuo and colleagues,[56] in a retrospective review of 3230 lumbar spine surgeries, found an incidence of deep wound spinal infections ranging from 0.33% to as high as 4.4% for revision instrumentation and fusion. *Staphylococcus aureus* was the most common isolated organism from postoperative wound cultures.

In regard to antimicrobial prophylaxis (AMP), studies show no difference in surgical site infection (SSI) when comparing postoperative antibiotics for 24 hours versus 7 days postoperative.[57] In a retrospective review of 1597 posterior lumbar surgeries, the SSI did not differ significantly between the single day and multiday (0.4% and 0.8%) prophylaxis.[57] A retrospective review of consecutive elective cases for general surgery, neurosurgery, and orthopedics cases for 3 months analyzed the risk factors for surgical site infections, and surgeons' adherence to infection prevention guidelines. These authors found 8.3% of the 216 surgeries to have had SSIs. A significant percent of the surgeries deviated to some degree from the recommended guidelines of AMP timing and duration less than 24 hours. Specific risk factors were use of a surgical drain for more than 3 days, as well as more than two prophylaxis variations made in a case.[58] Prolonged drain placement and the risk for postoperative infection were previously reported in the literature.

Spine trauma patients often lie recumbent without adequate skin hygiene waiting until surgery. Routine daily skin washing with chlorhexidine and alcohol solutions is becoming routine and has been shown to significantly reduce overall nosocomial infections including surgical site infections. The use of a 4% chlorhexidine dressing applied to the surgical site the night before and morning of surgery reduces skin bacteria counts at the incision and lowers the incidence of surgical site infections by 50% to 80% and can be easily adapted to the spine trauma patient.

Catheter-Associated Urinary Tract Infections

Seung-Lee and colleagues,[55] in a retrospective review of 355 patients older than 65 years who had either a prior laminectomy, fusion, and/or discectomy, evaluated urinary tract infection (UTI) as an independent risk factor for postoperative surgical site infection. A postoperative spine infection in 42 patients was identified based on their criteria.[55] In the same population, recognized risk factors such as diabetes, use of instrumentation, and multilevel surgery were significant ($P <$ 0.05) risk factors, whereas the presence of a UTI was not. One other reason why UTIs are important is the high prevalence of indwelling Foley catheters in the SCI patient.

Urinary-associated catheter infections are mostly associated with the duration of Foley catheter use. Therefore the catheter should be removed as soon as medically possible. For patients with neurogenic bladder from a spinal cord or cauda equina injury, "bladder training" can be used, which refers to intermittent catheterization guided by ultrasonic bladder volume estimation in tandem with patient cues.[59]

Acute Deep Venous Thrombosis

Acute deep venous thrombosis (DVT) is common in spinal surgery series but can occur at an alarmingly high rate in the SCI patient, approaching 100% in some studies. In addition to the multisystem injury, the prolonged immobilization places these patients at risk for DVT. In a systematic review, Christie and coworkers[60] analyzed the ideal time of initiation for DVT prophylaxis with low molecular weight heparin (LMWH). Comparing the use of LMWH administration before and after 72 hours, they found an incidence of DVT as detected by color Doppler ultrasonography of 26% in the late group (3 days) versus 2% in the early group. However, an additional RCT compared unfractionated heparin and compression stockings versus enoxaparin (LMWH).[61] Treatment was initiated within 3 days, holding prophylaxis the day of surgery and resuming treatment the following morning. These authors found the incidence of venous thromboembolism (VTE) to be similar between both treatment arms. Interestingly, the incidence of pulmonary embolism (PE) was statistically higher in the unfractionated heparin group, without an overall increase in morbidity.

Overall, spinal patients are at increased risk for acute DVT and prophylaxis should be used. Depending on the operative procedure and patient risk factors, treatment can vary from chemical prophylaxis, mechanical prophylaxis, to early mobilization.

Inferior Vena Cava Filter

In the postoperative setting, the use of anticoagulation for a DVT must be addressed on a case-by-case basis. This practice varies by physician. Inferior vena cava (IVC) filters are an option when the risks of VTE and bleeding complications from anticoagulation are elevated. In a prospective study, McClendon and coworkers[62] found a significant reduction in PEs in patients who underwent preoperative IVC filter placement prior to "major" spinal surgery. As previously mentioned, individual medical comorbidities are necessary to weigh risks and benefits.

Pseudarthrosis

Failure of implanted spinal hardware can be an indicator of pseudarthrosis, as the instrumentation is designed to provide an immobilizing force resisting body movements for a finite time period long enough for fusion usually within 6 months.[63] The single best modifiable risk factor for pseudarthrosis, as well as postoperative wound infection and healing, is tobacco usage. Other considerations should include the assessment and treatment of potential defects in bone mineral metabolism. In a survey of practicing spine surgeons, only 20% used preoperative bone mineral density workup prior to fusion

TABLE 38-2 *VITAMIN D_3 REFERENCE RANGES*

	25 Vitamin D_3 (ng/L)	Treatment
Normal	>30	1–2000 ng/L vitamin D_3 daily
Insufficiency	20–30	2000 ng/L vitamin D_3 daily
Deficiency	<20	50,000 ng/L vitamin D_2 3 times per week for 6 weeks, then recheck level

surgery, despite its association with the occurrence of nonunion.[64] Vitamin D deficiency is common especially in northern climates and is easily measured by 25-hydroxy vitamin D levels. Insufficiency is between 20 and 30 ng/L and deficiencies are less than 20 ng/L. Correction by replacement with oral vitamin D_3 based on serum levels is recommended and may improve bone healing as well as a host of other medical conditions (Table 38-2).

In a prospective study with a 3-year follow-up, Barsa and colleagues[65] compared multilevel and single-level anterior cervical discectomy and fusions (ACDFs) to determine if the pseudarthrosis rate increased with the length of the construct. They reported no statistically significant difference between one-level and two-level ACDFs.[65] The majority of these studies are in elective cases not involving trauma. Awareness of aforementioned patient predispositions to pseudarthrosis should be involved in the surgical planning process.

Neurologic Deterioration

Neurologic deterioration is among the most serious of complications. In the event of a postoperative decline in motor or sensory function, an immediate magnetic resonance imaging (MRI) scan is performed of the suspected levels after a neurologic examination and brief review of any current medical issues. In practice, it is uncommon that the authors have seen new-onset motor deficits in the postoperative setting to be caused by a nonsurgical lesion, such as a medication or metabolic abnormality. Still, this should be quickly ruled out and not delay definitive diagnosis with an MRI, with the intent of diagnosis of an expanding fluid collection or hematoma. T2-weighted imaging should be obtained initially to assess the space available to the spinal cord in the canal and can save the patient precious time if an urgent surgical decompression is indicated. If there is a concern for graft or screw-rod dislodgment or malpositioning, CT imaging is also obtained.

Decubitus Ulcer

SCI patients are at high risk for pressure ulcer formation because of immobilization and insensate skin.[66] Prevention must be addressed from the time immediately after the injury with frequent turning, mobilization, and identification of early skin breakdown. Identification of risk factors and attention to detail is key. Patients at an elevated risk include the obese, ASIA grade A spinal cord impairment, traumatic brain injury (TBI) patients, and the elderly.[67]

Controversy in Characterizing Spinal Cord Complications

As previously mentioned, often the biggest obstacle to reporting and comparing complications among different institutions and publications is the discrepancy in the very definition of a postoperative complication (Fig. 38-4). Lebude and colleagues[4] surveyed both neurosurgical and orthopaedic spine surgeons to define "complications in spinal surgery." Using a web-based utility, physicians were surveyed on a number of common complication vignettes and asked to determine the presence or absence of a complication, as well as the severity. Of the 229 respondents, mostly orthopaedic surgeons, consensus regarding the presence of a complication was only 70%. With almost one-third of surgeons not in agreement, this highlights the need for a greater consensus in determining the relevance of medical complications and the definition of major versus minor.[4]

Throughout the literature, prospective studies yielded a higher incidence of complications than retrospective studies because of recall bias, which may highlight the need for a prospectively collected database. Yadla and coworkers[30] reported this association where a prospective incidence of complication from spinal surgery was 53.2%, which was significantly greater than previously reported retrospective studies. With the use of prospective collection and more stringent classification, it is hoped these adverse events can be further minimized to improve patient outcomes.

CONCLUSION

Spinal trauma, especially that resulting in SCI, is a serious disease involving multidisciplinary care. Without a team-based approach, the surgeon will be ineffective in preventing adverse events preoperatively or postoperatively, as well as in the operating room. Regarding preoperative management, patient selection and an evidence-based algorithm are important in preventing intraoperative complications. SCI patients, because of immobilization, need diligent attention with

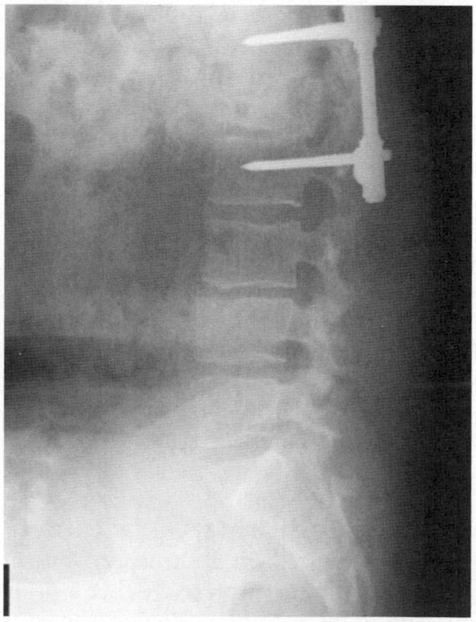

Figure 38-4. Lateral radiograph of the lumbar spine 6 months postoperatively, demonstrating progressive kyphosis and failure of the anterior column. Even among practicing spine surgeons, there is a lack of unanimity about whether this constitutes a procedural complication.

TABLE 38-3 *SUMMARY OF EVIDENCE*

Reference	Issue	Level of Evidence	Design	Conclusion
Peeters et al	Cervical collar in prevention of injury post trauma	Ib	Systematic review of efficacy of cervical orthoses in whiplash injury	Inconclusive trend toward favoring surgical intervention
Fehlings et al	Surgical timing in acute SCI study	Ib	Randomized, multicenter trial of early (<24 h) vs. delayed surgical stabilization of cervical spine fracture	Improvement in outcome favored in early surgical group (OR, 2.83)
Bracken et al	Use of methylprednisolone in acute SCI	Ib	RCT, early administration of methylprednisolone in acute SCI (<8 h)	Neurologic benefit of early administration, elevated pulmonary complications, sepsis
Hurlbert et al	Use of methylprednisolone in acute SCI	Ia	Review of RCTs, early administration (<8 h) of methylprednisolone	No neurologic benefit. Authors discourage use.
Christie et al	DVT prophylaxis in acute SCI	Ib	RCT, early vs. late (>3 days) administration of LMWH	Significant decrease in DVT in early group (2% vs. 26%)
Yadla et al	Method of measuring complications	II	Prospective vs. retrospective measurement of complications	Significantly higher complication rate in prospectively collected data (>50%) in spinal surgery

DVT, Deep venous thrombosis; *LMWH,* low molecular weight heparin; *OR,* odds ratio; *RCT,* randomized controlled trial; *SCI,* spinal cord injury.

frequent turning and DVT prophylaxis for the prevention of decubitus ulcers and VTE, respectively. Strict adherence to World Health Organization (WHO) protocols for the intravenous administration of antibiotics 1 hour prior to skin incision has led to a significant reduction in SSIs. A high suspicion for the underlying causes of postoperative neurologic deterioration can help reverse the deterioration by preventing an unnecessary delay in care. Prompt mobilization and care by an SCI rehabilitation team will help maximize functional outcomes (Table 38-3).[12,19,60,68,69]

KEY REFERENCES

The level of evidence (LOE) is determined according to the criteria provided in the preface.

8. Rampersaud YR, Moro ER, Neary MA, et al: Intraoperative adverse events and related postoperative complications in spine surgery: implications for enhancing patient safety founded on evidence-based protocols. *Spine* 31(13):1503–1510, 2006. LOE II
11. Benzel EC, Hadden TA, Saulsbery CM: A comparison of the Minerva and halo jackets for stabilization of the cervical spine. *J Neurosurg* 70(3):411–414, 1989. LOE III
15. Kirshblum SC, Burns SP, Biering-Sorensen F, et al: International standards for neurological classification of spinal cord injury (revised 2011). *J Spinal Cord Med* 34(6):535–546, 2011. LOE V Editorial highlighting the lack of definitive evidence for the acute surgical treatment of acute central cord injury.
20. Fehlings MG, Arvin B: The timing of surgery in patients with central spinal cord injury. *J Neurosurg Spine* 10(1):1–2, 2009. LOE V
21. Nesathurai S: Steroids and spinal cord injury: revisiting the NASCIS 2 and NASCIS 3 trials. *J Trauma* 45(6):1088–1093, 1998. LOE V
33. Magit DP, Hilibrand AS, Kirk J, et al: Questionnaire study of neuromonitoring availability and usage for spine surgery. *J Spinal Disord Tech* 20(4):282–289, 2007. LOE V Survey data highlighting the more common use of neuromonitoring in surgeons with higher levels of training after residency.
36. Ohlin A, Stromqvist B: [The risk of wrong-level or wrong-side spinal surgery not insignificant. Psychological trauma for both the patient and the surgeon]. *Lakartidningen* 105(9):642–643, 2008. LOE IV Discussion of survey data regarding the psychological damage caused by wrong-level surgery.
46. Huang AP, Chen CM, Lai HS, et al: Posterior transthecal approach for repair of cauda equina fibers and ventral dural laceration in lumbar burst fracture: a novel surgical technique. *Spine* 38(18):E1156–E1161, 2013. LOE V The authors describe this method for repair of ventral dural lacerations more common to high-velocity lumbar burst fractures.
50. Comer GC, Smith MW, Hurwitz EL, et al: Retrograde ejaculation after anterior lumbar interbody fusion with and without bone morphogenetic protein-2 augmentation: a 10-year cohort controlled study. *Spine J* 12(10):881–890, 2012. LOE II In this retrospective analysis of a prospective cohort controlled study, a statistically significant rate of retrograde ejaculation was found in the cohort exposed to rhBMP-2.
51. Carragee EJ, Mitsunaga KA, Hurwitz EL, et al: Retrograde ejaculation after anterior lumbar interbody fusion using rhBMP-2: a cohort controlled study. *Spine J* 11(6):511–516, 2011. LOE II In this retrospective analysis of a prospective cohort-controlled study, a statistically significant rate of retrograde ejaculation was found in the cohort exposed to rhBMP-2.
58. Young B, Ng TM, Teng C, et al: Nonconcordance with surgical site infection prevention guidelines and rates of surgical site infections for general surgical, neurological, and orthopedic procedures. *Antimicrob Agents Chemother* 55(10):4659–4663, 2011. LOE III A linear association was found between concordance with SSI prophylaxis guidelines and SSI incidence at a single institution.
60. Christie S, Thibault-Halman G, Casha S: Acute pharmacological DVT prophylaxis after spinal cord injury. *J Neurotrauma* 28(8):1509–1514, 2011. LOE III Systematic review of predominantly level II and III data in support for the prevention of VTE by the initiation of LMWH within 72 hr.
61. Prevention of venous thromboembolism in the acute treatment phase after spinal cord injury: a randomized, multicenter trial comparing low-dose heparin plus intermittent pneumatic compression with enoxaparin. *J Trauma* 54(6):1116–1124, discussion 1125–1116, 2003. LOE I VTE rates were not statistically different in groups treated with enoxaparin or unfractionated heparin.

The complete References list is available online at https://expertconsult.inkling.com.

Chapter 39

Principles of Orthotic Management

CHRISTOPHER S. BAILEY

The orthotic management of spinal trauma remains an essential treatment option. However, the indications for orthotic management are constantly changing because of the evolving concepts of stability, indications for surgery, and surgical techniques. The complications traditionally associated with the surgical management of certain spinal fractures have significantly decreased with the increasing prevalence of minimally invasive techniques. This influences the indications for orthotic use in some trauma scenarios. However, the principles and expectations of orthotic use remain constant and an important option in the treatment of spinal trauma. One must determine the stability of the injury and the stabilizing ability of the orthoses available when considering the appropriate orthotic. This decision-making process is, therefore, specific to the individual fractures and their respective level of injury.

Spinal orthoses can be used by a member of the emergency medical service to provide initial immobilization, as temporary management until the surgery is performed, as the definitive management, or as an adjunct to surgery. The principle of preventing motion in the adjacent joints, as used in the extremity, also applies to the spine. However, when using spinal orthoses, the goal is not only to immobilize the motion segments adjacent to the injured level but also the functional levels adjacent to the injured spinal region (i.e., occipitocervical or thoracolumbar). As such, when stabilizing the cervical spine, the head and the thoracic spine must be included so that the occipitocervical and cervicothoracic levels are immobilized or, when stabilizing the lumbar spine, the pelvis and the thoracic spine are immobilized. Compared with surgical management of spinal disorders, the use of orthoses may seem benign; however, it is not without risks and complications. These devices may be associated with skin irritation, muscular atrophy, osteopenia, joint stiffness, severe discomfort, and even death.

The purpose of this chapter is to review the different types and function of spinal orthoses, commonly encountered adverse effects, and the principles in their use for the nonoperative treatment of selected spinal trauma.

CERVICAL ORTHOSIS

The orthotic devices commonly used to immobilize the cervical spine after trauma are grouped into cervical collar, poster brace, cervicothoracic orthosis (CTO), and halo-vest device (Table 39-1). The unique anatomy within the upper cervical spine and subaxial spine makes immobilization challenging, and the choice of device remains dependent on the location of the injury. The stabilization of the cervical spine depends on the ability to immobilize the skull proximally (usually via occiput and the mandible) and the clavicle or thorax (or both) distally.[1] Hard contact against the mandible and occiput are associated with skin irritation and impairment of mandibular movement can interfere with mastication. Increased rigidity of the device can increase these adverse effects. Distal immobilization is challenging because the clavicle moves with shoulder motion and the soft tissues around the shoulder and the upper trunk are variable in size and shape. All of these factors, along with the degree of injury, must be taken into consideration. The clinician must choose a device that meets the patient's specific needs while minimizing adverse effects.

Cervical Collar

The cervical collar is generally categorized into soft and hard options; both extend between the occiput and the mandible down to the clavicle. The soft collar (Fig. 39-1) provides very little support or stability to the cervical spine. It has been shown to only reduce cervical motion by approximately 5% to 20%.[2-5] The primary purpose of the device is to provide some proprioceptive feedback to the patient. Although the least stabilizing of all the cervical collars, it is also the least expensive and is associated with minimal patient discomfort. Generally, patients with whiplash injuries and posttraumatic neck pain may be treated with a soft collar for a short time so as to limit the associated potential for deconditioning, increased stiffness, and psychological dependence. In postoperative patients, we may use cervical ruffs, made from stockinette filled with cotton padding, loosely tied around the patient's neck to provide proprioceptive feedback, reassurance, and a visual reminder to caregivers of the patient's postoperative state.

The hard cervical collars are the most commonly used cervical orthoses. There are many commercially available variants of the collar, the most common being the Philadelphia, Aspen, PMT, Cervmax, and Miami J (Fig. 39-2). Most of the collars consist of a plastic bivalved shell that is lined with removable pads (however, the Philadelphia collar consists of two plastic-reinforced Plastazote shells). The anterior shell encompasses the mandible and chin superiorly and rests on the anterior chest, sternum, and clavicles. The posterior shell lines the occiput around to below the ears and rests on the upper back and trapezium. The anterior and posterior shells are connected by Velcro straps. The hard cervical collars tend to be more effective in minimizing motion in the sagittal plane compared with lateral bend and axial rotation.[6-8] Multiple biomechanical studies have compared the effectiveness of these devices. Most commercially available cervical collars appear to be effective in immobilizing the spine, but some models may be more comfortable for the patient than others.[6-9] Importantly, the improper fitting of the hard collar, whether it is too small or too big, will have a significant effect on the ability of the collar to limit cervical motion in all planes

TABLE 39-1 *COMMON CERVICAL ORTHOSES*

Cervical Orthosis	Characteristics	Common Types
Soft collar	Proprioceptive feedback to the patient Reduced cervical motion by 5% to 20%	Serpentine, Form fit, Universal, Ruffs
Hard collar	Plastic bivalved shell, lined with removable pads, connected by Velcro straps More sagittal motion control than axial or lateral motion	Philadelphia, Aspen, PMT, Cervmax, Miami J
Cervicothoracic	Superior restriction of lateral and axial motion than collars Head controlled by padded mandibular and occiput supports; rigid uprights attach head to thoracic plates and straps	SOMI, Minerva, Guilford, poster brace
Halo vest	Most effective method of upper cervical and occipitocervical stabilization Halo ring around head secured to thoracic vest Subaxial snaking phenomena possible	

SOMI, Sternal-occipital-mandibular immobilizer.

(flexion-extension, axial rotation, and lateral bend).[7] These devices are commonly used to immobilize the cervical spine as part of cervical spine precautions in trauma patients until the cervical spine is safely cleared. Some of the rigid collars initially applied by the emergency medical service are often less padded than those described earlier. In all cases, it is important that these devices be removed as soon as injury to the cervical spine is excluded to limit the potential complications of skin irritation, difficulty with ingestion and speaking, and general discomfort. Furthermore, the use of rigid collars has the potential to increase intracranial pressure, which can be perilous in patients with traumatic brain injury.[10]

Cervicothoracic Orthosis and Poster Braces

Compared with the hard cervical collars, CTOs and poster braces provide better restriction of motion in axial rotation and lateral bend. CTOs are designed to be more effective in immobilization of the cervical spine than cervical collars because of the more extensive chest plates.[9,11,12] The poster brace and the CTO are similar devices with the CTO extending slightly more distal and incorporating more of the chest, usually with a circumferential strap. The poster brace is best described as a cervical collar with extension down to the chest and/or back. CTOs and poster braces control the head through padded mandibular platforms and supports at the back of the occiput. Rigid uprights then attach the head to the thorax via thoracic plates or straps. Examples of these orthoses include the Minerva brace (Fig. 39-3), the SOMI (sternal-occipital-mandibular immobilizer) brace (Fig. 39-4), and commercially available hard collars outfitted with extension pieces to both the skull and chest. The poster braces connect the mandibular and occipital pads to the torso by two or four metal struts.

The SOMI brace consists of a rigid anterior chest plate that extends over the shoulders and connects to the occipital pad. The chin piece is removable for eating and can be reinforced with a strap that spans across the forehead. Unlike the Minerva brace, the SOMI brace does not have a posterior chest plate so it is more comfortable for patients confined to bed. The SOMI brace has been extensively studied compared with a variety of hard collars.[2,4,5,11] There appears to be very little difference between the braces' ability to stabilize the cervical spine, except for flexion-extension, for which a difference has been shown favoring the SOMI brace. Johnson and colleagues demonstrated that the SOMI brace is significantly better at controlling flexion between C1 and C5 than the cervical hard collar (Philadelphia collar), CTO, and four-poster brace but was very poor at controlling extension in the same location.[4]

The addition of posters to the hard collar improves the control of flexion-extension, lateral bend, and rotation.[3,9] Apart from the halo-vest orthosis, the CTO, such as the Minerva and Guilford, is the best immobilizer for all planes of cervical motion.[4,13] It is important to note that all cervical orthoses are not particularly effective at limiting flexion-extension at the occipitocervical spine compared with segmental motion in the upper cervical and subaxial spine.[4] Improved immobilization comes at the expense of patient

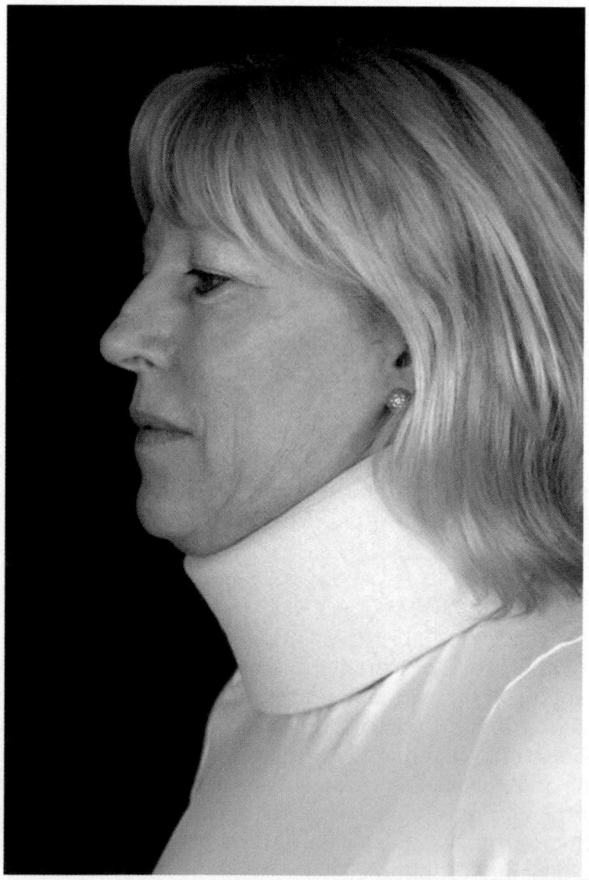

Figure 39-1. Soft cervical collar.

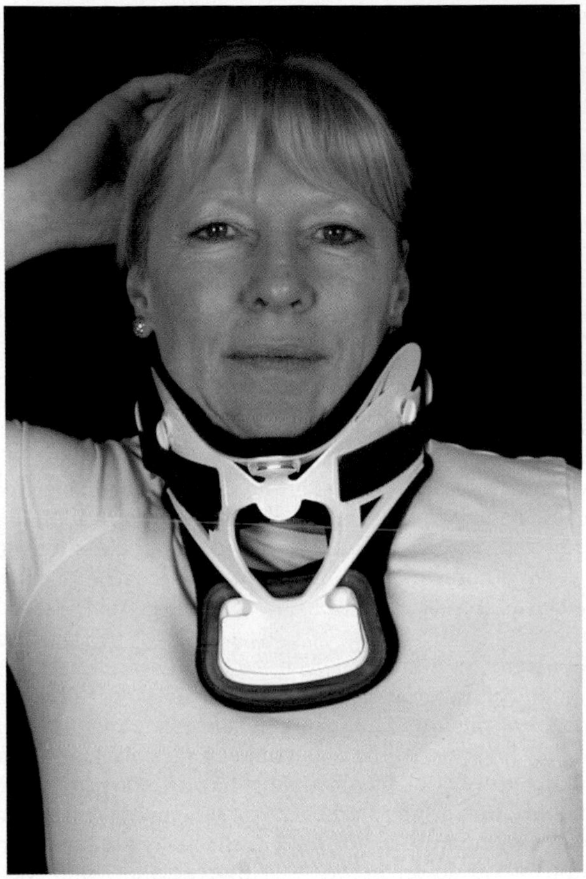

Figure 39-2. Miami J cervical collar.

comfort and the risk of skin breakdown. Use of these more rigid orthoses in cognitively impaired patients risks occipital and mandibular skin ulceration.

Halo-Vest Device

The halo fixator is a device that connects the head to the thorax. In adults, four pins are placed that pierce the outer table of the calvarium and secure the halo ring around the head. The halo vest device is generally accepted as the most effective method of upper cervical spine stabilization including the occipitocervical junction and is superior to all other orthotic devices discussed earlier.[2,4,13] However, some vertebral segmental motion, on average 7 degrees of angulation and 1.7 mm of translation, can be detected at the injured level in the majority of patients.[14] Furthermore, the halo-vest device can be associated with a snaking phenomenon, whereby neck muscle contraction causes translation of individual vertebrae in the midcervical spine producing focal kyphosis caused by immobilization of the upper and lower segments. The halo-vest device is commonly used to stabilize the cervical spine when the rigid collar and CTOs are deemed to be insufficient. When using this device, careful consideration must be given to patient selection to avoid complications. Absolute contraindications to the use of the halo ring include cranial fractures and infection or severe soft tissue injury at proposed pin sites. Relative contraindications include chest trauma, obesity, pregnancy, advanced age, and barrel-shaped chest.[15] The elderly population is particularly at high risk of halo vest–related complications with a mortality rate reported to be as high as 40%.[16-19] In this patient cohort, the mortality and major complication rates of those treated with halo-vest devices are significantly higher than compared with those treated with cervical collar.[19]

Recommended Orthoses for the Nonoperative Treatment of Selected Cervical Injuries

For all fractures, the potential for surgical intervention must be excluded before initiating conservative care. Indications for surgical intervention are discussed in detail within other chapters of this textbook.

C1 Ring Fracture

For minimally displaced fractures of the C1 ring, we commonly use a hard cervical collar because this injury pattern is relatively stable. For potentially unstable Jefferson fractures (i.e., C1 ring burst fractures), a halo-vest fixator or CTO if the halo vest is contraindicated can be used with the goal of preventing either C1-C2 instability caused by transverse ligament injuries or deformity secondary to C0-C1 or C1-C2 lateral mass malalignment.

Transverse Ligament Injuries

When an avulsion fracture has disrupted the integrity of the transverse ligament, management in a cervical orthotic may be considered. In this case, flexion at the C1-C2 level should be immobilized using either a CTO (a SOMI brace best controls upper cervical spine flexion) or halo-vest device.

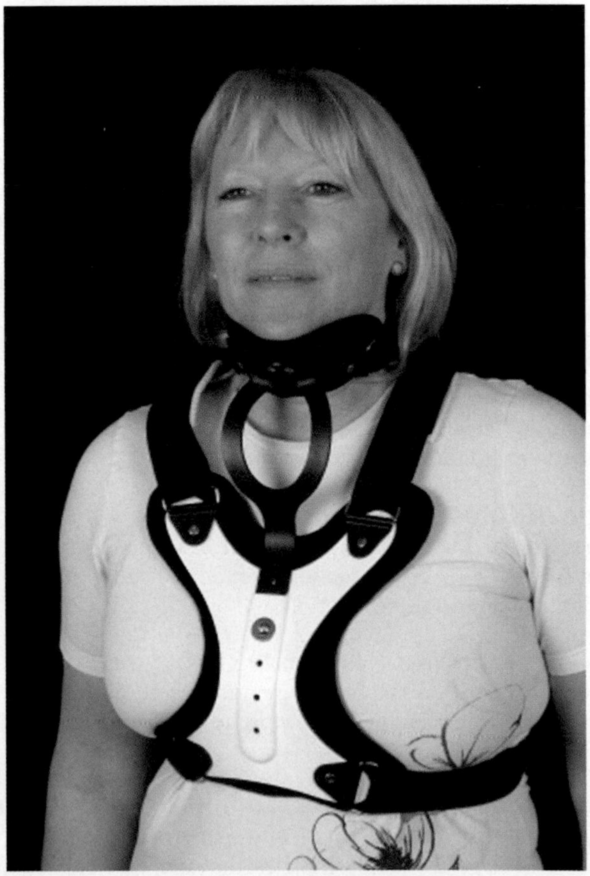

Figure 39-3. Minerva cervicothoracic orthosis.

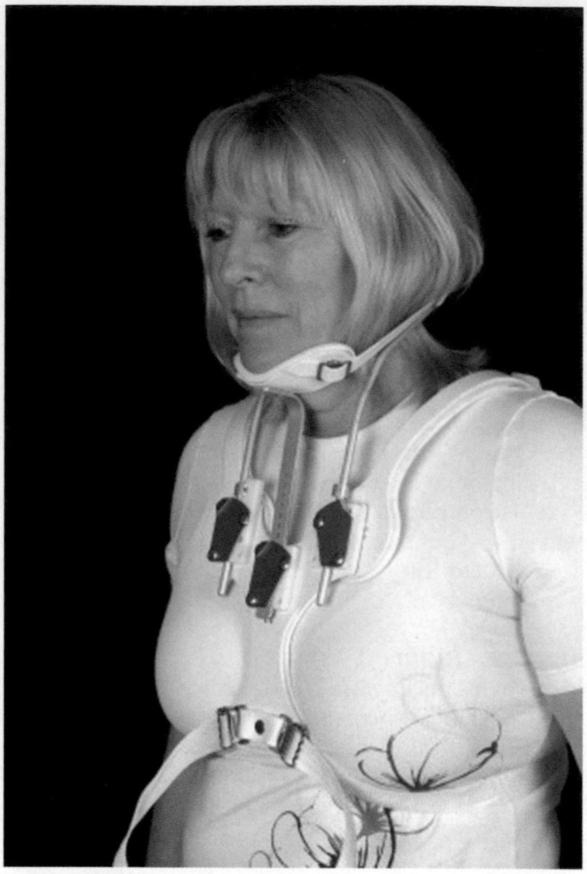

Figure 39-4. Sternal-occipital-mandibular immobilizer (SOMI) brace.

Type II Odontoid Fractures

If orthotic management of this fracture is selected, then the age of the patient will determine the type of orthotic selected. For patients younger than 65 years of age, the halo-vest device should be chosen to provide the best immobilization of this fracture. If the fracture pattern is noncomminuted and nondisplaced and in a reverse oblique fracture pattern (which predisposes the peg to anterior translation relative to the C2 body), then a SOMI brace may be considered. In the elderly population, we use the hard cervical collar if the fracture is to be treated nonoperatively. The expectation of this approach is to achieve a relatively stable fibrous nonunion, but not necessarily consolidation, of the fracture.[20-22]

Type III Odontoid Fractures

A hard collar for the elderly population is recommended for this fracture.[21] We recommend either a hard collar or CTO for the nonelderly adult population.

C2 Pars Fractures (Hangman's Fractures)

In the case of a stable hangman's fracture with no or minimal displacement, we recommend the use of a hard collar or CTO.

Spinous Process Fractures, Laminar Fractures, and Compression Fractures of the Subaxial Spine

These fractures are stable injuries that are well treated in a hard collar.

Facet Fractures of the Subaxial Spine

The CTO is most appropriate for this potentially unstable fracture.

THORACOLUMBAR ORTHOSIS

A number of fractures in the thoracolumbar spine, including wedge fractures, burst fractures, and seat belt injuries, are well treated using thoracolumbar orthotic devices. A variety of braces are available that extend from the upper thoracic spine across the thoracolumbar and lumbosacral junction to the pelvis. As with the cervical orthoses, thoracolumbar orthoses can be either hard or soft. The common types include the prefabricated or custom thoracolumbosacral spinal orthosis (TLSO), thoracolumbar hyperextension orthosis (i.e., Jewett brace), prefabricated or custom lumbosacral orthosis (LSO), and low back corsets (Fig. 39-5). In addition, occipital and mandibular extension can be added to TLSOs to cross the cervicothoracic junction; and, similarly, a hip extension can be added to stabilize lower lumbar and sacroiliac injuries.

Generally, fractures between T6 and L3 are treated with the thoracolumbar hyperextension orthosis or TLSO and fractures of the lower lumbar spine are treated with the LSO (Figs. 39-5 to 39-7). The soft lumbosacral corsets serve as a reminder to restrict trunk motion but do not provide rigid immobilization. Many studies have confirmed that a thoracolumbar and lumbosacral orthotic is effective in reducing gross motion of the lower spine.[23-29] However, the ability of the orthotic to control intervertebral mobility is controversial.[23,25] The more rigid the brace, the more effective it is in reducing spine motion.[26,27] Overall, the body cast is most effective in limiting motion in all planes in the thoracolumbar and lumbosacral spine. The Jewett hyperextension brace is effective in limiting instability in flexion but not in rotation or lateral bending and is ineffective in preventing progression of deformity in three-column injuries.[29,30] The custom-molded TLSO provides protection in all three planes and distributes the force over a large surface area.[25,27,29-31]

Recommended Orthoses for the Nonoperative Treatment of Thoracolumbar Injuries

If desired, compression fractures can be treated with an off-the-shelf TLSO, hyperextension, or LSO.[32] The stable thoracolumbar burst fracture is a well-studied fracture using conservative treatment. We recommend the use of a hyperextension brace to resist kyphosis in association with early ambulation. Some fracture collapse is expected, but this has not been shown to influence the patient-rated, subjective outcome.[33] When the fracture is also potentially unstable in the coronal plane, an off-the-shelf or custom-made TLSO should be used. Stable burst fractures have been shown to have equivalent outcomes when treated with or without the use of a TLSO.[34] Treating these fractures using early ambulation without a brace avoids the cost and patient deconditioning associated with a brace and complications and costs associated with long-term bed rest if a TLSO or body cast is not available. Flexion-distraction and Chance-type fractures may be treated nonoperatively using orthoses that control mainly hyperflexion forces such as a hyperextension brace or a TLSO.

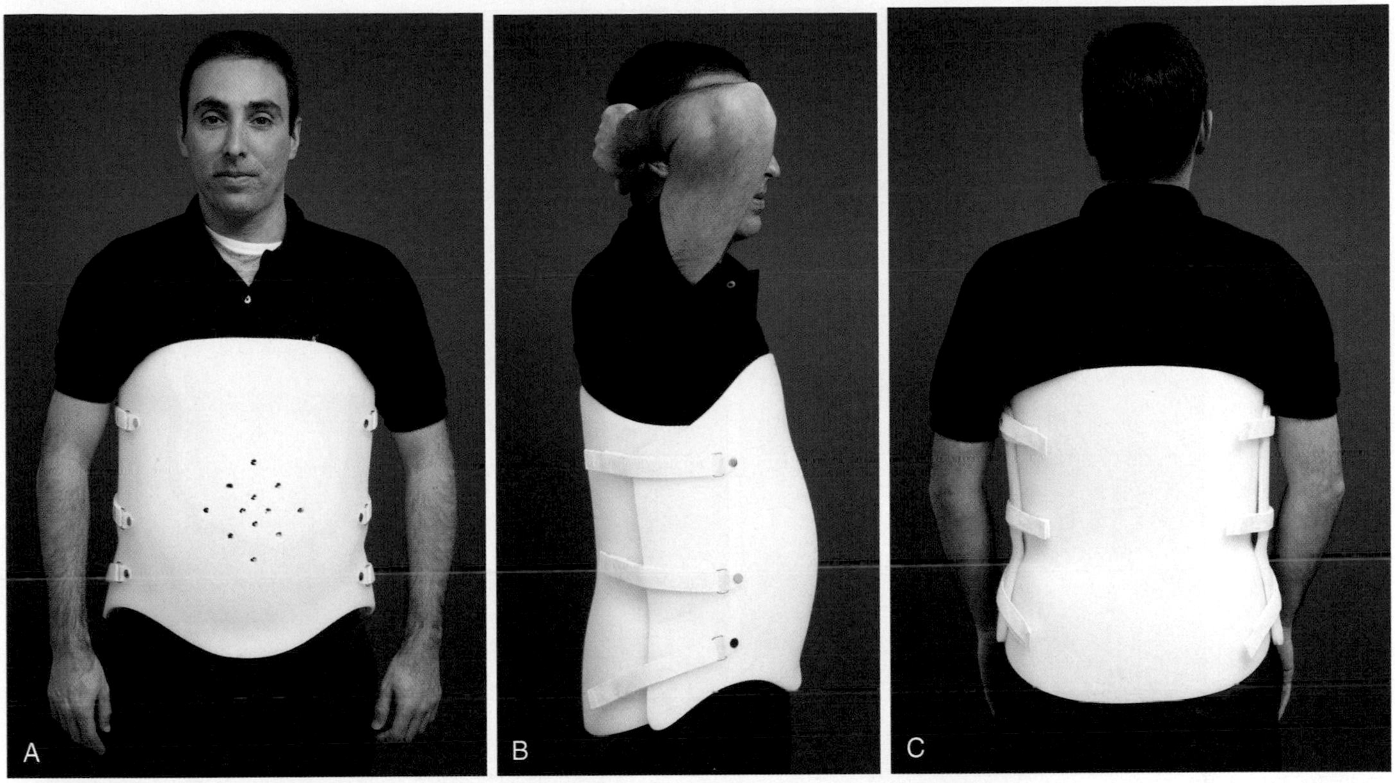

Figure 39-5. A thoracolumbar spinal orthosis (TLSO). **A** to **C,** The thoracolumbar orthosis, or body jacket, is the most rigid brace and is effective from T7 through L4. It is custom molded by an orthotist and is fabricated from polypropylene or ethylene plastic. It can be made as a two-piece clamshell, which is less rigid than the one piece, which opens in the front and has overlapping edges.

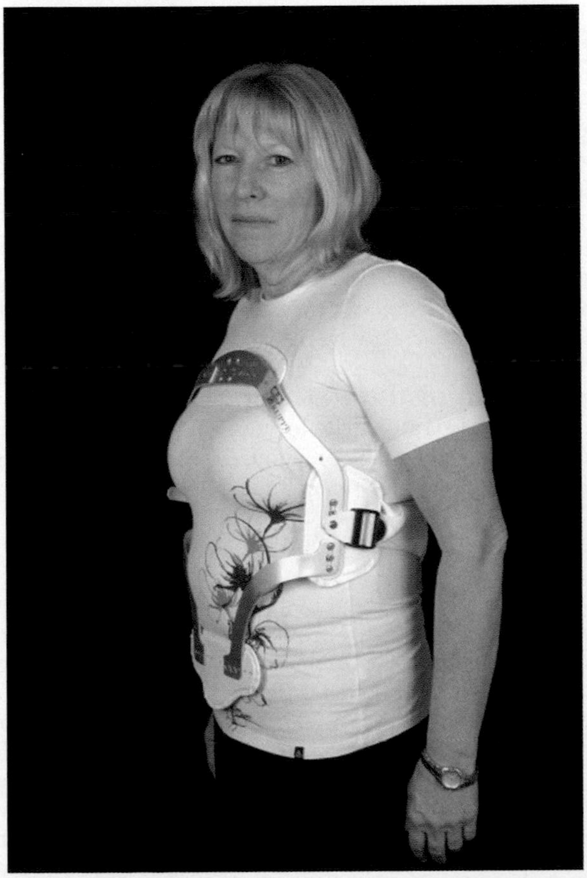

Figure 39-6. Jewett hyperextension orthosis.

Injuries below L4 are poorly treated with TLSO braces and require a hip extension. Similarly, when upper thoracic, cervicothoracic, or noncontiguous injuries are present in the cervical and thoracolumbar spine, use of a cervicothoracolumbosacral orthosis (CTLSO) would be appropriate. Practically, these orthoses have low patient acceptance and greater risk of skin breakdown, so they are used much less commonly today.

CLINICAL USE OF SPINAL ORTHOSIS IN TRAUMA

All spinal injuries treated nonoperatively with an orthotic device require frequent clinical and radiographic follow-up to exclude the development of progressive deformity, pain, or neurologic deficit. We ensure our patient receives "upright" (standing or sitting) imaging in the brace before discharge from the hospital and biweekly thereafter until consolidation of the fracture is well underway. This assures that the nonoperative treatment is effective. Alignment changes may occur slowly; therefore, comparison with initial upright radiographs should be performed. In addition, patients should be queried for skin complications and, if neurologically impaired, the skin should be directly visualized.

ADVERSE EVENTS

Adverse Events of Cervical Orthoses

The most commonly associated adverse effect of cervical orthoses usage is skin irritation and skin breakdown.[35] Risk

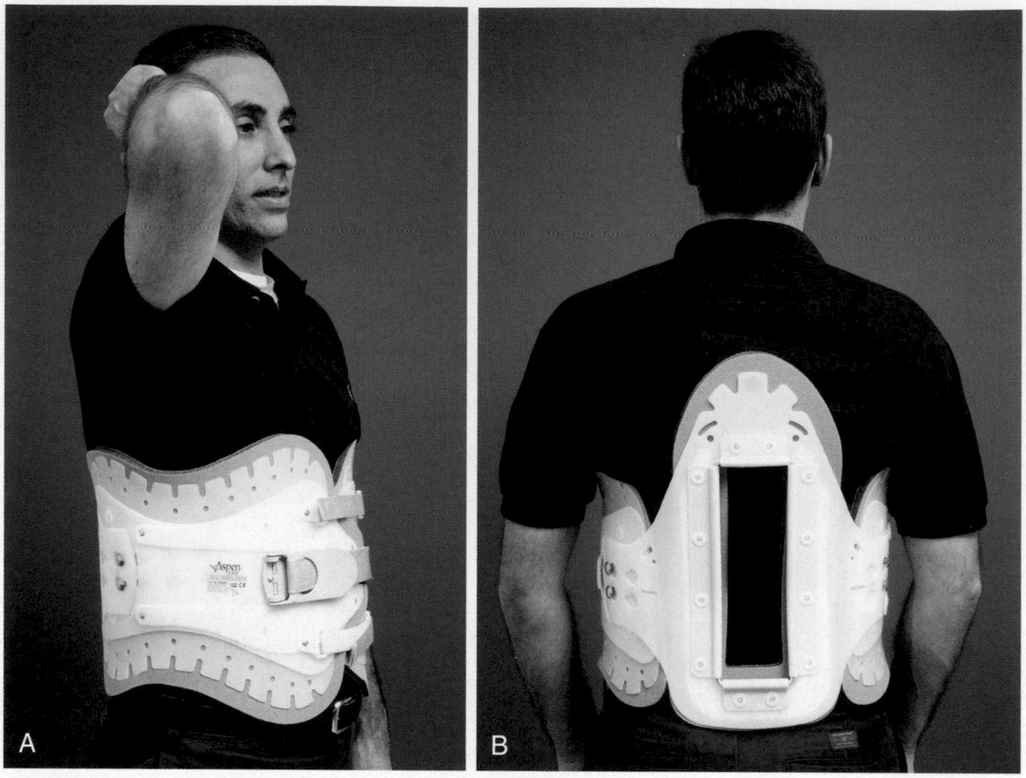

Figure 39-7. A lumbosacral orthosis (LSO). **A** and **B,** The Aspen lumbosacral orthosis has inner soft pads and an outer layer of plastic with buckles, straps, and bars that connect them together. The four bars, two anterior and two posterior, act as vertical struts. The buckles and straps allow for adjustments at several crucial connections to form a personal fit.

factors commonly associated with the development of collar-related decubitus ulceration include time to collar removal, intensive care unit admission, mechanical ventilation, and increased length of hospitalization.[36,37] Other difficulties include compliance, interference with ingestion and speaking, and general discomfort. Rigid collars have the potential to increase intracranial pressure.[10]

Adverse Events of the Halo-Vest Device

Complications of the halo-vest device include pin loosening (36%), loss of fixation requiring pin replacement, pin site infection (12%–20%), pin site discomfort (18%), skin necrosis, supraorbital nerve injury (2%), and dural penetration (1%).[38,39] Infected pins should be treated with local pin site care and systemic antibiotics, as well as pin tightening. Persistent pin site infections should be treated by removing the pin, continuing the antibiotics, and replacing the pin at an adjacent site.

Adverse Events of Thoracolumbar Orthoses

Adverse effects resulting from the use of an orthosis may include muscular atrophy, deconditioning, and skin irritation. The TLSO distributes the force exerted by the brace over a large surface area to decrease the chance of skin irritation and damage from pressure. Local nerve compression from the edge of the brace can occur to the lateral femoral cutaneous nerve or the brachial plexus. This nerve pressure may be specific to a particular position, such as sitting for the lateral femoral cutaneous nerve, and not present in other positions.

SURGICAL TECHNIQUE: PLACEMENT OF THE HALO VEST

Sizing of the Halo

A variety of halo ring designs are available, but the use of one that is magnetic resonance imaging compatible is recommended. Having an open ring eases placement compared with a closed ring. Rings are available in many sizes, and the correct size should have only 1 to 2 cm of clearance around the circumscribed skull. Similarly, the chest component of the system should be sized correctly by measuring the thoracic girth.

Localization of the Halo Ring

The halo ring is temporarily located with special positioning screws, holding it equally on all sides (Fig. 39-8). The ring is placed 1 cm above the pinna and just above the eyebrows.

Pin Placement

In adults, two pins are placed in the forehead and two into the posterolateral occiput (behind the ears and opposite the anterior pins) (Fig. 39-9). The frontal pins must be placed at or below the equator of the forehead (to prevent superior migration while tightening), lateral to the supraorbital nerve (the safe zone is 1 cm above the lateral third of the eyebrow), ensuring that eyebrow is not tethered and the eyelid can close (Fig. 39-10). The supraorbital and greater occipital nerves have been demonstrated to be safe when the halo pins are placed at sites 4.5 cm and 6.0 cm lateral to the anterior and posterior midlines, respectively.[40] In children, one should use a greater number of pins, evenly distributed around the ring (six to 10

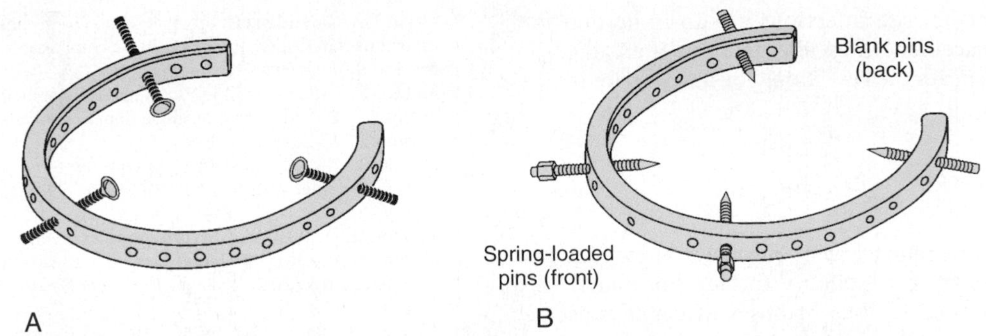

Figure 39-8. The halo ring is held in a temporary position equidistant from the patient's head, 1 cm above the eyebrows and 1 cm above the tip of the ears, with the use of blunt positioning pins (**A**). With the halo ring held in place, sharp halo pins are then placed just below the skull equator. Spring-loaded pins are placed in front and a blank pin on the back (**B**). The pins are inserted and tightened in a diagonal fashion.

depending on age) that are inserted with less torque to prevent skull penetration or deformation. A computed tomography scan is often ordered to evaluate the thickness of the skull to plan for proper pin positioning.

Skin Preparation

The hair at the intended pin sites should be shaved to allow screws to be turned freely and for future pin care. The skin is then prepared with chlorhexidine, and local anesthetic is placed in the skin and into the periosteum of the skull. Halo placement does not require general anesthesia but should be a consideration in pediatric patients.

Pin Insertion

All four pins are slowly advanced equally to maintain positioning. In adults, the pins are tightened to 8 inch-pounds of torque. Pins should never be torqued beyond 10 inch-pounds to minimize the risk of penetrating the cortex.[41] A locking nut is tightened on the pin threads against the ring to prevent inadvertent skull penetration. In children 2 to 5 inch-pounds of torque should be used.

Vest Attachment

The posterior vest is applied by carefully turning the patient using a three-person logroll to immobilize the spine and slip the posterior vest in place. The patient is then placed supine, and the anterior vest is applied and connected by straps to the posterior shell. The ring is then attached to a thoracic jacket via rigid bars. All connections are then tightened according to the manufacturer's recommendations. When connecting the vest to the ring, the alignment of the cervical spine should be considered so that fracture reduction can be achieved. After the halo vest has been applied, lateral supine radiographs are obtained, and, if needed, adjustments may be made to improve reduction and alignment. We recommend a follow-up upright radiograph to assure reduction is being maintained. More extensive versions of the halo-vest device connect the head to the body via plaster of Paris body casts or pins in the pelvis.

Halo-Vest Care

The pins should be retightened 2 to 3 days after the ring was applied. The patient should be reassessed every 2 to 3 weeks thereafter. Pins should be assessed for loosening, drainage, and infection. Drainage without evidence of infection may indicate pin loosening requiring pin tightening. Pin site infections should be treated with antibiotics, local pin site care, and possibly pin tightening. During pin retightening, if torque does not increase after 1 or 2 rotations, then the pin should be

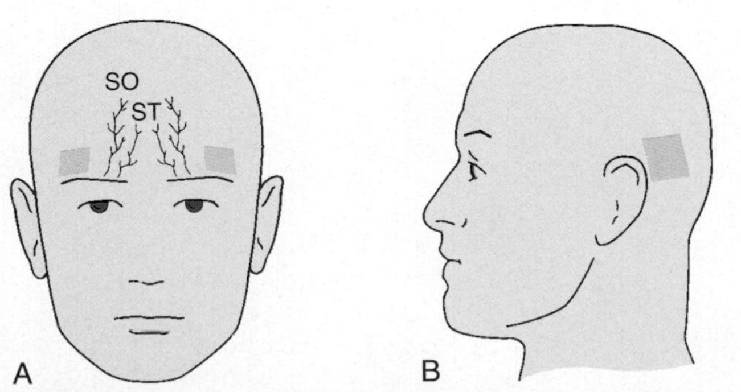

Figure 39-9. The safe zone for the anterior pins is located 1 cm superior and two-thirds lateral to the orbital rim, just below the greatest circumference of the skull. On the medial aspect of the safe zone are the supraorbital (SO) and supratrochlear (ST) nerves (**A**). The zone for the posterior pins is inferior to the widest portion of the skull yet superior enough to prevent ring or crown impingement on the upper helix of the ear (**B**).

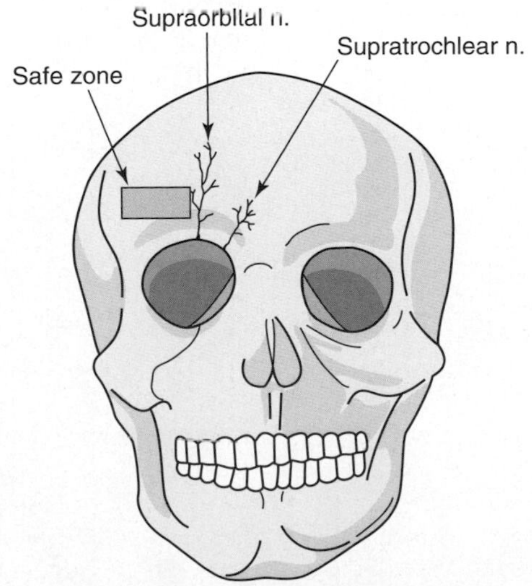

Figure 39-10. Anterior halo pins should be placed within the safe zone.

removed. Persistent pin site infections are an indication for pin removal and placement of an alternate pin at an adjacent site. The skin underneath the vest should be assessed for irritation or breakdown.

CONCLUSION

The successful orthotic management of spinal trauma requires the consideration of fracture stability and level of injury. The stabilizing ability of the various orthoses available must be matched to the relative stability of the spinal injury. Appropriate follow-up is necessary to ensure adequate fracture union while minimizing the occurrence of adverse events.

KEY REFERENCES

The level of evidence (LOE) is determined according to the criteria provided in the preface.

2. Bell KM, Frazier EC, Shively CM, et al: Assessing range of motion to evaluate the adverse effects of ill-fitting cervical orthoses. *Spine J* 9(3): 225–231, 2009.
4. Johnson RM, Hart DL, Simmons EF, et al: Cervical orthoses. A study comparing their effectiveness in restricting cervical motion in normal subjects. *J Bone Joint Surg Am* 59(3):332–339, 1977.
9. Gavin TM, Carandang G, Havey R, et al: Biomechanical analysis of cervical orthoses in flexion and extension: a comparison of cervical collars and cervical thoracic orthoses. *J Rehabil Res Dev* 40(6):527–537, 2003.
13. Richter D, Latta LL, Milne EL, et al: The stabilizing effects of different orthoses in the intact and unstable upper cervical spine: a cadaver study. *J Trauma* 50(5):848–854, 2001.
21. Harrop JS, Hart R, Anderson PA: Optimal treatment for odontoid fractures in the elderly. *Spine (Phila Pa 1976)* 35(21 Suppl):S219–S227, 2010. LOE V
32. Stadhouder A, Buskens E, Vergroesen DA, et al: Nonoperative treatment of thoracic and lumbar spine fractures: a prospective randomized study of different treatment options. *J Orthop Trauma* 23(8):588–594, 2009. LOE II
33. Thomas KC, Bailey CS, Dvorak MF, et al: Comparison of operative and nonoperative treatment for thoracolumbar burst fractures in patients without neurological deficit: a systematic review. *J Neurosurg Spine* 4(5):351–358, 2006. LOE V
39. van Middendorp JJ, Slooff WB, Nellestein WR, et al: Incidence of and risk factors for complications associated with halo-vest immobilization: a prospective, descriptive cohort study of 239 patients. *J Bone Joint Surg Am* 91(1):71–79, 2009. LOE I

The complete References list is available online at https://expertconsult.inkling.com.

SECTION THREE

Pelvis

EDITED BY CHRISTIAN KRETTEK

Section Outline

Chapter 40

Pelvic Ring Injuries

CARLO BELLABARBA • MARCEL WINKELMANN • SEBASTIAN DECKER • RICHARD JACKSON BRANSFORD • CHRISTIAN KRETTEK

INTRODUCTION

The pelvis is a key component of the axial skeleton that links the lower extremities with the rest of the body through the lumbosacral spine. Its ringlike structure allows it to surround and protect important inner organs, such as the urinary bladder, the lower intestines, and the reproductive organs, as well as major nerves and blood vessels. In patients with healthy bone, high-energy injuries are required to disrupt the integrity of the pelvic ring. However, because of age-related demographic changes in Western populations, injuries of the pelvic ring are increasingly being seen in elderly patients after minor trauma because of decreased bone mineral density, primarily caused by osteoporosis. However, the incidence of pelvic fractures under these circumstances (3%–5%) is relatively low compared with other fractures.

Because of the high-energy injury mechanisms required to sustain these injuries, patients with pelvic fractures have a high likelihood of associated injury to the abdominopelvic structures, including neurologic and vascular injuries, which can result in permanent neurologic deficits as well as severe life-threatening hemorrhage. Compared with other injuries, death after pelvic ring fractures is high, particularly because these injuries often occur in multiply injured patients.[1,2] In the long term, fractures of the pelvis may result in considerable morbidity because of deformity; chronic pain; and loss of lower extremity, bowel, bladder, and sexual function.

Treatment of pelvic ring injuries is challenging and requires in-depth knowledge of the complex pelvic anatomy as well as a high degree of surgical experience and skill. Because of the multiply injured nature of these patients, a coordinated multidisciplinary approach to treatment is essential. Treatment of the pelvic ring injury is often done in phases, which include a "damage control" phase that must be performed urgently to address concerns such as acute, life-threatening hemorrhage, followed by the final reconstruction of the pelvis and associated injuries after the patient has been appropriately resuscitated and physiologically stabilized. Proper identification of the specific injury patterns and their associated injuries can help guide both emergent treatment as well as definitive reconstruction. The principles behind damage control surgery should be familiar to every surgeon who deals with trauma patients. However, the definitive reconstruction of pelvic ring injuries should be reserved for appropriately experienced surgeons whenever possible. Final reconstruction of the pelvis is a potentially high-risk and sophisticated undertaking that requires intensive preoperative planning combined with experience and skill to optimize reduction and minimize complications.

ANATOMY

The pelvis has a ring-shaped structure that is formed by two innominate bones and the sacrum. The innominate bones are formed by the fusion of three ossification centers between the ilium, the ischium, and the pubis. These are linked through cartilaginous growth plates during childhood but coalesce with each other during adolescence at the triradiate cartilage of the acetabulum (Fig. 40-1). Familiarity with the anatomy of the ilium is also important for accurate iliac screw placement in lumbopelvic fixation techniques. The ilium provides a continuous bony channel, the sciatic buttress, that extends between the posterior superior iliac spine (PSIS) and the anterior inferior iliac spine (AIIS), with dimensions that readily accommodate iliac screws. The osseous sacral anatomy is composed of five kyphotically aligned, fused vertebral segments, with significant variability in upper sacral anatomy in the form of transitional vertebrae and sacral dysplasia. Because upper sacral variability results in significant alteration in the relationships between the sacrum, pelvis, and spinal column relative to their adjacent neurovascular structures, these variations must be recognized, particularly if surgical treatment of sacral fractures is being considered.[3,4]

The upper sacral body has the densest sacral cancellous bone, particularly adjacent to the superior S1 endplate. The ventral aspect of the upper S1 body that projects anteriorly and superiorly into the pelvis is termed the *sacral promontory*. The sacral ala, the lateral portion of the sacrum that articulates with the ilium through the sacroiliac (SI) joints, is largely cancellous and is formed by the coalescence of the sacral transverse processes. The cancellous alar bone is hypodense, particularly in older individuals, and an alar void is a consistent finding in middle-aged and older adults.[5,6] The relative difference in bone density between the upper and lower sacral body predisposes this area to fracture. The hypodense ala is predisposed, particularly in older and osteopenic patients, to fracture line propagation. This problem is accentuated by the relative strength of the SI joint ligaments. The suboptimal alar bone density must be taken into consideration when planning reconstructive procedures.

The posterior surface of the sacrum is convex and is formed by the coalescence of posterior elements. The middle sacral crest corresponds to the spinous processes, the intermediate sacral crests to the zygapophyseal joints, and the area in between to the lamina. The lowest one or two sacral segments have incompletely formed bony posterior elements, resulting in an aperture into the sacral spinal canal known as the sacral hiatus. Enlargement of the sacral hiatus may weaken the sacrum and predispose it to fracture, and it must also be

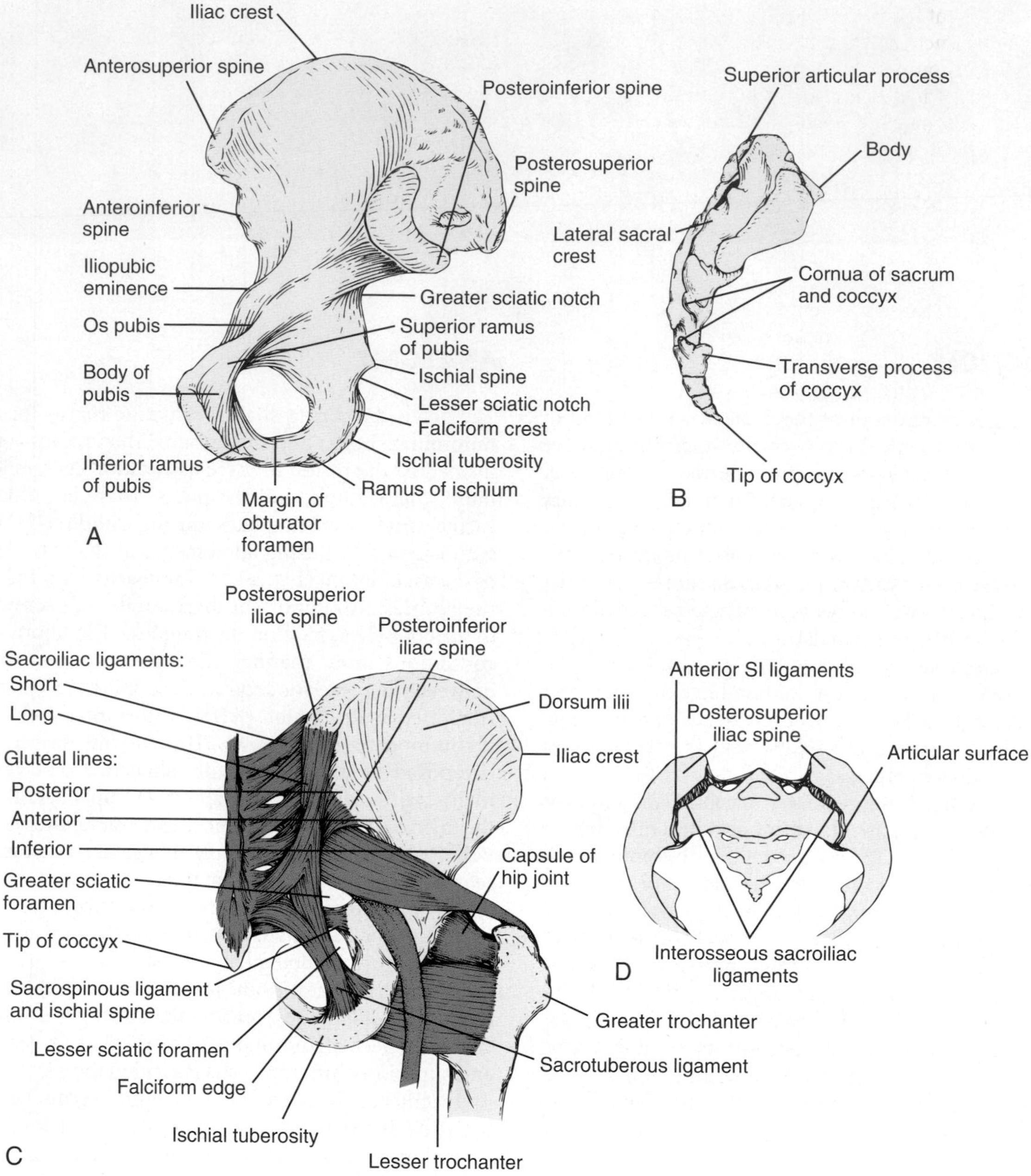

Figure 40-1. The sacroiliac (SI) joint. **A,** Iliac side of the SI joint, as well as the remainder of the innominate bone and the important bony landmarks. **B,** Sacral side. The two portions of the SI joint can best be appreciated on these views. The articular surface of the SI joint on the sacrum has a ridge and is covered by articular cartilage. The posterior portion is filled with ligamentous structures. **C** and **D,** Ligamentous complexes of the pelvis. **C,** Posteriorly, the major ligaments noted in the region of the SI joint are the posterior SI ligaments, both long and short. The long blend with the sacrospinous and the sacrotuberous ligaments. **D,** In cross-section, the orientation of the very thick posterior interosseous SI ligaments is noted.

recognized as a potential source of intraoperative iatrogenic sacral root injury.

The sacrum and the two innominate bones are linked by tenacious ligamentous structures that are the most essential in providing pelvic stability. Minimal mobility within the pelvic ring occurs between the innominate bones and the sacrum at three joints: two SI joints and the pubic symphysis. Rupture of the pubic symphysis as well as the ligaments forming the SI joint results in pelvic instability. The SI joint has two parts. The caudal portion consists primarily of the articular surface, and the upper, more dorsal portion, between the posterior tuberosity of the ilium and the sacrum contains the fibrous or ligamentous parts of the joint. The anterior portion of this synovial joint is covered with articular cartilage on the sacral side and fibrocartilage on the iliac side. The joint itself has a small ridge on the sacral side that provides minimal intrinsic stability. In general, SI joint stability is contingent on the integrity of a complex of anterior and posterior SI ligaments.

The pubic symphysis consists of two opposed surfaces of hyaline cartilage covered with intervening fibrocartilage surrounded by a thick band of fibrous tissue. The joint is further strengthened by the superior pubic ligament above and the arcuate pubic ligament below. Moreover, adjacent pelvic floor muscle insertions, such as that of the levator ani muscle, provide a minor amount of additional stability. The pubic symphysis is usually widest superiorly and anteriorly.

The pelvis is designed to ideally provide the necessary rigidity for upright gait and the transmission of forces between the lower extremities and the spine while providing for required mobility, such as during parturition. Because the forces that are transmitted from the lower extremities to the spine affect mainly the posterior pelvic ring, the integrity of the SI ligamentous complex is essential to pelvic stability.[7] The posterior SI ligaments are divided into two components, short and long. The short posterior ligaments are oblique and run from the posterior ridge of the sacrum to the posterior superior and posterior inferior spines of the ilium. The long posterior ligaments are longitudinal fibers that course from the lateral aspect of the sacrum to the PSIS and merge with the sacrotuberous ligament. The long ligaments lie posterior and superficial to the short ligaments. Anterior SI ligaments, which provide less stability than their posterior counterparts, also connect the ilium to the sacrum. The most important ligaments for pelvic ring stability are the posterior interosseous SI ligaments that join the sacrum and the tuberosities of the ilium in the transverse plane.

The above-mentioned ligaments are the most important for maintaining stability of the pelvic ring. Additional ligaments that do not directly span the joints but connect various portions of the pelvic ring also have important stabilizing roles. The sacrotuberous ligament is a strong band that runs from the posterolateral aspect of the sacrum and the dorsal aspect of the posterior iliac spine to the ischial tuberosity. Its medial border thickens to form a falciform tendon, which blends with the obturator membrane at the ischial tuberosity. It also merges into the posterior origin of the gluteus maximus. This ligament, in association with its ipsilateral posterior SI ligaments, is especially important in maintaining the vertical stability of the pelvis. The sacrospinous ligament is triangular and runs from the lateral margins of the sacrum and coccyx and the sacrotuberous ligament to insert onto the ischial spine. It serves as the border between the greater and lesser sciatic notches. The sacrospinous ligament may be important in maintaining rotational control of the pelvis if the posterior SI ligaments are intact.

Several ligaments extend from the spine to the pelvis and are important in providing spinopelvic stability. The iliolumbar ligaments originate from the L4 and L5 transverse processes and insert onto the posterior iliac crest, securing the pelvis to the lumbar spine. The lumbosacral ligaments run from the transverse process of L5 to the ala of the sacrum. They form a strong ridge anteriorly and abut the L5 root.

If its ligamentous structures are intact, the pelvis constitutes a stable ring. The sacrum forms the posterior aspect of the pelvic ring and serves as its keystone because it maintains stability while transmitting forces from the lumbosacral articulation across the SI joints to the pelvis. This keystone function is particularly true in the pelvic outlet plane, in which the orientation of the sacrum relative to the ilium is such that axial forces lock the sacrum into the pelvic ring and further stabilize the SI articulation. In the pelvic inlet plane, the sacrum is shaped like a "reverse keystone," which is more inherently unstable and therefore requires substantial intrinsic and extrinsic ligamentous stabilization of the SI joints while permitting required pelvic ring motion. The posterior SI ligaments create a posterior tension band for the pelvis. The transversely oriented ligaments, including the short posterior SI and the anterior SI ligaments along with the iliolumbar and sacrospinous ligaments, resist rotational forces. The vertically placed ligaments, including the long posterior SI, sacrotuberous, and lateral lumbosacral ligaments, help resist vertical shear and vertical migration.[8]

The pelvis contains two major anatomic regions. The false pelvis and the true pelvis are divided by the pelvic brim, which extends from the sacral promontory along the junction between the ilium and the ischium onto the pubic ramus. No major muscular structures cross the pelvic brim. Above the brim, the false pelvis (greater pelvis) is contained by the sacral ala and the iliac wings. The false pelvis is lined laterally by the iliopsoas muscle. It forms part of the abdominal cavity. The true pelvis (lesser pelvis) lies below the pelvic brim, and its lateral wall consists of portions of the pubis, ischium, and a small triangular portion of the ilium.

The obturator foramen, which is covered by muscles and a membrane, also defines the boundary of the true pelvis. The foramen opens superiorly and laterally for passage of the obturator nerve and vessels. An aberrant obturator artery is one of the many known vascular variants in the pelvis that is located near the pubic ramus to supply the musculature of the obturator foramen. Because of its location, it is often injured in pelvic ring disruptions.[9,10]

The obturator internus muscle originates from the obturator membrane and courses through the lesser sciatic notch to insert onto the proximal end of the femur. The obturator internus tendon is an important structure because it serves as an intraoperative guide to identify the posterior column. The piriformis originates from the lateral aspect of the sacrum and is key to identifying the sciatic nerve. A schematic illustration of the pelvic musculature is presented in Figure 40-2. Usually, the sciatic nerve exits the pelvis anterior to the piriformis muscle and enters the greater sciatic notch. Occasionally, the peroneal division exits either through or posterior to the piriformis. The floor of the true pelvis consists of the coccyx; the coccygeal and levator ani muscles; and the urethra, rectum, and vagina.

The dural sac typically ends at the S2 level, and the filum terminale attaches at its caudal end to the coccyx. Four paired ventral and dorsal neuroforamina are formed at the junction of the sacral body and ala, through which pass the ventral and dorsal rami of the sacral nerve roots. The relative space available to the sacral nerve roots in the ventral foramina is lowest at the S1 and S2 levels, where the nerve roots occupy one-third to one-fourth of the foraminal space compared with the S3 and S4 levels, where the nerve roots occupy one-sixth of the available foraminal space. The lower sacral roots are therefore less likely to be impinged upon in injuries involving displacement of the neuroforamina.[11]

The dorsal nerve roots exit through their respective posterior neuroforamina to supply motor branches to the paraspinal muscles and cutaneous sensory branches that form the cluneal nerves. Anteriorly, the L5 nerve root passes underneath the inferior edge of the sacrolumbar ligament and drapes over the anterosuperior aspect of the sacral ala. It anastomoses with the L4 ventral ramus to form the lumbosacral plexus at the level of the sacral promontory, approximately 12 mm lateral to the SI joint. The sacral roots join the lumbosacral plexus along the sacral ala as they exit through their

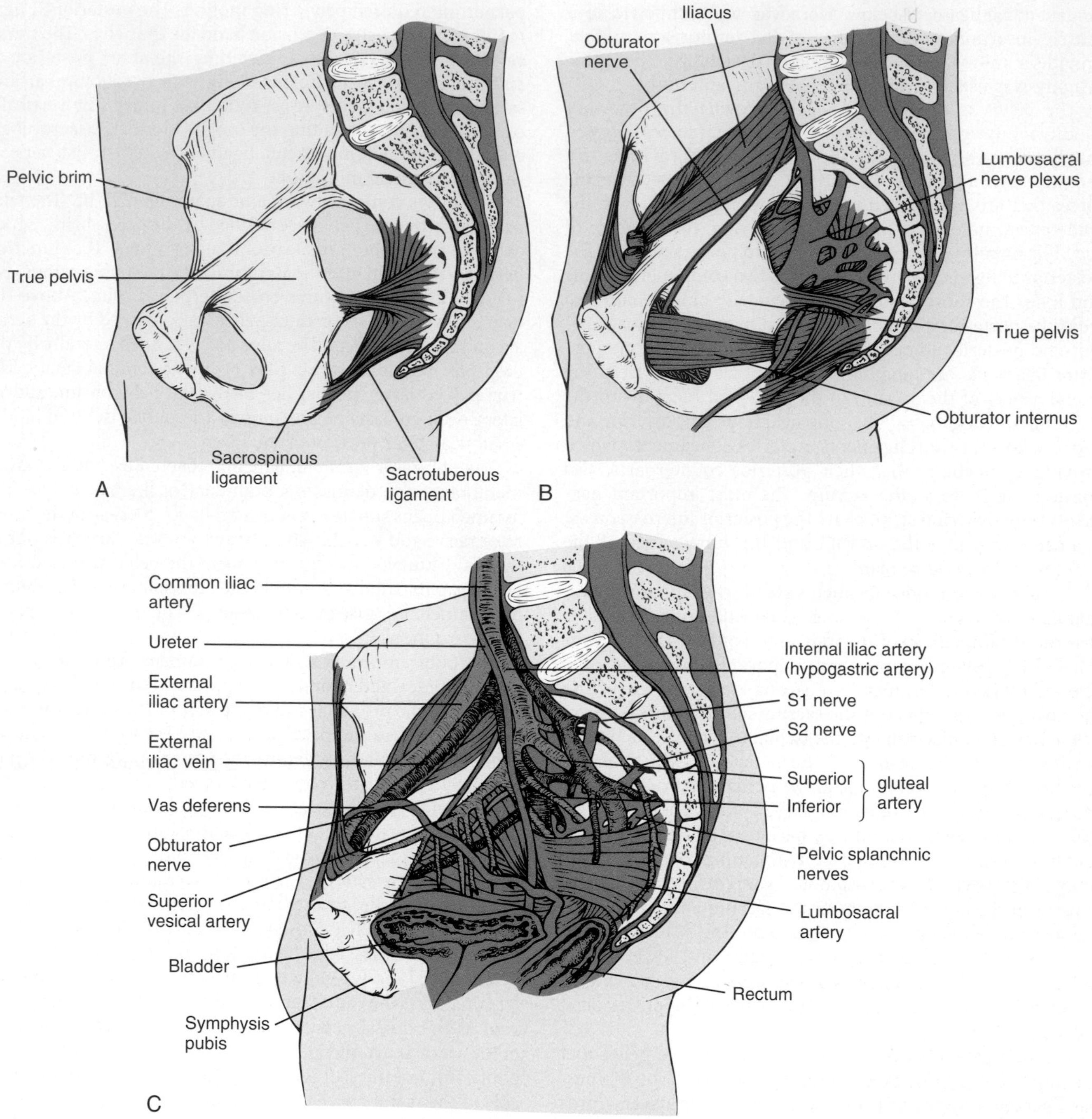

Figure 40-2. Internal aspect of the pelvis. **A,** The inner aspect of the pelvis consists of the true pelvis, which is below the pelvic brim, and the false pelvis above it. The sacrotuberous and sacrospinous ligaments are attached to their appropriate structures and form the basis of the pelvic floor. **B,** The major structures in the inner aspect of the pelvis are the lumbosacral plexus, which originates from the L5 and the sacral roots and leaves the pelvis through the greater sciatic notch as the sciatic nerve and the superior gluteal artery. The obturator internus originates from the obturator membrane and loops out through the lesser sciatic notch. Note that no muscles cross the pelvic brim. **C,** Internal aspect of the pelvis showing the great vessels and the lumbosacral plexus, as well as the pelvic floor, bladder, and rectum.

respective ventral sacral foramina.[12] The lumbosacral coccygeal plexus is made up of the anterior rami of T12 through S4. The L4 through S1 roots are most at risk of compromise due to pelvic injury or surgical intervention. Whereas the L4 and L5 roots enter the true pelvis from the false pelvis, the sacral roots originate in the true pelvis. The L4 and L5 roots course, on average, 17.9 and 18.4 mm lateral to the SI joint, respectively. The dual innervation of the perineal structures from both the left and right sacral plexus is somewhat protective of bowel, bladder, and sexual function. These functions are largely preserved in the event of unilateral transection of the sacral nerve roots, but bilateral transection causes complete loss of function.[13] Numerous nerve branches extend to the major muscles within the pelvis. The superior gluteal and inferior gluteal nerves exit the pelvis ventral to the piriformis and through the greater sciatic notch.

The major pelvic blood vessels lie along the inner wall of the pelvis. The bilateral common iliac arteries arise from the aorta at the level of L4 to L5 and give rise to the internal iliac arteries, which lie anterior to the SI joints and course beyond the pelvic brim into the true pelvis, giving off both superior and inferior lateral sacral arteries in the process. A branch of the internal iliac artery, the superior gluteal artery, crosses over the anterior and caudal portion of the SI joint to exit the greater sciatic notch. As it sweeps around the notch, it lies directly on bone. The external iliac artery runs cranial to the pelvic brim at the level of the pubic ramus, exiting the pelvis posterior to the inguinal ligament, where it becomes the common femoral artery. The presacral area has an extensive and highly variable vascular network. The middle sacral artery typically courses ventrally along the midline of the L5 vertebral body and the sacrum after branching from the aorta at the common iliac bifurcation. The superior lateral sacral artery arises from the internal iliac artery and courses caudally just lateral to the sacral foramina and supplies the spinal canal through the S1 and S2 ventral foramina, and the inferior lateral sacral artery traverses the inferior aspect of the SI joint before anastomosing with the middle sacral artery and giving off spinal arteries that pass through the S3 and S4 ventral foramina. The superior rectal artery, which is a continuation of the inferior mesenteric artery, lies posteriorly along the midline. All arteries are accompanied by correspondingly named veins. The internal iliac veins lie posteromedial to the internal iliac arteries and course caudally. They are located medial to the SI joint directly adjacent to the sacral ala. The internal iliac veins give rise to an extensive presacral venous plexus, formed by anastomoses between the lateral and middle sacral veins that communicate transforaminally with epidural veins in the spinal canal. This extensive vascular network renders anterior exposures to the sacrum impractical and perilous. The major arteries and veins are both at significant risk of injury during pelvic ring fractures and are a potential source of lethal hemorrhage. Data about the exact source of bleeding have been difficult to obtain. Nevertheless, only a minority of cases of lethal bleeding that result from pelvic ring fractures can be attributed to major arterial damage. Huittinen and colleagues reported only 11.1% of hemorrhage to be of arterial origin, with the rest being of venous origin.[14,15] The presacral venous plexus is of particularly high risk of rupture, leading to subsequent bleeding into the lesser and greater pelves.

Because of the substantial risk of injury to intrapelvic organs, which can occur from either the trauma itself or from surgical treatment, detailed anatomic knowledge of intrapelvic anatomy is crucial to the safety of patients. The bladder is situated immediately posterior to the symphysis pubis and cranial to the pelvic floor, which is formed by several different muscles, including the levator ani, transversus peroneus profundus, and coccygeal muscles. Similarly, the uterus in females is located behind the bladder and is connected to the ovaries through the fallopian tubes. The muscles of the pelvic floor arise in continuity from the ischial spines, obturator membranes, and pubis and insert into the coccyx and anal coccygeal raphe. They form a muscular diaphragm with a gap anteriorly, through which pass the urethra, vagina, rectum, and supporting ligaments. In contrast, the ureters course along the retroperitoneum from the kidneys into the pelvis and join the bladder after crossing over the external iliac arteries and veins. The fascia of the pelvic floor is loose and mobile. In males, the prostate lies between the bladder and the pelvic floor and is invested by a dense fascial membrane. The urethra passes through the prostate before exiting the pelvic floor. It is divided into five sections; the preprostatic urethra is the most cranial segment and is generally within the wall of the urinary bladder, depending on bladder fullness. The prostatic urethra courses through the prostate, transitioning to the membranous urethra, which passes through the external urethral sphincter. The part of the urethra that extends beyond the pelvic floor is divided into the bulbous and pendulous urethra. The junction between the prostate and the pelvic floor is strong, as is the membranous urethra. The weak link is the segment of urethra just below the pelvic diaphragm in its bulbous portion. Colapinto has shown that when the bladder is pulled forcefully, the urethra ruptures in its bulbous portion, which is the most common site of urethral rupture below the pelvic floor and a common associated injury in pelvic ring disruption.[16] In contrast, the urethral injury in females occurs most commonly near the neck of the bladder. Urinary continence depends on the external (striated muscle) sphincter at the level of the membranous urethra (midurethra in females) and the bladder neck (smooth muscle) in both males and females. Other structures that pass through the urogenital diaphragm include the pudendal arteries and veins, the pudendal nerve (S2–S4), and the autonomic nerves of the pelvis (S2–S4). These are all responsible for normal sexual function and are at risk of injury in pelvic trauma.

A considerable part of the intestine is located within the confines of the pelvis. The descending colon transitions into the sigmoid colon, which transitions to the rectum and finally the anus, formed by internal and external sphincter muscle layers. The rectum and anus are located behind the uterus in women and behind the bladder in men. The diversity of anatomic structures within such a confined space lends itself to a high potential for injury to a multitude of organ systems, either from the trauma itself or from surgical treatment.

PELVIC STABILITY AND BIOMECHANICS

Therapeutic management of pelvic ring fractures largely depends on pelvic stability. Stable fractures can typically be managed nonoperatively, but unstable fractures generally require surgery. Unfortunately, a clear distinction between stable and unstable has yet to be well defined. One should instead conceptualize a given injury as lying along a spectrum between the two extremes that are designated as stable and unstable.

For practical purposes, it is necessary to simplify the biomechanics of the pelvic ring into its basic elements. The articulations between the three bony elements (sacrum and two innominate bones) provide little in the way of inherent stability. As mentioned previously, the keystone function of the sacrum does provide some intrinsic stability in the outlet plane, but the reverse is true of the inlet plane. However, because of the above-mentioned ligamentous structures that stabilize the pelvic ring at the SI joints and pubic symphysis, under physiologic conditions the pelvis is stable, meaning that it can withstand physiologic loads without displacement. The unstable pelvis will therefore displace under minimal load.[17,18] However, because slight motion does occur at its three primary articulations under physiologic loads, the pelvic ring cannot

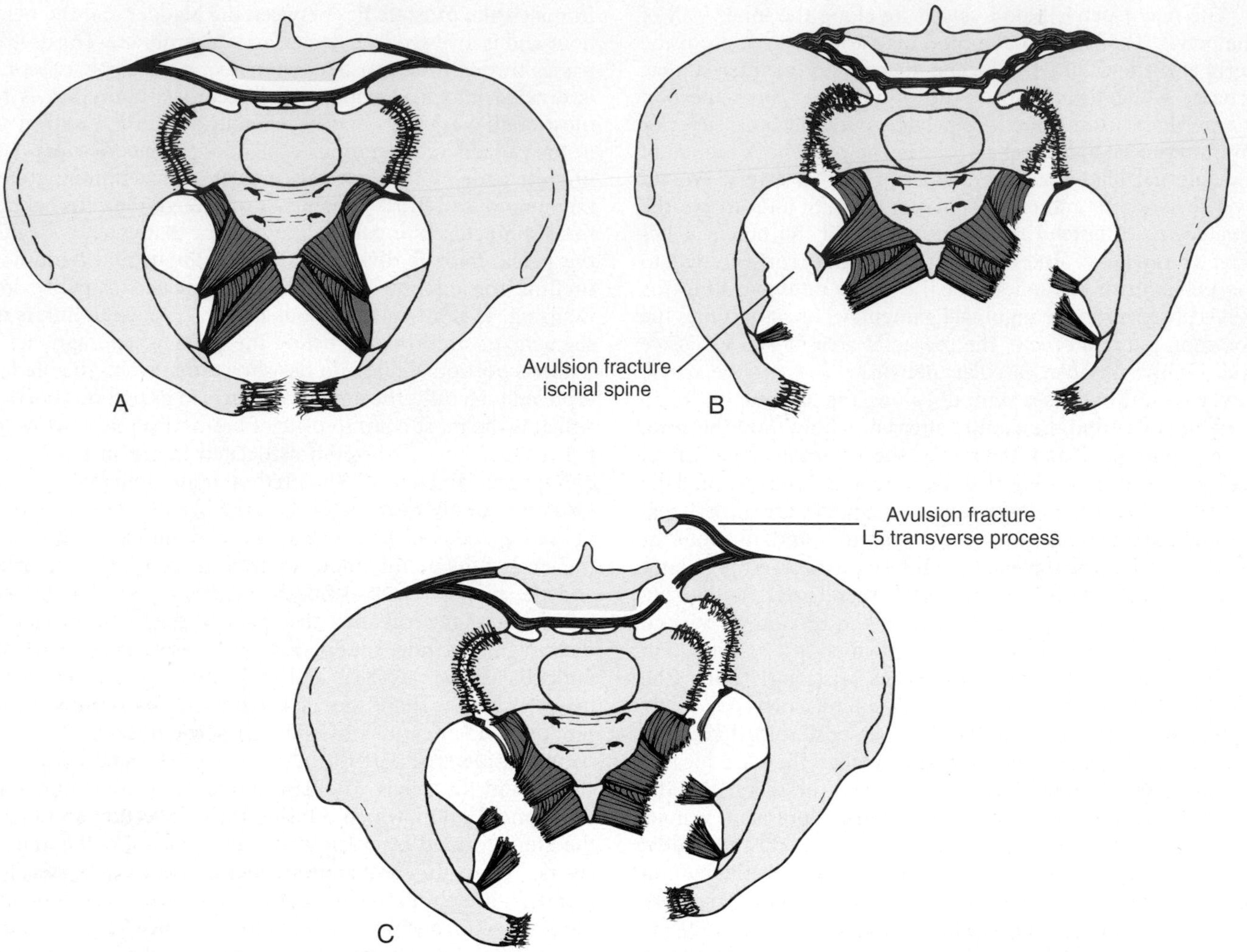

Figure 40-3. A, Division of the symphysis pubis allows the pelvis to open to approximately 2.5 cm with no damage to any posterior ligamentous structures. **B,** Division of the anterior sacroiliac (SI) and sacrospinous ligaments, either by direct division of their fibers *(right)* or by avulsion of the tip of the ischial spine *(left),* allows the pelvis to rotate externally until the posterior superior iliac spines abut the sacrum. Note, however, that the posterior ligamentous structures (e.g., the posterior SI and iliolumbar ligaments) remain intact. Therefore, no displacement in the vertical plane is possible. **C,** Division of the posterior band ligaments, that is, the posterior SI, as well as the iliolumbar ligaments, causes complete instability of the hemipelvis. Note that global displacement is now possible.

be considered a completely rigid construct. In the upright position, loading of the sacrum between the iliac wings causes approximately 5 degrees of dorsoventral rotation of the sacrum.[19] The innominate bones translate posteriorly and flexion occurs as the pubic rami rotate cranially relative to the posterior ring.[20] The physiologic motion at the symphysis pubis includes transverse and vertical translation of approximately 1 and 2 mm, respectively.[21] Tile and Hearn also demonstrated that with sitting or double-leg standing, whereas the symphysis pubis is loaded in tension, the posterior ring is loaded in compression. In single-leg stance, the symphysis is compressed, and the posterior complex is loaded under tension.[18] The ligaments, which maintain the integrity of the posterior ring, are among the strongest ligaments in the body.[18] When Miller and colleagues tested isolated SI joints, some specimens withstood loads of 1440 N without failing.[22] In addition, a normal pelvis can withstand vertical loads from 3630 to 5837 N without failing.[13]

To better understand the relative contribution of individual components of the pelvic ring to the spectrum of pelvic stability, Tile and Hearn, based on work by Pennal, studied the consequences of sequential sectioning of the pelvic ligaments.[18] Sectioning of the symphyseal ligaments alone resulted in symphyseal diastasis of no greater than 2.5 cm (Fig. 40-3, *A*), but the relationship of this value to the integrity of the anterior SI, sacrotuberous, and sacrospinous ligaments is weak.[23] The sacrospinous and anterior SI ligaments are thought to restrain further widening of the anterior pelvis. Additional sectioning of the sacrospinous and anterior SI ligaments results in increased diastasis (Fig. 40-3, *B*), but intact posterior longitudinal and sacrotuberous ligaments prevent vertical translation. In this situation, the pelvis is only rotationally unstable and can therefore be restored to its anatomic integrity by reduction and stabilization of the anterior ring only using the intact posterior ligamentous hinge as a fulcrum. Sectioning of the posterior ligaments only with an intact symphysis results in relatively little posterior instability because the posterior bony complex is loaded primarily in compression.[24] With sectioning of the symphyseal, sacrospinous, sacrotuberous, and posterior SI ligaments, the pelvis becomes globally unstable and is free to translate or rotate in any direction (Fig. 40-3, *C*). However, this description represents a simplification of the complex interaction between the ligaments and soft tissues investing the pelvis, and the functional interaction of all components of the pelvic ring has yet to be fully understood.[25] For example, although the sacrospinous and sacrotuberous ligaments were previously considered to have no effect on patterns of pelvic deformity, recent studies have suggested that they provide vertical load transfer, with resulting translation of the sacrum.[7] In general, decreased ligament stiffness increases SI joint stress and angular motion, with maximum strains occurring at the interosseous SI ligament.[26] However, increased sacrospinous and sacrotuberous ligament stiffness has been found to paradoxically increase SI motion.[7]

In addition to the instability induced by ligamentous insufficiency, bony injuries can produce equivalent degrees of pelvic instability. Fractures through the iliac wing, fracture-dislocations of the SI joint, or some complete fractures of the sacrum bypass the ligamentous structures and may therefore constitute globally unstable posterior injuries.

TRAUMA MECHANISM AND PATHOMECHANICS OF PELVIC INJURIES

Pelvic ring injuries usually occur because of high-energy trauma. Two different approaches allow for a better understanding of the relationship between the mechanism of injury and the pelvic fracture pattern. The more clinical way is to extrapolate from trauma mechanism to fracture pattern or severity because the mechanism usually is known from third-party history. On the other hand, a biomechanical approach to injury patterns allows one to deduce the mechanism of injury based on the fracture configuration.

TRAUMA MECHANISM

The medical history provides essential information about the mechanism of injury. Depending on the patient's age, it is possible to draw inferences about the severity of the pelvic injury from the trauma mechanism. In adult patients, high-energy trauma is usually necessary for pelvic ring disruption. Motor vehicle accidents and falls from a substantial height and industrial accidents are therefore the most common causes of severe pelvic fractures.

Motor Vehicle Accident

Motor vehicle accidents are the most common cause of complex pelvic trauma. One can distinguish among different accident mechanisms. Vehicle–pedestrian accidents are usually associated with low or moderate speed. There is a correlation between the speed of the automobile and the incidence and severity of pelvic fractures. A collision velocity of 30 mph (50 km/h) and above should raise the index of suspicion for pelvic ring injury. The collision type can also provide relevant clues in the suspicion of pelvic injuries. The risk of a pelvic injury is highest in side impact collisions on the same side as the victim followed by head-on collisions. Pedestrians, bicyclists, and motorcyclists have twice the risk of sustaining a pelvic fracture.[27,28]

Fall from a Height

A fall from a height (>4 m) is considered a high-energy trauma because the injury severity and pattern are directly correlated with the height of the fall. If the height is relatively low (<7 m), fractures of pelvis, upper limbs, lower limbs, and blunt thoracic trauma are the most common injuries. Above 20 feet (7 m), traumatic brain injuries and spinal fractures are the most frequent causes of mortality.[29-31]

Osteoporotic Pelvic Fractures of the Elderly

Demographic changes have been leading to an aging society and increased number of elderly patients. With increasing age, the risk for osteoporosis increases, especially in postmenopausal females. Conditions contributing to osteoporosis are often present, such as chronic corticosteroid use or a history of radiation therapy to the pelvis (Fig. 40-4).[32] In contrast to the adolescent and young adult pelvic ring, the compromised bone density in an elderly patient may result in pelvic fracture from minimal trauma, such as stumbling or falling from a low height such as from a standing or seated position. The precipitating event in insufficiency fractures is often not even identifiable. Usually, clinical signs of sacral and pelvic ring insufficiency fractures are rather vague and consist of poorly localized groin and low back pain in the region of the sacrum or SI joints that may be exacerbated by sitting and standing. Occasionally, radicular pain may be reported. The sacral component of these fractures is typically oriented vertically and occurs through the ala adjacent to the SI joint. There may also be a transverse component extending between bilateral vertical fractures, resulting in more complex U-fracture variants (see Fig. 40-4). Although neurologic deficits are uncommon under these circumstances,[33] cauda equina dysfunction has been reported, and neurologic status must be carefully evaluated.[34]

Magnetic resonance imaging (MRI)–based studies report a 25% incidence of occult pelvic ring fractures in elderly patients, of which two-thirds comprise injury of the posterior ring. One must therefore maintain a high index of suspicion to avoid overlooking these injuries.

Stress fractures of the pelvis, unlike insufficiency fractures, occur in bone that is not weakened by a pathologic process. They usually occur in individuals whose activity level causes repetitive stress that exceeds the bone's reparative ability. High-demand individuals such as endurance athletes and military recruits are particularly susceptible.

PATHOMECHANICS AND MECHANISM OF PELVIC INJURIES

From a biomechanical point of view, fracture patterns can be construed from the primary force vector because each applied force can result in characteristic deformities of the pelvic ring. Pennal postulated that three basic forces were responsible for traumatic pelvic deformities: anterior-posterior (AP) compression, lateral compression, and vertical shear, which, respectively, tend to open the pelvis like a book, collapse it toward the midline, or cause vertical translation.[18]

Anterior-Posterior Force Pattern

Anterior-posterior force patterns typically cause external rotation of the hemipelvis. Two different application points are

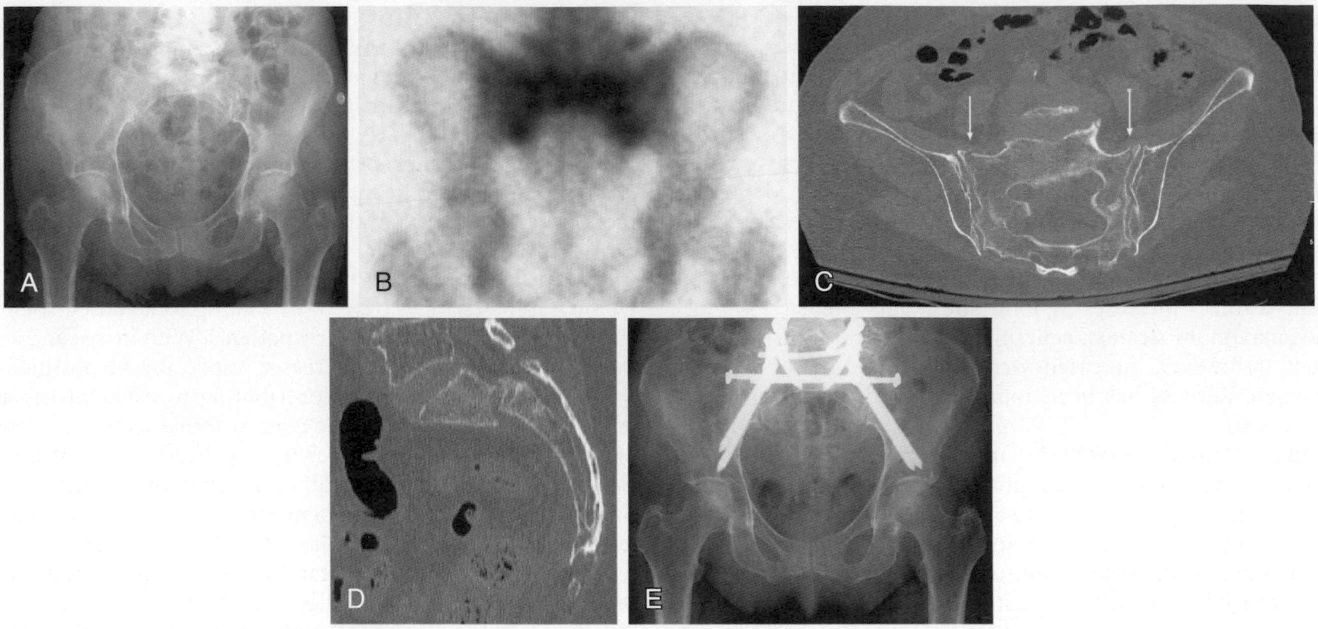

Figure 40-4. Anterior-posterior (AP) radiograph (**A**), technetium bone scan (**B**), axial computed tomography (CT) image (**C**), and sagittal CT image (**D**) of the pelvis of a 72-year-old woman with a history of radiotherapy to the pelvic region for treatment of endometrial carcinoma. She had begun experiencing severe low back and gluteal pain and symptoms of cauda equina dysfunction without any inciting trauma and could neither sit nor stand because of pain. Postoperative AP radiograph of the pelvis (**E**) after spinopelvic fixation. The patient was able to tolerate sitting and standing immediately after surgery and had gradual resolution of her preoperative symptoms.

possible. The most common is a direct posterior blow through the PSIS that leads to diastasis and disruption of the symphysis and, with increasing force, of the anterior SI ligaments as well. Direct forces applied to the anterior superior iliac spine (ASIS) also cause disruption of symphyseal and anterior SI ligaments and can tear the posterior SI ligament or cause correspondingly unstable fractures through the sacrum.

In general, this force pattern leads to rotational instability (open book) with the posterior SI ligament remaining intact (Fig. 40-3, *B*). If the force overcomes the integrity of the posterior ligamentous complex, the result is vertical instability.

Lateral Compressions Force Pattern

The most common force pattern causing pelvic fractures is lateral compression. Depending on the point of application and the magnitude of this force, different lateral compression injuries are seen.

If a force is applied to the posterior SI complex, it is typically parallel to the trabeculae of the sacrum, creating compression or impaction of the cancellous bone of the sacrum. It causes minimal soft tissue disruption because the posterior ligamentous structures relax as the hemipelvis is driven inward. Because the force of injury is essentially parallel to the ligament fibers and trabeculae of the bone, it produces a very stable fracture configuration.

If a force is applied to the anterior half of the iliac wing, it tends to rotate the hemipelvis internally, with the pivot point being the anterior SI joint or anterior ala. Consequently, the anterolateral portion of the sacrum adjacent to the SI joint sustains an impaction fracture, and injuries of the posterior SI ligament complex may follow.[35] Rather than involving the sacrum, fracture may involve the posterior ilium adjacent to the SI joint, producing relatively common patterns such as the "crescent" fracture. This injury becomes more unstable as disruptions of the posterior osseous or ligamentous structures become more severe. However, the sacrospinous and sacrotuberous ligaments remain intact along with the pelvic floor, thereby limiting translational instability. This force can continue to displace the hemipelvis across toward the opposite side, producing a lateral compression injury on the side of force application and an external rotation injury on the contralateral side.[36] The resulting anterior pelvic lesions may be any combination of ramus fractures or fracture-dislocations through the symphysis. The pubic ramus fractures are typically horizontal in orientation (Fig. 40-5).

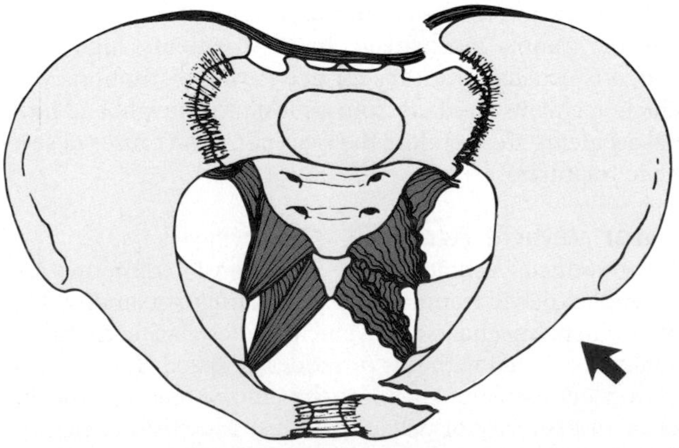

Figure 40-5. Lateral compression—unstable. In this mechanism, the force *(arrow)* is directed over the anterior aspect of the hemipelvis. The hemipelvis pivots around the anterior portion of the sacroiliac joint, thus compressing the sacrum or fracturing through the ilium (or both). Posteriorly, the posterior interosseous hinge is now disrupted, and the pelvis is unstable in internal rotation. It may exhibit some degree of vertical instability. Vertical instability is limited by the intact sacrotuberous ligaments.

Finally, if force is applied to the greater trochanteric region, this leads to a lateral compression injury, usually associated with an acetabular fracture.

External Rotation-Abduction Force Pattern

Because of its characteristic mechanism and direction, an external rotation-abduction force pattern is an independent force type. Nevertheless, there are several similarities with AP force pattern. This force is common in motorcycle accidents and usually applied indirectly through the femoral shafts and hips. The leg is caught and externally rotated and abducted, a mechanism that tends to tear the hemipelvis from the sacrum. Coincident femoral neck and shaft fractures are common.

Shear Force Pattern

Shear fractures are the result of high-energy forces, usually applied perpendicular to the bony trabeculae. These forces quite commonly lead to unstable fractures or dislocations or both. The exact fracture pattern depends on both the amount of force applied and the bone strength in relation to the ligamentous structures. In general, if bone strength is less than ligamentous strength, a shear force will result in vertically oriented sacral and rami fractures, as opposed to the horizontal pattern seen in lateral compression. Conversely, if the bone strength is relatively high, ligamentous injuries usually occur and manifest as symphysis and SI joint dislocations but often with some degree of bony avulsion.[37]

Traumatic hemipelvectomy, a rare injury, occurs most commonly because of an external rotation-abduction force followed by direct blow (e.g., ship's propeller). However, extreme shear forces can also lead to hemipelvectomy.

In conclusion, trauma mechanism can be obtained from personal or third-party history and may often be inferred from the pelvic fracture pattern.[38] The fracture pattern, displacement, deformity, and the clinical examination provide clues to pelvic stability. Subsequent diagnostic tests and classifications are aimed at categorization of the stability to enable appropriate treatment decisions.

RADIOLOGY OF THE PELVIS

Radiologic imaging is mandatory if the physician suspects that a patient has sustained a pelvic ring fracture and is generally dictated by standard trauma protocols in situations involving high-energy trauma. Pelvic imaging in the form of an AP radiograph of the pelvis is recommended in all polytrauma patients by the Acute Trauma Life Support (ATLS) guidelines published by the American College of Surgeons, highlighting the importance of excluding pelvic ring disruptions with potential lethal hemorrhage so that immediate damage control surgery can be initiated, if necessary.[39] A more conservative approach to imaging can be considered under specific circumstances, such as in the case of pregnancy, particularly in the case of a relatively minor trauma with a low risk of a pelvic ring injury. However, in the case of a high-energy injury with potentially unstable isolated pelvic ring injury or multiple trauma patients, even in pregnancy, the mother's safety should take priority over radiation exposure to the fetus. Unfortunately, there are few data on pelvic ring injuries in pregnancy.[40,41]

In general, a pelvic ring fracture has to be excluded after sufficient trauma has been sustained or if corresponding symptoms are suspicious of a fracture. Moreover, preoperative planning requires proper radiographic evaluation to minimize the rate of complications and to guarantee an optimal reduction during surgery. During the past decade, different planning tools and software have been established. These programs are mostly based on computed tomography (CT) imaging.[42] Whereas plain radiographs constituted the gold standard in former decades, trauma centers are increasingly turning to the routine use of abdominopelvic CT scans with reconstruction of the bony anatomy to establish the diagnosis of pelvic ring disruption while also being able to assess for visceral or vascular injuries. The different radiologic techniques are described in the following text.

Plain Radiographs

Three standard plain radiographic images are used to evaluate the pelvic ring: AP, inlet, and outlet views. In former decades, all of them had to be obtained for thorough radiographic evaluation. However, CT evaluation with multiple reformations has become the gold standard with possibly the use of three-dimensional (3-D) CT. Nevertheless, inlet and outlet views are still routinely used, both in the operating room during surgery to evaluate pelvic reduction and the placement of implants as well as during follow-up visits to evaluate pelvic alignment. This paradigm shift toward the use of CT imaging with 3-D reformations is illustrated by the ATLS guidelines, which recommend an AP view followed by CT of the pelvis.[39] However, in hemodynamically and mechanically stable polytraumatized patients suspected of pelvic ring fractures, there is evidence that the AP radiograph can be omitted in lieu of CT scan.[43,44] Because both the Young and Burgess classification as well as the Arbeitsgemeinschaft für Osteosynthesefragen (AO) classification modified by Tile refer to plain radiographs, this algorithm change also has an impact on the classification of pelvic injuries.[45-47]

Anterior-Posterior Radiograph

The AP radiograph (Fig. 40-6) gives an overview of the complete pelvis. Fractures of the superior and inferior pubic ramus can be visualized as well as disruption of the pubic symphysis. Although injuries of the posterior pelvic ring might be identified, further imaging is often required to properly evaluate for injuries to the iliac wing as well as the sacrum.[48] Useful indicators of sacral injuries include abnormalities in the contour of the sacral foramina and sacral arcuate lines and the presence of a "paradoxical inlet" view of the sacrum caused by an increase in sacral inclination that is so great as to give the appearance of an inlet view of the S1 vertebral body on the AP pelvic view. Their presence warrants CT evaluation of the sacrum. It is important to remember that in the supine position, the pelvis is anteverted 45 to 60 degrees relative to the long axis of the skeleton. This angulation pertains to pelvic tilt, the degree of which has considerable implications in the treatment of spine deformities and sacral fractures with spinopelvic dissociations. The pelvic tilt is, however, a flexible parameter that changes based on positioning.[49,50] Consequently, an AP radiograph is essentially an oblique radiograph of the pelvis. The acquisition technique is as follows: The patient is placed supine with symmetrical positioning of the legs and subtle abduction and internal rotation of the hips. The beam is

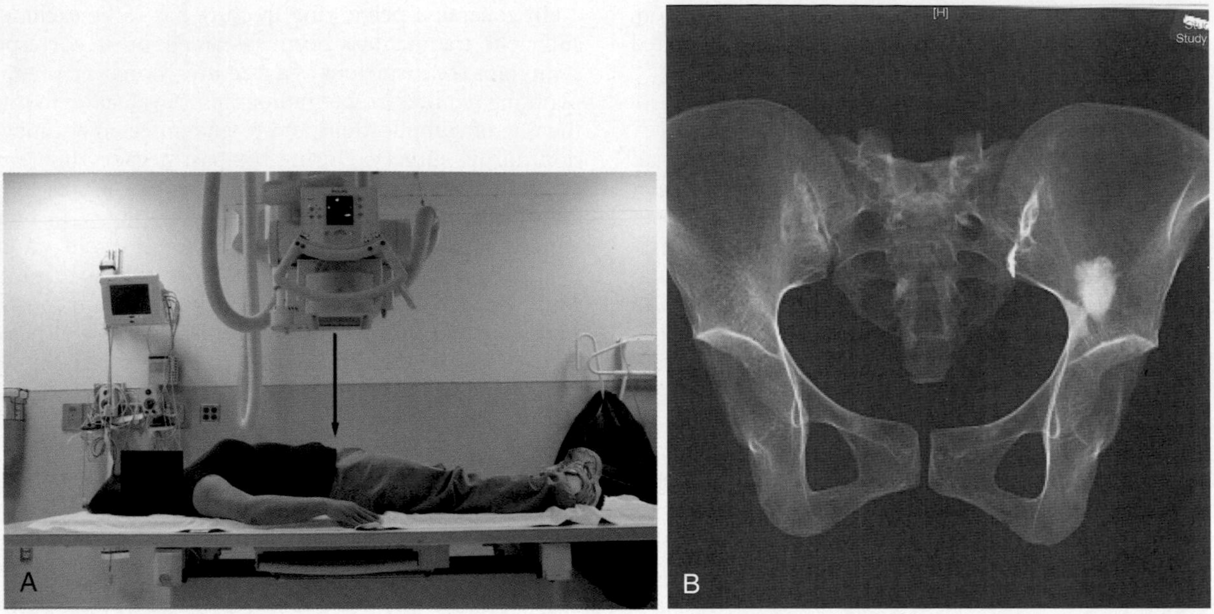

Figure 40-6. Anterior-posterior radiograph of the pelvis: direction of x-ray beam angulation (**A,** *arrow*) and resulting radiographic view (**B**).

directed perpendicular to the midpelvis, about 2 fingerbreadths above the pubic symphysis and the radiologic plate.[51]

Inlet Radiograph (Pennal I)

The inlet view (Fig. 40-7) allows for evaluation of the pelvic brim, the pubic rami, the SI joints, the sacral ala, and the body of the sacrum as well as the posterior iliac spine. Displacement of the hemipelvis in the transverse (axial) plane can be identified on this view. Fractures of the iliac wings and of the ala can be identified. The patient is positioned as described for the AP radiograph. The craniocaudal beam is directed at the level of the ASIS and the middle of the radiographic plate at an angle of approximately 40 degrees relative to the horizontal plane.[51,52]

Outlet Radiograph (Pennal II)

The outlet view (Fig. 40-8) is essentially the true “anterior” view of the pelvis and is orthogonal to the inlet view. The vertebral bodies of S1 and S2 can usually be clearly visualized. This view allows for evaluation of the symmetry of the SI joints

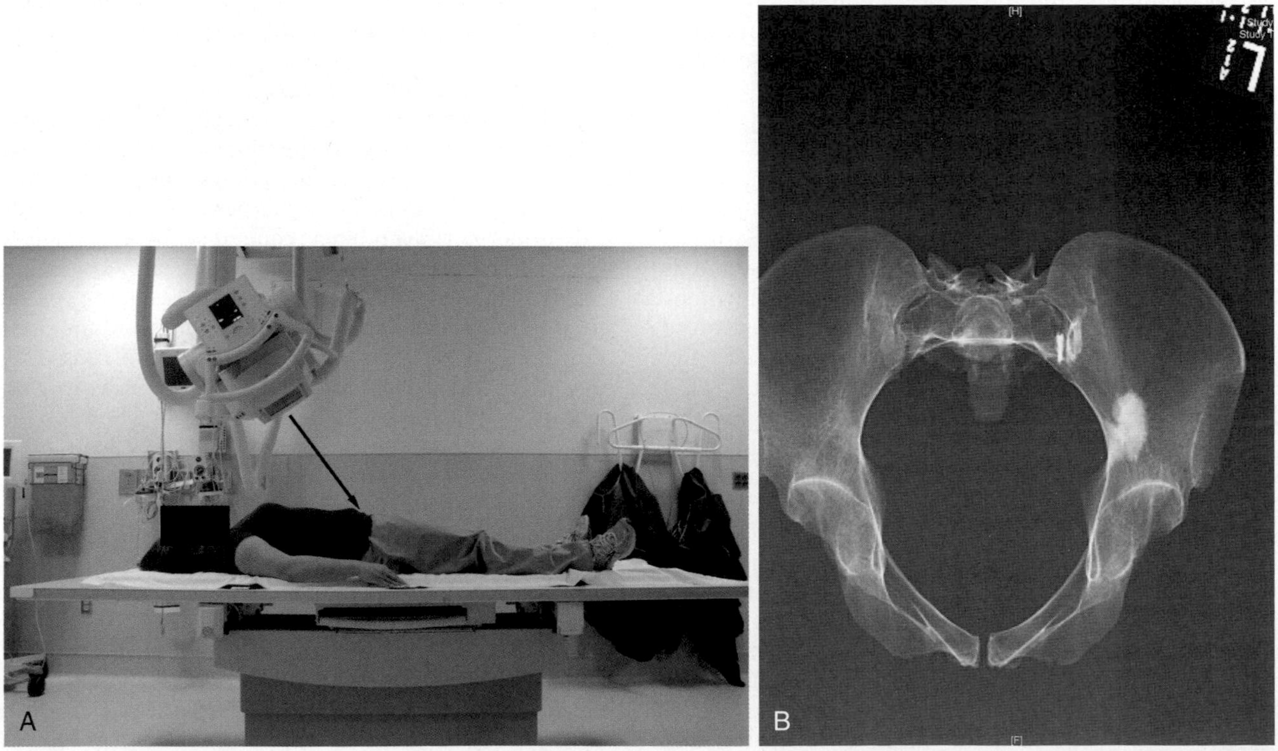

Figure 40-7. Inlet radiograph of the pelvis: direction of x-ray beam angulation (**A,** *arrow*) and resulting radiographic view (**B**).

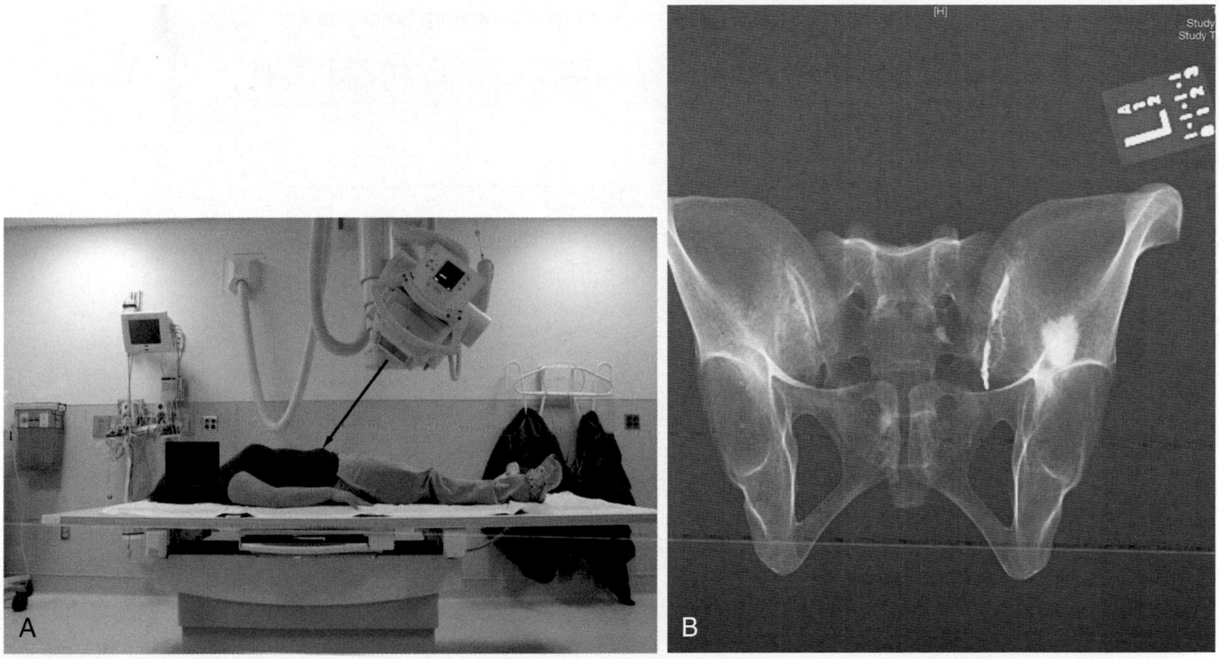

Figure 40-8. Outlet radiograph of the pelvis: direction of x-ray beam angulation (**A,** *arrow*) and resulting radiographic view (**B**).

and the pubic symphysis. Vertical displacement of the hemipelvis can be identified. Because the obturator foramen is brought into profile, fractures extending into the obturator foramen can be detected more easily than on the AP view. However, the inferior aspect of the SI joint may not be visualized clearly because it is superimposed on the superior pubic rami. The acquisition technique involves positioning as described for the AP and inlet radiographs. The caudocranial beam is focused 2 to 3 fingerbreadths below the pubic symphysis.[51,52]

Computed Tomography

Computed tomography is currently the accepted gold standard for the evaluation of pelvic fractures and is considered to be mandatory for the evaluation of patients who have sustained high-energy injuries or in whom a posterior pelvic injury is suspected for any reason.[43,53,54] The use of CT has especially revolutionized the assessment of posterior osseoligamentous pelvic structures and may detect up to 50% of occult fractures.[53,54] In fact, in a study that predates the routine use of abdominopelvic CT for the evaluation of trauma patients, Denis and colleagues found that in neurologically intact patients, the diagnosis of sacral fracture was made during the initial hospitalization only 51% of the time when using plain radiography. The presence of a neurologic deficit increased the diagnostic accuracy to only 70%.[11] The etiology of missed sacral fractures is multifactorial and includes difficulty identifying these fractures on screening AP pelvis radiographs because of the complex anatomy of the sacrum and pelvis; the presence of distracting injuries in the trauma patient; and low clinical suspicion in general, particularly in patients with insufficiency fractures. CT is mandatory for determining the exact nature of a posterior injury and can help determine whether an injury through the sacrum is a potentially stable impaction injury or a more unstable shear fracture with displacement. Establishing the extent of SI joint displacement is valuable in determining the stability of this posterior injury. Many pubic rami fractures that occur near the base of the anterior column involve the acetabulum, and CT imaging allows for appropriate assessment of these injuries.

It is currently recommended that polytraumatized patients should receive a CT scan of the pelvis.[43] Moreover, implementation of a similar diagnostic process after low-energy trauma has become increasingly common because osteoporotic fractures are happening with increasing frequency.[55] These insufficiency or pathologic fractures are often difficult to diagnose without CT (see Fig. 40-4).[56,57] CT imaging of the pelvis is therefore recommended if a patient presents with symptoms in the posterior pelvic region and a history that suggests a potential pelvic insufficiency fracture. If any fracture is identified on plain radiographs, the threshold to perform a pelvic CT should be low to properly delineate the fracture pattern for therapeutic purposes. High-energy pelvic ring fractures are often associated with life threatening hemorrhage, which can be evaluated with contrast CT scan and computed tomography angiography (CTA). Contrast extravasations establish the presence of vessel injury and allow for subsequent therapeutic steps such as embolization or surgical intervention.[58] However, potential sources of bleeding can be identified even without the use of contrast.[59-61] CT evaluation can also be used to predict the risk of death after pelvic fracture.[62] Two- and three-dimensional CT reconstructions may provide a more useful evaluation of fracture morphology and of the overall extent of pelvic fracture displacement than plain radiography. An important indicator of severe pelvic instability is a pelvic ring fracture associated with a fracture of the transverse process of L5, the attachment site of the iliolumbar ligament. Because this robust ligament serves as an important stabilizer of the spinopelvic junction, loss of its integrity caused by a transverse process fracture of L5 in the presence of a pelvic ring injury suggests severe instability of the posterior pelvic ring. Our algorithm for radiologic assessment of the acute trauma patient is shown in Figure 40-9.

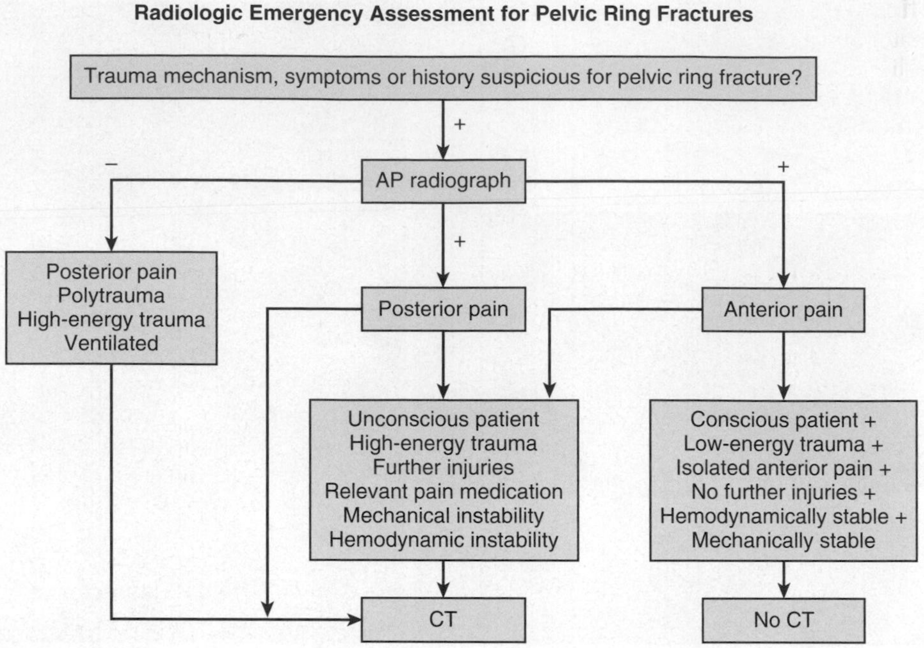

Figure 40-9. Algorithm for emergency assessment of pelvic ring fractures. *AP,* Anterior-posterior; *CT,* computed tomography.

Magnetic Resonance Imaging

Despite the high sensitivity of CT scans for diagnosing pelvic ring fractures, delayed diagnosis may occur, particularly in minimally or nondisplaced insufficiency fractures. Potential reasons include the presence of overlying intact cortical bone or microfractures that involve minimal compromise of trabecular bone only. In these cases, MRI may successfully diagnose occult fractures. Cabarrus and colleagues were able to detect 100% of sacral fractures using MRI versus 74.6% with CT.[63] Sensitivity has been shown to be much higher with MRI compared with CT.[64] In another recent study, MRI detected 96.3% of all pelvic ring fractures compared with 77% with CT. Sacral fractures in particular were more consistently detected using MRI (98.6%) compared with CT (66.1%).[65] However, MRI is not the imaging modality of choice in the acute trauma setting. Instead, it should be used primarily in cases with persistent posterior pelvic pain after trauma despite the absence of obvious fracture on CT scan.[66] MRI also has the advantage of allowing for evaluation of ligamentous integrity, which can be helpful in cases of persistent joint instability.[8]

Scintigraphy

Scintigraphy also offers a means for identifying occult pelvic ring fractures that cannot be seen on CT, with a sensitivity that approaches 100 percent (see Fig. 40-4) and a positive predictive value of approximately 92%. However, most reports deal with isolated sacral fractures only.[33,67,68] If CT findings are negative after trauma but pain persists, scintigraphy may be an alternative to MRI, especially if MRI is contraindicated or unavailable.

Special Imaging of the Symphysis

Bauman and colleagues published a study as to the ultrasonographic determination of pubic symphyseal disruption during focused assessment with sonography for trauma (FAST). All four of their patients who were diagnosed with pelvic fractures with widening of the symphysis pubis on subsequent AP radiographs had been previously identified using ultrasound during the FAST. All were detected by the ultrasound examination.[69] However, because a standard AP radiograph is routinely obtained per standard ATLS recommendations anyway, ultrasound diagnosis of symphysis pubis disruption saves little in the way of time and provides no additional information. This technique may, however, be of potential benefit in specific circumstances, such as during pregnancy.

CLASSIFICATION AND ITS IMPACT ON TREATMENT

Several different classification systems have been proposed for pelvic ring fractures. They can be divided into subgroups according to the mechanism of injury or based on an anatomic classification system that focuses primarily on the location and orientation of the fracture. Moreover, the AO published a classification that combined elements of both mechanism of injury and pelvic stability, the latter being specifically dependent on the anatomic location of the fracture. Because pelvic ring fractures are associated with a high risk of death, some authors have also tried to incorporate the presence of associated injuries or hemorrhage into their classification schemes.[70] In daily practice, surgeons should strive to describe the fracture according to both mechanism of injury as well as anatomic location to facilitate communication and rapid decision making in the acute "damage control" environment. Definitive surgical treatment requires a thorough comprehension of the injury and intensive preoperative planning. A potential limitation of the classification systems described below is that they were devised based on plain radiographic evaluation rather than the CT imaging with reformatting that is now more commonplace as a preliminary imaging study.

Anatomic Classifications

Several different anatomic classifications have been proposed.[71] Bucholz published a pathologic classification based on 47 autopsy studies. Five sites of injury were characterized: (1) anterior vertical fractures dividing the obturator ring or adjacent bodies of the pubis, (2) transiliac fractures extending from the crest of the greater sciatic notch, (3) transsacral fractures either outside or inside the foramina, (4) pure separation of the symphysis, and (5) pure disruption of the SI joint.[71]

Judet and Letournel suggested a more comprehensive classification system based on the site of injury. These included injuries to the posterior ring (i.e., sacral fractures, SI joint fracture-dislocations, SI joint dislocations, and iliac wing fractures), acetabulum, and anterior ring (rami fractures, pubic body fractures, and symphyseal disruptions) (Fig. 40-10).[72] Regardless of which classification scheme a surgeon subsequently uses, identifying the fracture site and pattern is an integral but not necessarily independently sufficient component of the evaluation. Although the classification by Judet and Letournel still serves as the most descriptive system, it is best used in conjunction with current mechanism-based classification schemes to define a specific patient's injury in a more sophisticated manner.

Mechanism of Injury Classification

The classification by Young and Burgess is based on mechanism of injury, which also suggests the most likely potential associated injuries and resuscitation requirements. It is among the most favored classifications of pelvic ring fractures.[47] It should be noted that Pennal and colleagues had previously published a classification of pelvic ring disruptions that was primarily contingent on the force applied at the time of injury.[73] The Burgess and Young classification has three major components (A–C) (Fig. 40-11). The mechanism of injury is divided into lateral compression (LC) (type A), AP compression (APC) (type B), and vertical shear stress and combined force injuries (type C). The first component of the Young and Burgess classification is the lateral compression injury. A lateral compression type I injury results from a posteriorly applied force that causes a stable sacral impaction fracture. However, the possibility of mechanical instability has recently been reported by Tosounidis and colleagues, who have therefore recommend surgical stabilization of these fractures.[74] Patients with these injuries usually have minimal problems with resuscitation. A lateral compression type II injury is caused by a more anteriorly directed force, with resultant injury to the posterior osseous–ligamentous structures, typically in the form of juxtaarticular fracture of the posterior ilium. Because of preservation of pelvic floor integrity, these injuries are generally rotationally unstable only. LCII injuries may be associated with an anterior sacral impaction injury and are often associated with head injuries and intraabdominal trauma. A lateral compression type III injury results from a laterally directed force that has continued to cross the pelvis to produce an external rotation injury to the contralateral hemipelvis. This is usually the result of an isolated direct impact (crush) to the pelvis. A common example is being run over by a car. The injury is usually isolated to the pelvis and has few significant associated injuries.

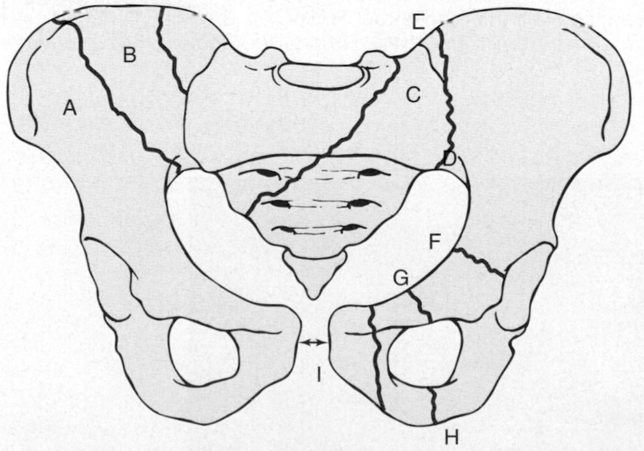

Figure 40-10. The Letournel and Judet classification of pelvic fractures is anatomic. **A,** Iliac wing fractures. **B,** Ilium fractures with extension to the sacroiliac (SI) joint. **C,** Transsacral fractures. **D,** Unilateral sacral fractures. **E,** SI joint fracture-dislocation. **F,** Acetabular fractures. **G,** Pubic ramus fractures. **H,** Ischial fractures. **I,** Pubic symphysis separation. Combinations of all of these injuries can occur.

The second component is the AP compression injury, which is also divided into three types. Type I is characterized by less than 2.5 cm of anterior ring diastasis and consists of vertical fractures of the pubic rami or disruption of the symphysis. Because there is no significant associated posterior injury, relatively few patients tend to require resuscitation. An AP compression type II injury has greater than 2.5 cm of anterior ring diastasis with widening of the anterior SI joints, resulting in rotational instability. An AP compression type III injury is a complete fracture of the anterior and posterior pelvic ring. APC type II and type III injuries have significant potential need for resuscitation because severe hemorrhage can occur from the presacral venous plexus. The type III fracture is globally unstable and should be interpreted as a vertically unstable or shear injury. A combined mechanism of injury is likely required to achieve this injury pattern, and the potential for retroperitoneal hemorrhage and major associated injuries is high.[47,75]

Similar to the classification by Young and Burgess, the classification by Müller as modified by Tile and published by the AO is widely used to classify pelvic ring fractures.[45,46] It combines the mechanism of injury and the degree of pelvic stability as well as the site of injury. It can also help to assess the prognosis as well as treatment options.[37,76] Determination of pelvic stability is based on the degree of rotational or global displacement and the mechanism of injury. The classification is completed with an assessment of associated injuries, especially soft tissue injuries such as the Morel-Lavallee lesion, and designation of the fracture as either open or closed.

The AO classification is partitioned into three groups (A–C), similar to the Young and Burgess classification, with greater attention given to the anatomic site of the fracture. Type A injuries are stable because the bony and ligamentous integrity of the posterior pelvic ring as well as the pelvic floor remains intact. Subtype A1 injuries (Fig. 40-12, *A*) consist of avulsions of the pelvic apophyses by a sudden muscular pull; these injuries usually require only symptomatic care. However, muscular dysfunction can be an indication for surgery, especially in young people. Subtype A2 injuries (Fig. 40-12, *B*) represent isolated iliac wing fractures without violation of the posterior osseous ligamentous hinge. This group includes a spectrum of injuries resulting from direct blows.

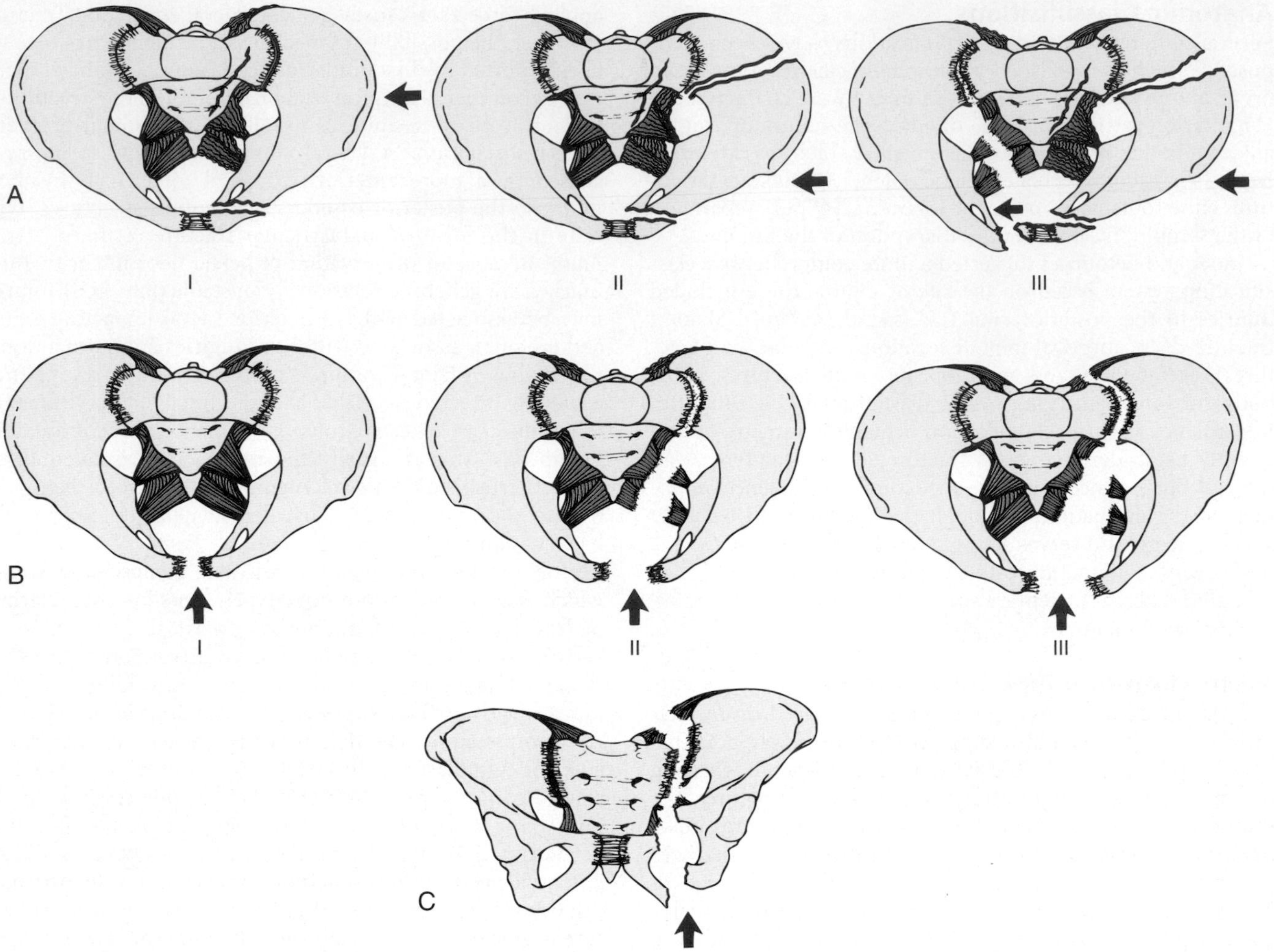

Figure 40-11. Young and Burgess classification. **A,** Lateral compression force. Type I, a posteriorly directed force causing a sacral crushing injury and horizontal pubic ramus fractures ipsilaterally. This injury is stable. Type II, a more anteriorly directed force causing horizontal pubic ramus fractures with an anterior sacral crushing injury and either disruption of the posterior sacroiliac (SI) joints or fractures through the iliac wing. This injury is ipsilateral. Type III, an anteriorly directed force that is continued and leads to a type I or type II ipsilateral fracture with an external rotation component to the contralateral side; the SI joint is opened posteriorly, and the sacrotuberous and spinous ligaments are disrupted. **B,** Anterior-posterior (AP) compression fractures. Type I, an AP-directed force opening the pelvis but with the posterior ligamentous structures intact. This injury is stable. Type II, continuation of a type I fracture with disruption of the sacrospinous and potentially the sacrotuberous ligaments and an anterior SI joint opening. This fracture is rotationally unstable. Type III, a completely unstable or a vertical instability pattern with complete disruption of all ligamentous supporting structures. **C,** A vertically directed force or forces at right angles to the supporting structures of the pelvis, leading to vertical fractures in the rami and disruption of all the ligamentous structures. This injury is equivalent to an AP type III or a completely unstable and rotationally unstable fracture. *(Redrawn from Young JWR, Burgess AR: Radiologic management of pelvic ring fractures, Baltimore, 1987, Urban & Schwarzenberg.)*

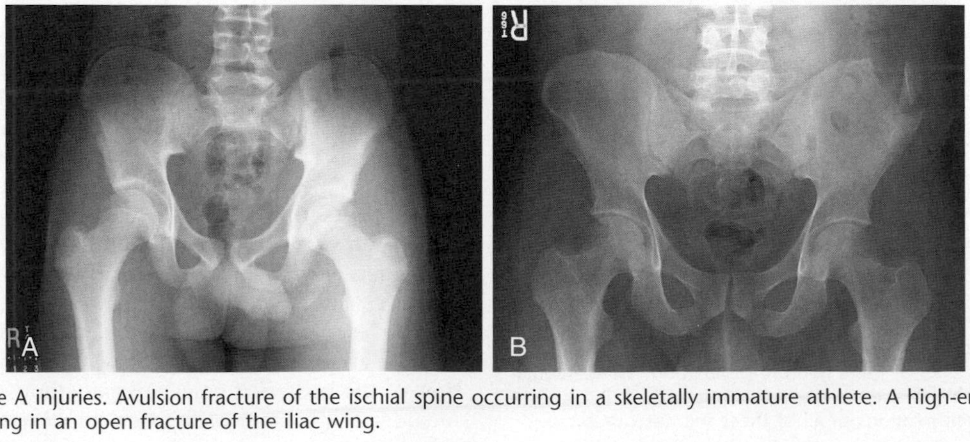

Figure 40-12. Type A injuries. Avulsion fracture of the ischial spine occurring in a skeletally immature athlete. A high-energy direct blow to the iliac wing resulting in an open fracture of the iliac wing.

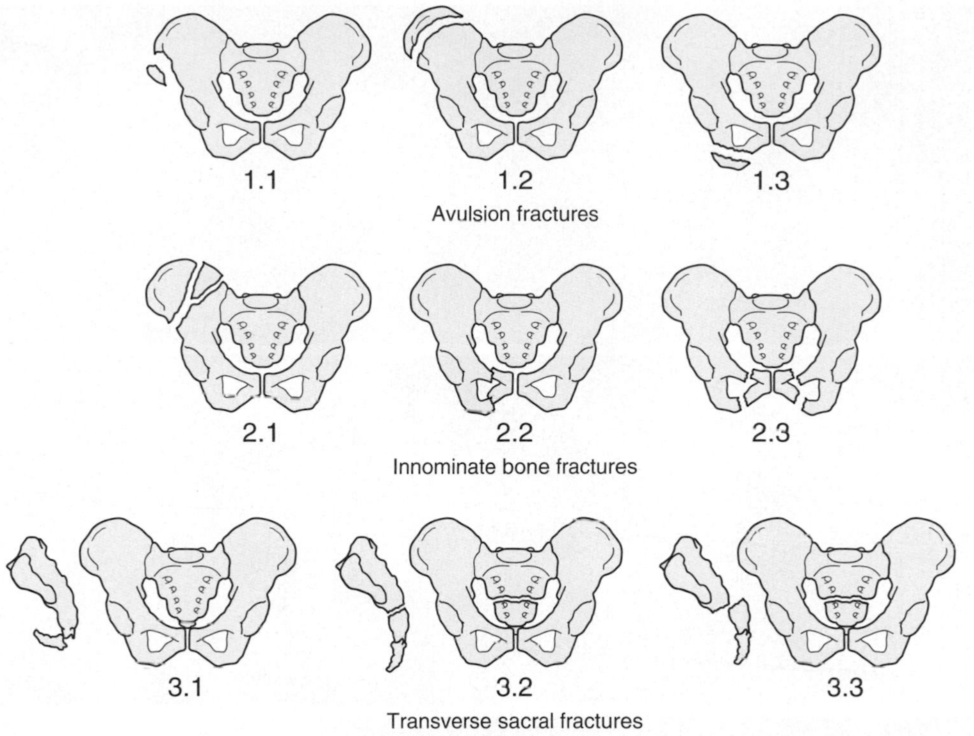

Figure 40-13. Modified Tile AO Müller classification. Type A, stable posterior arch with intact pelvic ring injuries. Group 1 represents avulsion fractures of the iliac spine (A1.1), iliac crest (A1.2), and ischial tuberosity (A1.3). Group 2 represents fractures of the innominate bone or injuries from direct blows: iliac wing (A2.1), unilateral anterior arch (A2.2), and bifocal anterior arch (A2.3). Group 3 represents transverse fractures of the sacrum caudal to S2: sacrococcygeal dislocation (A3.1), sacrum undisplaced (A3.2), and sacrum displaced (A3.3). *(Redrawn from Müller E, editor: Comprehensive classification of pelvis and acetabulum fractures, Bern, Switzerland, 1995, Maurice E. Müller Foundation.)*

They constitute isolated fractures of the anterior pelvic ring. Whereas nondisplaced low-energy injuries are usually seen in osteoporotic bone, high-energy direct blows are usually responsible in younger individuals. Isolated wing fractures do not require surgery unless they are open. Type A3 fractures involve the sacrum or coccyx below the SI joints (below S2), meaning that the integrity of the posterior pelvic ring and the spinopelvic junction are both preserved. Chronic pain is the main indication for surgery. In rare cases of sacral root symptoms, decompression of the sacral spinal canal is indicated, possibly with fracture stabilization. Assessment of neurologic deficits therefore is of great importance in the evaluation of type A3 pelvic ring fractures.[11] Type A pelvic ring fractures are illustrated in Figure 40-13. Type A fractures are generally treated surgically except type A2.2 and often the transverse sacral fractures.

Type B fractures are complete disruptions of the anterior pelvic ring combined with incomplete disruptions of the posterior arch that allow rotation of the hemipelvis. This fracture pattern therefore presents with rotational instability in the absence of vertical instability. Type B fractures, especially type B1, are at high risk for severe hemorrhage.[77] Surgery is usually required to prevent exsanguination and to reestablish pelvic ring stability. A B1 injury is a unilateral external rotation or tension failure fracture through the sacrum (B1.2). A variable degree of rotational instability may be present with these injuries (Fig. 40-14). Type B2 injuries are produced by lateral compression or internal rotation. A type B2.1 injury is caused by a force directed over the posterior iliac wing. This results in a sacral impaction injury and most commonly with horizontally oriented rami fractures (Fig. 40-15, *A*). As noted earlier, this does not result in injury to the posterior pelvic or pelvic floor ligaments. A B2.2 injury is produced by a lateral compression force and involves a partial fracture-subluxation of the SI joint, associated with anterior ring fractures or fracture-dislocations of the pubic symphysis. The typical posterior fracture pattern extends from the iliac wing into the SI joint, with ligamentous disruption of the caudal SI joint. A portion of the cranial iliac wing and SI joint remains attached to the sacrum (Fig. 40-15, *B*). These rotationally unstable injuries are the equivalent of the Young and Burgess lateral compression type II injuries. Because the force of injury is applied in an oblique fashion across the pelvis, the involved portion of the pelvis is flexed, adducted, and internally rotated, positioning the femoral head cranially; these can be associated with a leg length discrepancy. This clinical finding, however, is usually sufficiently subtle as to not be easily identifiable in the emergency setting unlike in the case of femoral neck fractures or inner hemipelvectomies (type C pelvic ring fracture). Less common anterior arch injuries associated with B2 injuries can be a locked symphysis or a tilt fracture (Fig. 40-16). A locked symphysis injury disrupts the symphysis rather than fracturing the rami as it drives one side of the symphysis behind the other. A tilt fracture is an unusual anterior variant associated with a lateral compression mechanism in which the superior pubic ramus is fractured at the pubic root near the acetabulum and through the ischial ramus; continued medial displacement of the hemipelvis causes dislocation of the symphysis or fracture of the pubic body, allowing the fragment to tilt caudally and anteriorly into the perineum. Tilt fractures

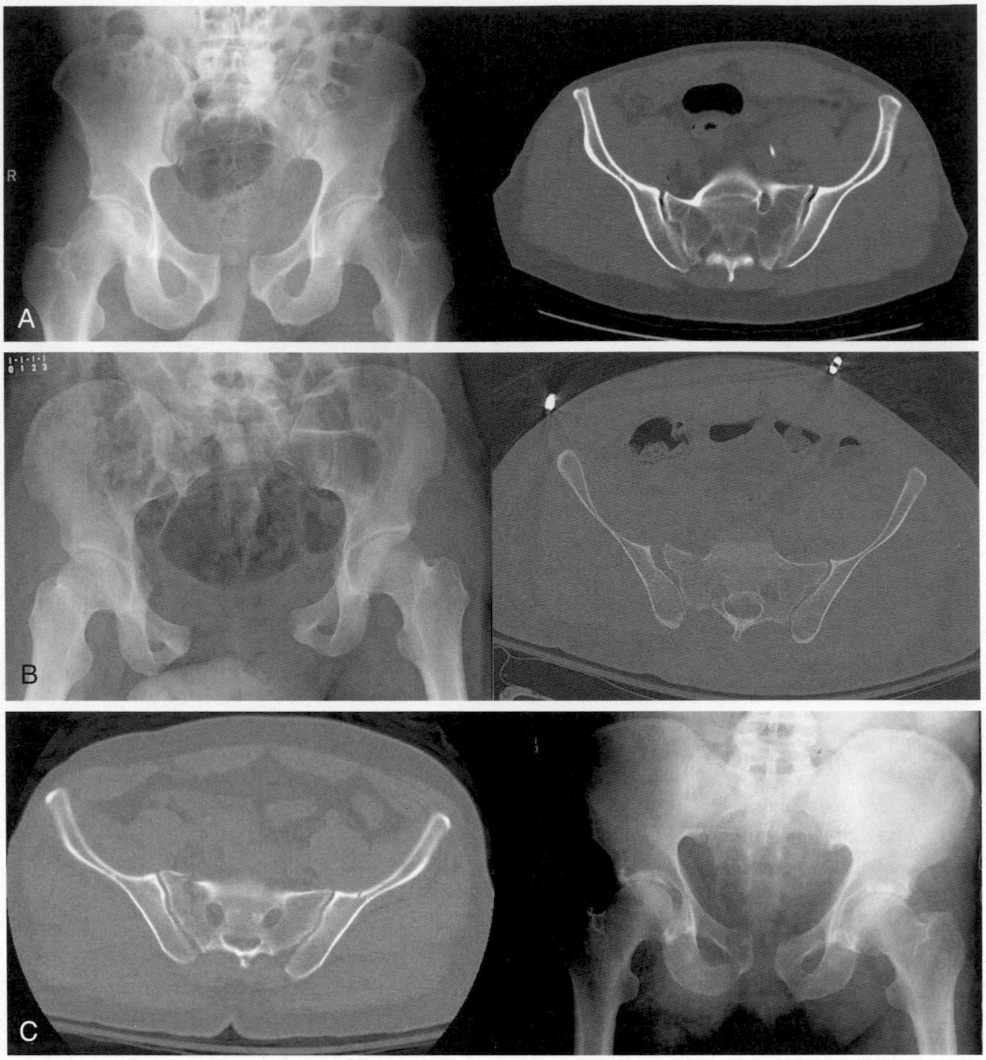

Figure 40-14. B-type injuries. **A,** Type B1.1 with injury to the anterior sacroiliac (SI) joint. Note air density within the joint, which may indicate rotational injury through the joint. Physical examination may confirm the instability. **B,** Type B1.1, injury with obvious instability. Computed tomography confirms unilateral injury through the SI joint with concomitant tensile sacral fracture. **C,** Type B1.2, posterior injury noted through the sacrum. The anterior border of the sacrum is typically a location for simple fracture caused by the tensile force creating the posterior injury.

are at high risk of harming the perineum. Type B3 injuries are bilateral posterior ring injuries with each side possibly having a different mechanism of injury, but in which neither side is vertically unstable. A type B3.1 injury is a bilateral external rotation injury with greater than 2.5 cm of symphyseal displacement (Fig. 40-17, *A*). Type B3.2 (Fig. 40-17, *B*) and 3.3 injuries are secondary to a lateral compression mechanism, respectively, causing either external rotation of the contralateral hemipelvis or a lateral compression mechanism bilaterally. Type B fractures are summarized in Figures 40-18 and 40-19. Rotational instability generally requires either external or internal fixation.

Type A fractures are considered stable, and type B fracture are partially stable with only rotatory instability. Fractures that present with rotatory as well as vertical instability are classified as type C injuries. These injuries are generally caused by high-energy trauma. Subdivision of type C fractures depends on the characteristics of the posterior fracture (Fig. 40-20). C1.1 is an iliac fracture, C1.2 is an SI joint dislocation or fracture-dislocation, and C1.3 is a fracture through the sacrum. C2 injuries are bilateral disruptions in which one hemipelvis is rotationally unstable (B types) and the other side is globally unstable (C types) (Fig. 40-21). C3 injuries represent bilateral, globally unstable hemipelves. Type C fractures are summarized in Figure 40-22.

Key characteristics of the AO classification fracture types are summarized in Table 40-1. A good review of indications for surgery and the impact of classification were given by Tscherne and colleagues.[78] This classification has been reported to have a high interobserver reliability and is predictive of injury severity and prognosis.[79-81] However, some authors have also stated that even though both the Young and Burgess as well as the Tile classifications are widely used, interobserver and intraobserver variability are low and might limit their validity.[82,83]

Fractures with Proper Names

A handful of fractures are often designated by proper names.

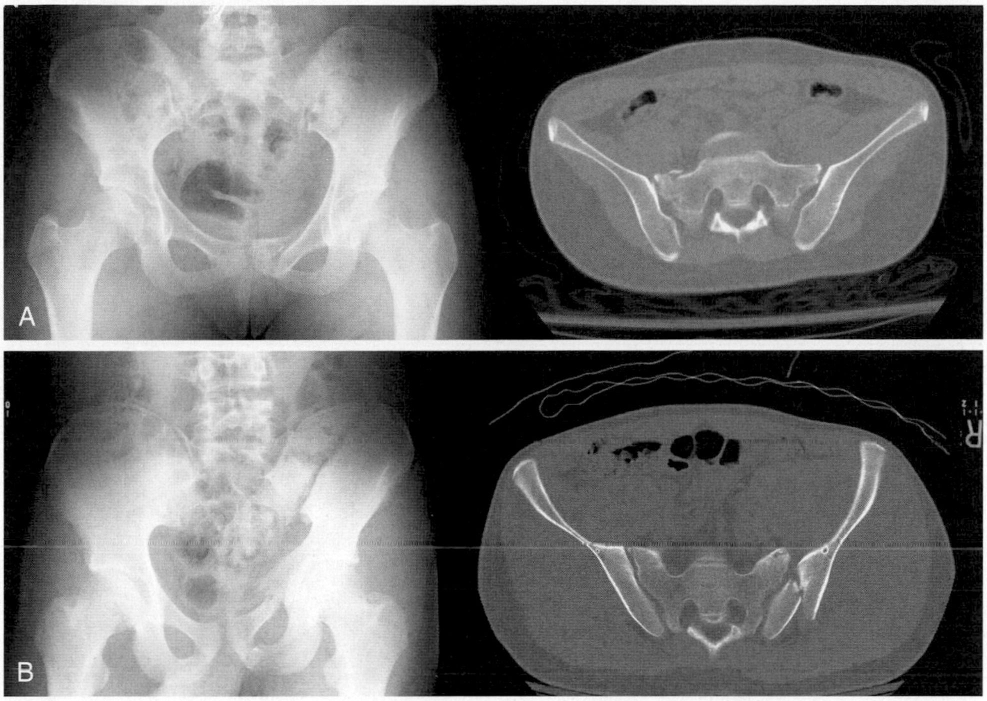

Figure 40-15. Clinical example of lateral compression-type injuries. **A,** Type B2.1, anterior sacral compression fracture associated with contralateral segmental parasymphyseal fracture. **B,** Crescent fracture. Note the fracture entering the caudal portion of the sacroiliac joint with dislocation.

Open Book Fracture

The open book fracture can be classified as type B1.1 and B1.2 according to the AO classification modified by Tile and AP compression type II in the Young and Burgess classification. The unilateral external rotation increases the volume of the true pelvis and often leads to severe hemorrhage.[77]

Malgaigne Fracture

The Malgaigne fracture was first characterized in 1847 and describes an injury with multiple ipsilateral vertically oriented anterior and posterior pelvic ring fractures, resulting in a type C pattern of rotatory and vertical instability. The original fracture description, however, specifically included a vertical fracture of the sacrum as well as a unilateral fracture of the superior and inferior pubic ramus.[84]

Hemipelvectomy

This is a very rare injury, which comprises fewer than 1% of all pelvic fractures. The osseous hemipelvis is completely disarticulated, with resulting disruption of nerves and vessels. The mortality rate is more than 50% in patients who reach the hospital, but most patients die at the site of injury.[85-87] This injury is classified as type C in the AO classification.

Duverney Fracture

This is a comminuted fracture of the iliac wing.[88]

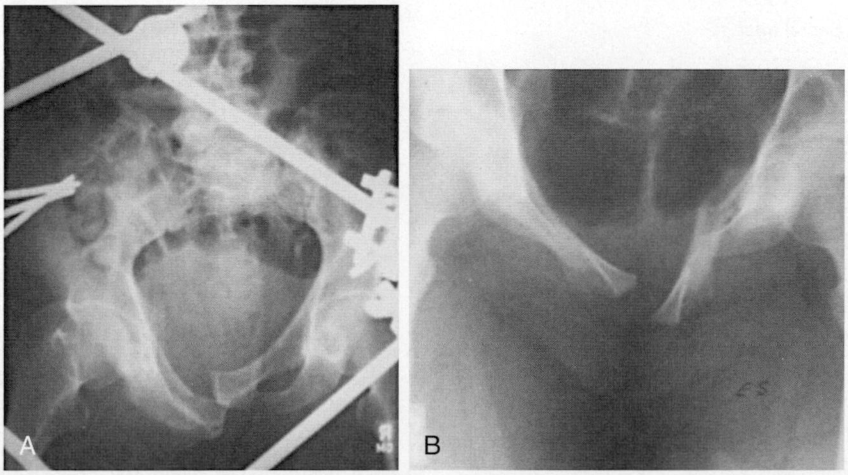

Figure 40-16. A, A locked symphysis with one pubic body displaced behind the other. **B,** A tilt fracture occurs when the superior pubic body has dislocated from the symphysis and rotates into the perineum around a fracture of the ipsilateral pubic root.

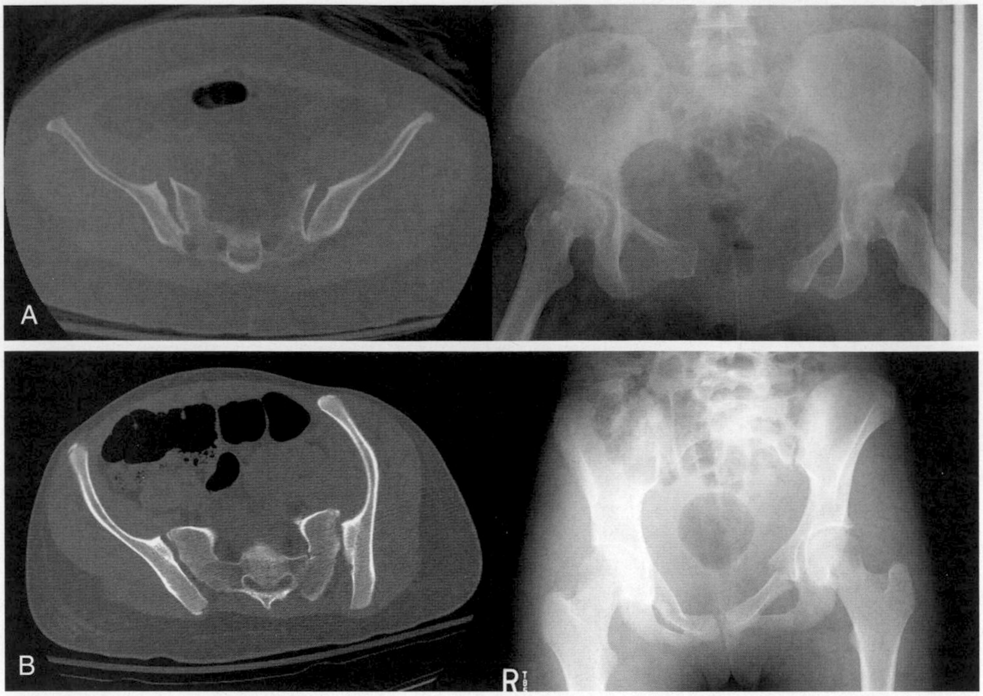

Figure 40-17. Clinical examples of B3 injuries. **A,** Type B3.1, bilateral rotational injuries occurring through both sacroiliac (SI) joints. **B,** Type B3.2, a windswept deformity with internal rotation of the left hemipelvis through the SI joint and partial disruption of the anterior right SI joint and external rotation of the hemipelvis.

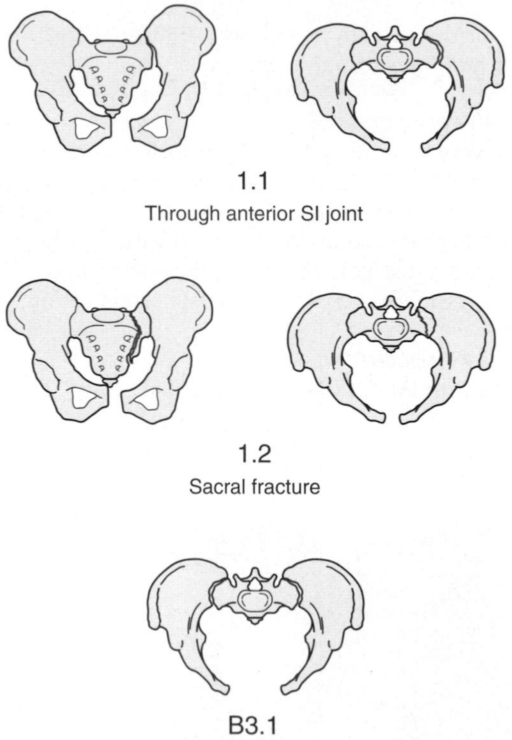

Figure 40-18. Examples of B-type injuries, all with anterior symphyseal disruptions. Anterior injuries can also include unilateral or bilateral rami fractures. *(Redrawn from Müller E, editor: Comprehensive classification of pelvis and acetabulum fractures, Bern, Switzerland, 1995, Maurice E. Müller Foundation.)*

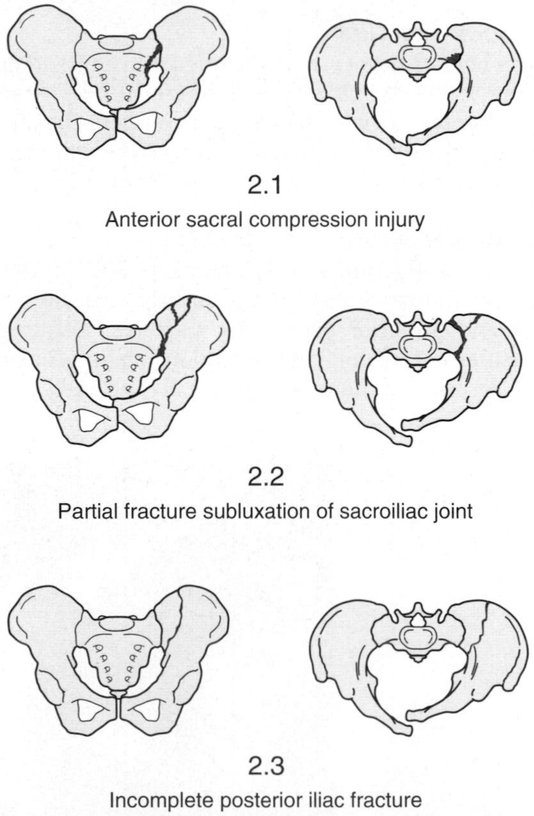

Figure 40-19. Modified Tile AO Müller classification. Type B, incomplete disruptions (internal rotation). Internally directed or lateral compression forces cause anterior sacral compression injuries (B2.1), partial fracture-subluxations of the sacroiliac joint (B2.2), and incomplete posterior iliac wing fractures (B2.3). *(Redrawn from Müller E, editor: Comprehensive classification of pelvis and acetabulum fractures, Bern, Switzerland, 1995, Maurice E. Müller Foundation.)*

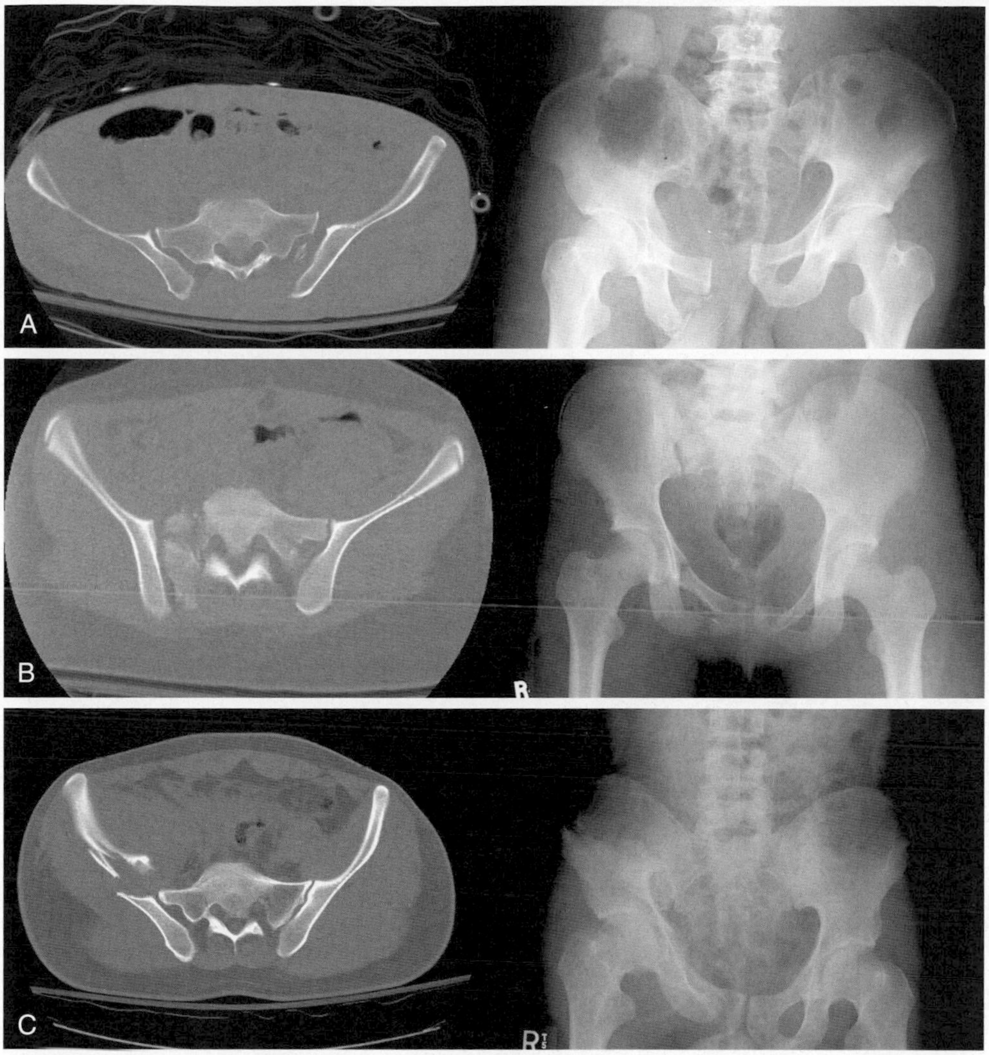

Figure 40-20. Examples of C1 injuries. **A,** Posterior injury occurring through the sacroiliac joint. **B,** Sacrum. **C,** Ilium.

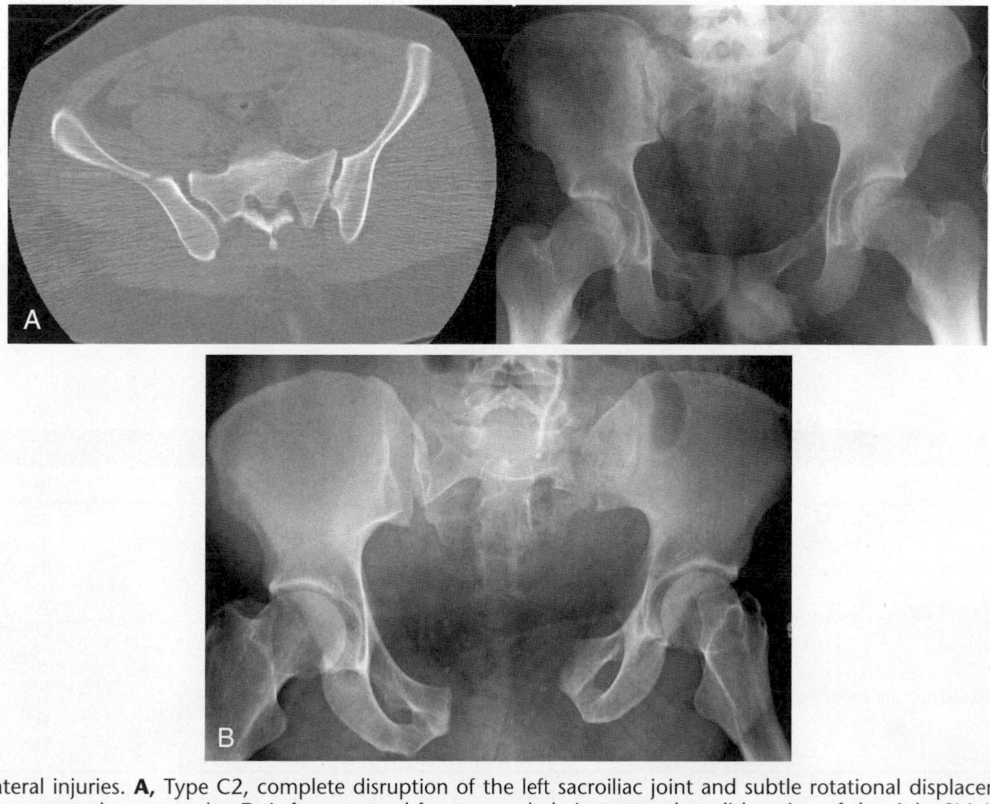

Figure 40-21. Bilateral injuries. **A,** Type C2, complete disruption of the left sacroiliac joint and subtle rotational displacement of the right SI joint, confirmed on computed tomography. **B,** Left transsacral fracture and obvious complete dislocation of the right SI joint; both injuries are globally unstable posteriorly.

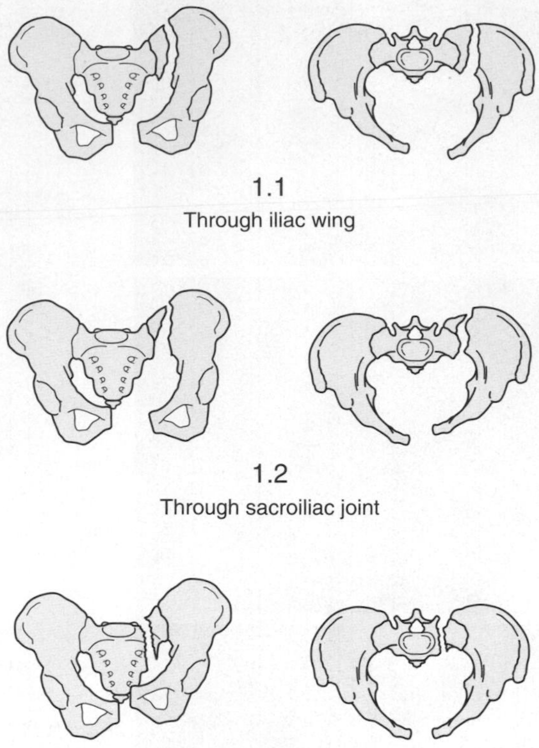

Figure 40-22. Modified Tile AO Müller classification. Type C, Complete disruptions. Complete disruptions can be unilateral or bilateral. Unilateral disruptions occur through the iliac wing (C1.1), through the sacroiliac joint (C1.2), and through the sacrum (C1.3). Bilateral injuries are combinations of incomplete, complete, and totally complete injuries and are not shown in this figure. *(Redrawn from Müller E, editor: Comprehensive classification of pelvis and acetabulum fractures, Bern, Switzerland, 1995, Maurice E. Müller Foundation.)*

Osteoporotic Pelvic Ring Fractures

Because of the relative aging of Western populations, the rate of fragility fractures appears to be progressively increasing.[55,86,89] These osteoporotic fractures generally occur secondary to low-energy mechanisms or even in the absence of any known injury. They are most often located in the pubic and ischial rami but can also occur in the sacrum.[33,90] In the posterior pelvic ring, the sacral ala are especially at risk for an osteoporotic fracture. Because fragility fractures of the pelvis are low-energy injuries that occur in the absence of ligamentous instability, fracture displacement is generally minimal compared with higher energy injuries in younger patients.[63,91] Classifying these injuries according to the AO and Young and Burgess classifications is therefore of limited value and results in misinterpretation of the biomechanical stability of these fractures. Rommens and Hofmann recently published a new classification system for fragility fractures of the pelvis, based on both plain radiographs as well as 3-D imaging using CT and MRI.[57] A total of 245 patients were included, who were only operated on after having failed nonoperative therapy. Fractures with significant displacement and complete bilateral fractures required surgical treatment. They proposed a new classification based on the degree of instability. Fracture patterns of this new classification are summarized in Table 40-2.

Sacral Fracture Classification

Sacral fractures play an integral role in pelvic ring stability, and are thus generally incorporated into the pelvic ring injury classifications described earlier. However, there is considerable value to looking at the sacral fracture location and configuration in a more isolated fashion for two reasons: (1) specific fracture patterns and location can have prognostic and treatment significance independent of the associated ring injury, and (2) some sacral fractures have little effect on overall pelvic ring stability.

Although several sacral fracture classification systems were proposed earlier, none was widely adopted until 1988 when Denis and colleagues described an anatomic classification that correlated fracture location with the presence of neurologic injury.[11] This classification divides the sacrum into three zones (Fig. 40-23). Zone I (alar zone) fractures remain lateral to the neuroforamina, zone II (foraminal zone) fractures involve one or more neuroforamina while remaining lateral to the spinal canal, and zone III (central zone) fractures involve the spinal canal. The likelihood of neurologic injury increases as fractures occur in more medial zones. In their series, zone I fractures had a 5.9% incidence of neurologic injury, primarily to the L5 nerve root as it courses over the ala. Zone II fractures had a 28.4% incidence of neurologic injury caused by either foraminal displacement with resulting impingement on the exiting nerve root or the "traumatic far-out syndrome" in which the L5 nerve root is caught between the L5 transverse process and the displaced sacral ala. Zone III fractures had a 56.7% incidence of neurologic deficits resulting from injury within the spinal canal, with 76.1% of these individuals having bowel, bladder, and sexual dysfunction.

TABLE 40-1 *AO CLASSIFICATION OF PELVIC FRACTURES*

Type	Instability	Characteristics	Indication for Surgery
A	None	A1 pelvic ring intact A2 minimally displaced anterior pelvic ring fracture A3 sacral fracture	Rarely Rarely Rarely
B	Rotatory	B1 open-book injury B2 unilateral B3 bilateral	Yes Often Often
C	Rotatory and vertical	C1 unilateral C2 bilateral: one type B and one type C C3 bilateral type C	Yes Yes Yes

TABLE 40-2 ***CLASSIFICATION OF FRAGILITY FRACTURES OF PELVIS***[57]

Type	Degree of Instability	Fracture Pattern	Posterior Displacement	Indication for Surgery
Ia	Stable	Isolated unilateral anterior fracture	None	No
Ib	Stable	Isolated bilateral anterior fracture	None	No
IIa	Moderate	Isolated sacral fracture	None	No
IIb	Moderate	Sacral crush with anterior fracture	None	Should be considered
IIc	Moderate	Sacral, iliosacral, or ilium fracture with anterior disruption	None	Should be considered
IIIa	High	Unilateral iliac fracture	Yes	Yes
IIIb	High	Unilateral iliosacral fracture	Yes	Yes
IIIc	High	Unilateral sacral fracture	Yes	Yes
IVa	Highest	Bilateral iliac or iliosacral fracture	Yes	Yes
IVb	Highest	Bilateral sacral fracture	Yes	Yes
IVc	Highest	Combination of posterior instabilities	Yes	Yes

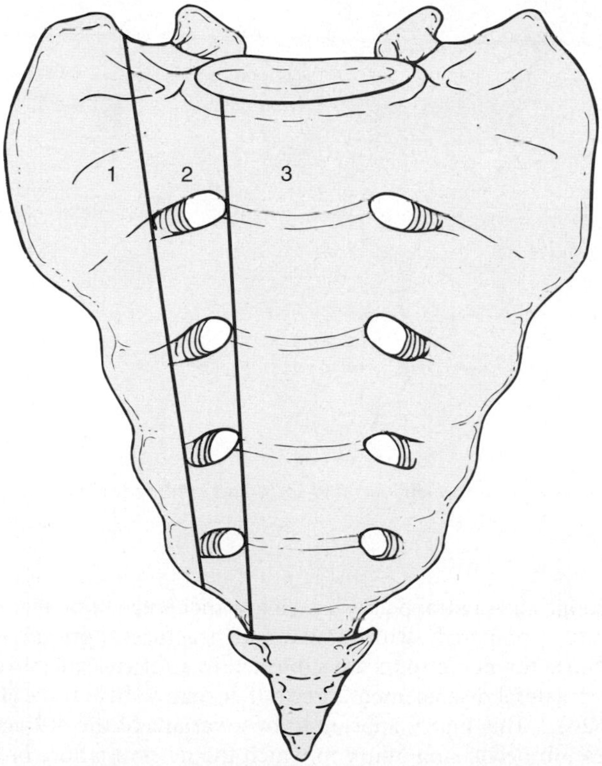

Figure 40-23. Denis and associates classified 236 fractures of the sacrum into zones. Zone 1 was the region of the ala, and fractures in this area occurred in 118 patients, 5.9% of whom had neurologic deficits. Zone 2 was the foraminal region, where the fracture line involved one or more foramina and exited without involvement of the central neural canal. This group consisted of 81 patients, 28.4% of whom had neurologic findings. The final group of patients had zone 3 injuries, or central canal involvement. This pattern was seen in only 21 patients, but they had an extremely high rate of neurologic deficit (56.7%). *(Redrawn from Denis F, Davis S: Comfort T. Sacral fractures: an important problem. Retrospective analysis of 236 cases, Clin Orthop Relat Res 227:67–81, 1988.)*

Denis and colleagues identified a broad spectrum of zone III sacral fracture-dislocations, which included the presence of both transverse and longitudinal fracture orientations. Because of their neurologic and biomechanical implications, zone III sacral fractures have been more formally characterized by several other investigators. Review of various series and case reports reveals a high likelihood of neurologic deficit characterized as cauda equina injury affecting the lower extremity as well as bowel and bladder function.[92]

Early case reports often characterized the zone III injury pattern as solely a transverse fracture, possibly because of imaging limitations. CT demonstrates that most transverse fractures of the upper sacrum have complex, 3-D fracture patterns. The majority of these injuries are now understood to consist of a transverse fracture of the sacrum with associated "longitudinal" or "vertical" transforaminal or alar fractures that extend rostrally to the lumbosacral junction to form the so-called "U" fracture and its variations (e.g., H, Y, and lambda fracture patterns) (Fig. 40-24). These fractures are also characterized by a high incidence of L5 transverse process fractures, indicating disruption of the iliolumbar ligament.[92]

Roy-Camille and coworkers reported a series of 13 patients with transverse sacral fractures, which they classified as type 1, flexion deformity of the upper sacrum (angulation alone); type 2, flexion deformity with posterior displacement of the upper sacrum (angulation and posterior translation); and type 3, anterior displacement of the upper sacrum without angulation (anterior translation alone). They hypothesized that whereas types 1 and 2 were caused by impact with the lumbar spine in flexion, type 3 fractures were caused by impact with the lumbar spine and hips in extension.[93] Strange-Vognsen and Lebech added the type 4 injury, theorizing that comminution of the upper sacrum without significant angulation or translation was caused by impact with the lumbar spine in the neutral position (Fig. 40-25).[94] A type 5 direct impalement type injury has recently been proposed by Schildhauer and coworkers.[95]

Other patterns of zone III sacral fractures have been identified as resulting from specific mechanisms or having predictable patterns of associated injuries. In contrast to transverse Denis zone III sacral fractures, midline longitudinal Denis zone III sacral fractures, in which the sacrum is disrupted

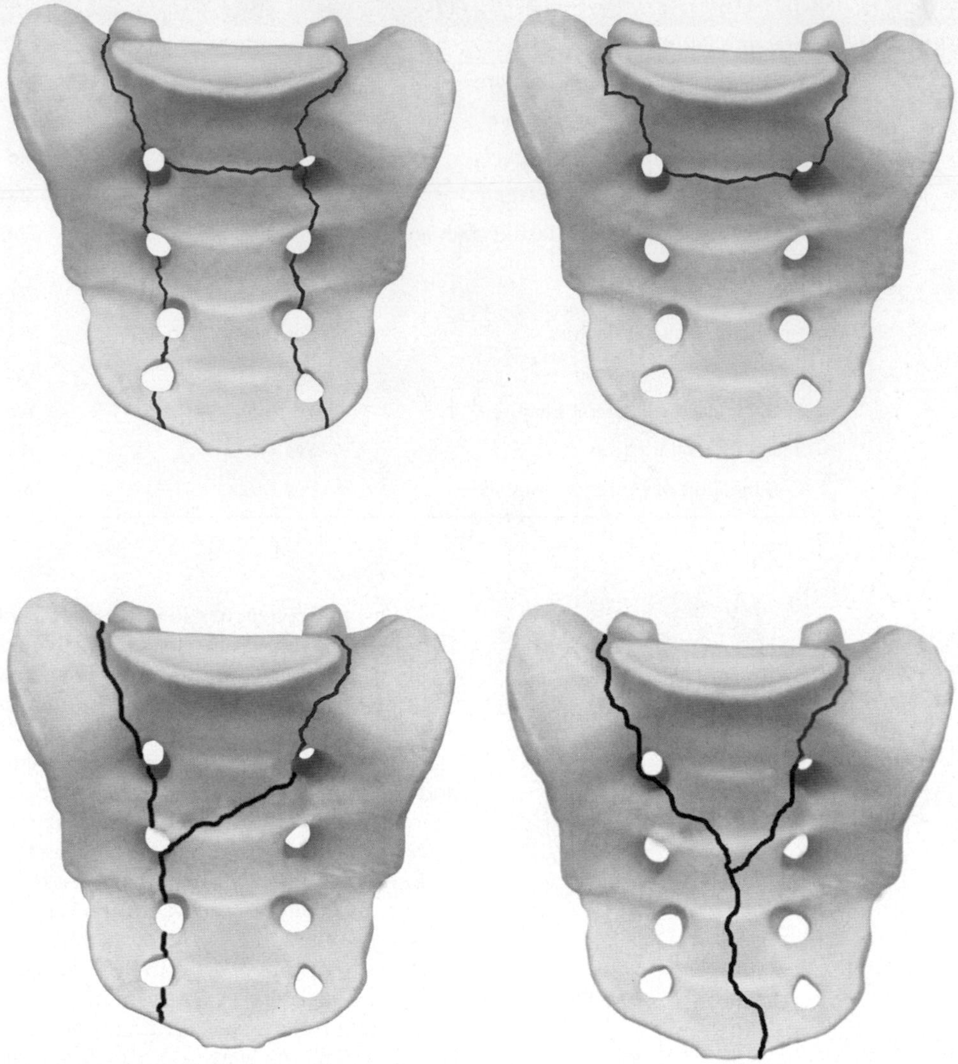

Figure 40-24. Colloquial classification of zone III sacral fractures. Clockwise from top left, sacral H, U, Y, and lambda fractures.

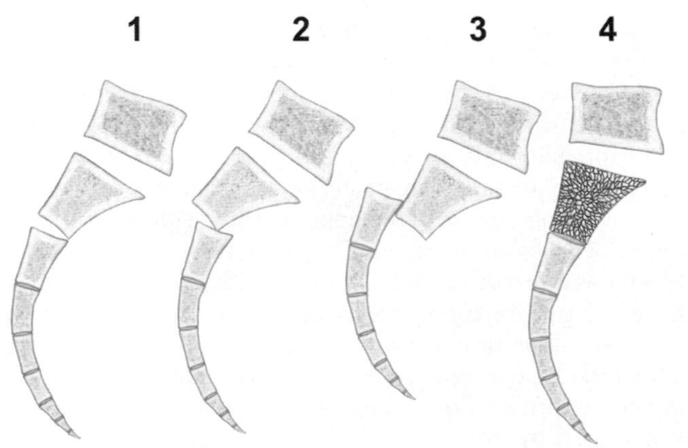

Figure 40-25. Roy-Camille[93] classification of Denis zone III injuries. Type 1, nondisplaced; type 2, flexion injury; type 3, extension injury; and type 4, comminuted upper sacral fracture *(modification by Strange-Vongsen and Lebech[94])*.

through the sagittal plane, have a low incidence of neurologic injury compared with transverse fractures, presumably because the nerve roots are subjected to a relatively less traumatic lateral displacement force rather than a shear force (Fig. 40-26).[96] This injury appears to be a variant of the AP compression pelvic ring injury in which the tension failure of the posterior ring occurs through the middle of the sacrum rather than at the SI joints or their juxtaarticular bone. Neurologic deficits are not usually seen in contrast to the high incidence of neurologic injury reported in patients with predominantly transverse sacral fractures involving the spinal canal.[96]

Isler demonstrated that even in the absence of a transverse fracture line, sacral fractures can be associated with spinal column instability. He described variations of longitudinal sacral fractures through the S1 and S2 neuroforamina that result in L5 to S1 instability because of facet joint disruption (Fig. 40-27).[97] Injuries with the fracture line lateral to the S1 articular process are not associated with instability of the lumbosacral articulation because the L5 to S1 articulation remains continuous with the stable component of the sacrum. Fractures that extend into or medial to the S1 articular process,

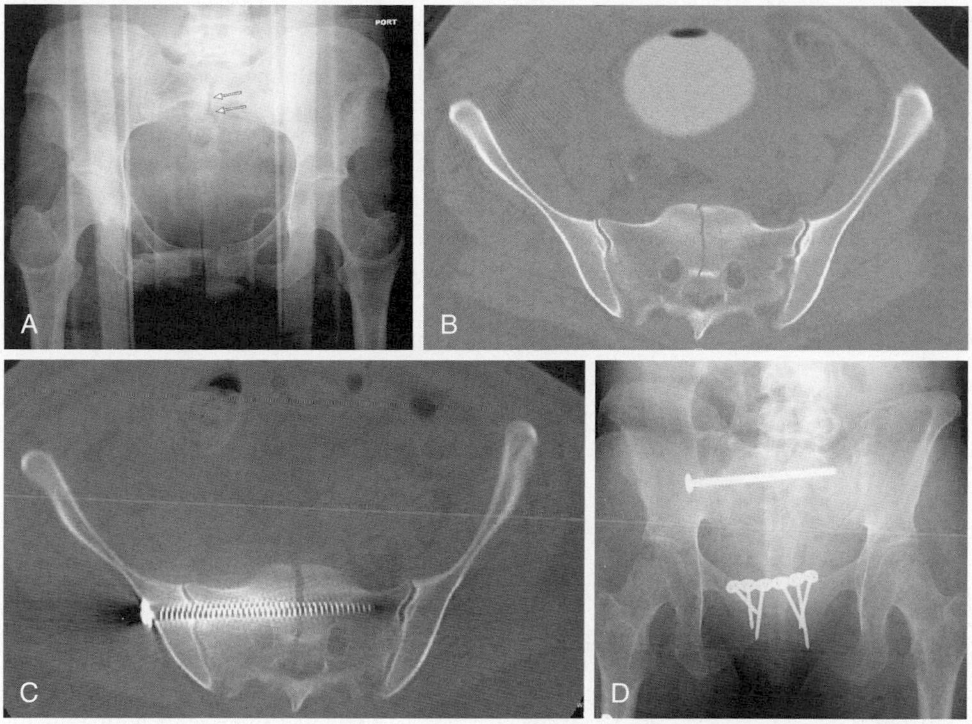

Figure 40-26. Midline longitudinal zone III sacral fracture. Unusual variant of zone III sacral fractures, which is the result of anterior-posterior (AP) compression mechanism with midline fracture of the sacrum, as seen on AP (**A**) and axial computed tomography (CT) (**B**) images of the pelvis. Postoperative axial CT (**C**) and outlet (**D**) views of the pelvis demonstrate treatment with plating of the symphysis pubis and percutaneous iliosacral screw fixation.

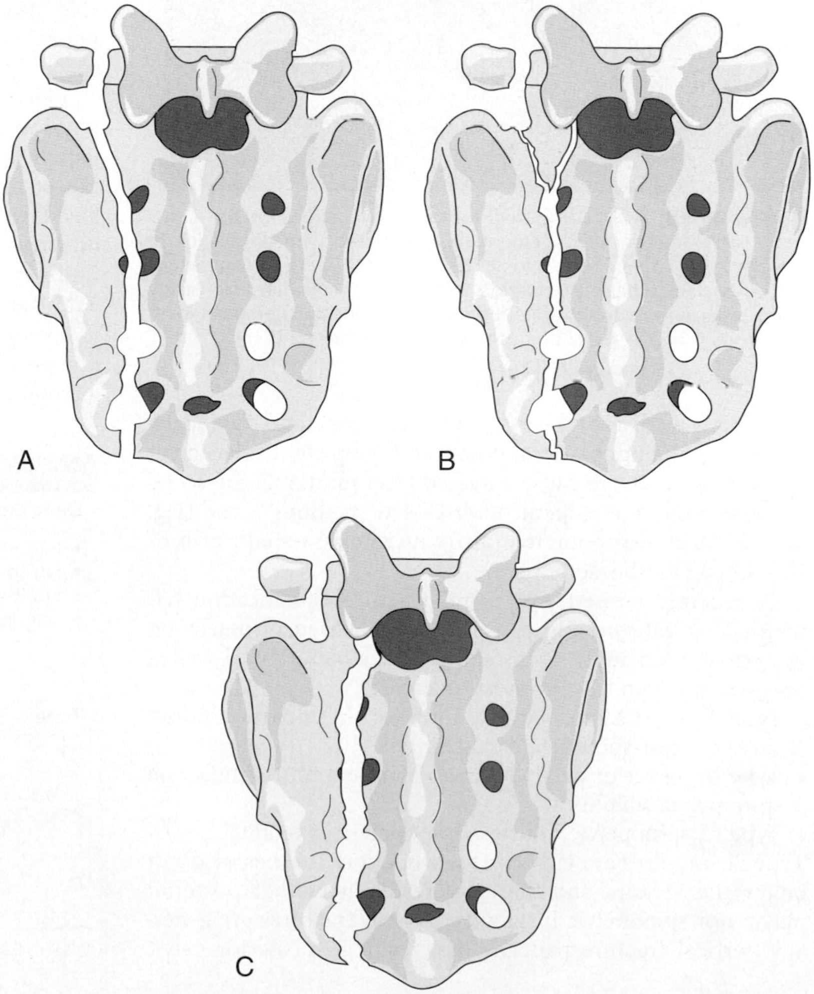

Figure 40-27. Classification of injuries involving the lumbosacral junction as proposed by Isler.[97] **A,** The fracture line goes lateral to the L5 to S1 facet and does not destabilize it. The L5 to S1 facet is destabilized when the fracture line either goes on both sides (**B**) or just medial to it (**C**).

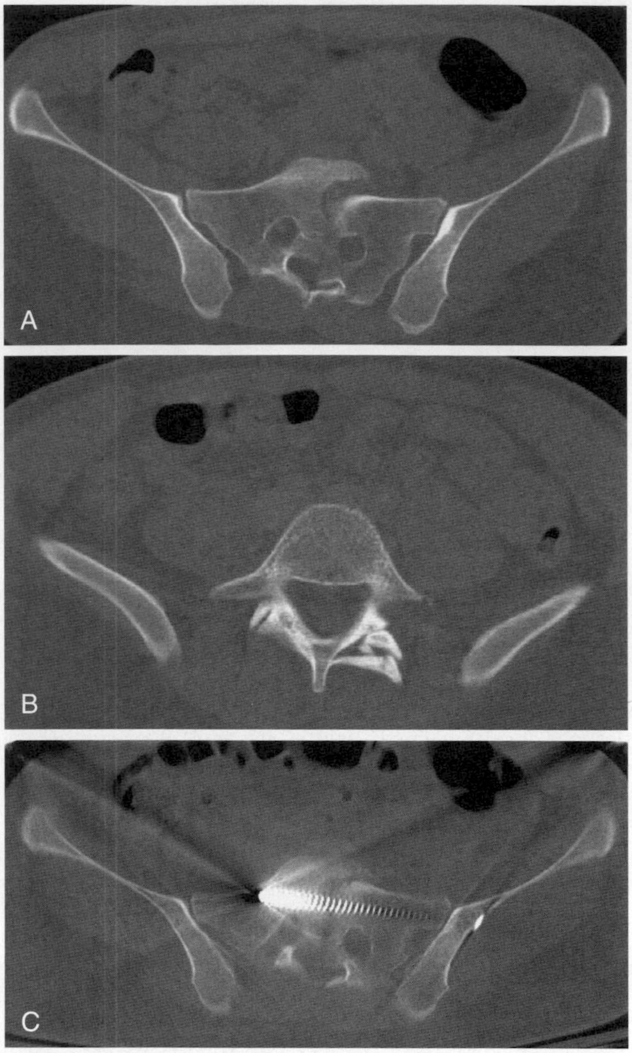

Figure 40-28. Axial computed tomography images of the pelvis show sacral fracture displacement (**A**) associated with dislocation of the ipsilateral L5 to S1 facet joint (**B**). This injury pattern is generally not amenable to closed reduction and percutaneous iliosacral screw fixation because, without open reduction of the dislocated facet joint, realignment of the sacral fracture cannot be achieved (**C**).

however, may disrupt the associated facet joint and potentially destabilize the lumbosacral junction. Complete displacement of the facet joint can cause a locked facet joint, making sacral fracture reduction difficult with closed methods alone (Fig. 40-28). Facet disruption may also cause posttraumatic arthrosis and late lumbosacral pain.

A recently revised AO sacral fracture classification has focused on categorizing sacral fractures based primarily on the extent and pattern of instability. It is a hierarchical system progressing from least to most unstable:

- Type A, lower sacrococcygeal injuries: No impact on posterior pelvic or spinopelvic instability
- Type B, posterior pelvic injuries: Minimal to no impact on spinopelvic stability
- Type C, spinopelvic injuries: Spinopelvic instability

Type A fractures are either inconsequential injuries or occur below the SI joint and therefore result in neither posterior pelvic nor spinopelvic instability. Type B fractures are generally vertical fracture patterns that result in posterior pelvic instability only. Type C injuries are complex sacral U fracture variants or bilateral vertical fractures that result in posterior pelvic and spinopelvic instability. Within each type there are three to four subtypes, categorized based on worsening potential prognosis or greater likelihood of operative intervention due to greater risk of neurologic deficit or of instability (Table 40-3).

ACUTE MANAGEMENT

Marcel Winkelmann, Sebastian Decker

Acute management of pelvic ring injuries is inextricably linked with management of multiple trauma (or polytrauma) because associated injuries are common because of its high-energy mechanism.

EARLY (PREHOSPITAL) MANAGEMENT

The initial evaluation and primary interventions follow ATLS protocols. Preclinical diagnosis of pelvic injury is based on personal or third-party history and clinical findings. Death in unstable pelvic fractures during the first 24 hours is caused by either associated injuries or by hemorrhage, and survival of multiply injured patients is negatively influenced by concomitant pelvic fracture. Therefore, fast and reliable diagnosis and appropriate, timely therapy are crucial to the patient's outcome. The emergency physician or paramedic should gather all available information about circumstances and the mechanism of injury. Pedestrians run over by motor vehicles, for example, sustain pelvic fractures in about 80% of cases.

During the initial evaluation of the patient, the emergency physician should get an idea of the injury pattern. An awake patient usually reports severe pain in the groin or lower back. Lower limb deformity or shortening without obvious associated lower extremity fracture or dislocation and pelvic motion on stress testing may be present. However, the lower extremity findings may only consist of subtle rotational asymmetry. Additional clinical signs are listed in Table 40-4.

Every examination should include an evaluation of peripheral perfusion, lower extremity motor function and sensation, a rectal examination to evaluate for sacral root injury and the

TABLE 40-3A *TYPE A: SACROCOCCYGEAL FRACTURES*

Definition

- Injuries below the SI joint
- No impact on posterior pelvic stability
- No impact on spinopelvic stability
- May have impact on neurology

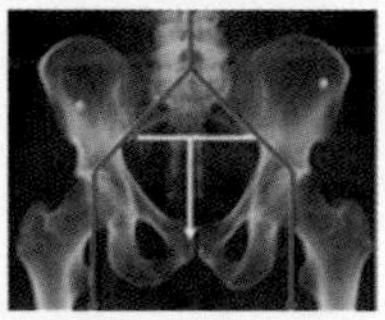

Type	Description
A1	• Coccygeal or sacral compression vs. ligamentous avulsion fractures
A2	• Nondisplaced transverse injuries below SI joint • Usually neurologically intact
A3	• Displaced transverse injuries below SI joint • Often have cauda equina injuries

SI, Sacroiliac.

TABLE 40-3B ***TYPE B: POSTERIOR PELVIC INJURIES***

Definition

- Unilateral longitudinal sacral fractures
- Primary impact is on posterior pelvic stability
- Minimal to no impact on spinopelvic stability (except B4 injuries extending in facet)
- Framework is variation of Denis zones I through III injuries
- Usually treated with SI screw fixation

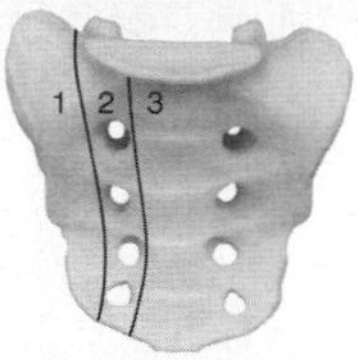

Type	Description	
B1	• **Central** fracture that involves spinal canal but with primarily longitudinal fracture pattern • **Longitudinal** injuries only; rare type of Denis zone III injuries • Does not have the same impact on spinopelvic stability nor same propensity for cauda equina injury as transverse fractures involving canal	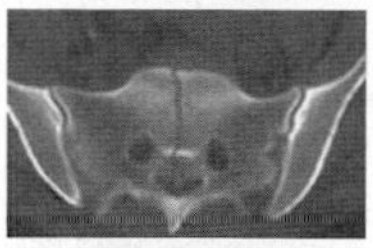
B2	• **Transalar** fracture: does not involve foramina or spinal canal • Denis zone I injury • ≈5% chance of neurologic injury	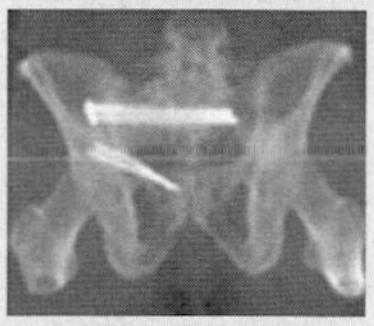
B3	• **Transforaminal** fracture: involves foramina but not spinal canal • Denis zone II injury • ≈25% chance of neurologic injury	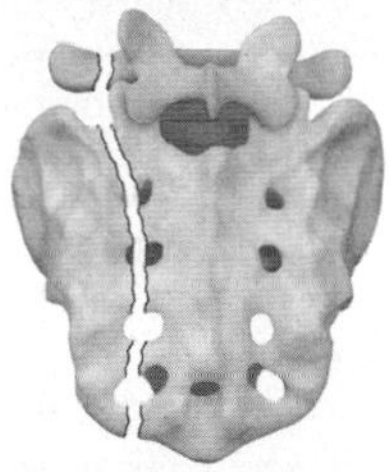 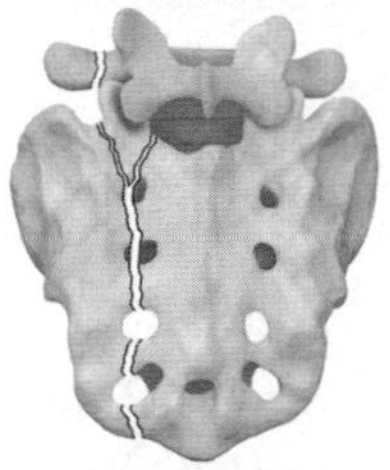 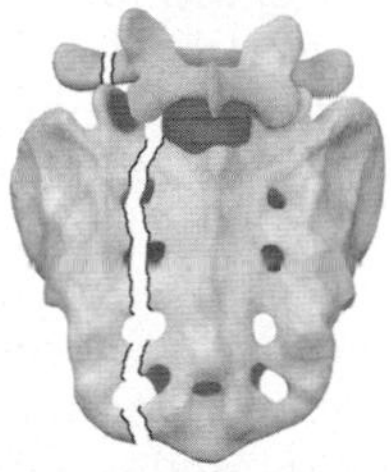
B4	• **Any** unilateral B subtype that involves fracture of ipsilateral L5–S1 facet joint • *May impact* spinopelvic stability (Isler), thus potentially most unstable of B subtypes	

SI, Sacroiliac.

presence of open fracture, and stability testing of the pelvic ring. Early detection of neurologic deficits is of paramount importance in patients with sacral fractures. It is particularly important to perform the rectal examination early in the evaluation of all multiply injured patients, even in the absence of obvious sensorimotor deficits in the extremities, to evaluate perianal sensation, anal sphincter tone, and voluntary perianal contraction, and to assess for the presence of anal wink and the bulbocavernosus reflex. A straight-leg raise test may detect lumbosacral entrapment in cognitively unimpaired patients. Extremity motor function is graded on a scale of 0 to 5 according to the American Spinal Injury Association (ASIA) scoring system, and a sensory level is obtained. For stability testing, the examiner applies lateral, medial, and anterior pressure to the iliac crests and palpates the pubic symphysis and sacral area. As a rule of thumb, an unstable pelvic ring fracture can be expected if a fingerbreadth gap of pubic symphysis can be palpated and if the iliac wings can be shifted with manual compression. Depending on the mechanism of injury, one must be aware of serial injuries (e.g., dashboard injury). Typical serial injuries concomitant with pelvic fractures include calcaneal, ankle, tibial shaft, proximal tibia, femoral shaft and neck, acetabular, and spinal fractures (lumbar and thoracolumbar spine).

TABLE 40-3C ***TYPE C: SPINOPELVIC INJURIES***

Definition

- Injuries resulting in spinopelvic instability

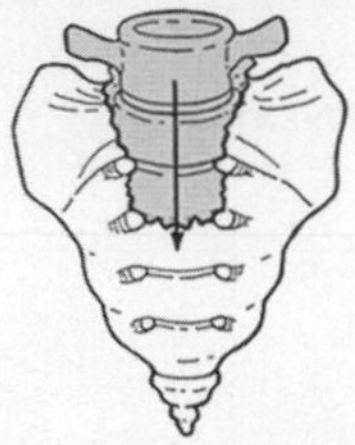

Type	Description
C1	• Nondisplaced sacral U-type fracture • Commonly seen as low-energy insufficiency fracture
C2	• Bilateral type B injuries without transverse fracture • More unstable and higher likelihood of neurologic injury than C1 but lower than C3
C3	• Displaced sacral U-type sacral fracture • Worst comminution on instability and likelihood of neurologic injury • Displaced transverse sacral fracture = canal compromise

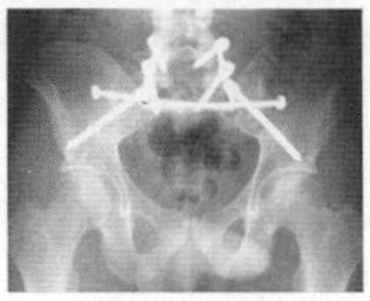

In accordance with ATLS protocols, immediate lifesaving measures (e.g., release of tension pneumothorax) should be undertaken as needed. Because the most common cause of death in patients with unstable pelvic ring injuries is hemorrhagic shock due to uncontrolled bleeding, an early focus on restoring hemodynamic stability is essential.

Trauma-induced hemorrhagic shock is a result of both obvious or occult bleeding and coincident extensive tissue damage, with the release of various inflammatory mediators. However, the initial injury itself usually does not lead to life-threatening bleeding, which appears to be more the result of injury-related coagulopathy, which triggers persistent, uncontrolled bleeding that maintains and intensifies shock. Compared with the established concept that characterizes hemorrhage as a combination of blood loss with dilution and disseminated intravascular coagulation, which is amplified by acidosis and hypothermia (lethal triad), trauma-induced coagulopathy is an independent disorder. Tissue damage and hypoperfusion (shock) endogenously lead to anticoagulant and fibrinolytic processes. Approximately one quarter of all multiply injured patients have a coagulopathy at the time of admission. Injury severity positively correlates with the risk of early coagulopathy, which likely accounts for more than 40% of patients with Injury Severity Scores (ISS) greater than 30 manifesting symptoms of shock. Early coagulopathy is an independent predictor of morbidity and mortality and is associated with a fourfold increased overall and eightfold increased early mortality (<24 hours) in the presence of multiple injuries.[98-100] The basic cause of trauma-induced coagulopathy is a function of the injury itself. Therefore, therapy and prevention of amplifying factors have to begin as soon as possible, ideally even before hospitalization.

If a pelvic ring injury is suspected and hemorrhagic shock is manifested, crucial therapeutic actions should be initiated at the scene of injury. Assessment of shock according to ATLS criteria can be challenging and often impossible in this environment, as suggested by data from the German trauma registry (TR-DGU).[101] Use of the shock index, the ratio of heart rate to systolic blood pressure, seems to be more suitable to adequately estimate hypovolemic shock.[102] Besides prevention of hypothermia and hypotension, control of hemorrhage is the major concern. Open wounds should be covered with sterile and compressive dressings whenever possible. An alternative, if compression is impossible (e.g., in the groin), is the use of topical hemostatics such as chitosan, a polysaccharide polymer based on chitin.[103] If pelvic ring injury is suspected, pelvic stabilization or even compression is reasonable. Different measures and devices are available. Internal rotation of the lower extremities can transmit an internal rotation force to the pelvis and therefore partially reduce the pelvic ring and diminish pelvic volume. Taping the knees and ankles with the limbs in this internally rotated position is therefore one option for temporary pelvic "stabilization." The tape should be neither applied for excessive periods nor circumferentially to protect the soft tissues and lower extremity perfusion.[104] Vacuum body splints are easy-to-use, time-saving devices. Their use is not limited to pelvic fractures because they can also be used with lower extremity and spine injuries, and they are usually available at the scene. They can be applied to the patient's flanks to maintain access to the abdomen and groin. Noninvasive pelvic circumferential compression devices (PCCDs) are targeted more specifically to the site of injury, and their use has increased over the past decade. A concern with the application of PCCDs has been the potential for soft tissue or visceral injury to pelvic structures such as the bladder, urethra, and vagina because of accentuation of lateral compression injury deformity. However, Bottlang and colleagues demonstrated that such injuries are not likely to occur.[105] Skin lesions have been reported after tight compression and a longer duration of PCCD application. Application of any PCCD is time saving and can be done relatively effortlessly by two people. PCCD results in only slight diminution in accessibility of the groin and lower abdomen. An expeditiously accomplished, improvised alternative is the use of a sheet, which is longitudinally folded and wrapped circumferentially around the pelvis, placed between the iliac crests and greater trochanters. It can be secured either by anterior clamping or by creating a knot with a stick used to twirl and thereby compress the pelvis.[106,107] Recent literature analysis suggests that PCCDs are effective in the early stabilization of unstable pelvic fractures, although the reasons for their effectiveness have not been fully explained. Although PCCDs may decrease the pelvic volume

TABLE 40-4 ***LOCAL SIGNS***

Pain	Deformity
Abrasions	Shortening of leg
Bruises	Pelvic asymmetry
Effusions	Blocking of hip joint
Discolorations	Pulselessness
Swelling	

of open-book injuries,[77] it is debatable whether they are actually able to exert a tamponade effect because the retroperitoneum is disrupted, and reduction in volume of the true pelvis is much less than expected. For example, a wide pubic diastasis of 10 cm only corresponds to a 35% increase in pelvic volume, or approximately half a liter.[108-110] Splinting of pathologic pelvic motion is more likely to be the mechanism that aids in hemostasis.[111] However, because nearly all studies are retrospective, prospective data concerning mortality rates and complications are lacking.[112,113] The oldest form of emergency pelvic stabilization is the pneumatic antishock garment (PASG). This inflatable garment is placed over the lower extremities and around the abdomen and inflated until blood pressure is stabilized. Major concerns pertain to lower extremity compartment syndrome caused by prolonged inflation times. Research done over the years has shown contradictory results, so no recommendation can be made regarding its use as a first-line therapy. Because simpler and lower priced alternatives are available, PASGs are used only rarely today and are mainly of historical interest.[114]

After noninvasive temporary pelvic stabilization has been performed and resuscitation is in progress, efficient transfer of the patient to a qualified trauma center is crucial. Appropriate interdisciplinary care, diagnostic evaluation of fracture pattern and associated injuries, and specialized surgical or interventional treatment options are generally available only at specialized hospitals. Whenever possible, direct transfer from the accident scene to a trauma center is preferred. However, if a hemodynamically unstable patient is at risk of not surviving a longer transport, the patient should be transported to the closest medical center and transferred as soon as possible to a trauma center after appropriate resuscitation and temporary hemodynamic stabilization,

Acute Management

A defined protocol for the treatment of multiply injured patients is useful and helps to facilitate and fast-track therapy. The trauma team is interdisciplinary and includes, depending on the health care system, a general or trauma or critical care surgeon, an emergency department physician, an anesthesiologist, and an orthopaedic surgeon. Clinicians from other disciplines join the team depending on specific associated injuries. Soon after admission, a complete survey of the patient is mandatory. Focusing on the pelvis, physical signs of pelvic instability include deformity of the lower extremity without obvious lower extremity fracture. This usually presents as shortening or malrotation of the limb ipsilateral to the unstable hemipelvis. Buttock or flank ecchymosis (Grey Turner sign) and swelling may herald significant retroperitoneal hemorrhage. Palpable hematoma above the inguinal ligament, on the proximal thigh, or over the perineum (Destot sign) may indicate a pelvic fracture with associated bleeding. Visual inspection of the posterior part of the pelvis is done when the patient is logrolled for examination of the spine. Palpation of the posterior aspect of the pelvis may reveal a closed degloving injury, a large hematoma, or more rarely a palpable displacement through a posterior ring injury site (ilium, SI joint, or sacrum). Similarly, palpation of the symphysis may lead to recognition of a gap. A single manual pelvic stress examination by an experienced surgeon may be useful if questions of pelvic stability persist after the survey. This examination should not be undertaken, however, if a circumferential sheet or PCCD has been applied and the patient remains hemodynamically unstable. Additional signs of potential instability include an open pelvic fracture, scrotal hematomas, and lower extremity neurologic deficits potentially attributable to lumbosacral plexus injury. Validity of the manual stability examination findings remains controversial. Sensitivity has been reported to be low (25%–45%), but specificity is high (90%–99%).[115-117] However, because of its high positive predictive value, this relatively simple examination should be an inherent part of the emergent evaluation of all high-energy injuries. As an adjunct to the survey, an AP radiograph of the pelvis is mandatory in all patients who are suspected of having multiple injuries or pelvic ring injury due to a trauma mechanism, who have a depressed level of consciousness, who complain of pain or tenderness on examination of the pelvis, or who fail to respond to fluids when no intraabdominal or thoracic source of bleeding is noted. Diagnosis of the likely source of hemorrhage, and distinction of an intraperitoneal from a retroperitoneal source of bleeding are necessary. FAST is a fast and noninvasive screening instrument for diagnosis of pericardial effusion and free fluid around abdominal organs (hemoperitoneum) and retroperitoneum (Fig. 40-29). Four areas are checked routinely:

1. Perihepatic space (Rutherford-Morison pouch)
2. Perisplenic space (Koller pouch)
3. Pericardium
4. Pelvis (rectouterine pouch, Douglas pouch, cul-de-sac, rectovesical excavation)

Sensitivity and specificity range from 25% to 80% and 87% to 96%, respectively.[118,119] Ultrasonography is useful because of its relatively high positive predictive value. If a patient is hemodynamically unstable and FAST shows free peritoneal fluid, it is a clear indication for early stabilization of pelvic ring fracture (e.g., external fixation or C-clamp) or diagnostic laparotomy. However, one must acknowledge that negative FAST findings do not exclude free peritoneal fluid, so that an additional CT should be considered.

Computed tomography angiography or multidetector computed tomography (MDCT) is currently the gold standard in pelvic fracture diagnostics. If possible, one should use multiplanar reconstruction (MPR) for better assessment of imaging. This increases the sensitivity of pelvic fracture detection compared with axial slices. In addition, CT is helpful in detecting pelvic hemorrhage, with a sensitivity of approximately 90%. It has primarily replaced diagnostic peritoneal lavage (DPL). When used alone in this patient population, DPL is associated with a high number of false-positive results and therefore a nontherapeutic laparotomy and negative impact on outcome.[120-122] Blackmore and colleagues state that the risk ratio for severe bleeding due to fracture-related hemorrhage is 4.8 in patients with more than 500 mL of extravasate compared with patients with less than 500 mL. Thus, one should assume a relevant hemorrhage in patients with more than 500 mL of intrapelvic fluid. By implication, one can exclude relevant hemorrhage in patients with less than 200 mL of intrapelvic fluid with 95% certainty.[123] In addition to fracture pattern and intraperitoneal as well as extraperitoneal bleeding, CT is essential in diagnosing associated injuries. Thus, every adult patient with pelvic fracture on the AP radiograph, suspected pelvic ring injury without obvious fracture on the AP radiograph, or multiple injuries should get a CT scan with one exception. Hemodynamically unstable patients who require

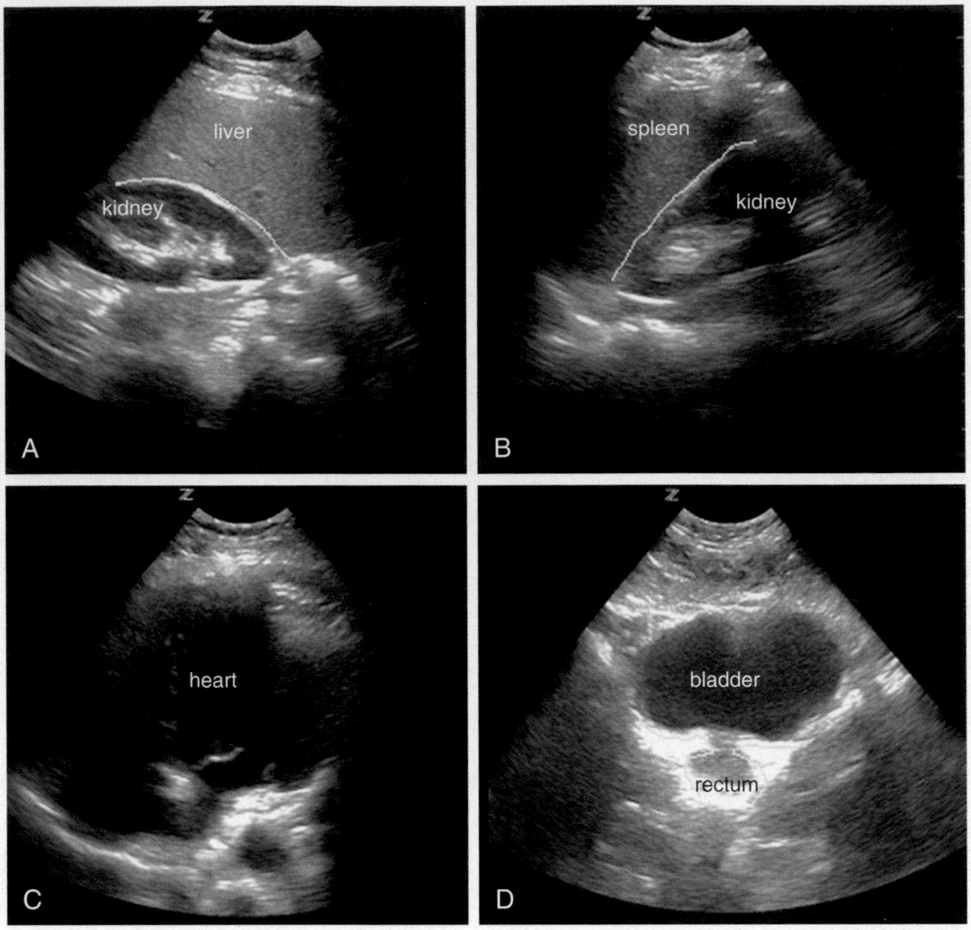

Figure 40-29. Examples of the organ systems that can be rapidly evaluated with the use of ultrasonography in a multiply injured patient.

further surgical or interventional bleeding control and are at highest risk of not surviving the additional delays required to obtain the CT scan should undergo surgical therapy according to the principles of damage control surgery without delay. When the patient is hemodynamically stable, CT scan can be obtained.

Immediately after admission, a blood sample should be taken to give further information about red blood cell count or hemoglobin, perfusion, and coagulation. Blood gas analysis should be available at the trauma room as point-of-care testing (POCT). The base excess allows better estimation of shock (hypoperfusion) and positively correlates with transfusion requirement and outcome.[124,125] Base excess values of −2 to −6 mmol/L indicate a mild, −6 to −10 mmol/L a moderate, and below −10 mmol/L a severe shock. Standard evaluation of the coagulation system includes partial thromboplastin time and prothrombin time (Quick, INR). However, these tests are time consuming, and values are usually only available a minimum of 30 minutes after sampling. Thrombelastography and thrombelastometry represent POCT that provides rapid and more complete information about the patient's actual hemostatic capabilities within minutes. Multiply injured patients and patients with unstable pelvic fractures with exsanguinating hemorrhage especially benefit from earlier targeted transfusion and clotting management.

For this purpose, the concept of damage control surgery was adapted to damage control resuscitation. It combines early and aggressive treatment of trauma-induced coagulopathy with surgical bleeding control. Although this approach arises from the military experience derived from Operations Iraqi and Enduring Freedom, the principles can be extrapolated to the civilian treatment of severe and multiply injured patients in industrialized nations and urban centers. Key concepts are permissive hypotension, preferred usage of blood products with a high ratio (1 : 1) of packed red blood cells and fresh-frozen plasma for transfusion, and early and fast correction of coagulopathy by administration of clotting factors.[126]

Associated Injuries

Because of its complex anatomy with proximity of multiple organs on the one hand and the high-energy causative mechanism of injury on the other, high-energy pelvic fractures are regularly associated with intrapelvic and extrapelvic injuries. Whereas significant pelvic hemorrhage may occur in up to 75% of patients, rupture of larger caliber pelvic vessels is verifiable in up to 27%, especially in run-over injuries and degloving or avulsion of skin.[85] Urogenital injuries may occur in 6.5% to 30% (urethra, 4%–15%; bladder, 5%–25%) and lumbosacral plexus injuries in about 8% to 25%, with increasing likelihood in globally unstable fractures.[16,127-134] The likelihood of aortic rupture is eight times greater in high-energy pelvic ring trauma than in blunt trauma injury overall.[135] About 60% to 80% of patients with high-energy pelvic fractures have associated musculoskeletal injuries. Up to 56% of the patients have concomitant thoracic trauma, and approximately one-third have a relevant traumatic brain injury. The mortality rate ranges from 10% to 40%.[1,136-140] Therefore, it is crucial to diagnose all concomitant injuries as early as possible to initiate appropriate therapy.

Damage Control Orthopaedics

After the patient is assessed and resuscitation is underway, the surgical team must be prepared to act efficiently if ongoing pelvic bleeding is observed or suspected. To summarize, persistent pelvic bleeding generally comes from three different sources: arterial bleeding from disruption of any pelvic artery; venous bleeding from tearing or shearing of pelvic veins, especially in the posterior (presacral) venous plexus; and bleeding directly from fractured cancellous bone. It is likely that pelvic hemorrhage results from injuries to both arteries and veins. Bleeding from a large vessel such as the common, external, or internal iliac is less likely to occur. Injury to large vessels is usually associated with rapid, massive bleeding and loss of distal pulses. Because it is rarely possible to determine the primary source of hemorrhage for a particular injury, it is important to address both the arterial and venous systems.[141] Furthermore, one has to consider different bleeding sources; the five areas of potential hemorrhage in multiply injured patients are external, thoracic, intraperitoneal, retroperitoneal, and from extremity fractures.

The primary aim of the trauma or orthopaedic surgeon in controlling pelvic bleeding is the stabilization of the unstable pelvic injury.[142-145] In terms of hemodynamically unstable patients with pelvic fractures, immediate surgical management follows the principles of damage control surgery or damage control orthopaedics to minimize the surgical insult to the patient.[146] The timing of operative acute pelvic stabilization depends on the need for resuscitation.

The key clinical correlates pertaining to injury type are the association of lateral compression and vertical shear injuries with major intraabdominal and head injuries.[132] Also, unstable AP compression injuries and completely unstable injuries have a far greater incidence of retroperitoneal hemorrhage than of intraabdominal bleeding. Given these correlations, it is reasonable to expect that few lateral compression injuries will benefit from emergency stabilization techniques. Unstable AP and vertical shear injuries, however, remain an important focus in the acute setting and can be managed by a variety of techniques. In cases in which prehospital administration of a PCCD has not been undertaken, this is a logical first step and has been shown to be safe and effective.[105] The duration of therapy with a PCCD is controversial. Some authors advocate its use for 1 to 2 days, mainly until the patient is hemodynamically stable and transfusion requirements have ceased, or until another intervention is required if the patient continues to bleed.[111,147] We propose the use of PCCD only as a short-term stabilizer for transport and early management in the trauma room, emergency department, and early part of admission. Because of facilitated patient care and the possibility of fairly long-term duration of external fixator or C-clamp, respectively, an early exchange seems reasonable.

In the case of a rotationally or vertically unstable pelvic disruption, emergency stabilization can be accomplished by anterior external fixation or a pelvic C-clamp. Anterior external fixation has been the default option for several decades.[148,149] It usually contains hemorrhage, theoretically by direct compression of bleeding vessels at the fracture site or SI joint disruption, but only if the posterior SI ligaments remain intact (rotational instability only). The amount of stability and hemorrhage control achieved in vertically unstable patterns with complete fracture of the posterior complex is limited.[150] Application of the fixator requires operative intervention, and it should be applied in the operating room under fluoroscopic guidance. The fixator location has to take into account the bony structure of the pelvis and accessibility of the abdomen in case further intervention is necessary. The pins can be placed in the iliac crest (Fig. 40-30), but we propose supraacetabular positioning because of better trabecular bone structure and enhanced abdominal accessibility (Fig. 40-31). However, there are no data available to suggest that this technique improves survival.[151-154]

Recently, the use of supraacetabular subcutaneous fixation using pedicle screw–based internal fixation devices has become increasingly popular (Fig. 40-32). It provides satisfactory biomechanical stability with a favorable risk-to-benefit profile. This technique facilitates mobilization and nursing care of the patient, improves stability relative to the external fixator because of a shorter distance between the bar and the pelvis, and theoretically decreases the risk of infection and associated loosening of pins. Although temporary irritation of the lateral femoral cutaneous nerve and asymptomatic heterotopic ossification around the implants are common, if done correctly, this technique does not appear to endanger major neurovascular structures.[155-158]

In selected cases, application of a specialized pelvic clamp (C-clamp, which derives from the C-shaped frame of a clamp device originally used to hold metal or wood) may be necessary (Fig. 40-33). The C-clamp can be applied in the trauma room, operating room, or intensive care unit. It is designed mainly for use in C-type injuries in hemodynamically unstable patients with significant displacement through a disrupted SI joint(s) or sacral fracture. It addresses the site of instability by a direct compressive force applied to the ilium lateral to the SI joints. Its use in transiliac injuries is contraindicated because of the risk of perforation of the tips of the clamp through the fracture zone and into the pelvis.[132,159] A rough landmark for surgical access, generally through a 2-cm incision, is the intersection of a line extending along the longitudinal axis of the femur and a perpendicular line originating from the ASIS (Fig. 40-34, *A* and *B*). Additionally, a depression of the lateral bone surface at the level of the SI joint can be palpated. One should start with the uninjured side. After incision, the pin is positioned and driven against the lateral ileum. Before positioning of the tip on the injured side, one must carry out a reduction maneuver consisting of internal rotation and traction of the leg (Fig. 40-34, *C*). After the second pin has been driven into position, one can apply the previously assembled clamp and close it by lateral compression. However, because of serious reported complications (fracture displacement, pin site perforation, nerve injury),[160,161] the C-clamp requires specific training for its successful application. Fluoroscopic control during application may be helpful, especially for the inexperienced user. In general, a C-clamp alone is seldom sufficient, since the anterior pelvic ring remains mobile. For this reason, one should combine a C-clamp with either a PCCD or anterior external fixator. As an alternative, application of a pelvic clamp to the anterior pelvis in the cancellous bone

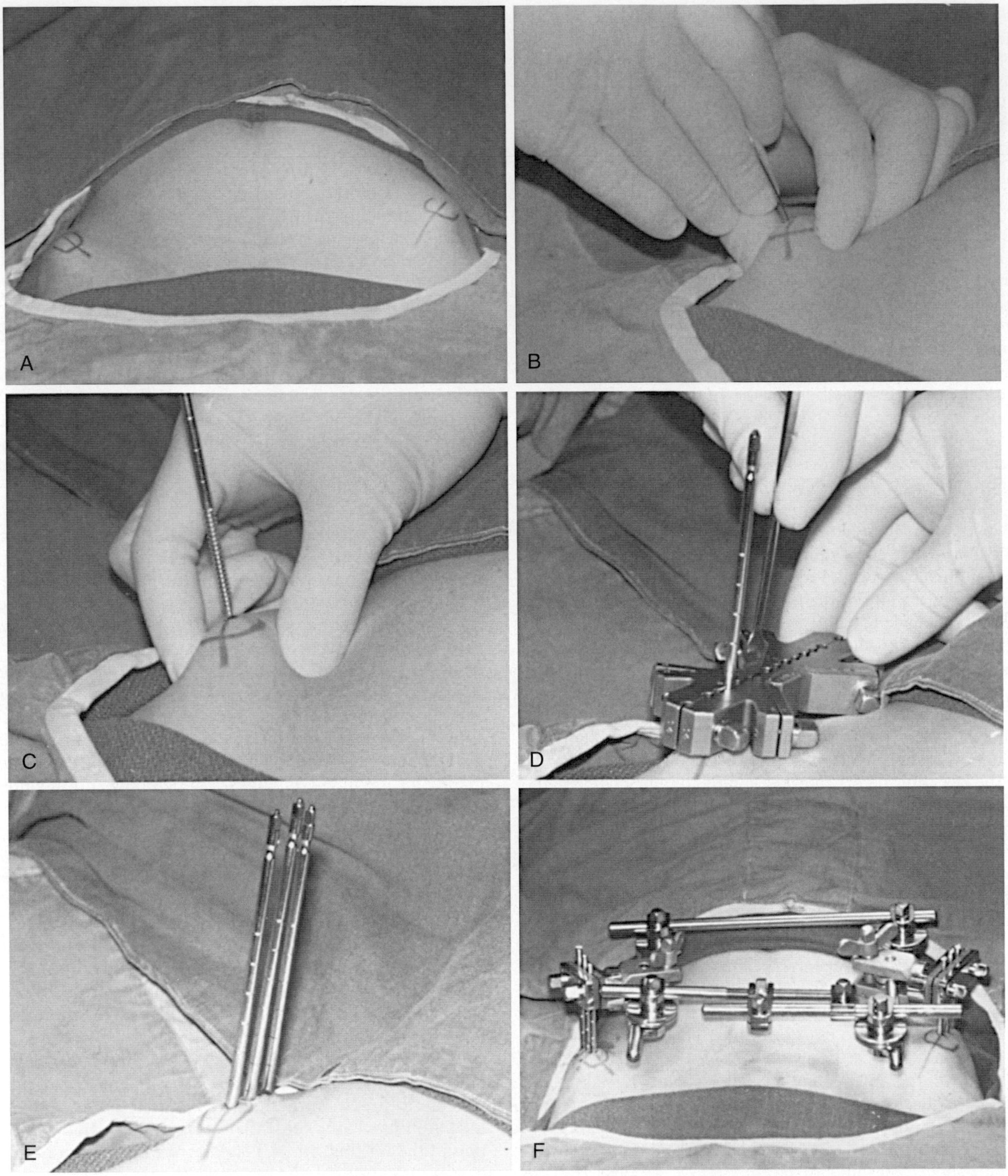

Figure 40-30. Application of external fixation to the pelvis. **A,** Landmarks are the iliac crest and the anterior superior iliac spine. **B,** The iliac wing is palpated to determine its orientation. It may also be determined by the use of an open technique or by spinal needles to outline both the inner and the outer aspects of the pelvis. **C,** Appropriate orientation of the iliac wing; note the pin orientation at an angle to the body.

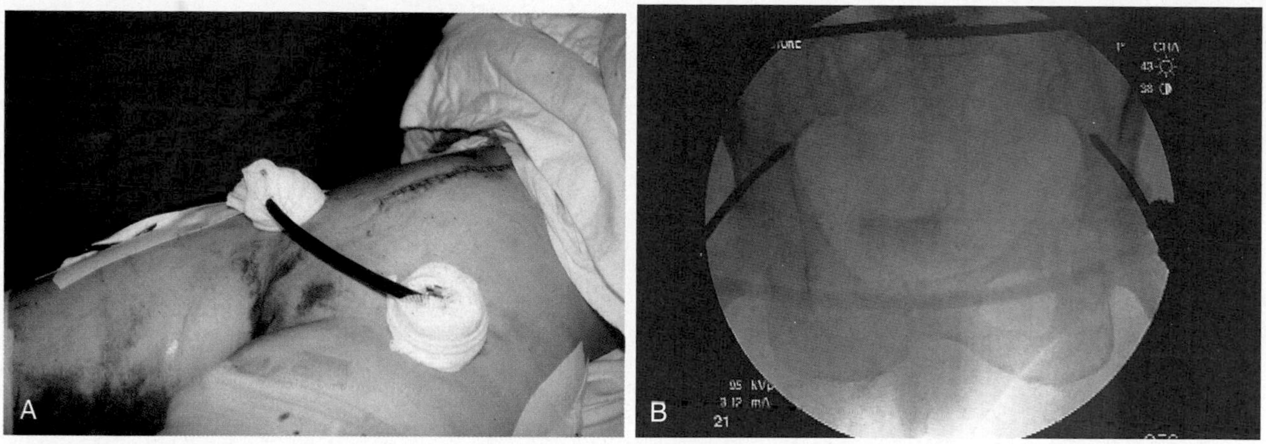

Figure 40-31. Clinical (**A**) and radiographic (**B**) images of pelvic external fixator constructed with 5.5-mm Schanz screws placed just cranial and lateral to the hip joint. These are connected by a curved carbon fiber rod, which is under tension as evidenced by the Schanz screw deflection. The bulky dressing minimizes soft tissue shear against the pins.

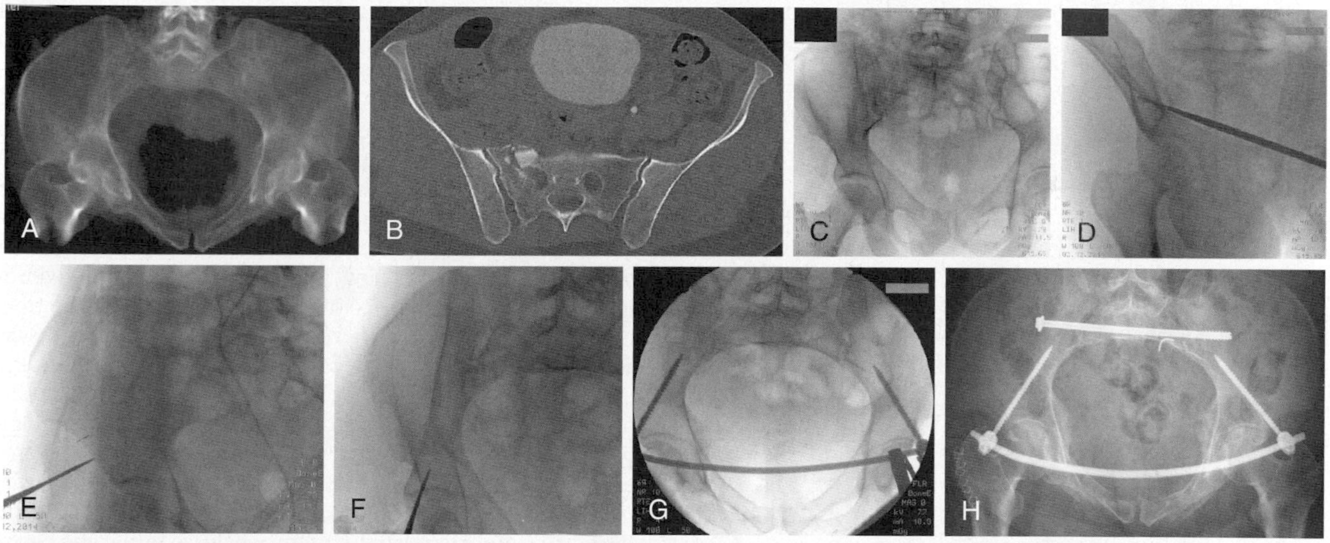

Figure 40-32. Fixation of rotationally unstable pelvic fracture with "INFIX" subcutaneous fixation. Inlet view (**A**) and axial computed tomography image (**B**) of rotationally unstable pelvic ring fracture with right zone II sacral fracture and bilateral pubic ramus fractures in a multiply injured patient. Intraoperative views demonstrate pelvic realignment with right lower extremity traction (**C**), obturator-outlet (**D**), iliac (**E**), and obturator inlet oblique (**F**) views of the pelvis to establish starting point for iliac screws, and the use of distraction across the anterior subcutaneous bar to reestablish pelvic ring alignment (**G**). Postoperative inlet view (**H**) shows the final INFIX construct. *(Courtesy of Tania Ferguson, MD.)*

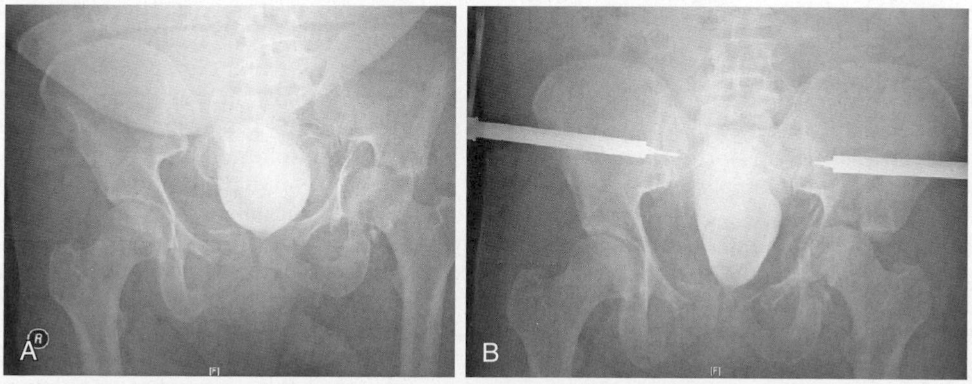

Figure 40-33. Clinical example for the use of a C-clamp. **A,** Anterior-posterior (AP) radiograph of a complex pelvic fracture with complete disruption of the right sacroiliac (SI) joint, transpubic fractures on both sides and anterior and posterior column acetabular fracture on the left side. Note the almost spherical bladder filled with contrast agent. **B,** AP radiograph after use of the C-clamp; the right SI joint is nearly closed. Note the compressed bladder as a result of the reduced intrapelvic volume.

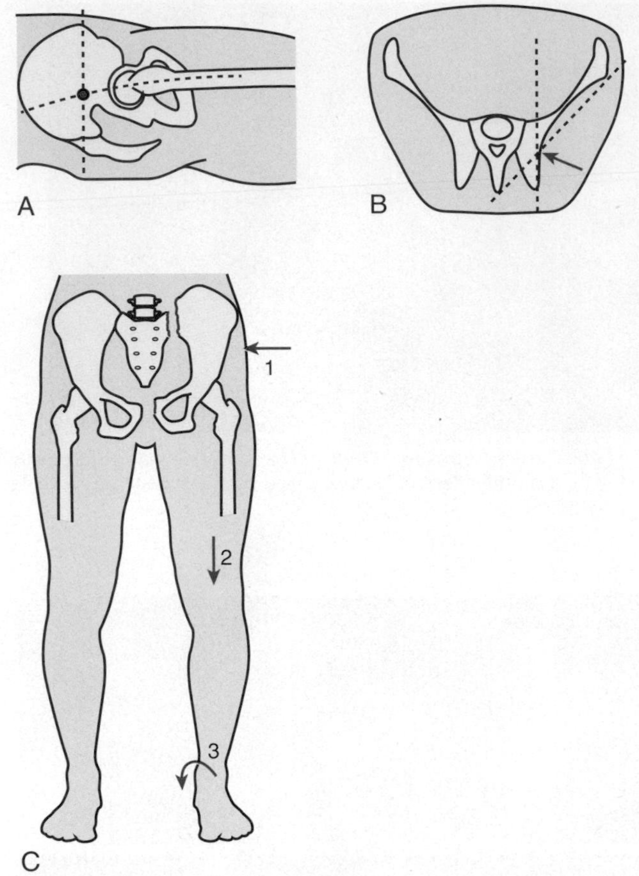

Figure 40-34. Landmarks for surgical access of a C-clamp. **A,** Intersection of extended longitudinal axis of the femur and perpendicular line from the anterior superior iliac spine. **B,** Depression of the lateral bone surface at the level SI joint. **C,** Repositioning maneuver with lateral compression of the pelvis combined with traction and internal rotation of the leg.

above the acetabulum or to the greater trochanter has been reported.[162,163]

Further therapeutic management of unstable pelvic injuries depends on the response to resuscitation measures. After appropriate resuscitation has been completed and pelvic stabilization has been applied, bleeding will cease in most patients. However, patients who remain hemodynamically unstable despite the aforementioned measures are of particular concern and require targeted therapeutic action. Nevertheless, the optimal therapeutic strategy remains controversial, with a bias in Europe toward extraperitoneal pelvic packing after external pelvic stabilization and in North America toward emergent pelvic angiography and external stabilization of the pelvis (Fig. 40-35).[111,164]

A positive test result for intraabdominal blood in a patient who fails to respond to standard resuscitation protocols mandates an exploratory laparotomy as part of a coordinated treatment plan. Crash laparotomy without further diagnostic procedures is recommended for patients in extremis who have either absent vital signs or severe shock caused by exsanguinating hemorrhage.[165-167] The treatment plan should provide for pelvic stability during the abdominal procedure. Because sheet wraps and PCCDs encroach on the surgical field, they should be moved distal to the proximal thighs and replaced by an external fixator, C-clamp, or occasionally percutaneous image-guided posterior ring fixation. During laparotomy, if the retroperitoneal hematoma is expanding, packing of the presacral area and retropubic space is carried out. If retroperitoneal hematoma is suspected to be a major source of bleeding, extraperitoneal pelvic packing should be carried out before laparotomy, thus preserving anatomic spaces. During laparotomy, in the presence of multiple massive sources of bleeding, local tamponade or aortic compression is possible. Temporary aortic clamping can be considered as a last resort. In case of hemodynamic impairment, complex reconstructive procedures in the abdomen should be avoided. A major splenic rupture usually necessitates splenectomy. In hepatic injuries, tamponade usually controls bleeding. Additionally, the Pringle maneuver can be applied in extreme situations. The need for partial liver resection is rare. Bowel injuries are clamped and covered, and definitive treatment is performed after the hemodynamic situation is stabilized.[168-172] In open pelvic fractures that are hemorrhaging through an open wound, packing of the area plus compressive dressing is needed to assist in the control of bleeding. Angiography should be performed immediately if the patient remains hypotensive despite emergent pelvic stabilization, control of abdominal bleeding, and retroperitoneal packing.

Transcatheter arterial embolization (TAE) has a reasonable safety profile despite several reported complications.[173,174] TAE appears to work by terminating arterial bleeding and allowing the hematoma to tamponade the venous component of the hemorrhage.[111] Advocates of this procedure emphasize that persistent arterial bleeding is the reason for hemodynamic instability in the majority of patients who remain hemodynamically unstable despite resuscitation, pelvic compression, and exclusion of associated injuries.[120,175,176] Critics counter that arterial bleeding can be ascertained in only 10% to 20% of cases.[15,177] However, diagnostic and therapeutic angiography in patients with pelvic hemorrhage is difficult even in experienced hands. Selective embolization is most effective in controlling bleeding from small-diameter vessels (i.e., $\leq$3 mm). Pelvic ring injury–related rupture of the external iliac artery is rare and requires surgical techniques to control bleeding and restore blood supply to the lower leg.[178] Angiography may assist in localizing large vessel bleeding but only if time and hemodynamic stability permit because the procedure is time consuming and simultaneous treatment of other injuries during this time is delayed. The mean time between admission and TAE has been reported to be 10 hours, and procedure times for TAE can average over 90 minutes.[169,176,179,180]

The use of extraperitoneal pelvic packing has become popular, especially in Europe and more recently in North America (Fig. 40-36). This technique requires external bony pelvic fixation followed by packing of the pelvic retroperitoneal space via an extraperitoneal route. The rationale for the technique is that most of the severe bleeding originates from the pelvic presacral venous plexus and from cancellous bone surfaces. Bleeding can therefore be effectively controlled by applying a direct tamponade. The procedure is performed through an 8-cm midline incision extending superiorly from the pubic symphysis. The peritoneum is left intact, and the space between the peritoneum and bony pelvis is bluntly dissected bilaterally. Three sponges are packed below the pelvic brim toward the SI joint bilaterally. The incision is then closed. Packing is removed at 24 to 48 hours, depending on the patient's hemodynamic stability. If hypotension persists after

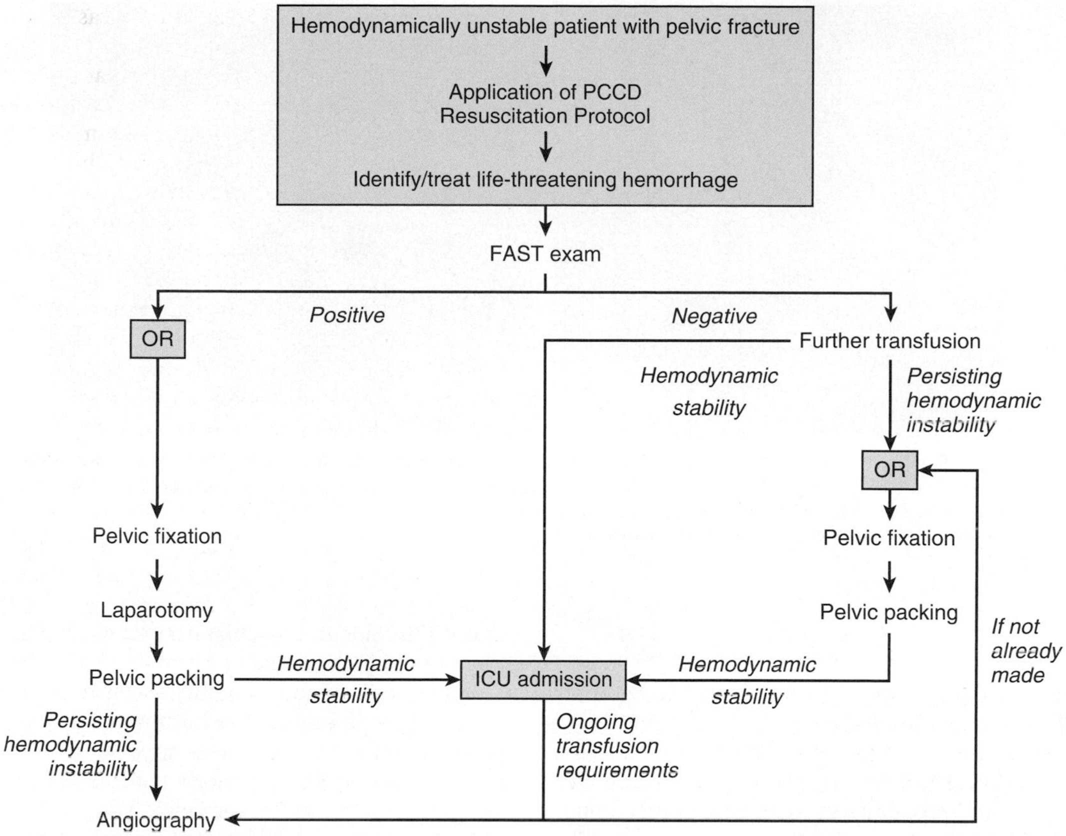

Figure 40-35. Algorithm for resuscitation after pelvic disruption. *FAST,* Focused assessment with sonography in trauma; *ICU,* intensive care unit; *OR,* operating room; *PCCD,* pelvic circumferential compression device.

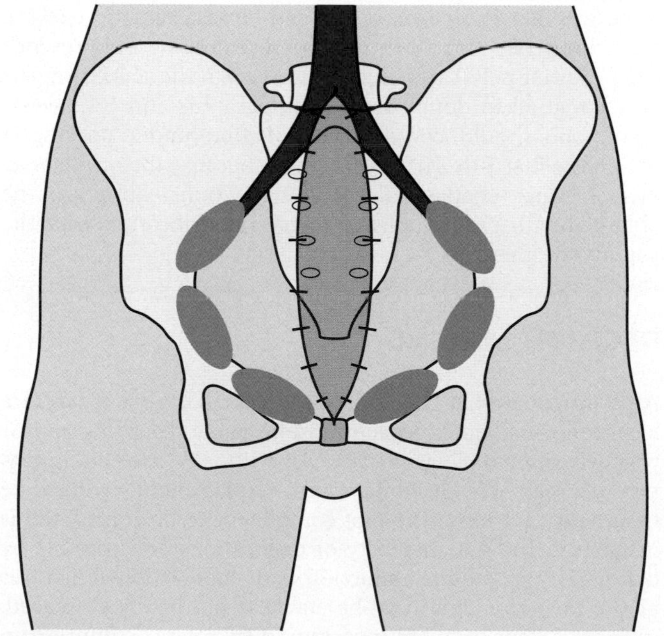

Figure 40-36. Landmarks for surgical access and placement of the sponges below the pelvic brim.

the packing, then angiography is performed.[181] The proponents of this technique believe that it is a more efficient use of resources and time than is the case with protocols that involve performing angiography first followed by surgery.

Because convincing prospective studies are lacking, no evidence supports that either approach is better. It is therefore up to the hospital trauma and orthopaedic surgeons to decide what protocol best fits their experience and resources.[111,169,178,181,182]

DEFINITIVE MANAGEMENT AND DECISION MAKING

Sebastian Decker, Marcel Winkelmann, Christian Krettek, Carlo Bellabarba

After stabilization of an acutely injured patient, assessment of multiple factors will help to determine definitive management. This evaluation is necessary to decide the appropriate management based on the balance between our ability to decrease the risk of late pain, malunion and nonunion after pelvic injuries, and the need to avoid complications of the injury or subsequent treatment.[35,183-185]

Recommendations for therapy are based primarily on two factors, (1) fracture pattern including pelvic stability and (2) patient factors such as associated injuries, soft tissue conditions within and around the zone of injury, and comorbidities. Besides radiographic assessment, which is elaborated in the paragraph on radiology of the pelvis, an accurate personal or third-party history and a thorough secondary survey are essential.

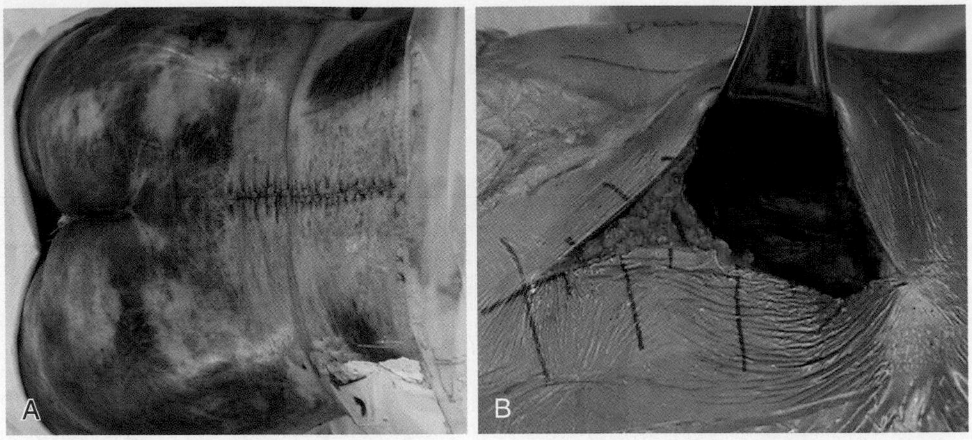

Figure 40-37. Internal degloving injuries. High-energy pelvic fractures are frequently associated with severe soft tissue injuries (**A**), which can best be described as variants of the Morel-Lavallée lesions seen with acetabular fractures. Incision through the skin and subcutaneous tissue in this patient who sustained a severe pelvic fracture with spinopelvic dissociation after fall from a height reveals degloving between the subcutaneous tissue and muscle fascia extending throughout the torso (**B**).

HISTORY

Accident site information, patient history, and radiographic data can all be used to help in determining the mechanism of injury. Direct application of force or crushing injuries to the pelvis can cause serious soft tissue disruption, which can lead to degloving lesions and possibly soft tissue or wound complications (Fig. 40-37). Indirectly applied force usually spares the soft tissue.

Knowledge of the patient's age, occupation, and expectations is necessary if the surgeon and the patient are to have a common treatment goal. Preexisting leg length discrepancies should be noted. Mobility before the injury can also influence treatment, especially in elderly patients. Comorbidities and medication are of particular interest because reduced immunologic competence can lead to serious complications and impaired outcome.

PHYSICAL EXAMINATION

After neurologic, cardiovascular, and respiratory issues have stabilized, a thorough secondary orthopaedic survey should be completed. Specifically regarding the pelvis, the surgeon should take into account prior abdominal interventions, including wound conditions. Suprapubic or transurethral indwelling catheters serve to monitor resuscitation or therapeutically address bladder and urethral injuries, respectively, because associated genitourinary injuries are common. Thus, specific diagnostic investigation is mandatory to avoid overlooking occult injuries. The paragraph on genitourinary injuries addresses these diagnostic and therapeutic approaches in depth. Evaluation of open pelvic wounds for location, contamination, and residuals of prior intervention should be noted. Scrotal or labial hematoma can be indicative of injury to the pelvic floor. Any leg length discrepancies should be measured and any internal or external rotational abnormalities evaluated. Areas of abrasions or ecchymosis may be associated with soft tissue degloving injuries. After inspection, palpation of the areas of injury should be carried out to determine soft tissue damage, bony gaps, and hematomas. A full neuromuscular and vascular examination of the lower extremities should be repeated.

The role of manual stability assessment is controversial.[111] If instability previously has been noted or temporary external pelvic stabilization has been applied, repeated examination should be avoided. In hemodynamically stable patients without pelvic stabilization or who have solely sheet wrap or PCCD, one can consider a new examination, always keeping the risk of bleeding recurrence in mind. Rotational instability can be assessed by pushing on the anterior superior iliac wings, with both external and internal rotation forces to determine whether the pelvis opens and closes. Palpation of the posterior pelvic ring is sensitive to determining the presence of a posterior pelvic ring injury. However, if the stability of the pelvis is at all in doubt despite radiographic and CT assessment, one should consider examination under anesthesia within the first 5 to 7 days after injury because the results may dictate major changes in treatment. Confirmation can be obtained with radiographs or image intensification with the patient anesthetized.[186]

DECISION MAKING

After the patient has been fully assessed and the pelvic fracture has been classified, a decision can be made regarding appropriate treatment (Fig. 40-38). As with any skeletal injury, two key factors—instability and displacement—will drive treatment decisions. The first component to be considered is instability. The vast majority of dislocations are unstable by definition and require reduction and stabilization. Fractures of the posterior ring may be stable if minimally displaced, especially impaction injuries caused by lateral compression forces, but will be mobile and heal in an unacceptable position if initial displacement is unacceptable. Nonsurgical treatment of pelvic ring injuries demands close early clinical and radiographic follow-up to identify instability or subsequent displacement.

B-type fractures that are stable include AP compression injuries with minor displacement (<2.5 cm) (subtype B1.1) and lateral compression injuries with sacral impaction

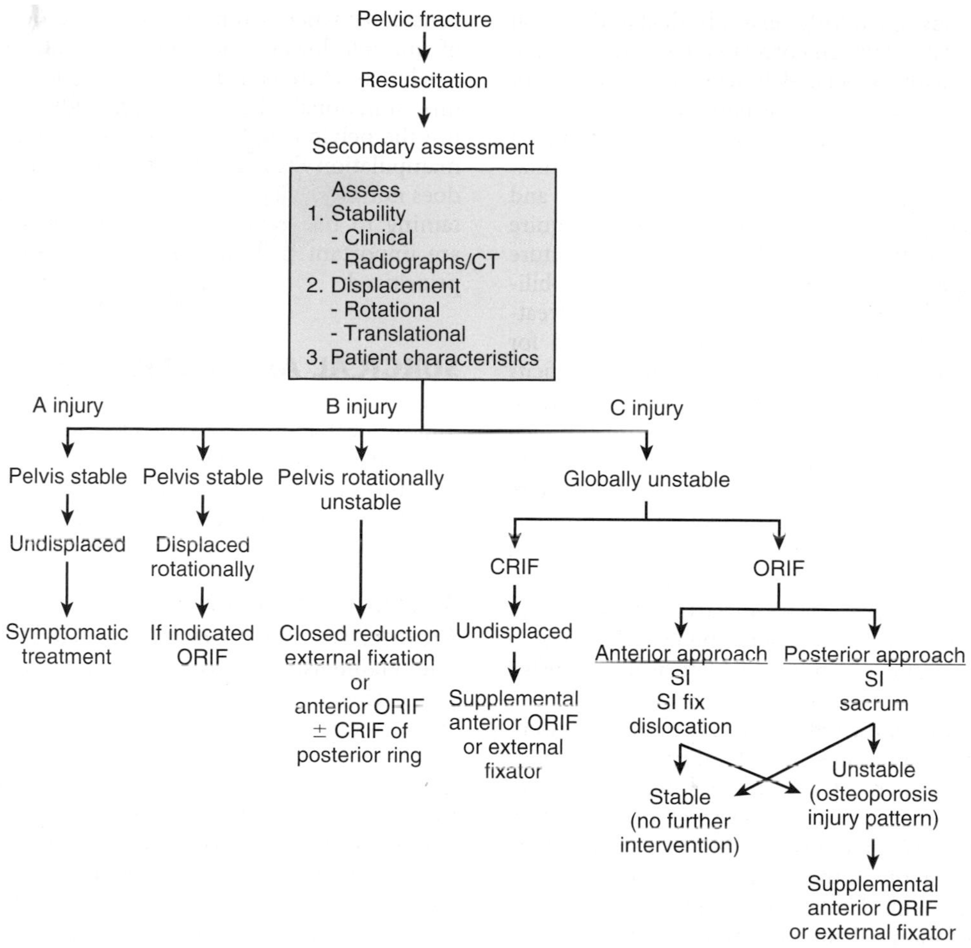

Figure 40-38. Algorithm for management of pelvic fractures. *CRIF,* Closed reduction and internal fixation; *CT,* computed tomography; *ORIF,* open reduction and internal fixation; *SI,* sacroiliac.

(subtype B2.1). It is unlikely that these injuries will displace farther, but imaging is only a static evaluation of a dynamic injury process, and recoil can lead to underestimation of initial displacement. Nonsurgical treatment is a process that requires adaptation if conditions change. Thus, if patients are difficult to mobilize, if there is significant internal rotation of the ring with associated injuries to the genitourinary system, or if an air density is detected in the SI joint along with possible anterior SI ligament injury, then anterior external fixation or evaluation under anesthesia may be considered, depending on the surgeon's preferences.

Major displacement of the symphysis pubis (>2.5 cm) is an indication for operative stabilization.[187] Fractures and dislocations through the SI joint have a high incidence of sequelae such as long-term pain, discomfort, and nonunion.[76,183,188] To reduce the likelihood of these problems, operative stabilization of the pelvis is indicated to ensure reduction and stability. Extraarticular SI joint fractures occurring through the iliac wing (C1.1) or sacrum are globally unstable and have the potential for further displacement. If initial displacement is acceptable, these may be closely monitored with radiographs as the patient is mobilized. If initial displacement is deemed unacceptable, fractures of the posterior ring should be treated operatively unless medically contraindicated. Significant displacement is defined as:

- Leg length discrepancy greater than 1 cm
- Significant internal rotation abnormality (>20 degrees as compared with the opposite side) with loss of external rotation of the lower extremity past neutral. Similarly, the lack of internal rotation past neutral in an external rotation-type fracture is significant.

Indications for surgical stabilization may be expanded if early patient mobilization because of the associated injuries is thought to be beneficial. It may be argued that this helps to diminish pain, instability, or subsequent displacement during early rehabilitation but has not been substantiated in the literature.

A tilt fracture (see Fig. 40-16) leads to a significant deformity, which can be particularly problematic in females because they may be subject to dyspareunia caused by the proximity of the displaced fragment to the vagina. If a stable fracture is significantly displaced, intervention may be required because subsequent surgical correction is more difficult after osseous healing.

In addition to the above factors, decision making in the treatment of sacral fractures in particular is primarily based on fracture pattern and neurologic status. Recently published functional outcome studies indicate that only a minority of sacral fracture patients were able to return to their preinjury vocational status more than 1 year after injury. The vast

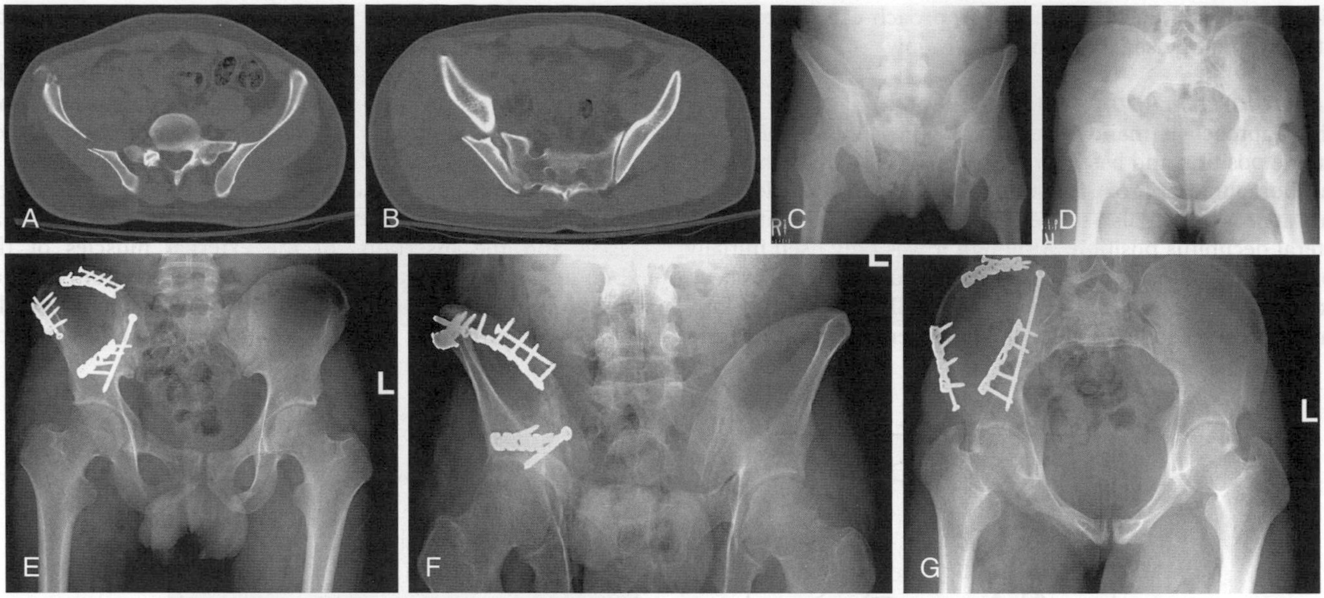

Figure 40-42. Iliac fracture with anterior extension stabilized through a lateral approach. Plates were placed on the tension side of the injury to protect interfragmentary fixation.

tissue medially, it is important to not incise medial to the iliac crest. The external oblique muscle is then incised medial to the ASIS for 3 to 5 cm and reflected caudally. The inguinal ligament is incised along this distance over the iliopsoas muscle, similar to the exposure of the lateral window of the ilioinguinal approach. This provides for improved exposure and visualization of the anterior SI joint. The SI joint can be seen after medial retraction of the iliopsoas muscle as well as the organs in the smaller and larger pelvis. The SI joint can best be seen after exposure by placing a Hohmann retractor posteriorly subperiosteally with the tip fixed at the pars lateralis of the sacrum. Subperiosteal placement is essential to protect the lumbosacral plexus. A second Hohmann retractor can be placed more caudally. The lateral femoral cutaneous nerve is located just medial to the anterior superior spine and must be protected in this approach. At this point, with flexion and internal rotation of the hip to relax the psoas and iliacus, careful dissection along the inner table of the iliac wing will bring the SI joint into view. Because the iliac wing usually displaces posteriorly, the sacrum is generally found anterior to the iliac wing. Care should be taken to avoid going through the iliacus onto the sacrum and damaging the L5 root. By following the displaced iliac wing, the articular cartilage of the SI joint can be identified, and by moving both superiorly and posteriorly, the sacral ala can be identified. Subperiosteal dissection is then carried along the ala. Care should be taken to gently retract the soft tissues medially, including the L4 and L5 roots. The L5 root normally courses 2 to 3 cm medial to the S1 joint in a small groove before passing over the anterior aspect of the sacrum to drop into the true pelvis. After the superior aspect of the sacral ala has been identified, dissection continues along the anterior aspect of the ala and the pelvic brim down inside the true pelvis to identify the notch. The surgeon must take care that the dissection remains subperiosteal and avoids injury to the superior gluteal artery. If bleeding does occur, packing of the area can usually control it. After the dislocation or fracture dislocation has been identified, the SI joint may be denuded of cartilage on its sacral side and the subchondral plate roughened if fusion of the joint is desired. If desired, bone graft can be harvested from the anterior iliac crest. The fracture or dislocation is then reduced. In addition to the SI joint, isolated iliac wing fractures can be addressed using the anterolateral approach. The anterolateral approach can be extended to the ilioinguinal approach by also opening the more medial two windows.

Lateral Approach

Most iliac fractures can be fixed using the anterolateral approach, which allows excellent visualization of the iliac fossa. Although few patients truly need a lateral approach, alone or in combination with medial fixation of the ilium, the lateral approach does remain an option for stabilization of fractures involving the ilium (Fig. 40-42). The patient is positioned either supine or in the lateral decubitus position, and the incision is placed along the iliac crest with sharp dissection of the subcutaneous tissue. The abductor muscles are detached from the iliac wing for subperiosteal exposure to the outer cortex of the ilium.[201]

Posterior Approaches

Compared with anterior approaches, posterior approaches are used relatively infrequently for ORIF of pelvic ring fractures.

Paramedian Approach (Fig. 40-43)

Of the posterior approaches to pelvic ring injuries, the paramedian approach, as described by Letournel, is the most utilitarian and can be used for SI joint fracture-dislocations, SI joint dislocations, and sacral fractures and has extensive utility in delayed reconstruction or repair of malunions and nonunions of the pelvic ring.[202]

The patient is placed in the prone position on a radiolucent table with the hip extended to neutral and the knees flexed to protect the sciatic nerve. Adequate fluoroscopic images are obtained before the preparation and draping. The gluteal cleft

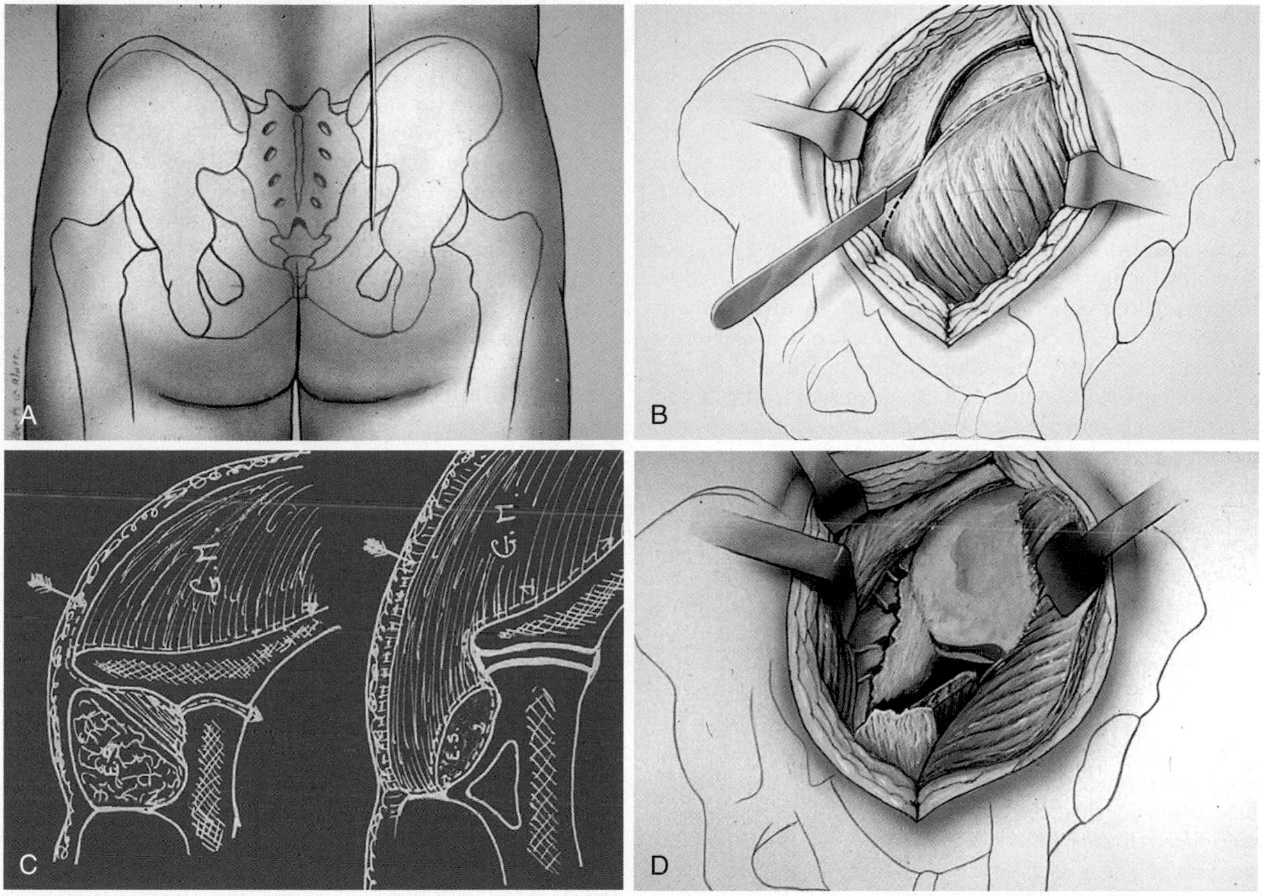

Figure 40-43. Posterior approach to the pelvic ring. **A,** Incision lateral to the posteroinferior iliac spine. **B,** Elevation of the gluteus from the posterior crest and midline. **C,** Cranial and caudal extent to gluteus maximus past the posterior iliac crest. **D,** Deep exposure after elevation of the glutei from the ilium and erector spinae from the sacrum, allowing access to all injuries of the posterior pelvic ring.[201]

is isolated from the operative field, and the skin is antiseptically prepared. Commercially available radiolucent tables and devices that facilitate anchoring of the stable hemipelvis to the table allow for longitudinal traction to the unstable hemipelvis without the potential for deformity introduced by the use of a perineal post. A longitudinal incision is made 2 cm lateral to the PSIS. It is important to not incise directly on top of the PSIS to avoid compression postoperatively when the patient lies in the supine position because wound healing disorders may occur. This incision may be curved slightly in its cephalad extent if more anterior exposure of the iliac crest is needed. Cutaneous flaps are then raised off the fascia of the gluteus maximus to the midline. The abductors are released from their origin on the posterior iliac crest to the PSIS. The origin of the gluteus maximus is released from the PSIS and the dorsal fascia of the multifidus. Care should be taken during the dissection to preserve this origin to facilitate later repair of the glutei. The glutei are then elevated as a flap based on the superior and inferior gluteal artery and nerve from the external surface of the ilium.[203] If not already disrupted by the injury, access to the SI joint and sacrum can be accomplished by elevation of the erector spinae from the dorsal sacrum. Entrance into the true pelvis through the greater sciatic notch is initially gained by release of the sacrotuberous and sacrospinous ligament attachments to the lateral sacrum. Care should be taken when dissecting along the lateral and ventral notch to protect the superior gluteal neurovascular pedicle.

A similar approach using the lateral position can provide more anterior iliac access for reduction and fixation of SI joint fracture-dislocations or iliac fractures. By placing the patient in the lateral decubitus position and carrying the incision along the iliac crest to the posterior tubercle and then distally as previously described, the surgeon can mobilize the gluteal mass from the outer aspect of the pelvic ring. Then, by detaching the abdominal musculature and iliacus from their attachments to the inner aspect of the iliac crest, the SI joint and sacral ala may be visualized. Care must be taken to not devascularize the iliac wing if both sides of the bone are elevated; in addition, detachment of the abductor mass has been associated with a higher incidence of heterotopic ossification.[204] Depending on the exact location of the injury, the approach can be modified and extended superiorly or inferiorly.

Excellent reviews about the surgical approaches to pelvic ring disruptions have recently been published by Becker and colleagues[205] and Lehmann and colleagues.[206]

DEFINITIVE TREATMENT

Logical decisions regarding the stabilization of pelvic injuries require knowledge of the mechanical stability of different internal and external techniques. A mechanical study showed that in bilateral unstable posterior injuries, the anterior external fixator frame does not afford enough stabilization to allow weight bearing because the posterior pelvic ring transmits load from the leg to the spine.[18] Mears and Rubash attempted to improve the mechanical stability of external fixation by using pelvic transfixation pins, but this technique led to insertional difficulties and problems with nursing care. By adding another cluster of pins to the anterior inferior spine region, Mears and Rubash achieved increased stability.[144] McBroom and Tile suspended a pelvis from the sacrum, which allowed full triplanar motion and showed that all existing external frames would stabilize the pelvic ring sufficiently to allow mobilization of the patient if the posterior osseous ligamentous hinge remained intact. With disruption of this posterior hinge, unstable pelvic injuries could not be stabilized with any of the existing external frames. The best external frame design was a rectangular construct mounted on two to three 5-mm pins spaced 1 cm apart and inserted into the iliac crest. Using a similar model, McBroom and Tile showed that internal fixation could significantly increase the force resisted by the pelvic ring when compared with external fixation.[207]

For unilateral SI dislocation, direct fixation across the joint with cancellous screws or anterior SI fixation with plates failed at similar loads.[208] Tile and Hearn showed that iliosacral lag screws have the best pull-out strength if they have a 32-mm thread length and are positioned in the sacral body.[18] Posterior iliosacral screws that have purchase in the sacral body (S1) constitute a suitable technique, but insertion may be complicated by neurologic or vascular injury. More recently, the transiliac-transsacral screw, a variation of the iliosacral screw, has been used increasingly as a method for percutaneous stabilization of the posterior pelvis.[209] These are effectively longer iliosacral screws with a slightly altered starting point and trajectory that allows them to traverse the entire upper sacrum from one outer cortex of the ilium to the other. Because they exit the contralateral iliac cortex, they may provide a greater degree of stability and serve to stabilize associated contralateral posterior pelvic injuries. Transiliac-transsacral screws may be particularly useful in patients at higher risk of iliosacral screw fixation failure, such as in the presence of osteoporosis, sacral comminution, significant posterior pelvic instability including spinopelvic dissociation, obesity, anticipated noncompliant behavior, and bilateral posterior pelvic injuries and as for the treatment of nonunion.

Anterior Pelvic Ring Fixation: Symphyseal Reduction and Stabilization

Because an external rotation force is required for symphyseal disruption, reduction of the deformity requires internal rotation of the hemipelvis to close the symphysis. These injuries can be addressed with either external fixators or symphyseal plating, the latter being the gold standard.[35]

Supraacetabular Fixator. However, for emergency stabilization, the supraacetabular external fixator can be recommended.[210] The patient is placed supine. Under fluoroscopic control, one pin is inserted with a starting point established at the AIIS superior to the acetabulum and directed approximately 70 degrees posteriorly and 30 degrees medially on each side to follow the robust column of bone above the sciatic notch and directed toward the PSIS (see Fig. 40-32, *D* to *G*). After identifying the supraacetabular bone, a 1- to 2-cm incision is made, and blunt dissection is carried down to the supraacetabular location. The intended screw trajectory is drilled, and the Schanz screw can then be inserted, with the goal of placing the tip as close as possible to the SI joint to maximize biomechanical stability. The Schanz screw should gently be turned by hand and allowed to seek its way between the inner and outer cortical tables of the innominate bone. Rotational reduction maneuvers followed by connection of the external fixation pins with a stabilizing bar completes the procedure. The pins can be used as a handle to assist the reduction maneuver, if necessary. Biomechanical stability of the supraacetabular construct has been shown to be better than that of the external fixator applied to the iliac crest.[151,153,211] Moreover conversion to ORIF is easier with the supraacetabular fixator.

Subcutaneous Anterior Internal Fixation Device (Fig. 40-32)

Although the above-described placement of the supraacetabular external fixator provides adequate stability of rotationally unstable but vertically stable pelvic injuries,[210] the disadvantages of this technique pertain to problems with positioning of the anterior fixation bar, which can cause difficulty with patient mobility and with sitting in particular, as well as with surgical access to the lower abdomen and pelvis. Application of this type of external fixation frame can also be challenging in obese patients because of a lack of acceptable clearance between the fixation bar and the underlying skin, making application of the external fixator potentially impossible versus resulting in decreased biomechanical stability because of increased distance of the bar from the pelvis and increased risk of infection and pin loosening contributed to by large, gaping pin tracts. One proposed method designed to mitigate these problems involves the placement of a subcutaneous, pedicle screw-based construct, which has been referred to as the "INFIX."[156] Because this technique is less efficient than the more routine external fixation technique, it should only be used on a more elective basis and is not indicated for emergent pelvic stabilization in the hemodynamically unstable patient.

Fluoroscopic imaging is used to identify the starting point of the screw in a manner similar to that described for the supraacetabular external fixator. The beam should be directed in the obturator-outlet direction to identify the teardrop-shaped column of bone from the AIIS to the PSIS. A 2- to 3-cm longitudinal incision is centered over the AIIS in line with the groin crease. The AIIS is identified on the iliac oblique view of the hemipelvis and is accessed with blunt dissection. The interval between the sartorius and tensor fascia lata muscles is developed to access the AIIS. The starting point for the supraacetabular pin is immediately proximal to the insertion of the rectus femoris tendon. Potential dangers include injury to the lateral femoral cutaneous nerve and injury to the hip capsule. Hohmann retractors are placed on either side of the iliac bone. A pedicle awl is used to establish the starting point, and either a drill or pedicle finder is then used to create the pedicle screw tract between the inner and outer tables of the ilium. The lateral or iliac oblique views can be used to confirm the starting point and to direct the screw tract toward the PSIS just above the sciatic notch. After measuring the depth of the tract, and, depending on the size of the patient, a screw that will lie 15 to 40 mm proud of the AIIS is selected. The screw head lies ideally at or just superficial to the level of the sartorius muscle. In some morbidly obese patients, this could be 30 to 40 mm away from the bone. Placement of the screw deeper than this level is not recommended because of the risk of compression of underlying structures by the bar after it is attached. The typical screw diameter is 7 to 9 mm, and the length of the screw may vary from 75 to 140 mm, depending on the habitus of the patient, with at least 60 mm of the screw being intraosseous. A rod is then contoured with an anterior convexity, cut to a length approximately 5 cm longer than the distance between the screws and tunneled just under the skin from one screw to the other, superficial to the sartorius muscle. The location of rod placement is at the superior border of what is known as the "bikini" area, formed by the groin creases on each side and superiorly by a fold of the abdominal tissue. Because this area does not change between sitting and standing, the rod does not interfere with these functions when positioned in this area. Compression or distraction can then be performed between the rod and screws in a manner similar to how this instrumentation is used in the spine, and the excess rod length can be trimmed after definitive tightening of connections between screws and rod. Hardware removal is usually done within 6 months.

Symphyseal Plating

Usually symphyseal plating is performed using a Pfannenstiel approach; however, it can also be done through a midline approach. After the exposure has been completed, a variety of reduction techniques can be used. The simplest and least invasive method uses a pointed reduction (Weber) clamp that can be applied through the soft tissues to the anterior pubic bodies just caudal and lateral to the pubic tubercle. The clamp can also be placed obliquely to address small vertical step-offs at the symphysis (Fig. 40-44). It is usually unnecessary to place clamps through the obturator externus muscle and membrane into the medial margin of the obturator foramen. A more powerful and invasive alternative is the Jungbluth clamp placed on the anterior pubic bodies, anchored to anterior-to-posteriorly positioned screws, usually accompanied by a nut on at least one side.

After a satisfactory reduction is achieved, an appropriate plate is contoured and applied to the superior aspect of the pubic bodies. The choice of plate depends on the type of associated ring injury as well as the presence and stability of posterior fixation. If the posterior osseous ligament hinge is intact (a stable AP compression injury), the use of a single plate placed on the superior aspect of the pubic bodies and crossing the symphysis is adequate. According to a recently published study, there is no difference in stability when comparing locked and unlocked plates for symphyseal plating.[212,213]

The symphysis cycles in tension and compression, depending on the patient's position. For this reason, both the surgeon and the patient need to be aware that all symphyseal fixation constructs ultimately loosen or fail. Clinically and radiographically, these failures are often subtle, but they can be more dramatic as well, particularly when mobilization limitations are exceeded.

We generally use a four- or six-hole 3.5-mm plate with a minimum of two screws placed on each side of the pubic symphysis. Although different plates are available, the one with the best fit should be used. After the plate is positioned, palpation of the posterior aspect of the pubic body determines the orientation of the drill so that the screw can be placed through the full length of the pubic body. Usually, a 50- to 60-mm screw can be placed into the body of the pubis. More

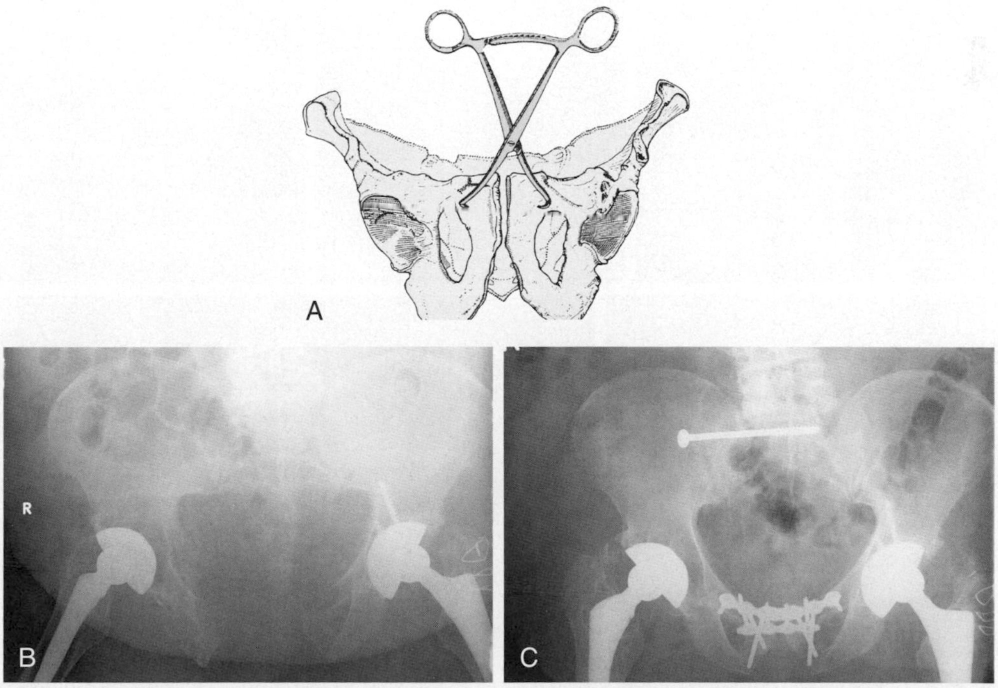

Figure 40-44. A, Typical positioning of pointed reduction forceps to achieve reduction of the anterior ring. More substantial reduction tools may be necessary in the setting of complete (C type) posterior injuries to effect reduction. **B,** Preoperative anteroposterior pelvic view of anterior-posterior compression injury with widening of the symphysis pubis. **C,** In the setting of poor bone material, typical cranially positioned plates may be supplemented with an anterior plate or posterior fixation (or both) to improve the mechanical stability of a rotational injury after reduction.

lateral screws are shorter, but they may be directed to engage the primary pubic body screw to provide additional fixation in osteoporotic bone. In the unusual setting in which a second plate is deemed useful, it can be contoured along the anterior aspect of the pubic bodies and the screws placed in an anterior-to-posterior direction between the superiorly placed plate screws. These screws must not be left proud, extending beyond the posterior pubic ramus, to avoid erosion into the bladder.

Anterior Pelvic Ring Fixation: Pubic Ramus

If a pubic ramus fracture occurs in combination with a symphyseal disruption and requires exposure as well as fixation, the ramus fracture can be fixed by extending the surgical exposure of the symphysis (Pfannenstiel approach) along the pubic ramus. If a modified Stoppa approach has been used before, this can also be extended to expose a pubic ramus fracture. The reduction can be accomplished, and stabilization of the symphysis will usually control displacement of the pubic ramus. If the displaced fracture is within 4 cm of the body of the pubis, a plate may be extended out laterally onto this area to achieve plate fixation. If an extensile approach is required for reduction and stabilization of a pubic ramus fracture, particularly more lateral injuries at the root of the acetabulum, it is accomplished through an ilioinguinal anterior approach. This approach allows adequate exposure of the whole anterior aspect of the pelvis and appropriate plate fixation with a well-contoured 3.5-mm reconstruction plate. Screws inserted at or lateral to the iliopectineal eminence will penetrate the hip joint and should therefore be avoided.

Usually isolated pubic ramus fractures do not have to be fixed, with the exception of some tilt fractures, because of possible associated injuries.[214] However B-type injuries with pubic ramus fractures anteriorly and incomplete disruption of the ipsilateral SI joint should be treated surgically. Here the supraacetabular fixator is an easy and less invasive tool for stabilization.[210] We generally leave it in place for 3 weeks and then loosen it and evaluate the pain. If the patient is pain free, it can be removed. On the other hand, if the patient still experiences pain, the fixator should be retightened and kept in place for 3 more weeks. Especially in elderly patients, the supraacetabular fixator has been shown to be successful in reducing pain during treatment of B-type pelvic ring fractures.[215] The INFIX technique also has potential application in this setting as an alternative to the supraacetabular external fixator. The Stoppa approach is useful, especially for the combination of acetabular fractures and anterior pelvic ring instability. Regardless of the approach used, the standard fixation technique for pubic ramus fractures is plate osteosynthesis.

Superior Ramus Screw Fixation

Intramedullary screw fixation of ramus fractures offers a percutaneous alternative to ORIF or external fixation for anterior pelvic ring fixation and can be extremely effective in skilled hands. Although the role of the pubic ramus screw has been poorly defined, it appears to provide adjunctive anterior ring stability, especially in rotationally unstable injuries.[216,217] Ramus screws can be placed in either a retrograde (starting at the symphysis and directed above the acetabulum) (Fig. 40-45)

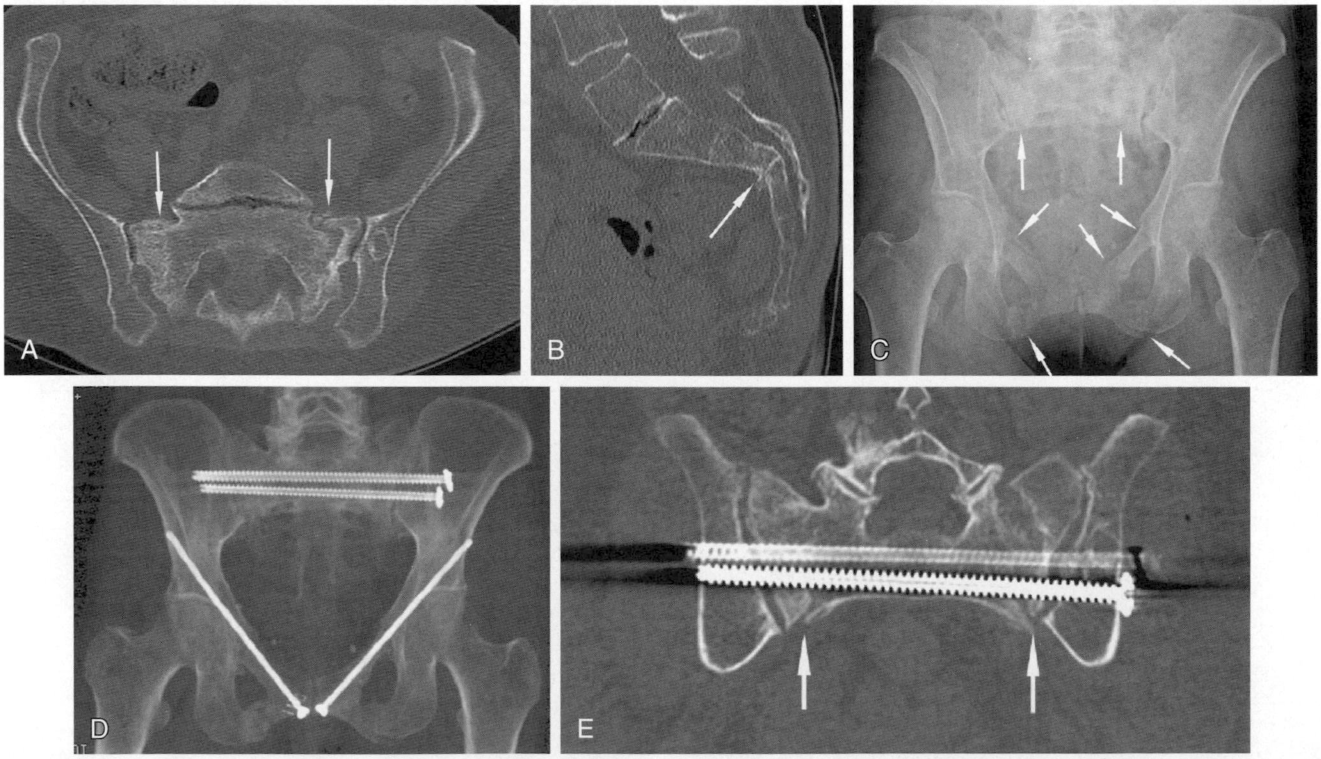

Figure 40-45. Axial (**A**) and sagittal (**B**) computed tomography (CT) images showing sacral U insufficiency fracture in patient with osteoporosis, causing back pain and loss of bowel and bladder function. These fractures are often associated with anterior pelvic ring fractures, as seen on the anterior-posterior (AP) radiograph of the pelvis (**C**). Depending on the circumstances, these injuries can be treated nonoperatively or operatively with either percutaneous or open techniques. In this medically frail patient with minimally displaced fractures, percutaneous transiliac transsacral and pubic ramus screw techniques were felt to be appropriate, as illustrated by postoperative AP (**D**) and axial CT (**E**) images of the pelvis. After treatment with decompression and lumbopelvic fixation, bowel and bladder function returned, and pain resolved.

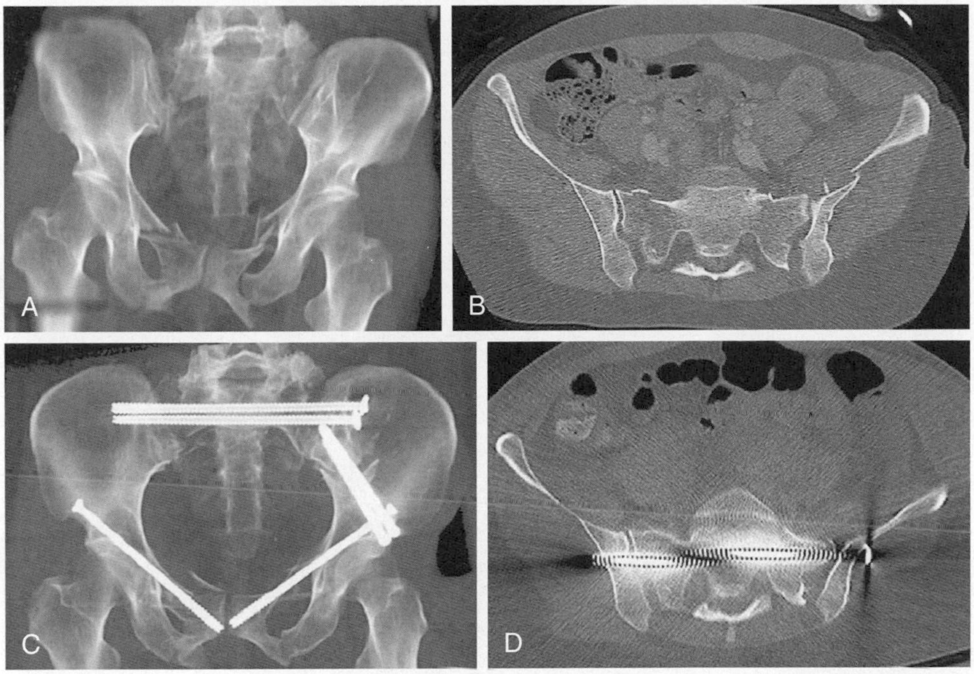

Figure 40-46. Lateral compression pelvic fracture treated with percutaneous techniques. Anterior-posterior (AP) (**A**) and axial computed tomography (CT) (**B**) images of pelvis of a pedestrian struck by a car demonstrate bilateral pubic ramus fracture, sacral fracture, and left iliac wing fracture. These injuries were amenable to percutaneous techniques with transsacral-transiliac, antegrade superior pubic ramus and iliac screw fixation, as illustrated on postoperative AP (**C**) and axial (**D**) CT images. *(Courtesy of M.L. Routt, Jr, MD.)*

or antegrade (starting on the ilium superolateral to the acetabulum and directed toward the symphysis) (Fig. 40-46) fashion. The patient is positioned supine with a bump beneath the buttocks to allow for mild hip extension, which facilitates clearance of the anterior thighs during retrograde screw insertion. If antegrade screw fixation is selected, the ipsilateral arm should be folded across the body. Antegrade screws can be more difficult because of the extent of the buttock musculature, but the desired trajectory of retrograde screws can be impeded by obesity or large thighs. Careful planning and review of preoperative imaging is essential because variations in pubic ramus anatomy, such as excessive curvature, may preclude the use of ramus screws. The two key fluoroscopic images used to direct the placement of ramus screws are the inlet and obturator-outlet views. For antegrade screws, it is easier to use a cannulated system, with appropriate starting point and trajectory established percutaneously by extrapolating along the pubic ramus from the two key fluoroscopic projections. For retrograde screws, a stab incision is made at the level of the contralateral pubic tubercle. Blunt dissection allows placement of the drill tip just lateral to the symphysis below the ipsilateral pubic tubercle. Drilling is done under fluoroscopic guidance to ensure intraosseous drilling and to avoid penetration of the hip joint.

Posterior Pelvic Ring Fixation: Iliac Wing Fractures and Sacroiliac (Fracture) Dislocations

Iliac wing fractures or SI joint injuries can be reduced and fixed both anteriorly and posteriorly.[202,206,218-220] Fixation is achieved by interfragmentary compression and the application of neutralization plates. Advantages of the anterior approach include better visualization of the cranial and anterior SI joint, which can then be reduced under direct visualization. It may be easier to denude the articular cartilage of the SI joint to facilitate the insertion of a bone graft for potential fusion of this joint. Reduction of the caudal portion of the SI joint may be difficult from the anterior approach when the SI joint is globally unstable. Careful CT evaluation of the SI articulation is imperative before SI joint reduction from an anterior approach. In a lateral compression mechanism, the anterior SI joint may be impacted and reduction and fixation made difficult or even impossible from an anterior approach. The advantages of the posterior approach are its surgical simplicity in exposing the iliac wing and SI joint. The decision regarding which approach to use is determined by the characteristics of the soft tissue injury and the fracture. A combination of approaches and techniques is often advantageous. The anterior approach is indicated for SI joint dislocations and fracture-dislocations involving the ilium, for iliac wing fractures, and when either of these injuries occurs in conjunction with an associated anterior pelvic ring injury that requires fixation.

Lateral compression injuries may also be amenable to closed reduction and percutaneous fixation techniques, both anteriorly and posteriorly (Fig. 40-46).

Sacroiliac (Fracture) Dislocations: Anterior Approach

The anterolateral approach is common for the anterior access to the SI joint. As previously discussed, the iliac wing usually displaces posteriorly, and the sacrum is generally found anterior to the iliac wing. If bleeding does occur, packing of the area can usually control it. After the dislocation or fracture-dislocation has been identified, the SI joint may be denuded of cartilage on its sacral side and the subchondral plate roughened if fusion of the joint is desired. A small bone graft can

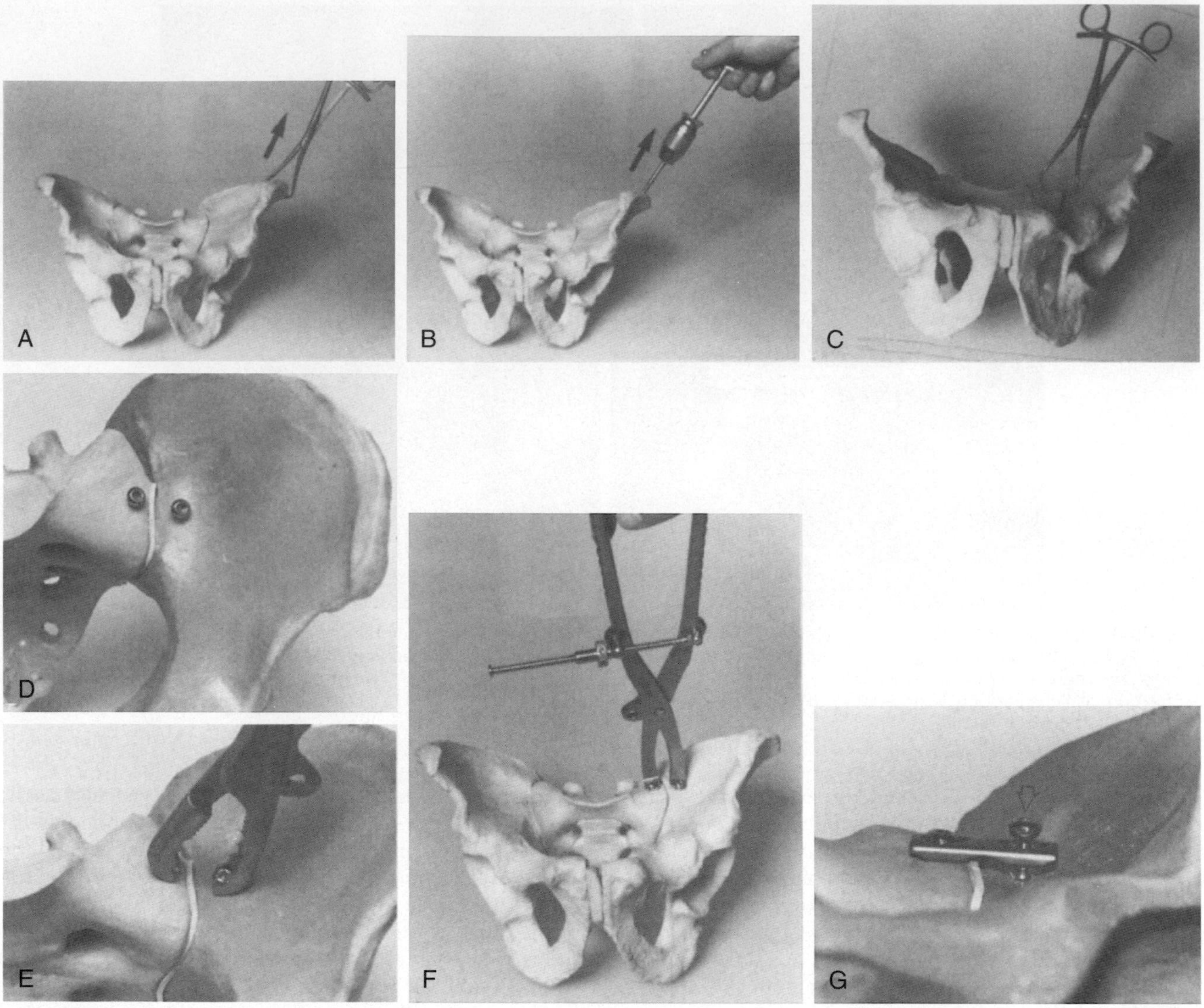

Figure 40-47. Reduction technique for sacroiliac (SI) dislocation—anterior approach. **A,** Use of a pointed reduction clamp to apply traction and control rotation. **B,** A Schanz screw in the iliac crest to apply traction, produce translation, and control rotation. **C,** A pointed reduction clamp may be used to maintain reduction through a previously drilled hole in the sacrum and the iliac wing, or a large asymmetric pointed clamp may be placed onto the anterior aspect of the sacrum, just medial to the SI joint, and then passed over the posterior aspect of the iliac crest (not shown). **D,** Preinsertion of two screws on either side of the sacral iliac joint. The reduction may be performed with a Farabeuf clamp. **E** and **F,** Pelvic reduction clamp. **G,** Reduction may also be achieved indirectly by using a plate attached to the sacrum with one screw and subsequently using a second screw to pull the pelvis up and in. The flat plate is inserted into the sacrum and fixed. A gap is left under the SI joint but will be reduced when the iliac screw *(arrow)* is tightened. *(From Tile M, editor: Fractures of the pelvis and acetabulum, ed 3, Baltimore, 1995, Williams & Wilkins.)*

be taken from the anterior iliac crest; however, in our experience, this is rarely needed. The fracture or dislocation is then reduced. Reduction is best accomplished by placing bone-holding forceps on the iliac wing through the interval between the ASIS and AIIS to grasp the hemipelvis and pull it forward. Five-mm Schanz pins in the iliac crest can be helpful as joysticks to obtain the correct rotational position of the hemipelvis. By pulling the pelvis anteriorly with the reduction clamp and rotating it with the Schanz pin, reduction is obtained at the level of the SI joint.

By using an asymmetrical pelvic reduction clamp, the SI joint can be reduced and stabilized provisionally. One arm of the clamp is placed on the posterior aspect of the iliac crest and the other on the anterior aspect of the sacral ala (Fig. 40-47). The direction of force is such that the joint is pushed anteriorly and closed down posteriorly. With a fracture through the iliac wing, this maneuver helps reduce the dislocation. Reduction may also be accomplished by placing one screw into the sacral ala and one into the iliac wing and then applying the pelvic reduction clamp. Provisional stabilization is achieved by placing a 3.2-mm Steinmann pin percutaneously through the iliac wing into the ala. Before reduction, this pin may be inserted through the ilium into the iliac side of the SI joint so that its position is confirmed under direct vision. A 3.5- or 4.5-mm three- or four-hole reconstruction plate is then contoured appropriately. In the case of associated iliac or acetabular fractures, longer plates can be chosen to bridge all fractures. One screw is placed into the sacral ala and directed parallel to the SI joint. The direction of the screw can be determined by placing a 1.6-mm Kirschner wire (K-wire) in the

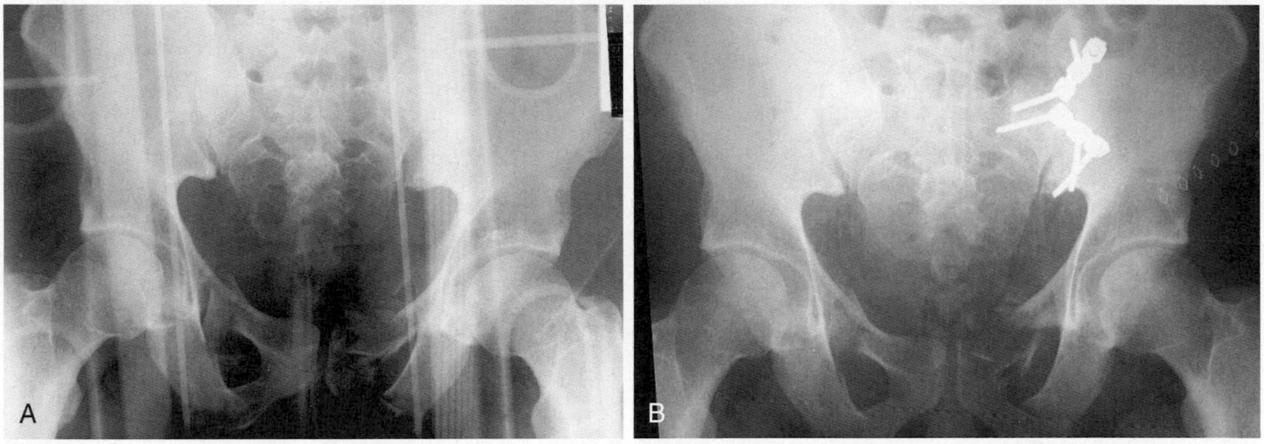

Figure 40-48. Rotational injury with complex anterior ring fractures is an indication for an anterior approach to the sacroiliac (SI) joint. **A,** Rotational injury to the left SI joint with multifragmentary bilateral rami fractures. **B,** Stabilization of the SI joint using an anterior approach.

joint at the time of reduction. These screws are usually 30 to 40 mm long. The plate is attached to the iliac wing by fully threaded cancellous screws, which usually traverse the length of the posterior tubercle (Fig. 40-48).

At times, a small ridge may overgrow the SI joint on either the iliac or the sacral side. This ridge may make reduction and plate fixation difficult and can be removed. A final way of stabilizing the joint after reduction is achieved is by insertion of a percutaneous cancellous screw into the sacral body and neutralization with a three- or four-hole 3.5- or 4.5-mm anterior SI plate.

Similar reduction and fixation techniques are used to reduce and stabilize the caudal portion of the SI joint component of a fracture-dislocation, if needed. This should be accomplished first because reduction of the joint should take precedence over fracture reduction. Reduction and interfragmentary fixation of accompanying fractures of the iliac wing followed by neutralization plating completes the fixation construct if there is a combination injury of SI dissociation and an iliac wing fracture (Fig. 40-49).

In our own practice setting, we try percutaneous reduction and screw fixation of the posterior pelvic ring whenever possible because of its effectiveness in stabilizing most posterior pelvic injuries and its lack of invasiveness. However, if an anterior approach is needed regardless, for example, because the patient received pelvic packing or has an anterior column acetabular fracture, anterior plating is, of course, considered to prevent further approaches.

Sacroiliac (Fracture) Dislocations: Posterior Approach (Fig. 40-50)

The paramedian approach is used most frequently for posterior reduction and reconstruction of SI joint dislocations or adjacent sacral fractures. After proper preparation, the bony structures can be manipulated for reduction and osteosynthesis. Use of a lamina spreader allows the joint or fracture to be distracted and débrided. After débridement of the joint or fracture, reduction is accomplished with the use of pointed reduction clamps, a femoral distractor, and pelvic reduction forceps. Reduction of the SI joint can be confirmed by palpation anteriorly and direct visualization of the caudal portion of the joint. Palpation along the superior border of the sacral ala and the iliac crest can also be carried out. Exposure of the caudal aspect of the sacrum at the level of the sciatic notch also provides a reliable reference point to assess the adequacy of the reduction by direct visualization and palpation. Confirmation of a satisfactory reduction by radiographs or image intensification is recommended. The cranial reduction of the SI joint dislocation can be performed with the use of a clamp from the sacrum to the posterior spine. Rotational reduction of the SI joint can be achieved with a Schanz pin in the posterior spine and held with an angled clamp placed through the greater notch.

After the SI dislocation has been reduced, iliosacral screw fixation is performed. As an open procedure, the guidewire or drill starts on the outer aspects of the iliac crest 1.5 cm anterior to a line from the posterior superior to the posterior inferior spine (crista glutea) and 2.5 cm above the greater sciatic notch (Fig. 40-51, *A* and *B*). The use of a specific point on the iliac wing demands that the SI joint be anatomically reduced and that there be minimal sacral dysmorphism. This position should be used merely as a guide to identifying an appropriate starting point. Before being advanced into the sacrum, the position of the starting point and trajectory of the drill or wire should be confirmed radiographically. AP and inlet views determine the AP position and angulation of the screw. The outlet view is used to determine the superoinferior starting position and angulation of the screw and to confirm that the guidewire or drill is being aimed into the sacral body (Fig. 40-51, *C*). The authors recommend using an oscillating drill and slowly advancing the tip using a subtle pistoning motion. This helps to ensure that the drill bit remains in bone and enhances the ability to identify an extraosseous trajectory as soon as possible. Unless a transiliac-transsacral screw is being placed (see later), three cortical barriers should be crossed for iliosacral screw placement (i.e., the outer iliac wing, the iliac side of the SI joint, and the sacral subchondral bone). If a fourth cortical barrier is encountered, the drill bit is about to leave the sacrum, with potential danger either to the cauda equina or to the anteriorly placed neurologic and vascular structures. If the position of the drill or guidewire is incorrect, it is withdrawn completely and redirected. In SI dislocations, cancellous screws with a 16- or 32-mm thread length and a 6.5- or 7.3-mm diameter are normally used.

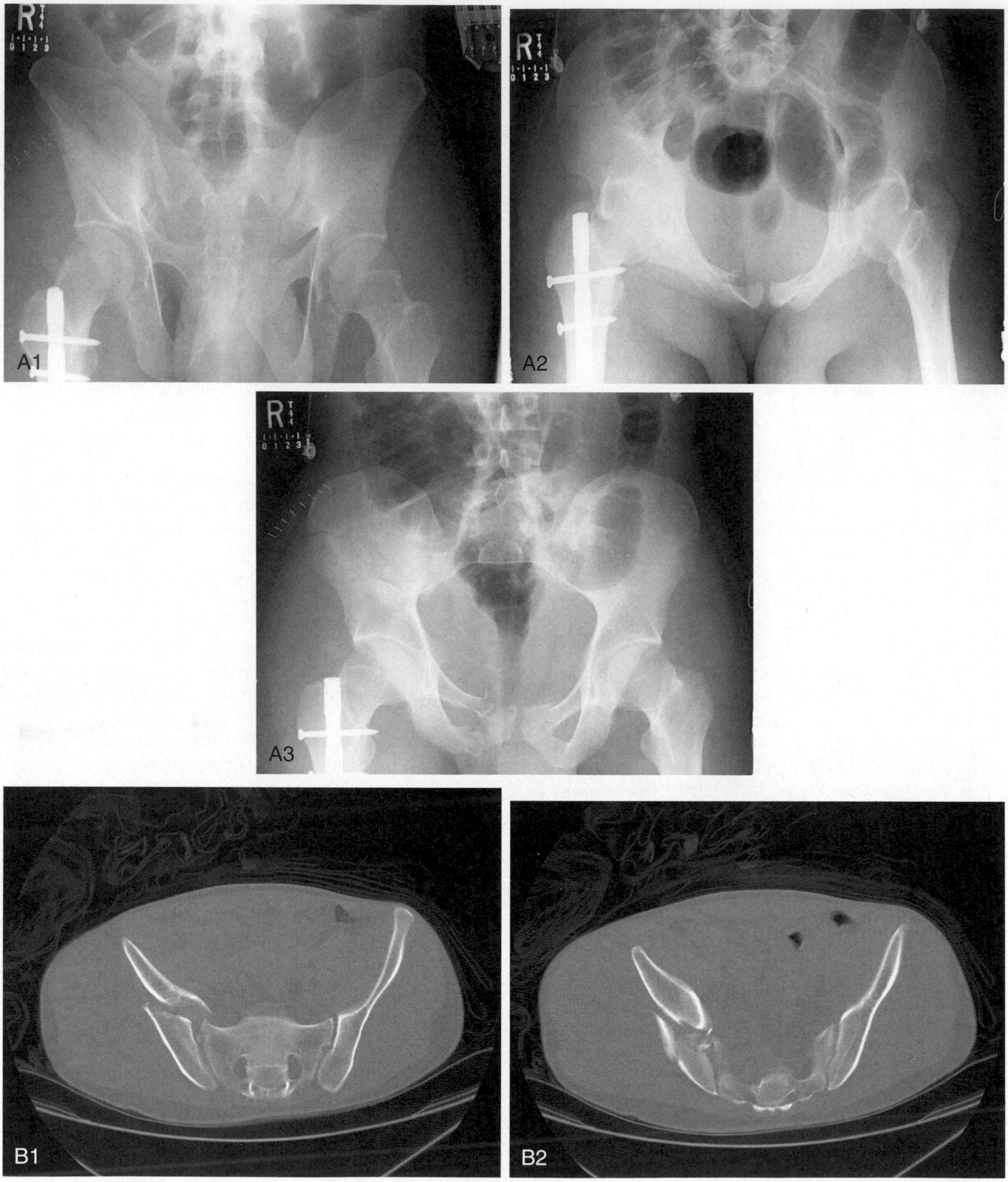

Figure 40-49. A, Sacroiliac (SI) fracture-dislocation with anterior extension. **B,** Note the sacral impaction on computed tomography.

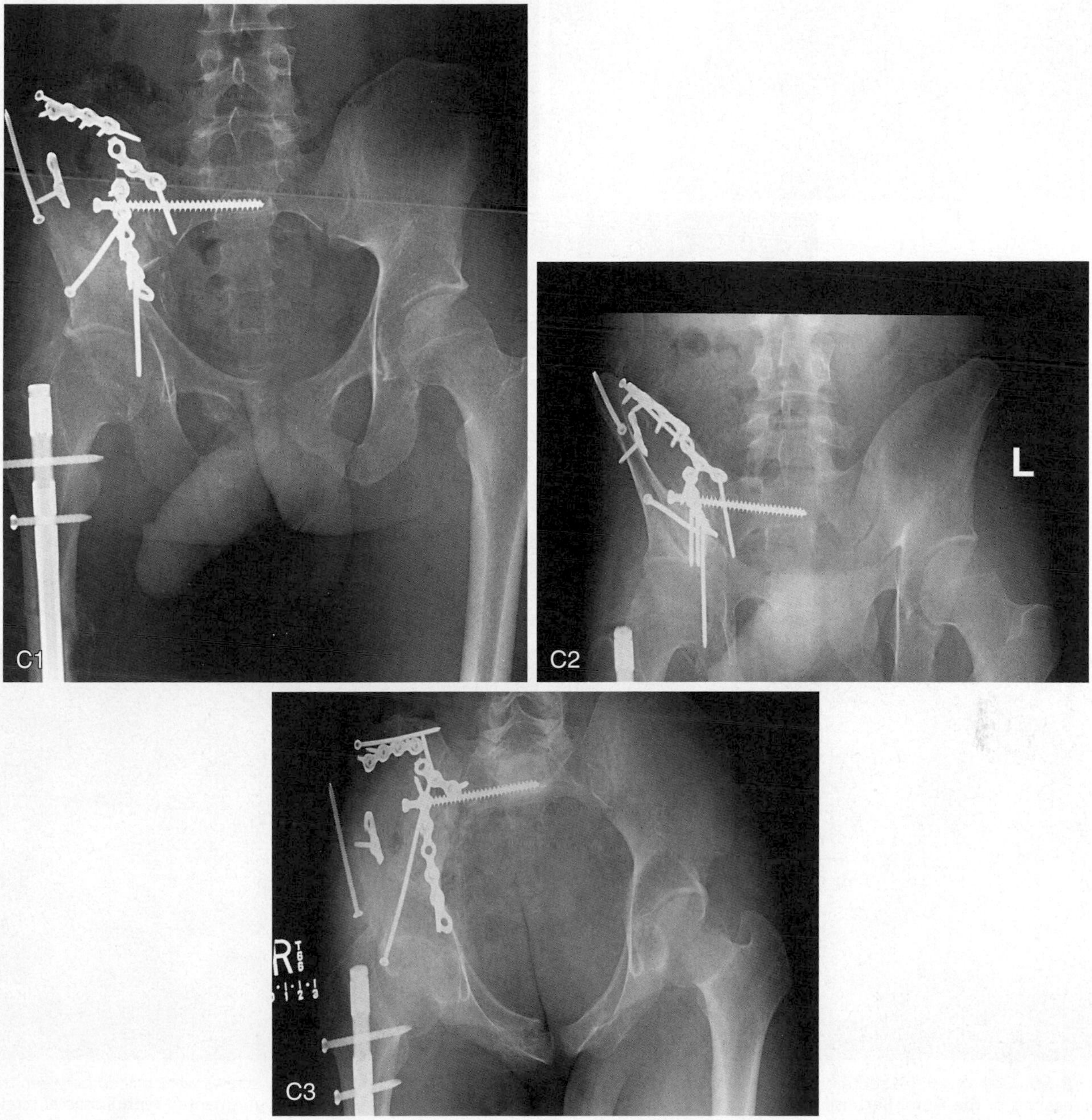

Figure 40-49, cont'd. C, SI reduction neutralized with a fully threaded cancellous screw caused by impaction of the sacrum. Screw and plate fixation of multifragmentary iliac component.

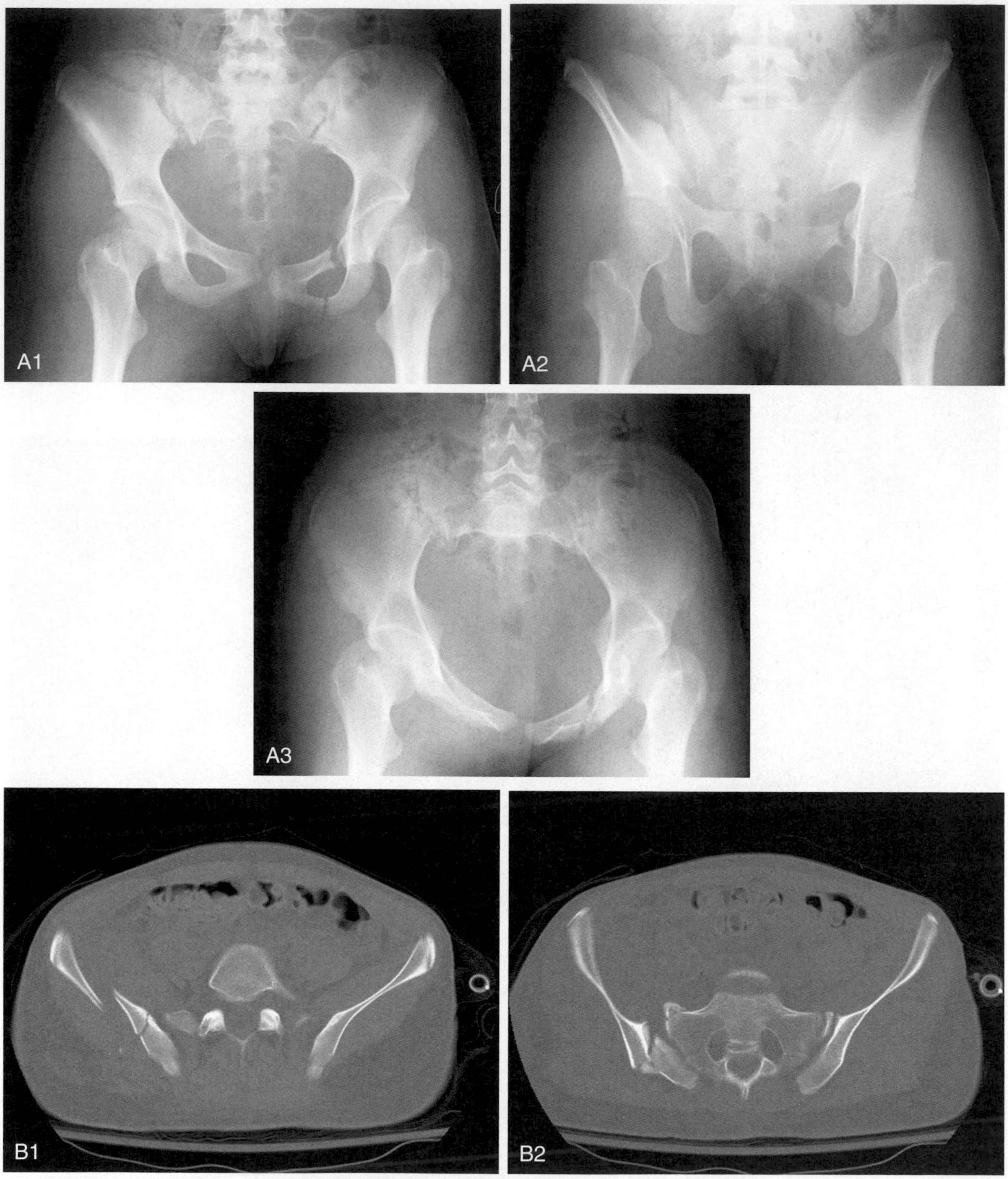

Figure 40-50. Fracture-dislocation approached and stabilized posteriorly. Note that the interfragmentary screws were placed between the inner and outer tables of the ilium. Because of a small intact cranial fragment of the intact ilium, fixation was augmented with iliosacral screws.

A small two- or three-hole plate can be applied to the outer aspect of the iliac wing, or a washer can be used to prevent intrusion of the screws into the iliac bone, which can significantly compromise screw fixation (Fig. 40-52, *A*). Tactile sensation alone in the case of percutaneous rather than open screw placement across the SI region is inadequate to determine that the screw head and washer are in contact with the posterior ilium. Routt and coauthors have recently described a technique that combines tactile sensation with radiographic assessment to prevent (versus recognize and salvage) iliosacral screw intrusion and to avoid inadequate seating of the screw, both of which have undesirable biomechanical consequences. The technique is based on obtaining optimal radiographic visualization of the position of the screw head and washer as they are being advanced against the lateral cortex of the ilium.[221] By rotating the C-arm between 20 and 40 degrees

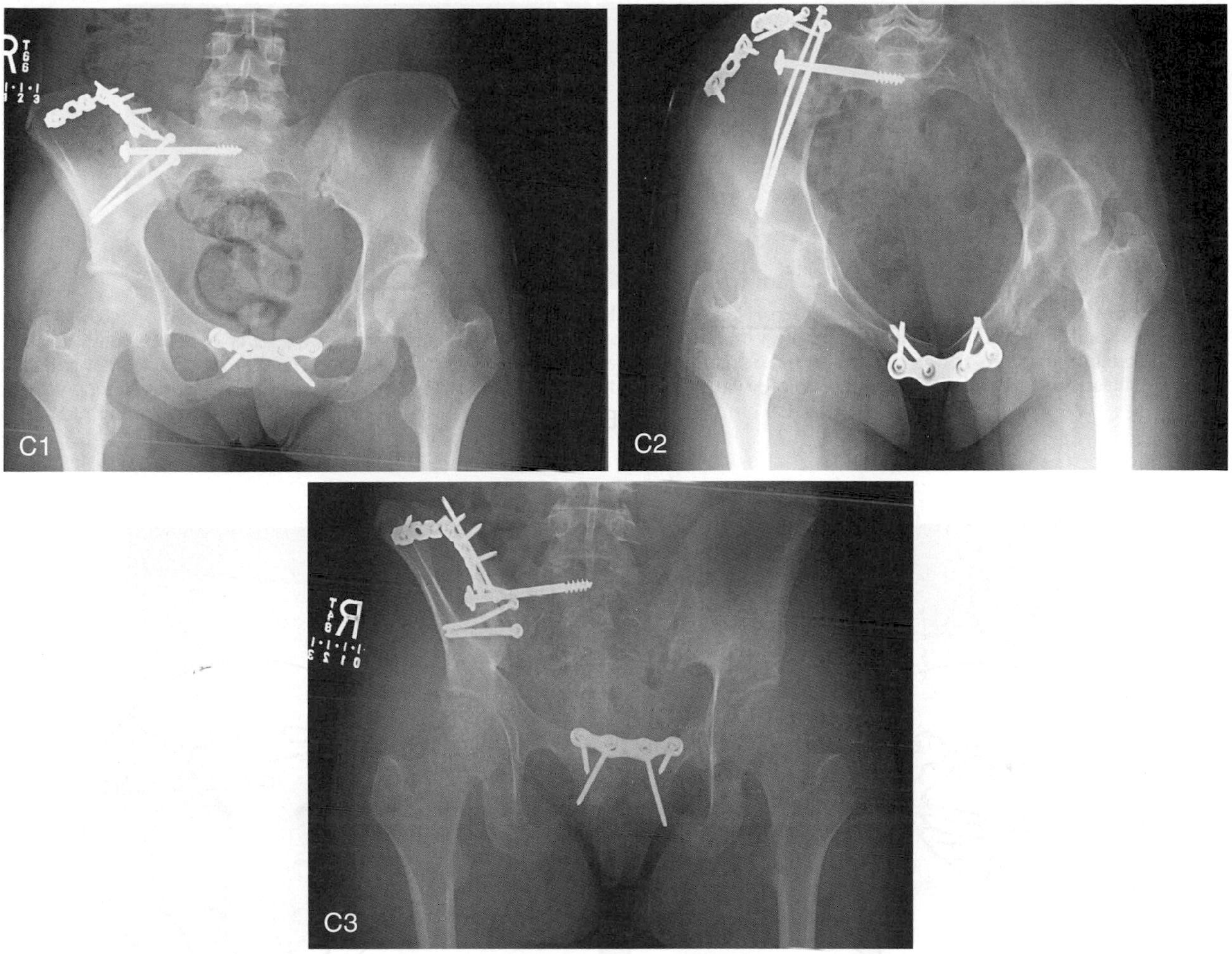

Figure 40-50, cont'd

toward the obturator oblique projection, with the exact amount determined by preoperative imaging, a patient-specific obturator oblique view can tangentially visualize the posterolateral iliac cortical surface (see Fig. 40-57) as the screw head and washer are being seated, allowing the engagement of the lateral cortex to be fine tuned radiographically (Fig. 40-52, *B*). Visualization can be further optimized by adjusting the pelvic tilt of the C-arm.

Percutaneous Posterior Pelvic Fixation

In contrast to this open iliosacral fixation procedure, we usually perform percutaneous iliosacral or transiliac-transsacral screw fixation.[155,217,222] This technique is suitable for stabilization of most SI joint dislocations and vertically oriented sacral fractures. Percutaneous iliosacral screw fixation techniques are most frequently used with closed reduction alone in the supine position. Prone positioning is usually reserved for situations in which open reduction is necessary. To use this method, the fracture must be adequately reduced to ensure acceptable alignment and preserve an acceptable safe zone for screw placement. The surgeon must have a clear understanding of the radiographic anatomy of the sacrum and the posterior iliac wing and the relationship of vital soft tissue structures, especially pertinent neurovascular anatomy. One approach to preoperative planning for percutaneous SI screw fixation is demonstrated in Figure 40-53.

Accurate iliosacral screw placement is critical to achieving maximal stability and avoiding complications. The screw must start on the outer aspect of the iliac wing, cross the SI joint, follow the S1 pedicle mass into the body of S1, and remain completely in bone. The percutaneous approach demands thorough understanding of sacral radiographic anatomy for safe screw placement (Fig. 40-54). The S1 pedicle is bordered inferiorly by the S1 root canal and foramen. The pedicle varies in size but averages approximately 28 mm in diameter. The superior surface of S1 slopes downward in a posterior-to-anterior direction at an angle of 45 degrees, with a gutter for the L5 root located 2 cm medial to the SI joint (Fig. 40-54, *C*). The internal iliac artery lies anterior to the ala and gives off its largest branch, the superior gluteal artery, anterior to the SI joint. These three structures are at risk of injury if the drill bit, guidewire, or screw penetrates through the ala. The body of the sacrum joins both ala through the pedicles and is surrounded by the cauda equina posteriorly, the pelvic viscera anteriorly, the L5 to S1 intervertebral disc superiorly, and the fused S1 to S2 disc space inferiorly. The S1 body has an anteriorly protruding bony prominence, the sacral promontory, which is anterior to the sacral ala. Screws aimed toward the promontory will course anterior to the more lateral aspects of the sacrum (in–out–in) and may cause injury to the neurovascular structures that lie anterior to the pedicle or ala. More than half of the S1 neuroforamen is filled by the S1 nerve root.

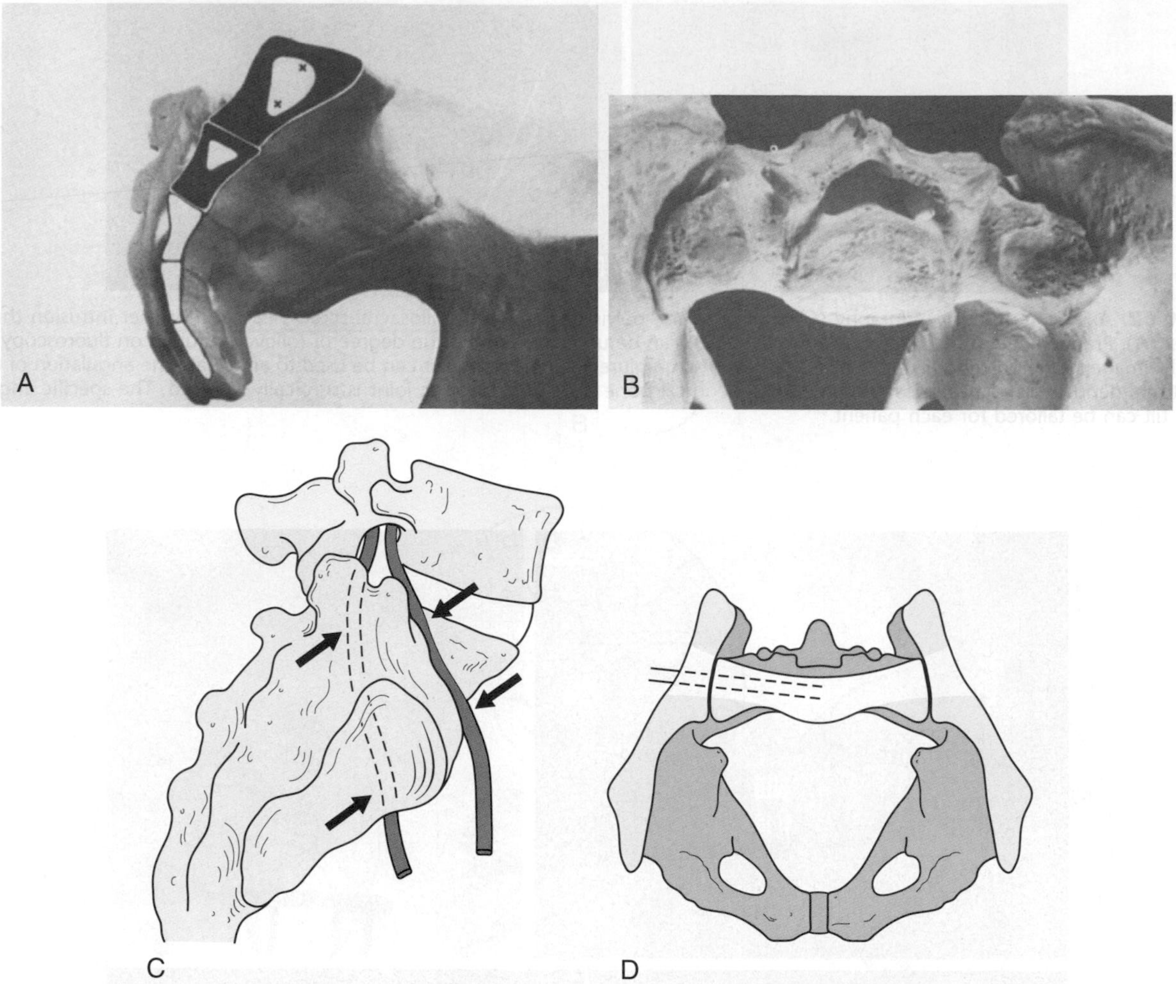

Figure 40-54. Anatomy of the upper part of the sacrum (S1–S2). **A,** This cross-section through the sacrum demonstrates the promontory of S1 and the concavity of the sacral ala. Safe placement of screws is marked by the *white area.* **B,** From above the promontory, the concavity of the ala can again be appreciated, as can the location of the posterior sacral wall. **C,** This diagram represents the course of the L5 root *(arrows)* going over the gutter of the sacral ala and descending in front of the sacroiliac joint and the course of the S1 root in a medial to lateral direction. One can see where the safe position is for screw placement. **D,** This diagram shows the area that must be taken into account for placement of a percutaneous screw from outside the iliac wing into the body of the sacrum. *(**A, B,** and **D** from Tile M, editor: Fractures of the acetabulum and pelvis, ed 2, Baltimore, 1995, Williams & Wilkins. **C** from Chip M, Chip L Jr, Simonian PT, et al: Radiographic recognition of the sacral alar slope for optimal placement of iliosacral screws: a cadaveric and clinical study, J Orthop Trauma 10:171–177, 1996.)*

It runs inferiorly and laterally to the anterior S1 foramen. Because of this inferior, sloping course, the posterior half of the body of S1 is not available for screw placement because the screw could traverse the S1 root canal. Only the middle portion of the S1 body is therefore left for screw placement near the upper S1 endplate. For safe placement of the screws, only the sacral landmarks should be used; the iliac landmarks are important to confirm reduction. The sacral landmarks are identified using fluoroscopy. Successful use of closed reduction and percutaneous fixation techniques for the posterior pelvic ring is predicated on good intraoperative imaging and the achievement of a satisfactory reduction. Osteoporosis also limits the stability of iliosacral screw fixation. This may warrant a modified mobilization plan or supplemental anterior ring internal or external fixation that would not be necessary in patients with normal bone density. Research is currently being done regarding this topic, with current trials involving cement augmentation of SI screws.[223] However, large prospective studies to evaluate the efficacy of augmented screws compared with regular screw fixation have yet to be conducted. Bilateral displaced injuries are generally not amenable to closed techniques, although it may be possible to carry out an open reduction on one side to restore a foundation for closed reduction of the contralateral hemipelvis. Last, the presence of sacral dysmorphism may complicate assessment of reduction and safe screw placement (Fig. 40-55).[4,224] Careful preoperative planning based on plain radiographs and CT with appropriate sagittal, coronal, and three-dimensional reconstructions is required to assess whether a safe corridor for screw placement exists in these cases. Closed reduction and percutaneous fixation is usually performed with the patient in the supine position because of the ease of reduction and to enable simultaneous anterior ring fixation when appropriate. Prone positioning is used if open reduction of the sacrum is anticipated or simply according to the surgeon's preference. For the supine

Text continued on p. 1080

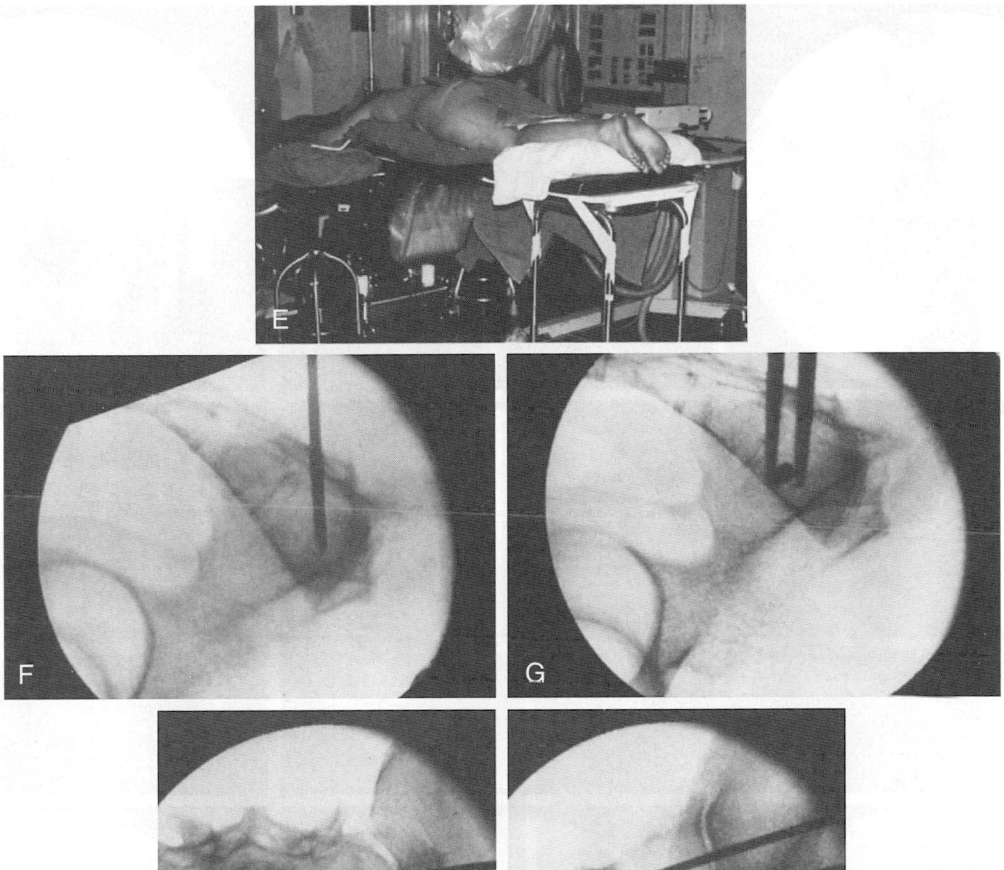

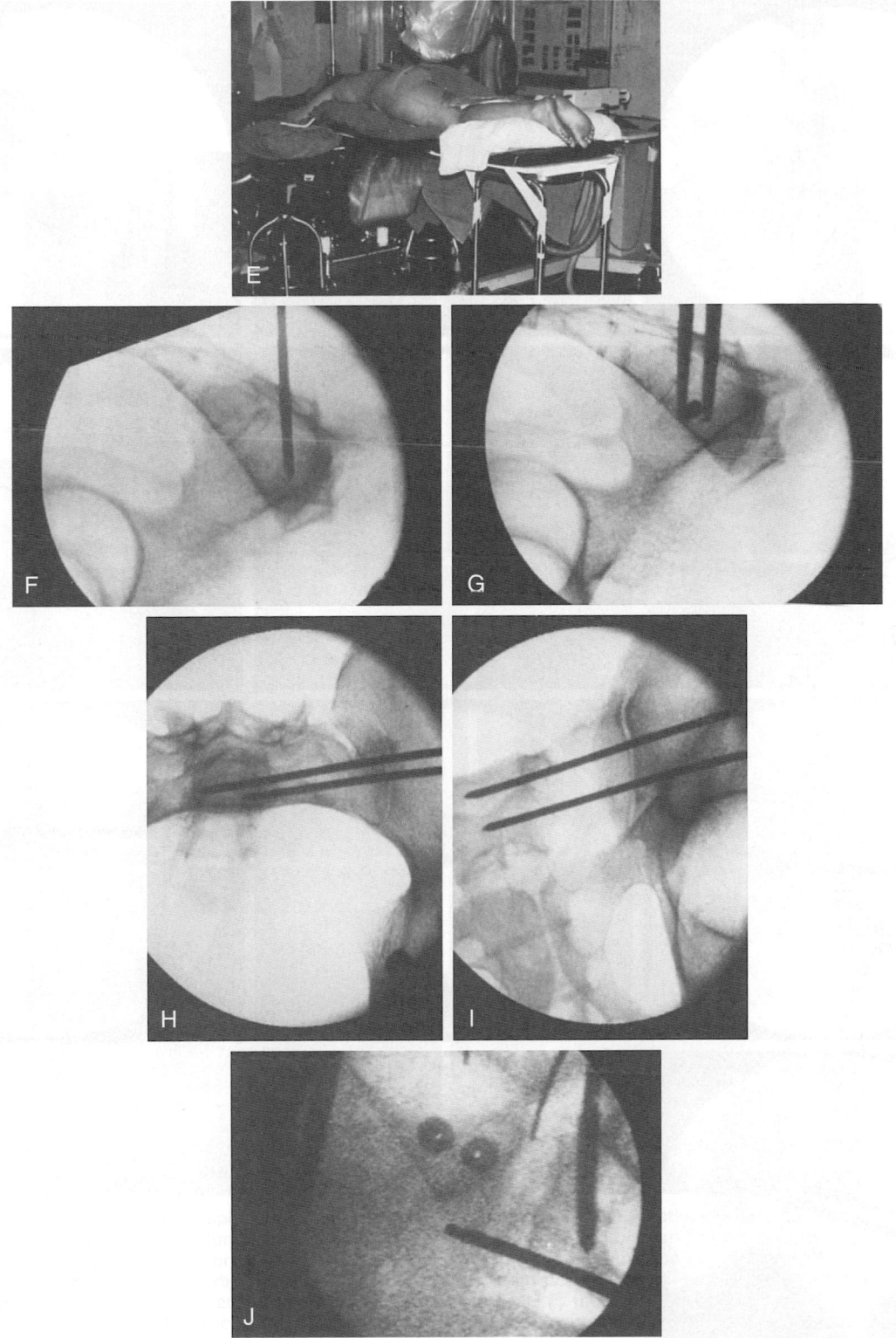

Figure 40-54, cont'd. Technique for insertion of percutaneous iliosacral screws. **E,** The prone position on a radiolucent table. Similarly, screw insertion may be accomplished with the patient in a supine position with access by the C-arm for all three views. **F** and **G,** Alignment of the guidewire or drill for placing a screw into the sacrum. Note that the alignment is behind the S2 cortex in the central portion of the body to avoid the pedicles and the promontory and is below the alar slope line. **H** and **I,** Inlet view with S1 and S2 superimposed to show the position of the guide pins in place and avoid penetration of the ala and the posterior cortex of the sacrum. The outlet view confirms the appropriate position in the S1 body to avoid the S1 foramen. **J,** Final placement of screws in the safe zone of the sacrum. *(From Tile M, editor: Fractures of the acetabulum and pelvis, ed 2, Baltimore, 1995, Williams & Wilkins.)*

Continued

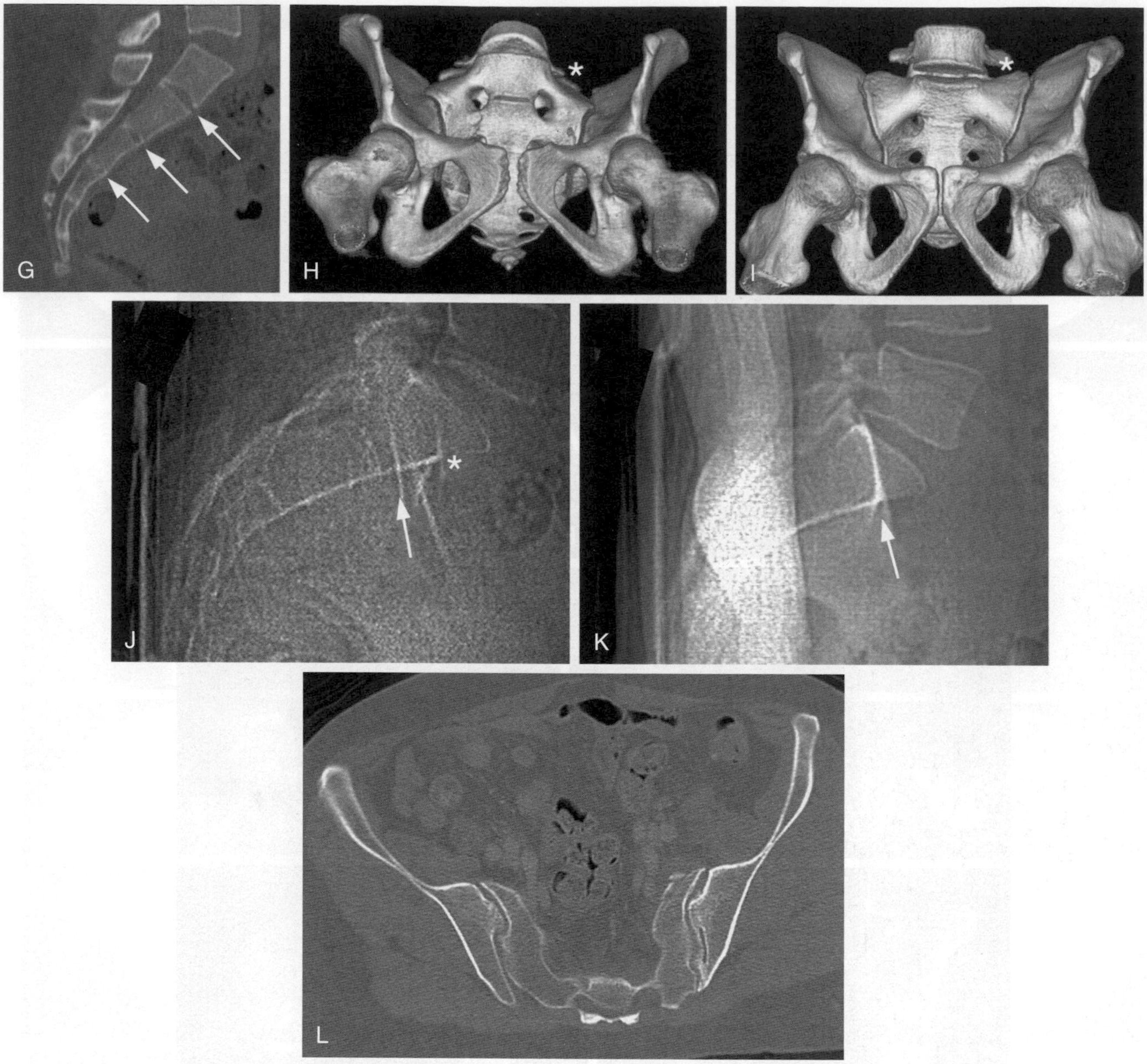

Figure 40-55, cont'd. G, Sagittal computed tomography (CT) scan of a dysmorphic sacrum demonstrating the presence of residual discs *(arrows).* **H,** Three-dimensional surface rendering of an outlet view of a dysmorphic sacrum demonstrating an acute alar slope *(asterisk).* **I,** Three-dimensional surface rendering of an outlet view of a normal sacrum demonstrating a flat alar slope *(asterisk).* **J,** Lateral CT scout radiograph of a dysmorphic sacrum with an acute alar slope *(asterisk)* that does not correlate with the iliac cortical density (ICD) *(arrow).* **K,** Lateral CT scout radiograph of a normal sacrum with an alar slope that corresponds with the ICD *(arrow).* **L,** Axial CT scan demonstrating a tongue-in-groove sacroiliac (SI) joint in a patient with sacral dysmorphism. Comparison of intraoperative fluoroscopic views obtained during screw insertion in a patient with a dysmorphic sacrum.

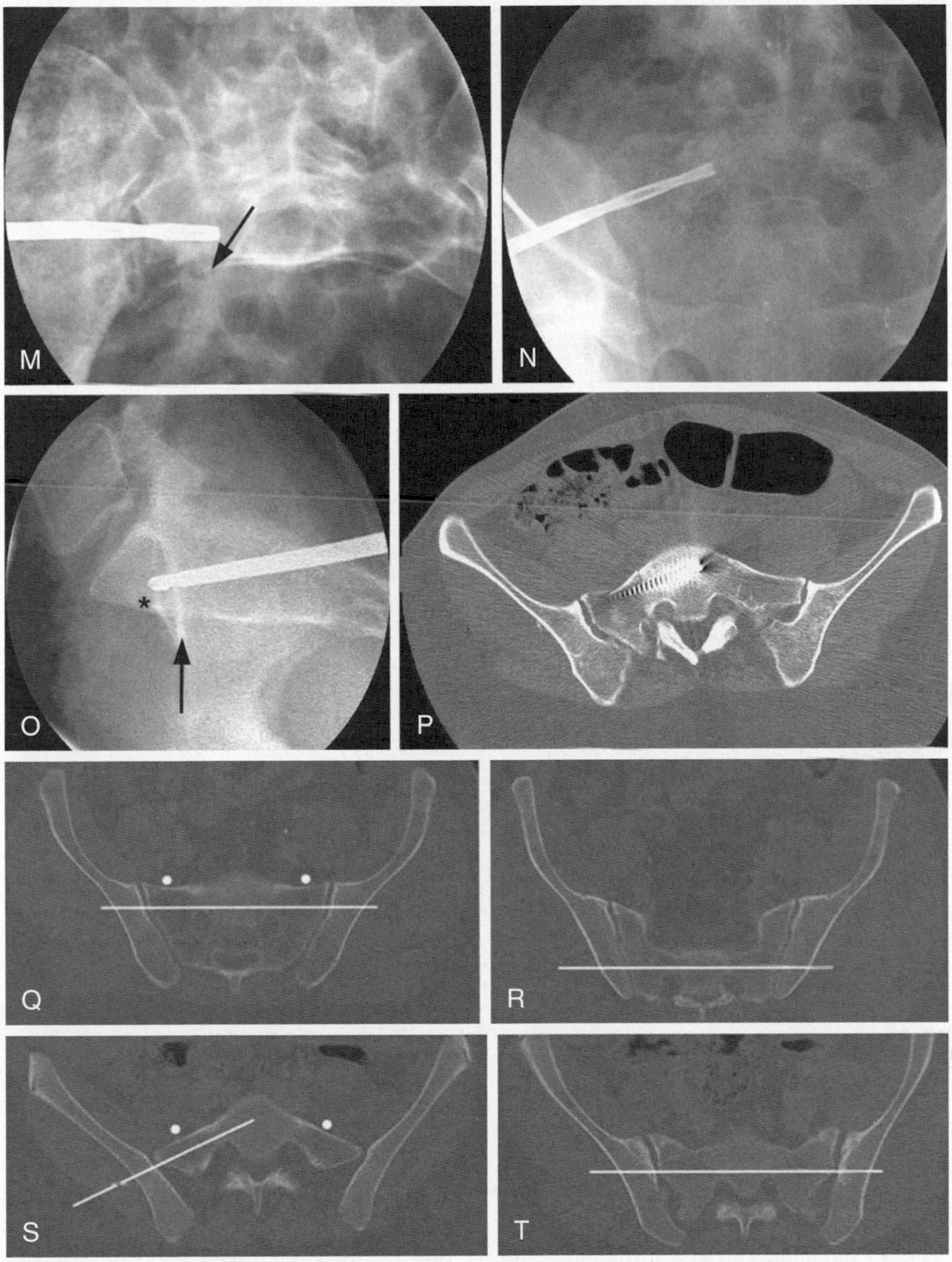

Figure 40-55, cont'd. M, Fluoroscopic inlet view with the drill located in the sacral ala and just lateral to the S1 nerve tunnel. The *arrow* represents the path of the S1 nerve root. **N,** Fluoroscopic outlet view with the drill located in the sacral ala and just lateral to the S1 nerve tunnel. **O,** Fluoroscopic lateral view with the drill located in the sacral ala and just lateral to the S1 nerve root tunnel (in the same location as in panel **M.** The drill tip lies just cranial and anterior relative to the iliac cortical density *(arrow)* but remains contained within the sacral alar bone because of the alar slope *(asterisk)*. **P,** Axial CT scan obtained to evaluate the screw trajectory. Upper (**Q**) and second (**R**) sacral segment axial CT scans in a normal sacrum. The *white lines* represent the transiliac-transsacral intraosseous pathway for fixation. Upper (**S**) and second (**T**) sacral segment axial CT scans in a dysmorphic sacrum. The *white lines* represent pathways for screw fixation. These images demonstrate that a transiliac-transsacral intraosseous pathway is available only at the second sacral segment. In panels **Q** and **S,** the *solid white circles* indicate the approximate locations of the nerve root.

Continued

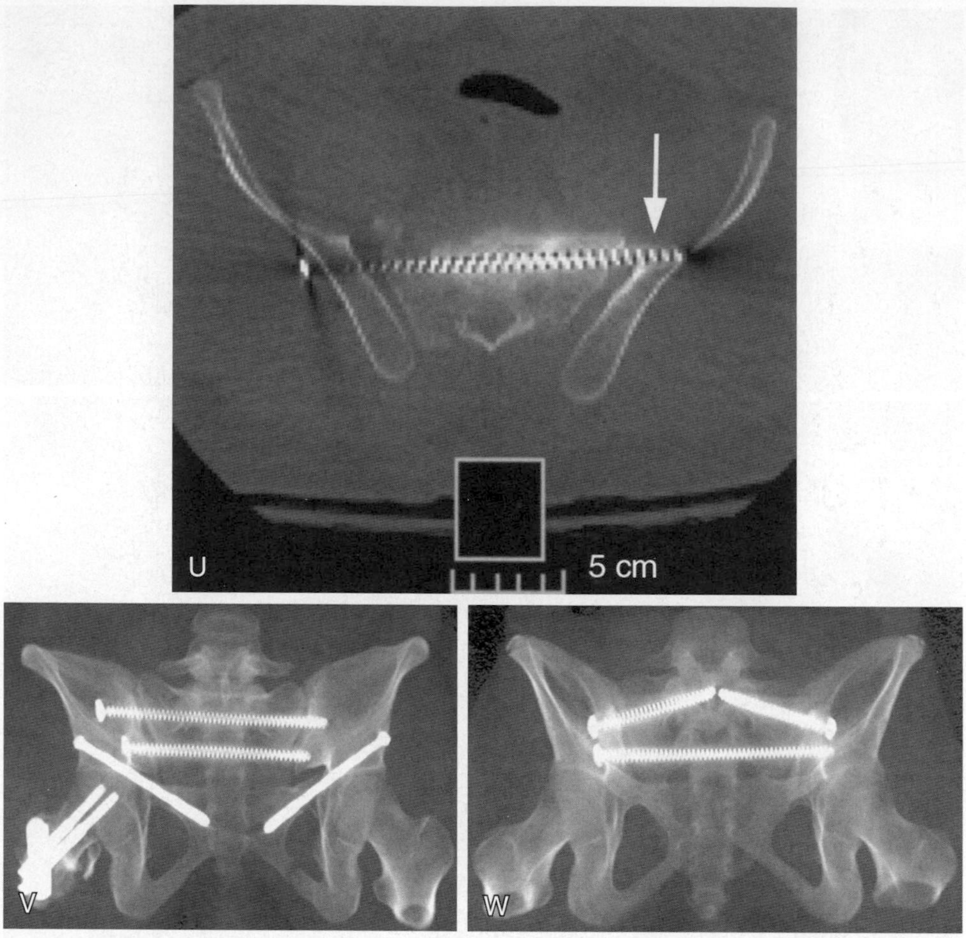

Figure 40-55, cont'd. U, Axial CT scan demonstrating malreduced SI injury with subsequent poor screw placement potentially leading to iatrogenic soft tissue injury anterior to the ilium in the region of the iliac cortical density. The screw *(arrow)* extrudes anterior to the ilium in this patient. **V,** Two-dimensional pelvic CT reconstruction of the screw fixation construct in a patient with a normal sacrum. This patient had a safe zone that permitted placement of one transiliac-transsacral screw in the upper sacral segment and one transiliac-transsacral screw in the second sacral segment. The patient also underwent percutaneous fixation of bilateral superior pubic ramus fractures. **W,** Two-dimensional pelvic CT reconstruction in a patient with a dysmorphic sacrum. This patient had a safe zone that permitted placement of SI-style screws in the upper sacral segment as well as one transiliac-transsacral screw in the second sacral segment. *(Images and legend from Miller AN, Routt ML Jr: Variations in sacral morphology and implications for iliosacral screw fixation, J Am Acad Orthop Surg 20(1):8–16, 2012.)*

position, the patient is placed on a soft radiolucent support beneath the lumbosacral spine to elevate the buttocks off the table and ensure access to the lateral aspect of the flank and buttock so that the starting point for the screw is not compromised. An entirely radiolucent table is preferred. The fluoroscopy unit is brought in on the side opposite the surgeon, and satisfactory inlet, outlet, and AP pelvis imaging as well as lateral sacral views centered on S1 are verified to be of satisfactory quality (Fig. 40-54, E to J). To obtain the inlet view, the C-arm is tilted so that the anterior cortex of S1 overlaps that of S2. If such visualization is not done, the concavity of the sacrum will not be appreciated, and the screw may exit anteriorly and place the neurovascular structures, namely L5, at risk (Fig. 40-56). However, the posterior cortex of S1 is best seen if the anterior cortex of S1 overlaps the coccyx. This projection is needed to ensure that the screw does not exit posteriorly. The outlet view is obtained by rotating the C-arm approximately 90 degrees so that the pubic tubercles lie just inferior to the S1 foramen and the symphysis overlies the midline of the sacrum. The floor positions for the fluoroscopy base and appropriate inlet and outlet angles are marked by the radiology technician for easy reproduction. After complete radiographic visualization has been obtained, fracture reduction can be undertaken and can be facilitated by the use of muscle relaxants. Closed reduction, which is usually possible within 2 to 5 days of the injury, requires knowledge of the axes of displacement of the fracture. A completely unstable hemipelvis is displaced cranially and posteriorly and is externally rotated. However, depending on the mechanism of injury, the displacement patterns may differ. Therefore, a preoperative review of the radiographic studies provides the basis for intraoperative reduction maneuvers.

The patient is prepared from the costal margins to the knees on both sides and down to the table on the involved side. The involved leg is prepared and draped free to allow manipulation. The first displacement to be corrected is the axial malposition, which is accomplished by longitudinal skeletal traction through a traction pin inserted in the distal femur. Traction counterforce may not be needed in the large patient or with early intervention. However, if greater force (>10–15 kg/25–35 lb) is required because of delay or if the patient is of small stature, stabilization of the uninvolved

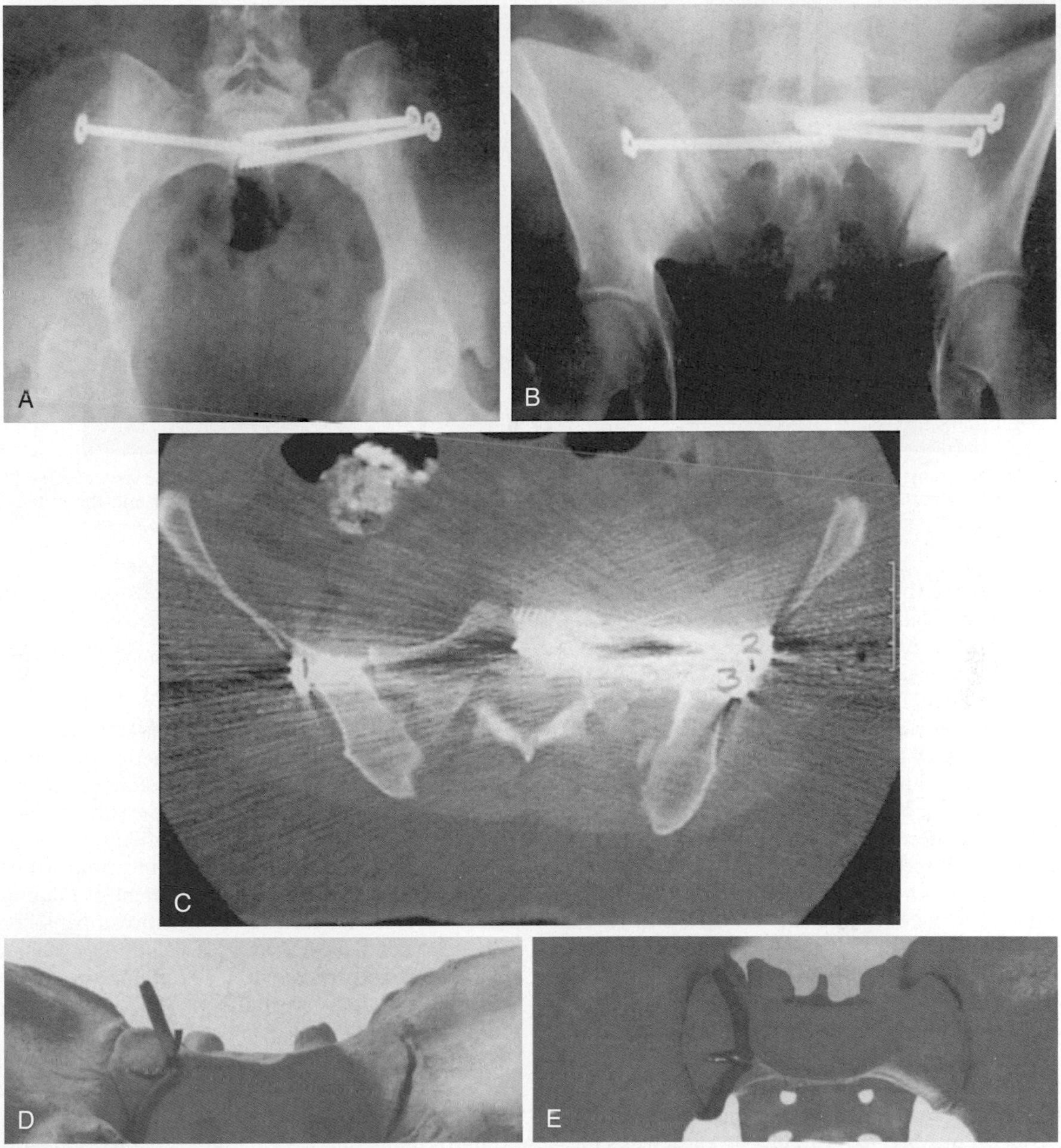

Figure 40-56. Penetration of the ala with screw placement. Inlet (**A**) and outlet (**B**) views of the pelvis show that the screw appears to be intraosseous. **C,** A postoperative computed tomography scan shows that the anterior cephalad screw is extraosseous. The patient's left L5 nerve root was injured. **D** and **E,** A plastic model shows how this injury can occur. *(**A** to **C**, from Chip M, Chip L Jr, Simonian PT, et al: Radiographic recognition of the sacral alar slope for optimal placement of iliosacral screws: a cadaveric and clinical study, J Orthop Trauma 10:171–177, 1996. **D** and **E**, from Tile M, editor: Fractures of the acetabulum and pelvis, ed 2, Baltimore, 1995, Williams & Wilkins.)*

hemipelvis may be needed. This can be done indirectly with a foot plate and soft thigh strap on the contralateral side as well as chest bolster on the side of the intervention. The most effective way to stabilize the intact pelvis to facilitate closed reduction is to secure the ilium and proximal femur to the table with a modified external fixation frame using iliac as well as proximal femoral Schanz screws. If the fracture is posteriorly displaced, the traction is directed anteriorly by flexing the hip. Rotational displacement is corrected by placing one or two Schanz screws into the involved iliac crest or supraacetabular area and using them to manipulate the hemipelvis into place. The external fixator or universal distractor can be used to reduce this component as well. These reduction maneuvers may require one or two assistants. Open reduction of a concomitant symphyseal disruption may also lead to at least a partial indirect reduction of the posterior ring. After the reduction is achieved, it is confirmed by C-arm visualization with the three views of the hemipelvis. Provisional fixation follows with a prepositioned K-wire inserted into the ala or S1 body. The superficial skin location for screw insertion is approximately 2 cm posterior to the intersection of a line extrapolated from the longitudinal axis of the femoral shaft and a line dropped from the ASIS. However, these coordinates may be distorted by soft tissue trauma or the change in position of the femur related to traction. The guidewire or drill bit is advanced through a punctate wound down to the

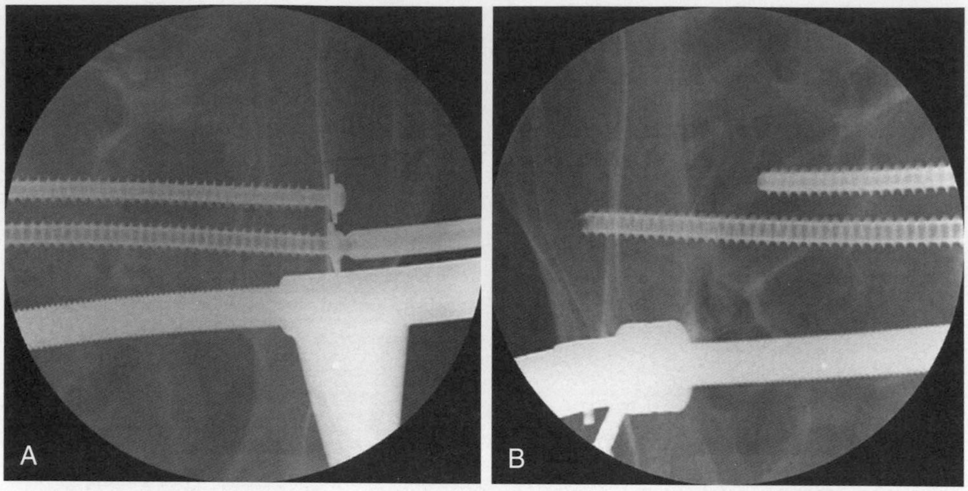

Figure 40-57. During transsacral-transiliac screw fixation, the intraoperative obturator-outlet oblique fluoroscopic view obtained tangential to the posterior iliac lateral cortical surface (see Fig. 40-52) allows visualization of the contact between the washer and the outer cortex of the ilium (**A**) and the desired screw length (**B**).[221]

posterolateral aspect of the ilium. The inlet and outlet views show that this device is aimed into the S1 body and perpendicular to the SI joint. At this point, the C-arm is used to visualize the lateral projection of the sacrum. The position of the drill bit or guidewire is confirmed to be in the middle of the S1 body. It is important to make sure that the screw is placed so that it is below the cortical projection of the sacral ala, which is seen only on the lateral view. If the position is correct, the incision can be enlarged to approximately 1 cm, and the drill bit or guidewire is advanced toward the body of S1. It is useful to halt insertion of the pin when the tip reaches the superior aspect of the lateral border of the first sacral foramen on the outlet view. A true lateral view of the sacrum is obtained again to confirm that the tip of the pin is in the alar safe zone (pedicle). The progress of the drilling is monitored on the three pelvic views. The drill bit or guidewire perforates three cortices (outer part of the ilium, inner iliac side of the SI joint, and sacral side of the SI joint). If a fourth cortex is encountered, insertion is stopped, and the drill bit or guidewire is realigned as necessary, according to radiographic evaluation. Usually, misdirected drill bits or guidewires must be completely removed and restarted to create a new tract. However, occasionally, it may be possible to reinsert through the same starting point and establish a new trajectory with the guidewire or drill in reverse and gentle medial pressure. After the position of the drill bit or guidewire is confirmed, its intraosseous length is confirmed, and an appropriately sized screw is inserted. A lag screw is used to fix an SI dislocation or zone I sacral fracture to achieve interfragmentary compression. We recommend the use of a washer, especially in osteoporotic bone. Screw head position is confirmed by rotating the anterior-posteriorly positioned C-arm 20 to 40 degrees toward the involved side (obturator oblique) to project along the axis of the outer cortex of the ilium so that the screw head is confirmed to abut the cortex (Fig. 40-57, *A*). This relationship can also be seen on the inlet view, centered on the screw head. Longer screw, placement past midline, is more difficult because of superimposition of the opposite-side alar cortical slope. Care must be taken if the screw is inserted past the midline to avoid the risk of perforation of the anterior sacral surface to not damage important local neurovascular structures.

We generally only place one screw on each side at the S1 level. If there is a need to place a second screw, this may be accomplished at the S2 level using the technique described earlier, at the S2 level.

Transiliac-Transsacral Screw Fixation

As a result of the deforming forces acting perpendicular to the implant axis, standard iliosacral screw fixation may not provide adequate stabilization, especially in more unstable injuries, obese or noncompliant patients, patients with compromised bone quality, or patients in whom stronger fixation is required, such as with the treatment of nonunion. Longer iliosacral screws that traverse the entire upper sacrum and exit the contralateral iliac cortex may improve fixation and also stabilize contralateral posterior pelvic injuries. These transiliac-transsacral screws are reliably safe to insert using routine intraoperative fluoroscopy, and they provide durable fixation. Their placement requires careful preoperative planning and more precise technical attention during insertion because they must pass through both sacral alar zones. The patient positioning, radiographic views, and general principles underlying the technique are similar to those already described for iliosacral screw fixation. Several specific technical considerations warrant extra attention when inserting screws across the entire sacrum and into the contralateral ilium. Longer guide pins are needed to accomplish this technique than are typically available, particularly in patients with truncal obesity. As one might expect, the transiliac-transsacral screw's starting point and trajectory are much more constrained, thus warranting careful planning. The starting point is established with a threaded guidewire inserted through the skin onto the lateral ilium and tends to be slightly anterior and superior relative to the typical iliosacral screw starting point. As with iliosacral screw placement, guide pin position and trajectory are evaluated and adjusted as needed using the pelvic inlet and outlet fluoroscopic views (Fig. 40-58). A true lateral sacral view is obtained before crossing both the near and far sacral nerve root tunnels to ensure safe placement. The intended trajectory is followed across the near SI joint and across the entire sacrum anterior to the S1 tunnels to the contralateral SI joint. If the flexible guidewire begins to stray off course, it can be

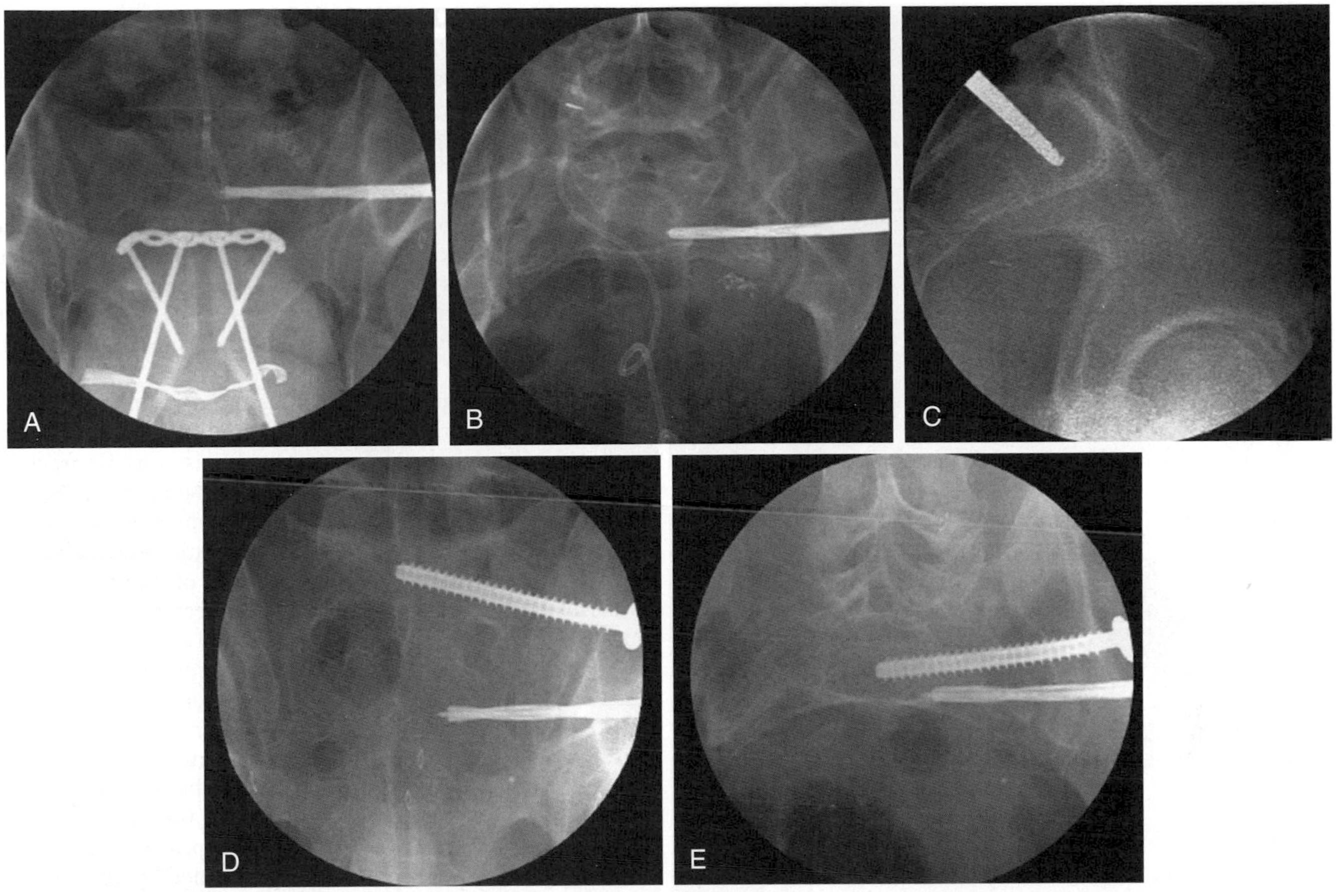

Figure 40-58. The starting trajectory for an upper sacral segment screw is exactly transverse and just cranial to the neural foramen on the intraoperative outlet view (**A**) and posterior to the ventral sacral cortex on the inlet view (**B**). The lateral sacral view (**C**) is essential to verify the appropriate position of the drill bit. Placement of an S2 screw follows similar principles based on the outlet (**D**) and inlet (**E**) views.

overdrilled and slightly corrected with the more rigid drill bit to establish the remainder of the drill path. Larger diameter guide pins (e.g., 3.2 mm) can minimize this risk. The guide pin is advanced until it is just short of exiting the contralateral iliac cortex so that an accurate length assessment can be obtained using either the cannulated screw system's pin-based depth gauge or another guide pin of equal length. The screw path is drilled and tapped along the guide pin, and a 7.3-mm cannulated screw of the appropriate length is inserted over the guide pin. Bilateral oblique fluoroscopic images along the plane of the posterior lateral iliac cortices can ensure that the screw is neither insufficiently seated nor intruded while also allowing for verification of screw length contralaterally (see Fig. 40-57).

The initial screw is positioned to allow for a second and parallel transiliac-transsacral screw. When possible, the second transiliac-transsacral screw is inserted at the same or an adjacent level to address residual rotational movement and further improve stability (see Fig. 40-45, *D*). Doing so from the same side is more efficient and saves operative time because the C-arm need not be moved to the contralateral side.[209]

Posterior plating of the sacrum (Fig. 40-59) can also be considered in pelvic ring fractures, especially in type C fractures as well as ring fractures that include comminuted sacral fractures (Fig. 40-60).[225,226] The paramedian approach should be used. The indication is the vertical unstable sacral fracture. After reduction, osteosynthesis should be performed using a 4.5-mm reconstruction plate. However, in the situation of an accompanying Morel-Lavallée lesion, the risk of infection may be increased.[225] An alternative to sacral plating is "triangular" or "distraction" osteosynthesis that uses fixed-angle screws that are placed in the PSIS and additional anchoring in one lumbar pedicle (Fig. 40-61).[226,227] Nevertheless, we generally try to avoid these techniques because most fractures can be addressed using iliosacral screw fixation, which is the less invasive technique. If additional stabilization is needed, spinopelvic stabilization techniques are appropriate, which will be described in the section dedicated to complex sacral fractures with spinopelvic instability. Sacral bars are also an appropriate option and have the advantage of requiring less dissection and being sufficiently distant from neural elements that there is low risk for neurologic complications, but the disadvantage of being less biomechanically robust than spinopelvic techniques. For placement of sacral bars, the patient is positioned prone, and bilateral modified paramedian approaches are performed with a slightly curved orientation lateral to the PSIS. After reduction and temporary fixation using either clamps or K-wires, one or two bars can be implanted at the level of the PSIS.[228]

Isolated Iliac Wing Fractures

These are uncommon injuries, most of which are avulsion fractures of the anterior superior spine after bone graft harvest from the iliac crest. The need for surgical reduction and

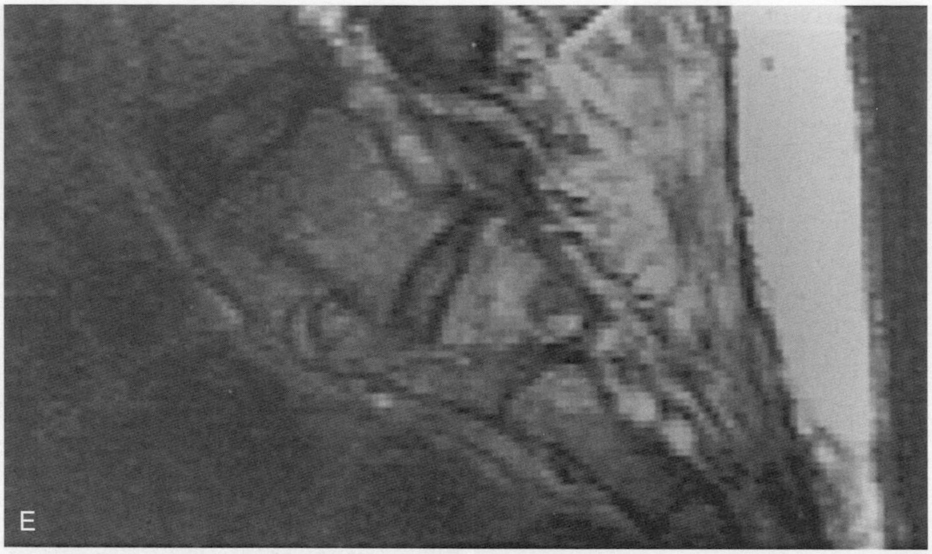

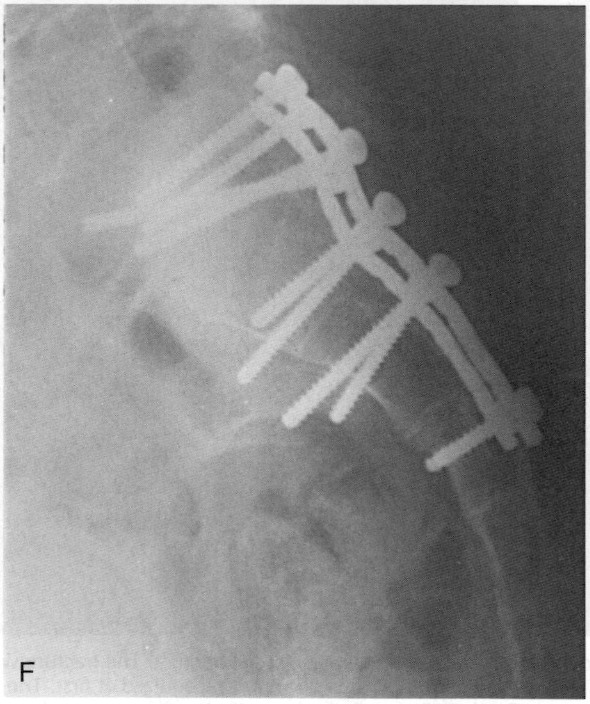

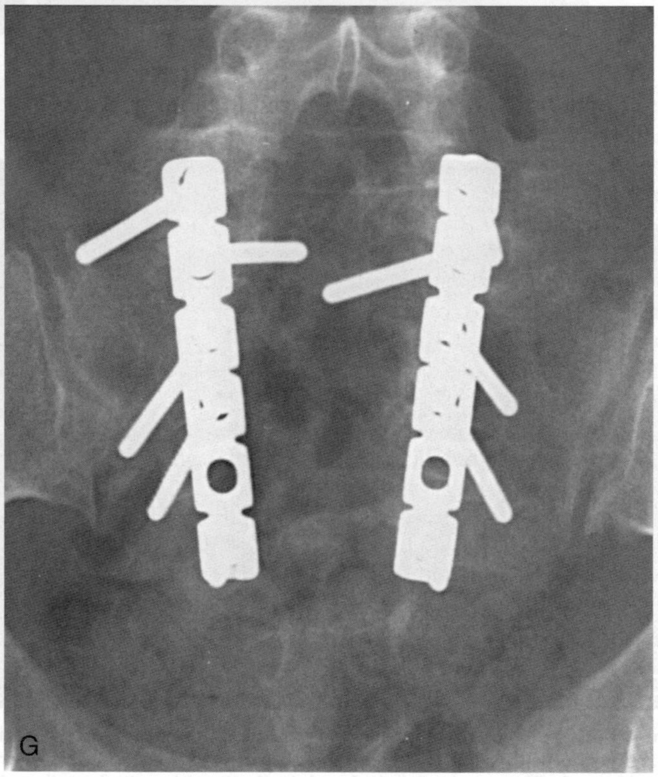

Figure 40-65, cont'd. E, The magnetic resonance image, however, shows an angulated fracture in the S2 region. The fracture was in kyphosis with the superior fragment displaced posterior to the inferior fragment. The patient underwent operative reduction and decompression with plate fixation as shown on lateral (**F**) and AP (**G**) views. The double-screw fixation in S1 stabilized the proximal fragment, with the cephalad screw directed medially and the next screw directed laterally. The patient regained bowel and partial bladder function and return of perineal sensation.

fixation also facilitates reduction of the posterior ring fracture because the anterior fixation acts as a fulcrum and prevents the compensatory anterior displacement that occurs with posteriorly applied reduction forces in these highly unstable injuries.

Spinopelvic fixation is performed through a dorsal approach with the patient in the prone position on a radiolucent frame. Unilateral sacral fractures are generally treated with unilateral fixation through a paramedian incision when this stabilization technique is used (see Fig. 40-61). The focus of this description, however, will be on bilateral fixation for sacral U variant fractures with spinopelvic instability, in which midline exposures are performed. The longitudinally oriented constructs are placed laterally, adjacent to the posterior iliac wings. The lateral placement also allows for posterior decompression of the neural elements as well as open reduction of the sacral fracture. Fixation is generally performed from L5 to the ilium, but L4 is occasionally included if there is concern about the adequacy of spinal fixation. S1 pedicle screws are not commonly placed because of compromised fixation caused by fracture comminution.

Subperiosteal exposure is performed to the lateral aspect of the transverse process of the lumbar vertebra to be instrumented as well as the sacral ala. The paraspinal musculature

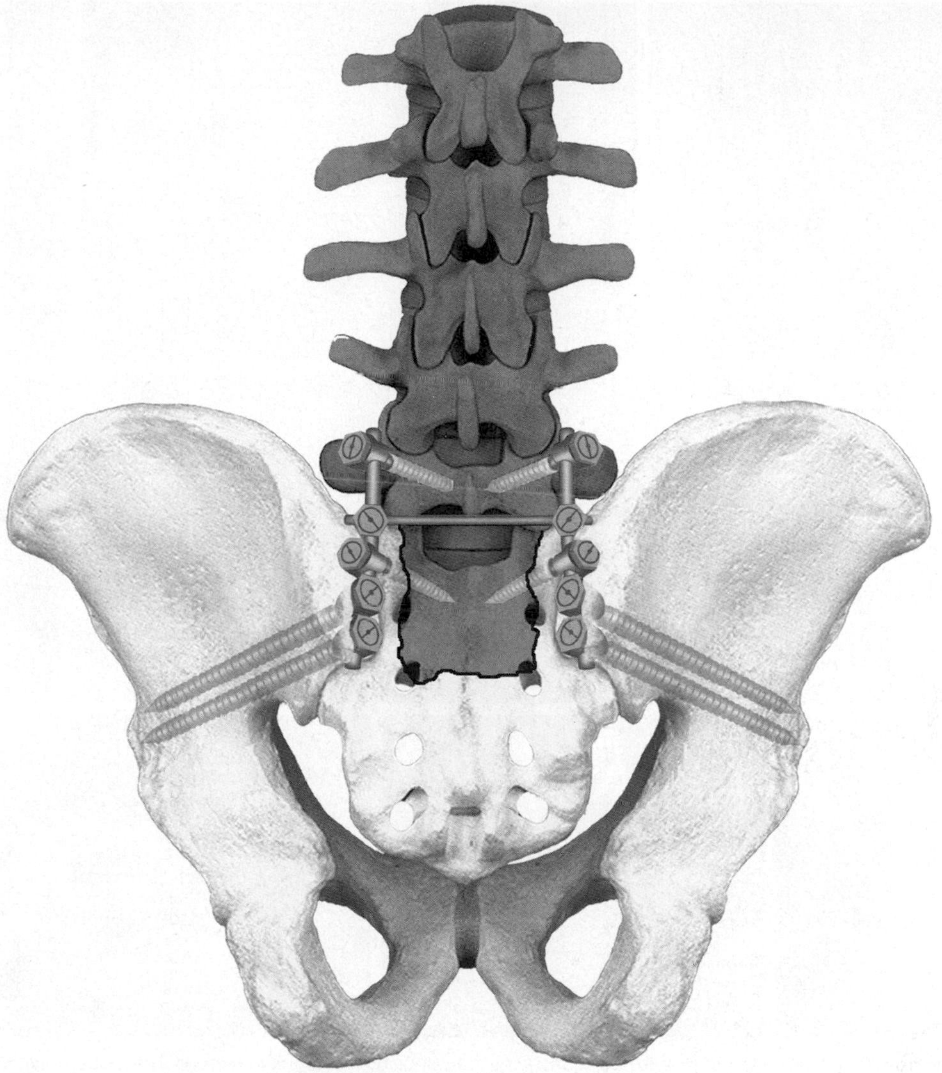

Figure 40-66. Spinopelvic fixation for sacral fractures with spinopelvic dissociation. L4 to ilium spinopelvic and lumbopelvic fixation for sacral U-type fracture-dislocation. The two primary fracture "fragments" are emphasized by different shading to illustrate how stabilization of the sacral fracture is achieved. Cross-connectors are useful to stabilize the longitudinal (vertical) components of the fracture, thus enhancing posterior pelvic stability.

is elevated to expose the posterior aspect of the ilium to the posterior inferior iliac spine (PIIS). In severe injuries, the muscle is often avulsed off one or both ilia. Reduction of the fracture is then performed using techniques already described for the "vertical" components of the injury. The transverse sacral fracture can be challenging to reduce because of limited access to the fracture and significant shortening. Length can be restored through bifemoral traction or the use of a femoral distractor (Fig. 40-68). Because length needs to be obtained between the pelvis and the lumbar spine, distractor pins are placed unilaterally in the L5 pedicle and the ipsilateral ilium using the same trajectory as the eventual screw fixation. Distraction is then achieved across the fracture site, generally providing a partial reduction. In fractures with significant displacement of the sacral fracture and neurologic compromise, a multilevel sacral laminectomy is performed using a high-speed burr. After the sacral roots are exposed, suture repair of dural tears is performed as needed and the degree of neural injury is noted. Access to the primary transverse sacral fracture line is achieved by gently retracting either the S2 or the S3 nerve root medially. The fracture is mobilized with an elevator, and a Schanz screw is placed through the posterior cortex of the upper central sacral fragment to joystick the fragment into the correct angular and translational alignment (see Figs. 40-62 and 40-63). After a satisfactory reduction has been achieved, one or more transiliac-transsacral screws are placed to obtain provisional fracture fixation. In our experience, the technique of spinopelvic fixation for sacral U variant fractures is most successful when the reduction has been achieved and provisionally stabilized before applying the spinopelvic construct, which serves primarily as a neutralization device. Pedicle and iliac screws are placed under lateral fluoroscopic guidance to ensure correct screw orientation. The L5 pedicle screws are placed by establishing a starting point at the junction of the inferolateral aspect of the superior facet and the corresponding transverse process, orienting the angle of the screw trajectory according to preoperative CT imaging. Care should be taken to avoid injuring the L4 to L5 facet joint. Two rods are then contoured into an S shape to accommodate the lumbar lordosis and sacral kyphosis. These are secured to the lumbar pedicle screws cranially and are positioned along the dorsal aspect of the sacrum caudally along the

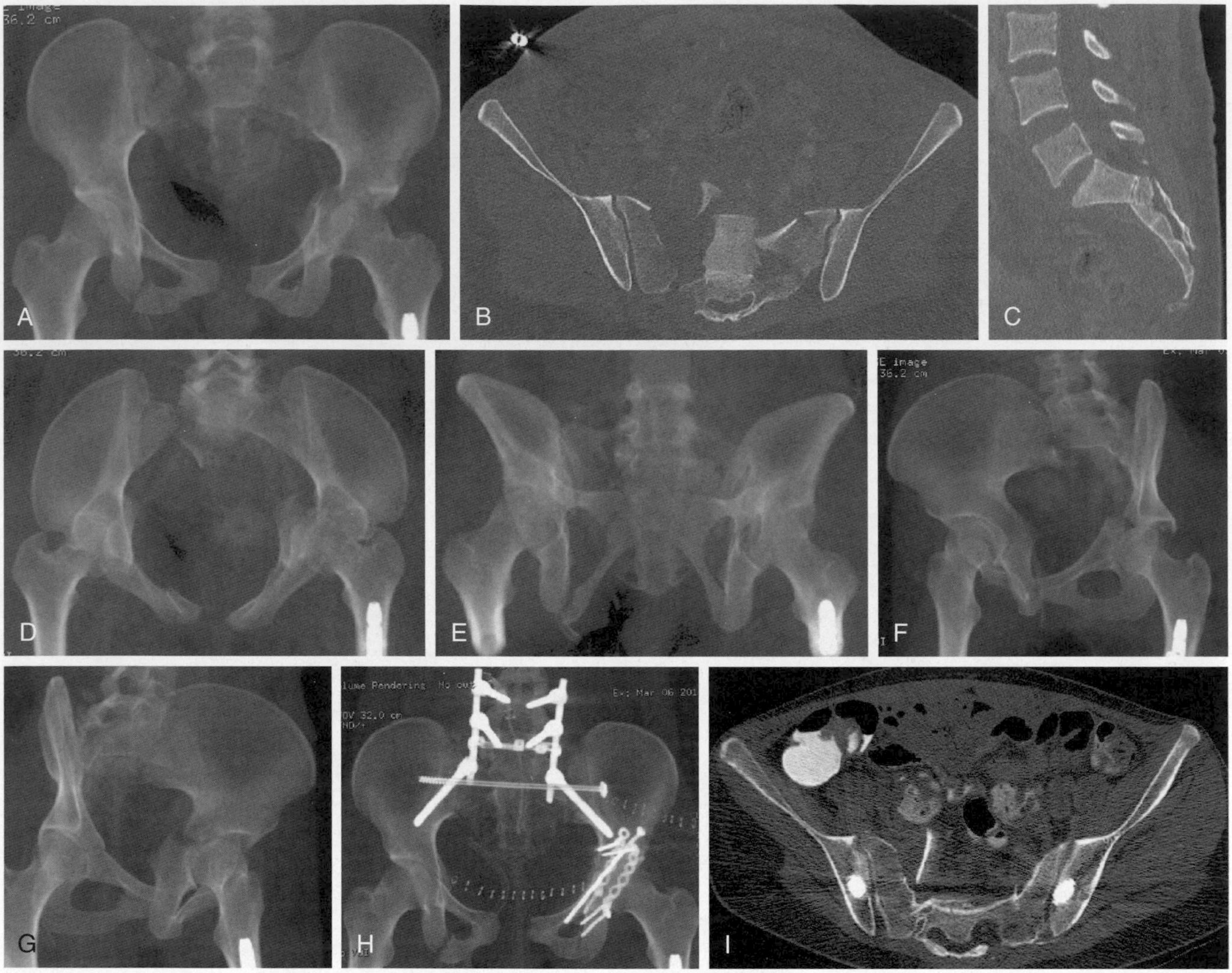

Figure 40-67. Complex open pelvic ring injury with zone III sacral fracture and acetabular fracture in a patient with cauda equina deficits: Anterior-posterior (AP) (**A**), axial computed tomography (CT) (**B**), sagittal CT (**C**), inlet (**D**), outlet (**E**), and Judet (**F** and **G**) views of the pelvis in a patient who sustained an open pelvic fracture secondary to high-speed motor vehicle collision, with right low anterior column acetabular fracture and left T-type with associated posterior wall acetabular fracture. The pelvis fracture consisted of a comminuted and displaced H-type, Roy-Camille type 2 sacral fracture posteriorly and complete symphysis pubis disruption anteriorly. The patient required emergent laparotomy to control life-threatening hepatic and splenic bleeding and bilateral tube thoracostomies for treatment of bilateral pneumothoraces. She also sustained left open tibial shaft and closed segmental femoral shaft fracture treated with intramedullary fixation and standard wound care before transfer. Temporary diverting colostomy was performed to address the open pelvic injury. When associated with acetabular fractures in which the joint reduction is highly dependent on rotational alignment of the ilium, the acetabular fracture should be addressed before definitive fixation of the pelvis, otherwise any malreduction of the ilium can make it impossible to obtain an anatomic reduction of the acetabulum, particularly when using more rigid forms of spinopelvic fixation. The patient underwent open reduction and internal fixation of her left acetabular fracture before open posterior reduction of the pelvis with sacral laminectomies and transiliac-transsacral screw with L4 to ilium spinopelvic fixation, as seen on postoperative AP (**H**), axial CT (**I**), sagittal CT (**J**), inlet (**K**), outlet (**L**), and Judet (**M** and **N**) images. Because of wound contamination issues, the symphysis pubis was not internally fixed, but an advantage to spinopelvic fixation is that it is generally sufficiently robust to support the absence of anterior pelvic ring stabilization. The patient has had an excellent functional recovery with only primarily well-compensated residual L5 nerve root deficits 2 years after surgery.

medial aspect of the posterior ilium. The use of a side-loading pedicle screw system allows for placement of the iliac screw after the rod has already been positioned in this manner. An acceptable lateral projection of the pelvis is then confirmed by perfect overlap of the two sciatic notches (Fig. 40-69, *A*). Iliac screws are typically placed caudal to the previously applied iliosacral or transiliac-transsacral screw(s). A starting point is established with a high-speed burr lateral to the rod, along the medial aspect of the posterior ilium, in a craniocaudal location that allows for a trajectory perpendicular to the rod and within the thick column of bone just above the sciatic notch between the PSIS or PIIS and AIIS (Fig. 40-69, *B*). Alternatively, if a top-loading system is used with more than a single lumbar instrumented level, a more medial starting point at the inferolateral aspect of the S1 dorsal foramen may be preferred because of a more colinear alignment with more rostrally placed screws, especially in cases that require multiple levels of pedicle screw fixation (Fig. 40-69, *C*). A pedicle awl is used to cannulate between the inner and outer tables to a length that extends at least to the anterior margin of the sciatic notch

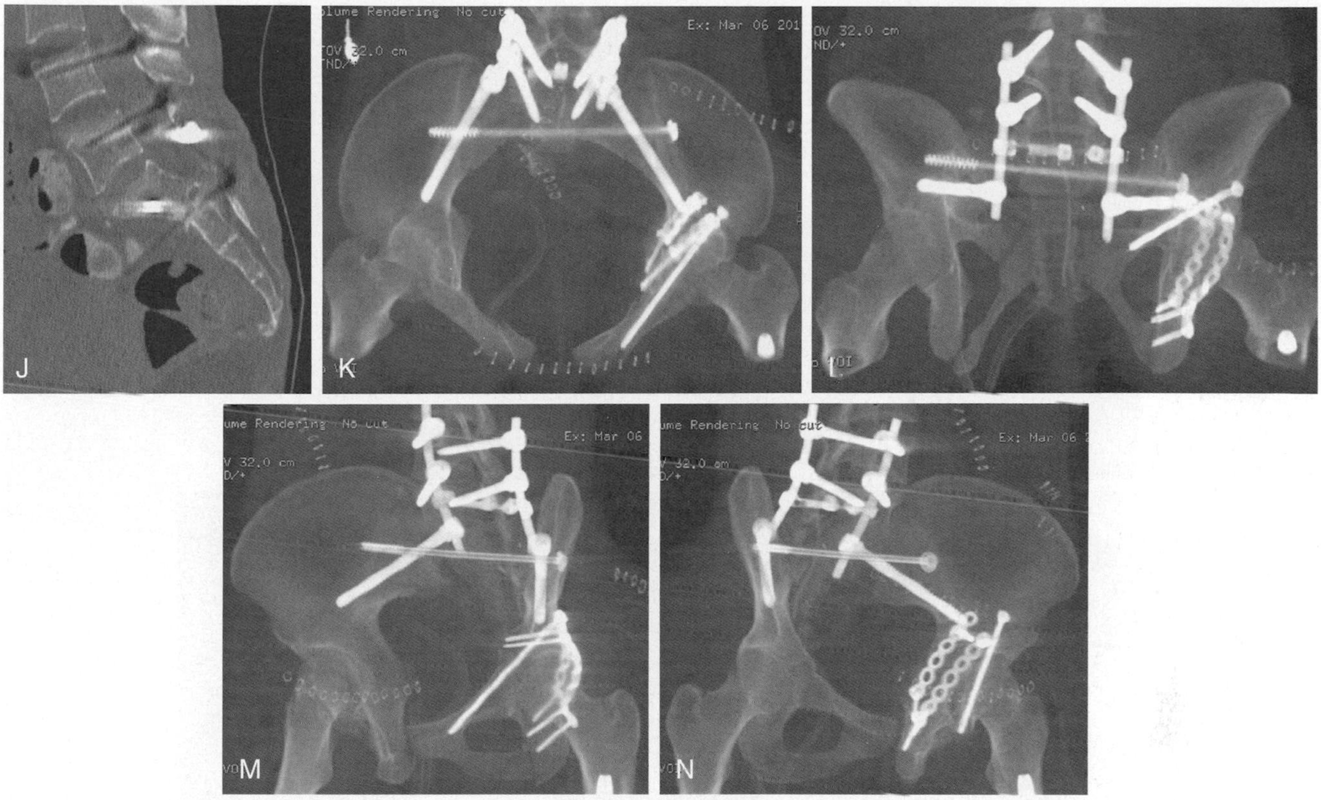

Figure 40-67, cont'd

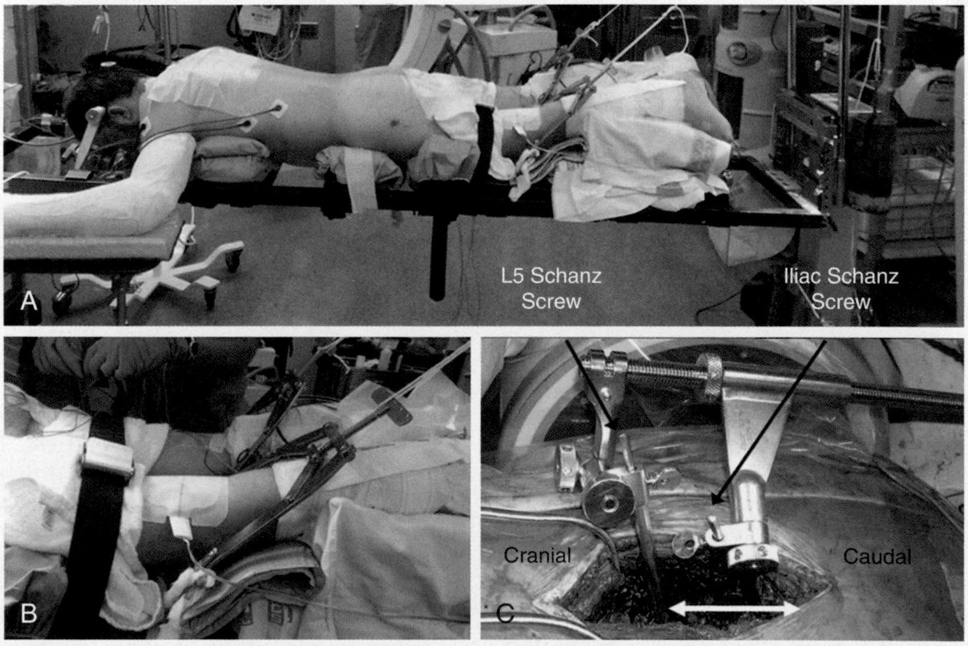

Figure 40-68. Techniques for achieving length when treating sacral U fracture variants with spinopelvic instability. **A** and **B,** Distal femoral traction. It is essential to extend the hip and flex the knee to minimize tension on the sciatic nerve and to be sure that the traction bow does not apply pressure to the perineal nerve in the region of the fibular head. **C,** Femoral distractor applied to the L5 pedicle in the cranial fracture "fragment" and to the ilium in the caudal fracture "fragment."

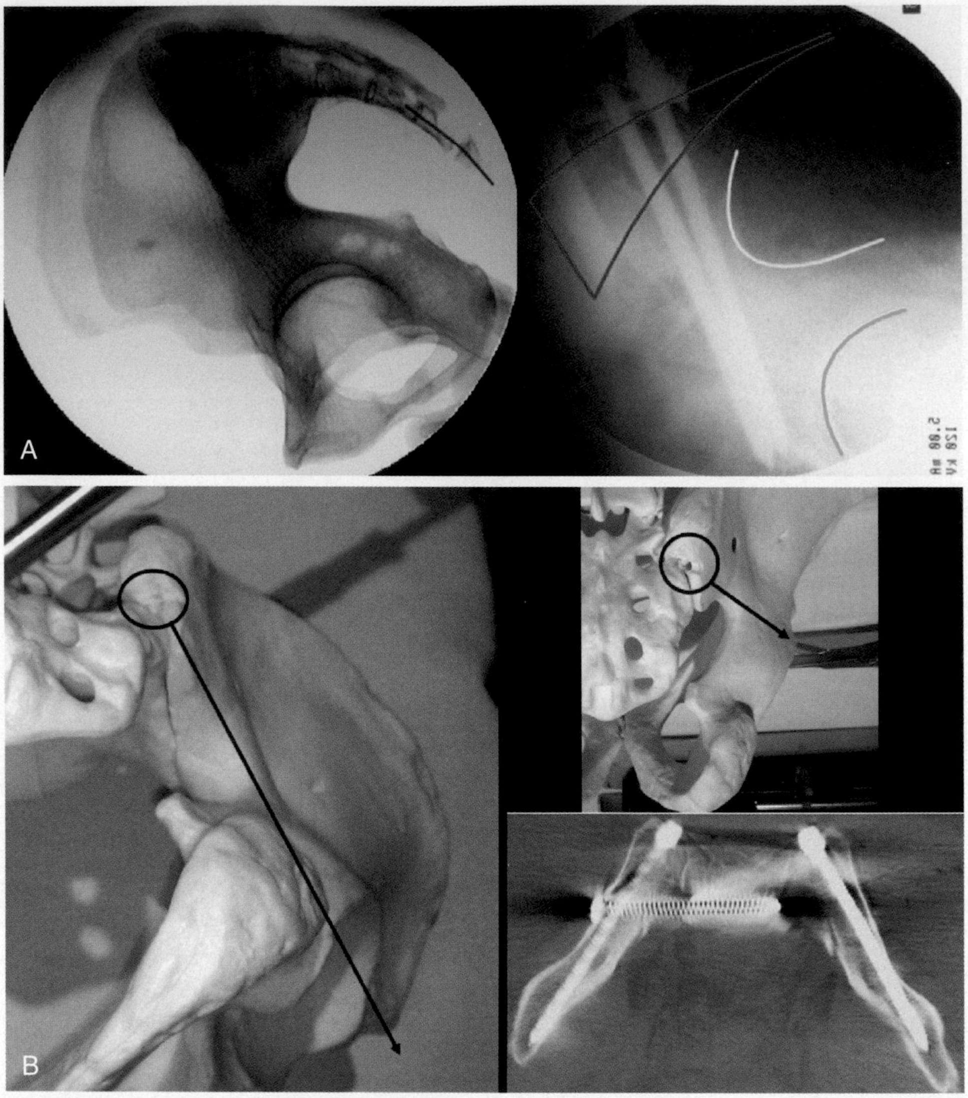

Figure 40-69. Intraoperative imaging for placement of iliac screws: The lateral fluoroscopic projection (**A**) of the pelvis provides the most useful radiologic guide for accurate iliac screw placement. Screws should be positioned superior to the sciatic notches and acetabuli. The best possible overlap of the sciatic notches should be obtained to ascertain a true lateral view. A starting point is made at the posterior inferior iliac spine, which generally aligns well with pedicle screw instrumentation and allows for countersinking of the screw heads anterior to the iliac crest to minimize screw prominence (**B**). Alternatively, a starting point can be established just inferolateral to the S1 dorsal foramen (**C**), for which screw trajectory that crosses the SI joint to reach the cancellous bone between the iliac cortices is required. Countersinking the screw heads anterior to the posterior iliac crest is helpful in preventing screw prominence-related complications (**D**). The obturator-outlet oblique view ("teardrop" view) (**E**) is a projection along the axis of the screws that is useful to confirm appropriate screw placement within the teardrop-shaped cross-section of bone above the sciatic notch (**F**). This view can also be useful during screw placement to confirm appropriate starting point location and intended screw trajectory. The obturator-inlet oblique view (**G**) is effectively perpendicular to the obturator-outlet oblique view and serves to confirm screw position within the cancellous bone between the iliac cortices. The iliac oblique view (**H**) confirms screw positioning above the sciatic notch and acetabuli and confirms acceptable screw length.

to extend beyond the axis of sagittal rotation of the pelvis. Medial-lateral angulation can be measured on preoperative CT imaging. After a fully intraosseous trajectory has been confirmed, an 8- or 9-mm-diameter screw of appropriate length is applied. Care is taken to advance the screw head so that it lies anterior to the posteriormost aspect of the posterior ilium to minimize screw prominence (Fig. 40-69, *B* to *D*). The connections between screws and rods are completed. A cross-connector is then applied between the two rods to further neutralize the bilateral longitudinal fractures' plane of instability. Appropriate screw placement is confirmed at least with lateral, AP, and obturator-outlet views (Fig. 40-69, *E* and *F*), the latter being used to confirm iliac screw positioning with the bony teardrop of the sciatic buttress. The obturator-inlet view (Fig. 40-69, *G*) serves as the orthogonal view to the obturator-outlet view and can also be helpful to confirm intraosseous screw position. An intraoperative iliac oblique fluoroscopic view (Fig. 40-69, *H*) can help confirm that the iliac screws have not penetrated the sciatic notch.

Layered wound closure is performed over a suction drain followed by placement of either a wound vacuum-assisted closure (VAC) or Tegaderm seal to keep the incision from being soiled with stool, particularly in the obtunded patient. Weight bearing from a spinopelvic standpoint is not restricted,

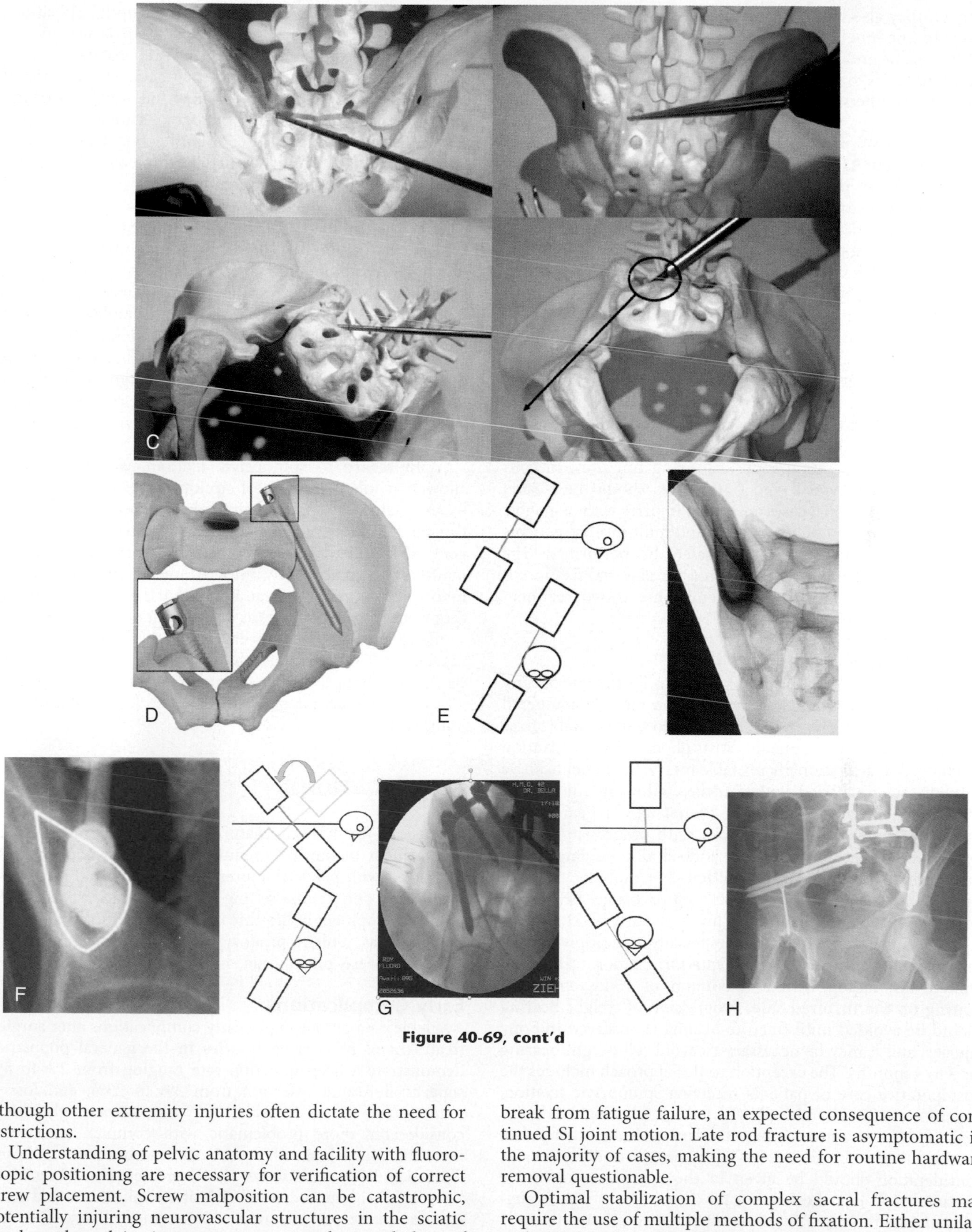

Figure 40-69, cont'd

although other extremity injuries often dictate the need for restrictions.

Understanding of pelvic anatomy and facility with fluoroscopic positioning are necessary for verification of correct screw placement. Screw malposition can be catastrophic, potentially injuring neurovascular structures in the sciatic notch or the pelvic viscera or penetrating the acetabulum. If placed correctly, the hardware profile is low. Infection and wound-related problems are common, however, and have been found to approach 20%.[239] A formal SI joint arthrodesis is not usually performed, and in many instances, the rods will break from fatigue failure, an expected consequence of continued SI joint motion. Late rod fracture is asymptomatic in the majority of cases, making the need for routine hardware removal questionable.

Optimal stabilization of complex sacral fractures may require the use of multiple methods of fixation. Either unilateral or bilateral lumbopelvic fixation can be combined with iliosacral screw fixation, the so-called triangular osteosynthesis technique, to obtain optimal fixation in the horizontal direction stabilizing the pelvic ring in addition to the vertical direction, along the weight-bearing axis.[227,238] Lumbopelvic fixation may also benefit from adjunctive sacral plating, used solely to fine tune fracture realignment and prevent recurrent displacement and canal compromise, while the lumbopelvic fixation's role is to neutralize the bulk of the loads being transferred across the sacrum.

Conservative Treatment of Pelvic Ring Fractures

Relatively little is understood regarding the nuances of conservative treatment of pelvic ring fractures because prospective randomized trials comparing different therapeutic regimens have not been conducted. Fell and colleagues published a case series of 114 patients with nonoperatively treated pelvic fractures. Whereas 60% of patients with stable type A fractures were pain free at the time of evaluation, only 15% of patients with type C injuries were pain free, and only 10% of them had no functional deficit. Clinical results with type B injuries were intermediate to those of type A and C injuries, with only 45% of patients being pain free and without functional deficit.[240] Based on these and similar results, as well as our own experience, only type A injuries should be treated conservatively, excluding some iliac wing fractures. In contrast, we believe type B and C fractures should be treated surgically. Exceptional cases are type B injuries with negligible displacement in compliant patients and multimorbid patients in whom osteosynthesis cannot safely be performed. The latter, however, should be considered for external fixation, if at all possible. We do not recommend conservative treatment for type C fractures.

Postoperative Plan

The postoperative plan for these patients is ideally one of early mobilization. However, such mobilization must be tempered by the quality of the bone and the ability to achieve stable fixation of the fracture. If bone quality is good and stable fixation is achieved in a rotationally unstable injury, the patient can be immediately mobilized with crutches, allowing full weight bearing on the uninvolved side. Partial weight bearing can be allowed between 3 and 6 weeks, with progression to full weight bearing at 8 to 10 weeks and off all ambulatory aids by 3 months if gait has normalized. For globally unstable injuries, however, a more cautious approach may be needed for all but spinopelvic fixation techniques. Early bed to reclining chair transfers are important, especially in multiply injured patients. Stable posterior and anterior fixation can allow limited ambulation with a maximum of 15 kg of weight bearing on the involved side. Progression of weight bearing should be avoided until fracture healing is observed in bony injuries, and it may be necessary to avoid full weight bearing for 3 to 4 months. The exception to this approach includes the postoperative care of patients receiving spinopelvic fixation, who in most cases can be allowed to bear full weight as tolerated. If there is concern that standard techniques of pelvic fixation are unstable because of injury pattern or bone density, consideration should be given to the use of postoperative traction to protect the fixation for 4 to 6 weeks versus augmentation with more robust yet often less soft tissue–friendly techniques such as spinopelvic fixation. The former is often not appropriate because of the risks associated with prolonged immobilization, particularly in polytrauma patients, and should therefore be considered as a salvage procedure only. The use of external fixation as a supplement to internal fixation may allow the patient to be in the upright position in bed or in a chair. Radiographic follow-up is usually done in the early postoperative phase before hospital discharge and at 6 weeks and 3 months after surgery. At 3 months, the healing is usually sufficient to allow full weight bearing in most patients, and no further radiographs are necessary until 6 months after surgery. After this interval, radiographs are necessary only if indicated by patient complaints. Pelvic internal fixation is not generally removed on a routine basis. The only locations in which fixation causes local irritation problems are at the iliac crest or the symphysis. In the case of spinopelvic fixation, the iliac screws are a relatively common source of symptomatic screw prominence.[239] Symptomatic fixation in these locations may require removal. Women of reproductive age may elect to have symphyseal fixation removed to avoid potential problems with labor, although the obstetric risk of retaining these implants has not been well established. Last, consideration should be given to iliosacral screw removal if significant posterior pelvic ring pain persists, particularly in the younger patient with obvious radiographic evidence of loosening.

With regard to spinopelvic fixation, weight bearing is allowed as tolerated in most circumstances unless restricted by associated lower extremity injuries. Because formal arthrodesis is frequently not undertaken, hardware removal is generally planned within 6 months of surgery, after CT confirmation of acceptable bony union. Many patients, however, opt to forego hardware removal. Because of the absence of fusion, they frequently experience asymptomatic rod breakage.

There are few objective data as to the best postoperative management of patients with pelvic ring injuries. Moreover, pelvic ring disruption often occurs in multiply injured patients whose management depends to a greater degree on associated injuries.

COMPLICATIONS

Because of the systemic nature of the injury and the wide spectrum of methods of required treatment, complications associated with pelvic fractures are common and potentially severe. The polytrauma setting makes the patient susceptible to the development of life-threatening nonorthopaedic conditions such as adult respiratory distress syndrome, thromboembolic disease, pneumonia, and multiple organ failure.

Early Complications

Available data pertaining to early complications after surgical treatment of pelvic ring injuries in the general population demonstrate a deep infection rate ranging from 2% to 8%, superficial wound infection from 3% to 23%, and loss of reduction of 0% to 10%.[201,233,241-243] Not surprisingly, this is considerably more problematic with complex spinopelvic reconstructions than with percutaneous techniques.[239] Obesity, defined as body mass index (BMI) greater than 30 kg/m^2, is associated with an increased risk of complications and reoperation. Obese patients are 6.9 times more likely to have a complication and 4.7 times more likely to undergo reoperation than patients with BMIs less than 30 kg/m^2.[244,245] This is of particular interest because obesity is pandemic, mainly affecting North America but increasingly also Europe and Southeast Asia.

Infection

Postoperative infection can occur after either external or internal fixation. The risk of infection correlates with patient-related factors (e.g., comorbidities) as well as iatrogenic factors. Minimizing iatrogenic postoperative infection necessitates time-saving, cautious, and preferably soft tissue–friendly surgical procedures with proper soft tissue handling techniques that involve limited subcutaneous dissection; creating a full-thickness, fasciocutaneous flap; and minimizing dead space.[246]

Infection with the use of external fixation devices usually occurs around the pin tracts. The incidence of pin tract infection averages 22% with no difference between anterior external fixation alone versus when combined with internal fixation of the posterior ring.[247] The dramatic differences in reported external fixation infection rates (0% vs. 33%) may indicate different definitions of pin tract infection (compared with soft tissue reaction and wound secretion) because similar differences in surgical infection rates have not been reported.[219,248] Nonetheless, regardless of the true incidence of pin tract infection, the need for surgical intervention to control the infection is nominal. Pin tract infection can generally be managed adequately by appropriate release of the skin surrounding the pins and by changing dressings as required to manage drainage from the pin sites. Antibiotic coverage may be appropriate if drainage is excessive or if cellulitis develops and is unresponsive to pin tract release and local dressing changes. Pin loosening may occur with persistent local infection; therefore, the clamps attached to the pins should be released and the pins checked for stability within the bone. If a pin is loose, it is inadvisable to reinsert it in the same location because of the localized infection. Consequently, the fixator may have to be removed, or alternative placement of the pins may be necessary. Most pin tract infections resolve with removal of the pins and local débridement of the pin tract itself.

Postoperative infections after internal fixation usually occur secondary to significant soft tissue integrity or healing problems.

Although some authors, especially in the 1980s, found unacceptably high complication rates,[143,249] contemporary studies on the posterior approach to the pelvis demonstrate acceptable complication rates, comparable to those reported with the anterior approach, with an incidence of deep wound infection ranging between 3.4% and 7.1%.[233,247,250-253] However, if a postoperative infection does develop in the presence of internal fixation, the same treatment principles apply as for acute postoperative infections after internal fixation elsewhere. Incision and drainage plus débridement must begin early. The wound should be covered with a VAC dressing that usually accelerates the secondary healing or the establishment of a well-vascularized wound surface that can be covered by a local flap. Additionally, the fixation is evaluated for stability. Stable fixation should generally be left in place, at least until healing takes place. If systemic infection is noted by either laboratory or clinical findings and is not responsive to intravenous antibiotics or if fixation is loose and therefore not maintaining stability, it must be removed and supplemented or changed to an alternative.

Pelvic osteomyelitis is a rare but serious complication.[254,255] Repetitive débridement is the only treatment method. In rare cases, it may be necessary to excise major portions of the iliac crest to control the osteomyelitis.

Loss of Fixation

Loss of fixation often occurs when the expected degree of healing cannot be achieved during the early phase of pelvic fixation. Fortunately, it occurs rather uncommonly, with an overall incidence ranging between 0% to 10%.[201,233,241-243] The average incidence is 8.5% if an anterior external fixator is used as a single stabilization device and 5% after combined anterior and posterior ring stabilization.[247] Particularly when an anterior external fixator is used, the wide variation in reported infection rates is remarkable. As mentioned previously, this may be due to differences in how a pin tract infection is defined across the various studies or because of different surgical techniques and heterogeneous patient populations. This wide variation in reported infection rates complicates our ability to reliably compare the outcomes of different approaches. Realistic assessment of the stability of the fixation must be made at the end of any surgical intervention. The use of external fixation or, in certain cases, traction to supplement internal fixation must be considered. If the adequacy of the fixation is uncertain, it can be beneficial to keep the patient on bed rest with external fixation or traction and to delay mobilization until bony union or ligamentous healing has occurred. However, this should be limited to specific cases in which lack of mobilization is considered acceptable. Late fixation failure (hardware breakage) is common after plate fixation of the pubic symphysis, although the need for revision surgery is rare because failure is largely asymptomatic (90%) and therefore clinically unimportant in most cases.[256] Failure of iliosacral screw fixation occurs uncommonly and can be treated by more biomechanically rigid fixation techniques such as spinopelvic fixation (Fig. 40-70).

Neurologic Injury

Concomitant neurologic injuries are common in pelvic fractures, ranging between 8% and 25% overall, and are most likely in C-type fractures. The incidence increases to 60% in SI separation and severe sacral fractures (zone III according to Denis classification).[11,192,243,257-259] The characteristic neurologic injury is a lumbosacral plexus injury in 70% to 80% of cases. Sciatic nerve injuries are more common in patients with isolated acetabular fractures.[260,261] As previously mentioned, fractures through or medial to the sacral foramina are associated with a high incidence of neurologic injury, as are transverse fractures of the sacrum with a kyphotic deformity.[192] Reduction and stabilization of these pelvic injuries may improve recovery.[238,239,243] Decompression of any sacral transverse fracture with a kyphotic deformity or of any burst fracture of the sacrum that appears to compromise the roots posteriorly may be of some value. However, there is no literature providing evidence or guidelines to help dictate the timing of surgical decompression.[238] Nerve recovery usually begins within 3 months of trauma and plateaus within 2 years. Complete recovery of cauda equina function is more likely in patients with continuity of all sacral roots and incomplete deficits. However, complete neurologic recovery in severe nerve injuries is uncommon.[238,258] Neuropathic pain resulting from injuries to the L5 or S1 root or to the sciatic nerve can be particularly difficult to manage, both acutely and on a long-term basis. Early and sufficiently dosed analgesic medication may help to prevent chronic pain. Consultation with pain management physicians should be carried out to determine an approach to minimize long-term disability. Epidural analgesia

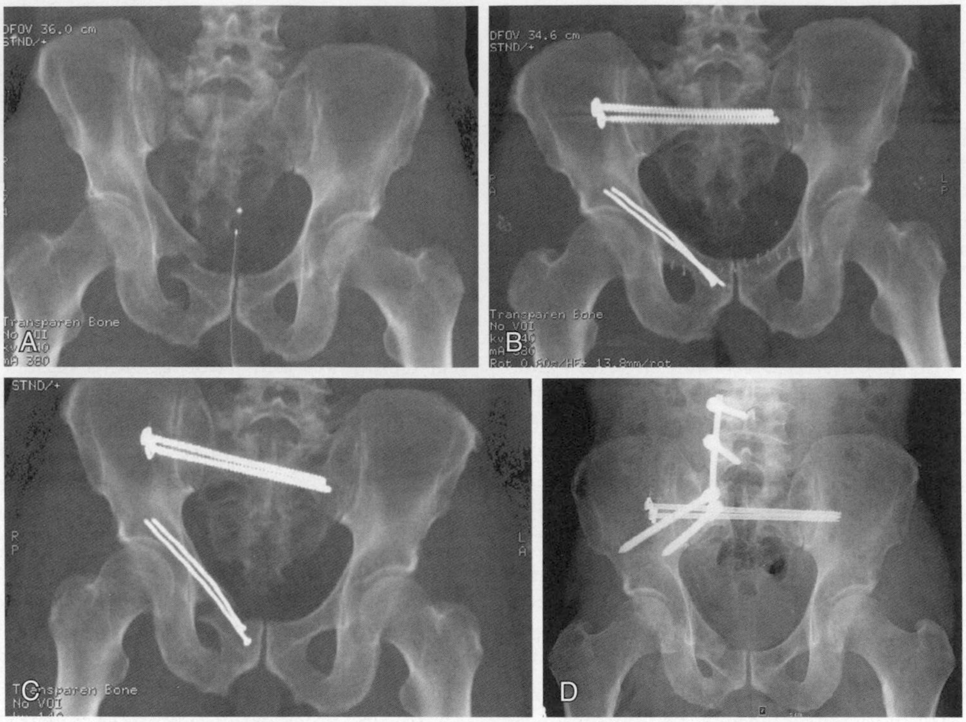

Figure 40-70. Right Denis zone II sacral fracture (**A**) treated with closed reduction and percutaneous iliosacral screw and superior pubic ramus fixation (**B**). Early fracture displacement (**C**) required revision with the triangular osteosynthesis variant of spinopelvic fixation (**D**).

has been shown to be beneficial in pelvic and lower extremity surgery.[262] In certain cases, lumbar sympathetic blockade may be of value in helping break the pain cycle.[263]

Neurologic damage should be managed with appropriate bracing and early rehabilitation. Surgical intervention should be carried out if indicated. Early surgical correction may be beneficial if malunion is presumed to cause nerve compression. Repair or decompression of the sciatic nerve has not yet shown a great deal of success. Repair of the femoral nerve, which has a shorter travel route than the sciatic nerve, may be indicated if the nerve has been lacerated.

Iatrogenic nerve injury may occur secondary to operative treatment. Its incidence has not been reliably decreased by intraoperative electrodiagnostic monitoring.[264,265] The use of electromyographic monitoring techniques might be beneficial, although randomized controlled data are lacking.[266,267]

Thromboembolism

Thromboembolic complications occur commonly in patients with a major pelvic disruption, especially those with associated lower extremity fractures.[268,269] The incidence ranges from 12% to 61%, depending on the use of prophylaxis and of adequate diagnostic screening (e.g., venography).[268-271] Pulmonary embolism is more frequent with pelvic injuries, and surgical fixation of the pelvis is an independent predictor of early pulmonary embolism (within the first 72 hours of admission).[271,272] Screening has not been successful in determining the at-risk group because most clots are located in the internal pelvic venous plexus, which is not amenable to standard screening methods. Because of the strikingly increased risk of thromboembolism, it seems logical to administer some form of prophylaxis. Many different protocols are used, but no single approach has proven to be reliably more effective or even better than the use of no prophylaxis in the prevention of fatal pulmonary emboli. The largely accepted early administration of low-molecular-weight heparin is, for instance, based on a single study with 100 subjects.[273,274]

Late Complications

Pain

Unfortunately, posttraumatic chronic pain is common and may have various sources such as malunion, nonunion, or osteoarthritis of the SI joint. The source of pain can often not be reliably be identified. Approximately 25% to 40% of patients have neuropathic pain, and 20% to 40% have musculoskeletal pain.[260] With regard to operative versus nonoperatively treated patients, there is no significant difference in the incidence of chronic pain. Although this constitutes a comparison of different injury types and patient populations, severe pain has a lower incidence in operatively treated patients, averaging 1% to 5% versus 27% in nonoperatively treated patients.[247] This supports the hypothesis that, with anatomic or near-anatomic reduction, 60% to 70% of patients can be expected to have successful outcomes with minimal pain.[275] Nonetheless, some patients continue to complain of discomfort despite having had anatomic reduction and adequate fracture union or even a fused SI joint. Pain is generally localized to the lower back over the SI joint. Therapeutic management is difficult and often limited to analgesic agents and physical therapy. However, careful evaluation of the lower lumbar spine must be carried out to ensure the absence of missed lumbosacral injuries, particularly lumbosacral facet injuries that are seen with relative frequency in association with pelvic fractures (see Fig. 40-28). Other causes of pain include significant soft tissue injury, particularly to the muscles and neurologic structures.

Malunion

Malunion of the pelvic ring is a common problem that can be a source of chronic pain and dysfunction. It occurs in 30% to 42% of cases after nonoperative treatment or after solely anterior fixation but in only 7% to 10% of cases after combined anterior and posterior fixation, probably because of more anatomic reduction and more stable fixation.[243,247] Both malunion and nonunion are extremely uncommon after spinopelvic fixation despite the complexity of the injuries for which this technique is used.[238,239]

Most clinical consequences of pelvic malunion stem from pelvic obliquity with accompanying sitting imbalance, compensatory scoliosis, relative leg length inequality, and secondary gait abnormalities. Deformities occurring through or adjacent to the SI joint appear to be the most disabling.

As already mentioned, pain is a common problem, localizing to the lower back or the SI joints. Additionally, pain may localize over the ischial tuberosities, which are at an unequal level and therefore subjected to excessive pressure with sitting. Occasionally, severely displaced lateral compression fractures (type B2) can result in an internal rotation deformity that can encroach on the vagina, bladder, or anterior soft tissue of the pelvis.

Careful evaluation of the patient's functional and physical disability is mandatory. Chronic pain sequelae are common and may require a multidisciplinary approach. Complex deformity correction often requires a multistage osteotomy approach with significant surgical risk. Pain relief and deformity correction are usually incomplete, but in carefully selected patients, the likelihood of improvements may warrant the risks. Symptomatic malunion of the SI joint with modest deformity is a more straightforward problem that is usually treated by SI fusion.

Nonunion

Compared with malunion, nonunion is rare but well recognized. Union rates after operative fixation range from 95% to 100% with relatively good data quality.[247] Regarding nonoperatively treated pelvic ring fractures, few data are available. Matta and colleagues recorded union rate of 83%.[201] Pelvic pain and instability are the most common initial symptoms of pelvic nonunion. However, some patterns of nonunion, such as anterior ramus nonunion caused by lateral compression injuries, tend to be relatively asymptomatic.

Complete evaluation of the patient's symptoms and bony pelvic abnormalities is mandatory. MRI may help to make the diagnosis but is not generally necessary. The principles of surgical treatment are to achieve stable pelvic ring fixation in proper alignment with débridement and bone grafting of the nonunion. The approach differs depending on the location of the nonunion and the degree of associated pelvic malalignment, but many cases may require takedown of the nonunion or osteotomy to allow for correction of the deformity followed by stable fixation both anteriorly and posteriorly.[276] Sacral fracture nonunions after iliosacral screw fixation techniques can be treated with débridement, bone grafting, and more rigid fixation such as spinopelvic techniques (see Fig. 40-70).

Genitourinary Injuries

The incidence of genitourinary injuries in association with pelvic trauma is high, ranging from 6.5% to 30%.[127,128,134] These injuries include bladder disruptions, injury to the bladder neck, and urethral injuries. Bladder ruptures occur in 5% to 16%, urethral injuries in 4% to 14%, and combined bladder and urethral injuries in 0.5% to 2.5% of patients.[277-280]

Assessment

Because there are no typical clinical signs, medical history is of particular importance. The mechanism of injury is helpful for establishing a suspicion of urologic injury. For adequate treatment, knowledge of preexisting renal conditions is necessary.[281-283] Clinical signs are varied and rarely specific. They range from external signs such as bruises, hematoma (e.g., suprapubic in case of bladder lesion) and swelling of the perineum, scrotum, or abdominal wall to abdominal pain and distention, urinary retention or voiding disorder, or suprapubic discomfort. The most suggestive sign is gross hematuria, which occurs in 80% of all bladder lesions but does not correlate with injury severity.[283,284]

A thorough whole-body examination that includes palpation of the abdomen and pelvic stability testing is mandatory. This should include vaginal examination to rule out open fracture, especially in case of tilt fractures. Urine should be collected and screened for hematuria in the early diagnostic phase. Although gross hematuria or microscopic hematuria are strong indicators of renal and bladder injury, the absence of hematuria does not exclude a relevant injury. Diagnostic imaging depends on the hemodynamic stability of the patient. In hemodynamically unstable patients with suspected intraperitoneal or retroperitoneal sources of bleeding, a laparotomy is indicated. Sonography (FAST) can help guide the surgical decision-making process.[285-288] The diagnostic gold standard for kidney and ureteral injury is a contrast-enhanced CT imaging, with 10 to 20 minutes of delay after the administration of contrast to allow for its excretion into the renal collecting system.[289-290] The standard diagnostic tool for detecting bladder injuries is CT cystography, which is almost 100% sensitive.[291-293] Suspicion of urethral injury warrants evaluation with retrograde urethrography.[294] When combined upper and lower urinary tract injuries are suspected, the upper tract contrast study should be performed before the cystogram because retained contrast dye in the abdomen or retroperitoneum can obscure upper tract pathology.[283]

Management

The treatment of bladder lesions is primarily nonoperative and involves transurethral catheterization for the majority of extraperitoneal injuries. In about 90% of such cases, healing occurs within 10 days.[291] Operative intervention is necessary in the case of an intraperitoneal lesion, penetrating bladder injury, injury to the bladder neck, presence of bone fragments in the vesical wall, or bony incarceration of the bladder.[295] The preferred standard of care is an open surgical repair with absorbable suture.[296]

The treatment of urethral rupture is more controversial. Three options exist: immediate exploration and realignment over a catheter, primary urethroplasty, and suprapubic cystostomy drainage with delayed urethroplasty. Endoscopic realignment has been shown to be feasible and effective with an acceptable risk profile.[297-299] The timing of surgery is dictated by the magnitude of the injury and complicating injuries to adjacent structures. The most important factor appears to be related to avoiding further surgical damage to the pelvic floor to keep the incidence of stricture and impotence as low as possible.

Results

Despite improved diagnostics and therapy, genitourinary sequelae are common. Urethral injuries may result in strictures and infection in men, pelvic organ prolapse and voiding disorder in girls and women, and urinary incontinence in both sexes. Sexual dysfunction is common and includes erectile dysfunction and persistent impotence in men and dyspareunia, anorgasmia, or painful orgasms in women.[134,278,279,300-304] Harvey-Kelly and colleagues reported an overall incidence of sexual dysfunction of 35.9% in men and 39.6% in women in their recent systematic review.[305] Dyspareunia is most likely in AP compression injuries and in symphyseal disruptions.[306] Urinary symptoms and dyspareunia are much more common in women with residually displaced pelvic fractures than with nondisplaced fractures.[307] Interestingly, sexual dysfunction is increasingly recognized in patients with no detectable genitourinary injury, thus raising the important question on how pelvic ring fractures can lead to sexual and genitourinary dysfunction apart from direct injury.[279,280,308-312]

OPEN PELVIC FRACTURES

An open pelvic fracture is among the most devastating possible injuries. It is defined as any fracture of the pelvic ring in which the fracture site is or has the potential for bacterial contamination because of communication with the external environment, of which the gastrointestinal and genital tracts are a part. It therefore comprises both a fracture site open to the external environment and a fracture site communicating with a vaginal or rectal laceration. About 2% to 5% of all pelvic fractures are deemed open.[313-317] A high-energy injury is usually necessary to cause this compound injury pattern, which leads to significant bony disruption and, more important, to severe soft tissue damage and resultant susceptibility to infection and late disability (Fig. 40-71). Not surprisingly, motor vehicle versus pedestrian and motorcycle injuries are the most common causes.[313,316,317] Although a decrease in mortality in past 2 decades has been reported, overall mortality remains high. In their compound data analysis, Grotz and colleagues reported an average mortality rate of 30.4% before 1990 and 18% from 1990 onward.[318] More recent studies confirm a mortality rate of approximately 20%.[319] The partly improved outcome may be related to advanced diagnostics (e.g., routine use of CT), altered resuscitation protocols, and a more widespread use of damage control laparotomy in patients with combined pelvic and abdominal injuries. Factors positively associated with death include age, injury severity (ISS), injury complexity, wound size, and transfusion requirements.[314,318,320] Early mortality is almost entirely due to exsanguinating hemorrhage.[314,316,321] Late mortality is most commonly due to sepsis, but complications related to associated injuries in these polytraumatized patients, such as traumatic brain injury or respiratory dysfunction, are frequently implicated.[314,316,317] A thorough and early evaluation and diagnosis is mandatory to commence specific and sufficient treatment.

Assessment

On top of the usual approach, assessment of the soft tissue is of particular importance in patients with open pelvic fractures. One method of determining the extent of soft tissue damage is to describe the exact injury. Anteriorly or laterally directed wounds in the flank usually occur through muscle and do not involve rectal or genitourinary contamination. Wounds that occur in the perineum with extension into the rectum posteriorly and wounds that extend into the rectal or genitourinary tracts are contaminated and have the potential for later contamination (Fig. 40-71, *C*).[322] Additionally, two systems are commonly used to assess the soft tissue injury. The Tscherne-Oestern classification of the extent of the soft tissue injury is most commonly used in Central Europe,[323] but the Gustilo-Anderson classification is more popular in England and North America.[324,325] Contamination of the wound from both external and internal (intestinal) sources must be determined.

Finally, rectal and vaginal examinations are mandatory in all patients with pelvic fractures. The presence of blood on either examination is an indication for visual inspection of that orifice to rule out an open injury.[131] Evaluation of neurologic status must also be undertaken immediately because concomitant axonal injury is common.[11,192,243,257-259]

After evaluation of the soft tissue injuries, appropriate radiographic and CT evaluation of the pelvic fracture must be undertaken.

Management

As previously mentioned, early mortality is almost entirely due to exsanguinating hemorrhage. Treatment of these patients must be well coordinated and meticulous and should involve temporary pelvic stabilization and compression dressing of open, bleeding wounds as soon as possible, preferably already prehospital. Rapid resuscitation and application of massive transfusion protocols are mandatory. Surgical bleeding control consists of fracture stabilization (temporary or definitive); damage control laparotomy; pelvic packing; and, in certain cases, arterial embolization. In cases of large vessel bleeding, surgical repair should be considered. These injuries may rarely represent internal traumatic hemipelvectomies and, in fact, conversion to an actual hemipelvectomy may be lifesaving in some patients. After hemodynamic stabilization has occurred, appropriate débridement of the wounds is necessary. This procedure may involve consultation with general surgeons, urologists, and gynecologists so that the wounds can be explored adequately. It comprises thorough débridement (up to healthy tissue with capillary bleeding), extensive irrigation (washout), and removal of foreign bodies and loose bony fragments. Wounds were historically left open; however, VAC dressings have been generally accepted as safe and effective for complex open wound management.[326-329]

One very serious injury that occurs to the soft tissues is the degloving injury, with shearing and avulsion of the skin and subcutaneous tissue from the underlying muscle fascia (see Fig. 40-37). In a sense, the skin has become devascularized by the loss of its deep blood supply. In these situations, a decision must be made regarding the extent of débridement required. These avulsions can be massive, and determination of their extent is usually guided by an evaluation of the skin and subcutaneous bleeding. All tissue that is dead and thought to be potentially nonviable must be removed. If débridement is inadequate and a large quantity of devitalized soft tissue remains, necrosis and subsequent sepsis may result and compromise the patient's outcome. However, skin necrosis is less likely to lead to rapid sepsis than, for instance, muscle necrosis

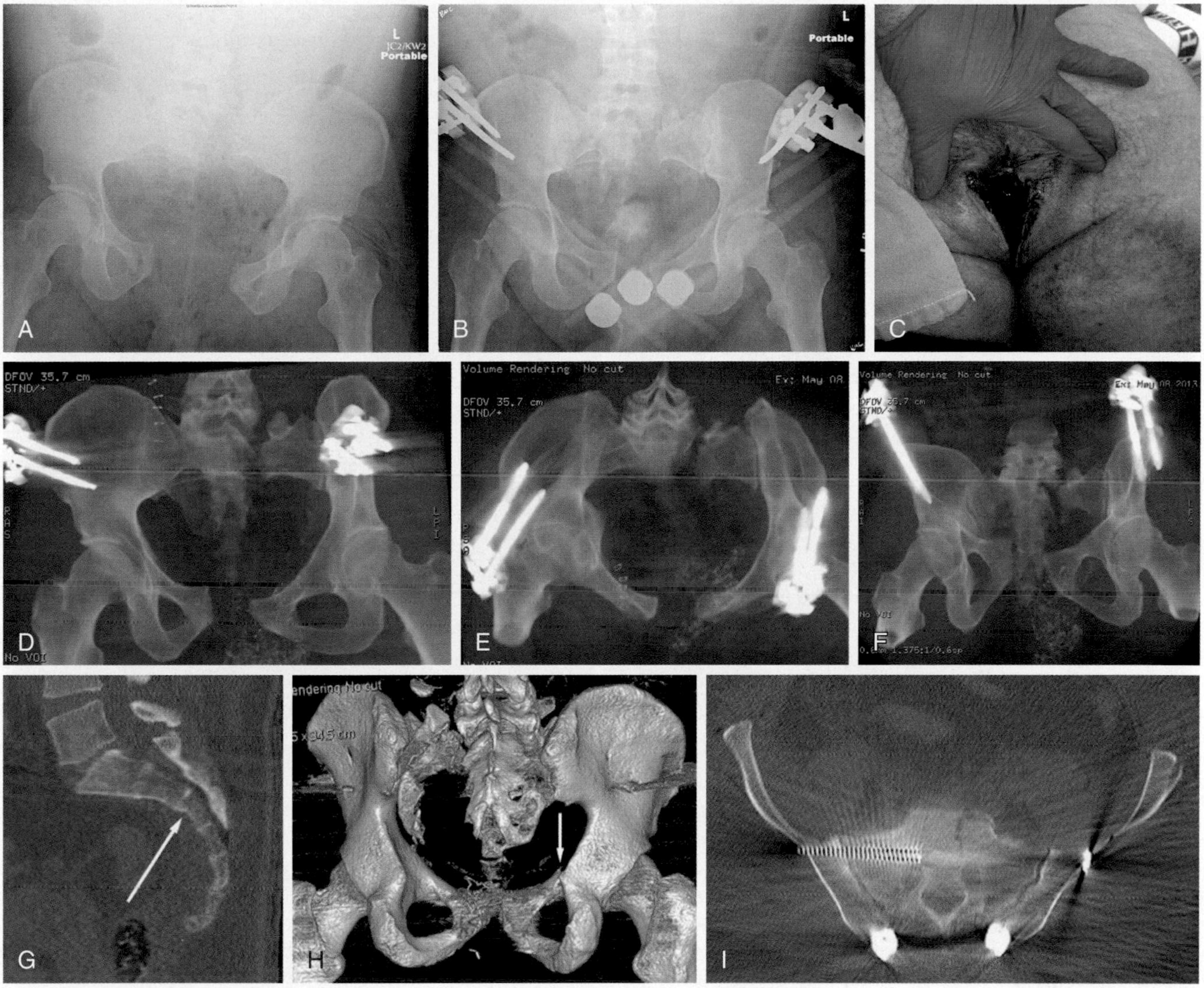

Figure 40-71. Open pelvic fracture: This multiply injured patient sustained a severely displaced pelvic fracture as seen on anterior-posterior (AP) radiograph (**A**), with an associated perineal wound and both bowel and bladder injuries. He was treated initially with closed reduction, provisional pelvic external fixation (**B**), and diverting colostomy. This approach allowed for débridement and care of his perineal wound, as seen 5 days after injury (**C**). The Denis zone III sacral fracture with pubic symphysis disruption is better appreciated after external fixation on AP (**D**), inlet (**E**), and outlet (**F**) pelvis reconstructions and sagittal computed tomography (CT) images (**G**). A previously underappreciated, nondisplaced right pubic ramus fracture, which displaced slightly during the reconstruction procedure, is better seen on three-dimensional CT reconstruction of the pelvis (**H**). The patient underwent a pubic symphysis plating followed by open reduction of his sacral fracture and posterior pelvic ring through a posterior approach, with transiliac-transsacral and spinopelvic fixation. Postoperative axial (**I**) and coronal (**J**) CT images demonstrate the postoperative alignment and fixation of the posterior pelvis. Postoperative AP (**K**), inlet (**L**), and outlet (**M**) images of the pelvis demonstrate the pelvic reconstruction.

Continued

and a more hesitant approach to débridement may be indicated. If the exact amount and extent of devitalized skin are not initially evident, repetitive débridement after allowing for the area of devascularization to more definitively declare itself is a reasonable approach.

If any wound enters the perineum, especially if it has rectal involvement, a diverting colostomy (e.g., loop colostomy) should be considered (see Fig. 40-71). However, fecal diversion does not appear to be associated with a lower incidence of abdominopelvic infectious complications and overall infection rate. Most authors assume that selected patients would benefit from colostomy, especially those with perineal wounds. Convincing data to support this assumption have yet to be obtained, and randomized controlled trials are required.[330,331] Broad-spectrum antibiotics with adequate coverage for bowel contamination should be started immediately and used prophylactically for 24 to 48 hours.

In fractures with significant contamination involving the perineum or rectum and in situations in which it is impossible to achieve a clean surgical wound, external fixation should be used.[332] Such fixation provides a relatively stable pelvic ring so that the patient can be mobilized and repeat débridement can be performed. After the soft tissues have demonstrated viability and healing has progressed, definitive stabilization can be carried out. However, percutaneous limited internal fixation has been shown to be a feasible alternative approach with an acceptable risk profile.[147,222,333-335] Primary internal fracture fixation is possible if the wound does not involve the perineum

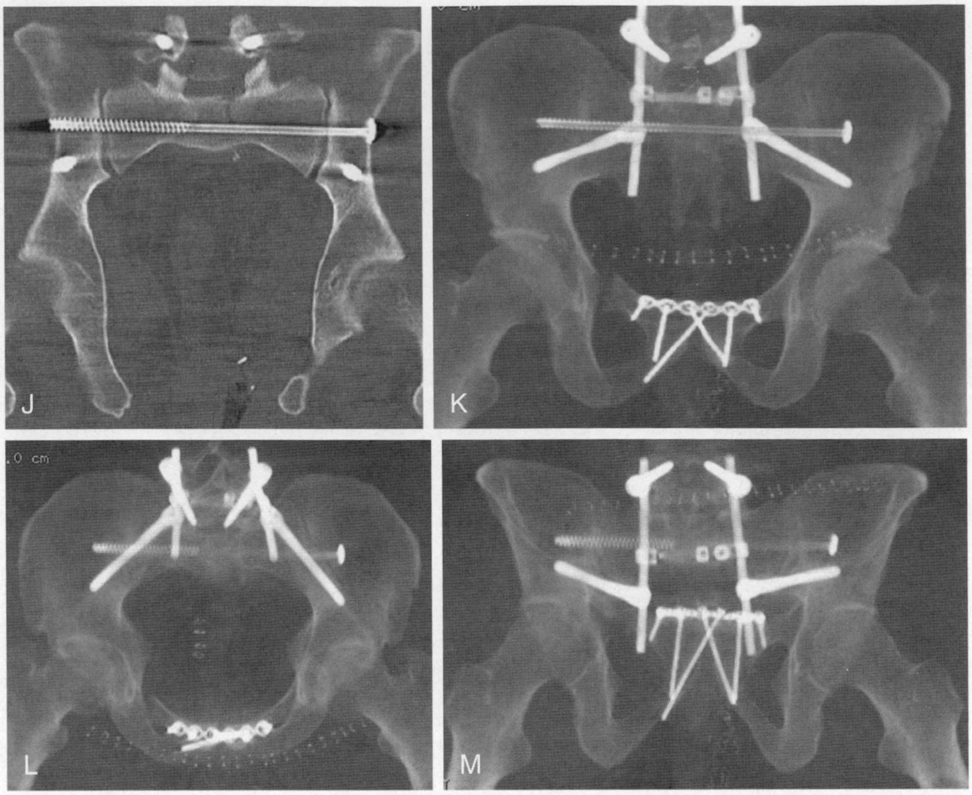

Figure 40-71, cont'd

and is not significantly contaminated and if a clean surgical wound can be achieved. The open wound may often allow reasonable access to areas requiring fixation. This technique can also be supplemented by external fixation. The use of minimal lag screw or percutaneous fixation along with external fixation may be the best method for obtaining stability with this type of injury.

If the urethra or bladder is injured and the abdomen has been opened, stabilization of the anterior injury can be done by internal fixation if the fracture pattern is amenable.

In females with an open fracture into the vagina, débridement of the open fracture, usually through the vagina, is all that is required. If the vaginal laceration is clean, it can be closed primarily. Any potentially contaminated vaginal wound should be left open to heal secondarily. In these settings, anterior stabilization of the pelvis in the acute phase is best accomplished by external fixation.

Follow-Up Care

After the patient is hemodynamically stable and the pelvis has been stabilized, definitive fracture care can be undertaken. Further soft tissue treatment can be carried out, such as repair of the genitourinary system, and any colostomy can be closed at 6 to 12 weeks after the soft tissue and rectal injuries have healed.[336,337]

With aggressive care of patients with pelvic fractures, historical mortality rates of up to 50% can be reduced to approximately 20%, which is equivalent to the mortality rate associated with a closed but completely unstable (type C) pelvic ring injury.[313]

Results

Our knowledge about the long-term results of pelvic ring fractures is still based on empirical findings, simply because no high-quality and reliable study data are available. However, previous research has provided some insight. The available literature suggests that, on average, 80% of operatively treated and 68% of nonoperatively treated patients have restoration of normal gait patterns. The discrepancy may be due to increased residual displacement of nonoperatively treated compared with operatively treated pelvic ring fractures but cannot be proven because of the absence of reliable comparative data. Relatively few studies have focused on return to previous employment, which has been reported as 68% without any significant difference in nonoperatively and operatively treated patients.[247]

Most authors agree that with anatomic or near-anatomic reduction, 60% to 70% of patients can be expected to have successful outcomes and that complications related to limb length discrepancy, sitting imbalance, and pelvic stability can be reliably avoided.* A recent outcome analysis by Papakostidis and colleagues[247] regarding pelvic ring disruption support this finding. Excellent or good results according to the Majeed score[340] were achieved in approximately 70% of patients, with no statistical difference in outcome between external and internal fixation. Additionally, the physical component score (PCS) and mental component score (MCS), the two components of Short Form 36 (SF-36), ranged from 55.5 to 75.3 and

*References 143, 148, 240, 249, 275, 338, 339.

from 64 to 74.8, respectively.[247] In summary, it can be stated that although the techniques of reduction and internal fixation of a disrupted pelvis are being refined, little objective proof has been presented that these techniques provide the patient with any better result than closed reduction and stabilization by external fixation. Dujardin and colleagues reviewed two consecutive cohorts of patients with unstable pelvic ring injuries by using anatomic measures and the validated pelvic outcome score of Majeed. One group was treated by external fixation and the other by internal fixation based on protocol. The overall functional result depended on the location of the posterior lesion and the ability to reduce it anatomically.[341] Pure SI joint dislocations fared poorly if anatomic reduction was not achieved. Fractures of the iliac wing or associated fracture-dislocations of the wing and SI joint did very well because they were easily reduced and stabilized. Sacral fractures did poorly despite good reduction because functional outcome was related to the associated nerve injury.

It has been demonstrated that although anatomic reduction and stable internal fixation are possible and lead to excellent anatomic and radiographic results, even in completely unstable pelvic ring injuries, the final functional outcome is usually determined by the associated soft tissue injury or other nonorthopaedic injuries.[35,241] In the rotationally unstable group, the results of internal fixation are much better, with up to 96% of patients having no pain on strenuous exercise.[36]

There is little disagreement that patients with unreduced SI joint injuries do not do well unless the injuries are reduced and stabilized, but it cannot be guaranteed that this result is as consistent as the results of operative treatment of SI joint fracture-dislocation or iliac wing fractures. Until a high-quality research trial is conducted to determine which method of treatment of sacral fractures, fracture-dislocations of the SI joint, and juxtaarticular fractures of the iliac wing (crescent fractures) is most effective, surgeons must treat the patient's injury with prompt recognition of any problems, reduction of the fracture displacement with restoration of pelvic alignment, and appropriate stabilization. If such treatment is not possible, referral for appropriate care to an institution that has sufficient resources to accomplish these goals is mandatory.

KEY REFERENCES

The level of evidence (LOE) is determined according to the criteria provided in the preface.

11. Denis F, Davis S, Comfort T: Sacral fractures, an important problem. Retrospective analysis of 236 cases. *Clin Orthop Relat Res* 227:67–81, 1988.
18. Tile M, Hearn T: Biomechanics. In Tile M, editor: *Fractures of the pelvis and acetabulum*, ed 2, Baltimore, 1995, Williams & Wilkins, pp 22–36.
35. Tornetta P, Matta JM: Outcome of operatively treated unstable posterior pelvic ring disruptions. *Clin Orthop Relat Res* 329:186–193, 1996.
111. White CE, Hsu JR, Holcomb JB: Haemodynamically unstable pelvic fractures. *Injury* 40(10):1023–1030, 2009.
192. Gibbons KJ, Soloniuk DS, Razack N: Neurologic injury and patterns of sacral fractures. *J Neurosurg* 72(6):889–893, 1990.
201. Matta JM, Saucedo T: Internal fixation of pelvic ring fractures. *Clin Orthop Relat Res* 242:83–97, 1989.
233. Templeman D, Goulet J, Duwelius PJ: Internal fixation of displaced fractures of the sacrum. *Clin Orthop Relat Res* 329:180–185, 1996.
238. Schildhauer T, Bellabarba C, Nork SE, et al: Decompression and lumbopelvic fixation for sacral-fracture dislocations with spino-pelvic dissociation. *J Orthop Trauma* 20(7):447–457, 2006.
239. Bellabarba C, Schildhauer TA, Vaccaro AR, et al: Complications associated with surgical stabilization of high-grade sacral fracture dislocations with spino-pelvic instability. *Spine (Phila Pa 1976)* 31(11 Suppl):S80–S88, 2006.
243. Lindahl J, Hirvensalo E: Outcome of operatively treated type C injuries of the pelvic ring. *Acta Orthop* 76:667–678, 2005.
247. Papakostidis C, Kanakaris NK, Kontakis G, et al: Pelvic ring disruptions: treatment modalities and analysis of outcomes. *Int Orthop* 33(2):329–338, 2009.
314. Dente CJ, Feliciano DV, Rozycki GS, et al: The outcome of open pelvic fractures in the modern era. *Am J Surg* 190(6):830–835, 2005.
316. Perry JP: Open pelvic fractures. *Clin Orthop* 151:41–45, 1980.

The complete References list is available online at https://expertconsult.inkling.com.

Chapter 41

Surgical Treatment of Acetabular Fractures

MILTON LEE (CHIP) ROUTT, JR. • JOSHUA L. GARY

Acetabular fractures are uncommon and quite complex injuries that usually result from high-energy traumatic events. The rarity of these fractures makes it difficult for most physicians to become familiar with them. These injuries challenge even the most experienced physicians because of their deep and complex anatomy and associated primary organ system injuries. Over the past 4 decades, a great deal of information has been gathered regarding these injuries and their treatments.

EPIDEMIOLOGY

Acetabular fractures occur when the lower extremity, specifically the proximal femur, is excessively loaded. The resultant acetabular fracture pattern details are determined by the hip position at impact, the local bone quality, and the force of the applied load. As the load is further transmitted, the acetabular fracture displaces, and the femoral head may dislocate from the hip joint in line with the applied force (Fig. 41-1). Two different age groups of patients typically sustain acetabular fractures.[1] Young adults with active and perhaps reckless lifestyles tend to be involved in high-energy traumatic accidents resulting in acetabular injuries. More senior but not necessarily less active patients sustain acetabular injuries from lower energy events such as falling from a standing height, and their frequency is increasing.[2] These injuries most likely result from insufficient bone quality. Acetabular fractures do occur in pediatric patients; however, these are rare.

The mechanisms of injury are usually automobile and motorcycle accidents, pedestrians struck by motor vehicles, falls from significant heights, and crush injuries. Legislation directed at seatbelt wear and enforcement has been shown to decrease the incidence and severity of acetabular injuries.[3] Conversely, some studies have suggested that mandatory helmet laws have improved patient survivability after motorcycle accidents and therefore increased the number and complexity of acetabular trauma.[4] A variety of ongoing projects are focused on automobile redesign for improved safety. These new safety features may decrease the incidence and severity of pelvic and acetabular fractures.[5]

OSTEOLOGY

Normal pelvic osteology is complex and can be quite confusing, and displaced acetabular fractures further complicate understanding. The acetabulum is a hemisphere-shaped recess located between the ilium, ischium, and pubis. It develops from the triradiate cartilage and matures into a variety of appearances. Some acetabuli are shallow and termed "dysplastic," and others are deeper and referred to as "normal." On radiographs, whereas the dysplastic acetabuli are situated peripherally relative to the ilium, deeper ones appear medially located. All of these anatomic factors are important when treating acetabular injuries. Other than the regions of the fossa acetabuli and the far acetabular rim, the concave acetabular surface is covered with hyaline cartilage and surrounded on its periphery by the labrum. The peripheral labrum is attached to both the acetabular rim and the joint capsule. The fossa acetabuli is filled with fat and anchors the ligamentum teres along with its blood vessels. The fossa acetabuli's cortical backing is the quadrilateral surface. The transverse acetabular ligament borders the caudal aspect of the acetabulum.

The articular regions of the acetabulum include the anterior wall, dome, and posterior wall. The anterior wall's chondral surface area is small relative to the other two articular regions. The cortical surface of the anterior wall area is actually that part of the superior pubic ramus referred to as the iliopectineal eminence (IPE). The IPE is a mound of corticocancellous bone that has the anterior wall articular cartilage surface as its base. The iliopsoas tendon passes lateral to the IPE and anterior relative to the anterior acetabular wall within a shallow longitudinal recess referred to as the iliopsoas gutter. The anterior acetabular wall's peripheral edge is concave at the site where the iliopsoas tendon passes across it, and a bursa surrounds the tendon protecting it from the anterior acetabular wall, labrum, and capsule as it courses anterior to the hip joint toward its insertion on the lesser trochanter of the femur. Medially, the dense cortical pelvic brim borders the anterior acetabular wall, and anteriorly the cortical surface of the pectineal sulcus neighbors the IPE and anterior wall area. The acetabular dome is the superior articular area located directly beneath the anterior inferior iliac spine (AIIS). The posterior wall region is the largest surface area of the three articular zones and comprises the remainder of the acetabular articular surface. Many surgeons include the acetabular dome area as a component part of the posterior acetabular wall. All three articular zones are backed by a topographically complex corticocancellous bony anatomy. Similar to tectonic plates, the surrounding bony "hills and valleys" represent the acetabular fault lines that allow fracture propagation (Fig. 41-2).

The acetabular two-column concept was introduced by Letournel. Using this conceptual model, the articular acetabulum is located between and as a part of two surrounding bony limbs representing an inverted Y shape. The anterior limb, or supporting column, includes the symphysis pubis, superior pubic ramus, anterior acetabular wall, anterior halves of the dome and fossa acetabuli, anterior half of the quadrilateral

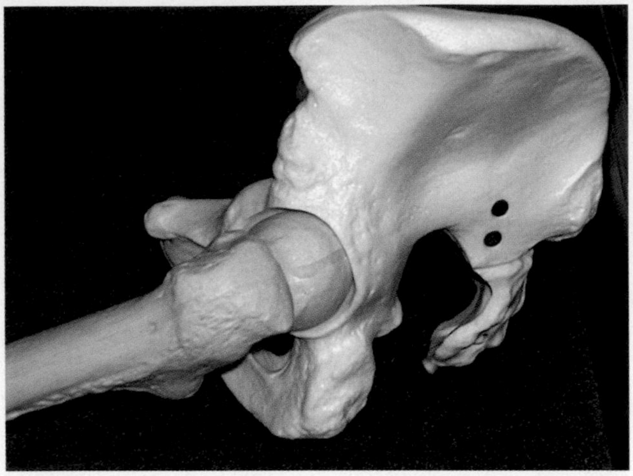

Figure 41-1. Acetabular fractures occur as a result of excessive loads applied to the bone via the proximal femur. The exact fracture characteristics and details are related to the position of the femur relative to the acetabulum, the bone quality, and the amount of force applied. In the model shown, a force applied at the knee region would produce a much different fracture pattern than if the force was applied through the greater trochanter.

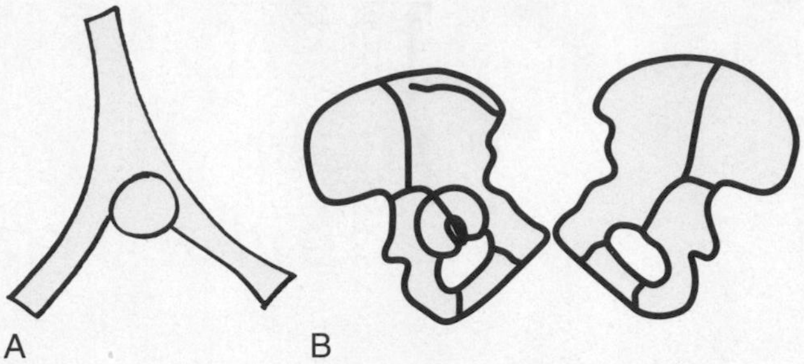

Figure 41-3. A, Letournel's two-column concept is demonstrated schematically by this illustration depicting the acetabulum between two supporting "columns" of an inverted Y shape. **B,** The anatomic correlation of the inverted Y model demonstrates the anterior column consisting of iliac and pubic components and the posterior column consisting of ischial components. The quadrilateral surface and fossa acetabuli are divided. The acetabulum is situated between the two limbs of the inverted Y-shaped support. The anterior and posterior wall regions are portions of their respective supporting columns.

surface, and anterior ilium (including both anterior iliac spines and crest). The posterior limb, or supporting column, includes the entire posterior wall, the posterior portions of the dome and fossa acetabuli, the caudal portion of the greater sciatic notch, the ischial spine, the entire lesser sciatic notch, and the posterior half of the quadrilateral surface (Fig. 41-3). Understanding the inverted Y conceptual model and corresponding acetabular structural supporting columns is the first step to learning acetabular osteology and leads to understand

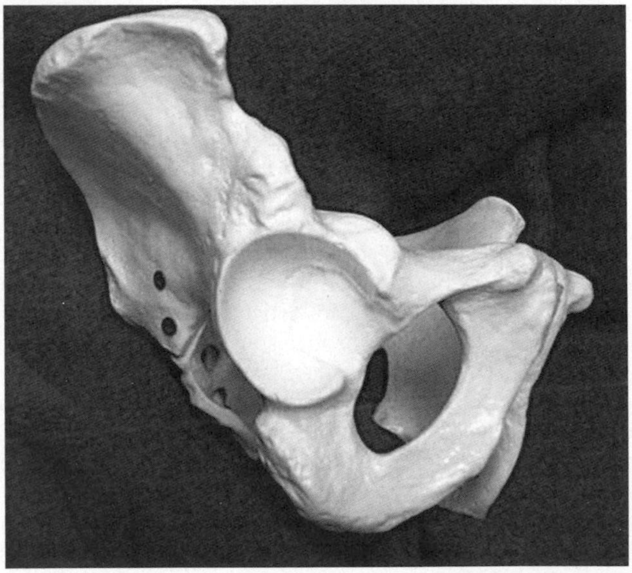

Figure 41-2. The acetabulum has a variable topography. The anterior wall articular surface is small and is the base of the iliopectineal eminence. The acetabular dome articular area is slightly larger than the anterior wall and is located caudal to the anterior inferior iliac spine and iliopsoas gutter. The posterior wall articular surface is the largest articular surface. The fossa acetabuli is a nonarticular corticated recess within the joint that is backed by the quadrilateral surface, bounded caudally by the transverse acetabular ligament, and contains fat and the ligamentum teres.

more complex issues such as the associated radiology and fracture patterns.

The two-column structural model was intended to simplify the acetabular osseous architecture so that clinicians could better understand the injury patterns. But for some, it became confusing, especially when the fracture patterns and classification scheme were defined using most of the same osteology terminology. In the two-column acetabular structural model, the anterior column area includes the anterior wall, and the posterior column area includes the entire posterior wall. This confuses some clinicians because the anterior and posterior walls are component parts of the supporting columns but separate from them as individual fracture patterns. For example, an elementary posterior column acetabular fracture pattern divides the area of the anatomic or bony posterior wall, extends through the greater sciatic notch, progresses through the quadrilateral surface, exits the caudal aspect of the fossa acetabuli, and fractures the inferior ramus. The osteologic, two-column model and fracture pattern terminologies use shared words yet are truly distinct from one another. To resolve the confusion, the anatomic acetabular areas, two-column model components, and the individual fracture patterns must be considered while respecting and consolidating all of this information (Fig. 41-4).

RADIOLOGY

Pelvic radiology is even more complex than pelvic osteology but is the essential key to understanding acetabular fractures. Acetabular fracture diagnosis and classification schemes are based on the radiographic findings and Letournel's two-column acetabular concept. An anterior-posterior (AP) plain pelvic radiograph taken early in the workup of a trauma patient often alerts the treating physician to the acetabular fracture. For this reason, certain radiographic osseous landmarks were introduced by Letournel and still serve as the foundation of acetabular imaging. Many clinicians evaluate the uninjured side initially to review the relevant landmarks and then compare them and their asymmetry with the injured side.

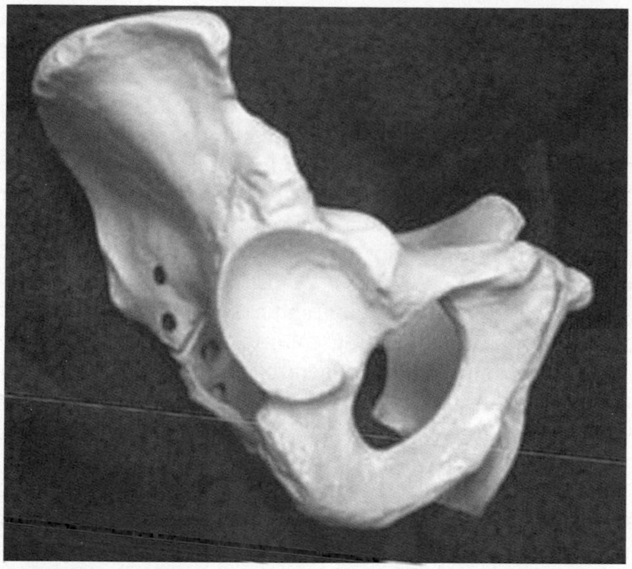

Figure 41-4. This model shows that the anterior wall area is a portion of the anterior column, and the posterior wall area is a portion of the posterior column.

The normal radiographic markers represent bony cortical edges revealed by tangential x-ray beams. These cortical lines include the peripheral edges of both the anterior and posterior walls; the dense line representing the pelvic brim and superior pubic ramus' posterior-cranial edge (iliopectineal line); the dense line representing the pelvic brim and quadrilateral surface (ilioischial line); the dome region's subchondral arc (sourcil); and the acetabular "teardrop" representing the fossa acetabuli, obturator sulcus, and a portion of the quadrilateral surface. These six radiographic markers help clinicians to better understand and mark the two walls, the two supporting columns, the weight-bearing dome, and the caudal joint (Fig. 41-5).

Clinicians should learn normal acetabular radiology first and while holding and handling a pelvic model. The osseous model helps correlate osteology and radiology. Three-dimensional (3-D) radiographic modeling and volume-rendered images capable of on-screen manipulation should also facilitate pelvic and acetabular radiographic correlations and learning. Normal radiology should be mastered first; then the clinician moves on to trying to comprehend displaced fracture imaging.

Normally, the anterior wall is medially located relative to the more peripheral posterior wall on the AP pelvic

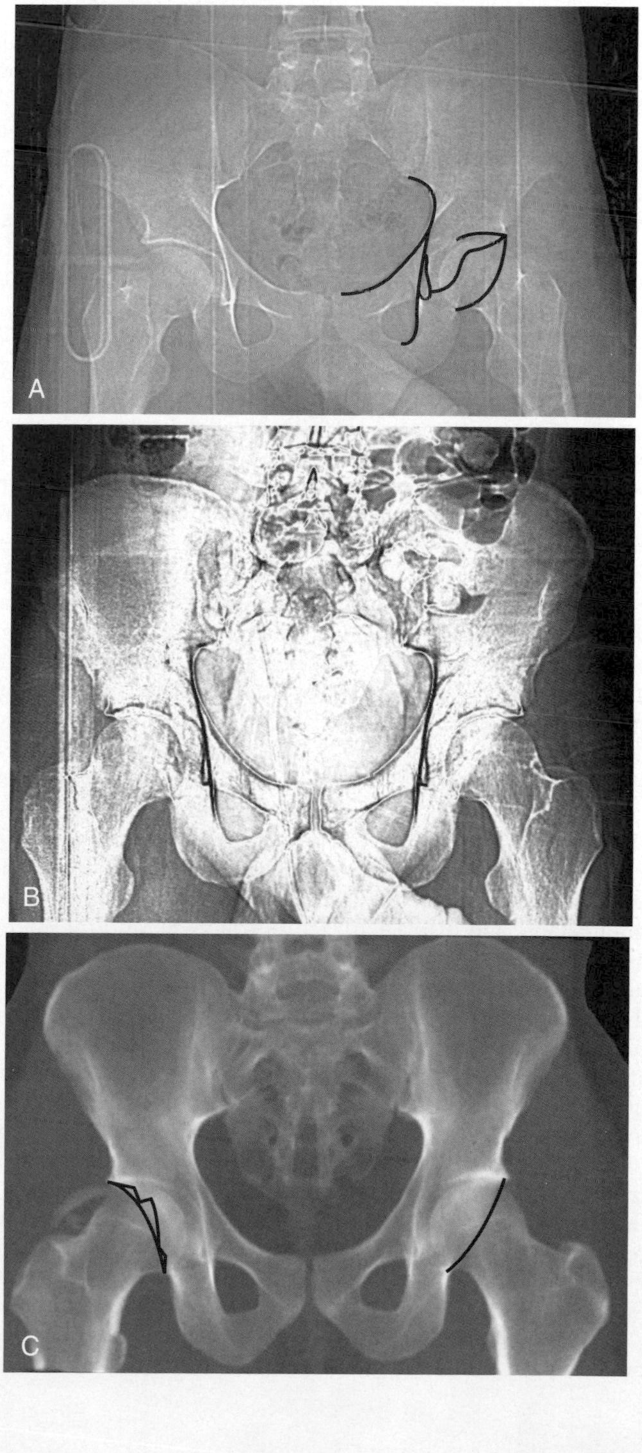

Figure 41-5. A, Plain pelvic anterior-posterior (AP) radiograph demonstrating the six important acetabular lines. The dome arc, the anterior wall, posterior wall, iliopectineal (or iliopubic) line, ilioischial line, and teardrop are noted. The dome line represents a subchondral region of the weight-bearing area. The anterior wall is medially located and undulating relative to the more peripheral and convex posterior wall. The anterior wall appears denser than the posterior wall because of the radiographic "bony stacking" or superimposition of the two walls and femoral head. The peripheral posterior wall only radiographically stacks the femoral head and posterior wall. The iliopectineal (or iliopubic) line is a condensation of cortical bone shadows from the greater sciatic notch and pelvic brim ("ilio-") and superior pubic ramus ("pectineal or pubic"). This line represents the supporting anterior column. The ilioischial line shares the "ilio-" component with the previous line but then diverges, representing the quadrilateral surface cortical bone imaged tangentially for its "ischial" component. The ilioischial line represents the structural posterior acetabular column. The teardrop is the last landmark; is located lateral to the ilioischial line; and indicates the fossa acetabuli, quadrilateral surface, and obturator sulcus. **B,** Image alteration of this AP pelvic radiograph accentuates the ilioischial lines and teardrops bilaterally. **C,** AP plain pelvic radiograph demonstrating the radiographic appearance of a displaced posterior wall acetabular fracture. Five landmark lines are intact, but the peripheral posterior wall line is lost because of the displaced fracture. Also, a radiolucency is noted in the area where the intact posterior wall density should be, and the displaced peripheral posterior wall fracture-displacement is seen.

radiograph. The anterior wall has an undulating edge anatomy attributed to the iliopsoas gutter, IPE, and pectineal cortical sulcus. Imaging of the anterior wall area reveals it to appear more radiodense than the posterior wall because of the superimposed osseous anatomy. The posterior wall edge anatomy is usually convex and located peripherally relative to the anterior wall. Knowing these anatomic details helps the treating physician to better understand the acetabular injury when evaluating the radiographs.

The anterior acetabular supporting column is represented on the AP pelvic radiograph by the iliopectineal (iliopubic) line. This radiodense line is formed from tangential imaging of the pelvic brim cortical bone as it extends from the sacroiliac (SI) area to the pubis. The superior and posterior cortical edge of the superior pubic ramus in continuity with the pelvic brim cortical bone forms the iliopectineal line. The iliopectineal line represents the supporting acetabular anterior column and is only imaged on the AP plain pelvic radiograph, not on oblique imaging.

The posterior acetabular supporting column is represented on the AP pelvic radiograph by the ilioischial line. This radiodense line is formed from the tangential imaging of the pelvic brim, quadrilateral surface, and medial ischial cortical bone. As with the iliopectineal line, the ilioischial line is only seen on the AP plain pelvic radiograph and not on oblique images.

When first learning Letournel's inverted Y model of the structural anterior and posterior acetabular columns, most students view the hemipelvis and acetabulum from a direct lateral side view. Learning the acetabular structural columnar osteology and its imaging on an AP view is more difficult because now the inverted Y and two supporting osseous columns and their representative radiographic landmarks are viewed obliquely, and they are superimposed on one another. With a pelvic model in hand and a high-quality AP pelvic image to study, the learning is enhanced. Understanding that the AP pelvic image reveals the structural acetabular columns obliquely and that they are superimposed on one another is the second step to learning the osteology, related radiography, and fracture patterns.

Normally, the acetabular dome's subchondral arc is seen cranial to and congruent with the femoral head. In its simplest form, it represents the weight-bearing area of the articular acetabulum and is vital to assessing hip joint congruity. A variety of acetabular fracture patterns will divide the dome area. In some patterns, the medial portion of the dome will be the unstable and displaced fracture fragment, and the lateral dome fragment will be the stable or intact part. In other fracture patterns, the medial dome will be the stable portion on the intact pelvis, and the lateral dome part will be the displaced and unstable fracture fragment. The dome area is also affected by impaction, almost always located on the intact side of the fracture just at the fracture's edge, although articular impaction can also occur more rarely on displaced fragments too. This crushed articular area along the fracture line is termed "marginal impaction." Fracture displacement through the acetabular dome region is important because accurate operative restoration of the dome articular surfaces and congruity with the femoral head correlate with improved long-term function and durability of the injured hip joint.[6]

The acetabular "teardrop" is probably the most difficult radiographic landmark of the six to understand, but its value is relevant, especially when assessing the accuracy of surgical repair. The medial cortical portion of the teardrop is formed by the obturator neurovascular sulcus and a portion of the quadrilateral surface. The lateral cortical boundary represents the cortical surface of the fossa acetabuli. For certain displaced fracture patterns, the teardrop is no longer recognizable on the AP pelvic radiograph. After operative acetabular fracture repair, the teardrop landmark should be symmetrical to the contralateral normal hip joint. If not, the reduction is not accurate.

These six AP pelvic radiographic acetabular markers represent acetabular supporting columns, walls, and the dome area. On the injured side, depending on the specific fracture details, the walls, columns, and dome arc may be divided by fracture lines, impacted, or displaced along with certain fracture fragments.[7]

After an acetabular fracture is identified, further radiographic assessments are indicated after any dislocations have been reduced. Biplanar imaging is obtained by placing the radiographic cassette beneath the patient's pelvis as for an AP image but then rolling the patient approximately 45 degrees onto the uninjured side for the film and then rolling similarly onto the injured side using the same imaging technique. Rolling the patient onto the injured acetabular side usually causes pain and should be performed last. These two biplanar images identify the columns and walls more specifically and are named according to the injured side. When the injured side is rolled up, the obturator foramen is relatively perpendicular to the x-ray beam, so the image is termed an "obturator oblique" (OO). The OO image demonstrates the structural anterior column and the posterior wall area. Similarly, when the injured side is rolled down, the iliac fossa is essentially perpendicular to the x-ray beam, and the image is named an "iliac oblique" view. The iliac oblique radiograph reveals the anterior wall area and the structural posterior column (Fig. 41-6).

Rolling the patient for the oblique images not only causes pain but often reveals fracture instability sites that may not have been apparent on the AP plain pelvic radiograph. The oblique acetabular images should not be obtained with the hip dislocated. The displaced fracture fragments and femoral head will obstruct important anatomic landmarks. Whenever the clinical situation allows it, routine reduction maneuvers should be performed before obtaining the oblique radiographs.

Other plain pelvic radiographs, such as inlet and outlet images, are indicated for those patients with pelvic ring injuries coupled with acetabular fractures. Combination pelvic ring–acetabular injuries are not uncommon, especially with high-energy injury mechanisms, and inlet and outlet plain pelvic views should be obtained if a concurrent pelvic ring injury is suspected. Certain acetabular fracture patterns such as transverse fractures disrupt the acetabular portion of the pelvic ring completely and will often have a related pelvic ring injury site.

Pelvic computed tomography (CT) imaging further delineates acetabular injuries. Two-dimensional (2-D) pelvic CT scans are usually obtained in 5-mm axial slices from the iliac crest to the acetabular dome. From the dome region through the caudal articular areas, 3-mm images are recommended, and then 5-mm axial slices through the ischium. 2-D pelvic CT imaging, including axial, coronal, and sagittal

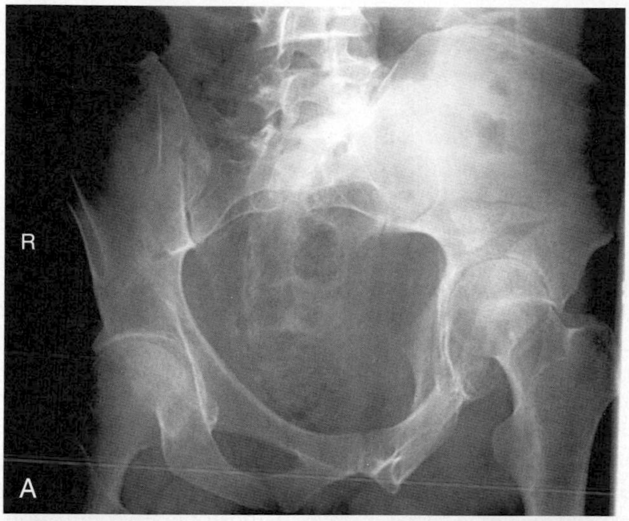

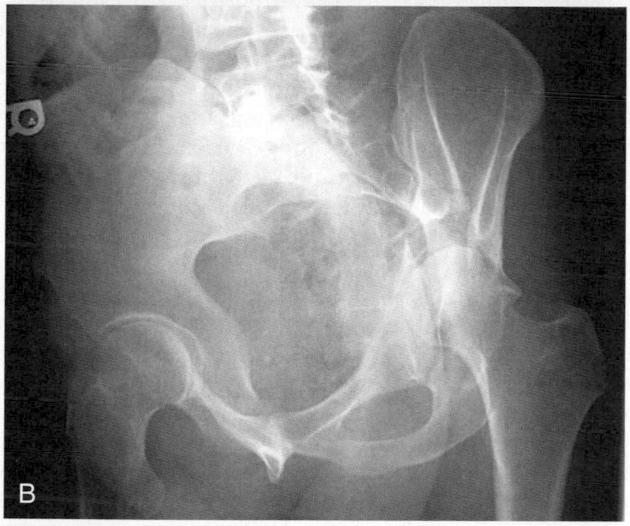

Figure 41-6. A, This patient has a significantly displaced left-sided acetabular fracture. On this oblique image, the patient's right side was rolled up and the injured left side down while the oblique radiograph was obtained. Because the x-ray beam is essentially perpendicular to the iliac fossa on the injured side, this is the iliac oblique image. The edge of the anterior wall and the outline of the posterior column are best seen on this view. The iliac oblique imaging can be very painful for the patient, so patients are often less rotated as a result. Alert patients complain as body weight is applied onto the injured side. **B,** The injured left side has been rolled up and the normal right side is down. On the injured left side, the obturator foramen is essentially perpendicular to the x-ray beam, making this an obturator oblique image. The area of the anterior acetabular column and the posterior wall region are best seen on this view. This patient has a seizure disorder, and his medications have diminished his bone quality. He fell from a standing height and sustained an unusual acetabular fracture with severe crush and intrusion of the femoral head because of his poor bone quality.

reformations, provides information regarding bone quality, body habitus, surrounding soft tissue injury, occult posterior pelvic injury, remote injuries, and other acetabular details.[8,9] Related local osseous findings may include acetabular or femoral head impaction injuries, intraarticular debris, and subtle incongruity, among other findings. If the patient has received an intravenous contrast agent before the scan, the fracture fragments' displacements and their relationships with the pelvic vascular structures will be highlighted as well as related bleeding sites and accumulations. Displaced anterior column fracture fragments often deform the iliac artery and vein (Fig. 41-7) Medial displacement of quadrilateral surface fracture fragments will usually impact the course of the obturator vessels and nerve. Fractures displaced through the cranial portion of the greater sciatic notch may injure the superior gluteal neurovascular complex. Vascular contrast on the pelvic CT scan also may reveal other relevant vascular anatomy such as the corona mortis vascular conduits and their relationship to the fracture fragments or anticipated surgical exposure. Numerous studies have demonstrated the need for CT when evaluating acetabular fractures.[10-15]

Recent computer imaging software allows the operator to produce "plain radiographs" from the data acquired during pelvic CT. These surface-rendered pelvic images can then be rotated and manipulated on the monitor to provide the necessary oblique images.[16] The treating physicians must remember that such computer-generated and rotated oblique radiographs are processed data acquired with the injured patient positioned supine in the CT scanner and are not obtained by rolling the patient as the routine oblique radiographs are performed. Because of this, subtle or occult fracture instability will not be identified as it is with the traditional oblique radiographs that apply positional body-weight clinical loading of the acetabular fracture (Fig. 41-8).

Three-dimensional pelvic CT techniques have been refined, thus improving the model quality and decreasing the radiographic exposure needed. The 3-D surface-rendered acetabular images provide the treating physician with a more realistic understanding of the overall acetabular pattern and fragment relationships. The displacements and fracture line specifics are revealed on a radiographic 3-D model.[17] Such modeling should facilitate understanding and treatment planning. Surface-rendered images allow the surgeon to plan for fracture site access and extent, clamp site application and vectoring, and implant locations. Many surgeons are lured by and may prefer the 3-D images solely for obvious reasons but must be aware that certain 3-D imaging software packages may smooth some fracture lines, and the radiography technician may also have digitally removed relevant anatomic features to improve the fracture assessment. 2-D pelvic CT remains the radiographic standard for acetabular fracture imaging and planning (Fig. 41-9).

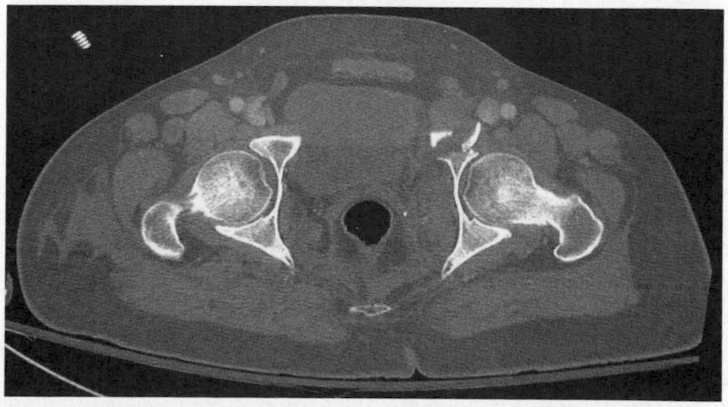

Figure 41-7. The injury pelvic computed tomography scan demonstrates bone and other details. In this patient, the displaced fracture fragment is located posterior to the iliac vein. Details such as this are important to know before surgery.

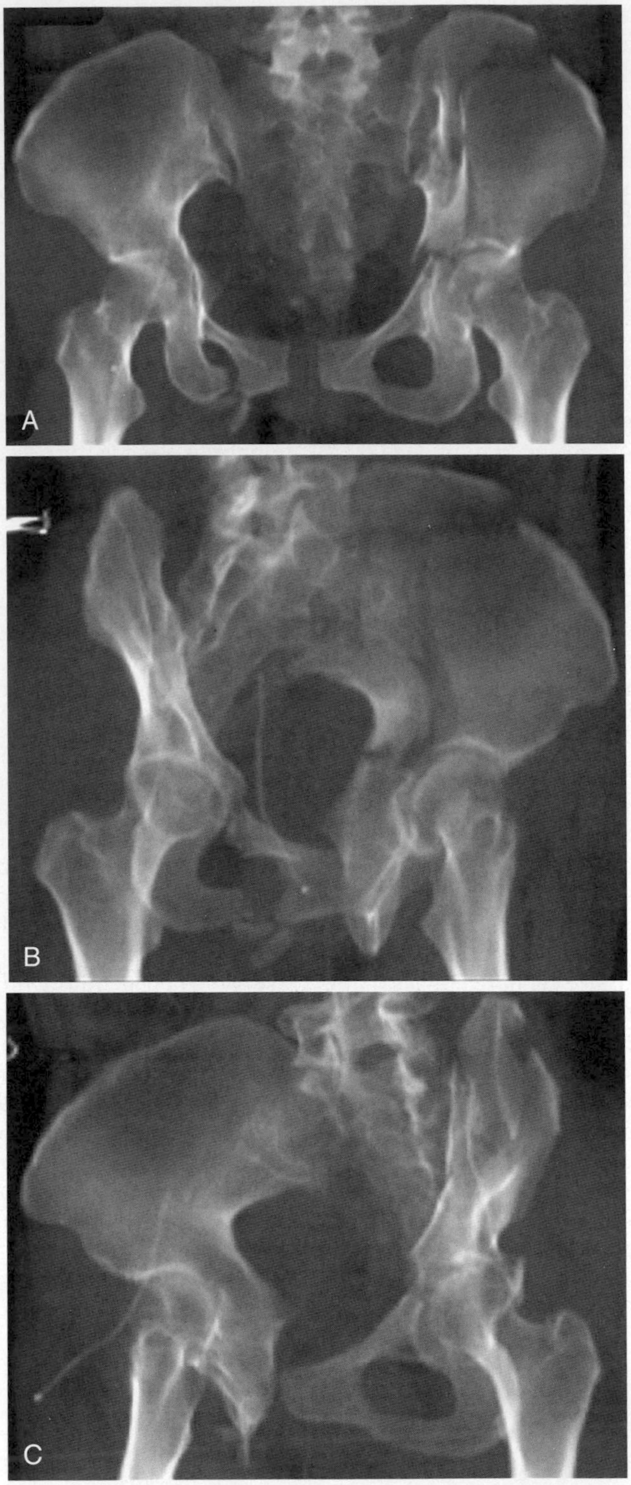

Figure 41-8. **A** to **C**, Anterior-posterior (AP) and biplanar oblique acetabular images generated from routine pelvic computed tomography (CT) data. Such computer-generated images do not reflect fracture instability because of patient positioning as routine oblique acetabular plain radiographs do because the acquired axial CT imaging information is acquired with the patient positioned supine and then manipulated to create these images. The AP image identifies the extensive injuries to both the pelvic ring and left acetabulum. The iliac oblique view shows the posterior column and anterior wall areas of injury. The obturator oblique identifies the posterior wall and anterior column areas of involvement.

Other radiographic studies have been advocated to better understand acetabular fractures. Dynamic acetabular imaging using angiographic fluoroscopic equipment was shown to improve understanding of certain complex fracture patterns. However, these methods were advocated before current CT imaging techniques.[18]

Pelvic angiography is indicated in hemodynamically unstable patients with acetabular fractures who have not responded to routine resuscitation techniques and evaluations. The angiographer should access the pelvic arterial tree using the contralateral side from the acetabular injury because fracture displacements may alter the groin vascular anatomy. Similarly, contrast agent leakage or hematoma in the ipsilateral groin area can cause significant dermatitis. These conditions in turn can adversely affect acetabular fracture treatment. Strategic embolizations can be lifesaving but also influence treatment decisions such as surgical exposure choice and have been associated with increased rates of postoperative infection.[19] The embolization procedure and its details should be documented in the permanent medical record. Radiodense metallic coils are commonly used to treat the injured artery, are visible on plain pelvic and CT imaging, and alert the surgeon to the prior embolization procedure. Conversely, other embolic substances are radiolucent and therefore not obvious on routine imaging. The treating surgeon should always consider the injured artery site as well as the level of embolization when planning for surgery. The treating surgeon should also remember that angiographic images are usually multiplanar and of the highest quality. These images should be reviewed whenever possible.

The angiography suite is often an ideal location for closed manipulative reduction of acetabular fracture-dislocations. Typically, the patients are amply sedated, and the reductions can be performed under real-time imaging if desired. Using the angiographic imaging equipment, the biplanar oblique plain radiographs can be obtained without moving the patient because the radiographic beam rotates around the patient. Coordinating the closed reduction in the angiography suite requires consent of the patient before anesthesia and consent of the angiography team.

Magnetic resonance imaging (MRI) has thus far had limited indications in patients with acetabular fractures caused by acute trauma. Insufficiency fractures of the peripheral pubic ramus and related acetabular stress fractures have been identified using MRI. Acetabular fracture nonunion rarely occurs after operative treatment but does occasionally complicate closed treatment. Pelvic MRI and CT scanning are both diagnostic for acetabular nonunion.

CLASSIFICATION

Acetabular fracture classification is a confusing diagnostic exercise because the same terms used to describe the anatomic walls and supporting columns are used again to define certain specific fracture patterns. Using the same terms to describe the supporting structures of the inverted Y conceptual model and the distinct fracture types confuses essentially every student trying to learn the Letournel-Judet acetabular fracture classification scheme. The treating physician must comprehend that anatomic areas and fracture patterns are related and similar but are not the same. An anatomic area is an

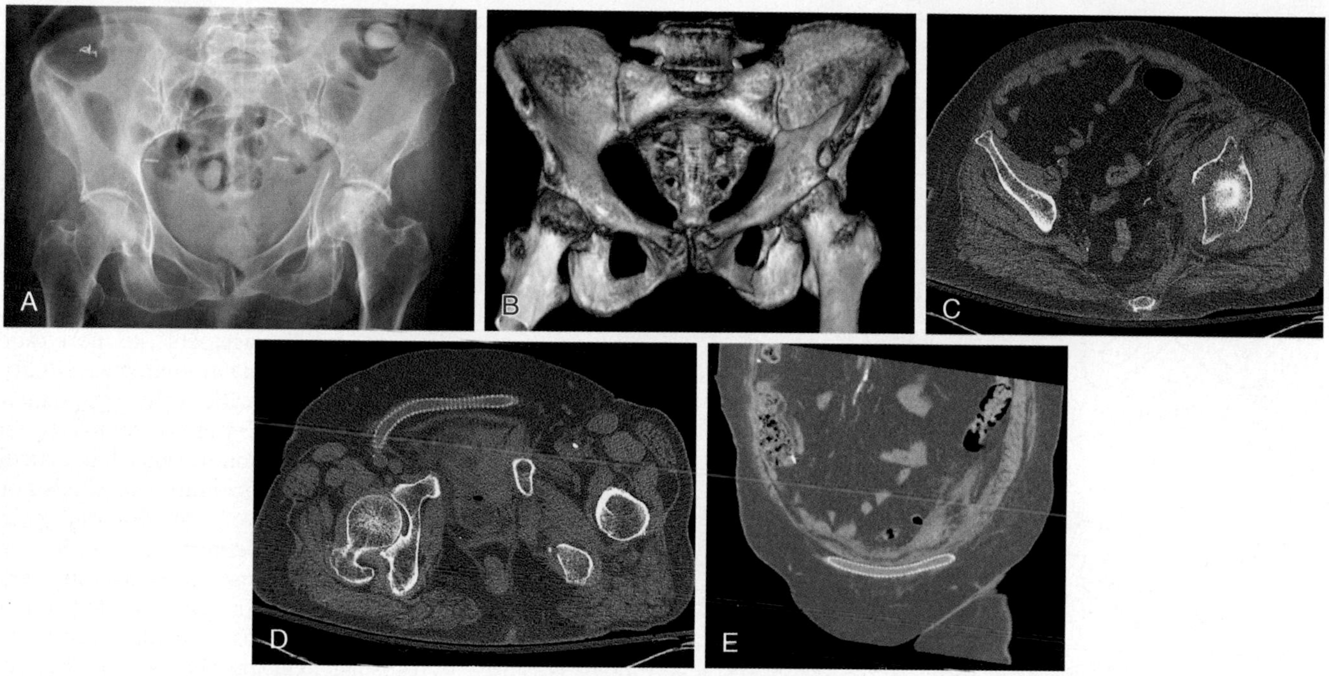

Figure 41-9. All of the images from the pelvic computed tomography (CT) scan must be examined before formulating a final treatment plan. This 63-year-old woman complained of left hip pain after falling from a standing height. She was unable to move her left hip because of pain, and passive range of motion attempts caused severe pain. She stated that she had prior abdominal surgeries but could not remember any details. She had several healed abdominal scars. Her plain pelvic anterior-posterior radiograph (**A**) and three-dimensional (3-D) modeled image (**B**) demonstrate her displaced acetabular fracture (**C** to **E**). The axial and coronal CT images revealed a femoral–femoral bypass graft. The radiology technician had "digitally erased" the bypass graft from the reconstructed 3-D images so it would not obstruct the fracture assessment. Nonoperative management was selected because of the patient's overall poor medical condition and in part because of the graft and its location.

anatomic area, and the named fracture pattern involves that anatomic area.

Classifications are assigned based on radiographic criteria.[7,20-23] The AP pelvic radiograph provides certain clues that are then refined on the oblique images and CT scans. When the iliopectineal line is disrupted or displaced but the ilioischial line is not on the AP pelvic plain radiograph, the acetabular fracture is likely an anterior column fracture pattern. The pelvic oblique views and CT images reveal the fracture details needed to define the classification pattern. When only the ilioischial line is disrupted or displaced on the AP radiograph, then a posterior column pattern is presumed and further investigated. Similarly, many fracture patterns involve the anterior and posterior wall anatomic areas but are not necessarily an anterior wall acetabular fracture pattern or posterior wall acetabular fracture pattern. For example, a transverse acetabular fracture pattern splits the acetabulum into two halves. The fracture line usually extends through the anterior wall area and then through the pelvic brim and along the quadrilateral surface, dividing the area of the posterior column usually through the greater sciatic notch, and exits through the area of the posterior wall. So even though all of those anatomic areas are injured by the fracture line, the fracture is best classified as a transverse pattern.

Letournel's acetabular classification scheme was devised to help surgeons select an appropriate surgical exposure for those fractures needing operative management.[7] The scheme is relatively inclusive and easy to remember but does not direct treatment nor is it prognostic.[24]

Ten common fracture patterns divided between two groups of five each were described. The "elementary" fractures included five different patterns, with the common theme being simplicity of the singular fracture plane. The elementary fractures include posterior wall, posterior column, anterior wall, anterior column, and transverse patterns. The transverse pattern is the only one of the five elementary patterns to not involve a single wall or single column. Instead, as described earlier, the transverse pattern fracture extends though the anterior wall and column areas as well as the pelvic brim and the posterior wall and posterior column areas. The transverse pattern is a single fracture surface, however, and for the reason of fracture "purity," it was placed in the elementary group.

The five "associated" fractures were more complicated fractures, combining some of the elementary patterns.[25] The associated patterns often have numerous fracture planes and details that make them distinct but are also more difficult to understand and sort. These five associated patterns are termed posterior column with associated posterior wall, transverse with associated posterior wall, anterior column with associated posterior hemitransverse, T-type, and associated both column. Simply from their individual names, it is clear that the five associated acetabular fracture patterns complicate the complexity level of the injury and therefore the evaluation and management. Similar to the transverse pattern being the outlier in the elementary group, the posterior column with associated posterior wall is the unusual member of the associated group in that it is the only associated fracture pattern that does not involve the two acetabular columns (Fig. 41-10).

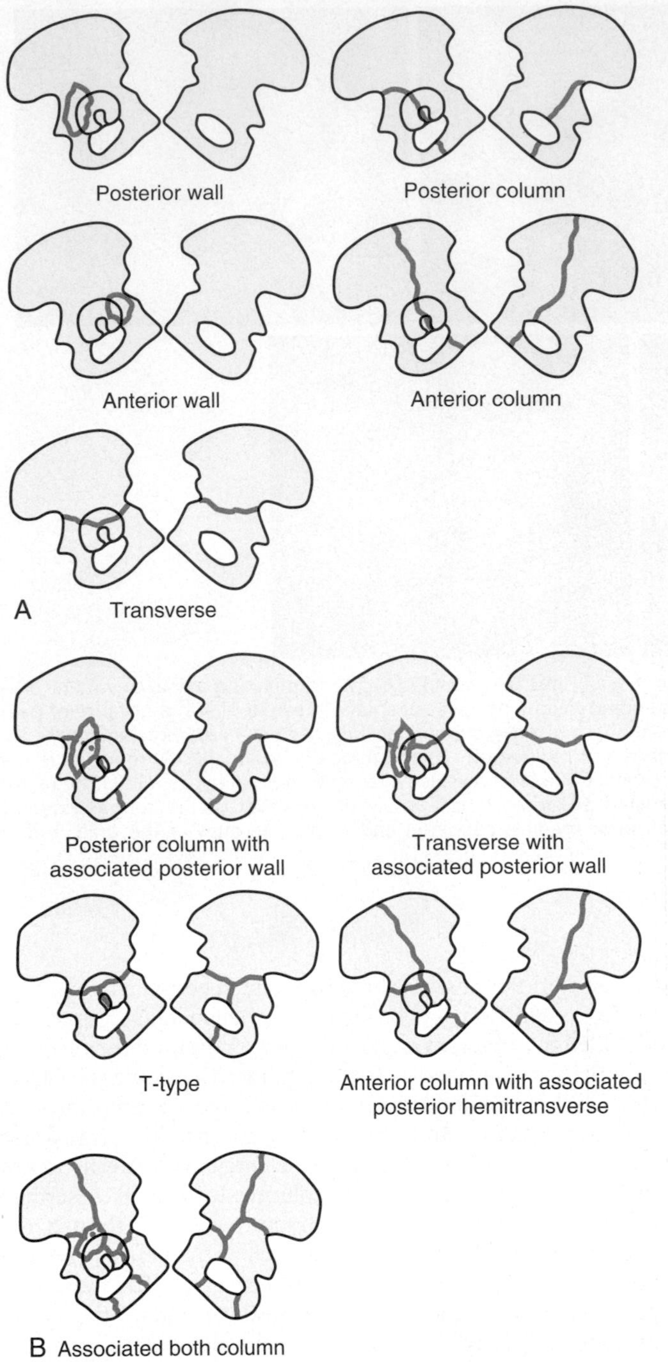

Figure 41-10. The five elementary (**A**) and five associated acetabular (**B**) fracture patterns.

Posterior Wall

The most common fracture pattern occurs in the posterior wall area.[7,26] These injuries tend to occur when the flexed hip loads the posterior wall and a portion of the posterior wall is displaced away from its intact base.[27] These injuries are often seen after automobile accidents when the seated motorist rapidly decelerates and the flexed knee contacts the dashboard, causing the flexed hip to load the posterior acetabular wall to failure. Because of this mechanism, knee-related injuries such as patellar fractures, traumatic arthrotomy, and posterior cruciate ligament injuries are associated with posterior wall acetabular fractures. In drivers contacting the steering mechanism with or without airbag protection, thoracic aortic injuries were previously identified and therefore must be ruled out.[28]

Similar to all acetabular fractures, posterior wall patterns have a variety of appearances, depending on the limb's position at load, the local bone quality, and the normal anatomy of the acetabulum.[29-31] Most surgeons would like to believe that "a posterior wall is a posterior wall, and they are simple," but nothing is further from the truth. Posterior wall acetabular injuries range from superior dome area wall displacements, to more common posterior wall displacements, to more caudal wall displacements, to "barn door" comminuted wall injuries, among other configurations and locations. In some patients, the posterior wall fragment fracture yields incompletely, and the femoral head crushes several chondrocancellous articular fragments into the intact posterior column cancellous bone, thereby producing an "intraarticular" posterior wall variant fracture-dislocation. Experienced clinicians recognize the variety of posterior wall injuries caused by impact loading as well as those seen with the more complex associated acetabular fracture patterns in which the posterior wall fracture fragment is caused by capsular avulsion (Fig. 41-11). Posterior wall fractures can be comminuted or associated with osteochondral impaction injuries along the fracture margin of the stable posterior column fragment, or they can involve both.[32] Marginal impaction is not the only local chondro-osseous problem related to these fractures. Displaced posterior wall fractures imply that the patient experienced an associated dislocation. For this reason, the femoral head should be evaluated for resultant impaction or cleavage injuries and the hip joint inspected for related bone or chondral debris.[33] Common sites for debris include the fossa acetabuli, between the femoral head and acetabular dome, in the cranial and caudal capsular recesses, and between the anterior femoral head and capsule. Debris can be fragments of cartilage, cancellous bone, cortical bone, or any combination of the three. Capsular and labral tissues may also be mislocated within the hip joint and cause joint incongruity. During surgery, these same tissues can obstruct accurate reduction of the bone fragments.

Routine posterior wall fractures are best identified on the OO image, especially when displaced. Usually, the displaced wall fragment yields in tension caudally along with tearing of the local capsule and labral tissues while the superoanterior labrum and capsule remain intact. The superior cortical aspect of the fracture is often comminuted because it yields in compression as the wall displaces. The displaced posterior wall fracture fragment damages the superior gemellus muscle and the portion of the gluteus minimus muscle caudal to the SGNVB as well. With more extensively displaced and dramatic injuries, the piriformis muscle belly can be injured and even transected by the displaced wall fragment's sharp cortical edge. In some instances, inspection of the buttock skin will reveal a circular ecchymotic area representative of the femoral head contusion (Fig. 41-12). Not surprisingly, the sciatic nerve may be damaged by direct injury from the displaced wall fragment, the extruded femoral head at the time of dislocation, or other direct or indirect factors. The piriformis anatomy is variable, and its relationship with the sciatic nerve bundles may also be responsible for nerve injury (Fig. 41-13). The sciatic nerve can also escape injury by the fracture-dislocation only to be injured by the reduction maneuver. In these unusual

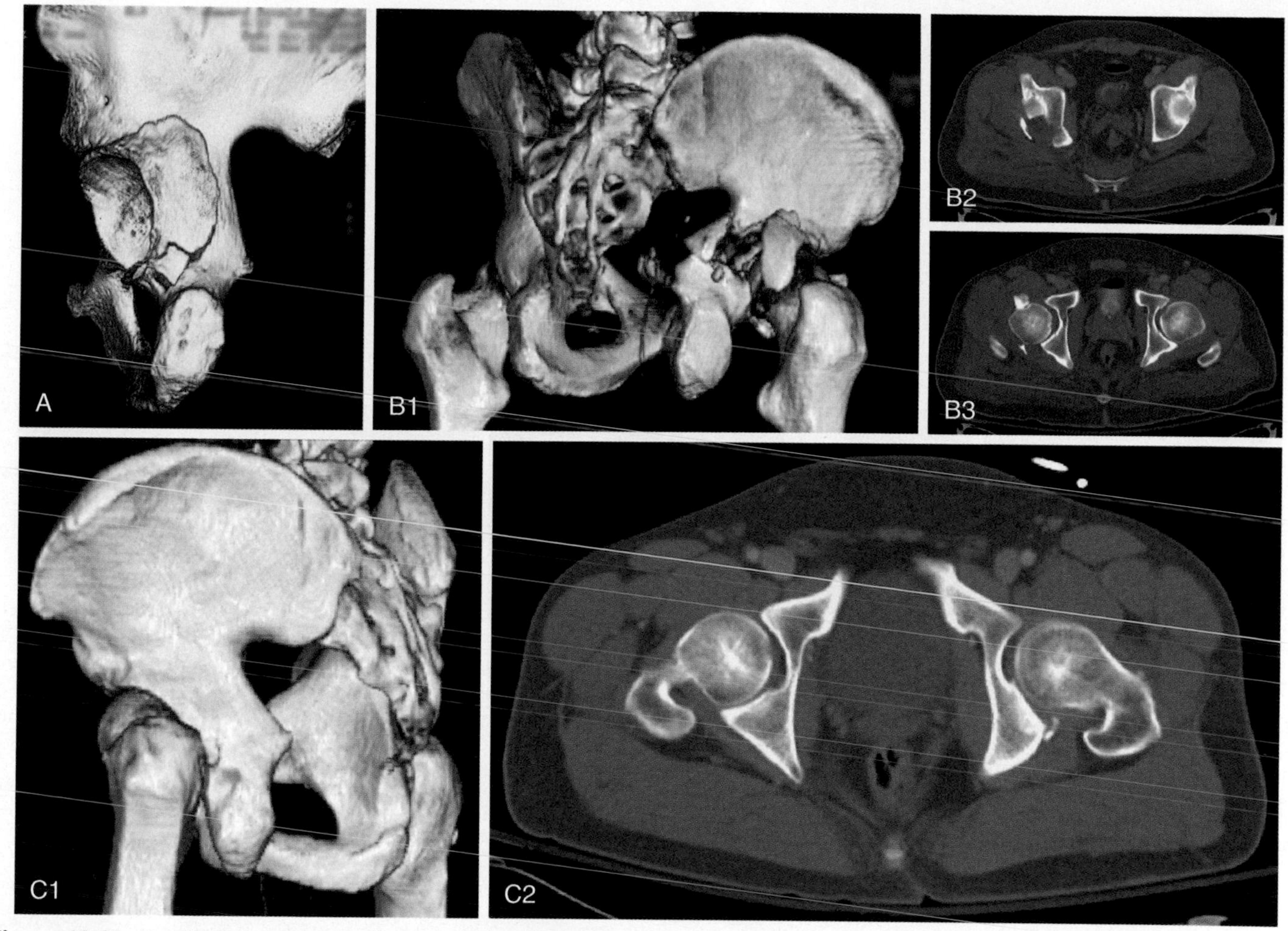

Figure 41-11. A variety of posterior wall acetabular injuries are represented by these images. There are commonly three different types of posterior wall acetabular fractures. The most common are elementary patterns associated with posterior hip fracture-dislocations. In these situations, the posterior wall fragment is "pushed off" by the femoral head as it dislocates. The next most common type occurs as a component of an associated both-column fracture pattern. In these situations, the posterior wall fragment is avulsed or "pulled off" as the femoral head displaces medially. The least common type occurs when the femoral head intrudes into the ischium, causing an impaction injury of the posterior wall area. The cortical posterior wall remains largely intact while the articular fragments are "pushed into" the underlying cancellous bone of the ischium. **A,** The elementary pattern common posterior wall is seen in this three-dimensional (3-D) model. The posterior wall primary fracture fragment is large and displaced. A small, comminuted fragment is noted caudally. During surgery, the hip capsule and labrum were both intact. For most displaced posterior wall fractures, the caudal labrum and adjacent hip capsule are torn, but the cranial labrum usually remains intact. **B1** and **B2,** This patient has a comminuted posterior wall acetabular fracture that extends into the greater sciatic notch. **B3,** On the axial computed tomography (CT) image, a large posterior wall articular fragment is located anteriorly relative to the femoral head. **C1,** This patient was crushed by a large metallic object, but states that his hip did not dislocate. **C2,** The 3-D model identifies a very small and caudally located posterior wall fracture. The axial image reveals that the posterior wall articular surface has been crushed into the cancellous bone of the ischium.

Continued

instances, the displaced wall fracture fragment follows the hip reduction, and the sciatic nerve becomes compressed between the posterior wall fragment and its base.

Posterior Column

Posterior column fractures occur infrequently but are relatively predictable in their appearance. As an elementary pattern, the fracture plane is singular, descending from the greater sciatic notch, with the lateral cortical disruption splitting the posterior column and posterior wall anatomic areas while the medial cortical line divides the quadrilateral surface. The fracture plane progresses through the dome area, exits the caudal posterior wall and fossa acetabuli, and terminates through the ischium–inferior ramus junction. It is not unusual for dome chondrocancellous pyramidal-shaped fragments to be displaced and associated with this pattern. Similarly, portions of the torn posterior labrum may be mislocated between the femoral head and weight-bearing dome with this fracture pattern. The displaced posterior column fracture fragment may injure the SGNVB, especially when the fracture line is located high in the greater sciatic notch. This is important to remember both before and during surgery because arterial injury may cause ongoing bleeding and require embolization. Buttock compartmental syndrome is rare but can also occur because of superior gluteal system bleeding. During surgery, the SGNVB should be visually identified to ensure that it is not displaced between the fracture fragments. If it is displaced, it should be either carefully retracted as the fracture is reduced and clamped, or the cortical spike of the greater sciatic notch should be removed to prevent crushing the neurovascular

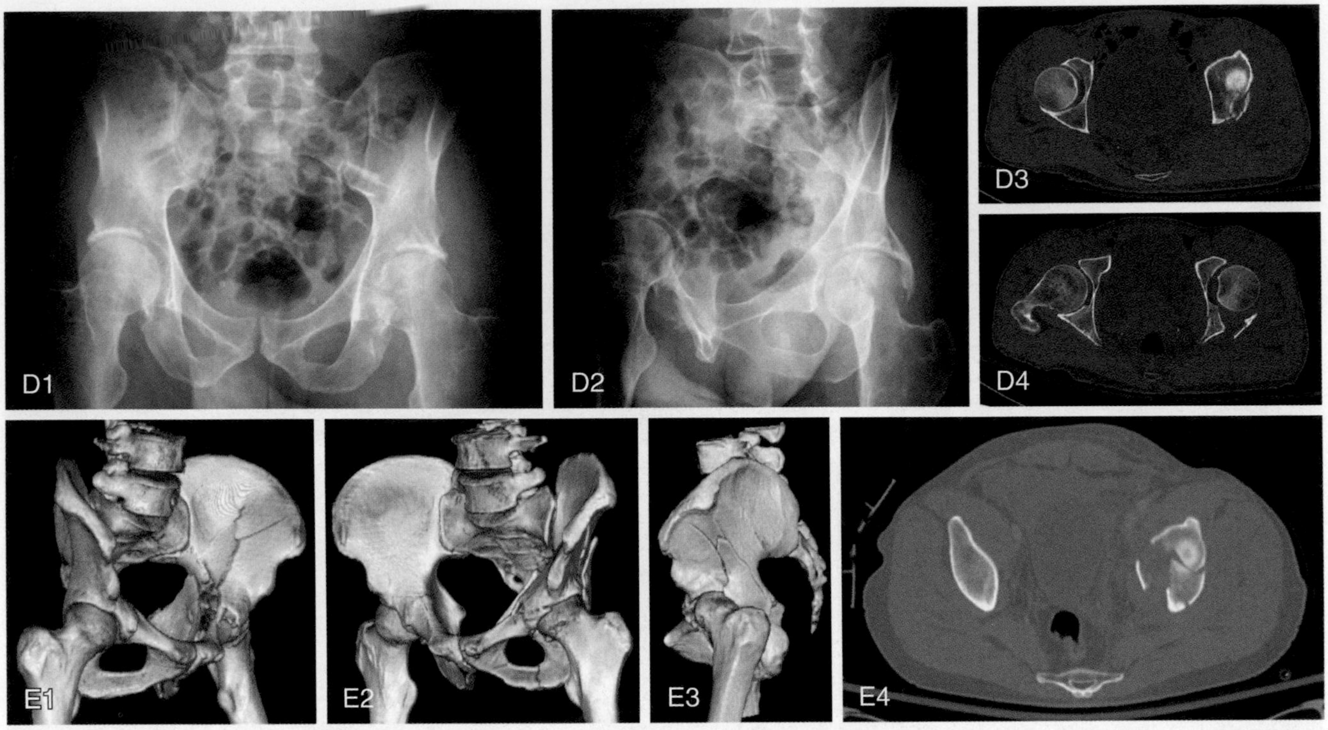

Figure 41-11, cont'd. D1 and **D2,** This patient has a comminuted and displaced posterior wall acetabular fracture, but the wall fragments are frail. **D3** and **D4,** The CT axial images identify two large regions of chondrocancellous "marginal" impaction. **E1** to **E4,** This patient has an associated both-column acetabular fracture pattern but with a large posterior wall fracture fragment as a part of it. The posterior wall fracture fragment has approximately one-third of the dome articular surface on it. In associated both-column acetabular fracture patterns, the posterior wall fragment is commonly large, not comminuted, and avulsed by the medial displacement of the overall fracture. When directly visualized via a posterior exposure at surgery, the capsule and labrum are usually completely intact posteriorly.

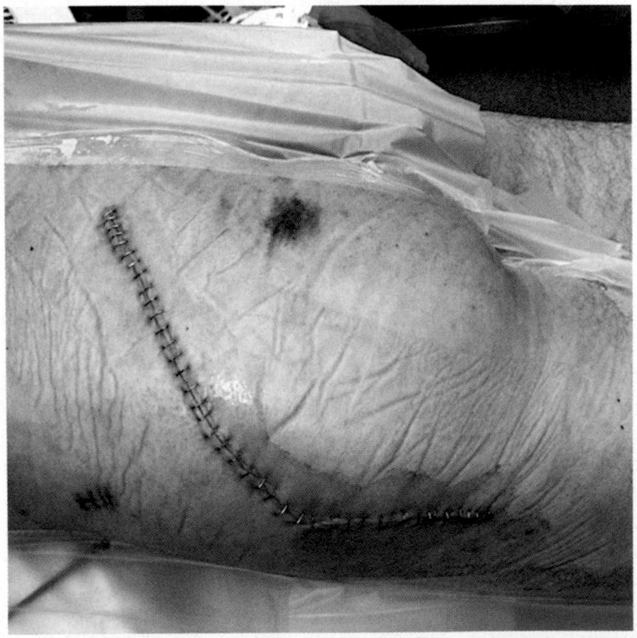

Figure 41-12. The circular bruise noted on this patient's left buttock was caused by the femoral head displacement at the time of fracture-dislocation. During the operation, a circular pathway was noted from the hip joint through the buttock muscles to the dermis.

bundle. Commonly, displaced posterior column fractures obstruct venous flow of the superior gluteal vein, causing its tributaries locally to engorge and dilate throughout the gluteal muscle bellies. These enlarged veins are fragile and often require ligation individually to control bleeding if they tear. It is important to spare the superior gluteal nerve during these ligations. The surgeon must resist the urge to simply apply a large vascular clip that could inadvertently damage the artery, vein, and nerve. Retraction of the proximal vascular bundle into the true pelvis caused by either a traumatic or iatrogenic injury usually obviates ligation, so packing is then recommended to attempt to control such bleeding. Venous bleeding and often arterial bleeding respond to packing. The packing material should be applied so that the superior gluteal and sciatic nerves are not inadvertently injured by overly aggressive packing. If the packing fails to control superior gluteal arterial bleeding, then prompt wound closure is performed, and urgent angiographic evaluation and embolization if possible are advised.

Similar to the superior gluteal neurovascular structures, the sciatic nerve can also be injured by displaced posterior column acetabular fractures. These are usually traction or contusion injuries noted at patient presentation. Some may be related to direct contusion or stretch, and some may be related to piriformis muscle anatomic abnormalities that divide and tether

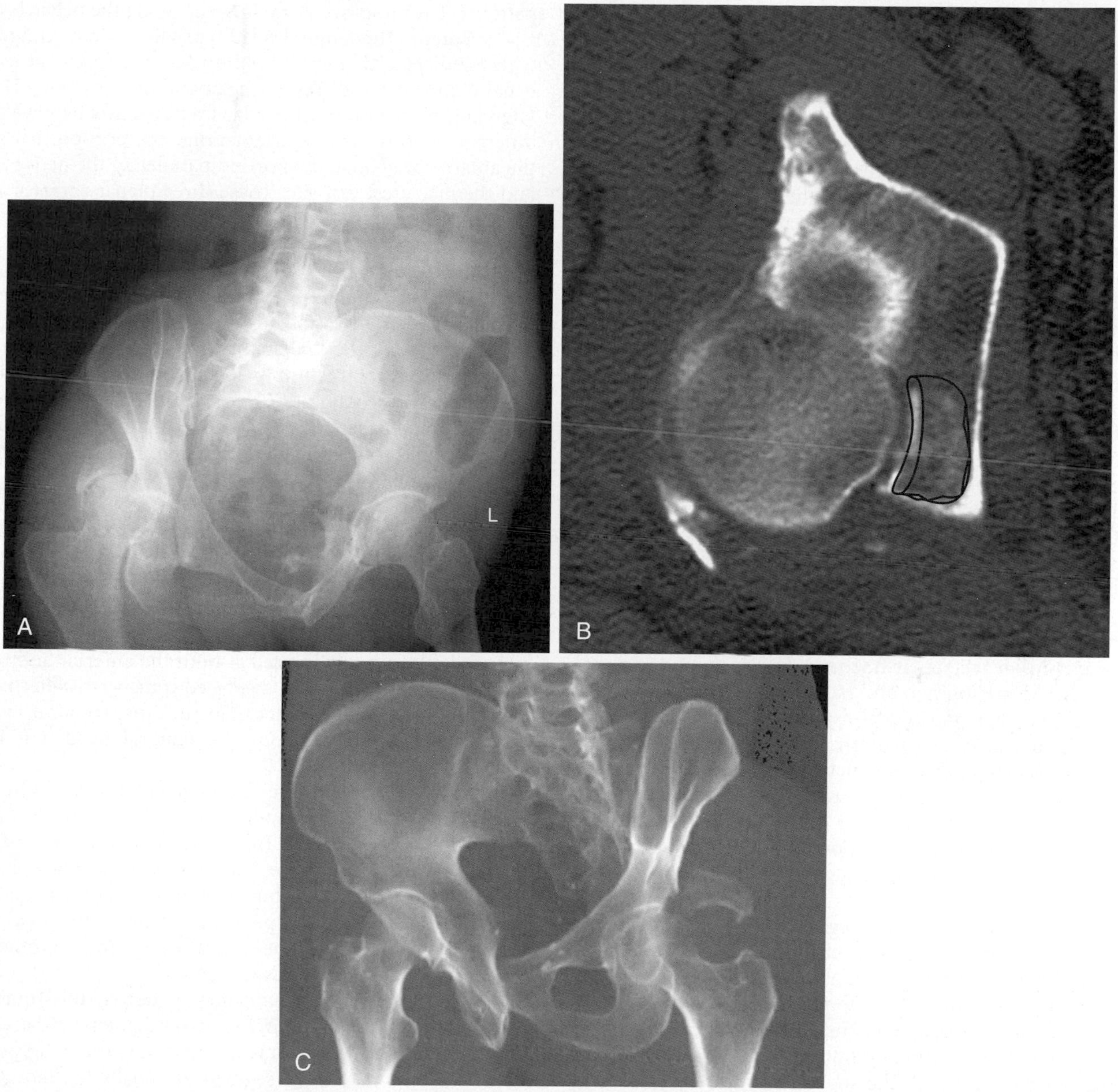

Figure 41-13. A, The obturator oblique plain pelvic image demonstrates a displaced posterior wall fracture-dislocation. This radiograph was obtained after a screening anterior-posterior radiograph had diagnosed the fracture-dislocation but before orthopaedic consultation. Manipulative reduction of the fracture-dislocation is recommended after diagnosis and before complete radiographic evaluation. **B,** The corresponding acetabular computed tomography image reveals marginal impaction of chondrocancellous fragments into the intact posterior column area. As the femoral head dislocates, these chondrocancellous impaction fractures occur along the fracture edge. Less frequently, the articular surface of the displaced posterior wall may have impaction or comminution. **C,** This patient has a left-sided displaced posterior wall acetabular fracture with a common displacement pattern.

the nerve, making it vulnerable with fracture fragment displacement. Sciatic nerve injury can also result from the closed reduction. This occurs because the sciatic nerve course parallels certain displaced posterior column fracture planes and can become trapped within the fracture line as the displaced fracture-dislocation is reduced. This happens rarely but must be remembered and not missed or justified as an injury-related occurrence. For this reason, the pre- and postreduction nerve assessments are carefully detailed and documented. If the sciatic nerve examination findings change after closed reduction of any acetabular fracture, then urgent exploration, neuroplasty, and fracture fixation are recommended.[34]

Posterior column acetabular fractures are best seen on the iliac oblique and AP plain pelvic radiographs. The pelvic CT scan reveals detailed displacement information; identifies comminution, dome fragmentation, and loose bodies within the joint; and shows impaction injuries that may occur along the fracture line.

Anterior Wall

Anterior wall acetabular fractures are the least common of all types. The unnatural lower limb and body positionings needed to load the anterior wall coupled with the tiny surface area of the anterior wall make this pattern the most unlikely. Simply because of their anatomy, these fractures are quite small and associated with anterior dislocations. The iliac vasculature, femoral nerve, and lateral femoral cutaneous nerve (LFCN) can be injured in association with anterior wall fracture-dislocations. In Letournel's original description, focal fractures of the anterior column involving the pelvic brim were included as anterior wall fractures. This continues to confuse surgeons. To remain consistent with the classification scheme, if the anterior acetabular fracture lines do not violate the iliopectineal line, then it is an anterior wall fracture pattern. If the anterior fracture disrupts the iliopectineal line and therefore involves the pelvic brim, then it is an anterior column fracture pattern.

The anatomic area of the anterior wall is often involved in pelvic ring fractures when the fracture lines of the peripheral superior pubic ramus extend into the anterior wall area. This pelvic ring injury, however, should not be misclassified as an anterior acetabular wall fracture.

Anterior wall acetabular fractures may involve a small portion of the iliopectineal line on the AP radiograph. Whereas the OO image may show subluxation of the femoral head, the iliac oblique demonstrates the anterior wall fragment displacement.

Anterior Column

Anterior column acetabular fractures disrupt the iliopectineal line on the AP radiograph and have a variety of appearances depending on their peripheral exit points and displacement extents. As an elementary pattern, the fracture plane is singular but may also have three distinct surface orientations. These fractures were subclassified according to their iliac exit site. "High" anterior column fractures include those in which the iliac crest is the peripheral exit point. "Intermediate" patterns have their exit points in the region of the anterior superior iliac crest, and "low" patterns exit adjacent to the AIIS. "Very low" patterns only involve the region medial to the IPE. The fracture displacement depends on the subclassification type. The high types have the tensor, abdominal obliques, gluteus medius, and sartorius muscle forces to cause displacement. Because of this displacement, the LFCN may be injured in association with this particular fracture type. On its other end, the fracture exits through the superior ramus. Displacement at the ramus region can injure or deform the iliac vessels and femoral nerve, as well as the obturator neurovascular bundle. It is not difficult to understand why femoral deep venous thrombosis (DVT) occurs for these fractures. The other patterns have variable deformities depending on the fracture specifics and related deforming forces. Displaced intermediate and low types risk associated femoral and obturator neurovascular injuries. In some patients, the anterior column fracture's exit at the iliac crest is incomplete and demonstrates plastic deformation. The incomplete fracture at the iliac exit site allows deformity but usually lends some degree of fracture stability. This incomplete fracture may need to be osteotomized at surgery to reduce the fracture accurately.

The iliac oblique image usually best demonstrates displaced anterior column acetabular fractures. These fractures are often missed on the screening AP radiograph because the fracture line along the pelvic brim's displacement is perpendicular to the radiographic beam, so the iliopectineal line's density appears nearly symmetrical. The iliac oblique radiograph reveals the peripheral exit points well, especially for the high patterns. The radiolucent fracture gap along the pelvic brim is also apparent. The femoral head typically remains congruent with the displaced anterior column fracture fragment, which usually indicates a disrupted ligamentum teres (Fig. 41-14). High anterior column acetabular fractures usually have three different fracture surface orientations: the portion that splits the anterior wall area, the portion paralleling the pelvic brim, and the iliac crest exit site. These three planar surfaces allow for strategic reduction clamp and implant applications.

Transverse

Transverse acetabular fractures often confuse clinicians because of their inclusion in the elementary fracture group despite involving the two supporting columns and two wall areas. Transverse fracture patterns occur in a variety of orientations and obliquities but remain a singular yet often complex fracture surface. Because of their singular fracture plane "purity," transverse fractures were included in the elementary group.

A common transverse fracture pattern begins at the anterior wall anatomic area, extends through the iliopsoas gutter and anterior wall articular surface, progresses across the pelvic brim and anterior column, through the quadrilateral surface dividing the upper and lower halves of the fossa acetabuli, and exits the posterior column and posterior wall's edge. The labrum is also usually injured at both the anterior and posterior exit sites, especially in displaced transverse patterns. The torn labrum or portions of it can intrude into the joint, causing further incongruity between the femoral head and intact dome region.[35,36]

Transverse fractures are the only elementary pattern to extend through the two wall areas and the two acetabular supporting column zones. The terminology can be confusing because the fracture involves "both of the acetabular columns" but is not an "associated both-column" fracture pattern. As previously stated, fracture patterns and anatomic areas share terminology but should not be confused with each other nor the terms used synonymously.

Just like the other elementary patterns, the transverse pattern splits the acetabulum into two fragments. Whereas the upper or cephalad fragment is almost always the stable portion of the fracture, the caudal segment is usually the mobile and displaced fragment. The caudal fragment mobility is due to the fracture plane and the fact that the symphysis pubis ligaments function as a hinge for it (Fig. 41-15).[37-39]

The acetabular dome is involved to some extent by the transverse fracture plane. Letournel subclassified transverse fractures depending on their dome involvement. Whereas transtectal transverse fractures involve the weight-bearing dome, juxtatectal transverse fractures preserve the dome and exit at the junction of the dome and fossa acetabuli. Infratectal transverse patterns divide the fossa acetabuli. Typically, more intact dome before fracture involvement correlates with improved hip stability, congruity, and outcome. In cadaveric mechanical evaluations, step malreductions of transverse acetabular fractures in the superior articular surface resulted in abnormally high contact forces that in clinical practice should predispose to the development of posttraumatic arthritis.[40,41]

Certain transverse acetabular fractures are associated with medial displacement of the femoral head along with the caudal fracture fragment. As the fracture displacement occurs, the

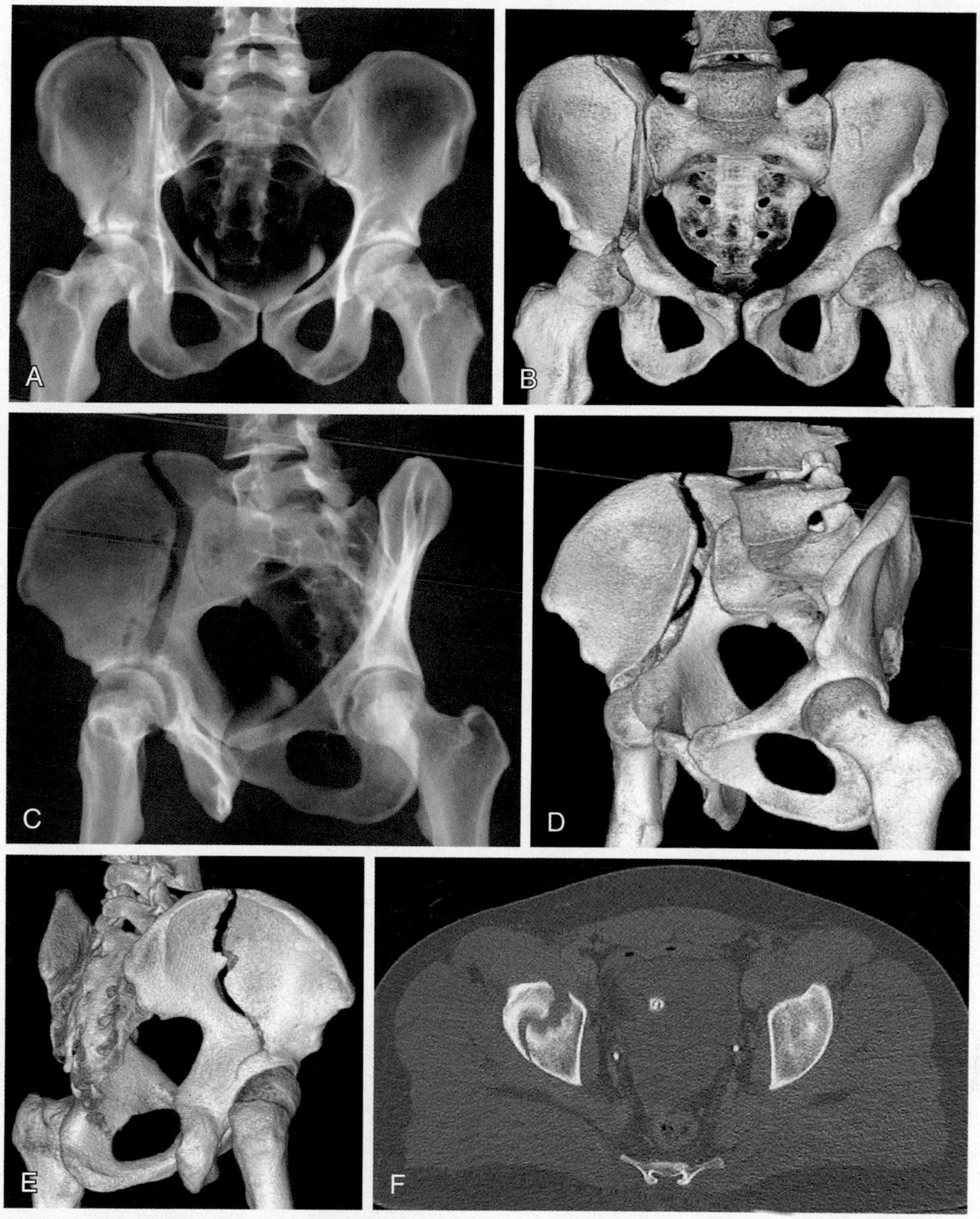

Figure 41-14. These images demonstrate a very high anterior column acetabular fracture pattern. The iliac exit point is posteriorly located. **A** and **B,** It is easy to see on the anterior-posterior pelvic image and three-dimensional (3-D) model how the fracture can be confusing because the iliopectineal line appears mostly intact. The fracture involves the anterior portion of the pelvic brim area, but the posterior portion remains intact and gives the appearance of an intact iliopectineal line in that area. However, the density is asymmetrical, indicating the fracture displacement. The different fracture surface angles are notable on these images. **C** and **D,** The iliac oblique image and 3-D model best demonstrate the iliac exit site, iliac involvement, and anterior wall area exit site. In this patient, the femoral head is displaced and remains congruent with the displaced anterior column fracture fragment. **E,** The posterior oblique 3-D model shows the lateral surface fracture line. **F,** The axial image at the dome level identifies the complex fracture orientation there.

femoral head can sustain a superolateral impaction fracture or the intact upper portion of the acetabular fracture line can be crushed.

In these fractures, the femoral head may remain beneath the weight-bearing dome or follow the caudal segment's displacement depending on several factors. For transtectal patterns, there may be insufficient intact dome laterally for the femoral head to remain stable. Muscular spasm, especially from the iliopsoas muscle, causes further displacement of the femoral head medially and superiorly through the fracture. As the intact dome coverage expands medially with juxtatectal and infratectal transverse patterns, femoral head stability improves.

Transverse acetabular fracture patterns or other associated fracture patterns with a transverse fracture component should alert the treating physician to potential associated pelvic ring injuries, especially ipsilateral SI joint injuries. Careful study of all preoperative imaging is imperative. If the commonly stable cranial fracture fragment is rendered unstable or is displaced because of an ipsilateral SI joint injury or sacral fracture, then both the upper and lower portions of the transverse fracture are unstable. The upper fracture fragment of such a transverse

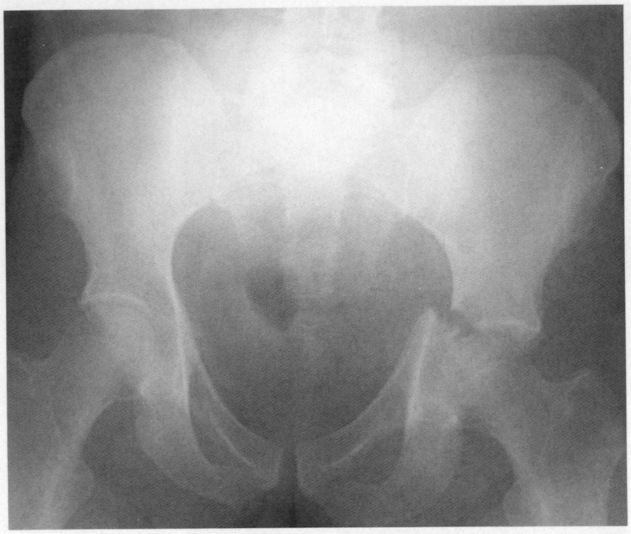

Figure 41-15. In transverse acetabular fracture patterns, the ilioischial and iliopectineal lines are disrupted on the anterior-posterior pelvic radiograph. The remaining amount of dome determines stability after closed reduction. The caudal fragment of most transverse acetabular fractures is the unstable portion hinging on the symphyseal ligaments. In this example, the femoral head is no longer congruent with the intact dome fragment and is displaced medially along with the displaced caudal segment. The related symphyseal injury for this patient is also noted. Impaction injuries of the superolateral femoral head as well as along the transverse acetabular fracture surface are noted with such fracture lines and displacement patterns.

acetabular fracture pattern is displaced and unstable because the ipsilateral SI joint is disrupted or an unstable ipsilateral sacral fracture is present. In this unusual scenario, the transverse acetabular fracture functions as an associated both-column acetabular pattern because there is no articular component in continuity with the intact hemipelvis.

Similar to certain posterior column acetabular fractures and their relationship with the sciatic nerve, transverse fractures can also be associated with sciatic nerve injury if the posterior column portion of the transverse fracture plane parallels the nerve pathway (Fig. 41-16).

Transverse Fractures with Associated Posterior Wall Involvement

Transverse with associated posterior wall acetabular fractures are common patterns combining the elementary transverse fracture plane with an additional displaced posterior wall component. The AP radiograph demonstrates both iliopectineal and ilioischial line disruptions along with the loss of the posterior wall convex edge because of its displacement. Often the displaced wall is noted superimposed on the dome area on this radiograph. If the radiograph is examined carefully, the transverse fracture plane's displacement through the anterior wall area is seen as a lucent gap. On the AP radiograph, the femoral head has several location options with these injuries. The simplest occurs when the femoral head is noted to be congruent with the dome. Another displacement pattern occurs when the femoral head follows the posterior wall displacement. Another pattern occurs when the femoral head follows the transverse caudal segment and is displaced medially. The oblique images are obtained after closed reduction of the femoral head beneath the dome. The iliac oblique image

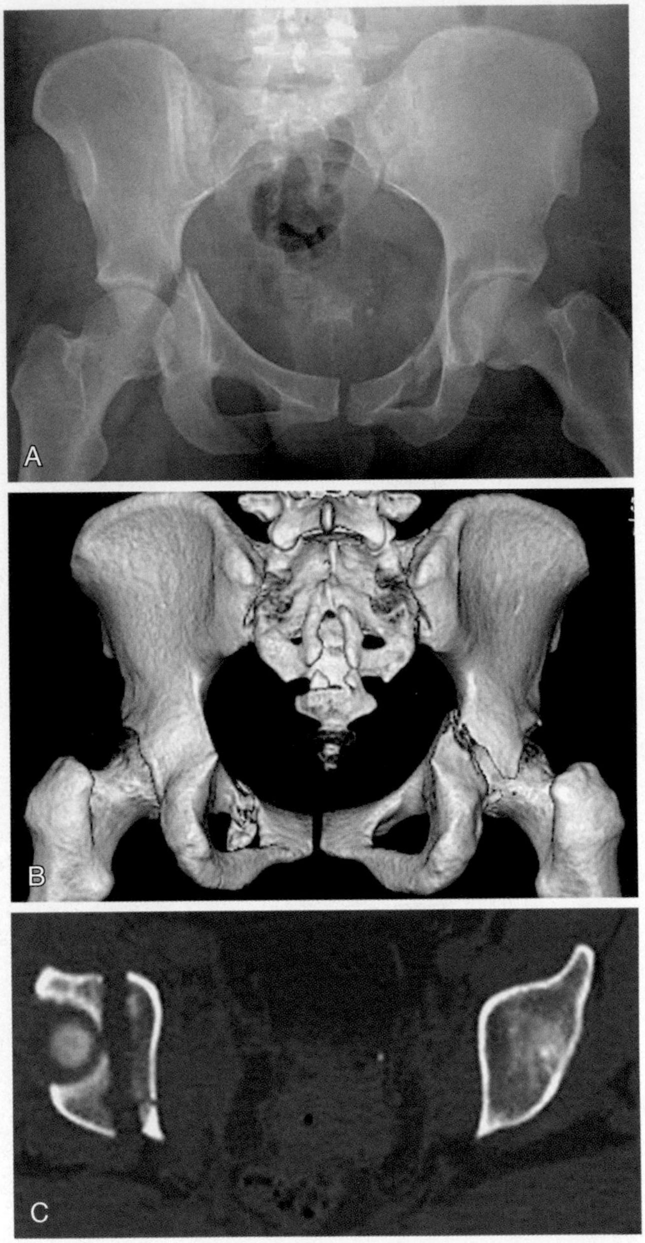

Figure 41-16. Depending on the fracture orientation through the area of the posterior column, transverse acetabular fractures can be associated with sciatic nerve injury. **A,** This woman was injured in an automobile accident, resulting in a displaced transverse acetabular fracture. She had sciatic nerve palsy on initial presentation. The anterior-posterior plain pelvic radiograph demonstrates that the posterior column component of the fracture parallels the sciatic nerve's course. **B,** The surface rendered posterior three-dimensional image also shows the fracture orientation in the area of the sciatic nerve. **C,** The sciatic nerve is seen on the axial computed tomography image to be located between the posterior fracture surfaces. A posterior surgical exposure was selected so the sciatic nerve could be explored. It was trapped between the fracture fragments and was in continuity but contused. A sciatic neuroplasty was performed, and then the fracture was cleansed, manipulated, reduced, clamped, and stabilized.

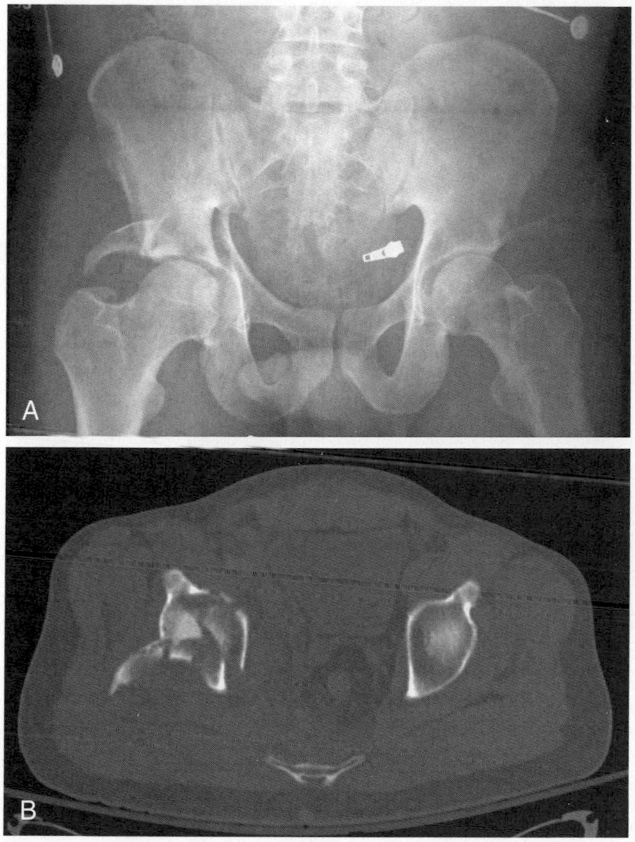

Figure 41-17. A and B, This patient has a transverse with associated posterior wall acetabular fracture. The iliopectineal and ilioischial lines are disrupted and the posterior wall fragment is displaced and also comminuted. The caudal portion of the transverse fracture is unstable and displaced on its symphyseal hinge. The dome has been split by the transverse fracture, so it is subclassified as a transtectal pattern.

shows the exit points of the transverse fracture line in the areas of the posterior column and anterior wall. The OO image demonstrates the anterior column exit point of the transverse fracture as well as the displaced posterior wall fracture fragment and the defect left because of its displacement. It is not unusual in unstable patterns for the femoral head to redislocate as the patient is turned for each image and the body weight or limb weight is applied onto the injury. After closed reduction, an AP radiograph in traction may reveal a previously missed superolateral femoral head impaction fracture. Just as for any fracture that includes a transverse fracture component, the ipsilateral SI joint and sacral areas should be carefully assessed on the radiographs for injuries and displacements.

The pelvic CT scan reveals the transverse fracture orientation, dome area involvement, and specific exit sites as well as any loose bodies within the joint or marginal impaction associated injuries. Posterior wall comminution is not always obvious on the plain images and is best seen on the CT scan. The CT scan may also confirm femoral head impaction lesions (Fig. 41-17).

Posterior Column Fracture with Associated Posterior Wall Involvement

In these uncommon injuries, the ilioischial line is disrupted, and the posterior wall defect and displacement are seen on the AP radiograph. The iliac oblique image shows the posterior column component's exit through the greater sciatic notch, but the OO view identifies the displaced posterior column fracture exit at the ischium and the displacement of the posterior wall fracture fragment. The pelvic CT scan should be examined not only for the specific fracture-related details but also for the local soft tissues. An injury to the superior gluteal artery or vein may cause deep buttock asymmetry or accumulated vascular contrast agent on the scan because of local bleeding. The details cited earlier regarding both posterior column and posterior wall fracture elementary patterns are also relevant here.

Anterior Column Fracture with Associated Posterior Hemitransverse Injury

Acetabular fracture patterns that involve the anterior column as well as associated posterior hemitransverse injuries combine any variety of anterior column fracture with an additional fracture line that splits the posterior column, usually through the greater sciatic notch. Both the iliopectineal and ilioischial lines are disrupted on the plain AP radiograph. The iliac oblique pelvic radiograph reveals the anterior column fracture component's exits both along the iliac crest and through the anterior wall area, as well as the posterior hemitransverse fracture component's exit point, usually through the greater sciatic notch. These injuries can be unstable although each fracture component and the oblique radiographs demonstrate the instability and displacement sites. Just like for anterior column elementary patterns, the anterior column component of the fracture is variable. The posterior hemitransverse component predictably divides the greater sciatic notch. These fractures are common in elderly patients (Fig. 41-18)

T-Type

The T-type acetabular fracture is simply a transverse acetabular fracture but with the unstable caudal segment split into two individual unstable segments. When viewed laterally, this

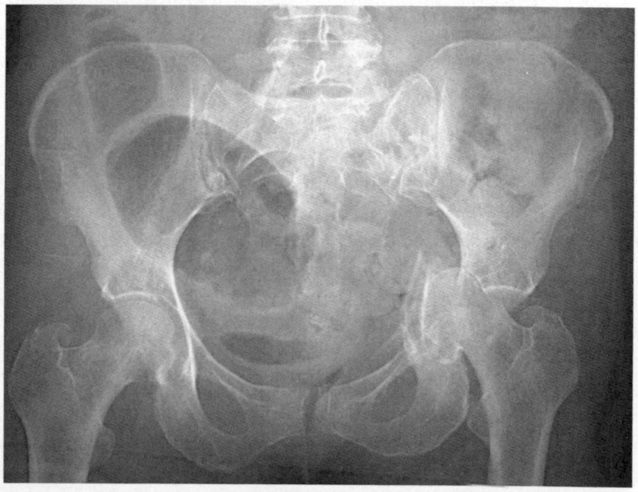

Figure 41-18. In this example of an anterior column with associated posterior hemitransverse acetabular fracture, the iliopectineal and ilioischial lines are disrupted. The acetabular dome remains a part of the intact ilium, and there is no obvious fracture of the inferior ramus or posterior wall on this anterior-posterior pelvic radiograph. The femoral head and acetabular fracture fragments are displaced medially, and the superolateral femoral head and medial acetabular dome region are both severely impacted.

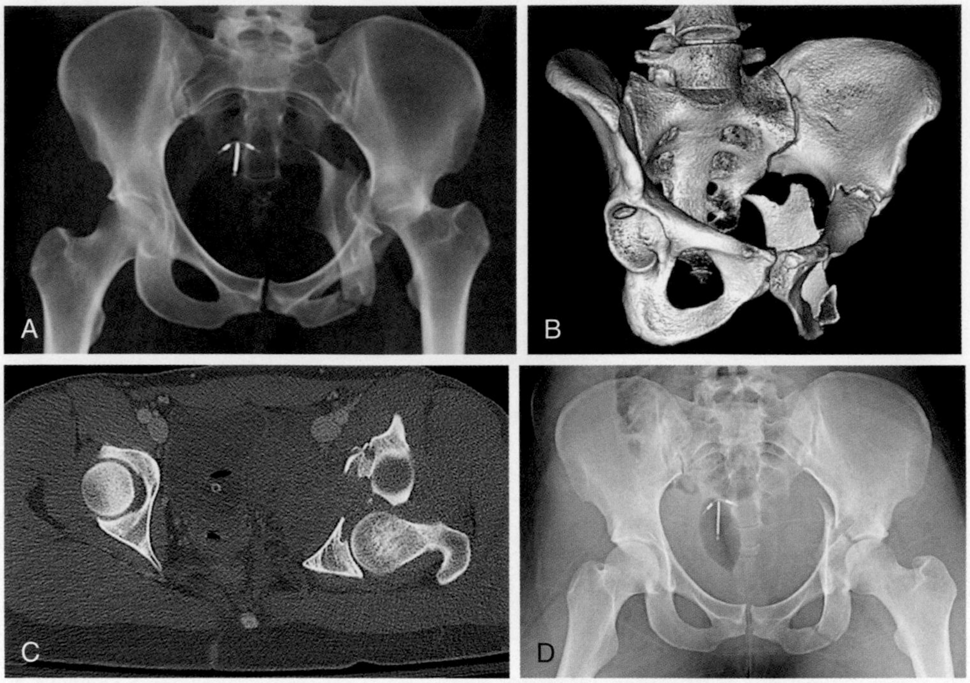

Figure 41-19. T-type acetabular fracture. The anterior column fracture is much less displaced than the posterior column fracture component. The femoral head remained congruent with the displaced posterior column component. Despite the severity and direction of the fragment displacement, the sciatic nerve and superior neurovascular bundle remained intact before and after closed reduction. **A,** On the anterior-posterior pelvic radiograph, the displaced posterior column fracture fragment and dislocated femoral head are easily seen. The ilioischial line is disrupted. The anterior column fracture is minimally displaced and therefore the iliopectineal line disruption is more difficult to identify, **B,** The iliac oblique three-dimensional model demonstrates the fracture surfaces and displacements, **C,** The dislocated femoral head remains congruent with the displaced posterior column fracture fragment. The local hematoma is notable as well on this axial image at the level of the intact acetabular dome, **D,** Identifying the T-type fracture lines is improved after closed reduction of the femoral head beneath the intact weight-bearing dome.

acetabular fracture patterns is shaped like the letter T. For example, the anterior column portion of the fracture line begins at the anterior wall area and extends along the iliopsoas gutter across the pelvic brim and descends the quadrilateral surface. The posterior column portion of the fracture line begins at the greater sciatic notch and descends to split the posterior wall area and meets the anterior column fracture line at the quadrilateral surface. The fracture line that divides the quadrilateral surface is a common fracture line. It is the vertical fracture line that descends from the transverse component to make this a T-type fracture pattern.

The anterior column component is unstable because of the symphyseal hinge. The posterior column component is tethered by the sacrospinous and sacrotuberous ligaments. These injuries often have central displacement of the femoral head between the fracture fragments, or the femoral head can remain attached to the posterior column fragment if the ligamentum teres is intact.

On the AP radiograph, both iliopectineal and ilioischial lines are disrupted, and the femoral head may be dislocated away from the intact dome. The ischial fracture may be minimally displaced and not always obvious. The iliac oblique image reveals that the posterior column exits at the greater sciatic notch and ischial ramus. The OO identifies the anterior column exit site and displacements. CT details each component's location (Fig. 41-19).

Associated Both-Column Fracture

The associated both-column acetabular fracture pattern is thought by many surgeons to be the most difficult of all 10 acetabular fracture types. In these injuries, the articular dome and all other articular fracture fragments are without connection to the intact hemipelvis. In all nine other patterns, at least some portion of the articular acetabulum remains attached to the intact hemipelvis. Because of this traumatic fracture-separation of the articular fragments from the stable ilium, some use the term "floating acetabulum" for these patterns. Because this term is misleading and not descriptive, most surgeons do not use it.

Associated both-column acetabular fractures have several consistent fracture fragments. The intact iliac piece is the stable component. Its caudal extent represents the "spur sign," so named because it resembles a cockspur on the OO image, as the unstable articular fragments displace from it medially. Such medial articular fragment displacements cause the intact ileum's caudal extent (the "spur") to appear prominent as it remains in its normal site. When seen on the OO radiograph, this spur sign is indicative of an associated both-column acetabular fracture. Inexperienced surgeons may confuse a displaced posterior wall acetabular fracture with the spur sign of an associated both-column fracture because both are seen on the OO image (Fig. 41-20).

When articular fragment displacement is minimal yet there is still no articular connection to the intact iliac segment, no spur sign is obvious, but an associated both-column acetabular fracture pattern is the correct diagnosis. In some patients, the intact iliac caudal extent is obvious even on the AP and iliac oblique radiographs, so it is possible to see the spur on these other images. It is easy for the clinician to see that which he or she knows to look for (Fig. 41-21).

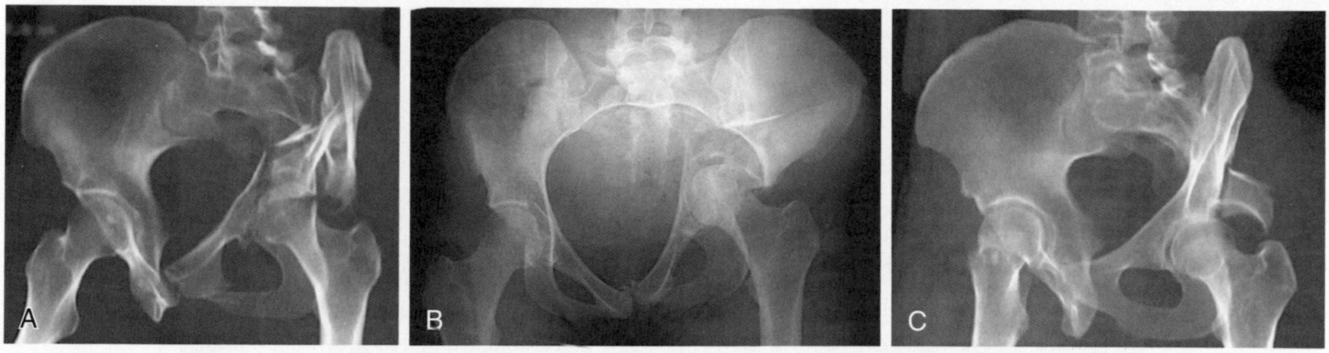

Figure 41-20. The "spur sign" represents the caudal portion of the intact ilium and is indicative of an associated both-column acetabular fracture pattern. **A,** Named for its similar appearance to a rooster's cockspur, the "spur sign" is seen best on the obturator oblique (OO) injury radiograph because the articular portions of the fracture displace medially leaving the intact ilium in profile. **B,** In this patient with severe fracture fragment displacement, the caudal aspect of the intact ilium (spur) is also notable on the anterior-posterior radiograph. **C,** This patient has a displaced posterior wall acetabular fracture. Similar to the "spur sign," in associated both-column fracture patterns, the displaced posterior wall fracture is also best seen on the OO image, but the two should not be confused.

Besides the intact iliac component, associated both-column fractures have several other consistent components. The upper anterior column fracture fragment usually contains the majority of the dome and may be incomplete at its iliac crest exit point, as previously described for anterior column fracture patterns. If so, the anterior column fragment may be displaced and relatively stable because of the deformed yet incomplete fracture along the crest. The lower anterior column fracture fragment typically includes the articular anterior wall and pubic ramus limbs. The posterior column component typically exits the greater sciatic notch and ischial areas. It is not unusual for the pelvic brim to have some degree of cortical comminution. In some patterns as detailed in the earlier section on posterior wall fracture, the posterior wall fracture component is an avulsion injury caused by medial displacement of the proximal femur.

Variant Patterns

Certain acetabular fractures do not fit Letournel's classification system (Fig. 41-22). These variant patterns exist and must be recognized after routine patterns have been ruled out. For example, a T-type fracture pattern may have an associated displaced posterior wall fracture. The "T-type with associated posterior wall" fracture pattern is not an option in the Letournel classification scheme, but this and other variant patterns do occur, and the treating physician needs to be aware of and able

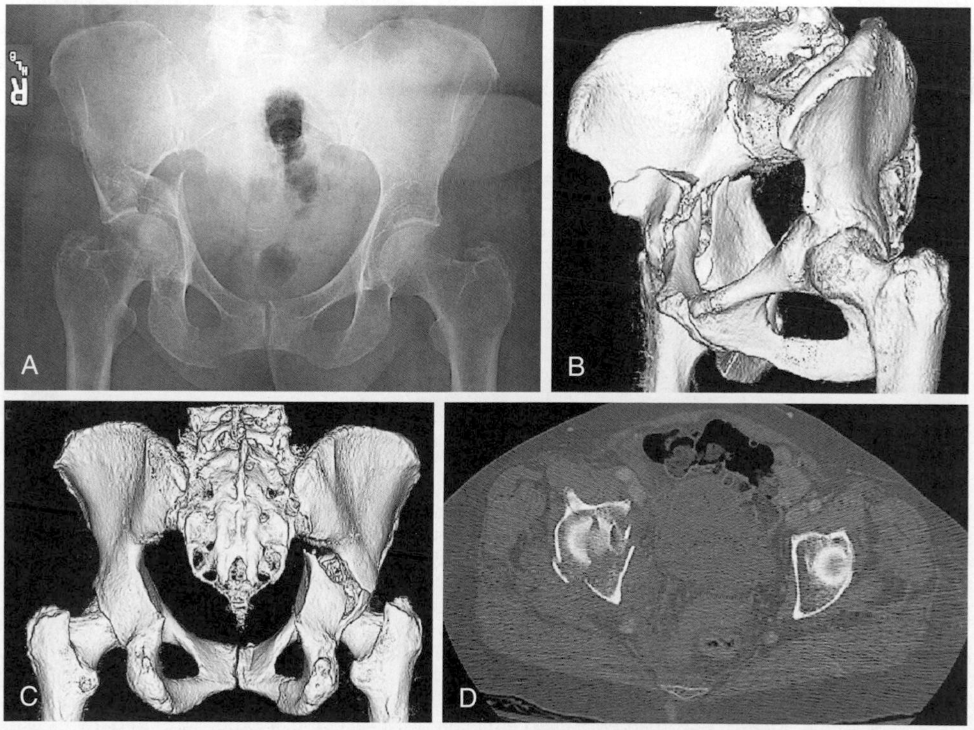

Figure 41-21. This patient has an associated both-column fracture that initially may seem to be an anterior column with associated posterior hemitransverse. The dome fragment is not in continuity with the intact iliac fragment, but this fact may not be entirely obvious on initial inspection. Further study of the anterior-posterior plain radiograph (**A**) shows the asymmetry and displacement of that fragment. **B** and **C,** The three-dimensional model when viewed posteriorly reveals the spur sign. **D,** The axial computed tomography image also shows the displacements.

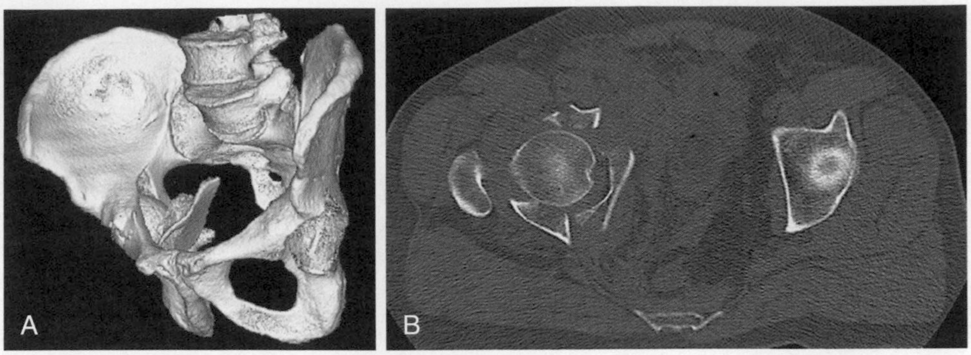

Figure 41-22. Not every acetabular fracture can be classified using Letournel's scheme of elementary and associated patterns. Some fractures, such as this one involving the quadrilateral surface, are best classified as variant patterns. **A,** The obturator oblique three-dimensional image demonstrates the quadrilateral surface fracture and medial displacement. **B,** The axial computed tomography image further demonstrates the fracture sites and displacement pattern.

to plan treatment for such variant and hybrid fracture patterns. Remember that the Letournel acetabular classification system was initially developed simply to guide the surgical exposure decision. Just as for the other fractures, the variant patterns' radiographic details will guide the operative planning. Unusual position of the lower extremity at injury, poor bone quality, or extreme loading conditions are responsible causes for these injuries. Variant patterns are assessed and managed routinely. Their fracture specifics may necessitate more detailed planning, more extensile exposure, or special fixation tools. Dramatic impaction injuries, for example, may demand allograft bone or other suitable material to fill the defects. Acetabular fractures in association with unstable pelvic ring injuries are included as variant patterns as well (Fig. 41-23).

Decision Making

The management goal for acetabular fractures is a painless and functional hip joint without complications.[42-46] Selecting the best treatment option is a complex clinical decision based on numerous factors related to the patient, the physician, the facility, and others.

The following questions arise when determining treatment:

1. Is the patient medically stable? If not, how can he or she be made stable? Would urgent operative management of the acetabular fracture actually help to stabilize the patient overall? Are there open wounds in communication with the fracture?
2. Could the patient withstand any planned operation, much less an extensive one?
3. Could the patient withstand traction management or prolonged bed rest?
4. Are there patient-related medical, physical, psychosocial, or other issues that adversely affect either operative or nonoperative management? For example, is noncompliant behavior anticipated despite the treatment choice?
5. Are the fracture fragments and hip joint stable or unstable?

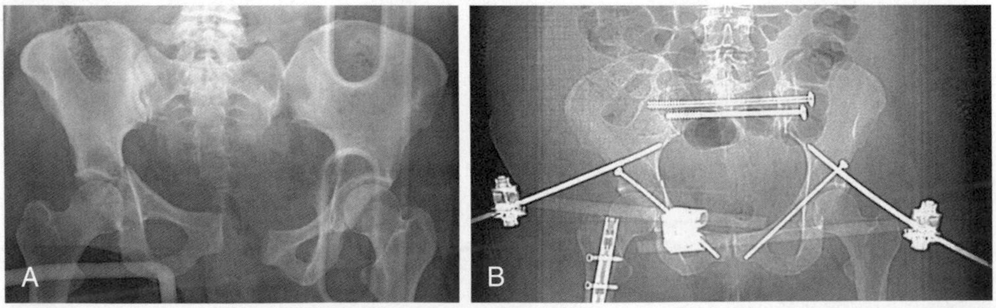

Figure 41-23. Acetabular fractures and pelvic ring disruptions can occur together, usually after high-energy traumatic events. Those acetabular fracture patterns that involve the two structural columns and thereby disrupt the pelvic ring through the acetabular region are the transverse, transverse with associated posterior wall, T-type, anterior column with associated posterior hemitransverse, and associated both-column fractures. **A,** In this patient, the right-sided juxtatectal transverse acetabular fracture is a component of the overall pelvic ring disruption along with the symphysis pubis, left pubic ramus, and left sacroiliac joint injuries. Subluxation of the right femoral head medially from beneath the weight-bearing dome is noted. The reduction sequence should prioritize the acetabular fracture whenever the patient's overall condition allows. Early pelvic ring reduction and stabilization procedures must respect the eventual need for acetabular fracture reduction and fixation. Initial malreductions of the other ring components will obviate eventual accurate acetabular reduction. **B,** Because of her overall clinical status upon presentation, the acetabular fracture and pelvic ring injuries were treated as a part of her overall resuscitation effort. The acetabular facture and the other pelvic ring injuries were treated with closed reduction, percutaneous screw fixations, and an anterior external fixation frame. The femur fracture was then stabilized with an antegrade, locked, and reamed nailing after the pelvic–acetabular procedure. In patients like this, the initial percutaneous fixation does not have to be definitive treatment, especially when the acetabular manipulative reduction is inaccurate. In this patient, the right transverse acetabular fracture closed reduction should have been revised to an open reduction with internal fixation after her overall condition was stable. Her right hip developed symptomatic arthrosis 3 years after injury, perhaps caused by the malreduction from percutaneous management.

6. Is the fracture displaced or not? If displaced, where specifically are the displacement sites and to what extent? Is the hip congruent? Does the femoral head remain beneath the intact weight-bearing dome during oblique imaging?
7. If displaced, is there sufficient relative (secondary) congruity of the fracture fragments with the femoral head?
8. Is there ample bone to allow routine reduction and stable fixation techniques, or are special considerations indicated?
9. Will the fracture pattern specifics allow for accurate reduction, or will fracture-related issues, such as extensive dome comminution or crush injury, prevent reduction or stable fixation?
10. Will associated femoral head traumatic issues such as superolateral or other zone impaction fractures adversely affect the result apart from the acetabular repair?
11. Are there prior hip issues such as arthritis, previous hip injury, aseptic necrosis, or others that would impact the treatment plan?
12. Does the surgeon, a colleague, or regional referral center have sufficient experience and expertise in treating similar acetabular fractures?
13. Does the medical facility have sufficient ancillary support (e.g., intraoperative imaging technicians) and the necessary equipment?

Even though clinicians would rather have some absolute radiographic measurement to guide their acetabular management decision, the individual patient's overall medical condition is the primary determinant. First and foremost, the patient must be able to endure the chosen treatment.[47-49] Although many clinicians begin with the specific fracture pattern when choosing a treatment plan, the overall patient condition guides treatment considerations. In some situations, the acetabular fracture is related to the patient's overall instability and urgent acetabular reduction and fixation are indicated as a part of the overall patient resuscitation. When the initial resuscitation of the patient is successful, the surgeon should focus on the fracture pattern and associated local soft tissue injuries. Fracture stability is related to several factors; the primary one is how much weight-bearing dome or intact acetabulum remains for the femoral head to articulate with. Biomechanical studies have shown that acetabular fracture stability decreases with higher applied loads across fracture surfaces and with a less intact dome. Because of this dome coverage issue, roof arc measurements can be used to quantify in three radiographic views and on CT scanning the amount of intact dome.

Roof arc angles are measured on the AP and two oblique radiographs. A line is first drawn on the radiograph to set the horizontal standard and correct for patient positioning error on the x-ray cassette. For elementary patterns, the ischial tuberosities on each side are reliable as long as the injured side remains uninvolved by the fracture-displacement. For example, in some elementary transverse and posterior column fracture patterns, the ischial area may be involved by the fracture to a degree that the tuberosities could not be used for the horizontal standard measurement. In these and the associated patterns, some other intact osseous landmark is used to set the horizontal standard. Next, a perpendicular vertical line is drawn from the horizontal standard line through the center of the hip joint, which, depending on its displacement, may or may not be the center of the femoral head. The next line is drawn from the center of the hip joint/femoral head to the acetabular fracture's articular edge on that particular view. The roof arc angle is measured between the vertical line and the articular edge line. As the roof arc angle expands, so does the acetabular dome coverage and in turn so does the hip joint congruity and perhaps stability. Mechanical and clinical studies have offered a variety of roof arc angle limits for improved results (Fig. 41-24).

The physician measuring the roof arc angles must remember that the center of the hip joint is not always the femoral head itself because the head may be displaced from the anatomic hip joint center. If this occurs, then the hip is incongruent, and the fracture is displaced sufficiently that roof arc measurements are in fact unwarranted because surgery is indicated.

Closed treatment of acetabular fractures should be based on hip congruity and fracture instability. Stability is determined from the history reflecting the energy of the traumatic event and from the radiographs. Commonly, unstable acetabular fractures will be easily identified on the oblique plain pelvic images. Even minimally displaced fractures seen on the AP image can be unstable and will show displacement and subluxation when body weight is applied to the fracture during oblique imaging. Final determination may require an examination of the fracture under anesthesia and real-time fluoroscopy. The fluoroscopic examination under anesthesia should be performed using the AP as well as both oblique views. The C-arm must be positioned correctly to view possible instability sites without obstructing the necessary limb positions and movements needed to challenge the fracture stability. For posterior wall acetabular assessment, the C-arm is positioned on the ipsilateral side to injury so the OO image is obtained and the unit does not obstruct hip flexion, adduction, and internal rotation. For fractures involving the posterior column, the C-arm unit is positioned on the opposite side to allow the iliac oblique view without obstructing limb movements. The AP view has limited use other than for medial instability assessment because the fluoroscope obstructs most limb movements other than central loading.

If the fracture is congruent and stable, protected weight bearing is chosen, and then serial pelvic radiographs are used in follow-up examinations to ensure no further displacement.[50,51] If the hip is congruent yet unstable without traction, then skeletal traction is used to maintain the reduction while the fracture heals (e-Fig. 41-1) or percutaneous fixation is used. The traction pin is best inserted during this same anesthetic examination using the C-arm to perfectly position the pin. A threaded pin of sufficient diameter is recommended when several weeks of traction is anticipated. The distal femoral traction pin is inserted to avoid the knee joint and local vascular structures.

If traction is selected, the patient is committed to a prolonged 6- to 8-week period of bed confinement. If traction is chosen, it is also important to know if the fracture reduction is maintained while the patient is upright in bed. A portable AP pelvic radiograph with the patient awake and in traction confirms this fact and ensures that the hip is not overdistracted by excessive weight (Fig. 41-25). An upright chest allows the patient to avoid problems associated with recumbency. Every patient in traction is at risk for aspiration, such that the traction is adjusted to allow head of the bed elevation while maintaining the fracture reduction.

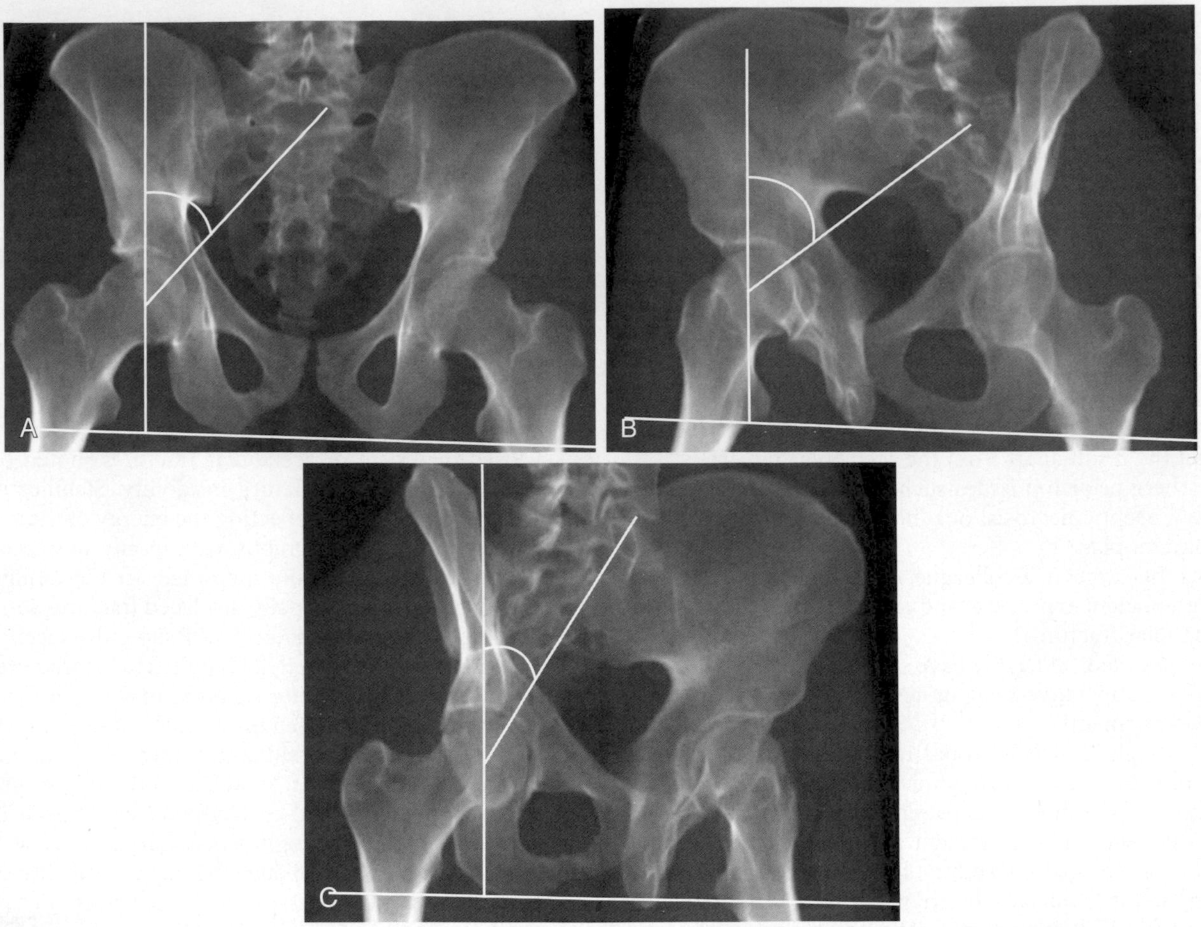

Figure 41-24. The measurements of acetabular fracture roof arc angles are shown on these three pelvic radiographs. **A,** On the anterior-posterior (AP) pelvic radiograph, the right ischial tuberosity is involved by the fracture, so the horizontal standard line must be estimated. The femoral head is slightly subluxated on the AP view, so the center hip joint determination accounts for this. A vertical perpendicular line is drawn from the horizontal standard line through the hip joint center. Next and from the hip center, a line is drawn to the acetabular fracture edge. The angle between the perpendicular vertical and fracture edge lines is the roof arc angle. **B** and **C,** The process is repeated for the iliac and obturator oblique images.

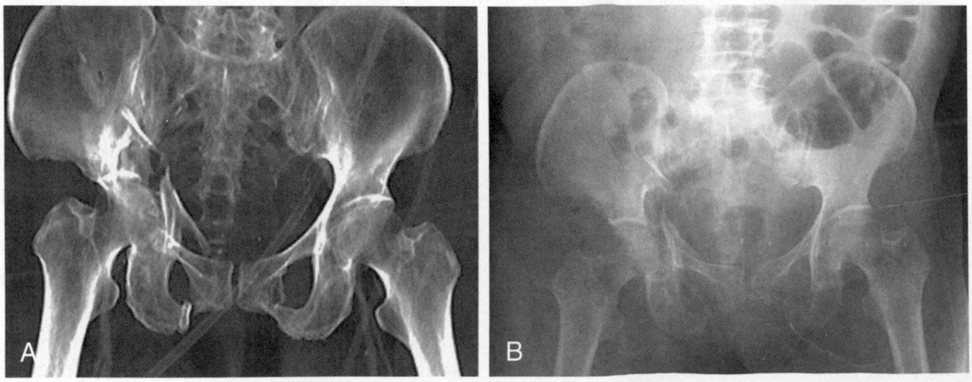

Figure 41-25. Traction was helpful in this elderly patient. **A,** The injury radiograph shows significant instability and displacement. **B,** Distal femoral skeletal traction was applied, and this anterior-posterior pelvic radiograph was then obtained with the patient in traction. It demonstrates improved reduction of the fragments. In many patients, skeletal traction improves realignment of the displaced fragments, combats muscle spasm, provides patient comfort, protects the femoral head and articular fragments from further damage, and reminds the nursing staff of the acetabular fracture.

Operative repair of acetabular fractures is difficult; can be extensive; and is associated with numerous problems, including operative bleeding. Because of this fact, the patient's cardiopulmonary and medical condition should be capable of withstanding surgery.

Some patients may refuse to receive blood or blood products based on their religious beliefs and therefore may not be candidates for open fracture reconstructive techniques. Blood salvage systems during surgery diminish this potential problem if the patient will allow such system to be used.[52,53]

If there are no patient-related issues, then the fracture pattern is evaluated for displacement and instability. Treating physicians must remember that displacement and stability are not necessarily linked. Certain displaced fractures may demonstrate relative stability, especially when the peripheral portions of the fractures are incomplete. Conversely, nondisplaced or minimally displaced fractures are not necessarily stable. For example, certain transverse acetabular fractures may have essentially no displacement on the AP radiograph, but the oblique radiographs reveal their displacements and instability. In these situations, the patient's body weight along with gravity cause fracture displacement. Examination of the hip under anesthesia and fluoroscopy can also identify dramatic fracture instability in minimally displaced injuries (Fig. 41-26).

For stable fractures, some clinicians measure roof arc angles on the pelvic plain radiographs and the subchondral

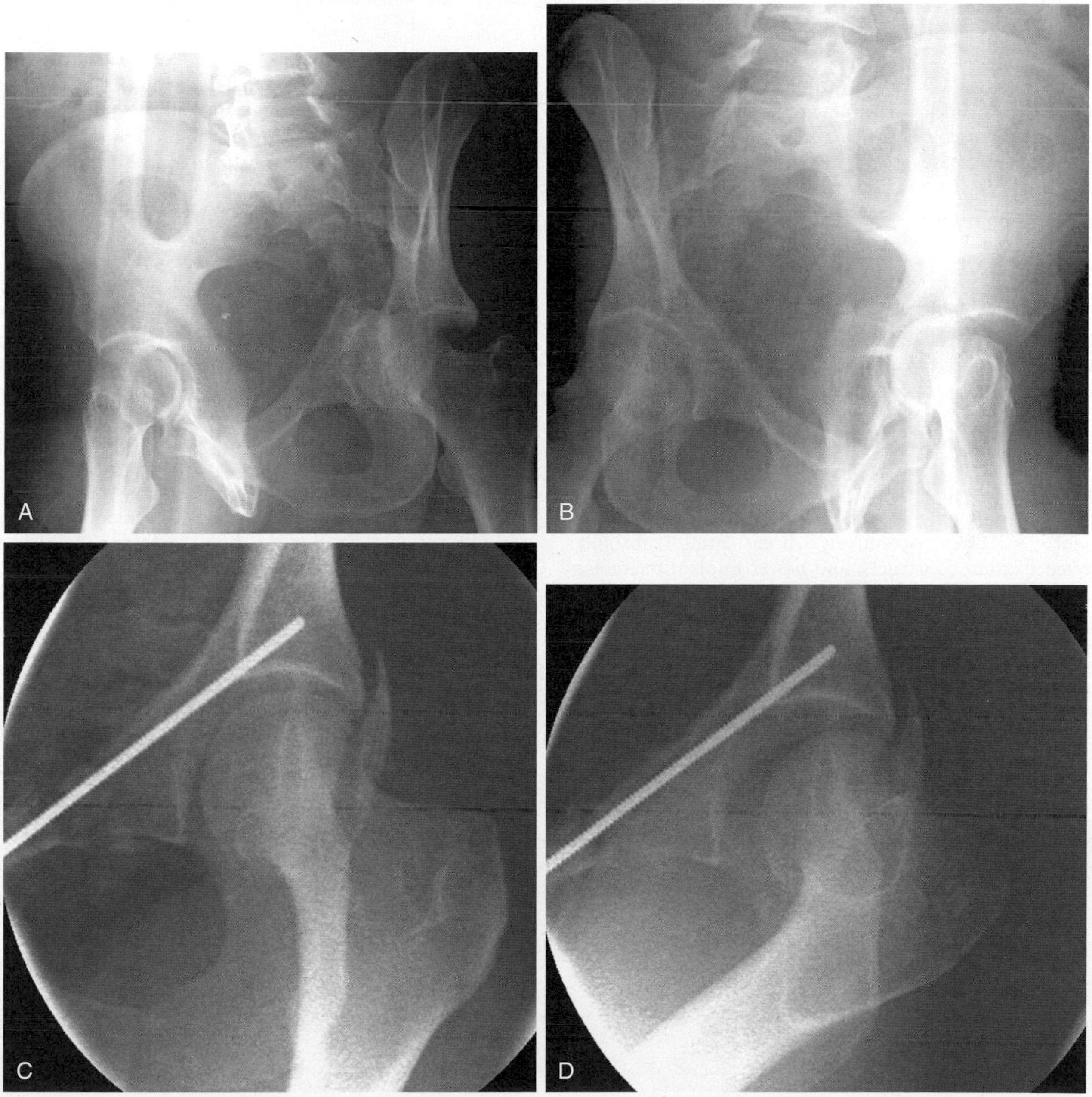

Figure 41-26. **A** and **B,** This acetabular fracture's instability is revealed by the oblique images. **C** and **D,** This patient had a small, peripheral posterior wall acetabular fracture and an unstable pelvic ring injury. During the same anesthetic session as the pelvic ring stabilization, the acetabular fracture was examined under fluoroscopy and noted to be unstable, with 30 degrees of passive hip flexion. The extraarticular medullary ramus screw is located posterior to the hip joint on this view.

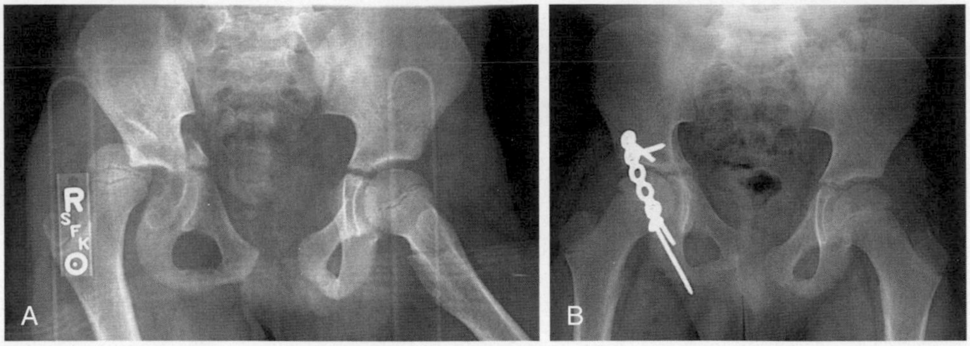

Figure 41-27. **A,** Acetabular fractures occur rarely in children but may involve the triradiate cartilage, as in this patient. **B,** Operative management is indicated for displaced and unstable fractures as in adult patients. The implant size must be adjusted to fit the patient. Physeal bar formation can result depending on the patient's age, fracture pattern, and hip development status at the time of injury. Early implant removal should be considered and serial radiographs are indicated to evaluate for physeal bar formation in younger patients.

arcs on the pelvic CT to determine congruity between the femoral head and acetabular dome region. As the intact dome area expands, thereby improving femoral head coverage, the roof arc angle increases, and better results are anticipated.

Bone quality issues are important factors to consider before surgery.[54] Usually this problem is seen most in elderly patients and those with other bone diseases such as osteogenesis imperfecta.[55-59] The cortical surfaces may not be sufficient to hold a reduction clamp and support fixation plates. Children and adolescent patients with acetabular fractures warrant special considerations also.[13,60-63] The triradiate cartilage is usually injured in younger patients, and standard sized implants may not fit younger pediatric patients. Depending on the status of the triradiate injury and the patient's age, the fixation implants may require removal after healing, and physeal bar formation is likewise evaluated radiographically in follow-up clinic visits (Fig. 41-27).

Special equipment has value when treating such "bone-deficient" fractures operatively. Bone graft substitutes, improved fixation constructs, and newer implant technology may all be needed to manage these injuries. Comminution of the quadrilateral surface; medial dome impaction injuries; significant crush or impaction, especially to the femoral head cranially; frail peripheral posterior wall fractures; and chondral damage are but a few of the nuisance clinical issues that complicate and frustrate successful acetabular fracture management. Specially designed or complex contouring of routine surface implants may be needed to stabilize some of these complex fracture patterns.

Articular chondrocancellous crush injuries along the primary fracture lines are difficult to reduce accurately. Small focal impaction fractures are elevated, reduced to the femoral head after the primary fracture lines are reduced and stabilized, and the defects are supported with bone graft. Extensive impaction fractures including more zones of injury and more comminution are more difficult to accurately reduce and support and therefore correlate directly with posttraumatic arthritic changes (Fig. 41-28).

Operative management restores articular congruity and provides stable fixation.[64] These factors should improve the clinical result by decreasing the incidence of posttraumatic arthritis and allowing early patient and joint mobility.

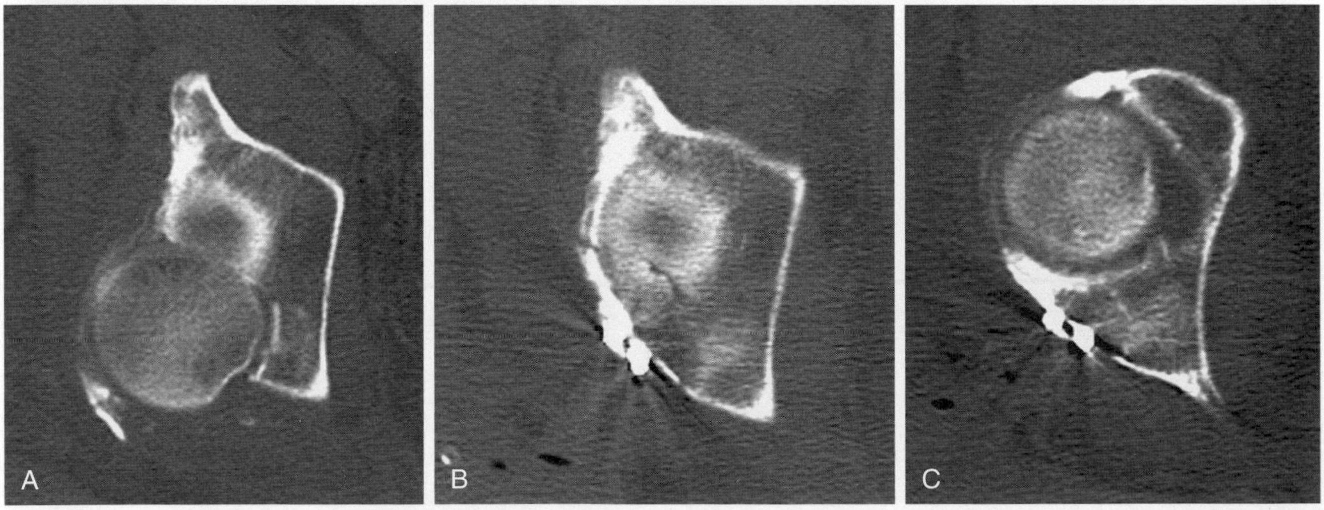

Figure 41-28. Marginal impaction is commonly associated with posterior wall acetabular fracture-dislocations. **A,** This axial image from the injury computed tomography scan demonstrates the chondrocancellous fragments on the fracture's edge that are crushed into the normal cancellous bone of the posterior column. **B** and **C,** After surgery, the posterior wall fracture reduction is shown as is the bone graft material used to support the reduced, previously impacted fragments.

Operative management is advocated for patients with displaced and unstable acetabular fractures who are appropriate surgical candidates.

Operative Timing

Operative treatment of an acetabular fracture occurs when the patient is medically stable, when the surgeon understands the fracture and its treatment details, and when the appropriate operative team is available. Usually this interval is between 1 and 5 days after injury.[65,66] Some surgeons believe that earlier operative intervention allows the fracture surfaces and local tissues to bleed more than if surgery occurs several days after injury. Delay for posterior approach is not associated with decreased blood loss or complications.[67] Recent evidence indicates immediate anterior approach in the appropriately resuscitated patient may be beneficial to the patient's overall physiology.[68] The surgeon must also remember that fracture surface cancellous bone bleeding halts when the fracture surfaces are reduced and stabilized. Knowing this, the surgeon performs the surgical exposure, prepares the fracture fragments for clamp and implant applications, and does so without disturbing the fracture surface clots. Removing the fracture surface clots immediately before reducing the fracture decreases operative blood loss. A blood salvage suction system is also advocated to recycle surgically related blood loss. Recent investigations suggest that blood salvage systems may not be worth the additional expense.[69]

Urgent operative management is recommended for unusual patients with open fractures, irreducible fracture-dislocations, nerve changes after closed reduction, and buttock or iliac compartmental syndrome (e-Fig. 41-2). Rarely, acetabular fracture reduction and fixation will be needed to diminish fracture-related bleeding as a part of the patient's ongoing resuscitation. Open acetabular fractures can be staged as an initial irrigation and débridement procedure followed by open reduction and fixation. The open wounds are commonly located in the iliac crest region or the inguinal area. The initial wound débridement is performed in consideration of the definitive surgical exposure. If the patient's condition and the overall situation are optimal, the reduction and fixation can be performed during the initial anesthetic or at a later date as a separate procedure, allowing the surgeon more time to plan the operative strategy. Certain fracture patterns are at risk for sciatic nerve changes after manipulative reduction. These include any pattern involving displacement through the posterior column or wall areas, especially when the fracture plane parallels the sciatic nerve's course. Compartmental syndrome is also unusual but can occur in the buttock and iliac areas. Buttock compartmental syndrome has been linked to superior gluteal vascular injury caused by displaced acetabular fractures involving the greater sciatic notch. The physical examination demonstrates buttock asymmetry and dramatic swelling. These findings are more difficult in obese patients, but the pelvic CT scan demonstrates the buttock asymmetrical swelling and soft tissue density. Before operative compartment release, angiographic evaluation, and embolization of the potentially injured artery should be considered. Patients with internal iliac compartmental syndrome caused by acetabular fracture usually have minimal fracture displacement but significant bleeding into the iliopsoas muscle or internal iliac fossa. They present with femoral and LFCN dysfunction, but otherwise their physical examination findings may be unremarkable. Pelvic CT demonstrates the asymmetrical swelling and soft tissue density. Before surgical release, a routine screening coagulation panel is obtained and any abnormalities corrected.

Delayed patient referrals delay operative management and should be avoided. Early referral of a patient with an acetabular fracture to an experienced surgeon and fully staffed medical center allows routine management to proceed. In some specialty centers dedicated to acetabular fracture care, aggressive early management of even complex acetabular fractures is standard and uncomplicated. Fracture reduction and fixation are easier when performed routinely and soon after injury. Early intervention avoids more extensile exposures. Dealing with fracture clots and mobile fragments several days after injury is much simpler than débriding fracture callus from relatively immobile fragments several weeks after injury. Early reduction and fixation of the acetabular fracture allows the patient to be upright and mobile so that the systemic adverse effects of recumbency and prolonged traction can be avoided. The patient's overall clinical status routinely improves after early operative management.

Initial Management

The initial management of acetabular fractures follows routine evaluation and resuscitation guidelines similar to those with pelvic ring injuries. The patient's airway is secured, oxygenation confirmed, and vital signs assessed. Volume resuscitation begins with intravenous fluids while laboratory evaluations proceed. Just as for pelvic ring injuries, laboratory testing for patients with acetabular fractures should include routine serology along with serial hematocrits and a hemorrhage panel, including blood typing. A toxicology screen may aid both initial and subsequent treatments.

As mentioned previously, pelvic angiography is indicated when the resuscitation is thorough and adequate, yet unexplained bleeding is noted. Certain acetabular fracture patterns, such as those involving the greater sciatic notch (superior gluteal) and pubic ramus (iliac–corona mortis–obturator) areas, have been associated with vascular injuries. Similarly, acetabular injuries can occur in association with pelvic ring injuries. Targeted angiographic embolization halts pelvic arterial bleeding but not venous or osseous sources.

For less dramatic injuries, initial management assumes that the diagnosis is recognized by the evaluating physician. The injury history may include a description of hip subluxation and spontaneous reduction or described dislocation that was reduced by an initial responder. Some acetabular fractures, such as certain anterior column patterns, may not be obvious on the screening AP plain pelvic radiograph. Most commonly, missed or delayed acetabular fracture diagnosis occurs for peripheral or minimally displaced posterior wall fracture patterns. These are missed because the displaced fracture fragments are superimposed on the normal anatomy and additional oblique radiographs are not obtained. The hip joint articular symmetry is lost on a plain AP radiograph when the femoral head is no longer located beneath the dome. This particular finding is an indication for further imaging including oblique radiographs and a pelvic CT scan.

After the diagnosis is confirmed, the femoral head should be located beneath the acetabular dome. This may require manipulative reduction. Adequate patient sedation and fluoroscopy facilitate the manipulative reduction and allow the physician to easily assess congruity and stability. Once reduced, skeletal traction can be used to maintain the reduction, offset local muscular spasm, and provide comfort, as well as alerting the medical personnel of the injury. A portable AP plain pelvic radiograph obtained with the patient in his or her hospital bed while in skeletal traction ensures that the reduction has been maintained and that the traction weight amount is appropriate (e-Fig. 41-3). Overdistraction of the hip joint either manually during manipulative reduction or while in traction is not recommended because it can cause injury to the surrounding nerves. The treating physician must remember that manipulative maneuvers reduce acetabular fracture-dislocations. Simply adding more and more weight to the skeletal traction device will not provide reduction for the majority of acetabular fracture-dislocations. Incomplete but displaced fracture fragments that include the dome can be confusing during the initial evaluation because reducing the femoral head to the displaced dome fracture fragment may not be possible. Prompt consultation with an orthopaedic surgeon is recommended to sort through such injury details so that the treatment is appropriate.

SURGICAL EXPOSURES

The selection of a surgical exposure is a very important factor in the operative management of acetabular fractures. The exposure must allow the surgeon to sufficiently see the fracture surfaces and their cortical edges so they can be thoroughly cleaned and then manipulated to an anatomic reduction. The surgical exposure must also allow the surgeon to then clamp the fracture reduction and apply definitive and stable fixation. The operative table, surgical exposure, and patient positioning are chosen so that intraoperative fluoroscopic imaging can be used to assess the reduction and implant safety in multiple planes.

Kocher-Langenbeck

The Kocher-Langenbeck exposure is recommended for posterior wall, posterior column, transverse, transverse with associated posterior wall, posterior column with associated posterior wall, and some T-type fractures. It provides direct surgical access to the lateral cortical surfaces of the posterior column and wall regions and with dissection through the greater sciatic notch, digital and clamp access to a majority of the quadrilateral surface. The exposure is best performed with the patient positioned prone, but the lateral position can also be used. Most orthopaedic surgeons will initially try to do the exposure with the patient positioned laterally because the approach in that position is more familiar because of their arthroplasty experiences; however, the lateral position has disadvantages when used for acetabular fractures. In the lateral position, a vacuum beanbag or other secure positioning device is needed to prevent patient movement during the surgery. Intraoperative routine acetabular iliac oblique imaging is obstructed by the vacuum beanbag or other positioning devices. In the lateral position, the dependent side of the torso and limbs requires careful positioning and special padding to avoid nerve stretch and skin pressure necrosis. Also, the weight of the injured limb and gravity act together to apply a constant medial displacement force on the injured hip. In certain fracture patterns, such as transverse fractures, the constant medial displacing force on the unstable fracture segment complicates reduction. Dissection, digital palpation, and clamp application through the greater sciatic notch are more difficult with a laterally positioned patient.

Prone patient positioning is demanding. The airway will be more difficult to readily access, so the position and security of the endotracheal tube must be assured before the patient is rolled into the prone position. Padded chest rolls are adjusted so the abdomen is suspended and the chest can expand freely. The patient's face is placed in a padded support with no pressure on the eyes, nose, and chin. The genitalia and urinary catheter are located so that pressure points are avoided. The perineum should be shaved, cleansed thoroughly, and then isolated from the sterile field with adhesive barrier drapes. The injured lower extremity will be included in the sterile field. The uninjured lower extremity is padded at the anterior thigh, the knee is flexed so the toes are suspended from the bed, and a soft support such as a pillow is placed anterior to the leg. The uninjured lower extremity is then secured to the bed so that inadvertent limb movement is prevented during the surgery. Sequential compression devices can be used when indicated on the well leg. The shoulders are supported anteriorly with rolled foam, and the upper extremities are positioned on articulated, padded arm boards to avoid brachial plexus stretch and pressure points. The ulnar nerve area at the medial elbow should be free of pressure. If the shoulders are stiff or the upper extremity is injured, it can be adducted, but this position denies the anesthesiologist easy access to that adducted upper extremity and could obstruct intraoperative imaging if not properly located relative to the injured hip. Just like the uninjured lower extremity, the upper extremities will be covered by the sterile drapes and should be securely held to the supporting arm boards. A standard radiolucent operating table is recommended (Fig. 41-29). Some surgeons prefer a traction table, but these are expensive; require a skilled, unscrubbed assistant to manipulate; and have been associated with a variety of complications, including pudendal nerve palsy and perineal pressure necrosis caused by the center post, well-limb compartmental syndrome, and other significant complications. If a traction table is selected, traction should be applied only when needed during the surgery to accomplish the reduction (Fig. 41-30).[70]

The injured extremity and both buttock areas are included in the sterile prepared area. Including the injured lower extremity in the sterile field allows the surgeon to manipulate the limb during surgery. For example, internal rotation of the hip moves the greater trochanter away from the posterior acetabular wall, improving the field of view and bone access. The lower portion of the exposure parallels the upper lateral femoral shaft and extends from slightly distal to the gluteus maximus muscle's femoral insertion to the level of the greater trochanter. At the greater trochanteric tip, the incision curves so that the upper incisional component is directed toward the posterior iliac spine. The skin and fat are divided, and the fascia lata incision is made anterior to the gluteus maximus muscle's femoral insertion. The fascia lata incision is continued superiorly and posteriorly to include the gluteus maximus fascia. The gluteus maximus muscle bundles are bluntly split manually, preserving crossing neurovascular bundles if possible. The caudal crossing bundle of the inferior gluteal nerve is often sacrificed during this portion of the dissection to allow retraction and improved exposure. In certain patients,

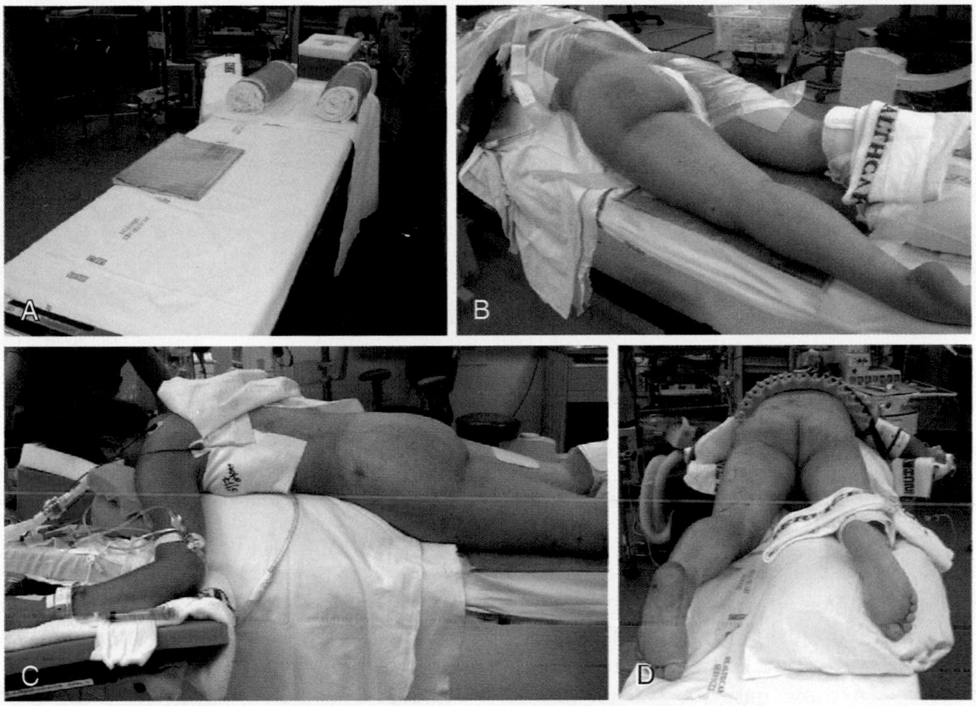

Figure 41-29. Prone positioning facilitates the Kocher-Langenbeck exposure but is demanding. **A,** The operating table is first prepared with articulated arm boards, and the padded chest rolls are sized and located to fit the patient. Before being rolled prone, the patient is intubated, and the endotracheal tube is firmly secured. Any skin leads or other anterior potential pressure points are removed. Then the face and eyes are placed in a face holder so they are relieved of pressure points. **B,** The patient is rolled onto the operating table and into the prone position. **C,** The chest rolls are positioned, and the upper extremities are placed on articulated arm boards to avoid brachial plexus stretch. **D,** The chest rolls are located to suspend the abdomen, allowing uncomplicated ventilation. The genitals are then adjusted to avoid compression, and the urinary catheter position avoids meatal pressure. The injured lower extremity will be prepped into the sterile field while the opposite lower extremity is padded anteriorly, positioned so the toes are suspended, and secured to the table. A well-leg sequential compression device is used as needed. The perineum is cleansed thoroughly, shaved, and then isolated using barrier drapes. Careful razor shaving of the buttock and perineal hair and then initial skin cleansing with isopropyl alcohol are used to thoroughly cleanse the area. A skin adherent is then applied topically to the surgical field's perimeter to improve the barrier drapes' function. Many patients with acetabular fractures have overdue bowel movements during anesthesia induction and positioning. The soiled laundry should be removed from the operating room.

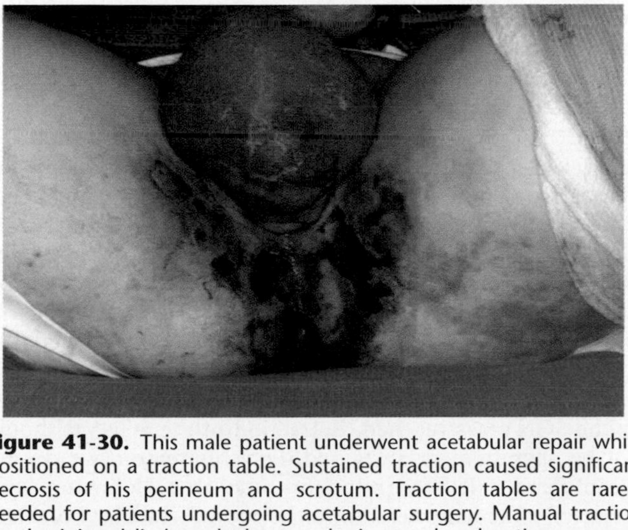

Figure 41-30. This male patient underwent acetabular repair while positioned on a traction table. Sustained traction caused significant necrosis of his perineum and scrotum. Traction tables are rarely needed for patients undergoing acetabular surgery. Manual traction on the injured limb and pharmacologic muscle relaxation are used only during the direct manipulation of the critical fracture fragments. Manual traction is usually necessary for those few seconds as the fracture fragment is manipulated into its reduced location just before clamp application.

retraction of the gluteus maximus muscle is difficult and perhaps slightly improved by incising its tendon at the insertion along the posterior proximal femur just medial to the vastus lateralis muscle's posterior fascial edge. This gluteus maximus tenotomy is rarely necessary and is later repaired before wound closure. The trochanteric bursa is divided, and the gluteus medius muscle is bluntly separated along its caudal edge from both the cranial aspect of the piriformis muscle and the underlying gluteus minimus muscle bellies. The gluteus medius muscle can then be retracted anteriorly and superiorly. Rarely in morbidly obese or patients with huge buttock musculature, the posterior portion of the gluteus medius tendon can be incised to improve retraction and exposure. This focal tenotomy is repaired before wound closure. The piriformis muscle is then further isolated cranially from the gluteus medius and minimus muscles, caudally from the superior gemellus muscle, and anteriorly from the hip capsule. Before piriformis muscle tenotomy, its relationship with the sciatic nerve must be known and seen. The sciatic nerve is then exposed distally within the wound usually dorsal to the quadratus femoris muscle and then carefully traced cranially to the piriformis muscle and the greater sciatic notch. The sciatic

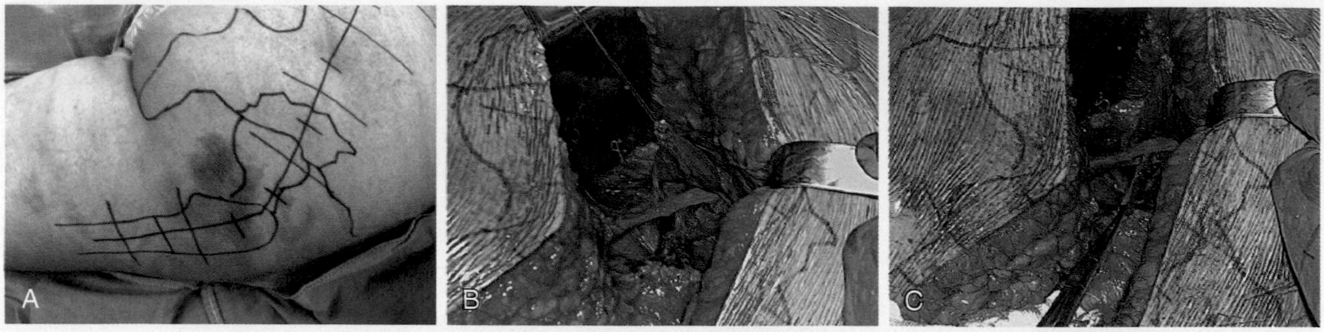

Figure 41-31. **A,** This patient has a right-sided posterior wall fracture, is positioned prone, and is being treated using a Kocher-Langenbeck exposure. **B,** The fascia lata and gluteus maximus muscle fascia has been incised, the gluteus maximus muscle bundles have been separated, and the posterior half is retracted medially by the larger retractor. The gluteus medius muscle is being retracted superiorly by the smaller retractor. The sciatic nerve is visible within the deeper aspects of the surgical field. The gemellus muscles are anterior to the nerve. This patient has two piriformis muscle bundles. One is posterior to the sciatic nerve and has been tenotomized in this image while the other anterior piriformis muscle bundle is penetrating through and dividing the sciatic nerve at that site. **C,** With the dorsal piriformis muscle bundle tagged and retracted medially by a suture, the anterior piriformis muscle is isolated and then excised so that it cannot harm the dorsal nerve bundle.

nerve and piriformis muscle have a variety of relationships, and the surgeon must identify it during surgery at this point. For most patients, the piriformis muscle is completely posterior to the sciatic nerve. In some patients, the piriformis muscle has an additional anterior muscle belly that penetrates through the sciatic nerve bundles yet shares a common insertion tendon with the normal dorsal piriformis muscle. These ancillary anterior muscle bellies should be excised to avoid inadvertent sciatic nerve injury when the piriformis is retracted (Fig. 41-31). The sciatic nerve should be freed bluntly from any local tethering tissues extending from the greater sciatic notch to the quadratus femoris muscle. This can be done easily by the surgeon's finger palpating the nerve along its anterior and lateral surfaces. Frequently, a small-diameter nerve is identified between the anterior sciatic nerve and the posterior hip capsule. This capsular nerve tethers the sciatic nerve and prevents safe retraction of the sciatic nerve. In these situations, the capsular nerve is divided at the capsule so the sciatic nerve can be safely mobilized and retracted. Many patients also have large-diameter veins coursing along the dorsal surface of the sciatic nerve as well as soft tissue vascular leashes located posterolateral relative to the sciatic nerve. These also must be ligated and released to allow for safe nerve manipulation during the surgery. Hip extension and knee flexion relax the sciatic nerve within the field of view during the procedure. For patients with a tight rectus femoris muscle, hip extension and knee flexion will inadvertently flex the hip, cause the femoral head to intrude medially if there is a transverse fracture, or extrude posteriorly if there is a posterior wall fracture. In these patients, sciatic neuroplasty is necessary so the knee can be extended to relax the rectus femoris muscle and eliminate its deforming effect on the fracture. After the sciatic nerve's relationship with the piriformis muscle is known and any tethering tissues released, the piriformis muscle can then be safely tenotomized 1 to 2 cm lateral to its insertion, tagged with a suture, and retracted superiorly and medially. Next the superior and inferior gemellus muscles are assessed. In many patients, especially those after posterior wall fracture-dislocations, the superior gemellus muscle has been destroyed by the injury. The remnants of the superior gemellus are débrided in these situations. The inferior gemellus muscle is larger than the superior gemellus muscle, and its caudal location protects it better from traumatic injury. Because of its size, the inferior gemellus muscle is often confused with the quadratus femoris muscle. The inferior gemellus muscle should be separated bluntly from the quadratus muscle. The quadratus femoris muscle has an important relationship with the medial femoral circumflex vessels and therefore is preserved and protected throughout the operation. Once isolated, the inferior gemellus muscle is noted to have a direct muscular femoral insertion approximately 1 cm in diameter. The inferior gemellus muscle is then incised near its femoral insertion, elevated from its origin adjacent to the lesser sciatic notch, separated from the obturator internus muscle tendon, and excised. The excision is recommended because the inferior gemellus muscle is essentially dead once it has been detached from its femoral insertion and then elevated from its origin in anticipation of subsequent fixation plate placement.

The obturator internus muscle tendon is then easily identified and is tenotomized 1 to 2 cm from its insertion. The adjacent superior and inferior gemellus muscle remnants are excised from the obturator internus tendon after they have been elevated with subperiosteal dissection from the ischial area adjacent to the lesser sciatic notch. The quadratus femoris muscle is not disturbed throughout this exposure to preserve the femoral head's blood supply.

The caudal portion of the gluteus medius muscle is retracted superiorly and anteriorly thereby exposing the caudal portion of the gluteus minimus muscle. Next the superior gluteal neurovascular bundle (SGNVB) is identified approximately 3 to 4 cm cranial to the gluteus minimus muscle's caudal edge. The SGNVB is isolated and protected from excessive retraction during the operation. Similar to the superior gemellus muscle, that portion of the gluteus minimus muscle tissue caudal to the SGNVB is often severely injured by the posterior fracture-dislocation and is excised until healthy muscle tissue is noted or the SGNVB is reached. Retraction of the SGNVB should not be aggressive or sustained. For this reason, we do not recommend a levered retractor such as a Hohmann style retractor to be hammered into the supraacetabular bone and then handed to an assistant. Sustained force from a levered retractor will injure the SGNVB and should be avoided.

The dissection continues if necessary through the greater sciatic notch. The periosteum along the edge of the greater sciatic notch is quite thick and dense, and excision of this tissue is recommended. The dissection proceeds superiorly within the notch to the level of the SGNVB and inferiorly to the ischial spine. With the sciatic nerve relaxed and carefully retracted medially, subperiosteal dissection through the greater sciatic notch of the obturator muscle belly away from the quadrilateral surface is safely accomplished.

For the Kocher-Langenbeck exposure, the cranial limit is the SGNVB, the posterior limit is the greater and lesser sciatic notches and the sciatic nerve, the caudal limit is the quadratus femoris muscle and hamstring muscle origin, and the lateral limit is the hip's labrum and capsule.

After reduction and fixation, multiplanar fluoroscopic imaging ensures the reduction quality and implant safety. The residual necrotic tissues are excised, the wound is irrigated, the tenotomies are repaired, and closure proceeds in layers.

One disadvantage of prone positioning for the Kocher-Langenbeck approach is the inability to perform an anterior surgical dislocation with a digastric trochanteric osteotomy. This requires lateral positioning to allow for hip flexion and external rotation after a Z-shaped capsulotomy is made.[71] This approach has gained popularity for treatment of femoral head fractures associated with posterior wall acetabular fractures.[72] Others have advocated the technique to improve direct articular visualization[73]; however, the technique has not been shown to improve the quality of fracture reduction nor long-term outcome.[74] Similar to many "new" techniques, the precise indications and related complications remain undefined.[73,75,76]

Ilioinguinal

The ilioinguinal exposure is an interesting exposure that can be divided into three main access intervals, or "windows"—lateral (iliac), middle (vascular), and medial (intrapelvic).[77,78] Anatomic terms are preferred because numbering these surgical intervals is confusing and not advocated. Via these surgical intervals, the ilioinguinal exposure provides direct access to the lateral sacral ala, anterior SI joint, the internal iliac fossa and iliac crest, the pelvic brim, the anterior acetabular wall, the superior pubic ramus, the symphysis pubis, and the upper half of the quadrilateral surface and greater sciatic notch. The ilioinguinal exposure is therefore indicated for anterior column and anterior wall fractures, anterior column with associated posterior hemitransverse patterns, certain T-type fractures, transverse fractures, and associated both-column acetabular fractures. If necessary, associated SI injuries are also addressed using this exposure. The exposure also allows access to the contralateral superior pubis ramus if necessary.

The ilioinguinal exposure should be performed with the patient positioned supine, preferably on a radiolucent operating table. The patient's pelvis should be elevated from the table approximately 4 to 6 cm on a soft lumbosacral support such as a folded blanket. Just like for the Kocher-Langenbeck surgical zone preparation, the perineal area should first be shaved and then cleansed completely with antiseptic solution such as isopropyl alcohol. The entire abdomen, bilateral flanks, and ipsilateral injured lower extremity are included in the sterile field. The upper extremities are usually abducted. The uninjured lower extremity is padded, and a sequential compression device is applied if indicated and then secured to the table. The initial barrier draping isolates the perineum but allows access to the pubis, inguinal area, and flank areas, as well as the entire ipsilateral lower extremity. This allows limb manipulation, including manual traction if needed. Hip flexion during the operation relaxes the iliopsoas muscle as well as the iliac-femoral vessels (Fig. 41-32).

As for the Kocher-Langenbeck exposure, traction tables are not recommended for the ilioinguinal exposure because of their expense, inventory, size, need for specially trained unscrubbed assistants to manipulate the table, imaging obstruction, and the potential for traction-related skin and nerve problems.[70]

It is important for the surgeon to identify both in the history and on physical examination if the patient has had previous inguinal operations such as hernia repair, appendectomy, cesarean section delivery, or open bladder procedures, among others. If so, prior infections are ruled out. Hernia repairs, especially those with mesh reinforcement, complicate the ilioinguinal exposure. Similarly, the preoperative examination and pelvic CT scan should be evaluated for inguinal hernia or other intrapelvic pathology (Fig. 41-33).

Before skin incision, the surgeon determines which surgical intervals or windows are needed to expose, clean, reduce, and stabilize the fracture. If all three windows are to be used, the skin incision begins at the ipsilateral iliac crest, parallels the inguinal ligament, and ends just above the symphysis pubis. Osseous landmarks are difficult to determine in obese patients and those with significant displacements of the iliac crest fracture fragments. The contralateral normal-sided osseous landmarks may be used for symmetry, or the fluoroscope can be used if needed. Some surgeons consider the ilioinguinal skin incision in three individual segments: a Pfannenstiel portion, an iliac portion, and a connecting inguinal portion.

The skin and subcutaneous fat are incised, and the spermatic cord or round ligament is identified and protected. Some surgeons prefer to place rubber drains around these structures in an attempt to protect them during the operation. Inadvertent or sustained retraction using the rubber drains can injure the spermatic cord, femoral vessels, and femoral nerve.

To open the lateral or iliac window, the abdominal oblique muscular insertions onto the iliac crest are incised, leaving a small stump for subsequent repair. Alternatively, the abdominal obliques are cauterized at their iliac crest insertions and then later repaired onto the tensor muscle fascia at closure. The external oblique insertion can be incised posteriorly around the iliac crest or its fascia split midway along the iliac crest and the posterior portion of the muscle left intact. The internal oblique and transversus abdominis insertions along the iliac crest are next divided from the anterior superior iliac crest to the posterior aspect of the crest. This dissection allows a two-layered closure and decreases the risk of wound hernia. Dissection of the abdominal oblique muscular insertion near the anterior superior iliac spine (ASIS) proceeds medially with care so that the LFCN is not inadvertently injured, especially if electrocautery is being used to elevate the abdominal oblique insertion from the iliac crest anteriorly. The lateral aspect of the inguinal portion of the dissection will subsequently meet with this iliac wound interval at the ASIS, and the LFCN is best identified as it penetrates the inguinal ligament during that portion of the exposure. The iliacus muscle is elevated subperiosteally and retracted medially. Hip flexion eases this

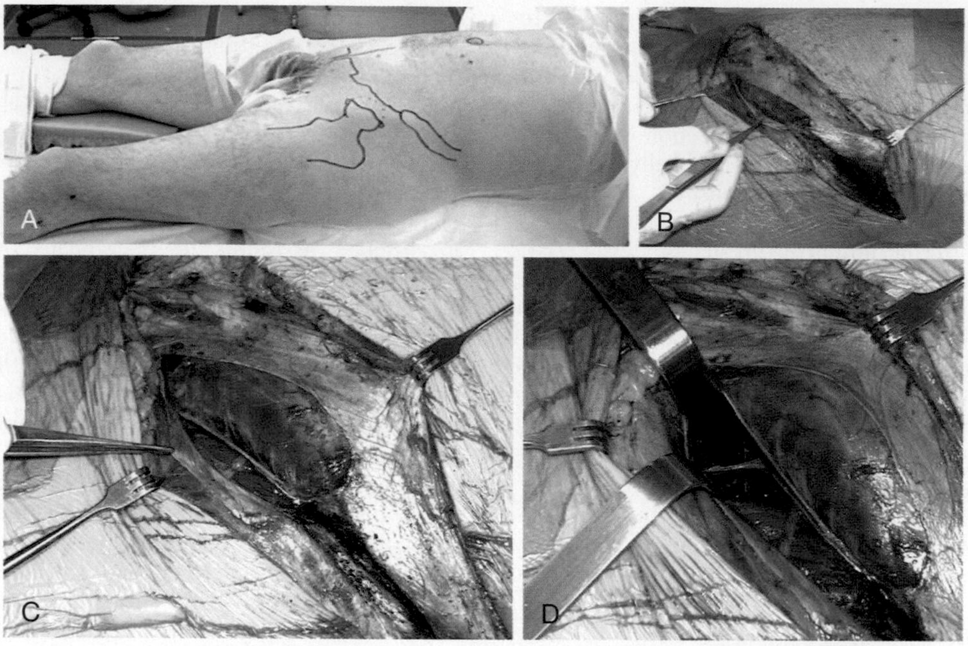

Figure 41-32. **A,** For ilioinguinal exposures, the patient is positioned supine and elevated on a padded support located posterior to the lumbosacral area. The perineum is cleansed and isolated. The upper extremities are abducted and secured on arm boards. The uninjured lower extremity is positioned on a soft pad and secured. The entire abdomen, bilateral flanks, and injured extremity are included in the sterile field. **B,** The lateral and middle surgical intervals are being developed. The abdominal oblique muscles have been cauterized along their iliac crest insertions. The anterior abdominal fascia has been sharply incised approximately 2 cm cranial to the palpable inguinal ligament, and then the caudal flap has been retracted to expose the ilioinguinal nerve and the inguinal ligament. The external inguinal ring has been spared. **C,** The inguinal ligament has been incised from the iliopectineal fascia (IPF) medially to the anterior superior iliac spine (ASIS) laterally. The lateral femoral cutaneous nerve (LFCN) is seen penetrating the cut inguinal ligament several centimeters medial to the ASIS. **D,** The IPF has been isolated. The medial retractor pulls the iliac artery and vein medially, and the lateral retractor pulls the iliopsoas muscle and femoral nerve laterally. This patient has an interesting blood vessel stemming from the iliac artery that penetrates the IPF and then enters the iliopsoas muscle. The vessel is ligated and controlled before the IPF is excised.

dissection by relaxing the iliopsoas muscle dramatically. This deep dissection involving exposure of the fracture surfaces should be delayed until the remainder of the exposure is performed because excessive bleeding from the iliac fracture components is common. It is best to wait until the entire ilioinguinal exposure is accomplished before exposing the fracture surfaces and removing their hematoma. In many situations, the fracture bleeding is only arrested by the fracture reduction, so the surgeon should resist the temptation to burrow into the iliac interval and begin working on the iliac fracture fragments until the remainder of the exposure and intervals are developed.

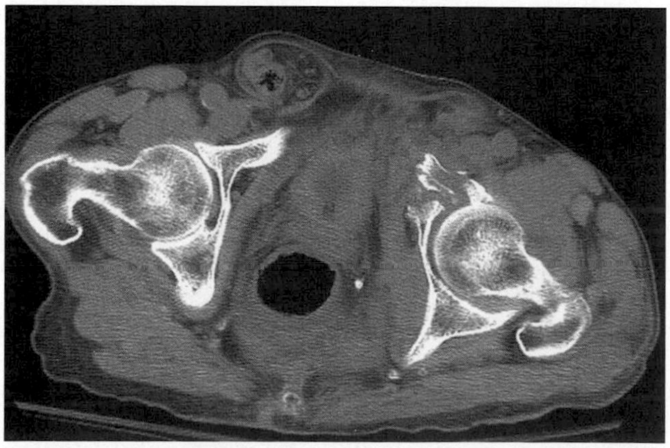

Figure 41-33. Computed tomography image demonstrating a notable inguinal hernia. The hernia repair was performed using the ilioinguinal exposure at the time of acetabular fracture operative reduction and fixation.

The medial window is simply a Pfannenstiel surgical exposure that can be extended to an intrapelvic exposure when needed. The midline rectus abdominis muscular raphe is divided superiorly from the pubis approximately 6 cm, and the local hematoma is removed from the space of Retzius. The ipsilateral rectus abdominis muscle is retracted anteriorly and laterally. The bladder is retracted posteriorly with a malleable retractor. The surgeon should stand on the uninjured side and use headlamp illumination for the deep pelvic dissection. The ipsilateral rectus abdominis muscle insertion is then progressively yet incompletely tenotomized beginning at the midline and progressing laterally and distally along the muscle insertion until sufficient visualization of the superior pubic ramus is achieved by the retraction. Visualization of the posterior surface of the injured-side superior pubic ramus will identify any communicating conduits between the obturator and inferior epigastric or iliac vascular systems.[79] These arteries and veins are ligated or cauterized depending on their diameter. The deep dissection should proceed after the inguinal dissection is complete, so the medial window is packed with a sponge.

The inguinal dissection is the portion of the procedure that intimidates most surgeons, but it should not. It simply connects the other two portions of the exposure, provides access to and liberates the iliac vascular structures as they cross the anterior pelvis, further mobilizes the iliopsoas muscle, and allows direct visualization of the superior pubic ramus and a portion of the quadrilateral surface. The inguinal interval provides another window for fracture surface cleaning, clamp placement, and implant application. Some surgeons believe that the inguinal interval is dangerous because it involves dissection adjacent to the iliac vessels.

The inguinal portion of the dissection begins simply by inspecting and assessing the anterior abdominal fascia's local condition. Often because of fracture-displacement and associated local trauma, this anterior abdominal fascia is contused and ecchymotic. It may even be frayed and its fascial bundles traumatically separated. The anterior abdominal fascia should be incised 1 to 1.5 cm cranial to and paralleling the underlying yet palpable inguinal ligament. This fascial incision can include or use bands of traumatic separation when necessary. This fascial incision extends from and connects with the prior abdominal oblique incision adjacent to the ASIS and then proceeds medially and caudally toward the pubis. This fascial incision extends to and can even include opening the external inguinal ring (EIR) if the surgeon chooses. Some surgeons note the diameter of the EIR before opening it sharply to facilitate its accurate repair at closure. Other surgeons realize that opening the EIR is unnecessary to complete a safe and effective inguinal window dissection. Whether the EIR is opened or spared is unimportant. What is important is to repair it accurately if you choose to open it. The abdominal fascial incision paralleling and just above the inguinal ligament should now expose the ilioinguinal nerve seen penetrating anteriorly through the deep tissues and traveling parallel to the inguinal ligament toward the spermatic cord or round ligament. The ilioinguinal nerve is interesting in that it is almost always exactly at the level and parallel to the optimal anterior abdominal fascia incision site. The surgeon must be aware of this fact and avoid heavy-handedness and electrocautery for this incision. The ilioinguinal nerve should always be identified, protected, and not forgotten, especially during retraction and then at closure of the abdominal fascial layer. The nerve can be inadvertently sutured during the inguinal ligament repair and also potentially during the anterior abdominal fascial closure.

The inguinal ligament becomes visible when the caudal flap of the abdominal fascia is retracted inferiorly. The inguinal ligament is almost always intact. The inguinal ligament is then divided. Some surgeons prefer to split it along the entire extent of its course from its pubic insertion to the ASIS origin. Others divide it only from the level of the iliopectineal fascia (IPF) to the ASIS. Regardless of the chosen technique, the inguinal ligament is divided at least to the IPF.

The LFCN directly penetrates through the inguinal ligament usually only millimeters medial to the ASIS. The LFCN has an accompanying vascular system. It is wise to seek the nerve carefully as the inguinal ligament surgical division proceeds near the ASIS. Not every patient has an LFCN several millimeters medial to the ASIS, but most do. Some have branches of the LFCN located more medially just superficial to the femoral nerve and iliac vascular system.[80] The surgeon should protect the LFCN when possible. The LFCN can be dissected proximally and distally to improve its retraction without stretch injury. The LFCN can also be segmentally excised during the initial exposure to avoid injury if significant stretch injury is anticipated because of retraction. The patient should be informed before operation that permanent thigh numbness will result if the nerve is excised, and chronic pain and dysesthesias may result if stretch injury occurs. Some patients with displacement of the anterior column fracture component or trauma-related contusion in the area of the ASIS have an abnormal LFCN examination on presentation that should be documented.

After the inguinal ligament is surgically divided, the IPF is next isolated. The IPF is a confusing oblique "curtain" of dense tissue that separates the false from the true pelvis. Lateral to this fascial curtain is the iliopsoas muscle and the femoral nerve while the iliac vessels and pelvic contents are medial to it. The IPF is attached to the inguinal ligament and anchored to pelvic brim by blending with the local periosteum there. It is isolated easily either by digital or blunt instrument dissection medially and laterally. During this dissection, the surgeon inspects for penetrating vessels from the iliac system into the iliopsoas muscle. These small-diameter yet high-flow conduits should be isolated and ligated as necessary. After the iliac vessels are carefully retracted medially and the iliopsoas muscle–femoral nerve unit is retracted laterally, the IPF is divided from inguinal ligament to the pelvic brim and then divided from or elevated along with the pelvic brim periosteum. In some displaced fracture patterns, the IPF may be very taut and almost horizontal in orientation because of the fracture fragment deformity. It is unnecessary to expose the iliac artery and vein directly. They simply should be mobilized as a unit to allow safe retraction for deep visualization of the acetabular anatomy. In some patients, the traumatic injury disrupts the iliac vessels surrounding soft tissues, and consequently, the vessels are obvious within the middle surgical wound interval. After the IPF has been divided, the surgeon should know that the periosteum that shrouds the IPE is thick. This thick periosteum is elevated and then excised from the middle surgical interval.

After the IPF is divided and elevated and the iliac vessels mobilized, the deep dissection of the medial intrapelvic window resumes. Standing again on the uninjured side, the surgeon detaches the rectus abdominis tendon incompletely from its anterior parasymphyseal insertion until sufficient visualization of the superior pubic ramus is achieved. It is not necessary to completely tenotomize the rectus abdominis insertion because incomplete release always provides excellent deep exposure and facilitates the later repair. With the rectus abdominis muscle retracted anterolaterally, the periosteum of the superior pubic ramus is inspected, especially its posterior surface. Communicating vessels between the iliac and obturator systems are isolated, ligated, and divided so they can be safely retracted. The superior pubic ramus periosteum is then elevated along with a portion of the pectineus muscle fascial origin. The iliac vessels are retracted carefully along with the rectus abdominis muscle. Ipsilateral hip flexion eases and improves the retraction and hence the deep exposure. The superior pubic ramus periosteal elevation proceeds laterally until it meets the site of the IPF elevation at the IPE previously accomplished via the middle surgical interval.

Progressing more deeply, the obturator neurovascular bundle is identified and retracted medially. This bundle is often displaced medially by the quadrilateral surface fracture fragment's displacement. Occasionally, the obturator neurovascular bundle is found within the fracture site and despite its contused and distorted appearance should be carefully removed from the fracture and protected thereafter. The quadrilateral surface is next exposed by elevating the obturator internus muscle subperiosteally. Medial displacement of the quadrilateral surface fracture fragment obstructs visualization of the intact ilium posterior and lateral to it. The surgeon can lateralize the fracture fragment using a spiked bone pusher together with gentle manual traction on the limb by an assistant. Subperiosteal elevation of the intact ilium cranial to the greater sciatic notch is important if an intrapelvic plate application is needed. The dissection is facilitated by medial retraction of the obturator internus muscle, obturator NVB, SGNVB, and sciatic nerve. A narrow, malleable retractor is effective for this purpose. If the iliacus muscle has not been completely elevated because of anticipated fracture-related bleeding, the surgeon should return to the injured side and do it via the iliac interval at this point so the three surgical intervals can be completed. Mobilization of the iliacus muscle, iliac vessels, obturator NVB, and urinary bladder along with excision of the IPF and periosteal tissues along the pelvic brim and superior pubic ramus provide an optimal exposure.

At this point in the operation, the three windows have been connected. The surgeon can stand on the uninjured side using the medial intrapelvic interval; retract the bladder posteromedially along with the obturator neurovascular bundle; retract the rectus abdominus muscle and iliac vessels anterolaterally; and directly visualize the upper half of the quadrilateral surface, the pelvic brim, the superior pubic ramus, the anterior wall, and symphysis pubis. By standing on the injured side using the inguinal interval, the surgeon can retract the iliac vessels medially; retract the iliopsoas and femoral nerve laterally; and directly visualize the anterior wall, midportion of the pubic ramus, the iliopsoas gutter, a portion of the internal iliac fossa, and the upper aspect of the quadrilateral surface. And standing on the injured side using the iliac window, the surgeon can retract the iliacus muscle medially and visualize the entire iliac crest, internal iliac fossa, pelvic brim, SI joint, iliopsoas gutter, and AIIS.

Several more details are also very relevant. The surgeon should sequence the deep interval dissections according to anticipated fracture bleeding so that the deep area of most anticipated fracture bleeding is exposed last. Similarly, fracture surface clots should be removed as the last phase of site preparation. After these clots are removed, the fracture surface bleeding is often impressive and can only be halted by fracture reduction. It is important to remember that fracture fragment displacements can alter the palpable anatomy of the iliac crest and pubis. Because of this fact, the skin incision should be located where these palpable landmarks should be rather than where they may be when displaced. Similar to scarring from prior local operations, displaced fracture fragments distort the soft tissue anatomy and thereby complicate the dissection. Identifying the appropriate anatomy is vital for a successful procedure. Mobilizing the iliac vessels is an important step in the ilioinguinal exposure and frightens many surgeons. The critical step is to isolate the IPF and then make sure to divide it and then elevate it from the pelvic brim and IPE. If the IPF is left even incompletely attached, then mobilization and retraction of the iliac vessels is compromised, adding to the surgical risk. Hip flexion during the dissection relaxes the local anatomy and eases retraction. The surgeon should also remember that the iliac vessels may have small branches that penetrate through the IPF before they enter or exit the iliopsoas muscle. Palpation along the IPF before blunt dissection reveals these penetrating small-diameter yet high-flow conduits. They should be controlled with ligation and then divided.

Avoid plunging fingers and retractors anterior and deep to the bladder. Such maneuvers are unnecessary and can disrupt the local anterior bladder venous plexus, causing bleeding that is often difficult to stop even with packing.

The communicating vessels between the obturator system and iliac or inferior epigastric system, the so-called corona mortis, also causes much surgical concern. These branches are quite common unless fracture comminution or displacement has destroyed them. The surgeon should simply look for them during the initial blunt dissection along the posterior surface of the superior pubic ramus via the medial intrapelvic interval. When seen, vessels of sufficient diameter should be isolated and controlled with ligation or clipping. Similarly, the obturator vascular bundle may be injured by fracture comminution at its sulcus beneath the lateral aspect of the superior pubic ramus. Fracture-related bleeding in this zone responds to local packing, but aggressive packing can injure the local blood vessels and potentially the nerve. Use the suction to first inspect the area to determine what is bleeding. If a vessel is identified, then it can be ligated or cauterized. If the fracture surface is bleeding, then expedient reduction is indicated. Rarely, the iliac vein can be injured on its posterior surface by displaced and sharp comminuted superior pubic ramus fracture fragments. This is usually apparent on the injury pelvic CT scan as a very large local hematoma or disturbed vein when contrast is used. The iliac vein injury is also identified during dissection as impressive venous bleeding into the wound via the middle vascular wound interval or medial intrapelvic wound interval dissection and is best controlled by manual or retractor pressure on the vein at the bleeding site or by simply applying manual pressure in the groin. The surgeon must take care to apply enough pressure to stop the iliac venous bleeding yet not apply too much pressure, causing further tearing of the friable vein hole and without disturbing arterial flow. Excessive and sustained pressure can cause arterial thrombus formation. Random clamping of the area will also potentially injure the vessel and is not recommended. Depending on the institution, vascular or general surgical consultation is recommended, and their special equipment is obtained so that it is available when they arrive. A blood salvage suction system is also recommended. The ilioinguinal exposure is not always familiar to the consultant, so it is helpful to orient him or her to the wound and its developed intervals. The iliac vein can then be exposed either via the intrapelvic or vascular interval; then vascular clamps are applied proximally and distally relative to the lesion, and the vessel is repaired without stenosis. After the iliac vein is repaired, the ipsilateral peripheral pulses should be monitored throughout the remainder of the operation (Fig. 41-34).

Extended Iliofemoral

This surgical exposure has been advocated for delayed acetabular reconstruction and for patterns that demand direct visualization of the articular surface during the repair.[81-84] Because the mobilized flap is based on the superior gluteal vascular supply, some angiographic studies advocate a preoperative assessment of these vessels to ensure their patency.[85-87] Clinical studies have not supported such preoperative angiography, citing few problems related to flap necrosis.[57,88]

For this extensile acetabular approach, the patient is positioned laterally, and the entire injured lower extremity and

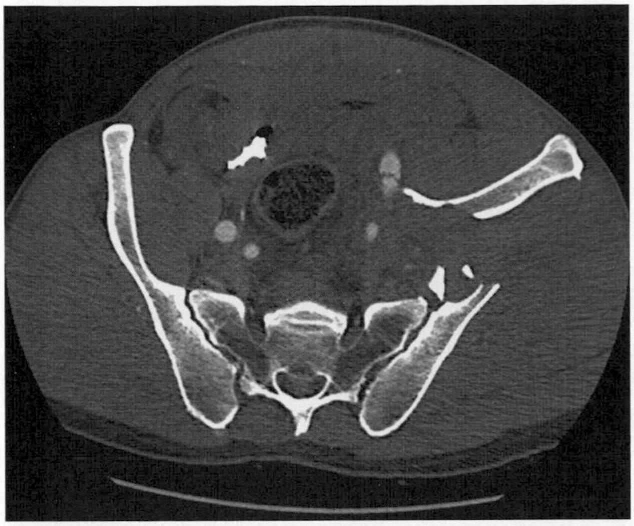

Figure 41-34. Axial computed tomography (CT) image demonstrating an iliac vein injury caused by the widely displaced anterior column fracture fragment of an associated both-column fracture pattern. During the ilioinguinal exposure, the vein injury required repair. A vascular surgeon was available and prepared for this portion of the operation. Iliac vascular injuries are rare but usually identifiable on the injury CT scan, especially those with contrast.

flank are prepared in the sterile field after the perineum is cleaned and isolated. The surgical incision parallels the iliac crest from posterior to anterior, curving at the ASIS and following the palpable interval between the sartorius and tensor muscles. The ascending branch of the lateral femoral circumflex vessels is ligated; the entire lateral ilium is elevated subperiosteally; and the gluteus medius, gluteus minimus, piriformis, and obturator internus muscles are tenotomized at their proximal femoral insertions. The hip abductor muscle mass is retracted carefully to protect the SGNVB and sciatic nerve. A hip joint capsulotomy is performed along its periphery at the labral edge, and the proximal femur is retracted to expose the articular fracture fragments. The proximal femur is retracted using a greater trochanteric bone hook or a sturdy pin inserted at the level of the lesser trochanter. The fracture reductions begin at the articular surfaces and proceed toward the iliac crest from central to peripheral. The fragments are cleaned, manipulated, clamped, and secured with lag screws and supporting plates applied to the lateral ilium and posterior column.

The closure is performed with the hip abducted to relax tension on the proximal femoral tendon insertion repairs and abductor origin repair along the crest. Prolonged operative times are related to flap swelling, which complicates closure. Some form of ectopic bone prophylaxis is advocated for this extensile exposure.

Combined Anterior and Posterior Exposures

Combined sequential and simultaneous anterior and posterior surgical exposures during the same anesthetic administration were designed to improve reduction quality of associated fracture patterns by improving fracture visualization.[89,90] With two surgeons working simultaneously, operative times were diminished. Unfortunately, the medial intrapelvic surgical interval of the ilioinguinal exposure cannot be developed with the patient placed in the mobile or "floppy" lateral position. Similarly, the Kocher-Langenbeck exposure cannot be developed to its full extent because of the positioning.

In some patients with associated or variant fracture patterns, sequential use of an initial ilioinguinal exposure with the patient positioned supine followed by a Kocher-Langenbeck exposure with the patient positioned prone has real merit.[91] For example, in a patient with an associated both-column acetabular fracture that has a large posterior wall component and an ipsilateral anterior SI joint disruption, the SI joint and primary column fractures are reduced and stabilized initially. Then the patient is turned prone either during the same anesthesia or subsequently for a prone Kocher-Langenbeck exposure to reduce and stabilize the posterior wall fracture (Fig. 41-35).

If this sequential exposure tactic is selected, the surgeon should not obstruct the subsequent reduction with initial procedure implants. All acetabular repairs should be carefully planned preoperatively, but sequential exposures demand the best planning because malreduced fracture fragments and poorly located screws applied during the initial procedure can obstruct the subsequent reductions and fixations.

Other Exposures

Several other exposures have been described for acetabular surgery.[75,80,92-105] The modified extended iliofemoral exposure employs an iliac crest osteotomy to improve visualization and therefore reduction–fixation while maintaining some local soft tissue attachments. Using this approach, both the inner and outer iliac areas are exposed.[36,103]

The Smith-Petersen surgical exposure is not often indicated for acetabular fractures, but certain variant fracture patterns involving the AIIS, anterior wall area, and cranial or extended posterior wall patterns are best treated using this exposure.

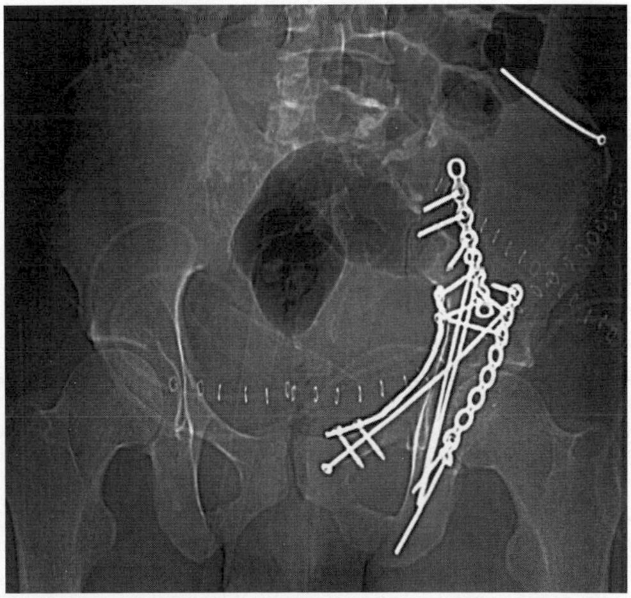

Figure 41-35. This patient had sequential ilioinguinal (supine) and then Kocher–Langenbeck (prone) exposures during the same anesthetic session to treat his displaced associated both-column acetabular fracture. There was a large posterior wall component of the fracture. The posterior column screws were inserted using the initial ilioinguinal exposure and positioned carefully so as to not obstruct the subsequent posterior wall reduction from the posterior exposure. Because of the associated risk of ectopic bone with two exposures, oral indomethacin was used for 6 weeks after surgery.

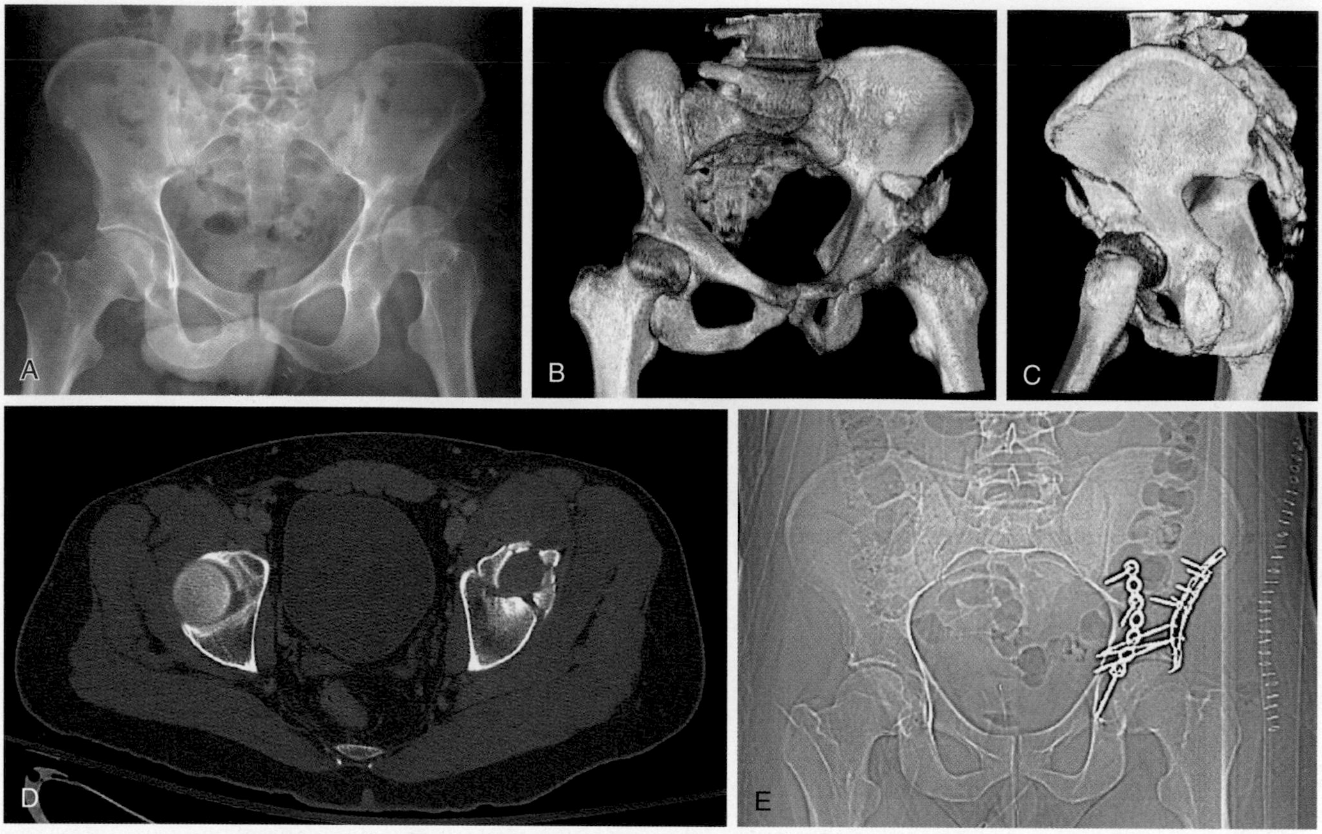

Figure 41-36. **A,** This patient sustained a variant pattern acetabular fracture with both anterior and posterior wall comminution involving the weight-bearing dome. **B** to **D,** The three-dimensional models and axial image further define the fracture details and comminution. **E,** The skin staples mark the anterior Smith-Petersen surgical exposure that was used to reduce and stabilize the fracture fragments. The fracture comminution and instability warranted the use of spring-hook plates to secure the peripheral fragments.

The patient is positioned and draped as for an ilioinguinal exposure. The skin incision measures approximately 15 to 20 cm and extends from the ASIS directed toward the lateral patella within the palpable interval between the tensor fascia lata and sartorius muscles. The ascending branches of the lateral femoral circumflex vessels are protected and preserved when possible. The rectus femoris muscle origin and common tendon may shroud the fracture area and require elevation or tenotomy. The iliopsoas muscle is retracted medially, and the gluteus medius and minimus muscles are retracted laterally as necessary to treat the fracture (Fig. 41-36). Subperiosteal elevation of the cortical surfaces of the intact bone and the fracture fragments are limited to areas needed for implant application to provide stable fracture fixation. Ectopic bone formation is associated with these injuries and this surgical exposure, so some form of prophylaxis is recommended.

MANIPULATIVE REDUCTION AND PERCUTANEOUS FIXATION

Some acetabular fractures may be amenable to percutaneous treatment, and some patients' overall medical condition demands it.[106-111] For these fractures, screws are inserted through small wounds across the fracture surfaces using aiming devices and intraoperative fluoroscopy or other imaging guidance systems.[112-114] This technique seems best suited for minimally displaced fractures that are unstable.[115,116] It may also have a role for medically unstable patients who cannot undergo more extensive operations or those with unsuitable soft tissues that prevent open procedures. Accurate fracture reduction without subluxation is required before percutaneous fixation. Intrapelvic clamps placed through minimal open approaches can be used to assist with reduction, but knowledge of anatomy is paramount because there is no direct visualization and protection of neurovascular structures nor is there cleaning of the fracture surfaces. A surgical field for a traditional open approach should be included because the surgeon must be prepared if there is failure to obtain an accurate reduction or other complications arise intraoperatively. The treating physician must also remember that fracture reduction quality is more important than screw insertion techniques. Malreductions should not be accepted only in order to use percutaneous fixation techniques.[117,118] Surgeon experience, patient selection, improved manipulative devices, and refined intraoperative imaging have allowed this technique to progress. Critical assessments of this technique and its true indications and complications are ongoing (Fig. 41-37).

EXPOSURE, REDUCTION, AND FIXATION BY FRACTURE PATTERN

Posterior Wall

Routine posterior wall fractures are reduced and stabilized using Kocher-Langenbeck exposures.[7,119,120] The displaced wall

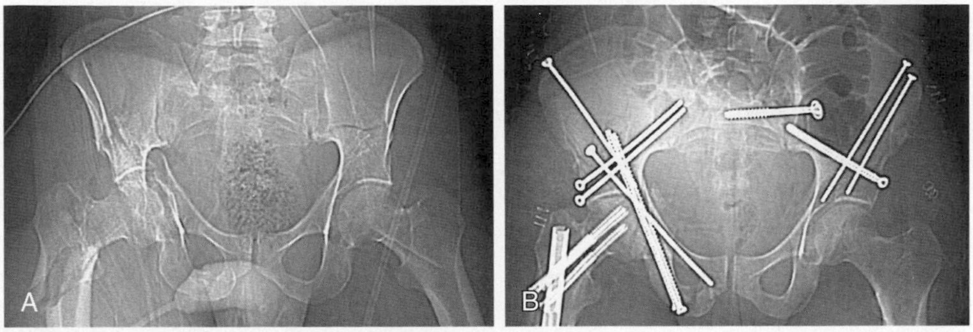

Figure 41-37. **A,** Percutaneous fixation after closed reduction was initially selected for this patient because of his overall medical condition. The femur fracture was stabilized first, and then 10 lb of distal femoral traction was applied bilaterally. The reduction was approved using a variety of intraoperative fluoroscopic images. **B,** All of the screws, except for the posterior column screws, were inserted with the patient positioned supine. The posterior column fixation screws were inserted with the patient positioned prone after the other fixation screws were initially inserted while the patient was supine.

fragment may contuse or stretch the sciatic nerve, may be impaled on the medial undersurface of the gluteus medius muscle, or may be extruded between the muscle intervals. Often the piriformis, obturator internus, and gemellus muscles are anteriorly located relative to the displaced posterior wall fragment. The necrotic portion of the gluteus minimus muscle located caudally relative to the SGNVB should be excised, preserving the neurovascular bundles.[121] The wall fragment edge and cancellous surface are cleansed of debris and hematoma, and then the fracture site is likewise prepared. The wall fragment often has a caudal labral remnant that can be used to manipulate the fragment somewhat or excised. This caudal labral remnant can obstruct the reduction if it becomes positioned between the femoral head and posterior wall fragment. The hip joint is distracted to remove bone fragments and chondral debris using either a bone hook on the greater trochanter or a hip distractor. The patient should be completely relaxed using anesthetic agents so the surgeon is not working against contracted muscles during the debris removal process. The bone hook must be positioned to avoid medial femoral circumflex vessel injury. If a hip distractor is needed, one pin is inserted into the proximal-lateral femur at the level of the lesser trochanter, and the supraacetabular pin is inserted caudal to the SGNVB near the greater sciatic notch in an area remote from anticipated fixation implants (Fig. 41-38). Before hip distraction, the surgeon must ensure that the sciatic nerve has been freed of any tethering tissues and is tension free. Hip distraction is limited to that amount needed to remove the known fragments from the joint. After the distraction is applied, the sciatic nerve is reinspected to ensure that it remains tension free. Knee flexion can relax the nerve but also stretches the rectus femoris muscle. In some patients with a tight rectus femoris muscle, knee flexion will either flex the hip or dislocate the femoral head into the posterior wall

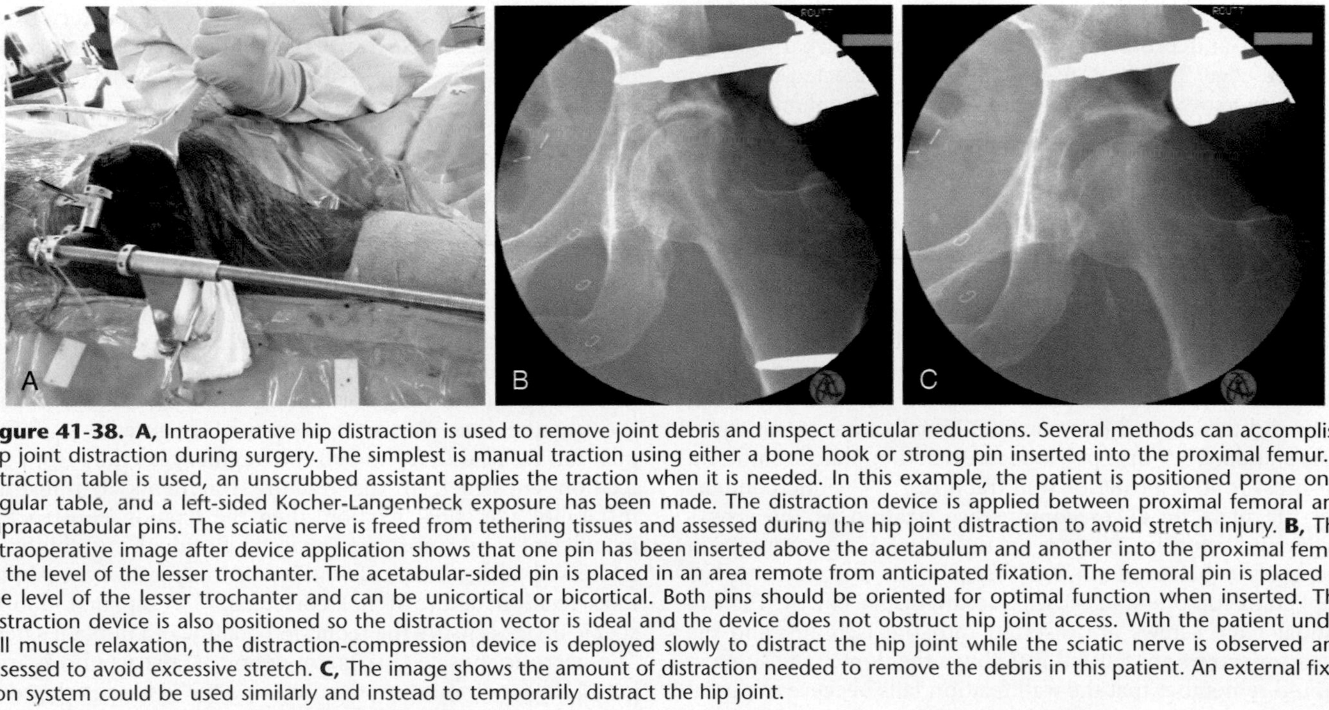

Figure 41-38. **A,** Intraoperative hip distraction is used to remove joint debris and inspect articular reductions. Several methods can accomplish hip joint distraction during surgery. The simplest is manual traction using either a bone hook or strong pin inserted into the proximal femur. If a traction table is used, an unscrubbed assistant applies the traction when it is needed. In this example, the patient is positioned prone on a regular table, and a left-sided Kocher-Langenbeck exposure has been made. The distraction device is applied between proximal femoral and supraacetabular pins. The sciatic nerve is freed from tethering tissues and assessed during the hip joint distraction to avoid stretch injury. **B,** The intraoperative image after device application shows that one pin has been inserted above the acetabulum and another into the proximal femur at the level of the lesser trochanter. The acetabular-sided pin is placed in an area remote from anticipated fixation. The femoral pin is placed at the level of the lesser trochanter and can be unicortical or bicortical. Both pins should be oriented for optimal function when inserted. The distraction device is also positioned so the distraction vector is ideal and the device does not obstruct hip joint access. With the patient under full muscle relaxation, the distraction-compression device is deployed slowly to distract the hip joint while the sciatic nerve is observed and assessed to avoid excessive stretch. **C,** The image shows the amount of distraction needed to remove the debris in this patient. An external fixation system could be used similarly and instead to temporarily distract the hip joint.

fracture defect. The distractor pins and device must be oriented to provide desired vector of longitudinal joint distraction. A blunt-tipped, long, curved vascular clamp is often useful to sweep the anterior joint region and deliver loose fragments from that area into the posterior aspects of the joint and wound for removal. The preoperative plan indicates the number, location, and size of the fragments that need to be removed from the joint. The fragments should be measured and quantified upon removal so the debris removal is known to be complete. Retracting the posterior wall fracture fragment improves visualization of the joint for debris removal as well. Large posterior wall fracture defects also improve joint visualization. The hip distraction is released after the debris has been removed from the joint. Ideally, fluoroscopy is used before debris removal to identify the fragments and then after removal to assure that all have been removed and that the joint is now congruent. After the femoral head is located beneath the dome, chondrocancellous impaction injuries are then elevated using the reduced femoral head and dome as templates. Next the loose chondrocancellous and other fragments that were previously removed from the joint or wound area are reduced to fit the cancellous defects and their chondral surfaces are matched with the femoral head articular surfaces. All of these fragments are supported with bone grafting into their related defects as needed. Narrow-diameter screws applied along the subchondral margin can be used to secure some of the larger chondrocancellous fragments. These screws should have their heads buried into the fragments so they are not prominent and obstruct reduction of the posterior wall fracture fragment. Bone grafting of the residual defects is recommended to support these small chondrocancellous fragments. The narrow-diameter screws should not be relied on solely to maintain their reduction.[15,32,122] Before reducing the wall fragment, the surgeon should mark the cranial and caudal articular limits of the joint to avoid inadvertent drilling into the joint during implant application (Fig. 41-39). After the wall is reduced, the upper and lower joint articular limits are not visible as they are when the wall is displaced. The wall fragment is reduced using the cortical edges to refine the reduction and protecting the sciatic nerve from the sharp fracture edge. The fracture is clamped or impacted and then held with extraarticular thin wires remote from planned plate application sites. Lag screws can be used individually or through the plate.[123] Unfortunately, the quadrilateral surface is not the sturdiest of bones, so these lag screws often have questionable fixation power and risk intraarticular penetration of the acetabular and femoral head chondral surfaces. A slightly undercontoured pelvic reconstruction plate is applied in a balanced location along the cortical surface of the wall fragment and secured above and below the joint with screws of appropriate length after predrilling and accurate depth assessment. A balanced plate is located between the labral edge and the cortical fracture line. Usually a seven- or eight-hole standard 3.5-mm pelvic reconstruction plate is sufficient for most routine posterior wall fractures.[124,125] Undercontouring the plate produces compressive fixation as the screws above and below the fracture are tightened. Plate compression demands a balanced implant because an unbalanced plate applied in compression causes fracture displacement. The two caudal plate screws are inserted into the ischium, and the superior screws are located just above the dome. The surgeon should remember that the wall fixation fails because of caudal

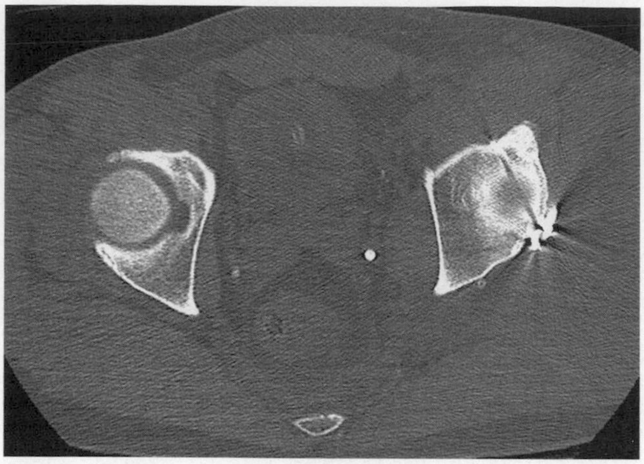

Figure 41-39. It is important to keep all of the operative instruments, including wires, drills, and screws, out of the joint. This patient had a posterior wall acetabular fracture treated operatively. During the plate application, a drill was used in the supraacetabular region without checking its relationship to the dome. The drill encountered more than expected resistance, but the surgeon persisted and did not check the drill's location relative to the dome. Intraoperative fluoroscopy identified a screw through the acetabular dome, and it was removed. A postoperative computed tomography scan shows the drill and screw path relative to the dome. Intraoperative fluoroscopy can be used to direct the drill and screw insertion away from the joint when necessary.

tension, so the lower screws must be securely fixated in the bone (Fig. 41-40). Similarly, if the plate is located too medially or not firmly applied, the wall fragment will displace from beneath the plate[82] (Fig. 41-41). Lag screw fixation alone is not recommended, so some form of plate fixation is needed for all posterior wall fractures. The plate function relies on its undersurface having intimate contact with the cortical surfaces of the posterior wall fracture fragment, as well as the intact bone above and below the fracture. To achieve such contact of plate and bone, the periosteum and soft tissues of the posterior wall fracture fragment's cortical surface are removed where the plate is to be applied. The plate's undersurface must uniformly contact the cortical bone to avoid fixation failures. The peripheral soft tissue attachments such as the capsule and labrum are preserved, but the more medial cortical bone at the site of plate application must be denuded for plate application (Fig. 41-42). For comminuted cortical fragments, two plates may be needed to support the overall reduction. Because the posterior column is narrowest caudally in the ischium at the lesser sciatic notch region, the initial plate must be located anticipating the second plate's location so they can both fit and not be stacked upon each other. The fixation construct is stressed by moving the hip through a full range of motion while directly observing the fracture line. For very peripheral fragments, a dental pick can be used to try to pull the fragment laterally from the fixation construct. If the fracture fragments demonstrate instability after final fixation, then the fixation construct is insufficient and must be revised. Residual instability is addressed immediately. Identified intraoperative instability risks fixation failure if not corrected.[126-128] Biplanar fluoroscopic images ensure the reduction quality and implant safety. The necrotic muscle tissues are débrided, the wound is irrigated, the tenotomies are repaired, and the wound is closed in

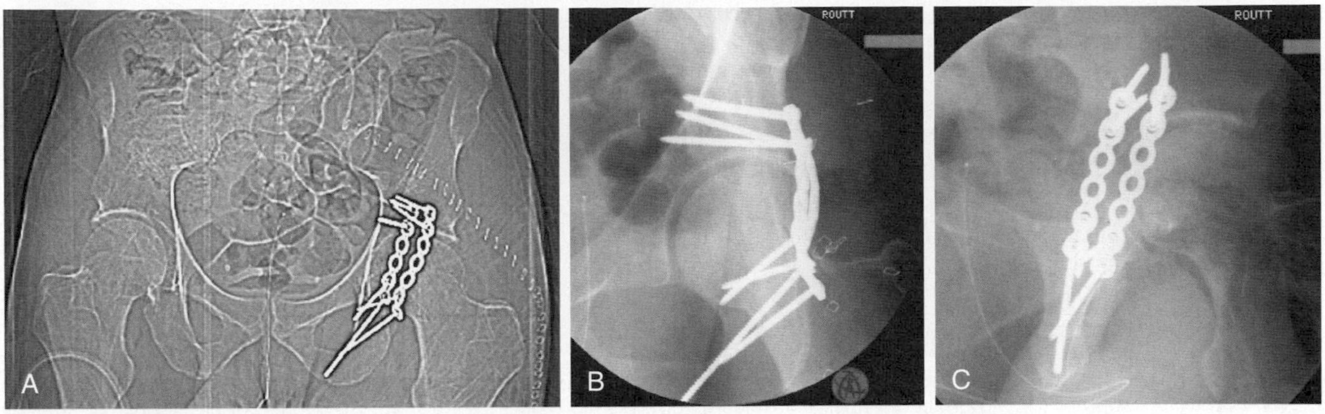

Figure 41-40. A, Posterior wall acetabular fractures are routinely stabilized with malleable pelvic reconstruction plates contoured to fit the cortical surfaces of the wall fracture fragments. The plates are located so they are equally balanced on the cortical surfaces of the fractures. This patient had a comminuted posterior wall fracture consisting of peripheral and medial fragments. Two plates were used to stabilize the fractures, and each plate was positioned in the middle of the dorsal cortical fracture surface. By locating the plate in a balanced manner between the fracture edges, uniform compression is applied as the screws are tightened. Lag screws through the plate are used to support the fragments when possible. During surgery, after fixation and before wound closure, intraoperative biplanar fluoroscopy is used to assess the reduction, assure the removal of all joint debris, and check the implant locations. **B** and **C,** The cranial plate screws are best noted to be out of the joint on the obturator oblique view, while the caudal plate screws are seen to be extraarticular on the iliac oblique image. The iliac oblique image also shows residual debris in the cranial and caudal capsular recesses.

layers. The traumatic capsular disruption can usually be repaired after the reduction and fixation and before layered wound closure.

Posterior Column

Posterior column acetabular fractures are reduced and stabilized using a Kocher-Langenbeck exposure with the patient positioned either lateral or prone. Prone positioning is preferred, and the dissection should allow digital access to the quadrilateral surface portion of the fracture via the greater sciatic notch. The sciatic and superior gluteal nerves are both at risk and therefore protected during the exposure, fracture manipulation for cleaning, reduction, and clamp application. The surgeon should first distract the primary fracture and anatomically reduce any chondrocancellous dome fracture fragments. The surgeon should include the peripheral fracture exit site through the posterior wall area to ensure that the torn posterior labrum is not obstructing the reduction. The

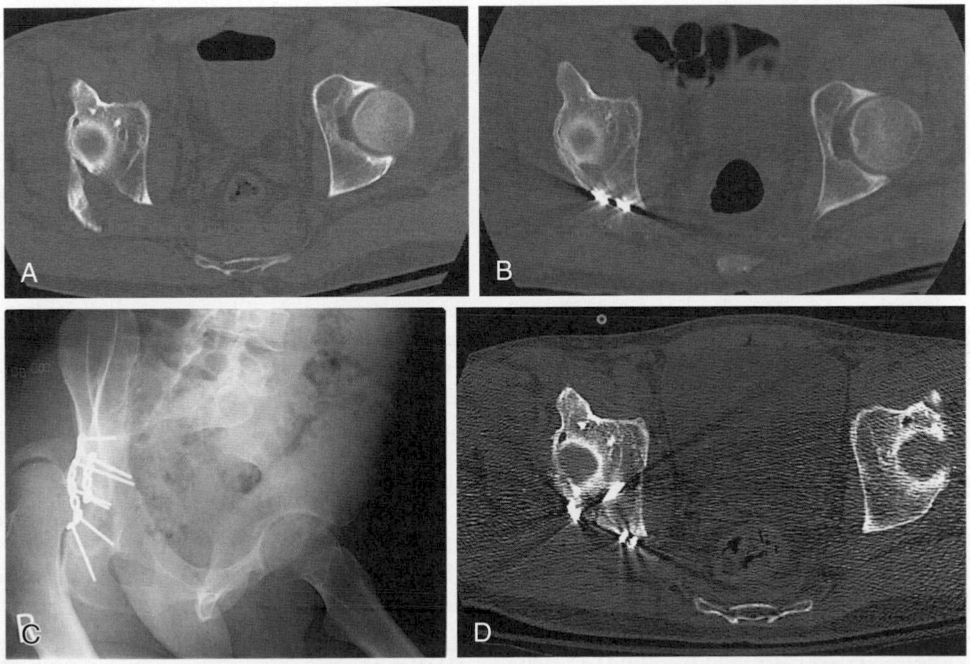

Figure 41-41. A and **B,** This posterior wall fracture-dislocation was treated operatively with an accurate reduction, but the plate was applied too medially and not in a balanced location along the wall fragment. **C,** Two weeks after surgery, the patient returned to clinic complaining of hip pain and limb deformity for 6 days. The wall fragment had displaced from beneath the misplaced plate, and the femoral head was dislocated. **D,** Reoperation included removal of the plate, open reduction of the femoral head and posterior wall fracture, and internal fixation with a more peripherally located and hence balanced plate.

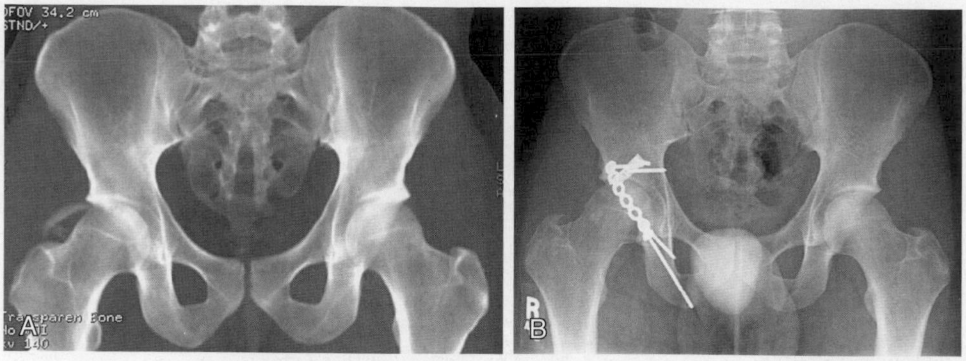

Figure 41-42. A, Even seemingly small and peripheral posterior wall acetabular fractures can be associated with hip instability. This patient underwent an examination of the hip under anesthesia and fluoroscopy. His hip dislocated with only 30 degrees of hip flexion. **B,** Stabilizing peripheral posterior wall fracture fragments while maintaining their labral and capsular attachments may require a spring-hook plate. The spring-hook plate is fashioned and then positioned so the tines hold the peripheral fracture in place without injuring the femoral head. The spring-hook plate alone is not sufficiently stable and is therefore reinforced with a pelvic reconstruction plate contoured to fit the wall fragment and accommodate the spring-hook plate.

posterior column fracture is then reduced with care taken to assure that the SGNVB is not in the fracture. The fracture is clamped through the greater sciatic notch according to the preoperative plan and based on the radiographic imaging. Half of the fracture reduction is visible in the surgical field from the posterior wall edge to the greater sciatic notch. The other half of the fracture is assessed by palpation through the greater sciatic notch. If the fracture reduction looks accurate along the visible fracture line but feels displaced along the quadrilateral surface, then it is not acceptable. The reduction must be improved, and the clamp should be oriented appropriately to maintain the reduction without harming the local soft tissues. Some surgeons use a reduction clamp anchored to the unstable fracture fragment and intact pelvis using two cortical screws. If applied properly, the clamp manipulates the unstable fragment and secures the reduction as the definitive implants are applied. It is important to locate the clamp remote from anticipated surgical implant sites and with extraarticular screws that are not inadvertently placed into the fracture plane or hip joint. The clamp should not cause tension on the sciatic nerve.

Lag screw fixation for a reduced posterior column fracture is usually difficult to accomplish safely because it is directed from the area of the greater sciatic notch anteriorly. This screw insertion requires significant medial retraction of the buttock tissues and sciatic nerve. A malleable pelvic reconstruction plate with or without lag screw is recommended for the posterior column fracture fixation, but remember that the screws into the caudal segment are important for stability (Fig. 41-43). Two plates are recommended for highly displaced and unstable fractures and for noncompliant patients. Lag screws can also be inserted percutaneously from the ischium to the pelvic brim.

Anterior Wall

Anterior wall acetabular fractures are exposed, cleaned, reduced, and stabilized using an ilioinguinal or Smith-Petersen exposure. In the ilioinguinal exposure, the middle (vascular) surgical interval reveals the fracture beneath the iliac vessels and iliopsoas tendon. The reduction is held with clamps or thin wires while the supporting plate fixation and lag screws are applied. The surgeon should take care when drilling and inserting screws using the middle surgical interval because the iliac vessels are medially located, the femoral nerve is laterally located, and the obturator neurovascular bundle is medial and deep to the joint. The surgeon should not plunge with the drill or depth gauge when aiming toward the obturator neurovascular bundle. A drill sleeve of sufficient length to protect the local soft tissues is recommended during drilling within this interval. The anterior wall has a limited cortical surface that makes fixation challenging. For some of these injuries, the Smith-Petersen exposure provides the optimal visualization for reduction and fixation. Fortunately, these are rare injuries.

Anterior Column

The ilioinguinal exposure is used for anterior column acetabular fractures, and commonly all three surgical intervals are recommended to sufficiently expose, clean, reduce, and stabilize the fracture. These fractures have several distinct planes as they divide the anterior wall, pelvic brim, and iliac crest. Understanding these fracture planes improves the exposure, visualization of the fracture surfaces, clamp applications, and fixation strategies. A manipulation pin in the iliac crest allows the surgeon to externally rotate the displaced fracture fragment to better clean the fracture surfaces. The pin can also be used to internally rotate and manipulate the fragment for subsequent reduction. Clamps are used at the anterior wall, pelvic brim, and iliac crest sites. Lag screws are applied along the pelvic brim into the superior ramus, posterior column, greater sciatic notch, posterior ilium, or iliac crest depending on the specific fracture details. Large-diameter (4.5 mm and greater) screws are recommended because smaller diameter screws can more easily fail in bending as the powerful hip abductor forces overpower them. A plate is used when necessary to support the lag screws, serve as a washer for the screws, and offset the deforming forces caused by the tensor muscle and hip abductors (Fig. 41-44).[129,130]

Transverse

Transverse acetabular fractures are difficult to group because of their variety. Patient factors such as obesity and fracture details such as impaction injuries dictate which exposure is selected.[131,132]

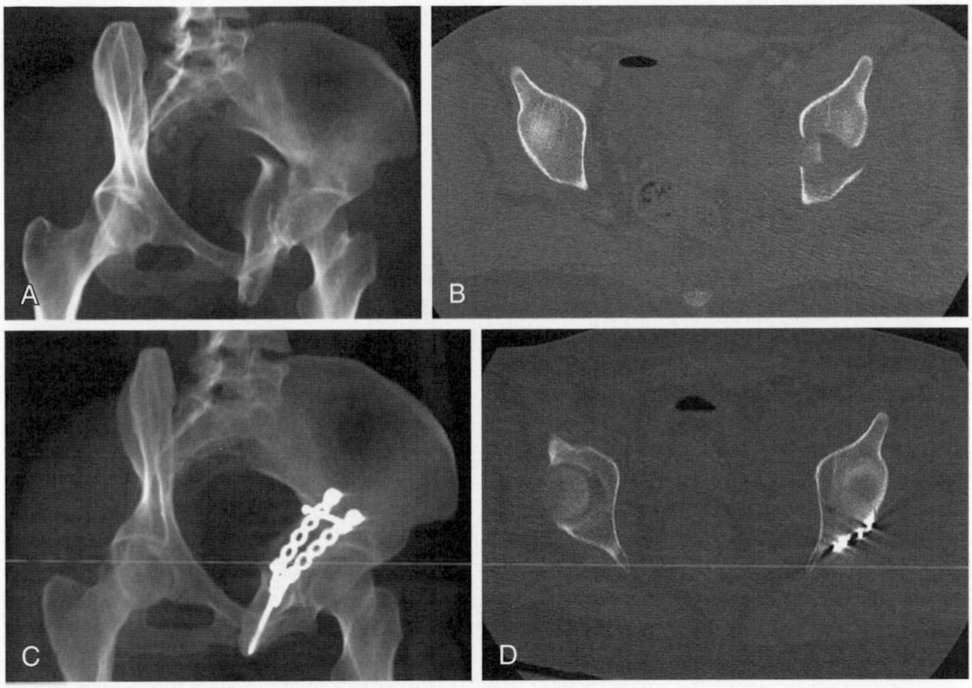

Figure 41-43. A, A displaced posterior column acetabular fracture is shown on this iliac oblique image. **B,** The injury computed tomography (CT) axial image reveals a large chondrocancellous dome fragment trapped between the primary fracture surfaces. A Kocher-Langenbeck exposure allowed distraction of the primary fracture initially, reduction of the dome fragment, and then reduction and fixation of the posterior column fracture. **C** and **D,** The postoperative iliac oblique and CT axial images demonstrate the reduction and fixation.

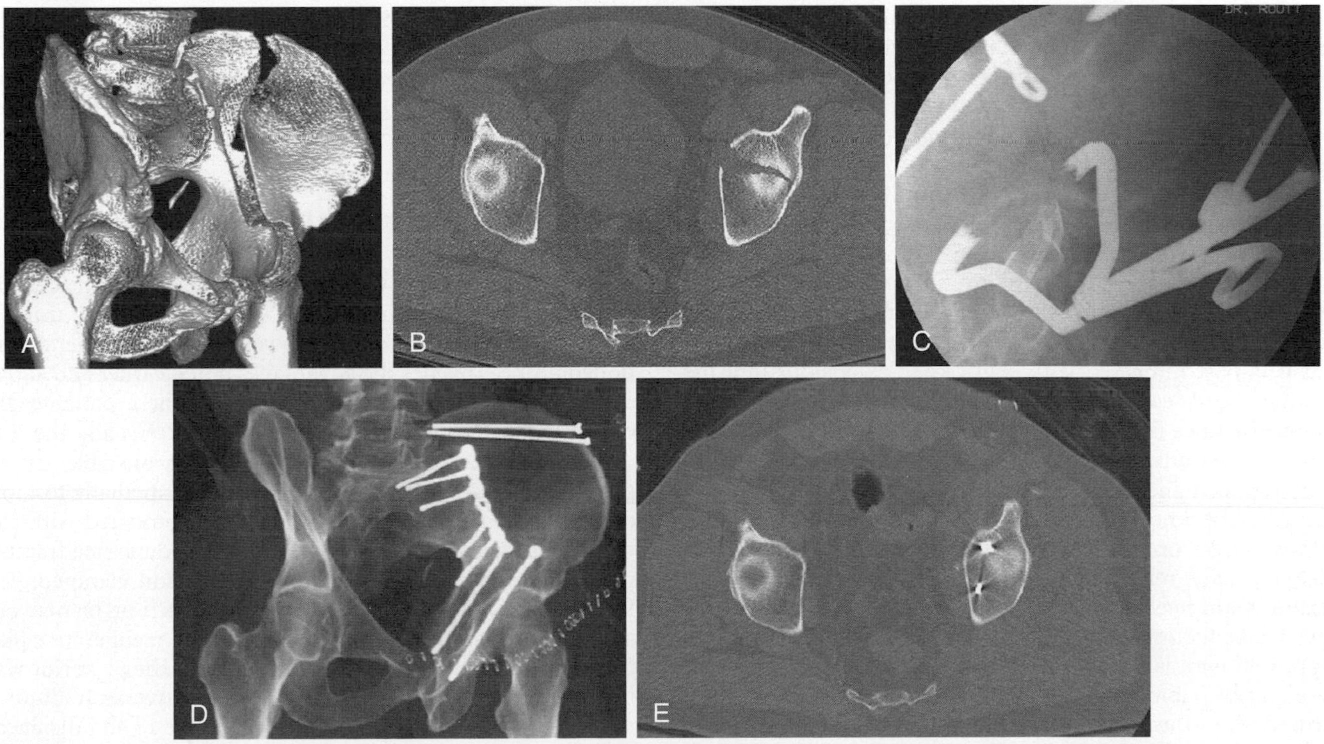

Figure 41-44. A, Displaced anterior column acetabular fractures are commonly treated operatively using an ilioinguinal exposure. The fracture surfaces are cleaned best using all three surgical intervals. The iliac oblique three-dimensional model shows the fracture surfaces. **B,** The pelvic computed tomography (CT) scan axial image at the dome level further reveals the fracture details that allow planning. **C,** The reduction clamp is applied via the intrapelvic interval onto the pelvic brim and the quadrilateral surface. The iliac oblique intraoperative image shows the clamp site and resultant reduction. **D,** The plate is located lateral to the sacroiliac joint along the pelvic brim and attached to the intact ilium with screws positioned between the cortical tables of the posterior ilium through the lateral surgical interval. Lag screws are then inserted toward the greater sciatic notch and ischium through the plate. The anterior wall fracture exit site is stabilized with a superior pubic ramus medullary screw. **E,** The postoperative CT image shows the reduction quality at the dome level.

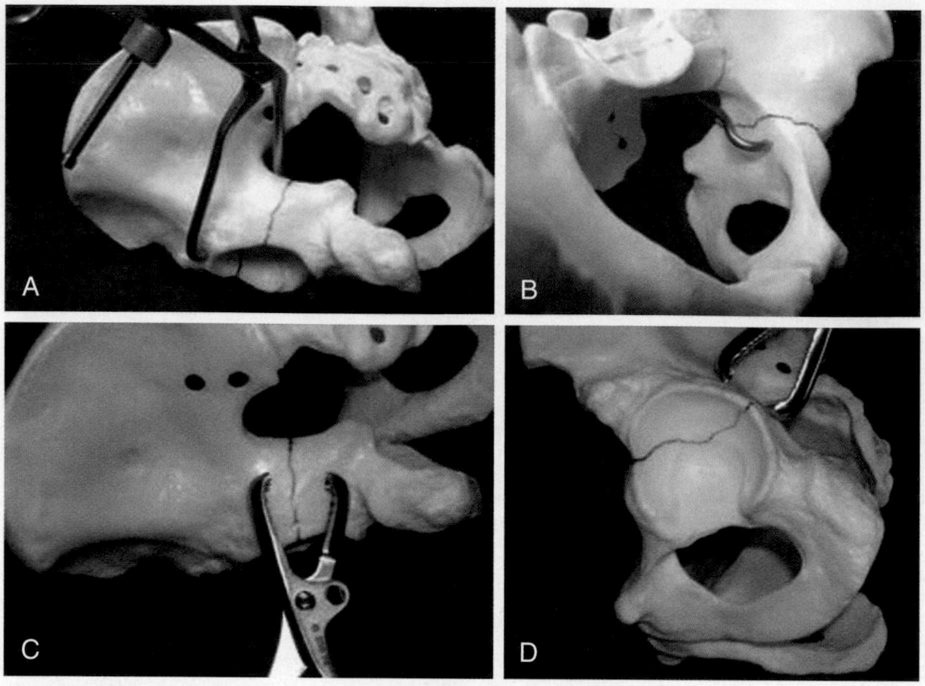

Figure 41-45. Various clamp applications are possible for transverse acetabular fractures. **A** and **B,** Using a Kocher-Langenbeck exposure with the patient positioned prone, the clamp can be positioned through the greater sciatic notch onto the quadrilateral surface, avoiding the sciatic and obturator nerves. **C** and **D,** A different reduction clamp that is applied dorsally using two independent screws is also shown. All clamps should be positioned to secure the reduction but not obstruct implant applications.

Many transverse acetabular fractures can be accurately reduced and stabilized using a Kocher-Langenbeck exposure with the patient positioned prone. The prone position eliminates the weight of the ipsilateral limb, causing unwanted displacement of the fracture, and facilitates dissection through the greater sciatic notch along the quadrilateral surface for fracture cleaning and clamp application. The prone position demands the hip to be in neutral position. In some patients, as the knee is flexed to relax the sciatic nerve, the rectus femoris muscle becomes taut and in certain fracture patterns causes the transverse fracture to further displace despite adequate pharmacologic muscle relaxation and traction. The surgeon must be alert to this potential problem and know that it is best remedied with slight knee extension until the femoral head easily reduces beneath the weight-bearing dome. The knee is supported in that position while the sciatic nerve is carefully retracted to allow the transverse fracture to be reduced and clamped. After it has been clamped satisfactorily, the knee can be flexed again to relax the nerve without effect on the reduction (Fig. 41-45). Sciatic neuroplasty usually releases the nerve sufficiently so that knee flexion is not needed.

After reduction and clamping, the transverse fracture is supported with lag screws from the supraacetabular area into the superior pubic ramus.[105,133] These screws are inserted either through the wound or more commonly percutaneously using fluoroscopic biplanar guidance. The transverse fracture is supported using a plate, the surgeon remembering that the caudal screws hold the unstable fracture along with the lag screw into the ramus (Fig. 41-46).

For some transverse patterns in certain patients, an ilioinguinal exposure is selected. The fracture is cleaned, reduced, clamped, and stabilized using lag screws, and a plate is applied along the anterior column. An intrapelvic plate is selected when medial displacement of the caudal fracture fragment is significant. The intrapelvic plate is anchored to the intact bone through the medial intrapelvic surgical interval just above the greater sciatic notch and to the unstable segment along the posterior superior aspect of the superior pubic ramus (Fig. 41-47).[134]

Transverse Fracture with Associated Posterior Wall Involvement

The transverse fracture with associated posterior wall acetabular involvement is usually reduced and stabilized using a Kocher-Langenbeck surgical exposure with the patient positioned prone. This has the advantages noted earlier and allows access to the displaced wall fracture. In these patients, the debris within the joint is removed initially. Usually the wall can be retracted superolaterally and the unstable caudal portion of the transverse fracture displaced medially to more easily remove intraarticular loose bodies compared with elementary posterior wall patterns. Then the transverse fracture plane is cleansed, manipulated, reduced, and clamped. The fracture surface access and cleaning, reduction maneuvers, and optimal clamp sites are all details of the preoperative plan based on the injury radiographs and scans. The posterior wall fracture fragment is displaced, so the transverse fracture is more difficult to accurately reduce because of the displaced wall defect. Similarly, a clamp using two independent screws to manipulate and hold the reduction is much more complicated to apply than simply clamping through the greater sciatic notch.

Just as with transverse patterns, knee flexion in these patients may also cause a tight rectus femoris muscle to displace the primary transverse fracture line and caudal fragment

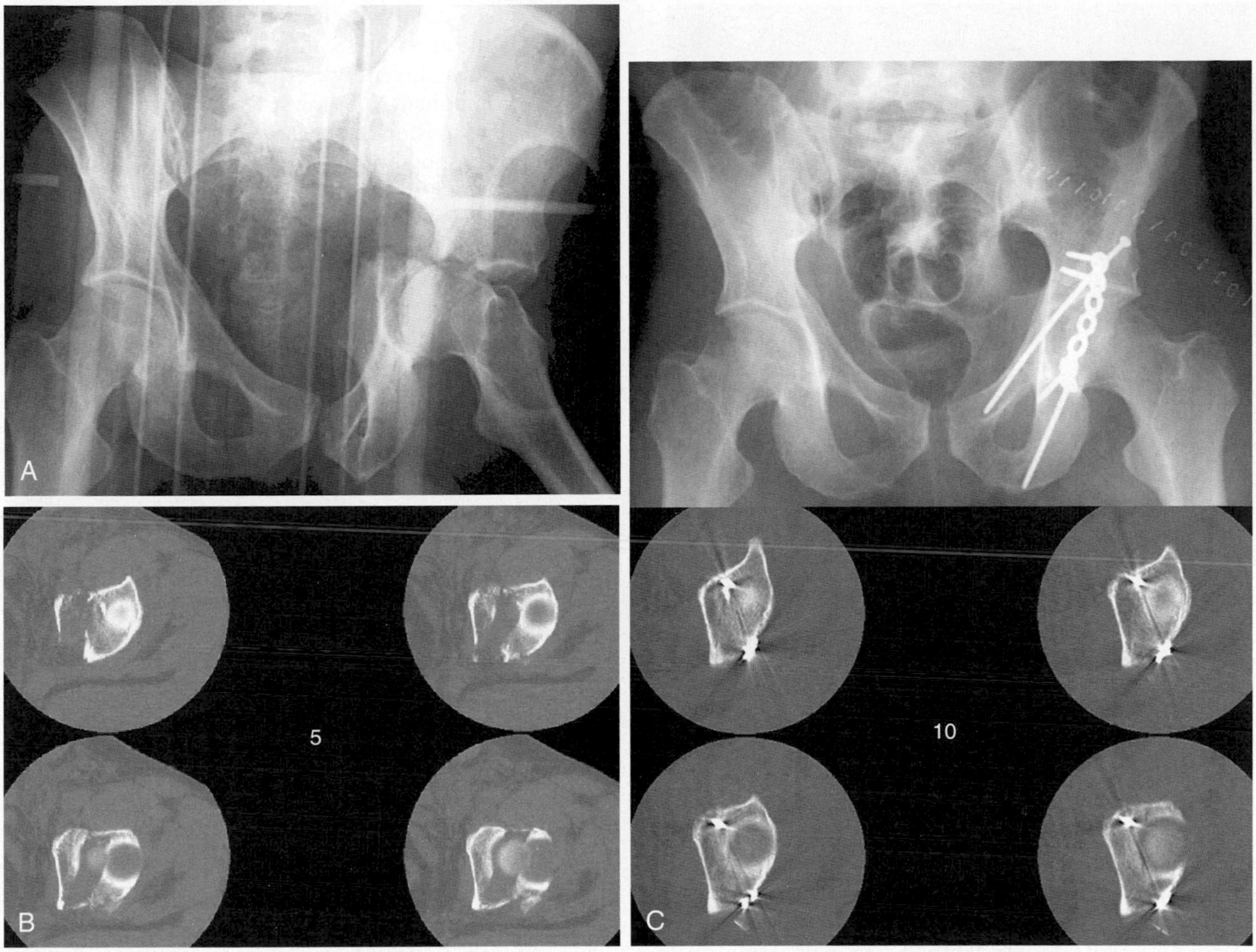

Figure 41-46. A and **B,** This displaced transverse acetabular fracture-dislocation was initially treated with manipulative reduction and skeletal traction. **C,** After the patient was medically cleared, open reduction was performed using a Kocher-Langenbeck exposure, and the fracture was clamped through the greater sciatic notch. The fluoroscopic inlet and obturator-outlet views were used to insert the medullary ramus screw through a separate stab incision, thereby securing the anterior column component of the transverse fracture initially. The plate further supports the fixation construct.

medially. The same remedy works for this pattern, and the transverse is reduced, clamped, and stabilized through its anterior column using a lag screw into the superior pubic ramus from the supraacetabular surface. With a displaced posterior wall associated fracture, the femoral head can now be distracted to visually assess the transverse plane reduction. This is not possible for elementary transverse patterns without a wall fracture. After the transverse fracture reduction is stabilized and approved, the wall fragment is cleansed; any impaction segments are elevated, reduced, and supported with bone graft; and the wall is reduced and held with thin wires or clamped. The surgeon should be aware that impaction fragments into the transverse fracture surface will also obstruct the transverse reduction.

If the wall fragment does not reduce perfectly, it is obstructed, usually by a malreduction of the transverse fracture, malreduction of the elevated impacted fragments, or too much graft material has been packed into the defects in supporting the impaction fragments. After it has been corrected and the reduction achieved, the wall and posterior column component of the transverse fracture line are stabilized using a contoured malleable pelvic reconstruction plate, just as described previously for posterior wall fracture patterns. Lag screws for the wall fracture are not needed if the reduction and plate application are excellent but can be applied through the plate or remote from it to further support the wall fracture if the surgeon chooses (Fig. 41-48). Two plates are recommended for highly unstable transverse fractures because a single malleable plate can deform in bending and torsion. Medullary screws inserted percutaneously can also be used to support the posterior column component from ischium to pelvic brim but will obstruct the subsequent plate screws needed for wall fixation.

Posterior Column Fracture with Associated Posterior Wall Involvement

Posterior column fractures with associated posterior wall involvement are treated using a Kocher-Langenbeck exposure with the patient positioned prone. The same details as noted earlier for the elementary posterior column pattern and elementary posterior wall pattern apply. Similar to the transverse fracture with associated posterior wall involvement, the posterior column reduction is complicated by the displaced wall defect at the time of posterior column reduction. Palpation through the greater sciatic notch along the quadrilateral surface cortical fracture line and intraoperative fluoroscopic

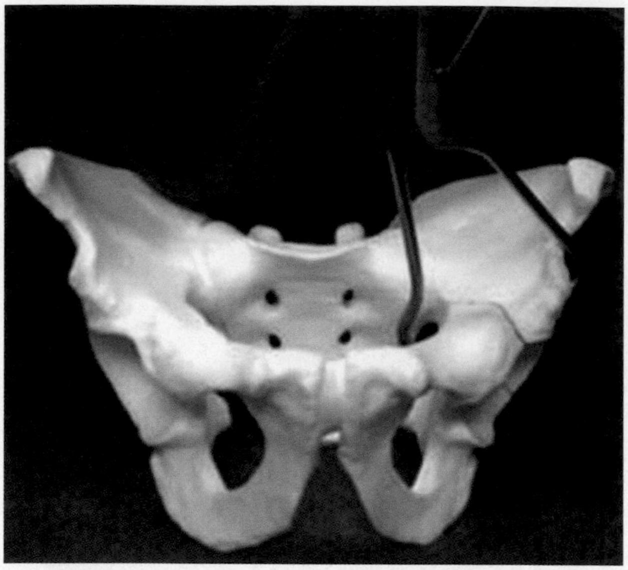

Figure 41-47. Clamp application for a transverse acetabular fracture using an ilioinguinal exposure. The clamp is applied to the quadrilateral surface through the middle surgical interval and lateral to the anterior inferior iliac spine. Anterior column medullary ramus screw(s) can be inserted using fluoroscopic imaging or under direct visualization. Interfragmentary screws from the internal iliac fossa into the ischium can also be used. It is difficult to apply plate fixation while the clamp is holding the reduction.

imaging are used to guarantee the reduction accuracy. The posterior column reduction is initially clamped, and then the wall fragment is reduced and clamped or held with thin wires. The fracture is stabilized usually with two supporting plates. Lag screws are applied as needed[135] (Fig. 41-49).

Anterior Column Fracture with Associated Posterior Hemitransverse Involvement

These fractures have a variety of appearances but can usually be reduced and fixed using an ilioinguinal exposure (e-Fig. 41-4). The anterior column component is reduced and stabilized initially with lag screws and plates (spanning from the intact ilium to the anterior column fracture fragment), but the surgeon is careful not to inadvertently place screws that obstruct the posterior hemitransverse fracture line. The posterior hemitransverse fracture is reduced using the middle vascular and medial intrapelvic surgical intervals, clamped, and then secured with screws inserted from the internal iliac fossa along the pelvic brim into the ischium. Biplanar fluoroscopy is recommended to guide insertion of these screws into the ischium and remote from the hip joint (Fig. 41-50).

T-Type

These fractures have many variables. When the anterior column fracture articular component is low and minimally displaced, a Kocher-Langenbeck exposure is selected to address the posterior column displaced fracture component.

When both fracture components are displaced and involve significant portions of the joint, an ilioinguinal exposure is used to reduce and stabilize them. Fixation implants are tailored to the fracture specifics and deformity pattern. Plates are positioned to buttress the bone fragments to avoid fixation failures.

In some patients, an initial supine ilioinguinal exposure addresses the anterior column component, and a subsequent prone Kocher-Langenbeck exposure is used for the posterior column component.[136] Some surgeons advocate simultaneous anterior and posterior surgical exposures, but the "floppy" lateral positioning limits the extent of each exposure, thereby potentially compromising the reduction, and gravity deforms the fracture (Fig. 41-51).

Associated Both-Column Fracture

Associated both-column acetabular fractures have numerous variables and details that determine the proper exposure or exposures necessary to achieve accurate reduction and stable fixation (e-Fig. 41-5). For fracture patterns in which the posterior column component is located in the upper portion of the greater sciatic notch, an ilioinguinal exposure is indicated. Typically, the anterior column fracture components are first reduced to the intact ilium. The dome articular anterior column fracture fragment may be incomplete at its iliac crest exit site and require local osteotomy to complete the fracture. This allows the fragment to be sufficiently mobilized for cleaning and reduction. Incomplete fractures cannot be accurately reduced without completing the fracture. When stabilizing the fracture components, the surgeon must be careful to locate the fixation screws so they do not obstruct the subsequent columnar fragment reduction.

The posterior column fracture surface is best seen either through the ilioinguinal's middle surgical interval or in some instances the medial intrapelvic interval. Using the medial intrapelvic interval, the posterior column fracture component can be manipulated using a spiked pusher while a clamp is applied to maintain the reduction. After the intruded posterior column fragment is reduced, the medial intrapelvic interval provides access to the intact ilium adjacent to and above the greater sciatic notch. This area of intact ilium is the site where an intrapelvic plate is securely attached when indicated. Rarely is this sturdy intact bone region involved in the fracture.

The posterior column fracture fragment is routinely reduced to the intact ilium and anterior column fracture together. Fixation is achieved using screws directed from the internal iliac fossa adjacent to the pelvic brim, posterior to the hip joint, and into the ischium. These screws anchor at both the intact ilium and anterior column fracture component, depending on the fracture details. Intraoperative fluoroscopy is used to ensure that these screws are located remote from the joint yet deep into the posterior column fracture fragment (e-Fig. 41-6). Abdominal obesity and the lower ribs occasionally interfere with aiming during the insertion of these screws. Plate fixation supports the reductions. Short-length plates support the interfragmentary screws and are easily contoured. Longer plates can span several fracture zones but are more difficult to accurately contour.

For certain associated both-column acetabular fracture patterns with low posterior column fracture planes or posterior wall components, other surgical exposures are selected. Sequential supine ilioinguinal followed by a subsequent prone Kocher-Langenbeck exposure may be indicated for such fractures.

The extended iliofemoral approach is selected for those patients with variant fracture patterns or delayed presentation.

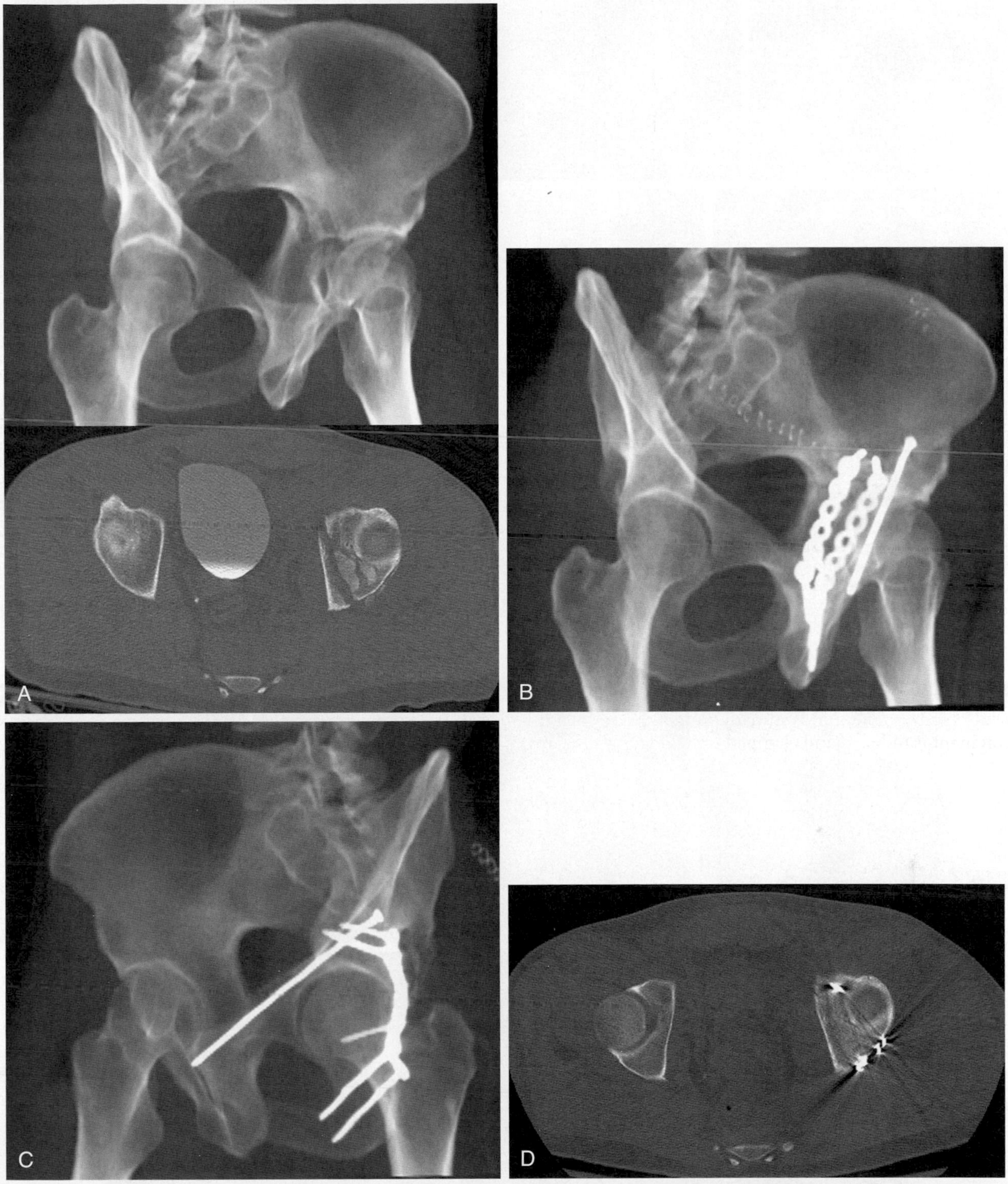

Figure 41-48. A, Patient with a transverse fracture with an associated posterior wall acetabular component with chondrocancellous impaction fractures along the fracture margin. The transverse fracture component is more displaced through the posterior than the anterior column. **B** to **D,** The Kocher-Langenbeck exposure was used with the patient positioned prone to reduce and stabilize the fracture. The debris was removed from the joint, the head was located beneath the dome, and the transverse fracture was reduced and stabilized with a medullary ramus screw. The impaction segments were then elevated to fit the femoral head and supported with greater trochanteric donor cancellous autograft. Then the wall fragment was reduced and the entire construct supported with plate fixation.

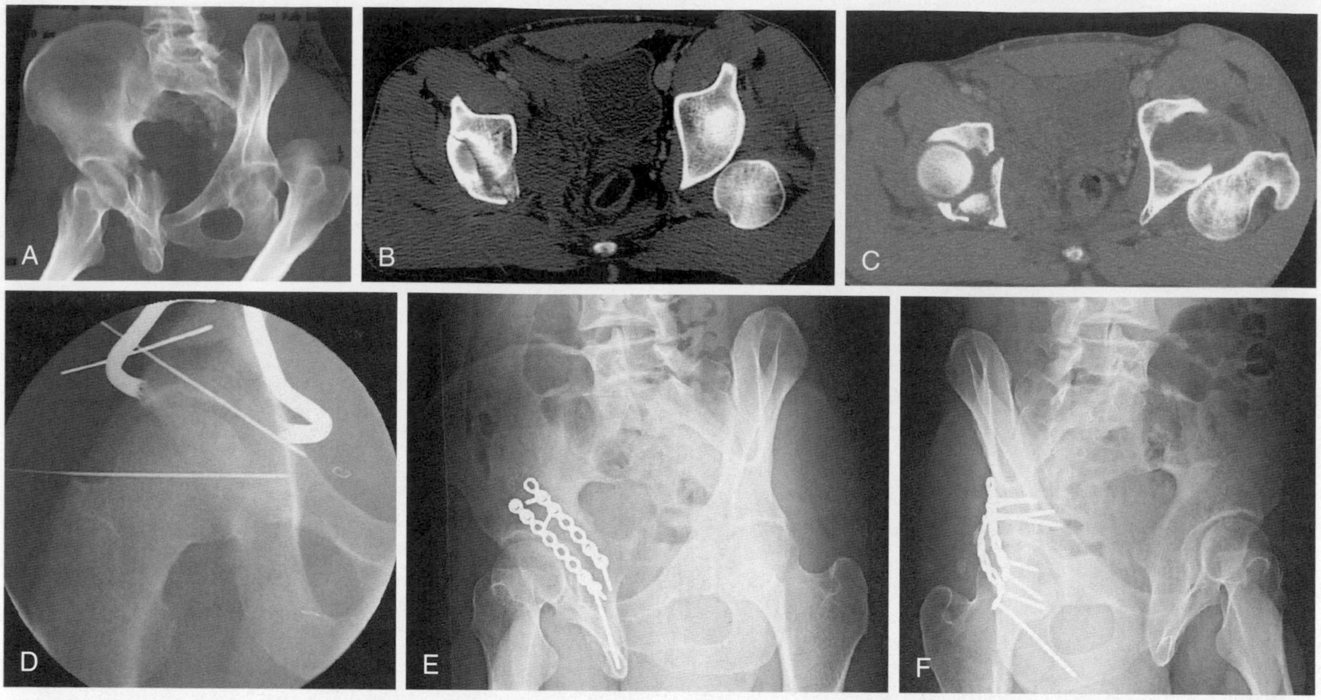

Figure 41-49. A to **C,** This patient had bilateral hip injuries after an automobile accident. The right-sided posterior column with associated posterior wall acetabular fracture is best noted on the iliac oblique and axial dome images. **D,** A Kocher-Langenbeck exposure was used. Initially, the posterior wall and posterior column fragments were further displaced so the intercalary chondrocancellous fragment could be reduced to the intact dome. Then the posterior column fragment was reduced and clamped, and finally the wall was reduced and held temporarily with thin diameter wires. **E** and **F,** The peripheral plate was contoured and located to support both the posterior wall and the posterior column fracture fragments. The medial plate stabilized the posterior column component.

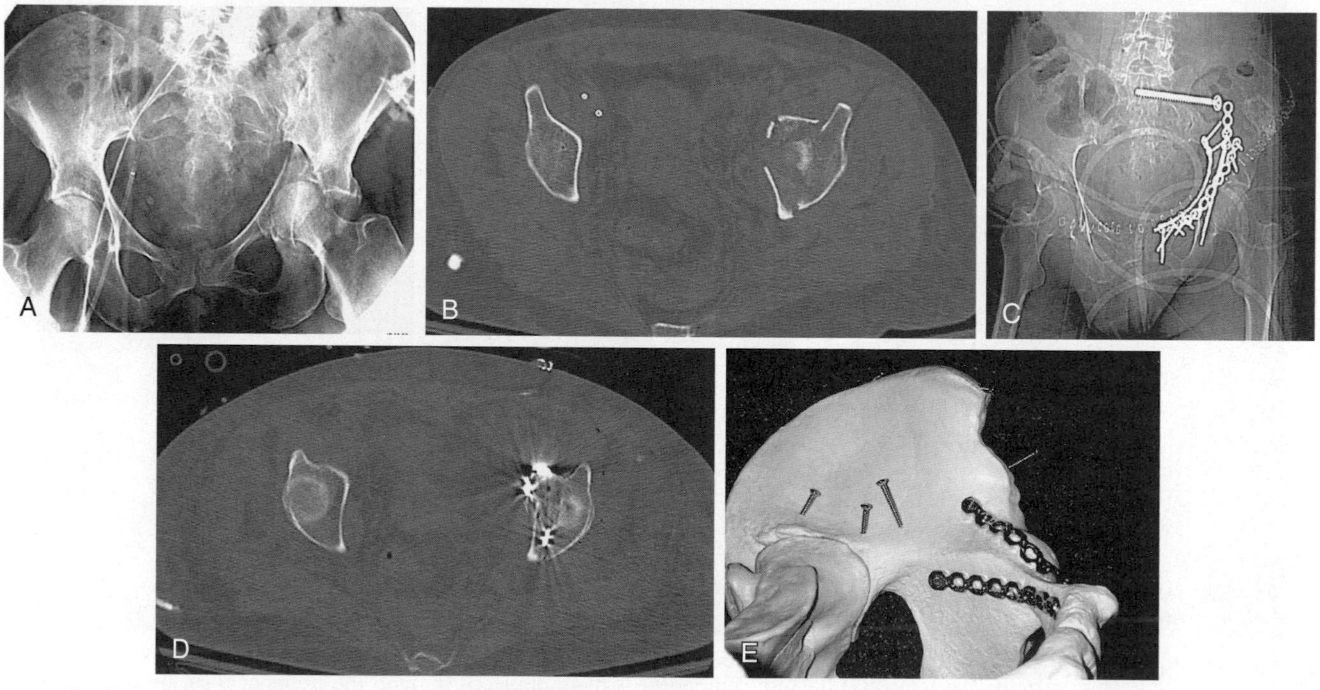

Figure 41-50. A, Buttressing plates and interfragmentary lag screws are effective implants used to stabilize acetabular fractures. This 68-year-old patient has a left acetabular fracture with medial displacement and a left sacral fracture. **B,** The axial image at the level of the dome shows the two major columnar fracture components and that the dome articular fragment is displaced from the other components as a chondrocancellous independent fragment. **C,** An ilioinguinal exposure was used to reduce and stabilize the fracture fragments. The dome fragment was reduced first through the two columnar fracture components, and then the columnar fracture fragments were reduced. A long intrapelvic plate was positioned to support both the anterior and posterior column fracture fragments and to decrease the risk of later medial displacement failure. A second long plate was applied to the anterior column to support that fracture fragment. A third short plate was used as a washer for interfragmentary lag screws inserted from the internal iliac fossa into the posterior column fracture fragment. An iliosacral screw was used to stabilize the sacral fracture. **D,** The postoperative computed tomography image indicates that the dome reduction is not completely accurate. Reduction of an independent dome fracture fragment is difficult using the ilioinguinal exposure but can be accomplished by further displacing the columnar fracture fragments initially. Buttressing plates are planned based on the injury images so the plate can be applied to the cortical fracture surfaces optimally and buttress the known displacement directions. **E,** Similar in location, the two buttressing plates are shown on the model. In our patient, the independent lag screw shown on the model directed toward the posterior column was inserted through a plate because of the poor cortical bone quality.

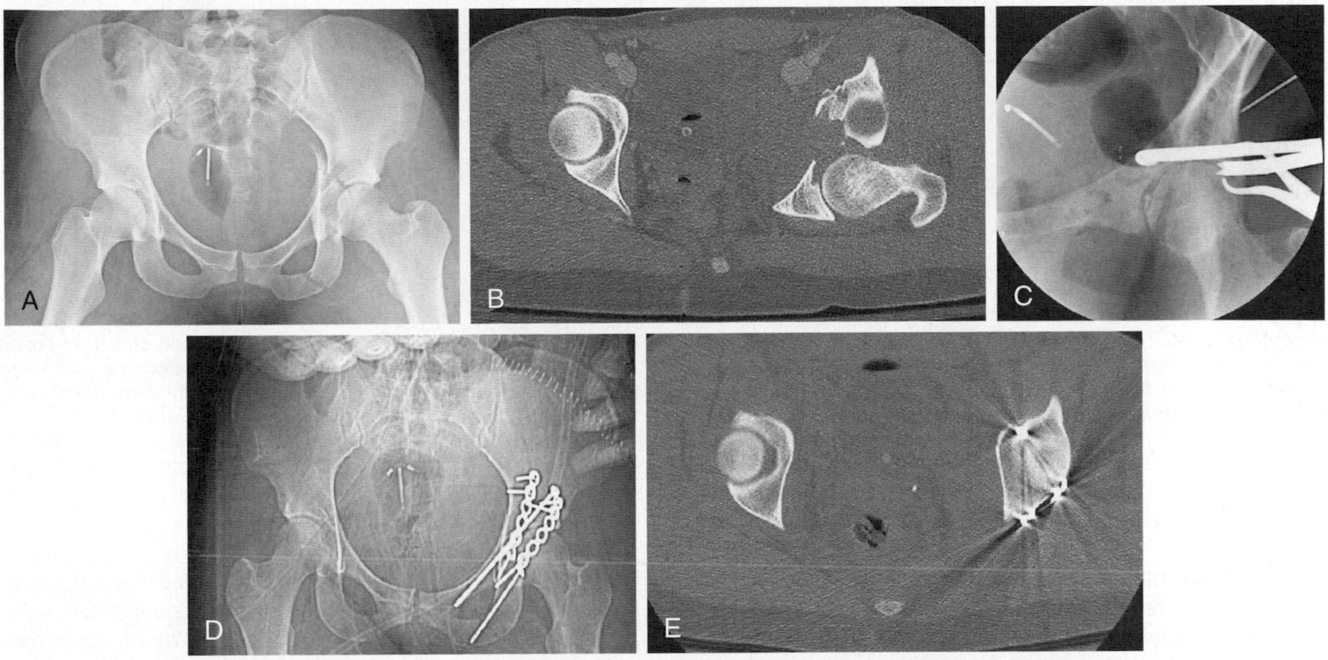

Figure 41-51. **A** and **B,** This displaced T-type acetabular fracture was treated using a Kocher-Langenbeck exposure with the patient positioned prone. **C,** The anterior column fracture was held with a clamp applied through the greater sciatic notch, and the posterior column was held with a tenaculum clamp positioned through unicortical drill holes. The intraoperative fluoroscopy image identified residual debris in the fossa acetabuli so the clamps were removed, the fracture fragments were displaced, and the debris was removed. Then the fracture was reduced and clamped again and stabilized. **D** and **E,** The anterior column fracture was held with a medullary screw, and the posterior column was stabilized with two plates.

Technical Note: Operative Management of a Transverse Fracture with Associated Posterior Wall Acetabular Component Using a Kocher-Langenbeck Exposure and the Patient Positioned Prone

After the exposure is completed, the fracture surfaces are cleansed of organizing hematoma and debris. With the patient relaxed, the hip joint can be distracted using either a bone hook placed at the greater trochanter or a distractor device applied through bone pins. If a distraction device is selected, one bone pin should be located above the joint yet adjacent to the greater sciatic notch remote from anticipated future fixation implants. The other pin is inserted into the femur at or just above the level of the lesser trochanter. The distraction device should be positioned so as not to obstruct wound access yet providing the needed joint visualization. The distraction should be applied carefully and without tension on the sciatic nerve. Ipsilateral knee flexion during the distraction process usually relaxes the nerve sufficiently but may be unnecessary if the sciatic neuroplasty is done appropriately. The amount and duration of distraction should be limited to that needed to remove loose bodies, clean the fracture surfaces, or assess the reduction. Distraction should never be sustained longer than several minutes unless reliable nerve monitoring is being used.

The dominant fracture surfaces are reduced after the joint debris is removed. The femoral head should be located beneath the stable weight-bearing dome fragment. The fracture fragments are maneuvered using a variety of techniques. A pointed dental pick or other similar device is useful for manipulating the fragments without disrupting their soft tissues excessively. Clamps or extraarticular wires temporarily stabilize the fracture until definitive lag screws or a contoured plate is applied. Impaction fractures are elevated and reduced using the femoral head articular surface as a mold. Elevation of marginal impaction fragments leaves a residual cancellous defect that is then filled with bone graft material to support the elevated osteochondral piece. Small volumes of cancellous autograft are available at the greater trochanter within the surgical exposure. The interval between the hip abductor muscular insertion and vastus lateralis muscular origin is exposed, and an elliptical corticotomy is predrilled and fashioned with a narrow osteotome. The corticotomy is sized according to the anticipated amount of graft material needed to pack the defect. The cancellous trochanteric donor bone graft is then packed into the acetabular juxtaarticular defect, preventing collapse of the elevated articular fragment.

After the primary fracture lines are reduced and the impaction fragments elevated and supported, the posterior wall fracture component is reduced and secured with wires. The temporary fixation wires should be located to maintain the reduction without interfering with subsequent definitive fixation. Wires are not used as definitive implants for acetabular fractures. Reports describe movement of acetabular wires primarily to the thorax.[122,137]

Malleable plates have the benefit of being easily contoured to fit the complex acetabular topography while maintaining stability when applied properly. For posterior wall fractures, the malleable plate must contact the cortical surface of the wall uniformly and be located in a balanced manner. Balancing the plate indicates that the implant is located equidistant between the labral edge and the cortical fracture line of the wall. The

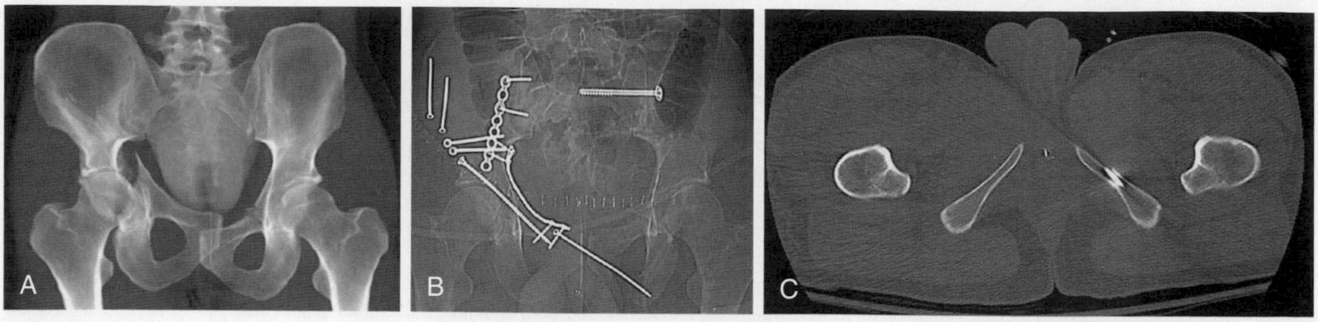

Figure 41-52. **A,** This patient sustained a complex acetabular fracture with associated pelvic ring disruption. **B,** The fixation construct consists of an antegrade medullary screw located within the anterior column acetabular osseus fixation pathway. The 4.5-mm-diameter cortical screw was inserted before the intrapelvic plate application because the medullary screw must be located within the anatomically demanding osseus pathway, while the plate screws can be aimed to dodge the medullary screw. The intrapelvic plate attaches to the stable ilium located cranial to the greater sciatic notch and then to the unstable fragment in the parasymphyseal area. Proper plate contouring is essential. **C,** The symphyseal injury was similarly stabilized using a transymphyseal screw positioned within the medullary space of the contralateral inferior pubic ramus pathway.

plate should be slightly undercontoured to provide compression as it is anchored above and below the fracture using extraarticular screws. The caudal plate fixation screws are directed deep into the ischium because they must resist tension failure, while the supraacetabular fixation screws are positioned just above the wall fracture line. Iliopsoas tendon irritation can result if the cranial plate screws are inserted too long.

Technical Note: Application of an Intrapelvic Plate to Support the Quadrilateral Surface Fracture Component

Intrapelvic plating is a demanding and detailed yet beneficial procedure.[134,138,139] The intrapelvic plate is applied using the medial intrapelvic interval of an ilioinguinal exposure and after the quadrilateral surface fracture component has been reduced and clamped. The technique requires that the iliac bone anterior to the SI joint and cranial to the greater sciatic notch be intact and stable because this is the attachment site for the implant (e-Fig. 41-7). The implant extends from this stable iliac area to the symphyseal region. A 9- or 10-hole 3.5-mm pelvic reconstruction plate is chosen for most adult patients and is slightly overcontoured to provide a buttressing effect after it has been applied. The implant can be contoured to a model pelvis preoperatively and sterilized during the procedure. The screws that attach the plate to the stable iliac bone are inserted obliquely simply because of the local soft tissue anatomy. For this reason, these two or three most proximal plate holes should be obliquely sculptured with a 3.5-mm drill to allow the eventual oblique screw insertions to occur without impinging on the plate and therefore being misdirected by the plate. The initial drill hole for the first screw is drilled in the perfect location for plate application before the implant is placed. This drill hole depth is measured, and several millimeters of additional length are added to accommodate the plate thickness. The plate is then placed, and the predrilled screw is inserted. As the initial oblique screw is tightened, the plate may rotate as the screw impinges on it; therefore, the plate should be held by a sturdy clamp to prevent this potentially dangerous plate movement. The plate flexion can be adjusted to fit the pelvic brim medially before the initial oblique screw is finally tightened into the stable iliac component. After the plate is adjusted, it is clamped to the parasymphyseal area. The implant's overcontouring produces compression along its contact with the quadrilateral surface, if well contoured and applied. Next the parasymphyseal screws are inserted after predrilling and accurate depth assessment. Another iliac area screw can be inserted at this point, and lag screw fixation is also used when needed through the plate (Fig. 41-52).

Technical Note: Acetabular Osseous Pathways for Screw Fixation

Pelvic osseous fixation pathways (POFPs) are predictable bony conduits throughout the pelvis that allow long fixation screw placement. These were initially noted and then popularized for the percutaneous treatment of pelvic ring disruptions. Four of these POFPs are useful and commonly used in the operative fixation of acetabular fractures.

Anterior Column Pathway. The superior ramus is a part of the anterior acetabular column. The acetabular osseous fixation pathway for the anterior column therefore extends from the symphysis pubis to the supraacetabular lateral iliac cortex and consists of the entire superior pubic ramus, anterior acetabular wall, and supraacetabular area. The critical limits of this potential fixation screw pathway include the superior pubic ramus, undulating surface of the anterior ramus, obturator neurovascular sulcus, pubic tubercle, and hip joint. The superior pubic ramus osteology is structurally and topographically complex. The superior pubic ramus radius of curvature is variable, and this fact makes straight implant (screw) insertion difficult, especially for patients with the most extreme curvatures. The superior pubic ramus' anterior surface anatomy is undulating because of the pubic tubercle, pectineus recess, IPE, and iliopsoas gutter. These "hills and valleys" are not apparent on routine intraoperative fluoroscopic imaging such that a medullary screw could possibly extrude from its cortical coverage without being obvious on the imaging. The posterior-medial superior pubic ramus cortical surface is flattened but also twists to an oblique orientation at the parasymphyseal region for most patients. The caudal cortical surface of the superior ramus is narrowed to a blunted apex and is recessed laterally by the obturator neurovascular sulcus. The acetabular dome subchondral bone is the peripheral caudal limit of this pathway, and just cranial to it is the iliopsoas tendon's cortical gutter. The superior pubic ramus cross-sectional anatomy is consequently variable depending on where any cut is made. At the parasymphyseal zone, it is elliptical; at the midramus medial to the IPE, it is triangular; at the eminence, it is circular; and at the iliopsoas gutter, it is ovoid and then triangular again in the anterior acetabular wall region. The cross-sectional anatomy assessment reveals that the cranial-posterior superior ramus cortical surfaces and therefore adjacent medullary space are consistent for imaging and implant insertion. The anterior acetabular column osseous pathway is narrowest between the iliopsoas gutter and obturator neurovascular sulcus.[16,17] Misplaced drills or screws in these two areas in particular are at risk of being extraosseous. The superior ramus is an arched structure so that there is a single point on the on the absolute concavity of the arch, similar to the vertex of a parabola, that is the cortical limit for any drill or screw. Where the surgeon chooses that point to be will therefore determine the screw insertion site, aim, eventual implant length, and overall safety.

Imaging of the superior pubic ramus OFP is confusing because of the superior ramus surface anatomy. Close inspection of this anatomy using a model alongside the imaging reveals the pectineus recess, iliopsoas gutter, and obturator neurovascular sulcus. By examining a pelvic model, it is obvious that a cranial-anterior located screw could be extraosseous but appear contained on the orthogonal imaging. It also becomes clear that the superior ramus curvature is variable. As a result, the safest region for insertion of a completely contained medullary screw is the cranial-posterior zone, and the imaging is then focused on that cranial-posterior ramus cortical edge.

The superior ramus is best imaged using two views: the pelvic inlet (PI) and combination obturator oblique–outlet (COOO) views. The C-arm fluoroscopy unit's tilt for an ideal PI image must be adjusted for each patient so that the superior pubic ramus' flattened posterior cortical surface is identifiable on tangent and viewed posterior relative to the inferior ramus. Superimposition of the superior and inferior ramus is not recommended to avoid confusion. Ramus separation on the PI imaging clarifies the anatomy. The PI view shows the anterior and posterior borders of the superior pubic ramus. The surgeon must be aware that the superior ramus' anterior cortical surface is visualized en face on this image; therefore, the posterior-cranial to anterior-caudal cortical slope must be understood so it can be "seen" on the image. For the COOO image, the C-arm unit tilt is adjusted so that the superior pubic ramus cranial cortical edge and acetabular dome have the maximum distance between them. Because of the ramus' anterior-caudal slope, the cranial-posterior edge and acetabular dome are the critical limits on the COOO image. The surgeon must also seek the image of the relatively radiolucent obturator neurovascular sulcus on the COOO.

Both antegrade (supraacetabular) and retrograde (pubic) insertion sites must accommodate the patient's pelvic osteology and body habitus. Genitalia, excessive thigh girth, and patient positioning are but a few of the confounding variables that negatively affect a retrograde insertion site. On the PI view, the insertion site for a retrograde screw is at the pubic tubercle zone but specifically depends on the planned screw length and aim. The COOO view helps the surgeon evaluate the cranial borders of the ramus as well as the proximity of any implant to the hip joint. The starting point for an antegrade screw on this view is 1 to 2 cm cranial to the acetabulum on the gluteus medius pillar.

It is very important for the surgeon to fully comprehend the superior pubic ramus cortical surface recesses for the iliopsoas and pectineus muscles and obturator neurovascular bundle. Orthogonal views of the anterior column and superior pubic ramus can give the false sense that there is bone in these areas when there actually is none. The ideal screw location is posterior on the PI view and cranial on the COOO image.

Antegrade screw insertions are accomplished percutaneously whether done along with a Kocher-Langenbeck exposure with the patient positioned prone or with an ilioinguinal exposure in a supine patient. Lateral positioning complicates imaging and is not recommended. For some thinner patients, the retrograde screw can be inserted via the ilioinguinal exposure. If a combination fixation construct using the anterior column medullary screw together with anterior column plating is planned, then the screw should be inserted before the plate is applied because the medullary screw demands the anatomy in order to be safe, and the plate screws can be oriented to dodge the medullary screw. We prefer stiff implants such as 4.5-mm cortical or 7-mm cannulated screws depending on the individual patient's osteology (Fig. 41-53).

Midpelvic Pathway: Anterior Inferior Iliac Spine to Posterior Ilium. The midpelvic/iliac OFP is located from the AIIS to the posterior ilium just above the greater sciatic notch and contained within the pelvic brim bone. The borders of the OFP are the concave inner and convex outer iliac cortical tables, the acetabular dome, the greater sciatic notch, and the SI joint. The medullary implants inserted within the pathway stabilize anterior column fracture fragments to the intact posterior ilium. Similar to the superior ramus medullary screw, the midpelvic pathway screw should be inserted before plates are applied because the plate screw insertions can dodge the midpelvic screw. The midpelvic screw may completely obstruct the insertion of a long posterior column pathway screw (see later discussion), so the preoperative planning must include this potential problem.

For the midpelvic OFP, four different images are used sequentially to ensure accurate screw insertion: the COOO, the combined obturator oblique–inlet (COOI), the iliac oblique (IO), and the OO views. The COOO view shows the medial, lateral, cranial, and caudal borders of the OFP and is used initially when establishing the appropriate starting point for an implant. On this COOO image, the midpelvic OFP is visualized parallel to its path and appears as a blunted triangle or "teardrop." Unfortunately for the surgeon, the required position of the C-arm unit for the COOO view obstructs access to the bone pathway. Therefore, the COOO image can be used to site the appropriate skin insertion site, but then the C-arm is repositioned to the COOI view. The COOI image guides the implant from the AIIS starting point between the iliac cortical tables into the posterior ilium lateral to the SI joint and medial to the lateral posterior iliac cortical surface. The IO view demonstrates the location of the greater sciatic notch and thereby directs cranial to caudal trajectory and reveals accurate depth assessment. The OO image is used to visualize the SI joint to ensure that the implant does not inadvertently proceed posteromedially beyond the ilium into the sacrum.

Iliac Crest Pathways. Iliac crest OFPs are superficial and extend along and within the iliac crest. The borders are defined by the inner and outer tables of the ilium, the iliac crest, and the unicortical bone of the iliac fossa. The iliac crest

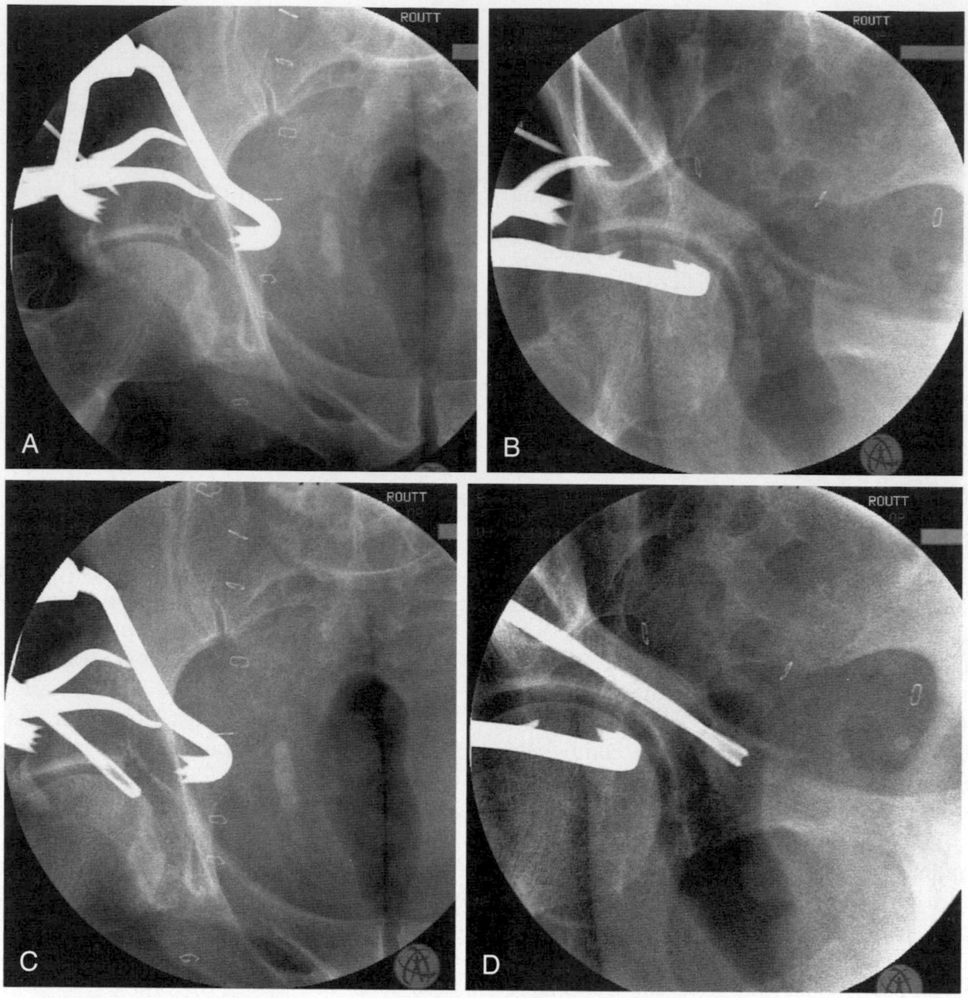

Figure 41-53. A to **I,** This patient has a displaced transverse with associated posterior wall acetabular fracture. A Kocher-Langenbeck exposure was used, and the transverse fracture was reduced and clamped first. A superior pubic ramus antegrade screw was inserted within the medullary pathway to stabilize the anterior column portion of the fracture. The superior ramus medullary osseous pathway is curved and has a variety of cortical surface orientations. The screw is straight and therefore must be precisely located in order to be safely contained within the curved osseous pathway. Sequential inlet and obturator oblique images are used to safely insert the screw. An initial thin-diameter wire is used to identify the optimal skin insertion site, screw trajectory, and bone insertion site. On the inlet image, the optimal osseous fixation pathway is just anterior relative to the flat and concave posterior cortical surface of the superior ramus. On the outlet image, the optimal osseous fixation pathway is just beneath the ramus' cranial cortical limit and just above the acetabular dome. The wire is slightly inserted into the bone. A skin incision is then made around the wire, and the cannulated drill is used to create a glide hole in the bone for the cortical lag screw. Next a calibrated small-diameter drill is used to prepare the medullary space for the screw in the caudal segment of the transverse fracture. The progress is halted when the cortical exit point is met by the oscillating drill point so an accurate depth can be determined. Another small diameter calibrated drill of equal length is then used to determine the pathway depth. The far cortex can be drilled if desired at this point. The cortical lag screw is then inserted and tightened. **J** and **K,** The posterior wall fracture can then be reduced and the stabilizing plates applied.

is curved from ASIS to posterior ilium and therefore has several component OFPs rather than one long pathway. The anterior iliac crest OFP extends from the ASIS to midcrest. The posterior iliac crest OFP includes the remaining crest posteriorly. The posterior iliac crest OFP is much narrower than the anterior one. This narrow area coupled with the crest curvature complicates screw insertion even when performed using an open surgical exposure. To avoid inadvertent posterior screw extrusion, the screw should be visible beneath the cortical bone of the internal iliac fossa. Because of the variable curvature, the imaging must be customized for the patient's crest osteology. An OO view with varying degrees of inlet and outlet tilt is used to define the inner and outer tables of the ilium while the iliac oblique view allows evaluation of implant length as well as cranial-caudal trajectory.

The iliac OFPs are used to stabilize the iliac crest exit sites of anterior column fractures, anterior column components of associated patterns, and osteotomies performed on incomplete anterior column fracture components. Screw insertion through the anterior iliac crest OFP can begin at the ASIS and be directed posteriorly or can be inserted at the midcrest and be directed toward the ASIS. If pointed reduction clamps are used, the surgeon must consider the depth of clamp tine intrusion because deep clamp tines can obstruct the crest screw. The surgeon must also consider the LFCN location and retraction when either inserting screws into or directing drills toward this region. We dissect the LFCN and protect it from injury during drilling, depth assessment, and screw insertion. We commonly use either 3.5- or 4.5-mm cortical screws and advocate an open technique to avoid injuring the LFCN. We

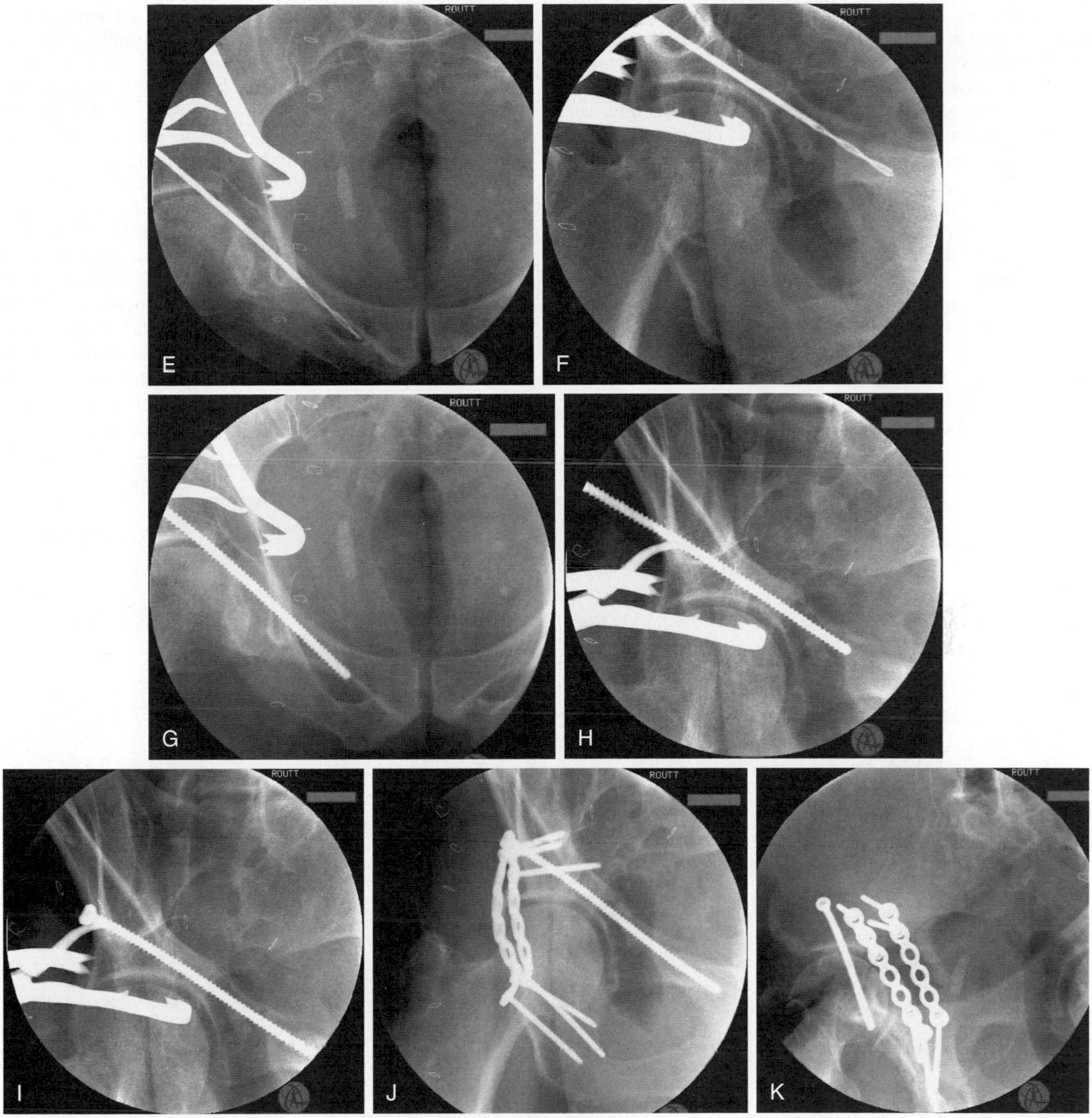

Figure 41-53, cont'd

insert the screw head slightly along the iliac crest to avoid prominence and symptoms related to the screw head after surgery. The screw can also be inserted from the midcrest and directed anteriorly to exit at the ASIS, but penetration by the drill or screw can injure the LFCN using this technique.

Posterior Acetabular Column Pathway. The posterior acetabular column OFP extends from the internal iliac fossa at the pelvic brim to the ischial tuberosity. The borders are defined by the ischium, quadrilateral surface, acetabulum, and internal iliac fossa and pelvic brim. Similar to the superior pubic ramus' surface contours, the cortical topography of this OFP are undulating because of the posterior acetabular wall. As a result, this OFP is located posteromedial to the acetabulum but, more important, just lateral relative to the quadrilateral surface. The posterior acetabular column OFP is best imaged using three views: the IO, pelvic outlet (PO), and lateral sacral (LS) views. The IO image reveals the greater and lesser sciatic notches and the acetabulum. The PO view shows the quadrilateral surface tangentially similar to the ilioischial line on an AP view. The PO view is preferred to the AP view because the C-arm unit position for the PO image does not obstruct screw insertion as it does when positioned for an AP view. If the surgeon prefers, the AP image can be used instead to more purely image the quadrilateral surface, but the C-arm unit must be positioned slightly toward the midline to allow the surgeon enough working room. The LS image demonstrates the pelvic brim and is used when the screw insertion begins at the ischium as for percutaneous treatment. In this application, the LS image reveals the pelvic brim so the accurate screw length can be verified. On the PO view, the optimal OFP is located just lateral to the ilioischial line. The IO view guides anterior to posterior implant trajectory within the posterior acetabular column and verifies that the hip joint is spared.

The posterior acetabular column OFP is used for fixation of acetabular fractures involving the posterior column and is most commonly accessed via the iliac window of the ilioinguinal approach. For maximal length, screws are inserted lateral to the pelvic brim and directed posterior relative to the acetabulum. In obese patients, the abdomen obstructs the drill aiming. Similarly for more senior patients, their caudal ribs interfere with directional aiming. We typically use 3.5- and 4.5-mm cortical screws, which, depending on the fracture pattern and overall fixation construct, can be incorporated into a pelvic reconstruction plate or used independently. As mentioned previously, a midpelvic OFP usually obstructs a posterior acetabular column OFP screw.

For select indications, minimally invasive retrograde screw insertion through the ischial tuberosity is also possible, although the thick hamstring muscle origin shrouds this insertional ischial region, making the percutaneous technique cumbersome. Patients can be positioned supine, lateral, or prone, but prone positioning is simplest. Regardless of positioning, slight hip flexion is important to best reveal the ischial tuberosity. A cannulated screw technique is helpful because finding the starting hole in the ischium can be difficult. It is important to obtain a length measurement before penetrating pelvic brim cortex because after this is done, all tactile feedback is lost and accurate length assessment compromised. The LS image helps to avoid pelvic brim penetration. Depending on patient anatomy, 4.5- or 7.0-mm cannulated screws are used (Fig. 41-54).

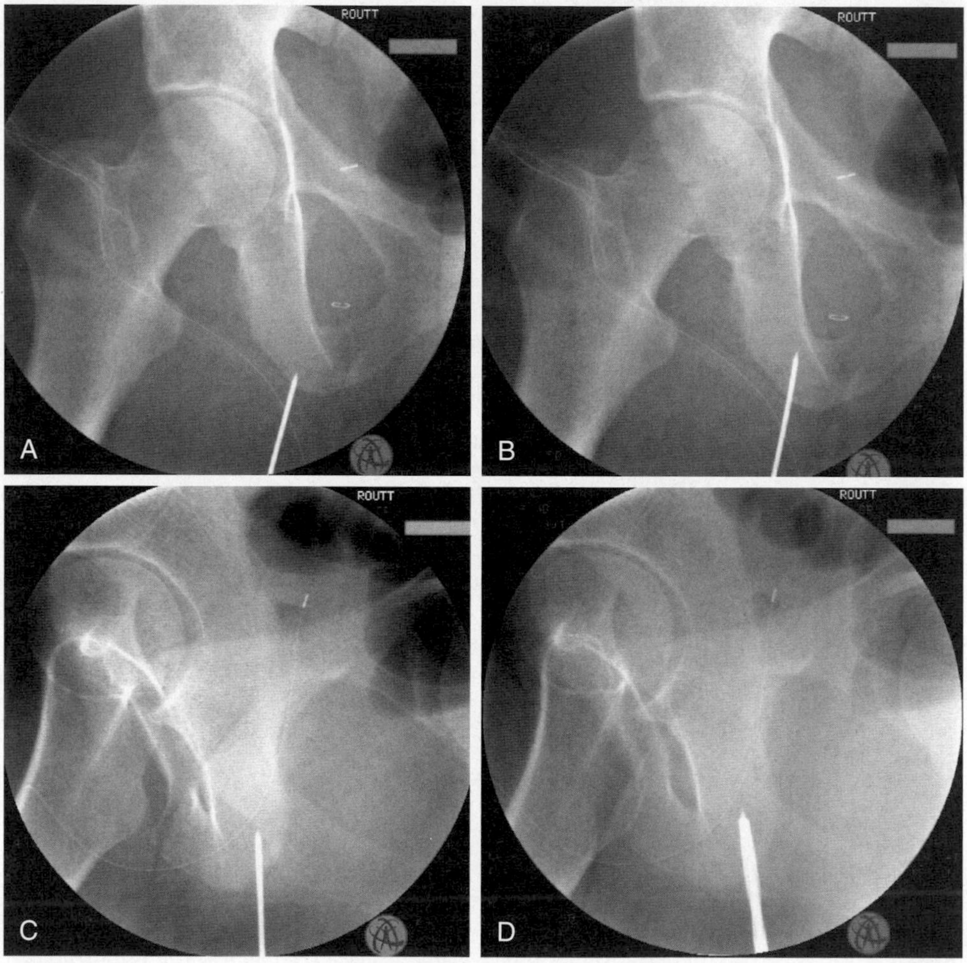

Figure 41-54. **A** to **C,** This patient underwent percutaneous treatment of his right acetabular fracture. He was positioned prone, and the buttock region was carefully prepped and draped after the anus was isolated from the surgical field using barrier drapes. Three images were used to insert the posterior column pathway medullary screw. The anterior-posterior (AP) view demonstrated the ilioischial line, the iliac oblique showed the hip joint and sciatic notches, and the true lateral showed the pelvic brim. A thin wire was adjusted to obtain the optimal ischial starting point and was inserted using an oscillating technique. **D** to **H,** A skin incision was made, and the cannulated drill was used to prepare the pathway. Using the iliac oblique image, the drill was directed between the hip joint and sciatic notches. The AP view was used to keep the drill just lateral to the ilioischial line. The lateral image was used to ensure that the drill did not penetrate the pelvic brim. **I,** The guide pin was then reinserted through the cannulated drill and impacted until it contacted the cortical bone of the pelvic brim. **J,** Another guide pin was used to determine the medullary pathway depth. **K** to **M,** The cannulated lag screw was inserted. Multiple images were obtained to ensure that the screw head was well approximated to the ischial cortical bone without intruding nor being prominent. The guide pin was removed and the wound was closed.

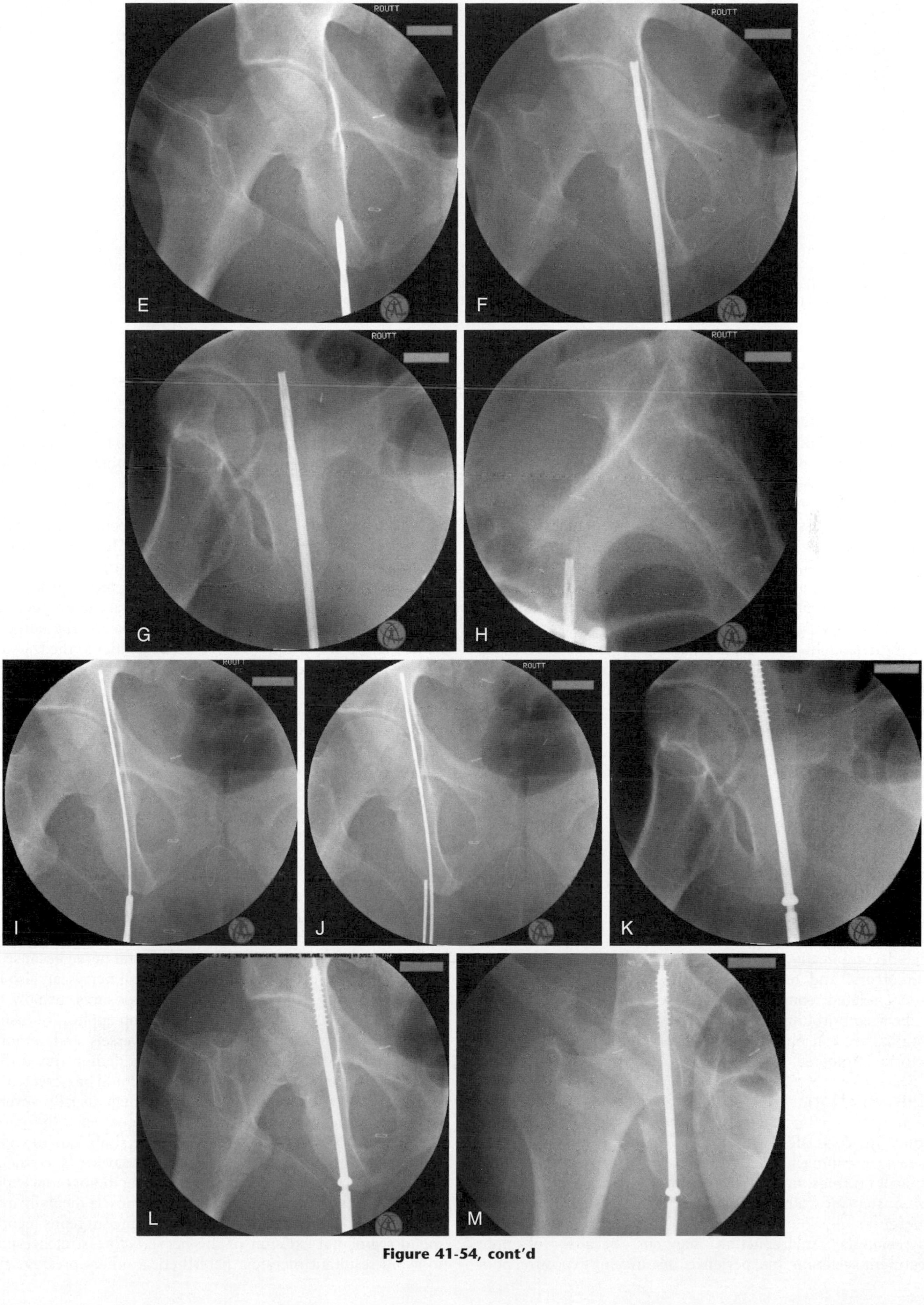

Figure 41-54, cont'd

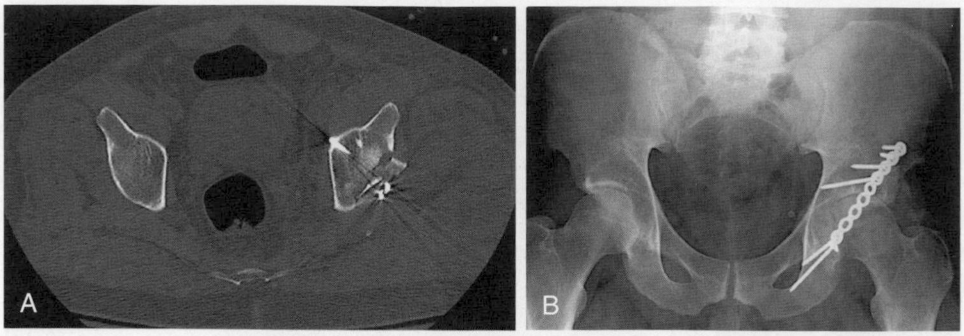

Figure 41-55. Comminuted posterior wall acetabular fractures are elementary patterns but certainly not simple to reduce accurately. **A,** This young adult patient had his acetabular repair performed by an inexperienced surgeon. The postoperative computed tomography scan axial image identifies a poor reduction of the posterior wall acetabular fracture, but it was not revised. **B,** Six months after surgery, the patient had a stiff and painful hip joint, and arthritic changes were noted on his plain pelvic anterior-posterior radiograph.

AFTERCARE

Rehabilitation after acetabular fracture depends on the injury details, patient condition, and selected treatment[140-142] (e-Fig. 41-8). A licensed physical therapist helps guide the prescribed rehabilitation program that is designed to not only restore hip range of motion and strength but also improve coordination and overall fitness. For the initial 6 weeks after injury, protected weight bearing using assistive devices such as crutches or a walker is indicated. Isometric exercises are used to maintain muscle strength. Passive range of motion exercises or devices usually provide patient comfort and may improve acetabular cartilage healing.[143,144] Progressive partial weight bearing and light resistance exercises are instituted 6 weeks after injury with the goal of independent ambulation 3 months after injury. After 3 months, most patients discontinue using ambulation assistance devices and increase their strengthening and conditioning programs accordingly.[145] Some patients, such as those with contralateral lower extremity injuries, are not able to ambulate because of their associated injuries. Rehabilitation programs are tailored to meet each patient's individual needs.

COMPLICATIONS

Complications related to acetabular fractures and their treatments are certainly not uncommon.[89,146,147] Surgeon-related complications include patient selection errors, decision errors, and technical mistakes, among others.[125,148-155] Patient-related complications often stem from associated medical comorbidities, other primary system injuries, noncompliance, and obesity.[156-159] Certain problems have multifactorial etiologies.[61,160-170]

Malreduction

In numerous clinical series, inaccurate acetabular fracture reduction correlates with poorer clinical results.[60,127,171-184] Cadaveric biomechanical studies have substantiated these clinical findings in that even 2 mm or more of articular dome step-off caused significant articular peak pressure differences.

Acetabular malreduction happens because of poor treatment selection, inexperience, insufficient exposure, poor fracture surface cleaning, misaligned clamp or implant application, delayed surgery, comminution, obesity, age, insufficient fixation, and other factors. Regardless of the reason, acetabular malreduction is directly related to hip degeneration (Fig. 41-55). Other than situations of significant impaction and comminution, malreduction should be avoidable. Simple solutions include developing a sufficient exposure, mobilizing and cleaning each fracture surface, and being patient with the reduction maneuvers and sequence. Inaccurate initial reductions are not acceptable, and the surgeon must take the time to correct such errors during the initial procedure. Intraoperative fluoroscopy confirms obvious malreductions but also identifies more subtle misalignments. The surgeon should adjust the C-arm beam to be tangential to the fracture surfaces to best assess the reduction quality. Oblique imaging of the fracture planes will not reveal gap and step displacements as well as adjusted images that are tangential to the fracture surfaces.

Nerve Injury

Several nerves surround the acetabulum and can be injured because of the acetabular fracture fragments' displacement or operative management. Anteriorly, the femoral, lateral femoral cutaneous, and ilioinguinal nerves are most at risk. The femoral nerve courses along with the iliopsoas muscle through the false pelvis and travels beneath the inguinal ligament as it enters the thigh bordered medially by the IPF. Certain acetabular fracture patterns involve the peripheral pubic ramus area and can injure the femoral nerve because of their anterior displacements.[185] The femoral nerve can also be damaged during ilioinguinal surgical exposures, usually by sustained or vigorous retraction and clamp application using the middle interval between the iliac vessels and femoral nerve. One study of femoral nerve injury demonstrated that good functional motor–sensory recovery could be expected.[186]

The LFCN pierces the inguinal ligament usually several millimeters medial to the ASIS. In some patients, the nerve is situated more medially. One anatomic study documented this variant location in 25% of the cadaveric specimens. This cutaneous nerve can be injured during ilioinguinal exposures. Routine retraction of the iliopsoas muscle medially may cause excessive stretching of the nerve. Some surgeons recommend segmental excision of the nerve before stretch injury to avoid resultant meralgia paresthetica; others preserve the

LFCN. The patient should be informed preoperatively about the LFCN and the potential for dysesthesias or numbness after surgery.

During the inguinal dissection of the ilioinguinal exposure, the ilioinguinal nerve is exposed as the deep fascia is incised. This nerve is at most risk during this portion of the exposure and then again at closure of the same fascia. The nerve is often adherent to the undersurface of the anterior abdominal fascia and should be freed from it before closure. This process avoids inadvertent suturing of the nerve during the fascial closure.

The obturator nerve travels deep within the pelvis located only a few millimeters medial to the quadrilateral surface. Displaced fractures through this zone injure the obturator nerve. It is difficult to examine the obturator nerve motor function in patients with acetabular fractures because hip adduction is painful, but the sensory evaluation of the medial thigh should be performed and noted, especially preoperatively. During ilioinguinal exposures using the medial intrapelvic interval, retraction of the obturator neurovascular bundle may be necessary to visualize, clean, and reduce the posterior column fracture lines and remove debris from the medial aspect of the fracture and hip. Excessive or sustained retraction can similarly injure the obturator nerve and should be avoided. Although it seems far-fetched, the nerve can likewise be injured from deep intrapelvic reduction clamp application through the greater sciatic notch via a posterior exposure. Some transverse and many transverse with associated posterior wall fracture patterns are treated operatively using a posterior exposure. The transverse fracture plane reduction is maintained using a clamp with one limb positioned through the greater sciatic notch onto the quadrilateral surface. The other clamp limb is located at the supraacetabular area. The clamp application onto the quadrilateral surface risks obturator nerve injury. The surgeon must make sure during application of the clamp onto the quadrilateral surface that the ONVB is located medially relative to the clamp. The other clamp limb must be situated to avoid stretching the sciatic nerve and SGNVB.

The pudendal nerve function should be examined upon admission because it can be injured from both the acetabular fracture displacement and the operative procedure, especially if traction tables are used during the surgery. The operative risk is decreased if the traction table's perineal post is appropriately padded and if sustained and excessive traction are avoided during surgery. Traction is only applied when needed during the operation to aid with the fracture reduction and then is released after the reduction is achieved and clamped securely.

The sciatic nerve is most at risk during posterior surgical exposures. The nerve may be traumatically injured by posterior fracture-dislocations from stretch or direct contusion. The sciatic nerve is very rarely lacerated by sharp fracture fragment edges. Sciatic nerve injuries have also been noted immediately after manipulative reduction of posterior wall fracture-dislocations caused by entrapment of the nerve between the posterior wall fragment and its posterior column fracture plane. Progressive sciatic nerve injuries are known to also occur in association with any fracture that has a vertical fracture through the posterior column, usually noted from the greater sciatic notch to the caudal posterior wall region paralleling the nerve's course. For these reasons, the function of the sciatic nerve is detailed before manipulative reduction maneuvers for all fractures and fracture-dislocations and should be monitored along with the patient's vital signs during each nursing shift. The sciatic nerve can also be injured during posterior acetabular repairs. Even in situations of the most dramatic displacements, the sciatic nerve can reliably be found on the dorsal surface of the quadratus femoris muscle and then traced and liberated progressing proximally to the greater sciatic notch. The piriformis muscle is commonly dorsal to the sciatic nerve, but variant muscle bundles of the piriformis are not unusual. For this reason, the nerve and its relationship with the piriformis are fully exposed. Any muscle bundles located anterior to the nerve or those piercing the nerve are completely excised to avoid injuring the nerve during retraction of the piriformis muscle. In comminuted posterior fractures, small bone and chondral fragments may be impaled within the nerve or its epineurium, especially anteriorly. In some patients with significant posterior wall region fracture comminution, the nerve can be almost surrounded with very tiny chondrocancellous fragments. These fragments are identified and removed before the nerve is manipulated or retracted. The sciatic nerve is relaxed during the operation by positioning the hip in extension and the knee in flexion. In some patients, the rectus femoris muscle is tight such that knee flexion will produce unwanted hip flexion. This can frustrate reduction because the hip flexion force is transferred to the acetabular fracture, allowing the femoral head to either subluxate through the posterior wall defect or displace the columnar fracture fragments. In such situations, the knee is extended, and the reduction proceeds, with care taken to avoid sciatic nerve stretch. Special retractors have been designed to "protect" the sciatic nerve during posterior acetabular exposures. The retractor is positioned in the lesser sciatic notch and oriented to be parallel to the sciatic nerve course. However, even specially designed retractors apply direct pressure and deformity to the nerve focally, especially at their edges. So the surgeon monitors the retractor position at all times because even minimal tilting of the retractor compresses the nerve. The nerve is visualized and protected during the exposure, fracture surface cleaning, reduction, clamp application, and implant placement. A concise preoperative plan outlining the operative details of reduction sequence and implant location diminish the amount of time that the sciatic nerve retraction is needed, further decreasing the risk of injury. Finally, the implants are positioned and located to avoid nerve injury. Screw-and-plate application, especially along the caudal aspect of the posterior column adjacent to the lesser sciatic notch and hamstring origin, should be done under direct visualization to avoid inadvertent sciatic nerve injury.

Intraoperative nerve monitoring has had mixed results in acetabular fracture surgery.[187-190] Most studies have focused on the sciatic nerve injury during surgery. Spontaneous electromyography (EMG) has been shown to be superior to somatosensory evoked potential monitoring in detecting intraoperative sciatic nerve compromise in acute acetabular surgery. Spontaneous EMG allows more rapid detection and therefore more rapid response to the offending maneuver that should prevent permanent nerve problems. One study demonstrated that routine visualization and protection of the sciatic nerve during surgery obviated the need for intraoperative electrodiagnostic modalities.[191]

The superior gluteal nerve is often forgotten in the grand scheme of acetabular surgery. Most surgeons tenotomize the piriformis muscle after they have ensured its normal dorsal relationship with the sciatic nerve, but they neglect to protect the superior gluteal nerve, especially from stretch injury. The superior gluteal nerve can be injured in a variety of ways. The simplest is caused by fracture displacements in the upper aspect of the greater sciatic notch. Frequently, the SGNVB is found in continuity but displaced into the fracture surface that has divided the greater sciatic notch. The surgeon can manipulate the unstable fracture fragment and protect the bundle as the fracture surfaces are reduced and clamped. The superior gluteal nerve can also be damaged by excessive or sustained retraction of the gluteus medius and gluteus minimus muscles anterosuperiorly within the surgical wound. This commonly occurs when broad, spiked retractors are hammered into the supraacetabular bone caudal to the hip abductors and then handed to an assistant on the other side of the injury to retract the hip abductors using a levered motion and sustained retraction. This type of levered retraction is not recommended. The surgeon should remember that when the assistant fatigues and retraction becomes insufficient that the muscles and nerve bundles being retracted are fatigued of being focally retracted as well. Excessive anterior or superior dissection beyond the supraacetabular region causes stretch injury of the superior gluteal nerve. Surgical exposure alternatives are used when anterosuperior acetabular access is necessary. As long as it does not adversely affect the fracture reduction, hip abduction during the surgical exposure and retraction is helpful to relax the superior gluteal nerve.

Deep Venous Thrombosis

Patients with acetabular fractures are at risk for DVT. Clinical examination seeking this diagnosis is performed at least daily. Special investigations such as venography, MRI venography, and duplex examinations have been advocated. Each method has its associated problems.[192-195]

The DVT risk is diminished with anticoagulant medications and with mechanical methods such as sequential pneumatic compression.[196] Low-molecular-weight heparin (LMWH), when begun without delay, is an effective method of thromboprophylaxis, especially in high-risk patients with acetabular fractures.[197] Continuation of chemoprophylaxis for a period of at least 10 to 14 days is recommended.[198] Some surgeons note increased wound problems in patients treated with LMWH after acetabular fracture surgery.

However, some patients have contraindications to systemic anticoagulation and cannot use sequential limb compression devices because of limb injuries or other reasons. Vena caval filters do not prevent or treat DVT but do decrease the risk of pulmonary embolus. Recent advances include easier insertion techniques and the development of temporary and removable vena caval filters. Removable filters protect the patients during their most vulnerable clinical phase and are then removed after the risk has normalized. The filters do require the risk of a second procedure for removal,[199,200] and life-threatening complications can include erosion through the vena caval wall, filter obstruction, migration, or filter fracture with migration into the cardiovascular system.[201] Retrieval rates have traditionally been poor.[202,203] With dedicated clinics for removal, retrieval rates have been shown to modestly improve to 60%.[204]

Infection

Fortunately, wound infections after acetabular operations are rare and are best avoided by thorough cleansing of the perineal, flank, buttock, and abdominal regions after anesthesia is instituted and before draping. Isolating the perineum from the surgical field with skin adherent and occlusive barrier drapes avoids contamination during the operation and perioperative antibiotic administration. Also, at the time of wound closure, if the traumatic capsule is reparable, it should be repaired. This maneuver coupled with anatomic reduction of the articular fragments will seal the hip joint from the rest of the wound in case superficial or deep infection occurs. If infection does result, it may be superficial or deep. Deep infections involving the joint are devastating when septic necrosis of the femoral head occurs. Hip irritability, wound erythema, and persistent drainage are clinical signs of deep infection involving the joint. Expeditious and thorough surgical wound débridement allows accurate cultures to be obtained. The wound is débrided of necrotic tissues and irrigated appropriately. In most circumstances, the wound is closed over drains, and specific antibiotic therapy is directed at the offending organism. The patient's overall medical condition is optimized. Some surgeons recommend halting physical therapy, including range of motion exercises, until the wound is sealed and secure. Before operative débridement, pelvic radiographs are obtained to rule out fixation failure related to the infection. If recurrent wound infection ensues after surgical débridement and appropriate antibiotics, the surgeon should repeat the wound cultures to assess the potential for superinfection (e-Fig. 41-9). Open wound management is used for rare patients with recurrent infections despite adequate débridement and specific antibiotic therapy. Open wound management of an infected ilioinguinal exposure is problematic because the abdominal oblique muscles must be repaired to the iliac crest with each débridement. If this repair fails, the muscles contract, and the iliac crest is exposed. Some form of flap coverage is needed and effective for these unusual situations. Fortunately, the middle surgical interval repair can usually be left intact for ilioinguinal wound infection débridements because the iliac and medial intrapelvic intervals provide excellent exposure for the débridements. Surgical implants may be colonized but should not be considered for removal until the fracture has healed (Fig. 41-56).

Ectopic Bone Formation

Regional ectopic bone formation after acetabular fracture surgery varies in its severity and location.[121,205-209] Craniocerebral trauma, extensile approaches, combined simultaneous surgical exposures, highly displaced fractures, and the Smith-Petersen exposure are often associated with symptomatic ectopic bone formation. Ectopic bone occurs rarely after ilioinguinal exposures alone. More severe forms of ectopic bone limit hip movement and therefore impair function. In some patients, ectopic bone forms around the sciatic nerve and may cause the nerve to be irritable or have altered function.

Clinical studies substantiate the use of oral indomethacin as ectopic bone prophylaxis after acetabular fracture surgery.[210-213] Similarly, targeted low-dose irradiation decreases the incidence and severity of ectopic bone formation after acetabular surgery.[214-217] Some patients are unable to take or tolerate oral indomethacin such that rectal administration is considered when appropriate. Irradiation is more costly and time consuming, and some clinicians are concerned about its short-term effect on wound healing and long-term oncogenic potential.[218]

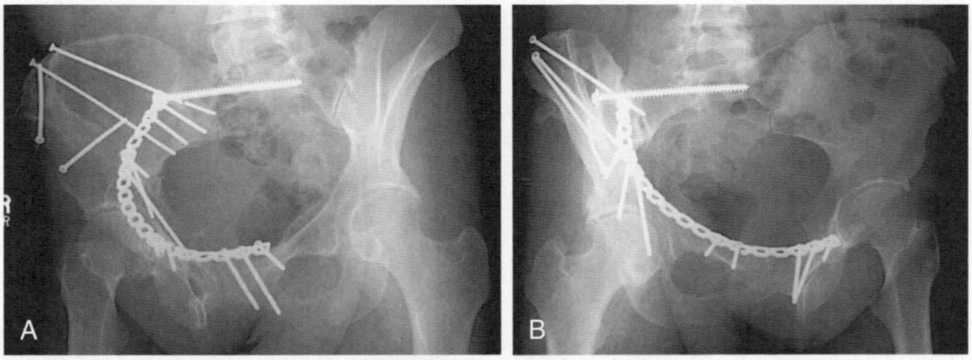

Figure 41-56. A and **B,** This woman had a displaced associated both-column acetabular fracture, ipsilateral sacral fracture, symphysis pubis disruption, and a torn urethra. On the night of injury, she underwent attempted urethral repair using a low midline exposure, but the repair failed. A suprapubic catheter was inserted. Three days later, she had open reduction and internal fixation of her acetabular fracture and symphysis pubis using an ilioinguinal exposure that transected the prior incision. The sacral fracture was stabilized using a percutaneously inserted iliosacral screw. The acetabular fracture consisted of five main fragments, and the articular reconstruction was anatomic. After surgery, the patient developed a polymicrobial deep infection that required numerous débridements. During the initial débridement, the middle surgical interval tissues had healed, and the deep infection could be easily accessed using the lateral and medial intrapelvic surgical intervals. During each débridement, the abdominal oblique muscle insertion could be repaired so that the iliac crest was covered. Intravenous antibiotics were administered, and the infection resolved. Despite the severity and extent of the deep polymicrobial infection, the hip joint was sealed by the reduction and never showed signs or symptoms of infection. These images were obtained 15 years later when the patient complained of intermittent low back pain. Her hip remains asymptomatic. Septic arthritis can be avoided if the joint fracture fragments are anatomically reduced, thereby isolating the joint surfaces from the rest of the wound before the wound infection occurs.

Early surgical excision of ectopic bone is recommended when functional hip range of motion is limited. Because acetabular and femoral head articular cartilage viability is dependent on joint movement, early surgical excision of offending ectopic bone is necessary. Special studies such as bone scans and blood tests to assess ectopic bone maturity before excision are not indicated in these patients. Similarly, when the nerve function is adversely affected by ectopic bone, the offending bone excision is not delayed so that a neuroplasty can be performed to liberate the nerve and regain function (Fig. 41-57).

Aseptic Necrosis of the Femoral Head

Aseptic femoral head necrosis is an unusual but significant problem after acetabular fracture, especially in young patients (Fig. 41-58). The unique femoral head blood supply is theoretically injured by the traumatic event, causing the necrosis. Hip dislocations and acetabular fracture-dislocations may damage the medial femoral circumflex or lateral epiphyseal vasculature and cause such necrosis.[219] Injury to these blood vessels can also occur during surgery. The quadratus femoris muscle contains the medial femoral circumflex vessels and must be protected and preserved during surgical exposures. During surgery, manipulative devices such as bone hooks along the femoral neck and greater trochanteric regions may also damage these vessels. Patients should be counseled regarding the potential development of aseptic necrosis and its clinical symptoms to improve early detection. MRI evaluations are compromised somewhat by the local acetabular fixation devices. Many patients, despite education about the symptoms of aseptic necrosis, will deny the symptoms and delay presentation in the clinic until the femoral head collapses or the femoral neck fractures because of the head necrosis.

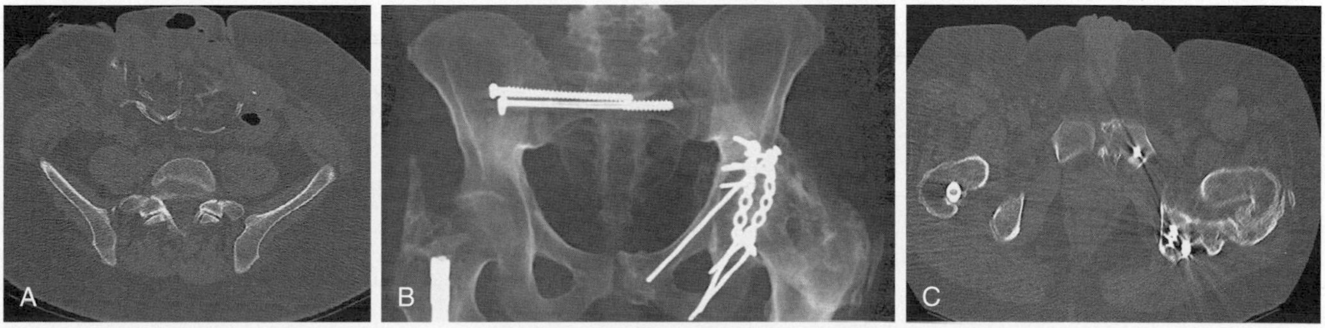

Figure 41-57. A, Ectopic bone formation may complicate acetabular surgery. Early excision is recommended when the ectopic restricts hip function or causes sciatic nerve symptoms. Multifocal ectopic bone formation was noted in this 25-year-old patient with numerous injuries. He formed symptomatic, excessive bone in his omentum, at the femur fracture, between his radius and ulna, and at the sites of his femoral nail and iliosacral screw insertions. The omental bone was removed initially. **B,** The Brooker class IV ectopic bone in the hip region prevented hip movement. **C,** He did not have sciatic nerve symptoms, but on the computed tomography axial images, the ectopic bone mass had semicircular indentations along its dorsal cortical surface that corresponded to the location of the sciatic nerve. The sciatic nerve was contained within this bony tunnel at operation. The excess bone was surgically excised at every site.

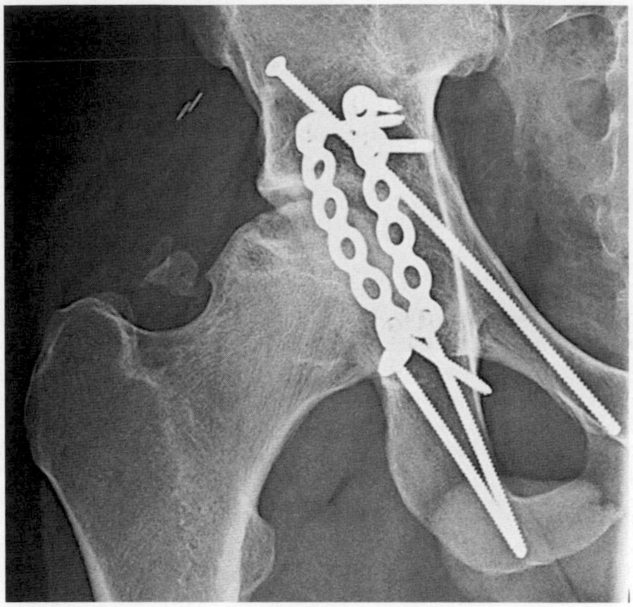

Figure 41-58. Aseptic necrosis is an uncommon complication after posterior acetabular fracture-dislocation. The femoral head blood supply can be damaged by the injury and during surgery. The surgeon should use techniques that protect the vessels that supply the femoral head with its critical blood flow. This patient noted symptomatic groin pain 10 months after injury.

Arthritis

Posttraumatic arthritis causes hip stiffness, pain, and a poor clinical result.[220] Most studies agree that improved fracture reduction decreases the incidence and severity of posttraumatic arthritis.[7,221,222] Chondral injury, especially of the acetabular dome, is directly related to arthritic changes (e-Fig. 41-10).

Fixation Error

Fixation errors usually follow insufficient exposure and reduction.[223-227] The mechanical features of each fixation construct should be planned preoperatively and then critically assessed before wound closure. It is often helpful to draw each fracture fragment and its related fixation construct on a sterile towel to ensure that each fracture fragment has achieved sufficient stability before closing the wound. The hip should be stressed under direct visualization to guarantee stability (Fig. 41-59).

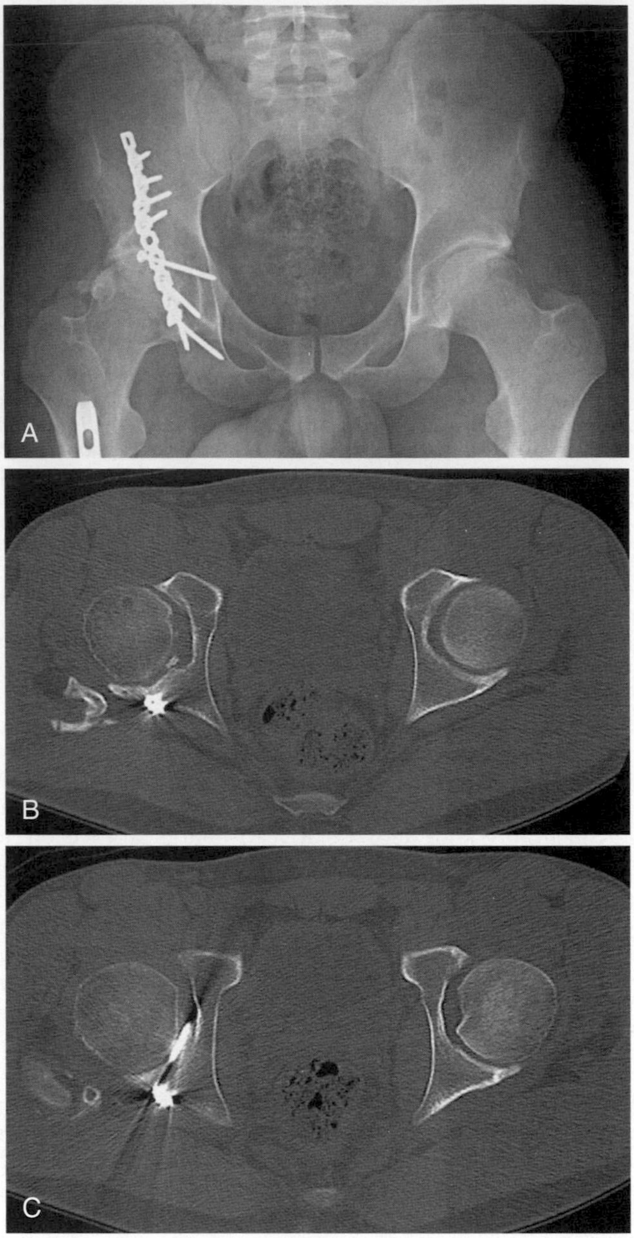

Figure 41-59. A, This patient had surgery for a posterior wall acetabular fracture. The patient complained of continued pain after surgery and eventually sought another opinion. **B** and **C,** The pelvic plain radiograph and computed tomography (CT) scan demonstrate fracture union, arthritic changes, ectopic bone formation, intraarticular bone debris, and a misdirected screw between the joint surfaces. These are all avoidable problems. Joint debris should be quantified and each fragment measured preoperatively on the CT scan to ensure complete removal during the surgery. Multiplanar intraoperative fluoroscopy will prove that each screw is out of the joint. If the screw cannot be shown to be extraarticular on at least one view, then it is an intraarticular screw and must be removed or redirected out of the joint before wound closure. Ectopic bone formation after posterior acetabular injury and surgery is common and should be excised when it interferes with hip mobility or affects nerve function.

SUMMARY

Acetabular fractures occur rarely and are quite variable. The anatomy and radiology are complex but critical to understanding the injuries and their classification. Early management follows routine resuscitation protocols, and fracture-dislocations should be reduced expediently. Operative reduction and stable fixation is advocated for displaced and unstable fractures. An appropriate surgical exposure facilitates an accurate fracture reduction, which is vital for improved outcomes. Stable fixation is mandatory to allow early rehabilitation of the joint and patient. A variety of complications are well known and should be avoided when possible. The treatment of acetabular fractures is challenging for orthopaedic surgeons in many ways, but experience and modern technologies should continue to advance this clinical area.

KEY REFERENCES

The level of evidence (LOE) is determined according to the criteria provided in the preface.

6. Tannast M, Najibi S, Matta J: Two to twenty year survivorship of the hip in 810 patients with operative treated acetabular fractures. *J Bone Joint Surg Am* 94:1559–1567, 2012. LOE II
7. Letournel E: Acetabulum fractures: classification and management. *Clin Orthop Relat Res* 151:81–106, 1980. LOE IV
67. Furey A, Karp J, O'Toole R: Does early fixation of posterior wall acetabular fractures lead to increased blood loss? *J Orthop Trauma* 27:2–5, 2013. LOE II
78. Letournel E: The treatment of acetabular fractures through the ilioinguinal approach. *Clin Orthop Relat Res* 292:62–76, 1993. LOE IV
83. Johnson E, Matta J, Mast J, et al: Delayed reconstructions of acetabular fractures 21-120 days following injury. *Clin Orthop Relat Res* 305:20–30, 1994. LOE IV
84. Matta J: Fractures of the acetabulum: accuracy of reduction and clinical results in patients managed operatively within three weeks after the injury. *J Bone Joint Surg Am* 78:1632–1645, 1996. LOE IV
121. Rath E, Russell G, Washington W, et al: Gluteus minimus necrotic muscle debridement diminished heterotopic ossification after acetabular fracture fixation. *Injury* 33:751–756, 2002. LOE III
170. Russell G, Nork S, Routt M: Perioperative complications associated with operative treatment of acetabular fractures. *J Trauma* 51:1098–1103, 2001. LOE II
192. Borer D, Starr A, Reinert C, et al: The effect of screening for deep vein thrombosis on the prevalence of pulmonary embolism in patients with fractures of the pelvis or acetabulum: a review of 973 patients. *J Orthop Trauma* 19:92–95, 2005. LOE II
197. Steele N, Dodenhoff R, Ward A, et al: Thromboprophylaxis in pelvic and acetabular trauma surgery. The role of early treatment with low-molecular-weight heparin. *J Bone Joint Surg Br* 87:209–212, 2005. LOE II

The complete References list is available online at https://expertconsult.inkling.com.

SECTION FOUR

Upper Extremity

EDITED BY JESSE B. JUPITER

SECTION OUTLINE

Chapter 42

Fractures and Dislocations of the Hand

DAVID E. RUCHELSMAN • RANDY R. BINDRA

Additional videos related to the subject of this chapter are available from the Medizinische Hochschule Hannover collection. The following videos are included with this chapter and may be viewed at https://expertconsult.inkling.com:

42-1. Thumb metacarpal base.
42-2. Metacarpal shaft placing.
42-3. Complex metacarpophalangeal joint dislocation.
42-4. Surgical treatment of infections at the hand.
42-5. Resection arthroplasty of the basal joint of metatarsal one.

Each unique anatomic region and its associated ligamentous and osseous injuries are discussed. Elucidation of the surgical anatomy, review of surgical techniques with associated pearls and pitfalls, and general postoperative rehabilitation protocols are presented. Evidence-based reviews of outcomes based on contemporary literature are provided.

THE THUMB RAY

The position of the thumb ray and its unique local anatomy at the carpometacarpal (CMC) and metacarpophalangeal (MCP) joints make it susceptible to well-defined ligamentous and osseous injuries. Dedicated thumb radiographs are imperative in evaluating injuries about the longitudinal axis of the thumb. Often, patients present with hand radiographs from the emergency department that do not allow for accurate assessment of joint reduction and fracture deformity. Anterior-posterior (AP) Roberts, lateral, and oblique views should be obtained. The Roberts view represents a true AP image obtained with hyperpronation of the forearm with the dorsal surface of the thumb against the radiograph plate and the beam directed perpendicular to the plate. When there is concern for articular involvement, computed tomography with sagittal and coronal plane reconstruction can be helpful in preoperative planning in select cases.

INTRAARTICULAR CARPOMETACARPAL FRACTURES OF THE THUMB METACARPAL

As proposed by Buchler,[1] fractures of the base of the thumb are conceptually divided into epibasilar extraarticular, partial articular (Bennett fracture), and complete articular (Rolando fracture) fractures based on the zone of articular involvement (Fig. 42-1). Because of the multiple deforming myotendinous forces at the thumb CMC joint and along the longitudinal axis of the thumb metacarpal, these fractures are inherently unstable. Predictable shaft displacement is caused by the unopposed pull of the abductor pollicis longus, flexor pollicis brevis (FPB), and the adductor pollicis on the distal fragment, creating an apex dorsal-radial deformity combined with shortening and supination of the shaft (Fig. 42-2).

Regional Anatomy

The double saddle-joint design of the thumb CMC joint allows for a wide range of flexion-extension, abduction-adduction, and pronosupination of the thumb. Four main ligaments stabilize this articulation during pinch and grasp. These include the anterior and posterior oblique ligaments, the dorsal-radial ligament, and the intermetacarpal ligament (Fig. 42-3). The volar oblique ligament is stout originating from the trapezium and inserting onto the volar beak of the thumb metacarpal. It resists dorsoradial subluxation. The thin dorsal capsule is reinforced by the aponeurosis of the abductor pollicis longus.

Examination

AP Robert, lateral, and oblique radiographs of the thumb are standard. Traction radiographs are beneficial for assessing the effect of ligamentotaxis on reduction, but are often reserved for the intraoperative setting.

Indications

Surgical indications include sagittal plane angulation greater than 30 degrees, joint subluxation, and articular incongruity (i.e., gap and depression) greater than 2 mm.

Surgical Exposures and Fixation Techniques

For epibasilar and proximal shaft metadiaphyseal fractures, closed reduction and percutaneous Kirschner wire (K-wire) fixation is attempted (Fig. 42-4). Given the short metaphyseal segment, transarticular fixation across the CMC joint with fixation into the trapezium is performed. A minimum of two K-wires (0.054 or 0.045 inch) are used. The K-wires are removed at 4 weeks postoperatively. Cast immobilization is used while the K-wires are in place.

When acceptable reduction cannot be achieved in a closed fashion or in combined injuries, open reduction through a dorsal approach is performed. Following elevation of skin flaps and protection of regional branches of the radial sensory nerve, the interval between the extensor pollicis brevis and longus is developed (Fig. 42-5). Meticulous subperiosteal dissection along the fracture may allow the periosteum to be

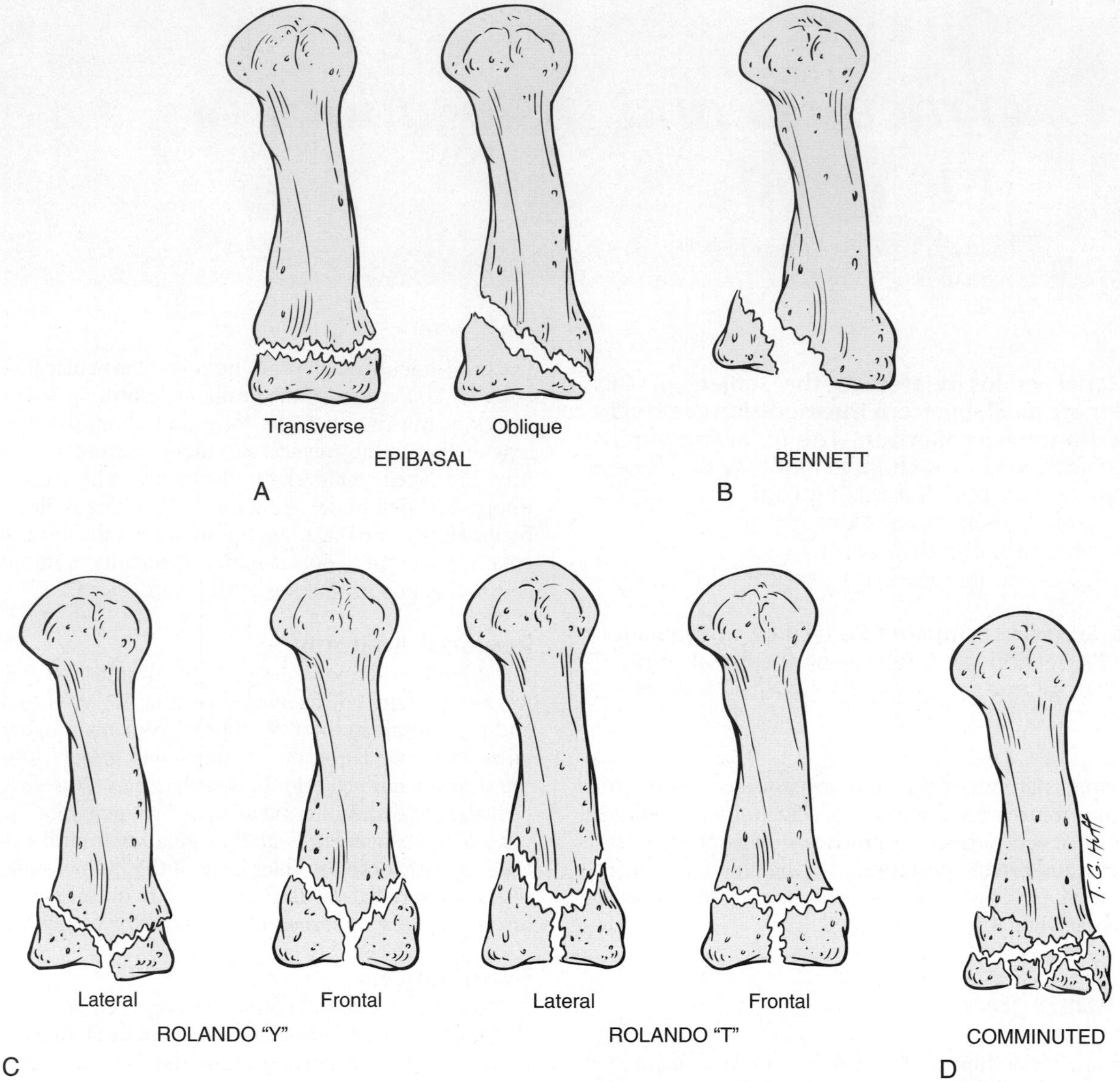

Figure 42-1. Fractures of the base of the thumb metacarpal can be grouped into four types: **A,** epibasal; **B,** Bennett; **C,** Rolando Y and T; **D,** comminuted.

closed over the plate and helps to minimize the potential for extensor tendon adhesions. Following fracture reduction, provisional K-wire fixation placed in the radial midaxial plane may be performed prior to plate application if the reduction is unstable. Given the short metaphyseal segment, a fixed-angle (i.e., condylar blade plate or locking plate) construct is preferred. In this area, 2- and 2.4-mm T- or Y-plates are often used (Fig. 42-6; Video 42-1). Localization of the trapeziometacarpal joint can be achieved by placing a K-wire through one of the locking sleeves before screw fixation begins to avoid intraarticular screw placement. If the epibasilar fracture is oblique, a nonlocking bicortical interfragmentary screw can be placed perpendicular to the obliquity. For transverse fractures, compression technique is followed. Bridge plating is used for comminuted and axially unstable fracture patterns.

Following open reduction and internal fixation, early functional rehabilitation is initiated within the first postoperative week. The patient is transitioned to a short or long opponens splint and thenar cone and tendon gliding exercises are begun. Pinch strengthening is initiated between 4 and 6 weeks postoperatively when there is evidence of clinical and early radiographic union.

For partial and complete articular fractures at the base of the thumb metacarpal, the volar-ulnar articular fragment is variably sized, but remains reduced by the stout volar-oblique ligament to the trapezium. Intraarticular fractures may consist of a small oblique fragment or a larger articular shear fracture. Meticulous assessment of the articular surface is needed following reduction to assess for any central articular impaction. Often, this is best assessed following an attempted closed reduction using a combination of longitudinal traction, direct reduction at the apex of the dorsoradial deformity, abduction, and pronation of the shaft under fluoroscopy. Articular impaction typically does not correct with closed reduction, and requires formal open reduction as described later to elevate the central impaction and restore joint congruity.

Congruent joint and fracture reduction is the goal regardless of operative technique selected. When the metacarpal

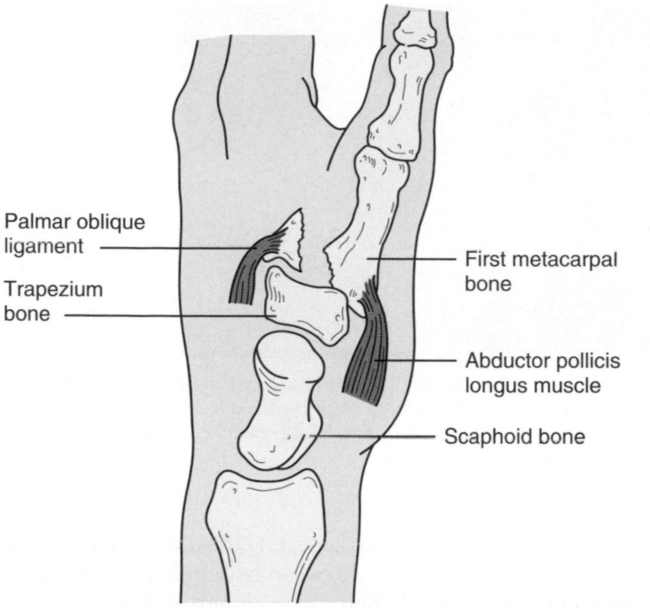

Figure 42-2. Patterns of force displacement leading to the typical carpometacarpal dislocation of a Bennett fracture. Note that the palmar oblique ligament holds the medial fragment anatomically aligned with the trapezium.

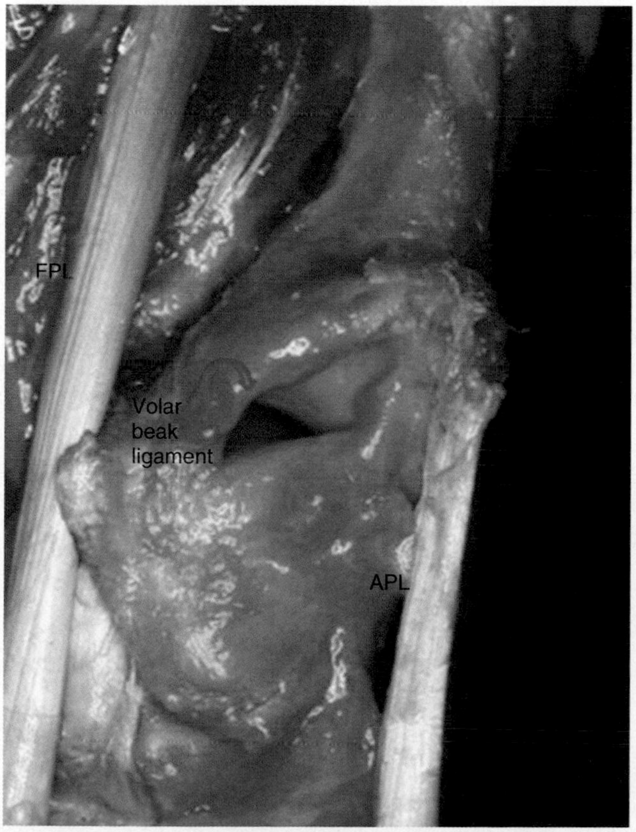

Figure 42-3. The volar oblique ligament is stout originating from the trapezium and inserting onto the volar beak of the thumb metacarpal. It resists dorsoradial subluxation. *APL*, Abductor pollicis longus; *FPL*, flexor pollicis longus.

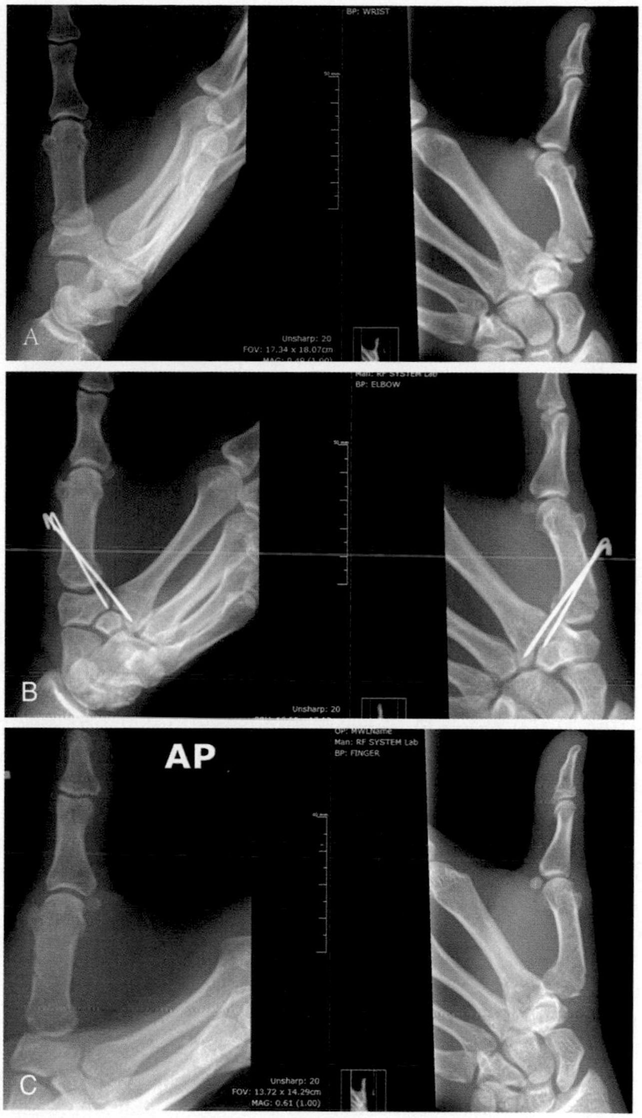

Figure 42-4. A, Comminuted epibasilar thumb metacarpal with sagittal plane deformity. **B,** Closed reduction and percutaneous Kirschner wire fixation performed for the epibasilar fracture. Transarticular fixation across the carpometacarpal (CMC) joint with fixation into the trapezium and index metacarpal is performed. **C,** Osseous union is achieved at 6 weeks. *AP,* Anterior-posterior

base subluxation can be reduced and articular congruency obtained with closed reduction, percutaneous K-wire fixation is performed using 0.054- and/or 0.045-inch wires. K-wire entry begins along the dorsoradial border of the thumb metacarpal. One of several configurations are acceptable. The K-wire does not need to cross the fracture site. Beginning in the dorsoradial aspect of the shaft will often allow one to advance the wire across the dorsal quadrant of the articular surface of the metacarpal to obtain transarticular fixation within the trapezium (Fig. 42-7). Alternatively, the wire can be advanced into the base of the index metacarpal. Two to three diverging K-wires are used to maximize stability of the construct. AP Roberts and lateral views confirm reduction and K-wire positions. Wires are routinely cut and bent outside of the skin. The K-wires are removed at 4 to 6 weeks postoperatively. Cast immobilization is used while the K-wires are in place.

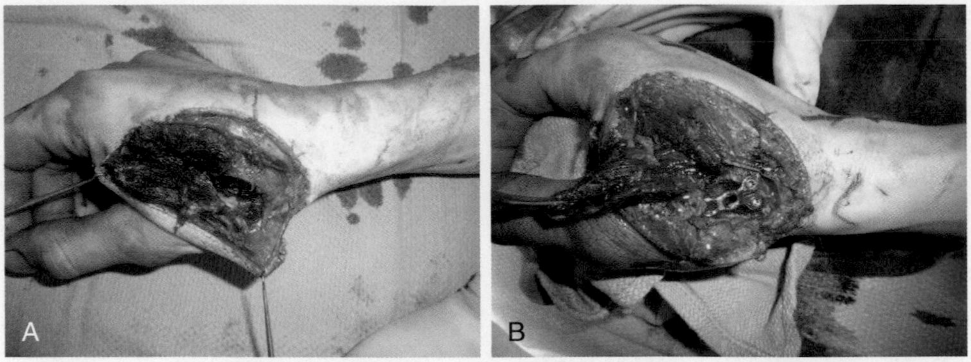

Figure 42-5. A, Partial thumb amputation at the level of the carpometacarpal (CMC) joint was sustained in a construction site accident. Lacerations of the extensor pollicis longus (EPL), extensor pollicis brevis (EPB), and the radial sensory nerve were repaired following open reduction and internal fixation (ORIF) of the underlying metaphyseal thumb metacarpal fracture. **B,** Stable internal fixation with a fixed-angle implant allowed for early functional rehabilitation of this combined injury, using dynamic extension splinting.

When acceptable reduction cannot be achieved, or the volar-ulnar fragment is larger than 20% to 30% of the articular surface, open reduction and internal fixation is performed (Fig. 42-8). A palmoradial Wagner incision is used, which extends from the distal wrist flexion crease overlying the flexor carpi radialis and extends distally along the shaft of the metacarpal at the junction of the glabrous and nonglabrous skin. Skin flaps are elevated and cutaneous branches of the palmar cutaneous, radial sensory, and lateral antebrachial cutaneous nerves are carefully mobilized and protected. The thenar intrinsic musculature is elevated extraperiosteally from the shaft segment. The insertion of the abductor pollicis longus (APL) is identified and protected. An arthrotomy is performed. Soft tissue attachments to the fracture are preserved.

Supination of the metacarpal shaft greatly facilitates fracture site exposure. For simple sagittal plane fractures, the shaft can be reduced with traction, abduction, and pronation and the articular fragment controlled with a dental pick and secured with a fine reduction forceps. A dorsal skin flap is elevated to facilitate provisional K-wire placement and modular lag screw insertion dorsal to the APL. They are typically placed from dorsal-radial to volar-ulnar to secure fixation of the articular fragment. Modular hand screw size and trajectory are selected based on size of the articular fragment and the obliquity of the fracture line. Modular hand screws, 1.1 to 2.4 mm, should routinely be available. K-wires of corresponding diameter to the screw core diameter are selected so that the provisional K-wires can be sequentially exchanged for bicortical screws. When the fragment is smaller, a single screw and K-wire or an additional 1.3- or 1.1-mm screw may be used. We favor two screws, even if this requires placement of a 1.3- or 1.1-mm screw.

Alternatively, an "inside-out" technique may be used. The shaft segment may be first hypersupinated to expose the cancellous surface of metacarpal fracture line and then drilled from volar to dorsal from "inside" the fracture site. This ensures that following fracture reduction and bicortical drilling from dorsal to volar the screw trajectory obtains maximal purchase in the articular fragment. Intraoperative fluoroscopy is essential in assessing joint reduction, articular congruency, and subchondral screw position.

Central impaction requires elevation using the trapezium as a template, and supplemental cancellous bone grafting may be needed in select cases. When the articular fracture line is vertical, shear forces should be neutralized prior to screw fixation. When there is an associated trapezial body fracture, reduction and fixation of the trapezium is performed prior to the metacarpal articular fracture.

Complete articular Rolando-type fractures are often the result of axial loading of the joint surface. Preoperative computed tomography (CT) scan may help elucidate the plane of the intraarticular fracture and help in the selection of

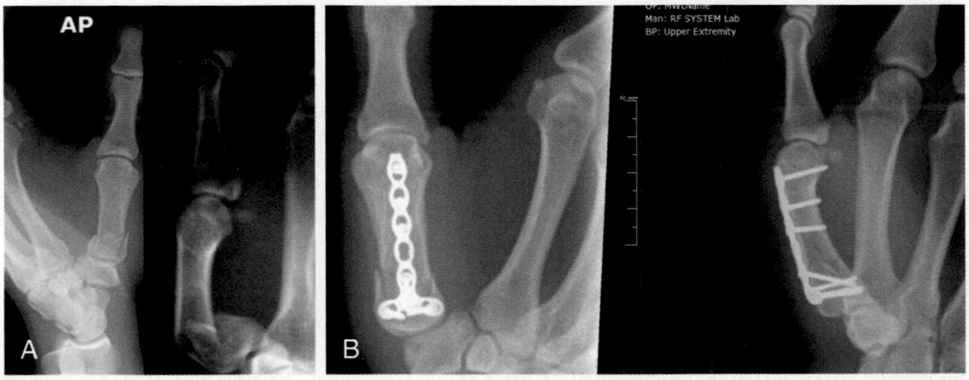

Figure 42-6. A, Comminuted thumb metacarpal metaphyseal epibasilar fracture. *AP,* Anterior-posterior. **B,** Open reduction was performed with a 2-mm Combi Hole plate to allow for fixed angular-stable fixation in the comminuted metaphyseal segment to facilitate early functional rehabilitation in this professional athlete.

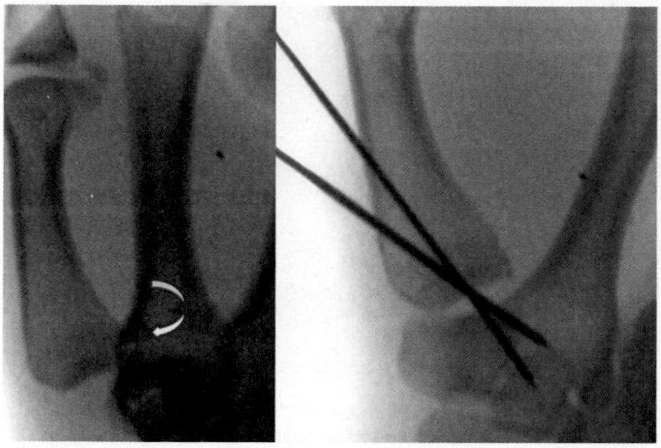

Figure 42-7. Bennett fracture with associated trapeziometacarpal joint subluxation. Closed reduction at percutaneous transarticular fixation restores joint congruency.

operative exposure. At times, these fractures may reduce with traction. Meticulous K-wire placement allows restoration of the joint surface. Additional K-wires are then used to secure the shaft to the articular segments.

Coronal and sagittal plane fracture lines impact the selection of surgical exposure. When the main fracture line is in the coronal plane, a dorsal exposure is used; when the articular split is in the sagittal plane, a palmoradial exposure is selected. Stepwise reduction of the articular surface and provisional K-wire fixation are performed. Articular fragments may be captured through independent modular hand lag screws or with screws placed through the plate. A fixed-angle construct is preferred and 2- to 2.4-mm condylar or locking plates are used. The transverse portions of the plate allow for stabilization of the basilar fragments. When the fracture line is in the coronal plane, eccentric placement of cortical screws in the T or Y portion of the locking plate creates interfragmentary compression. Plate contouring along the shaft is necessary to prevent residual deformity. Provisional plate fixation proximally and distally is helpful to avoid shaft malrotation. Care is taken to avoid convergence of the screws along the volar cortex and articular violation.

Following open reduction and stable internal fixation, early functional rehabilitation is begun within the first postoperative week. The patient is transitioned to a short opponens splint and thenar cone and tendon gliding exercises are begun. Pinch strengthening is initiated between 4 and 6 weeks postoperatively when there is evidence of clinical and early radiographic union.

Highly comminuted articular fractures may require limited-open reduction and internal fixation (ORIF) of the articular segment, bone grafting of the metaphyseal void, and supplemental bridging external fixation to maintain distraction across the trapeziometacarpal joint.[1-3] Various external fixation constructs may be used. Terminally threaded 1.1- to 1.25-mm K-wires may be placed in the thumb and index metacarpal to create a stable quadrangular construct that also maintains the first web space to minimize web space contracture.[1] Alternatively, K-wires may be placed in the thumb metacarpal combined with a trapezial wire to directly distract the trapeziometacarpal joint. The frame is removed between 4 to 6 weeks postoperatively.

Outcomes

Early literature favored nonoperative treatment of these articular fractures, and a single study[4] reported little evidence of symptomatic arthrosis following nonoperative treatment of partial articular fractures at the base of the thumb metacarpal. Contemporary series[5-8] demonstrated that clinical and radiographic outcomes are optimized when subluxation is corrected and there is less than 1 mm of articular gap following reduction and stabilization. Other clinical series confirmed that residual articular incongruity yields a higher incidence of symptomatic posttraumatic arthrosis.[6,8] Biomechanical evidence[9] supports the rationale for articular reduction as simulated Bennett malunion with a 2-mm stepoff created abnormal joint contact forces dorsoradially.

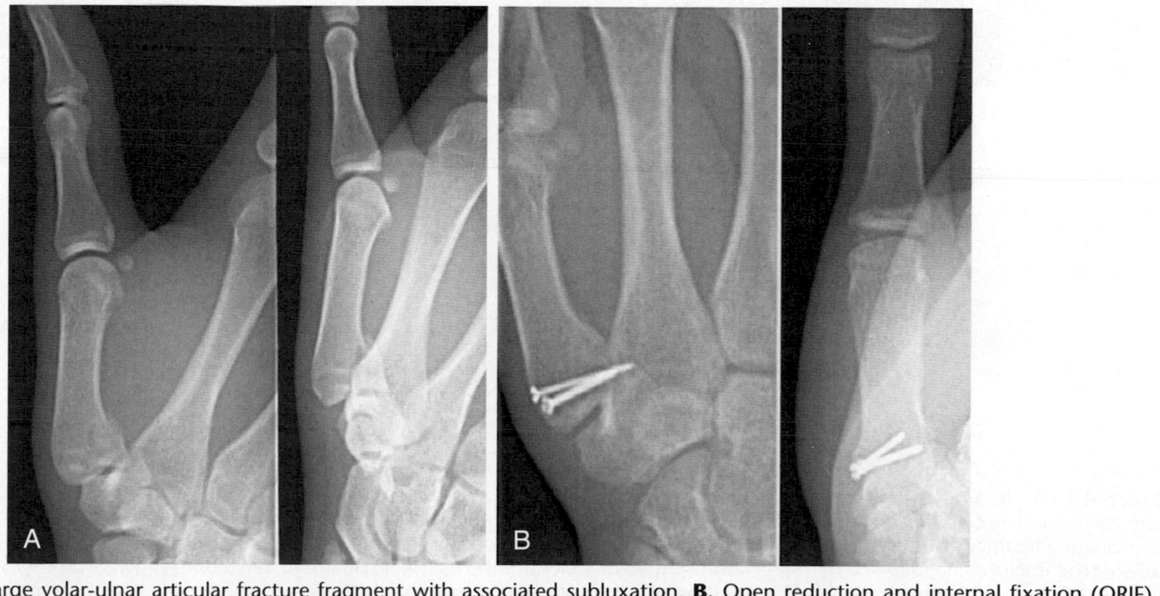

Figure 42-8. A, Large volar-ulnar articular fracture fragment with associated subluxation. **B,** Open reduction and internal fixation (ORIF) is achieved through a palmoradial incision using modular hand screws.

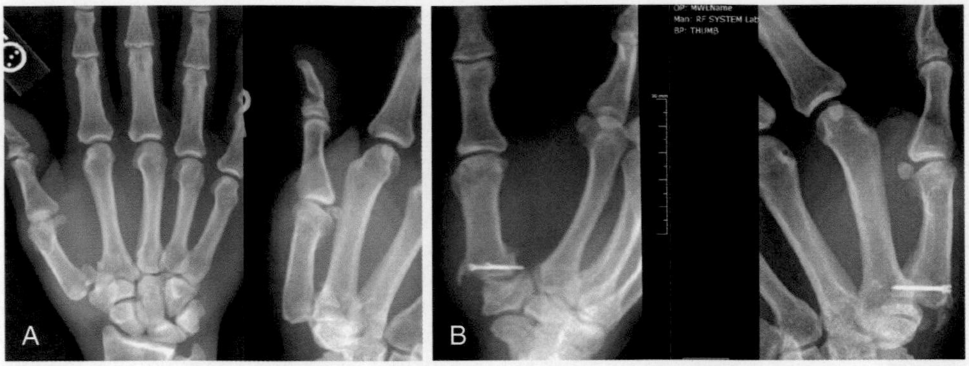

Figure 42-9. A, Large volar-ulnar articular fracture fragment with associated subluxation. **B,** Following open reduction and internal fixation (ORIF), progressive nonbridging periarticular heterotopic ossification is seen. Symmetric thumb opposition was achieved.

Sequelae

In the majority of cases, functional thenar motion and pinch strength is recovered. Residual stiffness rarely requires additional treatment. In some cases, extensor tenolysis with concomitant removal of hardware may be required and is performed 4 to 6 months postoperatively when the soft tissue envelope is supple and full osseous union confirmed. The risk of arthrosis is greater following complete articular fractures in this area. In the setting of a high-energy mechanism of injury and articular fracture-subluxation/dislocation, periarticular heterotopic ossification may be seen but no cases of bridging ankylosis have been reported (Fig. 42-9).

If intraarticular fractures are suboptimally reduced, the resulting articular malunion, especially if associated with persistent subluxation, may progress to trapeziometacarpal arthrosis. Corrective closing wedge or intraarticular osteotomy is indicated for persistent joint subluxation and instability if recognized before development of arthrosis. In these cases, preoperative CT scan may be helpful to define the fracture plane and to aid in osteotomy planning (Fig. 42-10). Once

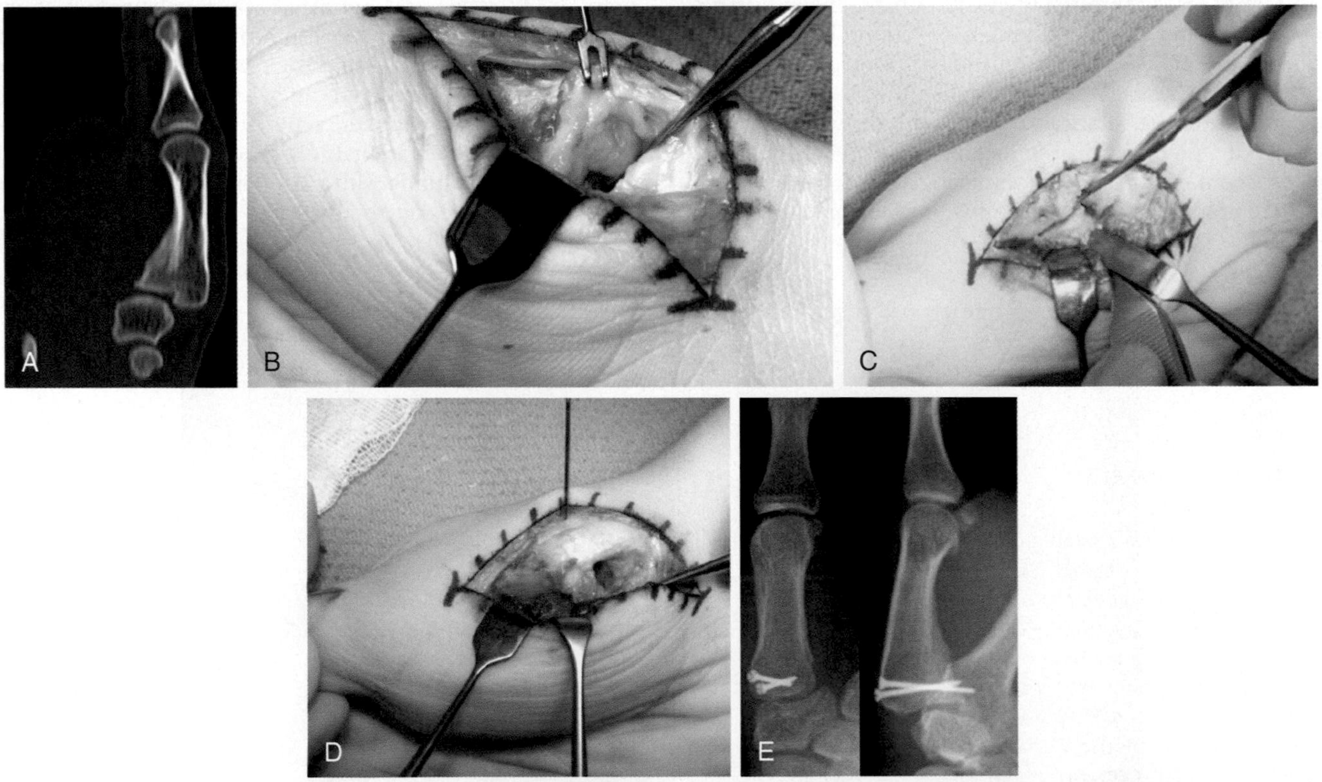

Figure 42-10. A, Missed Bennett fracture with delayed presentation in a high school athlete. Articular depression and subluxation is noted. Early degenerative changes are already present. **B,** Intraarticular osteotomy is performed through a palmoradial incision. Preservation of the volar oblique ligament on the malunited articular is essential during the arthrotomy. **C,** Multiple stacked fine K-wires were used to develop the plane of the fracture line followed by osteoclasis using a Freer elevator. **D,** Following anatomic reduction, provisional K-wire fixation is achieved. **E,** Final radiographs demonstrate union, restoration of joint congruency, and maintenance of the joint space without progressive degenerative changes.

degenerative arthrosis has developed, salvage options include arthroplasty and arthrodesis. Chronic pain and instability treated with arthrodesis tends to be less well tolerated than arthrodesis at the fourth or fifth CMC joints. Nonunion at the base of the thumb metacarpal is rare.

Future Directions

Some centers reported the use of small joint arthroscopy to aid in the reduction and fixation of thumb MCP and CMC articular fractures and collateral ligament avulsion fractures.[10,11] Culp and Johnson[11] described arthroscopically assisted reduction using a 1.9-mm arthroscope and percutaneous fixation of Bennett fractures. It remains unclear whether arthroscopically assisted reduction and stabilization offers superior clinical or radiographic outcomes, and in our practices, use of arthroscopy in the treatment of these injuries has a limited role.

EXTRAARTICULAR FRACTURES OF THE THUMB METACARPAL

The management principles of the thumb metacarpal neck, shaft, and extraarticular base fractures are similar to those in other metacarpals (discussed later). Shaft fractures are uncommon as stress is transmitted along the strong cortical shaft to the cancellous basilar region. Given the large range of motion in the basal joint, larger extraarticular deformity is tolerated. Apex dorsal sagittal plane angular deformity greater than 30 degrees leads to first web space narrowing and compensatory hyperextension at the MCP joint. A true lateral radiograph of the metacarpal is needed to demonstrate the degree of sagittal plane deformity.

Thumb spica casting or orthoplast splinting are the mainstays of nonoperative management. When open reduction and internal fixation is performed, a dorsal exposure and the interval between the extensor pollicis brevis and longus is used as described earlier. A radial midaxial exposure with elevation of the thenar musculature may be advantageous in select fracture patterns or treatment of combined injuries necessitating concomitant metacarpal fixation and extensor tendon and sensory nerve repairs and/or reconstructions.

LIGAMENTOUS INJURIES

Carpometacarpal Joint

Examination

Thumb CMC joint dislocations are rare, and reported dislocations have all been dorsal. The mechanism of injury consists of axial loading of the flexed metacarpal. There is typical clinical deformity consistent with the radiographic dislocation. A standard thumb radiographic series is performed. There remains disagreement with regard to which of the ligaments must be injured to allow complete dislocation of the CMC joint. Disruption of the capsule-ligamentous restraints may include midsubstance rupture, insertional avulsions, or subperiosteal stripping of the anterior oblique ligament from the metacarpal insertion.

If partial ligament tear is suspected, a stress examination under fluoroscopy may help detect dorsoradial subluxation of the metacarpal base. Comparison with the contralateral thumb CMC joint helps to differentiate laxity and instability. A stress posterior-anterior (PA) view of the thumbs parallel to the radiograph plate with the distal phalanges firmly pushed together along their radial borders will subluxate the metacarpal base radialward relative to the trapezium in the presence of capsule-ligamentous disruption. If the examination is equivocal, magnetic resonance imaging may be helpful in distinguishing partial and complete ruptures.

Posttraumatic tenderness localized to the CMC joint without frank clinical or radiographic instability is consistent with partial tears of the anterior oblique and/or dorsoradial ligaments. These injuries are managed with forearm-based thumb spica splinting or casting followed by functional rehabilitation.

Indications

If concentric closed reduction is obtained, but the CMC joint remains unstable, transarticular pinning is considered. Given the available data (level IV evidence) suggesting recurrent instability with this technique, indications for open reduction and ligament repair and/or reconstruction include irreducible dislocations (acute or chronic); reducible, but unstable joint (acute or chronic); and chronic symptomatic laxity or recurrent dislocation in cases without radiographic arthrosis. Arthrosis is a contraindication to ligament reconstruction.

Surgical Exposures and Technique

Frank dorsal dislocations are initially managed with closed reduction. Stability is assessed. If a closed reduction is congruous and stable, closed treatment with thumb spica casting is initiated together with close serial radiographic follow-up.

There is no consensus for optimal treatment of persistent or recurrent clinical or radiographic instability. Options include closed reduction and percutaneous transarticular trapeziometacarpal K-wire fixation, Eaton-Littler[12,13] anterior oblique ligament reconstruction, and open reduction and repair of the dorsoradial ligament complex comprised of the dorsoradial and posterior oblique ligaments.[14]

Anterior oblique ligament reconstruction is performed using the volar-radial Wagner exposure and volar CMC capsulotomy to inspect the articular surfaces, followed by utilization of the flexor carpi radialis to reconstruct the anterior oblique and dorsal-radial ligamentous complex. The distally based autograft is passed through a volar-to-dorsal subchondral intraosseous channel, secured to the dorsal periosteum, passed deep to the APL and secured to the dorsal capsule, weaved through the ulnar one-half of the flexor carpi radialis (FCR), and then secured back to the radial capsule (Fig. 42-11). There is no consensus whether the reconstruction requires supplemental transarticular pinning. Postoperative cast immobilization is used for approximately 4 to 6 weeks, and then patients are transitioned to a custom Orthoplast long opponens splint, which is removed for range of motion exercises. Thenar cone strengthening is initiated at 2 months postoperatively followed by pinch and grasp strengthening. Associated trapezial body fractures are treated with ORIF (Fig. 42-12).

Combined repairs of the dorsoradial ligamentous complex and anterior oblique ligament supplemented with transarticular K-wire fixation for 6 weeks with the CMC in the "screw-home-torque opposition" position is advocated by Edmunds.[14]

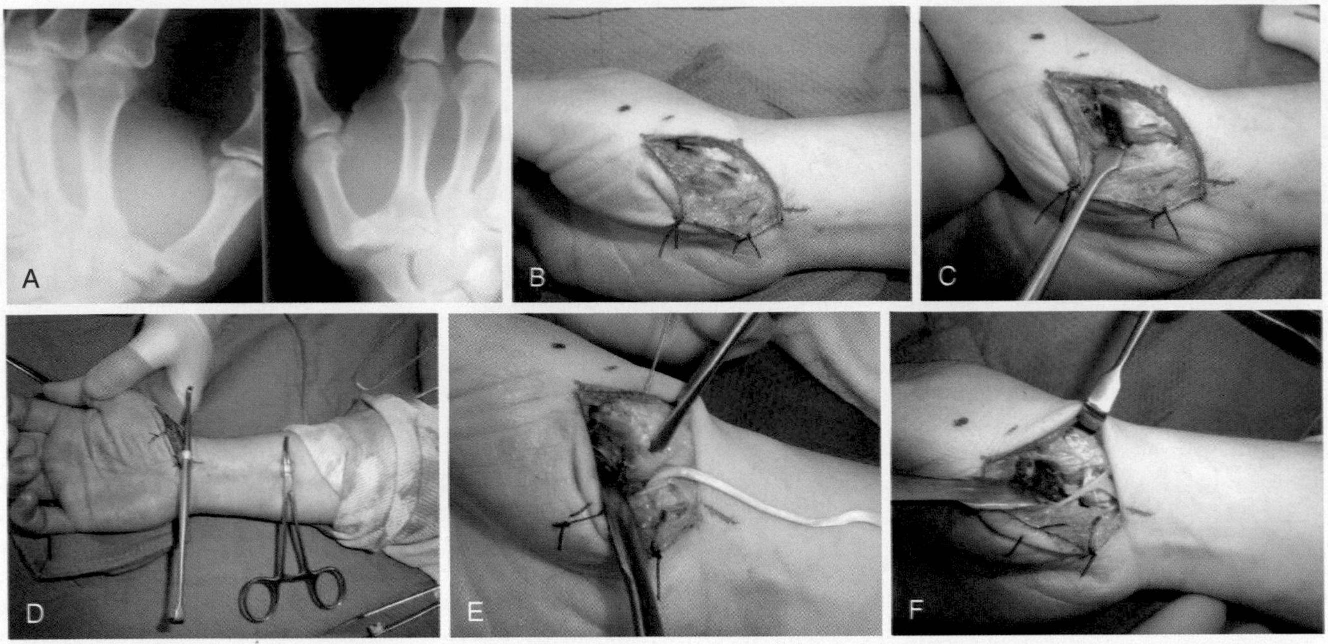

Figure 42-11. A, Thumb trapeziometacarpal dislocation with associated trapezial body fracture. **B,** Anterior oblique ligament reconstruction is performed using the volar-radial Wagner exposure. **C,** The thenar musculature is elevated from the volar carpometacarpal (CMC) capsule. **D,** The flexor carpi radialis is harvested to reconstruct the anterior oblique and dorsal radial ligamentous complex. **E,** The distally based autograft is passed through a volar-to-dorsal subchondral intraosseous channel. **F,** The graft is then secured to the dorsal periosteum, passed deep to the abductor pollicis longus (APL) and secured to the dorsal capsule, weaved through the ulnar one-half of the flexor carpi radialis (FCR), and then secured back to the radial capsule.

Cadaveric biomechanical studies[15,16] support the importance of the dorsoradial ligamentous complex in CMC stability and this surgical approach. When the dorsal-radial complex is irreparable, Eaton-Littler reconstruction is performed.

Ozer[17] described a new surgical technique performed through a dorsal approach using half of the extensor carpi radialis brevis (ECRB) to reconstruct all four stabilizing ligaments of the trapeziometacarpal joint. Superficial branches of the radial nerve and the deep branch of the radial artery are mobilized after cauterizing dorsal capsular perforating branches. A dorsal arthrotomy allows inspection of the articular surfaces. Following trapezial and metacarpal drill holes, a distal and radially based strip of the ECRB is sequentially passed:

1. The ECRB tendon is passed from ulnar hole to palmar hole at the base of the first metacarpal.
2. The tendon is passed from the palmar to dorsal direction through the trapezium tunnel after traversing the palmar aspect of the CMC joint.
3. The tendon is passed along the dorsal surface of the CMC joint, and passed from dorsal through the radial hole of the thumb metacarpal.
4. The tendon is then sutured to itself on the dorsal surface of the trapezium using 2-0 nonabsorbable suture. The authors did not include transarticular pinning in this report.

Appropriate tensioning of these described ligament reconstructions remains challenging. Reconstructions performed

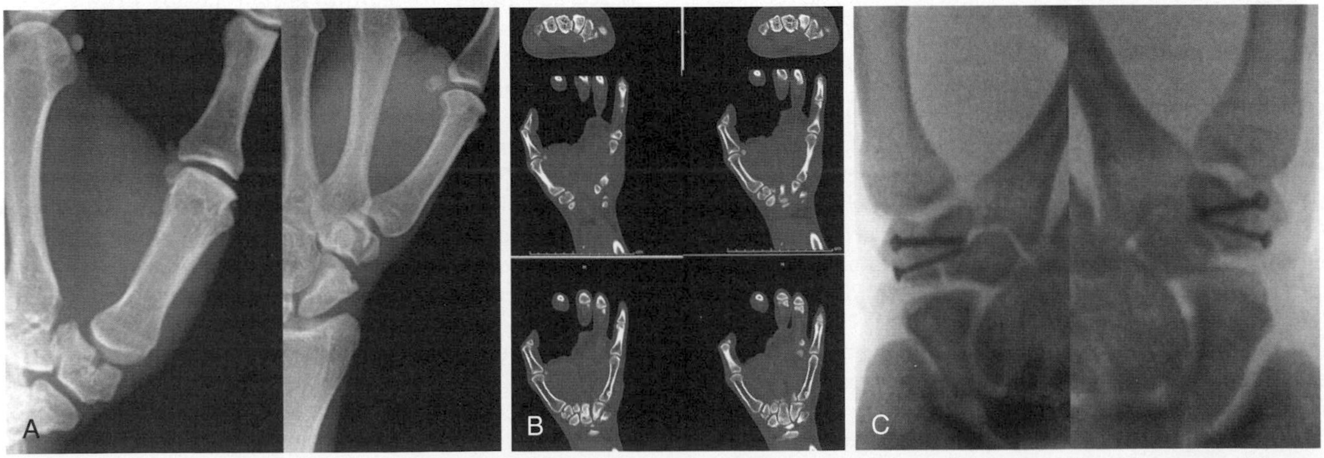

Figure 42-12. A, Isolated trapezial body fracture. **B,** Computed tomography (CT) scan demonstrating plane of major fracture line. **C,** Open reduction and internal fixation (ORIF) with modular hand screws.

too tautly will limit CMC motion and may predispose to early arthrosis. Laxity in the reconstruction will result in persistent laxity and dysfunction.

Outcomes

Only a single retrospective clinical series (level IV evidence) reported by Simonian and Trumble[18] compared available treatment options for traumatic dislocation of the thumb CMC joint. Four of eight patients treated with closed reduction and pinning had unsatisfactory results, and three required revision surgery for recurrent instability. In the nine patients treated with early (i.e., mean 7 days following injury) open reduction and FCR ligament reconstruction, improved clinical, functional, and radiographic outcomes were reported at a minimum year follow-up. These authors concluded that early ligament reconstruction following traumatic dislocation decreases the incidences of recurrent instability and symptomatic posttraumatic arthrosis. Fontes' results also support the role for acute ligament reconstruction.[19]

Sequelae

Despite reduction and stabilization of the CMC joint, patients are counseled about the potential for stiffness, recurrent instability, incomplete restoration of pinch and grip strength, and posttraumatic arthrosis.

Future Directions

Level I randomized controlled trials assessing available treatments are needed to elucidate an optimal treatment strategy for these injuries in order to maximize functional and radiographic outcomes. Multicenter collaboration would help achieve this goal given the low incidence of these injuries.

Thumb Metacarpophalangeal Collateral Ligament Injuries

Regional Anatomy

The thumb MCP joint is diarthrodial, with a dominant sagittal plane arc of motion (i.e., flexion/extension). The magnitude of thumb MCP motion is highly variable and dependent on the morphology of the metacarpal head.[20,21] Compared with the finger metacarpals, the thumb metacarpal head is less spherical and its cartilage is wider but more limited on the dorsal aspect.

Thumb MCP joint stability in pinch and grasp is derived from the osseous and soft tissue dynamic and static stabilizers. The sesamoids are embedded in the lateral margins of the volar plate and incorporate the tendinous insertions of the FPB radially and the adductor pollicis ulnarly. The tendinous and aponeurotic insertions are stout on the ulnar aspect of the joint, where the adductor pollicis myotendinous junction spans the ulnar sesamoid, volar plate, and extensor pollicis longus (EPL). The extrinsic myotendinous units providing dynamic stability include the EPL, extensor pollicis brevis (EPB), and flexor pollicis longus. The intrinsic stabilizers include the abductor pollicis brevis (APB), FPB, and adductor pollicis. The ulnar collateral ligament (UCL) and radial collateral ligament (RCL) each consist of a proper (dorsal) and accessory (volar) collateral ligament. The proper component originates from the middle of the collateral recess and continues to the proximal volar aspect of the proximal phalanx. The accessory collateral is contiguous with the proper and attaches to the phalanx and volar plate at the critical corner. On average, the center of the origin of the UCL is 3 mm from the dorsal border of the metacarpal head, and 7 mm from the joint. The insertion is a mean 3 mm from the joint, and 3 mm from the palmar border.[22]

In flexion, both proper collateral ligaments are taut and confer lateral stability in the presence of coronal plane stresses. In extension, both accessory collateral ligaments and the volar plate are taut. Therefore, in the setting of suspected collateral ligament injuries, the MCP joint is examined in terminal extension and 30 degrees of flexion to ascertain the injured portion of the collateral complex, and to distinguish partial and complete tears. The dorsal capsule together with the collateral ligaments resists the net volar moment on the MCP joint created by flexor pollicis longus and thenar intrinsics.[23]

While the majority of UCL tears are distal, Coyle[24] confirmed that the RCL tear site is more variable with proximal tears in 55%, distal tears in 29%, and midsubstance tears in 16% in his large cohort.

Examination

Injury to the collateral ligaments are caused by an acute, forceful coronal plane stress. Following acute injuries, tenderness over the collateral ligament and dorsal capsule, swelling, and ecchymosis are often present in combination with decreased motion. Chronic complaints include deformity and loss of pinch strength. The MCP joint may rest with appreciable coronal plane deviation of the proximal phalanx away from the incompetent collateral ligament, and is more commonly seen following complete RCL injuries. A palpable, tender mass on the ulnar side is pathognomic of a Stener lesion,[25,26] the displaced distal end of the UCL lying above the proximal edge of the adductor aponeurosis (Fig. 42-13). In a prospective study of 24 consecutive patients with posttraumatic instability of the thumb MCP joint, Abrahamsson and colleagues[27] confirmed that the presence of discrete soft tissue prominence at the level of the UCL predicted a Stener lesion in seven of eight thumbs and was an indication for surgical exploration. RCL injuries present with pain with ulnar stress on the thumb MCP joint, and when complete, are more often associated with sagittal, coronal, and rotatory instability.[28]

Examination aims to determine whether the injury is incomplete (grade 1 or 2) or complete (grade 3). Grade 1 injury is a sprain with no joint instability. Grade 2 is an incomplete tear with asymmetric joint laxity, in which instability does not meet the criteria for a complete tear. Grade 3 injury involves complete tear with joint instability.

Criteria for diagnosis of grade 3 collateral ligament injuries vary. In a clinical study (level II evidence), Heyman and colleagues[26] determined that the presence of valgus instability of more than 35 degrees with the joint in extension and 30 degrees of flexion was predictive of a complete UCL tear. A Stener lesion was present in 15 of 17 cases. The diagnostic characteristics of these examination findings included sensitivity, 94%; specificity, 57%; accuracy, 83%; positive predictive value, 83%; and negative predictive value, 80%. Bowers and Hurst (level III evidence)[29] demonstrated that preoperative stress angulation greater than 30 degrees was predictive of a complete rupture of the UCL noted intraoperatively. An alternative criterion for instability is relative opening of greater than 10 to 15 degrees compared with the contralateral side with the MCP joint in extension and 30 degrees of flexion. However, in a study of 100 asymptomatic persons, a variation of greater than 10 degrees

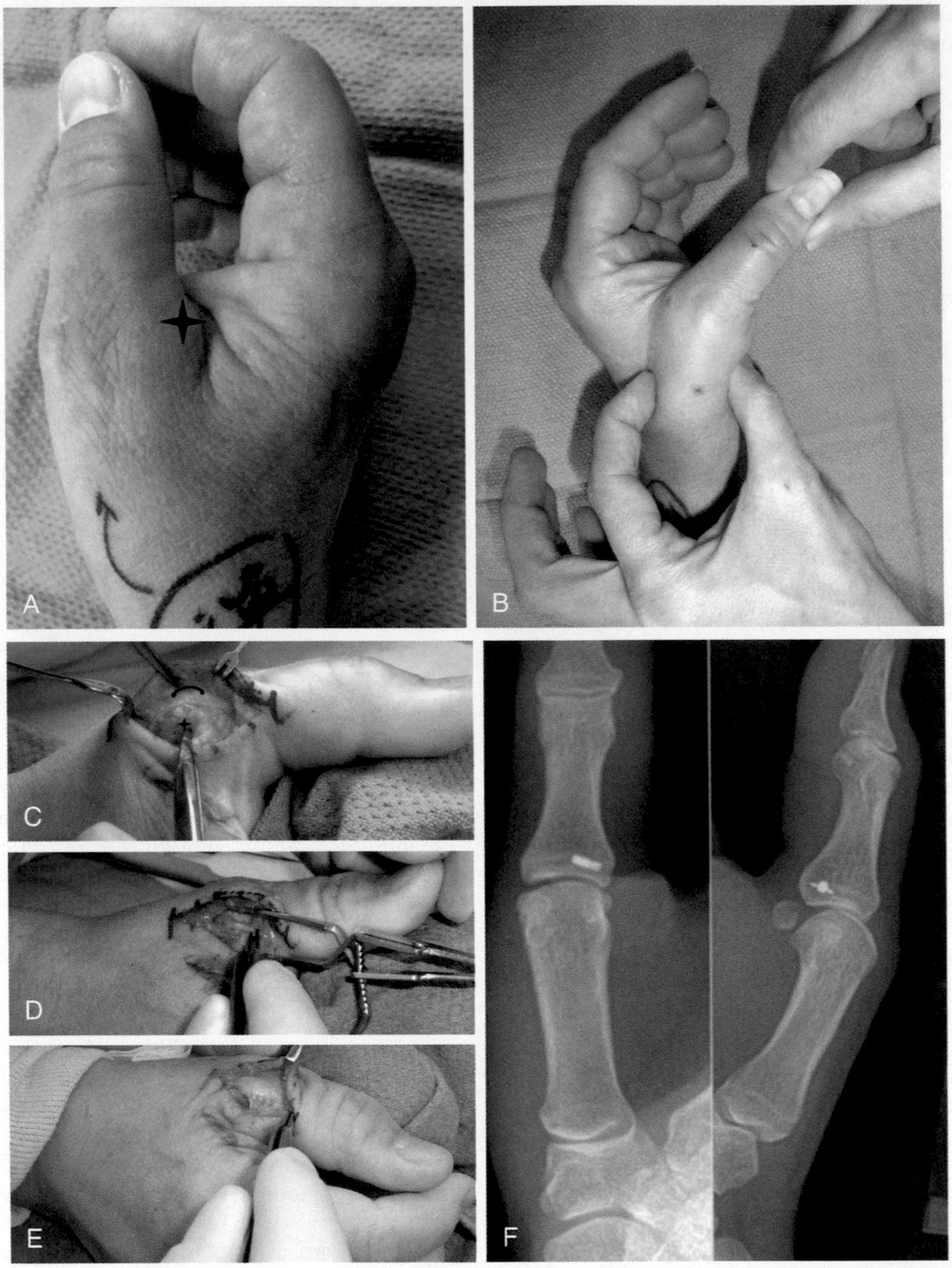

Figure 42-13. A, Thumb metacarpophalangeal (MCP) ulnar collateral ligament (UCL) avulsion with underlying Stener lesion. The *asterisk* overlies the clinically apparent soft tissue prominence overlying the adductor aponeurosis. **B,** Stress examination demonstrates instability of the UCL complex with loss of end point. **C,** Stener lesion defined by the distal UCL avulsion with the terminal end of the collateral ligament lying above the leading edge of the adductor aponeurosis. The dorsal-ulnar sensory branch of the radial sensory nerve is identified and protected. **D,** Following division of the adductor aponeurosis and mobilization of the UCL, the terminal portion of the collateral ligament can be reapproximated to its insertional footprint. **E,** Anatomic repair of the adductor aponeurosis following primary repair of the UCL. **F,** Primary repair completed with nonabsorbable suture anchors placed at the anatomic footprint of the UCL insertion in the volar-ulnar quadrant at the base of the proximal phalanx.

was found between their uninjured thumbs. Testing the MCP joint in extension may be more reliable as testing in flexion may yield a false-positive grade 3 diagnosis due to rotation of the metacarpal. Lack of a firm end point rather than degree of angulation between thumbs is most frequently used to determine the presence of complete collateral ligament ruptures. If guarding by the patient precludes an accurate stress examination, local anesthetic (i.e., intraarticular or digital block) may be used to improve the diagnostic accuracy.[30]

A dedicated radiographic series of the thumb is performed prior to stress examination to assess for a collateral ligament avulsion fracture fragment. It is important to note that the location of the avulsion fracture does not always predict joint stability. Volar subluxation of the proximal phalanx is more common with complete RCL injuries than with UCL injuries.

Routine use of ultrasound and magnetic resonance imaging (MRI) in the setting of acute injuries is not recommended.

Three level I studies[31-33] investigating the efficacy of ultrasound in the diagnosis of complete UCL tears reported moderate mean diagnostic characteristics. No level I studies assessed the efficacy of MRI in diagnosing acute UCL injuries. Level III series[34,35] reported that MRI yields superior diagnostic capabilities. Only one study directly compared ultrasonography with MRI in the evaluation of UCL injuries, and found MRI to be superior with regard to sensitivity and specificity.[36] Dedicated extremity (wrist or digit) coils are preferred as they improve diagnostic resolution.[37]

Indications

Partial collateral ligament injuries (grade 1 or 2) may be treated nonoperatively with immobilization. Variety exists among hand surgeons with regard to type of immobilization. Options include long and short opponens splinting or casting with or without the interphalangeal joint included. Full-time immobilization is continued for approximately 4 weeks, followed by an additional 2 to 4 weeks during sport and while beginning active range of motion exercises. At 6 to 8 weeks, thenar cone strengthening is initiated based on resolution of tenderness along the collateral complex.

Indications for surgical repair of thumb collateral ligament tears include instability greater than 30 degrees, 15 degrees greater than the contralateral MCP joint, lack of an appreciable end point with stress examination in the coronal plane, palmar subluxation greater than 3 mm, or persistent pain after nonsurgical treatment. Nonoperative treatment of grade 3 UCL tears is not consistently successful.[38] Therefore, surgical repair of complete UCL tears with or without a Stener lesion is recommended. Treatment for grade 3 RCL tears is controversial, although more recent literature favors surgical fixation. Some authors[39-41] recommended casting for acute complete thumb RCL tears. The rationale[42] for nonsurgical treatment of grade 3 RCL tears is the lack of an analogous interposing abductor aponeurosis to prevent healing. However, a single case of a radially sided Stener-type lesion has been reported.[24] Recent literature supports surgical treatment of complete RCL tears.[24,43-45] The ulnar force vector of the EPL maintains ulnar deviation of the MCP joint following RCL tears and may allow the ligament to heal elongated. Patients with acute unstable UCL and RCL injuries may develop late symptomatic instability or possibly degenerative joint disease of the MCP joint.[43]

Controversy exists regarding optimal treatment of collateral ligament avulsion fractures. Satisfactory results may be obtained with nonoperative treatment when the joint is stable with stress examination.[46] When there is instability or the avulsion fragment is displaced and malrotated, surgical fixation or fragment excision and ligament advancement is recommended.[38]

Ligament reconstruction is indicated in a patient with symptomatic, chronic collateral ligament insufficiency when the thumb MCP joint is without arthrosis. If there is arthrosis present, arthrodesis is performed. Fixed instability of a chronically subluxated MCP joint which cannot be reduced without release of the RCL is a contraindication to graft reconstruction.

Surgical Exposures and Repair Techniques

Acute Ulnar Collateral Ligament Repairs. An apex volar chevron, lazy-S, or longitudinal midaxial skin incision centered over the ulnar aspect of the MCP joint may be used. The dorsal ulnar sensory branch of the radial sensory nerve is mobilized and protected. In the subacute setting, it may be scarred along the adductor aponeurosis and requires careful neurolysis. The proximal edge of the adductor aponeurosis is inspected for the presence of a Stener lesion. The adductor aponeurosis is incised 2 to 3 mm volar to the extensor pollicis longus and reflected volarward. The presence of a dorsal ulnar capsular tear is noted. A dorsal longitudinal arthrotomy is performed and the articular surfaces examined. Proximal, midsubstance, or distal rupture of the UCL is determined (see Fig. 42-13).

Suture anchor repair is most commonly performed for insertional ruptures or proximal ligamentous avulsions from the collateral recess.[47,48] Other techniques, including transosseous nonabsorbable suture, bone tunnels, and buttons, have been described. Biomechanical analyses have demonstrated that nonanatomic repair alters ultimate MCP motion.[22] The origin or insertional sites are cleared of organized hemarthrosis and fibrosis. Suture anchors are placed just distal or proximal to the articular surface. Horizontal mattress sutures are passed through the ends of the ligament for repair. If the ligament is broad and stout, it may accommodate a running locking suture repair. Occasionally, a second anchor, or double-loading the anchor eyelet with an additional nonabsorbable suture allows for a double-row horizontal mattress repair. Midsubstance tears are repaired with interrupted figure-of-8 or horizontal mattress sutures using nonabsorbable braided synthetic suture. In some scenarios, primary repair of acute midsubstance rupture is not possible, and acute primary graft reconstruction may be needed.

At the completion of the repair, an absorbable suture loaded on an "UCL needle" can be placed between the distal volar portion of the repaired ligament and the volar plate to restore the critical corner of the three-dimensional ligamentous complex. The dorsal capsular tear is repaired, especially in the setting of preoperative joint subluxation. K-wire transarticular pinning is not routinely performed. Its use varies among hand surgeons and is a current topic of study among the membership of the American Society of Surgery of the Hand. Following ligament repair, the adductor aponeurosis is repaired anatomically with 4-0 nonabsorbable suture. The thumb MCP joint is typically immobilized in a thumb spica cast for 4 to 6 weeks postoperatively. Inclusion of the interphalangeal (IP) joint varies among hand surgeons. We favor exclusion of the IP joint so that the patient may begin IP motion to minimize adhesions along the EPL. A short opponens splint is worn for an additional 2 to 4 weeks in between range of motion exercises. Pinch strengthening is initiated at approximately 10 weeks postoperatively.

Chronic Ulnar Collateral Ligament Reconstructions. Most commonly, chronic thumb MCP UCL insufficiency is treated with a static reconstruction using free tendon graft reconstruction (Fig. 42-14). Graft options include the palmaris longus, and in its absence, use of the extensor indicis proprius, strip of the ipsilateral FCR, bone-tendon grafts, and allografts. Satisfactory results have been reported by several groups.[23,49] Figure-of-eight,[50] rectangular,[51] and triangular[52,53] (apex distal or apex proximal) configurations have been described for static graft reconstructions. Bone tunnels are created using appropriately sized drill bits or a series of handheld gouges. The ends of the tendon graft are whipstitched

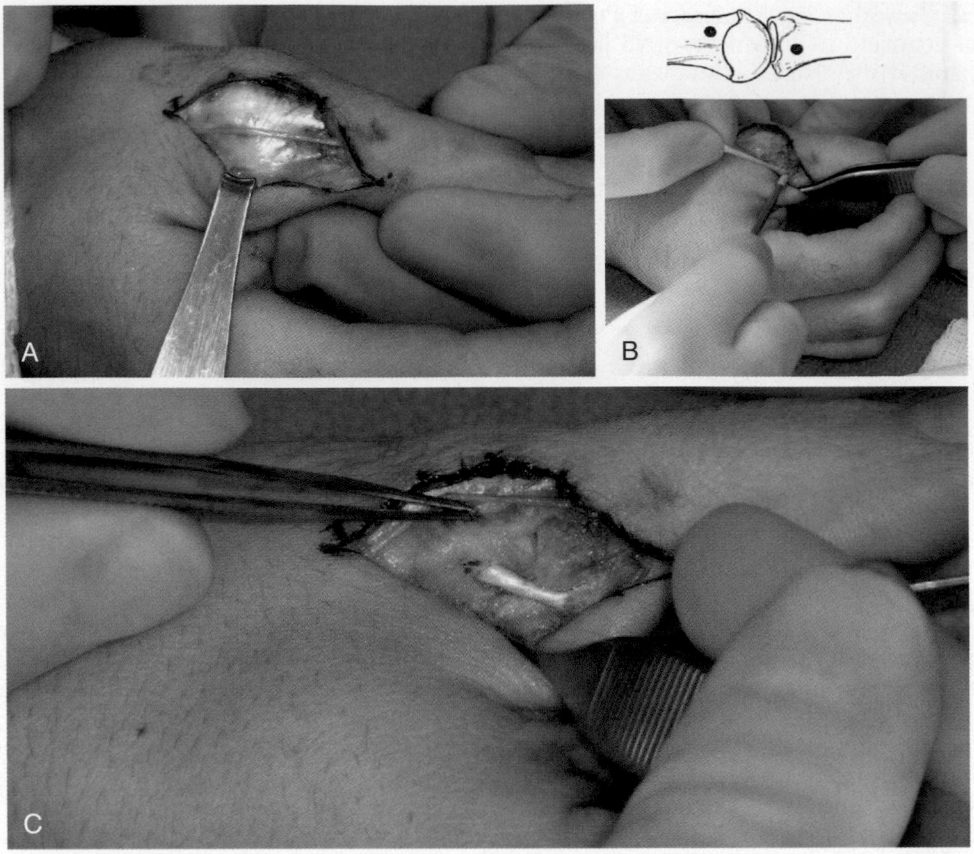

Figure 42-14. **A,** Chronic ulnar collateral ligament (UCL) insufficiency. The dorsal ulnar sensory branch of the radial sensory nerve is identified and protected as it runs along the adductor aponeurosis. **B,** Following division of the adductor aponeurosis and excision of the deficient UCL remnant, ipsilateral palmaris longus autograft reconstruction is performed with biotenodesis screw fixation. Distal fixation is performed first at the volar-ulnar base of the proximal phalanx. **C,** Proximal fixation is then performed.

with nonabsorbable suture and then shuttled through the transosseous tunnels using 28-gauge stainless steel wire. Multiple graft fixation options exist including transosseous nonabsorbable sutures tied over a bone bridge or button, graft ends sutured to each other over a bone bridge, aperture fixation using Bio-Tenodesis screws, and combinations of aperture fixation and suture anchors. Transarticular pinning is usually performed in the setting of graft reconstruction. Surgeon bias dictates whether the joint is transfixed before or after graft tensioning. The rationale for transfixion prior to graft tensioning is that joint position is first fixed and therefore, avoids overtightening the graft. Alternatively, tensioning can only be adjusted if performed prior to transfixion.

Dynamic stabilization with adductor advancement from the ulnar sesamoid to the proximal phalanx base was advocated by Nevasier and colleagues.[54] Success with dynamic tendon transfers using the extensor indicis proprius (EIP)[41] and extensor pollicis brevis (EPB)[55] have also been reported.

Acute Radial Collateral Ligament Repairs. Skin incision options for RCL repair mirror those for the UCL. Superficial branches of the radial nerve must be protected to avoid postoperative neuritis or painful neuromas. A longitudinal incision is made in the abductor aponeurosis volar to the EPB, leaving a rim of aponeurosis for closure. With the abductor aponeurosis retracted volarward, a dorsal-radial arthrotomy is performed and the RCL is examined. A decision is made as to whether to repair or reconstruct the ligament.

Acute ligament avulsions from the origin or insertion are repaired to their respective osseous footprints using one of many commercially available small bone anchors. At the volar radial base of the proximal phalanx, the anchor is placed in the volar half of the lateral tubercle 3 to 5 mm distal to the articular surface, and in the metacarpal head, the anchor is placed 1 to 2 mm dorsal to the central axis of the lateral condyle.[56] For midsubstance tears, one can attempt an end-to-end repair, but primary ligament reconstruction may be needed.[57] If the torn ligament is attenuated or cannot be advanced due to fibrosis, then a reconstruction is performed.

The dorsal-radial capsular tear is repaired, but care is taken to not overtighten the capsular closure to minimize loss of flexion.[43] When there is preoperative MCP joint volar subluxation, the MCP is transfixed with a 0.045-inch K-wire to protect the repair and neutralize the adductor pollicis.[24]

A short-arm thumb spica cast is worn for 4 to 6 weeks following surgery. The thumb IP joint is left free to minimize extensor tendon adhesions and IP joint contracture. Following pin removal, the patient is transitioned to a removable hand-based thumb splint for an additional 2 weeks during which thenar cone motion is initiated. Strengthening of the thenar muscles and pinch is begun at 3 months.

Chronic Radial Collateral Ligament Reconstructions. Treatment options for reconstruction of chronic radial instability include delayed primary ligament repair, abductor

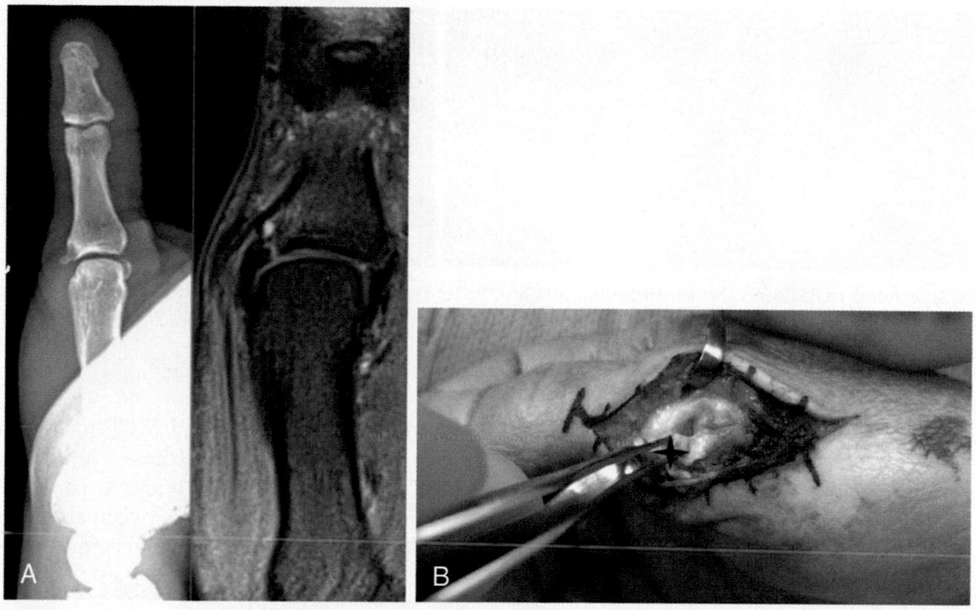

Figure 42-15. A, Symptomatic chronic radial collateral ligament (RCL) insufficiency secondary to nonunion of osseous avulsion at the RCL insertion. Preoperative magnetic resonance imaging (MRI) *(right panel)* confirms that the RCL insertion remains attached to the nonunited fragment. **B,** The nonunited fragment *(asterisk)* is excised and the ligament advanced and repaired with suture anchor technique.

advancement, and free tendon grafting (Fig. 42-15). Abductor advancement is similar to the adductor advancement technique described by Neviaser, and may be performed alone or in combination with repair or reefing of the RCL remnant and capsule. This represents dynamic reconstruction of a static restraint. Posner and Retaillaud[57] noted that ligament reconstruction using a tendon graft was necessary in 33% of cases with chronic RCL injury versus 69% of cases with chronic UCL injury.

When graft reconstruction is needed, the RCL remnants are excised and the proximal phalangeal subluxation and pronation is corrected in preparation for the transosseous tunnels in the proximal phalanx. The transosseous tunnels are created using appropriately sized drill bits or a series of handheld gouges. Free graft options include the palmaris longus, extensor indicus proprius, and a strip of the FCR. The orientation of the graft restores support of the dorsal capsule and the proper collateral ligament.[43] As discussed in UCL reconstruction, the graft may be tensioned before or following MCP K-wire transfixion. The graft tails may be tied together on the ulnar side or secured with suture anchors and/or Bio-Tenodesis screws. The dorsal limb of the reconstruction may limit MCP joint flexion if it is made too tight. The conjoined tendon of insertion of the APB and the radial head of the FPB can be tightened for additional stability.

Open Reduction and Internal Fixation of Collateral Ligament Avulsion Fracture. Collateral ligament avulsion fracture is not uncommon. Treatment depends on joint stability, as well as the size of the fragment. If the fragment is small (<10% to 15% of the articular surface), it may be excised, and the ligament advanced into the defect and secured with a pullout suture or anchor. If the fragment is large, it is reduced anatomically. Fixation constructs available include tension band suture or wire, K-wires, and one or more modular hand screws (Fig. 42-16). Displaced Salter-Harris

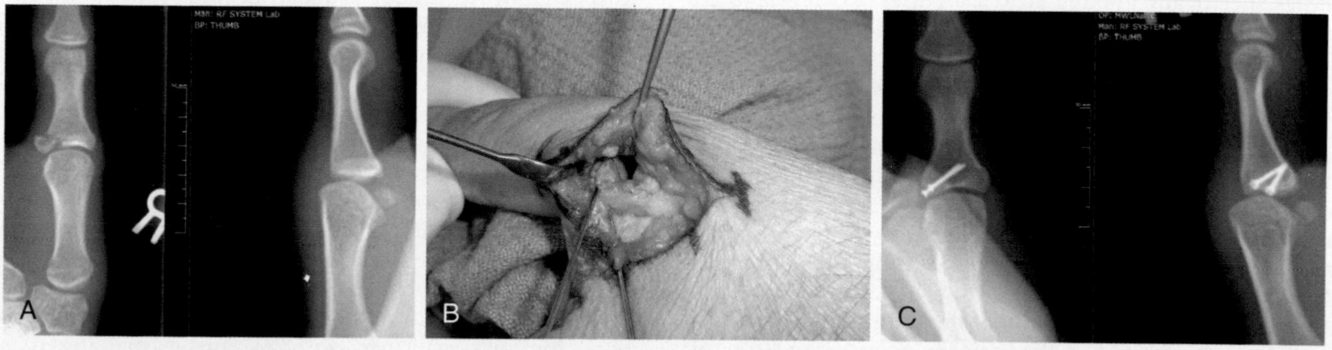

Figure 42-16. A, Displaced and malrotated ulnar collateral ligament (UCL) avulsion fracture. **B,** Open reduction and internal fixation (ORIF) is performed through the same surgical exposure as UCL repair. Intraoperative reduction is performed with preservation of the UCL insertion of the displaced fracture fragment. Anatomic reduction is directly visualized. Provisional fixation is performed with fracture fragment size-appropriate K-wires. **C,** The wires are then sequentially exchanged for modular hand screws.

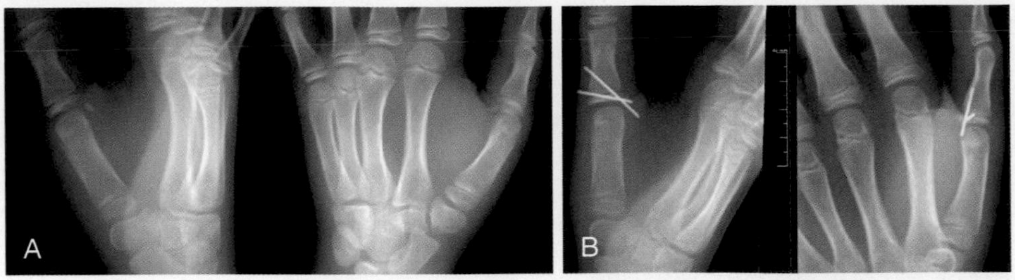

Figure 42-17. A, Displaced and malrotated thumb proximal phalanx Salter-Harris type III epiphyseal fracture. **B,** Open reduction and internal fixation (ORIF) with buried smooth K-wires is performed to restore physeal anatomy, ligamentous stability, and joint congruency.

type III epiphyseal fractures in the skeletally immature hand require ORIF to restore physeal anatomy, ligamentous stability, and joint congruency (Fig. 42-17).

Outcomes

Ulnar Collateral Ligament. Several cohort studies have shown that acute surgical treatment of complete UCL tears yields good to excellent results in 90% or more of cases.[23,45,48,58-60] Satisfactory results have also been reported following graft reconstruction.[23,49] Glickel[52] reported satisfactory results in 24 of 26 patients following free graft reconstructions, but results in the chronic setting have not been as uniform as in the acute repair setting.[61] Complications in both the acute and chronic setting include dorsal ulnar sensory nerve neurapraxia, stiffness, and persistent or recurrent instability.

Katolik and coworkers[47] reported improved range of motion and pinch strength following bone anchor repair compared to pullout suture techniques. Jarrett and colleagues[62] reported stronger resistance to 2-mm gap formation at the repair site when using newer PushLock suture anchors, but similar load to failures when compared to traditional suture anchors. In a cadaveric model, Harley and colleagues[63] suggested that a controlled active motion protocol following UCL repair with suture anchors may be safe from a biomechanical perspective.

Radial Collateral Ligament. Durham and colleagues[44] reported a 94% subjective satisfaction rate at a mean 6-year follow-up following repair and/or reconstruction of acute and chronic RCL injuries. The acute repair group had an 11% decrease in MCP joint motion, whereas the chronic cohort experienced a 23% loss of joint motion compared to the contralateral side. More recently, there have been several studies specifically looking at RCL injuries. Coyle[24] reported on a series of patients comprised of grade 3 RCL injuries (overall 89% late or chronic injuries) treated with RCL soft tissue sleeve advancement with bony reattachment treated at a mean of 10.8 months after injury. At a mean follow-up of 4 years, 87% were symptom free, 92% regained normal pinch and grip strength, and 79% had full MCP and IP joint motion. No recurrent symptomatic MCP joint instability was noted. Three patients (8%) had mild residual asymptomatic MCP joint volar subluxation. One patient had progression of preexisting degenerative joint changes. This suggests that acute and chronic grade 3 RCL instability of the thumb MCP joint can be successfully treated in the majority of cases by RCL soft tissue sleeve advancement and bony reattachment alone without the need for other soft tissue reinforcement. Reefing of the abductor may tether the MCP joint dorsal hood, limiting both IP and MCP joint motion. Catalano and colleagues[43] compared outcomes of acute repairs and reconstructions of grade 3 RCL tears. At latest follow-up, there were no important differences between the groups with regard to MCP or IP joint motion, grip or pinch strength, or MCP joint stability.

Future Directions

Larger cohorts with long-term follow-up are needed to assess the incidence of degenerative arthrosis following nonoperative and operative treatment of MCP joint collateral ligament injuries. Outcome differences between acute repairs and static and dynamic reconstructions will help define optimal treatment strategies. Repair techniques continue to evolve and may ultimately facilitate earlier postoperative functional rehabilitation. The role of MCP joint transfixion, and the type and duration of postoperative immobilization remain areas of study by the American Society for Surgery of the Hand.

The role and indications for arthroscopic-assisted ligament and fracture reduction and fixation in the MCP joint continue to expand. Ryu and Fagan[64] treated eight Stener lesions successfully by using MCP joint arthroscopy to reduce the ligament followed by joint transfixion. Rozmaryn and Wei[65] detailed the technical aspects of MCP joint arthroscopy for treating juxtaarticular and intraarticular fractures. Badia[66] reported encouraging results with arthroscopic-assisted reduction and internal fixation of bony UCL avulsion fractures.

Thumb Metacarpal-Phalangeal Joint Dislocations

The thumb MCP joint is similar to the MCP joints of the other fingers. However, unique articular geometry makes the MCP joint of the thumb more hingelike than multiaxial. Sesamoids lie anterior to the metacarpal head and are embedded in the volar plate. The FPB and APB muscles partially insert into the sesamoids. Collateral ligament anatomy in the thumb MCP joint is similar to the other digits.

The mechanism of dorsal dislocation is one of hyperextension, with resultant rupture of the volar plate, capsule, and at least a portion of the collateral ligaments. Rupture of the volar plate usually occurs proximally, but may be intrasubstance or distal to the sesamoids. Under local anesthetic or joint insufflation, closed reduction for dorsal dislocations of the thumb MCP joint is performed with the metacarpal flexed and adducted and then the MCP is hyperextended. Manual pressure is applied from dorsal to volar on the base of the proximal phalanx to translate the phalanx and its attached volar plate over the metacarpal head. Coronal and sagittal plane stability are then assessed clinically, and reduction is confirmed with dedicated radiographs of the thumb.

When there is grade 1 to 2 collateral laxity, a thumb spica cast is applied with the MCP joint in mild flexion, and the IP joint may be left free. Motion is initiated at 3 to 4 weeks. Some prefer dorsal block splinting in 10 degrees more flexion than the point of sagittal plane instability followed by weekly reduction of the dorsal block. If there is grade 3 collateral ligament rupture, operative repair or reconstruction is considered.

Closed reduction is more often successful in the thumb than the other fingers.[67,68] This phenomena may in part be due to the absence of a deep transverse intermetacarpal ligament in the thumb that may maintain the volar plate dorsally.

Irreducible dorsal dislocations in the thumb are often due to interposition of the volar plate, sesamoids, or flexor pollicis longus.[69,70] Irreducible dorsal thumb MCP dislocations are treated with open reduction through a dorsal exposure between the EPL and EPB. Open dorsal dislocations typically present with a volar wound, which is then extended to allow for débridement and open reduction. Volar plate repair can be performed through this volar exposure. In the subacute or chronic setting, a combined approach may be needed. Volar dislocations are rare, and more often require open reduction.

MCP stiffness is a common sequela of dislocation. Patients are counseled that recovery of motion can be slow, and that stability is more essential than full motion. Symptomatic chronic volar plate insufficiency is uncommon. When it occurs, reconstructive options include proximal advancement of the volar plate to the retrocondylar fossa and volar capsulodesis with suture anchor fixation and joint transfixion for 3 to 4 weeks; APB/FPB distal advancement along the volar-radial aspect of the proximal phalanx; and graft reconstructions for multidirectional instability.

METACARPAL FRACTURES (EXCLUDING THE THUMB)

Regional Anatomy

The metacarpals are structurally divided along their longitudinal axes into a *base, shaft, neck,* and *head.* The bases create the foundation and are approximately twice as wide as the shaft in the coronal plane. The congruent articulations and stout capsule-ligamentous condensations about the trapezoid, capitate, and corresponding index and long finger metacarpals are responsible for the relative rigidity in these CMC joints. In contrast, the sagittal plane mobility in the ring and small finger metacarpals allowing for power grip is derived from the modified saddle joint between the hamate articular facets and the corresponding bases of the ring and small finger metacarpals. The distal articular surface of the hamate contains two concave facets separated by a sagittal ridge. The base of the fifth metacarpal consists of a concave-convex facet that articulates with the hamate and a flat radial facet that articulates with the fourth metacarpal base. The ulnar CMC joints therefore not only accommodate a 20- to 30-degree flexion-extension arc, but also a slight rotatory motion that aids in allowing the small finger to contact the thumb. There is now expanding anatomic and kinematic data on the finger through small finger CMC joints. Viegas and colleagues[70] detailed the osseous anatomy of the CMC joints. Nakamura and colleagues[71] highlighted the ligamentous anatomy, which is reviewed in the following section. El-Shennawy and colleagues[72] elucidated the three-dimensional kinematics of the index through small finger CMC joints and their clinical relevance.

The metacarpals are tubular bones extending from the carpal arch to form the breadth of the hand. They extend distally with a dorsal convexity. Their coronal and sagittal plane geometry create the longitudinal and transverse arches of the hand. The sagittal plane bow and transverse arch must be understood and restored when performing percutaneous transmetacarpal pinning.

The concave palmar cortex is denser and experiences compressive loads with functional loading. Plating is usually performed dorsally along the tensile side of the metacarpals. The rigid central pillar projects through the index and long finger metacarpals. The thumb and ring and small finger metacarpals and their respective CMC joints form the mobile borders of the palm.

The metacarpal neck represents the transitional zone between the shaft and articular head. The metacarpal head represents a curve of increasing diameter from the dorsal to volar. Additionally, the articular head in the coronal plane is wider on the palmar aspect, creating a "pear-shape" to the head. The dorsal corridor of the metacarpal head is in line with the medullary canal, and this anatomic relationship has implications when performing percutaneous and open longitudinal intramedullary fixation of shaft and neck fractures.

The collateral ligaments originate dorsal to axis of MCP flexion from their respective radial and ulnar collateral recesses of the metacarpal head and insert broadly along the volar aspects of the proximal phalangeal base. Their eccentric origin and coronal and sagittal plane asymmetry of the head account for the collateral ligaments being more lax in extension and taut in flexion (i.e., cam effect) (Fig. 42-18). This phenomenon is the rationale for splinting of the MCP joints in flexion to minimize capsuloligamentous contracture and stiffness. Similar to the IP joints, there is a dorsal proper collateral and a more palmar accessory collateral ligament.

An understanding of the intricate extrinsic and intrinsic anatomy elucidates expectant osseous deformity following fracture, the impact of osseous deformity on myotendinous imbalance between the intrinsic and extrinsic systems, and surgical exposures at various levels along the longitudinal axis of the metacarpals. The dorsal and palmar interossei fill their corresponding intermetacarpal spaces. Isolated diaphyseal fractures may have inherent stability because of the origins of the dorsal and palmar interossei and the stabilizing effect of transverse intermetacarpal ligaments distally. The extrinsic flexor and extensor tendons contribute deforming forces. On the dorsal surface of the hand lie the extensor tendons of the fourth and fifth extensor compartments (i.e., extensor digitorum communis [EDC] of index through small fingers, extensor indicis proprius, and extensor digiti minimi). A potential subaponeurotic space exists between the undersurface of the extensor tendons and investing fascia of the dorsal interossei. Additionally, the radial wrist extensors of the second compartment (i.e., extensors carpi radialis longus and brevis) and the extensor carpi ulnaris of the sixth compartment insert at the base of the index, long, and small finger metacarpals, respectively, and may be deforming forces in fractures about these CMC joints.

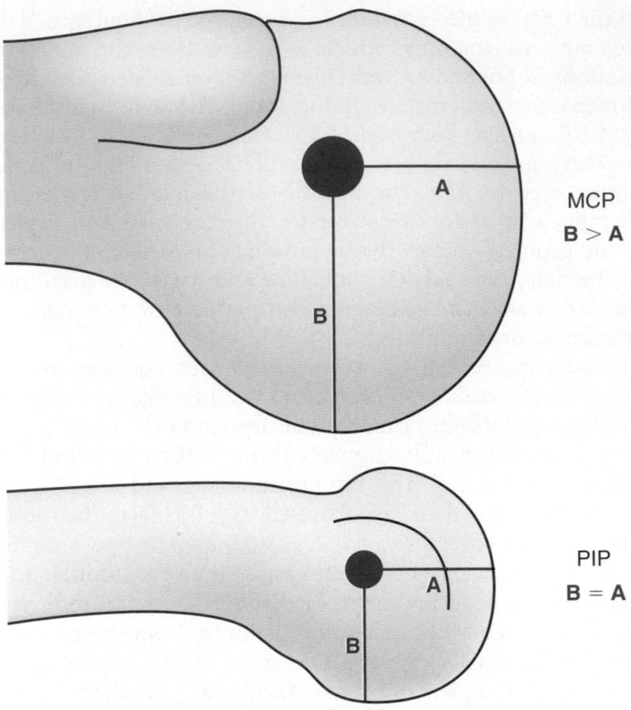

Figure 42-18. Metacarpophalangeal (MCP) joint collateral ligament anatomy: The collateral ligaments originate dorsal to the axis of MCP flexion from their respective radial and ulnar collateral recesses. Their eccentric origin and coronal and sagittal plane asymmetry of the head accounts for the collateral ligaments being more lax in extension and taut in flexion (i.e., cam effect). *PIP,* Proximal interphalangeal.

The communis tendons are joined distally near the MCP joints by fibrous interconnections, juncturae tendineae. The juncturae tendineae orientation changes during MCP joint motion. While the juncturae are oblique in MCP extension, they adopt a transverse orientation during MCP extension and contribute stability to the extensor hood. The extrinsic extensors join the dorsal aponeurosis at the level of the MCP joints. The radial and ulnar sagittal *bands* of the extrinsic system pass volarward from the extensors and insert onto the volar plate and volar base of the proximal phalanx and aid in MCP extension. The intimate association of the central extensor tendon and its articular fibers with the dorsal capsule at the level of the metacarpal neck and dorsal articular margin creates challenges during ORIF of metacarpal neck and subcapital fractures. Placement of fixation to the level of the articular margin can create extensor tendon adhesions and capsular contracture (Fig. 42-19).

The transverse and oblique *fibers* are located distal to the sagittal *bands,* and are part of the intrinsic system. They arise from the lateral bands and arch dorsally and aid in phalangeal flexion. The contributions to each lateral band by the volar and dorsal interossei (deep head) and lumbricals vary by finger. The interossei pass dorsal to the deep transverse metacarpal ligament, while the lumbricals pass volar. The intricate extrinsic and intrinsic extensor tendon anatomy responsible for IP joint extension is reviewed in the section on phalangeal fractures and IP joint injuries. For a detailed discussion of the intrinsic system of the hand, the reader is referred to the classic works of Emanuel Kaplan, MD,[73] and Richard J. Smith, MD.[74]

Examination

Examination of the hand reveals swelling and ecchymosis. Diaphyseal fractures typically present with apex dorsal deformity, which can be appreciated clinically. The soft tissue envelope is inspected for associated abrasions, lacerations, and fracture blisters. The cascade is examined with active motion if the patient can tolerate it, and with the tenodesis maneuver to assess for angular and rotational deformities. Combined injuries are examined for flexor and extensor function and associated neurovascular injuries.

A complete radiographic series of the hand includes PA, lateral, and oblique views. When involvement of the ring and small finger metacarpal bases and intraarticular extension to the CMC joints is suspected, an AP view with the forearm pronated 30 to 60 degrees from full supination is helpful in assessing joint congruity in this area.[75] CT scanning with coronal and sagittal plane reconstructions is helpful in assessing articular impaction, displacement, and subtle joint subluxation not readily visible on standard plain films. These criteria impact the decision for operative intervention. The Brewerton view[76] is obtained when evaluating metacarpal head fractures. CT scans for these articular fractures are also helpful. MRI is rarely indicated, except in select cases of collateral ligament avulsions.

Metacarpal Base and Carpometacarpal Fractures of the Digits

Over the last decade, clinical anatomic studies have provided a better understanding of the regional anatomy of the CMC joints and the associated pathomechanics of fracture-dislocations in this area. Viegas and colleagues,[70] followed by Nakamura and colleagues,[71] detailed the osseoligamentous details of the second through fifth CMC joints. Multiple dorsal and volar ligaments were identified. A single intraarticular ligament was identified between the third and fourth metacarpals and their capitohamate articulations. Multiple distinct facets forming the articulations between the metacarpal bases and the distal carpus were common. Five different articular subtypes were identified between the fourth metacarpal and the capitate and/or the hamate. El-Shennawy and colleagues[72] elucidated the three-dimensional kinematics of the index through small finger CMC joints and their clinical relevance.

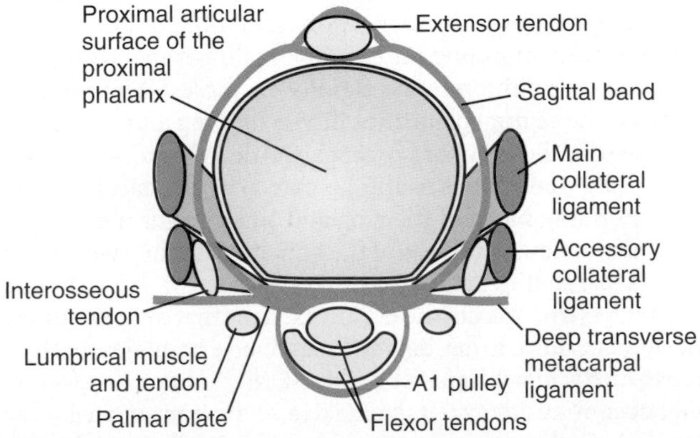

Figure 42-19. Extrinsic and intrinsic anatomy of the extensor hood at the level of the metacarpophalangeal (MCP) joint. *(Source: From Singh M, Singh R, Singh D: Sagittal bands: are they really sagittal? Internet J Hand Surg 2(1), 2008.)*

A fist blow (i.e., axial load) is the most commonly described mechanism of trauma resulting in a constellation of intraarticular CMC fractures, CMC dislocations, or fracture-dislocations. Cain and colleagues[77] proposed a classification of ulnar CMC fracture-dislocations. Type IA injuries included subluxation or dislocation of the small finger metacarpal base with dorsal CMC ligamentous disruption. Type IB injuries included a dorsal hamate fracture. Type II fracture-dislocations were defined by dorsal hamate comminution. A larger coronal plane fracture of the hamate comprised type III injuries. Similar to fractures at the base of the thumb metacarpal, these fractures can be conceptually divided into epibasilar, two-part (reverse Bennett), three-part, and comminuted with impaction.

Yoshida and colleagues[78] detailed the pathomechanics of ring and small finger CMC joint injuries using a custom jig for axial loading of 20 fresh-frozen cadaver upper extremities with the ring and small finger CMC joints fixed at 20 degrees and 30 degrees of flexion, respectively. The most common fractures were a dorsal capitate fracture and a middle metacarpal dorsal base fracture. The most common combinations of fractures were dorsal capitate and dorsal hamate fractures. Multiple fractures often were identified in a number of locations including dorsally: the capitate, hamate, and index through small metacarpal bases; and volarly: the hook of the hamate and the middle through the small metacarpal (MC) bases. Based on anatomic dissections, the patterns of injuries encountered at the ring and small CMC joints were explained by the direction and force of the applied load, position of the CMC joint at the time of loading, and the constraints imposed by specific CMC ligaments. These results highlight that ring and small CMC fracture-dislocations are a more complex combination of fractures than identified by plain radiographs alone. A combination of axial load and shear stresses creates variable carpal fractures and ligament avulsion fractures, as well as frank fracture-dislocations. This study, and our experience, suggests that CT with coronal and sagittal plane reconstructions is the preferred diagnostic imaging method for complete assessment of these injuries. CT identifies occult fractures, and allows assessment of articular impaction, displacement, and subtle joint subluxation not readily visible on standard plain films. Multiple CMC dislocations and fracture-dislocations represent high-energy injuries, and multiple combinations have been reported (i.e., convergent, divergent).

Indications

Extraarticular fractures of the base of the metacarpals are managed with similar principles to shaft fractures as reviewed later. There is little consensus on the optimal management of isolated CMC joint intraarticular base fractures, and the amount of acceptable joint impaction is not well defined. The rationale for operative reduction is based on the belief that anatomic joint reduction will optimize clinical, functional, and radiographic outcomes. In the absence of CMC joint instability (i.e., subluxation/dislocation), nonoperative treatment with splint immobilization followed by early motion is reasonable.[5,79] Restoration of articular congruency and reduction of coronal or sagittal plane joint subluxation either by closed reduction and percutaneous fixation or ORIF[80] is recommended (Fig. 42-20). When fracture-dislocation of the CMC joint is seen more than 10 to 14 days following the trauma, often open reduction is required. In chronic CMC dislocations, expectant management may be considered and salvage procedures (i.e., arthrodesis or interpositional arthroplasty) are performed for symptomatic arthrosis or pain. Other indications for open reduction and stabilization include delayed presentation, multiple CMC fractures-dislocations, and associated hamate coronal shear fractures.

Fracture-dislocations of the fifth CMC joint are inherently unstable, and closed reduction and casting is prone to recurrent instability and re-dislocation. If closed treatment is pursued, close serial radiographic follow-up is needed, but reliable imaging is challenging to achieve due to osseous overlap and plaster artifact. For these injuries, closed reduction and percutaneous pinning (CRPP) is preferred.

The fifth CMC joint is more commonly dislocated than the ring finger CMC joint. Pure dislocation of the small finger CMC joint has previously been reported as associated with an apparently isolated ring finger metacarpal shaft fracture.[81] The CMC joints should be examined carefully clinically and radiographically in the presence of adjacent metacarpal diaphyseal fractures.

Isolated intraarticular fractures of the base of the index and long finger metacarpals are rare because of the lack of motion at these CMC joints. These fractures are usually the result of a fall on a flexed wrist or a wrist-jamming injury resulting in dorsal avulsion fractures. Although most may be managed nonoperatively, surgical indications include reattachment of the extensor carpi radialis longus or brevis insertion,[82] restoration of the articular surface of the CMC joint, and excision of a fracture fragment that may cause attritional extensor tendon rupture.[83]

Fracture of a preexisting carpal boss is seen in high-level athletes and can often be managed nonoperatively in season with splint immobilization, lidocaine injections to facilitate return to play, and customized CMC boss splints that fit inside sport-specific gloves during competition. If they remain symptomatic, off-season surgery is scheduled with excision of the nonunited fragment with preservation of the radial wrist extensor insertion.

Surgical Exposures and Fixation Techniques

Extraarticular fractures of the metacarpal bases may be amendable to closed reduction and transarticular fixation into the carpus. Low-profile precontoured periarticular locking plates (2 to 2.4 mm) allow for rigid ORIF and early postoperative mobilization (see Fixed-Angle Constructs) (Fig. 42-21; see Video 42-1).

In reverse (baby) Bennett fractures,[84] approximately 25% to 30% of the radial base of the small finger metacarpal remains reduced to the hamate and ring finger. The deforming force of the extensor carpi ulnaris is responsible for the proximal dorsal-ulnar subluxation of the shaft and dorsal articular surface. Articular comminution and impaction are common. Closed reduction includes longitudinal traction of the small and ring fingers and volar-directed pressure to the dorsally subluxated base. If fluoroscopy confirms shaft reduction, percutaneous K-wire fixation is performed under fluoroscopic guidance. A transmetacarpal K-wire (0.054 or 0.045 inch) is placed above the metaphyseal flare of the small finger metacarpal and distal to any metaphyseal or impacted articular fragments. Additional cortical purchase can be obtained by advancing the K-wire into the long finger metacarpal. As discussed later, in transmetacarpal pinning for shaft and neck

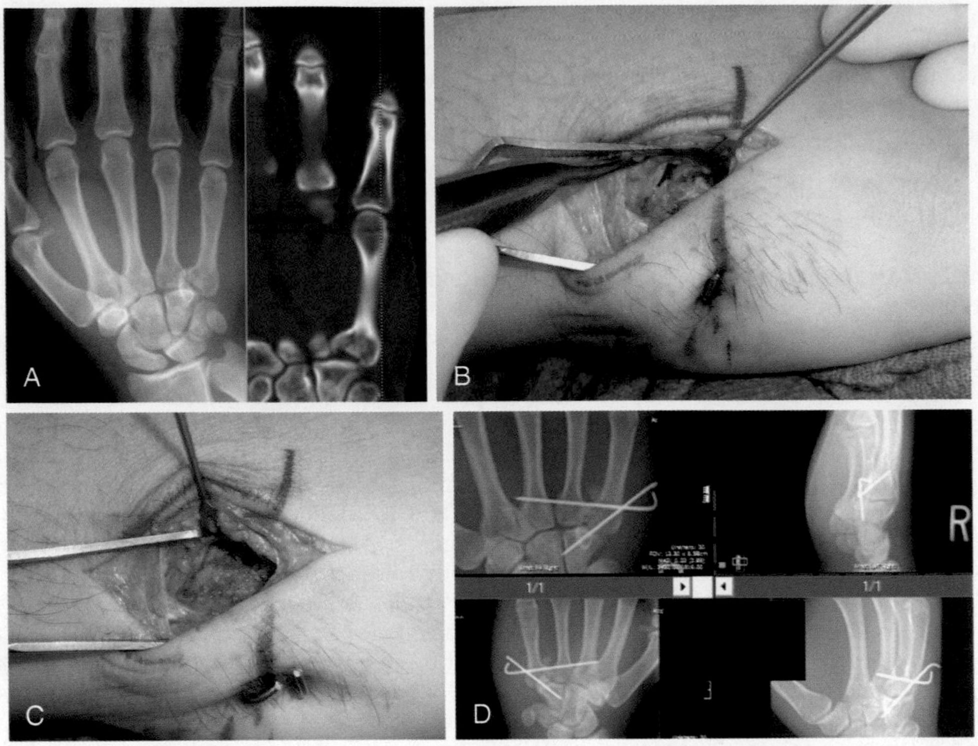

Figure 42-20. **A,** Small finger metacarpal base articular impaction fracture with associated carpometacarpal (CMC) subluxation as demonstrated on plain film. Preoperative computed tomography (CT) scan allows appreciation of the magnitude of articular impaction. **B,** Open reduction is performed after mobilization of the extensor digitorum communis (EDC) to the ring finger (radialward) and the EDQ (ulnarward) followed by dorsal arthrotomy. The subluxation is corrected and transmetacarpal pinning of the small finger to the adjacent ring/long finger metacarpals (4 to 6 cortices) is performed under fluoroscopic guidance distal to the zone of metaphyseal involvement. **C,** Thereafter, the articular impaction is reduced using the hamate as a template, followed by subchondral bone grafting. **D,** An additional oblique K-wire is placed from the small finger metacarpal metaphysis into the body of the hamate. Care is taken to not violate the volar cortex of the hamate in the region of the hook of hamate.

fractures, one must account for the concavity of the transverse metacarpal arch to ensure bicortical fixation in the ring and long fingers, respectively. A second more distal parallel transmetacarpal wire may be placed for additional stability. If a congruous articular reduction is obtained with the closed reduction maneuver, an oblique transarticular K-wire is advanced from a midaxial starting point at the metadiaphyseal junction of the small finger metacarpal into the body of the hamate. Saing and colleagues[85] demonstrated the close proximity of the deep motor branch of the ulnar nerve to the volar cortex of the hamate in a cadaveric study. Care is taken to confirm there is no violation of the volar cortex of the hamate or hook region using multiplanar fluoroscopy.

If the articular base of the small finger metacarpal remains impacted and incongruous, limited-open articular reduction is performed through a dorsal-ulnar incision centered over the CMC joint to reduce the articular impaction. The open reduction may be performed following shaft reduction and stabilization with a transmetacarpal wire (see Fig. 42-20). Branches of the dorsal sensory branch of the ulnar nerve are mobilized and protected. The EDC to the ring finger and the EDC to small finger and extensor digiti quinti (EDQ) are mobilized radialward and ulnarward, respectively. The traumatic arthrotomy is extended and the joint irrigated. The impacted articular segment(s) is reduced directly to the template of the hamate facet maintaining as much subchondral cancellous bone on the articular fragments as possible. The reduction is maintained with an oblique transarticular K-wire into the body of the hamate or modular screws if there is sufficient cortex available dorsally and volarly. The metaphyseal void is then filled with autograft (i.e., distal radius or olecranon), allograft cancellous bone chips, or commercially available bone graft substitutes. When ORIF is performed for cases of isolated articular impaction, the K-wires may be left outside the skin and removed between 4 and 6 weeks postoperatively. When there is associated joint subluxation or dislocation, we prefer to bury the K-wires and remove them at 8 weeks postoperatively. Supplemental casting is routinely used while the wires are in place. We favor immobilizing the MCP joints in the intrinsic plus position to minimize skin motion about the K-wire sites.

Extensive intraarticular comminution may preclude stable internal fixation. In these cases, intraoperative use of a small joint distractor during joint reduction, K-wire fixation, and bone grafting is helpful. The distractor may be left in place postoperatively or replaced with a static ulnar-based 1.6-mm mini external fixator with pin fixation in the hamate and small or ring finger metacarpals in order to off-load the CMC joints for 6 weeks. Alternatively, a joint-spanning locked fixed-angle plate and/or screw construct to create an "internal-external fixator" may be selected.[86] Following provisional joint reduction, the transarticular bridge plate is secured with screws in the carpus and metacarpal shaft. In the index or long finger CMC joints, the implant does not require routine removal

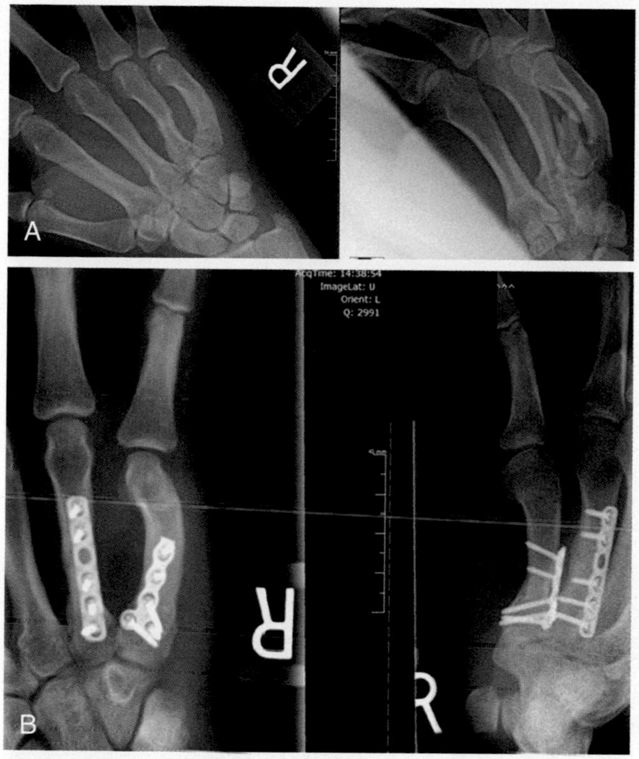

Figure 42-21. A, Widely displaced ring finger metacarpal shaft fracture and small finger epibasilar fractures. Note preexisting diaphyseal deformity in the small finger metacarpal. **B,** Open reduction and internal fixation (ORIF) is performed with 2 modular plate/screw system. A low-profile precontoured periarticular locking plate was used in the small finger for angular stable fixation in the small periarticular segment. Early functional rehabilitation resulted in restoration of full wrist and digital motion.

given the relatively fixed motion at these joints. In contrast, the implant is removed when placed across the mobile ulnar CMC joints.

ORIF through the described dorsal-ulnar approach is preferred when there is a large associated dorsal hamate shear fracture (Fig. 42-22). The dorsal CMC interosseous ligaments are carefully preserved on the dorsal hamate fracture fragment. If there is an associated capitate fracture, it must be reduced and stabilized prior to reduction of the hamate fracture. The ring and small finger metacarpal bases are reduced concurrently with the hamate shear fracture. Anatomic reduction and fixation of the fourth CMC joint typically results in spontaneous reduction of the fifth CMC joint. One to two transmetacarpal K-wires may be first placed from the ulnar border of the small finger metacarpal into the long finger metacarpal to neutralize the tendency of the metacarpal bases to redislocate during hamate fixation. The hamate shear fracture is fixed with bicortical modular hand screws, and screw lengths confirmed under fluoroscopy. We prefer to leave the transmetacarpal wires to neutralize dorsal shear forces on hamate fixation for 4 to 6 weeks.

For multifragmentary articular CMC fractures, primary arthrodesis may be considered, especially in the setting of open or complex injuries in which maximal stability postoperatively is desired to facilitate early functional hand rehabilitation. Primary arthrodesis is more readily considered in the index and long finger CMC joints given their inherent stiffness. Articular preservation of the ulnar CMC joints is attempted given the mobility of these joints.

Multiple CMC dislocations represent high-energy injuries. Closed reduction and percutaneous pinning to the carpus and/or ORIF through dorsal longitudinal incisions are performed as needed, as closed reduction alone is not reliable with these injury patterns.[87] Reduction of multiple CMC fracture-dislocations begins with the "keystone" third CMC joint.

Outcomes

Petrie and Lamb[79] treated 14 fracture-dislocations of the fifth CMC joint with immediate motion. Despite metacarpal shortening and articular incongruity at 4.5 years following injury, only one patient reported pain-limiting function. Lundeen and Shin[88] reported good-to-excellent results in 20 of 22 patients treated with closed reduction and cast immobilization for intraarticular fractures of the base of the fifth metacarpal at a mean 3.5 years following injury. In this retrospective study (level IV evidence), fracture type, degree of subluxation or articular step-off, or the presence of arthrosis did not influence clinical outcome. At latest follow up, there was no evidence of CMC arthrosis in 13 patients, and 9 demonstrated mild arthrosis. Kjaer-Petersen and colleagues[5] reported that regardless of the method of treatment (closed, percutaneous, or open), 19 of 50 (38%) patients reported intermittent pain with grip at a median follow-up of 4.3 years.

In contrast, Bora and Didizian[75] believed that loss of grip strength was due to residual CMC malreduction, and recommended percutaneous fixation. Goedkoop and colleagues[89] recommend reduction and stabilization of reverse (baby) Bennett fractures to minimize pain, reduced grip strength, and posttraumatic arthrosis. Papaloizos and colleagues[90] reported that pain following osteosynthesis of fractures at the base of the small finger metacarpal correlated with the presence of degenerative changes.

Combined ring–small finger CMC fracture-dislocations have been treated successfully with both closed reduction and K-wire fixation and formal ORIF. Schortinghuis and Klasen[91] reported success with temporary bridge plating of combined ring and small finger CMC fracture-dislocations. Complex divergent CMC fracture-dislocations are exceedingly rare, and may require a combination of techniques.[92,93]

Wharton and colleagues[94] reported superior functional and radiographic outcomes following rigid internal fixation of coronal plane hamate fractures associated with CMC subluxation as compared to K-wire fixation.

Prokuski and Eglseder[95] reported satisfactory results in 12 patients following ORIF with K-wires of multiple dorsal dislocations and fracture-dislocations of the index through small finger CMC joints. Three patients underwent staged planned secondary index and long finger CMC arthrodesis. Delay of ORIF up to 4 weeks did not adversely affect results.

Sequelae

Symptomatic posttraumatic arthrosis of the ulnar CMC joints has been reported as a sequela of these injuries. Clendenin and Smith[96] reported symptom relief with arthrodesis of the hamate–small finger CMC joint when using an iliac crest inlay bone graft. Arthrodesis may be performed using K-wires

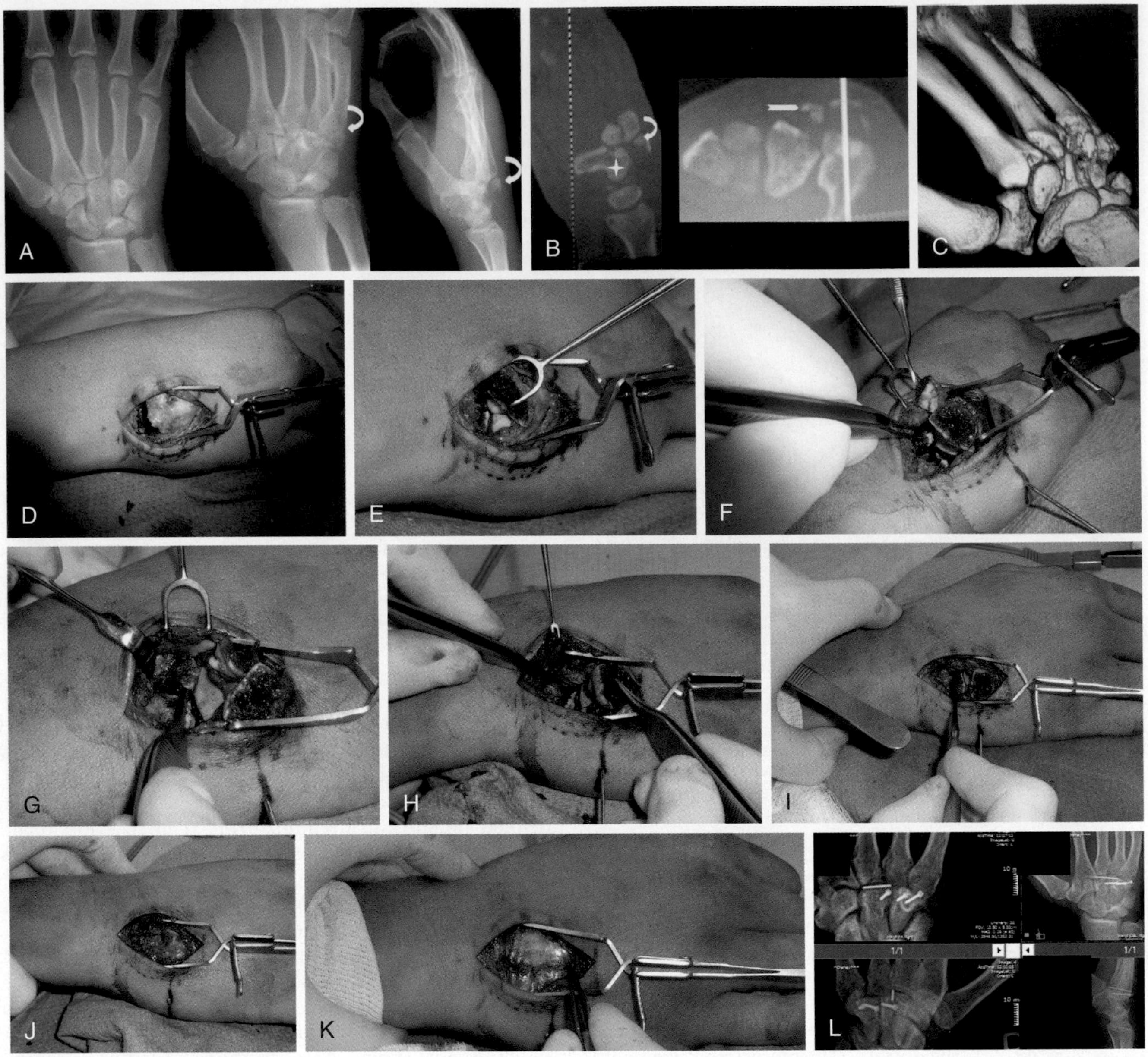

Figure 42-22. A, Ring and small finger complex carpometacarpal (CMC) fracture-dislocation with associated dorsal hamate coronal shear fracture *(arrows)*. **B,** Preoperative computed tomography (CT) scan demonstrates the large hamate shear fracture *(left panel, curved arrow),* the central hamate articular impaction *(left panel, asterisk),* and the concomitant articular capitate fracture *(right panel, chevron)* involving the capitohamate articulation and the capitate–ring finger articular facet. **C,** Three-dimensional (3-D) computed tomography (CT) reconstruction of the complex CMC injury. **D,** Open reduction and internal fixation (ORIF) through a dorsal exposure is performed. The dorsal CMC interosseous ligaments are carefully preserved on the dorsal hamate fracture fragment. **E,** Fracture reduction then proceeds by working through the dorsal hamate shear fracture. The dorsal hamate shear fracture is carefully reflected to appreciate the dorsally dislocated ring and small finger metacarpal bases and the articular impaction in the central portion of the hamate. **F,** The dorsally dislocated ring and small finger metacarpal bases are first reduced and held with a transmetacarpal K-wire. Note the associated comminuted articular capitate fracture fragments. **G,** In this case, the capitate fracture fragments are first reduced and stabilized prior to reduction of the hamate fracture. The intercalary capitate head fracture is fixed with an intraosseous K-wire cut flush with cancellous surface. **H,** The remainder of the ulnar aspect of the capitate head (at the capitohamate articulation and the capitate-ring finger articular facet) is then reduced and fixed with a modular hand screw. **I,** The central hamate articular impaction is elevated followed by subchondral bone grafting, using the bases of the ring and small finger metacarpals as templates. **J,** The dorsal hamate shear fracture is then reduced and stabilized with two additional modular hand screws. One to two transmetacarpal K-wires are placed from the ulnar border of the small finger metacarpal into the long finger metacarpal to neutralize hamate fixation and dorsal shear forces on hamate fixation. **K,** Retinacular closure following ORIF. **L,** Final radiographs demonstrating anatomic reduction of the CMC joints and the capitate and dorsal hamate shear fractures.

or plate and screw constructs. Gainor and colleagues[97] used tendon interpositional arthroplasty to address posttraumatic arthritis of the ulnar CMC joints. At 5-year follow-up, motion preservation and a mean 30% increase in grip strength was reported.

Following multiple CMC fracture-dislocations, patients are counseled regarding the potential for autofusion and the requirement for secondary surgical arthrodesis for symptomatic posttraumatic arthrosis.

Future Directions

The series reporting outcomes following articular fractures at the CMC joints are limited to retrospective cohorts (level IV evidence) without use of accepted outcome measures of hand and wrist function. Additionally, the magnitudes of articular impaction, diastasis, and subluxation present were not uniformly detailed. Instruments that capture subtle deviation from normal hand function will aid in defining best practice for these fractures. Larger randomized clinical series are needed to determine the magnitude of articular incongruity and subluxation that impact long-term clinical, functional, and radiographic outcomes. The role of arthroscopic-assisted reduction and fixation of ulnar CMC fracture-dislocations may continue to expand.[98]

Metacarpal Shaft Fractures

Indications

Metacarpal diaphyseal fractures can be broadly classified as transverse, oblique, spiral, and comminuted. Central *transverse diaphyseal fractures* may remain minimally displaced or nondisplaced secondary to the adjacent interossei and proximal and distal interosseous ligaments. Apex dorsal deformity with volar angulation is secondary to the deforming forces of the interossei and commonly seen in the border metacarpals. Increased volar angulation can create myotendinous imbalance, compensatory MCP joint hyperextension, and decreased proximal interphalangeal (PIP) extension. The mobility of the ring and small finger CMC joints facilitates functional compensation for some sagittal plane deformity in contrast to the fixed CMC joints of the index and long fingers. For diaphyseal fractures in the ring and small fingers, greater than 20 to 30 degrees of apex dorsal deformity warrants reduction and stabilization. Angular deformity greater than 10 degrees in the index and long metacarpals is corrected.

Oblique fractures tend to shorten. Shortening of 2 to 3 mm is usually well tolerated so long as there is no associated rotational or angular deformity. Strauch and colleagues[99] suggested that 2 mm of shortening would result in a 7-degree extensor lag. The functional effect in the clinical setting is unclear, so absolute indications for surgical fixation based on shortening alone do not exist. Spiral fractures secondary to torsional stress malrotate. Minor degrees of diaphyseal malrotation may have significant effect on the digital cascade. Royle[100] demonstrated that as little as 10 degrees of malrotation can lead to 2 cm of fingertip overlap. Rotation is best assessed during digital flexion, and angulation during extension. Correction of malrotation and angular deformity is recommended.

Additional indications for operative fixation include multiple metacarpal fractures, comminuted and segmental fractures, open fractures, concomitant extremity fractures and polytrauma, and combined injuries.

Nonoperative Treatment

Isolated, minimally displaced metacarpal fractures without rotational or angular deformity may be treated in a cast or custom rigid orthosis with the wrist in 30 to 40 degrees of extension and the MCPs in intrinsic plus (80 to 90 degrees of flexion) for 3 to 4 weeks. When a central metacarpal is involved, we routinely include all four digits. For proximal diaphyseal fractures, one may choose to leave the MCP joints free on a case-by-case basis. Close serial radiographic follow-up is recommended to assess for interval displacement.

Surgical Exposures and Fixation Techniques

Optimal surgical fixation of metacarpal shaft and neck fractures will limit surgical exposure of the fracture site, allow for early postoperative mobilization to regain full MCP joint motion and extensor excursion,[101] expedite return to activities of daily living and work or sport, and minimize the need for removal of hardware and other secondary procedures.

Various percutaneous and open fixation techniques[102-105] have been described for the reduction and stabilization of displaced, malrotated, and significantly angulated metacarpal shaft fractures. Each technique has its own inherent advantages and disadvantages. Selection of technique is often based on fracture characteristics and surgeon preference.

Although percutaneous K-wire techniques limit soft tissue dissection, 3 to 4 weeks of postoperative immobilization is required to minimize the risk of superficial and deep pin tract infections that can necessitate early K-wire removal and additional procedures. Formal ORIF may achieve rigid fixation and facilitate early postoperative functional rehabilitation, but complications are well described.[106,107]

Closed Reduction and Percutaneous Techniques

Transmetacarpal Pinning. Transmetacarpal pinning is indicated for isolated mid or distal diaphyseal transverse metacarpal fractures of the border digits amendable to closed reduction. Under fluoroscopic guidance, 0.054- or 0.045-inch K-wires are sequentially placed and advanced from the fractured border metacarpal into the adjacent intact metacarpal. Appreciation for the transverse arch of the palm and the dorsal bow of the metacarpals is necessary to successfully obtain four cortices of fixation with each K-wire. One to two K-wires are placed proximal and distal to the fracture site (Fig. 42-23).

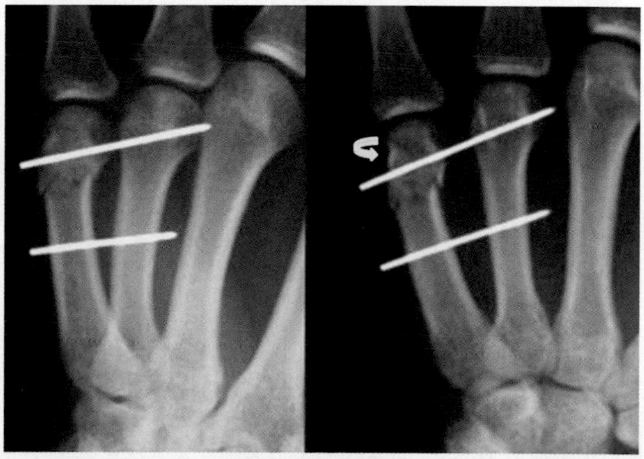

Figure 42-23. Closed reduction and percutaneous pinning (CRPP) with transmetacarpal technique. Care is taken to avoid the collateral recesses *(arrow)*.

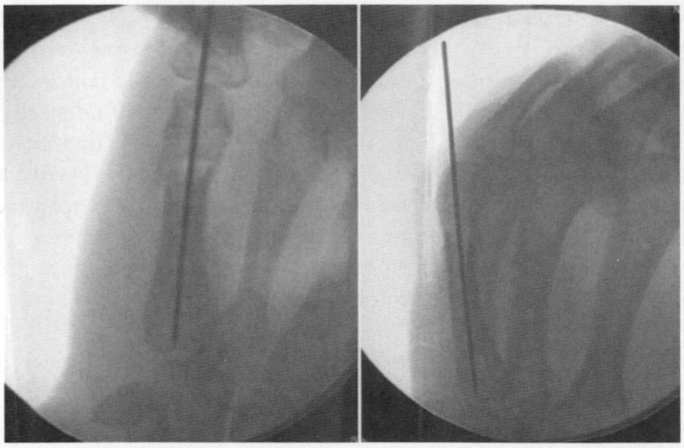

Figure 42-24. Closed reduction and percutaneous pinning (CRPP) of distal metacarpal shaft and neck fracture with retrograde longitudinal intramedullary fixation.

Bending stiffness of this construct approaches that of a plate and screw construct.[108] Care is taken to ensure adequate distance is left between the K-wires on each side of the fracture site when more than one is placed. Although this is an acceptable technique for distal shaft and neck fractures, the collateral recesses should not be violated with the distal wire. Incarceration of the collaterals creates ligament and capsular contracture, and risks intraarticular sepsis if a superficial pin tract infection occurs. As with all percutaneous techniques, the K-wires may be cut and buried beneath the skin or left protruding through the skin where the tip is bent. Supplemental postoperative casting is used for 3 to 4 weeks.

RETROGRADE TECHNIQUES

RETROGRADE LONGITUDINAL INTRAMEDULLARY FIXATION. A single 0.062- or 0.054-inch K-wire may be advanced in a retrograde fashion through the metacarpal head following closed reduction. The MCP joint is maximally flexed, and with the reduction maintained, the wire is advanced under fluoroscopic control down the intramedullary canal, across the fracture site, and obtains purchase in metaphysial subchondral bone (Fig. 42-24). While this technique is straight forward, it too, requires several weeks of postoperative immobilization.

Given the articular starting point, there is a risk of deep sepsis (i.e., septic arthritis, osteomyelitis) if a superficial pin tract infection occurs. Alternatively, the K-wire can be advanced with the wrist flexed until it exits proximally through the base of the metacarpal or CMC joint, and then it is withdrawn until the distal portion of the wire lies in the subchondral zone of the metacarpal head. The proximal end is cut beneath the skin. While this modification avoids leaving the wire at the MCP joint, its presence proximally can cause irritation of the adjacent extensor tendons.

RETROGRADE CROSSED PINNING. For distal shaft and neck fractures, retrograde crossed pinning has been described. K-wires are placed radial and ulnar to the extensor and advanced either into the intramedullary canal or obliquely to obtain bicortical purchase in the diaphysis proximal to the fracture line (Fig. 42-25). Care again is taken to avoid the collateral recess if possible. Inherent disadvantages with this technique are similar to those with longitudinal intramedullary K-wire fixation.

RETROGRADE LIMITED-OPEN INTRAMEDULLARY HEADLESS SCREW FIXATION. Intramedullary headless screw fixation of subcapital and metacarpal neck fractures has previously been described.[109,110] Retrograde intramedullary fixation using a cannulated headless screw can be achieved using a limited-open extensor-splitting approach and small dorsal arthrotomy. This technique represents only one additional step beyond percutaneous longitudinal intramedullary retrograde K-wire wire fixation. Expanded indications in our practice now include select cases of symptomatic nascent malunions and axial-stable acute transverse distal diaphyseal fractures that are reducible with closed manipulation. The technique and postoperative protocol are reviewed in the "Metacarpal Neck Fractures" section.

ANTEGRADE TECHNIQUES. Antegrade longitudinal intramedullary fixation of shaft and neck fractures can also be performed through a limited-open approach to the metaphyseal flare distal to the CMC joint. A cortical window is made with a drill bit. A single K-wire under fluoroscopic control is advanced into the medullary canal and across the fracture site. Bouquet pinning consists of multiple K-wires advanced into the canal and across the fracture site to enhance rotational stability (Fig. 42-26).[102,111,112] Orbay[113] introduced flexible intramedullary nails with a proximal locking pin to enhance fixation of transverse fractures. With the rotational control afforded by the locked nail construct, expansion of the

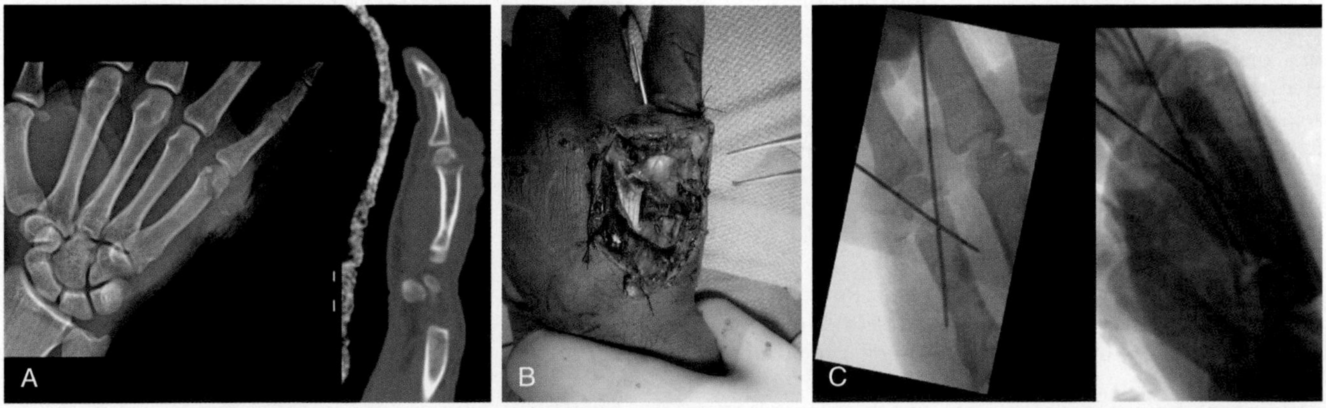

Figure 42-25. A, Combined injury including an open distal small finger metacarpal neck fracture with distal metaphyseal bone stock and overlying extensor tendon laceration to ring and small finger. **B,** Following incision and drainage (I&D) of the soft tissue and osseous injuries, retrograde crossed pinning was performed followed by extensor tendon repairs. **C,** Intraoperative fluoroscopy demonstrates fracture reduction.

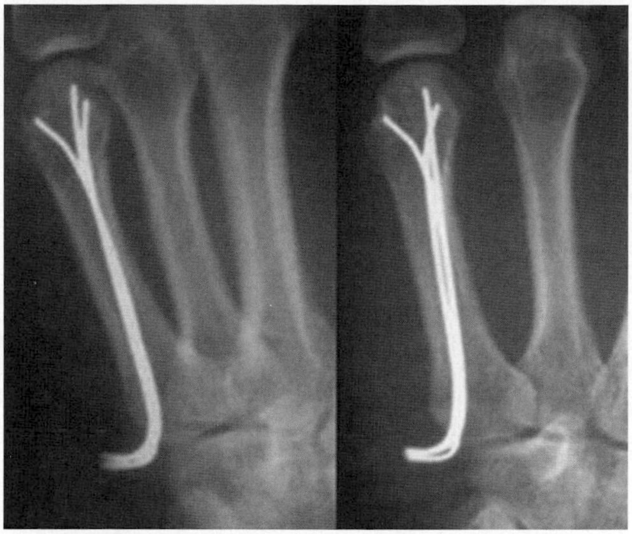

Figure 42-26. When closed reduction of metacarpal shaft or neck fractures is possible, multiple K-wires may be advanced into the canal through a limited open incision and unicortical drill hole across the fracture site.

surgical indications to include spiral and comminuted fractures can be considered. When the antegrade wires are buried under the skin, removal is required following osseous union.

Open Reduction and Internal Fixation. When ORIF is selected, extensile longitudinal incisions are used. The border metacarpals may be approached through a more radial or ulnar-based incision and the corresponding extensor tendon gently retracted. When central metacarpals are involved, an incision over the intermetacarpal space is used. When multiple metacarpal fractures require plate fixation, two longitudinal parallel incisions are designed between the second and third metacarpals and between the fourth and fifth metacarpals (Fig. 42-27). Proximal or distal Y-shaped extensions may be used when additional exposure is needed. Following retraction of the extensors, the juncturae tendineae may require division if distal exposure is needed. These can be repaired anatomically during closure. Subperiosteal exposure of the fracture site is performed, which facilitates mobilization of the adjacent interossei while preserving their origins. At times, interossei muscle may be interposed in the fracture site preventing reduction and a limited débridement is required. In lower energy fractures and with meticulous surgical technique, the periosteum can be closed over the implant and this may minimize extensor adhesions. The goal of ORIF is to achieve rigid fixation to allow for early postoperative functional range of motion and edema control.

Oblique and Spiral Fractures. These fracture patterns are often unstable following an attempt at closed reduction. Percutaneous K-wire techniques obtain limited control of these rotationally unstable fracture patterns. Interfragmentary compression screws (i.e., lag screws, 1.5 to 2.4 mm) are recommended and provide rigid fixation that resists shear and rotational stresses (Fig. 42-28).[114] Fracture length should be a minimum of twice the metacarpal diameter. Following exposure of the proximal and distal apices of the fracture, the fracture is "booked open" to not only débride fracture site hematoma, but to help fully understand the changing obliquity of the fracture line(s) so that interfragmentary screws may be placed perpendicular to the plane of fracture continuously along its course. Anatomic reduction is then obtained and held with fine bone reduction forceps. When there are

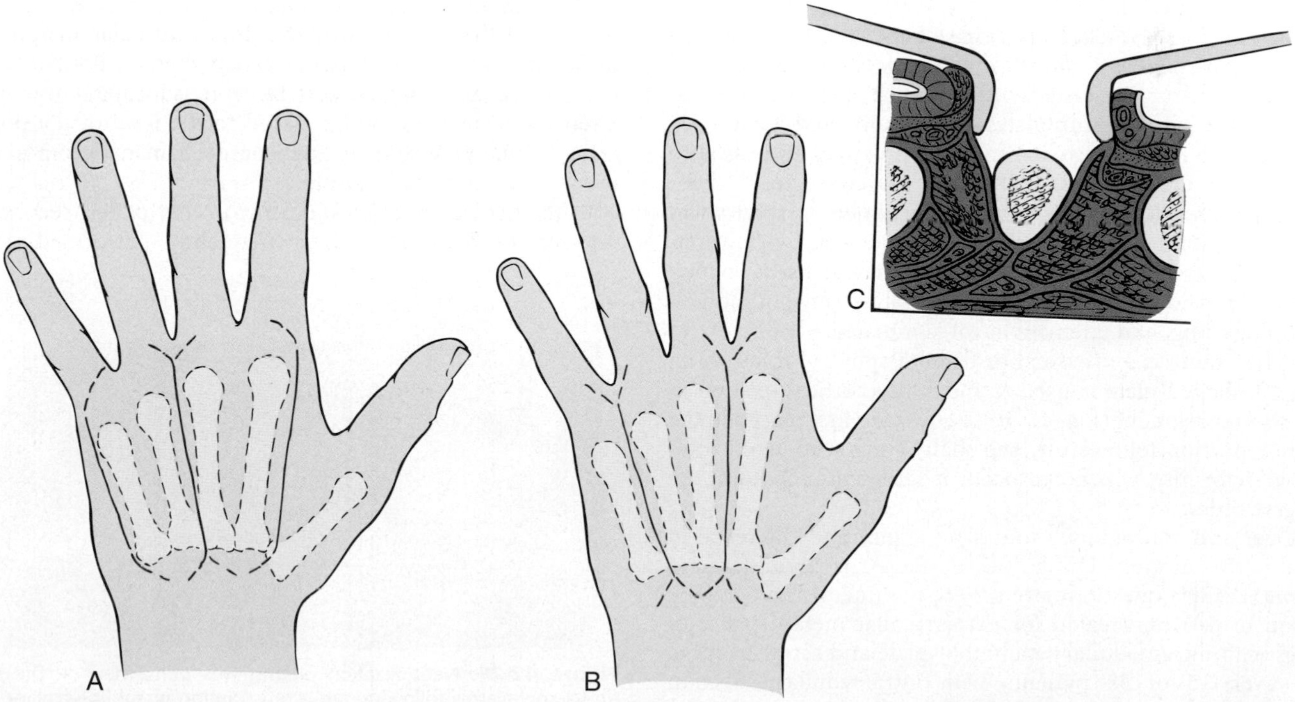

Figure 42-27. Surgical approaches to the metacarpals. **A,** Incisions for exposure of individual metacarpals. **B,** Incisions for exposure of all four metacarpals. **C,** Exposure of the metacarpal is subperiosteal on the dorsal surface, with care taken to minimize elevation of the interosseous muscles.

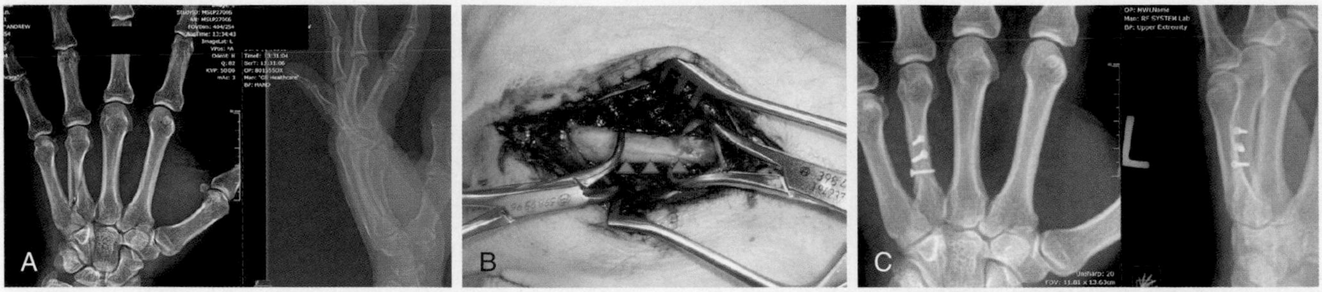

Figure 42-28. **A,** Displaced and malrotated ring finger metacarpal diaphyseal fracture. **B,** Following fracture site débridement, anatomic reduction *(arrows)* is obtained and secured with bone reduction forceps during sequential bicortical screw fixation along the plane of the fracture. **C,** Osseous union following screw fixation.

associated butterfly fragments, these smaller fragments may require smaller screws (1.3 to 1.5 mm). In some cases, following reduction, terminally threaded K-wires may be used to secure provisional fixation and then sequentially exchanged for appropriately sized modular hand screws. Fragmentation at the apices of the fracture is to be avoided. At the apical zones, appropriately sized screws are selected so that there is a minimum of two screw diameters from the apex of the fracture. When stable interfragmentary fixation is obtained, early postoperative range of motion is initiated. Roth and Auerbach[115] have reported successful treatment of 37 metacarpal and phalangeal fractures with bicortical modular screw fixation without formal compression lag technique. If stable screw fixation is not achieved, tendon band wiring[116] and interosseous wiring[117] are alternative techniques that may achieve fixation stable enough to permit functional rehabilitation without postoperative casting. Short oblique fractures are often amenable to a single interfragmentary compression screw. *Neutralization plating* is required to resist postoperative shear and rotational stresses and avoid failure of interfragmentary screw fixation (Fig. 42-29).

Simple Transverse Diaphyseal Fractures. These fractures are amendable to *dorsal compression plating* using Arbeitsgemeinschaft für Osteosynthesefragen (AO) technique. Low-profile 2- to 2.4-mm plates are typically used. Four to six cortices of fixation are recommended proximal and distal to the fracture (Video 42-2).[118-120] Black and colleagues[121] demonstrated that dorsal plating with or without lag screws was more rigid than crossed K-wire and interosseous wiring constructs. Double compression technique may be used. Following compression plating, early postoperative range of motion, tendon gliding, and edema control is initiated.

When there is a proximal or distal diaphyseal fracture, an L- to T-shaped plate is used to maximize cortical fixation in the shorter segment (Fig. 42-30). Screws are first placed in the T or L portion followed by the shaft segment to avoid rotational deformity, which can occur if screws are placed in the reverse order.

Ozer and colleagues[122] found no significant difference in total active motion, Disabilities of the Arm, Shoulder, and Hand (DASH) questionnaire scores, or time to radiographic union in patients treated for extraarticular metacarpal fractures with intramedullary nailing or plate and screw fixation. However, 15 of 38 patients with intramedullary fixation required secondary removal of hardware, whereas only 2 of 14 patients treated with plate fixation underwent secondary surgery.

Sequelae

Two large series[123,124] reported similar overall complication rate (16%) following percutaneous K-wire fixation of various hand and wrist fractures. Major complications included osteomyelitis, tendon rupture, nerve injury, and pin tract infection. Pin tract infection rates were similar in both series (6%[123] and 5.1%[124]). Buried K-wires may reduce the incidence of infection,[125-127] but potentially increases the risk of a tendon rupture[128] or necessitates return to the operating room for removal.[126]

Complications following plate fixation are also well described.[106,107] In a series of 129 patients with 157 metacarpal fractures treated by open reduction and internal plate fixation, Fusetti and colleagues[106] reported complications in more than one-third of the cohort, including delayed union, extensor adhesions and stiffness, fixation failure, complex regional pain syndrome, and deep infection. Page and Stern[107] found a similar major complication rate of 36% in 105 metacarpal and/or phalangeal fractures stabilized with plates. While newer precontoured angular-stable (i.e., locking plates) plates available in customized configurations (i.e., T-, Y-, L-shaped plates) may avoid the need to abut the dorsal articular margin for distal shaft and neck fractures, when there is limited distal bone stock and metaphyseal bone in subcapital fractures, often the plate needs to be placed to the level of the dorsal articular margin where the extensor mechanism becomes confluent with the dorsal capsule.

With the newer generation low-profile plates, secondary removal of hardware is less frequently performed. Plate

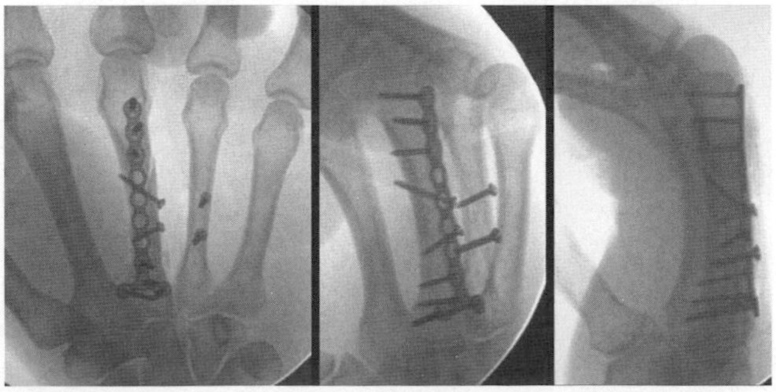

Figure 42-29. Neutralization plating was performed on the long finger metacarpal following lag screw fixation of the intercalary butterfly fracture fragment to resist postoperative shear and rotational stresses and avoid failure of interfragmentary screw fixation. Lag screw fixation was stable in the ring finger.

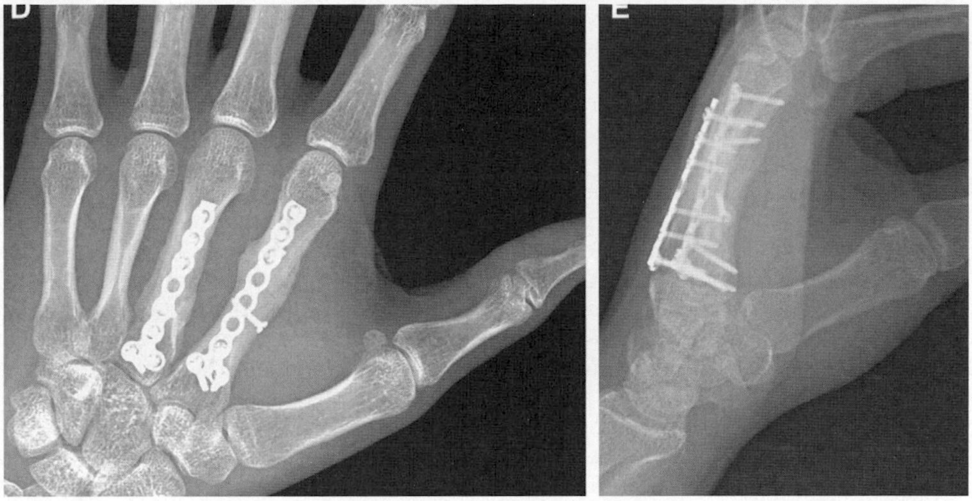

Figure 42-30. A periarticular T-plate is used in the long finger proximal diaphyseal metacarpal fracture to maximize bicortical purchase in the proximal segment.

removal is performed when extensor tenolysis and/or MCP extensor contracture release is needed.

Future Directions

Optimal surgical fixation of metacarpal and phalangeal fractures will limit surgical trauma, allow for early postoperative mobilization to regain full joint motion and tendon excursion, expedite return to activities of daily living and work or sport, and minimize the need for removal of hardware and other secondary procedures. Although metal implants remain the gold standard, early clinical results with second-generation bioabsorbable implants derived from copolymers of trimethylene carbonate, polyglycolic, and polylactic acid are promising. In a series of 14 displaced unstable metacarpal fractures, Dumont and colleagues[129] reported clinical and radiographic union within 6 weeks and a mean total arc of motion of 234 degrees. There were no major complications of wound dehiscence, infection, pseudarthrosis, sinus formation, or osteolysis. There were two cases of loss of reduction necessitating revision fixation using a titanium implant. Givissis and colleagues[130] found uneventful osseous union in 12 unstable metacarpal fractures. Four patients experienced histologically confirmed foreign-body reactions during the second postoperative year and required surgical débridement to remove implant remnants. Two other patients reported a transient local swelling that subsided without treatment.

Metacarpal Neck Fractures

These fractures (i.e., boxer's fractures) are one of the most common injuries in the hand. They typically occur in the ring and small finger, and assume an apex dorsal angulation secondary to the deforming forces of the interossei creating flexion of the metacarpal head. The volar cortex of the neck is relatively weak and volar cortical comminution and volar metaphyseal impaction are common. The mechanism is usually a direct impact on the metacarpal head with the hand in a clenched-fist position.

Indications

The vast majority of metacarpal neck fractures can be treated nonoperatively, as apex dorsal angulation can be functionally compensated for in the ring and small fingers as a result of the 20 to 30 degrees of motion at the CMC joints. There is no consensus regarding the degree and magnitude of acceptable angulation in the ring and small finger metacarpal necks. Volar angulation between 30 and 70 degrees has been reported as acceptable in small clinical series.[131-133] Biomechanical cadaveric studies suggest that at greater than 30 degrees of apex dorsal deformity at the metacarpal neck there is decreased functional length of the intrinsics and reduced efficiency in the flexor system during MCP joint motion.[134] In contrast, given the rigid nature of the index and long finger CMC joints, reduction and stabilization of neck fractures in these metacarpals is considered for sagittal plane deformity greater than 10 to 15 degrees.

A true lateral radiograph is necessary to measure the magnitude of sagittal plane angulation. The oblique radiograph may exaggerate the magnitude of deformity.[135] The interobserver and intraobserver reliability of metacarpal neck angulation measurements on plain films remains variable.[135,136]

Indications for operative management include unstable, widely displaced, and markedly angulated neck fractures (greater than 50 degrees volar angulation/apex dorsal deformity). Reduction and stabilization is also indicated when clinical examination reveals pseudoclawing (i.e., compensatory MCP joint hyperextension with PIP flexion with attempted composite digital extension), which represents a dynamic imbalance of the extrinsic and intrinsic musculature. Rotational deformity is not commonly seen with neck fractures, but if present, should be corrected. Open and combined injuries are treated with débridement and internal fixation.

Sagittal plane deformity creates loss of the knuckle contour. More importantly, the associated prominence of the metacarpal head in palm may create discomfort in select patient populations, such as laborers and elite athletes. In all cases, the surgeon should use careful judgment and discussion to determine whether conservative or operative management is the most appropriate approach to achieve maximum function and return to work or play.

Nonoperative Treatment and Outcomes

There is no consensus regarding type and duration of immobilization. Several prospective, randomized trials have compared splint or cast immobilization with early mobilization of neck fractures. Braakman and colleagues[137] reported similar mean radiographic deformities and clinical outcomes at 6 months in patients treated with ulnar gutter casting or immediate buddy taping and motion. Kuokkanen and colleagues[132] reported minimal differences in motion and grip at 3 months in patients treated with 4 weeks of splinting or an elastic bandage for 1 week prior to mobilization. Mean angulation was 29 degrees in the splint group and 42 degrees in the bandage group. Statius Muller and colleagues[131] reported similar clinical and radiographic outcomes and patient satisfaction rates with ulnar gutter casting for three weeks or a compression bandage for 1 week for neck fracture with mean angulation of 39 degrees. Hofmeister and colleagues[138] found similar clinical, functional, and radiographic outcomes in patients treated with a short-arm volar outrigger cast or a short-arm cast extending to the PIP joint for neck fractures with less than 45 degrees of angulation. Although hand surgeons have previously recommended that the MCP joints be immobilized in the intrinsic plus position (i.e., MCP joints in maximal flexion), there is now evidence that metacarpal neck fractures may be immobilized in extension.[138] When the IP joints are included in the splint or cast, they are maintained in extension. We often leave the IP joints free. Poolman and colleagues[139] performed a systematic review of randomized controlled studies of nonoperative treatment of metacarpal neck fractures and concluded that based on limited studies and cohort sizes that there was no superior treatment modality.

Surgical Exposures and Fixation Techniques

Percutaneous and open techniques available to treat displaced and markedly angulated metacarpal neck and subcapital fractures are identical to those described for metacarpal shaft fractures, namely antegrade (i.e., single intramedullary or multiple bouquet pinning),[102] retrograde (i.e., longitudinal intramedullary fixation, crossed collateral recess K-wires),[103] transmetacarpal K-wire constructs,[104] as well as plate fixation.[105] When retrograde techniques are selected, the MCP joint is flexed to expose the articular surface of the metacarpal head. As discussed previously, each technique has its own advantages and disadvantages. External fixation has been described, but pin loosening and extensor tendon impalement are pitfalls of this technique.[140]

For percutaneous and limited-open techniques, the apex dorsal angulation is corrected using the Jahss maneuver.[141] The proximal phalanx is flexed 90 degrees on the metacarpal head and it is used to deliver a dorsal force on the head while using counterpressure of the dorsal aspect of the proximal fragment. With the reduction maintained, K-wire fixation is performed.

Retrograde Limited-Open Intramedullary Headless Screw Fixation. Retrograde intramedullary fixation using a cannulated headless screw can be achieved using a limited-open extensor-splitting approach and small dorsal arthrotomy (Fig. 42-31). This technique represents only one additional step beyond percutaneous longitudinal intramedullary retrograde K-wire fixation. This technique is achieved through a small extensor-split and dorsal arthrotomy. Closed reduction with the Jahss maneuver is confirmed under fluoroscopic guidance and a 1.1-mm smooth K-wire is then inserted under direct visualization for provisional fixation through the center of the dorsal corridor of the metacarpal head in line with the medullary canal. It is then overdrilled and replaced with a 2.4- or 3-mm cannulated headless compression screw (HCS) based on preoperative templating of the dimensions of the isthmus of the intramedullary canal. Although clinical concerns remain regarding the articular starting point, three-dimensional CT analyses of this technique have demonstrated that subchondral head volume occupied is minimal, surface-area violation is least during clinically relevant maximal sagittal plane arc of motion, and the dorsal starting point is in line with the medullary canal and avoids engagement of the center of the articular base through a majority of sagittal plane motion.[110]

Limited-open retrograde intramedullary headless screw fixation offers clinical advantages over K-wire fixation and other open techniques. Countersunk intramedullary fixation with isthmal purchase *(relative stability)* allows early active and active-assisted motion within the first postoperative week. A removable hand-based ulnar-gutter splint with the metacarpal-phalangeal joints in intrinsic plus position and the IP joints free is worn until suture removal and then is gradually weaned. This technique obviates concerns for pin tract infections or adhesions following extensor tendon mobilization with formal ORIF. When neck comminution is present, the screw is inserted without the compression sleeve. Potentially, direct visualization of the starting point additionally eliminates multiple attempts at achieving the correct starting point during percutaneous K-wire insertion for retrograde longitudinal or crossed K-wire intramedullary fixation. Increasing clinical experience with this technique may allow for expanded indications in select cases to include symptomatic nascent malunions and axial-stable acute transverse middiaphyseal fractures that are reducible with closed manipulation.

Open Reduction and Internal Fixation. ORIF is rarely needed. Indications include irreducible fractures, multiple metacarpal or hand fractures, open, and combined injuries. Plating of metacarpal neck fractures has been associated with stiffness as fixation often needs to extend to the dorsal articular margin where the extensor mechanism is confluent with the dorsal capsule. For distal shaft and neck fractures where there is limited distal bone stock and metaphyseal bone, low-profile locked fixed-angle plates are advantageous (Fig. 42-32). Newer precontoured angular-stable plates with polyaxial locking screws available in customized configurations (i.e., T-, Y-, L-shaped plates) may avoid the need to abut the dorsal articular margin. Lateral plate application can also be considered, but fixation should not impinge on the collateral recess. An alternative fixation construct includes tension band wiring around two K-wires. When stable internal fixation is obtained, early postoperative mobilization is initiated including tendon gliding and intrinsic stretching exercises.

Surgical Outcomes. There is no consensus on an optimal treatment modality for significantly angulated metacarpal neck fractures. Wong and colleagues[142] reported similar outcomes for neck fractures with greater than 30 degrees of angulation treated with closed reduction and percutaneous transmetacarpal wires or intramedullary K-wires. In a series by Winter and colleagues,[143] there was a greater total arc of motion and active MCP joint motion in patients treated with intramedullary wires compared to transmetacarpal pinning.

In a prospective series of 39 consecutive patients (23 neck, 11 shaft, and 5 nascent malunions) with a mean age of 28 years and mean sagittal plane deformity of 48 degrees treated

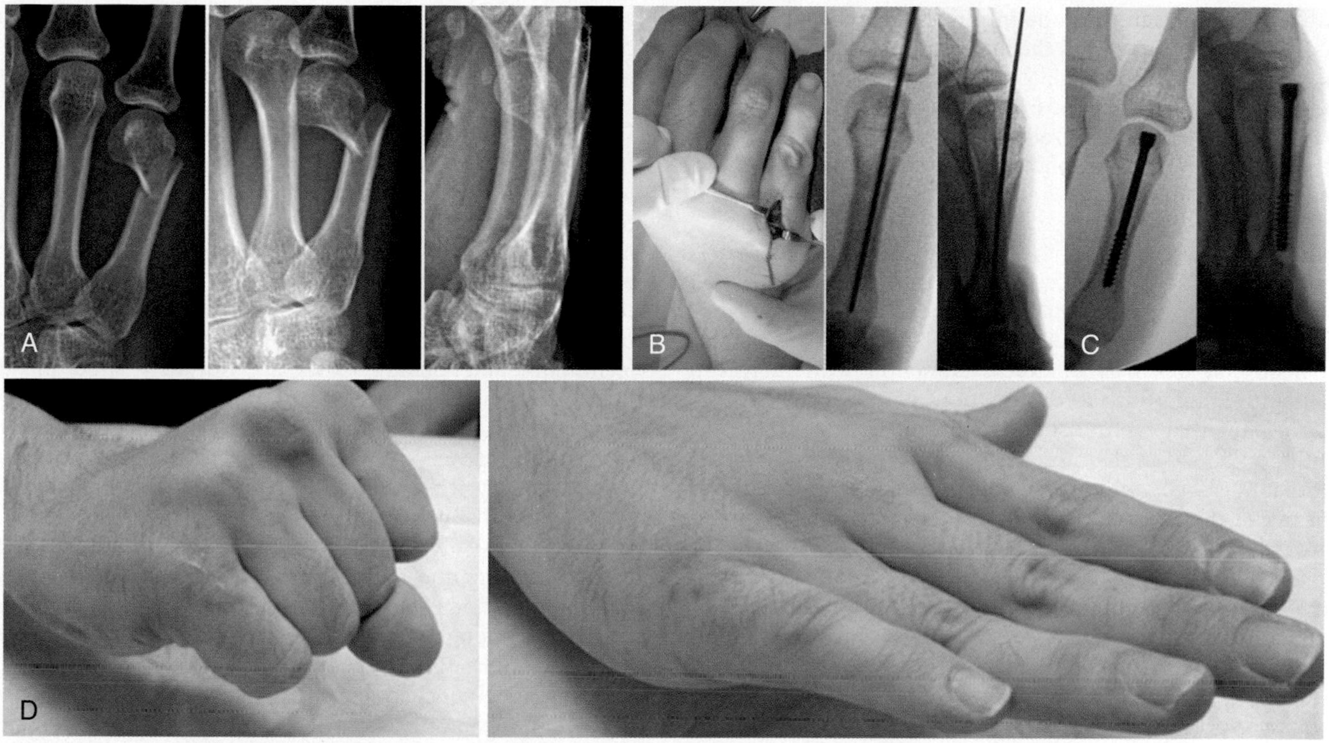

Figure 42-31. A, Displaced and angulated small finger metacarpal neck fracture. **B,** Retrograde intramedullary fixation using a cannulated headless screw can be achieved using a limited-open extensor-splitting approach *(left panel)* and represents only one additional step beyond longitudinal intramedullary retrograde Kirschner wire fixation. **C,** The guidewire is overdrilled with a cannulated drill, and the headless screw is advanced and countersunk beneath the articular surface. **D,** Internal fixation allows for early postoperative joint motion and facilitates recovery of functional motion within the first month postoperatively.

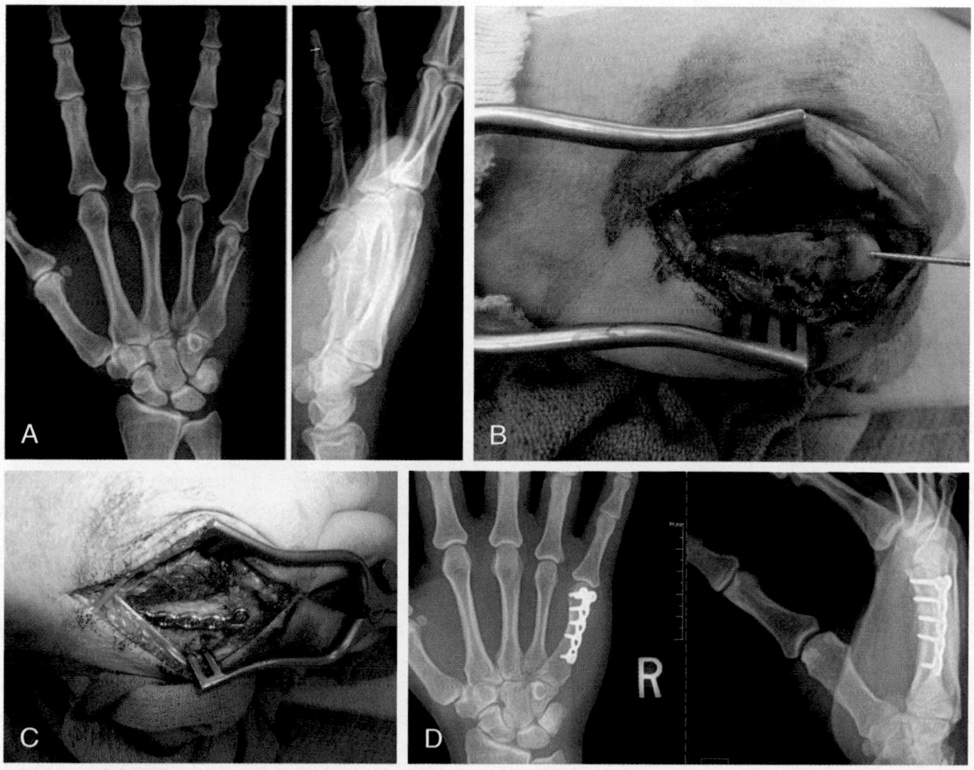

Figure 42-32. A, Unstable comminuted small finger metacarpal distal shaft and neck fracture. **B,** Closed reduction was not obtainable due to interposed soft tissue. Open reduction was required. Anatomic reduction along remaining cortical keys was obtained followed by provisional longitudinal K-wire fixation. **C,** Open reduction and internal fixation (ORIF) with fixed-angle plate-locking screw construct followed by early motion. **D,** Osseous union is achieved.

with limited-open retrograde intramedullary headless screw fixation and motion within the first postoperative week, excellent results were reported.[144] All fractures achieved union and full composite flexion. Extensor lag resolved at approximately 3.5 weeks postoperatively. No secondary procedures were required. At latest follow-up, there was no evidence of arthrosis.

Future Directions

Optimal treatment of these fractures remains to be defined. Accurate and reproducible measurement of angulation remains elusive. Correlation between biomechanical data on intrinsic and extrinsic tendon dysfunction with increasing angulation and clinical dysfunction is needed. Outcome instruments that capture subtle deviation from normal hand function will aid in defining best practice for these fractures. Ultimately, large randomized clinical series are needed to determine the magnitude of angulation and shortening that impact hand function.

Fixed-Angle Implants

Conventional nonlocked plate and screw constructs rely on frictional force created between the plate and bone surface in order to neutralize the axial, torsional, and three-point bending forces experienced by the plate-screw-bone construct.[145] Fixed-angle implants in the hand were introduced more than 20 years ago by Büchler and Fisher.[146] These authors reported their initial experience with the mini condylar plate (Synthes, Paoli, PA) for periarticular metacarpal and phalangeal fractures. The design of this fixed-angle implant was predicated on larger blade plates used extensively for periarticular fractures in other anatomic locations. Fixed-angle plate and screw constructs function as an "internal-external fixator" and extraperiosteal application preserves periosteal vascularity while maintaining fixation by locking the fixation screws to the plate, which may be placed extraperiosteally.[145,147,148] Locked screws act together in parallel, whereas conventional screws act in series.[147] As a result, the fixed-angle construct leads to a mechanism of screw-purchase failure that is fundamentally different from that of conventional unlocked screws.

Fixed-angle technology continues to be refined by the AO/Association for the Study of Internal Fixation (ASIF) group.[149-153] The evolution of small locking plates for hand applications may minimize the complications reported with mini condylar plates. Fixed-angle locking subarticular buttress pins represent an alternative to the use of the mini condylar blade plate. The AO/ASIF group (Synthes, Paoli, PA) developed the minifragment and modular hand locking compression plate (LCP) fixation systems. The LCP plates are unique in that they offer sequential Combi Holes that afford either cortical or locking screw fixation through the same hole and are available in 2.7 through 1.5 mm. Plates are available in straight, Y-, T-, and H-shaped configurations. Notched plates facilitate plate cutting and additional contouring. These low-profile plates (plate thickness range, 0.7 to 1.25 mm[119]) make periosteal closure around the implant easier. Further, novel plate and screw locking mechanisms continue to emerge. A proliferation of locked-plate designs by several manufacturers continues and has recently led to the introduction of polyaxial locking capabilities. Biomechanical analyses in cadaveric specimens validated the use of these low-profile plates.[154-156] Studies reporting clinical and radiographic outcomes following dedicated use of the current systems are needed in order to further define their applications.

Open Reduction and Internal Fixation in Special Circumstances

In the setting of comminuted and multifragmentary diaphyseal or periarticular fractures with or without segmental bone loss, multiple metacarpal and/or phalangeal fractures, open and volar and/or dorsal combined injuries, open reduction and rigid internal fixation is selected to facilitate early functional rehabilitation. In these settings, indirect reduction techniques and locking plates appropriately sized for the injured region (i.e., 2 to 2.7 mm) are applied using a *bridge-plating technique* to restore metacarpal length, rotation, and alignment (Fig. 42-33). Intraoperatively, transmetacarpal or intramedullary wires or a mini external fixator may be used to provisionally maintain metacarpal length prior to plate application.[157-161] Bridging the comminuted area avoids periosteal stripping and preserves vascularity of the intercalary comminuted fracture fragments. Relative stability is achieved and allows enough strain at the fracture site to promote secondary bone healing with callus formation.[162]

Alternatively, locked screws can be used to augment a standard compression plate and screw construct to create hybrid fixation (i.e., nonlocked and locked screws). In a hybrid construct, it is essential to apply compression across the fracture site using standard techniques prior to insertion of the locked screws. The use of hybrid fixation with bicortical locking screws is advantageous in osteopenic bone, and in select fracture patterns in which one aspect of the fracture would benefit from anatomic reduction and compression (i.e., simple intraarticular component), whereas another fracture component would benefit from bridging fixation (i.e., comminuted metadiaphyseal portion). If corticocancellous bone graft is indicated, additional screw fixation can be placed in order to secure the graft. In the border metacarpals, plate application may be dorsal or lateral for fracture fixation.

In cases of combined injuries, early soft tissue and skeletal reconstruction minimizes disability. Freeland and colleagues reported excellent results with reconstruction performed within 10 days of the initial injury.[163] In the settings of infection or significant dorsal soft tissue loss, external fixation allows for provisional stabilization during planned serial débridements. Definitive fixation is performed at the time of soft tissue coverage and tendon and osseous reconstruction.[163,164] When there is osteomyelitis and/or segmental bone loss, consideration is given to the use of antibiotic-impregnated cement spacers[165-167] to provide a high-concentration local elutant and minimize contracture of the soft tissue envelope space to facilitate staged placement of autograft bone.

Metacarpal Head Fractures

Metacarpal head fractures are uncommon injuries. In a series by Hastings and Carroll,[168] only 16 of 250 articular fractures of the hand were metacarpal head fractures. McElfresh and Dobyns[169] divided partial articular fractures of the metacarpal head into sagittal, coronal, and transverse fracture patterns according to the obliquity of the fracture line. Comminuted head fractures were found in almost one-third of their series, and the index metacarpal head was most frequently involved. Nonarticular collateral ligament avulsion

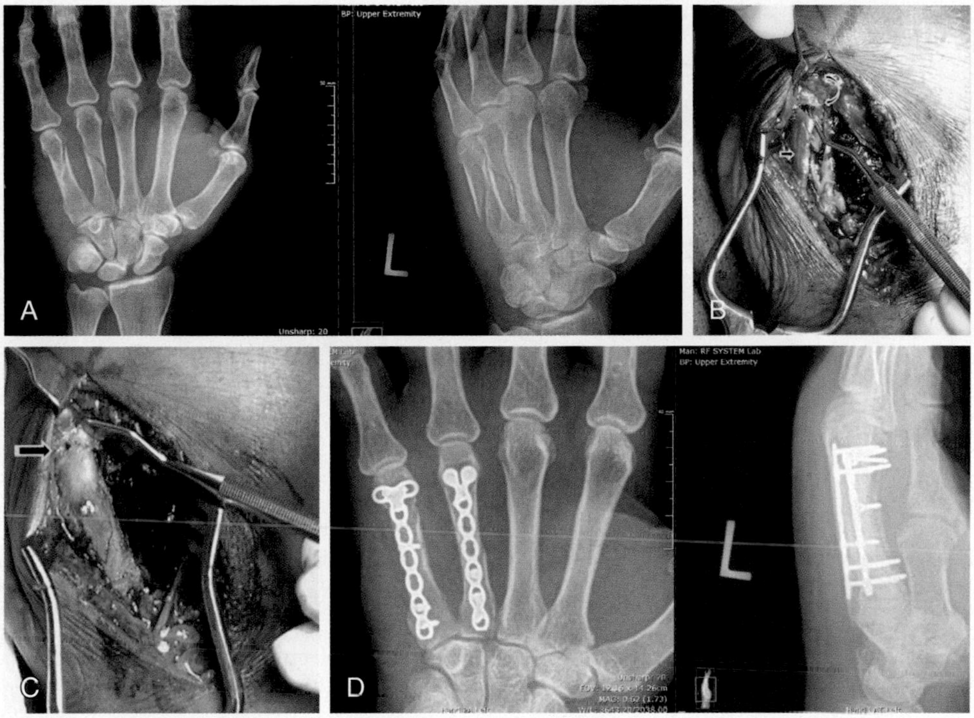

Figure 42-33. **A,** Unstable multifragmentary small finger metacarpal fracture and adjacent ring finger metacarpal fracture. **B,** Intraoperative photo of the multifragmentary fracture. The dorsal intercalary fracture fragment *(straight arrow)* extends to the dorsal articular margin of the metacarpal head *(curved arrow)*. **C,** The dorsal intercalary fragment is first fixed to the proximal diaphyseal segment with interfragmentary screw fixation, followed by anatomic reduction of the subcapital segment *(arrow and dental pick)*. **D,** Periarticular locked plating is performed given the limited distal metaphyseal bone stock.

fractures are discussed in the section reviewing MCP joint ligamentous injuries.

These articular fractures may be difficult to appreciate on standard plain films of the hand. The Brewerton view[170] (MCP joint flexed 60 to 70 degrees with the dorsal surface of the digits flat on the radiograph cassette and the radiograph tube angled 15 degrees ulnar-to-radial) may be helpful in demonstrating the articular involvement. We routinely perform CT scans with coronal and sagittal plane reconstruction to elucidate the fracture plane, magnitude of articular surface involvement, and the presence of articular involvement.

Articular head fractures may also be seen associated with fight bites. Small, stellate, or transverse lacerations over the dorsum of the MCP joints incurred during a fistfight are typically consistent with open wounds secondary to contact with a human tooth. There is usually an associated injury to the extensor mechanism and an underlying traumatic arthrotomy. Urgent irrigation and débridement of wounds and involved joints and antibiotics are recommended to minimize the risks of septic arthritis and/or osteomyelitis (Fig. 42-34). When these present early and are treated expeditiously, early internal fixation is performed. When serial débridements are anticipated, delay of definitive fixation may be considered.

Indications

Displaced articular fractures require ORIF.

Nonoperative Treatment

When the articular head fracture is nondisplaced and there is no mechanical block to motion or resultant angular or rotational deformity, nonoperative management is selected. A hand-based radial or ulnar gutter intrinsic plus splint is worn for 3 weeks followed by gradual progressive motion. In this setting, weekly serial clinical and radiographic examinations are performed to assess for interval displacement.

Surgical Exposures and Fixation Techniques

A dorsal curvilinear incision followed by division of the ulnar sagittal band and dorsal arthrotomy is used. Meticulous repair of the sagittal band fibers is performed following fixation. Alternatively, a dorsal extensor-splitting approach and longitudinal arthrotomy may be used (Video 42-3).

The articular fragment(s) are reduced with a dental pick and provisionally reduced with fine smooth K-wires. Cancellous autograft may be needed for subchondral support once the articular segment is elevated and reduced. Headless compression screws countersunk beneath the articular surface are the implant of choice for these fracture patterns. Variable diameter, both cannulated and noncannulated, headless screws are commercially available. Countersunk cortical modular hand screws (1 to 1.5 mm) may also be used. Biodegradable screws and pins are also available. In multifragmentary fractures with articular involvement and shaft extension, the articular surface is reconstructed and then reduced to the shaft segment with a fixed-angle plate and screw construct. The metaphyseal locking screws provide additional subchondral support.

Highly comminuted articular head fractures may be better addressed with distraction and external fixation. In select cases, acute hemiarthroplasty or arthrodesis may be considered.

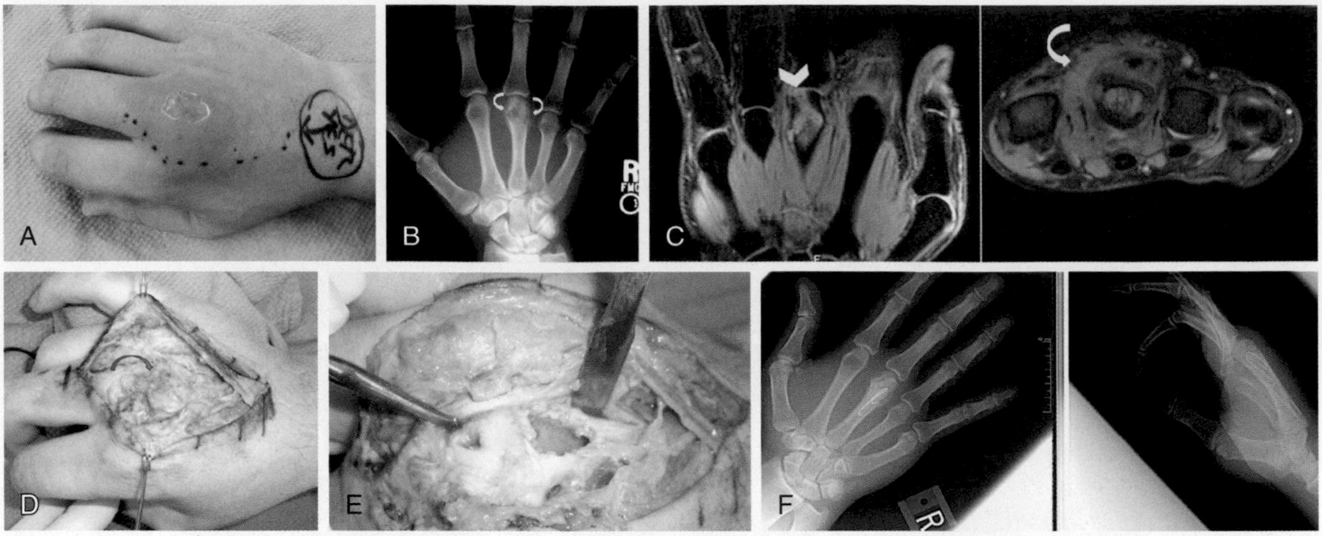

Figure 42-34. A, Delayed presentation following fight bite overlying the metacarpophalangeal (MCP joint of the middle finger. **B,** Preoperative radiographs with evidence of multifocal lysis within the metacarpal head and periosteal reaction about the metacarpal neck consistent with chronic osteomyelitis. **C,** Preoperative magnetic resonance imaging (MRI) demonstrates marrow replacement, enhancement, and edema throughout the metacarpal head and neck with erosive lesion through the articular surface *(chevron)* and periarticular soft tissue phlegmon *(arrow)*. **D,** Intraoperative finding of soft tissue peritendinous and periarticular phlegmon and abscess. **E,** Metadiaphyseal corticotomy and bony débridement of the subcapital and neck region. **F,** Antibiotic-impregnated cement packing is inserted for local elution of broad-spectrum antibiotics and for subchondral support.

Outcomes

Stiffness,[168] arthrofibrosis, osteonecrosis, chondrolysis, and posttraumatic arthrosis may occur following metacarpal head fractures.

Complications of Metacarpal Fractures

Nonunions and malunions of the metacarpals and phalanges continue to represent unique challenges for the treating hand surgeon. Angular and rotational deformities with functional deficits are indications for surgical correction. Prior scars, and tendon adhesions may make exposure challenging, and the presence of soft tissue contractures may increase the stress on the fixation. In the setting of these complex nonunion and malunions, angular-stable fixation may allow early functional rehabilitation following concomitant tenolysis, arthrolysis, and capsulectomy.

Nonunions of the tubular bones of the hand remain uncommon. Nonunions are addressed surgically when associated with disability and functional limitations. There are limited reports of the results of treatment of metacarpal and phalangeal nonunions and malunions.[171,172] Jupiter and colleagues,[171] in a series of 25 nonunions and delayed unions, found plate and screw fixation achieved a more functional digit as compared to several other techniques. Implant selection will depend on the location and direction of the nonunion or malunion within the longitudinal axis of the involved bone. Diaphyseal corrections are amendable to straight plates or extended H-plates. In transverse nonunions, cortical screws can be used to achieve compression across the nonunion site prior to placing locking screws. Mini condylar plates are used for metaphyseal, juxtaarticular, or combined metadiaphyseal reconstructions. As a general rule, in the setting of these reconstructions, implants one size larger than would be required for an acute fracture at the same level should be considered (i.e., 2.4-mm plates in the metacarpal and 2-mm plates in the proximal phalanx). The need for intercalary structural corticocancellous grafting is determined preoperatively. Additional locking screws can be used to stabilize the graft at the nonunion or osteotomy site. In the case of hypertrophic nonunions, bone grafting may not be needed, and all that is needed is stable fixation.

Malunions of hand fractures are not uncommon. Malrotation and excessive angulation result in functional impairment. Preoperative planning followed by templating includes localization of the malunion (extraarticular, intraarticular, combined, epiphyseal, metaphyseal, or diaphyseal); assessment of the plane of deformity (uni-, bi-, multiplanar); examination of associated soft tissue contracture or deficiency and neurovascular deficits; and evaluation of skeletal maturity. When corrective osteotomy is performed at the site of the original fracture, multiplanar deformity can be completely addressed while simultaneously performing tenolysis and arthrolysis. Büchler and colleagues[173] reported good-to-excellent results in 96% of patients following corrective osteotomy for isolated posttraumatic phalangeal malunions; however, this rate dropped to 64% when soft tissue structures were also involved. In this setting, rigid fixation is required in order to allow for early postoperative rehabilitation to optimize outcome.

In general, corrective osteotomy is performed at the site of deformity. For pure angular uniplanar deformities, a unicortical opening wedge osteotomy reliably restores length and tendon balance. When length is less of a concern, a closing wedge osteotomy is performed. Pure rotational deformities are addressed with complete osteotomy at the site of deformity. Some advocate derotational osteotomy at the metacarpal level.[172,174-176] Intraarticular osteotomies for articular nonunion and malunions are technically challenging. Alternatives to osteotomy include arthrodesis, implant arthroplasty, and resection of impinging osteocartilaginous areas. Articular malunions of Bennett fractures may result in subluxation of the trapeziometacarpal joint. Articular osteotomy is recommended prior to the onset of arthrosis (see Fig. 42-10).

Joint contractures (extension and flexion) and stiffness due to tendon adhesion are relatively frequent complications of phalangeal fractures. Tendon adhesions occurring after closed metacarpal fractures are uncommon. More commonly, adhesions follow combined or crush injuries. Initial management includes static and dynamic splinting. If initial treatment fails, tenolysis with or without capsulotomy is indicated when the soft tissue envelope is supple. Preoperative examination is essential in differentiating capsular contracture and extrinsic and intrinsic tightness. As outlined by Jupiter and colleagues,[177] the correction of soft tissue–related stiffness begins with clinical examination of the active and passive flexion and extension of the finger. Four questions are asked during clinical examination to help in preoperative planning:

1. Can the finger be flexed passively?
2. Can the finger flex actively?
3. Can the finger be extended passively?
4. Can the finger extend actively?

By definition, fingers that lack passive motion in a particular direction also lack active motion in the same direction. The answers to these questions reliably reveal the location of the abnormal tissue as well as the surgical approach needed to address it. Six possible permutations of finger stiffness are seen clinically.

Posttraumatic arthrosis at the MCP joints can be addressed with implant arthroplasty as arthrodesis is not well tolerated at this level. Symptomatic arthrosis at the CMC joints is most reliably treated with arthrodesis, although interpositional arthroplasties have been described. The CMC joint of the thumb may be treated with either trapeziectomy-ligament interpositional arthroplasty or arthrodesis based on patient-specific considerations. Various fixation techniques have been described for arthrodesis in the hand.

METACARPOPHALANGEAL JOINT LIGAMENTOUS INJURIES

Regional Anatomy

The articular surfaces form a condyloid joint with a shallow and concave proximal phalanx congruent with the large metacarpal head, which is asymmetric in the coronal and sagittal planes. The articular geometry allows for multiplanar motion. The dorsal capsule extends from the metacarpal neck to the base of the proximal phalanx and is reinforced by the collateral ligaments that course obliquely from dorsal-proximal to palmar-distal. The proper collateral ligaments insert into the base of the proximal phalanx, and the accessory collateral ligaments insert onto the volar plate. The volar plate is comprised of a thick fibrocartilaginous portion distally and a membranous portion proximally devoid of the strong proximal checkrein ligaments seen at the PIP joints. This anatomic difference allows for relative hyperextension of the MCP joint. The flexor tendons and A1 pulley lie directly volar to the volar plate. The dorsal capsule is relatively thin and is comprised of areolar tissue. The extrinsic extensor tendons are intimately associated with the capsule. The extrinsic tendons are supported by the sagittal bands of the extensor hood which connect with the transverse intermetacarpal ligament. The common digital neurovascular bundles lie palmar to the lumbricals. This position places the bundle at risk during traumatic dorsal dislocation as well as during a volar surgical approach to the joint.

Dislocations

Dorsal dislocations are more frequent than volar dislocations.[178] The index finger is most frequently involved, followed by the thumb. As the joint is hyperextended, the volar plate is avulsed proximally from its attachment on the metacarpal neck. In a simple (i.e., reducible) dislocation, the volar plate is not interposed within the joint, and the base of the proximal phalanx remains in contact with the articular surface of the metacarpal head. The collateral ligaments may be torn, depending on the magnitude and vector of the traumatic forces. Volar dislocations may occur through hyperflexion or hyperextension injuries.

In complex (i.e., irreducible) dorsal dislocations, the interposed volar plate prevents reduction. Kaplan[179] described entrapment of the metacarpal head between the displaced natatory ligament (distally), the superficial transverse metacarpal ligament (proximally), lumbrical (radially), and the flexor tendons (ulnarly). This circumferential tendinous noose tightens with attempted closed reduction. Complex volar dislocations may be due to interposed dorsal capsule, distal volar plate or collateral ligament, juncturae tendineae, interossei, and sesamoids.

Reduction with simple distraction is usually unsuccessful. Following local anesthetic or joint insufflation, the wrist and PIP joint are flexed to relax the flexor tendons. Direct dorsal-to-volar pressure is applied to translate the base of the proximal phalanx and the attached volar plate. When closed reduction is successful, coronal and sagittal plane stability is tested. Dorsal block splinting to prevent extension beyond neutral and early motion is begun with gradual reduction in the extension block.

When open reduction is required, a dorsal or volar approach may be used. The dorsal approach[180,181] allows one to reduce the interposed volar plate with a lower risk of injury to the displaced neurovascular bundle[182] and address associated metacarpal head fractures (see Video 42-3). The volar plate is incised longitudinally and retracted to either side allowing for gentle reduction of the metacarpal head. Others favor the volar approach as described by Kaplan.[179] The metacarpal head causes palmar displacement of the digital neurovascular bundles, which may come to lie directly beneath the tented subcutaneous tissues. Following mobilization of the neurovascular bundles, the A1 pulley is released. This exposure allows treatment of associated collateral ligament injuries and incarcerated flexor tendons. The palmar incision may be extended along midaxial lines as needed for treatment of collateral ligament injuries. Combined exposures may be needed for chronic (>3 weeks) injuries.

Stiffness is the most common complication related to MCP joint dislocations. Joint contracture release and/or tenolyses may be necessary to improve motion. Delayed diagnosis and/or treatment portend suboptimal outcomes including posttraumatic arthrosis or osteonecrosis of the metacarpal head.

Collateral Ligament Injuries

Isolated MCP joint RCL ruptures are more common the UCL injuries.[183] The typical mechanism of injury is forced ulnar deviation of the flexed MCP joint. It is common for these patients to present in a delayed fashion with persistent discomfort and swelling along the injured collateral ligament. The collaterals are examined in extension and midflexion, and end points are assessed in comparison to adjacent and contralateral digits. Treatment is based on the grade of injury: grade 1 (tenderness over collateral but without instability), grade 2 (laxity compared to the contralateral digit with a definite end point), or grade 3 (laxity without end point). Grade 1 and 2 injuries are treated with early protected range of motion and use of buddy taping. If there is marked discomfort, osteoarthritis hand-based splint maintaining the MCP joint in midflexion is used for 3 weeks. Patients should be counseled that even when MCP stability is restored, discomfort and soreness may persist with terminal MCP flexion and gripping activities for 1 year. For persistent symptoms without instability, a therapeutic cortisone injection may be considered if the integrity of the collateral is confirmed. If instability or pain persist, despite an appreciable end point, surgical repair or reconstruction may be considered.

Treatment recommendations for acute complete grade 3 tears are based on patient age, occupational demands, digit involved, and activity level. For grade 3 injuries seen early (<4 weeks) a trial of casting or full-time splint immobilization can be attempted with close clinical follow-up and serial exams to assess for any restoration of stability. In the higher demand patient and in border digits, acute surgical repair may be preferred. It is unclear whether acute repair yields superior outcomes to delayed repairs and reconstructions.[183,184] In a recent series, Kang and colleagues[184] reported failure of an initial trial of conservative treatment in 9 of 12 patients seen acutely for grade 3 RCL tears of the index finger MCP joint. Similar outcomes were reported following acute and delayed primary repairs. In contrast, Gaston and Lourie[183] reported fair-to-poor results in grade 3 injuries treated late.

A dorsal incision is made and the extensor hood is divided and the extensor mobilized. Following capsulotomy, the site of ligament disruption is identified, and a suture anchor repair performed with the repair tensioned with the MCP joint in at least 45 degrees of flexion. The joint is immobilized for 5 to 6 weeks in midflexion.

If degenerative arthrosis is already present, arthrodesis or arthroplasty combined with ligament reconstruction depending on patient age and demand are considered.

Metacarpophalangeal Collateral Ligament Avulsion Fractures

Treatment of collateral ligament avulsion fractures at the collateral recess origin or insertion is based on joint stability, size of the fragment, and the finger injured. Nonoperative treatment is recommended for small, collateral ligament avulsion fractures of the nonarticular head when the MCP joint is stable on clinical examination. If there is instability and fragment is small (<10% to 15% of the articular surface), it may be excised, and the ligament advanced into the defect and secured with a suture anchor or pullout suture technique. If the fragment is large, it is reduced anatomically. Fixation constructs available include tension band suture or wire (Figs. 42-35 and 42-36), K-wires, and one or more modular hand screws.

PHALANGEAL FRACTURES AND INTERPHALANGEAL JOINT INJURIES

Phalangeal Fractures

Fractures of the Distal Phalanx

Distal phalangeal fractures are the most commonly encountered fracture in the hand due to the propensity for fingertip injuries. Distal phalangeal fractures can be classified into the more common tuft fractures, shaft fractures, and articular injuries of the distal interphalangeal (DIP) joint.

A clinically relevant way to classify distal phalangeal fractures is by mechanism of injury.

- Crush injuries
- Bending force
- Avulsion injuries
- Impaction injuries

Tuft fractures are bony injuries confined to the distal flare of the distal phalanx and are a result of a crushing injury. These injuries are, by default, associated with some element of disruption of the nail bed as the latter constitutes the dorsal periosteum. Subungual hematoma contained beneath the nail plate can result in significant discomfort. Pain can be successfully and immediately relieved by perforating the overlying nail plate using a sterile 18-gauge hypodermic needle or a battery-powered electrocautery. A tip-protector splint is worn for comfort for a period of 2 to 3 weeks until tenderness and sensitivity subside. If the radiographs demonstrate sagittal plane displacement extending into the shaft, consideration must be given to reduction of the fragments in order to perform the more important task of reapproximation of the overlying nail matrix. The nail plate is removed to allow visualization of the nail matrix and manipulation of the fragments. Fragment fixation is achieved by 1 to 2 fine K-wires followed by careful reapproximation of the nail matrix with fine resorbable undyed sutures or Histoacryl glue.

Some comminuted tuft fractures may never achieve radiographic union due to compromised vascularity of the bone fragments. The resulting fibrous union or nonunion is rarely symptomatic due to stability provided by the regenerated nail plate and soft tissue envelope.

Axial force injuries to the tip of the finger can result in transverse fractures of the distal phalanx. Nail bed injury is implied in displaced fractures and the latter should be treated with nail plate removal, open reduction, and K-wire fixation followed by nail bed repair. Occasionally there is angulation of the distal phalanx without displacement. The need for intervention in these cases is determined by clinical appearance. If the finger angulation is not aesthetically acceptable, reduction should be considered. Closed reduction can be achieved in most cases presenting early. In some cases, removal of the nail plate may be required for reduction as the nail splints the fracture. Reduction should be secured with an intramedullary K-wire.

Marginal fractures off the dorsal (Fig. 42-37) or volar lip (Fig. 42-38) of the distal phalanx should raise concerns of extensor or flexor tendon injury. Careful clinical examination must be performed to ensure active flexion and extension at the DIP joint as part of the assessment of distal phalanx fractures. Large fragments may result in joint instability and subluxation and require reduction and fixation (transarticular, dorsal block pinning, or formal open reduction and internal fixation). When there is no subluxation, nonoperative

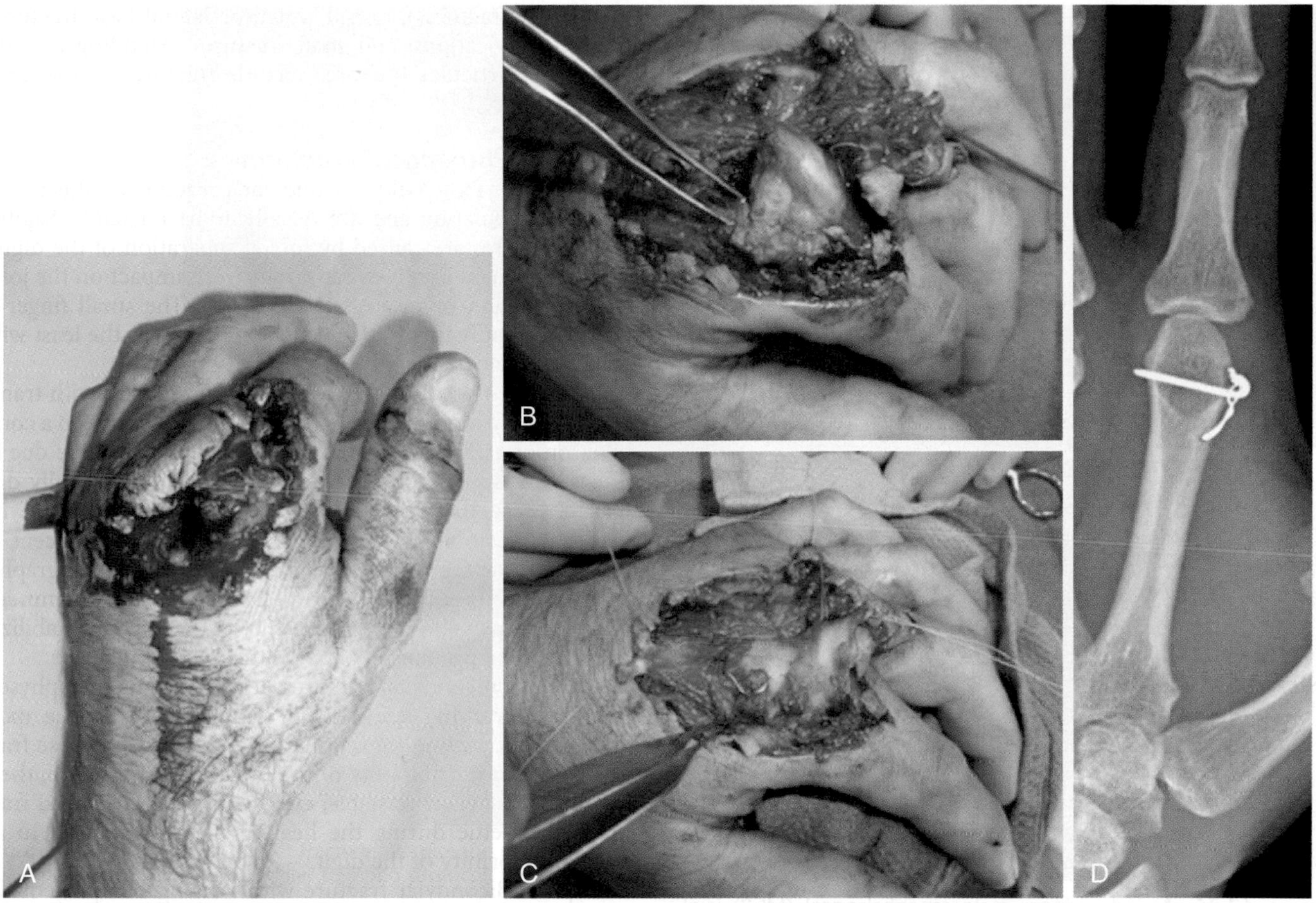

Figure 42-35. A, Combined injury with extensor lacerations and metacarpal fracture. **B,** The bony origin of the index finger radial collateral ligament (RCL) at the metacarpophalangeal (MCP) joint is avulsed creating instability. **C,** K-wire tension band technique restores RCL stability. **D,** Postoperative radiographs.

treatment is usually preferred. The treatment of small avulsion fragments is directed toward the tendon injury.

Closed epiphyseal avulsion fractures (Salter-Harris type III) of the distal phalanx are relatively common and are managed in a similar fashion to their adult variants. "Seymour" fractures represent epiphyseal separations, result from hyperflexion of the digit from axial impact or bending force such as getting the fingertip caught in a door, and represent open physeal injuries when there is associated nail plate avulsion. The terminal extensor tendon retains its attachment to the epiphysis while the flexor profundus flexes the distal fragment resulting in a mallet-like deformity of the digit. The overlying nail is usually avulsed at the proximal nail fold with increasing severity with worsening fracture displacement. Avulsion of the proximal nail plate from the eponychial fold with concomitant matrix root avulsion or laceration renders this an open injury with subsequent risk of superficial, and deep osseous infection if not treated urgently with irrigation and débridement, fracture reduction and stabilization, and matrix repair. If these injuries present in a delayed fashion, it is not uncommon for the finger to be painful and swollen. Osteomyelitis remains a concern, as does premature physeal closure.

Primary management can be performed in the emergency department if there are facilities for conscious sedation of the child along with digital nerve block. Often these injuries are managed in the operating room. The nail plate is carefully elevated from the underlying matrix. Matrix tissue interposed in the fracture site is carefully freed. The bone is irrigated through the matrix laceration or root avulsion without disturbing the physis. The fracture is reduced and often requires K-wire fixation. The matrix is repaired with absorbable sutures. The nail plate may be replaced. With suspected infection or delayed presentation, a formal irrigation and débridement should be performed.

Complications. Symptomatic nonunion of distal phalangeal fractures is uncommon. Small painful nonunited tuft fragments may be excised. Corticocancellous grafting and screw and K-wire fixation through a midaxial or palmar midline approach may be performed for diaphyseal nonunions (Fig. 42-39). Diaphyseal malunions of the distal phalanx may require osteotomy in select cases of significant clinical deformity.

Fractures of the Middle and Proximal Phalanges

Middle and proximal phalanges are short "long" bones and they exhibit similar fracture patterns with cortical shaft fractures that are subject to displacement and/or rotation and metaphyseal and/or articular fractures subject to compression and displacement. In the hand "form follows function," and restoration of alignment is important to maintain range of motion. Reduction and immobilization of unstable phalangeal fractures with closed techniques is challenging. Loss of motion

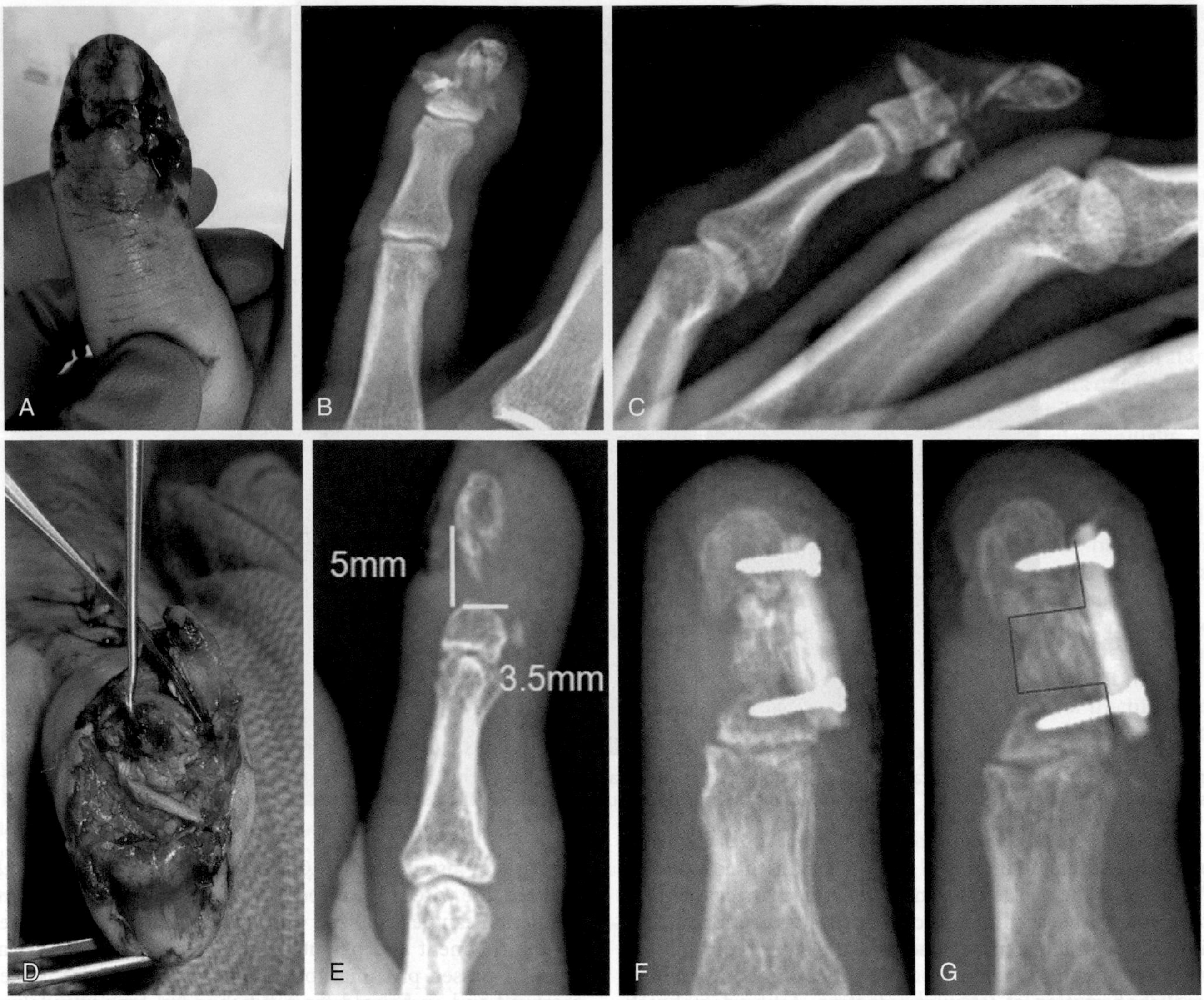

Figure 42-39. **A,** Severe crush injury of the small finger. **B** and **C,** Comminuted underlying distal phalanx fracture with segmental bone loss. **D,** Segmental bone loss and nail matrix avulsion. **E,** Symptomatic unstable atrophic diaphyseal nonunion developed with intact terminal extensor and flexor digitorum profundus. **F,** Through a radial midaxial incision the nonunion site was débrided and a distal radius corticocancellous bone was harvested and fashioned to fill the diaphyseal defect using the distal radius cortex as a structural strut through which 1.3-mm modular hand screws were placed to fix the autograft. **G,** Healed nonunion.

TABLE 42-1 *FACTORS AFFECTING OUTCOME OF PHALANGEAL FRACTURES*

Patient Factors	Injury Characteristics	Treatment and Rehabilitation
Age	Soft tissue crush	Appropriate evaluation
Comorbidities (e.g., diabetes, osteoporosis)	Associated nerve and/or tendon injury	Early reduction and stabilization
Preinjury range of motion	Articular fracture	Joint reduction and articular alignment
Motivation	Unstable fracture pattern (i.e., spiral, oblique, comminuted)	Soft tissue management, edema control
Compliance	Open injury Comminuted fracture or bone loss Multiple injuries	Timely mobilization and rehabilitation Recognition and treatment of complications

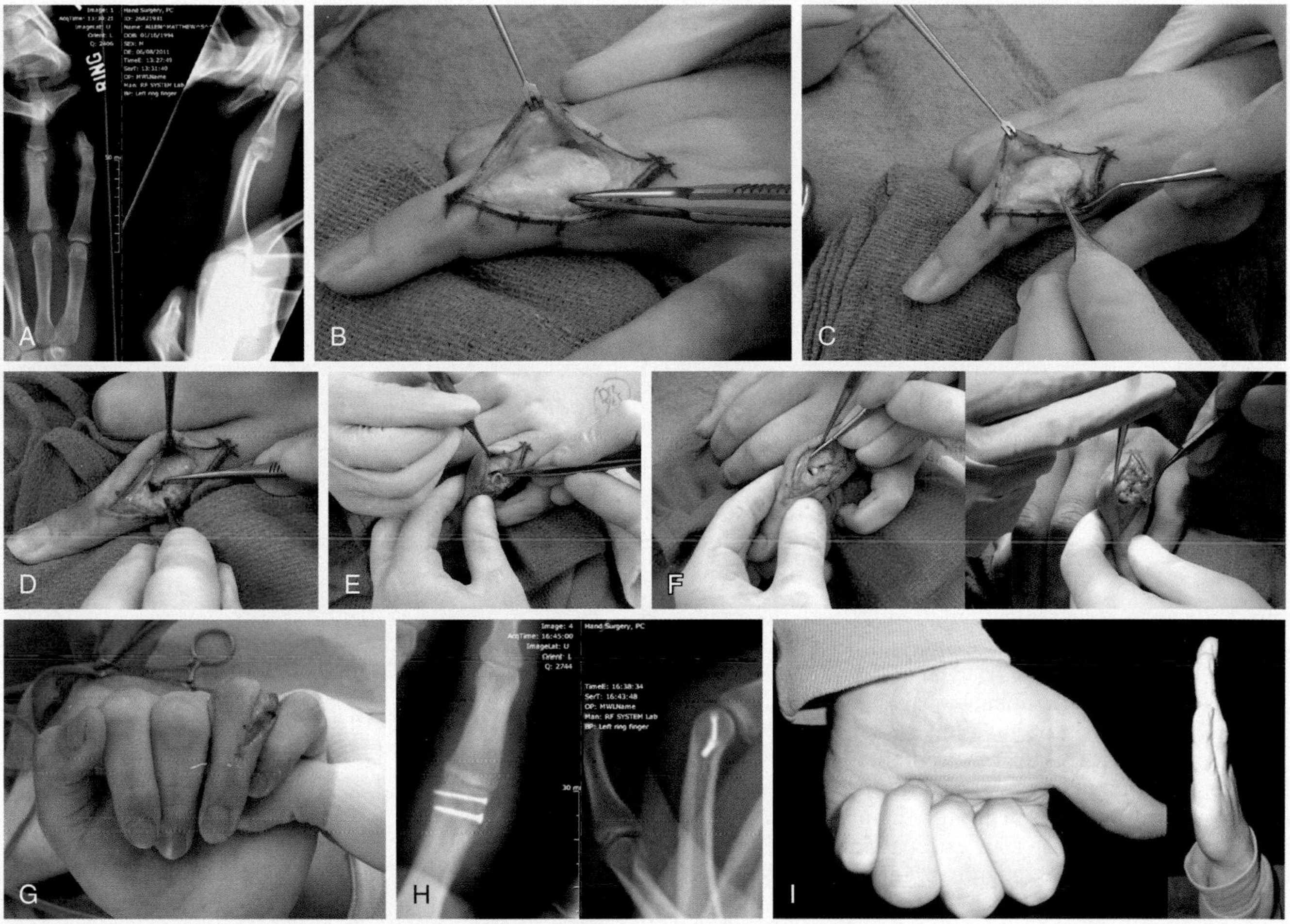

Figure 42-40. **A,** Preoperative radiographs demonstrate malrotated ulnar condylar fracture. Computed tomography (CT) was used in this case to better define the fracture plane. **B,** A dorsal curvilinear incision is used, followed by elevation of a full thickness cutaneous flap. **C,** Division of the transverse retinacular ligament. **D,** Division of the transverse retinacular ligament allows retraction of the ipsilateral conjoined lateral band and central extensor followed by dorsal capsulotomy and fracture mobilization. **E,** Complete malrotation of the condylar fracture fragment on the ipsilateral collateral ligament is seen. **F,** Articular reduction and fixation with two modular hand screws. **G,** Tenodesis demonstrates restoration of the digital cascade. **H,** Final postoperative radiographs. **I,** Final clinical outcome at 6 months' follow-up.

fragment is not rendered stable in the sagittal plane by a single fixation point. Following stable fixation, active and active-assisted motion and reverse-blocking exercises are initiated within the first postoperative week. A hand-based intrinsic plus splint is used in between range of motion sessions.

Coronal condylar fractures pose the biggest management challenge. While clinical deformity is not immediately obvious due to limited motion, a rotational deformity of the digit becomes obvious when mobility is regained later as the middle phalanx rotates when flexed onto a depressed condyle. Displaced fractures lead to joint instability in flexion and, left untreated, can lead to nonunion or malunion with significant joint stiffness. Nonoperative treatment is ineffective as the condylar fragment is devoid of soft tissue attachments and cannot be manipulated into position. The fracture is best exposed through a lateral approach. The fragment is gently manipulated back into position and can be fixed with a K-wire passed from dorsal to volar. The wire can be cut close to bone and left buried with minimal risk of late migration. Alternatively, the wire is passed through a stab incision from intact dorsal skin and can be left outside for removal at 3 weeks. Screw fixation of these small fragments is difficult but obviates problems associated with wires and provides for better stability. The screw is inserted from dorsal to volar using lag screw technique. Screw length is critical as a long screw will protrude through the articular surface of the condyle on the volar surface and cause discomfort during terminal flexion.

Open reduction of bicondylar fractures requires good visualization of and access to the entire distal articular surface of the proximal phalanx. A curved dorsal skin incision is made over the PIP joint and the extensor mechanism is elevated in one of two ways: by making an incision between the lateral and extensor slip on either side, or by elevating the extensor mechanism and creating a distally based V-shaped flap with the apex of the V situated at the proximal third of the proximal phalanx (i.e., reverse Chamay[189] extensor tenotomy). A transverse capsulotomy will allow visualization of the joint. The articular surface is first restored and held with a K-wire. The articular fragments are then stabilized to the shaft with an oblique K-wire (Fig. 42-41). While this fixation will maintain reduction it will not permit early motion, and consideration must be given to stable internal fixation with a plate, either a dorsal T-plate or a laterally applied mini condylar plate. Although insertion of a lateral condylar plate is technically

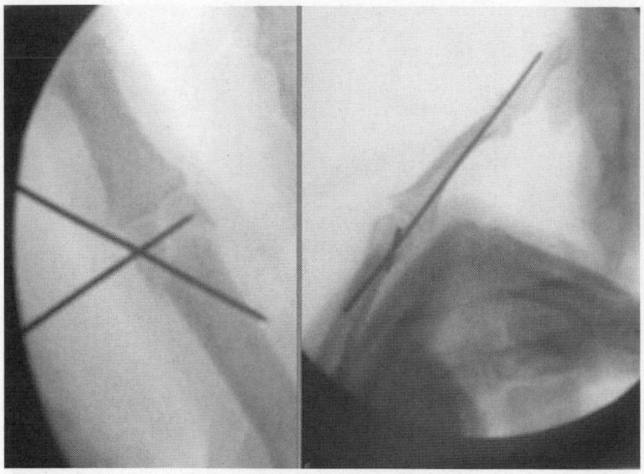

Figure 42-41. K-wire fixation of bicondylar proximal phalangeal fracture.

more challenging, it causes least interference with the extensor mechanism. Laterally applied modular fixed-angle plates have begun to replace mini condylar blade plates. The extensor tendon is repaired with nonabsorbable sutures. Controlled active mobilization is started within a week.

Alternative forms of treatment should be considered in extensively comminuted phalangeal head fractures. In these cases, conservative treatment with longitudinal traction applied through the nail or an external fixator may be used to maintain length and alignment of the digit. Primary joint replacement arthroplasty may be considered in elderly low-demand individuals when the articular surface is not reconstructible or poor bone quality precludes stable fixation (Fig. 42-42).

Phalangeal Base Fractures

Dorsal Base Fractures. Isolated dorsal base fractures occur in the middle phalanx and represent avulsion fractures of the central slip of the extensor mechanism. These injuries are usually part of a volar dislocation of the proximal IP joint. Treatment of the injury depends on alignment of the fragment after reduction of the joint and splinting in full extension. Operative treatment is indicated if the fragment remains displaced by 2 mm or more, if the joint is incongruent due to angulation of a large fragment, or if there is joint subluxation.

Small, minimally displaced or nondisplaced dorsal base fractures not associated with a volar dislocation or extensor lag may be treated with a short arc of motion protocol[190] with the understanding that close serial clinical follow-up is needed to ensure that an extensor lag does not develop.

Pinning the PIP joint in full extension will usually restore satisfactory alignment when the avulsion fragment is small. Open reduction and screw fixation via a dorsal approach may be considered for displaced, large fragments with residual joint subluxation (Fig. 42-43). An alternative method of fixation consists of tension band and cerclage wiring applied through transverse metaphyseal drill holes in the base of the middle phalanx and passed deep to the central slip (Fig. 42-44). Supplemental transarticular K-wire for 3 to 4 weeks is necessary to protect the fixation.

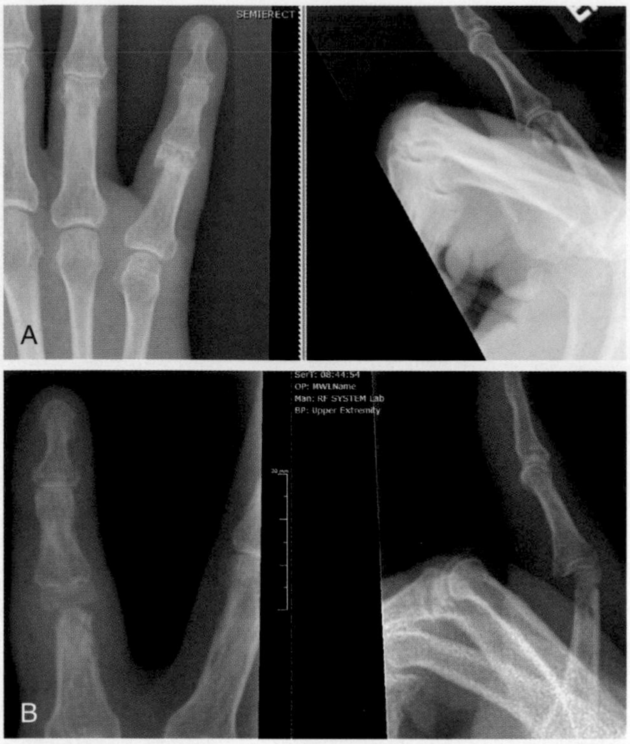

Figure 42-42. **A,** Complex complete articular fracture of the head of the proximal phalanx. **B,** Silicone implant arthroplasty performed as the articular surface was not reconstructible.

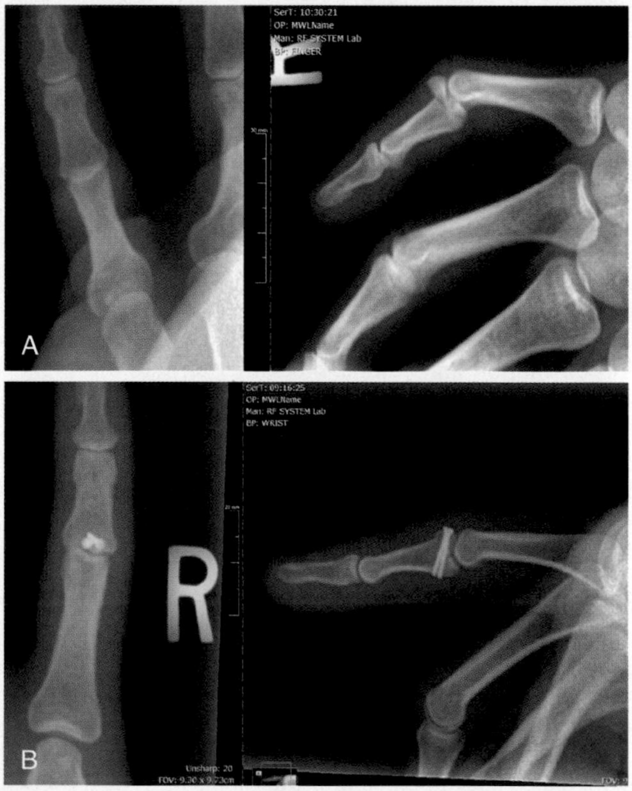

Figure 42-43. **A,** Large, displaced central slip avulsion fracture with resultant volar rotatory subluxation of the proximal interphalangeal joint. **B,** Open reduction and internal fixation (ORIF) via dorsal approach using modular screw fixation. Postoperative rehabilitation consisted of an active short arc of motion protocol with progressive reduction of the proximal interphalangeal (PIP) flexion block.

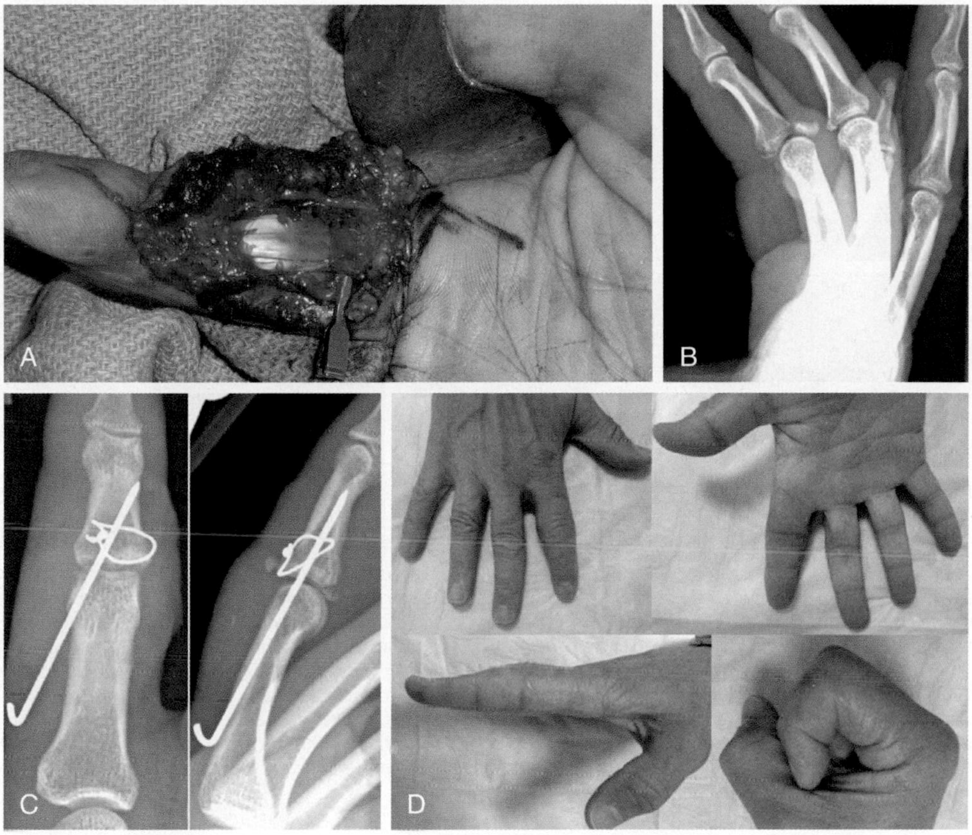

Figure 42-44. **A,** Severe digital crush injury with dysvascular digit and (**B**) open, large, displaced central slip avulsion fracture. **C,** Postoperative posterior-anterior (PA) and lateral radiographs following open reduction and internal fixation (ORIF) with cerclage wire transarticular fixation. Revascularization was performed following bony fixation. **D,** Final clinical outcome.

Volar Lateral Fractures. Fractures of the lateral volar base of the proximal or middle phalanx result from collateral avulsion and may be associated with joint dislocation. Minimally displaced lateral corner fractures that do not compromise joint stability or result in an incongruous articular surface can be treated by splinting followed by early protected motion with buddy taping to the digit adjacent to the fracture when pain and swelling have subsided. Significantly displaced lateral corner fractures or large fragments may compromise joint stability and require internal fixation. A volar approach to the joint allows direct access to fragment that can be compressed against the phalanx with a lag screw.[191] A palmar approach to the joint involves a chevron incision centered over the joint flexion crease. The interval between the neurovascular bundle and the flexor tendon sheath is developed. The cruciate-synovial window between the A2 and A4 pulleys is reflected. The flexor tendons are reflected laterally exposing the volar plate. The volar plate is then incised and reflected distally. By maintaining traction on the digit to counteract displacing forces, the fragment can be elevated to its normal position and fixed with temporary wires while the reduction is confirmed by radiography. One or preferably two screws are inserted. If secure fixation is achieved, protected motion can be started as soon in a few days after the initial pain and swelling are controlled (Fig. 42-45).

Plateau Fractures

Compression injuries can cause impaction of the radial or ulnar plateaus at the base of the middle phalanx or proximal phalanx. The radiographic findings may be subtle. Clinical examination under local anesthesia will demonstrate angular deformity as the phalangeal condyle engages the articular impaction. These injuries require open reduction from a dorsal or lateral approach with elevation of the articular fragment and bone grafting of the resulting metaphyseal void. Additional buttress plate should be considered if the fracture is felt to be unstable.[192]

Volar Central Fracture-Dislocations

Palmar lip fractures are classified based on the stability of the IP joint, which is predicated on the size of the articular marginal fracture (Fig. 42-46). In most cases, the PIP remains stable in the coronal and sagittal planes with smaller palmar lip avulsion fractures (<30% articular surface) due to hyperextension injuries, and are treated with early protected motion protocols. Splinting these injuries in flexion is not necessary and will risk flexion contracture of the joint. Occasionally, the marginal fracture may be significantly displaced or malrotated, but the PIP joint remains stable. Displaced volar marginal fractures may limit IP joint flexion and may be excised when joint stability is not compromised (Fig. 42-47). Extrusion of the fragment into the flexor sheath has been described.[193]

Cadaveric analyses demonstrated that when the articular fragment measures more than 40% of the articular surface, the IP joint becomes unstable as the insertional footprint of the collateral ligaments remains with the volar articular fragment(s).[168] Unstable, dorsal, intraarticular fracture-dislocations and pilon fractures (middle phalangeal complete

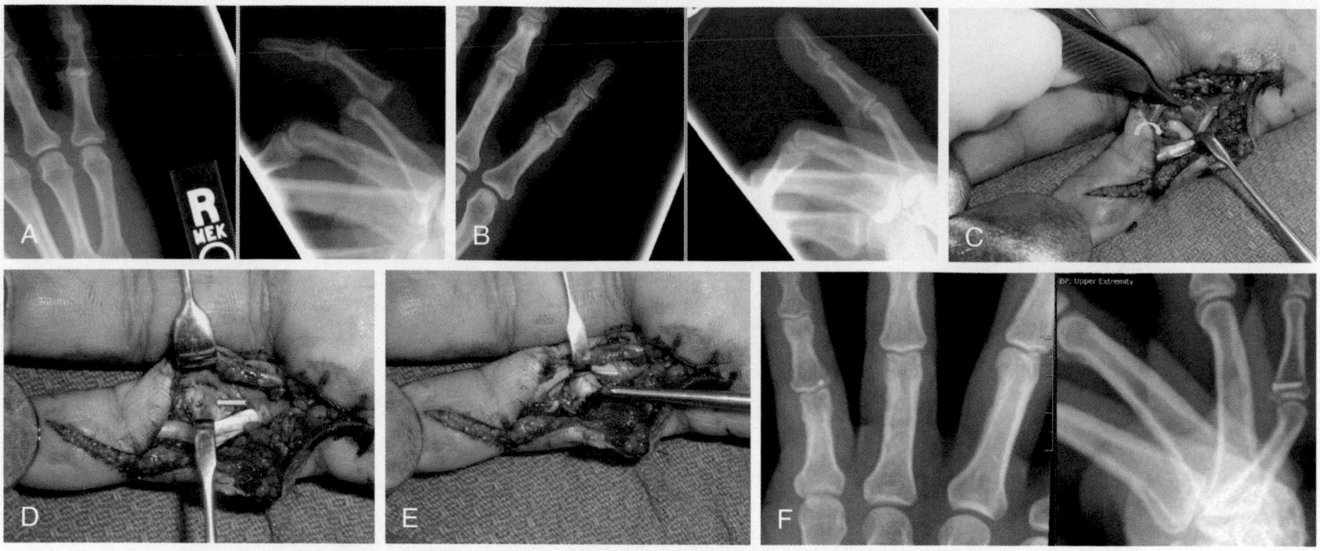

Figure 42-45. **A,** Small finger open dorsal proximal interphalangeal (PIP) fracture-dislocation. **B,** Under digital anesthetic, the open wound was first irrigated followed by closed reduction. Postreduction radiographs demonstrate a large displaced and malrotated volar-radial marginal fracture at the base of the middle phalanx. **C,** Open reduction is performed via palmar exposure through the open palmar wound. The A2 and A4 pulleys are preserved and the flexor tendons are retracted ulnarward. The volar plate remains attached to the volar-radial marginal fracture fragments (forceps). The metaphyseal donor site at the volar-radial margin of the middle phalangeal base is visualized *(arrow)*. **D,** The articular fragments are anatomically reduced and internal fixation performed with a 1.3-mm modular hand screw while preserving the volar plate attachment on the articular fragment *(arrow)*. **E,** The volar plate is repaired to the ulnar critical corner (dental probe) following fixation of the volar-radial margin. Postoperative rehabilitation included early active motion with gradual reduction of a dorsal block splint. **F,** Final postoperative radiographs demonstrate preservation of joint space and maintenance of a congruous reduction. Full composite flexion was achieved. A small residual PIP flexion contracture did not require further treatment.

articular fractures) of the PIP joint are difficult to treat and often lead to long-term pain, stiffness, functional deficits, and arthrosis. The goals of treatment of unstable PIP joint dorsal fracture-dislocations include reestablishing articular congruity and providing a stable and concentric joint, thereby permitting early motion to minimize joint stiffness and contracture.

For larger fractures with associated dorsal instability, closed reduction by traction, volar translation, and flexion of the PIP joint may be successful if seen within a few days after injury. Fluoroscopy is helpful to assess joint congruency following reduction. In unstable injuries, the joint dislocates as the digit is brought into extension and it is important to document the position at which this occurs. Immobilization of the PIP joint in extreme flexion will stabilize the joint but lead to severe flexion contracture and morbidity. Therefore, if a position of more than 30 degrees of flexion is necessary to maintain a congruous reduction, alternative methods of stabilization are selected.

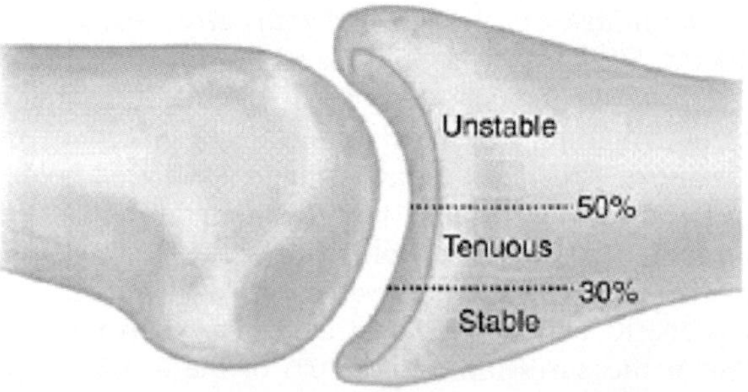

Figure 42-46. Proximal interphalangeal (PIP) joint palmar lip fracture classification. *(Source: From Kang R, Stern PJ: Fracture dislocations of the proximal interphalangeal joint, J Am Soc Surg Hand 2:2, 2002.)*

Extension Block Splinting

Extension block splinting[194] is applicable to cases when a closed, congruous reduction can be achieved. The dorsal block splint prevents extension of the PIP joint to the point of redislocation, while permitting further flexion. Custom splinting is initiated at 10 degrees more than the angle of PIP stability and the middle phalanx is left free for active flexion exercises of the PIP joint. The amount of flexion is reduced on a weekly basis by about 25% and full extension is delayed for about 4 weeks followed by buddy taping for an additional 2 weeks. Acceptable outcomes have been achieved with short periods of immobilization with the finger in as much as 50 to 60 degrees of flexion. Close follow-up with frequent radiographic examination is warranted to ensure that congruous reduction is maintained.

Extension Block Pinning

Extension block pinning[195] is used when the reduced PIP cannot be adequately stabilized in a dorsal block splint. The PIP joint is reduced by applying manual traction and placing the joint into maximal possible flexion. A smooth K-wire is then introduced percutaneously to engage the distal articular surface of the proximal phalanx and advanced in an intramedullary fashion to engage the volar cortex of the proximal phalanx. The wire is left long outside the skin and limits terminal PIP extension. Pin placement should avoid incarceration of the central slip. Gentle active range of motion exercise

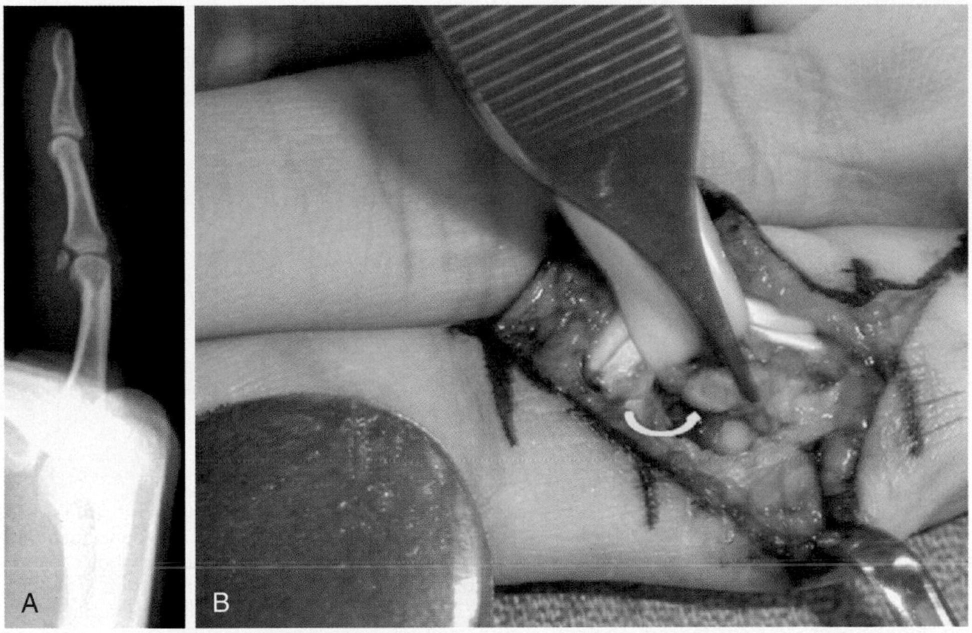

Figure 42-47. A, Displaced volar marginal fracture limiting interphalangeal joint flexion but without associated proximal interphalangeal (PIP) instability. **B,** The fracture fragment was found extruded into the flexor sheath *(arrow)*.

is initiated, and the K-wire is removed at 3 to 4 weeks. Pin care is recommended to avoid synovial fistula and superficial or deep infection.

Closed Reduction and Percutaneous Fixation

Closed reduction and percutaneous pinning (CRPP) of unstable singular volar central articular fractures has been described with parallel percutaneous K-wires.[196]

Open Reduction and Internal Fixation

ORIF of unstable fracture-dislocations of the PIP joint is reserved for fracture-dislocations with a large, noncomminuted volar articular fragment amendable to screw fixation or in cases with delayed presentation when closed reduction or traction techniques are unsuccessful. Reduction and stabilization of the volar lip fracture of the middle phalanx restores adequate stability to allow early active motion and rehabilitation.[197-199] A palmar exposure using either Bruner or midaxial incisions is performed from the proximal digital crease to the distal IP joint flexion crease. The flexor tendon sheath is opened between the A2 and A4 pulleys and reflected laterally. Often the sheath is ruptured in this region and can be excised without significant functional loss. The flexor profundus tendon is retracted to one side and the natural split between the slips of the sublimis tendon is extended to expose the traumatized volar plate. The volar plate is mobilized by releasing its lateral attachments to the collateral ligaments. It is left attached to the volar articular fragment (see Fig. 42-45). The articular fragment is reduced and provisionally held size-appropriate K-wires. The reduction is assessed fluoroscopically and the K-wires can then be sequentially exchanged for modular hand screws (usually two to three screws ranging from 1.1 to 1.3 mm). Rarely, a buttress plate for comminuted fractures may be needed. In chronic cases with an irreducible joint, the attachments of the collateral ligaments to the base of the middle phalanx are partially released in a volar to dorsal direction and the digit is gently hyperextended until it is fully "shotgunned." The volar fragment is then fully visualized. Small comminuted fragments are removed and the major volar fragment is elevated, reduced, and held either with a circumferential wire loop or with lag screws passed from volar to dorsal.[200]

External Fixation

Unstable, acute, comminuted volar central fractures, pilon fractures, and subacute and/or chronic PIP fracture-subluxations are complex articular injuries. Continuous dynamic skeletal traction can be applied to the digit through several transosseous proximal and middle phalangeal K-wire configurations and with addition of force-coupling wires.[201] Alternative forms of external fixators include K-wires bent in tension,[202] wires coiled into springs,[203] hinged devices,[204] force-couple devices,[205] parallel spring-framed systems,[206] and pins and rubber bands.[207] Static external fixators also may be used. If adequate reduction of the articular surface of the middle phalanx is not achieved by traction alone, the articular surface can be manipulated percutaneously or by open reduction. The fragments are then stabilized with multiple small K-wires and traction is then applied.[208] The variable configurations are all based on the concept of joint reduction through soft tissue distraction around the articular base of the middle phalanx. These fixators are designed to allow some degree of active motion to allow the concave articular surface to remodel around the convex condyles of the proximal phalanx while the joint is unloaded from compressive and shear forces.

Volar Plate Arthroplasty

When the volar central base is comminuted and cannot be stabilized, volar plate interpositional arthroplasty (Fig. 42-48) to resurface the volar articular surface of the middle phalanx is indicated when less than 40% of the joint is involved.[209] Dionysian and Eaton have reported on midterm outcomes

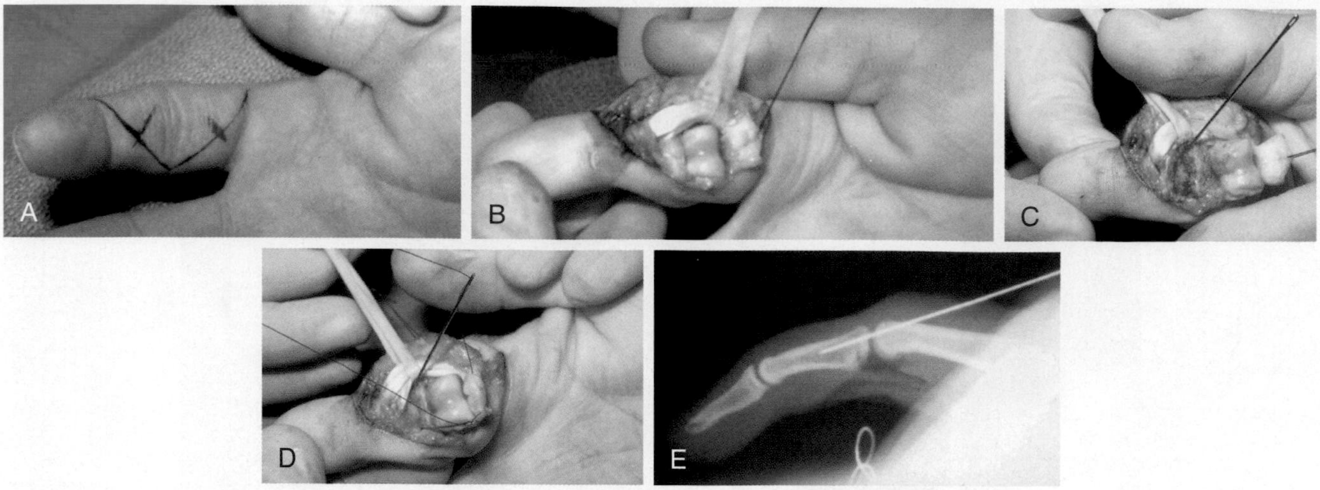

Figure 42-48. **A,** A radially based volar flap is used. **B,** A cruciate synovial window between A2 and A4 is used and flexor tendons are retracted. The collateral ligaments are released proximally. The volar plate is reflected proximally. The proximal interphalangeal (PIP) joint is then "shotgunned." **C,** The base of the middle phalanx is then débrided to create a symmetric transverse groove. Drill holes with 0.045-inch K-wires are placed at the periphery of the defect. **D,** 2-0 Prolene suture is passed through the distal edge and the suture limbs are then passed volar to dorsal using straight thin Keith needles. **E,** The PIP joint is transfixed in 20 to 30 degrees of flexion. The volar plate is then advanced and the Prolene sutures are tied dorsally over a pullout button. The critical corners of the three-dimensional ligamentous box supporting the PIP joint is restored when the volar plate is sutured to the collateral ligament insertions.

following volar plate arthroplasty (VPA).[210] At a mean of 11.5 years postoperatively, patients treated with VPA within 4 weeks of injury attained a mean 85-degree active arc of PIP motion compared to 65 degrees in patients treated with VPA at greater than 4 weeks. Four of seventeen patients showed some degree of joint narrowing at the follow-up examination.

Hemi-Hamate Arthroplasty

Hemi-hamate osteochondral autograft (HHA) reconstruction of the volar base of the middle phalanx has augmented the armamentarium of treatment options for previously irreconstructible articular injuries.[211-213] HHA is indicated for comminuted, unstable PIP palmar lip fracture-dislocations. Comminuted, lateral plateau fractures that cause angular deformity and are not large enough for ORIF are also appropriate for HHA. HHA is also a satisfactory salvage option for patients who have re-dislocated after external fixation, ORIF, or VPA (Fig. 42-49). At a mean 4.5 years following HHA, Calfee and colleagues reported a mean 70-degree arc of PIP motion with a 19-degree flexion contracture and the mean DASH score indicated little functional impairment.[213] HHA is contraindicated when there is advanced articular changes already present on the head of the proximal phalanx. In these cases, arthrodesis or implant arthroplasty are considered.

Nonarticular Fractures of the Phalanges

Phalangeal Neck Fractures

Isolated subcondylar fractures of the neck of the phalanx are almost exclusively seen in children with the majority occurring in toddlers. The mechanism of injury is usually from crush injury (i.e., digit getting caught in a door) and the fracture displaces as the child pulls the finger away.

Al-Qattan[214] has divided pediatric phalangeal neck fractures into nondisplaced, minimally displaced with partial contact of the bony fragments and completely displaced with loss of any contact of the distal fragment with the metaphysis. The distal fragment can be displaced dorsally or volarly and also may rotate completely on its transverse axis. Minimally displaced or nondisplaced phalangeal neck fractures are easily overlooked in the emergency department when suboptimal orthogonal radiographs are obtained. A true lateral radiograph is required to appreciate more subtle phalangeal neck fractures. In this view, displacement of the capital fragment or condylar malrotation is best visualized.

K-wire stabilization for approximately 4 weeks is recommended for all but the nondisplaced fractures to avoid late displacement and malunion. Nondisplaced neck fractures are followed with serial radiographs to confirm maintenance of reduction. Following closed reduction, the fracture is stabilized with either a transarticular or oblique K-wires (Fig. 42-50). Fractures of the middle phalangeal neck that are significantly angulated can be reduced by hyperextending the joint to line up the distal phalanx with the angulated fragment. The fragment is then transfixed with a longitudinal retrograde wire passed through the fingertip. The distal fragment is then maneuvered into a reduced position and the wire advanced into the middle phalanx. Limited-open incisions may be necessary to facilitate anatomic reduction prior to percutaneous pinning. Because of the narrow area of contact and lack of any soft tissue attachment to the distal fragment, these fractures are inherently unstable and displaced fractures cannot always be reduced with closed techniques alone (Fig. 42-51).

Sagittal plane malunion may result in loss of motion due to an altered arc of motion. Dorsal displacement leads to an osseous block at the subcondylar fossa. Displacement in the coronal plane leads to angular deformity of the digit. As the injury is distant to the growth plate, it is believed that remodeling potential is limited. There is more recent clinical evidence that remodeling in the sagittal plane may occur even in older patient who remain skeletally immature.[215-217] Remodeling in the coronal and axial planes is less predictable. Waters and colleagues[218] have proposed a treatment algorithm for skeletally immature phalangeal neck fractures that present in a

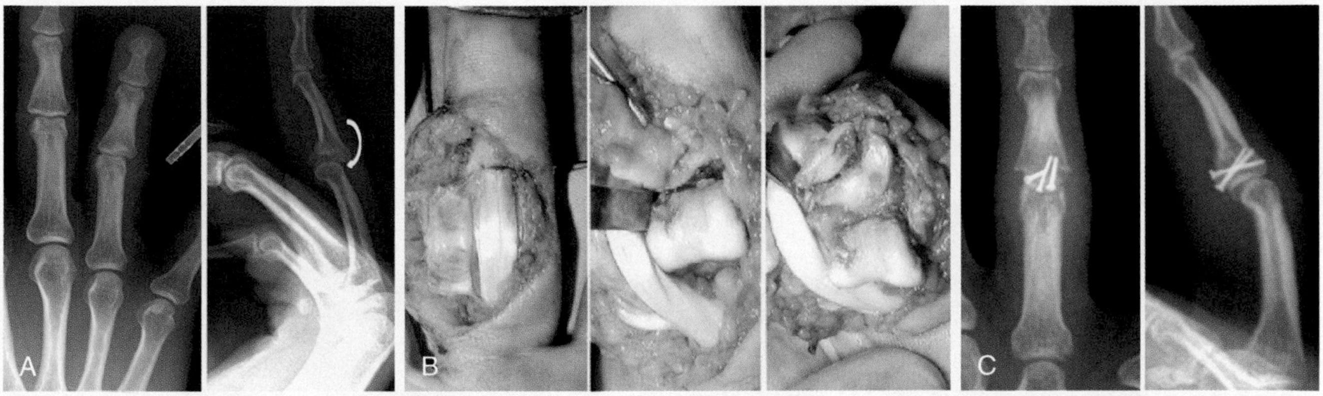

Figure 42-49. A, Preoperative radiographs demonstrating comminuted impacted volar central and lateral plateau articular fractures of the middle phalanx with dorsal subluxation of the proximal interphalangeal (PIP) joint (V-sign; *arrow*). **B,** Intraoperative exposure as previously described. **C,** Postoperative radiographs following hemi-hamate osteochondral autograft (HHA) demonstrating restoration of articular congruency.

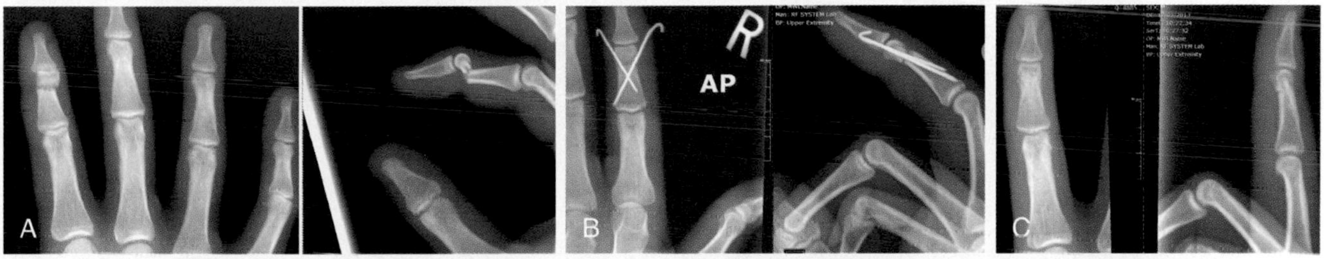

Figure 42-50. A, Widely displaced and angulated phalangeal neck fracture. **B,** Closed reduction and percutaneous pinning with crossed K-wire technique. *AP,* Anterior-posterior. **C,** Well-healed phalangeal neck fracture at 6 weeks.

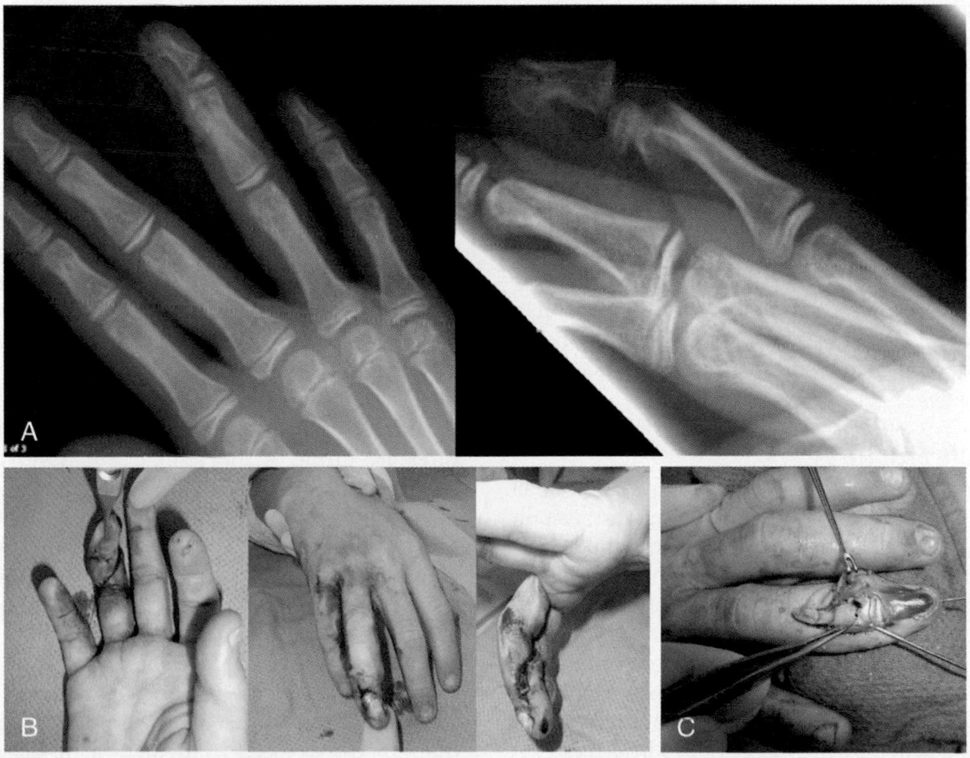

Figure 42-51. A, Skeletally immature patient with severe crush injury and complex combined injury. The skeletal injury included an open distal phalanx transphyseal separation with an open comminuted displaced middle phalangeal neck fracture. The phalangeal neck fracture was extremely unstable secondary to comminution and severe soft tissue injury. **B,** Clinical photos demonstrate a volar-radial soft tissue degloving injury off of the flexor sheath and the dorsal-ulnar extension of the soft tissue injury. The digital arteries were lacerated requiring revascularization, and the digital nerves contused. **C,** Reduction was obtained using the remaining cortical keys along the dorsal ulnar neck (forceps). Bone grafting of the radial metaphyseal void was performed. The avulsed terminal extensor was repaired.

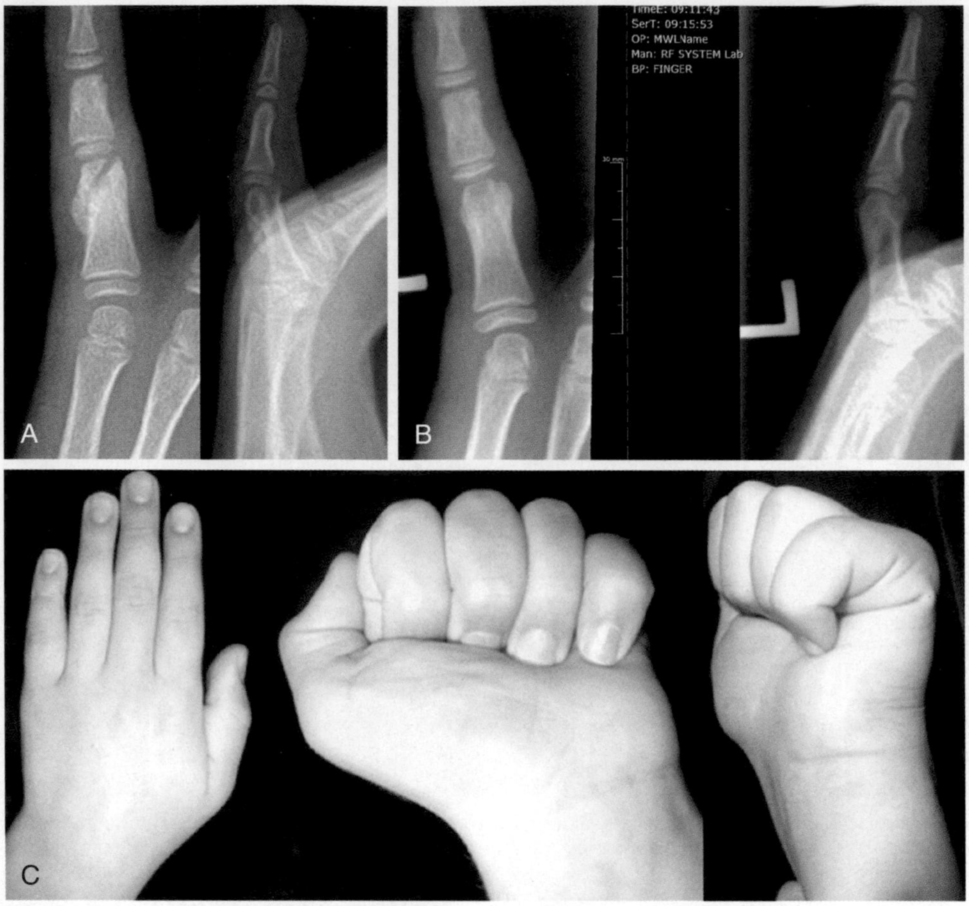

Figure 42-52. A, Skeletally immature patient with a proximal phalangeal neck nascent malunion. Delayed presentation at 1 month after injury. Sagittal plane displacement and abundant callus is noted at presentation. Expectant management was selected because there was minimal fracture site tenderness at presentation, no malrotation, and satisfactory early active (60 degrees) and passive (90 degrees) flexion. **B,** Remodeling noted at the phalangeal neck at 1 year following initial fracture. **C,** Clinical examination demonstrated full motion at latest follow-up.

delayed fashion. Subacute fractures with residual tenderness at the fracture site may be amendable to percutaneous osteoclasis, reduction, and fixation. Open treatment is associated with increased risk of osteonecrosis. Neck fractures with delayed presentation, minimal residual fracture site tenderness, and satisfactory PIP joint motion are potentially better managed with observation and subcondylar recession if a block to flexion ensues (Fig. 42-52).

Phalangeal Shaft Fractures

Phalangeal fractures may be transverse, oblique, spiral, or comminuted and multifragmentary. The latter are usually associated with significant soft tissue injury even if the overlying skin envelope is intact and the injury is technically a closed one. Spiral and oblique fractures are more common in the proximal phalanx diaphysis and transverse fractures tend to be more common in the middle phalanx and proximal third of the proximal phalanx. Transverse proximal phalangeal fractures tend to collapse into an apex volar angulation, with the proximal metaphysis flexed by the interosseous insertion. The remainder of the phalanx then collapses into extension due to the longitudinal pull of the extrinsic extensor. Angulation of middle phalangeal fractures is generally apex dorsal as the sublimis insertion along the distal fragment draws the distal fragment into flexion.

Management of phalangeal fractures depends on the following factors: displacement, fracture geometry, soft tissue injury, and patient characteristics and requirements. Treatment should be tailored to the individual, taking into consideration fracture characteristics.

Oblique and spiral fractures are prone to shortening and malrotation when treated nonoperatively. Periarticular oblique fractures may involve the collateral recess or subcondylar fossa and affect function (Fig. 42-53). Comminuted fractures are prone to shortening, soft tissue adhesions, delayed healing, and stiffness.

Closed Reduction and Immobilization

Closed reduction of phalangeal fractures may be achieved in the first few days after injury under digital block anesthesia. The MCP joint is flexed maximally and the distal fracture fragment of the proximal phalanx reduced to the metaphyseal segment. Fractures that are stable after reduction can be treated nonoperatively with immobilization. In general, less than 10 degrees of malangulation in the coronal or sagittal plan is acceptable. Following reduction, the finger is buddy strapped to the adjacent digit and the hand is immobilized in a hand-based "intrinsic-plus" splint with the MCP joints in 70 degrees of flexion and the IP joints in neutral extension for approximately 3 to 4 weeks. Initiation of mobilization is based

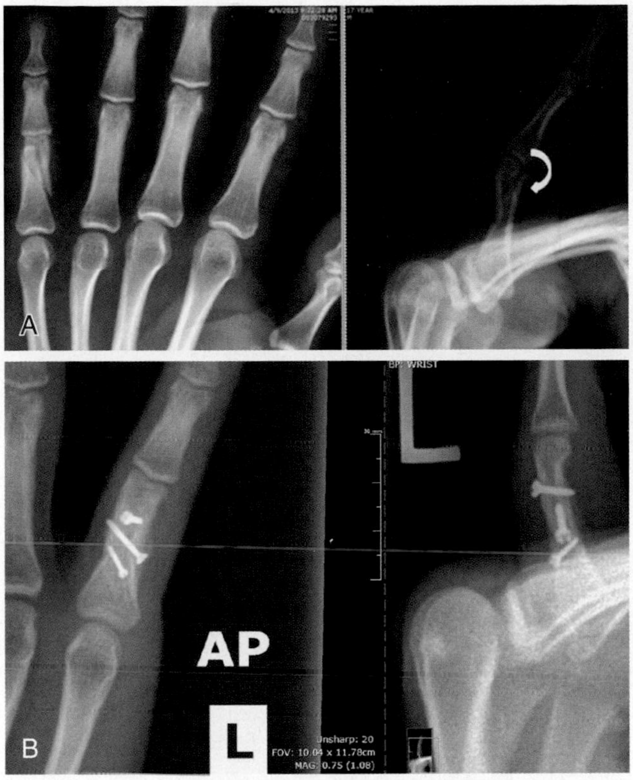

Figure 42-53. A, Proximal phalangeal nascent malunion of diaphysis. Disruption of the subcondylar fossa *(arrow)* creates an osseous block to motion. **B,** Osteotomy and open reduction and internal fixation (ORIF) yields union and full functional arc of motion. *AP,* Anterior-posterior.

on clinical tenderness as early clinical union precedes radiographic union. Early mobilization of reduced stable fractures in a functional splint or cast is facilitated by extending the dorsal aspect past the PIP joint but leaving the palmar aspect of the fingers free to allow active finger flexion. The extensor apparatus overlying the proximal phalanx acts as a tension band, and gliding of the flexors and extensors minimizes risks of flexor tendon adhesions and stiffness. A recent report has suggested that wrist immobilization is not necessary.[219]

Closed Reduction and Percutaneous Pinning

Percutaneous K-wire fixation is the most common method of operative stabilization of unstable proximal and middle phalangeal shaft fractures once satisfactory reduction has been achieved. Care is taken to try and avoid violation of the extensor hood, central extensor tendon, and neurovascular bundles. Early range of motion following percutaneous K-wire fixation is often limited as skin motion at the pin sites may lead to superficial and/or deep pin site infections.

K-wire placement depends on the fracture pattern, configuration, and bone quality. Proximal metaphyseal fractures at the base of the proximal phalanx usually demonstrate dorsal cortical comminution with apex volar angulation. Multiple adjacent fingers can fracture in this fashion in the elderly osteoporotic individual after a fall. Imaging of the phalangeal base is difficult especially after an acute injury. While these fractures are reducible with digital flexion, they are inherently unstable. These fractures may also extend proximally and involve the articular surface. Antegrade crossed K-wires beginning at the periphery of the articular margin are often used to stabilize these fractures (Fig. 42-54). Alternatively, these fractures can be stabilized with a longitudinal wire passed antegrade through the metacarpal head into the medullary cavity of the proximal phalanx.[220] Additional pins may be inserted to provide rotational stability especially in more distal fractures. Each technique has inherent advantages and disadvantages. Patients are counseled regarding the potential for extensor and/or flexor tendon adhesions at the level of the metaphyseal fracture corresponding to the A2 pulley. Following clinical union (typically 4 to 6 weeks postoperatively), a digital block may be performed in the office when there is early postoperative digital stiffness followed by active digital motion to attempt tenolysis and facilitate recovery of digital motion. Sagittal plane malunion may result in clinical pseudo-claw deformity and extensor imbalance with resultant extensor lag.

Oblique and spiral fractures may be fixed with two or more K-wires passed percutaneously perpendicular to the fracture plane, but it is imperative to use fluoroscopy to ensure that the wires truly engage in a bicortical fashion and in the plane perpendicular to the plane of the fracture (Fig. 42-55). Transverse or short oblique wires can be fixed with crossed K-wires (Fig. 42-56). As crossing K-wires tends to distract the fracture, manual compression must be applied to the digit at the time of insertion of the second wire. The fracture is usually immobilized for approximately 3 weeks and the wires are then removed followed by protected motion with buddy taping.

Newer fixation systems with self-tapping miniscrews allow for percutaneous screw fixation through small incisions after reduction. Percutaneous screw fixation achieves interfragmentary compression and may allow for earlier motion.

Open Reduction and Internal Fixation

Open reduction is indicated for irreducible phalangeal fractures, open fractures, and combined injuries. Stable internal fixation facilitates early postoperative functional rehabilitation to try and minimize digital stiffness due to tendon adhesions.

A dorsal curvilinear or lateral and midaxial incisions are most frequently used for proximal phalangeal exposure. Several deep surgical exposures exist. For diaphyseal fractures of the proximal phalanx, the interval between the central extensor tendon and lateral band may be incised, or the extensor may be mobilized together with the ipsilateral conjoined lateral band (Fig. 42-57). For metadiaphyseal fractures, a unilateral intrinsic resection of the lateral band and obliques fibers of the MCP joint facilitates mobilization and reflection of the central extensor tendon in a supraperiosteal fashion (Fig. 42-58).[221] The periosteum is incised along the obliquity of the fracture to allow for anatomic reduction and internal fixation. This exposure is especially useful for plate fixation of unstable proximal phalanx fractures. Lateral plate application minimizes interference with extensor tendon excursion. Furthermore, biomechanical analyses[222,223] suggested that midlateral plate positioning may have superior biomechanical properties. Alternatively, the extensor may be split in its midline for wide exposure of the fracture.

Fractures of the distal third of the proximal phalanx can be exposed in a limited fashion for screw placement without incising the extensor mechanism by retracting the lateral bands dorsally following division of the transverse

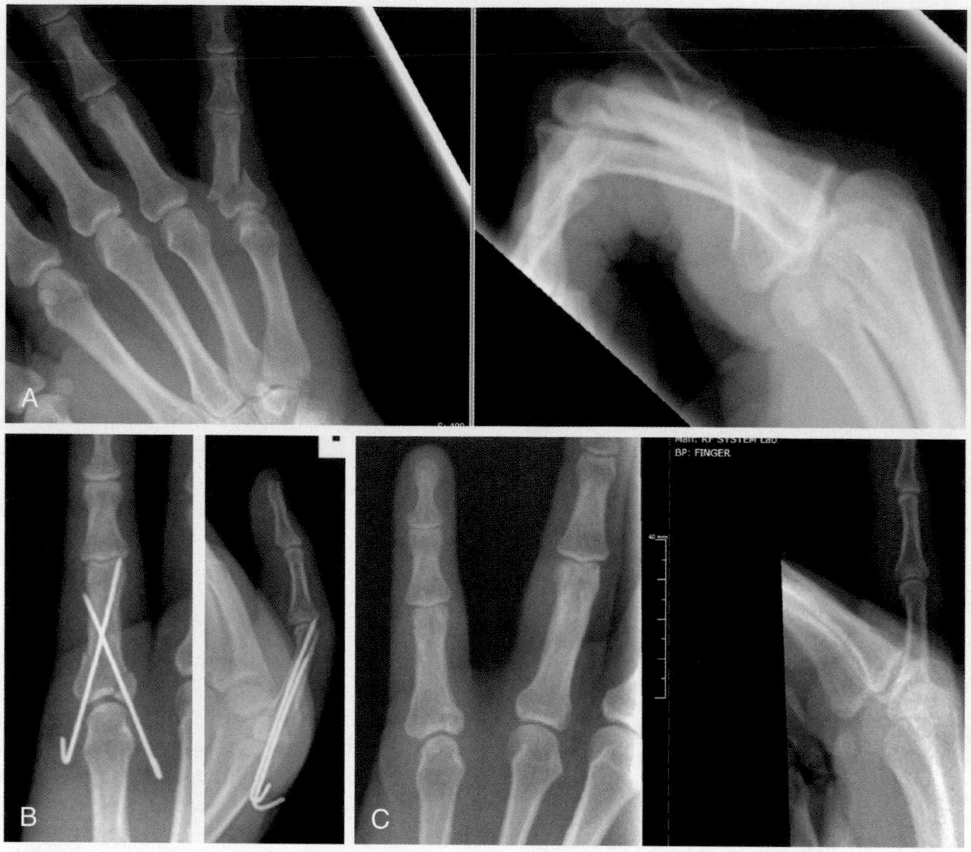

Figure 42-54. A, Proximal phalangeal metaphyseal fracture with articular extension. Apex volar angulation is seen. **B,** Closed reduction and percutaneous crossed K-wire fixation is achieved. **C,** Osseous union with anatomic articular and metadiaphyseal alignment.

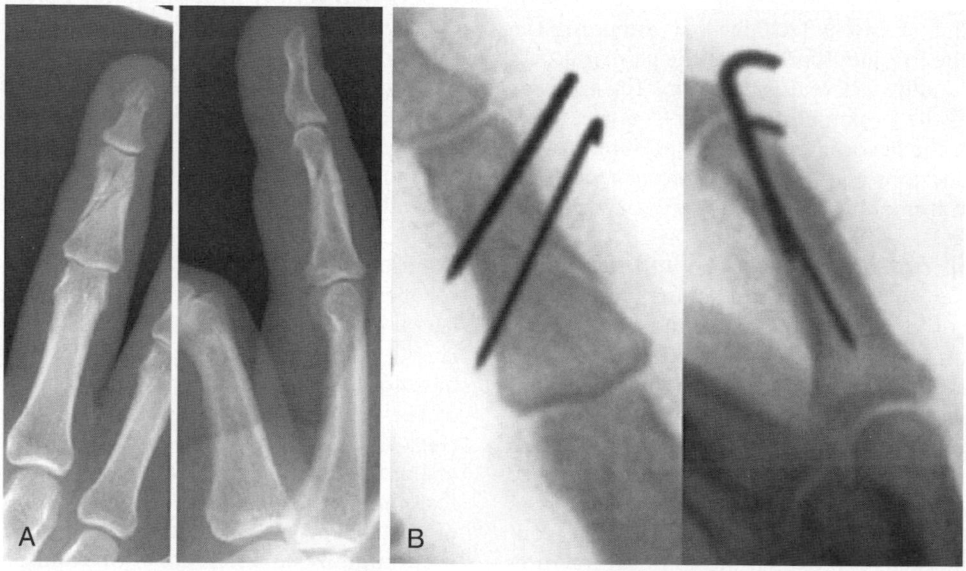

Figure 42-55. A, Rotationally unstable middle phalanx oblique diaphyseal fracture. **B,** Closed reduction and percutaneous parallel K-wires perpendicular to the plane of the fracture. Postoperatively, a distal interphalangeal (DIP) joint tip protector splint is used while early proximal interphalangeal (PIP) joint motion is initiated.

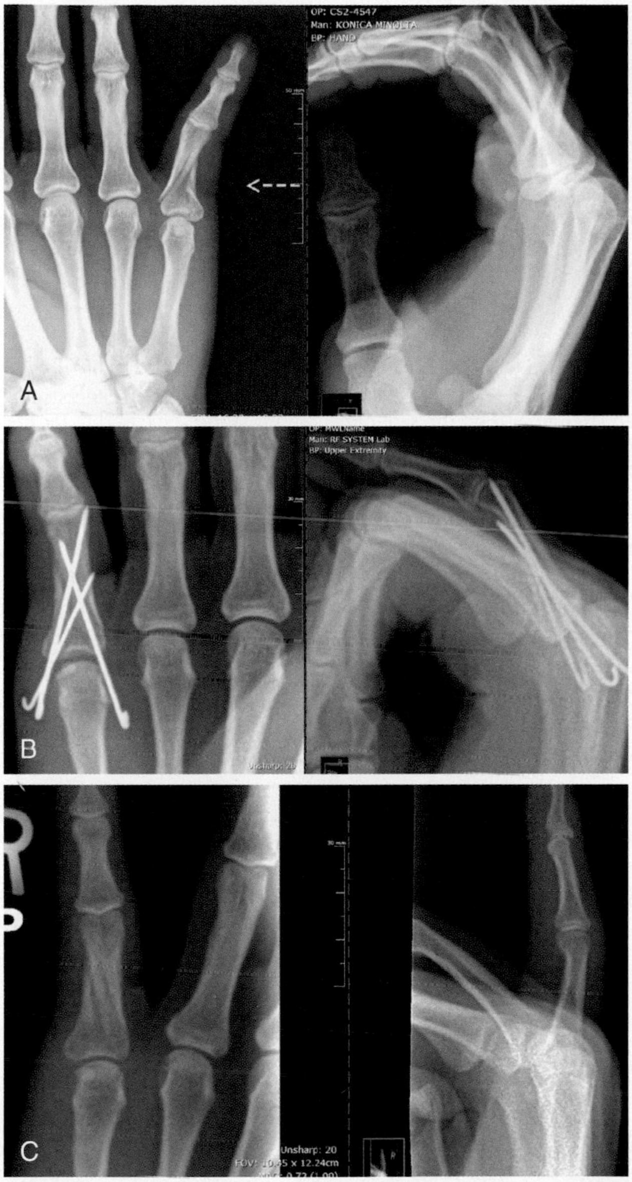

Figure 42-56. **A,** Proximal phalangeal metadiaphyseal fracture with rotational and sagittal plane deformity. **B,** Closed reduction and percutaneous crossed K-wire fixation is achieved. **C,** Osseous union with anatomic articular and metadiaphyseal alignment. Full motion was achieved at latest follow-up.

retinacular ligament as is performed for fixation of unicondylar fractures.

Independent of deep exposure selected, the entire length of the fracture must be exposed, especially with spiral fractures, prior to reduction. The apices must be visualized to confirm anatomic reduction. Once the fracture is provisionally reduced with bone reduction forceps or K-wires, tenodesis maneuver is performed to confirm restoration of the digital cascade. Fixation construct is then selected.

An attempt is always made to repair the periosteum over the implants. When an extensor split is used, the extensor is approximated with a running or interrupted nonabsorbable suture. Extensor adhesion is minimized by encouraging early active motion, reverse blocking exercises, functional splinting, and edema control.

Open Reduction and Wire Fixation

K-wire fixation is acceptable for nearly all fracture configurations but most suited for oblique and spiral fractures when placed perpendicular to the fracture line. Additional compression can be achieved by looping a stainless steel wire around the pins and over the dorsal cortex of the phalanx. When used for transverse fractures, crossed wires can distract the fracture and delay healing especially in the shaft. Compression in transverse fractures can be achieved by passing a cerclage wire through transverse holes in either fragment parallel to the fracture line. The fracture is then reduced and fixed with a single oblique wire prior to tensioning the cerclage wire to achieve fracture compression[224]; 90-90 wiring also achieves compression across a transverse fracture.[225] Coronal and sagittal plane stainless steel wires are passed at the fracture site for bending and rotational stability. This technique requires extensive soft tissue stripping and is usually reserved for replantation.

Screw Fixation

Interfragmentary screws enhance stability by and allow earlier rehabilitation than wire fixation alone. Screws alone are best indicated for the stabilization of oblique and spiral fractures when the length of the fracture is more than twice the diameter of the bone to allow placement of at least two screws (Fig. 42-59). Obtaining bicortical fixation is more imperative than true lag compression.[115] When planning screw placement, care should be taken to stay a minimum of two screw diameters

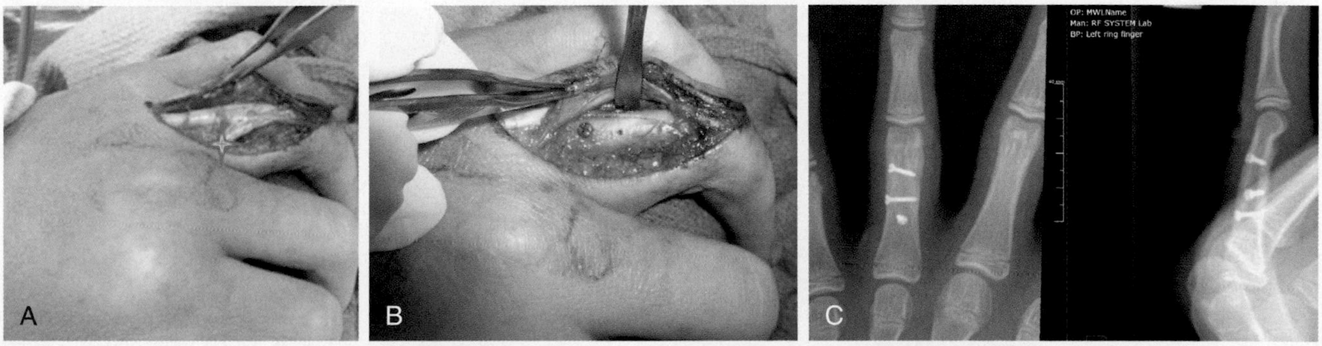

Figure 42-57. **A,** For diaphyseal fractures of the proximal phalanx, a dorsal curvilinear incision is used followed by mobilization of the central extensor in a supraperiosteal fashion together with the ipsilateral conjoined lateral band *(star)*. **B,** Following mobilization of the extensor, the fracture is exposed and anatomically reduced along cortical keys, followed by interfragmentary screws. **C,** Anatomic reduction and osseous union is achieved. A small residual extensor lag at the proximal interphalangeal (PIP) joint is expected.

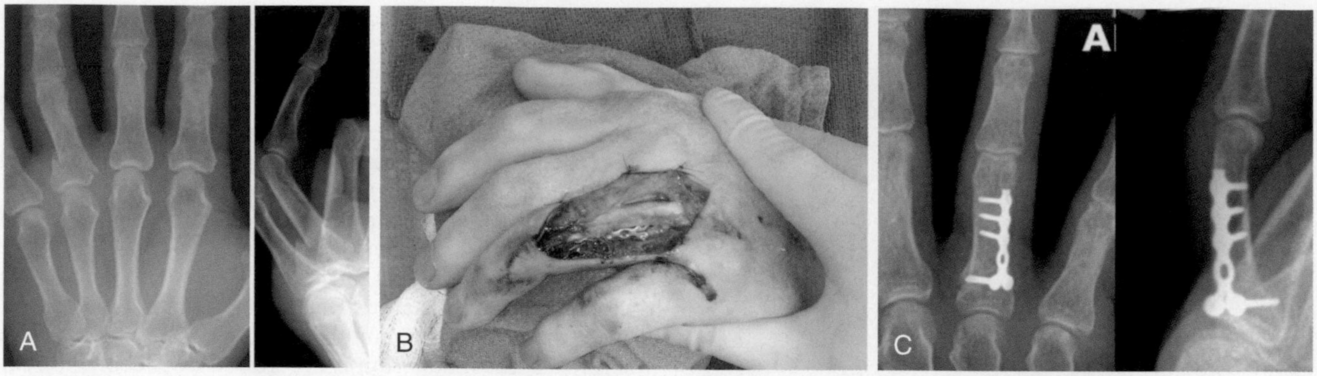

Figure 42-58. **A,** Unstable and displaced ring finger proximal phalangeal metaphyseal fracture. Following elevation of a full-thickness subcutaneous flap from the peritenon of the central extensor tendon, the conjoined lateral band on the side of plate application is excised to facilitate fracture site exposure and reduction. **B,** Ulnar (lateral) plate application following excision of the ulnar conjoined lateral band and fracture reduction. A periarticular locking plate is selected based on the metaphyseal location of the primary fracture line. **C,** Final radiographs demonstrate osseous union.

away from the fracture margin to prevent cortical failure. Generally, 1.3- and 1.5-mm screws are used depending on fragment size and comminution (Fig. 42-60). Care is taken to visualize occult nondisplaced fracture lines that may preclude screw fixation. In the setting of malunited phalangeal fractures with resultant deformity and digital dysfunction, one may consider osteotomy at the level of the malunion if the prior fracture plane can be identified (Fig. 42-61). Alternatively, a derotational osteotomy at the level of the metacarpal is performed for mature digital malunions.[226]

Plate Fixation

Plate and screw stabilization of phalangeal fractures has the advantage of providing stable fixation and permitting early

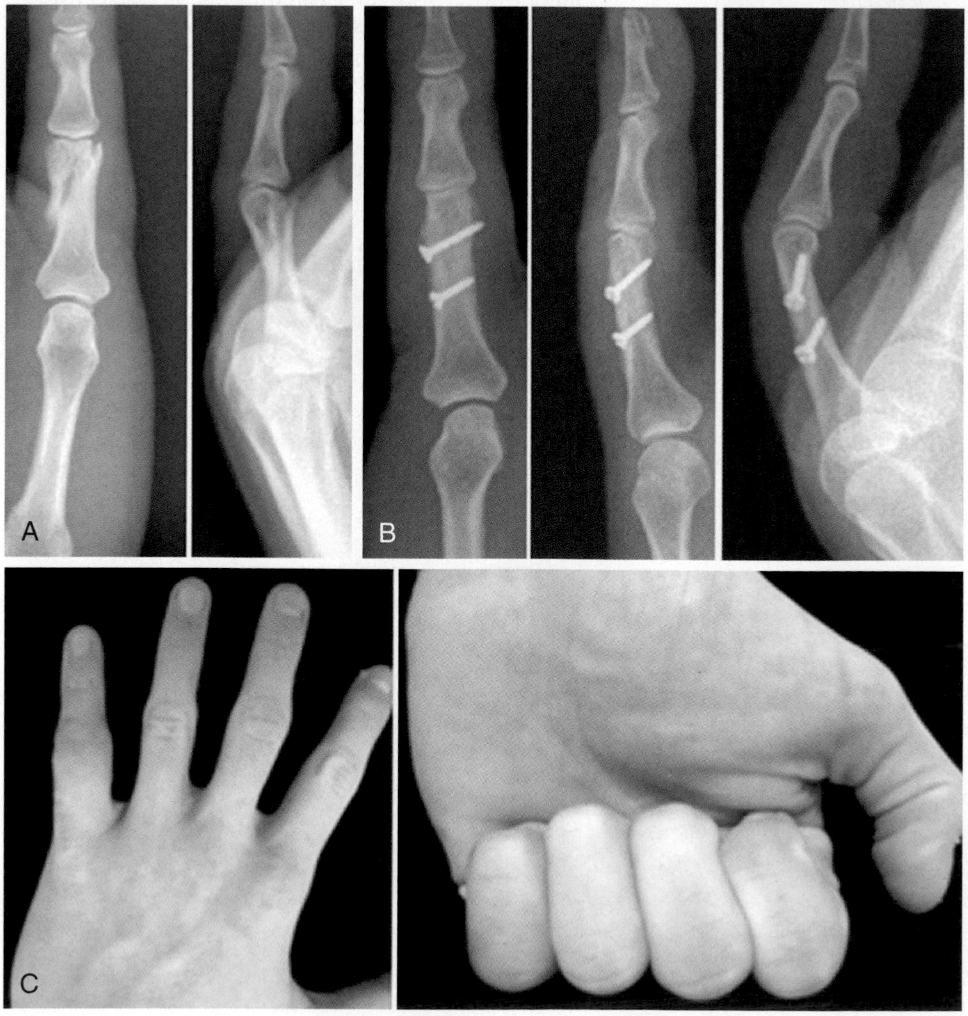

Figure 42-59. **A,** Long oblique proximal phalangeal fracture with shortening and disruption of the subcondylar fossa. **B,** Open reduction and internal fixation (ORIF) with two interfragmentary screws. **C,** Final clinical outcome demonstrates full composite digital flexion and extension.

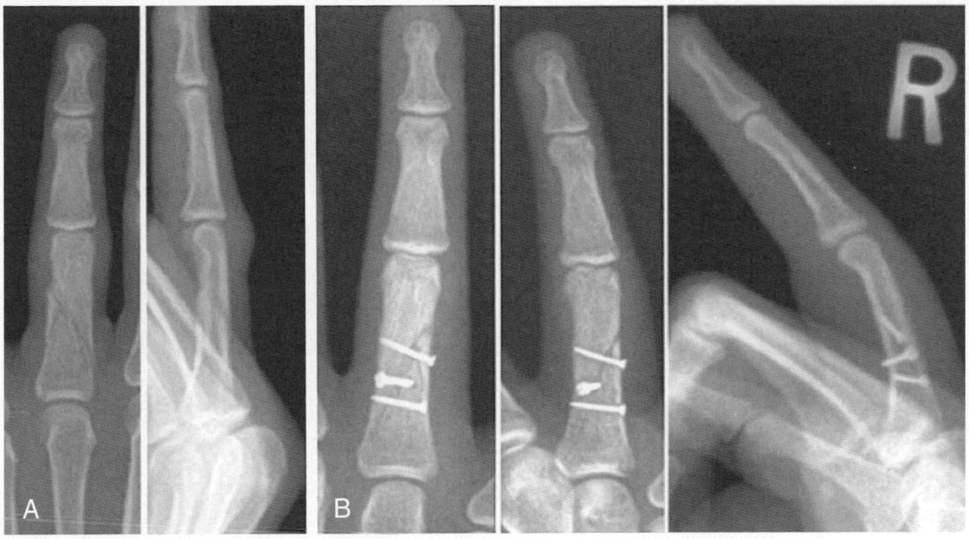

Figure 42-60. A, Multifragmentary ring finger proximal phalangeal fracture. **B,** Appropriately sized interfragmentary screws were used to secure fixation of this multiplanar fracture.

range of motion. Complications of plate fixation are related to their use in more complex cases and open fractures rather than the technique itself.[107] Plate fixation is indicated when K-wire or lag screw fixation is inadequate as in fractures with comminution, articular fractures with extension into the shaft, and for reconstruction of nonunions and malunions. Additionally, there are some fractures, such as transverse fractures of the midshaft, which are amenable to compression plating.

Plates can be placed dorsally (Fig. 42-62) or laterally (Fig. 42-63) based on fracture pattern and direction of displacement. While extensor irritation is less likely with lateral plate placement, the latter is also more technically demanding due to the limited area of bone surface available. Generally a minimum of four cortices should be fixed on either side of the fracture.

Several recent technical advances in plate and screw design have facilitated the application of plates to the phalanges and may reduce complications. New plates are lower profile with varying shapes, thicknesses, and recessed screw heads. A particularly important advance is locking screw technology that

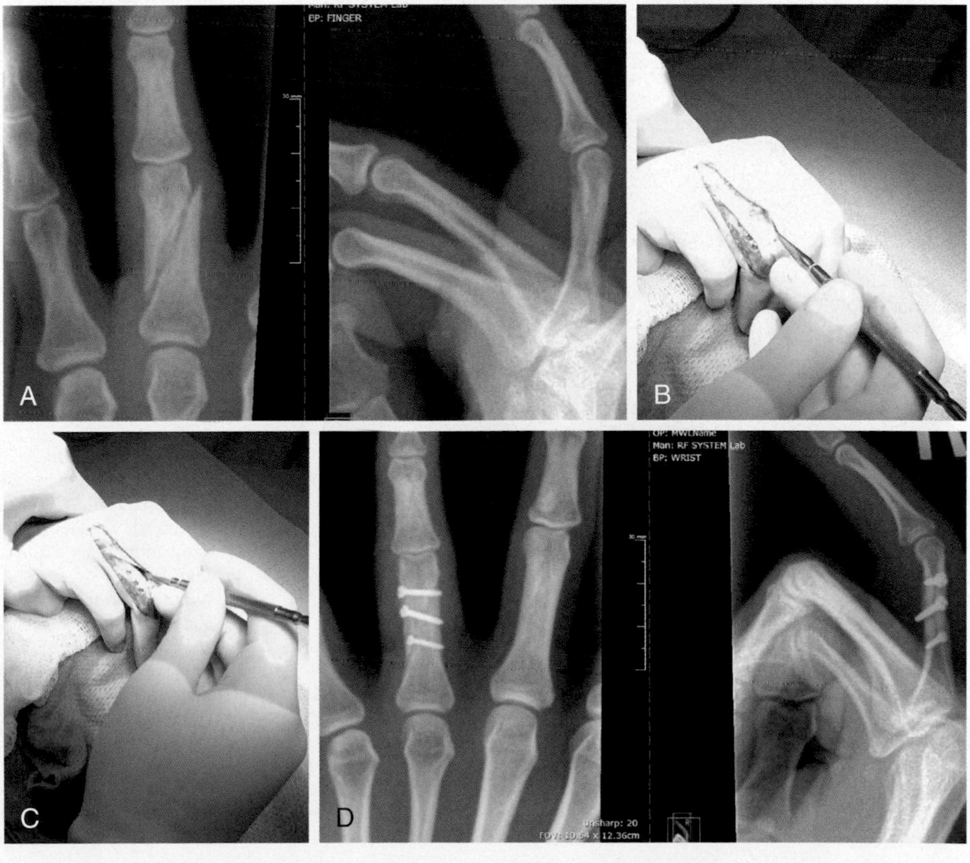

Figure 42-61. A, Proximal phalangeal nascent malunion with rotational deformity. **B,** Osteotomy was performed for the malunited spiral fracture. The ulnar conjoined lateral band was excised. **C,** The extensor was mobilized and the apices of the malunited fracture were identified. The primary fracture plane was identified and osteotomy performed. Reduction and stabilization with three bicortical modular hand screws was performed. **D,** Final radiographs demonstrate anatomic alignment and union.

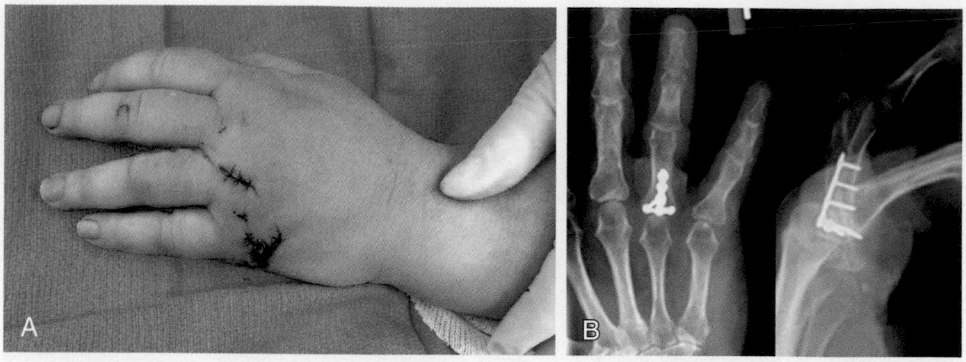

Figure 42-62. A, Ring finger proximal phalangeal fracture secondary to crush injury. **B,** Given the location of the wound and the underlying combined extensor tendon injury, dorsal plating was performed. Ultimately, extensor tenolysis, hardware removal, and proximal interphalangeal (PIP) joint capsulectomy were required.

allows the screw to thread into the plate hole for added stability. Locking plates are particularly useful for osteopenic bone, comminuted fractures, and periarticular fractures where the locking screws buttress the articular surface.[227]

External Fixation

The main indications for the use of external fixation are highly comminuted diaphyseal fractures precluding stable internal fixation, combined injuries with bone and soft tissue loss, and management of infected nonunions necessitating staged reconstruction. External fixation avoids additional soft tissue dissection and fragment devascularization. Various unilateral fixators are available and multidirectional clamps allow fine tuning of fracture reduction following pin placement.

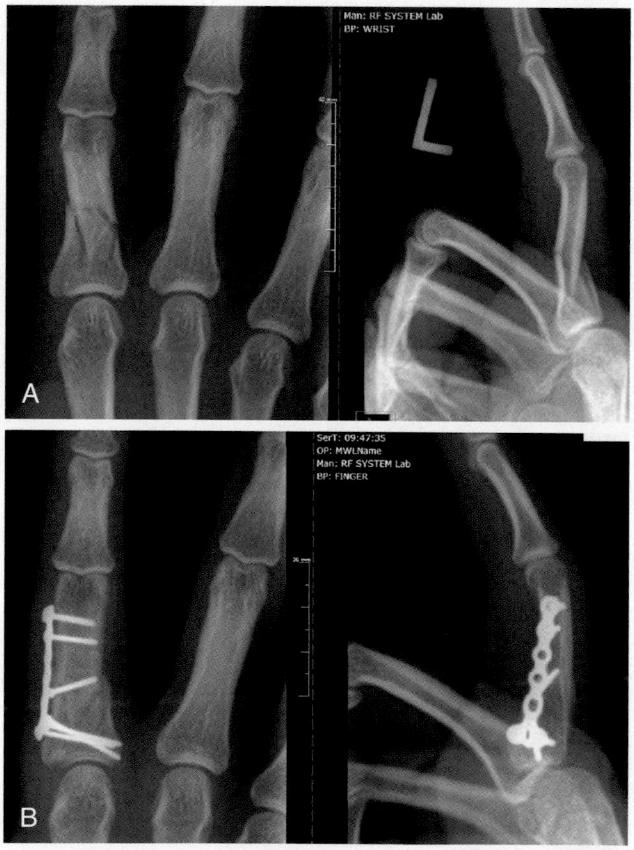

Figure 42-63. A, Mal-angulated comminuted index finger proximal phalangeal fracture. **B,** Following excision of the radial conjoined lateral band, fracture reduction and stabilization was performed using a hybrid fixation construct. A single interfragmentary screw secured an intercalary butterfly fragment, followed by lateral application of a 1.5-mm periarticular locking plate based on the comminuted metaphyseal nature of this fracture.

KEY REFERENCES

The level of evidence (LOE) is determined according to the criteria provided in the preface.

13. Eaton RG, Lane LB, Littler JW, et al: Ligament reconstruction for the painful thumb carpometacarpal joint: a long-term assessment. *J Hand Surg Am* 9(5):692–699, 1984. LOE IV
18. Simonian PT, Trumble TE: Traumatic dislocation of the thumb carpometacarpal joint: early ligamentous reconstruction versus closed reduction and pinning. *J Hand Surg Am* 21(5):802–806, 1996. LOE III
26. Heyman P, Gelberman RH, Duncan K, et al: Injuries of the ulnar collateral ligament of the thumb metacarpophalangeal joint: biomechanical and prospective clinical studies on the usefulness of valgus stress testing. *Clin Orthop Relat Res* 292:165–171, 1993. LOE III
43. Catalano LW III, Cardon L, Patenaude N, et al: Results of surgical treatment of acute and chronic grade III tears of the radial collateral ligament of the thumb metacarpophalangeal joint. *J Hand Surg Am* 31:68–75, 2006. LOE IV
107. Page SM, Stern PJ: Complications and range of motion following plate fixation of metacarpal and phalangeal fractures. *J Hand Surg Am* 23:827–832, 1998. LOE IV
123. Hsu LP, Schwartz EG, Kalainov DM, et al: Complications of K-wire fixation in procedures involving the hand and wrist. *J Hand Surg Am* 36: 610–616, 2011. LOE IV
138. Hofmeister EP, Kim J, Shin AY: Comparison of 2 methods of immobilization of fifth metacarpal neck fractures: a prospective randomized study. *J Hand Surg Am* 33(8):1362–1368, 2008. LOE I
146. Büchler U, Fischer T: Use of a minicondylar plate for metacarpal and phalangeal periarticular injuries. *Clin Orthop Relat Res* 214:53–58, 1987. LOE IV
157. Orbay JL, Touhami A: The treatment of unstable metacarpal and phalangeal shaft fractures with flexible nonlocking and locking intramedullary nails. *Hand Clin* 22:279–286, 2006. LOE IV
159. Ashmead D IV, Rothkopf DM, Walton RL, et al: Treatment of hand injuries by external fixation. *J Hand Surg Am* 17:956–964, 1992. LOE IV
171. Jupiter JB, Koniuch MP, Smith RJ: The management of delayed union and nonunion of the metacarpals and phalanges. *J Hand Surg Am* 10(4):457–466, 1985. LOE IV
173. Büchler U, Gupta A, Ruf S: Corrective osteotomy for post-traumatic malunion of the phalanges in the hand. *J Hand Surg Br* 21(1):33–42, 1996. LOE IV
186. Weiss APC, Hastings H: Distal unicondylar fractures of the proximal phalanx. *J Hand Surg Am* 18:594–599, 1993. LOE IV
197. Hamilton SC, Stern PJ, Fassler PR, et al: Mini-screw fixation for the treatment of proximal interphalangeal joint dorsal fracture-dislocations. *J Hand Surg Am* 31(8):1349–1354, 2006. LOE IV

208. Sarris I, Goitz RJ, Sotereanos DG: Dynamic traction and minimal internal fixation for thumb and digital pilon fractures. *J Hand Surg Am* 29A:39–43, 2004. LOE IV

210. Dionysian E, Eaton RG: The long-term outcome of volar plate arthroplasty of the proximal interphalangeal joint. *J Hand Surg Am* 25(3):429–437, 2000. LOE IV

213. Calfee RP, Kiefhaber TR, Sommerkamp TG, et al: Hemi-hamate arthroplasty provides functional reconstruction of acute and chronic proximal interphalangeal fracture-dislocations. *J Hand Surg Am* 34(7):1232–1241, 2009. LOE IV

214. Al-Qattan MM: Phalangeal neck fractures in children: classification and outcome in 66 cases. *J Hand Surg Br* 26:112–121, 2001. LOE IV

220. Belsky MR, Eaton RG, Lane LB: Closed reduction and internal fixation of proximal phalangeal fractures. *J Hand Surg Am* 9(5):725–729, 1984. LOE IV

221. Freeland AE, Sud V, Lindley SG: Unilateral intrinsic resection of the lateral band and oblique fibers of the metacarpophalangeal joint for proximal phalangeal fracture. *Tech Hand Up Extrem Surg* 5(2):85–90, 2001. LOE V

The complete References list is available online at https://expertconsult.inkling.com.

Chapter 43

Fractures and Dislocations of the Carpus

CHARLES CASSIDY • †LEONARD K. RUBY

The following videos are included with this chapter and may be viewed at https://expertconsult.inkling.com:

43-1. Volar approach to the scaphoid.
43-2. Dorsal approach to the scaphoid.
43-3. Acute scapholunate dissociation.
43-4. Four-corner fusion of the wrist.
43-5. Wrist joint arthrodesis.
43-6. Operative technique of dorsopalmar plate osteosynthesis.
43-7. Surgical treatment of scaphoid nonunion.
43-8. Operative technique of palmar plate osteosynthesis.
43-9. Operative technique of the radioscapholunate fusion.
43-10. Antegrade and retrograde screw osteosynthesis of the scaphoid.
43-11. Indications and techniques of arthroscopy of the wrist.
43-12. Corrections of deformities in rheumatoid arthritis.
43-13. Indications for surgery, approaches.
43-14. Operative technique of dorsal plate osteosynthesis.
43-15. MRI of lesions of the wrist.
43-16. Carpal instability and carpal fractures.

FRACTURES OF THE SCAPHOID

Introduction: Scope and Purpose

Almost exclusively, scaphoid fractures occur in young, vigorous men. They account for 60% to 80% of all carpal bone fractures[1] and are second only to fractures of the distal radius in the frequency of wrist fractures. One recent study[2] estimates the frequency of scaphoid fractures to be approximately 21,500 per year in the United States, which is a magnitude less than previous reports.[3] Nevertheless, the potential impact of these injuries is significant. The diagnosis may be challenging. The course of treatment is often protracted and even under the best of circumstances has a significant impact on these patients, many of whom are engaged in the most productive years of their lives. One European study[4] demonstrated that the average time off work after a scaphoid fracture was 6 months. Even with proper treatment, at least 5%[5,6] of these fractures fail to unite. There is a consensus that displaced fractures and fractures of the proximal pole of the scaphoid should be managed surgically. Controversy exists regarding the optimal treatment of nondisplaced scaphoid fractures.

†This, the fifth edition of the carpal fractures and dislocations chapter, is written in memory of Professor Leonard K. Ruby, who was passionate about the subject.

Mechanism of Injury and Biomechanics

The scaphoid functions as a link between the proximal and the distal carpal rows via strong ligamentous connections, leaving the scaphoid waist susceptible to fracture.[7-11] Two different mechanisms can produce fracture of the scaphoid. By far, the more common mechanism appears to involve hyperextension and bending. In elucidating the pathomechanics, Weber and Chao[12] consistently produced scaphoid waist fractures in cadaver wrists by applying an axial load to the radial half of the palm while the wrist was stabilized in 95 to 100 degrees of extension. It is surmised that the proximal pole of the scaphoid becomes fixed in this position by the radius proximally, dorsally, and radially; by the capitate and lunate ulnarly; and by the long radiolunate ligament and the radioscaphocapitate ligament volarly. At the same time, the distal pole is free to translate dorsally with the distal row of carpal bones, which results in fracture, usually through the waist of the scaphoid. The palmar aspect of the bone fails in tension, and the dorsal aspect fails in compression. Smith and colleagues[11] showed that osteotomy of the waist of the scaphoid in cadaver specimens causes a 27-degree volar angulation of the scaphoid, with consequent collapse deformity of the wrist with extension of the proximal row of carpal bones. This study confirmed the stabilizing link function of the scaphoid—between the proximal and the distal rows—that has been assumed by most investigators based on the anatomy of the scaphoid and on clinical experience.[7,9-11,13]

A less common mechanism of scaphoid waist fracture, termed the puncher's scaphoid, was documented recently by Horii and colleagues.[14] In this instance, with the wrist positioned in neutral or slight flexion, force is transmitted axially along the second metacarpal, through the trapezium and trapezoid, resulting in a flexion moment through the distal pole of the scaphoid. The investigators noted a high incidence of open metacarpal head fractures in these patients. Wrist pain in this setting should therefore raise a high index of suspicion for scaphoid fracture.

Evaluation

Examination

A high index of suspicion is the key to early diagnosis.[7-11] Scaphoid fractures may produce surprisingly little pain, swelling, or limitation of motion.[15] Therefore, if a young adult man has a history of a fall on the palm of his hand and pain and

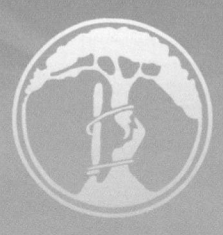

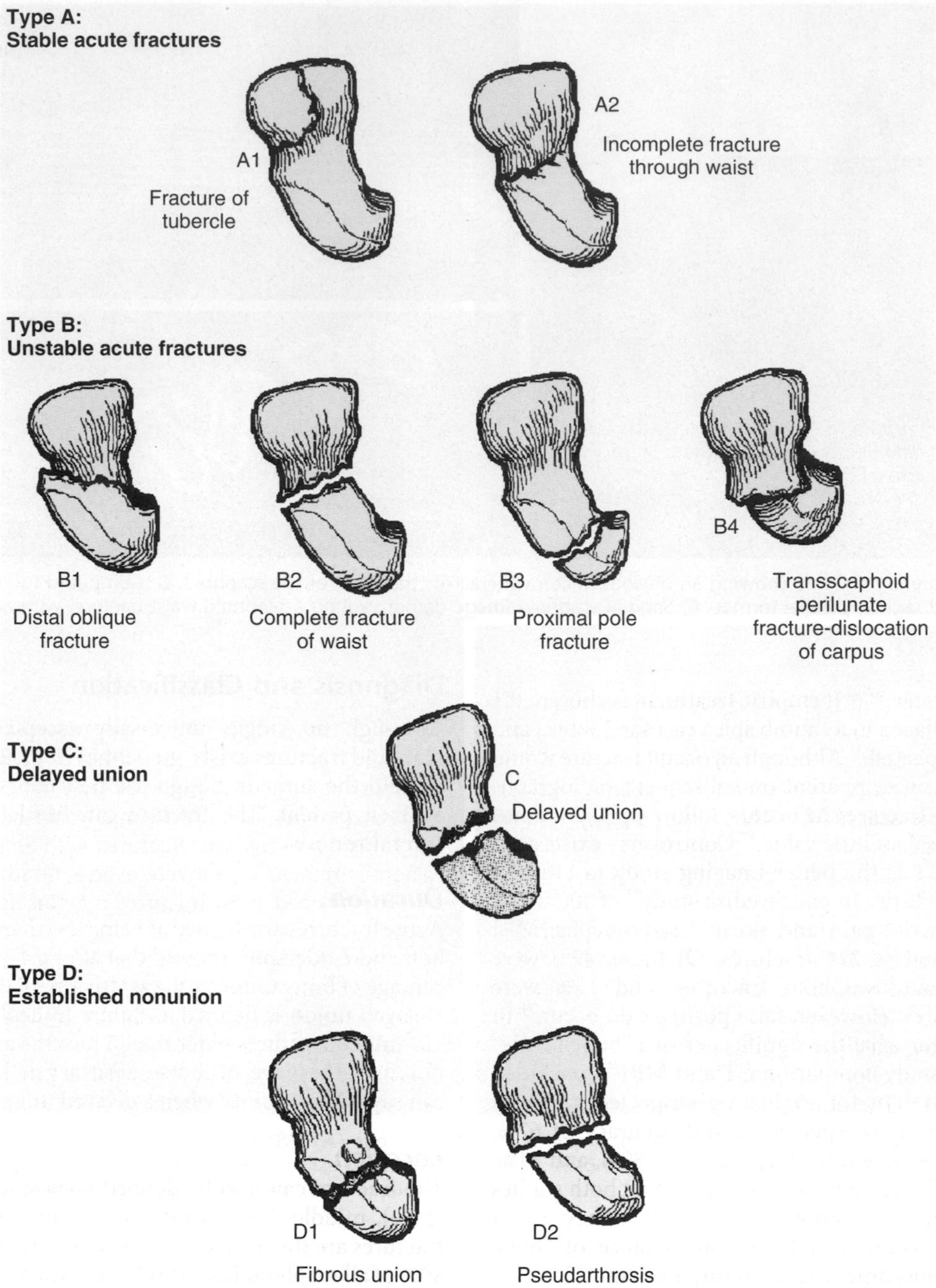

Figure 43-4. Herbert classification (Herbert and Fisher, 1984) of scaphoid fractures. *(Reproduced with permission from Amadio PC, Taleisnik J: Fractures of the carpal bones. In Green DP, editor: Operative Hand Surgery, 4th ed, New York, 1999, Churchill Livingstone, pp 809–864.)*

major blood supply is from branches of the radial artery that enter the bone at or distal to the waist at the dorsal ridge. This blood supply accounts for 70% to 80% of the total intraosseous vascularity and 100% of the proximal pole (Fig. 43-5). The osteonecrosis rate for proximal pole fractures approaches 100%.

Orientation

Russe[42] (Fig. 43-3) and later Herbert and Fisher[45] (Fig. 43-4) suggested that the plane of the fracture is important and described horizontal oblique, vertical oblique, and transverse fractures; they concluded that vertically oriented fractures are less stable and, consequently, less likely to heal.

Displacement

Cooney and colleagues[39] and Weber[22] emphasized fracture stability as defined by displacement. Fractures with more than 1-mm stepoff on any view, a scapholunate angle of more than 60 degrees, a lunocapitate angle greater than 15 degrees, or a lateral intrascaphoid angle of more than 20 degrees are considered displaced. Displacement has been shown to affect healing dramatically in conservatively treated scaphoid waist fractures,[39] with nonunion rates as high as 92% being reported.[46]

Comminution

Comminuted fractures are inherently unstable.

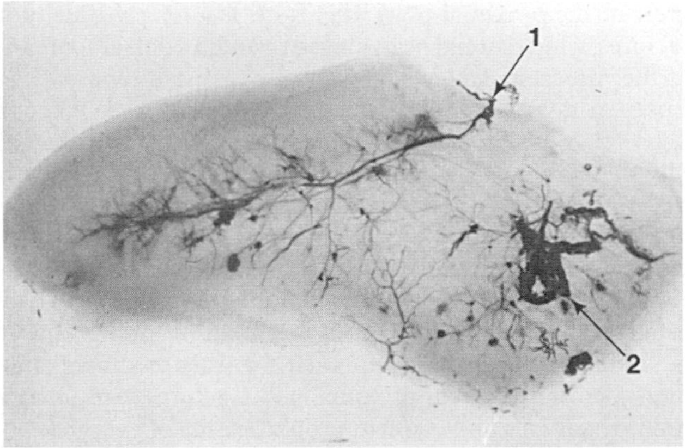

Figure 43-5. Sagittal section of the scaphoid with the proximal pole oriented to the left. *1,* The dorsal scaphoid branch of the radial artery; *2,* the volar scaphoid arterial branch. *(From Gelberman RH, Menon J: The vascularity of the scaphoid bone, J Hand Surg Am 5:508–513, 1980.)*

Associated Injuries

Scaphoid fractures commonly accompany perilunate dislocations. These unstable injuries require open reduction and internal fixation (ORIF). The specifics of management are discussed in the carpal dislocations section.

Approximately 5% of distal radius fractures are associated with fracture of the scaphoid.[47] These high-energy injuries usually require surgery.

Patient Factors

Smoking has a deleterious effect on the outcome of surgery for scaphoid nonunions.[48] Although there are no conclusive data that smoking affects the healing of acute scaphoid fractures, we nevertheless advise patients to discontinue smoking. Depending on his or her perspective, the surgeon may be more or less inclined to operate on an acute scaphoid fracture in a smoker. The potential economic impact of cast immobilization on the individual is also a factor and may be the principal determinant for surgery in some instances.

We agree that displacement and angulation are more important indicators of prognosis than is the plane of the fracture. However, plain radiographs may not be sufficient to determine whether a scaphoid fracture is truly nondisplaced. Some researchers[49,50] recommend obtaining a scaphoid CT for all waist fractures, citing the high incidence of nonunion, malunion, and avascular necrosis (AVN) associated with fracture displacement. Their rationale is that the treating physician is obligated to prove that the scaphoid fracture is truly nondisplaced before recommending nonoperative treatment.

In summary, poor prognostic factors for successful nonoperative treatment of scaphoid fractures include late diagnosis, proximal location, displacement or angulation, and possibly obliquity of the fracture line. Scaphoid fractures associated with perilunate dislocations are unstable and require internal fixation.

Management

Disorder or Injury

Treatment clearly remains the most controversial aspect regarding scaphoid fractures.[51-54] The advent of percutaneous methods of stabilizing the fractured scaphoid, combined with early mobilization, has made surgical management more appealing to patients and some surgeons. However, the concept of surgical treatment of even nondisplaced scaphoid fractures is not new. In 1954, McLaughlin advocated open treatment of all scaphoid waist fractures, acknowledging "the almost universal refusal of surgeons who advocate prolonged immobilization to submit their own fractured naviculars to the 'long enough' requisite of this plan of treatment."[55] The treating physician must weigh these issues with the fact that the vast majority of nondisplaced scaphoid fractures will heal without surgery.

Emergent Treatment

The majority of scaphoid fractures can be treated electively. As noted, immobilization initiated within the first 4 weeks appears to result in satisfactory outcomes for nondisplaced scaphoid fractures. The most common indications for emergent treatment include scaphoid fractures associated with perilunate dislocations (transscaphoid perilunate dislocation) and those associated with dense or worsening median neuropathy. Other indications for emergent treatment include open scaphoid fractures (exceedingly rare) and those associated with vascular injury.

Indications for Definitive Care

Given the potential difficulty in obtaining union, all scaphoid fractures require treatment with some form of immobilization, fixation, or both. Distal pole fractures are generally treated nonoperatively. Proximal pole fractures, comminuted fractures, and scaphoid fractures with associated injuries are generally treated operatively, even if nondisplaced. Treatment of nondisplaced waist fractures remains controversial.

Nonoperative Treatment

Nondisplaced Fractures. Cast immobilization remains the mainstay of treatment for nondisplaced scaphoid fractures.[40,50,56] The particular type of cast, however, has been the subject of much debate. Almost every wrist position has been advocated, including flexion,[12,57] extension,[58] radial deviation,[12] ulnar deviation,[57] neutral,[42] and various combinations. Most investigators have recommended including the thumb,[59,60] but others have included the thumb, index, and middle fingers (three-digit cast).[61] Yet others believe that a simple short arm cast is sufficient.[62-64]

Undoubtedly, the most controversial aspect of cast immobilization has been the long arm versus short arm debate.[40,41,57] The most frequently cited study in this regard was performed by Gellman and colleagues,[41] who concluded that the time to union was faster (9.5 vs. 12.7 weeks; $P < 0.05$) and the nonunion rate lower (0 vs. 8.7%, not significant) when a long arm thumb spica cast was used for the first 6 weeks of treatment. However, a recent cadaver study demonstrated only 0.2 mm of scaphoid fracture motion throughout full forearm rotation in a short arm thumb spica cast.[65] Furthermore, another researcher concluded that long arm casts can be detrimental to scaphoid healing because they prevent normal forearm rotation and potentially increase radiocarpal rotation as the patient attempts to use the hand.[66]

Part of this diversity in cast immobilization treatment may be because of the consistently successful results (94%–98.5%) reported by several investigators with varying cast treatment of fresh undisplaced fractures.[67] It appears that the exact type of cast is not a critical factor in successful treatment.[68] Consequently, we favor a well-fitting short arm thumb spica fiberglass cast starting just below with the wrist in neutral position. The cast is usually changed at 2-week intervals to ensure that it fits snugly. PA, lateral, and ulnar deviation PA radiographs are performed at 6 weeks. If the radiographs are equivocal for healing, a short arm thumb spica cast is reapplied, and a scaphoid CT is obtained. If radiographs do not show that the fracture is healed, regardless of the absence of pain or tenderness, a below-elbow cast is applied for 6 more weeks. If after a total of 12 weeks of immobilization, radiographic examination fails to show unequivocal healing, a CT scan is performed.

Some evidence indicates that cast immobilization accompanied by electrical stimulation may promote union of un-united scaphoid fractures.[69] However, recent literature suggests that this modality is not effective in hastening union of acute scaphoid fractures.[70] Our experience with electrical stimulation in this setting is anecdotal.

Surgical Treatment

NONDISPLACED FRACTURES. Although the majority of surgeons remain satisfied with cast treatment for nondisplaced scaphoid fractures, there appears to be a growing interest in internal fixation of these fractures. Herbert and Fisher[45] reported a 50% failure rate with nonoperative treatment and suggested that early internal fixation was appropriate for many patients, especially young manual laborers and professional athletes who would not tolerate prolonged cast immobilization. This position was supported by Rettig and associates,[71] whose patients returned to athletics within 6 weeks after scaphoid fixation through a volar approach. More recently, percutaneous scaphoid fixation using a cannulated screw through either a dorsal[72] or volar[51,73-75] approach has gained popularity. Union rates of 100% have been reported in several series.[51,72,74,75] Furthermore, return to function may be hastened.[76] In one series of percutaneous scaphoid fixation in military personnel, patients achieved union 5 weeks earlier and returned to full duty 1 month sooner than with cast treatment[51]; similar results were subsequently demonstrated in the civilian population.[77] Whether such an approach is considered overtreatment is controversial.[53] Two meta-analyses of randomized controlled studies on the subject demonstrated earlier time to union in the surgical group but conflicting results on the frequency of union and complications.[78,79] Although the early studies reported virtually no complications from percutaneous scaphoid fixation, a recent study demonstrated a sobering complication rate of 29%, including nonunion, hardware problems, and postoperative fracture of the proximal pole of the scaphoid.[80]

In considering the surgical approaches for percutaneous scaphoid fixation, potential advantages of the volar approach include (1) higher surgeon level of comfort because the traditional open approach for waist fractures is volar, (2) easier ability to obtain proper radiographs because the obligatory wrist extension places the long axis of the scaphoid parallel to the radius, (3) one-step placement of the guidewire, and (4) potentially less likelihood of displacing the fracture. Potential disadvantages of the volar approach include injury to cutaneous nerves and the scaphotrapezial joint and possibly biomechanically inferior fixation because it is more difficult to place the screw tip in center of the proximal pole. The major advantage of the dorsal approach is that it is easier to center the screw in the proximal pole. This is critical for proximal pole fractures, which should be managed through a dorsal approach. Furthermore, if an arthroscopically assisted approach is chosen, a dorsal approach to fixation is preferred. Potential drawbacks of the dorsal approach include (1) it is more technically demanding than the volar approach, (2) injury to the extensor tendons, (3) damage to the articular surface of the proximal pole of the scaphoid, and damage to the radius if the screw is prominent, and (4) fracture displacement resulting from the acute wrist flexion required to place the guidewire. In instances in which percutaneous scaphoid fixation is chosen, the authors favor a volar approach for waist fractures and a mini-open approach for proximal pole fractures to protect the extensor tendons and confirm proper seating of the screw.

PERCUTANEOUS SCAPHOID FIXATION

VOLAR PERCUTANEOUS SCAPHOID FIXATION TECHNIQUE (Fig. 43-6). We prefer to wrap the wrist with sterile Coban to maintain the wrist in extension. In this way, the guidewire will be inserted parallel to the radius and approximately 45 degrees toward the ulna. A 0.45-in guidewire is advanced percutaneously from the radial aspect of the distal pole of the scaphoid into the center of the proximal pole. Proper pin placement is then confirmed fluoroscopically on multiple views. An antirotation pin is then placed parallel to the first pin. A 1-cm incision is made at the guidewire entry site, and a second guidewire is advanced to the distal pole by hand, parallel to the guidewire, to measure proper screw length. After measurement, the cannulated drill is advanced by hand under fluoroscopic control. An Acutrak (Acumed, Beaverton, OR) screw measuring 2.5 mm shorter than the measured length is then advanced. Maintenance of the reduction is confirmed fluoroscopically, as is proper screw length. The guidewire is withdrawn before final seating. The skin is approximated with a single 5-0 nylon suture, and a sterile dressing and radial gutter splint are applied. At the 2-week follow-up, the suture is removed, and a removable splint is applied. Wrist motion is encouraged, although strengthening is not. Radiographs are obtained at 6 weeks after surgery and then monthly if necessary. Unrestricted activity is permitted once the scaphoid fracture is bridged.

DORSAL PERCUTANEOUS SCAPHOID FIXATION. The following has been adapted from Slade and colleagues.[72,81,82] (Fig. 43-7). The wrist is flexed 45 degrees and pronated until the proximal and distal scaphoid poles overlap radiographically. The entry site is determined, and a small incision is made directly overlying it. The extensor tendons are protected, and a small capsulotomy is made. For proximal pole fractures, proper reduction is confirmed. A 0.045-in guidewire is placed in the center of the overlapping scaphoid rings and is advanced through the volar skin adjacent to the trapezium. The wire is then withdrawn distally to obtain high-quality radiographs by extending the wrist. After proper placement and reduction are confirmed, the wrist is flexed, and the guidewire is advanced dorsally and then withdrawn so that the tip is at the level of the subchondral plate of the distal scaphoid pole. The screw length is then measured, and a screw 4 mm shorter than the measured length is selected to maintain the screw within the bone. The guidewire is then readvanced volarly so that that it may be retrieved in the event of breakage. An antirotation pin may be necessary. The guidewire is then overdrilled from proximal to distal by hand with the cannulated reamer. Proper depth of the drill is confirmed fluoroscopically, the drill is removed, and the screw is advanced over the guidewire until

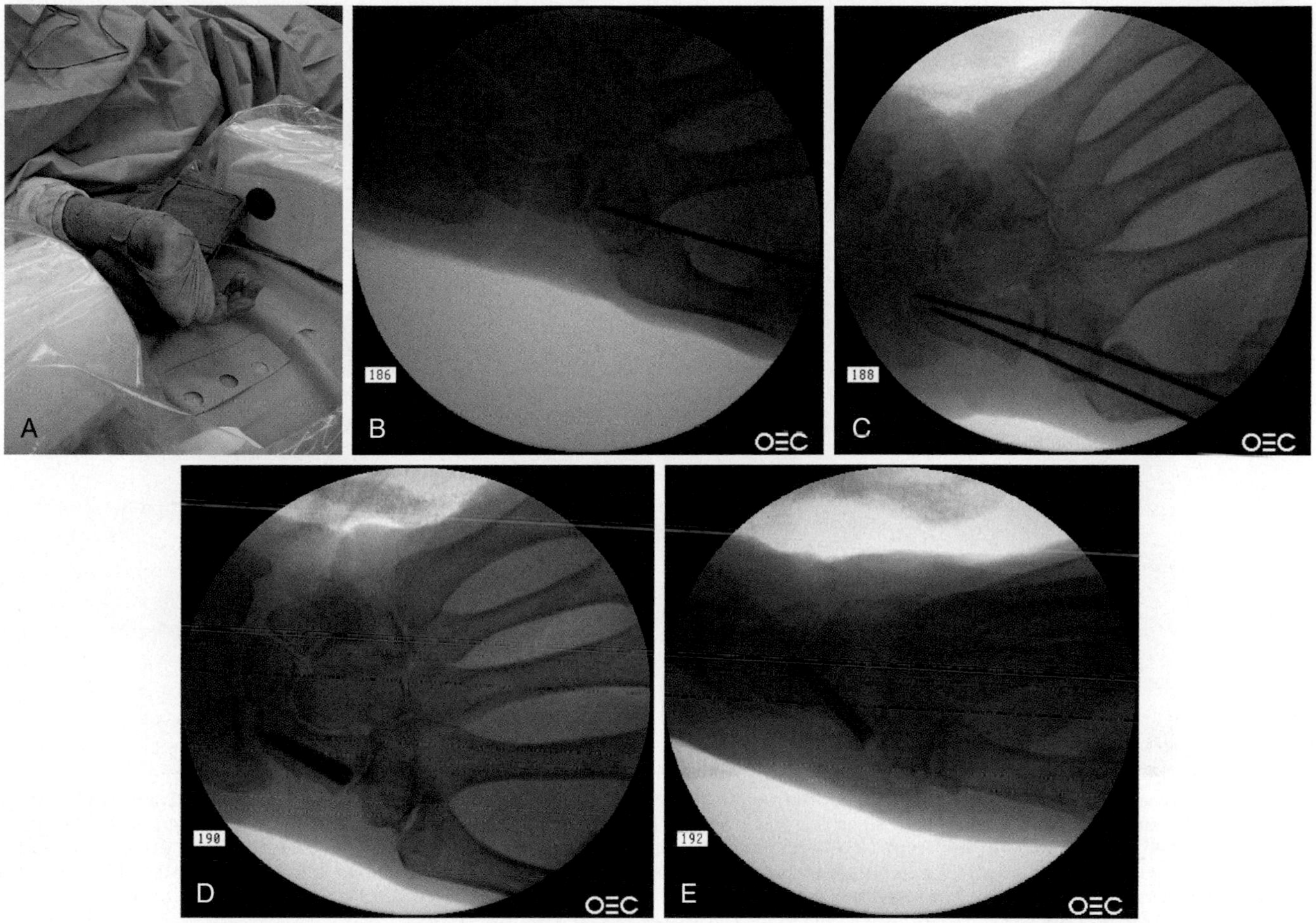

Figure 43-6. Volar percutaneous scaphoid fixation with an Acutrak screw (fracture depicted in Fig. 43-1). **A,** The wrist is maintained in an extended position with sterile Coban wrap. The mini C-arm is placed horizontally. A 0.045-in guidewire is inserted percutaneously from distal to proximal, roughly parallel to the radius and 45 degrees toward the ulna. **B,** The proper starting point is identified fluoroscopically. **C,** The guidewire and an antirotation pin have been placed. Multiple views must be taken to confirm proper guidewire placement. **D** and **E,** Final screw position.

the trailing end is under the articular cartilage. The remainder of the procedure and postoperative care are the same as for the volar approach.

Displaced or Unstable Fractures

The management of acute, displaced scaphoid fractures is far less controversial. These fractures require surgical treatment. Options include closed reduction and percutaneous pin or screw fixation,[83-85] arthroscopically assisted pin or screw fixation,[72,84,86,87] and open reduction with either pin[88] or screw fixation.[31,45,89] Our preference is ORIF with a cannulated screw. In general, the screw will be inserted from the smaller fragment into the larger fragment. The dorsal approach is reserved for proximal pole fractures. The volar approach is safer for waist or distal one-third fractures because the primary blood supply to the scaphoid is dorsal.[44] Bone graft, when necessary, can usually be obtained from the distal radius.

Open Volar Approach (Fig. 43-8 and Video 43-1). A rolled towel under the wrist will facilitate exposure. A 4- to 5-cm zigzag volar incision is made directly over the flexor carpi radialis (FCR) tendon ending distally at the tuberosity of the scaphoid. One should be careful in dividing the skin to not injure the palmar cutaneous branch of the median nerve, which often lies in the skin flap adjacent to FCR tendon. The FCR tendon is mobilized and retracted ulnarward, and the radial artery is retracted radialward. The small crossing superficial branch of the radial artery is identified and is usually ligated and divided. The posterior wall of the FCR sheath is divided longitudinally, and the underlying pericapsular fat is exposed. This too is divided, and the multiple vessels in this layer are cauterized with a bipolar instrument. The scaphoid tuberosity is exposed, and dissection is carried proximally through the volar capsular ligaments, incising only as much as is necessary to adequately visualize the fracture site. Depending on the interval from injury, early callus may need to be curetted from the fracture. K-wires may be placed as joysticks, with care to avoid the projected path of the screw. Typically, the distal pole rests in flexion and pronation, and the proximal pole rests in extension. The fracture is then reduced and stabilized provisionally with a distal-to-proximal axial K-wire, radial to the projected path of the screw. Proper reduction and pin placement are confirmed fluoroscopically. The volar lip of the trapezium adjacent to the scaphotrapeziotrapezoid joint (STT) joint is removed with a rongeur to facilitate guidewire placement. In most instances, we will supplement the fixation with a headless screw inserted from the distal pole of the scaphoid.

With the Acutrak system, a 0.045-in guidewire is then inserted in a distal to proximal direction. After the proper angle of insertion is confirmed fluoroscopically, the guidewire is advanced into the subchondral plate of the proximal pole.

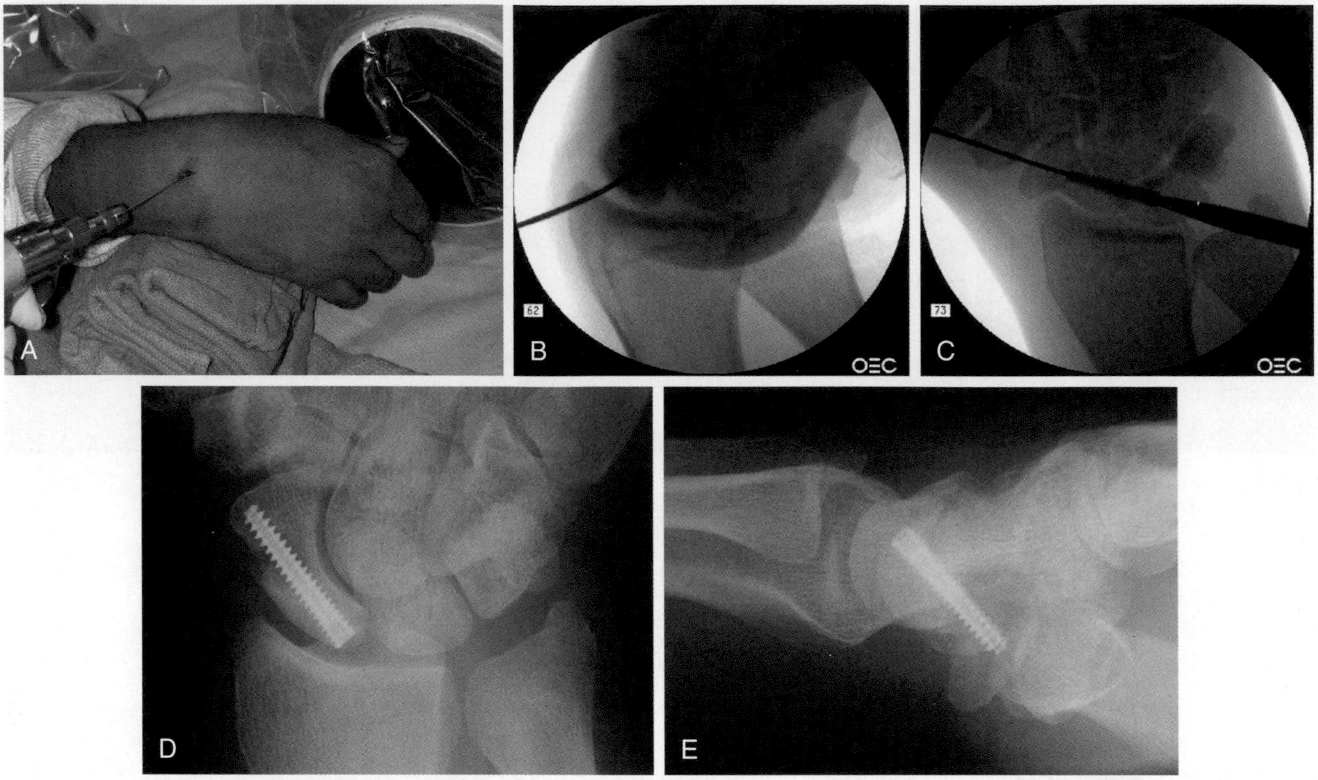

Figure 43-7. Dorsal percutaneous scaphoid fixation with Acutrak screw. **A,** The wrist is flexed and pronated. The mini C-arm is placed horizontally. The guidewire is inserted through a small incision over the proximal scaphoid pole. **B,** Fluoroscopic image demonstrating proper guidewire placement in the center of the "ring," overlapping the proximal and distal scaphoid poles. **C,** Proper guidewire placement has been confirmed and measured. The guidepin has been advanced through the thenar eminence and withdrawn, and the cannulated drill is advanced under fluoroscopic control. **D** and **E,** Final screw placement.

Proper guidewire placement must be confirmed fluoroscopically in multiple planes. Ideally, the guidewire should traverse the central third of the proximal pole. The proper screw length is then measured over the guidewire, with care to ensure that the depth gauge is contacting the scaphoid. In general, we select a screw that is 2.5 mm shorter than the measured length for several reasons: the scaphotrapezial joint is oblique to the screw insertion angle, which can result in screw impingement on the trapezium; the leading end of the screw must not be allowed to penetrate into the radioscaphoid joint; and the Acutrak screw is tapered and cannot be withdrawn without compromising the fixation. Before the guidewire is overdrilled, a 0.045-in antirotation pin is inserted across the fracture. The guidewire is then overdrilled by hand under fluoroscopic control until the tip of the drill reaches the anticipated final screw position. Failure to drill completely may result in distraction of the fracture as the screw is advanced. The screw is then inserted over the guidepin while the surgeon inspects the fracture site for rotation or gapping. The guidepin is withdrawn before final seating of the screw to prevent incarceration. Stability is checked by moving the wrist and checking the fracture site, and final radiographs are obtained. If there is any concern about fracture stability, the antirotation pin is left in place and cut beneath the skin. Proper reduction and

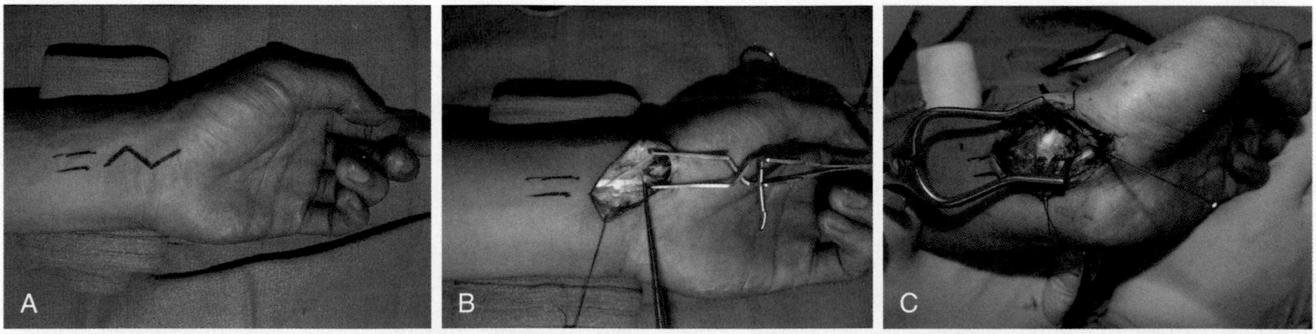

Figure 43-8. Volar approach to scaphoid fixation. **A,** Zigzag incision is centered over flexor carpi radialis (FCR) tendon, with distal limb directed toward the thumb. **B,** The superficial branch of the radial artery (draped over probe) crosses over the FCR at the wrist crease and may need to be ligated. Note the cutaneous nerve crossing obliquely from medial to lateral across the FCR tendon. **C,** FCR tendon retracted ulnarward; distal capsulotomy exposes the scaphoid waist fracture. Proximal capsular exposure is limited to protect capsular ligaments. The incision has been extended proximally to harvest a bone graft from the radial metaphysis. Joystick in distal scaphoid pole.

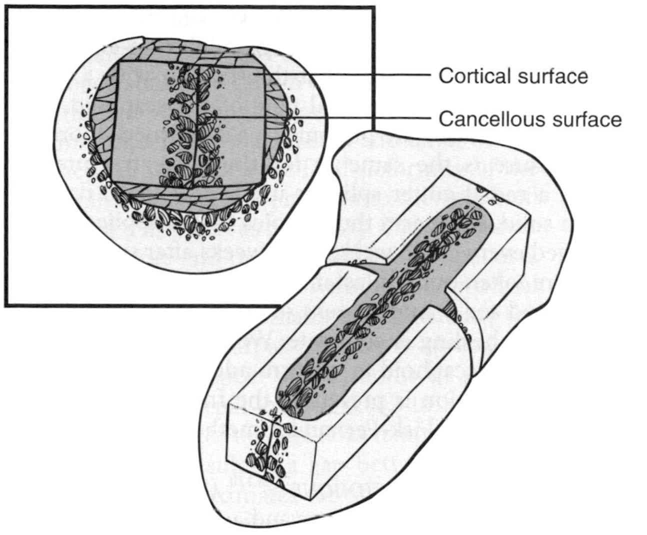

Figure 43-10. Russe's latest technique using Matti's excavation concept but incorporating corticocancellous graft for improved fixation and a volar approach. *(From Green DP: The effect of avascular necrosis on Russe bone grafting for scaphoid nonunion, J Hand Surg Am 10:597–605, 1985.)*

be used.[121] Green[110] pointed out that the Matti-Russe technique has a lower success rate when the proximal pole is avascular, as documented by no bleeding of the bone at surgery. In his experience, he had a failure rate of 100% in five patients in whom there was no bleeding of the proximal pole at the time of surgery. He and others have shown that radiographic avascularity is not a reliable indicator of actual vascularity. Our experience with the Matti-Russe method is consistent with that of most investigators, and 80% to 90% healing rates can be expected.[97]

Vascularized Bone Grafts. Over the past 2 decades, increasing attention has been paid to the use of vascularized bone grafts in the management of difficult nonunions. These have included the volar pronator pedicle graft[122]; the dorsal Zaidemberg 1,2 intercompartmental artery pedicle graft[123] (Fig. 43-11); the Fernandez vascular bundle implant[124]; the free vascularized iliac crest graft[125]; and, most recently, the free vascularized medial femoral condyle graft.[126,127] In general, the results using these techniques have been equivalent to those of more conventional nonvascularized methods. A study from the Mayo Clinic concluded that the dorsal-based Zaidemberg graft may not be capable of predictably correcting humpback deformities,[128] which may be better managed with a nonvascularized corticocancellous or a vascularized medial femoral condyle graft through a volar approach. We believe that the structural requirements of the graft are more important in graft selection than its vascularity. There clearly does appear to be a role for the dorsal pedicle grafts in the management of well-aligned, proximal pole nonunions associated with AVN. The vascularized medal femoral condyle graft is reserved for the disastrous scaphoid nonunion associated with carpal collapse and AVN or failure of prior surgery.

Modified Matti-Russe Technique[42,117] (Video 43-1). The volar approach for scaphoid nonunion is the same as for the acute fracture (see Open Volar Approach and Video 43-1). Only as much of the volar capsular ligaments is incised as necessary to adequately visualize the nonunion site. At this point, the radioscaphoid joint and the majority of the volar surface of the scaphoid are exposed. The fracture site is usually obvious, but on occasion, a wrinkle in the articular cartilage of the scaphoid may be the only clue. Fingertrap traction and wrist extension will optimize the exposure. An opening is made in the volar nonarticular cortex of the scaphoid at the level of the fracture. The opposing cavities of the two fragments are then excavated. Russe advocated using only hand

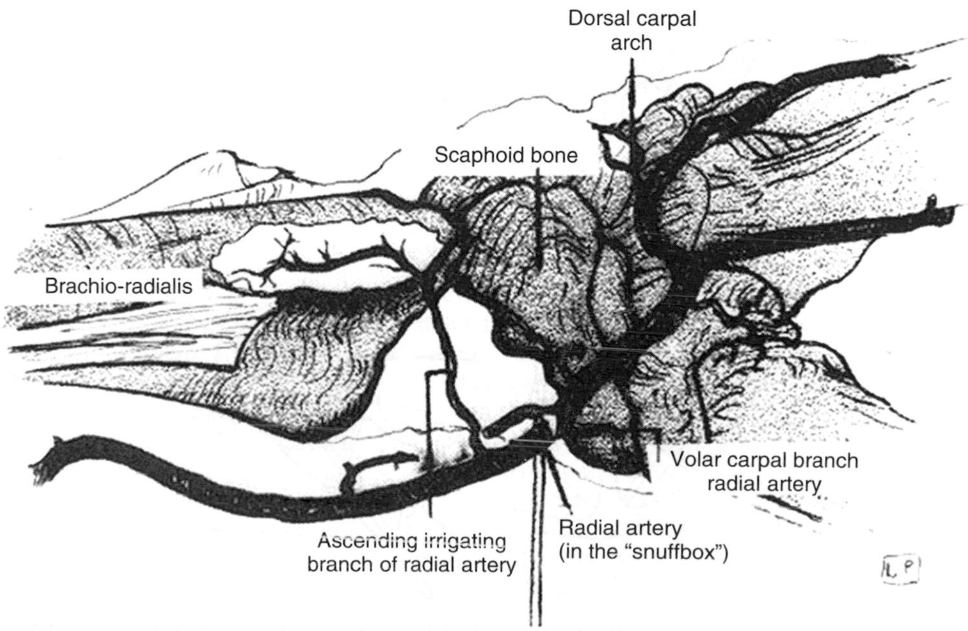

Figure 43-11. Original drawing of the Zaidemberg 1,2 intercompartmental artery pedicle graft, referred to as the ascending irrigating branch of the radial artery. *(From Zaidemberg C, Siebert JW, Angrigiani C: A new vascularized bone graft for scaphoid nonunion, J Hand Surg Am 16:474–478, 1991.)*

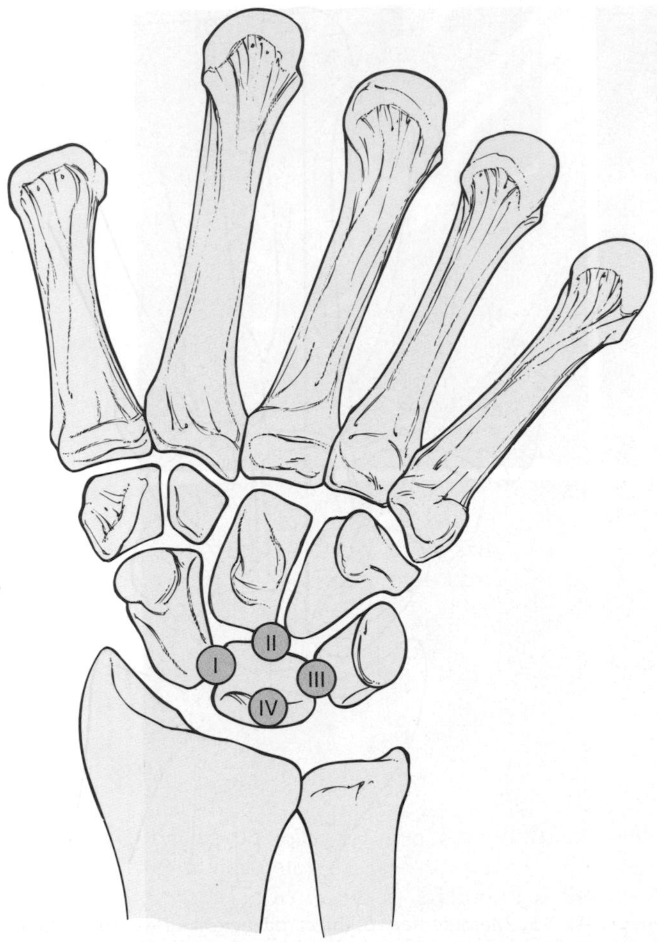

Figure 43-36. The pathomechanics and progressive perilunar instability pattern demonstrated by Mayfield and colleagues. *I,* Scaphoid instability with respect to the lunate; *II,* scaphoid plus capitate instability with respect to the lunate; *III,* scaphoid plus capitate plus triquetrum instability with respect to the lunate; *IV,* lunate dislocation. *(From Mayfield JK, Johnson RP, Kilcoyne RK: Carpal dislocations: pathomechanics and progressive perilunar instability, J Hand Surg Am 5:226–241, 1980.)*

The midcarpal shift test has been described by Lichtman and Wroten[257] to diagnose nondissociative midcarpal instability. While stabilizing the forearm in pronation, the examiner exerts a palmarly directed force onto the patient's wrist and ulnarly deviates the wrist maximally. Feinstein and colleagues have graded the degree of instability based on the degree of palmar midcarpal translation and the degree of "clunking."[258]

Although none of these physical examination maneuvers is difficult to perform, it takes a great deal of experience to interpret the results. It is very helpful to examine the normal wrist first as a baseline.

Imaging

Radiography is the mainstay of diagnosis. When ordering diagnostic studies for wrist instability, remember that the views generally represent static images of a dynamic problem.

Routine Views. Routine views should include PA, true lateral, and a 45-degree pronation view. The third metacarpal should be perfectly aligned with the radius in all views. Bellinghausen and associates[259] pointed out that three smooth lines (Gilula lines) can be drawn on a normal PA view of the wrist. If these lines are broken, instability can be suspected. The proximal line describes the proximal articular surfaces of the proximal row, the middle line describes the distal articular surfaces of the proximal row, and the distal line outlines the proximal articular surfaces of the distal row (Fig. 43-40). On the PA view, increased overlap of a carpal bone, especially the lunate, to the capitate should be sought. If the lunate presents a triangular as opposed to a quadrilateral appearance, perilunate instability may be suspected. The scaphoid normally appears elongated. If it appears foreshortened and demonstrates a "ring" bicortical density, it has become abnormally vertical with respect to the radius, as occurs in both scapholunate dissociation and VISI. The examiner should check also for increased space in the scapholunate interval (>3 mm in scapholunate dissociation) and should assess carpal height[248] (Fig. 43-35). On the lateral view, as has been discussed (see Figs. 43-33 and 43-34), any disruption of the normal colinear relationship of the capitate, lunate, and radius should be

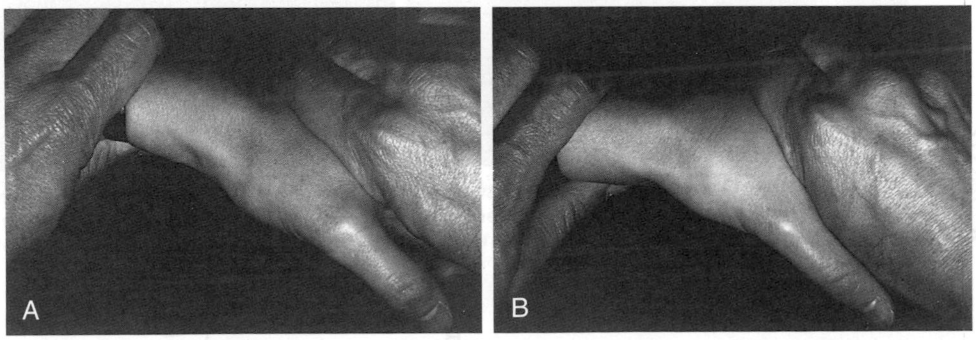

Figure 43-37. A, Volar shift test. The examiner stabilizes the distal forearm and simultaneously pushes the hand in the volar direction. Normally, a painless "shift" is felt by the examiner and patient. This generally represents midcarpal laxity and should be tested against the normal side. **B,** Dorsal shift test. The examiner stabilizes the distal forearm with one hand and simultaneously pushes the hand dorsally. Normally, very little motion is felt. In patients with dorsal intercalated segment instability, increased motion or pain, or both, compared with the findings on the normal side, is a positive finding.

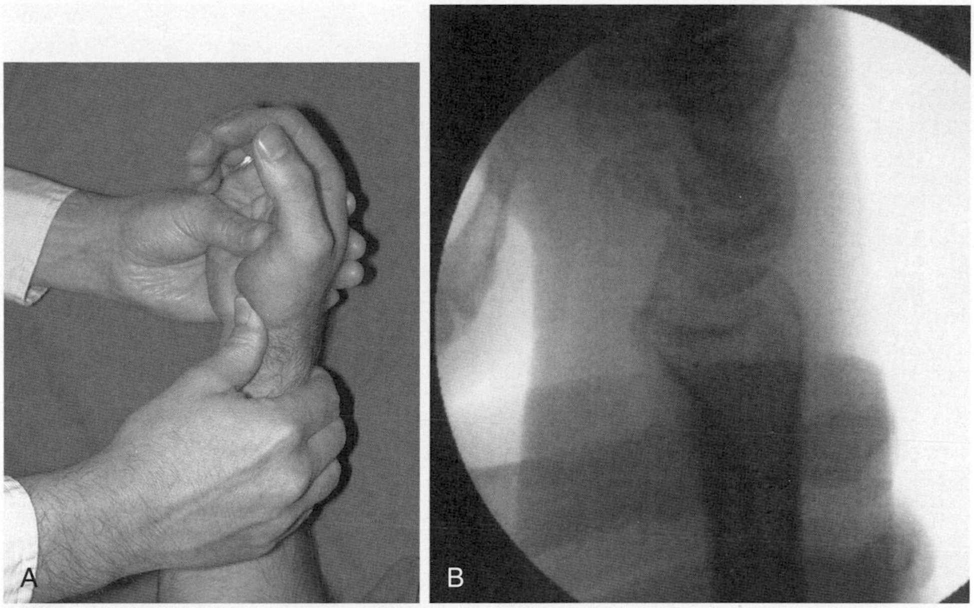

Figure 43-38. Scaphoid shift test (Watson et al., 1988).[252] **A,** Dorsally directed pressure is applied to the scaphoid tuberosity with the examiner's thumb as the wrist is moved from ulnar to radial deviation. With scapholunate instability, the proximal pole is thought to sublux dorsally out of the scaphoid fossa. When the pressure on the scaphoid is released, the scaphoid abruptly reduces back into the fossa, and a "clunk" is felt. **B,** Lateral stress radiograph demonstrating dorsal subluxation of the scaphoid.

noted.[260] Additionally, the scapholunate angle should be measured to check for scapholunate dissociation (angle >60 degrees) or VISI pattern (angle <30 degrees). It must be emphasized that because of the normal flexion and extension of the proximal row in radial and ulnar deviation, all measurements must be made on radiographs in which the third metacarpal is aligned parallel to the long axis of the radius in all planes.

Supplemental Views. If the results of the routine radiographs are normal and the clinician suspects an instability, a stress or motion series may be helpful.[260] These views include a PA view in radial deviation, neutral, and ulnar deviation; a clenched fist AP view (which accentuates scapholunate diastasis); and a lateral in radial deviation, neutral, and ulnar deviation. These additional views are often routinely obtained when instability is subtle. However, Levinsohn and Palmer[261] reported a 65% false-negative rate even with this complete series. It is important to note that a LT stepoff with radial deviation may be a normal finding.[262]

Other Studies

Cineradiography. Cineradiography can be helpful when the static film results are normal or suspicious but not conclusive.[263] These views are most useful when performed by the surgeon, who has a clear idea of what is being looked for. The

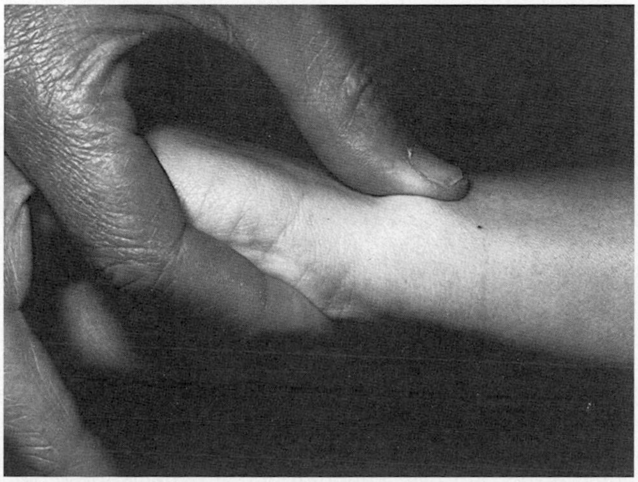

Figure 43-39. Ulnar carpal shift test. The examiner pushes down on the ulnar head and up on the pisiform. If the test result is positive, pain is felt by the patient in the extensor carpi ulnaris and flexor carpi ulnaris interval. This may be found in cases of ulnar–carpal impingement.

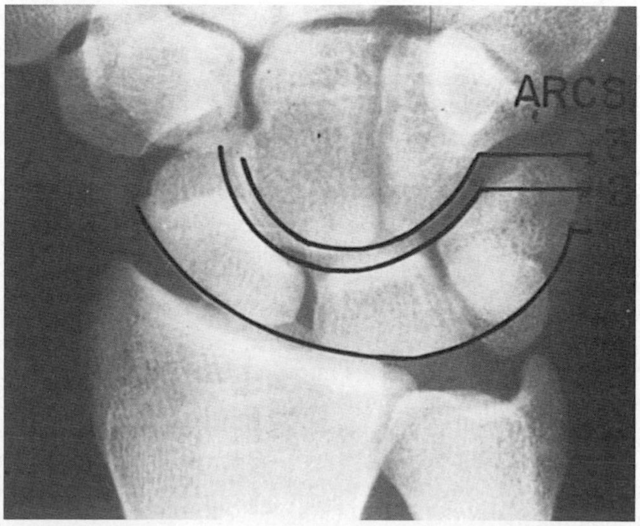

Figure 43-40 In a normal wrist, three smooth arcs can be drawn on an anterior-posterior radiograph. If there is a break in any of these three lines, an intracarpal malalignment should be strongly suspected. *(From Bellinghausen HW, Gilula LA, Young LV, Weeks PM: Post-traumatic palmar carpal subluxation: report of two cases. J Bone Joint Surg Am 65:999, 1983.)*

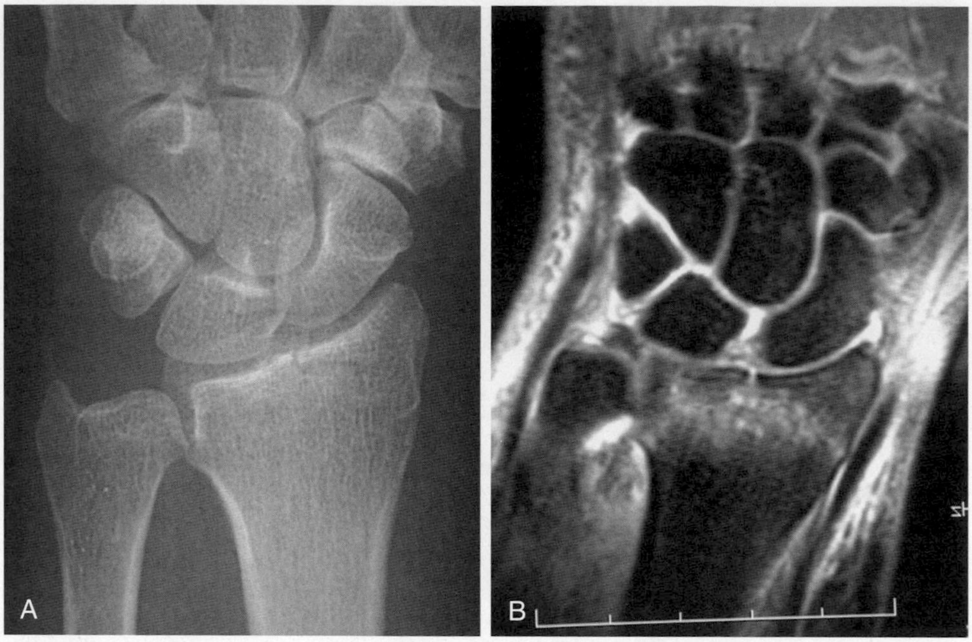

Figure 43-41. Indirect magnetic resonance (MR) imaging. **A,** Posterior-anterior radiograph demonstrates minimally displaced articular split between scaphoid and lunate facets. **B,** Indirect MR fat suppression coronal image shows scapholunate ligament tear in addition to distal radius fracture.

wrist is actively or passively moved in radial and ulnar deviation and examined in the PA, lateral, and oblique planes. Evidence of dyssynchronous motion is sometimes found. Traction and stress views performed under fluoroscopy may help clarify subtle findings.

Magnetic Resonance Imaging. Given the anatomic detail seen in the images, wrist MR has obvious appeal in the evaluation of suspected wrist instability. However, several limitations are apparent. Foremost, MR is a static study potentially being used to identify a dynamic problem. Second, the demonstration of an interosseous ligament communication ("tear") by MR does not necessarily mean that the patient's symptoms are related to these findings or that a "leak" is mechanically significant. This is partly because the interosseous ligaments have a thin membranous central portion that probably does not contribute significantly to ligament stabilizing function. After the age of 50 years, these tears become increasingly common,[264] making interpretation that more difficult. Third, although the specificity is relatively high, unenhanced MR appears to be unreliable in excluding interosseous ligament tears.[265] Johnstone and colleagues[266] reported a sensitivity of 37% and 0% in identifying scapholunate and LT interosseous ligament tears, respectively. Indirect and direct MR arthrographic techniques have been developed in an effort to improve the accuracy of wrist MR. Indirect MR arthrography involves an intravenous injection of gadolinium, some of which diffuses into the wrist synovial fluid, yielding an arthrographic appearance on the study. Compared with unenhanced MR, indirect MR arthrography is more sensitive at demonstrating scapholunate tears (69% vs. 38%) but no better for evaluating the TFCC or LT ligament[267] (Fig. 43-41). Direct MR arthrography involves injecting gadolinium or saline directly into the wrist. In one European center, three-compartment MR arthrography using a dedicated coil was reported to have a sensitivity of 97% in detecting full-thickness ligament tears.[268] Most centers, however, perform single-compartment (radiocarpal) MR arthrography. At the minimum, a 1.5-Tesla magnet and dedicated wrist coil are necessary to study the wrist. Magnets are becoming more sophisticated, and the 3-Tesla magnet intuitively will provide more accurate information. Using a 3-Tesla magnet without contrast, one recent study demonstrated a specificity of 100% and a sensitivity of 89% and 82% for scapholunate and LT tears, respectively, which improved to 100% with contrast.[269] Interestingly, there were several false positives in the contrast group, in which microperforations were identified arthroscopically.

Computed Tomography. Computed tomography alone is not of much value in the diagnosis of wrist instability. It clearly is most useful in diagnosing fractures, evaluating fracture displacement, and scaphoid nonunions.[270] It may be useful for measuring more clearly subtle changes in the capitolunate and radiolunate angles on the lateral views.[271] When combined with arthrography, multiplanar, multidetector CT arthrography may be superior to unenhanced MR in detecting scapholunate and LT ligament tears.[272] Motion artifact is potentially much less given the short duration of the study compared with MR. However, the CT studies do subject the patient to radiation.

Arthroscopy. Wrist arthroscopy has become the gold standard diagnostic study[273] for wrist instability.[274-277] Ruch and colleagues[278] devised an arthroscopy-based classification of wrist ligament injuries. Several researchers have also described treatment of wrist instabilities using the arthroscope.[279-281]

Our experience with wrist arthroscopy has been very favorable, with few complications and a high degree of success in diagnosing obscure causes of wrist pain. The physician should examine the wrist under anesthesia before introducing the arthroscope. Through the radiocarpal 3,4 portal, the surgeon should inspect for osteochondral injury, damage to the volar extrinsic ligaments, and tears or redundancy in the scapholunate interosseous ligament. The LT ligament is best visualized from one of the ulnar portals; our preference is the 6R portal. Although interosseous ligament tears are seen in the radiocarpal joint, the instability resulting from the tears is best seen

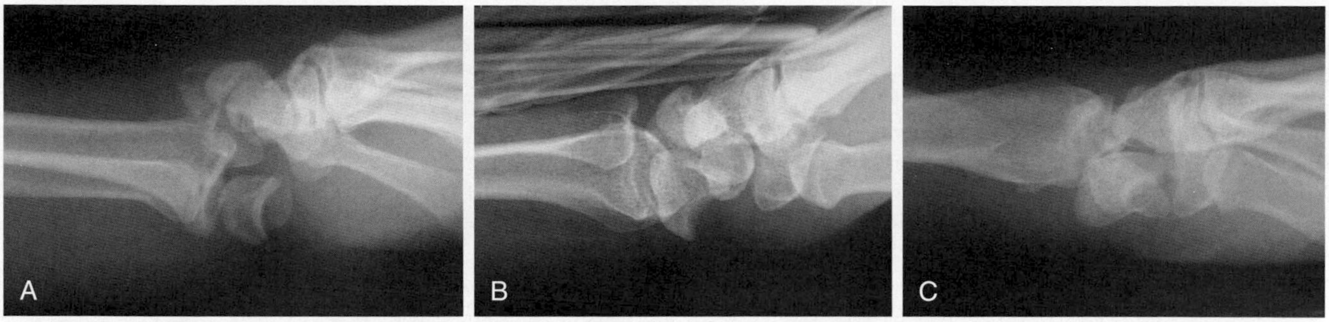

Figure 43-42. In a patient with a carpal dislocation, the initial lateral radiograph may depict a configuration at any point in the spectrum of injury. **A,** Dorsal transstyloid, transscaphoid perilunate dislocation. **B,** An intermediate state. **C,** Volar lunate dislocation in a patient with multiple hereditary exostoses.

from the midcarpal joint, such as gapping, rotation, and stepoff between the carpal bones. Although valuable as a diagnostic tool, arthroscopic management of wrist instability is largely limited to débridement of partial-thickness ligament tears.[276] We have had some encouraging early results with arthroscopically assisted thermal shrinkage of ligaments and capsule for mild forms of nondissociative midcarpal instability. However, the long-term benefit of this technique remains unproven.

In summary, our present approach to the patient with wrist pain is a systematic history and physical examination, paying particular attention to the magnitude and location of the pain, and includes the various stress tests. Next, we perform plain radiographs and, if we suspect a subtle instability, stress radiographs. If the diagnosis is a symptomatic partial tear, wrist arthroscopy is usually the next step. If the diagnosis is still i n doubt, an MR arthrogram is ordered. If we suspect AVN, MRI is the next examination. If we suspect fracture, a CT scan is ordered.

Perilunate Dislocations and Fracture-Dislocations

As described earlier, these injuries[282,283] represent the ultimate stage in perilunate instability (Mayfield stage IV) (Fig. 43-42). Perilunar instability may be purely ligamentous (lesser arc injury) or a combination of osseous and ligamentous injuries (greater arc injuries). If the force of injury traverses a carpal bone, resulting in fracture, the prefix trans- is used. Therefore, dorsal perilunate, volar lunate, transradial styloid, transscaphoid, transscaphoid transcapitate, and transtriquetral perilunate dislocations are variations of the same injury. The most common of these is the transscaphoid perilunate dislocation, accounting for 60% of all perilunate dislocations.[13] All of the soft tissue structures connecting the lunate to the rest of the carpus are torn. The short radiolunate and ulnolunate ligaments remain intact. The capitate and the rest of the carpus come to lie dorsal to the lunate. Depending on the degree of injury, the lunate either is in its normal position with respect to the radius and the rest of the carpus dorsal (dorsal perilunate dislocation) or is anteriorly displaced and rotated, with the capitate and other carpal bones in more or less normal relationship to the radius (lunate dislocation).

Diagnosis. Perilunate dislocations result from high-energy trauma, such as a motor vehicle accident or a fall from a significant height. These patients often have associated injuries, and it is not uncommon for the wrist injury to be overlooked. When seen acutely, the wrist is swollen, and wrist and digital motion are limited. Median nerve dysfunction is common, especially with a lunate dislocation. When seen late, patients complain of wrist pain but may exhibit a remarkable degree of wrist motion. In addition to median neuropathy, late findings may include ulnar neuropathy and flexor tendon ruptures.[38]

Standard wrist radiographs are sufficient to make the diagnosis, although the dislocation may be missed by the uninitiated because the PA view may appear to be relatively normal. As pointed out by Green and O'Brien,[284] the lateral radiograph is the key, with the finding being loss of colinearity of the radius, lunate, and capitate. In a dorsal perilunate dislocation, the capitate rests on top of the lunate. In a volar lunate dislocation, the lunate pivots around the intact short radiolunate ligament and faces anteriorly, a finding termed the spilled teacup sign.[284] The capitate migrates proximally and sits in the lunate fossa. On the PA view, overlap of the carpal bones and loss of carpal height are evident. The lunate assumes a triangular shape as it flexes. Associated fractures may be identified. Traction radiographs obtained before reduction may provide additional information about the extent of injury.

Treatment. In the acute setting, early closed reduction is mandatory. Reduction reduces pain and minimizes swelling, digital stiffness, and the risk of median nerve dysfunction. Definitive treatment, however, remains controversial. Treatment options include cast immobilization; arthroscopically assisted percutaneous pin fixation[285]; and ORIF through a dorsal,[286-289] volar,[290,291] or combined dorsal and volar[13,229,292] approach. Reports of cast treatment for perilunate dislocations date back to the 1920 to 1940 era. There is now general consensus that the risk of late instability from cast treatment alone is unacceptably high. Percutaneous fixation has been advocated by some, but precise reduction is difficult to achieve by closed manipulation. Osteochondral fragments with loose bodies are also frequently present. In addition, some investigators[282] believe that ligament repair is a necessary element of treatment. In our opinion, percutaneous pinning has a role in treating severely injured patients in whom open management is contraindicated.

ORIF is the preferred method of treatment of many investigators, including ourselves. However, there has been controversy regarding the best surgical approach. Campbell and colleagues[287] reported using a dorsal approach in nine patients and a volar approach in four patients, all without the complication of AVN. These investigators preferred the dorsal approach, noting that (1) it is usually necessary to remove scar tissue in the lunate space, and (2) it is easier to visualize and align the carpal bones through a dorsal approach. Linscheid and colleagues[229] advocated a dorsal and volar approach to repair the volar ligaments. Green and O'Brien[293] and Taleisnik[291] also recommend a volar approach to effect ligament repair. Adkinson and Chapman[286] reported good results with a dorsal approach only, indicating that it is not necessary to suture the volar ligaments if bony reduction is achieved and maintained with K-wires.

Our preference is to treat these injuries using ORIF with K-wires or screw fixation (or both) through a dorsal approach. If the patient has a median neuropathy, we also perform a volar incision to release the transverse carpal ligament, explore the nerve, and repair the volar wrist capsule. However, in our experience, the dorsal approach alone is adequate to reduce and fix the dislocation, and suture repair of the volar ligaments is not absolutely necessary.

OUTCOME. The end result is influenced by the timing of reduction, and earlier is better. Although successful results have been reported in isolated cases as late as 4 to 5 months after injury,[293] the best results are seen when definitive treatment is performed within 1 to 2 weeks. Most patients regain approximately 50% of normal motion, and some stiffness is the rule.[292,293] Almost one-third of patients develop radiographic arthritis, although it does not necessarily correlate with clinical outcome.[294] Outcomes may be somewhat better with a transscaphoid variant; a recent study using screw fixation of the scaphoid and a LT ligament repair through a dorsal approach yielded 91% of normal motion and 80% of grip strength.[289]

CLOSED REDUCTION TECHNIQUE. Closed reduction is best accomplished under regional or general anesthesia. Longitudinal traction is applied for 10 minutes using finger traps with 10 to 15 lb of counterweight on the upper arm. We prefer to use the wrist arthroscopy setup with 6 kg of weight applied to the thumb, index, and middle fingers by finger traps through the shoulder holder (Dyonics, Andover, MA) (Fig. 43-43). Alternatively, end-of-the-table traction can be used. Green and O'Brien[293] recommend PA and lateral radiographs at this point to better delineate the extent of injury. The finger traps are then removed, and a closed reduction maneuver as described by Tavernier is performed.[295]

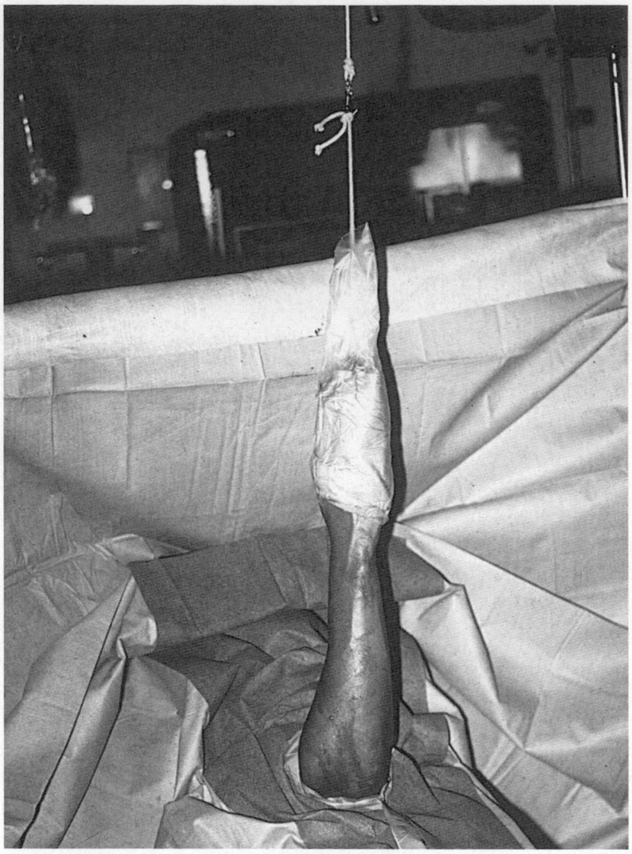

Figure 43-43. The patient is supine with the upper arm taped to an arm board. The hand is suspended through finger traps to an overhead pulley system, and weight (2.25–3.15 kg) is applied.

The surgeon simultaneously applies longitudinal traction and extends the wrist with one hand while stabilizing the lunate volarly using the thumb of the other hand. The wrist is then gradually flexed, pushing the capitate over the dorsal pole of the lunate. Mini C-arm fluoroscopy may facilitate reduction. A short arm thumb spica cast is applied with the wrist in slight flexion, and postreduction radiographs are obtained. The arm is then put in a short arm thumb spica cast with the wrist in slight palmar flexion, and postreduction radiographs are obtained.

OPEN REDUCTION INTERNAL FIXATION TECHNIQUE. Use the straight dorsal approach already described in the Fracture Treatment section. After the extensor pollicis longus is retracted radially, the entire dorsal carpus is in view because the dorsal capsule has been torn and stripped off the radius by the injury. The proximal pole of the scaphoid and capitate are easily visualized, and the lunate is hidden underneath. Reduction is obtained by applying traction through the hand and pushing up on the lunate anteriorly after clearing the lunate space of soft tissue. Reduction of the lunate can be facilitated by placing a blunt periosteal elevator between the capitate head and the lunate and levering the lunate up dorsally. Any small osteochondral fragments are removed. Next, before reduction, a long 0.062-in K-wire is driven antegrade from the head of the capitate, exiting in the second intermetacarpal space. The capitolunate relationship is then aligned by translating the capitate volarly and radially deviating the capitate on the lunate approximately 10 degrees. The second intermetacarpal pin is then driven retrograde into the lunate with the lunate maintained in a neutral position. The scaphoid is reduced to the lunate by pushing down firmly on the proximal pole of the scaphoid and radially deviating the wrist. K-wires can be used as joysticks, clamping a bone reduction forceps around them to close the scapholunate gap. One 0.062-in K-wire is driven through the scaphoid into the capitate, and a second wire is driven through the scaphoid into the lunate. Another wire is passed from the triquetrum into the lunate. Radiographs are taken to assess reduction and pin placement. One of the authors (CC) prefers to repair the scapholunate ligament with suture anchors. Closure is accomplished in routine fashion, although the dorsal capsule may be badly damaged and irreparable. A short arm splint is applied with the wrist in neutral position and is changed to a short arm thumb spica cast at 1 week. The cast is changed at 2- to 3-week intervals for a total of 10 to 12 weeks of immobilization. After pin removal, intensive therapy is begun. Motion is emphasized initially followed by strengthening exercises.

Transscaphoid Perilunate Dislocation

Transscaphoid perilunate dislocation (Fig. 43-44) occurs by a mechanism very similar to that in dorsal perilunate

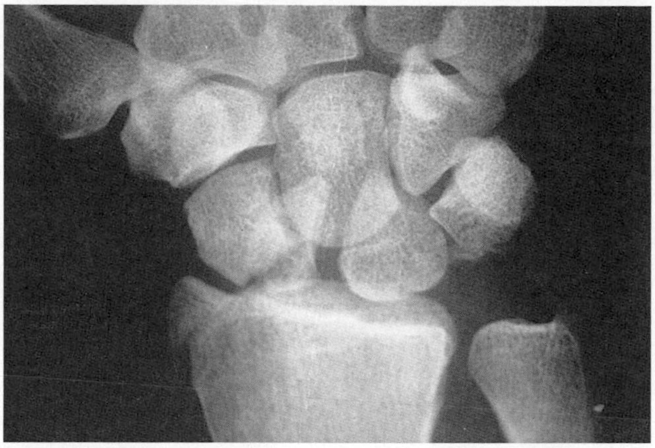

Figure 43-44. A transscaphoid perilunate dislocation with an associated radial styloid fracture.

dislocation, except the energy is transmitted through the waist of the scaphoid instead of through its ligamentous attachments to the lunate. The technique of closed reduction is the same as that for dorsal perilunate–volar lunate dislocation and usually requires less force. Unfortunately, even with excellent initial reduction, the scaphoid usually angulates, and the wrist collapses into DISI, with the proximal row and proximal pole of the scaphoid angulated dorsally and the distal pole of the scaphoid and distal row angulated volarly. Consequently, we agree with other investigators[287,288,293,296] that early ORIF is the treatment of choice.

The specific technique is controversial. As with simple perilunate dislocations, volar, dorsal, and combined approaches have been recommended. We use a dorsal approach just as for the dorsal perilunate dislocation and for the same reasons. The disadvantage of this method is that if there is comminution of the volar cortex of the scaphoid, it is difficult to add a bone graft to maintain scaphoid alignment after reduction. Also, the volar ligaments cannot be repaired. Often, just as in a dorsal perilunate–volar lunate dislocation, the question becomes moot because a carpal tunnel release must be done to decompress the median nerve.

Technique—Dorsal Approach. A straight dorsal incision is made, centered a few millimeters ulnar to Lister tubercle. The extensor pollicis longus is retracted radially, and the dorsal wrist capsule is mobilized radially and ulnarly. (It will have been stripped off the carpus and distal radius by the injury.) The head of the capitate will come into view with the distal pole of the scaphoid. Hematoma is removed from the scapholunate fossa, and traction is applied to the hand. The lunate and the attached proximal pole of the scaphoid are pushed up (dorsal), and the capitate and distal scaphoid fragment are pushed down (volar) over the dorsal pole of the lunate. Again, this maneuver can be facilitated with a blunt periosteal elevator placed in the fracture site and used as a lever. Reduction and stability are checked clinically by radially and ulnarly deviating the wrist. The scaphoid is then stabilized using a headless screw (Fig. 43-45) inserted from proximal to distal. We also repair the LT ligament with bone anchors if necessary and pin the LT joint with 0.062-in K-wire. If scaphoid comminution or a concomitant scapholunate injury is present, a capitolunate pin is also placed. For significant scaphoid comminution, a combined volar–dorsal approach with bone graft may be necessary. After radiographs confirm anatomic reduction of the carpus and proper placement of the hardware, the wound is closed, and a short arm splint is applied for 1 week. This is followed by a short arm thumb spica cast for 6 weeks. The cast is converted to a removable splint when radiographs demonstrate healing of the scaphoid. The wires usually are removed at 10 to 12 weeks.

Technique: Volar Approach for Scaphoid Fixation. A skin incision is made over the FCR tendon, which is exposed and retracted ulnarly. The radial artery is protected. The dorsal sheath of the FCR is incised longitudinally, and pericapsular fat is divided. The anterior capsule of the wrist is divided, and the proximal pole of the scaphoid and the lunate are visualized. Hematoma is removed from the fracture surface and dorsally as far as possible by placing traction on the hand. This should expose the distal fragment of the scaphoid and the head of the capitate. The proximal fragment is pushed dorsally while the distal fragment is pulled volarly. If reduction is successful, internal fixation or bone graft, or both, can be performed. We recommend bone graft if the volar cortex of the scaphoid is sufficiently comminuted to preclude anatomic reduction and adequate fixation. Because a volar approach does not allow good visualization of the critical scapholunate–capitate relationship, radiologic assessment or a dorsal incision will have to be made. Internal fixation is then performed by using a headless screw technique as already described in the treatment of scaphoid fractures. Closure is

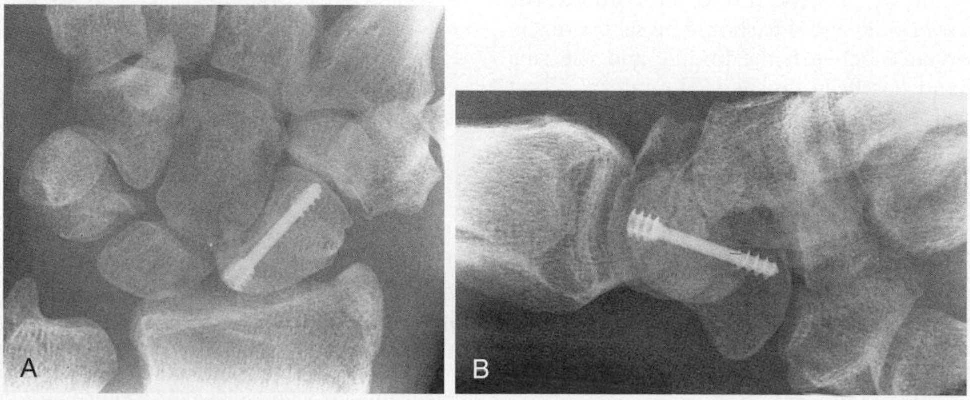

Figure 43-45. Anterior-posterior (**A**) and lateral (**B**) postoperative radiographs demonstrating a Herbert screw used to fix the scaphoid fracture in a patient with a transscaphoid perilunate dislocation. The screw has been placed in retrograde fashion through the dorsal approach without the jig.

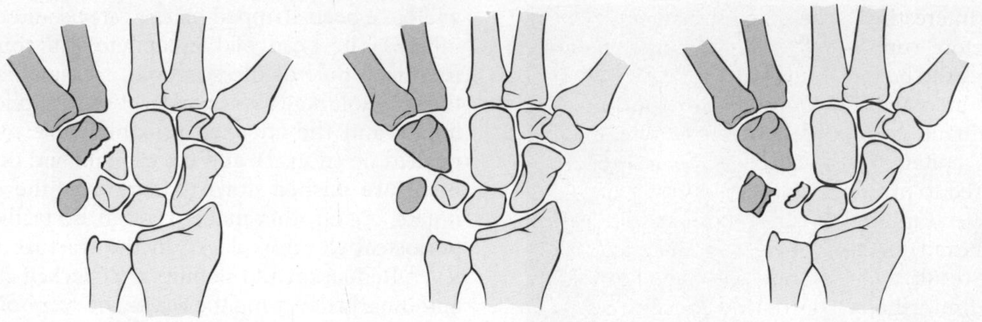

Figure 43-46. The three patterns of capitate–hamate diastasis described by Garcia-Elias and colleagues.[28] *(Redrawn from Garcia-Elias M, Abanco J, Salvador E, et al: Crush injury of the carpus, J Bone Joint Surg Br 67:289, 1985.)*

routine, and aftercare is as already described for the dorsal approach. Again, stiffness is a common sequela of these injuries, so vigorous and prolonged rehabilitation is necessary.

Although the carpal tunnel can be released through a trans-FCR approach, we favor the standard extended carpal tunnel release approach to manage concomitant carpal tunnel syndrome or an irreducible lunate dislocation.

It is not rare to have an accompanying radial styloid fracture, in which case these injuries are termed transradial transscaphoid fracture-dislocations. If the radius fracture is large and in one piece, it should be treated by internal fixation because it may contribute to ligamentous and bony stability of the radiocarpal joint. If it is small or comminuted, excision is a reasonable option.

Transtriquetral Perilunate Fracture-Dislocation

In some carpal dislocations, the plane of injury propagates ulnarly not between the lunate and triquetrum but through the triquetrum. The proximal portion of the triquetrum stays with the lunate, and the distal fragment displaces dorsally with the capitate and distal row analogous to the transscaphoid perilunate dislocation. Treatment is the same as for the perilunate dislocation, and the triquetral fracture will be reduced automatically. We recommend ORIF of the fracture and the carpus through a dorsal approach.

Capitate–Hamate Diastasis

If a hand is severely crushed, a cleavage plane may be created between the capitate and hamate and the third and fourth metacarpals (Fig. 43-46). This injury propagates proximally through the triquetrum or between it and the hamate. The diagnosis is easy to overlook, and one should be suspicious in a patient with divergence between the middle and the ring fingers when the hand has been crushed. The injury is best visualized on a PA view. It is important to reduce and fix this diastasis because failure to do so destroys the transverse arch of the hand and causes rotational malalignment of the fingers. Primiano and Reef[297] performed carpal tunnel release and internal fixation in four patients. Garcia-Elias and colleagues[28] summarized all 13 cases reported in the literature up to 1985, including four of their own patients, and concluded that closed reduction produced good long-term results.

Scapholunate Dissociation

This entity may be defined as dyssynchronous movement of the scaphoid with respect to the lunate. Although the scaphoid is the most mobile bone in the proximal row, its motions are normally similar in direction and amplitude to those of the lunate and triquetrum.[230] If this synchronous motion with respect to the lunate is lost, scapholunate dissociation is said to exist.[229] Although several ligaments, including the scapholunate interosseous ligament, the dorsal radiotriquetral ligament, the DIC ligament, and the scaphotrapezial ligament, contribute to scapholunate stability, there is general agreement that the scapholunate interosseous ligament is the most important of these.

The scapholunate interosseous ligament is composed of three distinct regions: a relatively thin palmar ligament, a fibrocartilaginous proximal (membranous) portion, and a thick dorsal ligament[298] (Fig. 43-47). Of these, the dorsal fibers are the strongest and clinically the most important.[299] As previously described, the mechanism of injury usually involves hyperextension, ulnar deviation, and intercarpal supination. In the scapholunate interval, the force of injury propagates from the palmar to the dorsal direction. Disruption of the palmar and proximal regions alone produces only minor alterations in

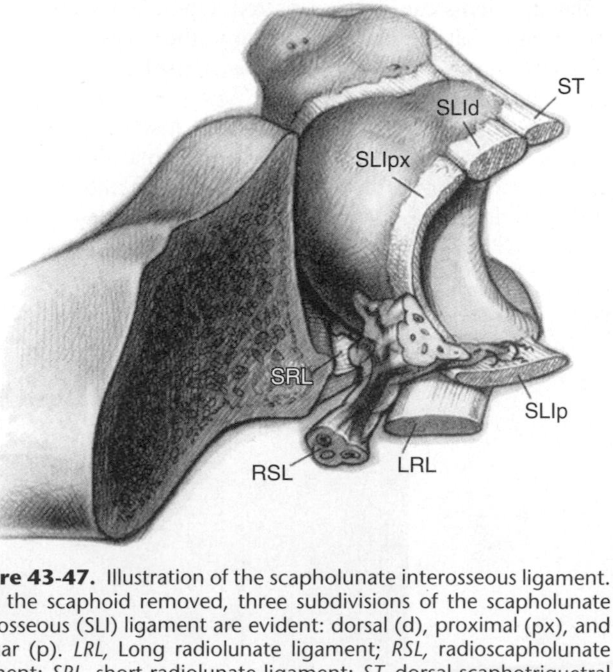

Figure 43-47. Illustration of the scapholunate interosseous ligament. With the scaphoid removed, three subdivisions of the scapholunate interosseous (SLI) ligament are evident: dorsal (d), proximal (px), and palmar (p). *LRL,* Long radiolunate ligament; *RSL,* radioscapholunate ligament; *SRL,* short radiolunate ligament; *ST,* dorsal scaphotriquetral (or intercarpal) ligament. *(Reproduced with permission from Berger RA: The gross and histologic anatomy of the scapholunate ligament, J Hand Surg Am 21:170–178, 1996.)*

wrist kinematics. Interestingly, the scapholunate ligament can elongate 100% before rupturing[300]; consequently, an injured ligament may appear to be intact intraoperatively even though it is functionally incompetent. Complete disruption of the scapholunate ligament, combined with incompetence of the volar radioscaphocapitate or the scapho-trapezial-trapezoidal ligament, is required to produce static deformity.

With a complete scapholunate tear, the scaphoid assumes a more vertical (flexed) position, and the lunate and triquetrum extend. As a result, overall contact between the scaphoid and the radius is diminished,[301] becoming concentrated at the distal pole and radial styloid and the proximal pole and dorsal lip of the radius. These are the initial sites for the development of arthritis. Abnormal contact between the capitate and lunate eventually results in arthritis at that articulation.

Watson and colleagues[302,303] have classified the spectrum of scapholunate instability into four types: predynamic, dynamic, static, and scapholunate advanced collapse.[151] Predynamic instability is defined as localized pain over the scapholunate joint with a positive scaphoid shift test result (see stress tests) and normal radiographic results, including stress views. The existence of this entity remains controversial. In dynamic instability, abnormalities are seen only on stress radiographs or arthroscopy. This would be seen, for example, with a partial scapholunate tear. In static instability, the diagnosis is clear on plain radiographs. Long-standing static instability results in extensive degenerative arthritis or a scapholunate advanced collapse (SLAC) wrist.

Scapholunate dissociation can also be seen in conjunction with distal radius fractures. Arthroscopically, the incidence has been found to be as high as 31%.[304] Radiographically, the incidence is probably about 5%[305] (Fig. 43-48). Cast treatment alone does not appear to be adequate in this setting.[6]

Diagnosis. A wide spectrum of symptoms and findings may be present, depending on the age and severity of the injury and associated problems.[229] A history of a hyperextension injury is sought, although it is not always found. Symptoms include radial dorsal wrist pain, weakness of grip, limited motion, and a clicking or popping sensation with use. Swelling may be present. Tenderness is localized to the dorsal scapholunate interval or dorsal rim of the radius. There will often be a positive dorsal shift test result with increased pain at the capitate head as it subluxates dorsally out of the lunate concavity. The scaphoid shift test[252,254] should produce pain and demonstrate instability.

Radiographs should include a PA and lateral in neutral wrist position, with the third metacarpal parallel to the radius. Comparison radiographs are often helpful, although interestingly, widened scapholunate intervals and increased scapholunate angles may be seen in as many as 80% of asymptomatic contralateral wrists.[306] A mildly increased scapholunate interval without DISI may be a normal variant and is usually evident on the unaffected wrist as well.[307] Findings of static instability on the PA radiograph (see Fig. 43-48, *A*) include the following:

1. An increased scapholunate joint space (the so-called Terry Thomas sign). A gap of more than 3 mm is suspicious, and a gap of more than 5 mm is diagnostic of a scapholunate tear.[308]
2. The "scaphoid ring" sign.[307] When the scaphoid is flexed, the tuberosity is superimposed on the waist, producing a cortical ring or oval. To be considered positive, the distance between the ulnar corner of the scaphoid and the edge of the ring should be less than 8 mm.[309] This finding indicates only that the scaphoid is abnormally flexed and is therefore not specific for a scapholunate tear.
3. Reduction in carpal height. The carpal height ratio is decreased (<0.54).
4. Increased overlap of the lunate on the capitate with a more triangular shape of the lunate.
5. The triquetrum is also dorsiflexed, giving it a wider appearance.

Findings on the lateral view include the following (see Fig. 43-48, *B*):

1. The scapholunate angle is greater than 60 degrees.[229]
2. The lunate and triquetrum are extended with respect to the radius and capitate (DISI). The lunate–capitate angle is reversed from the normal 0 to 15 degrees of palmar flexion of the lunate. An angle of more than 10 degrees dorsal is considered abnormal.
3. The V sign of Taleisnik. Normally, the palmar margins of the scaphoid and radius assume a C shape. When the scaphoid is abnormally flexed, these cortical surfaces form a V shape.[178]

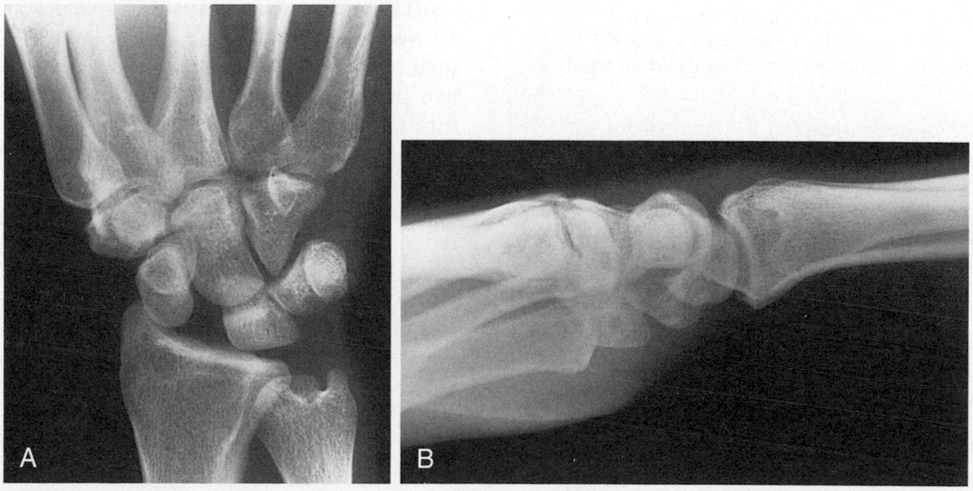

Figure 43-48. Anterior-posterior (**A**) and lateral (**B**) radiographs of scapholunate diastasis with dorsal intercalated segment instability deformity.

If the diagnosis is not evident from the results of the routine radiographs, a stress series is ordered. This includes a radial and ulnar deviation PA view and an AP clenched fist view. The latter view places the opposing facets of the scaphoid and lunate parallel to the x-ray beam, accentuating any scapholunate gap. Other stress radiographs include the "pencil grip PA" view[310] and the carpal stretch test.[311] The pencil grip view is obtained while the patient is making tight fists around a pencil and has the added benefit of simultaneously visualizing the unaffected wrist. The carpal stretch view is a PA obtained while applying traction to the thumb and index fingers and may demonstrate a scapholunate stepoff. Additional studies include cineradiography, arthrography, MRI, and arthroscopy. Cineradiography may help to clarify confusing physical findings. Arthrography can be helpful in younger patients; its limitations have been highlighted earlier. The sensitivity of the routine MRI in detecting scapholunate tears is poor (37%)[266]; we have not found unenhanced MRI to be useful in this setting. As noted earlier, indirect or direct MR arthrography may be of some value.

Wrist arthroscopy has become the diagnostic procedure of choice to confirm clinically suspected dynamic scapholunate instability.[277,312] The scapholunate interosseous ligament, radioscapholunate ligament; radiolunate ligament; and scaphoid, lunate, and radial proximal articular surfaces can all be directly visualized through the radiocarpal 3,4 portal. As already noted, the midcarpal portal often provides the best view of a scapholunate gap (or stepoff). The degree of instability is classified according to the method of Geissler and colleagues[304] (Table 43-2).

Treatment. This issue is best considered in terms of management of the acute or chronic condition because the methods and prognosis for each differ.[235] It should also be pointed out that two of the most prominent authorities on the wrist, Linscheid and Dobyns, stated that "treatment of this condition is seldom satisfactory."[313] Unfortunately, our own experience supports their conclusion.

Acute Scapholunate Dissociation. These injuries are often missed and in fact may be relatively asymptomatic initially. If, however, one does see an acute injury, most investigators, including these authors, recommend open repair. In our hands, closed reduction has never succeeded. The difficulty of closed reduction in this injury is probably owing to the paradox of the scaphoid.[239] To close the scapholunate gap, radial deviation of the wrist, which compresses the scapholunate joint, should be done. However, this causes the scaphoid to assume a more vertical position, thereby increasing scapholunate angulation. Conversely, to align the scaphoid more horizontally, ulnar deviation of the wrist should be performed, which distracts the scapholunate joint, increasing the gap. Nonetheless, it may be possible to accomplish closed reduction with the maneuvers described later.

TABLE 43-2 *ARTHROSCOPIC CLASSIFICATION OF TEARS OF THE INTRACARPAL LIGAMENTS*

Grade	Description
I	Attenuation or hemorrhage of the interosseous ligament as seen from the radiocarpal space. No incongruency of carpal alignment in the midcarpal space.
II	Attenuation or hemorrhage of the interosseous ligament as seen from the radiocarpal space. Incongruency or stepoff of carpal space. There may be a slight gap (less than the width of the probe) between carpal bones.
III	Incongruency or stepoff of carpal alignment as seen from both the radiocarpal and midcarpal space. Probe may be passed through the gap between carpal bones.
IV	Incongruency or stepoff of carpal alignment as seen from both the radiocarpal and midcarpal space. There is gross instability with manipulation. A 2.7-mm arthroscope may be passed through the gap between carpal bones.

Reproduced with permission from Geissler WB, Freeland AE, Savoie F.H, et al: Intracarpal soft-tissue lesions associated with an intra-articular fracture of the distal end of the radius, J Bone Joint Surg Am 78:357–365, 1996.

Several researchers[283,314] have advocated closed reduction and percutaneous pin fixation using the image intensifier. Others[280,315] have recommended arthroscopically assisted reduction and pinning. In Whipple's series,[315] clinical and radiographic success was achieved in 85% of the patients when the symptoms were of fewer than 3 months' duration and the preoperative scapholunate gap was less than 3 mm more than that of the normal side. Otherwise, only 53% had an acceptable result. We believe that wrist arthroscopy is useful in the diagnosis and management of dynamic scapholunate instability associated with partial scapholunate ligament tears. Acute, complete scapholunate tears are best treated with ORIF.

Closed Reduction and Percutaneous Pinning Technique. After adequate axillary block or general anesthesia, the capitolunate joint is reduced by volar translation and radial deviation of the capitate on the lunate by pushing volarly and radially on the patient's hand while stabilizing the forearm. This is very similar to the volar shift test (see Fig. 39-37, *A*). The assistant then drives a 0.062-in smooth K-wire across the capitolunate joint, and its position is checked by fluoroscopy. Next, the scaphoid is reduced by 15 to 20 degrees of radial deviation, and simultaneous downward (anteriorly directed) pressure is applied over the proximal pole of the scaphoid. A second 0.062-in smooth K-wire is introduced across the scaphocapitate joint and a third wire across the scapholunate joint. If the reduction is difficult, temporary K-wires may be placed into the dorsal aspects of the lunate and scaphoid for use as "joysticks." Again, reduction and wire placement are checked radiologically. The wires are cut under the skin. After an initial 1 week of U-shaped thumb spica splinting, a solid, short arm thumb spica cast is applied and continued for 8 to 10 weeks and changed at 2- to 3-week intervals. Alternative methods of wire placement have been described, including two pins through the scaphoid to the capitate and two pins through the scaphoid to the lunate.[283] Dobyns and colleagues[227] suggest one pin through the radius into the lunate and a second pin through the radius into the scaphoid.

Authors' Preferred Method. Our preference is open reduction through a dorsal approach and pin placement as described previously for closed reduction and percutaneous pinning. In addition, if there is significant scapholunate interosseous ligament to repair, No. 0 nonabsorbable horizontal mattress sutures are placed, if possible, through bone tunnels in the scaphoid to repair the scapholunate interosseous ligament.[227] This technique is especially useful if the scapholunate interosseous ligament is avulsed from its attachment to the rim of the scaphoid, as it often is. Alternatively, a bone anchor can be placed into the proximal pole of the scaphoid to reinforce the repair. We combine this with a dorsal capsulodesis, securing the DIC ligament to the dorsal scapholunate area. Aftercare is the same as for closed reduction and percutaneous fixation.

Chronic Scapholunate Dissociation. The dividing line between acute and chronic is not distinct but is arbitrarily drawn at 3 weeks by some[291] and at 3 months by others.[314] The majority of scapholunate tears fall into this category. Rather than focus on time, Lavernia and colleagues[316] have suggested that we consider the quality of the ligament, the reducibility of the joint, and the presence of arthritis as the critical factors in determining the feasibility of ligament repair. The treatment of subacute and chronic scapholunate dissociation remains controversial and difficult, and the results are unpredictable. No single procedure has been uniformly successful in treating this problem.[290] Numerous soft tissue and bony techniques have been recommended.

Soft Tissue Methods. These include scapholunate ligament repair, capsulodesis, and tendon grafts. The preferred option for treatment of chronic instability is the same as that for acute instability—open reduction through a dorsal approach, pinning of the three key carpals (i.e., capitate, lunate, and scaphoid), and repair of the scapholunate interosseous ligament. However, the ligament is often of poor quality.

Direct Ligamentous Repair. Lavernia and associates[316] described a combination ligament repair and dorsal capsulodesis. Following the prerequisites of good quality ligament, reducibility, and minimal arthritis, they found that the interval between injury and surgery was not important. They had 90% good to excellent results in 21 patients, with the major limitation being a 15-degree loss of wrist flexion. These remarkable results have not been duplicated by other authors. Attention to detail, with anatomic reduction of the carpus and meticulous repair of the ligament, is essential.

Dorsal Capsulodesis. Blatt[309] described a soft tissue technique that does not rely on reconstruction of the scapholunate ligament and re-creation of the scapholunate linkage that Linscheid recommended.[314] Rather, the Blatt procedure creates a dorsal capsulodesis that realigns, or “horizontalizes,” the scaphoid with respect to the radius (Fig. 43-49). The wrist is exposed through a dorsal approach, dissecting a proximally based 1-cm wide flap of dorsal capsule. The scaphoid is then reduced and pinned to the capitate with a single 0.045-in K-wire. A trough is created in the distal dorsal pole of the scaphoid, and the flap is attached with a suture anchor or a pullout wire led volarly. Motion is begun when the cast is removed at 2 months. The K-wire is removed at 3 months. Recent modifications of the dorsal capsulodesis procedure have been developed that use the DIC ligament.[89,317] We believe that dorsal capsulodesis may have a role in the management of dynamic scapholunate instability. We have no experience with this technique for chronic scapholunate dissociation.

Tendon Grafts. Various ligament reconstructions using tendon grafts have been described. These are complicated, technically demanding procedures with unpredictable results. Dobyns and Linscheid and their colleagues[227,318] described a method using drill holes in the scaphoid and lunate through which is passed a strip of extensor carpi radialis brevis or longus tendon in an attempt to reconstruct the scapholunate interosseous ligament and restore the scapholunate linkage. They emphasize several technical points: (1) careful drilling of the holes to avoid fractures, (2) passage of good quality tendon graft, (3) over-reduction of the radiolunate–capitate

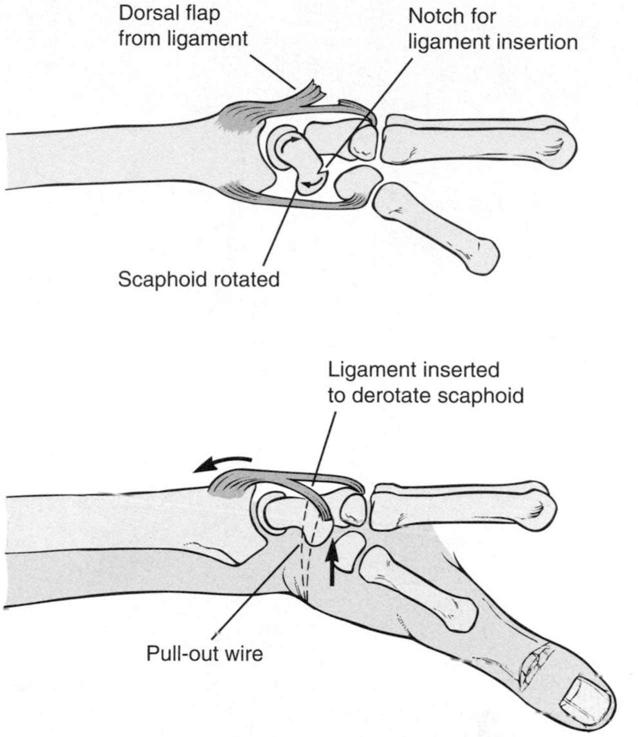

Figure 43-49. Blatt’s technique of dorsal capsulodesis for chronic rotary subluxation of the scaphoid. *(Redrawn from Blatt G: Capsulodesis in reconstructive hand surgery: dorsal capsulodesis for the unstable scaphoid and volar capsulodesis following excision of the distal ulna, Hand Clin North Am 3:81–102, 1987.)*

and scaphoid joints and using three K-wires to maintain reduction, and (4) postoperative immobilization with the K-wires for 6 to 8 weeks followed by part-time splinting for an additional 6 weeks.

Another type of tendon graft has been proposed by Brunelli and Brunelli[319] that uses half of the FCR. They believe that incompetence of the scapho-trapezial-trapezoidal ligaments is a critical feature of scapholunate instability that must be addressed in ligament reconstruction. Consequently, the distally based graft is passed volarly over the scapho-trapezial-trapezoidal joint and then through the scaphoid tuberosity. The graft exits dorsally and is attached to the dorsal aspect of the distal radius. A modification by Van Den Abbeele[320] anchors the tendon to the lunate rather than the radius. K-wires are removed after 30 days, at which time motion is begun.

A ligament reconstruction technique by Garcia-Elias and colleagues.[321] that holds some promise is three-ligament tenodesis (Figs. 43-50 and 43-51). This uses elements of the most popular ligament reconstructions.[227,318,319] The intent is to replicate the action of the dorsal scapholunate ligament, the dorsal radiotriquetral ligament, and the scaphotrapezial ligament. In their series of 38 patients, carpal collapse, advanced arthritis, or both were seen in a total of four patients. This has become our (CC) preferred technique for chronic, reducible static scapholunate dissociation when direct repair is not possible.

Bone–Ligament–Bone Grafts. Extrapolating from the success of such constructs in knee reconstruction, several investigators[322,323] have developed bone–ligament–bone techniques for scapholunate ligament reconstruction. Donor

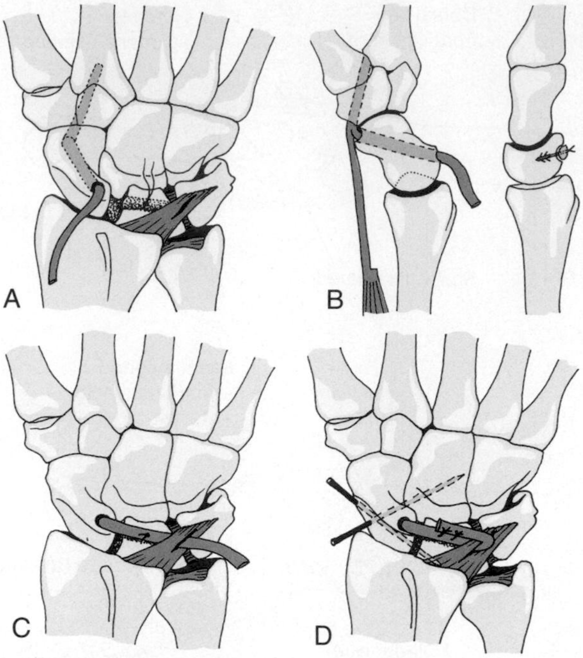

Figure 43-50. The 3LT technique. **A,** A strip of flexor carpi radialis tendon is passed obliquely from the palmar scaphoid tuberosity to the dorsal ridge of the scaphoid where the dorsal scapholunate ligament (SL) normally inserts. **B,** The tendon graft is set across the SL joint to be buried in a trough created on the dorsum of the lunate by means of an anchor suture. **C,** To obtain adequate graft tension, a slit at the distal portion of the dorsal radiotriquetral ligament (RTq) ligament is made, through which the tendon is passed. **D,** The graft finally is sutured onto itself while two K-wires neutralize both the SL and scaphocapitate ligament joints. Unlike in Brunelli's tenodesis, the tendon graft does not cross the radiocarpal joint. *(From Garcia-Elias M, Lluch AL, Stanley JK: Three-ligament tenodesis for the treatment of scapholunate dissociation: indications and surgical technique, J Hand Surg Am 31:125–134, 2006.)*

sites have included extensor retinaculum over Lister tubercle,[322] and the navicular–first cuneiform ligament.[323] In one series,[322] only two of five patients with static instability had significant improvement. Long-term follow-up suggests that these, similar to many scapholunate reconstructive procedures, are prone to fail radiographically over time.[324]

INTERCARPAL ARTHRODESIS. Because of the difficulty with and variable results of soft tissue procedures, some investigators have proposed various limited intercarpal arthrodeses to stabilize the wrist.

Scapholunate Arthrodesis. This procedure appears to be a logical solution to the problem of chronic scapholunate dissociation because it addresses the key feature of this instability directly. Unfortunately, several surgeons who have had experience with it report low arthrodesis rates.[325,326] Nonetheless, clinical improvement and radiologic reduction can be achieved even in the face of nonunion. In common with all surgery for chronic scapholunate dissociation, no large series have reported uniformly good results.

Technique. Expose the proximal half of the scaphoid, lunate, and capitate through a dorsal approach. Using a power burr or hand instrument, create cavities in the adjacent articular surfaces of the scaphoid and lunate. Reduce or over-reduce the capitate to the lunate as described for reduction of acute dissociation. Pin this joint with a 0.062-in K-wire from capitate to lunate. Reduce the scaphoid to the lunate and pin this joint and the scaphocapitate joint with 0.062-in K-wires. Alternatively, a scapholunate screw can be used. Follow this by tightly packing the scapholunate joint with cancellous bone graft harvested from either the distal radius or the iliac crest. Close in routine fashion and apply a U-shaped above-elbow splint for 1 week followed by a short arm cast for 10 weeks that should be changed at 2- to 3-week intervals. Then remove the wires and begin range of motion exercises followed by strengthening exercises. Total rehabilitation usually takes 4 to 6 months.

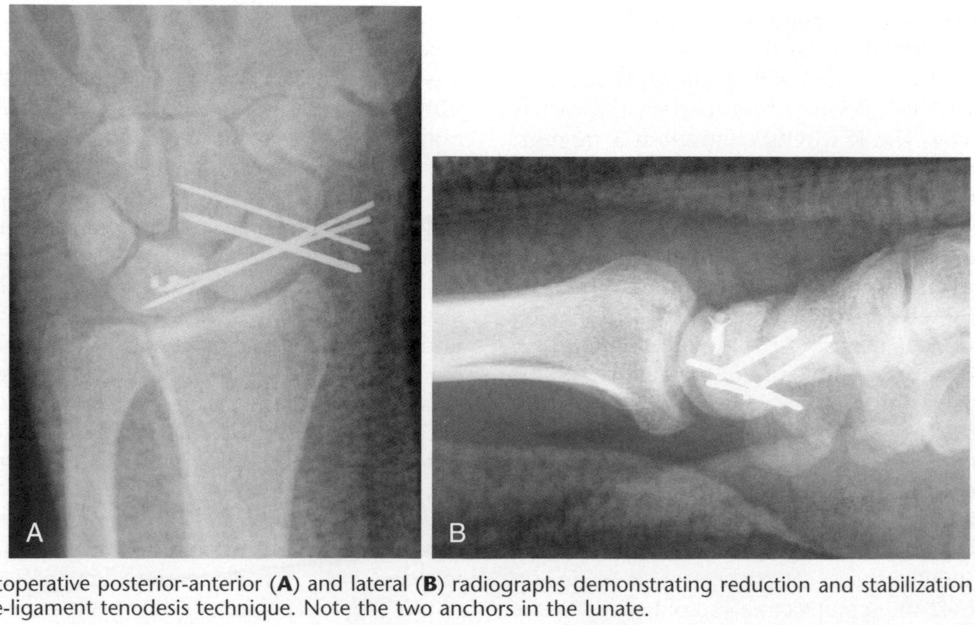

Figure 43-51. Postoperative posterior-anterior (**A**) and lateral (**B**) radiographs demonstrating reduction and stabilization of the scapholunate joint using the three-ligament tenodesis technique. Note the two anchors in the lunate.

Scapholunate-Capitate Arthrodesis.[327] This technique improves the fusion rate and solves the instability problem. However, there is at least a 50% loss of motion, and late changes may occur at the nonarthrodesed joints. In our hands, total intercarpal fusion, including the scaphoid, lunate, capitate, triquetrum, and hamate, has added nothing to the morbidity and has been predictable over the short term.

Technique. Expose the wrist through a dorsal third compartment subperiosteal approach, as already described, being careful not to expose the common digital extensor tendons. Remove cartilage and subchondral bone to expose cancellous bone at all the intercarpal joints. Reduce the wrist, taking care to preserve anatomic alignment of the proximal articular surface of the proximal row and preserve the external dimensions of the wrist. Stabilize all the intercarpal joints with 0.062-in smooth K-wires. Pack all the denuded surfaces tightly with cancellous bone harvested from the iliac crest. Close in layers over a drain. Place the wrist in a U-shaped above-elbow splint, which should be changed at 48 hours. Apply a solid short arm cast at 1 week and change it every 2 to 3 weeks until 6 to 8 weeks have passed or radiography has confirmed that solid union has occurred; then begin rehabilitation. It will require 3 to 6 months for the patient to return to heavy activity.

Scapho-Trapezial-Trapezoid Arthrodesis. This is a bony method to treat the vertical collapse pattern of the scaphoid. As with Blatt's technique, there is no attempt to restore scapholunate linkage. Watson and Hempton[106] popularized this arthrodesis, although it was first described by Peterson and Lipscomb[328] in 1967. Both Watson and Hempton[106] and Kleinman and associates[329] described acceptable clinical results with this technique. Kleinman[330] emphasized the change in wrist kinematics that occurs and reported 11 complications in his series of 41 patients. As with the Blatt dorsal capsulodesis procedure, the rationale is to prevent the scaphoid from assuming the vertical position that allows the proximal pole to sublux dorsally out of the radial facet, with consequent arthritis and midcarpal collapse. More experience with this procedure is reported than with any of the other arthrodesis operations,[331-333] but our personal experience has not been uniformly satisfactory, and we no longer use it.

The Watson Technique.[334] This begins with a transverse incision made over the dorsoradial aspect of the wrist over the scaphoid. Nerves and tendons are retracted, and the scaphoid, trapezium, and trapezoid are exposed with a transverse incision through the wrist capsule. The articular surfaces of the distal scaphoid, proximal trapezium, proximal trapezoid, and trapezial trapezoid joints are denuded of cartilage. Bone graft is harvested from the distal radius through a second transverse incision between the first and the second extensor compartments. The three bones are then aligned properly with the scaphoid at 45 degrees to the long axis of the radius, and the normal external configuration at the three bones is preserved. At least three 0.045-in K-wires are prepositioned: one to cross each prepared articular surface and left protruding at the joint surface. To secure proper scaphoid position, two more K-wires are driven across the scaphoid into the capitate after aligning the proximal pole to the lunate. Cancellous bone is packed into the joints, and the wires are driven across. Cortical bone is added. Radiographs are taken to confirm proper alignment and wire placement. No pins should cross into the radius or ulna. The wires are cut under the skin, and a bulky dressing is applied with a long arm splint. At 10 days, a long arm cast is applied, including the index and middle fingers. Four weeks after surgery, this is removed, and a short arm cast is applied. Finger motion is encouraged. At 8 weeks, if radiographs demonstrate satisfactory healing, the pins are removed, and a light volar splint is applied. Range of motion of the wrist is begun. At 9 weeks, all immobilization is stopped, and full activity is begun.

Reduction Association of the Scapholunate Joint (RASL)[335] A novel technique for stabilizing the scapholunate interval in the setting of inadequate ligament has been termed the RASL technique. The technique involves open reduction and placement of a cannulated headless screw from the scaphoid into the lunate. Prerequisites include a reducible joint and minimal arthritis. Preliminary results are promising, with reduction of pain and improvement in radiographic alignment.[336] Concerns about the longevity of this construct have tempered its wide adoption.

Authors' Preferred Methods. For a patient with acute scapholunate instability, we prefer open reduction and soft tissue repair to attempt to restore the scapholunate linkage, as described by Linscheid and others. For the subacute and chronic problem, we also attempt a soft tissue reconstruction of the scapholunate linkage using locally available ligament. This usually means placing drill holes in the scaphoid and threading No. 0 nonabsorbable sutures in horizontal mattress fashion into the ligament remnant on the lunate. The capitolunate relationship is reduced and pinned with a single 0.062-in K-wire. The scaphoid is reduced to the lunate and fixed with two pins: one from the scaphoid to the capitate and one from the scaphoid to the lunate. A 0.062-in K-wire is also placed from the capitate into the reduced lunate. The sutures are tied. A dorsal capsulodesis is performed by imbricating the dorsal radiotriquetral ligament as part of the closure. The pins are cut off under the skin and left in place for 3 months. Protected radiocarpal motion is begun at 6 weeks, and full motion is encouraged after the pins are removed at 12 weeks. If the ligament is inadequate for direct repair but the carpus remains reducible without significant arthritis, we (CC) prefer the three-ligament tenodesis procedure. Obviously, this is an intraoperative decision, and the surgeon and patient must be prepared before surgery for another salvage procedure if necessary. If the patient is young and has a high-demand wrist and the carpus is irreducible or arthritic, we perform a total intercarpal arthrodesis (LKR) or scaphoid excision and four-corner fusion (CC) not including the radiocarpal or carpometacarpal joints. Total wrist arthrodesis is a fairly reliable solution in a multiply operated wrist.

Lunotriquetral Dissociation

Disruption of the LT ligament complex may be seen in several settings. As mentioned earlier, LT dissociation occurs in perilunate and lunate dislocations. In this instance, the LT tear is addressed as part of the global instability (see Perilunate Dislocations and Fracture-Dislocations). At the other end of the spectrum, LT tears may be seen in the setting of chronic atraumatic ulnar-sided wrist pain. When associated with a relatively long ulna (ulnar-positive variance), repetitive overload to the ulnar side of the wrist leads to degeneration of the TFC, chondromalacia of the ulnar head and ulnar aspect of the lunate, and LT tear. This condition has been termed *ulnar impaction syndrome*. Surgical management should include ulnar shortening or a wafer procedure.[337]

Finally, acute LT ligament complex injury may occur as an isolated finding. The mechanism for LT tears appears to be different from that of perilunate dislocation. In fact, the combination of wrist extension, ulnar deviation, and intercarpal pronation has been termed the *reverse perilunate mechanism*.[256] Three stages of LT instability have been described.[250] When the injury is limited to the LT membranous ligament, no instability is seen. Accompanying injury to the volar and dorsal LT ligament results in dynamic instability. Extension of the tear into the dorsal radiotriquetral ligament results in static VISI.

DIAGNOSIS. Clinically, there may be a history of a hyperextension or twisting injury to the wrist followed by ulnar-sided wrist pain. On physical examination, there is point tenderness over the LT joint and a positive stress test result. This test, as described by Reagan and colleagues,[256] consists of stabilizing the lunate with one hand while shifting the triquetrum dorsally and palmarly with the other. Pain is elicited, and increased motion or crepitus may be perceived by the examiner. Other causes of ulnar-sided wrist pain should be considered, including a TFC injury, triquetral impaction fracture, and extensor carpi ulnaris tendonitis.

Routine radiographic results are normal in the majority of cases. Even with complete tears, an LT gap is not seen. Occasionally, however, the PA view may demonstrate a stepoff at the proximal and distal LT joints (Fig. 43-52). This represents a break in the proximal row line, as described by Gilula and Weeks,[260] accentuated by ulnar deviation. Ulnar variance should be measured. On the lateral view, a VISI pattern may be seen. Noncontrast MRI is a poor study to detect LT tears (Fig. 43-53). MR arthrography with a dedicated wrist coil improves the sensitivity from 0% to 70%, although it tells nothing about the kinematic consequences of the tear.

Wrist arthroscopy remains the study of choice to confirm clinically suspected LT tears.[338] The LT tear is best visualized through the radiocarpal 4,5 or 6R portal. An LT stepoff may be seen through the midcarpal portal. The degree of instability is classified according to the method of Geissler and colleagues[304] (see Table 43-2).

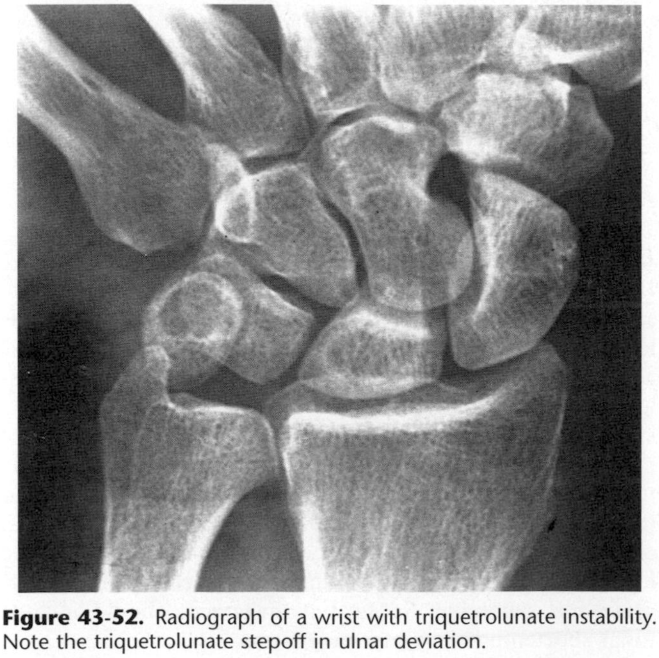

Figure 43-52. Radiograph of a wrist with triquetrolunate instability. Note the triquetrolunate stepoff in ulnar deviation.

TREATMENT. In the absence of static deformity, suspected acute LT tears are initially treated nonoperatively with cast immobilization.[256] This treatment appears to be successful in the majority of cases. For refractory pain, wrist arthroscopy and débridement of the membranous LT ligament with[338] or without[280,281] LT pinning is 80% to 100% successful.

For chronic LT-related pain (without VISI) refractory to arthroscopic débridement, several surgical options are available, including capsulodesis,[309,339] LT arthrodesis,[340-342] ligament reconstruction,[256,343] and ulnar shortening osteotomy.[342,344,345] A recent paper reported excellent results with DRC ligament capsulodesis.[339] Attempts at LT arthrodesis have produced variable results. Pseudarthrosis rates as high as 57% have been reported,[340,341,344,346] even using screw fixation.[347] Furthermore, successful LT fusion does not guarantee pain relief.[341,342] A 20% to 30% loss of wrist motion is expected. Our personal experience with LT arthrodesis has been disappointing.

Lunotriquetral ligament reconstruction has been recommended by several investigators.[256,343] One version[343] of this technically demanding procedure uses a distally based strip of extensor carpi ulnaris, weaving this through drill holes in the triquetrum and lunate. The investigators of this technique reported excellent pain relief in eight of nine patients, and the range of motion actually improved 9%. Ulnar shortening osteotomy is a popular alternative for LT tears without static instability.[342,344,345] This procedure offers several advantages: (1) it is an extraarticular procedure; (2) the resultant tightening of the ulnar carpal ligaments may help stabilize the LT joint; (3) a 2.5-mm shortening decreases the ulnocarpal joint force from 20% to 4%[233]; and (4) decompression of the ulnar aspect of the wrist may alleviate symptoms referable to TFC tears and lunatomalacia, which often accompany LT tears. Ulnar shortening has proved to be a predictable procedure in our hands.

AUTHORS' PREFERRED METHOD. For acute traumatic ulnar-sided wrist pain with normal radiographic results, we prefer cast immobilization with clinical reevaluation at 2-week intervals. In the rare instance when an acute complete LT injury (without VISI) is highly suspected, we perform arthroscopically assisted percutaneous LT pinning with two or three 0.045-in smooth K-wires under radiographic control. The pins are left in place for 6 to 8 weeks. For subacute instability, we prefer arthroscopic LT ligament débridement without pinning. For chronic instability, especially in the setting of ulnar-positive or ulnar-neutral variance, we prefer ulnar shortening osteotomy using the method of Rayhack and associates.[198] If VISI is present, we prefer scaphoid–capitate–lunate–triquetrum–hamate (total midcarpal) arthrodesis (LKR) or scaphoid excision and four-corner arthrodesis (CC).

Midcarpal Instability

Lichtman[236,257,258,348] and Dobyns[227] and their colleagues pointed out that in some patients, especially those with lax ligaments, there is a sudden shift of the entire proximal row into extension during wrist ulnar deviation and into flexion in radial deviation. There is no evidence of dissociation (no interosseous ligament disruption) within the proximal row. They termed this condition nondissociative carpal instability (CIND; or carpal instability nondissociative). The underlying pathology is thought to be incompetence of the ulnar limb of the volar arcuate complex, the dorsal radiotriquetral ligament, or both. Clinically, patients may complain of a painful "clunk"

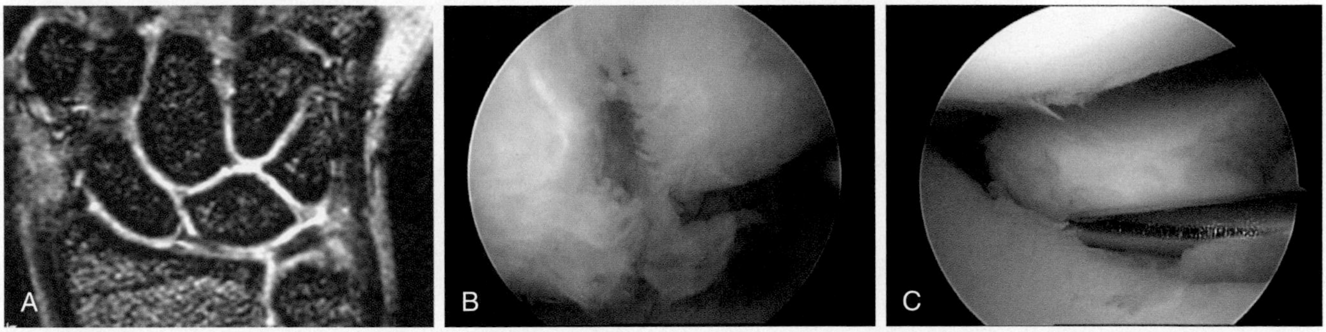

Figure 43-53. Lunotriquetral ligament tear. **A,** Coronal magnetic resonance image of the wrist was read as normal lunotriquetral ligament. **B,** Arthroscopic view through the radiocarpal 6R portal demonstrating a tear of the membranous portion of the lunotriquetral ligament. **C,** View from the radial midcarpal portal demonstrating a lunotriquetral stepoff (triquetrum in background).

(termed the catch-up clunk) with ulnar deviation and pronation and may be able to voluntarily demonstrate it. Generalized ligamentous laxity is a common finding. The midcarpal shift test[236] reproduces their symptoms. Routine radiographic results may be normal or may demonstrate a static VISI deformity (Fig. 43-54). Cineradiology is of potential value in equivocal cases. Arthrography results will be normal; MRI may occasionally demonstrate nonspecific dorsal midcarpal synovitis.[349] Variants of nondisocciative midcarpal instability include dorsal CIND and combined volar and dorsal CIND. In dorsal CIND, the capitate abruptly translates dorsally on the lunate in ulnar deviation. This is thought to be due to a combination of underdevelopment or attenuation of the DIC ligament and the volar ligaments that border the space of Poirier[350] (The symptoms of dorsal CIND are similar to volar CIND except that they tend to occur in supination.) The diagnostic maneuver, called the dynamic dorsal displacement test,[351] involves dorsally directed pressure on the scaphoid tubercle while the wrist is slightly flexed and ulnarly deviated. In combined volar and dorsal CIND, global wrist laxity is present.[352] The classic patient is a young female gymnast who presents with wrist pain after a relatively minor injury. Videofluoroscopy can help to differentiate these forms of instability from dynamic scapholunate instability.

Treatment at present remains challenging. Most investigators favor a trial of splinting, forearm strengthening, and activity modification. The ideal splint is custom molded in ulnar deviation, supporting the pisiform to counteract the VISI posture.[353] For refractory symptoms, surgical management options include joint-leveling procedures, soft tissue stabilization, and radiolunate or intercarpal arthrodesis. Radial shortening or ulnar lengthening is an option for the ulnar-minus patient with mild symptoms, the theory being that the ulnar head–TFC will support the ulnar side of the wrist.[354] We have no experience with the procedure in this setting. Soft tissue procedures include arthroscopic[355] and open volar[350] and combined volar–dorsal[236] capsulorrhaphy. Johnson and Carrera[350] described a volar soft tissue repair technique in

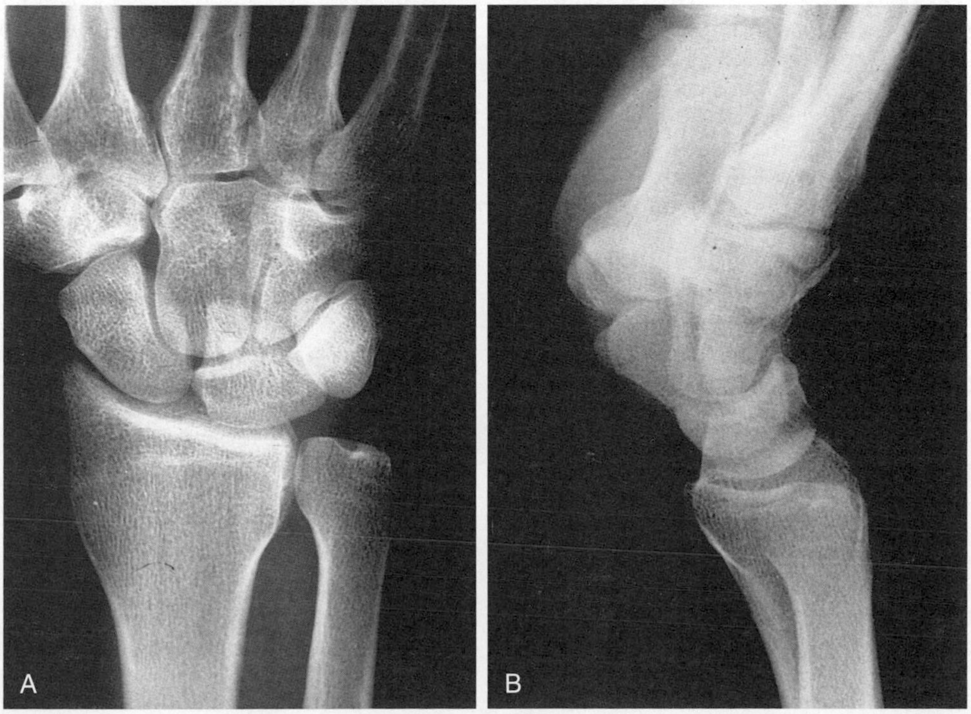

Figure 43-54. A and **B,** Volar intercalated segment instability, nondissociated (volar midcarpal instability).

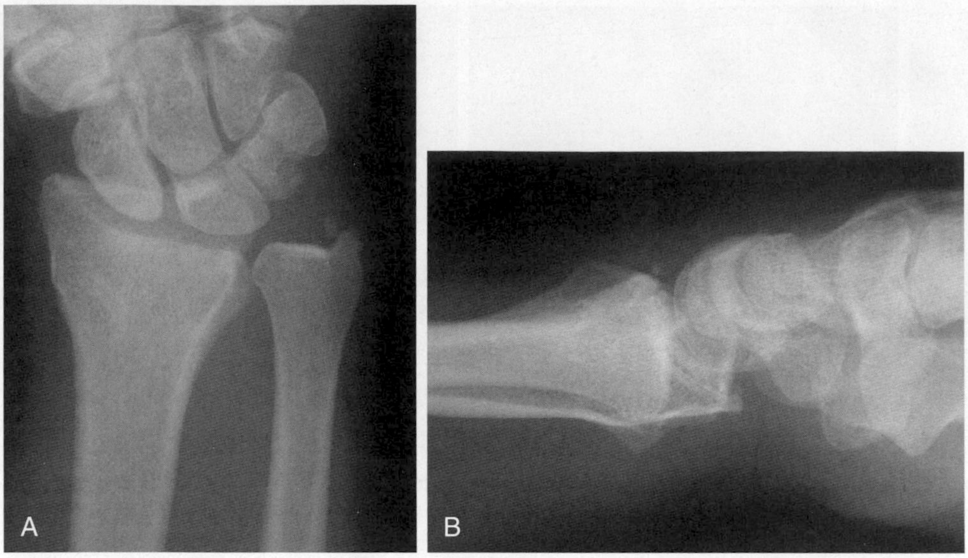

Figure 43-55. Adaptive midcarpal instability secondary to distal radius malunion. Posterior-anterior (**A**) and lateral (**B**) radiographs demonstrating dorsal tilt of the distal radius and dorsal intercalated segment instability pattern.

which the interval between the radioscapholunate and the radiolunotriquetral is tightened, obliterating the space of Poirier. Lichtman and associates[236] described repair of the dorsal and volar arcuate (V) ligaments. As Lichtman and colleagues point out,[257,258] these soft tissue procedures are destined to fail in moderate to severe cases. Good early results have been obtained with arthroscopic thermal capsulorrhaphy,[355] although there are obvious concerns about the long-term consequences of thermal injury. Limited intercarpal arthrodesis procedures have included triquetrum–hamate or four-corner fusions.[356] Midcarpal arthrodesis should be curative in this condition but may be excessively aggressive. Radiolunate arthrodesis[357] has the theoretical advantage of preserving the dart thrower's motion.

Authors' Preferred Approach. We recommend extensive nonoperative treatment, concentrating on forearm strengthening and avoidance of aggravating activities. If this fails, we suggest a soft tissue reconstruction first except in severe cases. In our experience, patients with mild forms of this instability can be successfully treated with arthroscopy and thermal capsulorrhaphy of the DRC capsule and volar midcarpal capsule followed by 6 weeks of cast immobilization. Conversely, soft tissue procedures will invariably fail if the patient can voluntary "clunk" the wrist. Total midcarpal arthrodesis or scaphoid excision and four-corner fusion are recommended for refractory cases.

Secondary (Adaptive) Midcarpal Instability

Another form of nondissociative midcarpal instability, termed secondary or adaptive DISI, may result from malunion of the distal radius.[358] In the setting of dorsal tilt, the entire proximal carpal row extends to accommodate to the radius malposition (Fig. 43-55). No interosseous ligament tear is present. As a result of alteration of contact forces, the patient may complain of weakness or pain and may possibly develop arthritis.[261] In patients with underlying ligamentous laxity, as little as 10 degrees' dorsal tilt can result in an adaptive DISI pattern.[359] Treatment for symptomatic adaptive DISI involves an opening wedge distal radius osteotomy.[360] We currently perform this through a volar approach with a locking plate in order to correct the dorsal tilt and radial height; cancellous autograft or bone graft substitute is used to fill the defect.

KEY REFERENCES

The level of evidence (LOE) is determined according to the criteria provided in the preface.

68. Doornberg JN, Buijze GA, Ham SJ, et al: Nonoperative treatment for acute scaphoid fractures: a systematic review and meta-analysis of randomized controlled trials. *J Trauma* 71:1073–1081, 2011. doi: 10.1097/TA.0b013e318222f485. LOE I
128. Chang MA, Bishop AT, Moran SL, et al: The outcomes and complications of 1,2-intercompartmental supraretinacular artery pedicled vascularized bone grafting of scaphoid nonunions. *J Hand Surg [Am]* 31:387–396, 2006. LOE IV
171. Kienböck R: Concerning traumatic malacia of the lunate and its consequences: degeneration and compression fractures. Translation of 1910 article. *Clin Orthop Relat Res* 149:4–8, 1980. LOE V
229. Linscheid RL, Dobyns JH, Beabout JW, et al: Traumatic instability of the wrist. *J Bone Joint Surg Am* 54:1612–1632, 1972. LOE V
236. Lichtman DM, Schneider JR, Swafford AR, et al: Ulnar midcarpal instability: clinical and laboratory analysis. *J Hand Surg [Am]* 6:515–523, 1981. LOE IV
240. Berger RA, Garcia Elias M: General anatomy of the wrist: Ligamentous anatomy. In An KN, Berger RA, Cooney WP, III, editors: *Biomechanics of the wrist joint*, New York, 1991, Springer-Verlag, pp 5–14. LOE V
248. Mayfield JK, Johnson RP, Kilcoyne RK: Carpal dislocations: pathomechanics and progressive perilunar instability. *J Hand Surg [Am]* 5:226–241, 1980.
302. Watson HK, Ottoni L, Pitts EC, et al: Rotary subluxation of the scaphoid: a spectrum of instability. *J Hand Surg [Br]* 18:62–64, 1993. LOE III
312. Cooney WP III: Evaluation of chronic wrist pain by arthrography, arthroscopy, and arthrotomy. *J Hand Surg [Am]* 18:815–822, 1993. LOE IV
316. Lavernia CJ, Cohen MS, Taleisnik J: Treatment of scapholunate dissociation by ligamentous repair and capsulodesis. *J Hand Surg [Am]* 17:354–359, 1992. LOE IV
340. Kirschenbaum D, Coyle MP, Leddy JP: Chronic lunotriquetral instability: diagnosis and treatment. *J Hand Surg [Am]* 18:1107–1112, 1993. LOE IV
359. Fernandez DL: Corrective osteotomy for extra-articular malunion of the distal radius. In Saffar P, Cooney WP III, editors: *Fractures of the distal radius*, London, 1995, Martin Dunitz, pp 104–117. LOE V

The complete References list is available online at https://expertconsult.inkling.com.

Index

Page numbers followed by *f* indicate figures, *t* indicate tables, and *b* indicate boxes.

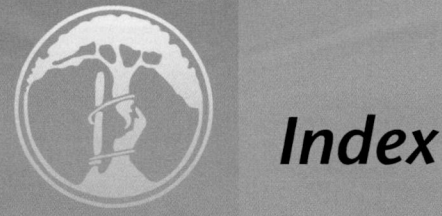

B

C

D

E

J

K

L

M

O

Q

R

S

T